Shackelford's
SURGERY *of the* ALIMENTARY TRACT

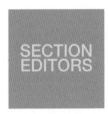

SECTION EDITORS

VOLUME 1

VOLUME 2

Jeffrey H. Peters, MD

Seymour I. Schwartz Professor and Chairman
Department of Surgery
University of Rochester School of Medicine and
Dentistry
Rochester, New York

Section I **Esophagus and Hernia**

David W. McFadden, MD

Professor and Chairman
Department of Surgery
University of Connecticut
Farmington, Connecticut

Section II **Stomach and Small Intestine**

Jeffrey B. Matthews, MD

Dallas B. Phemister Professor and Chairman
Department of Surgery
University of Chicago
Chicago, Illinois

Section III **Pancreas, Biliary Tract, Liver, and Spleen**

John H. Pemberton, MD

Professor of Surgery
Mayo Clinic College of Medicine
Consultant in Colon and Rectal Surgery
Mayo Clinic and Mayo Foundation
Rochester, Minnesota

Section IV **Colon, Rectum, and Anus**

Shackelford's
SURGERY *of the*
ALIMENTARY
TRACT

SEVENTH
EDITION

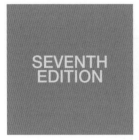
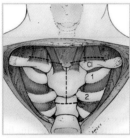
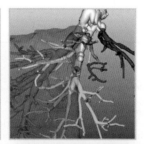
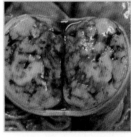
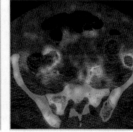

VOLUME
2

Charles J. Yeo, MD

Samuel D. Gross Professor and Chairman

Department of Surgery

Thomas Jefferson University

Philadelphia, Pennsylvania

ELSEVIER
SAUNDERS

1600 John F. Kennedy Blvd.
Ste 1800
Philadelphia, PA 19103-2899

SHACKELFORD'S SURGERY OF THE ALIMENTARY TRACT

ISBN: 978-1-4377-2206-2
Vol 1 PN: 9996084701
Vol 2 PN: 9996084760

Notices

Knowledge and best practice in this field are constantly changing. As new research and experience broaden our understanding, changes in research methods, professional practices, or medical treatment may become necessary.

Practitioners and researchers must always rely on their own experience and knowledge in evaluating and using any information, methods, compounds, or experiments described herein. In using such information or methods they should be mindful of their own safety and the safety of others, including parties for whom they have a professional responsibility.

With respect to any drug or pharmaceutical products identified, readers are advised to check the most current information provided (i) on procedures featured or (ii) by the manufacturer of each product to be administered, to verify the recommended dose or formula, the method and duration of administration, and contraindications. It is the responsibility of practitioners, relying on their own experience and knowledge of their patients, to make diagnoses, to determine dosages and the best treatment for each individual patient, and to take all appropriate safety precautions.

To the fullest extent of the law, neither the Publisher nor the authors, contributors, or editors assume any liability for any injury and/or damage to persons or property as a matter of products liability, negligence or otherwise, or from any use or operation of any methods, products, instructions, or ideas contained in the material herein.

Library of Congress Cataloging-in-Publication Data

Shackelford's surgery of the alimentary tract / [edited by] Charles J. Yeo.—7th ed.
    p. ; cm.
  Surgery of the alimentary tract
  Includes bibliographical references and index.
  ISBN 978-1-4377-2206-2 (2 v. set : hardcover : alk. paper)
  I. Yeo, Charles J.   II. Title: Surgery of the alimentary tract.
  [DNLM: 1. Digestive System Surgical Procedures—methods.   2. Digestive System Diseases—surgery. WI 900]
  617.4′3—dc23

                                                    2012011563

Global Content Development Director: Judy Fletcher
Content Development Manager: Maureen Iannuzzi
Publishing Services Manager: Anne Altepeter
Associate Project Manager: Jessica L. Becher
Design Direction: Teresa McBryan

Printed in China

Last digit is the print number: 9 8 7 6 5 4 3 2 1

Contributors

Andrea M. Abbott, MD, MS
Surgical Resident, Department of Surgery, University of Minnesota, Minneapolis, Minnesota
Small Intestine

Herand Abcarian, MD
Professor of Surgery, University of Illinois; Chairman, Division of Colon and Rectal Surgery, John H. Stroger, Jr. Hospital of Cook County, Chicago, Illinois
Complete Rectal Prolapse

Wasef Abu-Jaish, MD
Assistant Professor, Department of Surgery, University of Vermont College of Medicine, Fletcher Allen Health Care, Burlington, Vermont
Internal Hernias: Congenital and Acquired

David B. Adams, MD
Professor and Chief, Division of Gastrointestinal and Laparoscopic Surgery; Co-Director, Digestive Disease Center, Medical University of South Carolina, Charleston, South Carolina
Biliary Dyskinesia and Sphincter of Oddi Dysfunction

Julie E. Adams, MD
Associate Professor of Surgery, Vascular Surgery, University of Vermont College of Medicine, Fletcher Allen Health Care, Burlington, Vermont
Aortoenteric Fistula and Visceral Artery Aneurysms

Andrew S. Akman, MD
Assistant Professor of Radiology, Department of Radiology, Interventional Radiology Division, The George Washington University Medical Center, Washington, DC
Imaging and Intervention in the Biliary System

Steven R. Alberts, MD, MPH
Professor, Division of Medical Oncology, Mayo Clinic College of Medicine, Rochester, Minnesota
Adjuvant and Neoadjuvant Therapy for Colorectal Cancer

Hisami Ando, MD
Professor, Chairman, and Chief of Pediatric Surgery, Department of Pediatric Surgery, Nagoya University Graduate School of Medicine, Nagoya, Japan
Cystic Disorders of the Bile Ducts

Leonard Armstrong, MD, MS
Surgical Resident, Department of Surgery, University of Minnesota, Minneapolis, Minnesota
Small Intestine

Vivian A. Asamoah, MD
Board Certified Gastroenterologist, Division of Medicine, Cypress Fairbanks Medical Center, Houston, Texas
Approach to the Patient With Abnormal Hepatic Laboratory Tests

Theodor Asgeirsson, MD
Assistant Director, Outcomes Research, Department of Colorectal Surgery, Spectrum Health, Grand Rapids, Michigan
Hemorrhoids

Stanley W. Ashley, MD
Chief Medical Officer, Brigham and Women's Hospital; Frank Sawyer Professor of Surgery, Harvard Medical School, Boston, Massachusetts
Operations for Peptic Ulcer

Dimitrios Avgerinos, MD
Clinical Fellow in Cardiothoracic Surgery, Department of Cardiothoracic Surgery, New York-Presbyterian Hospital, Weill Cornell Medical College, Memorial Sloan-Kettering Cancer Center, New York, New York
Abdominoperineal Resection of the Rectum for Cancer

H. Randolph Bailey, MD
Clinical Professor and Deputy Chief, Department of Surgery, Division of Colon and Rectal Surgery, Weill Cornell Medical College, Methodist Hospital, Houston, Texas
Pilonidal Disease

Humayun Bakhtawar, MBBS, MD
General Surgery Resident, Department of General Surgery, West Virginia University School of Medicine, Morgantown, West Virginia
Anatomy and Physiology of the Mesenteric Circulation

Santhoshi Bandla, PhD
Post-Doctoral Research Associate, Department of Surgery, University of Rochester Medical Center, James P. Wilmot Cancer Center, Rochester, New York
Genetics of Esophageal Cancer

John M. Barlow, MD
Assistant Professor, Department of Radiology, Mayo Clinic College of Medicine, Rochester, Minnesota
Imaging in Esophageal Disease

Todd H. Baron, Sr., MD
Professor, Department of Gastroenterology and Hepatology, Mayo Clinic College of Medicine, Rochester, Minnesota
Colonoscopy

Juan Camilo Barreto Andrade, MD
Surgical Oncology Fellow, Department of General Surgery, University of Chicago, Pritzker School of Medicine, Chicago, Illinois
Management of Secondary Hepatic Neoplasms

Lokesh Bathla, MD
Clinical Fellow, Abdominal Transplantation, Department of Surgery, University of Nebraska Medical Center, Omaha, Nebraska
Laparoscopic Inguinal Hernia Repair

Jennifer S. Beaty, MD
Assistant Professor of Surgery, University of Nebraska Medical Center, Creighton University School of Medicine, Omaha, Nebraska
Anal Sepsis and Fistula

David E. Beck, MD
Professor and Chairman, Department of Colon and Rectal Surgery, Ochsner Clinic, New Orleans, Louisiana; Ochsner Clinical School, The University of Queensland School of Medicine, Brisbane, Australia
Miscellaneous Disorders of the Rectum and Anus

David Beddy
Mayo Clinic College of Medicine, Rochester, Minnesota
Anatomy and Physiology of the Rectum and Anus Including Applied Anatomy

Alec C. Beekley, MD
Associate Professor, Department of Surgery, Thomas Jefferson University, Philadelphia, Pennsylvania
Operations for Morbid Obesity

Kevin E. Behrns, MD
Edward R. Woodward Professor and Chairman, Department of Surgery, University of Florida College of Medicine, Gainesville, Florida
Gastric Resection and Reconstruction

Kfir Ben-David, MD
Assistant Professor, Department of Surgery, University of Florida College of Medicine, Gainesville, Florida
Gastric Resection and Reconstruction

Jacques Bergman, MD, PhD
Professor of Gastrointestinal Endoscopy, Department of Gastroenterology and Hepatology, Academic Medical Center, Amsterdam, The Netherlands
Endoscopic Evaluation of the Esophagus

Marc Besselink, MD, PhD
Department of Surgery, University Medical Center Utrecht, Utrecht, The Netherlands
Acute Pancreatitis

Adil E. Bharucha, MBBS, MD
Professor, Department of Medicine, Mayo Clinic College of Medicine; Consultant, Department of Gastroenterology and Hepatology, Mayo Clinic, Rochester, Minnesota
Physiology of the Colon and Its Measurement

Adrian Billeter, MD
Ferguson Fellow, Price Institute of Surgical Research, University of Louisville, Louisville, Kentucky
Traumatic Colorectal Injuries, Foreign Bodies, and Anal Wounds

Sylvester M. Black, MD, PhD
Clinical Fellow, Abdominal Transplantation and Hepato-Pancreato-Biliary Surgery, Department of Surgery, University of Toronto, Toronto, Ontario, Canada; Department of Surgery, University of Minnesota, Minneapolis, Minnesota
Liver Abscess

Jeffrey A. Blatnik, MD
General Surgery Resident, Dudley P. Allen Research Scholar, Department of Surgery, University Hospitals Case Medical Center, Cleveland, Ohio
Ventral Herniation in Adults

Ronald Bleday, MD
Chief, Section of Colon and Rectal Surgery, Department of Surgery, Brigham and Women's Hospital; Associate Professor, Department of Surgery, Harvard Medical School, Boston, Massachusetts
Local Excision of Rectal Cancer

Brendan J. Boland, MD
Liver Transplant and Pancreaticobiliary Surgery, Cedars-Sinai Medical Center, Los Angeles, California
Perioperative Management and Nutrition in Patients With Liver and Biliary Tract Disease

Scott J. Boley, MD
Professor of Surgery and Pediatrics, Albert Einstein College of Medicine, Montefiore Medical Center, Bronx, New York
Colonic Bleeding and Ischemia

Luigi Bonavina, MD
Professor and Chairman, Department of Surgery, University of Milano Medical School, Milano, Italy
Surgical Management of Esophageal Diverticula

Eduardo A. Bonin, MD
Research Fellow, Developmental Endoscopy Unit, Mayo Clinic, Rochester, Minnesota; Professor, Minimally Invasive Surgery Graduate Program, Positivo University, Curitiba, Paraná, Brazil
Endoscopic Antireflux Repairs
Colonoscopy

Sarah Y. Boostrom, MD
Consultant, Colon and Rectal Surgery, Mayo Clinic, Rochester, Minnesota
Colonic Bleeding and Ischemia
Resection and Ablation of Metastatic Colorectal Cancer to the Liver

Thomas C. Bower, MD
Chair, Department of Vascular and Endovascular Surgery, Gonda Vascular Center, Mayo Clinic College of Medicine, Rochester, Minnesota
Colonic Bleeding and Ischemia

Jan Brabender, MD
Professor of Surgery, Chief, Department of General Surgery, St. Antonius Hospital, Cologne, North Rhine-Westphalia, Germany
Epidemiology, Risk Factors, and Clinical Manifestations of Esophageal Cancer

Malcolm V. Brock, MD
Associate Professor of Surgery and Oncology, Division of
Thoracic Surgery, Johns Hopkins University School of
Medicine, Baltimore, Maryland
Benign Tumors and Cysts of the Esophagus

Jill C. Buckley, MD
Trauma and Reconstructive Surgery, Department of Urology,
Lahey Clinic Medical Center, Burlington, Massachusetts;
Assistant Professor, Tufts University School of Medicine,
Boston, Massachusetts
Rectovaginal and Rectourethral Fistulas

William J. Bulsiewicz, MD
Fellow, Gastrointestinal Outcomes Training Program, Division
of Digestive Diseases, University of North Carolina Hospitals,
Chapel Hill, North Carolina
*Clinical Features and Endoscopic Therapy for Dysplastic
Barrett Esophagus*

Adele Burgess, MD
Colorectal Surgeon, Head, Colorectal Surgery, Department of
Surgery, Austin Hospital, Heidelberg, Victoria, Australia
Pelvic Floor Dysfunction

Sathyaprasad C. Burjonrappa, MD
Assistant Professor of Surgery and Pediatrics, Westchester
Medical Center, Valhalla, New York
Basic Features of Groin Hernia and Its Repair

Angel M. Caban, MD
Assistant Professor, Department of Surgery, University of
Florida College of Medicine, Gainesville, Florida
Gastric Resection and Reconstruction

Jason A. Call, MD
Department of Radiation Oncology, Mayo Clinic College of
Medicine, Rochester, Minnesota
Adjuvant and Neoadjuvant Therapy for Colorectal Cancer

Mark P. Callery, MD
Associate Professor of Surgery, Harvard Medical School;
Chief, Division of General Surgery, Beth Israel Deaconess
Medical Center, Boston, Massachusetts
*Prevention and Management of Complications of
Pancreatic Surgery*

John L. Cameron, MD
Alfred Blalock Distinguished Service Professor, Johns Hopkins
University School of Medicine, Department of Surgery,
Baltimore, Maryland
Pancreatic and Periampullary Cancer

Michael Camilleri, MD
Atherton and Winifred W. Bean Professor, Professor of
Medicine and Physiology, Mayo Clinic College of Medicine;
Consultant, Gastroenterology and Hepatology, Mayo Clinic,
Rochester, Minnesota
Physiology of the Colon and Its Measurement

Peter W.G. Carne, MBBS
Senior Lecturer, Department of Surgery, Cabrini Monash
University, Malvern, Victoria, Australia
Rare Colorectal Malignancies

Jennifer C. Carr, MD
Resident, Department of General Surgery, University of Iowa
Hospitals and Clinics, Iowa City, Iowa
Small Bowel Diverticula

Emily Carter Paulson, MD
General Surgery, Division of Colorectal Surgery, Hospital of
the University of Pennsylvania, Philadelphia, Pennsylvania
*Evidence-Based Decision Making in Colon and Rectal
Surgery*

Riaz Cassim, MD
Associate Professor, Department of Surgery, West Virginia
University School of Medicine, Morgantown, West Virginia;
Chief of Surgery, Louis A. Johnson Veterans Affairs Medical
Center, Clarksburg, West Virginia
Short Bowel Syndrome

Donald O. Castell, MD
Professor of Medicine, Medical University of South Carolina,
Charleston, South Carolina
Physiology of the Esophagus and Its Sphincters
Multichannel Intraluminal Impedance

Peter Cataldo, MD
Professor of Surgery, University of Vermont College of
Medicine, Fletcher Allen Health Care, Burlington, Vermont
Ileostomy
Ostomy Management

Samuel Cemaj, MD
Assistant Professor, Creighton University School of Medicine,
Omaha, Nebraska
Basic Features of Groin Hernia and Its Repair

Parakrama T. Chandrasoma, MD
Professor of Pathology, University of Southern California,
Keck School of Medicine; Director, Anatomic and Surgical
Pathology, University of Southern California Medical Center,
Los Angeles, California
Pathology of Gastroesophageal Reflux Disease

George J. Chang, MD
Associate Professor, Department of Surgical Oncology,
Associate Medical Director, Colorectal Center, Director,
Clinical Operations, Minimally Invasive and New Technology
in Oncologic Surgery Program, The University of Texas MD
Anderson Cancer Center, Houston, Texas
Surgery in the Immunocompromised Patient

Vivek Chaudhry, MBBS
Head, Surgical Endoscopy, Clerkship Director, Department of
Surgery, John H. Stroger, Jr. Hospital of Cook County;
Clinical Assistant Professor of Colon and Rectal Surgery,
University of Illinois, Chicago, Illinois
Complete Rectal Prolapse

Herbert Chen, MD
Layton F. Rikkers MD Chair in Surgical Leadership,
Chairman and Professor, Division of General Surgery,
Department of Surgery, University of Wisconsin, Madison,
Wisconsin
Gastrointestinal Carcinoid Tumors

Clifford S. Cho, MD
Assistant Professor, Section of Surgical Oncology, University of Wisconsin School of Medicine and Public Health, Madison, Wisconsin
Biliary Tract Tumors

Eugene A. Choi, MD
Assistant Professor, Department of Surgery, Section of General Surgery, University of Chicago, Pritzker School of Medicine, Chicago, Illinois
Chronic Pancreatitis

Karen Chojnacki, MD
Associate Professor, Residency Program Director, Department of Surgery, Thomas Jefferson University, Philadelphia, Pennsylvania
Operative Management of Bile Duct Strictures

Michael A. Choti, MD
Jacob C. Handelsman Professor of Surgery, Vice-Chair, Department of Surgery, Johns Hopkins University School of Medicine, Baltimore, Maryland
Management of Malignant Hepatic Neoplasms Other Than Hepatocellular Carcinoma

John D. Christein, MD
Associate Professor, Department of Surgery, University of Alabama at Birmingham, Birmingham, Alabama
Autologous Islet Cell Transplantation

Donald O. Christensen, DO
Chief, Anatomic Pathology, Medical Director, Transfusion Services, Department of Pathology, Carl R. Darnall Army Medical Center, Fort Hood, Texas
Anatomy and Physiology of the Spleen

Chike V. Chukwumah, MD
Fellow, Department of Endoscopic Surgery, University Hospitals Case Medical Center, Cleveland, Ohio
Diagnostic and Therapeutic Endoscopy of the Stomach and Small Bowel

Albert K. Chun, MD
Assistant Professor of Radiology, Department of Radiology, Interventional Radiology Division, The George Washington University Medical Center, Washington, DC
Imaging and Intervention in the Biliary System

Robert R. Cima, MD, MA
Associate Professor, Department of Surgery, Division of Colon and Rectal Surgery, Mayo Clinic College of Medicine, Rochester, Minnesota
Inflammatory Bowel Disease

Clancy J. Clark, MD
Hepatobiliary and Pancreatic Surgery Fellow, Department of Surgery, Division of Gastroenterology and General Surgery, Mayo Clinic, Rochester, Minnesota
Prevention and Management of Iatrogenic Bile Duct Injury

Pierre-Alain Clavien, MD, PhD
Professor and Chairman, Swiss Hepato-Pancreato-Biliary and Transplantation Center, Department of Surgery, University Hospital Zurich, Zurich, Switzerland
Benign Hepatic Neoplasms

Alfred M. Cohen, MD
Chief Medical Officer, Cancer Prevention Pharmaceuticals, Tucson, Arizona
Operations for Colorectal Cancer: Low Anterior Resection

Jeffrey Cohen, MD
Clinical Professor, Department of Surgery, University of Connecticut, Farmington, Connecticut; Lead Physician, Surgical Institute, Chief, Division of Colorectal Surgery, Hartford Hospital, Hartford, Connecticut
Diverticular Disease

Steven D. Colquhoun, MD
Associate Professor, Department of Surgery, University of California Los Angeles; Director, Liver Transplant Program, Cedars-Sinai Medical Center, Los Angeles, California
Perioperative Management and Nutrition in Patients With Liver and Biliary Tract Disease
Hepatic Transplantation

Willy Coosemans, MD, PhD
Clinical Head, Department of Thoracic Surgery, University Hospital Gasthuisberg, Leuven, Belgium
Pathophysiology and Treatment of Zenker Diverticulum

Gene F. Coppa, MD
John D. Mountain MD Professor and Chairman of Surgery, Hofstra North Shore-Long Island Jewish School of Medicine, New York, New York
Anatomy and Physiology of the Liver
Anatomy and Physiology of the Spleen

Edward E. Cornwell, III, MD
LaSalle D. Leffall Jr., MD Professor and Chairman of Surgery, Howard University College of Medicine; Surgeon-in-Chief, Howard University Hospital, Washington, DC
Pancreatic Trauma

Daniel A. Cortez, MD
Surgical Pathology Fellow, Department of Pathology, University of Southern California Medical Center, Los Angeles, California
Pathology of Gastroesophageal Reflux Disease

Mario Costantini
Department of Surgical and Gastroenterological Sciences, University of Padua, Padua, Veneto, Italy
Laparoscopic Esophageal Myotomy: Techniques and Results

Daniel A. Craig, MD
Assistant Professor of Radiology, Mayo Clinic College of Medicine; Staff Radiologist, Mayo Clinic, Rochester, Minnesota
Imaging in Esophageal Disease

Peter F. Crookes, MD
Associate Professor of Surgery, University of Southern California, Keck School of Medicine, Los Angeles, California
Esophageal Caustic Injury

Joseph J. Cullen, MD
Professor, Department of Surgery, University of Iowa Hospitals and Clinics, Iowa City, Iowa
Small Bowel Diverticula

Alexandre d'Audiffret, MD
Associate Professor of Surgery, Section of Vascular and Endovascular Surgery, West Virginia University School of Medicine, Robert C. Byrd Health Science Center, Morgantown, West Virginia
Anatomy and Physiology of the Mesenteric Circulation

Herbert Decaluwé, MD
Joint Clinical Head, Department of Thoracic Surgery, University Hospital Gasthuisberg, Leuven, Belgium
Pathophysiology and Treatment of Zenker Diverticulum

Georges Decker, MD
Staff Surgeon, Department of Thoracic Surgery, University Hospital Gasthuisberg, Leuven, Belgium
Pathophysiology and Treatment of Zenker Diverticulum

Thomas C.B. Dehn, MD
Consultant, Upper Gastrointestinal Surgeon, Department of Surgery, Royal Berkshire Hospital, Reading, Berkshire, United Kingdom
Palliative Treatment of Cancer of the Esophagus

Paul De Leyn, MD, PhD
Chairman, Department of Thoracic Surgery, University Hospital Gasthuisberg, Leuven, Belgium
Pathophysiology and Treatment of Zenker Diverticulum

Steven R. DeMeester, MD
Associate Professor of Cardiothoracic Surgery, University of Southern California, Keck School of Medicine, Los Angeles, California
Pathophysiology of the Columnar-Lined Esophagus

Tom R. DeMeester, MD
Professor and Chairman Emeritus, Department of Surgery, University of Southern California, Keck School of Medicine, Los Angeles, California
Perspectives on Esophageal Surgery
The Gastroesophageal Barrier

Aram N. Demirjian, MD
Assistant Professor, Division of Hepatobiliary and Pancreas Surgery, University of California, Irvine, Irvine, California
Diagnostic Operations of the Liver and Techniques of Hepatic Resection

Anthony L. DeRoss, MD
Assistant Professor of Surgery and Pediatrics, Department of Surgery, Division of Pediatric Surgery, Rainbow Babies and Children's Hospital, Cleveland, Ohio
Surgical Diseases of the Stomach and Duodenum in Infants and Children

Eduardo de Santibañes, MD, PhD, MAAC
Professor and Chairman, General Surgical Service and Liver Transplant Unit, Italian Hospital of Buenos Aires, Buenos Aires, Argentina
Anatomy and Physiology of the Liver

John H. Donohue, MD
Professor, Department of Surgery, Mayo Clinic College of Medicine, Rochester, Minnesota
Splenectomy for Conditions Other Than Trauma

Eric J. Dozois, MD
Professor of Surgery, Division of Colon and Rectal Surgery, Mayo Clinic College of Medicine, Rochester, Minnesota
Retrorectal Tumors

Brian J. Dunkin, MD
Professor of Clinical Surgery, Weill Cornell Medical College; Head, Section of Endoscopic Surgery, Methodist Hospital; Medical Director, Methodist Institute for Technology, Innovation, and Education, Houston, Texas
Intubation of the Stomach and Small Intestine

Stephen P. Dunn, MD
Chief, Pediatric Surgery and Solid Organ Transplantation, Alfred I. duPont Hospital for Children; Professor of Surgery, Jefferson Medical College, Wilmington, Delaware
Biliary Atresia, Biliary Hypoplasia, and Choledochal Cyst

Christy M. Dunst, MD
Director, Research and Education, Division of Gastrointestinal and Minimally Invasive Surgery, The Oregon Clinic, Portland, Oregon
Partial Fundoplications

Andre Duranceau, MD
Professor of Surgery, Division of Thoracic Surgery, University of Montreal Hospital Center, Montreal, Quebec, Canada
Disorders of the Pharyngoesophageal Junction

Noreen Durrani, MD
Assistant Professor, Department of Surgery, Division of Acute Care Surgery, University of Florida College of Medicine, Jacksonville, Florida
Gastric, Duodenal, and Small Intestinal Fistulas

Philipp Dutkowski, MD
Professor of Surgery, Swiss Hepato-Pancreato-Biliary and Transplantation Center, Department of Surgery, University Hospital Zurich, Zurich, Switzerland
Benign Hepatic Neoplasms

Barish H. Edil, MD
Assistant Professor of Surgery and Oncology, Department of Surgery, Johns Hopkins University School of Medicine, Baltimore, Maryland
Pancreatic and Periampullary Cancer

Jonathan E. Efron, MD
Associate Professor, Mark M. Ravitch Endowed Professorship in Surgery, Chief, Ravitch Division, Johns Hopkins University School of Medicine, Baltimore, Marlyand
Neoplasms of the Anus

Yousef El-Gohary, MD
Pediatric Surgical Research Fellow, Department of Pediatric
Surgery, Children's Hospital of Pittsburgh, Pittsburgh,
Pennsylvania
Anatomy, Physiology, and Embryology of the Pancreas

E. Christopher Ellison, MD
Robert M. Zollinger Professor and Chair, Department of
Surgery, Ohio State University, Columbus, Ohio
Zollinger–Ellison Syndrome

Scott A. Engum, MD
Professor of Surgery, Section of Pediatric Surgery, Indiana
University School of Medicine, Riley Hospital for Children,
Indianapolis, Indiana
Anorectal Anomalies

Warren E. Enker, MD
Director, Department of Surgery, Gastrointestinal Institute,
Beth Israel Deaconess Medical Center; Associate Director,
Beth Israel Cancer Centers, New York, New York
Abdominoperineal Resection of the Rectum for Cancer

David A. Etzioni, MD, MSHS
Associate Professor, Department of Surgery, Mayo Clinic
College of Medicine, Phoenix, Arizona
Laparoscopic Colorectal Surgery

Douglas B. Evans, MD
Professor and Chairman, Department of Surgery, Medical
College of Wisconsin, Milwaukee, Wisconsin
Unusual Pancreatic Tumors

Victor W. Fazio, AO, MBBS
Rupert Turnbull Professor of Surgery, Department of
Colorectal Surgery, Chairman Emeritus, Digestive Disease
Institute, Cleveland Clinic Lerner College of Medicine, Case
Western Reserve University, Cleveland, Ohio
Reoperative Pelvic Surgery

Edward L. Felix, MD
Director, Center for Hernia Repair, Fresno, California
Femoral Hernia

Aaron S. Fink, MD
Chief Surgical Consultant, Veterans Affairs Southeast Network
7; Attending Surgeon, Veterans Affairs Medical Center,
Decatur, Georgia; Professor of Surgery, Emory University
School of Medicine, Atlanta, Georgia
Anatomy and Physiology of the Duodenum

James Fisher, MD
General Surgery Residency, Mayo Clinic, Rochester,
Minnesota
Fulminant Hepatic Failure and Liver Support Systems

Robert J. Fitzgibbons, Jr., MD
Harry E. Stuckenhoff Professor and Associate Chairman,
Creighton University School of Medicine; Chief, Division of
General Surgery, Department of Surgery, Creighton
University Medical Center, Omaha, Nebraska
Basic Features of Groin Hernia and Its Repair
Laparoscopic Inguinal Hernia Repair

Evan L. Fogel, MD
Professor of Clinical Medicine, Division of Gastroenterology
and Hepatology, Indiana University School of Medicine,
Indianapolis, Indiana
Endoscopic Retrograde Cholangiopancreatography in the
Evaluation and Management of Hepatobiliary and
Pancreatic Disease

Yuman Fong, MD
Murray F. Brennan Chair in Surgery, Memorial Sloan-
Kettering Cancer Center; Professor, Department of Surgery,
Weill Cornell Medical College, New York, New York
Biliary Tract Tumors

Debra H. Ford, MD
Associate Professor and Vice-Chairman, Department of
Surgery, Head, Section of Colon and Rectal Surgery, Howard
University College of Medicine, Washington, DC
Pilonidal Disease

Patrick Forgione, MD
Associate Professor of Surgery, Director, Bariatric and
Metabolic Surgery, University of Vermont College of
Medicine, Fletcher Allen Health Care, Burlington, Vermont
Internal Hernias: Congenital and Acquired

John B. Fortune, MD
Professor and Vice-Chair, Department of Surgery, Medical
Director, Trauma Services, University of Vermont College of
Medicine, Fletcher Allen Health Care, Burlington, Vermont
Injuries to the Stomach, Duodenum, and Small Bowel

Danielle M. Fritze, MD
Resident, Department of Surgery, University of Michigan,
Ann Arbor, Michigan
Hepatic Cyst Disease

Karl-Hermann Fuchs, MD
Professor of Surgery, Department of General,
Gastrointestinal, and Thoracic Surgery, Agaplesion Markus
Krankenhaus, Frankfurt am Main, Germany
Tests of Gastric Function and Their Use in the Evaluation
of Esophageal Disease

Brian Funaki, MD
Professor of Radiology, Chief, Vascular and Interventional
Radiology, University of Chicago Medical Center; Editor-in-
Chief, Seminars in Interventional Radiology, Chicago, Illinois
Imaging and Radiologic Intervention in the Pancreas

Thomas R. Gadacz, MD
Professor Emeritus, Past Chairman, Department of Surgery,
Georgia Health Sciences University, St. Petersburg, Florida
Anatomy, Embryology, Anomalies, and Physiology

Susan Galandiuk, MD
Professor of Surgery, Director, Division of Colon and Rectal Surgery and Price Institute of Surgical Research, University of Louisville, Louisville, Kentucky; Honorary Professor of Translational Surgical Research, Blizard Institute of Cell and Molecular Science, Barts and the London School of Medicine and Dentistry, The Queen Mary University of London, London, United Kingdom
Traumatic Colorectal Injuries, Foreign Bodies, and Anal Wounds

David Geller, MD
Richard L. Simmons Professor of Surgery, University of Pittsburgh School of Medicine, Pittsburgh, Pennsylvania
Minimally Invasive Techniques of Hepatic Resection

George K. Gittes, MD
Professor of Surgery, Division of Pediatric Surgery, University of Pittsburgh School of Medicine; Surgeon-in-Chief, Children's Hospital of Pittsburgh, Pittsburgh, Pennsylvania
Anatomy, Physiology, and Embryology of the Pancreas

Christopher A. Gitzelmann, MD
Associate Professor of Surgery, Division of Pediatric Surgery, Golisano Children's Hospital, University of Rochester Medical Center, Rochester, New York
Congenital Disorders of the Esophagus

Tony E. Godfrey, PhD
Associate Professor of Surgery and Biomedical Genetics, University of Rochester Medical Center, James P. Wilmot Cancer Center, Rochester, New York
Genetics of Esophageal Cancer

Matthew I. Goldblatt, MD
Associate Professor of General Surgery, Department of Surgery, Medical College of Wisconsin, Milwaukee, Wisconsin
Appendix

Hein G. Gooszen, MD, PhD
Professor of Surgery, Department OR, MITeC, Evidence Based Surgery, Radboud University Nijmegen Medical Center, Nijmegen, The Netherlands
Acute Pancreatitis

Gregory J. Gores, MD
Reuben R. Eisenberg Professor of Medicine, Department of Gastroenterology and Hepatology, Mayo Clinic, Rochester, Minnesota
Primary Sclerosing Cholangitis

Yogesh Govil, MD
Attending Physician, Division of Gastroenterology and Nutrition, Department of Medicine, Albert Einstein College of Medicine, Montefiore Medical Center, Philadelphia, Pennsylvania
Medical Therapy for Gastroesophageal Reflux Disease

Kimberly Grant, MD
Research Fellow, Department of Surgery, Division of Thoracic and Foregut Surgery, University of Southern California, Keck School of Medicine, Los Angeles, California
Surgical Treatment of Cancer of the Esophagus and Esophagogastric Junction

Sarah E. Greer, MD, MPH
Instructor, Department of Surgery, Dartmouth Medical School, Hanover, New Hampshire; Resident, Department of Surgery, Dartmouth-Hitchcock Medical Center, Lebanon, New Hampshire
Foreign Bodies and Bezoars of the Stomach and Small Intestine

Jay L. Grosfeld, MD
Lafayette Page Professor Emeritus of Pediatric Surgery, Section of Pediatric Surgery, Indiana University School of Medicine, Riley Hospital for Children, Indianapolis, Indiana
Anorectal Anomalies

José G. Guillem, MD, MPH
Attending Surgeon, Department of Surgery, Memorial Sloan-Kettering Cancer Center; Professor of Surgery, Weill Cornell Medical College, New York, New York
Colorectal Polyps and Polyposis Syndromes

Jeffrey A. Hagen, MD
Associate Professor of Surgery, Chief, Division of Thoracic Surgery, Director, General Surgery Residency, University of Southern California, Keck School of Medicine, Los Angeles, California
Surgical Treatment of Cancer of the Esophagus and Esophagogastric Junction

Jason F. Hall, MD
Surgeon, Department of Colon and Rectal Surgery, Lahey Clinic Medical Center, Burlington, Massachusetts; Assistant Professor, Department of Surgery, Tufts University School of Medicine, Boston, Massachusetts
Colonic Intussusception and Volvulus

Christopher L. Hallemeier, MD
Department of Radiation Oncology, Mayo Clinic College of Medicine, Rochester, Minnesota
Adjuvant and Neoadjuvant Therapy for Colorectal Cancer

Peter T. Hallowell, MD
Assistant Professor, Department of Surgery, University of Virginia Health System, Charlottesville, Virginia
Reoperative Surgery of the Stomach and Duodenum

Amy P. Harper, ACNP-BC
Department of Radiology, Interventional Radiology Division, The George Washington University Medical Center, Washington, DC
Imaging and Intervention in the Biliary System

Ioannis S. Hatzaras, MD, MPH
Chief Resident, General Surgery, Department of Surgery, Ohio State University, Columbus, Ohio
Zollinger–Ellison Syndrome

Elliott R. Haut, MD
Associate Professor of Surgery, Anesthesiology and Critical Care Medicine, and Emergency Medicine, Division of Acute Care Surgery, Department of Surgery, Johns Hopkins University School of Medicine; Director, Trauma and Acute Care Surgery Fellowship, Johns Hopkins Hospital, Baltimore, Maryland
Pancreatic Trauma

William S. Havron, III, MD
Assistant Professor, Department of Surgery, University of Oklahoma Health Sciences Center, Oklahoma City, Oklahoma
Vagotomy and Drainage

Richard F. Heitmiller, III, MD
Chief of Surgery, Union Memorial Hospital, Baltimore, Maryland
Benign Tumors and Cysts of the Esophagus

J. Michael Henderson, MB, ChB
Chief Quality Officer, Professor, Department of Surgery, Cleveland Clinic, Cleveland, Ohio
Multidisciplinary Approach to the Management of Portal Hypertension

H. Franklin Herlong, MD
Associate Professor of Medicine, Division of Gastroenterology, Johns Hopkins University School of Medicine, Baltimore, Maryland
Approach to the Patient With Abnormal Hepatic Laboratory Tests

O. Joe Hines, MD
Professor and Chief, Division of General Surgery, Director, Surgery Residency Program, Department of Surgery, University of California Los Angeles, David Geffen School of Medicine, Los Angeles, California
Anatomy and Physiology of the Stomach

Fuyuki Hirashima, MD
General Surgery Resident, University of Vermont College of Medicine, Fletcher Allen Health Care, Burlington, Vermont
Aortoenteric Fistula and Visceral Artery Aneurysms

Wayne L. Hofstetter, MD
Associate Professor, Director, Esophageal Surgery, Department of Thoracic and Cardiovascular Surgery, The University of Texas MD Anderson Cancer Center, Houston, Texas
Multimodality Treatment for Potentially Resectable Esophageal Cancer

Arnulf H. Hölscher, MD
Professor of Surgery, Chairman, Department of General, Visceral, and Cancer Surgery, University of Cologne, Cologne, Germany
Epidemiology, Risk Factors, and Clinical Manifestations of Esophageal Cancer

Roel Hompes, MD
Senior Clinical and Research Fellow, Department of Colon and Rectal Surgery, Churchill Hospital, Oxford, United Kingdom
Transanal Endoscopic Microsurgery

Toshitaka Hoppo, MD, PhD
Research Assistant Professor, Department of Cardiothoracic Surgery, Division of Thoracic and Foregut Surgery, University of Pittsburgh Medical Center, Pittsburgh, Pennsylvania
Endoscopic Antireflux Repairs

Philip J. Huber, Jr., MD
Colon Rectal Surgeon, Medical City Dallas Hospital, Dallas, Texas
Fissure-in-Ano

Tracy Hull, MD
Professor of Surgery, Holder, Shafran Family Charitable Trust Endowed Chair, Department of Colon and Rectal Surgery, Digestive Disease Institute, Cleveland Clinic, Cleveland, Ohio
Pelvic Floor Dysfunction

Eric S. Hungness, MD
Assistant Professor, Department of Surgery, Northwestern University Feinberg School of Medicine, Chicago, Illinois
Management of Common Bile Duct Stones

John G. Hunter, MD
Mackenzie Professor and Chair, Department of Surgery, Oregon Health & Science University; Editor-in-Chief, World Journal of Surgery, Portland, Oregon
Laparoscopic and Open Nissen Fundoplication

James E. Huprich, MD
Associate Professor of Radiology, Department of Radiology, Mayo Clinic College of Medicine, Rochester, Minnesota
Imaging in Esophageal Disease

Hero K. Hussain, MD
Associate Professor, Chief, Body Magnetic Resonance Imaging, Director, Clinical Magnetic Resonance Imaging Services, University of Michigan Health System, Ann Arbor, Michigan
Hepatic Cyst Disease

Neil Hyman, MD
Samuel B. and Michelle D. Labow Green and Gold Professor of Surgery, Co-Director, Digestive Disease Center, University of Vermont College of Medicine, Fletcher Allen Health Care, Burlington, Vermont
Ostomy Management

Jennifer L. Irani, MD
Division of Colon and Rectal Surgery, Department of Surgery, Brigham and Women's Hospital; Instructor of Surgery, Harvard Medical School, Boston, Massachusetts
Local Excision of Rectal Cancer

Emily T. Jackson, ACNP-BC
Department of Radiology, Interventional Radiology Division, The George Washington University Medical Center, Washington, DC
Imaging and Intervention in the Biliary System

Danny O. Jacobs, MD, MPH
David C. Sabiston Jr. Professor and Chair, Duke University School of Medicine; Department of Surgery, Duke University Hospital, Durham, North Carolina
Volvulus of the Stomach and Small Bowel

Eric H. Jensen, MD
Assistant Professor, Department of Surgery, University of Minnesota, Minneapolis, Minnesota
Small Intestine

Catherine Jephcott, BM, BCh, MRCP, MA
Department of Oncology, Peterborough City Hospital, Bretton Gate, Peterborough, United Kingdom
Palliative Treatment of Cancer of the Esophagus

Blair A. Jobe, MD
Sampson Family Endowed Professor of Thoracic Oncology, Department of Cardiothoracic Surgery, Division of Thoracic and Foregut Surgery, University of Pittsburgh Medical Center, Pittsburgh, Pennsylvania
Endoscopic Antireflux Repairs

Michael Johnston, MD
Director, Colorectal Clinic, Department of Colorectal Surgery, St. Vincent's Hospital, University of Melbourne, Melbourne, Victoria, Australia
Rare Colorectal Malignancies

Jeffrey Jorden, MD
Assistant Professor of Surgery, Division of Colon and Rectal Surgery, University of Louisville, Louisville, Kentucky
Traumatic Colorectal Injuries, Foreign Bodies, and Anal Wounds

Paul Joyner, MD
Integrated General Surgery Residency Program, University of Connecticut, Farmington, Connecticut
Diverticular Disease

Lucas A. Julien, MD
Colorectal Fellow, Department of Surgery, Creighton University School of Medicine, Omaha, Nebraska
Anal Sepsis and Fistula

Peter J. Kahrilas, MD
Gilbert H. Marquardt Professor, Department of Medicine, Northwestern University Feinberg School of Medicine, Chicago, Illinois
Techniques of High-Resolution Esophageal Manometry, Classification and Treatment of Spastic Esophageal Motility Disorders

Ronald Kaleya, MD
Professor of Clinical Surgery, Department of Surgery, Albert Einstein College of Medicine, Montefiore Medical Center, Bronx, New York
Colonic Bleeding and Ischemia

Elika Kashef, MBBS, MRCS
Attending Physician, Department of Radiology, Imperial College Healthcare NHS Trust, London, United Kingdom
Hepatocellular Carcinoma

Philip Katz, MD
Chairman, Division of Gastroenterology, Albert Einstein College of Medicine, Montefiore Medical Center, Bronx, New York; Clinical Professor of Medicine, Jefferson Medical College, Philadelphia, Pennsylvania
Medical Therapy for Gastroesophageal Reflux Disease

Tara Kent, MD
Department of Surgery, Beth Israel Deaconess Medical Center; Instructor of Surgery, Harvard Medical School, Boston, Massachusetts
Prevention and Management of Complications of Pancreatic Surgery

Nadia J. Khati, MD
Assistant Professor, Department of Radiology, The George Washington University School of Medicine and Health Sciences, Washington, DC
Imaging and Intervention in the Biliary System

Jonathan C. King, MD
Resident, Department of Surgery, University of California Los Angeles, Los Angeles, California
Anatomy and Physiology of the Stomach

Nicole A. Kissane, MD
Assistant in Surgery, Division of General and Gastrointestinal Surgery, Massachusetts General Hospital, Boston, Massachusetts
Paraesophageal and Other Complex Diaphragmatic Hernias

Andrew S. Klein, MD
Director, Comprehensive Transplant Center, Professor and Vice-Chair, Department of Surgery, Esther and Mark Shulman Chair, Transplant Medicine and Surgery, Cedars-Sinai Medical Center, Los Angeles, California
Hepatic Transplantation

Dean E. Klinger, MD
Associate Professor, Department of Surgery, Medical College of Wisconsin; Staff Surgeon, Department of Surgery, Zablocki Veterans Affairs Medical Center, Milwaukee, Wisconsin
Small Bowel Obstruction

Jennifer Knight, MD
Assistant Professor of Trauma and Surgical Critical Care, Department of Surgery, West Virginia University School of Medicine, Morgantown, West Virginia
Mesenteric Arterial Trauma

Issam Koleilat, MD
General Surgery Resident, Department of Surgery, Albany Medical Center, Albany, New York
Gastrointestinal Lymphomas

Robert Kozol, MD
Professor, Department of Surgery, University of Miami; Program Director, Department of Surgery, University of Miami Regional Campus, Atlantis, Florida
Miscellaneous Benign Lesions and Conditions of the Stomach, Duodenum, and Small Intestine

Seth B. Krantz, MD
Research Fellow, Department of Surgery, Robert H. Lurie Comprehensive Cancer Center, Northwestern University Feinberg School of Medicine, Chicago, Illinois
Ablative Therapies for Hepatic Neoplasms

Daniela Ladner, MD, MPH
Assistant Professor of Surgery, Division of Transplant Surgery, Northwestern University Feinberg School of Medicine, Chicago, Illinois
Neuroendocrine Tumors of the Pancreas

Alexander Langerman, MD
Assistant Professor of Surgery, Section of Otolaryngology, Head, and Neck Surgery, University of Chicago Medical Center, Chicago, Illinois
Epidemiology, Pathophysiology, and Clinical Features of Achalasia

David W. Larson, MD
Associate Professor, Department of Surgery, Mayo Clinic College of Medicine; Consultant, Mayo Clinic, Rochester, Minnesota
Surgery for Inflammatory Bowel Disease: Crohn Disease

Simon Law, MBBChir
Professor and Chief, Division of Esophageal and Upper Gastrointestinal Surgery, Department of Surgery, University of Hong Kong, Pokfulam, Hong Kong
Esophageal Cancer: Current Staging Classifications and Techniques

Leo P. Lawler, MD
Mater Misericordiae University Hospital, Dublin, Ireland
Minimally Invasive Surgical and Image-Guided Interventional Approaches to the Spleen

Konstantinos N. Lazaridis, MD
Associate Professor of Medicine, Division of Gastroenterology and Hepatology, Mayo Clinic College of Medicine, Rochester, Minnesota
Primary Sclerosing Cholangitis

Yi-Horng Lee, MD
Assistant Professor, Department of Surgery, Golisano Children's Hospital, University of Rochester Medical Center, Rochester, New York
Congenital Disorders of the Esophagus

Yoori Lee, MD
Division of Colorectal Surgery, Department of Biostatistics and Computational Biology, University of Rochester Medical Center, Rochester, New York
Lumbar and Pelvic Hernias

Jérémie H. Lefèvre, MD
Associate Professor, Department of General and Digestive Surgery, Hospital Saint-Antoine, Pierre and Marie Curie University, Paris, France
Coloanal Anastomosis and Intersphincteric Resection

Glen A. Lehman, MD
Professor of Medicine and Radiology, Division of Digestive and Liver Disorders, Indiana University Medical Center, Indianapolis, Indiana
Endoscopic Retrograde Cholangiopancreatography in the Evaluation and Management of Hepatobiliary and Pancreatic Disease

Toni Lerut, MD, PhD
Professor of Surgery, University of Leuven Medical School, Chairman Emeritus, Department of Thoracic Surgery, University Hospital Gasthuisberg, Leuven, Belgium
Pathophysiology and Treatment of Zenker Diverticulum

David M. Levi, MD
Professor of Clinical Surgery, Miami Transplant Institute, DeWitt Daughtry Family Department of Surgery, University of Miami, Miller School of Medicine, Miami, Florida
Vascular Diseases of the Liver

Anne Lidor, MD, MPH
Assistant Professor, Department of Surgery, Johns Hopkins University School of Medicine, Baltimore, Maryland
Management of Splenic Trauma in Adults

Dorothea Liebermann-Meffert, MD
Professor of Surgery, Department of General Surgery, Rechts der Isar Hospital, Technical University of Munich, Munich, Germany
Human Foregut Anatomy, Adjacent Structures, and Their Relation to Surgical Approaches
Clinically Related Prenatal Foregut Development and Abnormalities in the Human

Joseph Lillegard, MD, PhD
Instructor of Surgery, Department of Gastrointestinal and General Surgery, Mayo Clinic College of Medicine, Rochester, Minnesota
Fulminant Hepatic Failure and Liver Support Systems

Keith D. Lillemoe, MD
W. Gerald Austen Professor, Harvard Medical School; Surgeon-in-Chief, Massachusetts General Hospital, Boston, Massachusetts
Pseudocysts and Other Complications of Pancreatitis

Virginia R. Litle, MD
Associate Professor, Department of Surgery, University of Rochester Medical Center, Rochester, New York
Genetics of Esophageal Cancer

Donald C. Liu, MD, PhD
Mary Campau Ryerson Professor and Surgeon-in-Chief, University of Chicago, Comer Children's Hospital; Vice-Chairman, Department of Surgery, University of Chicago, Pritzker School of Medicine, Chicago, Illinois
Management of Splenic Trauma in Children

Edward V. Loftus, Jr., MD
Professor of Medicine, Director, Inflammatory Bowel Disease Interest Group, Division of Gastroenterology and Hepatology, Mayo Clinic College of Medicine, Rochester, Minnesota
Inflammatory Bowel Disease

Miguel Lopez-Viego, MD
General and Vascular Surgery, University of Miami, Miller School of Medicine, Miami, Florida
Miscellaneous Benign Lesions and Conditions of the Stomach, Duodenum, and Small Intestine

Reginald V.N. Lord, MD
Department of Surgery, St. Vincent's Hospital, University of
New South Wales, Sydney, Australia
History and Definition of Barrett Esophagus

Val J. Lowe, MD
Department of Radiology, Mayo Clinic, Rochester, Minnesota
Imaging in Esophageal Disease

Georg Lurje, MD
Chief Resident, Swiss Hepato-Pancreato-Biliary and
Transplantation Center, Department of Surgery, University
Hospital Zurich, Zurich, Switzerland
Benign Hepatic Neoplasms

Calvin Lyons, Jr., MD
Research Fellow, Methodist Institute for Technology,
Innovation, and Education, Methodist Hospital, Houston,
Texas
Intubation of the Stomach and Small Intestine

Robert L. MacCarty, MD
Professor Emeritus, Department of Diagnostic Radiology,
Mayo Clinic College of Medicine, Rochester, Minnesota
Imaging in Esophageal Disease

Robert D. Madoff, MD
Stanley M. Goldberg, MD, Chair in Colon and Rectal Surgery,
Chief, Division of Colon and Rectal Surgery, Professor,
Department of Surgery, University of Minnesota, Minneapolis,
Minnesota
Diagnosis and Management of Fecal Incontinence

Anurag Maheshwari, MD
Institute for Digestive Health and Liver Disease, Mercy
Medical Center, Baltimore, Maryland
Drug-Induced Liver Disease

Najjia N. Mahmoud, MD
Associate Professor, Department of Surgery, University of
Pennsylvania, Philadelphia, Pennsylvania
*Evidence-Based Decision Making in Colon and Rectal
Surgery*

David M. Mahvi, MD
James R. Hines Professor, Chief, Gastrointestinal and Surgical
Oncology, Department of Surgery, Northwestern University
Feinberg School of Medicine, Chicago, Illinois
Ablative Therapies for Hepatic Neoplasms

Massimo Malagó, MD
Professor, Department of Surgery and Interventional
Sciences, University College London; Consultant Surgeon,
Royal Free Hospital, London, United Kingdom
Anatomy and Physiology of the Liver

Patrick Mannal, MD
General Surgery Resident, University of Vermont College of
Medicine, Fletcher Allen Health Care, Burlington, Vermont
*Adenocarcinoma of the Stomach, Duodenum, and Small
Intestine*

Michael R. Marohn, DO
Associate Professor, Department of Surgery, Johns Hopkins
University School of Medicine, Baltimore, Maryland
*Minimally Invasive Surgical and Image-Guided
Interventional Approaches to the Spleen*

David J. Maron, MD
Staff Surgeon, Department of Colorectal Surgery, Cleveland
Clinic Florida, Weston, Florida
Surgical Treatment of Constipation

Joseph E. Martz, MD
Director, Colon and Rectal Surgery, Department of Surgery,
Beth Israel Deaconess Medical Center, New York, New York
Abdominoperineal Resection of the Rectum for Cancer

Kellie L. Mathis, MD
General Surgery, Mayo Clinic College of Medicine, Rochester,
Minnesota
Recurrent and Metatstatic Colorectal Cancer

Douglas Mathisen, MD
Hermes C. Grillo Professor of Surgery, Chief, Division of
Thoracic Surgery, Massachusetts General Hospital, Boston,
Massachusetts
Techniques of Esophageal Reconstruction

Jeffrey B. Matthews, MD
Dallas B. Phemister Professor and Chairman, Department of
Surgery, University of Chicago, Chicago, Illinois
Chronic Pancreatitis

Laurence E. McCahill, MD
Director, Department of Surgical Oncology, Richard J. Lacks
Cancer Center, Saint Mary's Health Care; Professor of
Surgery, Michigan State University, College of Human
Medicine, Grand Rapids, Michigan
Gastrointestinal Stromal Tumors

David A. McClusky, III, MD
Assistant Professor, Associate Chief-of-Surgery, Section Chief,
General Surgery, Atlanta Veterans Affairs Medical Center;
Department of Surgery, Emory University School of Medicine,
Atlanta, Georgia
Anatomy and Physiology of the Duodenum

David W. McFadden, MD
Professor and Chairman, Department of Surgery, University
of Connecticut, Farmington, Connecticut
*Adenocarcinoma of the Stomach, Duodenum, and Small
Intestine*

Lee McHenry, Jr., MD
Professor of Medicine, Department of Medicine, Division of
Gastroenterology and Hepatology, Gastrointestinal Cancer
Program, Melvin and Bren Simon Cancer Center, Indiana
University School of Medicine; Medical Director, Indiana
University Health Springmill Medicine Clinics, Indianapolis,
Indiana
*Endoscopic Retrograde Cholangiopancreatography in the
Evaluation and Management of Hepatobiliary and
Pancreatic Disease*

Paul J. McMurrick, MBBS
Associate Professor of Surgery, Frolich-West Chair of Surgery, Head, Cabrini Monash University, Malvern, Victoria, Australia
Rare Colorectal Malignancies

Anthony S. Mee, MD
Consultant Gastroenterologist, Royal Berkshire Hospital, Reading, Berkshire, United Kingdom
Palliative Treatment of Cancer of the Esophagus

John E. Meilahn, MD
Director, Bariatric Surgery, Associate Professor, Department of Surgery, Temple University School of Medicine, Philadelphia, Pennsylvania
Motility Disorders of the Stomach and Small Intestine

Fabrizio Michelassi, MD
Lewis Atterbury Stimson Professor, Chairman, Department of Surgery, Weill Cornell Medical College; Surgeon-in-Chief, New York-Presbyterian Hospital, New York, New York
Crohn Disease: General Considerations, Medical Management, and Surgical Treatment of Small Intestinal Disease

Robert C. Miller, MD
Professor, Department of Radiation Oncology, Mayo Clinic College of Medicine, Rochester, Minnesota
Adjuvant and Neoadjuvant Therapy for Colorectal Cancer

Thomas A. Miller, MD
Ammons Distinguished Professor of Surgery, Department of Surgery, Virginia Commonwealth University School of Medicine; Chief of General Surgery, Hunter Holmes McGuire Veterans Affairs Medical Center, Richmond, Virginia
Postgastrectomy Syndromes

J. Michael Millis, MD
Professor of Surgery, Director, University of Chicago Transplant Center; Chief, Section of Transplantation, Liver Transplantation, and Hepatobiliary Surgery, University of Chicago, Chicago, Illinois
Pancreas and Islet Allotransplantation

Ryosuke Misawa, MD, PhD
Associate Research Scientist, Department of Surgery, University of Chicago, Chicago, Illinois
Pancreas and Islet Allotransplantation

Sumeet Mittal, MBBS
Associate Professor, Department of Surgery, Creighton University School of Medicine; Director, Esophageal Center, Creighton University Medical Center, Omaha, Nebraska
Reflux Strictures and Short Esophagus

Ernesto P. Molmenti, MD, PhD
Vice-Chairman, Department of Surgery, Director, Transplant Program, North Shore University Hospital, Manhasset, New York; Professor of Surgery and Medicine, Hofstra North Shore-Long Island Jewish School of Medicine, New York, New York
Anatomy and Physiology of the Liver
Anatomy and Physiology of the Spleen

John R.T. Monson, MD
Professor of Surgery and Oncology, Chief, Division of Colorectal Surgery, Vice-Chairman, Department of Surgery, University of Rochester Medical Center, Rochester, New York
Lumbar and Pelvic Hernias

Jesse Moore, MD
Fellow, Department of Colon and Rectal Surgery, Mayo Clinic, Rochester, Minnesota
Ileostomy

Katherine A. Morgan, MD
Associate Professor, Section of Gastrointestinal and Laparoscopic Surgery, Medical University of South Carolina, Charleston, South Carolina
Biliary Dyskinesia and Sphincter of Oddi Dysfunction

Christopher R. Morse, MD
Instructor of Surgery, Division of Thoracic Surgery, Massachusetts General Hospital, Boston, Massachusetts
Techniques of Esophageal Reconstruction

Neil J. Mortensen, MB, ChB, MA, MD
Professor of Colorectal Surgery, Department of Colorectal Surgery, Oxford University Hospitals, Churchill Hospital, Oxford, United Kingdom
Anatomy and Embryology of the Colon
Transanal Endoscopic Microsurgery

Melinda M. Mortenson, MD
Surgical Oncology, Department of Surgery, Kaiser Permanente Medical Group, Sacramento, California
Unusual Pancreatic Tumors

Ruth Moxon, MSc
Upper Gastrointestinal Clinical Nurse Specialist, Royal Berkshire Hospital, Reading, Berkshire, United Kingdom
Palliative Treatment of Cancer of the Esophagus

Michael W. Mulholland, MD, PhD
Professor of Surgery, Department of Surgery, University of Michigan, Ann Arbor, Michigan
Hepatic Cyst Disease

Ido Nachmany, MD
Hepato-Pancreato-Biliary and Transplantation Clinical Fellow, Starzl Transplantation Institute, University of Pittsburgh Medical Center, Pittsburgh, Pennsylvania
Minimally Invasive Techniques of Hepatic Resection

Philippe Nafteux, MD
Clinical Head, Department of Thoracic Surgery, University Hospital Gasthuisberg, Leuven, Belgium
Pathophysiology and Treatment of Zenker Diverticulum

David M. Nagorney, MD
Professor of Surgery, Department of Surgery, Mayo Clinic College of Medicine, Rochester, Minnesota
Splenectomy for Conditions Other Than Trauma
Resection and Ablation of Metastatic Colorectal Cancer to the Liver

Govind Nandakumar, MD
Assistant Professor, Department of Surgery, Weill Cornell
Medical College, New York, New York
*Crohn Disease: General Considerations, Medical
    Management, and Surgical Treatment of Small
    Intestinal Disease*

Bala Natarajan, MBBS
Surgery Resident, Creighton University Medical Center,
Omaha, Nebraska
Basic Features of Groin Hernia and Its Repair

Heidi Nelson, MD
Fred C. Andersen Professor of Surgery, Chair, Division of
Surgery Research, Department of Surgery, Mayo Clinic
College of Medicine, Rochester, Minnesota
Recurrent and Metastatic Colorectal Cancer

Jeffrey M. Nicastro, MD
Assistant Professor of Surgery, Vice-Chairman, Department of
Surgery, Chief, Division of Acute Care Surgery, Hofstra North
Shore-Long Island Jewish School of Medicine, New York, New
York
*Anatomy and Physiology of the Liver
Anatomy and Physiology of the Spleen*

Ankesh Nigam, MD
Associate Professor of Surgery, Director, Surgical Oncology
Program, Department of Surgery, Albany Medical College,
Albany, New York
Gastrointestinal Lymphomas

Nicholas N. Nissen, MD
Comprehensive Transplant Center, Center for Liver Diseases
and Transplantation, Cedars-Sinai Medical Center, Los
Angeles, California
Hepatic Transplantation

Jeffrey A. Norton, MD
Professor of Surgery and Chief of General Surgery, Stanford
University School of Medicine, Stanford, California
Neuroendocrine Tumors of the Pancreas

Michael Nussbaum, MD
Professor and Chair, Department of Surgery, University of
Florida College of Medicine; Surgeon-in-Chief, Shands
Jacksonville Medical Center, Jacksonville, Florida
Gastric, Duodenal, and Small Intestinal Fistulas

Scott Nyberg, MD, PhD
Professor of Surgery, Department of Surgery, Mayo Clinic
College of Medicine, Rochester, Minnesota
Fulminant Hepatic Failure and Liver Support Systems

Stefan Öberg, MD, PhD
Department of Surgery, Lund University Hospital, Lund,
Sweden
Esophageal pH Monitoring

Daniel S. Oh, MD
Assistant Professor of Surgery, University of Southern
California, Keck School of Medicine, Los Angeles, California
Pathophysiology of the Columnar-Lined Esophagus

Jill K. Onesti, MD
Clinical Instructor, Department of Surgery, Michigan State
University, College of Human Medicine, Grand Rapids,
Michigan
Gastrointestinal Stromal Tumors

Robert W. O'Rourke, MD
Associate Professor of Surgery, Co-Director, Bariatric Surgery
Program, Department of Surgery, Oregon Health & Science
University, Portland, Oregon
Laparoscopic and Open Nissen Fundoplication

Aytekin Oto, MD
Professor of Radiology and Surgery, Chief, Abdominal
Imaging and Body Magnetic Resonance Imaging, University
of Chicago, Pritzker School of Medicine, Chicago, Illinois
Imaging and Radiologic Intervention in the Pancreas

Mary F. Otterson, MD
Professor, Department of Surgery, Associate Professor,
Department of Physiology, Medical College of Wisconsin;
Staff Surgeon, Department of Surgery, Zablocki Veterans
Affairs Medical Center, Milwaukee, Wisconsin
Small Bowel Obstruction

James R. Ouellette, DO
Associate Professor, Department of Surgery, Chief, Division of
Surgical Oncology, Director, Hepatobiliary and Pancreatic
Surgery Program, Wright State University Boonshoft School
of Medicine, Dayton, Ohio
*Perioperative Management and Nutrition in Patients With
    Liver and Biliary Tract Disease*

Charles N. Paidas, MD
Professor of Surgery and Pediatrics, Chief, Pediatric Surgery,
Associate Dean for Graduate Medical Education, Executive
Associate Dean for Clinical and Extramural Affairs, University
of South Florida, Health Morsani College of Medicine,
Tampa, Florida
Pancreatic Problems in Infants and Children

John E. Pandolfino, MD
Associate Professor of Medicine, Department of Medicine,
Northwestern University Feinberg School of Medicine,
Chicago, Illinois
*Techniques of High-Resolution Esophageal Manometry,
    Classification and Treatment of Spastic Esophageal
    Motility Disorders*

Harry T. Papaconstantinou, MD
Vice-Chairman, Department of Surgery, Chief, Section of
Colorectal Surgery, Scott & White Healthcare; Associate
Professor of Surgery, Texas A&M Health Science Center,
College of Medicine, Temple, Texas
Fissure-in-Ano

Theodore N. Pappas, MD
Professor of Surgery, Department of Surgery, Vice-Dean for
Medical Affairs, Duke University School of Medicine,
Durham, North Carolina
Operative Management of Cholecystitis and Cholelithiasis

Yann Parc, MD, PhD
Professor, Department of General and Digestive Surgery, Hospital Saint-Antoine, Pierre and Marie Curie University, Paris, France
Coloanal Anastomosis and Intersphincteric Resection

Susan C. Parker, MD
Retired, Division of Colon and Rectal Surgery, Department of Surgery, University of Minnesota, Minneapolis, Minnesota
Diagnosis and Management of Fecal Incontinence

Marco G. Patti, MD
Professor of Surgery, Director, Center for Esophageal Diseases, University of Chicago, Pritzker School of Medicine, Chicago, Illinois
Epidemiology, Pathophysiology, and Clinical Features of Achalasia

Walter Pegoli, Jr., MD, MHS
Surgeon-in-Chief, Department of Surgery, Golisano Children's Hospital, University of Rochester Medical Center, Rochester, New York
Congenital Disorders of the Esophagus
Hernias and Congenital Groin Problems in Infants and Children

John H. Pemberton, MD
Professor of Surgery, Mayo Clinic College of Medicine; Consultant in Colon and Rectal Surgery, Mayo Clinic and Mayo Foundation, Rochester, Minnesota
Anatomy and Physiology of the Rectum and Anus Including Applied Anatomy
Surgery for Inflammatory Bowel Disease: Chronic Ulcerative Colitis

Jeffrey H. Peters, MD
Seymour I. Schwartz Professor and Chairman, Department of Surgery, University of Rochester School of Medicine and Dentistry, Rochester, New York
Assessment of Symptoms and Approach to the Patient With Esophageal Disease
The Gastroesophageal Barrier
Treatment of Barrett Esophagus
Genetics of Esophageal Cancer
Perforation of the Esophagus

Thai H. Pham, MD
Assistant Professor, Department of Surgery, North Texas Veterans Affairs Medical Center, University of Texas Southwestern Medical Center, Dallas, Texas
Laparoscopic and Open Nissen Fundoplication

Lakshmikumar Pillai, MD
Associate Professor and Chief, Division of Vascular and Endovascular Surgery, Department of Surgery, West Virginia University Medical Center, Morgantown, West Virginia
Anatomy and Physiology of the Mesenteric Circulation

Carlos E. Pineda, MD
Resident, Department of Surgery, Stanford University School of Medicine, Stanford, California
Surgery in the Immunocompromised Patient

Henry A. Pitt, MD
Professor and Vice-Chairman, Department of Surgery, Indiana University School of Medicine, Indianapolis, Indiana
Anatomy, Embryology, Anomalies, and Physiology

Jeffrey L. Ponsky, MD
Oliver H. Payne Professor and Chairman, Department of Surgery, Case Western Reserve University School of Medicine; Surgeon-in-Chief, University Hospitals Case Medical Center, Cleveland, Ohio
Diagnostic and Therapeutic Endoscopy of the Stomach and Small Bowel
Management of Splenic Abscess

Mitchell C. Posner, MD
Thomas D. Jones Professor and Vice-Chairman, Department of Surgery, Chief, Section of General Surgery and Surgical Oncology, University of Chicago, Pritzker School of Medicine, Chicago, Illinois
Management of Secondary Hepatic Neoplasms
Adenocarcinoma of the Colon and Rectum

Russel G. Postier, MD
John A. Schilling Professor and Chairman, Department of Surgery, University of Oklahoma Health Sciences Center, Oklahoma City, Oklahoma
Vagotomy and Drainage

Sangeetha Prabhakaran, MD
Surgical Resident, Department of Surgery, University of North Dakota, Grand Forks, North Dakota
Liver Abscess

Vivek N. Prachand, MD
Associate Professor, Department of Surgery, University of Chicago, Pritzker School of Medicine, Chicago, Illinois
Endoscopic and Minimally Invasive Therapy for Complications of Acute and Chronic Pancreatitis

Florencia G. Que, MD
Associate Professor, Department of Surgery, Mayo Clinic College of Medicine, Rochester, Minnesota
Resection and Ablation of Metastatic Colorectal Cancer to the Liver

Arnold Radtke, MD, PhD
Associate Professor, Department of General and Thoracic Surgery, University of Schleswig-Holstein, Lubeck, Germany
Anatomy and Physiology of the Liver

Rudra Rai, MD
Assistant Professor of Medicine, Johns Hopkins University School of Medicine; Medical Director, Gastro Center of Maryland, Baltimore, Maryland
Drug-Induced Liver Disease

Jan Rakinic, MD
Associate Professor, Department of Surgery, Chief, Section of Colorectal Surgery, Program Director, Colorectal Surgery Training Program, Southern Illinois University School of Medicine, Springfield, Illinois
Antibiotics, Approaches, Strategy, and Anastomoses

David W. Rattner, MD
Professor of Surgery, Harvard Medical School; Chief, Division of General and Gastrointestinal Surgery, Massachusetts General Hospital, Boston, Massachusetts
Paraesophageal and Other Complex Diaphragmatic Hernias

Daniel P. Raymond, MD
Department of Thoracic and Cardiovascular Surgery, Cleveland Clinic, Cleveland, Ohio
Perforation of the Esophagus

Thomas W. Rice, MD
Professor of Surgery, Cleveland Clinic Lerner College of Medicine; Daniel and Karen Lee Chair of Thoracic Surgery, Head, Section of General Thoracic Surgery, Department of Thoracic and Cardiovascular Surgery, Cleveland Clinic, Cleveland, Ohio
Endoscopic Esophageal Ultrasonography

J. David Richardson, MD
Professor and Vice-Chair of Surgery, University of Louisville, Louisville, Kentucky
Management of Hepatobiliary Trauma

Martin Riegler, MD
Associate Professor of Surgery, Manometry Lab; University Clinic of Surgery, Medical University Vienna, Vienna General Hospital, Vienna, Austria
Epidemiology and Natural History of Gastroesophageal Reflux Disease

John Paul Roberts, MD
Chief, Division of Transplant, Department of Surgery, University of California, San Francisco, San Francisco, California
Hepatocellular Carcinoma

Patricia L. Roberts, MD
Chair, Department of Colon and Rectal Surgery, Lahey Clinic Medical Center, Burlington, Massachusetts; Professor of Surgery, Tufts University School of Medicine, Boston, Massachusetts
Rectovaginal and Rectourethral Fistulas

David A. Rodeberg, MD
Assistant Professor of Surgery, University of Pittsburgh School of Medicine; Assistant Director, Trauma and Injury Prevention, Children's Hospital of Pittsburgh, Pittsburgh, Pennsylvania
Pancreatic Problems in Infants and Children

Kevin K. Roggin, MD
Associate Professor of Surgery and Cancer Research, Director of General Surgery Residency Program, University of Chicago, Pritzker School of Medicine, Chicago, Illinois
Management of Secondary Hepatic Neoplasms

Rolando Rolandelli, MD
Professor of Surgery, University of Medicine and Dentistry of New Jersey, Chairman, Department of Surgery, Morristown Medical Center, Morristown, New Jersey
Suturing, Stapling, and Tissue Adhesives

Sabine Roman, MD, PhD
Associate Professor, Digestive Physiology, Université Claude Bernard Lyon 1, Lyon, France
Techniques of High-Resolution Esophageal Manometry, Classification and Treatment of Spastic Esophageal Motility Disorders

Ernest L. Rosato, MD
Professor of Surgery, Chief, Division of General Surgery, Department of Surgery, Thomas Jefferson University, Philadelphia, Pennsylvania
Pseudocysts and Other Complications of Pancreatitis

Michael J. Rosen, MD
Associate Professor of Surgery, Department of Surgery, University Hospitals Case Medical Center, Cleveland, Ohio
Ventral Herniation in Adults

Andrew Ross, MD
Director, Therapeutic Endoscopy Center of Excellence, Digestive Disease Institute, Virginia Mason Medical Center, Seattle, Washington
Endoscopic and Minimally Invasive Therapy for Complications of Acute and Chronic Pancreatitis

Amy P. Rushing, MD
Assistant Professor, Department of Surgery, Division of Acute Care Surgery, Trauma, and Surgical Critical Care, Johns Hopkins Hospital, Baltimore, Maryland
Pancreatic Trauma
Management of Splenic Trauma in Adults

Adheesh Sabnis, MD
Co-Director, Minimally Invasive and Laparoscopic Surgery, Good Samaritan Hospital, Baltimore, Maryland
Management of Splenic Abscess

Theodore J. Saclarides, MD
Professor of Surgery, Department of General Surgery, Head, Section of Colon and Rectal Surgery, Rush University Medical Center, Chicago, Illinois
Radiation Injuries to the Rectum

Peter M. Sagar, MD, MB, ChB
Consultant Surgeon, John Goligher Department of Colorectal Surgery, General Infirmary at Leeds, West Yorkshire, United Kingdom
Surgery for Inflammatory Bowel Disease: Chronic Ulcerative Colitis

George H. Sakorafas, MD
Associate Professor of Surgery, Fourth Department of Surgery, Athens University Medical School, Athens, Greece
Primary Pancreatic Cystic Neoplasms

Leonard B. Saltz, MD
Acting Chief, Gastrointestinal Oncology Service; Head, Colorectal Oncology Section, Memorial Sloan-Kettering Cancer Center, New York, New York
Adenocarcinoma of the Colon and Rectum

Shawn N. Sarin, MD
Assistant Professor of Radiology, Department of Radiology, Interventional Radiology Division, The George Washington University Medical Center, Washington, DC
Imaging and Intervention in the Biliary System

Michael G. Sarr, MD
James C. Masson Professor of Surgery, Department of Surgery, Mayo Clinic College of Medicine, Rochester, Minnesota
Primary Pancreatic Cystic Neoplasms

Kennith Sartorelli, MD
Professor, Department of Surgery, University of Vermont College of Medicine, Fletcher Allen Health Care, Burlington, Vermont
Surgical Conditions of the Small Intestine in Infants and Children

Jeannie F. Savas, MD
Associate Professor, Department of Surgery, Virginia Commonwealth University School of Medicine; Interim Chief of Surgery, Hunter Holmes McGuire Veterans Affairs Medical Center, Richmond, Virginia
Postgastrectomy Syndromes

Bruce Schirmer, MD
Stephen H. Watts Professor of Surgery, Department of Surgery, University of Virginia Health System, Charlottesville, Virginia
Reoperative Surgery of the Stomach and Duodenum

Christine Schmid-Tannwald, MD
Department of Radiology, University of Chicago, Pritzker School of Medicine, Chicago, Illinois
Imaging and Radiologic Intervention in the Pancreas

John G. Schneider, MD
Chief Resident, Department of Surgery, University of Vermont College of Medicine, Fletcher Allen Health Care, Burlington, Vermont
Surgical Conditions of the Small Intestine in Infants and Children
Mesenteric Ischemia

Paul M. Schneider, MD
Professor, Department of Surgery, University Hospital Zurich, Zurich, Switzerland
Epidemiology, Risk Factors, and Clinical Manifestations of Esophageal Cancer

Thomas Schnelldorfer, MD
Assistant Professor of Clinical Surgery, Department of Surgery, University of Pennsylvania, Philadelphia, Pennsylvania
Primary Pancreatic Cystic Neoplasms

David J. Schoetz, Jr., MD
Professor of Surgery, Chief Academic Officer, Academic Dean, Designated Institutional Official, Graduate Medical Education, Chairman Emeritus, Department of Colon and Rectal Surgery, Tufts University School of Medicine, Lahey Clinic Medical Center, Burlington, Massachusetts
Colonic Intussusception and Volvulus

Sebastian Schoppmann, MD
Department of Surgery, University of Vienna, Vienna, Austria
Epidemiology and Natural History of Gastroesophageal Reflux Disease

Wolfgang Schröder, MD
Department of General, Visceral, and Cancer Surgery, University of Cologne, Cologne, Germany
Epidemiology, Risk Factors, and Clinical Manifestations of Esophageal Cancer

Richard D. Schulick, MD
Professor of Surgery and Oncology, John L. Cameron Professor of Alimentary Tract Surgery, Chief, Division of Surgical Oncology, Johns Hopkins University School of Medicine, Baltimore, Maryland
Pancreatic and Periampullary Cancer
Diagnostic Operations of the Liver and Techniques of Hepatic Resection

Anthony Senagore, MD
Chief, Professor and Clinical Scholar, Division of Colorectal Surgery, Charles W. and Carolyn Costello Chair, Colorectal Diseases, University of Southern California, Keck School of Medicine, Los Angeles, California
Hemorrhoids

Boris Sepesi, MD
Cardiothoracic Surgery Fellow, Department of Thoracic and Cardiovascular Surgery, The University of Texas MD Anderson Cancer Center, Houston, Texas
Perforation of the Esophagus

Nicholas J. Shaheen, MD, MPH
Professor of Medicine and Epidemiology, Director, Center for Esophageal Diseases and Swallowing, University of North Carolina School of Medicine, Chapel Hill, North Carolina
Clinical Features and Endoscopic Therapy for Dysplastic Barrett Esophagus

Stuart Sherman, MD
Professor, Departments of Medicine and Radiology, Gastrointestinal Cancer Program, Melvin and Bren Simon Cancer Center, Indiana University School of Medicine, Indianapolis, Indiana
Endoscopic Retrograde Cholangiopancreatography in the Evaluation and Management of Hepatobiliary and Pancreatic Disease

Irene Silberstein, MD
Department of Surgery, Atlantic Health System Hospitals, Morristown, New Jersey
Suturing, Stapling, and Tissue Adhesives

Clifford L. Simmang, MD
Texas Colon and Rectal Surgeons, Dallas, Texas
Fissure-in-Ano

George Singer, MD
Department of General Surgery, Rush University Medical Center, Chicago, Illinois
Radiation Injuries to the Rectum

Douglas P. Slakey, MD
Professor and Chair, Department of Surgery, Tulane
University, New Orleans, Louisiana
Cysts and Tumors of the Spleen

Jason Smith, MD, PhD
Assistant Professor, Department of Surgery, Department of
Physiology and Biophysics, University of Louisville, Louisville,
Kentucky
Management of Hepatobiliary Trauma
Traumatic Colorectal Injuries, Foreign Bodies, and Anal
Wounds

Jessica K. Smith, MD
Assistant Professor, Department of Surgery, Gastrointestinal,
Minimally Invasive, and Bariatric Surgery, University of Iowa
Hospitals and Clinics, Iowa City, Iowa
Small Bowel Diverticula

Christopher W. Snyder, MD, MSPH
General Surgery Residency Program, University of Alabama at
Birmingham, Birmingham, Alabama
Autologous Islet Cell Transplantation

Christopher J. Sonnenday, MD, MHS
Assistant Professor of Surgery, Assistant Professor of Health
Management and Policy, Hepatobiliary, Pancreatic, and
Transplant Surgery, University of Michigan, Ann Arbor,
Michigan
Pseudocysts and Other Complications of Pancreatitis

Nathaniel J. Soper, MD
Loyal and Edith Davis Professor and Chair, Department of
Surgery, Northwestern University Feinberg School of
Medicine, Chicago, Illinois
Management of Common Bile Duct Stones

George C. Sotiropoulos, MD, PhD
Professor of Surgery and Transplantation, Department of
General, Visceral, and Transplantation Surgery, University of
Duisburg-Essen Medical School, University Hospital Essen,
Essen, Germany
Anatomy and Physiology of the Liver

Stuart Jon Spechler, MD
Professor of Medicine, University of Texas Southwestern
Medical Center; Chief, Division of Gastroenterology, Veterans
Affairs North Texas Healthcare System, Dallas, Texas
Endoscopic Evaluation of the Esophagus

Andrew Stanley, MD
Chief, Division of Vascular Surgery, Department of Surgery,
University of Vermont College of Medicine, Fletcher Allen
Health Care, Burlington, Vermont
Mesenteric Ischemia

Mindy B. Statter, MD
Associate Professor of Clinical Surgery, Division of Pediatric
Surgery, Albert Einstein College of Medicine, Montefiore
Medical Center, Bronx, New York
Management of Splenic Trauma in Children

Kimberley E. Steele, MD
Assistant Professor of Surgery, Director, Surgical Simulation
and Education, Johns Hopkins Bayview Medical Center;
Director, Adolescent Bariatric Surgery, Johns Hopkins Center
for Bariatric Surgery, Baltimore, Maryland
Minimally Invasive Surgical and Image-Guided
Interventional Approaches to the Spleen

Emily Steinhagen, MD
Clinical Research Fellow, Department of Surgery, Colorectal
Service, Memorial Sloan-Kettering Cancer Center, New York,
New York
Colorectal Polyps and Polyposis Syndromes

Luca Stocchi, MD
Staff Surgeon, Department of Colorectal Surgery, Digestive
Disease Institute, Cleveland Clinic, Ohio
Anatomy and Embryology of the Colon
Anatomy and Physiology of the Rectum and Anus
Including Applied Anatomy

Gary Sudakoff, MD
Department of Radiology, Medical College of Wisconsin,
Zablocki Veterans Affairs Medical Center, Milwaukee,
Wisconsin
Small Bowel Obstruction

Abhishek Sundaram, MD
Resident, Department of Surgery, Creighton University
School of Medicine, Omaha, Nebraska
Reflux Strictures and Short Esophagus

Magesh Sundaram, MD
Chief, Division of Surgical Oncology, Associate Professor,
Department of Surgery, West Virginia University School of
Medicine, Morgantown, West Virginia
Radiation Enteritis

Lee L. Swanström, MD
Professor of Surgery, University of Strasbourg, Strasbourg,
France; Clinical Professor of Surgery, Oregon Health &
Science University, Portland, Oregon
Partial Fundoplications

Daniel E. Swartz, MD
Director, Central California Institute of Minimally Invasive
Surgery, Fresno, California
Femoral Hernia

Tadahiro Takada, MD
Professor Emeritus, Department of Surgery, Teikyo University
School of Medicine, Tokyo, Japan
Cystic Disorders of the Bile Ducts

Eric P. Tamm, MD
Department of Radiology, The University of Texas MD
Anderson Cancer Center, Houston, Texas
Unusual Pancreatic Tumors

Ali Tavakkolizadeh, MD
Assistant Professor of Surgery, Harvard Medical School;
Department of Minimally Invasive and Gastrointestinal
Surgery, Brigham and Women's Hospital, Boston,
Massachusetts
Operations for Peptic Ulcer

Gordon L. Telford, MD
Professor of Surgery, Medical College of Wisconsin;
Chairman, Division of Surgery, Zablocki Veterans Affairs
Medical Center, Milwaukee, Wisconsin
Appendix

Julie K. Marosky Thacker, MD
Assistant Professor, Department of Surgery, Duke University
School of Medicine, Durham, North Carolina
Volvulus of the Stomach and Small Bowel
Diagnosis of Colon, Rectal, and Anal Disease

Dimitra G. Theodoropoulos, MD
Attending Surgeon, Department of Surgery, North Shore
University Hospital, Manhasset, New York
Ultrasonographic Diagnosis of Anorectal Disease

Michael S. Thomas, MD, PhD
Surgical Resident, Department of Surgery, Tulane University,
New Orleans, Louisiana
Cysts and Tumors of the Spleen

Alan G. Thorson, MD
Clinical Professor of Surgery, University of Nebraska Medical
Center, Creighton University School of Medicine, Omaha,
Nebraska
Anal Sepsis and Fistula

Kristy Thurston, MD
Resident, Department of General Surgery, University of
Connecticut, Farmington, Connecticut
Diverticular Disease

David S. Tichansky, MD
Associate Professor, Department of Surgery, Thomas Jefferson
University, Philadelphia, Pennsylvania
Operations for Morbid Obesity

Yutaka Tomizawa, MD
Barrett's Esophagus Unit, Division of Gastroenterology and
Hepatology, Mayo Clinic College of Medicine, Rochester,
Minnesota
Endoscopic Management of Early Esophageal Cancer

L. William Traverso, MD
Clinical Professor of Surgery, University of Washington,
Seattle, Washington; Director, Center for Pancreatic Disease,
St. Luke's Hospital System, Boise, Idaho
Prevention and Management of Iatrogenic Bile Duct
Injury

Thadeus Trus, MD
Associate Professor, Department of Surgery, Minimally
Invasive Surgery, Dartmouth-Hitchcock Medical Center,
Lebanon, New Hampshire
Foreign Bodies and Bezoars of the Stomach and Small
Intestine

Susan Tsai, MD, MHS
Assistant Professor, Division of Surgical Oncology,
Department of Surgery, Medical College of Wisconsin,
Milwaukee, Wisconsin
Unusual Pancreatic Tumors

Vassiliki Liana Tsikitis, MD
Assistant Professor, Department of Surgery, Division of
General and Gastrointestinal Surgery, Oregon Health &
Science University, Portland, Oregon
Operations for Colorectal Cancer: Low Anterior Resection

Steven Tsoraides, MD
General Surgery, Peoria Surgery Group, Illinois Medical
Center, Peoria, Illinois
Antibiotics, Approaches, Strategy, and Anastomoses

Radu Tutuian, MD, PhD
Clinical Lead, Outpatient Services and Gastrointestinal
Function Laboratory, Division of Gastroenterology, University
Clinic for Visceral Surgery and Medicine, Bern University
Hospital, Bern, Switzerland
Physiology of the Esophagus and Its Sphincters
Multichannel Intraluminal Impedance

Andreas G. Tzakis, MD, PhD
Professor of Surgery, Founding Director, Miami Transplant
Institute, DeWitt Daughtry Family Department of Surgery,
University of Miami, Miller School of Medicine, Miami,
Florida
Vascular Diseases of the Liver

Daniel Vallböhmer, MD
Associate Professor, Department of General, Visceral, and
Pediatric Surgery, University of Dusseldorf, Dusseldorf,
Germany
Epidemiology, Risk Factors, and Clinical Manifestations of
Esophageal Cancer

Dirk Van Raemdonck, MD, PhD
Department of Thoracic Surgery, University Hospital Leuven,
Gasthuisberg, Belgium
Pathophysiology and Treatment of Zenker Diverticulum

Hjalmar van Santvoort, MD, PhD
Clinical Research Fellow, Resident, General Surgery,
Department of Surgery, University Medical Center Utrecht,
Utrecht, The Netherlands
Acute Pancreatitis

Anthony C. Venbrux, MD
Professor of Radiology and Surgery, Director, Cardiovascular
and Interventional Radiology, The George Washington
University Medical Center, Washington, DC
Imaging and Intervention in the Biliary System

Selwyn M. Vickers, MD
Jay Phillips Professor and Chair, Department of Surgery,
University of Minnesota, Minneapolis, Minnesota
Liver Abscess

Hugo V. Villar, MD
Professor Emeritus, Department of Surgery, University of Arizona, Tucson, Arizona
Anatomy and Physiology of the Spleen

Leonardo Villegas, MD
Hepatobiliary and Surgical Oncology, Duke University Medical Center, Durham, North Carolina
Operative Management of Cholecystitis and Cholelithiasis

James R. Wallace, MD, PhD
Professor, Department of Surgery, Medical College of Wisconsin, Milwaukee, Wisconsin
Appendix

William D. Wallace, MD
Colorectal Fellow, Department of Surgery, Cabrini Monash University, Melbourne, Victoria, Australia
Rare Colorectal Malignancies

Huamin Wang, MD, PhD
Associate Professor of Pathology, Department of Pathology, The University of Texas MD Anderson Cancer Center, Houston, Texas
Unusual Pancreatic Tumors

Kenneth K. Wang, MD
Professor of Medicine, Director, Advanced Endoscopy Group, Division of Gastroenterology and Hepatology, Mayo Clinic College of Medicine, Rochester, Minnesota
Endoscopic Management of Early Esophageal Cancer

James L. Watkins, MD
Associate Professor of Clinical Medicine, Division of Gastroenterology and Hepatology, Indiana University School of Medicine, Indianapolis, Indiana
Endoscopic Retrograde Cholangiopancreatography in the Evaluation and Management of Hepatobiliary and Pancreatic Disease

Thomas J. Watson, MD
Associate Professor of Surgery, Chief, Thoracic Surgery, Division of Thoracic and Foregut Surgery, University of Rochester Medical Center, Rochester, New York
Esophageal Replacement for End-Stage Benign Esophageal Disease

Irving Waxman, MD
Professor of Medicine and Surgery, Center of Endoscopy Research and Therapeutics, University of Chicago, Pritzker School of Medicine, Chicago, Illinois
Endoscopic and Minimally Invasive Therapy for Complications of Acute and Chronic Pancreatitis

Martin R. Weiser, MD
Associate Member, Memorial Sloan-Kettering Cancer Center; Associate Professor, Department of Surgery, Weill Cornell Medical College, New York, New York
Adenocarcinoma of the Colon and Rectum

John Welch, MD
Senior Attending Surgeon, Department of Surgery, Hartford Hospital, Hartford, Connecticut; Clinical Professor, Department of Surgery, University of Connecticut, Farmington, Connecticut; Adjunct Professor, Department of Surgery, Dartmouth Medical School, Hanover, New Hampshire
Diverticular Disease

Mark L. Welton, MD, MHCM
Professor and Chief, Colon and Rectal Surgery, Department of Surgery, Stanford University School of Medicine; Vice-Chief of Staff, Stanford Hospital and Clinics, Stanford, California
Surgery in the Immunocompromised Patient

Steven D. Wexner, MD
Chief Academic Officer and Chief-of-Staff Emeritus, Cleveland Clinic Florida, Weston, Florida; Professor and Chair, Department of Colorectal Surgery, Associate Dean for Academic Affairs, Florida Atlantic University College of Medicine; Affiliate Dean for Clinical Education, Florida International University College of Medicine, Miami, Florida
Surgical Treatment of Constipation

Rebekah R. White, MD
Assistant Professor, Department of Surgery, Duke University School of Medicine, Durham, North Carolina
Volvulus of the Stomach and Small Bowel

Elizabeth C. Wick, MD
Assistant Professor of Surgery, Johns Hopkins University School of Medicine, Baltimore, Maryland
Neoplasms of the Anus

Alison Wilson, MD
Associate Professor, Chief, Trauma and Acute Care Surgery, West Virginia University School of Medicine, Morgantown, West Virginia
Mesenteric Arterial Trauma

Emily Winslow, MD
Assistant Professor, Section of Surgical Oncology, Department of Surgery, University of Wisconsin School of Medicine and Public Health, Madison, Wisconsin
Gastrointestinal Carcinoid Tumors

Piotr Witkowski, MD, PhD
Assistant Professor, Department of Surgery, University of Chicago, Pritzker School of Medicine, Chicago, Illinois
Pancreas and Islet Allotransplantation

Bruce G. Wolff, MD
Professor of Surgery, Mayo Clinic College of Medicine; Chair, Division of Colon and Rectal Surgery, Mayo Clinic, Rochester, Minnesota
Surgery for Inflammatory Bowel Disease: Crohn Disease

Christopher L. Wolfgang, MD, PhD
Associate Professor of Surgery, Pathology, and Oncology, Director, Pancreatic Surgery Section, Co-Director, Pancreatic Cancer Multidisciplinary Clinic, Cameron Division of Surgical Oncology, Johns Hopkins Hospital, Baltimore, Maryland
Pancreatic and Periampullary Cancer

†W. Douglas Wong, MD
Professor of Surgery, Weill Medical College; Chief, Colorectal Service, Department of Surgery, Memorial Sloan-Kettering Cancer Center, New York, New York
Ultrasonographic Diagnosis of Anorectal Disease

Jonathan Worsey, MBBS
San Diego Colon and Rectal Surgeons; Staff Surgeon, Scripps Memorial Hospital, La Jolla, California
Reoperative Pelvic Surgery

Cameron D. Wright, MD
Visiting Surgeon, Division of Thoracic Surgery, Massachusetts General Hospital; Professor of Surgery, Harvard Medical School, Boston, Massachusetts
Complications of Esophagectomy

Bhupender Yadav, MD
Department of Diagnostic Imaging and Radiology, Children's National Medical Center, Washington, DC
Imaging and Intervention in the Biliary System

Charles J. Yeo, MD
Samuel D. Gross Professor and Chairman, Department of Surgery, Thomas Jefferson University, Philadelphia, Pennsylvania
Pseudocysts and Other Complications of Pancreatitis
Operative Management of Bile Duct Strictures

Trevor M. Yeung, MBBChir, MRCS, DPhil
Academic Clinical Lecturer, Department of Colorectal Surgery, Churchill Hospital, Oxford, United Kingdom
Anatomy and Embryology of the Colon

Max Yezhelyev, MD
Surgical Service, Atlanta Veterans Affairs Medical Center; Department of Surgery, Emory University School of Medicine, Atlanta, Georgia
Anatomy and Physiology of the Duodenum

Kyo-Sang Yoo, MD, PhD
Department of Gastroenterology and Hepatology, Hallym University Sacred Heart Hospital, Hallym University College of Medicine, Anyang, South Korea
Endoscopic Retrograde Cholangiopancreatography in the Evaluation and Management of Hepatobiliary and Pancreatic Disease

Yi-Qian Nancy You, MD, MHSc
Assistant Professor, Department of Surgical Oncology, Division of Surgery, The University of Texas MD Anderson Cancer Center, Houston, Texas
Splenectomy for Conditions Other Than Trauma

Tonia M. Young-Fadok, MD
Professor, Department of Surgery, Mayo Clinic College of Medicine; Chair, Division of Colon and Rectal Surgery, Mayo Clinic, Phoenix, Arizona
Laparoscopic Colorectal Surgery

Johannes Zacherl, MD
Department of Surgery, Medical University of Vienna, Vienna, Austria
Epidemiology and Natural History of Gastroesophageal Reflux Disease

Giovanni Zaninotto, MD
Professor, Department of Surgical, Oncological, and Gastroenterological Sciences, University of Padova Padova, Italy; Chairman, General Surgery, Public Hospital, Venice, Italy
Laparoscopic Esophageal Myotomy: Techniques and Results

Merissa N. Zeman, MD
Department of Radiology, Interventional Radiology Division, The George Washington University Medical Center, Washington, DC
Imaging and Intervention in the Biliary System

Pamela Zimmerman, MD
Assistant Professor of Surgery, Division of Vascular and Endovascular Surgery, West Virginia University School of Medicine, Robert C. Byrd Health Science Center, Morgantown, West Virginia
Anatomy and Physiology of the Mesenteric Circulation

Gregory Zuccaro, Jr., MD
Department of Gastroenterology and Hepatology, Cleveland Clinic, Cleveland, Ohio
Endoscopic Esophageal Ultrasonography

---

†Deceased.

Preface

The time has come to release the seventh edition of the classic textbook *Shackelford's Surgery of the Alimentary Tract*. This publication has served as an important resource for surgeons, internists, gastroenterologists, residents, medical students, and other medical professionals over the past 57 years. I hope that you will find the seventh edition brimming with new information, beautifully illustrated, up to date, and educationally fulfilling.

BRIEF HISTORY

The first edition of *Surgery of the Alimentary Tract* was written solely by Dr. Richard T. Shackelford, a Baltimore surgeon, and was published in 1955. Following the success of the first edition, the book's publisher, W.B. Saunders Company, urged Dr. Shackelford to produce a second edition. Time passed. A second edition was released, as separate five-volume tomes, between 1978 and 1986, with Dr. Shackelford enlisting the assistance of Dr. George D. Zuidema, the Chairman of the Department of Surgery at Johns Hopkins, as co-editor. It was the second edition that served as my "bible" for alimentary tract diseases during my surgical residency and early faculty appointment.

The third edition, edited by Dr. Zuidema, was published as a five-volume set in 1991 and proved to be a major tour de force. The field of alimentary tract surgery had advanced, new research findings were included in the edition, and emerging techniques were illustrated. For the third edition, Dr. Zuidema enlisted the help of a guest editor for each of the five volumes.

The fourth edition, again headed by Dr. Zuidema, was published in 1996, and remained encyclopedic in scope, breadth, and depth of coverage. The textbook had become a classic reference source for surgeons, internists, gastroenterologists, and other healthcare professionals involved in the care of patients with alimentary tract diseases.

The fifth edition was published in 2002. At that time, Dr. Zuidema asked me to join him as a co-editor. The fifth edition remained a five-volume set, and was filled with new operative techniques, advances in molecular biology, and noninvasive therapies. It marked progress in the co-management of patients by open surgical, laparoscopic surgical, and endoscopic techniques.

In 2007, the sixth edition of *Shackelford's Surgery of the Alimentary Tract* was published. The look of the sixth edition was changed. The book went from five volumes to two volumes, deleting outdated material, and included a four-color production scheme, emphasizing new procedures and focusing on advances in technology.

THE SEVENTH EDITION

The seventh edition maintains the exterior changes and look of the sixth edition. However, the seventh edition has been carefully planned by me and the four expert section editors to represent the current state of alimentary tract surgery as practiced throughout the world. This edition has been completed with an enormous amount of assistance from my four colleagues, who have served as editors for the four major sections of the book. These section editors have worked tirelessly, planning, organizing, and developing this massive textbook. They have incorporated numerous changes in surgical practice, operative techniques, and noninvasive therapies within the text. Although each area does retain sections on anatomy and physiology, the numerous advances in genomics, proteomics, laparoscopic techniques, and even robotics are mentioned. The seventh edition includes the contributions of two new and two retained section editors, providing both innovation and stability.

Section I, Esophagus and Hernia, is again edited by Dr. Jeffrey H. Peters, the Seymour I. Schwartz Professor and Chairman of the Department of Surgery at the University of Rochester School of Medicine and Dentistry in Rochester, New York. Dr. Peters is an internationally known expert who brings his detailed knowledge of the esophagus and esophageal diseases to the textbook. Dr. Peters' reputation has been recently elevated by his being named as an associate editor of one of the most prominent surgical journals, the *Annals of Surgery*. He has enlisted new authors for many chapters and has again put together a spectacular section on esophageal diseases, including pathology and ambulatory diagnostics, extensive sections on gastroesophageal reflux disease, esophageal motility disorders, and esophageal neoplasia.

Dr. David W. McFadden has taken over as the editor for Section II, Stomach and Small Intestine. For most of the time during this edition's preparation, Dr. McFadden served as the Stanley S. Fieber Professor and Chairman of the Department of Surgery at the University of Vermont, in Burlington, Vermont. As of January 2012, Dr. McFadden has started a new position, at the University of Connecticut in Farmington, Connecticut, serving as the Professor and Chairman of the Department of Surgery. Dr. McFadden is an expert in alimentary tract diseases, surgical research, and education. He has served for many years as the co-editor-in-chief of the *Journal of Surgical Research*, and he has served as the president of the Society for Surgery of the Alimentary Tract. He has done a superb job of enlisting new chapter authors so as to present a modern, new, updated section regarding the luminal structures of the upper gastrointestinal system. Dr. McFadden's section is an outstanding contribution to this area.

For Section III, Pancreas, Biliary Tract, Liver, and Spleen, we have another new section editor, Dr. Jeffrey B. Matthews, the Dallas B. Phemister Professor and Chairman of the Department of Surgery at the University of Chicago, in Chicago, Illinois. Dr. Matthews' surgical career has focused on diseases of the nonluminal structures of the alimentary tract, and he has done a superb job in enlisting new contributors and reorganizing this section. Dr. Matthews' credentials include serving as the co-editor-in-chief of the *Journal of Gastrointestinal Surgery*, and he is soon to be the president of the Society for Surgery of the Alimentary Tract. This section has been carefully redone and serves as an outstanding contribution to the field.

Finally, Section IV, Colon, Rectum, and Anus, has once again been expertly edited and supervised by Dr. John H. Pemberton, Professor of Surgery at the Mayo Clinic College of Medicine in Rochester, Minnesota. Dr. Pemberton is an internationally known figure in his field, and his section has been wonderfully redone. Included are various new developments in the field, updates on pelvic floor anatomy and physiology, new therapies for inflammatory bowel disease, increased emphasis on laparoscopic interventions, and new chapters dealing with both surgical outcomes and an overview of colorectal surgery.

ACKNOWLEDGMENTS

The seventh edition would have been impossible to complete without the expertise, dedication, and hard work of each of these four expert section editors. They have been helped immensely by their colleagues, staff, and all the chapter contributors. I would like to thank each of these section editors for their vision, dedication, expertise, and incredible hard work in bringing this project to fruition.

As is often the case with printed works of this size, hundreds of individuals have contributed chapters to this edition. In fact, more than 400 contributors are listed in the Contributors section. We understand how difficult it is to produce superb chapters, and I wish to recognize these individuals and thank them for their dedication and commitment. Most of these contributors are nationally and internationally known leaders in their fields, and I am deeply indebted to them for sharing their knowledge and enthusiasm about their topic, culminating in an outstanding overall product.

I would also like to thank the production team at Elsevier, who again have been instrumental in making this edition a reality. My thanks go out to Judith Fletcher, Jessica Becher, Marie Clifton, Teresa McBryan, and Maureen Iannuzzi, and many others who have been involved in overseeing this project. This edition represents an enormous amount of new work, and thousands of hours have been spent on its production. These professionals have made it a labor of love to work on this project.

Finally, I must thank individuals who have helped me during this new edition process over the past four years. Here in my office at Jefferson Medical College, accolades go out to Claire Reinke and Dominique Marsiano, who have been outstanding assistants in bringing this work to fruition. Even in the current day and age of electronic mail and electronic manuscript management systems, there is much that still gets done using paper and writing implements!

Charles J. Yeo, MD

Contents

VOLUME 2

SECTION III

Pancreas, Biliary Tract, Liver, and Spleen

Section Editor: Jeffrey B. Matthews

PART ONE

Pancreas

SECTION **IV**

Colon, Rectum, and Anus

Section Editor: John H. Pemberton

PART ONE

Anatomy, Physiology, and Diagnosis of Colorectal and Anal Disease

†Deceased.

SECTION **III**

Pancreas, Biliary Tract, Liver, and Spleen

Jeffrey B. Matthews

PART ONE

Pancreas

CHAPTER 87

Anatomy, Physiology, and Embryology of the Pancreas

Yousef El-Gohary | George K. Gittes

The term *pancreas* is derived from Greek meaning "all flesh,"[1] and developmental biologists have been intrigued for years with the fascinating embryologic development of the pancreas. It is an endodermally derived organ, consisting of two morphologically distinct tissues, the exocrine and endocrine pancreas (Figure 87-1). Some have even described it as "two organs in one" because of the disparate function and organization of these two tissues (exocrine and endocrine) within the pancreas.

Given the importance of a better understanding of the embryologic and molecular biologic mechanisms of pancreatic development, we hope in the future to design strategies to generate therapeutically useful tissue (e.g., pancreas or β-cells) from stem cells as well as better understand differentiation pathways that may lead to pancreatic cancer.

The morphologic development of the pancreas is dictated by its two major functions, which are the production of digestive enzymes by the exocrine tissue, and the production of metabolically active hormones by the endocrine tissue. These two tissues exist together within the pancreas despite their contrasting morphology and function. The endocrine pancreas, which comprises only 2% of the adult pancreatic mass, is organized into islets of Langerhans consisting of five cell subtypes, α, β, δ, ε, and PP cells secreting glucagon, insulin, somatostatin, ghrelin, and pancreatic polypeptide hormones, respectively. The exocrine tissue, on the other hand, which forms nearly 98% of the adult pancreatic mass, is composed of acinar and ductal epithelial cells.[1] We will be reviewing in this chapter the basic physiology, anatomy, and embryology of the pancreas.

BASIC ANATOMY

The human pancreas is a long, tapered glandular organ, divided into four anatomic domains, the head, neck, body, and tail, along with one accessory lobe or "uncinate process," with the head nestled within the curve of the second part of the duodenum. It is situated in a retroperitoneal position, lying obliquely across and behind the stomach with a firm and lobulated smooth surface, extending transversely toward the hilum of the spleen, measuring between 12 and 15 cm long in adults. The digestive enzymes and bicarbonates are secreted by the exocrine-acinar tissue. The acini (the name stems from Greek for grape [acinus]) are an accumulation of acinar cells at the termination of ducts, and then drain into a centrally located acinar space connected to tiny pancreatic tubular ductal networks. These ducts eventually join to form the main pancreatic ducts (ducts of Wirsung and Santorini) to drain into the duodenum via the major (ampulla of Vater) and minor duodenal papilla. There is a main pancreatic duct (derived from the ventral anlage to become the duct of Wirsung and dorsal anlage as the distal duct of Santorini), and there is usually an accessory pancreatic duct (derived from the proximal duct of Santorini). Incomplete division of the dorsal and ventral pancreatic ducts results in pancreas divisum, which is the most common congenital pancreatic ductal anatomic variant, occurring at 4% to 14% in autopsy series, but many anatomic variations of the pancreatic ductal drainage system do exist (Figure 87-2).[2]

The endocrine hormones are produced in the islets of Langerhans, which are scattered throughout the pancreas and are drained by a network of capillaries that invade the islet.[3] The distribution of endocrine cells within the islet is species-dependent. In rodents, the core of the islet is occupied by the β-cells surrounded in the periphery by a ring of α-cells, whereas in humans and monkeys all the endocrine cell types are intermingled with each other (Figure 87-3).[4] Nonendocrine cells also exist in the islet, including endothelial cells, neurons, dendritic cells, macrophages, and fibroblasts.

Pancreatic surgery requires a good knowledge of the anatomic relationship of the pancreas to other

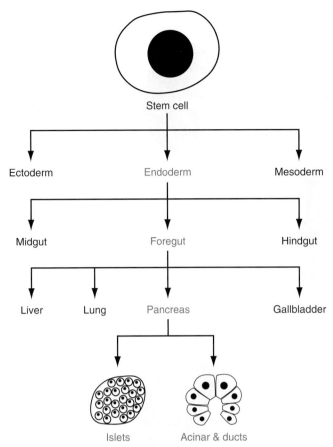

FIGURE 87-1 Cell lineage schematic for pancreatic development from a multipotent progenitor stem cell.

structures. The pancreatic head lies in front of the inferior vena cava, right renal artery, both renal veins, and the superior mesenteric vessels, whereas the uncinate process lies posterior to the superior mesenteric vessels. The neck of the pancreas lies directly over the portal vein and vertebral bodies L1 and L2; this region is where the splenic vein unites with the superior mesenteric vein to form the portal vein. The splenic vein receives the inferior mesenteric vein near the tail of the pancreas. Anterior-posterior blunt trauma can thus lead to pancreatic tissue damage as well as ductal injury. The common bile duct passes in a deep groove on the posterior aspect of the pancreatic head until it joins the main pancreatic duct at the ampulla of Vater in the pancreatic parenchyma. The stomach lies anterior to the body and tail of the pancreas, whereas the aorta, left adrenal gland, and left kidney lie posterior to the body of the pancreas. The tail lies in the hilum of the spleen with the splenic artery, which is often tortuous, running along the superior border of the pancreas (Figure 87-4).

The major blood supply to the pancreas arises from multiple branches of the celiac trunk and superior mesenteric arteries, which form arterial arcades within the body and tail of the pancreas. The splenic and common hepatic arteries arise from the celiac trunk. The dorsal and greater pancreatic arteries branch from the splenic artery, whereas the gastroduodenal artery branches from the common hepatic artery, then dividing around the head of the pancreas into anterior and posterior superior

pancreaticoduodenal branches that anastomose with the anterior and posterior branches of the inferior pancreaticoduodenal artery, which are branches of the superior mesenteric artery (Figure 87-5). Approximately one in every five patients has variations in the arterial anatomy, such as having the right hepatic artery, which usually originates from the celiac trunk, arising from the superior mesenteric artery (also known as a replaced right hepatic artery) traveling posterior to the pancreatic head toward the liver. Discerning this arterial anomaly is important in preoperative computed tomography (CT) scans to avoid injury (see Figure 87-5). The vascularization of the pancreatic islets will be discussed in greater detail later in the chapter. Venous drainage of the pancreas mainly flows into the portal system, with the head and neck draining primarily through the superior and inferior pancreaticoduodenal veins, whereas the body and tail drain into the splenic vein. The pancreas is drained by multiple lymph node groups. The body and tail drain mostly into pancreaticosplenic nodes, whereas the head and neck drain more widely into nodes along the superior mesenteric, hepatic, and pancreaticoduodenal arteries. The pancreas is innervated by both the sympathetic and parasympathetic fibers of the autonomic nervous system. Celiac plexus ablation or block can improve chronic pain arising from inoperable pancreatic tumors or chronic pancreatitis.

PHYSIOLOGY

Despite the disparate function between the endocrine and exocrine part of the pancreas, the two different components coordinate with each other in order to regulate food digestion by secreting different hormones as well as digestive enzymes, with a regulatory feedback system in place. The pancreas regulates the body's energy metabolism through the endocrine islet cells of Langerhans. This regulation is delicately balanced through the actions of the hormones insulin and glucagon. Insulin is the hormone of energy storage, which induces an increase in amino acid uptake as well as facilitating glucose uptake into cells, increasing protein synthesis, decreasing lipolysis and glycogenolysis, especially postprandially or in a hyperglycemic state. Glucagon is viewed as the hormone of energy release, stimulating higher blood glucose levels by the stimulation of hepatic gluconeogenesis, glycogenolysis, and lipolysis in the setting of hypoglycemia, thus counteracting the effects of insulin.

β-cells secrete insulin based on blood glucose levels as well as neural and humoral factors. The stimulus for insulin release into the bloodstream is far greater when glucose is ingested enterally compared to the parenteral route, indicating that a "feed-forward" mechanism in the digestive tract is activated, anticipating the rise in blood glucose. This anticipation is mediated by *incretins*, which account for up to 60% of postprandial insulin release in healthy individuals. There are two main incretin hormones, glucose-dependent insulinotropic peptide, also known as gastric inhibitory peptide (GIP), and glucagon-like peptide-1 (GLP-1). Both are secreted by endocrine cells located in the intestinal epithelium, and when the luminal concentration of glucose increases in the

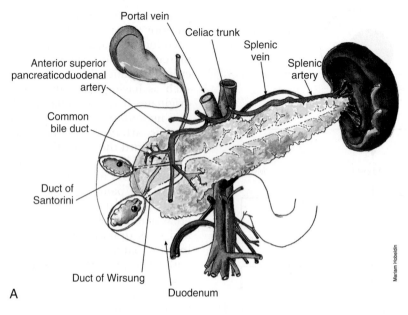

A

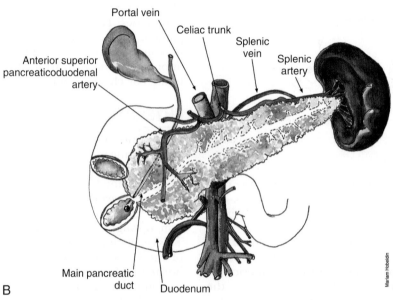

B

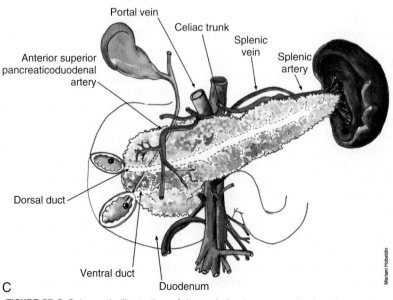

C

FIGURE 87-2 Schematic illustration of the variation in pancreatic ductal anatomy.

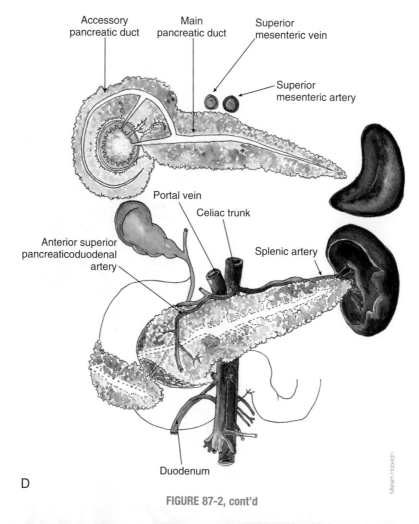

Accessory
pancreatic duct

Main
pancreatic duct

Superior
mesenteric vein

Superior
mesenteric artery

Portal vein

Celiac trunk

Anterior superior
pancreaticoduodenal
artery

Splenic artery

Duodenum

D

Miriam Hobdon

FIGURE 87-2, cont'd

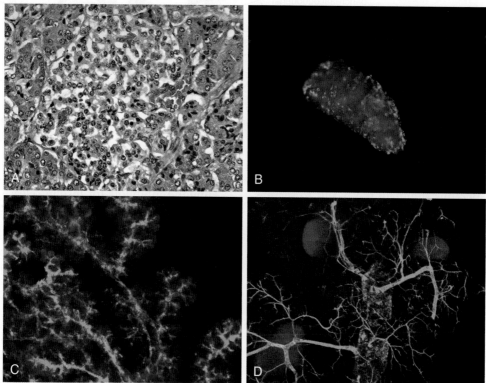

FIGURE 87-3 Standard histologic section of a human pancreas specimen **(A)** illustrating a small, relatively pale-staining cell known as the islet of Langerhans, which is embedded in darker-stained exocrine tissue. **B,** Adult mouse pancreas whole-mount image showing an isolated islet stained with insulin, with glucagon in the periphery. **C,** Whole-mount image of embryonic day (E)16.5 pancreas illustrating close relationship between insulin cells and pancreatic ducts. **D,** Whole-mount image of an adult mouse pancreas stained with insulin and dolichos biflorus agglutinin (DBA) for pancreatic ducts.

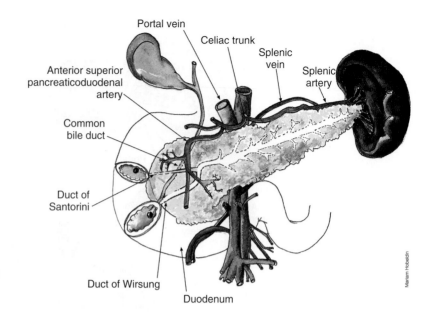

FIGURE 87-4 Schematic illustration of the anatomic relationship of the pancreas in relation to other anatomic structures.

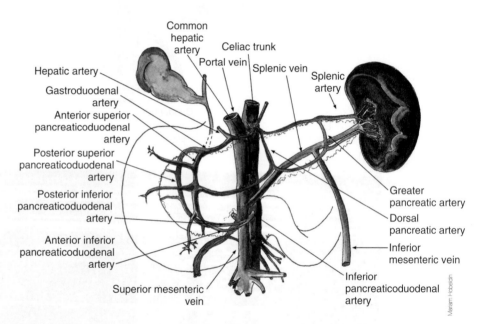

FIGURE 87-5 Arterial and venous blood supply of the pancreas, superimposed.

digestive tract, incretins stimulate the β-cells to secrete "more" insulin. Hence, there is great interest in the pharmaceutical industry to develop incretin-based therapies to treat diabetes because of its potent secretagogue effect on β-cells. Unlike traditional medications that stimulate β-cells to secrete insulin regardless of blood glucose level, incretins augment the β-cell response to blood glucose levels in a glucose-dependent manner.[5,6]

A peculiar phenomenon observed in type 2 diabetic patients undergoing Roux-en-Y gastric bypass surgery is that they experience a dramatic amelioration of blood glucose homeostasis and insulin sensitivity even before weight loss. The underlying mechanism behind this dramatic improvement is not fully understood. The dumping of nutrients into the distal small intestine stimulates an exaggerated GLP-1 release from intestinal endocrine L-cells into the portal vein, stimulating insulin release.[7]

Humoral inhibitors for insulin release include somatostatin, amylin, leptin, and pancreastatin. The vagus nerve generally stimulates insulin release, whereas the sympathetic nervous system inhibits it, mediated by various peptidergic molecules secreted from nerve fibers such as substance P, VIP, and neurotensin.

The exocrine pancreas consists of two morphologically distinct structures: acinar cells, which secrete digestive enzymes, and duct cells, which mainly secrete bicarbonate-rich fluid. The total external secretion of the pancreas consists of clear, colorless, bicarbonate-rich alkaline solution of about 2.5 L per day. Acinar cells, the functional unit of the exocrine pancreas, make up the majority of the pancreas. They are specialized to synthesize, store, and then secrete digestive enzymes. Secretion occurs in response to neurohormonal control via cholecystokinin (CCK) and parasympathetic vagal stimulation.

In many species, CCK binds directly to the acinar cells; however, in humans it is thought to act through the vagal cholinergic pathway as humans have no receptors for CCK on their acinar cells.[8] Acinar cells have a basal nucleus with abundant rough endoplasmic reticulum, where the digestive enzymes are synthesized and then packaged in the Golgi apparatus as zymogen granules. These zymogen (precursor enzymes) granules are located mainly at the apex of acinar cells. On stimulation, the zymogen granules migrate toward the cell surface and release their contents into the acinar lumen, which is drained by pancreatic ducts. Proximal ducts near the acini are lined by centroacinar and intercalated duct epithelial cells, with the latter two secreting bicarbonate (in exchange for chloride) when stimulated by secretin.

The process of electrolyte secretion by the duct cell occurs when carbon dioxide at the basal membrane of the duct cell is converted to carbonic acid via carbonic anhydrase. Carbonic acid dissociates into bicarbonate and protons, with the latter diffusing out the basal side of the cell. Secretin stimulation through cAMP accelerates chloride ion secretion through the apical membrane. Cystic fibrosis transmembrane conductance regulator (CFTR), which is defective in cystic fibrosis (CF), has been identified as the ion channel at the apical membrane of duct cells supplying chloride ions to the lumen. The exchange of cellular bicarbonate for luminal chloride results in net bicarbonate secretion from the apical cell membrane of the duct cell.

CFTR plays a significant role in transcellular secretion of bicarbonates, thus maintaining fluid secretion of ductal epithelial cells, which aids in flushing digestive enzymes out of the ducts and into the duodenum. The human pancreas in CF patients has the defective CFTR at the apical membrane of duct cells, which results in poor clearance of digestive enzymes because of the impaired bicarbonate secretion. This trapping of enzymes results in premature activation of the digestive enzymes with inflammation leading to pancreatic insufficiency.[9] Under physiologic conditions, bicarbonate is secreted into the duct lumen at a concentration five times higher than that of plasma, and thus helps to neutralize gastric acid, and provides an optimum pH environment for digestive enzymes in the duodenum.[9] The digestive enzymes secreted by the acinar cells can be secreted in their active form such as with amylase and lipase or may be secreted in an inactive zymogen form such as with proelastase, trypsinogen, and chymotrypsinogen. The brush-border enzyme enteropeptidase in the duodenum subsequently activates trypsinogen to form trypsin, which then activates other zymogens into their active forms. This cascade helps to prevent autodigestion of the pancreas by its proteolytic enzymes.

BASIC PANCREATIC EMBRYOLOGY

The embryonic pancreas is known to pass through three stages of development.[1] The first is the undifferentiated stage where the endoderm evaginates to initiate pancreatic morphogenesis, with only insulin and glucagon genes being expressed at this stage. The second phase involves epithelial branching morphogenesis with simultaneous formation of primitive ducts. This stage involves the separation of islet progenitors beginning to differentiate and losing their attachments to the basement membrane. The third and final stage begins with the formation of acinar cells at the apices of the ductal structures, with the development of zymogen granules containing enzymes. Acinar cells usually commence enzyme secretion shortly after birth.[1]

During early embryonic development, the pancreas is initiated with the regional specification of the undifferentiated primitive endodermal foregut tube by transcription factors Pdx1 (pancreatic and duodenal homeobox 1), which marks the prepancreatic endoderm and by PTF1a (pancreas transcription factor), where both are expressed in multipotent pancreatic progenitor cells.[10] The pancreas first appears morphologically as a mesenchymal condensation at the level of the duodenal anlagen, distal to the stomach on the dorsal aspect of the foregut tube at embryonic day (E) 9.0 in mice. All cells expressing Pdx1 and PTF1a in the endoderm will eventually give rise to all of the epithelial cells in the adult pancreas, which includes endocrine, acinar, and duct cells.[1] At around E9.5 gestation in mice and the 26th day of gestation in humans, the dorsal bud begins to evaginate into the overlying mesenchyme while retaining luminal continuity with the gut tube. Approximately 12 hours later in mice, and 6 days after dorsal bud evagination in humans, the ventral bud begins to arise. Gut rotation will bring the ventral lobe dorsally, ultimately fusing with the dorsal pancreatic bud (this event corresponds to around the 6th to 7th week of gestation in humans and E12 to E13 in mice) contributing to the formation of the uncinate process and inferior part of the head of the pancreas, while the rest of the pancreas arises from the dorsal pancreatic bud. The entire ventral pancreatic duct and the distal part of the dorsal pancreatic duct fuse together to form the main pancreatic duct of Wirsung. The remaining proximal part of the dorsal pancreatic duct is either obliterated or persists as a small accessory pancreatic duct of Santorini.[11] This fusion and evagination of the two buds is followed by elongation of the pancreatic bud stalk region (precursor to the main pancreatic duct) and branching morphogenesis of the apical region of the bud. Unlike the usual branching morphogenesis growth patterns seen in the developing kidney, lung, and salivary gland, in which the branching morphogenesis occurs at 90-degree angles, the pancreas grows in an acute-angled branching pattern, which leads to the exclusion or "squeezing out" of mesenchyme from between the closely apposed branches of epithelium (Figure 87-6). This exclusion of mesenchyme may influence epithelial-mesenchymal interactions and lineage selection. The pancreas then undergoes major amplification of the endocrine cell population through two distinct waves of differentiation within the pancreatic epithelium during embryogenesis, an early primary wave (pre-E13.5 in mice), followed by the secondary wave of differentiation (E13.5-E16.5 in mice).[1] Over a similar gestational window, the exocrine pancreatic precursors undergo an exponential increase in branching morphogenesis and acinar cell differentiation.

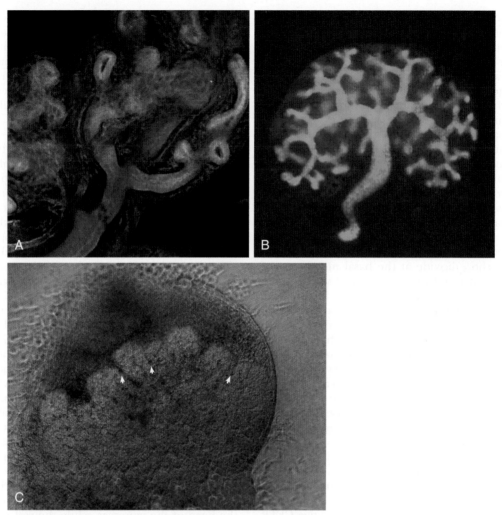

FIGURE 87-6 Pancreatic branching morphogenesis is different from that of other organ systems such as lung and kidney. **A,** Whole-mount of E12.5 lung stained for Ecad, PGP9.5 (a neuronal marker), and CD31. **B,** E11.5 kidney cultured for 3 days and stained with the epithelial marker calbindin-D28k, both demonstrating 90-degree branching pattern. **C,** E11 whole pancreas from CD-1 cultured for 5 days revealing acute branching pattern mesenchymal exclusion zones *(arrowheads)*. Mesenchyme contains factors that regulate pancreatic growth and differentiation.

DORSAL AND VENTRAL PANCREATIC BUD DEVELOPMENT

It is important to note that although the morphologic development of the ventral and dorsal pancreatic buds may be similar, they differ markedly at the molecular level, with various lines of evidence suggesting that there are differences in the specification between both pancreatic rudiments, with the notochord playing a key role. Sonic hedgehog (Shh), which is a potent intercellular patterning molecule and is expressed along the entire foregut, is noticeably absent in the prospective pancreatic endoderm. This suppression of Shh appears to be necessary for dorsal pancreatic development, permitting the expression of pancreas-specific genes including pdx1 and insulin. Deletion of the notochord in chick embryo cultures leads to ectopic Shh in the pancreatic region of the foregut endoderm, with subsequent failure of the pancreas to develop.[12] Activin-βB (a member of the transforming growth factor-β family) and FGF2 (fibroblast growth factor) both mimic notochord activity

in inducing pancreatic genes.[12] In stark contrast to the dorsal bud, developmental gene expression in the ventral pancreatic anlage is not affected when the notochord is removed.[13] The ventral pancreas, on the other hand, develops under the control of signals from the overlying cardiogenic mesenchyme, which also produces prohepatic signals (FGFs) to induce liver formation. Lack of prohepatic FGF signaling in regions of the cardiogenic mesenchyme will lead to the endoderm by "default" differentiating into ventral pancreas.[14] When ventral foregut endoderm is cultured in the absence of cardiac mesoderm or FGF, it fails to activate liver-specific genes, with pdx1 being expressed instead. Cardiac mesoderm, through FGF, induces liver formation from the ventral endoderm and simultaneously inhibits pancreatic development.[14] Further differences between ventral and dorsal pancreas are demonstrated in Hlxb9 mutant mice. The homeobox gene Hlxb9 is transiently expressed in the endoderm in the region of the dorsal and ventral pancreatic anlage. When it is inactivated in mice, only dorsal pancreatic development is blocked. Hex1 is an early

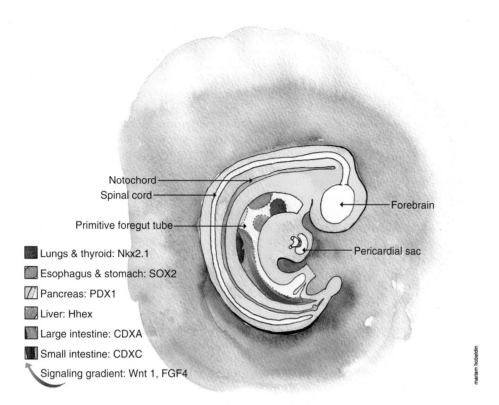

Notochord
Spinal cord
Primitive foregut tube

Forebrain
Pericardial sac

Lungs & thyroid: Nkx2.1
Esophagus & stomach: SOX2
Pancreas: PDX1
Liver: Hhex
Large intestine: CDXA
Small intestine: CDXC
Signaling gradient: Wnt 1, FGF4

mariam hobeldin

FIGURE 87-7 Schematic representation for the regional specification of the primitive foregut tube (~E8.5) with the various transcription factors. Wnt and FGF4, which are secreted from the posterior mesoderm in a gradient, repress foregut fate and promote hindgut development. Wnt and FGF4 inhibition in the anterior endoderm promotes foregut fate.

marker of the anterior endoderm and is expressed at E7.0 in the cells that will subsequently give rise to the ventral pancreas and liver. Hex null mutant embryos have specific failure of ventral pancreatic bud development, with the dorsal bud developing normally.[15] These examples underscore the significantly different molecular controls governing dorsal and ventral pancreatic bud development.

INITIATION OF THE PANCREAS WITH ENDODERMAL PATTERNING

The signaling molecules that govern the specification of the primitive gut tube into different specialized domains remains yet to be fully elucidated.[10] The pancreas and other endoderm-derived organs develop through a series of reciprocal interactions between the endoderm and the surrounding mesenchyme, which is a critical step in initiating organ specification or "*endodermal patterning*" along the anterior-posterior axis of the foregut endoderm. Endodermal patterning is manifested by the regional expression of transcription factors in the primitive gut tube; for example, Hex1 (hematopoietically expressed homeobox1, an early marker of anterior endoderm) and Nkx2.1 (also known as thyroid transcription factor 1) are expressed at E8.5 in defined foregut domains along the anterior-posterior axis of the primitive gut tube, giving rise to liver and lung/thyroid, respectively. Pdx1 and PTF1a are coexpressed in the foregut-midgut endoderm boundary, defining the pancreas and duodenum, whereas Cdx1, and Cdx4 (early markers of

posterior endoderm) are expressed in the posterior midgut and hindgut domains that will give rise to the small and large intestines. Thus, various domains of the primitive gut tube are specified (Figure 87-7).[16]

The primitive gut tube is divided into three domains, foregut, midgut and hindgut regions, each of which will give rise to specialized structures.[10] This subdivision into presumptive gut tube domains is governed by different molecular markers in the gastrula-stage endoderm (E7.5).[10,17] The endoderm toward the anterior side of the embryo generates the ventral foregut, which will later give rise to the liver, lung, thyroid, and the ventral pancreas. The dorsal region of the definitive endoderm, on the other hand, contributes to the formation of the esophagus, stomach, dorsal pancreas, duodenum, and intestines. The pancreas has been found to form as a result of the actions of some key specific transcription factors and signaling pathways. For example, FGF4 and Wnt signaling from the posterior mesoderm are specifically inhibited in the anterior endoderm to allow foregut development. FGF signaling is required to initially determine, and then to maintain, gut tube domains, as demonstrated with cultured mouse endoderm and by in vivo studies in chick embryos. FGF4 is normally expressed in the mesoderm and ectoderm adjacent to the developing midgut-hindgut endoderm, and when isolated mouse endoderm is cultured in the presence of high concentrations of FGF4, a posterior (intestinal) endoderm was induced. On the other hand, lower concentrations of FGF4 induced a more anterior (pancreas-duodenal) cell fate. Similarly, in chick embryos in vivo, when treated with FGF4, the Hex1 (anterior endodermal marker) expression domain was reduced, whereas CdxB (posterior endodermal marker) expression expanded anteriorly, inhibiting the development of the foregut.[16] Therefore, FGF4 plays a critical role in endodermal patterning by repressing anterior (foregut) fate and promoting posterior (intestinal) endoderm fate. Another molecular pathway that has linked endodermal patterning to the initiation of pancreatic development is Wnt/β-catenin signaling, as demonstrated in frog (*Xenopus*) studies.[18] β-Catenin repression in the anterior endoderm is specifically necessary to initiate liver and pancreas development, and to maintain foregut identity. Conversely, forcing high β-catenin activity in the posterior endoderm promotes intestinal development and inhibits foregut development. McLin et al[18] demonstrated that forced β-catenin expression in the anterior endoderm (where β-catenin is usually repressed) led to downregulation of Hhex, as well as other foregut markers for liver (*for1*), pancreas (*pdx1*), lung/thyroid (*nkx2.1*) and intestine (*endocut*), resulting in inhibition of foregut fate, namely liver and pancreas formation. Repressing β-catenin in the posterior endoderm (future hindgut that normally expresses β-catenin) induced ectopic liver and pancreas markers (hhex, pdx1, elastase, and amylase) with subsequent ectopic liver bud initiation and pancreas development.[18] The homeobox-containing gene Hhex is a direct target of β-catenin and is one of the earliest foregut markers and is essential for normal liver and ventral pancreas development in mice.[15] *Hex* expression was noted to have an important role in the specification and differentiation of the ventral pancreas, where Hex[−/−] null-mutant mouse embryos lacked a ventral pancreas, and lacked liver, thyroid, and parts of the forebrain.[15,19]

Targeted disruption of the Pdx1 gene in mice also prevented pancreatic development.[20] A critical role for Pdx1 in pancreatic initiation and patterning of foregut endoderm in mice was further demonstrated by humans with Pdx1 mutations being apancreatic.[21] Despite our growing knowledge of many molecular signals mediating crosstalk between the pancreatic mesenchyme and the epithelium, most pathways remain poorly understood.

PANCREATIC MESENCHYME

The pancreatic mesenchyme, which envelops the pancreatic epithelium after regional specification, contains important factors that are pivotal for pancreatic morphogenesis. These factors promote growth and differentiation of the developing pancreas, specifically inducing growth of the endocrine cell population and rapid branching morphogenesis.[1] The pancreatic mesenchyme helps regulate pancreatic epithelial lineage selection between the endocrine and exocrine lineages during early stages of pancreatic development. This interaction between pancreatic mesenchyme and epithelium is a vital process for pancreatic development. Pure pancreatic epithelium (E11) cultured without its mesenchyme failed to develop at all. However, the epithelium grew into a fully differentiated pancreas (acinar, ductal, and endocrine structures) when cultured with its mesenchyme. The pancreatic mesenchyme has a proexocrine

effect on the epithelium through cell-cell contact, and then also a pro-endocrine effect, mediated by diffusible factors secreted from the mesenchyme.[1] Mesenchymal contact with the epithelium both enhances notch signaling (Hes1), which favors the acinar lineage, and also inhibits neurogenin 3 (Ngn3) expression leading to the suppression of endocrine differentiation. The "default" differentiation of the pancreatic epithelium in the absence of mesenchyme is endocrine. Interestingly, culturing pure pancreatic epithelium in a basement membrane–rich gel, without its mesenchyme, led to the predominant formation of ductal structures. These results suggest that the basement membrane has factors or components which are conducive to ductal development.[1] To further illustrate the importance of the mesenchyme and mesenchymal signaling in embryonic and organ development, when the normal embryonic separation that occurs between the spleen and the pancreas-associated mesenchyme does not occur in Bapx1 null mutant embryos, the dorsal pancreatic bud becomes intestinalized.[22] Activin A, which is expressed in the splenic mesenchyme, is a possible mediator for this transdifferentiation since exposing pancreatic buds to activin A in an in vitro culture system, leads to intestinalization.[23]

Some signaling pathways have been implicated in mediating this epithelial-mesenchymal interaction, such as the FGFs. Specifically, FGFs 1, 7, and 10, which are expressed in the pancreatic mesenchyme, mediate their effects through FGF receptor 2B (FGFR2B), which is expressed in the pancreatic epithelium. Mesenchymal FGF signaling has been shown to induce epithelial proliferation.[24] Similarly, null mutation for the receptor FGFR2B or the ligand FGF10 leads to blunting of early branching pancreatic morphogenesis, with inhibition of proliferation of endocrine progenitor cells and premature endocrine differentiation, indicating that FGF10 normally induces proliferation of epithelial cells and prevents endocrine differentiation.[25,26] Despite the positive role that FGF plays in dorsal pancreatic development, it seems to play a different role in ventral pancreatic bud development. FGFs secreted from the cardiogenic mesenchyme inhibit ventral pancreatic bud formation and favor liver development.[14] BMP ligands in pancreatic mesenchyme induce epithelial branching and inhibit endocrine differentiation.[27]

KEY SIGNALING MOLECULES
Notch Signaling

One of the key decisions that a pancreatic progenitor cell must make is whether to enter the endocrine or the exocrine lineage selection. Notch signaling has been identified as a master regulator of this fate decision switch.[28] Activation of the Notch receptor leads to the activation of HES1 (Hairy-Enhancer of Split 1) and repression of genes such as Ngn3 (neurogenin 3, a prerequisite marker for pancreatic endocrine lineage development).[28] Notch also serves to maintain cells in an undifferentiated progenitor-like state. Impairing Notch signaling leads to premature differentiation of pancreatic progenitor cells into endocrine cells. However, the exact mechanism for Notch signaling in pancreatic lineage selection remains elusive, and ambiguity still surrounds the exact role of Notch signaling in pancreatic development.

Hedgehog Signaling

The mammalian hedgehog family consists of sonic hedgehog (Shh), desert hedgehog (Dhh), and Indian hedgehog (Ihh). Shh signaling is essential for foregut differentiation toward a gastrointestinal fate[29] and its suppression in the prospective pancreatic endoderm is a prerequisite for pancreas formation. However, hedgehog signaling in pancreatic development appears to be complex. Targeted deletion of Shh in the foregut of mice does not lead to an expanded pancreatic field as would be expected. Null mutant mice for Ihh develop a small pancreas, indicating a propancreatic role for Ihh.[30] Furthermore, combining an Shh null mutation with a heterozygous mutation for Ihh results in an annular pancreas (see Figure 87-2, D).

There appears to be a link between aberrant Hh signaling and pancreatic exocrine neoplasia, with the upregulation of Shh ligand being observed in noninvasive lesions preceding pancreatic adenocarcinoma.[31] In addition, it has been demonstrated that Shh ligand secreted by pancreatic cancer epithelium binds to stromal cells in a paracrine fashion, causing proliferation and "desmoplasia."[32-34] Clinical trials are in place to neutralize and target Hh molecules in patients with pancreatic adenocarcinoma.[35] Shh was not thought to be expressed in the normal pancreas[12] until recently when Strobel et al[31] identified expression in a specialized compartment within the proximal ductal system, known as the pancreatic duct glands (PDGs), which are blind-ending outpouches, that specifically produce Shh ligand. When exposed to chronic injury, PDGs grow, associated with an upregulation of Shh expression (along with gastric mucins [Muc6 and Muc5ac] and other progenitor markers such as pdx1 and hes1). This process leads to an Shh-mediated mucinous gastrointestinal metaplasia with features of a pancreatic intraepithelial neoplasia (PanIN). PanINs are pancreatic cancer precursor lesions of unclear origin that are known to aberrantly express Shh and gastrointestinal mucins. They are thought to arise from ducts, and thus PDGs may be the missing link between Shh, mucinous metaplasia, and neoplasia.[29]

ENDOTHELIAL CELLS AND OXYGEN TENSION

It has been shown that cells exposed to low oxygen tensions go through adaptive changes such as anaerobic metabolism, increased angiogenesis, and erythropoiesis.[36] In pancreatic development, β-cell differentiation seems to be influenced by oxygen tension. A key mediator for this adaptive response by cells is hypoxia-inducible factor (HIF).[37] HIF1α is expressed strongly in the rat pancreatic epithelium and mesenchyme at E11.5, then gradually decreases and is virtually undetectable by birth. Hypoxia leads to the stabilization of HIF1α, resulting in absent Ngn3 expression and thus arresting β-cell differentiation. Increasing oxygen tension leads to upregulation of β-cell differentiation with degradation of HIF1α, and restoration of Ngn3. Similarly, inhibiting the

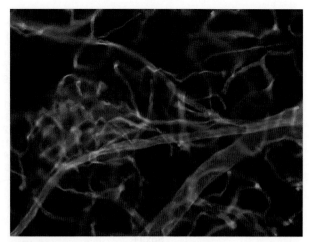

FIGURE 87-8 Whole-mount adult mouse pancreas, stained with CD31 and insulin demonstrating the complex microcapillary network within the islet.

degradation of HIF1α resulted in the repression of Ngn3 and arrest of β-cell differentiation, even in normoxia.[37]

Endothelial Cells

Pancreatic islets are highly vascularized, embedded in a capillary network that is 5 to 10 times denser than that of the exocrine pancreas, and allow efficient secretion of islet hormones into the bloodstream (Figure 87-8).[38] Islet transplantation entails an enzymatic digestion process that also removes some intraislet endothelial cells. This endothelial removal may take away an important vascular niche for the β-cells. During development, β-cells aggregate to form islets, and express high levels of vascular endothelial growth factors (VEGFs) to attract endothelial cells.[39] β-cells deficient in VEGF-A form islets with fewer capillaries, and experimental overexpression of VEGF-A has improved islet graft vascularization.[39] Thus, there is an intimate relationship between blood vessels and the pancreatic cells during embryonic development. As the embryonic pancreas progresses through the different developmental stages, it receives signals from different adjacent structures, including notochord, cardiac mesoderm, and the dorsal aorta. Removal of the dorsal aorta from *Xenopus* embryos led to the absence of pancreatic endocrine development.[40] In addition, aortic endothelial cells can induce dorsal pancreatic bud and β-cell formation in vitro from the endoderm. Interestingly, ventral pancreas development seems not to be dependent on the endothelium, despite its proximity to the vitelline veins. This difference was corroborated in a human with aortic coarctation. The patient lacked the pancreatic body and tail, but not the head of the pancreas, with the latter arising from the ventral bud, which develops independently of the aortae.[41] Here, the prospective pancreatic endoderm presumably lost the inducing signal from the "narrowed" aorta, leading to dorsal pancreatic agenesis.

GLUCAGON

The first detectable endocrine cells during pancreatic development are the glucagon-containing cells at around E9 in the mouse, and recent studies have shown that glucagon signaling is necessary for early differentiation

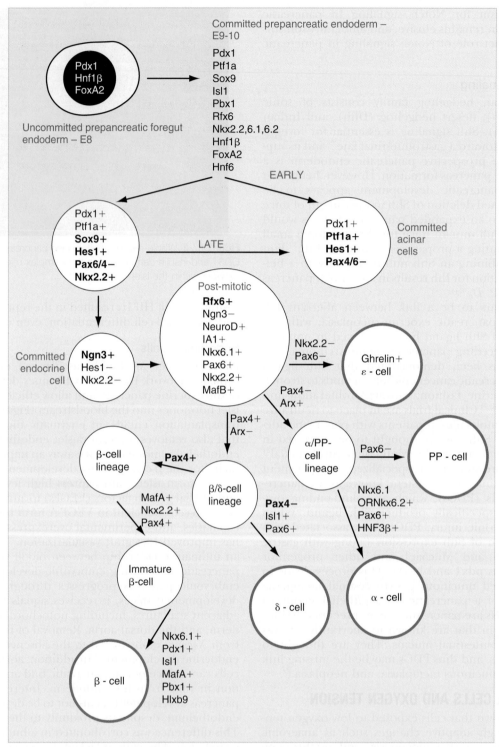

FIGURE 87-9 Overview of the pancreatic endocrine and exocrine cell lineage.

of insulin-expressing cells, which appear at E10 to E13.[1] Glucagon is generated from proglucagon by the action of prohormone convertase 2 (PC2). When PC2 or the glucagon receptor is knocked out, mutant mice lack glucagon and have delayed islet cell differentiation and maturation, but still show the large amplification of insulin-positive cells ("secondary wave") later in gestation. Furthermore, exogenous addition of exendin-4, a glucagon-like peptide-1 (GLP-1) analogue, was able to rescue the delay in early insulin differentiation and was shown also to be able to convert AR42J cells and ARIP cells into insulin-expressing cells.[42,43] These studies strongly support the role of glucagon signaling, through its receptor, in initiating early insulin differentiation. Recently it has been demonstrated that the glucagon-producing α-cells can be reprogrammed to form new β-cells during regeneration after ablating nearly 99% of the existing β-cells.[44]

TRANSCRIPTION FACTORS

Transcription factors are key elements to orchestrating the formation of all endocrine and exocrine cell lineages, and their roles have been extensively studied in pancreatic development. The most heavily studied transcription factor is pdx1, one of the earliest markers for pancreatic progenitors that later is expressed only in β-cells. It is expressed in the prepancreatic region of the primitive foregut tube at E8.5, then expands to be expressed in distal stomach, common bile duct, and duodenum by E10.5 to 11.5.[1] Pdx1 is initially expressed throughout the epithelium; however, its expression becomes suppressed in cells as they commit to the endocrine lineage or ducts. It then reappears as cells differentiate to the insulin-positive β-cell lineage. Pdx1 null mutant mice and humans that lack pdx1 gene have pancreatic agenesis.[21] Delayed pdx1 inhibition using a tetracycline regulatable transgenic knock-in system demonstrated severe blunting of pancreatic development with complete absence of acini and β-cells,[45] indicating that pdx1 continues to have a role in pancreas development beyond early regional specification during endodermal patterning.

PTF1a

Pancreas-specific transcription factor 1a (PTF1a) is an early marker of pancreatic progenitor cells, expressed slightly later than pdx1 at around E9.5 in mouse, and then becomes localized to the acini by E18.5. PTF1a null mutant mice develop severe pancreatic hypoplasia and absent acini and ducts, an observation that is similar to that seen in pdx1 null mutant mice; however, endocrine cells still develop and, interestingly, the endocrine cells migrate out through the pancreatic mesenchyme to form islets in the spleen.[1] A PTF1a nonfunctioning mutation has been seen in humans, where they are born without a pancreas.[46]

Ngn3

Ngn3 is one of the earliest markers specific to the pancreatic endocrine lineage and is required for endocrine lineage development. It is first expressed at E9.0, and then peaks at around E15.5, and is thought to be antagonized by Notch signaling through Hes1 in cells with an acinar fate.[47] Ngn3 cells proliferate, giving rise to postmitotic endocrine progenitor cells expressing transcription factors neuroD, nkx6.1, and pax6. Ngn3 shuts off at around E17.5.[47] When Ngn3 is deleted from cells, it leads to the absence of the four endocrine cell types (α, β, δ, and PP) that produce glucagon, insulin, somatostatin, and pancreatic polypeptide, respectively.[48] Thus, Ngn3 appears to be a critical and essential factor for pancreatic endocrine differentiation acting as a proendocrine gene. However, how exactly Ngn3 controls the subsequent specification of different endocrine subtypes remains to be fully elucidated.

Rfx6

Rfx6 is a transcription factor downstream of Ngn3 that has been identified as a key proendocrine regulator that directs islet cell differentiation. It is initially expressed broadly in gut endoderm, particularly in Pdx1-positive cells in the prospective pancreatic region, and then becomes restricted to the endocrine lineage, in postmitotic islet progenitor cells. Mice that are null-mutant for Rfx6 fail to generate all islet cell types except pancreatic polypeptide cells (insulin, glucagon, somatostatin, and ghrelin). A human syndrome of neonatal diabetes (patients lack pancreatic endocrine cells) with bowel atresia was shown to have mutations in the Rfx6 gene.[49] Thus, Rfx6 is dependent on Ngn3 and is a unique regulator of islet cell development.

MafA/B

There are two distinct waves of amplification of the endocrine cell population in the mouse, primary (pre-E13.5) and secondary (E13.5 to E16.5) transition periods. MafB is expressed in endocrine cells during both waves. As insulin-positive cells form into mature β-cells, MafB turns off and the cells then express MafA.[50] MafA is first expressed only in the secondary wave β-cells and in adult β-cells. MafA is a critical regulator of the insulin gene and is viewed as the only transcription factor specific to β-cells as well as a marker of a mature β-cell. However, it is not absolutely necessary for β-cell formation because mafA null-mutant mice have a normal proportion of insulin-positive cells at birth (Figure 87-9).[51]

REFERENCES

1. Gittes GK: Developmental biology of the pancreas: A comprehensive review. *Dev Biol* 326:4, 2009.
2. Yu J, Turner MA, Fulcher AS, et al: Congenital anomalies and normal variants of the pancreaticobiliary tract and the pancreas in adults: Part 2. Pancreatic duct and pancreas. *AJR Am J Roentgenol* 187:1544, 2006.
3. Gray S, Russo K: *Gray's anatomy*. Woodstock, Ill., 2008, Dramatic Publishing, p 69.
4. Kim A, Miller K, Jo J, et al: Islet architecture: A comparative study. *Islets* 1:129, 2009.
5. Baggio LL, Drucker DJ: Biology of incretins: GLP-1 and GIP. *Gastroenterology* 132:2131, 2007.
6. Scheen AJ, Radermecker RP: Addition of incretin therapy to metformin in type 2 diabetes. *Lancet* 375:1410, 2010.
7. Vahl TP, Tauchi M, Durler TS, et al: Glucagon-like peptide-1 (GLP-1) receptors expressed on nerve terminals in the portal vein mediate the effects of endogenous GLP-1 on glucose tolerance in rats. *Endocrinology* 148:4965, 2007.

8. Owyang C, Logsdon CD: New insights into neurohormonal regulation of pancreatic secretion. *Gastroenterology* 127:957, 2004.

9. Park HW, Nam JH, Kim JY, et al: Dynamic regulation of CFTR bicarbonate permeability by [Cl-]i and its role in pancreatic bicarbonate secretion. *Gastroenterology* 139:620, 2010.

10. Moore-Scott BA, Opoka R, Lin SC, et al: Identification of molecular markers that are expressed in discrete anterior-posterior domains of the endoderm from the gastrula stage to mid-gestation. *Dev Dyn* 236:1997, 2007.

11. Sadler TW, Langman J: *Langman's medical embryology,* ed 10. Philadelphia, 2006, Lippincott Williams & Wilkins, p xiii, 371.

12. Hebrok M, Kim SK, Melton DA: Notochord repression of endodermal Sonic hedgehog permits pancreas development. *Genes Dev* 12:1705, 1998.

13. Kim SK, Hebrok M, Melton DA: Notochord to endoderm signaling is required for pancreas development. *Development* 124:4243, 1997.

14. Deutsch G, Jung J, Zheng M, et al: A bipotential precursor population for pancreas and liver within the embryonic endoderm. *Development* 128:871, 2001.

15. Bort R, Martinez-Barbera JP, Beddington RS, et al: Hex homeobox gene-dependent tissue positioning is required for organogenesis of the ventral pancreas. *Development* 131:797, 2004.

16. Dessimoz J, Opoka R, Kordich JJ, et al: FGF signaling is necessary for establishing gut tube domains along the anterior-posterior axis in vivo. *Mech Dev* 123:42, 2006.

17. Grapin-Botton A: Antero-posterior patterning of the vertebrate digestive tract: 40 years after Nicole Le Douarin's PhD thesis. *Int J Dev Biol* 49:335, 2005.

18. McLin VA, Rankin SA, Zorn AM: Repression of Wnt/beta-catenin signaling in the anterior endoderm is essential for liver and pancreas development. *Development* 134:2207, 2007.

19. Martinez Barbera JP, Clements M, Thomas P, et al: The homeobox gene Hex is required in definitive endodermal tissues for normal forebrain, liver and thyroid formation. *Development* 127:2433, 2000.

20. Ahlgren U, Jonsson J, Edlund H: The morphogenesis of the pancreatic mesenchyme is uncoupled from that of the pancreatic epithelium in IPF1/PDX1-deficient mice. *Development* 122:1409, 1996.

21. Stoffers DA, Zinkin NT, Stanojevic V, et al: Pancreatic agenesis attributable to a single nucleotide deletion in the human IPF1 gene coding sequence. *Nat Genet* 15:106, 1997.

22. Asayesh A, Sharpe J, Watson RP, et al: Spleen versus pancreas: Strict control of organ interrelationship revealed by analyses of Bapx1$^{-/-}$ mice. *Genes Dev* 20:2208, 2006.

23. van Eyll JM, Pierreux CE, Lemaigre FP, et al: Shh-dependent differentiation of intestinal tissue from embryonic pancreas by activin A. *J Cell Sci* 117:2077, 2004.

24. Elghazi L, Cras-Meneur C, Czernichow P, et al: Role for FGFR2IIIb-mediated signals in controlling pancreatic endocrine progenitor cell proliferation. *Proc Natl Acad Sci U S A* 99:3884, 2002.

25. Bhushan A, Itoh N, Kato S, et al: Fgf10 is essential for maintaining the proliferative capacity of epithelial progenitor cells during early pancreatic organogenesis. *Development* 128:5109, 2001.

26. Pulkkinen MA, Spencer-Dene B, Dickson C, et al: The IIIb isoform of fibroblast growth factor receptor 2 is required for proper growth and branching of pancreatic ductal epithelium but not for differentiation of exocrine or endocrine cells. *Mech Dev* 120:167, 2003.

27. Ahnfelt-Ronne J, Ravassard P, Pardanaud-Glavieux C, et al: Mesenchymal bone morphogenetic protein signaling is required for normal pancreas development. *Diabetes* 59:1948, 2010.

28. Apelqvist A, Li H, Sommer L, et al: Notch signalling controls pancreatic cell differentiation. *Nature* 400:877, 1999.

29. Maitra A: Tracking down the hedgehog's lair in the pancreas. *Gastroenterology* 138:823, 2010.

30. Hebrok M, Kim SK, St Jacques B, et al: Regulation of pancreas development by hedgehog signaling. *Development* 127:4905, 2000.

31. Strobel O, Rosow DE, Rakhlin EY, et al: Pancreatic duct glands are distinct ductal compartments that react to chronic injury and mediate Shh-induced metaplasia. *Gastroenterology* 138:1166, 2010.

32. Yauch RL, Gould SE, Scales SJ, et al: A paracrine requirement for hedgehog signalling in cancer. *Nature* 455:406, 2008.

33. Bailey JM, Swanson BJ, Hamada T, et al: Sonic hedgehog promotes desmoplasia in pancreatic cancer. *Clin Cancer Res* 14:5995, 2008.

34. Olive KP, Jacobetz MA, Davidson CJ, et al: Inhibition of Hedgehog signaling enhances delivery of chemotherapy in a mouse model of pancreatic cancer. *Science* 324:1457, 2009.

35. Hidalgo M, Maitra A: The hedgehog pathway and pancreatic cancer. *N Engl J Med* 361:2094, 2009.

36. Semenza GL: Life with oxygen. *Science* 318:62, 2007.

37. Heinis M, Simon MT, Ilc K, et al: Oxygen tension regulates pancreatic beta-cell differentiation through hypoxia-inducible factor 1alpha. *Diabetes* 59:662, 2010.

38. Eberhard D, Kragl M, Lammert E: "Giving and taking": Endothelial and beta-cells in the islets of Langerhans. *Trends Endocrinol Metab* 21:457, 2010.

39. Lammert E, Gu G, McLaughlin M, et al: Role of VEGF-A in vascularization of pancreatic islets. *Curr Biol* 13:1070, 2003.

40. Lammert E, Cleaver O, Melton D: Induction of pancreatic differentiation by signals from blood vessels. *Science* 294:564, 2001.

41. Kapa S, Gleeson FC, Vege SS: Dorsal pancreas agenesis and polysplenia/heterotaxy syndrome: A novel association with aortic coarctation and a review of the literature. *JOP* 8:433, 2007.

42. Prasadan K, Daume E, Preuett B, et al: Glucagon is required for early insulin-positive differentiation in the developing mouse pancreas. *Diabetes* 51:3229, 2002.

43. Zhou J, Wang X, Pineyro MA, et al: Glucagon-like peptide 1 and exendin-4 convert pancreatic AR42J cells into glucagon- and insulin-producing cells. *Diabetes* 48:2358, 1999.

44. Thorel F, Nepote V, Avril I, et al: Conversion of adult pancreatic alpha-cells to beta-cells after extreme beta-cell loss. *Nature* 464:1149, 2010.

45. Holland AM, Hale MA, Kagami H, et al: Experimental control of pancreatic development and maintenance. *Proc Natl Acad Sci U S A* 99:12236, 2002.

46. Sellick GS, Barker KT, Stolte-Dijkstra I, et al: Mutations in PTF1A cause pancreatic and cerebellar agenesis. *Nat Genet* 36:1301, 2004.

47. Jensen J, Heller RS, Funder-Nielsen T, et al: Independent development of pancreatic alpha- and beta-cells from neurogenin3-expressing precursors: A role for the notch pathway in repression of premature differentiation. *Diabetes* 49:163, 2000.

48. Gradwohl G, Dierich A, LeMeur M, et al: Neurogenin3 is required for the development of the four endocrine cell lineages of the pancreas. *Proc Natl Acad Sci U S A* 97:1607, 2000.

49. Smith SB, Qu HQ, Taleb N, et al: Rfx6 directs islet formation and insulin production in mice and humans. *Nature* 463:775, 2010.

50. Artner I, Hang Y, Mazur M, et al: MafA and MafB regulate genes critical to β cells in a unique temporal manner. *Diabetes* 59:2530, 2010.

51. Nishimura W, Bonner-Weir S, Sharma A: Expression of MafA in pancreatic progenitors is detrimental for pancreatic development. *Dev Biol* 333:108, 2009.

Acute Pancreatitis

Marc Besselink | Hjalmar van Santvoort | Hein G. Gooszen

Acute pancreatitis is a relatively common, potentially life-threatening disease. It is the third most common gastrointestinal disorder requiring acute hospitalization in the United States, with annual costs exceeding $2 billion.[1,2] Approximately 20% of patients develop severe acute pancreatitis, defined by organ failure or necrotizing pancreatitis.[3] Severe pancreatitis is associated with a mortality of 15% to 30%, whereas the mortality of mild pancreatitis is only 0% to 1%.[4] Organ failure is the most important determinant for mortality in acute pancreatitis.[4] Sterile pancreatic necrosis and sterile peripancreatic collections can usually be treated conservatively. However, in approximately 30% of patients, secondary infection of necrosis occurs, mostly 3 to 4 weeks after the onset of disease.[4] If left untreated, mortality of infected necrosis approaches 100%.[3] This chapter describes current insights in the pathophysiology and treatment of acute pancreatitis. Throughout this chapter the highest available evidence is presented.

ETIOLOGY

In most Western countries, gallstones are the most frequent cause of pancreatitis, in approximately 50% of patients, followed by alcohol in 20%. In approximately 20% of cases, the cause remains unknown (idiopathic). The remaining 10% constitutes a rather large group of possible causes of acute pancreatitis. These causes include hypercalcemia, hypertriglyceridemia, medications, hereditary causes, sphincter of Oddi dysfunction, pancreas divisum, pancreatic neoplasms, and others. Before settling on a final diagnosis of "idiopathic" pancreatitis, it is important to make efforts with various imaging modalities to detect causative lesions that may have therapeutic implications (such as an underlying neoplasm requiring resection).

CLINICAL PRESENTATION AND DIAGNOSIS

CLINICAL PRESENTATION

The diagnosis of acute pancreatitis is based on two or more of the following criteria: (1) severe abdominal pain, (2) serum amylase or lipase more than three times higher than the institution's upper limit, and (3) contrast-enhanced computed tomography (CECT) findings of acute pancreatitis. Usually, the first two criteria are present, and CECT is not required for diagnosis. In the first 72 to 96 hours of disease, a CECT will often fail to demonstrate pancreatic necrosis and peripancreatic collections. A CECT scan has a place in patients who present after several days of abdominal pain when the amylase and lipase levels may have normalized or in patients with organ failure of unknown origin.

LABORATORY INVESTIGATION

The etiology of acute pancreatitis is best determined at admission as this may be the only time when laboratory abnormalities are detectable because they may normalize within days in the course of pancreatitis. Laboratory investigation should include liver function tests, and calcium and triglyceride levels. The latter two are easily forgotten, but hypercalcemia (usually related to hyperparathyroidism) and hypertriglyceridemia (arbitrarily >15 mmol/L) are both well-documented causes and represent easily treatable causes of acute pancreatitis. Triglyceride levels may be increased secondarily during acute pancreatitis in patients who do not otherwise have an underlying lipid disorder.

IMAGING

The most important imaging modality at admission is transabdominal ultrasound in order to detect gallstones or sludge in the gallbladder or in the common bile duct. When gallstones or sludge are visualized, a diagnosis of biliary pancreatitis can be presumed. In the absence of gallstones or sludge, a dilated common bile duct (>8 mm if the patient is 75 years or younger; >10 mm if the patient is older than 75 years) or elevation of serum alanine aminotransferase (ALT) greater than 100 U/L with ALT level greater than aspartate aminotransferase (AST) level strongly suggests the disease is of biliary origin. These levels are not absolute cutoff points, but they provide good guidance for the diagnosis of biliary pancreatitis. If the etiology remains unknown, endoscopic ultrasound can be used to detect gallstones or sludge in the gallbladder or common bile duct.

CECT is used to diagnose peripancreatic collections and pancreatic parenchymal or peripancreatic fat necrosis. A CECT scan has to be performed in patients who do not improve after the first week of symptoms. The terminology for describing morphologic changes in and around the pancreas has been the subject of debate and has undergone considerable changes in the revised Atlanta classification. A common pitfall in the description of peripancreatic collections is to use the term *pseudocyst* for a homogeneous peripancreatic fluid collection that contains not only fluid but also considerable amounts of pancreatic or peripancreatic necrosis. This misnomer is caused by the inability of CECT to discriminate solid components (necrosis) within a predominantly fluid collection (Figure 88-1). Magnetic resonance imaging (MRI) or ultrasonography are the only modalities capable of demonstrating the presence or absence of necrosis in

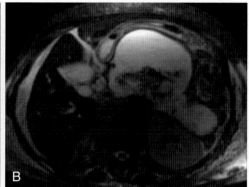

FIGURE 88-1 CT and MR images of a patient with necrotizing pancreatitis made within 2 days. **A,** CT scan with a typical peripancreatic collection. The collection appears homogeneous without necrosis. Often, such a collection is misdiagnosed as a "pseudocyst." **B,** T2-weighted MR image shows clearly a large amount of necrosis in the collection. This is, therefore, no pseudocyst.

such collections. The absence of necrosis is a prerequisite for the collection to be called a pseudocyst.[5] A true pseudocyst in the initial 4 weeks of acute pancreatitis is very rare.

CLASSIFICATION OF SEVERITY

Because of limitations with the 1992 Atlanta classification of acute pancreatitis and the improved understanding of the pathogenesis of acute pancreatitis, the 1992 classification has recently been updated. The updated classification includes, among many other adaptations, a clinical subdivision into *mild* and *severe* disease. In the early phase, this subdivision is based on clinical parameters, whereas in the weeks to follow, this subdivision is based on a combination of clinical parameters and morphologic complications prolonging hospitalization, either requiring active intervention (surgical, endoscopic, radiologic) or other supportive measures (such as need for pressors, ventilatory support, or renal dialysis). The qualifications of "severe" and "necrotizing" do not fully overlap.

Necrotizing pancreatitis is defined as the presence of parenchymal necrosis and/or necrosis of peripancreatic fat. The updated Atlanta classification includes patients with peripancreatic necrosis only (that is, without necrosis of the pancreatic parenchyma) in the category of necrotizing pancreatitis. Edematous interstitial pancreatitis usually runs a mild clinical course, but a small subset of patients suffer a fulminant course and die within 2 to 5 days; these patients clearly have severe disease, but do not meet criteria to have their disease be classified as necrotizing. In this chapter, for practical reasons, patients have been classified with severe pancreatitis when suffering from organ failure, necrotizing pancreatitis or both, mainly because most recent studies apply this definition. Future studies should ideally adhere to updated Atlanta classification criteria to ensure comparability in reporting.

PREDICTING SEVERITY

The clinical course of acute pancreatitis is highly unpredictable and may vary from full recovery within a single day to multiorgan failure and mortality within hours or a few days. Although predictive scores initially have been designed to guide clinicians in the initial management

TABLE 88-1 Commonly Used Predictive Laboratory Scoring Systems in Acute Pancreatitis and Their Cutoff for Predicted Severe Pancreatitis

Predictive Score	Cutoff
APACHE II	≥8 in first 24 hours
BISAP	≥3 in first 24 hours
Modified Glasgow (or Imrie)	≥3 in first 48 hours
Ranson	≥3 in first 48 hours
Urea at admission	>60 mmol/L
C-reactive protein	>150 U/L in first 72 hours

APACHE, Acute Physiology and Chronic Health Evaluation; *BISAP,* bedside index for severity in acute pancreatitis.

and the level of care or observation needed in each patient, their value for day-to-day clinical practice is only limited. The most used scores and cutoff points are listed in Table 88-1.

If a patient meets a certain cutoff value, this only means that a patient can at that stage of disease, temporarily, be classified as having "predicted severe pancreatitis." The clinical value of this label, however, is limited, as the positive predictive value (the chance of truly developing severe pancreatitis) is generally in the order of 50% to 70%. Actually, these classifications are most useful in excluding patients at risk for severe pancreatitis, because with a negative predictive value of 85% to 90%, patients with predicted mild pancreatitis run a 10% to 15% risk of developing the severe form of the disease.

Most clinical studies only include patients with predicted severe pancreatitis, so the reader should be aware that study findings are only applicable to this subgroup of patients and do not necessarily apply to the complete cohort of patients with acute pancreatitis.

EARLY AND LATE ORGAN FAILURE

Acute pancreatitis typically runs a biphasic course. The first phase is characterized by a systemic inflammatory response syndrome (SIRS) and lasts about 2 weeks. The second phase is characterized by a counteractive antiinflammatory response syndrome (CARS), characterized by a state of immunosuppression. Organ failure in the SIRS phase is considered not to be related to infection but

TABLE 88-2 Treatment of Acute Pancreatitis in Various Clinical Scenarios

Clinical Situation	Advice	Exception
WEEKS 1-2		
Predicted severe pancreatitis	Fluid supplementation based on urine production, enteral nutrition, adequate pain control. Not useful: routine antibiotic prophylaxis antioxidants, and oral probiotics.	
Abdominal compartment syndrome	Decompression laparotomy without accessing the retroperitoneum	Large amounts of intraabdominal fluid. In these cases percutaneous catheter drainage may be used but should lead to immediate clinical improvement.
Sterile necrosis (collections) and multiple organ failure	Treat organ failure. No evidence that necrosectomy and/or drainage of collections will improve outcome. There is evidence that drainage will increase the risk of infection.	Abdominal compartment syndrome, bowel ischemia, bleeding
WEEK 3 AND THEREAFTER		
Infected necrosis (collections) without or with only partial encapsulation	If possible, postpone intervention using antibiotics	Rapid deterioration without treatable cause
Infected walled-off necrosis (collections)	Intervention according to the "step-up" approach, starting with (retroperitoneal) catheter drainage. If needed, followed by (minimally invasive) necrosectomy.	Lack of experience; if so, transfer the patient to a more experienced center

rather to severe systemic inflammation. Organ failure in the CARS phase is related to secondary infections, such as infected necrosis. Infections, however, do occur in the SIRS phase, but bacteremia and (ventilator-associated) pneumonia are the most prominent types. This was found in a large series of acute pancreatitis patients where it was demonstrated that these infections were most often diagnosed in the first week of admission.[4]

Organ failure may affect all organ systems, but the pulmonary and the cardiovascular systems are dominant. The gastrointestinal system also suffers from the state of low flow and SIRS, but signs and symptoms are much more difficult to trace and quantify than oxygen exchange, blood pressure, and urine output. Organ failure in the SIRS phase is diagnosed at a median of 2 days after admission but may already be present at admission. Half of the patients who die from acute pancreatitis suffer from organ failure but not infected necrosis. A recent systematic review of cohort studies demonstrated that 32% of patients who develop organ failure eventually die.[6] Mortality in patients with both organ failure and infected necrosis was 43%.

The clinical course of necrotizing pancreatitis is highly variable, and there may be a continuum between the SIRS and CARS phases. Discrimination into three scenarios is potentially helpful to understand the underlying pathophysiologic processes at hand:

1. Early-onset organ failure (week 1), intensive care admission, followed by improvement with supportive measures and intensive care treatment (weeks 2 through 3). In the weeks to follow (weeks 3 through 5), clinical deterioration occurs. This sequence of events is highly indicative of infection of necrosis.

2. Without early organ failure, clinical stability is suddenly complicated by deterioration in weeks 3 through 4 of admission. Again, the chances of infected necrosis as the cause of clinical deterioration are high.

3. Early-onset organ failure does not improve, even after 2 to 3 weeks of supportive treatment in the intensive care unit. In this scenario, a fine-needle aspiration (FNA) of one of the collections has a place to differentiate between persistent SIRS or infected necrosis and to determine the need for intervention. If, however, gas bubbles are present on CECT scan, no further diagnostic procedures are required, and intervention to treat the source of infection needs to be planned.

See Table 88-2 for a summary on treatment of acute pancreatitis in various clinical scenarios.

TREATMENT

CONSERVATIVE MANAGEMENT

Systemic Inflammatory Response Syndrome Phase

Adequate fluid resuscitation forms the mainstay of initial treatment together with adequate pain relief. A diuresis-guided fluid regimen (goal: 1 mL/kg/hr urine production) is required in the initial phase, as long as organ failure is not present yet. Close monitoring and intravenous fluid supplementation in the initial 24 hours of severe pancreatitis are most important; crystalloid resuscitation volumes as high as 20 L may be required. Unrestricted fluid resuscitation may, however, be harmful. A recent Chinese randomized trial demonstrated that very rapid fluid supplementation aimed at keeping hematocrit levels less than 35% over the first 48 hours was associated with increased mortality.[7]

In this phase of the disease, there is no room for intervention (either radiologically, endoscopically, or surgically) for the pancreatic necrosis. Some indications for emergency intervention are discussed later.

Counteractive Antiinflammatory Response Syndrome Phase and Thereafter

If the patient does not improve or deteriorates after initial improvement, infection of pancreatic necrosis and peripancreatic collections needs to be ruled out. To anticipate possible further deterioration, some authors advocate weekly FNA of the collection to prove or disprove infection. Many others (including our group) do not support this strategy, because of the possibility of false-negative FNA and the risk of introducing infection. Moreover, in cases of clinical deterioration, a negative FNA should not deter intervention. A recent randomized controlled trial (RCT) that based intervention in patients with necrotizing pancreatitis on clinical grounds rather than on routine FNA indicated that 92% of patients had infected necrosis at the time of initial intervention.[8] Gas bubbles in peripancreatic collections are considered pathognomonic for infected necrosis, and FNA is not required.

PREVENTION OF INFECTION

As infection is associated with increased mortality in acute pancreatitis, numerous prophylactic strategies have been explored in the past two decades. Enteral bacteria are considered responsible for the majority of these infections, and the current concept is that these bacteria pass through the mucosal barrier in the first 24 hours of disease. In a recent multicenter study of all the infections diagnosed in the course of the disease, the first (usually a bacteremia or ventilator-associated pneumonia) was diagnosed at a median of 8 days after admission.[4] Infection of necrosis was only diagnosed at a median 26 days. Mortality from each individual infection (i.e., including pneumonia, bacteremia) was 30%. Bacteremia increased the risk of infection of necrosis from 38% to 65%. In multivariate analysis, persistent organ failure (odds ratio [OR], 18) and bacteremia (OR, 3.4) were the strongest predictors of mortality.

Systemic intravenous antibiotics, enteral nutrition, systemic intravenous antibiotics, selective bowel decontamination, and enteral probiotics all have been tried to lower the rate of infection.

Enteral Nutrition

Enteral nutrition is hypothesized to reduce small bowel bacterial overgrowth and to improve intestinal mucosal barrier function, theoretically thereby reducing bacterial translocation and resultant infectious complications. A recent randomized trial has demonstrated that in patients with mild pancreatitis, oral feeding can be started as early as the day of admission or the day thereafter.[9] In predicted severe pancreatitis, it is now generally advised to start enteral nutrition by nasojejunal feeding tube within approximately 3 days, if the patient is not expected to quickly resume a normal diet. A recent metaanalysis

demonstrated that in patients with predicted severe pancreatitis, enteral nutrition reduces both infections and mortality compared to the administration of total parenteral nutrition.[10] There are no clinically relevant differences in outcome between the various enteral nutrition formulations including glutamine supplementation.[11]

The optimal route for the administration of enteral feeding—through a nasojejunal or a nasogastric feeding tube—has yet to be established. Two relatively small randomized trials including 80 patients found no difference in tolerance for feeding and complication rates. The overall mortality was rather high, and the studies may have failed to show relevant differences in complications, such as aspiration, because of their small size. Results of ongoing larger studies should be awaited before using nasogastric feeding routinely in patients with severe acute pancreatitis.

Systemic Intravenous Antibiotics

Many studies have addressed the effect of systemic antibiotic prophylaxis in lowering the rate of infectious complications in (predicted) severe acute pancreatitis. The initial, nonblinded, non-placebo-controlled, randomized trials showed somewhat positive effects. In the past years, however, three placebo-controlled trials have failed to demonstrate a reduction of infections and/or mortality. A German multicenter trial stressed an increased risk of antibiotic resistance and fungal infections. In a recent analysis, a relationship between methodologic quality and the effect on mortality was documented: "the better the trial the less the positive effect."[12] A recent updated metaanalysis clearly demonstrated no beneficial effect in the routine use of systemic antibiotic prophylaxis.[13] So, based on current literature, there is no longer support for the routine prophylactic use of antibiotics.

Selective Bowel Decontamination

If the gut is indeed the source of bacteria responsible for the infectious complications in acute pancreatitis, it might seem a rational approach to administer antibiotics enterally. Many intensive care units nowadays use routine selective bowel decontamination (SBD) or selective oropharyngeal decontamination for a variety of indications. Only one RCT studied the value of SBD in acute pancreatitis[14] and compared the effect of SBD (norfloxacin, colistin, amphotericin) with no SBD in patients with severe acute pancreatitis. A reduction in (corrected) mortality in the SBD group, caused mostly by a reduction of gram-negative infections of pancreatic necrosis, was found. Yet, this study has not been repeated, and the strategy has not gained wide acceptance, but the data suggest that the concept of early intervention in the cascade of events—small bowel bacterial overgrowth, mucosal barrier failure, bacterial translocation, systemic infection—deserves further exploration.

Probiotics

Some placebo-controlled RCTs have shown that prophylactic enteral administration of probiotics is capable of reducing the incidence of infectious complications in pancreas and liver surgery.[15] Two small RCTs from Hungary suggested a beneficial effect of prophylactic use of probiotics in predicted severe pancreatitis. In the large Dutch probiotics trial in patients with predicted severe acute pancreatitis, however, no effect on infectious complications was found, but a more than twofold higher mortality rate (16% vs. 6%) was shown in the patients receiving probiotics. So far, no satisfactory answer to this puzzling finding has been presented, in spite of several follow-up studies, clinically and experimentally. At this stage, prophylactic probiotics are not recommended for patients with predicted severe acute pancreatitis.

INTERVENTIONAL TREATMENT

Systemic Inflammatory Response Syndrome Phase (First and Second Weeks)

Intervention in this phase of the disease should aim at treatment of acute life-threatening complications or prevention of further deterioration. Currently, the only means to prevent deterioration in acute pancreatitis is endoscopic retrograde cholangiopancreatography (ERCP) with sphincterotomy, although its exact place in the therapeutic armamentarium has yet to be established.

The only RCT on surgical necrosectomy in this phase was performed in 1989. In this study, intervention within 72 hours ("early") was compared with operation after 12 days ("late").[16] The authors terminated this study prematurely because of a much higher, not yet statistically significant, mortality for surgery within 72 hours (58% vs. 27%). Based on these findings, early operation to remove necrosis was essentially abandoned. The lessons from the past decades are that in the early phase the clinical picture is dominated by systemic inflammatory responses rather than by the presence or absence of infection of necrosis. Consequently there is no benefit to be expected from surgical exploration if removal of infected necrosis is the sole indication for exploration.

Indications for Acute Interventions. The only acute complications justifying very early intervention are abdominal compartment syndrome, bowel ischemia or perforation, and severe bleeding unresponsive to angiographic coiling.

According to the 2007 international consensus meeting, abdominal compartment syndrome is defined by an intraabdominal pressure higher than 20 mm Hg with signs of new organ failure.[17] Although the optimal treatment strategy for abdominal compartment syndrome remains to be defined, a consensus meeting suggested that percutaneous drainage can be used as an initial step if intraabdominal drainable fluid is present. If drainage does not immediately lower the pressure or if there is no (more) drainable fluid, laparotomy for decompression is advised. The pancreas should not be explored because it is too early to remove necrosis safely, and there is a risk to introduce infection into the necrosis.

Percutaneous drainage of noninfected collections is not indicated as sterile collections may become iatrogenically contaminated by the percutaneous drains. A recent randomized study, actually advocating the strategy of draining sterile collections, reported on a significant increase in infected necrosis caused by the practice of routine drainage.[18,19]

Intervention to Prevent Further Deterioration: Early Endoscopic Retrograde Cholangiopancreatography and Sphincterotomy in Biliary Pancreatitis. The current concept of the etiopathogenesis of acute biliary pancreatitis is that a gallstone, released from the gallbladder into the common bile duct, causes temporary obstruction at the level of the papilla of Vater, leading to obstruction of the pancreatic duct with obstructed flow of pancreatic juice and secondary damage to the exocrine cells with autodigestion of the exocrine pancreas. Theoretically, early relief by ERCP with endoscopic biliary sphincterotomy may stop this process at an early phase and reduce the risk of progression to complications. However, a recent metaanalysis concluded that there is no benefit of routine ERCP in patients with predicted severe biliary pancreatitis in the absence of cholangitis.[20] A recent prospective multicenter study demonstrated that ERCP with endoscopic sphincterotomy reduces the complication rate in patients with predicted severe biliary pancreatitis and cholestasis (arbitrarily defined as bilirubin >2.3 mg/dL [>40 µmol/L] and/or dilated common bile duct).[21]

Intervention in the Second Counteractive Antiinflammatory Response Syndrome Phase: Intervention for Treatment of Infected Necrosis

During the CARS phase or second phase, the patient is threatened by yet another episode of systemic infection or sepsis, caused most often by secondary infection of (peri)pancreatic necrosis. Documented or suspected infection of pancreatic or peripancreatic necrosis with signs of sepsis therefore is the most accepted indication for intervention, radiologically, endoscopically, or surgically. In this phase, less frequent indications for intervention include abdominal compartment syndrome, bleeding, gastric outlet obstruction, common bile duct obstruction, and bowel perforation. Once the threshold for intervention has been reached, the choice is between open laparotomy with necrosectomy and (minimally invasive) surgical, endoscopic, and radiologic percutaneous techniques. The use of these latter techniques is rapidly expanding, but the exact place and indication for any of these three options has not been established.

Timing of Intervention for Infected Necrosis: Third Week and Thereafter

Timing and choice of the type of intervention are best guided by an experienced multidisciplinary team. A systematic review of cohort studies concluded that postponing intervention until the intra- and/or extrapancreatic collections have become encapsulated, a process that usually takes 4 weeks, is beneficial.[22] Such encapsulated collections may be referred to as "walled off necrosis."

In the three clinical scenarios described earlier, encapsulation of the collection may not have been completed, when clinical deterioration occurs. Administration of antibiotics to allow for further encapsulation, under close guidance of the clinical developments and CECT scan, performed at regular intervals to prevent bacteriemia or sepsis, is a valid option to postpone surgical intervention. In the review mentioned earlier, necrosectomy was performed at a median of 27 days after onset of disease, with a mortality rate of 25%. If intervention was performed in the first 2 weeks, mortality was 75%. Based on the current literature, postponing of intervention, preferably until 4 weeks after onset of disease, is widely accepted as the strategy of choice. The length of the interval is mainly determined by the completeness of encapsulation and the clinical condition of the patient. This policy is obviously only applicable to the subset of patients who survive the initial phase of SIRS and develop infection of necrosis with signs of sepsis, in the CARS phase.

Types of Intervention

Catheter Drainage. Catheter drainage is the least invasive technique for treating infected necrosis. This drain can be placed percutaneously through the (left) retroperitoneum or transabdominally, but also through the wall of the stomach or duodenum, simply summarized as "transluminal." A recent systematic review suggested that in approximately 55% of patients with necrotizing pancreatitis, percutaneous catheter drainage can be the only intervention needed for cure. In this review, the technical success rate was 99%, the rate of preoperative organ failure was 77%, and the mortality rate was 17%.[23] Accordingly, a multicenter series from the United States and Canada found that 25% of 40 patients with infected necrotizing pancreatitis can be treated with percutaneous drainage only.[24] Finally, a randomized multicenter trial demonstrated that catheter drainage is feasible in 99% of patients.[8]

In patients who do not improve after technically adequate drainage, necrosectomy should be performed as the next step. The percutaneous drain can be used as a roadmap for (minimally invasive) necrosectomy. This two-step approach—drainage as the first step, followed by drain-guided minimally invasive necrosectomy—is called the *step-up approach* and is now considered by many, but not all, experts the standard of care in patients with infected necrosis.

Minimally Invasive Necrosectomy. In the United States and the Netherlands, the most frequently used minimally invasive surgical intervention is the video-assisted retroperitoneal debridement (VARD) procedure.[25,26] This technique is depicted in Figure 88-2.

The first step of the procedure consists of the placement of a left-sided percutaneous retroperitoneal drain through the left flank (Figure 88-2, *A*), if the collection can be reached through this route. The patient is placed in a supine position with the left side slightly elevated. Guided by the drain, a 5 to 7 cm incision is made, and the necrotic collection is opened (Figure 88-2, *B*). The initial pus and necrosis are removed blindly (Figure 88-2, *C*). Next, a 0-degree laparoscope is introduced in order to remove all the necrosis in reach, under direct vision (Figure 88-2, *D*). Only loosely adherent pieces of necrosis are removed to reduce the risk of bleeding. It is not the goal to remove all necrosis. In contrast to purely percutaneous necrosectomy techniques, VARD allows for the removal of large pieces of necrosis (Figure 88-2, *E*) In general, the more complete the encapsulation, the easier the necrosectomy can be performed. A video of this procedure is available at http://www.youtube.com/watch?v=XicI4a7Q768 (or search YouTube for VARD

pancreatitis). Following near-complete debridement, two large-bore surgical drains are placed into the empty cavity, one at the deepest point and one more shallow. Postoperatively, the drains are continuously lavaged with increasing amounts (2, 4, then 6 L) of 0.9% saline per day in the first 3 days.

In a recent Dutch multicenter randomized controlled trial[8] in patients with documented or suspected infection of necrosis, the minimally invasive step-up approach and primary open necrosectomy were compared. A significant difference in major complications and costs was observed, all in favor of the step-up approach, and there was no significant difference in mortality.

A purely percutaneous minimally invasive retroperitoneal necrosectomy using an operating nephroscope has been described by Carter at al from Glasgow and, later, by the group from Liverpool. A recent series by the latter group suggested a decrease in mortality when using this technique compared to historical controls.[27]

Endoscopic Transluminal Necrosectomy. If VARD is technically not feasible because the infected necrosis does not reach far enough left, then endoscopic transluminal/transgastric necrosectomy may be a viable option. Since the first description of the transgastric approach by Seifert in 2000, this technique has been increasingly adopted by expert endoscopists, usually gastroenterologists. Results are promising, with success rates ranging from 80% to 93% and mortality from 0% to 6%.[28-30] Controlled studies are needed, as selection bias may have influenced these results, and in several series the rate of infection of the necrosis was low.

The theoretical advantages are that no abdominal incision(s) are required, and consequently, external pancreatic fistula should not occur, because an internal fistula to the stomach is instead created. Incisional hernia, often difficult to treat after open necrosectomy, is also avoided. The need for repeated, multiple procedures to remove sufficient amounts of necrosis is a distinct disadvantage for the transgastric technique.

A summary of the advantages and disadvantages of these techniques is presented in Table 88-3.

Open Necrosectomy. Until the results of the PANTER trial were published, primary open necrosectomy was considered the reference standard of treatment in patients with infected necrotizing pancreatitis. One of the most frequently used techniques of open necrosectomy for infected necrosis is laparotomy with placement of a retroperitoneal lavage system after complete necrosectomy has been performed.[31] In this technique, initially described by Beger, drains are placed in the lesser sac after necrosectomy. These drains are continuously lavaged with increasing amounts (2, 4, then 6 L) of saline per day. Lavage may serve a number of purposes such as mechanical debridement, prevention of tube obstruction, and dilution of pancreatic juice, although the precise benefit is speculative. The mortality of this technique is approximately 25%.[31,32]

Another open approach is open necrosectomy and closed packing. The group from Boston reported an 11% mortality rate in 167 patients.[33] Their transmesenteric technique of open necrosectomy is depicted in Figure 88-3. Necrosis is approached through the transverse

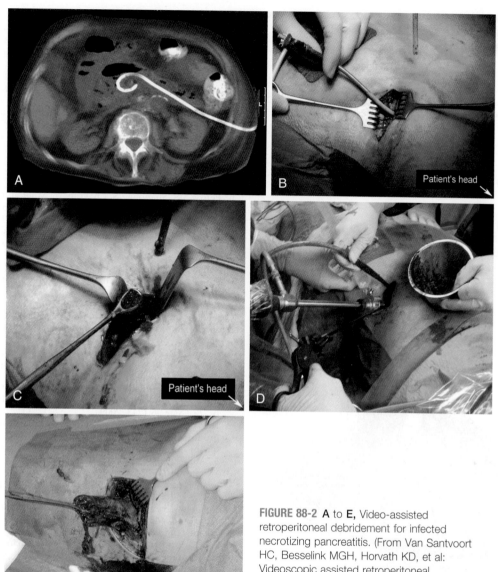

FIGURE 88-2 **A** to **E,** Video-assisted retroperitoneal debridement for infected necrotizing pancreatitis. (From Van Santvoort HC, Besselink MGH, Horvath KD, et al: Videoscopic assisted retroperitoneal debridement in infected necrotizing pancreatitis. *HPB (Oxford)* 9:156, 2007.)

mesocolon and debrided bluntly, with the goal of removing all necrotic tissue and particulate debris. The resulting cavity is then packed with gauze-stuffed Penrose drains that are removed one by one after a week.

Some groups continue to use an open abdomen strategy with regular, planned relaparotomies as a routine every 3 to 5 days. As the mortality of this procedure is approximately 70%, it is advised to use this only as a rescue strategy, when it is technically impossible to close the abdomen.[31]

PREVENTION OF RECURRENT PANCREATITIS

If gallstones are the cause of pancreatitis, cholecystectomy with bile duct clearance is required to prevent recurrent biliary pancreatitis. The optimal timing of cholecystectomy is subject to debate. Most authors perform the cholecystectomy during the index admission for mild biliary pancreatitis, although others claim that this may be technically more difficult, and they perform cholecystectomy at a 6-week interval. Controlled data are needed to make a final choice. Nealon demonstrated that early cholecystectomy in patients with severe pancreatitis (i.e., necrotizing pancreatitis) may be harmful, as collections may become infected secondary to cholecystectomy with a negative impact on outcome.[34]

SUMMARY

Acute pancreatitis remains an unpredictable, potentially lethal disease with a high mortality. Recent advances include

- More detailed knowledge on the pathophysiology of the disease.
- Routine use of nasojejunal nutrition in predicted severe disease.
- Postponed intervention to facilitate safe necrosectomy and improve prognosis.

TABLE 88-3 Techniques for Treating Infected Necrotizing Pancreatitis

	Minimally Invasive	No Open Necrosectomy Needed	Mortality
Percutaneous drainage	++++	25%-55%	17%
Endoscopic transgastric necrosectomy	+++	80%-93%	0%-6%
Percutaneous retroperitoneal necrosectomy	++	86%	19%
Video-assisted retroperitoneal debridement	+	93%	19%
Open necrosectomy (reference standard)	–	–	11%-39%

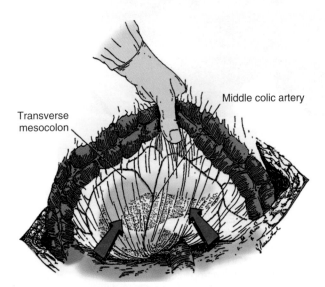

Middle colic artery

Transverse mesocolon

FIGURE 88-3 Technique for open debridement. The lesser sac can be approached through the base of the mesocolon; attention should be paid to avoid injury to the middle colic artery. (From Del-Castillo F, Warshaw A, Rattner D: Closed packing and drainage following débridement for necrotizing pancreatitis. *Probl Gen Surg* 13:127, 1996.)

- Catheter drainage as the first therapeutic step in cases of suspected or documented infected necrotizing pancreatitis is the procedure of choice; (minimally invasive) necrosectomy is no longer the first step in patients with infected (peri)pancreatic necrosis.
- The best technique for necrosectomy has yet to be established. After retroperitoneal percutaneous catheter drainage, it seems reasonable to perform a drain-guided VARD procedure.

ACKNOWLEDGMENT

Karen Horvath, MD, University of Washington Medical Center, edited a previous version of this chapter.

REFERENCES

1. Fagenholz PJ, Fernandez-del Castillo C, Harris NS, et al: Direct medical costs of acute pancreatitis hospitalizations in the United States. *Pancreas* 35:302, 2007.
2. Shaheen NJ, Hansen RA, Morgan DR, et al: The burden of gastrointestinal and liver diseases, 2006. *Am J Gastroenterol* 101:2128, 2006.
3. Banks PA, Freeman ML: Practice guidelines in acute pancreatitis. *Am J Gastroenterol* 101:2379, 2006.
4. Besselink MG, Van Santvoort HC, Boermeester MA, et al: Timing and impact of infections in acute pancreatitis. *Br J Surg* 96:267, 2009.
5. UK guidelines for the management of acute pancreatitis. *Gut* 54:iii1, 2005.
6. Petrov MS, Shanbhag S, Chakraborty M, et al: Organ failure and infection of pancreatic necrosis as determinants of mortality in patients with acute pancreatitis. *Gastroenterology* 139:813, 2010.
7. Mao EQ, Tang YQ, Fei J, et al: Fluid therapy for severe acute pancreatitis in acute response stage. *Chin Med J (Engl)* 122:169, 2009.
8. Van Santvoort HC, Besselink MG, Bakker OJ, et al: A step-up approach or open necrosectomy for necrotizing pancreatitis. *N Engl J Med* 362:1491, 2010.
9. Eckerwall GE, Tingstedt BB, Bergenzaun PE, et al: Immediate oral feeding in patients with mild acute pancreatitis is safe and may accelerate recovery: A randomized clinical study. *Clin Nutr* 26:758, 2007.
10. Petrov MS, Zagainov VE. Influence of enteral versus parenteral nutrition on blood glucose control in acute pancreatitis: A systematic review. *Clin Nutr* 26:514, 2007.
11. Petrov MS, Loveday BP, Pylypchuk RD, et al: Systematic review and meta-analysis of enteral nutrition formulations in acute pancreatitis. *Br J Surg* 96:1243, 2009.
12. De Vries AC, Besselink MGH, Van der Kraats CIB, et al: Antibiotic prophylaxis in acute necrotizing pancreatitis: Methodological quality of randomised controlled trials in relation to outcome. *Gut* 54:A38, 2005.
13. Wittau M, Mayer B, Scheele J, et al: Systematic review and meta-analysis of antibiotic prophylaxis in severe acute pancreatitis. *Scand J Gastroenterol* 46:261, 2011.
14. Luiten EJ, Hop WC, Lange JF, et al: Controlled clinical trial of selective decontamination for the treatment of severe acute pancreatitis. *Ann Surg* 222:57, 1995.
15. Van Santvoort HC, Besselink MG, Timmerman HM, et al: Probiotics in surgery. *Surgery* 143:1, 2008.
16. Mier J, Luque-de León E, Castillo A, et al: Early versus late necrosectomy in severe necrotizing pancreatitis. *Am J Surg* 173:71, 1997.
17. Cheatham ML, Malbrain ML, Kirkpatrick A, et al: Results from the International Conference of Experts on Intra-abdominal Hypertension and Abdominal Compartment Syndrome. II. Recommendations. *Intensive Care Med* 33:951, 2007.
18. Besselink MG, Van Santvoort HC, Bakker OJ, et al: Draining sterile fluid collections in acute pancreatitis? Primum non nocere! *Surg Endosc* 25:331, 2011.
19. Zerem E, Imamovic G, Omerovic S, et al: Randomized controlled trial on sterile fluid collections management in acute pancreatitis: Should they be removed? *Surg Endosc* 2009 May 15. [Epub ahead of print].
20. Petrov MS, Van Santvoort HC, Besselink MG, et al: Early endoscopic retrograde cholangiopancreatography versus conservative management in acute biliary pancreatitis without cholangitis: A meta-analysis of randomized trials. *Ann Surg* 247:250, 2008.
21. Van Santvoort HC, Besselink MG, De Vries AC, et al: Early endoscopic retrograde cholangiopancreatography in predicted severe acute biliary pancreatitis: A prospective multicenter study. *Ann Surg* 250:68, 2009.
22. Besselink MG, Verwer TJ, Schoenmaeckers EJ, et al: Timing of surgical intervention in necrotizing pancreatitis. *Arch Surg* 142:1194, 2007.
23. Van Baal MC, Van Santvoort HC, Bollen TL, et al: Systematic review of percutaneous catheter drainage as primary treatment for necrotizing pancreatitis. *Br J Surg* 98:18, 2011.
24. Horvath K, Freeny P, Escallon J, et al: Safety and efficacy of video-assisted retroperitoneal debridement for infected pancreatic

collections: A multicenter, prospective, single-arm phase 2 study. *Arch Surg* 145:817, 2010.

25. Horvath KD, Kao LS, Wherry KL, et al: A technique for laparoscopic-assisted percutaneous drainage of infected pancreatic necrosis and pancreatic abscess. *Surg Endosc* 15:1221, 2001.

26. Van Santvoort HC, Besselink MGH, Horvath KD, et al: Videoscopic assisted retroperitoneal debridement in infected necrotizing pancreatitis. *HPB (Oxford)* 9:156, 2007.

27. Raraty MG, Halloran CM, Dodd S, et al: Minimal access retroperitoneal pancreatic necrosectomy: Improvement in morbidity and mortality with a less invasive approach. *Ann Surg* 251:787, 2010.

28. Papachristou GI, Takahashi N, Chahal P, et al: Peroral endoscopic drainage/debridement of walled-off pancreatic necrosis. *Ann Surg* 245:943, 2007.

29. Seifert H, Biermer M, Schmitt W, et al: Transluminal endoscopic necrosectomy after acute pancreatitis: A multicentre study with long-term follow-up (the GEPARD Study). *Gut* 58:1260, 2009.

30. Voermans RP, Bruno MJ, van Berge Henegouwen MI, et al: Review article: Transluminal endoscopic debridement of organized pancreatic necrosis—the first step towards natural orifice transluminal endoscopic surgery. *Aliment Pharmacol Ther* 26:233, 2007.

31. Besselink MG, De Bruijn MT, Rutten JP, et al: Surgical intervention in patients with necrotizing pancreatitis. *Br J Surg* 93:593, 2006.

32. Rau B, Bothe A, Beger HG. Surgical treatment of necrotizing pancreatitis by necrosectomy and closed lavage: Changing patient characterics and outcome in a 19-year, single-center series. *Surgery* 138:28, 2005.

33. Rodriguez JR, Razo AO, Targarona J, et al: Debridement and closed packing for sterile or infected necrotizing pancreatitis: Insights into indications and outcomes in 167 patients. *Ann Surg* 247:294, 2008.

34. Nealon WH, Bawduniak J, Walser EM. Appropriate timing of cholecystectomy in patients who present with moderate to severe gallstone-associated acute pancreatitis with peripancreatic fluid collections. *Ann Surg* 239:741, 2004.

Chronic Pancreatitis

Eugene A. Choi | Jeffrey B. Matthews

Chronic pancreatitis is a progressive inflammatory disorder that leads to irreversible destruction of the exocrine and endocrine tissue of the pancreas. Fibrotic replacement of the normal pancreas may be associated with persistent abdominal pain, the development of exocrine insufficiency, and ultimately, diabetes mellitus. Inflammation may lead to local complications, including biliary and gastrointestinal obstruction, ascites, mesoportal-splenic thrombosis, pseudocyst formation, hemorrhage, and sepsis. Despite multiple consensus conferences, there are no uniformly satisfactory criteria for the diagnosis, classification, and staging of chronic pancreatitis. In its advanced stages, chronic pancreatitis is readily apparent clinically, typically associated with pancreatic duct stricture and ductal dilation, stones and diffuse parenchymal calcification, and the digestive and metabolic effects of organ insufficiency. However, recognition of patients with early and mild disease remains a difficult challenge. The absence of a clinically relevant classification system for chronic pancreatitis contributes to inconsistencies in the treatment of the disease. Treatment decisions, ideally taken after appropriate multidisciplinary input from surgical, endoscopic, and radiologic experts, are better made in the context of individual circumstances such as patient symptoms and anatomic findings rather than classification systems based on etiology or morphologic severity.

DEFINITION: CHRONIC PANCREATITIS

Acute pancreatitis generally refers to a single episode of acute inflammation of the organ, typically associated with histopathologic changes that may include edema, fat necrosis, and hemorrhage. Although often fully reversible, the acute injury may be so severe as to result in permanent parenchymal damage, local or remote complications, or death. Chronic pancreatitis generally refers to an ongoing inflammatory and fibrosing disorder characterized by irreversible morphologic changes, progressive and permanent loss of exocrine and endocrine function, and a clinical pattern of either recurrent acute exacerbation or persistent pain. In reality, however, acute and chronic pancreatitis represent more of a spectrum of inflammatory and fibrosing conditions of the pancreas than the two dichotomous terms would otherwise imply. Recurrent episodes (or even a single episode) of acute pancreatitis may lead to chronic changes within the pancreas, although the timing and extent to which such changes merit a change in nomenclature to chronic pancreatitis is somewhat arbitrary. The histopathologic changes of chronic pancreatitis comprise fibrosis, a reduced number of acinar cells and islets of Langerhans, and development of strictures and dilation of pancreatic ducts as well as calcium calculi (pancreatic duct stones). The morphologic/structural changes of chronic pancreatitis can occur years before any clinical symptoms are present. One hypothesis envisions the activation of pancreatic stellate cells, which induce desmoplasia, as the key pathogenetic "switch" that leads to the transition to chronic pancreatitis.[1]

Efforts to establish consensus for uniform terminology of pancreatitis began with an international conference held in Marseille in 1963, during which participants agreed that acute pancreatitis should refer to acute organ inflammation characterized by interstitial edema, peripancreatic fat necrosis, and hemorrhage, which resolves if the primary cause or risk factor is removed. Chronic pancreatitis was distinguished by irreversible focal, segmental, or diffuse destruction of the exocrine tissue along with dilation or focal strictures of the main pancreatic duct. However, these definitions failed to address the functional or clinical dimensions of acute or chronic pancreatitis. At a second meeting in Marseille held in 1984,[2,3] the definition of acute pancreatitis was modified to address the clinical presentation of acute abdominal pain along with an increase in serum or urine pancreatic enzymes, occurring either as a single attack or as recurrent episodes. Chronic pancreatitis was subclassified as chronic pancreatitis with focal or segmental or diffuse fibrosis, and chronic pancreatitis with or without stones, and obstructive chronic pancreatitis was listed as a distinct form. Patients with chronic pancreatitis present with recurrent episodes of pain or with painless progressive loss of exocrine or endocrine insufficiency. To help define changes associated with clinical risk factors, a 1988 meeting in Rome added the morphologic distinction of chronic calcifying pancreatitis that is characterized by intraductal calcifications and protein plugs, and chronic inflammatory pancreatitis that is characterized by dense infiltration of mononuclear inflammatory cells.[4] A consensus conference in Cambridge in 1984 defined the distinction between acute and chronic pancreatitis as the reversibility of the morphologic and functional changes of inflammation.[5] The Cambridge meeting proposed a classification system of chronic pancreatitis based on radiographic findings on endoscopic retrograde cholangiopancreatography (ERCP) (Table 89-1) and ultrasonography (US) or computed tomography (CT). Criteria for chronic pancreatitis from the Japan Pancreas Society focused on findings from an array of diagnostic approaches including US, CT, ERCP, secretin stimulation, and histologic examination of pancreatic tissue. The presence of certain criteria such as pancreatic stones on CT or US is considered definitive evidence of chronic pancreatitis, whereas others such as pancreatic deformity with irregular contour are considered only probable or

TABLE 89-1 Cambridge Conference Classification of Chronic Pancreatitis: ERCP

Terminology	Main Duct	Abnormal Side Ducts	Additional Features
Normal	Normal	None	
Equivocal	Normal	<3	
Mild changes	Normal	≥3	
Moderate changes	Abnormal	>3	
Marked changes	Abnormal	>3	1 or more of large cavity, obstruction, filling defects, severe dilation, or irregularity

Modified from Sarner M, Cotton PB: Classification of pancreatitis. *Gut* 25:756, 1984.

TABLE 89-2 Etiologic Risk Factors Associated With Chronic Pancreatitis: TIGAR-O

Toxic-metabolic	Alcoholic, tobacco smoking, hypercalcemia (hyperparathyroidism)
	Hyperlipidemia
	Chronic renal failure
	Medications, toxins
Idiopathic	Tropical
Genetic	Cationic trypsinogen
	CFTR, SPINK1
Autoimmune	Isolated or associated with autoimmune disorders
Recurrent acute and severe	Postnecrotic (severe acute pancreatitis)
	Recurrent acute pancreatitis
	Vascular disease/ischemic
	Postirradiation
Obstructive	Pancreatic divisum
	Sphincter of Oddi disorders
	Duct obstruction (tumor)
	Posttraumatic pancreatic duct scars
	Preampullary duodenal wall cysts

Modified from Etemad B, Whitcomb DC: Chronic pancreatitis: Diagnosis, classification, and new genetic developments. *Gastroenterology* 120:682, 2001.

possible evidence in support of the disease.[6] The shortcoming of all of these consensus approaches has been the inability to establish a definitive diagnosis in the earliest stages of disease. Moreover, no classification system has proven practical applicability in guiding decisions for therapy.

RISK FACTORS

The pathogenesis of chronic pancreatitis remains poorly understood. Most hypotheses are more associative and speculative than mechanistic. An association between alcohol and acute and chronic pancreatitis has been noted for over half a century. Sarles et al demonstrated that the relative risk of chronic pancreatitis increases directly with mean daily alcohol consumption.[4] However, even relatively moderate alcohol intake can cause chronic pancreatitis, and the duration of alcohol consumption can be relatively short before the onset of disease. In alcohol-induced acute pancreatitis, it has been postulated that by-products of alcohol metabolism induce acinar cell injury, which produces pancreatic enzyme (trypsin, chymotrypsin, and phospholipase A) activation and local tissue damage by autodigestion and recruitment of inflammatory cells. In chronic pancreatitis, alcohol is thought to increase the protein concentration in pancreatic juice, which causes intraductal calcium stone formation, ductal epithelial ulceration, inflammation, and fibrosis. Yet it is only a small percentage (5% to 10%) of alcoholics that develop pancreatic disease, suggesting that alcohol is more of a risk factor than a causative agent for pancreatitis in patients who are susceptible for various unknown or poorly defined reasons. Different disease processes causing similar-appearing injury to the pancreas may follow different clinical courses. Thus, rather than classifying pancreatitis based on the presumed causative agent, Whitcomb et al proposed a system to classify risk factors that may interact to predispose an individual patient to produce pancreatitis.[7] According to this framework, risk factors are grouped as **T**oxic/Metabolic, **I**diopathic, **G**enetic, **A**utoimmune, **R**ecurrent Acute, and **O**bstructive (Table 89-2).

TOXIC/METABOLIC

Almost 70% of chronic pancreatitis cases are associated with chronic alcoholic intake in Western countries.[8] The prevalence is significantly higher in men compared with women. Tobacco use is associated with the early presentation of alcoholic chronic pancreatitis and is associated with the presentation of calcifications and the development of diabetes. It is unknown whether tobacco initiates the disease[9]; however, tobacco is thought to potentiate the progression of chronic pancreatitis. In a preclinical model, investigators demonstrated that tobacco exposure increases the risk of pancreatic cancer in chronic pancreatitis patients.[10] Hyperparathyroidism and hypercalcemia are also associated with chronic pancreatitis. Pancreatitis has been reported to be the first manifestation of patients with multiple endocrine neoplasia 2A (MEN2A). Patients with chronic renal failure have a higher risk of chronic pancreatitis. Certain medications, including statins, steroids, oral contraceptives, and interferon, as well as clinical hyperlipidemia can be associated with chronic pancreatitis, but they are more often associated with acute or recurrent acute pancreatitis in high-risk patients, including the elderly and patients with cancer.

IDIOPATHIC

Historically, no environmental or metabolic risk factor can be identified in approximately 20% of patients who are therefore categorized as having idiopathic acute, recurrent acute, or chronic pancreatitis. Patients with idiopathic disease typically fall into a bimodal age distribution, presenting either between the ages of 10 and 20 or after age 50 years. However, many of these patients are increasingly recognized to have underlying genetic mutations and polymorphisms and may be more appropriately recategorized into the genetic subgroup. To better understand the interactions among genetic, environmental, and metabolic factors predisposing to chronic pancreatitis, a consortium (North American Pancreatitis Study 2) has been established to collect patient questionnaires and blood for genomic DNA and biomarker studies.[11]

GENETIC

Although hereditary pancreatitis was recognized as a distinct clinical entity in the 1950s, it was not until 1996 that its genetic basis began to be understood. The inheritance pattern of hereditary chronic pancreatitis is autosomal dominant and has roughly a 78% penetrance rate. Genetic linkage analysis established a locus for hereditary chronic pancreatitis on chromosome 7q, a region that encodes eight different zymogen genes including various trypsins and carboxypeptidase A. Whitcomb et al performed mutational screening analyses for each of the encoding regions of the cationic and anionic trypsinogen genes and discovered a single G to A transition mutation in the cationic trypsinogen gene (PRSS1).[7] This transition mutation resulted in an Arg (CGC) to His (CAC) (R122H) substitution that did not change the structure or catalytic activity of the enzyme but led to an unusually stable protein. The R122H mutation produces a proteolytic-resistant trypsinogen favoring inappropriate activation within the pancreas, leading to autodigestion. Other mutations in PRSS1 have been identified in various kindreds, although these are less well studied.[12-15] Patients with hereditary pancreatitis, especially those bearing the R122H mutation of PRSS1, have an estimated 35% lifetime risk of developing pancreatic cancer,[16] a risk that is roughly doubled by smoking.

Variations in a number of other genes have been associated with chronic pancreatitis. Witt et al studied 96 unrelated children and adolescents with idiopathic chronic pancreatitis and identified frequent mutations in the serine protease inhibitor, Kazal type 1 (SPINK1), a pancreatic trypsin inhibitor.[17] SPINK1 is colocalized with trypsinogen within zymogen granules and is thought to prevent inappropriate intrapancreatic protease activation. The most frequent mutation associated with chronic pancreatitis is an N34S amino acid substitution in exon 3. Mutations in SPINK1 or in PRSS1 lead to an imbalance toward intrapancreatic trypsin activation, thereby leading to autodigestion of the pancreas and inflammation. It is postulated the SPINK1 mutations are not directly responsible for pancreatitis but may lower the threshold for the disease from other risk factors.[18]

Chronic pancreatitis is also associated with mutations in the cystic fibrosis transmembrane conductance regulator gene (CFTR). Cystic fibrosis is an autosomal recessive disorder that has been linked to mutation of the CFTR gene, which encodes a cyclic adenosine monophosphate–regulated chloride channel located in the apical domain of epithelial cells lining the proximal ducts of the pancreas. More than 1000 mutations have been characterized with a wide range of impact on the characteristics of the channel function. The most common mutation results in a deletion of single amino acid, phenylalanine, at position 508 (DF508). The clinical manifestations are dependent on the specific mutation and the impact on the functional characteristic of the chloride channel. Sharer et al found that CFTR mutations were more common in patients with idiopathic rather than alcoholic chronic pancreatitis.[19] The CFTR mutation is not a direct cause of chronic pancreatitis but may contribute to the disease. Mutation of the CFTR may lead to a decrease in bicarbonate secretion, impaired fluid secretion and formation of protein plugs, and pancreatic insufficiency. Alternatively, the CFTR mutation may alter vesicular sorting and granule trafficking or cause membrane lipid imbalance. Chronic pancreatitis also has been associated with mutations in the anionic trypsinogen (PRSS2) and chymotrypsin C (CTRC). PRSS2 has a lower incidence of mutations in chronic pancreatitis; a variant of PRSS2 with a glycine to arginine change at codon 191 appears to have a protective effect against chronic pancreatitis.[20]

AUTOIMMUNE

Autoimmune pancreatitis, also known as lymphoplasmacytic sclerosing pancreatitis, is a rare cause (1%) of chronic pancreatitis.[21] Gland enlargement, diffuse duct narrowing, and stenosis of the intrapancreatic portion of the bile duct characterize the disease. Histologic examination of the tissue demonstrates pancreas parenchyma infiltrated by both CD4+ and CD8+ lymphocytes and IgG4 plasma cells, with interstitial fibrosis and acinar cell atrophy. Patients with autoimmune pancreatitis have antibodies directed against a peptide that is homologous with the sequence of the plasminogen-binding protein (PBP) of *Helicobacter pylori* and with the ubiquitin-protein ligase E3 component n-recognin 2 which is expressed in the acinar cells of the pancreas.[22] Autoimmune pancreatitis can be associated with other autoimmune diseases including Sjögren syndrome, primary sclerosing cholangitis (PSC), and inflammatory bowel disease. Primary treatment for autoimmune pancreatitis is steroid treatment. Focal inflammation seen with this disease can often mimic a pancreatic mass, which may be difficult to differentiate from a pancreatic malignancy on imaging studies.

RECURRENT ACUTE

Recurrent episodes of acute pancreatitis of any etiology can cause chronic pancreatitis. This mechanism is poorly understood but likely involves the accumulated effects of postinflammatory scarring and necrosis as well as the priming of pancreatic stellate cells to induce fibrosis. In addition, radiation and ischemia may contribute to irreversible histopathologic changes and inflammation characteristic of chronic pancreatitis.

OBSTRUCTION

Obstructive pancreatitis can be congenital, functional, or acquired. Causes of pancreatic obstruction include pancreatic or ampullary tumors, and postinjury pancreatic duct fibrosis. Elevated basal pressures at the sphincter of Oddi are thought by some to lead to relative outflow obstruction from the proximal duct and thereby contribute to pancreatitis, although direct evidence for this hypothesis is lacking and no convincing mechanism for progression to chronic disease has been proposed.

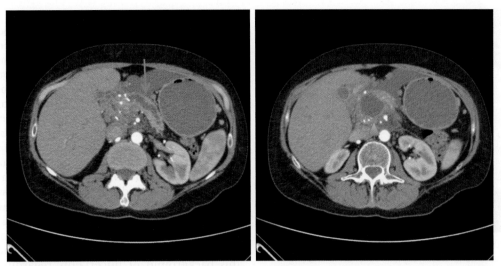

FIGURE 89-1 Chronic pancreatitis in a 48-year-old woman with a history of alcohol use. Axial cross-section abdominal computed tomography demonstrating dilated pancreatic duct *(arrow)* and a pseudocyst in the head of the pancreas communicating with the main duct *(arrowhead).*

Patients may also have anatomic variations in the pancreatic ductal system that predispose for obstruction, most notably pancreas divisum. Pancreas divisum occurs when the ventral and dorsal aspects of the pancreatic ducts fail to fuse during development and, consequently, the drainage of the pancreatic body and tail occurs through the dorsal duct and the minor papilla. Insufficient caliber of the dorsal duct is thought to induce relative obstruction to outflow that could lead to pancreatitis. However, the vast majority of patients with pancreas divisum are asymptomatic; thus, the anatomic variation may predispose to pancreatitis in combination with other risk factors rather than initiating pancreatitis directly.

CLINICAL MANIFESTATIONS

The most common symptom of chronic pancreatitis is abdominal pain (90%), although the pattern of pain is highly variable. In some patients, particularly early in the course of the disease, pain may be a minor feature. The pain may be episodic and minimal or absent in between acute exacerbations, but it often is noted to gradually become more constant. In late phases of the disease, pain may disappear ("burnout"), a transition that is often associated with the development of diabetes and exocrine insufficiency. The pain is most frequently localized to the epigastrium, often radiates to the back, and is typically associated with nausea and vomiting. Overall, the course of chronic pancreatitis is highly unpredictable and variable. Lankisch et al followed 335 patients with chronic pancreatitis, and despite a long-term observation period of more than 10 years, a majority of patients continued to experience pain.[23] Because eating can exacerbate pain, patients may avoid regular meals, leading to weight loss and malnutrition. Between 4% and 30% of patients have significant exocrine insufficiency and report bloating, flatulence, or steatorrhea (foul smelling, oily, and loose stools). Malabsorption leads to weight loss and deficiencies in micronutrients, especially fat-soluble vitamins A, D, and E. Endocrine insufficiency or diabetes mellitus

develops later in the course of the disease, typically when 90% of the parenchyma is replaced by fibrosis. Diabetes develops more often in those patients with alcohol-associated chronic calcifying pancreatitis than in hereditary forms of the disease.

EXTRAPANCREATIC COMPLICATIONS OF CHRONIC PANCREATITIS

A subset of patients develops symptoms of gastrointestinal and biliary obstruction. Duodenal, colonic, and bile duct obstruction can occur as a result of significant fibrosis of the head of the pancreas or the development of large pseudocysts (Figure 89-1). The incidence of biliary obstruction is approximately 3% to 23% among patient diagnosed with chronic pancreatitis, and is even higher (15% to 60%) among patients who require surgery.[24] The incidence of duodenal obstruction/stenosis is 2% in all patients, and again is higher (12%) in patients who require operative therapy. The majority of patients with splenic vein thrombosis are asymptomatic; the incidence of thrombosis varies anywhere from 4% to 45% depending on the population surveyed, but very few patients present with gastric variceal bleeding.[25,26]

Epidemiologic and preclinical studies demonstrate that chronic pancreatitis is associated with the development of pancreatic cancer. Lowenfels et al presented a multicenter historical cohort study of 2015 patients with chronic pancreatitis followed for at least 2 years.[27] The standardized incidence risk ratio for the development of pancreatic cancer was 16.5 and 14.4 at 2 and 5 years' followup, respectively, for the risk of developing pancreatic cancer. The incidence of pancreatic cancer was equally high in patients who presented with pancreatitis associated with chronic alcohol use and those with other risk factors. In a preclinical murine model, Guerrra et al reported that inflammation associated with chronic pancreatitis is essential for induction of pancreatic cancer by the oncogene K-ras (Figures 89-2 and 89-3).[28]

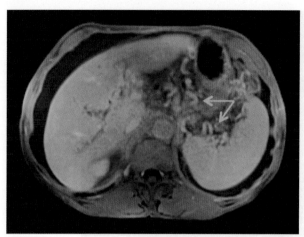

FIGURE 89-2 Chronic pancreatitis in a 50-year-old man with a history of extensive alcohol use. Magnetic resonance imaging demonstrates thrombosed splenic vein with extensive varices involving the splenic hilum and pancreatic tail *(arrows)*.

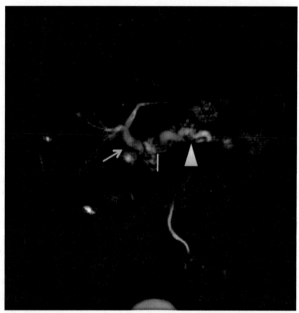

FIGURE 89-3 Chronic pancreatitis in a 52-year-old man with a history of extensive alcohol use. Magnetic resonance cholangiopancreatography demonstrates a dilated common bile duct up to intrapancreatic portion *(arrow)*, irregularity of and dilation of the pancreatic duct and sides *(arrowhead)*, and intraluminal filling defects at the level of the pancreatic head *(line)*.

MECHANISM OF PAIN IN CHRONIC PANCREATITIS

A number of mechanisms have been proposed to account for the pain of chronic pancreatitis. However, the correlation between the hypothetical cause of the pain and the clinical results of therapies directed at that cause is imperfect at best. Obstruction of the main pancreatic duct in some circumstances is thought to lead to increased ductal pressure (that may in turn be transmitted to secondary ducts and the surrounding parenchyma), leading to pain through stretch-activated neural pathways. Ductal obstruction may also induce missorting

and mistargeted basolateral secretion of pancreatic enzymes, triggering protease-activated nociceptive pathways. Relief of main duct obstruction via decompressive surgical procedures (see later) is often effective treatment for pain in these circumstances but is far from universally successful either in the short run or in extended followup. Chronic inflammation of the pancreas may lead to fibrosis of the peripancreatic capsule and perilobular parenchyma, which has been proposed to impair regional and local blood flow, thereby producing pain through ischemia and consequent tissue acidosis.[29] Parenchymal fibrosis has also been likened to a "compartment syndrome" of sorts, associated with impaired venous drainage.[30] Chronic inflammation associated with chronic pancreatitis may also induce visceral hyperalgesia through neural remodeling of local, spinal, or central nociceptive pathways.[31,32] Superimposed on this background of uncertainty regarding the cellular, organ, and systemic basis of pain is the confounding influence of narcotic addiction that afflicts many affected individuals.

DIAGNOSIS OF CHRONIC PANCREATITIS

The diagnosis of chronic pancreatitis is based on the combination of history and physical examination, blood tests, functional tests, and radiographic studies. The clinician should elicit a clear description of the pain, the recurrent nature of the episodes, and the presence of risk factors for the disease, including alcohol consumption and family history. Because the natural history of pain is highly variable and 20% of patients have painless chronic pancreatitis, it is not unusual that the diagnosis may be delayed. On physical examination, there may be evidence of malnutrition such as temporal wasting and decreased stores of subcutaneous fat. During acute episodes of inflammation, patients may sit upright and lean forward and present with epigastric tenderness. Abdominal fullness may suggest the presence of a pancreatic pseudocyst.

There are no perfect tests for chronic pancreatitis, particularly in its earliest stages. Serum amylase and lipase, as well as fasting serum glucose and glycosylated hemoglobin (HbA1c) may be helpful. Serum amylase and lipase levels may be elevated during an acute exacerbation of chronic pancreatitis, but with disease progression and pancreatic parenchymal fibrosis, these levels may remain normal even during an episode of acute inflammation. Blood glucose may be elevated in patients with advanced disease as endocrine function deteriorates. Stool samples can be examined for levels of fat. Stool is collected for a 72-hour period and fat content greater than 7 g per day is abnormal. Pancreatic exocrine function can also be assessed by analysis of duodenal bicarbonate concentration before and after stimulation with secretin during an upper endoscopy procedure[33] or by measurement of fecal elastase. However, fecal elastase levels may be insensitive in mild to moderate chronic pancreatitis. For patients with autoimmune pancreatitis, serum IgG4 protein levels, antinuclear antibodies, rheumatoid factor, and erythrocyte sedimentation rate (ESR) may help establish the diagnosis.[34]

Plain radiographs may demonstrate calcifications suggesting the diagnosis of chronic pancreatitis, but are otherwise not helpful and not routinely recommended. Similarly, transabdominal US is usually limited by patient body habitus and is operator dependent. Other imaging studies are more useful in chronic pancreatitis. The modality most often used is intravenous contrast-enhanced CT, which is effective in demonstrating late changes of the disease including ductal and parenchymal calcifications, ductal dilation and stricture, and parenchymal atrophy, as well as complications such as pseudocysts, vessel thrombosis, and pseudoaneurysms. A triphasic, thin-cut scan protocol is particularly helpful. ERCP and magnetic resonance cholangiopancreatography (MRCP) can complement CT imaging by better visualizing the pancreatic ductal system. Before the widespread use of magnetic resonance imaging, ERCP was the gold standard approach study to confirm early chronic pancreatitis in which CT findings were nondiagnostic. ECRP sensitivity and specificity for the diagnosis of chronic pancreatitis has been reported to be 70% to 90%, and 90% to 100%, respectively. Currently, ERCP is not routinely performed purely for diagnostic purposes because it is invasive and can induce acute pancreatitis; its use is largely restricted to situations where endoscopic therapy is contemplated, such as for stone removal. MRCP is noninvasive and avoids the use of nonionizing radiation and contrast media. MRCP with intravenous secretin administration may augment visualization of pancreatic side ducts and provide qualitative and semiquantitative information regarding the exocrine capacity of the pancreas, but it is limited in detecting calcifications. A few studies have demonstrated that endoscopic ultrasound (EUS) may detect early changes/features characteristic of chronic pancreatitis such as ductal wall echogenicity, focal echogenicity, and increased duct branches before changes are seen with CT scan, MRCP, and ERCP.[35] However, the criteria used to make the diagnosis of chronic pancreatitis with endoscopic US are controversial and some of these findings can be identified in individuals without clinical symptoms or known pancreatic disease. Risk factors for nonspecific changes in the pancreas include male gender, older age, increased body mass index, and history of smoking and alcohol consumption.

TREATMENT OPTIONS FOR CHRONIC PANCREATITIS

For patients with chronic pancreatitis, treatment usually begins with lifestyle changes. Patients should cease alcohol intake. Continuous exposure to alcohol may precipitate recurrent episodes of pancreatitis and exacerbate pain. Patients should stop smoking. Patients with pain may need to change their diet and eating patterns. Patients may need to eat six small low-fat meals during the day and increase fluid intake. Oral pancreatic enzyme supplementation with meals may help both with malabsorption and with pain associated with exocrine insufficiency. Scheduled dosing of uncoated enzyme preparations (rather than the more widely available coated preparations) may also reduce pain in chronic

TABLE 89-3 Pain Management Strategy Reflects Presumed Mechanism

Diagnosis	Proposed Treatment
Local inflammation	Pharmacotherapy (pancreatic enzymes, analgesics, narcotics)
Ductal hypertension	Decompression (Puestow, endoscopic stenting)
Organ hypertension	Resection (Whipple, Frey procedures)
Retroperitoneal damage	Neuroablation (celiac block, splanchnicectomy)
Altered nociception	Psychosocial intervention (counseling, detoxification)

pancreatitis according to several small randomized trials, although the efficacy of this approach is controversial. Patients developing type 1 diabetes may require insulin replacement.

One of the greatest challenges in treating patients with chronic pancreatitis is pain control. Patients with persistent pain despite diet modification may require fasting for several days with intravenous fluids, enteral feedings via nasojejunal feeding tubes, or parenteral nutrition via central catheter. A few limited studies suggest that antioxidants, octreotide, and antidepressants may help relieve pain and reduce the risk of exacerbation.[36] Nonsteroidal antiinflammatory drugs, such as ibuprofen, may be used early in the course of the disease. However, a regimen of a combination of long-acting and short-acting narcotics may be needed for refractory pain. For patients who are not candidates for endoscopic or surgical options, a celiac plexus nerve block may be performed percutaneously or endoscopically. The block relieves pain in about half of the patients who undergo the procedures; pain relief typically lasts for 2 months. However, for durable pain relief, patients may require additional treatment 2 to 6 months after the first treatment; however, these are usually ineffective. A variety of agents have been used for the nerve block, including neurolytic agents (alcohol), antiinflammatory agents (steroids), and anesthetics. Alternatively, thoracoscopic denervation of splanchnic nerves has been reported to achieve short-term pain relief. Implantable pumps for intrathecal infusion of narcotics have also been reported (Table 89-3).[37]

ENDOSCOPIC MANAGEMENT

Pancreatic endoscopic therapy may be used for patients with pain and radiographic evidence of duct obstruction by calcified stones.[38] Pancreatic sphincterotomy permits the introduction of endoscopic equipment in order to dilate pancreatic duct strictures either by balloon dilation or coiled wire stent removal device. Endoscopic polyethylene stents, ranging in size from 5.0 to 11.5 French, can be placed across areas of stricture to maintain ductal patency. Opening of strictures allows for the unobstructed flow of pancreatic juice to improve both pain and nutrient absorption. Unfortunately, the patency of the stents is relatively short-lived, usually 2 to 4 months. Stents can occlude from the calcific debris and

TABLE 89-4 Surgical Treatments for Chronic Pancreatitis

Resection	Decompression	Hybrid
Pancreaticoduodenectomy (Kausch-Whipple procedure)	Duval procedure	Frey procedure
Pylorus-preserving pancreaticoduodenectomy (Traverso-Longmire)	Puestow-Gillesby procedure	Hamburg modification
Beger procedure	Partington-Rochelle procedure (Puestow)	Berne modification
Near total or total pancreatectomy	Izbicki procedure	

TABLE 89-5 Surgical Treatment Options Based on Pancreas Morphology

	Dilated Pancreatic Duct	Small or Nondilated Duct
No focal mass	1. Decompressive: Partington-Rochelle procedure (Puestow) 2. Hybrid procedure: Frey	1. Observation 2. Resection: pancreaticoduodenectomy, total pancreatectomy 3. Decompressive: Izbicki procedure
Focal mass	1. Resection: pancreaticoduodenectomy, Beger procedure 2. Hybrid procedure: Frey	1. Resection: pancreaticoduodenectomy, Beger procedure

proteinaceous material, or migrate within the pancreatic duct. Stent occlusion and migration can exacerbate pain and lead to suppurative infection. Long-term stenting can paradoxically worsen periductal inflammation, fibrosis, and stricturing. Ductal stents are routinely removed after a period of time (2 to 4 months) and if the pain is improved, patients are observed and given pancreatic enzyme supplementation.

Stones may form within the pancreatic duct, in the duct wall, or in the pancreatic parenchyma, frequently in the segment of the duct proximal to a stricture, exacerbating ductal obstruction and inflammation. Intraductal stones can be removed with Dormia-type baskets. Stones larger than the pancreatic duct orifice can be broken into smaller pieces by mechanical lithotripsy. Extracorporeal shock wave lithotripsy (ESWL) can help remove stones not accessible by basket or mechanical lithotripsy. Endoscopic therapy can also be used to treat biliary strictures associated with chronic pancreatitis. Duodenal obstruction can be relieved in nonoperative candidates by endoscopic placement of expandable coated metallic stents. In addition, symptomatic pseudocysts can be drained transgastrically or transduodenally in appropriately selected patients to achieve relief of pain.

SURGICAL MANAGEMENT

Surgical management is generally reserved for otherwise unmanageable symptomatic chronic pancreatitis. Most patients are managed initially by nonoperative medical therapy. Current indications for surgery include intractable abdominal pain, secondary complications of chronic pancreatitis including biliary stricture, duodenal stenosis, pseudocyst, and suspected pancreatic neoplasm. The goals of surgical management are to relieve pain and address complications such as biliary or duodenal obstruction, while preserving as much as possible exocrine and endocrine function. The specific choice of surgical procedure is usually determined by anatomic findings, although there may be several reasonable alternatives in any given scenario (Tables 89-4 and 89-5). Useful features in considering surgical options are the presence of so-called large duct versus small duct disease as well as the presence and location of an inflammatory mass.

In many patients, inflammation and parenchymal abnormalities appear most prominently within the head of the pancreas. Longmire et al proposed that the head of the organ was also the prime source of pain in chronic pancreatitis.[39] In view of this notion, and because the three major ductal systems of Wirsung, Santorini, and the uncinate course through the head of the pancreas, it is often said that the head of the pancreas is the "pacemaker" of the disease. Patients may less commonly present with isolated inflammation in the tail of the pancreas, or with only ductal dilation and stricture without focal fibrosis or dominant inflammatory mass.

RESECTION

For patients with focal disease largely confined to the head of the pancreas without duct dilation, a Whipple procedure (pancreaticoduodenectomy [PD]) is generally the preferred option (Figure 89-4).[40] The procedure involves the resection of the head of the pancreas with the distal common bile duct, distal stomach, duodenum, and proximal jejunum. Removal of the head of the pancreas also addresses bile duct stricture and duodenal obstruction, if present, and improves drainage of the upstream proximal (main) pancreatic duct and its tributaries. The reconstruction after resection of the Whipple specimen includes a two-layered end-to-side pancreaticojejunostomy (Figure 89-5), an end-to-side hepaticojejunostomy, and a gastrojejunostomy. Pain relief, either complete or partial, is usually achieved in approximately

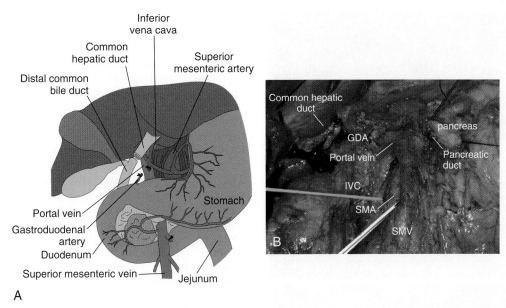

FIGURE 89-4 A, Pancreaticoduodenectomy (Classic Whipple procedure). The procedure involves the resection of the head of the pancreas with the distal common bile duct, distal stomach, duodenum, and proximal jejunum. **B,** The features of the retroperitoneum after the Whipple specimen has been removed. (Reprinted with permission from Ahmad SA, Wray CJ, Rilo HR, et al: Chronic pancreatitis: Recent advances and ongoing challenges. *Curr Probl Surg* 43:184, 2006.)

85% of patients. Following PD, new-onset diabetes is uncommon in patients with otherwise normal glucose tolerance preoperatively, although up to 50% of patients will develop diabetes during the subsequent 10 years.[41] Postoperative exocrine insufficiency requiring enzyme supplementation develops in nearly half of patients. Mortality associated with the procedure is generally less than 5% and near zero in experienced centers, although the overall rate of postoperative complications is relatively high, typically reported between 30% and 40%. Traverso and Longmire introduced a pylorus-preserving pancreaticoduodenectomy (PPPD), an operation that was intended to improve functional digestive outcomes and quality of life by preserving the physiologic gastric emptying mechanism.[42] Long-term followup studies show no meaningful differences in functional outcome or maintenance of weight, and PPPD may in fact be associated with a slightly higher incidence of early postoperative delayed gastric emptying than classic PD.

Beger introduced duodenum-preserving pancreatic head resection (DPPHR) as an alternative to PD or PPPD.[43] The procedure includes division of the neck of pancreas overlying the confluence of the splenic and superior mesenteric veins and removal of the head of the pancreas, leaving a small rim of pancreatic tissue along the duodenum. The procedure is completed with end-to-end and side-to-side Roux-en-Y pancreaticojejunostomy (Figure 89-6). DPPHR maintains gastrointestinal and biliary continuity, and achieves similar pain relief[43-45] and improvement in quality of life[46] as PD. Key steps in the procedure include identification and preservation of the posterior branch of the gastroduodenal artery and the intrapancreatic portion of the common bile duct. Gloor et al described a modification of the DPPHR, known as the Berne procedure, that involves excavation of the central portion of the head without formal division of the neck.[47]

DECOMPRESSION

For patients with large duct disease and no focal inflammatory mass, duct-enteric drainage is the preferred treatment. In 1954, Duval described drainage of the tail of the pancreas with a Roux-en-Y limb of jejunum as a procedure for chronic pancreatitis. This operation often failed because it did not address disease in the proximal pancreas. Puestow and Gillesby introduced a modified procedure to drain the entire pancreatic duct along the body and tail of the pancreas laterally into a Roux-en-Y limb of jejunum, which was initially described in conjunction with splenectomy and the distal pancreatectomy.[48] Partington and Rochelle simplified the Puestow technique by eliminating splenectomy and pancreatic resection.[49] The Puestow procedure or the lateral pancreaticojejunostomy involves a retrocolic side-to-side Roux-en-Y pancreaticojejunostomy (Figure 89-7). Typically, patients with large duct disease experience relief of pain in more than 80% of cases, although in long-term studies the durability of relief has been questioned.

HYBRID PROCEDURES

Some patients present with not only large duct disease but also significant inflammatory disease within the head of the pancreas, and Puestow-type lateral pancreaticojejunostomy may be insufficient to address potential sources of pain within the pancreatic head. Frey introduced a procedure that combines duodenum-sparing resection of the pancreatic head, without formal division of the neck of the pancreas, combined with longitudinal pancreaticojejunostomy of the dorsal duct.[50] The Frey procedure appears to be an acceptable surgical alternative to achieve durable long-term pain relief and decrease opiate dependence in selected patients. In the experience of a number of series, 75% or greater success in relief of pain and gain of weight was seen after the Frey

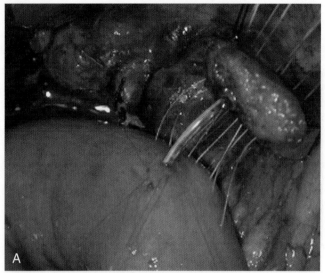

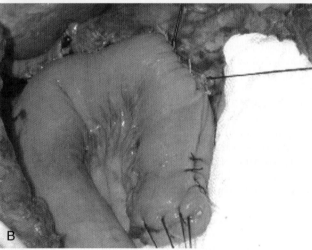

FIGURE 89-5 A, The reconstruction after resection of Whipple specimen involves a two-layered end-to-side pancreaticojejunostomy using a 5 French pediatric feeding as a pancreatic duct stent. **B,** The completed pancreaticojejunostomy anastomosis. (Reprinted with permission from Ahmad SA, Wray CJ, Rilo HR, et al: Chronic pancreatitis: Recent advances and ongoing challenges. *Curr Probl Surg* 43:185, 2006.)

procedure.[51,52] For patients with an inflammatory head mass but small duct disease, Izbicki introduced a procedure that combines excavation of the pancreatic head with a V-shaped longitudinal wedge resection, followed by lateral decompressive pancreaticojejunostomy of the pancreatic body and tail.[53] Complete pain relief was reported in 92% of the patients, and improvements were seen in physical status, working ability, and emotional and social functioning to varying degrees, with postoperative morbidity and mortality similar to other procedures for chronic pancreatitis.

TOTAL PANCREATECTOMY WITH ISLET AUTOTRANSPLANTATION

Patients with small duct disease and diffuse parenchymal inflammation or minimal change disease, hereditary syndromes, and failures of prior pancreatic operations present a particular challenge for treatment. These patients may have no discrete lesions that can be addressed by conventional endoscopic or surgical therapy. Options include near total or total pancreatectomy for end-stage or refractory disease. The initial attempts at total pancreatectomy were complicated by high postoperative complication rates, most notoriously poor long-term glycemic control, and severe exocrine insufficiency.[54] The introduction of long-acting insulin and more effective pancreatic enzyme replacement, as well as advances in islet isolation and preservation, has renewed interest in total pancreatectomy with islet autotransplantation. The first total pancreatectomy with islet cell autotransplantation was performed in 1977. A number of centers have now reported results with this procedure[55-57] in selected patient populations and typically report complete or near complete pain relief in about 75% of patients, with 60% to 70% achieving narcotic independence. Although a significant minority of patients (40%) is initially insulin-independent after islet autotransplantation, there is a steady drop-off of transplanted islet function over time. However, insulin requirements tend to be small and, overall, postoperative diabetes after islet autotransplantation appears to be facilitated and less vulnerable to wide swings in serum glucose, particularly severe hypoglycemia. The indications and timing for total pancreatectomy with islet autotransplantation is controversial, but potential candidates include those who have failed prior operation, patients with small duct disease without conventional surgical alternatives, and patients with hereditary pancreatitis syndromes.

RESULTS OF SURGICAL AND ENDOSCOPIC PROCEDURES

Interventional therapy should be considered in selected patients who are otherwise refractory to risk modification (cessation of alcohol and tobacco), dietary modification, and analgesics pain medication, diet modification, and endoscopic treatment. Surgical and endoscopic treatments carry significant risk of morbidity, and it is not unusual for patients to experience reductions in the pattern of pain relief as the disease progresses ("burnout") without invasive therapy. Ammann et al prospectively followed 245 patients with chronic pancreatitis. Of the patients with alcoholic relapsing pancreatitis, 53% did not require surgery and the number of patients who reported durable pain relief were similar in the operated and nonoperated group of patients.[58] However, numerous retrospective studies suggest that patients who are managed surgically may ultimately require fewer interventions and hospitalizations with an overall better quality of life.[59]

Despite the tendency to consider endoscopic intervention as "less invasive," there have now been two prospective randomized trials comparing surgery versus endoscopy that indicate a clear superiority of surgical intervention. Dite et al randomized 72 patients to surgery (resection or drainage) or endoscopic therapy including sphincterotomy, stent placement, and/or stone removal. Surgery provided better long-term pain relief and increase in weight gain.[60] A second study randomized 39 patients with distal obstruction of the pancreatic duct without inflammatory to pancreaticojejunostomy or

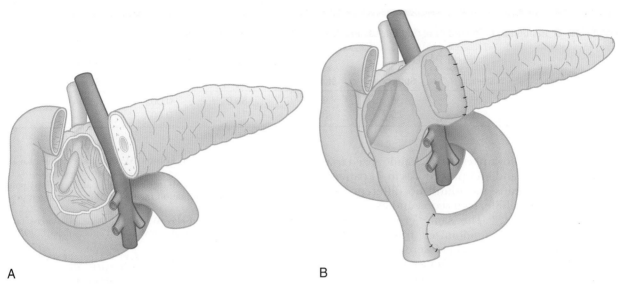

A   B

FIGURE 89-6 The duodenum-preserving pancreatic head resection (DPPHR) introduced by Beger. **A,** Procedure includes division of the neck of the pancreas, leaving a small rim of pancreatic tissues along the duodenum. **B,** The procedure is completed with end-to-end and side-to side Roux-en-Y pancreaticojejunostomy. (Reprinted with permission from Beger HG, Buechler M: Duodenum-preserving resection of the head of the pancreas in chronic pancreatitis with inflammatory mass in the head. *World J Surg* 14:83, 1990; and Beger HG, Krauztberger W, Bittner R, et al: Duodenum-preserving resection of the head of the pancreas in patients with severe pancreatitis. *Surgery* 97:467, 1985.)

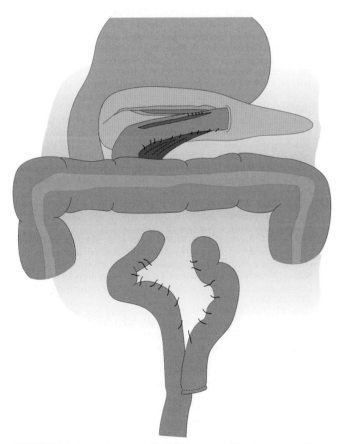

FIGURE 89-7 Lateral pancreaticojejunostomy (Puestow procedure). An illustration of a retrocolic side-to-side Roux-en-Y pancreaticojejunostomy.

endoscopic duct drainage. After a median followup of 24 months, surgical patients had lower pain scores, better physical health summary scores, and durable relief of pain (75% to 32%). Patients randomized to endoscopic therapy required more repeat treatments (Table 89-6).[61] Surgery for patients with large duct or focal inflammation may be appropriate earlier in the evolution of the disease. The optimal treatment of symptomatic patients with small duct disease and mild to moderate pain remains controversial.

Significant long-term pain relief along with weight gain and decreased narcotic dependence are achieved in a majority of patients who undergo operative therapy.[42] The postoperative mortality rate is usually reported to be below 3% and complication rates are typically 10% to 40%. However, the optimal choice of specific surgical alternatives in various settings is less clear. There have been some randomized comparison trials. In general, PD and PPPD are associated with higher complication rates than DPPHR and drainage procedures. However, there are no significant differences in pain relief and control of complications to adjacent organs.

Izbicki et al reported a randomized control trial comparing extended drainage with PPPD. The latter procedure had a higher rate of complication (53.3% vs. 19.4%), and the drainage procedure provided a better quality of life. Both procedures were equally effective in terms of pain relief and resolution of complications to adjacent organs.[62] Koninger et al presented results of a randomized study comparing the original Beger procedure with the Berne modification. Sixty-five patients were randomized and followed for 24 months. Operative time and median hospital stay were shorter in patients who underwent the Berne modification. Quality of life was similar in both groups 2 years after the surgery.[63] Strate et al

TABLE 89-6 Randomized Trials Comparing Endoscopic Stenting to Surgical Management

Author	Year	NO. OF PATIENTS		% WITH DURABLE RELIEF			MEAN NO. OF PROCEDURES	
		Stenting	Surgery	Stenting	Surgery	P-value	Stenting	Surgery
Dite[60]	2003	36	36	61.4	85.9	0.002	NA	NA
Cahen[61]	2007	19	20	32	75	0.007	8	3

reported long-term followup results of a randomized trial comparing the Beger and Frey procedures in 74 patients with chronic pancreatitis and found no differences in late mortality, quality of life, pain score, and exocrine or endocrine insufficiency.[64] The same group reported long-term followup of a randomized trial comparing PPPD and the Frey procedure. There were no differences in quality of life and pain control after a median followup of 7 years. Müller et al reported long-term followup of a randomized trial comparing the Beger procedure with PPPD.[65] The results demonstrate that both procedures were similar in pain control and exocrine and endocrine pancreatic function. In many instances, surgeon preference based on individual experience and training will determine the choice of operation.

CONCLUSIONS

Chronic pancreatitis results in the progressive and irreversible destruction and replacement of the normal pancreatic parenchyma with fibrosis, ultimately leading to exocrine and, later, endocrine insufficiency. There is no simple unifying mechanism of pathogenesis. Rather, it is the interaction among risk factors including environmental exposure, genetic factors, and anatomic anomalies that appears to predispose to the development of chronic pancreatitis. Recognition of chronic pancreatitis in its earliest stages continues to pose a challenge despite improvements in diagnostic testing and imaging. Treatment decisions should be guided by patient presentation but are hampered by the lack of consensus guidelines and by clinician bias. Therapeutic options include risk modification, analgesic therapy, diet, endoscopic therapy, and surgical therapy. Patients may be best treated in high-volume centers with radiologic, endoscopic, and surgical expertise, as well as an ancillary system of social workers, dietitians, and psychologists.

REFERENCES

1. Masamune A, Watanabe T, Kikuta K, et al: Roles of pancreatic stellate cells in pancreatic inflammation and fibrosis. *Clin Gastroenterol Hepatol* 7:S48, 2009.
2. Singer MV, Gyr K, Sarles H: Revised classification of pancreatitis. Report of the Second International Symposium on the Classification of Pancreatitis in Marseille, France, March 28-30, 1984. *Gastroenterology* 89:683, 1985.
3. Banks PA, Bradley EL 3rd, Dreiling DA, et al: Classification of pancreatitis—Cambridge and Marseille. *Gastroenterology* 89:928, 1985.
4. Sarles H, Adler G, Dani R, et al: Classifications of pancreatitis and definition of pancreatic diseases. *Digestion* 43:234, 1989.
5. Sarner M, Cotton PB: Classification of pancreatitis. *Gut* 25:756, 1984.
6. Homma T, Harada H, Koizumi M: Diagnostic criteria for chronic pancreatitis by the Japan Pancreas Society. *Pancreas* 15:14, 1997.
7. Whitcomb DC, Gorry MC, Preston RA, et al: Hereditary pancreatitis is caused by a mutation in the cationic trypsinogen gene. *Nat Genet* 14:141, 1996.
8. Irving HM, Samokhvalov AV, Rehm J: Alcohol as a risk factor for pancreatitis. A systematic review and meta-analysis. *JOP* 10:387, 2009.
9. Lin Y, Tamakoshi A, Hayakawa T, et al: Cigarette smoking as a risk factor for chronic pancreatitis: A case-control study in Japan. Research Committee on Intractable Pancreatic Diseases. *Pancreas* 21:109, 2000.
10. Song Z, Bhagat G, Quante M, et al: Potential carcinogenic effects of cigarette smoke and Swedish moist snuff on pancreas: A study using a transgenic mouse model of chronic pancreatitis. *Lab Invest* 90:426, 2010.
11. Whitcomb DC, Yadav D, Adam S, et al: Multicenter approach to recurrent acute and chronic pancreatitis in the United States: The North American Pancreatitis Study 2 (NAPS2). *Pancreatology* 8:520, 2008.
12. Teich N, Ockenga J, Hoffmeister A, et al: Chronic pancreatitis associated with an activation peptide mutation that facilitates trypsin activation. *Gastroenterology* 119:461, 2000.
13. Gorry MC, Gabbaizedeh D, Furey W, et al: Mutations in the cationic trypsinogen gene are associated with recurrent acute and chronic pancreatitis. *Gastroenterology* 113:1063, 1997.
14. Witt H, Luck W, Becker M: A signal peptide cleavage site mutation in the cationic trypsinogen gene is strongly associated with chronic pancreatitis. *Gastroenterology* 117:7, 1999.
15. Nishimori I, Kamakura M, Fujikawa-Adachi K, et al: Mutations in exons 2 and 3 of the cationic trypsinogen gene in Japanese families with hereditary pancreatitis. *Gut* 44:259, 1999.
16. Felderbauer P, Stricker I, Schnekenburger J, et al: Histopathological features of patients with chronic pancreatitis due to mutations in the PRSS1 gene: Evaluation of BRAF and KRAS2 mutations. *Digestion* 78:60, 2008.
17. Witt H, Luck W, Hennies HC, et al: Mutations in the gene encoding the serine protease inhibitor, Kazal type 1 are associated with chronic pancreatitis. *Nat Genet* 25:213, 2000.
18. Pfützer RH, Barmada MM, Brunskill AP, et al: SPINK1/PSTI polymorphisms act as disease modifiers in familial and idiopathic chronic pancreatitis. *Gastroenterology* 119:615, 2000.
19. Sharer N, Schwarz M, Malone G, et al: Mutations of the cystic fibrosis gene in patients with chronic pancreatitis. *N Engl J Med* 339:645, 1998.
20. Weiss FU, Sahin-Toth M: Variations in trypsinogen expression may influence the protective effect of the p.G191R PRSS2 variant in chronic pancreatitis. *Gut* 58:749, 2009.
21. Finkelberg DL, Sahani D, Deshpande V, et al: Autoimmune pancreatitis. *N Engl J Med* 355:2670, 2006.
22. Frulloni L, Lunardi C, Simone R, et al: Identification of a novel antibody associated with autoimmune pancreatitis. *N Engl J Med* 361:2135, 2009.
23. Lankisch PG, Löhr-Happe A, Otto J, et al: Natural course in chronic pancreatitis. Pain, exocrine and endocrine pancreatic insufficiency and prognosis of the disease. *Digestion* 54:148, 1993.
24. Vijungco JD, Prinz RA: Management of biliary and duodenal complications of chronic pancreatitis. *World J Surg* 27:1258, 2003.
25. Heider TR, Azeem S, Galanko JA, et al: The natural history of pancreatitis-induced splenic vein thrombosis. *Ann Surg* 239:876, discussion 880, 2004.
26. Agarwal AK, Raj Kumar K, Agarwal S, et al: Significance of splenic vein thrombosis in chronic pancreatitis. *Am J Surg* 196:149, 2008.

27. Lowenfels AB, Maisonneuve P, Cavallini G, et al: Pancreatitis and the risk of pancreatic cancer. International Pancreatitis Study Group. *N Engl J Med* 328:1433, 1993.
28. Guerra C, Schuhmacher AJ, Cañamero M, et al: Chronic pancreatitis is essential for induction of pancreatic ductal adenocarcinoma by K-Ras oncogenes in adult mice. *Cancer Cell* 11:291, 2007.
29. Patel AG, Reber PU, Toyama MT, et al: Effect of pancreaticojejunostomy on fibrosis, pancreatic blood flow, and interstitial pH in chronic pancreatitis: A feline model. *Ann Surg* 230:672, 1999.
30. Ebbehoj N, Svendsen LB, Madsen P: Pancreatic tissue pressure: Techniques and pathophysiological aspects. *Scand J Gastroenterol* 19:1066, 1984.
31. Ceyhan GO, Demir IE, Rauch U, et al: Pancreatic neuropathy results in "neural remodeling" and altered pancreatic innervation in chronic pancreatitis and pancreatic cancer. *Am J Gastroenterol* 104:2555, 2009.
32. Bockman DE, Buchler M, Malfertheiner P, et al: Analysis of nerves in chronic pancreatitis. *Gastroenterology* 94:1459, 1988.
33. Laugier R: Dynamic endoscopic manometry of the response to secretin in patients with chronic pancreatitis. *Endoscopy* 26:222, 1994.
34. Okazaki K, Uchida K, Ohana M, et al: Autoimmune-related pancreatitis is associated with autoantibodies and a Th1/Th2-type cellular immune response. *Gastroenterology* 118:573, 2000.
35. Wiersema MJ, Hawes RH, Lehman GA, et al: Prospective evaluation of endoscopic ultrasonography and endoscopic retrograde cholangiopancreatography in patients with chronic abdominal pain of suspected pancreatic origin. *Endoscopy* 25:555, 1993.
36. Bhardwaj P, Garg PK, Maulik SK, et al: A randomized controlled trial of antioxidant supplementation for pain relief in patients with chronic pancreatitis. *Gastroenterology* 136:149 e2, 2009.
37. Kongkam P, Wagner DL, Sherman S, et al: Intrathecal narcotic infusion pumps for intractable pain of chronic pancreatitis: A pilot series. *Am J Gastroenterol* 104:1249, 2009.
38. Rösch T, Daniel S, Scholz M, et al: European Society of Gastrointestinal Endoscopy Research Group. Endoscopic treatment of chronic pancreatitis: A multicenter study of 1000 patients with long-term follow-up. *Endoscopy* 34:765, 2002.
39. Briggs JD, Jordan PH Jr, Longmire WP Jr: Experience with resection of the pancreas in the treatment of chronic relapsing pancreatitis. *Ann Surg* 144:681, 1956.
40. Whipple AO: Radical surgery for certain cases of pancreatic fibrosis associated with calcareous deposits. *Ann Surg* 124:991, 1946.
41. Sakorafas GH, Farnell MB, Nagorney DM, et al: Pancreatoduodenectomy for chronic pancreatitis: Long-term results in 105 patients. *Arch Surg* 135:517, discussion 523, 2000.
42. Traverso LW, Tompkins RK, Urrea PT, et al: Surgical treatment of chronic pancreatitis. Twenty-two years' experience. *Ann Surg* 190:312, 1979.
43. Beger HG, Schlosser W, Friess HM, et al: Duodenum-preserving head resection in chronic pancreatitis changes the natural course of the disease: A single-center 26-year experience. *Ann Surg* 230:512, discussion 519, 1999.
44. Izbicki JR, Bloechle C, Knoefel WT, et al: Complications of adjacent organs in chronic pancreatitis managed by duodenum-preserving resection of the head of the pancreas. *Br J Surg* 81:1351, 1994.
45. Prinz RA, Kaufman BH, Folk FA, et al: Pancreaticojejunostomy for chronic pancreatitis. Two- to 21-year follow-up. *Arch Surg* 113:520, 1978.
46. Bloechle C, Izbicki JR, Knoefel WT, et al: Quality of life in chronic pancreatitis—results after duodenum-preserving resection of the head of the pancreas. *Pancreas* 11:77, 1995.
47. Gloor B, Friess H, Uhl W, et al: A modified technique of the Beger and Frey procedure in patients with chronic pancreatitis. *Dig Surg* 18:21, 2001.
48. Puestow CB, Gillesby WJ: Retrograde surgical drainage of pancreas for chronic relapsing pancreatitis. *AMA Arch Surg* 76:898, 1958.
49. Partington PF, Rochelle RE: Modified Puestow procedure for retrograde drainage of the pancreatic duct. *Ann Surg* 152:1037, 1960.
50. Frey CF, Smith GJ: Description and rationale of a new operation for chronic pancreatitis. *Pancreas* 2:701, 1987.
51. Frey CF, Amikura K: Local resection of the head of the pancreas combined with longitudinal pancreaticojejunostomy in the management of patients with chronic pancreatitis. *Ann Surg* 220:492, discussion 504, 1994.
52. Negi S, Singh A, Chaudhary A: Pain relief after Frey's procedure for chronic pancreatitis. *Br J Surg* 97:1087, 2010.
53. Izbicki JR, Bloechle C, Broering DC, et al: Longitudinal V-shaped excision of the ventral pancreas for small duct disease in severe chronic pancreatitis: Prospective evaluation of a new surgical procedure. *Ann Surg* 227:213, 1998.
54. Braasch JW, Vito L, Nugent FW: Total pancreatectomy of end-stage chronic pancreatitis. *Ann Surg* 188:317, 1978.
55. Sutton JM, Schmulewitz N, Sussman JJ, et al: Total pancreatectomy and islet cell autotransplantation as a means of treating patients with genetically linked pancreatitis. *Surgery* 148:676, discussion 685, 2010.
56. Garcea G, Weaver J, Phillips J, et al: Total pancreatectomy with and without islet cell transplantation for chronic pancreatitis: A series of 85 consecutive patients. *Pancreas* 38:1, 2009.
57. Ahmad SA, Lowy AM, Wray CJ, et al: Factors associated with insulin and narcotic independence after islet autotransplantation in patients with severe chronic pancreatitis. *J Am Coll Surg* 201:680, 2005.
58. Ammann RW, Akovbiantz A, Largiader F, et al: Course and outcome of chronic pancreatitis. Longitudinal study of a mixed medical-surgical series of 245 patients. *Gastroenterology* 86:820, 1984.
59. Rutter K, Ferlitsch A, Sautner T, et al: Hospitalization, frequency of interventions, and quality of life after endoscopic, surgical, or conservative treatment in patients with chronic pancreatitis. *World J Surg* 34:2642, 2010.
60. Díte P, Ruzicka M, Zboril V, et al: A prospective, randomized trial comparing endoscopic and surgical therapy for chronic pancreatitis. *Endoscopy* 35:553, 2003.
61. Cahen DL, Gouma DJ, Nio Y, et al: Endoscopic versus surgical drainage of the pancreatic duct in chronic pancreatitis. *N Engl J Med* 356:676, 2007.
62. Izbicki JR, Bloechle C, Broering DC, et al: Extended drainage versus resection in surgery for chronic pancreatitis: A prospective randomized trial comparing the longitudinal pancreaticojejunostomy combined with local pancreatic head excision with the pylorus-preserving pancreatoduodenectomy. *Ann Surg* 228:771, 1998.
63. Köninger J, Friess H, Müller M, et al: Duodenum-preserving pancreatic head resection—a randomized controlled trial comparing the original Beger procedure with the Berne modification (ISRCTN No. 50638764). *Surgery* 143:490, 2008.
64. Strate T, Taherpour Z, Bloechle C, et al: Long-term follow-up of a randomized trial comparing the Beger and frey procedures for patients suffering from chronic pancreatitis. *Ann Surg* 241:591, 2005.
65. Müller MW, Friess H, Martin DJ, et al: Long-term follow-up of a randomized clinical trial comparing Beger with pylorus-preserving Whipple procedure for chronic pancreatitis. *Br J Surg* 95:350, 2008.

Pseudocysts and Other Complications of Pancreatitis

Ernest L. Rosato | Christopher J. Sonnenday | Keith D. Lillemoe |

Charles J. Yeo

Complications following acute pancreatitis and the associated profound inflammatory response include: pseudocyst formation, acute fluid collections, pancreatic abscess and infected necrosis, pancreatic ascites, pancreatic-pleural effusion, as well as pancreaticoenteric and pancreatic-cutaneous fistulas. Many of these complications are the result of damage to, and alterations in, the normal pancreatic duct anatomy. Modern imaging techniques have facilitated earlier diagnosis of these complications and help to select patients who may benefit from less invasive treatment modalities, which include endoscopic and percutaneous duct stenting and drainage. Surgery remains an important tool in the treatment algorithm for pseudocysts and other complications of pancreatitis. Minimally invasive surgical techniques have been adapted to treat pancreatitis-related complications and offer the advantages of open surgery without the morbidity of extensive incisions and the associated systemic inflammatory response.

PANCREATIC PSEUDOCYSTS

A *pancreatic pseudocyst* is a localized collection of pancreatic secretions surrounded by a wall of fibrous or granulation tissue that arises as a result of acute or chronic pancreatitis, pancreatic trauma, or obstruction of the pancreatic duct by a neoplasm (Figures 90-1 and 90-2). Pseudocysts account for between 50% and 75% of cystic lesions of the pancreas. They are distinguished from other peripancreatic fluid collections (cystic neoplasms and congenital, parasitic, and extrapancreatic cysts) by their lack of an epithelial lining, a high concentration of pancreatic enzymes within the pseudocyst, and formation at least 4 weeks after an episode of pancreatitis or pancreatic trauma (Box 90-1). Pseudocysts are formed by the inflammatory response that occurs after extravasated pancreatic secretions are walled off by the surrounding structures. The capsule of the pseudocyst can be thin fibrous tissue, which can progressively thicken as the pseudocyst matures. Frequently, the liquid contents of the pseudocyst are gradually resorbed by the body, and the pseudocyst resolves, findings indicating that the communication between the pseudocyst and the pancreatic duct has closed. Persistence of a pseudocyst implies ongoing communication with the pancreatic ductal system, regardless of whether the ductal system can be demonstrated radiographically or pathologically.

TERMINOLOGY

Because pseudocysts may resemble other collections of fluid that can arise as a complication of acute pancreatitis, clear terminology is required to discriminate these different clinical entities. The International Symposium on Acute Pancreatitis, held in 1992 in Atlanta, established consensus definitions for pseudocyst, acute fluid collection, and pancreatic abscess.[1]

Acute fluid collections form early in the course of acute pancreatitis and lack a discrete wall of fibrous or granulation tissue (Figure 90-3). They are common in patients with severe pancreatitis and occur in 30% to 50% of cases.[2] The majority of these lesions regress spontaneously without specifically directed therapy or drainage. Most acute fluid collections do not represent a communication with the pancreatic duct. Instead, they are a serous or exudative reaction to pancreatic inflammation and trauma. Because they lack true communication with the pancreatic duct, acute fluid collections are also referred to as *pseudopseudocysts*. A fluid collection that persists for more than 4 weeks, that is usually surrounded by a well-defined wall, and that may communicate with the pancreatic ductal system is termed a *pancreatic pseudocyst*.

A *pancreatic abscess* is a circumscribed collection of purulent infected fluid that contains little or no necrotic material and arises as a complication of acute pancreatitis or trauma. A pancreatic abscess typically occurs late in the course of severe acute pancreatitis, often 4 or more weeks after the onset of symptoms. Patients have signs and symptoms of infection. The presence of a purulent exudate, a positive culture for bacteria or fungi, and little or no necrotic pancreatic material differentiate a pancreatic abscess from *infected pancreatic necrosis*, a catastrophic complication that often occurs earlier in the course of severe pancreatitis. This distinction is crucial because the mortality associated with infected pancreatic necrosis is double that of pancreatic abscess and the specific therapy for each condition is markedly different. A pancreatic abscess may be treated by percutaneous drainage in many cases, whereas infected pancreatic necrosis typically requires operative debridement.

ETIOLOGY

Pseudocysts have historically been thought to occur in 5% to 10% of patients with acute pancreatitis. As imaging techniques have improved, particularly computed tomography (CT), our knowledge of their prevalence and

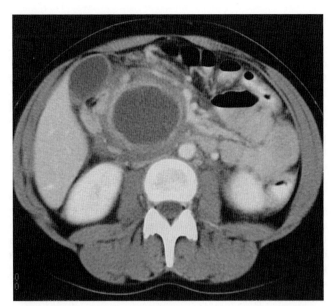

FIGURE 90-1 Computed tomographic scan of a patient with a pancreatic pseudocyst in the head of the pancreas. The patient had symptoms of abdominal pain and nausea. The gallbladder appears distended, although the results of liver function tests were normal.

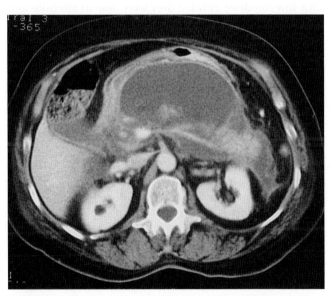

FIGURE 90-2 Computed tomographic scan of a patient with a large retrogastric pancreatic pseudocyst. The patient had symptoms of abdominal pain, back pain, nausea, and early satiety.

BOX 90-1 Cystic Lesions of the Pancreas and Peripancreatic Region

Pancreatic pseudocyst
Pancreatic pseudopseudocyst (acute fluid collection)
Pancreatic abscess
Cystic neoplasms of the pancreas
   Serous cystadenoma
   Mucinous cystadenoma/cystadenocarcinoma
   Cystic islet cell tumor
   Acinar cell cystadenocarcinoma
   Cystic choriocarcinoma
   Cystic teratoma
Parasitic cysts
   Echinococcal cyst
   Taenia solium cyst
Congenital cysts
   Simple cyst
Polycystic disease
   Isolated to the pancreas
   Associated with polycystic kidney disease
   Associated with von Hippel-Lindau disease
   Associated with cystic fibrosis
Extrapancreatic cysts
   Duplication cyst
   Mesenteric cyst
   Splenic cyst
   Adrenal cyst

Modified from Yeo CJ, Sarr MG: Cystic and pseudocystic diseases of the pancreas. *Curr Probl Surg* 31:165, 1994, with permission.

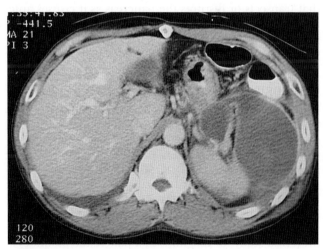

FIGURE 90-3 Computed tomographic scan of a patient with an acute fluid collection 10 days after an episode of acute alcoholic pancreatitis. The collection is located anterior to the spleen and appears to have a thin wall. The acute fluid collection was not causing symptoms and gradually resolved with observation.

---

natural history has improved. Pseudocysts are believed to occur in 10% to 20% of patients with acute pancreatitis and in 20% to 40% of patients with chronic pancreatitis.[3] Pseudocysts occur more commonly in males than in females, a finding that perhaps reflects the frequent occurrence of these lesions in patients with alcoholic pancreatitis. Forty-five percent to 50% of pseudocysts occur in or around the head of the pancreas, whereas the remainder are evenly distributed along the neck, body, and tail of the gland. Pseudocysts are most often

solitary round or ovoid collections, but 15% of patients may have multiple pseudocysts. As mentioned, alcohol appears to be the cause of 65% of pancreatitis-related pseudocysts, and gallstones are the origin of another 15% of cases.[4,5] Trauma causes 5% to 10% of pseudocysts, and other less common causes of pancreatitis account for the remainder of cases.

CLINICAL FEATURES

Abdominal pain, the most common symptom in patients with a pseudocyst, occurs in up to 90% of patients. Pseudocysts that follow an episode of acute pancreatitis are often characterized by persistence or recurrence of upper abdominal pain weeks after the initial attack. A pseudocyst may also be the source of increased or refractory pain in a patient known to have chronic pancreatitis. Other common symptoms include early satiety, nausea and vomiting (50% to 70%), weight loss (20% to 50%), jaundice (10%), and low-grade fever (10%).[6,7] Physical examination reveals upper abdominal tenderness in the majority of patients, and 25% to 45% will have a palpable abdominal mass. The symptoms of early satiety, nausea, and vomiting may be secondary to gastroduodenal obstruction caused by a mass effect of the pseudocyst. Rarely, patients with pseudocysts may not seek medical attention until a secondary complication occurs. Such complications include sepsis secondary to infection, hypovolemic shock secondary to pseudocyst-associated hemorrhage, jaundice secondary to common bile duct obstruction, and severe acute abdominal pain as a result of intraperitoneal rupture of a pseudocyst.

Patients with a pseudocyst secondary to trauma may have similar symptoms at a time remote from the trauma. Pancreatic trauma is uncommon, but it may occur after blunt or penetrating injury. The ductal disruption contributing to pseudocyst formation may occur as a direct result of penetrating trauma or, more commonly, as a result of blunt trauma to the upper part of the abdomen that transects or disrupts the pancreas as it crosses anterior to the vertebral column. These injuries may be missed during initial radiologic evaluation or laparotomy, and the diagnosis of a pseudocyst is often made weeks after the initial injury.

DIAGNOSIS

No definitive laboratory findings are available to establish a diagnosis of pancreatic pseudocyst. Elevated serum amylase and lipase concentrations may occur in half these patients. In fact, persistently elevated amylase after resolution of acute pancreatitis should prompt investigation for a pseudocyst. A few patients with a pseudocyst have mild leukocytosis, whereas others have elevated liver function test results, which may indicate some compression of the biliary tree. An abdominal CT scan is the preferred study for diagnosis of a pancreatic pseudocyst. Ultrasound examination also demonstrates many pseudocysts, and it is a less invasive test that may be used to

monitor a known pseudocyst for interval size changes.[8] The use of magnetic resonance imaging (MRI) has been advocated to predict whether solid debris within a pseudocyst will prevent adequate percutaneous drainage.[9] Conventional MRI also has the potential advantage of being coupled with magnetic resonance cholangiopancreatography (MRCP) to help define pancreatic ductal anatomy relative to a pseudocyst.[10] Magnetic resonance pancreatography has shown high specificity and diagnostic accuracy in the evaluation of duct strictures and filling defects.[11] More experience is needed in the use of MRI and MRCP for the evaluation of pseudocysts.

Differentiating pseudocysts from other cystic lesions of the pancreas can be challenging. Several groups have advocated the use of percutaneous aspiration to aid in the differentiation of these structures. Lewandrowski et al evaluated the intracystic fluid from 26 cystic lesions for amylase content, cytology, relative viscosity, and the serologic markers carcinoembryonic antigen (CEA) and cancer antigen 125 (CA-125).[12] The nine pseudocysts were found to have high amylase levels, negative cytologic findings, low viscosity, and low levels of CEA and CA-125. Mucinous cystic neoplasms had variable amylase concentrations, usually positive cytologic findings, high viscosity, and variably high levels of the serologic markers (Table 90-1). Serous cystic neoplasms produced fluid with intermediate results; they were low in viscosity and CEA but had elevated CA-125 levels. The few cystadenocarcinomas in the group had high viscosity, high CEA and CA-125 levels, and positive cytologic findings. The Cooperative Pancreatic Cyst Study prospectively evaluated cyst fluid tumor markers and final pathology in 112 patients. Cyst CEA (>192 ng/mL) demonstrated 79% accuracy in differentiating mucinous from inflammatory cysts.[13] A European pooled analysis of cyst fluid results showed that a CEA level less than 5 ng/mL suggested a pseudocyst or serous cystadenoma with 95% specificity.[14] Furthermore, low cancer antigen 19-9 (CA 19-9) cyst fluid levels were strongly predictive of a nonmucinous cyst. Although these results indicate that some conclusions may be made about the type of cystic lesion based on cyst fluid sampling, percutaneous aspiration is not usually necessary for differentiation between pseudocysts and cystic neoplasms. Many authors advocate the use of endoscopic retrograde cholangiopancreatography (ERCP) for the diagnosis and treatment planning of patients with pancreatic pseudocysts.[15-18] The obvious advantage of ERCP is the ability to define pancreatic ductal anatomy, which is of particular benefit in evaluating a pseudocyst in a patient with chronic pancreatitis.

TABLE 90-1 Cyst Fluid Parameters Useful in Diagnosis

Diagnosis	Amylase	Cytology	Viscosity	CEA/CA-125	CA 19-9
Pseudocyst	High	Negative	Low	Low/low	Variable
Serous cystic neoplasm	Variable	Negative	Low	Low/variable	Variable
Mucinous cystic neoplasm	Variable	Usually positive	Usually high	High/variable	High

Modified from Lewandrowski KB, Southern JF, Pins MR, et al: Cyst fluid analysis in the differential diagnosis of pancreatic cysts: A comparison of pseudocysts, serous cystadenomas, mucinous cystic neoplasms, and mucinous cystadenocarcinoma. *Ann Surg* 217:41, 1993, with permission.
CA 19-9, Cancer antigen 19-9; *CA-125,* cancer antigen 125; *CEA,* carcinoembryonic antigen.

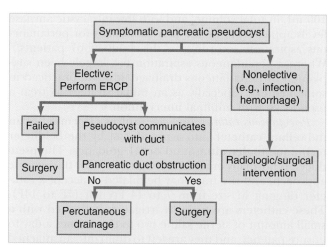

FIGURE 90-4 Treatment algorithm retrospectively applied to patients with pancreatic pseudocysts. *ERCP*, Endoscopic retrograde cholangiopancreatography. (From Ahearne PM, Baillie JM, Cotton PB, et al: An endoscopic retrograde cholangiopancreatography [ERCP]-based algorithm for the management of pancreatic pseudocysts. *Am J Surg* 163:111, 1992.)

TABLE 90-2 Pseudocyst Size Compared With Eventual Management			
Pseudocyst Size (cm)	No. of Patients	Operated (%)	Not Operated (%)
0-2	3	33	67
2.1-4	19	37	63
4.1-6	20	45	55
6.1-8	8	63	37
8.1-10	14	64	36
>10	11	73	27

From Yeo CJ, Bastidas JA, Lynch-Nyhan A, et al: The natural history of pancreatic pseudocysts documented by computed tomography. *Surg Gynecol Obstet* 170:411, 1990, with permission.

Nearly all patients with pseudocysts have some abnormality in their pancreatic ductal system, and 2% to 50% may have abnormal cholangiograms as well. A prospective study by Nealon et al of ERCP in patients with pseudocysts found that ERCP findings changed operative management in 24 of 41 patients undergoing surgery for a pseudocyst.[19] Nineteen of the patients in the study underwent longitudinal pancreaticojejunostomy for drainage of the pancreatic duct. Unfortunately, this study had no matched controls, and therefore no conclusions can be made regarding an outcome advantage for patients who underwent preoperative ERCP.

ERCP has also been advocated as a method to determine which patients with pseudocysts are candidates for percutaneous drainage. Ahearne et al, in a 1992 study, assumed that pseudocysts associated with disruption of or communication with the main pancreatic duct required surgical drainage, whereas those without these ERCP findings could be drained percutaneously.[20] This assumption may not be true. In retrospective fashion, the authors showed that patients treated according to an algorithm based on their stated assumption had fewer adverse outcomes (12%) than did patients treated in a manner that did not follow the algorithm (43% adverse outcomes). This study indicates that use of an ERCP-based algorithm can lower the incidence of adverse outcomes in patients with pancreatic pseudocysts (Figure 90-4).

NATURAL HISTORY

Appropriate management of a patient with a pancreatic pseudocyst requires knowledge of the natural history of these lesions. Before the widespread use of ultrasonography and CT, determination of the natural history of pancreatic pseudocysts relied on other, less accurate diagnostic modalities, such as upper gastrointestinal series, physical examination, and operative and autopsy findings. Data based on these methods indicated that pseudocysts rarely regress spontaneously and that complications occur in up to half of all patients. Therefore, nonoperative, conservative therapy was not advocated in patients with known pancreatic pseudocysts.

A series of studies based on improved imaging techniques increased our understanding of the natural history of pancreatic pseudocysts and led to the era of nonoperative management of the majority of these lesions. In 1979, Bradley et al reported on the natural history of pseudocysts as followed by ultrasonography.[21] Pseudocysts present for less than 6 weeks were found to resolve spontaneously in 40% of cases, although they had a 20% risk for complications. However, pseudocysts documented to be present for longer than 12 weeks did not resolve and were associated with a complication rate of 67%.

In 1990, Yeo et al reported data from the Johns Hopkins Hospital in Baltimore that evaluated the natural history of pseudocysts by CT scan.[22] Seventy-five patients with pseudocysts were monitored with interval CT scans of the abdomen. All patients with asymptomatic pseudocysts, regardless of size, were initially managed nonoperatively. Operative intervention was performed only for persistent abdominal pain, pseudocyst enlargement, or pseudocyst complications. Nearly half (48%) of these 75 patients were successfully managed nonoperatively. At a 1-year mean followup, 60% of patients had complete resolution of the pseudocyst, whereas the remaining 40% had pseudocysts that remained stable or decreased in size. The only significant difference between the two groups by CT criteria was pseudocyst diameter, with pseudocysts in the nonoperative group averaging 5.8 ± 0.8 cm and pseudocysts in the operative group averaging 7.4 ± 0.6 cm ($P < .05$). Pseudocyst size correlated with the eventual need for surgery: 67% of patients with pseudocysts larger than 6 cm required operative intervention, whereas 40% of patients with pseudocysts 6 cm or smaller required surgical treatment (Table 90-2). Of the patients with pseudocysts larger than 10 cm, 27% were successfully managed nonoperatively.

These data suggested that many patients with pancreatic pseudocysts can be managed nonoperatively with careful clinical and radiologic followup, a practice that was confirmed by a study reported from the Mayo Clinic in Rochester, Minnesota.[23] Vitas and Sarr described 68 patients treated nonoperatively, 6 (9%) of whom had a severe complication and only 24 (35%) required operative management. The likelihood of eventual operative intervention did increase with pseudocyst size, although no strict size cutoff could be demonstrated. The success of nonoperative management was independent of the cause of the pseudocyst. The experience of these large centers and others has led to the practice of initial nonoperative management in the majority of patients with pancreatic pseudocysts. According to these data, more than 50% of patients can be expected to require no further intervention. To qualify for conservative, nonoperative management, patients should have no symptoms referable to the pseudocyst, no pseudocyst-related complications, and a stable or decreasing pseudocyst size. Patients who do not meet any of these criteria at followup evaluation should undergo appropriate intervention (surgical, endoscopic, or percutaneous).

MANAGEMENT

Patients who do not meet the criteria for conservative, nonoperative management require intervention for the pseudocyst. Associated conditions, such as ductal disruption, biliary obstruction, and chronic pancreatitis, may require concomitant intervention. The recommended management strategies for patients with pancreatic pseudocysts have changed and continue to evolve as more long-term followup becomes available for specific procedures. Current management options for a patient with a pseudocyst include percutaneous drainage, endoscopic drainage, operative internal or external drainage, and resection (Box 90-2).

Percutaneous approaches to pseudocyst drainage have been reported since the early 1980s. Although many early studies claimed excellent results, extended followup information has revealed that recurrence and failure rates for percutaneous techniques are higher than initially documented. An important distinction should be made between percutaneous aspiration and percutaneous drainage. *Percutaneous aspiration* is aimed at aspirating all pseudocyst fluid at one procedure, without leaving an indwelling drainage catheter. On reviewing the literature to date, less than 50% of patients undergoing this technique will have complete resolution of their pseudocyst.[24] The remaining patients will require repeat aspiration or a second technique (endoscopic or operative drainage). One study attempted to determine which factors could predict successful pseudocyst management with percutaneous aspiration. Patients with pseudocysts in the tail of the pancreas, with pseudocysts less than

100 mL in total volume, and with low intracystic amylase levels appeared to be the best candidates for percutaneous aspiration according to this study of 67 patients.[25] Whereas percutaneous aspiration has largely been supplanted by percutaneous drainage, it is still practiced in some centers, especially as an initial strategy to treat a pseudocyst with minimal intervention.

Percutaneous catheter drainage involves placement of an indwelling catheter into a pseudocyst by the Seldinger technique under ultrasound or CT guidance. The pseudocyst is normally entered through a flank or transgastric approach, and the tract may be dilated to accept a catheter ranging in size from 7 to 14 French (7F to 14F). These catheters are typically irrigated or flushed with a small amount of sterile saline two to three times a day to ensure patency, and they are left to drain into an attached bag by gravity. Contraindications to percutaneous drainage include the presence of significant pancreatic necrosis or solid debris in the pseudocyst, lack of a safe access route, pseudocyst hemorrhage, and complete obstruction of the main pancreatic duct (a controversial contraindication). One review of percutaneous drainage series reported a total recurrence rate of 7%, with 16% of patients counted as treatment failures because of the eventual need for drainage by other techniques.[26] Although most of the studies included in this review consisted of small, selected groups of patients, a large retrospective review from a single center compared patients managed percutaneously, operatively, and expectantly.[24] This review found that only 42% of patients who underwent percutaneous drainage did not require other intervention, whereas 88% of patients undergoing operative intervention had a successful outcome. Ninety-three percent of the patients in the expectant group required no intervention. Patients in the expectant group had on average smaller pseudocysts (4 cm vs. 7 to 9 cm in the percutaneous and operative groups), but no other significant differences. Although these data conflict with previous series reporting the success of percutaneous drainage, they do emphasize the need for an adequate period of expectant management and careful patient selection before any intervention. The authors rightly called for a prospective study comparing percutaneous and operative intervention in comparable patients. The only prospective study to date has been reported by Lang et al. In this study of severe acute pancreatitis, patients were alternately assigned to either percutaneous or operative drainage.[27] Both procedures had similar rates of success, with 88% of pseudocysts ablated by operative management and 77% through percutaneous drainage. Until this study can be repeated in a more diverse group of patients, percutaneous drainage should continue to be considered an effective method of pseudocyst drainage in selected patients. Furthermore, it is a safe procedure. Most series have reported complication rates of less than 20%, with infection of the drain tract, persistent or recurrent pseudocyst, and pancreatic-cutaneous fistula being the most common complications.[24,26] A recent population-based study reviewed outcomes in 14,914 patients treated by surgical or percutaneous drainage. Although selection bias was present in the study, patients treated by percutaneous drainage exhibited increased

---

BOX 90-2 Management Options for Pancreatic Pseudocysts

Observation
Percutaneous aspiration/drainage
Endoscopic aspiration/drainage
Transpapillary endoscopic drainage or stenting
Operative approaches (open or laparoscopic)
    Internal drainage
    External drainage
    Resection

complications and a longer length of hospital stay. In the modern era of health care cost containment, these issues will certainly play a role in future treatment algorithms.[28]

Endoscopic approaches to the treatment of pseudocysts have also evolved substantially.[29] As with percutaneous methods, long-term followup is now becoming available. Current techniques involve the use of flexible upper endoscopy to localize and drain pseudocysts by creating a fistulous tract between the pseudocyst and the stomach or duodenum. This communication is created with electrocautery, and an endoprosthesis is left in place to stent the fistula open. Endoscopic drainage usually requires that the pseudocyst be located in the head or body of the pancreas and that it be well apposed to and bulging into the intestinal lumen. *Endoscopic ultrasound* (EUS) can be used to visualize the pseudocyst and to choose a site for drainage Risks associated with this procedure include hemorrhage from the gastric or duodenal wall and free perforation. Endoscopic and percutaneous techniques have been combined to localize and drain pseudocysts that are adjacent to the gastric wall but do not bulge into the lumen.[30]

Traditional *transmural endoscopic drainage* has a success rate that compares favorably with that of percutaneous and operative drainage. One literature review by Beckingham et al summarized a series of pseudocysts drained endoscopically from 1987 to 1997.[31] The review found that approximately 50% of pseudocysts were amenable to transmural drainage based on location and relation to the stomach or duodenum. Successful initial drainage was achieved in 86% of patients, whereas 11% had a recurrence requiring further intervention. About half the recurrences, or 5% of the total group, eventually required operative intervention. Endoscopic cystoduodenostomy was found to be slightly more effective than cystogastrostomy, with fewer recurrences, a finding that most likely relates to the longer patency rates of cystoduodenostomy and the smaller size of these pseudocysts. Complications after both routes of endoscopic drainage were extremely uncommon, with significant bleeding, infection, or perforation occurring in less than 2% of cases. Factors associated with successful endoscopic transmural drainage include location in the head and body of the pancreas, pseudocyst wall thickness less than 1 cm, and pseudocysts secondary to chronic pancreatitis or trauma.[32] Pseudocysts associated with severe necrotizing pancreatitis do not respond well to endoscopic drainage because solid debris obstructs the endoprosthesis.

Experience with the use of *transampullary pancreatic stents* also continues to increase, a development that has applications in the treatment of chronic pancreatitis, pancreatic ductal disruption, pancreatic fistulas, and pseudocysts. Drainage of a pseudocyst via the transampullary (transpapillary) route has been attempted in selected patients with pseudocysts shown to have an obvious communication with the main pancreatic duct by ERCP. Several groups published initial series and described similar techniques and results.[33-35] When possible, stents are placed through the ampulla, along the pancreatic duct, and into the lumen of the pseudocyst. When it is not possible to direct the stent into the

pseudocyst, the tip of the stent can be placed as close as possible to the communication between the pancreatic duct and the pseudocyst; one must take care to cross any intervening strictures of the pancreatic duct. Complications associated with this procedure are rare and have included mild postprocedure pancreatitis, bleeding, and abscess formation secondary to stent obstruction. Mean followup in the three reported series varied from 15 to 37 months. Some patients underwent traditional transmural endoscopic drainage in addition to transampullary drainage. Initial pseudocyst drainage was successful in 81% to 94%, with 76% to 78% of patients free of recurrence and requiring no further intervention through the period of followup. Endoscopic transpapillary nasopancreatic drain placement for pseudocysts that develop in atypical locations (mediastinal, intrahepatic, intrasplenic, pelvic) was recently reported. All patients had partial disruption of the pancreatic duct, which was successfully stented with resolution of the pseudocysts in 91% of patients.[36] Clearly, transampullary drainage and pancreatic stenting may play a role in pseudocyst drainage in select patients. Prolonged followup of these patients for recurrence and duplication of these excellent results in other centers may lead to more widespread use of this technique.

Although favorable results may be obtained with both percutaneous and endoscopic management of pancreatic pseudocysts, not all patients have pseudocysts that are amenable to these techniques. Furthermore, patients in whom these less invasive techniques fail may require *operative intervention* for definitive treatment of their pseudocyst. Complications associated with endoscopic and percutaneous pseudocyst drainage were reviewed by Nealon and Walser.[37] Seventy-nine patients with complications following endoscopic or percutaneous pseudocyst drainage were analyzed. Sepsis was the most common problem encountered in 91% of patients, followed by clinical shock (65%), hemorrhage (20%), renal failure (20%), and ventilator-dependent respiratory failure (24%). Eighty-four percent of these patients subsequently required operative management of their pseudocysts. Many of these failures of percutaneous/endoscopic drainage were predictable by ERCP, which detected disruption or stricture of the main pancreatic duct. A system to categorize pancreatic ductal abnormalities in pancreatic pseudocysts and direct therapy was proposed (Figure 90-5). Duct anomalies type I and II can be managed by percutaneous drainage with expected high rates of resolution. Types V to VII should be managed by surgical or endoscopic internal drainage, or surgical resection, because of the complicated duct strictures and stones associated with these variants of chronic pancreatitis. Types III and IV may be managed by either modality; however, percutaneous drainage alone may be associated with higher rates of recurrence because of the underlying duct strictures. Surgical salvage procedures following failed percutaneous and endoscopic drainage techniques include cyst debridement and external drainage, internal pseudocyst drainage, and pancreatic resection.[38] Surgical morbidity following salvage procedures was significant in 56% of patients; hemorrhage, wound infection, and pulmonary complications were most frequently observed.

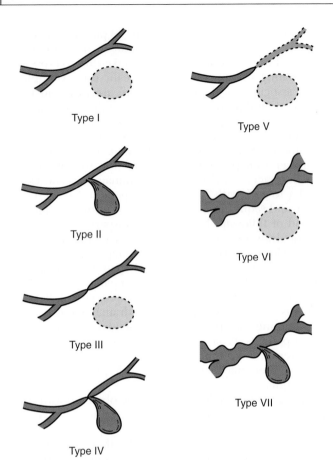

FIGURE 90-5 Schematic representations of the categories of ductal abnormalities in patients with pseudocysts: Type I—normal duct/no communication with cyst; type II—normal duct with cyst communication; type III—normal duct with stricture/no duct or cyst communication; type IV—normal duct with stricture and cyst communication; type V—normal duct with complete cutoff/no cyst communication; type VI—chronic pancreatitis/no cyst communication; type VII—chronic pancreatitis/communication between cyst and duct. (Adapted from Nealon WH, Walser E: Main pancreatic ductal anatomy can direct choice of modality for treating pancreatic pseudocysts [surgery versus percutaneous drainage]. *Ann Surg* 235:751, 2002.)

This study reinforces the need to appropriately choose patients for endoscopic and percutaneous drainage of pseudocysts. Operative intervention also provides the opportunity for biopsy of the pseudocyst wall, a procedure that is necessary to exclude the possibility of a cystic neoplasm.

The preferred operative approach for most uncomplicated pseudocysts requiring surgical intervention is *internal drainage.* The three standard options include cystojejunostomy to a Roux-en-Y jejunal limb, cystogastrostomy, and cystoduodenostomy. *Cystojejunostomy* is the most versatile technique of operative drainage and is particularly appropriate when a pseudocyst is located at the base of the transverse mesocolon and is not adherent to the posterior gastric wall (Figure 90-6). *Cystogastrostomy* is a faster and less technically demanding procedure that is used when the pseudocyst is adherent to the posterior

wall of the stomach (Figure 90-7). The least frequently used technique is *cystoduodenostomy*, which is appropriate only for pseudocysts in the pancreatic head or uncinate process that lie within 1 cm of the duodenal lumen. Cystoduodenostomy is best performed in a fashion similar to that for cystogastrostomy (i.e., by opening the lateral wall of the duodenum and creating a communication between the pseudocyst and the duodenum through a medial duodenotomy). The risk for duodenal leak and subsequent fistula makes cystoduodenostomy the least attractive method of internal drainage and thus reserved for rare use. Cystojejunostomy and cystogastrostomy have comparable morbidity, mortality, and recurrence rates.[26,39] Operative mortality in some series ranges from 0% to 5%. Cystojejunostomy has a slightly lower recurrence rate (7% vs. 10%), but it is associated with significantly more blood loss and operative time. Many authors have advocated cystogastrostomy because of these technical advantages. However, Johnson et al reported life-threatening postoperative complications, as well as two deaths, in patients with large pseudocysts (>15 cm) that were treated by cystogastrostomy.[40] These complications were attributed to incomplete emptying of the pseudocyst, a finding emphasizing that complete dependent drainage is critical in any internal drainage procedure and that any solid material lining a pseudocyst should be thoroughly debrided at the time of internal drainage.

In addition to the conventional open techniques of internal drainage of pancreatic pseudocysts, several centers have performed *laparoscopic drainage procedures.* Large retrogastric pseudocysts can be drained internally by endogastric approaches, as well as by laparoscopic transgastric and laparoscopic extragastric approaches. Each allows for biopsy of the cyst wall and the opportunity for cyst debridement. Laparoscopic cystojejunostomy can be performed in select patients for better dependent drainage. A recent review of laparoscopic internal drainage revealed an operative success rate of 89% with complications occurring in approximately 7% of patients (Figure 90-8).[41,42]

Natural Orifice Transluminal Endoscopic Surgery (NOTES) cystogastrostomy has recently been described as an endoscopic method to achieve the technical results similar to open and laparoscopic cystogastrostomy surgery. Six patients with mature pseudocysts (8 to 23 cm in diameter) underwent EUS-guided pseudocyst drainage combined with transoral cystogastrostomy anastomosis using a powered surgical stapler delivered via a flexible endoscopic shaft. Technical success was achieved in all patients; however; one patient was readmitted for recurrent pancreatitis, and one required dilation of the anastomosis for complete resolution of the cyst.[43] Additional series have described NOTES techniques for the debridement of infected pancreatic necrosis with excellent resolution of the particulate debris associated with these cavities.[44] Advances in these NOTES techniques and the development of advanced endoscopic tools may open the way to transoral endoscopic pseudocyst drainage, which offers the efficacy of an open surgical anastomosis, and the ability to directly debride any particulate matter in the cyst (Figure 90-9).

Text continued on p. 1158.

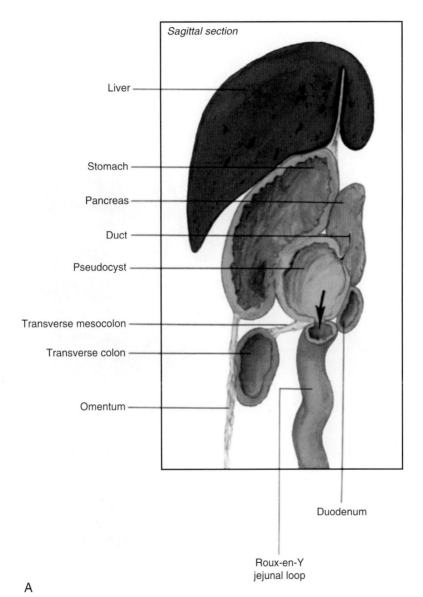

Liver

Stomach

Pancreas

Duct

Pseudocyst

Transverse mesocolon

Transverse colon

Omentum

Sagittal section

Duodenum

Roux-en-Y
jejunal loop

A

FIGURE 90-6 Cystojejunostomy for a pancreatic pseudocyst. **A,** Schematic of a sagittal section showing the final anatomy.

Continued

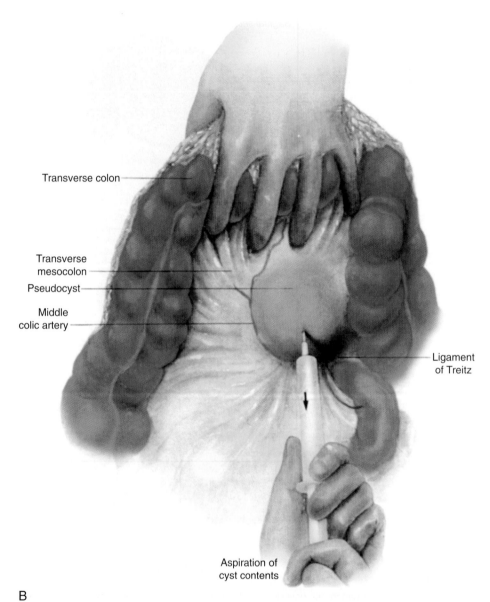

Transverse colon

Transverse mesocolon

Pseudocyst

Middle colic artery

Ligament of Treitz

Aspiration of cyst contents

B

FIGURE 90-6, cont'd B, Aspiration of a portion of the pseudocyst contents through the transverse mesocolon.

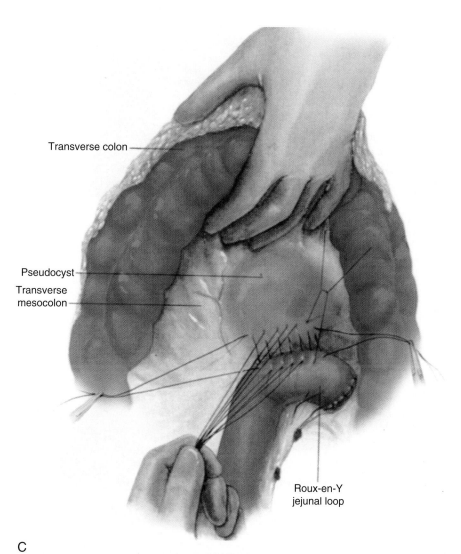

C

FIGURE 90-6, cont'd C, Creation of the posterior outer layer of the anastomosis with interrupted silk suture.

Continued

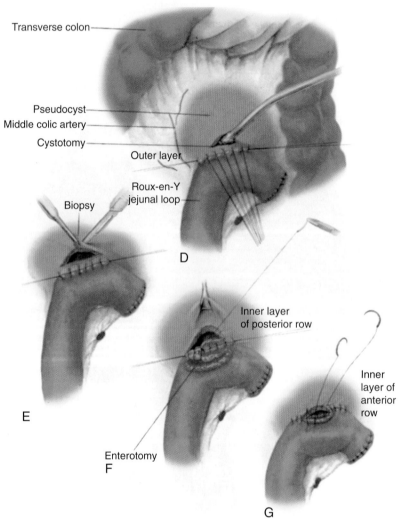

FIGURE 90-6, cont'd **D,** Opening into the pseudocyst. **E,** Biopsy of the pseudocyst wall. **F,** Suturing the posterior inner layer of the anastomosis. **G,** Completing the anterior inner row of the anastomosis.

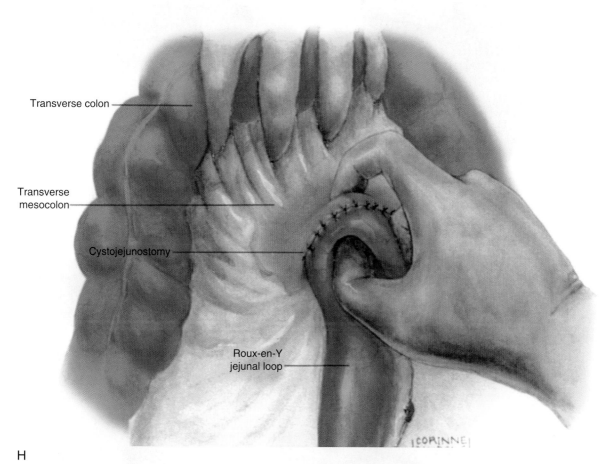

Transverse colon

Transverse
mesocolon

Cystojejunostomy

Roux-en-Y
jejunal loop

H

FIGURE 90-6, cont'd H, After closure with an anterior outer layer of interrupted silk, the orifice of the anastomosis between the pseudocyst cavity and the Roux-en-Y jejunal loop is gently palpated. (From Cameron JL: *Atlas of surgery*, vol 1, Toronto, 1990, BC Decker, p 373.)

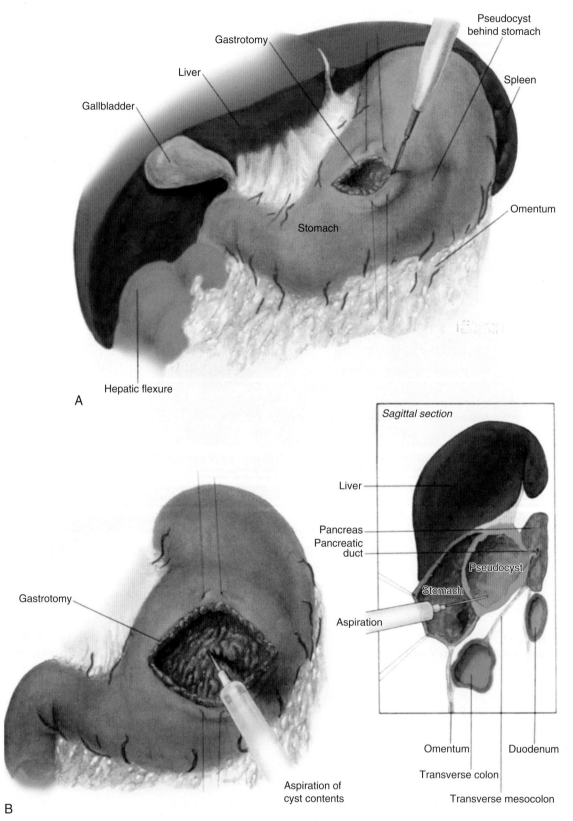

FIGURE 90-7 Cystogastrostomy for a pancreatic pseudocyst. **A,** An anterior gastrotomy is performed. **B,** Aspiration of a portion of the pseudocyst contents through the posterior gastric wall. The *inset* shows sagittal section anatomy.

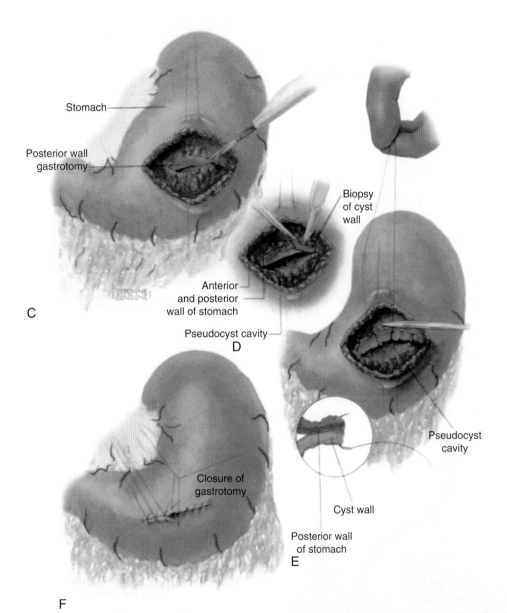

FIGURE 90-7, cont'd C, A posterior gastrotomy creates a communication between the pseudocyst and the stomach. **D,** Biopsy of the pseudocyst wall. **E,** A running locking suture is used for hemostasis and to maintain apposition of the pseudocyst wall to the posterior wall of the stomach. **F,** Closure of the anterior gastrotomy. (From Cameron JL: *Atlas of surgery,* vol 1, Toronto, 1990, BC Decker, p 381.)

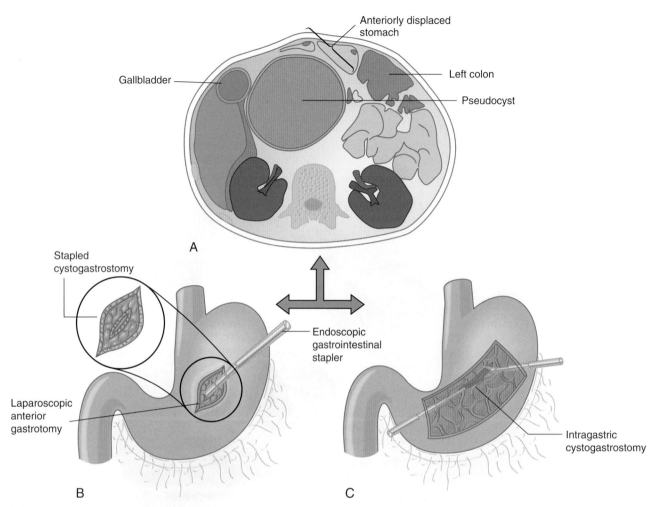

FIGURE 90-8 Large pancreatic pseudocyst (10 cm in size) located in the body of the pancreas **(A)**. Laparoscopic cystogastrostomy may be performed via anterior gastrotomy **(B)** or intraluminal cystogastrostomy **(C)**. (From Fernandez-Cruz L, Cesar-Borges G, Lopez-Boado MA, et al: Minimally invasive surgery of the pancreas in progress. *Langenbecks Arch Surg* 390:342, 2005.)

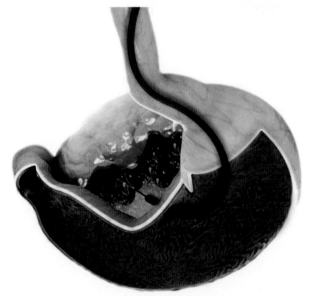

FIGURE 90-9 Transoral endoscopic pancreatic necrosis debridement technique. (From Escourrou J, Shehab H, Buscail L, et al: Peroral transgastric/transduodenal necrosectomy: Success in the treatment of infected pancreatic necrosis. *Ann Surg* 248:1074, 2008.)

A small proportion of pseudocysts are best treated by *pancreatic resection.* Most commonly, this operation involves distal pancreatectomy for pseudocysts located in the body or tail of the gland. Peripancreatic and peripseudocyst inflammation can make distal pancreatectomy a technically challenging procedure in this setting. After distal pancreatectomy, a Roux-en-Y pancreaticojejunostomy to the remnant pancreas may be required to decompress an obstructed or abnormal proximal pancreatic duct. In a few patients with symptomatic pseudocysts in the head of the pancreas associated with an inflammatory mass, excisional therapy may require *pancreaticoduodenectomy.* In this case, pylorus-preserving pancreaticoduodenectomy is the procedure of choice. Less commonly performed procedures, such as duodenum-preserving resection of the head of the pancreas, may be applicable in some patients.

External drainage of a pancreatic pseudocyst through an operative approach is indicated when gross infection is found at the time of surgery or when an immature, thin-walled pseudocyst is encountered that will not allow for safe internal drainage. When the pseudocyst is initially aspirated, purulent material is retrieved. At this time, the pseudocyst is isolated from the remaining abdominal viscera with moist packs, and the pseudocyst cavity is opened with the electrocautery device. The contents of the pseudocyst cavity are then completely evacuated, and the cavity is closely inspected to ensure adequate hemostasis. At least one closed-suction drainage catheter is then placed into the cavity and brought out through the abdominal wall. Appropriate antibiotic therapy should be instituted, and followup CT scans are obtained to ensure that the pseudocyst is entirely drained. External drainage may lead to the development of pancreaticocutaneous fistulas, most of which heal spontaneously as long as the proximal pancreatic duct is not obstructed. Total parenteral nutrition and octreotide therapy (50 to 250 µg subcutaneously three times per day) may assist in closure of a persistent pancreaticocutaneous fistula.[45] Nealon and Walser reported their experience with lateral pancreaticojejunostomy for pseudocysts associated with dilated pancreatic ducts (>7 mm) in patients with chronic pancreatitis. Forty-seven patients were treated by lateral pancreaticojejunostomy alone as pseudocyst management. Long-term pain relief was achieved in 90% of patients, with pseudocyst recurrence being observed in less than 1%.[46] This unique approach requires preoperative pancreatic duct evaluation by ERCP and appears to offer excellent results in select patients.

COMPLICATIONS

A review of the literature reveals that complications develop in up to 40% of patients with untreated pseudocysts, although most series report complication rates of 10% to 20%.[21-23,26,47,48] The most frequently reported complications include infection, hemorrhage, obstruction or compression of adjacent structures, and rupture.

Infection

An important distinction should be made between pseudocysts that are colonized or contaminated and those that are truly infected. Some pseudocysts contain small amounts of bacteria that are evident on Gram stain or culture, but the fluid from these pseudocysts is not purulent, and patients do not have clinical evidence of infection. However, in a few patients with pseudocysts (<5%), true *infection* can develop, as marked by fever, leukocytosis, and increased pain.[22,23] Aspiration of purulent fluid from the pseudocyst confirms the presence of an infection. The most recent Atlanta International Symposium defined these patients as having a *pancreatic abscess* and recommended that use of the term *infected pseudocyst* be avoided.[1] The bacteriology of a pancreatic abscess is highly variable, but up to 60% of these lesions contain gram-negative aerobic and anaerobic organisms.[49]

A pancreatic abscess is one clinical situation in which percutaneous drainage is clearly the treatment of choice. Success rates of up to 85% have been reported in multiple series.[50-52] Retrospective studies have shown similar success rates when comparing percutaneous and operative drainage procedures. Furthermore, the mortality rate is lower with percutaneous drainage, and a major open operative procedure is avoided. However, operative external drainage may become necessary in some patients. Percutaneous catheters often do not allow for rapid drainage of thick, purulent material or may not completely address multiloculated collections. Techniques used by interventional radiologists include upsizing drainage catheters to 20F to 30F diameters, biweekly imaging, and aggressive manipulation to break up loculations.[53] These techniques are not always successful. In these cases, open operative drainage allows for complete evacuation of all infected material, and external drains may be placed under direct vision. Most recently, percutaneous endoscopic techniques have enabled debridement of necrotic tissue under direct endoscopic vision. Using previous percutaneous drainage tracts, ureteroscopes are advanced into the retroperitoneum and devitalized tissues removed under direct vision while the cavity is continually irrigated. Experience is limited to a few select centers,[54,55] with promising early results and minimal stress to the patient (Figure 90-10). Because it is not often possible to predict which pseudocysts or abscesses will be successfully drained percutaneously, patients undergoing percutaneous drainage need to be closely monitored for evidence of resolution, both by clinical parameters and by followup imaging techniques. Recent reports have suggested that transampullary drainage, alone, for pancreatic abscesses is not an effective means for decompression of these more viscous, infected fluid collections, and additional percutaneous or endoscopic drainage was required to achieve complete abscess resolution in all studied patients.[56] Trevino et al reviewed 110 patients who underwent endoscopic transmural or nasocystic drainage of pseudocysts, necrosis, or abscesses combined with transampullary stenting of the pancreatic duct. Multivariable analysis revealed a significant improvement in treatment success in patients who underwent successful pancreatic duct stenting (36%) compared to transmural or nasocystic drainage alone.[57]

In patients who do not show clinical improvement or who have further progression of their symptoms and in patients who have collections that do not respond to reasonable attempts at percutaneous drainage, operative drainage should be performed.

Hemorrhage

Arterial hemorrhage may occur in up to 10% of patients with pancreatic pseudocysts.[22,23,58] The most common source of pseudocyst-associated bleeding is the splenic artery (up to 50%), with the gastroduodenal and pancreaticoduodenal arteries also accounting for a significant number of hemorrhagic events.[59] Bleeding may also occur from the portal, superior mesenteric, or splenic veins, although such bleeding occurs less commonly. The pathogenesis of arterial hemorrhage seems to follow a predictable sequence, with erosion of the vessel wall leading to pseudoaneurysm formation and eventual rupture. Massive hemorrhage is often preceded by a sentinel hemorrhage. Therefore, any degree of bleeding associated with a pseudocyst should be aggressively investigated. CT scan with intravenous contrast is an appropriate confirmatory test in a stable patient, but angiography may be necessary for diagnosis and provides a mode of treatment.

Initial management of a hemodynamically stable patient is attempted embolization of the pseudoaneurysm or source vessel, a technique performed by most

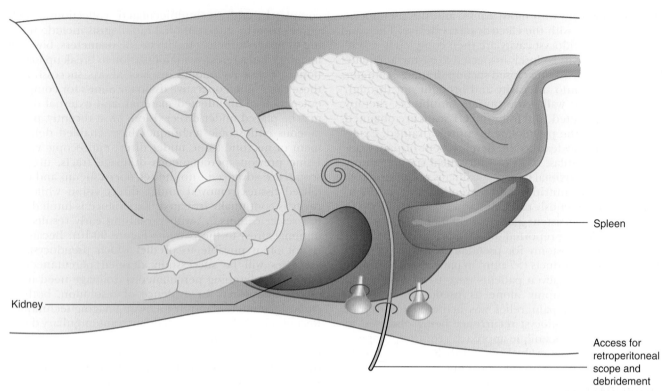

FIGURE 90-10 Retroperitoneal access to pancreatic necrosis. (From Fernandez-Cruz L, Cesar-Borges G, Lopez-Boado MA, et al: Minimally invasive surgery of the pancreas in progress. *Langenbecks Arch Surg* 390:342, 2005.)

skilled interventional radiologists. Most of these hemorrhages may be effectively controlled by current embolic techniques.[60-63] However, patients in whom embolic therapy fails, who rebleed, or who are hemodynamically unstable require emergency surgical exploration. Control of arterial bleeding may require associated pancreatic resection because oversewing vessels in the setting of the chronic inflammation and enzymatic erosion associated with pseudocysts is often unsuccessful. When the responsible blood vessel can be effectively ligated, the associated pseudocyst should be externally drained with large-bore catheters. If resection is required, distal pancreatectomy, splenectomy, and splenic artery ligation are the most common procedures. Rarely, emergency pancreaticoduodenectomy may be necessary.

Obstruction

Pancreatic pseudocysts may become symptomatic as a result of the mass effect that they exert on other structures. Although *duodenal obstruction* is the most common manifestation of mechanical obstruction secondary to pseudocyst formation, obstruction of the stomach, esophagus, jejunum, and colon may be identified.[64-68] Obstruction of the mesenteric vasculature and the portal venous system (particularly the splenic vein) may lead to extrahepatic portal hypertension and subsequent splenomegaly and gastric varices.[69] Pseudocysts have also been described as obstructing other retroperitoneal structures, such as the inferior vena cava and the ureters.[70,71] In addition, reports have described pseudocysts with mediastinal and pleural extension impeding cardiac performance secondary to obstruction of preload or

increased afterload.[72,73] Congestive heart failure secondary to cardiac compression by a mediastinal pseudocyst has also been reported.[74] Mechanical obstruction of any structure is a relative indication for intervention. At present, no prospective data are available on which to base recommendations for percutaneous, endoscopic, or surgical techniques.

Biliary obstruction secondary to pseudocyst formation is also well described, and it leads to such complications as jaundice, cholangitis, and biliary cirrhosis. Although biliary obstruction may be caused by direct compression of the bile duct by a pseudocyst, most patients have an associated stricture of the intrapancreatic portion of the bile duct that does not improve with pseudocyst drainage alone.[75] Evaluation of any patient with biliary obstruction and a pancreatic pseudocyst requires cholangiography before planning pseudocyst drainage. Treatment of a biliary stricture caused by concomitant chronic pancreatitis may require biliary-enteric bypass, either choledochoduodenostomy or choledochojejunostomy.

Rupture

Spontaneous rupture, the least common complication of pseudocyst formation, occurs in less than 3% of patients, but it may give rise to dramatic clinical manifestations. Spontaneous rupture of a pseudocyst into the peritoneal cavity may lead to severe acute abdominal pain as a result of chemical peritonitis. Such patients are often treated as a surgical emergency, especially those without a known pseudocyst. In patients with a known history of pseudocyst, acute abdominal pain should raise the possibility of free intraperitoneal rupture or rupture into an associated hollow viscus, most commonly a segment of the gastrointestinal tract. Rupture may be secondary to progressive expansion, but it may also indicate the presence of an infected or hemorrhagic pseudocyst. Patients with rupture and sepsis are likely to have either transenteric disruption or an infected pseudocyst that leads to contamination of the peritoneum with enteric bacteria.

Silent rupture of a pseudocyst may also occur. Some pseudocysts are presumed to resolve by rupture or fistulization into an associated portion of the stomach or small bowel, similar to operative or endoscopic enteric drainage. No further therapy is needed in these circumstances. Pseudocysts that rupture silently anteriorly into the peritoneal cavity or posteriorly into the pleural cavity may lead to the development of pancreatic ascites or pancreatic pleural effusion, respectively.[76] Management of these patients is discussed later.

PANCREATIC DUCTAL DISRUPTION

Pancreatic ductal disruption is an event leading to complications of chronic pancreatitis. Ductal disruption is most often described as creating an internal pancreatic fistula (as in pancreatic ascites, pancreatic pleural effusion, and pancreaticoenteric fistula) or an external pancreatic fistula that communicates with the skin. Pseudocysts of the pancreas are also the result of disruptions of the pancreatic duct, as discussed earlier.

PANCREATIC ASCITES AND PLEURAL EFFUSIONS

The first report of *pancreatic ascites* occurred in 1953,[77] and it was followed by individual case reports of other patients over the subsequent 15 years. In 1967, Cameron et al published the first review of 13 patients with pancreatic ascites.[78] The review established diagnostic criteria for pancreatic ascites and was followed by larger series of patients because the diagnosis was made more frequently. To date, more than 300 reports of pancreatic ascites have been published in the world literature. Parekh and Segal reported on 23 patients with pancreatic ascites or pleural effusions in 1992 and described factors that helped determine which patients would be likely to respond to conservative therapy.[79] Sankaran and Walt described 26 patients with pancreatic ascites and noted that pancreatic ascites occurred in 15% of patients with pseudocysts at their institution.[80] Lipsett and Cameron reported the Johns Hopkins Hospital experience with internal pancreatic fistulas over a 27-year period.[81] Fifty patients were included in the series, including 34 with pancreatic ascites and 7 with pancreatic ascites and pleural effusion.

Pancreatic pleural effusions have been described more recently. In an initial review of internal fistulas from the Johns Hopkins Hospital in 1967, five patients with pleural effusions were reported.[78] A subsequent update described 16 patients with pancreatic pleural effusions.[81] Most authors argue that pancreatic pleural effusions are often unrecognized because the effusions may be attributed to associated cardiac, pulmonary, or hepatic disease without fluid sampling for diagnostic studies. In fact, patients with pancreatic effusions often do not have symptoms of

pancreatitis but instead have pulmonary symptoms and respiratory compromise.

The diagnostic criteria for pancreatic ascites and effusion were initially proposed by Cameron et al in 1967.[78] Correct diagnosis requires sampling of the fluid and assessment of amylase and albumin levels. Amylase levels are elevated relative to serum values in all patients, and fluid albumin levels are elevated to levels of 3 g/100 mL or more. Serum amylase levels may also be elevated in up to 90% of patients with pancreatic effusions or ascites, a finding that may reflect absorption of amylase from the pleural and peritoneal surfaces rather than active pancreatic inflammation.[82] Patients with markedly depressed serum albumin levels secondary to malnutrition may have fluid albumin levels less than 3 g/100 mL. The fluid of pancreatic effusion or ascites is most often clear or straw colored, but it may appear thick, chylous, or even bloody. The differential diagnosis of these internal pancreatic fistulas often includes ascites secondary to cirrhosis and malignant ascites or effusion. Patients with cirrhotic ascites generally have fluid albumin levels less than 1.5 g/100 mL and most often have low amylase levels. Distinguishing pancreatic effusion or ascites from malignant fluid may be difficult cytologically because pancreatic enzymes appear to be capable of producing metaplastic changes in serosal cells and therefore of creating false-positive results.

The pathogenesis of both pancreatic pleural effusion and ascites involves a disruption of the pancreatic duct and creation of an internal fistula into the retroperitoneum,[82] which then tracks posteriorly into the pleural space (Figure 90-11) or anteriorly into the peritoneal cavity (Figures 90-12 to 90-15) At times, the fistula may be contained by adjacent structures and lead to the formation of a pancreatic pseudocyst. Pancreatic ductal disruptions are most commonly a result of

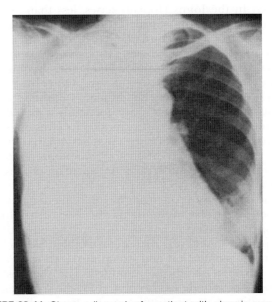

FIGURE 90-11 Chest radiograph of a patient with chronic massive right-sided pancreatic pleural effusion. (From Cameron JJ, Kieffer RS, Anderson WJ, et al: Internal pancreatic fistulas: Pancreatic ascites and pleural effusions. *Ann Surg* 184:587, 1976.)

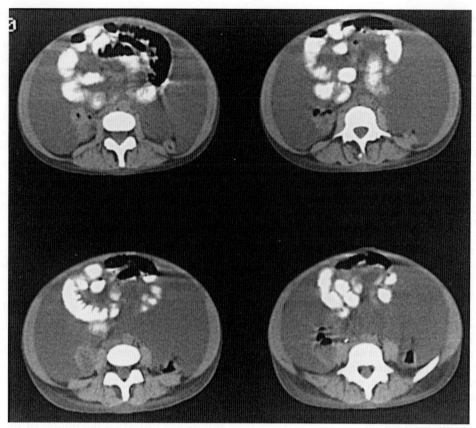

FIGURE 90-12 Four computed tomographic scans showing extensive pancreatic ascites in a young female patient with alcoholism. The small bowel loops float centrally, and ascitic fluid fills the abdomen.

alcoholic pancreatitis, but they may be secondary to blunt or operative trauma, gallstone pancreatitis, or other causes of pancreatitis. Pancreatic ductal injury in children is most commonly the result of trauma.

Most patients with pancreatic ascites or effusions have an indolent illness that may not suggest pancreatic disease. In the Johns Hopkins series, less than 50% of patients had a history of pancreatitis.[81] Only 12% had an acute attack of pancreatitis, whereas 42% gave no history suggestive of pancreatic disease. Patients with pancreatic ascites most often have painless abdominal swelling, frequently associated with weight loss. Other causes of ascites, such as cirrhosis, Budd-Chiari syndrome, tuberculous peritonitis, and carcinomatosis, should be excluded. Patients with pancreatic pleural effusions often complain of shortness of breath that has progressed over time, as well as other respiratory symptoms. Approximately 15% of patients have both pancreatic ascites and pleural effusion.

The diagnosis of pancreatic ascites or pleural effusion is based on the diagnostic criteria discussed earlier. Initial nonoperative management is advocated in all patients. The patient should be strictly denied oral intake to limit pancreatic stimulation and exocrine secretions. Parenteral nutrition should be instituted. The somatostatin analogue octreotide has been used for the treatment of pancreaticocutaneous fistulas, and a few small studies suggest that octreotide may be effective for pancreatic ascites.[83-85] Segal et al demonstrated that octreotide was able to lead to resolution of pancreatic ductal disruption

in a small group of patients in whom conservative therapy had failed.[83] However, no prospective randomized studies have yet been performed to evaluate the use of octreotide in these conditions.

One of the principles of conservative therapy is to encourage the approximation of serosal surfaces and to limit accumulation of ascitic or pleural fluid. Paracentesis or thoracentesis should be performed intermittently to empty the pleural or peritoneal cavity. If repeated high-volume thoracentesis is necessary, tube thoracostomy may be appropriate. A trial of nonoperative therapy should be limited to 3 weeks. In a report from the Johns Hopkins Hospital, limiting the initial nonoperative phase of therapy for pancreatic ascites to 3 weeks resulted in only a single death (in a patient who refused surgery).[81] Pancreatic pleural effusions may also be treated nonoperatively for 3 weeks. Parekh and Segal attempted to identify which pancreatic fistulas will close without surgical intervention.[79] Patients in whom treatment had failed had significantly lower serum sodium and albumin levels, and the ratio of total fluid protein to serum protein was significantly higher in the treatment failures than in patients who responded to conservative therapy. ERCP was also found to be an important predictor of response to nonoperative therapy. Patients with pancreatic ductal changes indicative of severe chronic pancreatitis had a 10% or less chance of resolving their internal fistulas without surgical intervention.

Patients in whom conservative therapy fails should have their pancreatic anatomy more clearly defined. CT

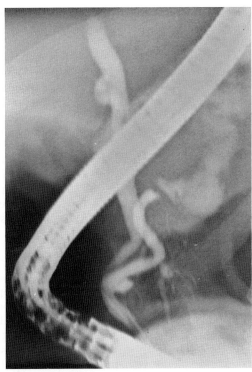

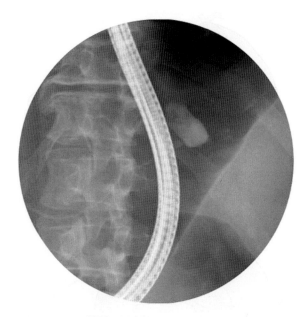

FIGURE 90-15 Endoscopic retrograde cholangiopancreatography revealing pancreatic–pleural fistula tract into left pleural space.

FIGURE 90-13 Endoscopic retrograde cholangiopancreatogram from the patient with pancreatic ascites whose computed tomographic scan is shown in Figure 90-12. Contrast extravasates from the proximal portion of the pancreatic duct into the peritoneal cavity. The visualized portion of the extrahepatic biliary tree is normal.

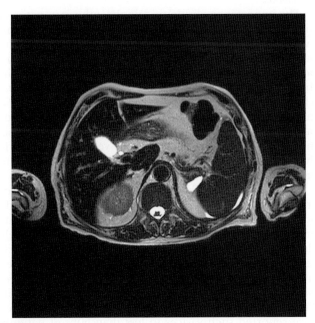

FIGURE 90-14 Pancreatic–pleural fistula tract from pancreatic tail via left crus into left pleural space.

or MRI/MRCP should be performed to assess the extent of pancreatic inflammation and to locate any pseudocysts associated with the ductal disruption. ERCP or MRCP is necessary to evaluate the pancreatic ductal anatomy and to identify the location of the leak. ERCP may identify

patients who may be treated by pancreatic duct stenting. Pancreatic duct stents bridging the ductal disruption have shown promise as a method to heal internal pancreatic fistulas. In the small number of reported cases, many stenting procedures have been successful, without complications.[86-92] As experience accumulates with these techniques, operative therapy may be avoided for all but the most complicated ductal disruptions. Anecdotal reports also exist of percutaneous pancreatic duct stents placed under ultrasound and fluoroscopic guidance. These techniques are unlikely to supplant the less demanding endoscopic approaches.

The choice of operative therapy is guided by pancreatic ductal anatomy. Distal pancreatic duct leaks may be addressed by *distal pancreatectomy*, a procedure that can be performed with low expected morbidity and mortality and eliminates the need for a pancreatic anastomosis. In some cases when proximal pancreatic ductal disease is present, the pancreatic remnant should be drained with a *Roux-en-Y loop*. If a direct duct leak is identified, the ductal disruption can be drained internally as a *Roux-en-Y pancreaticojejunostomy* (Figure 90-16). When ductal disruptions are associated with a pseudocyst, the pseudocyst may be drained either by a Roux-en-Y loop or into the stomach as a *cystogastrostomy*. These internal drainage techniques are always preferable to placement of external drains. Da Cunha et al showed that external drainage procedures are commonly complicated by infection and may require reoperation in up to 50% of cases.[93] Internal drainage, in contrast, has a greater than 90% chance of success. Although early series reported high mortality rates in patients undergoing operative therapy, many of these deaths could be attributed to poor nutritional status and less refined techniques in pancreatic surgery. More recent series report a mortality rate of less than 2%.[81,93,94]

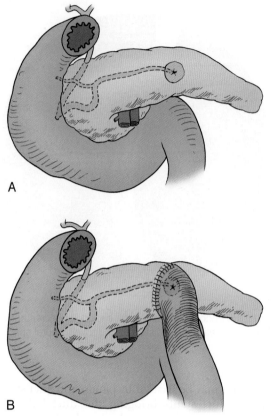

FIGURE 90-16 Schematic of pancreatic duct disruption **(A)** and pancreatic ascites treated by anastomosing a Roux-en-Y jejunal loop to the duct leak **(B)**. (From Cameron JJ, Brawley RK, Bender HW, et al: The treatment of pancreatic ascites. *Ann Surg* 170:668, 1969.)

EXTERNAL PANCREATIC FISTULA

Pancreaticocutaneous fistulas may be the result of trauma, surgical resection, necrotizing and chronic pancreatitis, or percutaneous drainage of a pseudocyst associated with pancreatic duct obstruction or disruption. Most fistulas will close spontaneously with adequate nutrition, resolution of the underlying pancreatic inflammatory process, and adequate local wound care. Refractory pancreaticocutaneous fistulas warrant further evaluation with ERCP or sinograms (or both) to delineate ductal abnormalities that may preclude spontaneous closure. Broadie et al reported on 38 patients evaluated by ERCP for pancreaticocutaneous fistulas. Fistulas originating from the side of the main pancreatic duct closed spontaneously within 11 weeks in 86% of patients. Side fistulas with continued pancreatic inflammation were less likely to close, with a 53% closure rate by 23 weeks. No end fistulas closed.[95]

Surgical treatment of persistent fistulas includes Roux-en-Y fistula tract–jejunostomy, pancreaticojejunostomy, or pancreatic resection. Fistula tract–jejunostomy is viewed as the safest option because it allows internal drainage in an operative field that is distant from the inflamed pancreatic bed. Best results are achieved in a stable patient with a mature fistula tract. A recent review of surgical treatment for pancreatic fistulas found that surgical closure was achieved in 90% of patients; however, operative mortality was noted in roughly 6.3% of the population.[96]

Endoscopic pancreatic duct stenting has been reported as a treatment option for refractory fistulas. Pancreatic stents successfully closed 55% of fistulas in a recent series of 97 patients with duct disruption.[97] Endoscopic transpapillary nasopancreatic drainage was recently reported for management of pancreatic fistulas following surgical and radiologic interventions. Ninety-one percent of patients with a partial pancreatic duct disruption were healed within 2 to 8 weeks, whereas only 33% of complete duct disruptions closed with this transpapillary technique.[98] These techniques may prove to be effective, minimally invasive approaches for fistula closure as technology and experience improve.[99,100]

SPLENIC VEIN THROMBOSIS

The splenic vein lies posterior to and closely approximated to the body of the pancreas, and it runs from the pancreatic tail to the neck of the gland. Immediately dorsal to the neck, the splenic vein joins with the superior mesenteric vein to form the portal vein. This location makes the splenic vein particularly susceptible to involvement by inflammatory diseases of the pancreas. Invasive neoplastic or inflammatory disease may lead to intrinsic damage to the venous intima or extrinsic compression secondary to edema, fibrosis, mass lesions, or lymphadenopathy. In either case, stasis of splenic vein blood flow occurs and may eventually lead to *splenic vein thrombosis.*

The importance of splenic vein thrombosis in patients with chronic pancreatitis is not completely known. Commonly used imaging techniques (particularly CT scan) have led to an increased diagnosis of splenic vein thrombosis in patients with chronic pancreatitis. Splenic vein thrombosis is clinically silent in the majority of patients. The incidence appears to be approximately 7% to 15% in patients with chronic pancreatitis, with 2% to 5% of patients having extension of the splenic vein thrombosis into the portal vein.[101,102] Splenic vein thrombosis is thought to be a relatively late complication of chronic pancreatitis.

Splenic vein thrombosis causes complications secondary to the development of extrahepatic, "left-sided" portal hypertension. Obstruction of splenic venous outflow leads to the enlargement of collateral vessels along the short gastric and gastroepiploic veins, which results in the formation of *gastric varices* along the greater curvature and fundus of the stomach, as well as *esophageal varices* secondary to increased flow to the coronary vein. These varices do not form in all patients, and some series have reported such varices in less than 50% of patients with documented splenic vein thrombosis.[101-104] *Splenomegaly* is a related common finding in patients with splenic vein thrombosis. The most common complication of splenic vein thrombosis is *upper gastrointestinal hemorrhage* secondary to gastric or esophageal varices, which occurs in less than 10% of patients with known thrombosis.[101] Patients may also have abdominal pain or, rarely, ascites. Another important manifestation of splenic vein thrombosis is excessive *intraoperative blood loss* as a result of the enlarged venous collateral vessels. Splenic vein thrombosis should be carefully noted in patients with chronic pancreatitis who are to undergo operative therapy.

As the diagnosis of *asymptomatic splenic vein thrombosis* has increased, more information has been obtained about the natural history of this process and the indications for intervention. In a prospective study by Bernades et al, 266 patients with chronic pancreatitis were monitored for a mean period of 8.2 years.[101] These patients were screened with ultrasound for splenic vein thrombosis, which was confirmed by CT or angiography. The incidence of splenic or portal vein thrombosis was 13.2%, with varices occurring in 17% of these patients. One patient required surgery for variceal bleeding. Twenty-three patients with splenic vein thrombosis underwent no therapy, and no episodes of bleeding occurred in more than 2½ years of observation.

Treatment of patients with bleeding gastroesophageal varices secondary to splenic vein thrombosis is *splenectomy*. This operation eliminates splenic artery inflow and venous outflow, with an attendant immediate reduction in variceal blood flow. Moosa and Gadd reported a cure rate of greater than 90% in patients undergoing splenectomy at a mean followup of 11 months.[105] "*Nonsurgical splenectomy*" via splenic artery embolization is a nonoperative intervention that may be appropriate for selected patients with extensive comorbidity. These patients are at risk for splenic abscess. Clearly, asymptomatic splenic vein thrombosis deserves no specific intervention. Splenectomy is the treatment of choice in most patients with symptomatic gastroesophageal varices.

REFERENCES

1. Bradley EL III: A clinically based classification system for acute pancreatitis. *Arch Surg* 128:586, 1993.
2. Bradley EL, III, Gonzalez AC, Clements JL, Jr: Acute pancreatic pseudocysts: Incidence and implications. *Ann Surg* 184:734, 1976.
3. Grace P, Williamson R: Modern management of pancreatic pseudocysts. *Br J Surg* 80:573, 1993.
4. Imrie CW, Buist LJ, Shearer MG: Importance of cause in the outcome of pancreatic pseudocysts. *Am J Surg* 156:159, 1988.
5. Nguyen BLT, Thompson JS, Edney JA, et al: Influence of the etiology of pancreatitis on the natural history of pancreatic pseudocysts. *Am J Surg* 162:527, 1991.
6. Ephgrave K, Hunt JL: Presentation of pancreatic pseudocysts: Implications for timing of surgical intervention. *Am J Surg* 151:749, 1986.
7. Mullins RJ, Malangoni MA, Bergamini TM, et al: Controversies in the management of pancreatic pseudocysts. *Am J Surg* 155:165, 1988.
8. Wilford ME, Foster WL, Halvorsen RA, et al: Pancreatic pseudocyst: Comparative evaluation by sonography and computed tomography. *AJR Am J Roentgenol* 140:53, 1983.
9. Morgan DE, Baron TH, Smith JK, et al: Pancreatic fluid collections prior to intervention: Evaluation with MR imaging compared with CT and US. *Radiology* 203:773, 1997.
10. Barishma MA, Yucel EK, Ferrucci JT: Magnetic resonance cholangiopancreatography. *N Engl J Med* 341:258, 1999.
11. Varghese JC, Materson A, Lee MJ: Value of MR pancreatography in evaluation of patients with chronic pancreatitis. *Clin Radiol* 57:393, 2002.
12. Lewandrowski KB, Southern JF, Pins MR, et al: Cyst fluid analysis in the differential diagnosis of pancreatic cysts: A comparison of pseudocysts, serous cystadenomas, mucinous cystic neoplasms, and mucinous cystadenocarcinoma. *Ann Surg* 217:41, 1993.
13. Brugge W, Lewandrowski K, Lee-Lewandrowski E, et al: Diagnosis of pancreatic cystic neoplasms: A report of the Cooperative Pancreatic Cyst Study. *Gastroenterology* 126:1330, 2004.
14. Vanderwaaij L, Van Dullemen H, Ponte R: Cyst fluid analysis in the differential diagnosis of pancreatic cystic lesions: A pooled analysis. *Gastrointestinal Endosc* 65:383, 2005.
15. Kolars JC, Allen MO, Ansel H, et al: Pancreatic pseudocysts: Clinical and endoscopic experience. *Am J Gastroenterol* 84:259, 1989.
16. Laxon LC, Fromkes JJ, Cooperman M: Endoscopic retrograde cholangiopancreatography in the management of pancreatic pseudocysts. *Am J Surg* 150:683, 1985.
17. O'Connor M, Kolars JC, Ansel H: Preoperative endoscopic retrograde cholangiopancreatography in the management of pancreatic pseudocysts. *Am J Surg* 151:18, 1986.
18. Walt AJ, Sugawa C: Endoscopic retrograde cholangiopancreatography in the surgery of pancreatic pseudocysts. *Surgery* 86:639, 1975.
19. Nealon WH, Townsend CM, Thompson JC: Preoperative endoscopic retrograde cholangiopancreatography in patients with pancreatic pseudocysts associated with resolving acute and chronic pancreatitis. *Ann Surg* 209:532, 1989.
20. Ahearne PM, Baillie JM, Cotton PB, et al: An endoscopic retrograde cholangiopancreatography–based algorithm for the management of pancreatic pseudocysts. *Am J Surg* 163:111, 1992.
21. Bradley EL III, Clements JL, Jr, Gonzalez AC: The natural history of pancreatic pseudocysts: A unified concept of management. *Am J Surg* 137:135, 1979.
22. Yeo CJ, Bastidas JA, Lynch-Nyhan A, et al: The natural history of pancreatic pseudocysts documented by computed tomography. *Surg Gynecol Obstet* 170:411, 1990.
23. Vitas GJ, Sarr MG: Selected management of pancreatic pseudocysts: Operative versus expectant management. *Surgery* 111:123, 1992.
24. Heider R, Meyer AA, Galanko JA, et al: Percutaneous drainage of pancreatic pseudocysts is associated with a higher failure rate than surgical treatment in unselected patients. *Ann Surg* 229:781, 1999.
25. Duvnjak M, Duvnjak L, Dodig M, et al: Factors predictive of the healing of pancreatic pseudocysts treated by percutaneous evacuation. *Hepatogastroenterology* 45:536, 1998.
26. Lehman GA: Pseudocysts. *Gastrointest Endosc* 49:S81, 1999.
27. Lang EK, Paolini RM, Pottmeyer A: The efficacy of palliative and definitive percutaneous versus surgical drainage of pancreatic abscesses and pseudocysts: A prospective study of 85 patients. *South Med J* 84:55, 1991.
28. Morton J, Brown A, Galanko J, et al: A national comparison of surgical versus percutaneous drainage of pancreatic pseudocysts: 1997-2001. *J Gastrointest Surg* 9:15, 2005.
29. Vitale GC, Lawhorne JC, Larson GM, et al: Endoscopic drainage of the pancreatic pseudocyst. *Surgery* 126:616, 1999.
30. Dunkin BJ, Ponsky JL, Hale JC: Ultrasound-directed percutaneous endoscopic cyst-gastrostomy for the treatment of a pancreatic pseudocyst. *Surg Endosc* 12:1426, 1998.
31. Beckingham IJ, Krige JEJ, Bornman PC, et al: Endoscopic management of pancreatic pseudocysts. *Br J Surg* 84:1638, 1997.
32. Beckingham IJ, Krige JEJ, Bornman PC, et al: Long term outcome of endoscopic drainage of pancreatic pseudocysts. *Am J Gastroenterol* 94:71, 1999.
33. Barthet M, Sahel J, Bodiou-Bertei C, et al: Endoscopic transpapillary drainage of pancreatic pseudocysts. *Gastrointest Endosc* 42:208, 1995.
34. Catalano MF, Geenen JE, Schmalz MJ, et al: Treatment of pancreatic pseudocysts with ductal communication by transpapillary pancreatic duct endoprothesis. *Gastrointest Endosc* 42:214, 1995.
35. Binmoeller KF, Seifert H, Walter A, et al: Transpapillary and transmural drainage of pancreatic pseudocysts. *Gastrointest Endosc* 42:219, 1995.
36. Bhasin DK, Rana SS, Nanda M, et al. Endoscopic management of pancreatic pseudocysts at atypical locations. *Surg Endosc* 24:1085, 2010.
37. Nealon WH, Walser E, Surgical management of complications associated with percutaneous and/or endoscopic management of pseudocyst of the pancreas. *Ann Surg* 241:948, 2005.
38. Evans KA, Clark CW, Vogel SB, et al: Surgical management of failed endoscopic treatment of pancreatic disease. *J Gastrointest Surg* 12:1924, 2008.

39. Newell KA, Liu T, Aranha GV, et al: Are cystogastrostomy and cystojejunostomy equivalent operations for pancreatic pseudocysts? *Surgery* 108:635, 1990.

40. Johnson LB, Rattner DW, Warshaw AL: The effect of size of giant pancreatic pseudocysts on the outcome of internal drainage procedures. *Surg Gynecol Obstet* 173:171, 1991.

41. Bhattacharya D, Ammori B: Minimally invasive approaches to the management of pancreatic pseudocysts: Review of the literature. *Surg Laparosc Endosc Percutan Tech* 13:141, 2003.

42. Teixeira J, Gibbs KE, Vaimaikis S, et al: Laparoscopic Roux-en-Y pancreatic cyst-jejunostomy. *Surg Endosc* 17:1910, 2003.

43. Pallapothu R, Earle DB, Desilets DJ, et al: Notes stapled cystgastrostomy: A novel approach for surgical management of pancreatic pseudocyst. *Surg Endosc* 25:883, 2011.

44. Escourrou J, Shehab H, Buscail L, et al: Peroral transgastric/transduodenal necrosectomy: Success in the treatment of infected pancreatic necrosis. *Ann Surg* 248:1074, 2008.

45. Yeo CJ: Pancreatic pseudocyst, ascites, and fistulas. *Curr Opin Gen Surg* 4:55, 1994.

46. Nealon W, Walser E: Duct drainage alone is sufficient in the operative management of pancreatic pseudocyst in patients with chronic pancreatitis. *Ann Surg* 237:614, 2003.

47. Crass RA, Way LW: Acute and chronic pancreatic pseudocysts are different. *Am J Surg* 142:660, 1981.

48. O'Campo C, Alejandro O, Zandalazini H, et al: Treatment of acute pancreatic pseudocysts after severe acute pancreatitis. *J Gastrointest Surg* 11:357, 2007.

49. Barthet M, Bugallo M, Moreira LS, et al: Management of acute pancreatic pseudocysts: A retrospective study of 45 cases. *Gastroenterol Clin Biol* 16:853, 1992.

50. von Sonnenberg E, Wittich GR, Casola G, et al: Percutaneous drainage of infected and noninfected pseudocysts: Experience in 101 patients. *Radiology* 170:757, 1989.

51. Grosso M, Gandini G, Cassinis MC, et al: Percutaneous treatment of 74 pancreatic pseudocysts. *Radiology* 173:493, 1989.

52. Adams DB, Harvey TS, Anderson MC, et al: Percutaneous catheter drainage of infected pancreatic and peripancreatic fluid collections. *Arch Surg* 125:1554, 1990.

53. Horvath K, Brody F, Davis B, et al: Minimally invasive management of pancreatic disease. *Surg Endosc* 21:367, 2007.

54. Connor S, Ghaneh P, Raraty M, et al: Minimally invasive retroperitoneal pancreatic necrosectomy. *Dig Surg* 20:270, 2003.

55. Lakshmanan R, Ganpathi I, Lee VT, et al: Minimally invasive retroperitoneal pancreatic necrosectomy in the management of infected pancreatitis. *Surg Laparosc Endosc Percutan Tech* 20:e11, 2010.

56. Shinozuka N, Okada K, Torii T, et al: Endoscopic pancreatic duct drainage and stenting for acute pancreatitis and pancreatic cyst and abscess. *J Hepatobiliary Surg* 14:569, 2007.

57. Trevino JM, Tamhane A, Varadarajulu S: Successful stenting in ductal disruption favorably impacts treatment outcomes in patients undergoing transmural drainage of peripancreatic fluid collections. *J Gastroenterol Hepatol* 25:526, 2010.

58. Adams DB, Zellner JL, Anderson MC: Arterial hemorrhage complicating pancreatic pseudocyst: Role of angiography. *J Surg Res* 54:150, 1993.

59. Stabile BE, Wilson SE, Debas HT: Reduced mortality from bleeding pseudocysts and pseudoaneurysms caused by pancreatitis. *Arch Surg* 118:45, 1983.

60. Huizinga WKH, Kalideen JM, Bryer JV, et al: Control of major hemorrhage associated with pancreatic pseudocysts and pseudoaneurysms caused by pancreatitis. *Br J Surg* 71:133, 1984.

61. Steckman ML, Dooley MC, Jaques PF, et al: Major gastrointestinal hemorrhage from peripancreatic blood vessels in pancreatitis: Treatment by embolotherapy. *Dig Dis Sci* 29:486, 1984.

62. Balachandra S, Siriwardena AK: Systematic appraisal of the management of the major vascular complications of pancreatitis. *Am J Surg* 190:489, 2005.

63. Bergert H, Dobrowolski F, Caffier S, et al: Prevalence and treatment in bleeding complications in chronic pancreatitis. *Langenbecks Arch Surg* 389:504, 2004.

64. Aranha GV, Prinz RA, Greenlee HB, et al: Gastric outlet and duodenal obstruction from inflammatory pancreatic disease. *Arch Surg* 119:833, 1984.

65. Propper DJ, Robertson EM, Bayliss AP, et al: Abdominal pancreatic pseudocyst: An unusual case of dysphagia. *Postgrad Med J* 65:329, 1989.

66. Winton TL, Birchard R, Nguyen KT, et al: Esophageal obstruction secondary to mediastinal pancreatic pseudocyst. *Can J Surg* 29:376, 1986.

67. Woods CA, Foutch PG, Waring JP, et al: Pancreatic pseudocyst as a cause for secondary achalasia. *Gastroenterology* 96:235, 1989.

68. Landreneau RJ, Johnson JA, Keenan RJ, et al: "Spontaneous" mediastinal pancreatic pseudocyst fistulization to the esophagus. *Ann Thorac Surg* 57:208, 1994.

69. McCormick PA, Chronos N, Burroughs AK, et al: Pancreatic pseudocyst causing portal vein thrombosis and pancreatico-pleural fistula. *Gut* 31:561, 1990.

70. Browman MW, Litin SC, Binkovitz LA, et al: Pancreatic pseudocyst that compressed the inferior vena cava and resulted in edema of the lower extremities. *Mayo Clin Proc* 67:1085, 1992.

71. Stone MM, Stone NN, Meller S, et al: Bilateral ureteral obstruction: An unusual complication of pancreatitis. *Am J Gastroenterol* 84:49, 1989.

72. Baranyai Z, Jakab F: Pancreatic pseudocyst propagating into retroperitoneum and mediastinum. *Acta Chir Hung* 36:16, 1997.

73. Singh P, Holubka J, Patel S: Acute mediastinal pancreatic fluid collection with pericardial and pleural effusion: Complete resolution after treatment with octreotide. *Dig Dis Sci* 41:1966, 1996.

74. Lee FY, Wang YT, Poh SC: Congestive heart failure due to a pancreatic pseudocyst. *Cleve Clin J Med* 61:141, 1994.

75. Warshaw AL, Rattner DW: Facts and fallacies of common bile duct obstruction by pancreatic pseudocysts. *Ann Surg* 193:33, 1980.

76. Lipsett PA, Cameron JL: Internal pancreatic fistula. *Am J Surg* 163:216, 1992.

77. Smith EB: Hemorrhagic ascites and hemothorax associated with benign pancreatic disease. *Arch Surg* 67:52, 1953.

78. Cameron JL, Anderson RD, Zuidema G: Pancreatic ascites. *Surg Gynecol Obstet* 125:328, 1967.

79. Parekh D, Segal I: Pancreatic ascites and effusions: Risk factors for failure of conservative therapy and the role of octreotide. *Arch Surg* 127:707, 1992.

80. Sankaran S, Walt AJ: Pancreatic ascites. *Arch Surg* 111:430, 1976.

81. Lipsett PA, Cameron JL: Internal pancreatic fistula. *Am J Surg* 163:216, 1992.

82. Cameron JL: Chronic pancreatic ascites and pancreatic pleural effusions. *Gastroenterology* 74:134, 1978.

83. Segal I, Parekh D, Lipschitz J, et al: Treatment of pancreatic ascites and external pancreatic fistulas with a long-acting somatostatin analog (Sandostatin). *Digestion* 54:53, 1993.

84. Oktedalen O, Nygaard K, Osnes M: Somatostatin in the treatment of pancreatic ascites. *Gastroenterology* 99:1520, 1990.

85. Gislason H, Gronbech JE, Cerate O: Pancreatic ascites: Treatment of continuous somatostatin infusion. *Am J Gastroenterol* 86:519, 1990.

86. Kozarek RA, Ball TJ, Paterson DJ, et al: Endoscopic transpapillary therapy for disrupted pancreatic duct and peripancreatic fluid collections. *Gastroenterology* 100:1362, 1991.

87. Saeed ZA, Ramirez FC, Hepps KS: Endoscopic stent placement for internal and external pancreatic fistulas. *Gastroenterology* 105:1212, 1993.

88. Kiil J, Ronning H: Pancreatic fistula cured by an endoprosthesis in the pancreatic duct. *Br J Surg* 80:1316, 1993.

89. Holst T, Grille W, Asbeck F: Endoscopic therapy of a pancreatic effusion caused by chronic pancreatitis. *Z Gastroenterol* 36:893, 1998.

90. Bracher GA, Manocha AP, DeBarto JR, et al: Endoscopic pancreatic duct stenting to treat pancreatic ascites. *Gastrointest Endosc* 49:710, 1999.

91. Bhasin DK, Rana SS, Siyad I, et al: Endoscopic transpapillary nasopancreatic drainage alone to treat pancreatic ascites and pleural effusion. *J Gastroenterol Hepatol* 21:1059, 2006.

92. Varadarajulu S, Noone TC, Tutuian R, et al: Predictors of outcome in pancreatic duct disruption managed by endoscopic transpapillary stent placement. *Gastrointest Endosc* 61: 568, 2005.

93. da Cunha JE, Machado M, Bacchella T, et al: Surgical treatment of pancreatic ascites and pancreatic pleural effusions. *Hepatogastroenterology* 42:748, 1995.

94. Ihse I, Larrson J, Lindstrom E: Surgical management of pure pancreatic fistulas. *Hepatogastroenterology* 41:271, 1994.

95. Howard T, Stonerock C, Sarker J, et al: Contemporary treatment strategies for external pancreatic fistulas. *Surgery* 124:627, 1998.

96. Alexis N, Sutton R, Neoptolemus J: Surgical treatment of pancreatic fistula. *Dig Surg* 21:262, 2004.

97. Varadaraulu S, Noone T, Tutuian R: Predictors of outcome in pancreatic duct disruption managed by endoscopic transpapillary stent placement. *Gastroint Endosc* 61:568, 2005.

98. Rana SS, Bhasin DK, Nanda M, et al: Endoscopic transpapillary drainage for external fistulas developing after surgical or radiological pancreatic interventions. *J Gastroenterol Hepatol* 25:1087, 2010.

99. Cicek B, Parlak E, Oguz D, et al: Endoscopic treatment of pancreatic fistulas. *Surg Endosc* 20:1706, 2006.

100. Halttunen J, Weckman L, Kemppainen E, et al: The endoscopic management of pancreatic fistulas. *Surg. Endosc* 19:559, 2005.

101. Bernades P, Baetz A, Levy P, et al: Splenic and portal vein obstruction in chronic pancreatitis. *Dig Dis Sci* 37:340, 1992.

102. Sakafovas GH, Sarr MG, Farley DR, et al: The significance of sinistral portal hypertension complicating chronic pancreatitis. *Am J Surg* 179:129, 2000.

103. Evans GR, Yellin AE, Weaver FA, et al: Sinistral (left-sided) portal hypertension. *Am Surg* 56:758, 1990.

104. Warshaw AL, Jin G, Ottinger LW: Recognition and clinical implications of mesenteric and portal vein obstruction in chronic pancreatitis. *Arch Surg* 122:410, 1987.

105. Moosa AR, Gadd MA: Isolated splenic vein thrombosis. *World J Surg* 9:384, 1985.

Endoscopic and Minimally Invasive Therapy for Complications of Acute and Chronic Pancreatitis

Andrew Ross | Irving Waxman | Vivek N. Prachand

Although acute pancreatitis (AP) and chronic pancreatitis (CP) have historically been approached as separate clinical entities, in the past decade, advances in the understanding of the pathogenesis of both diseases has led to the recognition that acute, recurrent acute, and CP represent a disease continuum resulting from the inhibition of apical exocytosis of pancreatic enzymes, ultimately resulting in pancreatic autodigestion and an inflammatory response. This pancreastasis may be triggered by environmental factors (e.g., alcohol, smoking), ductal obstruction, or oxidative stress, particularly in the setting of a genetic predisposition. Although the initial clinical presentation of both entities may be similar, the complete resolution of symptoms, histologic changes, and return of normal endocrine and exocrine pancreatic function differentiates AP from CP. A subset of patients with AP, however, will go on to develop CP, particularly if the factors contributing to pancreastasis persist or recur. Although the initial clinical management of AP and CP is generally supportive and pharmacologic, invasive therapies can be necessary to treat their complications. As with many procedures, therapies that are less invasive in nature, because they utilize endoscopic, percutaneous, and laparoscopic approaches, have been developed in an effort to reduce the morbidity associated with traditional open surgical techniques. With rare exceptions, however, there is a paucity of long-term level I evidence favoring one approach over the other, and given the heterogeneity of clinical manifestations, local technical expertise, and anatomic variation, the therapies chosen should be individualized, preferably within the context of a multidisciplinary team of surgeons, gastroenterologists, and radiologists, taking into account the natural history and pathophysiology of the disease process.

INFECTED PANCREATIC NECROSIS

Acute pancreatitis accounts for more than 240,000 hospitalizations annually in the United States and has increased in incidence nearly 30% over the last two decades.[1] Although most AP is mild and resolves without sequelae, up to 20% of all cases of acute pancreatitis present as severe acute pancreatitis (SAP), defined clinically by the presence of multiple organ dysfunction, as well as local complications, such as pancreatic necrosis, with mortality rates reaching as high as 17%.[2] About half of SAP-related mortality occurs within 2 weeks of admission, usually related to a vigorous systemic inflammatory response, while late deaths are typically related to local complications, such as infected pancreatic

necrosis (IPN) resulting in sepsis and multiple organ dysfunction.[3]

The cornerstone of management of SAP is supportive care, typically in the intensive care unit (ICU), with more invasive treatments, such as surgical, percutaneous, or endoscopic debridement, reserved for patients with IPN, which may develop in nearly 50% of patients with pancreatic necrosis.[4] IPN is suspected by the presence of gas in a pancreatic or peripancreatic fluid collection on CT or failure to respond to maximal ICU support and confirmed by aspiration or drainage and culture of the collection. Approximately 25% of SAP patients develop IPN, which left untreated, has a mortality rate that approaches 100%. The historical gold standard for the treatment of IPN has been surgical debridement with the goal of removal of all infected tissues. The significant mortality (11% to 39%) and complication rates (34% to 95%) associated with open necrosectomy,[5,6] including the development of pancreaticocutaneous and enterocutaneous fistulas, incisional hernia, and exocrine and endocrine pancreatic insufficiency, have led to the development and implementation of less-invasive techniques, such as endoscopic necrosectomy, percutaneous drainage, and combined-modality therapy. Regardless of approach, because demarcation and organization of necrotic tissues requires several weeks and surgical mortality may be greater following early intervention, it is preferable to defer debridement of IPN for at least 3 weeks following the onset of SAP.

ENDOSCOPIC NECROSECTOMY

For patients with an organized pancreatic necrosis located within close proximity (approximately 1 cm) to the gastric or duodenal wall, endoscopic necrosectomy has emerged as a therapeutic alternative to surgery. The technique for endoscopic necrosectomy involves initial guidewire access to the necroma either via direct puncture (in the case of a visible luminal bulge) or through the use of endoscopic ultrasound-guided needle puncture and subsequent wire guide access (Figure 91-1). Once access is secured, the tract is dilated either using a graduated dilating catheter, needle knife sphincterotome, or cystotome, and subsequent dilation to 15 to 20 mm is performed using a balloon dilator to allow passage of an upper endoscope into the necroma. Debridement is then performed using a combination of endoscopic accessories. Maintenance of the tract is achieved by the placement of two or more pigtail stents or a fully covered, self-expanding metal stent into the cavity across the gastric or duodenal wall. This allows for repeat access and debridement following initial

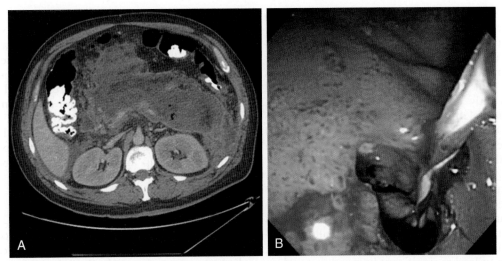

FIGURE 91-1 Endoscopic infected necroma drainage. **A,** CT scan demonstrating walled-off infected pancreatic necrosis. Note the gas bubbles present in the collection **B,** Endoscopic image demonstrating a transduodenal view into necroma.

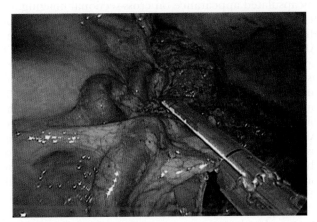

FIGURE 91-2 Perigastric varices caused by splenic vein thrombosis in chronic pancreatitis. Vascular stapler cartridges are used to divide the gastrosplenic ligament in preparation for laparoscopic distal pancreatectomy with splenectomy in a patient with hypersplenism and symptomatic chronic pancreatitis localized to the pancreatic tail.

necrosectomy. Placement of a nasocystic drain may be required for continuous lavage in select cases.

Several case series have reported the initial results of patients undergoing endoscopic necrosectomy for SAP. Although successful in avoiding surgery and pancreatico-cutaneous fistulas, there are several drawbacks to the technique. The largest series to date reported a procedure-related morbidity rate of 26% with a mortality rate of 7%, including two deaths directly related to the procedure.[7] In some cases, the necroma may not be adherent to the gastric wall. In such cases, air introduced during endoscopic insufflation can dissect freely into the lesser sac and may place the patient at increased risk for air emboli. In addition, large-diameter balloon dilation across the gastric wall may increase the risk of procedure-related bleeding, especially in the presence of left-sided portal hypertension and unrecognized gastric varices (Figure 91-2). Another drawback to endoscopic necro-sectomy is its resource-intensive nature, as this technique may require multiple procedures performed on consecutive days in the same patient,[4,8] which may not be feasible in a busy endoscopy unit with limited availability of fluoroscopy-equipped endoscopy suites.

PERCUTANEOUS DRAINAGE AND COMBINED-MODALITY THERAPY

Another method for drainage of IPN includes the CT-guided placement of large-caliber percutaneous drainage into the necroma. Drains are progressively upsized to a maximum of 30 French (F) to allow drainage and modest debridement of predominantly liquefied necrotic tissue. A single-center review of this technique found a less than 10% need for "rescue" surgical necro-sectomy with disease-related mortality rates of less than 10%.[9-11] Aside from the need for frequent radiographic tube checks and drain changes, as well as relatively inef-fective debridement of particulate necrotic tissues, a major drawback to this technique is the high rate of associated chronic pancreaticocutaneous fistula forma-tion. This is especially true in patients with the discon-nected duct syndrome—percutaneous drains placed into the disconnected segment of pancreas will almost uni-formly result in the formation of a chronic pancreatico-cutaneous fistula. As such, when disconnected duct syndrome is suspected based on central necrosis with normally perfused distal pancreatic tissue, endoscopic or magnetic resonance pancreatography should be per-formed prior to percutaneous drainage.

A combined-modality approach to draining IPN has been described.[12] In this technique, large-caliber percu-taneous drains are placed into the necroma followed immediately by endoscopic placement of double pigtail stents across the gastric or duodenal wall into the necrotic cavity. The pigtail stents are placed not for the purpose of endoscopic access into the necrosum, but rather as an attempt to create an internal fistula. As the cavity resolves over weeks to months of percutaneous drainage and debridement, the transenteric stents allow for redirec-tion of pancreatic juice into the GI tract. In patients with the disconnected duct syndrome, this technique is intended to prevent chronic pancreaticocutaneous fistula formation.

A recent retrospective comparison of standard percutaneous drainage versus combined-modality therapy for infected or symptomatic organized pancreatic necrosis demonstrated that the latter technique was associated with a significantly decreased length of hospital stay, duration of external drainage, and radiographic resource utilization.[13] Of the 23 patients undergoing combined drainage, none developed a pancreaticocutaneous fistula compared to three of the 43 patients undergoing standard drainage. There was no procedure-related mortality in the combined drainage group. Compared to endoscopic necrosectomy, the low procedure-related mortality rate associated with combined-modality therapy is likely secondary to the lack of large-caliber balloon dilation and passage of the endoscope into the necrosum, both of which can lead to significant hemorrhage and air emboli. A major consideration for combined-modality drainage is that it can only be used in patients in whom the necrosum is confined to the lesser sac where the cavity is within close proximity (<1 cm) to the gastric or duodenal wall.

MINIMAL ACCESS RETROPERITONEAL PANCREATIC NECROSECTOMY

Minimal access retroperitoneal pancreatic necrosectomy is an approach rapidly gaining favor for the treatment of IPN involving the pancreatic body and tail.[14] Several days following percutaneous placement of an 8F to 12F pigtail catheter to access the necroma, typically via CT guidance through a retroperitoneal window in the left flank between the kidney and splenic flexure, during which IPN is confirmed and appropriate antibiotics initiated, the patient is brought to the operating room, anesthetized, and placed in partial or full right lateral decubitus position. A guidewire is introduced through the drain under fluoroscopy, the drain removed, the skin incised and the tract dilated with Amplatz dilators to 30F to 45F diameter, the depth of dilation determined by preoperative CT. Through a nephroscope or a 15-mm laparoscopic cannula passed through the dilated tract and using a 5-mm laparoscope, graspers, and suction/irrigation devices, the necrotic tissues that are easily removed are gently debrided. After completion, a drain is placed into the cavity, maintaining access should further debridement be required based on clinical and radiographic findings. The skin is protected from pancreatic fluid injury through the use of a urostomy appliance. The drain is gradually withdrawn in 2- to 4-cm weekly increments until fully removed. Following removal, patients should be followed long-term for development of a pancreatic pseudocyst.

A recent multicenter randomized prospective trial (PANTER) of 88 Dutch patients comparing open debridement to a "step-up" approach to IPN treatment has been completed.[15] In this trial, minimal access retroperitoneal pancreatic necrosectomy was performed if two consecutive percutaneous drainage procedures failed to achieve clinical or radiographic improvement, with a primary outcome endpoint that included new organ system failure, perforation, enterocutaneous fistula, and death.

The step-up approach was associated with reduced incidence of a primary endpoint (40% vs. 69%), ICU admission (16% vs. 40%), incisional hernia (7% vs. 24%), new-onset diabetes (16% vs. 38%), and use of pancreatic enzyme supplements (7% vs. 33%). Interestingly, 35% of the step-up approach patients responded to percutaneous drainage alone and did not require minimal access retroperitoneal pancreatic necrosectomy. There was no difference in mortality (17% vs. 16%), and the total costs were $16,000 less per patient in the step-up group. As such, the step-up approach appears to have significant advantages over open necrosectomy.

PANCREATIC PSEUDOCYST

In patients with both AP and CP, disruption of the main pancreatic duct (PD) or its side branches can lead to the leakage of amylase-rich fluid into the peripancreatic tissues and retroperitoneum. Collections that persist for longer than 6 weeks with a characteristic round, encapsulated appearance on cross-sectional imaging are termed *pseudocysts* because of the absence of a true epithelium lining the cyst wall. Those that arise following AP are termed *acute pseudocyst*, while those following CP are termed *chronic pseudocyst*. Although they are often asymptomatic, pseudocysts can become infected, dissect into adjacent vascular structures, and obstruct the gastric outlet, as well as cause significant abdominal pain. The presence of these symptoms is an indication for drainage. Although size alone is not a criterion for drainage, larger pseudocysts tend to be the most symptomatic because of their space-occupying nature and resultant compression onto, or erosion into, contiguous structures. As with IPN, sufficient time to allow the robust development of the pseudocyst wall is required before drainage is contemplated.

Pseudocyst drainage can be accomplished through a variety of methods, including surgery (open and laparoscopic), interventional radiology, and endoscopy. There are no robust data to suggest the superiority of any of these modalities, and the choice of technique is typically based on local expertise. Endoscopic drainage can be performed with or without the use of endoscopic ultrasound (EUS) and can be approached through a transenteric or transpapillary approach. There are a number of series that have looked at either EUS or standard luminal endoscopy, or surgery for pseudocyst drainage.[16-19] Varadarajula et al randomized various endoscopic techniques of pseudocyst drainage and concluded that EUS procedures were more successful.[20] This same group demonstrated in a retrospective review that EUS-facilitated procedures had comparable efficacy and complications when compared to open pseudocystogastrostomy, although endoscopically treated patients had statistically significant decreased costs and resource utilization as compared to patients treated with open surgery.[21] In a systematic review comparing endoscopic and laparoscopic pseudocyst drainage, however, the laparoscopic approach appeared to have a higher success rate and lower risk of complications and recurrence, although the heterogeneity of the reporting within the various studies limited the ability to perform a direct comparison.[22]

Endosonographic guidance is typically required in cases where a bulge is not visible within the gastric or duodenal lumen, although three-dimensional imaging has changed this from an absolute to a relative requirement. In the presence of a luminal bulge, the wall of the pseudocyst can be punctured using a sclerotherapy needle, following which contrast is injected under fluoroscopic control to ensure that the lesion has been entered. A needle knife or cystotome can then be used to access the pseudocyst and allow for guidewire placement. Subsequent to this, the tract is enlarged using graduated dilating catheters and/or through the scope balloon dilators. The cystgastrostomy or cystduodenostomy is then maintained by the placement of at least two transenteric double-pigtail stents. When EUS is required, the cyst is initially accessed using a 19-gauge fine-needle aspiration needle through which a guidewire is placed. Dilation and stent placement can then proceed as described previously, either using the echoendoscope or exchanging for a therapeutic upper endoscope or duodenoscope. Novel devices for EUS-guided cystgastrostomy including a single-step access and dilation platform have been recently introduced into clinical practice. Transpapillary drainage can be accomplished in cases where the pseudocyst communicates directly with the main PD. A guidewire and subsequent stent are placed directly into the pseudocyst cavity across the major or minor papilla. Small pseudocysts associated with a PD leak may resolve following transpapillary stent placement to bridge the ongoing leak and decrease transpapillary pressures.

In cases where transenteric drainage is performed, pancreatography—either endoscopic or magnetic resonance—should be performed so as to define ductal anatomy and to determine the presence of leaks or strictures, the treatment of which may allow quicker and more durable resolution of pseudocysts. Pancreatography in the setting of pancreatic pseudocysts also helps to define the duration of transenteric stent placement. In patients in whom there is no communication between the pseudocyst and the main PD, transenteric stents can likely be removed 6 to 8 weeks after the pseudocyst has been completely drained. In cases where there is communication with the main PD, drainage is required for as long as the duct leak persists.[23]

The major complications associated with endoscopic pseudocyst drainage—infection, bleeding, stent migration, and perforation—occur in up to 37% of patients.[24-26] Infection is by far the most common complication seen, and as such, periprocedural prophylactic antibiotics are typically administered. Infection typically occurs as a result of incomplete evacuation of the cyst cavity, particularly when stents become blocked, or because of inadvertent drainage of organized pancreatic necrosis.[27,28] The former typically can be avoided through the placement of at least two large-caliber double-pigtail stents into the cyst cavity, while misidentification of a necroma for a pseudocyst can occur with radiologist inexperience or inadequate-quality imaging studies. It is imperative to review high-resolution cross-sectional imaging—typically a contrast-enhanced CT scan—with an experienced radiologist prior to drainage. Collections that are debris filled, irregular in appearance, or have thick septations are more likely to be organized pancreatic necrosis or even cystic neoplasms rather than pseudocysts, and therefore are at high risk for infection with transenteric drainage alone.

Bleeding associated with pseudocyst drainage is usually a result of puncture of blood vessels during the drainage procedure. Patients at high risk are those with concomitant gastric varices in whom the use of EUS with color Doppler can theoretically reduce the risk of inadvertent puncture of adjacent blood vessels. The use of electrocautery to create the internal fistula may also elevate the bleeding risk for small vessels within the duodenal or gastric wall. Another potentially severe (but rare) cause of bleeding with endoscopic pseudocyst drainage is inadvertent puncture of an unsuspected pseudoaneurysm. In most cases, however, bleeding is mild and can be treated using endoscopic techniques such as infiltration with epinephrine, heater probe application or hemoclip placement. In cases of severe hemorrhage, use of electrocautery applied through a 10F cystotome, angiography, or surgery may be required.[29]

Other complications of endoscopic therapy, such as free abdominal perforation and stent migration, are rare. Free perforation is usually seen when the pseudocyst is located more than 1 cm away from the gastric or duodenal wall. On occasion, the cyst wall may not be fully mature and cyst contents may leak into the abdominal cavity following puncture. Surgical consultation is advisable when perforation is encountered, although some cases may be managed conservatively with bowel rest, antibiotics, and, if necessary, percutaneous drainage.

Laparoscopic approaches to pseudocyst drainage have been well-described and are identical to those of open surgery, in that drainage can be achieved via pseudocystogastrostomy, Roux-en-Y cystojejunostomy, or cystoduodenostomy, according to the anatomic topography of the cyst, dependently positioned if feasible to facilitate drainage. Although more invasive than endoscopic therapies, laparoscopic (and open) procedures allow for concomitant debridement of remaining pancreatic necrosis within the pseudocyst, improved assessment and control of bleeding from the enteric or pseudocyst wall, opportunity to obtain adequate biopsy of the pseudocyst wall to rule out malignancy, and positioning of the common opening to facilitate dependent drainage. The simplest laparoscopic technique for a lesser sac pseudocyst is cystgastrostomy via an anterior approach (Figure 91-3). After making a 2- to 3-cm anterior gastrotomy, the pseudocyst can usually be seen bulging against the posterior wall of the stomach, confirmed by inserting a gallbladder aspiration needle through the posterior gastric wall into the pseudocyst cavity. If it is not readily apparent, laparoscopic ultrasound can be used to localize the pseudocyst. The opening into the pseudocyst is widened with monopolar, bipolar, or ultrasonic energy source to accommodate passage of a laparoscopic stapling device, with a portion of the wall excised and sent to pathology to rule out malignancy. The choice of staple height requires surgical judgment based on the thickness of the common wall of the stomach and pseudocyst to achieve appropriate tissue compression for hemostasis without excessive

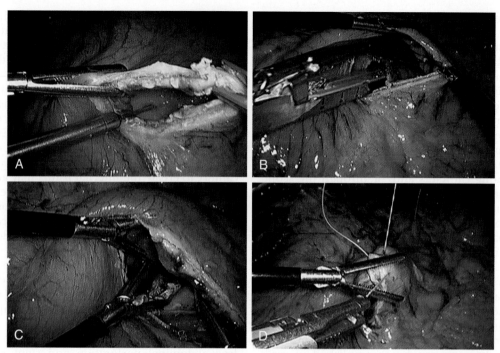

FIGURE 91-3 Laparoscopic cystgastrostomy. **A,** Needle aspiration of pseudocyst through posterior gastric wall via anterior gastrotomy. **B,** Thick-tissue stapler used to create common opening between posterior stomach and cyst wall. **C,** Debridement of residual necrotic pancreatic debris within cyst cavity. **D,** Sutured closure of anterior gastrotomy.

tissue necrosis. If the tissue thickness exceeds the capacity for stapling, the opening is extended and a running, slowly absorbable monofilament suture is used to approximate the edges of the opening. The pseudocyst cavity is explored, and any remaining necrotic tissues are gently debrided. The anterior gastrotomy is closed, and the patient can typically be started on liquids later that evening. Cystgastrostomy can also be performed via a lesser sac approach, which may be advantageous in allowing better dependent drainage as compared to the anterior approach, after opening the gastrocolic omentum, although the space can be obliterated because of prior pancreatitis episode(s).

Laparoscopic Roux-en-Y cystojejunostomy may be preferable to cystgastrostomy when a large pseudocyst extends inferior to the stomach. In this setting, the pseudocyst can be seen bulging through the transverse mesocolon when viewed from the infracolic perspective. A window is made through the mesocolon to the pseudocyst wall, avoiding injury to the middle colic vessels and inferior mesenteric vein, and following transection of the proximal jejunum 40 cm distal to the ligament of Treitz, the Roux limb is approximated to the pseudocyst wall using interrupted nonabsorbable or slowly absorbable suture with the stapled edge of the bowel and mesentery facing toward the patient's left side, and a stapled or sutured cystojejunostomy is performed as described earlier. The jejunojejunostomy is then performed at least 50 to 60 cm distally to reduce enteric reflux into the cavity.

Laparoscopic cystoduodenostomy for symptomatic pseudocysts in the pancreatic head can be performed when endoscopic drainage is inadequate, although this option should be used with caution so as to avoid injury to the ampulla as well as the risk of a side leak of the duodenal wall if healing of the anastomosis is inadequate—Roux limb drainage may be preferable if the anatomy and local tissue conditions do not clearly favor drainage into the duodenum.

PANCREATIC DUCT DISRUPTION

Disruption of the main PD or its side branches can be seen in both AP and CP. Virtually every case of acute pancreatitis involves some form of duct leak, which may or may not persist. Persistent leaks in the setting of acute pancreatitis can lead to pancreatic ascites and high amylase pleural effusions, pancreaticobiliary fistula, as well as the disconnected duct syndrome. In patients with CP, leaks are invariably associated with a downstream calculus or stricture. Endoscopy plays a significant role in the management of duct leaks in each of these clinical scenarios.

There are now several published series reporting transpapillary stents for ductal disruptions in the setting of pancreatic ascites and high amylase pleural effusions[30,31] in which more than 90% of patients resolve their fluid collection without complication or recurrence. Patients may require simultaneous large-volume paracentesis or concomitant pseudocyst drainage. It is likely that transpapillary stenting works less by leak occlusion than by bypassing potential areas of downstream obstruction and converting the duodenum to the path of least resistance to flow of pancreatic juice. Pancreaticobiliary fistulas almost invariably respond to concomitant pancreaticobiliary stenting[32] for 4 to 6 weeks, assuming that the fistula does not arise from the upstream portion of a disconnected gland. In this setting, it may be feasible to drain the segment into the fourth portion of the duodenum using EUS-guided stent placement,[33] although surgical therapy with Roux-en-Y drainage or distal pancreatectomy–splenectomy may ultimately be required, both of which can potentially be performed laparoscopically, although this has not yet been described. The former approach (internal drainage) was shown in one small series to have less operative time and blood loss, and has the theoretical advantage of preserving the endocrine function of the otherwise resected pancreatic segment.[34]

PANCREATIC DUCT STRICTURE

Strictures arising within the main PD are typically the result of chronic pancreatic inflammation or relapsing bouts of acute pancreatitis. Pancreatic malignancy is also a part of the differential diagnosis of PD strictures in the appropriate clinical setting. More than one stricture may be present at any given time with varying levels of symptomatology. In patients with CP, strictures may be associated with a ductal calculus. Once malignancy has been excluded by one or more methods (cross-sectional imaging, biopsy, EUS, cytology, or pancreatoscopy), a variety of therapeutic interventions can be employed in an attempt to alleviate symptoms such as pain and steatorrhea, which may be associated with chronic ductal strictures.

The endoscopic approach to managing PD strictures begins with guidewire access into the PD following a pancreatic sphincterotomy. There are a variety of methods for stricture dilation, including graduated dilating catheters and controlled radial expansion polyethylene balloons. Balloons are used most frequently; the size of balloon selected should approximate that of the PD downstream from the stenosis so as to avoid rupture of the more normal portion of the duct. Dilation is performed to waist effacement.

In strictures that are acutely angulated or impassable by graduated dilating catheters or balloon dilators, the use of a Soehendra stent extractor may be initially required to "drill through" the stricture prior to dilation. This is often the case with large PD calculi. Following dilation, most endoscopists attempt to place a 5F to 10F polyethylene stent approximating the downstream diameter of the duct. In patients who are symptomatically improved, prostheses are retrieved at 2 to 3 months followed by redilation and upsizing of the stent, if possible. This process is repeated several times over the course of a year, and if there is no stricture or symptom resolution and the patient becomes stent dependent, surgical therapy should be considered.

A recent single-center randomized prospective study comparing open surgical pancreaticojejunostomy to transampullary endoscopic therapy of 39 patients with symptomatic main duct strictures with a dilated (>5 mm) proximal duct suggested improved pain scores and better physical health summary scores in the surgically treated group, with 75% complete or partial pain relief versus 32% in the endoscopically treated group. Complication rates, length of stay, and changes in pancreatic function were similar between the two groups, although the endoscopically treated group required more procedures than the surgery group (median of eight vs. three). The trial was stopped early because of these findings.[35] In this study, a single 10F stent without side holes was used. In contrast, it has been our practice to place multiple, parallel 5F to 7F prostheses into the PD following stricture dilation. Although there are no clinical data to suggest that this is superior to a single larger stent, anecdotal experience suggests that this approach allows continued drainage between stents at the time of inevitable stent occlusion, which is nearly universal within 8 weeks after placement. In turn, this likely reduces the risk of both obstructive pancreatic infections and recurrent obstructive pancreatitis in the setting of stent occlusion. The recent introduction of fully covered self-expanding metal stents into clinical endoscopic practice has raised the possibility of using these larger-caliber devices as a removable endoprosthesis for benign strictures of the pancreaticobiliary tree. Additional study is required prior to advocating the routine use of these significantly more costly devices for benign PD strictures.

Several published series now exist that demonstrate a 60% to 80% reduction in attacks of relapsing pancreatitis following endotherapy for PD strictures.[36-42] Although a decrease in or resolution of chronic pain has also been suggested, this claim must be qualified by the fact that few studies have used true objective measurements, such as quality of life indices, reproducible pain scales, or pre- and posttreatment analgesic requirements. Furthermore, PD stenting is not without its own risk of iatrogenic complications. Side-branch occlusion, parenchymal atrophy, and glandular fibrosis are all possibilities when stents are placed into relatively normal ducts.[43,44] Moreover, inflammation or "ductitis" induced by a stent side flap or pressure from the internal stent tip can lead to further fibrosis and ductal stenoses. Additionally, because pancreatic stents are associated with bacterial colonization of the duct,[45] stent occlusion can lead to infectious complications, such as abscess formation and pancreatic sepsis, in addition to recurrence of pancreatic symptoms and duct blowout with formation of pseudocysts. As such, stenting must be used judiciously, preferably following multidisciplinary discussion of the therapeutic options.

The existing literature shows at best a 50% rate of resolution when PD strictures are endoscopically treated for 1 year, with most series suggesting rates closer to 20% to 30%.[46-50] It is important to recognize, however, that the presence of a stricture does not imply symptoms and, indeed, 60% to 80% of patients become asymptomatic following endoscopic therapy, even in the presence of a residual stenosis. Why this occurs remains unclear, however; increased flow of pancreatic juice, accelerated CP in side-branch parenchyma with resultant diminution of pain from capsular distention, and resolution of small upstream stenoses have all been hypothesized.

ENDOSCOPIC ULTRASOUND–GUIDED RENDEZVOUS

In some patients, the PD cannot be accessed through either the major or minor papilla because of a severe stenosis or calculus in the head of the pancreas. In cases where the main PD is dilated upstream from the stenosis, transpapillary access can often be obtained through the use of an EUS-guided "rendezvous" procedure.[51,52] A 19-gauge needle can be passed under EUS control into the dilated PD through which a slick 0.025-inch or 0.035-inch guidewire can be passed in an antegrade fashion through the stricture into the duodenum. After exchanging for a duodenoscope, cannulation can be achieved alongside the guidewire or the wire can be grasped using a snare or forceps and brought out through the accessory channel of the duodenoscope over which therapeutic accessories can subsequently be passed. This technique can also be used in patients with altered anatomy who require pancreatic intervention. One such group of patients are those who have undergone pancreaticoduodenectomy in whom an anastomotic stricture has developed at the pancreaticojejunostomy.

In cases where transpapillary access cannot be achieved in an antegrade fashion using the rendezvous technique, transgastric drainage of the PD has been reported.[50] A guidewire is left coiled within the dilated PD over which the tract is dilated either using a needle knife, cystotome, graduated dilating catheter, or Soehendra stent extractor. A pigtail or straight stent can then be passed over the guidewire into the dilated PD to allow for drainage into the stomach.

PANCREATIC DUCT STONES

As opposed to their biliary counterparts, PD calculi represent a more vexing clinical problem. Several factors contribute to this, including a significantly harder composition than bile duct stones as a consequence of the predominance of calcium carbonate, in addition to commonly being located upstream from a PD stricture. Indeed, less than half of patients with PD calculi have stones that are amenable to endoscopic extraction alone; the other 50% require some form of lithotripsy to facilitate removal. Finally, the PD upstream from impacted calculi can be markedly dilated; the resultant intraductal hypertension can lead to ductal disruption and the development of pancreatic pseudocysts, ascites, and pleural effusions.

Like other complications arising from CP, the management of PD calculi begins with obtaining high-quality cross-sectional imaging in the form of CT or MRI/magnetic resonance cholangiopancreatography. This allows for preprocedural planning and estimation of stone size, as well as the identification of sequelae of ductal disruption. Smaller stones can be removed by standard extraction techniques using an extraction balloon or basket passed alongside or over a hydrophilic guidewire. Dilation of ductal strictures, using a graduated dilating catheter or hydrostatic balloon, is required when stones are impacted upstream from a stenosis. In the case of severe stenosis that will not allow passage of a catheter or balloon dilator, the stricture and stone can be "drilled" through using a Soehendra stent extractor. In the majority of cases, endoscopic pancreatic sphincterotomy is performed to facilitate stone extraction. In some cases of obstructive CP, a "pseudodivisum" may be present in which the ventral PD is obstructed by a large stone or severe stricture. In such cases, access and drainage must typically be achieved through the minor papilla.

PANCREATIC LITHOTRIPSY

A majority of patients will require some form of lithotripsy to facilitate stone extraction. Mechanical lithotripsy can be difficult with PD stones, especially in the presence of a PD stricture, as the basket must be passed upstream from the calculus to allow for full deployment and stone capture. Probe-based lithotripsy—either electrohydraulic or laser—can be performed at the time of pancreatoscopy. The fragility of the instruments required, as well as the need to pass a pancreatoscope into an often strictured PD to access the stone, make this a more difficult, if not less attractive, option. Owing to the difficulties associated with both mechanical and probe-based lithotripsy, the majority of patients with large PD stones initially undergo extracorporeal shock wave lithotripsy (ESWL) for fragmentation prior to endoscopic extraction. Stone localization is required prior to ESWL, although some calculi will be evident on plain abdominal film. For those that are not, placement of a PD stent or nasopancreatic drain can be performed, the latter having the advantage of allowing for a pancreatogram to be performed to ensure fragmentation (stone diameter <2 mm) following a lithotripsy treatment. It is our practice to perform endoscopic retrograde cholangiopancreatography (ERCP) immediately following ESWL, at which time a PD sphincterotomy and stone extraction are performed. Both saline lavage at the time of post-ESWL ERCP, and nasopancreatic drain placement at the time of endoscopic retrograde pancreatography, seem to facilitate stone fragment passage and may preclude the need for multiple ERCPs. Regardless of whether ESWL was performed, placement of one or more endoprostheses into the PD is performed at the time of ERCP to allow for passage of additional stone fragments and allow for ductal decompression and prevention of pancreatitis secondary to edema from the performance of pancreatic endoscopic sphincterotomy (Figure 91-4). Interestingly, a randomized, prospective, controlled trial comparing ESWL to ESWL combined with endoscopic therapy demonstrated pain relapse (38% vs. 45%), reduction in pain episode frequency (3.8 vs. 3.7), and reduction in PD diameter (1.7 mm) that were not significantly different from one another, although the ESWL with endoscopy group had treatment costs three times greater than the ESWL group, suggesting that endoscopic therapy may not always be necessary following ESWL.[53] Furthermore, the patients were not blinded to their treatment group, which one might suspect would actually favor the combined therapy group because of placebo/suggestive effect of the additional intervention. It should also be noted, however, that nearly a third of ESWL-only treated patients did require subsequent ERCP.

Although there are data to suggest that endoscopic stone extraction leads to clinical improvement,[54,55] not all patients with chronic calcific pancreatitis should undergo attempted stone extraction. Poor candidates include those with a major burden of small stones within the pancreatic head (pseudotumor); patients without a dilated PD upstream from the calculus; stones in side branches or the distal tail; ductal calculi within the setting of a disconnected duct; and concomitant presence of an

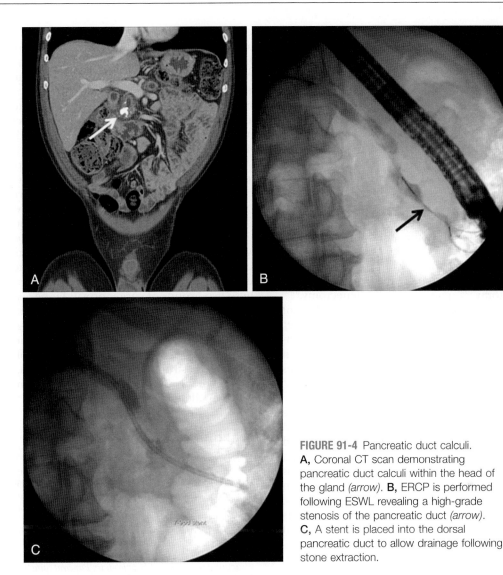

FIGURE 91-4 Pancreatic duct calculi. **A,** Coronal CT scan demonstrating pancreatic duct calculi within the head of the gland *(arrow)*. **B,** ERCP is performed following ESWL revealing a high-grade stenosis of the pancreatic duct *(arrow)*. **C,** A stent is placed into the dorsal pancreatic duct to allow drainage following stone extraction.

inflammatory mass in the pancreatic head. Such individuals should be considered for surgical treatment[56] or managed medically.

Most recent series suggest that approximately two-thirds of patients who have successful stone removal from the main PD will have a significant improvement in chronic pain and a decrease or elimination of attacks of relapsing pancreatitis.[57,58] One large series reported the results of ESWL pre- or post-ERCP in 40 patients with obstructing PD stones over a 5-year period.[59] Patients required an average of just over two ERCPs to completely clear the PD of stones. Complications occurred in 20% of the patients and included GI bleeding, exacerbation of pancreatitis, and bacteremia. At a mean followup of 2.5 years, 80% of patients avoided surgery and there was a statistically significant decrease in pancreatitis-related hospitalization and narcotic use, and improvement in an analogue pain scale. Despite this success and that of others, the requirement for careful patient selection cannot be emphasized enough. Those who are poor candidates for endoscopic therapy (see earlier), and those in whom repeated ERCP is required over a number of years to manage complications, should be strongly

considered for surgery. Even in an era of effective endoscopic therapy for CP and its associated complications, there are reasonable data to conclude that, in the appropriate candidate, surgical decompression or resection is superior to endotherapy in the long-term management of pain in patients with chronic obstructive pancreatitis.[60]

LAPAROSCOPIC DECOMPRESSION AND RESECTION IN CHRONIC PANCREATITIS

Abdominal pain is the predominant symptom in 85% to 90% of CP patients, and despite the advances in endoscopic interventions for the complications of CP (strictures, stones, pseudocysts), nearly half of CP patients continue to have progressively worsening pain, develop strictures of adjacent structures (bile duct, duodenum), or are noted to have radiographic lesions suspicious for neoplasia. As such, surgical intervention continues to play an important role in disease management. Because the pain in CP has multiple etiologies (ductal/tissue hypertension, neurogenic inflammation, visceral/central nerve sensitization, tissue ischemia),[61] surgical therapies for pain relief are thought to achieve their effects through decompression (lateral pancreaticojejunostomy, cystoenterostomy), resection (Beger procedure, Berne procedure, pancreaticoduodenectomy, distal pancreatectomy, total pancreatectomy), or a combination of the two (Frey procedure, Hamburg procedure). Details of these procedures and their outcomes are described elsewhere in this textbook. Procedure selection is based on the presence or absence of an inflammatory mass in the pancreatic head, dilated PD (with a diameter ≥7 mm considered to be "large duct"), extent of gland involvement, suspicion for cancer, and previous pancreatic procedures. Surgical therapy should achieve pain relief, address complications of adjacent structures if present, improve quality of life, and preserve endocrine and exocrine pancreatic function in a safe and durable manner. Minimally invasive surgical treatment of CP has been shown to be technically feasible with good short-term results: laparoscopic lateral pancreaticojejunostomy,[62-64] distal pancreatectomy,[65,66] pancreaticoduodenectomy,[67-69] and Frey procedure have all been described. Most of these series are relatively small, however, and the larger series are predominantly oncologic resections. Furthermore, there are no data comparing laparoscopy to open surgery in treating CP, nor are long-term outcomes regarding pain relief, quality of life, and endocrine/exocrine function available.

Nonetheless, laparoscopic pancreatic surgery has the potential to substantially reduce the morbidity associated with the midline or bilateral subcostal incisions utilized to perform the procedures listed previously. Given that most surgical candidates already have pain that is difficult to medically manage, reduced incisional pain following laparoscopy may be distinctly advantageous. Furthermore, the relative malnutrition of these patients may increase the risk of wound infection and incisional hernia, both of which are substantially reduced with laparoscopy. On the other hand, the inflammation, edema, and dense scar found in CP substantially increase the degree of difficulty of these procedures, whether performed open or laparoscopically, and should be taken into consideration. Additionally, in most of these procedures, the trauma caused by access to the abdomen is substantially outweighed by the surgical trauma of the procedure itself; indeed, the term *minimally invasive pancreaticoduodenectomy* is a significant semantic paradox.

From a technical standpoint, the Beger procedure appears to be the least amenable to laparoscopy, given the need to perform two pancreaticojejunostomies, dissect the portosplenic confluence in the setting of CP, and palpate the head of the pancreas to assess the depth of resection. Laparoscopic intraoperative ultrasound may be of utility for the latter, and is a mandatory skill, in addition to facility with intracorporeal suturing using fine suture and needles, in performing any of these procedures laparoscopically. The latter skills can be facilitated using robotic-assisted approaches. In contrast to the Beger procedure, lateral pancreaticojejunostomy, cystoenterostomy, and distal pancreatectomy are more readily performed laparoscopically, as they generally avoid the potentially hazardous major vascular dissection in the setting of CP and the required anastomoses are less technically challenging. The Frey and Berne procedures

represent an intermediate level of laparoscopic technical difficulty given the resection of the pancreatic head, though its resection is somewhat less extensive than that of the Beger procedure. The Hamburg procedure replicates the pancreatic head resection of the Beger procedure, increasing the laparoscopic degree of difficulty, although its lateral pancreaticojejunostomy is more amenable to laparoscopic suturing than the Beger procedure.

There are currently only a handful of pancreatic surgeons who have and regularly use the advanced laparoscopic skills necessary to effectively perform procedures for CP that require pancreaticoenteric reconstruction. There are correspondingly very few advanced laparoscopists who have adequate familiarity with the clinical management of CP and who regularly operate in the anatomic region of the duodenum and pancreatic head and neck. As such, collaboration and bilateral education between these two groups of surgeons will be necessary to bridge this gap so that patients may safely and maximally benefit from the available minimally invasive surgical therapies for CP. Similarly, given the need for individualized management of CP, a cooperative, multidisciplinary team of surgeons, gastroenterologists, radiologists, pain specialists, and dieticians is necessary for the optimal treatment of this challenging disease.

REFERENCES

1. DeFrances CJ, Hall MJ, Podgornik MN: 2003 National hospital discharge survey. Advance data from vital and health statistics No. 359. Hyattsville, Md, 2005, National Center for Health Statistics.
2. Lund H, Tonnesen H, Tonnesen MH, et al: Long-term recurrence and death rates after acute pancreatitis. *Scand J Gastroenterol* 41:234, 2006.
3. Gloor B, Muller CA, Worni M, et al: Late mortality in patients with severe acute pancreatitis. *Br J Surg* 88:975, 2001.
4. Hartwig W, Werner J, Uhl W, et al: Management of infection in acute pancreatitis. *J Hepatobiliary Pancreat Surg* 9:423, 2002.
5. Rau B, Bothe A, Beger HG: Surgical treatment of necrotizing pancreatitis by necrosectomy and closed lavage: Changing patient characteristics and outcome in a 19-year, single-center series. *Surgery* 138:28, 2005.
6. Connor S, Alexakis N, Raraty MG, et al: Early and late complications after pancreatic necrosectomy. *Surgery* 137:499, 2005.
7. Seifert H, Biermer M, Schmitt W, et al: Transluminal endoscopic necrosectomy after acute pancreatitis: A multicentre study with long-term follow-up (the GEPARD Study). *Gut* 58:1260, 2009.
8. Seewald S, Groth S, Omar S, et al: Aggressive endoscopic therapy for pancreatic necrosis and pancreatic abscess: A new safe and effective treatment algorithm (videos). *Gastrointest Endosc* 62:92, 2005.
9. Fotoohi M, D'Agostino HB, Wollman B, et al: Persistent pancreatocutaneous fistula after percutaneous drainage of pancreatic fluid collections: Role of cause and severity of pancreatitis. *Radiology* 213:573, 1999.
10. Fotoohi M, Traverso LW: Pancreatic necrosis: Paradigm of a multidisciplinary team. *Adv Surg* 40:107, 2006.
11. Fotoohi M, Traverso LW: Management of severe pancreatic necrosis. *Curr Treat Options Gastroenterol* 10:341, 2007.
12. Ross A, Gluck M, Irani S, et al: Combined endoscopic and percutaneous drainage of organized pancreatic necrosis. *Gastrointest Endosc* 71:79, 2010.
13. Gluck M, Ross A, Irani S, et al: Endoscopic and percutaneous drainage of symptomatic walled-off pancreatic necrosis reduces hospital stay and radiographic resource. *Clin Gastroenterol Hepatol* 8:1083, 2010.
14. Raraty MG, Halloran CM, Dodd S, et al: Minimal access retroperitoneal pancreatic necrosectomy: Improvement in morbidity and mortality with a less invasive approach. *Ann Surg* 251:787, 2010.

15. van Santvoort HC, Besselink MG, Bakker OJ, et al: A step-up approach or open necrosectomy for necrotizing pancreatitis. *N Engl J Med* 362:1491, 2010.

16. Johnson MD, Walsh RM, Henderson JM, et al: Surgical versus non-surgical management of pancreatic pseudocysts. *J Clin Gastroenterol* 43:586, 2009.

17. Melman L, Azar R, Beddow K, et al: Primary and overall success rates for clinical outcomes after laparoscopic, endoscopic, and open pancreatic cystgastrostomy for pancreatic pseudocysts. *Surg Endosc* 23:267, 2009.

18. Kahaleh M, Shami VM, Conaway MR, et al: Endoscopic ultrasound drainage of pancreatic pseudocyst: A prospective comparison with conventional endoscopic drainage. *Endoscopy* 38:355, 2006.

19. Varadarajulu S, Wilcox CM, Tamhane A, et al: Role of EUS in drainage of peripancreatic fluid collections not amenable for endoscopic transmural drainage. *Gastrointest Endosc* 66:1107, 2007.

20. Varadarajulu S, Christein JD, Tamhane A, et al: Prospective randomized trial comparing EUS and EGD for transmural drainage of pancreatic pseudocysts (with videos). *Gastrointest Endosc* 68:1102, 2008.

21. Varadarajulu S, Lopes TL, Wilcox CM, et al: EUS versus surgical cyst-gastrostomy for management of pancreatic pseudocysts. *Gastrointest Endosc* 68:649, 2008.

22. Aljarabah M, Ammori BJ: Laparoscopic and endoscopic approaches for drainage of pancreatic pseudocysts: A systematic review of published series. *Surg Endosc* 21:1936, 2007.

23. Deviere J, Bueso H, Baize M, et al: Complete disruption of the main pancreatic duct: Endoscopic management. *Gastrointest Endosc* 42:445, 1995.

24. Antillon MR, Shah RJ, Stiegmann G, et al: Single-step EUS-guided transmural drainage of simple and complicated pancreatic pseudocysts. *Gastrointest Endosc* 63:797, 2006.

25. Baron TH, Harewood GC, Morgan DE, et al: Outcome differences after endoscopic drainage of pancreatic necrosis, acute pancreatic pseudocysts, and chronic pancreatic pseudocysts. *Gastrointest Endosc* 56:7, 2002.

26. Cahen D, Rauws E, Fockens P, et al: Endoscopic drainage of pancreatic pseudocysts: Long-term outcome and procedural factors associated with safe and successful treatment. *Endoscopy* 37:977, 2005.

27. Baron TH, Thaggard WG, Morgan DE, et al: Endoscopic therapy for organized pancreatic necrosis. *Gastroenterology* 111:755, 1996.

28. Hariri M, Slivka A, Carr-Locke DL, et al: Pseudocyst drainage predisposes to infection when pancreatic necrosis is unrecognized. *Am J Gastroenterol* 89:1781, 1994.

29. Gambiez LP, Ernst OJ, Merlier OA, et al: Arterial embolization for bleeding pseudocysts complicating chronic pancreatitis. *Arch Surg* 132:1016, 1997.

30. Kaman L, Behera A, Singh R, et al: Internal pancreatic fistulas with pancreatic ascites and pancreatic pleural effusions: Recognition and management. *Austr N Z J Surg* 71:221, 2001.

31. Gomez-Cerezo J, Barbado Cano A, Suarez I, et al: Pancreatic ascites: Study of therapeutic options by analysis of case reports and case series between the years 1975 and 2000. *Am J Gastroenterol* 98:568, 2003.

32. Kozarek RA, Jiranek GC, Traverso LW: Endoscopic treatment of pancreatic ascites. *Am J Surg* 168:223, 1994.

33. Zhong N, Topazian M, Petersen BT, et al: Endoscopic drainage of pancreatic fluid collections into fourth portion of duodenum: A new approach to disconnected pancreatic duct syndrome. *Endoscopy* 43:E45, 2011.

34. Howard TJ, Rhodes GJ, Selzer DJ, et al: Roux-en-Y internal drainage is the best surgical option to treat patients with disconnected duct syndrome after severe acute pancreatitis. *Surgery* 130:714; discussion 719, 2001.

35. Cahen DL, Gouma DJ, Nio Y, et al: Endoscopic versus surgical drainage of the pancreatic duct in chronic pancreatitis. *N Engl J Med* 356:676, 2007.

36. Topazian M, Aslanian H, Andersen D: Outcome following endoscopic stenting of pancreatic duct strictures in chronic pancreatitis. *J Clin Gastroenterol* 39:908, 2005.

37. Ponchon T, Bory RM, Hedelius F, et al: Endoscopic stenting for pain relief in chronic pancreatitis: Results of a standardized protocol. *Gastrointest Endosc* 42:452, 1995.

38. Binmoeller KF, Rathod VD, Soehendra N: Endoscopic therapy of pancreatic strictures. *Gastrointest Endosc Clin N Am* 8:125, 1998.

39. Rosch T, Daniel S, Scholz M, et al: Endoscopic treatment of chronic pancreatitis: A multicenter study of 1000 patients with long-term follow-up. *Endoscopy* 34:765, 2002.

40. Boerma D, Huibregtse K, Gulik TM, et al: Long-term outcome of endoscopic stent placement for chronic pancreatitis associated with pancreas divisum. *Endoscopy* 32:452, 2000.

41. Delhaye M, Arvanitakis M, Verset G, et al: Long-term clinical outcome after endoscopic pancreatic ductal drainage for patients with painful chronic pancreatitis. *Clin Gastroenterol Hepatol* 2:1096, 2004.

42. Cremer M, Deviere J, Delhaye M, et al: Stenting in severe chronic pancreatitis: Results of medium-term follow-up in seventy-six patients. *Endoscopy* 23:171, 1991.

43. Smith MT, Sherman S, Ikenberry SO, et al: Alterations in pancreatic ductal morphology following polyethylene pancreatic stent therapy. *Gastrointest Endosc* 44:268, 1996.

44. Kozarek RA: Pancreatic stents can induce ductal changes consistent with chronic pancreatitis. *Gastrointest Endosc* 36:93, 1990.

45. Kozarek R, Hovde O, Attia F, et al: Do pancreatic duct stents cause or prevent pancreatic sepsis? *Gastrointest Endosc* 58:505, 2003.

46. Topazian M, Aslanian H, Andersen D: Outcome following endoscopic stenting of pancreatic duct strictures in chronic pancreatitis. *J Clin Gastroenterol* 39:908, 2005.

47. Ponchon T, Bory RM, Hedelius F, et al: Endoscopic stenting for pain relief in chronic pancreatitis: Results of a standardized protocol. *Gastrointest Endosc* 42:452, 1995.

48. Binmoeller KF, Rathod VD, Soehendra N: Endoscopic therapy of pancreatic strictures. *Gastrointest Endosc Clin N Am* 8:125, 1998.

49. Rosch T, Daniel S, Scholz M, et al: Endoscopic treatment of chronic pancreatitis: A multicenter study of 1000 patients with long-term follow-up. *Endoscopy* 34:765, 2002.

50. Boerma D, Huibregtse K, Gulik TM, et al: Long-term outcome of endoscopic stent placement for chronic pancreatitis associated with pancreas divisum. *Endoscopy* 32:452, 2000.

51. Shami VM, Kahaleh M: Endoscopic ultrasonography (EUS)-guided access and therapy of pancreatico-biliary disorders: EUS-guided cholangio and pancreatic drainage. *Gastrointest Endosc Clin N Am* 17:581, 2007.

52. Larghi A, Waxman I: Endoscopic ultrasound-guided rescue of an uncovered self-expanding metallic stent causing biliary obstruction. *Endoscopy* 38:857, 2006.

53. Dumonceau JM, Costamagna G, Tringali A, et al: Treatment for painful calcified chronic pancreatitis: Extracorporeal shock wave lithotripsy versus endoscopic treatment: A randomised controlled trial. *Gut* 56:545, 2007.

54. Smits ME, Rauws EA, Tytgat GN, et al: Endoscopic treatment of pancreatic stones in patients with chronic pancreatitis. *Gastrointest Endosc* 43:556, 1996.

55. Brand B, Kahl M, Sidhu S, et al: Prospective evaluation of morphology, function, and quality of life after extracorporeal shockwave lithotripsy and endoscopic treatment of chronic calcific pancreatitis. *Am J Gastroenterol* 95:3428, 2000.

56. Kozarek RA: Endoscopic treatment of chronic pancreatitis. *Indian J Gastroenterol* 21:67, 2002.

57. Smits ME, Rauws EA, Tytgat GN, et al: Endoscopic treatment of pancreatic stones in patients with chronic pancreatitis. *Gastrointest Endosc* 43:556, 1996.

58. Brand B, Kahl M, Sidhu S, et al: Prospective evaluation of morphology, function, and quality of life after extracorporeal shockwave lithotripsy and endoscopic treatment of chronic calcific pancreatitis. *Am J Gastroenterol* 95:3428, 2000.

59. Kozarek RA, Brandabur JJ, Ball TJ, et al: Clinical outcomes in patients who undergo extracorporeal shock wave lithotripsy for chronic calcific pancreatitis. *Gastrointest Endosc* 56:496, 2002.

60. Deviere J, Bell RH Jr, Beger HG, et al: Treatment of chronic pancreatitis with endotherapy or surgery: Critical review of randomized control trials. *J Gastrointest Surg* 12:640, 2008.

61. Demir IE, Tieftrunk E, Maak M, et al: Pain mechanisms in chronic pancreatitis: Of a master and his fire. *Langenbecks Arch Surg* 396:151, 2011.

62. Kurian MS, Gagner M: Laparoscopic side-to-side pancreaticojejunostomy (Partington-Rochelle) for chronic pancreatitis. *J Hepatobiliary Pancreat Surg* 6:382, 1999.

63. Tantia O, Jindal MK, Khanna S, et al: Laparoscopic lateral pancreaticojejunostomy: Our experience of 17 cases. *Surg Endosc* 18:1054, 2004.

64. Khaled YS, Ammori MB, Ammori BJ: Laparoscopic lateral pancreaticojejunostomy for chronic pancreatitis: A case report and review of the literature. *Surg Laparosc Endosc Percutan Tech* 21:e36, 2011.

65. Cuschieri A: Laparoscopic surgery of the pancreas. *J R Coll Surg Edinb* 39:178, 1994.

66. Patterson EJ, Gagner M, Salky B, et al: Laparoscopic pancreatic resection: Single-institution experience of 19 patients. *J Am Coll Surg* 193:281, 2001.

67. Gagner M, Pomp A: Laparoscopic pylorus preserving pancreatoduodenectomy. *Surg Endosc* 8:408, 1994.

68. Palanivelu C, Jani K, Senthilnathan P, et al: Laparoscopic pancreaticoduodenectomy: Technique and outcomes. *J Am Coll Surg* 205:222, 2007.

69. Kendrick ML, Cusati D: Total laparoscopic pancreaticoduodenectomy: Feasibility and outcome in an early experience. *Arch Surg* 145:19, 2010.

Imaging and Radiologic Intervention in the Pancreas

Aytekin Oto | Brian Funaki | Christine Schmid-Tannwald

Cross-sectional imaging modalities, such as computed tomography (CT), magnetic resonance imaging (MRI), and ultrasonography, are commonly used for diagnosis of pancreatic diseases. CT has been the most commonly used technique as it can provide high-resolution images of the pancreas and depict even small lesions and calcifications. With the advent of multidetector row spiral computed tomography (MDCT) technology, the acquisition speed and image quality have significantly improved. The development of 64-, 128-, 256-, and 320-slice scanners provides images with isotropic voxels on different phases of enhancement. MRI combined with magnetic resonance cholangiopancreatography (MRCP) has a growing role in imaging of the pancreas and biliary ducts. It allows evaluation of the pancreatic parenchyma, biliary, and pancreatic ducts and vessels during a single examination. The lack of ionizing radiation is an important advantage of MRI, making it an excellent choice for serial imaging. Transabdominal ultrasonography is often the primary diagnostic imaging modality in patients with suspicion of pancreatic/biliary disease. Contrast-enhanced ultrasonography may improve the accuracy in detecting pancreatic diseases but is not widely used in the United States. Even with the use of contrast agents, ultrasonography still has its own limitations. Visualization of the entire pancreas is often not possible because of overlying gas or obesity and the quality of examination is dependent on the experience of the operator. This chapter reviews the MDCT, MRI, and ultrasound imaging features of congenital, inflammatory, and neoplastic diseases of the pancreas, and the role of interventional radiologic procedures in their management.

CONGENITAL DISEASE

PANCREAS DIVISUM

Pancreas divisum is the most frequent congenital pancreatic abnormality. It may be asymptomatic; however, it is frequently associated with acute or chronic pancreatitis.[1] It is very difficult to diagnose pancreas divisum on CT because the pancreatic duct is difficult to visualize in its entirety on CT, especially when it is normal in size.

On the other hand, MRCP highlights the ducts and allows demonstration of separate entries of dorsal and ventral pancreatic ducts into duodenum in patients with pancreas divisum. Because pancreatic divisum is a key consideration in patients with pancreatitis of unknown etiology, MRI plays an important role in the imaging evaluation of these patients. Occasionally, the pancreatic duct is not visualized as a result of its small size or edema of the pancreas. In these cases, MRCP following secretin

administration can improve delineation of the pancreatic ductal anatomy (Figure 92-1).[2,3]

ANOMALOUS PANCREATICOBILIARY DUCTAL JUNCTION

In anomalous pancreaticobiliary ductal junction, the main pancreatic and common bile ducts join within the duodenal wall and form a common, usually more than 15 mm long, channel before the sphincter of Oddi.[4,5] Because anomalous pancreaticobiliary ductal junction is associated with pancreatitis and biliary carcinogenesis, its recognition is critical. Although endoscopic retrograde cholangiopancreatography is the most reliable method for evaluation, endoscopic sonography and MRCP are also useful for diagnosis. MRCP noninvasively detects the anomalous union between the common bile duct and pancreatic duct. MRCP can also reveal associated choledochal cysts, biliary dilation, and pancreatitis or biliary malignancy (common bile duct or gallbladder carcinoma).[6]

FATTY INFILTRATION

The distribution of fatty infiltration of the pancreas is generally diffuse but can also be focal and mimic a hypoattenuating mass on CT.[7,8] In these cases, MRI can provide correct diagnosis by using the chemical shift technique,[7,8] which unambiguously demonstrates fatty infiltration.

On CT, diffuse fatty infiltration appears as a separation of parenchymal tissue by intermixed, low attenuating areas. Fatty focal infiltration is seen as decreased-attenuation, nonenhancing fat interposed between normal pancreatic tissue. The focal sparing of fatty infiltration appears as a hyperdense, plate-like or triangular area,[8] compared to fatty infiltrated areas of the pancreas. On MRI, areas of focal fatty infiltration demonstrates loss of signal intensity on opposed-phase gradient-echo T1-weighted images, compared to in-phase T1-weighted images caused by the presence of intracellular lipid in these focal areas. Unlike pancreatic adenocarcinoma, focal fatty infiltration does not cause upstream pancreatic ductal dilation or displacement of adjacent vessels.

CONTOUR ABNORMALITIES

Annular pancreas is a rare congenital abnormality that may require surgical treatment, depending on the degree of duodenal obstruction.[9,10] CT and MRI demonstrate the normal pancreatic tissue encircling and encasing the second part of the duodenum. Immediate postcontrast images can be helpful to differentiate pancreatic tissue from the duodenum because of its early and significant enhancement and to demonstrate circumferential thickening of the duodenal wall. In addition, MRCP provides

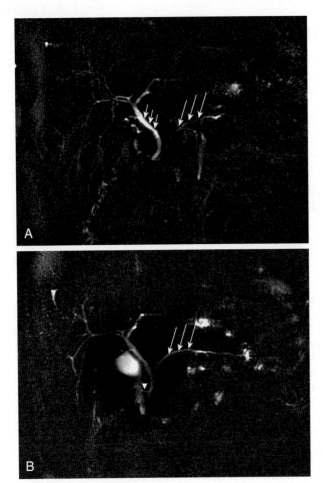

FIGURE 92-1 Pancreas divisum. **A,** Thick-slab MRCP image before secretin administration vaguely demonstrates the pancreatic duct *(long arrows)*. *(Short arrows* indicate common bile duct.) **B,** Following secretin administration, the pancreatic duct *(long arrows)* becomes much better defined as a result of distention and its separate opening to the duodenum *(arrowhead)* via the minor papilla becomes more prominent.

the depiction of course and drainage of the pancreatic and bile duct system.[9,10]

ACUTE PANCREATITIS

Acute pancreatitis is defined as an acute inflammatory process of the pancreas with involvement of adjacent organs and classified into edematous (70% to 80%) or necrotizing acute pancreatitis (20% to 30%).[11] The initial diagnosis is based on clinical features, but imaging may play a vital role in confirming the diagnosis, determining the severity, and detecting the complications of acute pancreatitis.[12] Ultrasound is frequently the first imaging modality and may identify underlying factors such as gallstones and biliary dilation. However, visualization of the pancreas is usually limited on ultrasonography. Contrast-enhanced CT is a fast and readily available imaging technique for diagnosis of pancreatitis.[13,14] MRI should be considered, especially in younger patients and in patients with risk factors for iodine contrast agents, and for followup.[12] MRCP allows evaluation of the entire

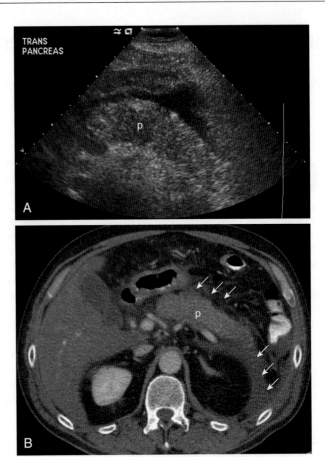

FIGURE 92-2 Acute pancreatitis. **A,** On ultrasound, pancreas *(p)* is enlarged and hypoechoic compatible with acute pancreatitis. A small amount of peripancreatic fluid is also noted. **B,** Contrast-enhanced CT image demonstrates edematous, enlarged pancreas *(p)* with peripancreatic fluid and inflammatory changes *(short arrows)* consistent with acute pancreatitis.

biliary and pancreatic ductal system and can be helpful in determining the etiology of acute pancreatitis.

The pancreas may appear normal on CT or MRI in mild cases of pancreatitis. Imaging features of the pancreas in acute pancreatitis include diffuse or focal enlargement with indistinct borders, heterogeneous, decreased signal on CT and T1-weighted images, and diminished enhancement because of edema. Peripancreatic inflammatory changes include stranding of surrounding fat and peripancreatic fluid (Figure 92-2). As the severity of the pancreatitis increases, nonenhancing areas of pancreas indicating necrosis can be seen.[12,13] Approximately half of the fluid collections, which do not resolve spontaneously, may become infected and evolve into pseudocysts or abscesses.[12] On MRI, peripancreatic fluid is best shown on T2-weighed images with fat saturation as high-signal-intensity collections.[11,12]

Complications of acute pancreatitis include infected necrosis, hemorrhagic fluid, pancreatic abscess, and pseudocysts (Figure 92-3, *A* and *B*).[11,12] Infected necrosis is a serious development often associated with complications and open surgical treatment and/or, increasingly, percutaneous drainage. The presence of gas within necrotic areas of pancreatic tissue suggests infected necrosis. Pseudocysts occur at last 4 weeks after the acute

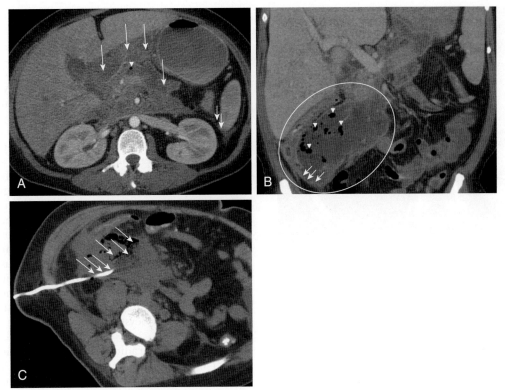

FIGURE 92-3 Necrotizing pancreatitis. **A,** Axial contrast-enhanced CT image demonstrates nonenhancing pancreas and peripancreatic fluid collections (pseudocysts) extending into the left upper quadrant *(long arrows)* with foci of air *(arrowhead)*. Free fluid is shown in the left anterior pararenal space *(short arrows)*. **B,** Coronal contrast-enhanced CT image demonstrates infected pseudocyst extending inferiorly into the right paracolic gutter *(circle)* with multiple foci of air *(arrowheads)* and enhancing wall *(short arrows)*. **C,** CT-guided drainage of the infected pseudocyst. Under CT guidance, pigtail catheter *(small arrows)* was placed into the collection and the fluid collection *(long arrows)* was drained.

onset of pancreatitis. They are usually round or oval in configuration and demonstrate rim enhancement representing a fibrous wall. Most of them are asymptomatic and remain stable or resolve spontaneously (40%).[12] If they are complicated by hemorrhage or infection, they may be drained percutaneously. On MRI, they appear hypointense on T1-weighted images, hyperintense on T2-weighted images, and show a progressive enhancement of their wall over time. Pancreatic abscesses have thick, enhancing walls.

Interventional radiology plays an increasingly important role in management of acute pancreatitis. Ultrasound or CT-guided percutaneous drainage or aspiration of fluid collections, abscesses, or pseudocysts is performed to exclude/confirm the diagnosis of infection or for definitive treatment.[12,15] Common access routes include a retroperitoneal approach through the lateral flank or an anterior approach through the peritoneum (see Figure 92-3, *C*).[15] Often, multiple large-bore drainage catheters (at least 12 French [F] to 14 F) with multiple side holes are necessary to drain viscous fluid collections. After placement of a drainage catheter, followup CT scans are required. By minimally invasive necrosectomy, a flexible endoscope can be placed in to the necrotic tissue cavity using an endoscopic or percutaneous approach, and necrotic material may be removed using irrigation, snares, and baskets. Emergency angiography and embolization may be required in patients

with vascular complications such as hemorrhage or pseudoaneurysms.[12]

CHRONIC PANCREATITIS

MRI, in combination with MRCP, is the most helpful noninvasive test for diagnosis of chronic pancreatitis. MRI allows evaluation of both parenchymal signal changes, atrophy, and pancreatic ductal changes. CT, on the other hand, is excellent for demonstrating characteristic pancreatic calcifications (Figure 92-4).

As early findings of chronic inflammation, abnormal pancreatic tissue signals are observed. Late findings include dilation and stenosis of the pancreatic and biliary ducts, intraductal calcifications, and parenchymal atrophy or enlargement.[16] Fibrosis is shown by a diminished signal on ultrasound, CT, and T1-weighted images on MRI. In patients with chronic pancreatitis, the pancreas demonstrates decreased enhancement compared to the normal pancreas.

Focal pancreatic enlargement as a result of acute/subacute pancreatitis may be difficult to distinguish from cancer. Distinguishing findings include the "duct-penetrating sign" (i.e., visualization of the normal duct in the focal abnormal pancreatic segment) and the presence of calcifications.

Complications of chronic pancreatitis include gastrointestinal obstruction caused by pseudocysts, pancreatic

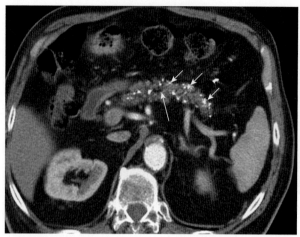

FIGURE 92-4 Chronic pancreatitis. Axial postcontrast CT image demonstrates atrophic pancreas with multiple calcifications (*short arrows*) and dilated pancreatic duct (*long arrow*) consistent with chronic pancreatitis.

abscess, vascular complications (e.g., portal vein or splenic vein thrombosis and arterial pseudoaneurysm), which may require radiologic interventions. MRCP with secretin stimulation allows evaluation of exocrine function of the pancreas. Negative oral contrast agents should be administered before secretin MRCP for accurate evaluation of pancreatic function.

AUTOIMMUNE PANCREATITIS

The diagnosis of autoimmune pancreatitis requires a multidisciplinary approach. Imaging modalities, especially CT and MRI, can confirm clinical suspicion and are helpful in monitoring the response to treatment.

In autoimmune pancreatitis, pancreatic parenchymal changes and abnormalities of the biliary and pancreatic ducts may be observed. Autoimmune pancreatitis leads to a diffuse ("sausage-shaped") or, more rarely, a focal ("mass-like") enlargement of the pancreas. The pancreas appears hypointense on T1-weighted images and hyperintense on T2-weighted images. Following intravenous contrast material injection, pancreatic enhancement can be delayed and peripancreatic rim enhancement can be appreciated. Irregular narrowing, strictures, and dilations of the pancreatic main duct and of the branch ducts may be best seen on MRCP. Other findings may include biliary strictures, retroperitoneal adenopathy, and bilateral, multiple, small hypodense/hypointense renal lesions.

Focal involvement of the pancreatic head must be distinguished from pancreatic cancer. Differentiation is extremely challenging but of paramount importance. In some cases, differentiation may be very difficult or impossible based on imaging findings alone. Identification of normal pancreatic duct within the suspicious, focal segment is an important imaging finding suggestive of a benign etiology, and should be actively sought, especially on MRCP. Irregular, but gradual tapering obstruction of the main pancreatic duct within the lesion, normal upstream duct, and normalization of the pancreatic

gland after steroid therapy all suggest the diagnosis of autoimmune pancreatitis.[17,18]

TRAUMA

Management of pancreatic injury is greatly influenced by the grade of the injury, especially the integrity of the main pancreatic duct and the presence of associated abdominal injuries.[19,20] CT is the modality of choice with sensitivity and specificity for pancreatic injuries greater than 85%.[21] Other imaging modalities are not as sensitive or specific and/or the examination (as for MRI) takes too long or is not available in most emergency settings.

On CT, imaging features include parenchymal laceration (i.e., areas of low intrapancreatic attenuation), fracture of the pancreas with or without separation of the fracture segments, hemorrhage, free fluid collections, thickening of anterior renal fascia, and associated injuries in the left upper quadrant structures.[19,20] Often, followup scans are required to exclude/monitor complications such as pancreatitis, pancreatic fistula, pancreatic abscess, or pseudocysts, which may require interventional management.

On abdominal radiograph, altered psoas shadow, mass effect indicating hematoma, or free air are significant findings, but occur in only 18% to 20% of patients with pancreatic injury.[22] Ultrasound is very limited in evaluation of pancreatic injuries. MRI provides not only the visualization of the entire pancreas but also the evaluation of the pancreatic duct. This may be useful, if a fracture of the pancreatic duct cannot be excluded by CT scan. On T1-weighted images the pancreatic tissue shows variable decreased signal intensity and enhances heterogeneously after gadolinium administration.[19,20] Fluid collections are best seen on T2-weighted fat-suppressed images as hyperintense areas.

NEOPLASM

ADENOCARCINOMA

Pancreatic ductal adenocarcinoma is characterized by its relatively rapid growth, early invasion of surrounding tissue, and early hepatic and lymphatic metastases. Criteria for unresectability include infiltration of the celiac trunk, superior mesentery artery or common hepatic artery, or distant metastases.

CT traditionally is the most commonly utilized method for diagnosing and staging pancreatic malignancy. MRI combined with MRCP and magnetic resonance angiography also provides the detection and characterization of pancreas lesions.[23] Ultrasonography is very limited in detection of focal pancreatic lesions and differentiation between cancer and chronic pancreatitis.

Both on CT and MRI, imaging at the pancreatic phase (i.e., approximately 45 seconds after contrast administration) and at the portal venous phase (i.e., approximately 70 seconds after contrast administration) is critical for detection of pancreatic adenocarcinoma, which is typically hypodense/-intense on these modalities following intravenous contrast administration (Figure 92-5, *A*). Mass effect of tumor involving the head of the pancreas

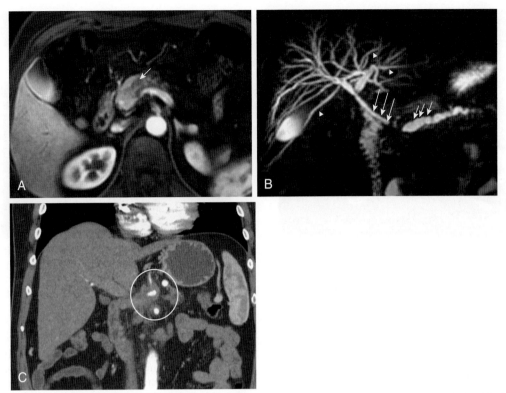

FIGURE 92-5 Adenocarcinoma of the pancreas. **A,** On contrast-enhanced T1-weighted image, hypointense, ill-defined lesion within the pancreatic head *(arrow)* consistent with adenocarcinoma of the pancreas. **B,** Coronal maximum-intensity projection MRCP image demonstrates "double-duct sign" caused by mass effect of the tumor involving the head of the pancreas: prestenotic dilation of the pancreatic *(short arrows)* and common bile duct *(long arrows)* and dilation of the intrahepatic biliary duct system *(arrowheads)*. **C,** Coronal contrast-enhanced CT image in the arterial phase demonstrates encasement of the celiac trunk and the superior mesentery artery *(circle)* by pancreatic adenocarcinoma.

causes upstream pancreatic and biliary ductal dilation ("double-duct sign") (Figure 92-5, *B*). Grading systems for diagnosing and assessing vascular invasion include the extent of contiguity with the vessels, morphologic deformation of vessels, dilation of peripancreatic veins, and the "teardrop sign" (Figure 92-5, *C*).[24,25] MRI is one of the most sensitive imaging modalities for detection and characterization of liver lesions.[26] The presence of malignant lymphadenopathy is often assessed by using size criteria, with a cutoff nodal diameter of 10 mm.[24] Ascites, abnormal peritoneal enhancement, and omental thickening can be indicators of peritoneal metastases. Liver metastases are hypovascular, hypointense on T1-weighted images, minimally hyperintense on T2-weighted images, and show an irregular rim enhancement on postgadolinium images.[23] Recently, diffusion-weighted MRI has been shown to improve detection of liver and peritoneal metastatic lesions.[27]

PANCREATIC ENDOCRINE TUMORS

The role of imaging in functioning pancreatic endocrine tumors is primarily for the detection and verification of the number and localization of lesions. Intraoperative ultrasound may play a particularly important role for the surgical planning by defining their number and localization. CT and MRI are also useful in monitoring and followup of patients with malignant neuroendocrine tumors. Insulinoma and gastrinoma are the two most common functioning endocrine neoplasms of the pancreas. Insulinomas are typically small (<2 cm) when diagnosed, richly vascularized, and appear as well-defined, round lesions. On unenhanced images, insulinomas generally demonstrate a low signal on CT and on T1-weighted magnetic resonance images, and increased signal on T2-weighted images. After contrast administration, they enhance avidly at the arterial phase and remain hyperdense/-intense on delayed-phase images (Figure 92-6). Liver metastases are also hypervascular and show a peripheral rim enhancement or enhance homogeneously, particularly when they are small.[28]

Gastrinomas may be relatively large (with a mean size of 4 cm) when diagnosed.[28] They occur most frequently in the gastrinoma triangle, which is defined as the neck and body of the pancreas medially, the confluence of the cystic and common bile ducts superiorly, and the second and third portion of the duodenum inferiorly. Gastrinomas are not as hypervascular as insulinomas. They appear as an isodense mass on nonenhanced CT scan and have a diminished signal on T1-weighted fat-suppressed magnetic resonance images, and an increased signal on T2-weighted images. After contrast media administration, they may show mild enhancement, but may also have low-attention areas.[29] Liver metastases are hyperintense on T2-weighted fat-suppressed images and have well-defined margins. The majority of gastrinomas are malignant and the evaluation of locoregional

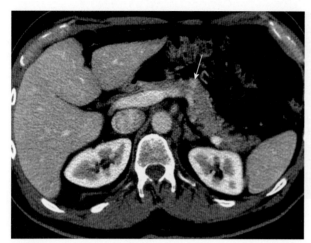

FIGURE 92-6 Insulinoma. Axial contrast-enhanced CT image of the pancreas shows small, well-defined, round lesion in the pancreatic body *(arrow)*. The lesion is hyperdense compared to normal pancreas, a typical CT finding for pancreatic neuroendocrine tumors.

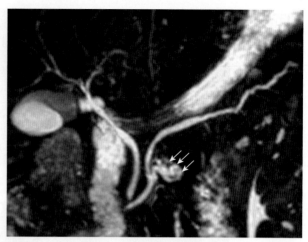

FIGURE 92-7 BD-IPMN. Coronal maximum-intensity projection MRCP demonstrates oval-shaped, lobulated, cystic mass in the uncinate process of the pancreas *(arrows)*, communicating with the main pancreatic duct. This mass is consistent with a BD-IPMN.

infiltration and distant metastases is critical for patient management.

Nonfunctioning pancreatic endocrine tumors are generally large at presentation. Consequently, the main role of imaging is not only their detection but their characterization, especially their differentiation from pancreatic adenocarcinoma.[30] Given that nonfunctioning pancreatic endocrine tumors are often malignant and generally, patients present with liver metastases at initial presentation, accurate staging and followup are required. Nonfunctioning pancreatic endocrine tumors are mostly solid and hypervascular. Typically, they have sharp margins and capsule. They may show cystic or necrotic changes. The presence of hemorrhagic content and central calcifications mostly depends on tumor size[31] and results in complex echogenicity on ultrasound and inhomogeneous enhancement after contrast application on CT and magnetic resonance images.

CYSTIC NEOPLASMS OF THE PANCREAS

The vast majority of cystic pancreatic neoplasms consist of intraductal papillary mucinous neoplasm (IPMN), serous cystadenoma, or mucinous cystadenoma/carcinoma. Cystic neoplasms of the pancreas are being diagnosed with increasing frequency as a result of technologic advances in cross-sectional imaging. In addition to detection and followup of these lesions, imaging is also done to differentiate malignant and nonmalignant cystic lesions, which can be challenging because of overlapping features. The following imaging features are important in differentiation of benign and malignant cystic lesions: uni- or multilocular nature of the lesion; its communication with the pancreatic duct; the size of the tumor and the pancreatic duct; the presence of thick septations or mural nodules; and the signal of the tumor on T1-weighted images. A history of pancreatitis and the lack of an epithelial lining make a pseudocyst most likely, whereas the presence of central calcifications, septations, and solid components is more indicative of a cystic neoplasm.[32] The advantage of CT over MRI is its ability to detect

central calcifications, whereas MRI provides a better soft-tissue contrast and a better depiction of the relationship between the tumor and the pancreatic duct. In addition, MRCP images can be useful for anatomic evaluation of the pancreatic duct system and its relation with the cystic lesion. MRI is also an ideal modality for followup imaging because of its lack of ionizing radiation.

Intraductal Papillary Mucinous Neoplasm

IPMNs are divided into three groups: main duct type, branch duct type (BD-IPMN), and mixed type.[33,34] The risk for malignancy depends on the type of IPMN. In 58% to 92% of main duct IPMN, malignancy has been reported,[33] whereas the risk for malignancy in BD-IPMN is much lower, with rates ranging from 6% to 46%. Thus an important challenge for diagnostic imaging is the differentiation between the types of IPMN and the detection of imaging features associated with malignancy. IPMN can be detected on MDCT; however, three-dimensional high-resolution contrast-enhanced MRI with high-resolution MRCP may be more accurate for demonstrating communication with the main pancreatic duct, showing main duct involvement and identification of small BD-IPMN.[35,36]

BD-IPMNs can be seen in any segment of the pancreas but are most commonly located in the uncinate process. They appear as oval-shaped cystic masses communicating with the branch ducts of the pancreas (Figure 92-7). Especially when small, they can mimic cystic changes in chronic pancreatitis. Imaging features of combined-type IPMN are the presence of BD-IPMN and a dilation of the pancreatic duct greater than 6 mm. The main-duct type IPMN may appear as a segmental or diffuse (but significant) dilation of the main pancreatic duct.

Imaging features associated with malignancy include mural nodules, dilated main pancreatic duct (greater than 8 to 10 mm), thick septae, intraluminal calcifications (best seen on CT scan), ductal filling defects on MRCP, bulging papilla, local invasion, and signs of invasive cancer, such as dilation of the common bile duct.[36]

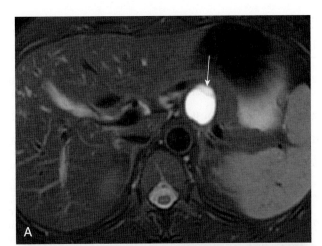

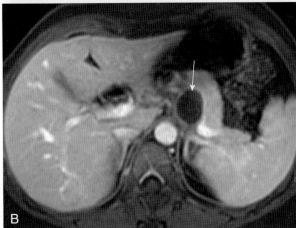

FIGURE 92-8 Mucinous cystadenoma. **A,** T2-weighted image with fat saturation demonstrates large, unilocular cystic lesion *(long arrow)*, which does not communicate with the pancreatic duct. **B,** After contrast administration, wall enhancement *(small arrows)* of the mucinous cystadenoma *(arrow)* is shown on T1-weighted image.

Serous Cystadenoma

One percent to 2% of all pancreatic tumors and 25% of all cystic pancreatic neoplasms are serous tumors. They are distributed evenly throughout the pancreas.[33] Serous cystadenomas are benign and can be classified into micro- and macrocystic, oligo- or unilocular.[37,38] Typically, they appear as a pancreatic mass with numerous, mostly small, serous, fluid-filled or solid, grape-like cysts. They may have a central stellate scar and sunburst pattern of calcifications.[37,38] Serous tumors never communicate with the main pancreatic duct. Small, discrete calcifications can best be visualized on CT, whereas MRI provides a better visualization of the small grape-like cysts and its content. After injection of contrast media, thin-walled septae enhance and produce the typical "honeycomb appearance." In addition, MRI and CT images may reveal the late enhancing central scar.

Mucinous Cystadenoma/Cystadenocarcinoma

Mucinous cystic neoplasms of the pancreas represent 2% of all pancreatic neoplasms.[33] Mucinous cystadenomas are described pathologically as having borderline malignant potential and need to be differentiated from serous cystadenomas. Most are localized in the pancreatic body or tail and their size ranges up to 35 cm.[33] They are characterized by the formation of large unilocular or multilocular cysts with enhancing septations (Figure 92-8).[34] Mucin production leads to high signal intensity of these tumors and of their liver metastases (in cases of mucinous cystadenocarcinoma) on T1- and T2-weighted images.[28] Hemorrhagic content is a strong predictor for mucinous cystic neoplasm and shows a high signal on CT, T1-, and T2-weighted images. Mucinous cystadenomas are well circumscribed and encapsulated, whereas mucinous cystadenocarcinoma infiltrates adjacent organs or structures. The appearance of solid nodules, irregularity/thickening of the cyst wall, size larger than 6 cm, presence of metastatic lesions, and peripheral eggshell calcifications are further criteria suggesting malignancy.

REFERENCES

1. Fulcher AS, Turner MA: MR pancreatography: A useful tool for evaluating pancreatic disorders. *Radiographics* 19:5, 1999.
2. Motosugi U, Ichikawa T, Araki T, et al: Secretin-stimulating MRCP in patients with pancreatobiliary maljunction and occult pancreatobiliary reflux: Direct demonstration of pancreatobiliary reflux. *Eur Radiol* 17:2262, 2007.
3. Sandrasegeran K, Lin C, Akisik FM, et al: State-of-the-art pancreatic MRI. *AJR Am J Roentgenol* 195:42, 2010.
4. Yu Z, Zhang L, Fu J, et al: Anomalous pancreaticobiliary junction: Image analysis and treatment principles. *Hepatobiliary Pancreat Dis Int* 3:136, 2004.
5. Funabiki T, Matsubara T, Miyakwa S, et al: Pancreaticobiliary maljunction and carcinogenesis to biliary and pancreatic malignancy. *Langenbecks Arch Surg* 394:159, 2009.
6. Kamisawa T, Tu Y, Egawa N, et al: MRCP of congenital pancreaticobiliary malformation. *Abdom Imaging* 32:129, 2007.
7. Isserow JA, Siegelman ES, Mammone J: Focal fatty infiltration of the pancreas: MR characterization with chemical shift imaging. *AJR Am J Roentgenol* 173:1263, 1999.
8. Kawamoto S, Siegelman SS, Bluemke DA, et al: Focal fatty infiltration of the head of the pancreas: Evaluation with multidetector computed tomography with multiplanare reformation imaging. *J Comput Assist Tomogr* 33:90, 2009.
9. Sandrasegaran K, Patel A, Fogel EL, et al: Annular pancreas in adults. *AJR Am J Roentgenol* 193:455, 2009.
10. Jadvar H, Mindelzun RE: Annular pancreas in adults: Imaging features in seven patients. *Abdom Imaging* 24:174, 1999.
11. Balci NC, Bieneman BK, Bilgin M, et al: Magnetic resonance imaging in pancreatitis. *Top Magn Reson Imaging* 20:25, 2009.
12. Koo BC, Chinogureyi A, Shaw AS: Imaging acute pancreatitis. *Br J Radiol* 83:104, 2010.
13. Vijayaraghavan G, Kurup D, Singh A: Imaging of acute abdomen and pelvis: Common acute pathologies. *Semin Roentgenol* 44:221, 2009.
14. Stevens T, Parsi MA, Walsh RM: Acute pancreatitis: Problems in adherence to guidelines. *Cleve Clin J Med* 76:697, 2009.
15. Segal D, Mortele KJ, Banks PA, et al: Acute necrotizing pancreatitis: Role of CT-guided percutaneous catheter drainage. *Abdom Imaging* 32:351, 2007.
16. Miller FH, Keppke AL, Wadhwa A, et al: MRI of pancreatitis and its complications: Part 2, Chronic pancreatitis. *AJR Am J Roentgenol* 183:1645, 2004.
17. Carbognin G, Girardi V, Biasiutti C, et al: Autoimmune pancreatitis: Imaging findings on contrast-enhanced MR, MRCP and dynamic secretin-enhanced MRCP. *Radiol Med* 114:1214, 2009.
18. Manfredi R, Graziani R, Cicero C, et al: Autoimmune pancreatitis: CT patterns and their chances after steroid treatment. *Radiology* 247:435, 2008.
19. Chrysos E, Athanasakis E, Xynos E: Pancreatic trauma in the adult: Current knowledge in diagnosis and management. *Pancreatology* 2:365, 2002.

20. Tkacz JN, Anderson SA, Soto J: MR imaging in gastrointestinal emergencies. *Radiographics* 29:1767, 2009.
21. Ahmed N, Vernick JJ: Pancreatic injury. *South Med J* 102:1253, 2009.
22. Balasegaram M: Surgical management of pancreatic trauma. *Curr Probl Surg* 16:1, 1979.
23. Vachiranubhap B, Kim YH, Balci NC, et al: Magnetic resonance imaging of adenocarcinoma of the pancreas. *Top Magn Reson Imaging* 20:3, 2009.
24. Grenacher L, Klauss M: Computed tomography of pancreatic tumors. *Radiologe* 49:107, 2009.
25. Kinney T: Evidence-based imaging of pancreatic malignancies. *Surg Clin North Am* 90:235, 2010.
26. Ba-Ssalamah A, Uffmann M, Saini S, et al: Clinical value of liver-specific contrast agents: A tailored examination for a confident non-invasive diagnosis of focal liver lesions. *Eur Radiol* 19:342, 2009.
27. Low RN: MR imaging of the peritoneal spread of malignancy. *Abdom Imaging* 32:267, 2007.
28. Ku YM, Shin SS, Lee CH, Semelka RC: Magnetic resonance imaging of cystic and endocrine pancreatic neoplasm. *Top Magn Reson Imaging* 20:11, 2009.
29. Horton K, Hruban RH, Yeo C, et al: Multi-detector-row CT of pancreatic islet cell tumors. *Radiographics* 26:453, 2006.
30. Graziani R, Brandalise A, Bellotti M, et al: Imaging of neuroendocrine gastroenteropancreatic tumors. *Radiol Med* 115:1047, 2010.
31. Dörffel Y, Wermke W: Contrast medium sonography of neuroendocrine tumors of the gastroenteropancreatic system. *Radiologe* 49:206, 2009.
32. Sand J, Nordback I: The differentiation between pancreatic neoplastic cysts and pancreatic pseudocyst. *Scand J Surg* 94:161, 2005.
33. Verbesey JE, Munson JL: Pancreatic cystic neoplasms. *Surg Clin North Am* 90:411, 2010.
34. Brambs HJ, Jucherns M: Cystic tumors of the pancreas. *Radiologe* 48:740, 2008.
35. Baiocchi GL, Portolani N, Missale G, et al: Intraductal papillary mucinous neoplasm of the pancreas (IPMN): Clinico-pathological correlations and surgical indications. *World J Surg Oncol* 8:25, 2010.
36. Augustin T, VanderMeer TJ: Intraductal papillary mucinous neoplasm: A clinicopathologic review. *Surg Clin North Am* 9:377, 2010.
37. Friedman AC, Liechtenstein JE, Dachman AH: Cystic neoplasms of the pancreas: Radiological-pathological correlation. *Radiology* 149:45, 1983.
38. Martin DR, Semelka RC: MR imaging of pancreatic masses. *Magn Reson Imaging Clin N Am* 8:787, 2000.

Pancreatic and Periampullary Cancer

Christopher L. Wolfgang | Barish H. Edil | Richard D. Schulick |

John L. Cameron

Pancreatic and periampullary carcinomas include a group of malignant neoplasms arising in or near the ampulla of Vater or in the pancreas. The initial pattern of symptoms is determined by the location of the primary lesion. Lesions growing in the periampullary region tend to cause obstructive jaundice, whereas pancreatic lesions that grow in the body or tail tend to be manifested as pain or a mass effect. The great majority of tumors that occur in these areas are adenocarcinomas arising from either the pancreas, ampulla of Vater, distal common bile duct, or duodenum. Less common neoplasms of the pancreas include pancreatic neuroendocrine neoplasms, acinar cell cancer, intraductal papillary mucinous neoplasms, mucinous cystic neoplasms, and solid pseudopapillary neoplasms.

INCIDENCE

The incidence of periampullary cancers is relatively low in comparison to colorectal, breast, and lung cancers. However, as a result of their lethal nature, they are a major cause of mortality. For example, pancreatic cancer is the ninth most common cancer in occurrence in the United States, but ranks fourth in number of deaths.[1] The majority of periampullary cancers are composed of adenocarcinomas. The most common periampullary adenocarcinoma is pancreatic followed, in order, by ampullary, distal cholangiocarcinoma, and duodenal. In the United States, the incidence of pancreatic cancer rose dramatically from the 1930s until the 1970s, nearly doubling. Since the mid-1970s, the incidence has remained stable at about 8 to 9 cases per 100,000 population. In the United States, demographic risk factors for pancreatic cancer include age, with the majority of patients in or beyond their sixth decade of life; sex, with a slight male preponderance; and race, with African American men having the highest overall incidence.

In Europe, pancreatic cancer is the sixth leading cause of cancer death, and the incidence is similar to that in the United States. The incidence in Europe has also remained stable during the past 3 decades. The Japanese, however, have seen a dramatic increase in the incidence of pancreatic cancer over the past 3 decades, although the overall incidence is still less than that observed in the West. India and parts of the Middle East have the lowest recorded incidence of pancreatic cancer. Worldwide, more than 200,000 people die of pancreatic cancer every year.[2]

Ampullary carcinoma has an overall incidence of 6 cases per 1 million or approximately 1800 cases per year

in the United States.[3] Although it constitutes between 7% and 19% of periampullary carcinomas, it accounts for a higher percentage of operative cases because these lesions are more amenable to complete resection.[4,5] Distal bile duct carcinoma and periampullary duodenal carcinoma occur less frequently than pancreatic and ampullary carcinoma. The actual incidence of these two carcinomas is much more difficult to estimate because they occur less frequently and are often lumped together with other malignancies. For example, distal bile duct carcinomas are often combined with all cholangiocarcinomas (perihilar and intrahepatic), as well as with gallbladder carcinoma. Likewise, periampullary duodenal carcinomas are often combined with all duodenal carcinomas or all small bowel carcinomas.

PATHOLOGY

Pathologic examination of resected pancreaticoduodenectomy specimens reveals that approximately 40% to 60% are performed for adenocarcinoma of the pancreas, 10% to 20% are performed for adenocarcinoma of the ampulla, 10% are performed for bile duct adenocarcinoma, 5% to 10% are performed for duodenal adenocarcinoma, and 10% to 20% of specimens contain only benign disease.[6,7] Because these data represent resected specimens and the resectability of pancreatic periampullary cancer is much lower, it is reasonable to assume that the pancreas is the primary site in 80% to 90% of periampullary cancers.

Although the periampullary region can harbor a diverse array of pathologic entities, pancreatic ductal adenocarcinoma (tubular) is by far the most common malignant histology. In addition, variants of adenocarcinoma exist, such as colloid carcinoma (mucinous noncystic), adenosquamous, and osteoclastic and are associated with unique biologies as evidenced by the difference in survival following resection. More than two thirds of pancreatic adenocarcinomas arise in the pancreatic head, neck, or uncinate process. Other histologic types that are encountered include pancreatic neuroendocrine neoplasms, acinar cell cancer, and solid pseudopapillary neoplasms.

Cystic neoplasms of the pancreas are more commonly identified in recent times because of the more widespread use of cross-sectional imaging. The majority of these lesions are benign and harbor essentially no malignant potential, such as serous cystadenomas (microcystic adenomas). There have been approximately 10 reported cases in the English literature documenting what appears to be a malignancy arising from a serous cystadenoma.[8] Mucin-producing cysts include mucinous cystic neoplasms (MCNs) and intraductal papillary mucinous neoplasms (IPMNs) and represent precursor lesions to invasive ductal adenocarcinoma similar to adenomatous colon polyps, which are precursors to invasive colorectal cancer. In a single-institution report of 136 pancreatic resections performed for IPMN over a 6-year period, 38% had evidence of invasive cancer.[9] Noninvasive IPMNs are classified based on their degree of dysplasia as low grade, intermediate grade, or high grade, and are also classified as carcinoma in situ (CIS). The mean age of patients with IPMN with low-grade dysplasia was 63.2 years; with intermediate- or high-grade dysplasia, 66.7 years; and with invasive cancer, 68.1 years, thus suggesting a sequential progression.

Nonfunctional pancreatic neuroendocrine neoplasms are usually detected because of their space-occupying characteristics. Obstructive jaundice is uncommon with small pancreatic endocrine neoplasms, even in the head of the pancreas, but can occur when the lesion is malignant.

Various sarcomas, including gastrointestinal stromal tumors (GISTs), fibrosarcomas, leiomyosarcomas, hemangiopericytomas, and histiocytomas, may also arise in the periampullary region. It is important to distinguish whether the lesion represents a GIST because of the availability of targeted therapeutics such as imatinib (Gleevec), which has a very high response rate. Thousands of patients worldwide with advanced GIST have been treated with imatinib and have achieved significant response rates, prolongation of survival, and improvement in quality of life.[10] The area around the porta hepatis, as well as the pancreas, is rich with lymphatic tissues. Lymphomas can occur in these areas and usually have ill-defined margins when compared with typical adenocarcinomas. Finally, the periampullary region may harbor sites of metastatic disease from kidney, breast, lung, melanoma, stomach, colon, and germ cell primaries, as well as from other primary sites of disease.

RISK FACTORS

More is known about the risk factors for pancreatic adenocarcinoma than for ampullary, bile duct, and duodenal adenocarcinoma.

PANCREATIC ADENOCARCINOMA

The known and suspected risk factors for pancreatic adenocarcinoma can be broadly classified as established, associated, and possible. Tobacco and inherited susceptibility are considered established. Chronic pancreatitis, type 2 diabetes mellitus, and obesity are consistently found to be associated with pancreatic cancer and are generally considered weak risk factors. Possible risk factors include physical inactivity, certain pesticides, and high carbohydrate/sugar intake, but the data are inconsistent and inconclusive. Cholecystectomy, cholelithiasis, coffee consumption, and alcohol have been sporadically associated with the development of pancreatic cancer but are unlikely to be true risk factors (Table 93-1).

TABLE 93-1 Risk Factors for Pancreatic Adenocarcinoma

Established	Tobacco
	Inherited susceptibility
Associated	Chronic pancreatitis
	Diabetes mellitus type 2
	Obesity
Possible	Physical inactivity
	Certain pesticides
	High carbohydrate/sugar intake

Environmental Factors and Pancreatic Adenocarcinoma

The evidence linking cigarette smoking to pancreatic adenocarcinoma is strong and may account for up to 25% of pancreatic cancers. Most studies have found that smoking results in about a twofold increased risk for pancreatic cancer.[11-14] Most studies also confirm the anticipated finding of a dose–response relationship, with higher rates of pancreatic cancer being linked to heavier smoking exposure. In a 50-year followup study of British physicians, pancreatic cancer rates in nonsmokers, ex-smokers, and current smokers were 21, 31, and 39 per 100,000 person-years, respectively.[15] Human autopsy studies have revealed increased hyperplastic changes with atypia in the pancreatic cells of cigarette smokers.[16]

Data reviewing the relationship of diet and pancreas adenocarcinoma are often conflicting.[11,17,18] Some studies have demonstrated an association with increased intake of total calories, as well as carbohydrates, cholesterol, meat, salt, dehydrated food, fried food, refined sugar, and nitrosamines. Fat, β-carotene, and coffee are of unproven risk, with studies demonstrating both the presence and the absence of increased risk. Some foods may have a protective effect, such as consumption of a diet high in fiber, vitamin C, fruits, vegetables, and unprepared food, but these relationships are not yet established.

Alcohol, coffee, and radiation do not seem to be significant risk factors for the development of pancreatic adenocarcinoma. Findings obtained from numerous prospective cohort and case–control studies on alcohol consumption and pancreatic cancer risk have been inconsistent, with many confounding variables present in various investigations.[19] Three case–control studies from Europe failed to demonstrate an increased risk for pancreatic cancer with coffee consumption,[11] in contrast to two earlier reported series linking an increased risk for pancreatic cancer with coffee consumption.[20,21] Ionizing radiation also does not seem to be associated with an increased incidence of pancreatic cancer. Survivors of the atomic bombing of Hiroshima and Nagasaki have not demonstrated an increased risk for pancreatic cancer.[22,23]

Host Factors and Pancreatic Adenocarcinoma

Familial clustering of pancreatic cancer accounts for approximately 10% of all cases.[2] Some of this clustering may represent shared environmental risk factors, but the majority of cases are due to underlying genetic susceptibility traits. Only 20% of familial pancreatic cancer cases occur as part of a named syndrome or have a defined underlying genetic defect.[24] The best characterized of these include BRCA2/Fanconi anemia pathway defects, familial atypical multiple mole melanoma (FAMMM) syndrome and Puetz–Jeghers syndrome. Germline mutations of BRCA2 are associated with increased risk of breast, ovarian, prostate, and pancreatic cancer.[3,4] The prevalence of BRCA2 mutation is about 1% in Ashkenazi Jews but can run in any family. Individuals with a mutation of this gene carry an increased risk of developing pancreatic cancer of 3.5- to 10-fold.[3,4] The defining features of FAMMM include multiple nevi, multiple atypical nevi, and an increased risk of melanoma. Approximately 30% of pancreatic cancers that develop in patients with this syndrome are associated with the mutation of p16/CDKKN2A.[5-7] The risk of pancreatic cancer in these individuals has been reported to range from 9- to 47-fold.[6] The least common of this group is Puetz–Jeghers syndrome but carries a 132-fold increased risk of developing pancreatic cancer.[8] Interestingly, the same gene (STK11/LKB1) that is responsible for the development of Puetz–Jeghers is also involved in the pathogenesis of IPMNs.[9] Individuals with Puetz–Jeghers are characterized by melanocytic macules (freckles) on the lips and hamartomatous polyps throughout the gastrointestinal tract.

The risk of an individual developing pancreatic cancer based on family history alone has been well established based on several large studies.[10,11] In these individuals, the strong family history is a surrogate of a defined genetic defect yet to be discovered. An individual with one first-degree relative with pancreatic cancer has a 2.3-fold increased risk of developing pancreatic cancer. With two first-degree affected relatives the risk is 6.4-fold, and with three first-degree relatives the risk increases to 32-fold. A first-degree relative is defined as a parent–child or sibling–sibling relationship. Using these and other studies, a risk prediction calculator has been developed called PancPRO.[12] This tool is available free online at http://astor.som.jhmi.edu/BayesMendel/pancpro. html (accessed November 21, 2010).

Chronic pancreatitis has been associated with pancreatic adenocarcinoma, but it is difficult to determine whether there is a common risk factor for the two diseases or whether chronic pancreatitis may represent an indolent manifestation of pancreatic adenocarcinoma.[11,25-27] In similar fashion, type 2 diabetes mellitus is often associated with pancreatic adenocarcinoma.[28,29] For both of these host factors, it is difficult to ascertain whether they are sequelae of the malignancy or whether they are truly causative factors.

Genetic Alterations and Pancreatic Cancer

Pancreatic cancer is among the best characterized cancers at the genetic level. A major contribution to the understanding of the genetics is the recent determination of the entire pancreatic cancer genome.[30] In this landmark study, the mutational status of more than 22,000 genes was assessed in 24 patients and approximately 1100 non-silent associated genetic alterations were identified. Of these mutations, 148 were found to occur more than once. Not surprisingly, the prevalence of mutations in

genes already known to be frequently mutated in pancreatic cancer was consistent with other published reports. For example, in an analysis of pancreatic adenocarcinoma specimens, 100% had mutations in the proto-oncogene K-ras, and 82%, 76%, 53%, and 10% had mutations in the tumor suppressor genes *p16*, *p53*, *DPC4*, and *BRCA2*, respectively.[31] These frequencies are similar to those found in the global sequencing project. The average number of genetic alterations in any given pancreatic cancer is 63. Despite the large number of genetic alterations, essentially all fell within 12 core signaling pathways that are known to be important in cell growth and differentiation.

This is very different from the genetic sequencing of neuroendocrine tumors. A completely different set of mutations in the following genes were found, with MEN I (44%), DAXX/ATRX (43%), and genes in the mTor pathway (15%) found mutated with this type of pancreatic cancer.[32]

These findings open the opportunity for future therapies developed to target one or more of these pathways. For example, everolimus, an mTor inhibitor, has been found to have a prolongation in median progression-free survival in neuroendocrine tumors, and 15% of neuroendocrine tumors have a mutation in the mTor pathway. Moreover, a significant number of these alterations occur in proteins that are predicted to be secreted on the basis of their leader sequence and thus may be useful in serum- or tissue fluid–based early detection tests.

NONPANCREATIC PERIAMPULLARY ADENOCARCINOMA

Ampullary, distal common bile duct, and periampullary duodenal adenocarcinomas are less common than pancreatic adenocarcinoma and are also less well characterized in terms of their risk factors and genetic alterations. All demonstrate an increasing incidence with age.[33] Ampullary and duodenal adenocarcinomas occur with increased frequency in patients with hereditary polyposis syndromes, including hereditary nonpolyposis colorectal cancer, Peutz–Jeghers syndrome, familial adenomatous polyposis, and Gardner syndrome. Distal common bile duct cancers make up approximately 30% of all cholangiocarcinomas, including perihilar and intrahepatic lesions. Cholangiocarcinomas are associated with several known risk factors, including age, inflammatory bowel disease, sclerosing cholangitis, choledochal cysts, and choledocholithiasis.[34,35]

DIAGNOSIS AND PREOPERATIVE EVALUATION

The diagnosis of a periampullary cancer is usually made on the basis of clinical findings, laboratory data, and radiologic imaging. In some cases of pancreatic or distal bile duct adenocarcinoma, a tissue diagnosis is available, but the delay in definitive treatment is seldom indicated to obtain histologic confirmation of malignancy. Biopsy of a duodenal or ampullary lesion, such as a soft polypoid growth, may sometimes be of benefit if it proves to be benign and local resection is being contemplated. If the clinical findings, laboratory data, and radiologic imaging are suspicious for a malignancy, the majority of patients brought to resection will indeed have a cancerous lesion. Additionally, a negative biopsy of a periampullary mass has a significant rate of being falsely negative for carcinoma. Confirmatory biopsy is relevant if the lesion is unresectable or if neoadjuvant therapy is being contemplated.

CLINICAL FINDINGS

Symptoms depend on the location of the lesion, with most patients having vague symptoms early in the course of their disease. Patients with lesions that occur near the bile duct, such as those near the ampulla, head of the pancreas, and uncinate process, are much more likely to present with obstructive jaundice. Those with lesions in the body or tail of the pancreas are more likely to complain of epigastric or back pain, early satiety, and weight loss.

The majority of patients with a head of the pancreas, ampullary, distal bile duct, or periampullary duodenal adenocarcinoma have the classic constellation of jaundice, pruritus, acholic stools, and tea-colored urine. Patients with a distal common bile duct or ampullary adenocarcinoma are the most likely to have obstructive jaundice because the lesion does not need to grow to a very large size before it completely obstructs the bile duct. In addition to the classic symptoms, vague upper abdominal discomfort often develops and sometimes radiates to the back. Late in the course of the disease, this pain can progress to become very debilitating. Other general symptoms include anorexia, fatigue, malaise, and weight loss. Nausea and vomiting can be a sign of gastric outlet obstruction from duodenal involvement. Patients may also have acute pancreatitis secondary to obstruction of the pancreatic duct. Elderly patients with acute pancreatitis but without a history of alcohol use or gallbladder stones should be screened for a neoplasm.

Patients with pancreatic adenocarcinoma involving the body or tail of the gland are more likely to have weight loss and abdominal pain as their initial complaints. These lesions can grow to a larger size before producing symptoms and are often diagnosed at a later stage with a poorer prognosis.

Physical findings on examination include scleral icterus, jaundice, and a palpable gallbladder (Courvoisier sign). Signs of advanced disease include cachexia, palpable metastatic lesions within the liver, palpable disease in the left supraclavicular fossa near the confluence of the subclavian vein and thoracic duct (Virchow nodule), palpable periumbilical metastatic disease (Sister Mary Joseph nodule), and pelvic metastatic disease palpable anteriorly on rectal examination (Blumer shelf nodule).

LABORATORY FINDINGS

In addition to the clinical signs and symptoms, patients early in the course of their disease may have subtle laboratory findings such as mildly elevated liver function test results, mildly elevated bilirubin levels, or elevated alkaline phosphatase levels, or they may have new-onset diabetes or anemia. If the disease has progressed and jaundice is apparent, patients generally have elevated serum levels of bilirubin and alkaline phosphatase, usually associated with only a mild elevation in liver transaminases. Ongoing obstruction of the biliary tree may lead to an inability to absorb vitamin K and resultant coagulopathy because of the lack of intrinsic pathway clotting factors. It is important to replete vitamin K in these patients.

There are no definitive serum markers for any of the pancreatic or periampullary adenocarcinomas. Markers that tend to be used are carbohydrate antigen 19-9 (CA 19-9) and carcinoembryonic antigen (CEA). CA 19-9 is elevated in up to 75% of patients with pancreatic adenocarcinoma, but levels are also elevated in benign conditions of the pancreas, liver, and bile ducts, as well as in smokers. CEA levels may be elevated with any of the periampullary adenocarcinomas, but more typically with bile duct and duodenal adenocarcinoma. Because nearly 100% of pancreatic adenocarcinomas have a mutation in K-ras, several groups have tried to detect these mutations from aspirates obtained by endoscopic techniques or in stool.[36-38]

IMAGING STUDIES

The imaging modalities most frequently used for patients with suspected periampullary cancer are right upper quadrant ultrasound (RUQ US), CT, MRI, including magnetic resonance cholangiopancreatography (MRCP), endoscopic retrograde cholangiopancreatography (ERCP), and percutaneous transhepatic cholangiography (PTC). The benefit of positron emission tomography (PET) has not been clearly defined. During the past 20 years there has been a general trend away from invasive imaging studies (ERCP and PTC) toward noninvasive imaging studies. This trend has occurred for two reasons. First, there have been studies that have documented an increased rate of both preoperative and postoperative complications with the routine use of these modalities.[39,40] Second, surgeons have become more willing to operate on jaundiced patients as long as they are not septic or malnourished from their biliary obstruction.

Right Upper Quadrant Ultrasound

RUQ US is usually available at all times, especially in emergency departments. It is very sensitive for the detection of gallstones, dilation of the biliary tree, pericholecystic fluid, and gallbladder wall thickening. The sonographer can also test for the presence of a sonographic Murphy sign, in which the patient experiences the most tenderness when the probe is pushed directly on the gallbladder fundus. RUQ US can also detect more ominous signs of advanced periampullary adenocarcinoma, including hepatic metastases, peripancreatic and hilar lymphadenopathy, and ascites. The sensitivity for actually demonstrating a pancreatic or periampullary mass is not high, and the absence of one on this imaging modality does not rule it out.

Computed Tomography

Multidetector spiral CT is probably the single most useful diagnostic and staging modality (Figure 93-1).[41] This study gives information about the immediately adjacent

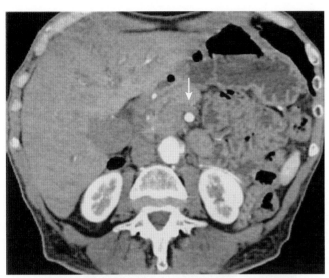

FIGURE 93-1 Axial computed tomography scan showing a 3-cm mass arising from the head of the pancreas. Arterial-phase axial images demonstrate loss of the periarterial plane over 90 degrees of the superior mesenteric artery *(arrow)*. (From House MG, Yeo CJ, Cameron JL, et al: Predicting resectability of periampullary cancer with three-dimensional computed tomography. *J Gastrointest Surg* 8:280, 2004.)

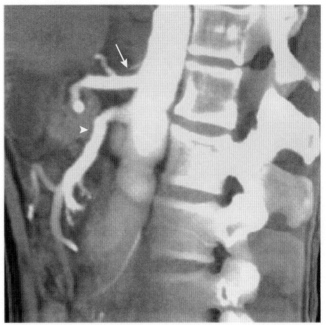

FIGURE 93-2 Sagittal three-dimensional computed tomographic image confirming the intimate relationship of the pancreatic mass *(arrowhead)* with the superior mesenteric artery in the same patient as in Figure 93-1; however, the vessel remains completely patent. The mass does not involve the origin of the celiac axis *(arrow)*. This patient underwent a margin-negative resection for pancreatic adenocarcinoma. (From House MG, Yeo CJ, Cameron JL, et al: Predicting resectability of periampullary cancer with three-dimensional computed tomography. *J Gastrointest Surg* 8:280, 2004.)

vascular structures, such as the portal and superior mesenteric veins, as well as the superior mesenteric artery and celiac axis. Three-dimensional reconstructions of these vessels aid in visualizing the anatomic relationships between the vessels and the mass.[42] Most importantly, the presence of tissue planes and the degree of circumferential involvement can be determined (Figures 93-2 and 93-3). Additionally, information on the presence of distant metastatic disease can be evaluated at the same setting if the entire abdominal and thoracic cavities are scanned. These images can sometimes reveal the presence of peritoneal dissemination, hepatic involvement, or pulmonary involvement. The presence of ascites, seen most readily in pelvic cuts, is usually an ominous sign.

Magnetic Resonance Imaging

When distal bile duct obstruction is suspected but no discrete mass is present on CT scan, cholangiography may be of benefit. MRCP is commonly used in this situation to image the biliary tree as well as the pancreatic duct (Figure 93-4). It is completely noninvasive and avoids the potential complications associated with the more invasive cholangiography modalities. MRCP has no potential for therapeutic maneuvers, such as extraction of stones or stenting, or for invasive diagnostic maneuvers, such as brushings or biopsies. Gadolinium enhancement can be used in T1-weighted sequences to study the vascular structures, which can also be three-dimensionally reconstructed. MRI and MRCP (potentially performed in a single session on the scanner) thus have the ability to provide information about tumor location, size, and extent; biliary and pancreatic ductal anatomy; and vascular involvement.

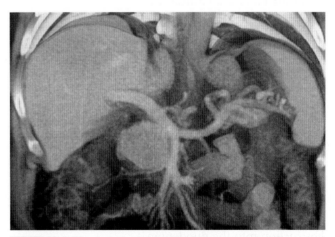

FIGURE 93-3 Three-dimensional axial oblique reconstruction showing a low-density mass within the head of the pancreas that abuts but does not encase the superior mesenteric vein or portal vein. The vessels appear patent with no evidence of displacement. This pancreatic adenocarcinoma was resected without the need for partial superior mesenteric vein or portal vein resection. (From House MG, Yeo CJ, Cameron JL, et al: Predicting resectability of periampullary cancer with three-dimensional computed tomography. *J Gastrointest Surg* 8:280, 2004.)

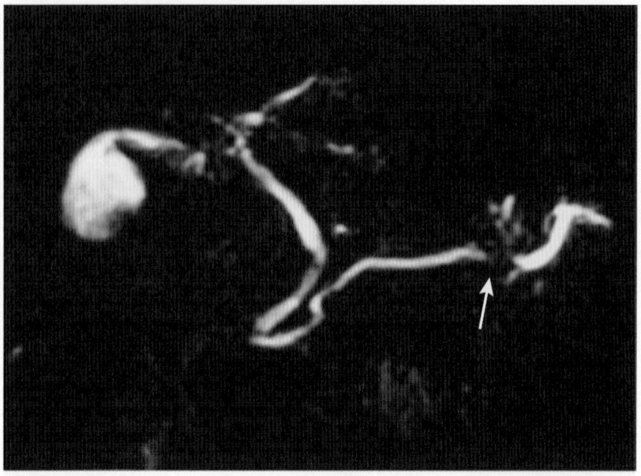

FIGURE 93-4 Magnetic resonance cholangiopancreatogram demonstrating stenosis of the main duct in the pancreatic body. (From Saisho H, Yamaguchi T: Diagnostic imaging for pancreatic cancer: Computed tomography, magnetic resonance imaging, and positron emission tomography. *Pancreas* 28:273, 2004.)

Endoscopic Retrograde Cholangiopancreatography

ERCP is sometimes required to decompress an obstructed biliary tree that is causing sepsis. The resulting images may solidify the suspected diagnosis of a pancreatic or periampullary adenocarcinoma. The classic finding of a long, irregular stricture in the pancreatic duct with distal dilation or a cutoff of both the genu of the pancreatic duct and the distal bile duct is pathognomonic of pancreatic cancer (Figure 93-5). With the current imaging capabilities of CT and MRI, diagnostic ERCP is rarely necessary to guide treatment; however, many patients still show up in the surgery clinic already having had ERCP performed and a stent inserted.

Percutaneous Transhepatic Cholangiography

PTC is another means of defining the biliary anatomy, albeit by an invasive approach. When compared with ERCP, it better defines the proximal biliary anatomy above the level of obstruction. During the cholangiogram, a percutaneous biliary drain may be inserted to drain the proximal biliary tree (Figure 93-6). PTC is perhaps even more invasive than ERCP, and complications include intraabdominal bleeding as well as hemobilia. The pancreatic duct and the most distal portion of the bile duct are not usually well visualized as with ERCP. For patients in whom canalization of the bile duct is not possible by ERCP, PTC is often successful in accessing the biliary tree and allows placement of a stent across the obstruction into the duodenum.

Upper Endoscopy and Endoscopic Ultrasound

Ampullary and duodenal cancers may be directly visualized through an endoscope, and it is relatively easy to obtain a biopsy specimen for tissue diagnosis. Endoscopic ultrasound (EUS) may be performed during upper endoscopy. The duodenum, ampulla, head of the pancreas, and uncinate process of the pancreas are acoustically accessible with a probe positioned in the duodenum,

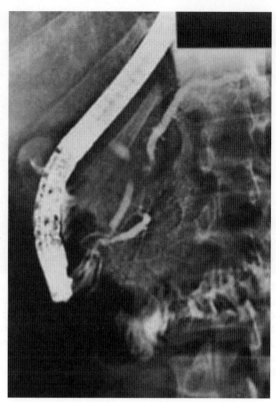

FIGURE 93-5 An endoscopic retrograde cholangiopancreatogram in a patient with obstructive jaundice reveals a classic double-duct sign. There is evidence of tumor at the genu of the common bile duct and the pancreatic duct. (From Yeo CJ, Cameron JL: Pancreatic cancer. *Curr Probl Surg* 36:59, 1999.)

whereas the body and tail of the pancreas are acoustically accessible with a probe positioned in the stomach. EUS may give information about vascular involvement (Figure 93-7), but the decision regarding whether to explore a patient should not rely solely on this test. Fine-needle aspiration of any suspected lesions can be performed at the same time as EUS if tissue diagnosis is of benefit.

Positron Emission Tomography

The role of PET scanning is not well defined at present for pancreatic and periampullary adenocarcinoma. Some recent reports support the use of PET imaging in patients with pancreatic cancer. In a comprehensive review of the PET literature, a report suggests the value of this test.[43,44] PET imaging, however, is not routinely used presently in patients suspected of having a pancreatic or periampullary adenocarcinoma.

TISSUE DIAGNOSIS

The use of either percutaneous (US- or CT-guided) or EUS-guided pancreatic biopsy to evaluate a patient who appears to have a resectable pancreatic mass is somewhat controversial. Biopsy can usually be performed with rare complications, including fistula, pancreatitis, hemorrhage, abscess, tumor seeding, and death. However, a negative biopsy in a patient with a lesion that is consistent with pancreatic cancer should not alter the decision to resect. Biopsy should be performed in patients whose

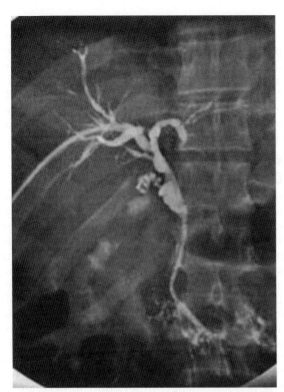

FIGURE 93-6 Cholangiogram obtained after placement of an internal–external percutaneous transhepatic biliary drainage catheter. The catheter traverses the obstruction in the head of the pancreas. The tip of the catheter resides in the duodenum, distal to the ampulla. (From Yeo CJ, Cameron JL: Pancreatic cancer. *Curr Probl Surg* 36:59, 1999.)

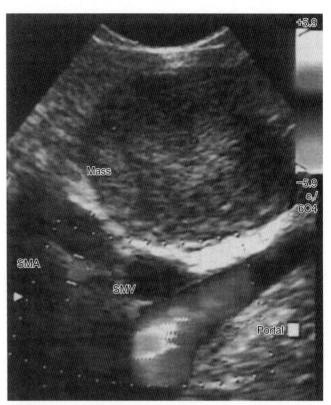

FIGURE 93-7 Endoscopic ultrasound image, with a linear-array echoendoscope, demonstrating a mass in the head of the pancreas with no vascular invasion of the superior mesenteric artery (SMA), superior mesenteric vein (SMV), or portal vein (Portal). (From Yeo CJ, Cameron JL: Pancreatic cancer. *Curr Probl Surg* 36:59, 1999.)

disease is unresectable, who are being considered for palliative therapy, or in whom neoadjuvant therapy is being considered in the hope of shrinking the lesion. In special circumstances in which there is suspicion of lymphoma or metastatic disease from another site, biopsy may be of benefit, especially if the disease is best managed without resection.

Tissue diagnosis of ampullary and duodenal cancer is usually straightforward and can easily be obtained through an endoscope. The ability to obtain large and deep biopsy specimens allows better sampling. The histologic finding of a benign villous adenoma with or without dysplasia cannot reliably rule out malignancy, but it may be appropriate to perform local ampullary resection or duodenal polypectomy first and proceed to the more radical resection if visual appearance and frozen-section pathologic examination support doing so. "Clamshell" or brush biopsy of distal common bile duct lesions is sometimes performed during ERCP or PTC to obtain a histologic diagnosis; however, it is often difficult to preoperatively ascertain the diagnosis because false-negative rates are near 50%.

PREOPERATIVE STAGING

There is substantial overlap between diagnosis and preoperative staging, with the goal being to determine the optimal treatment of each individual patient. The mainstay of preoperative staging is multidetector spiral CT with intravenous contrast performed in both the arterial and portal venous phase. Three-dimensional reconstruction of CT scans has increased the potential to predict resectable disease because of the ability to focus on the mesenteric blood vessels commonly involved. In a study of 115 patients with periampullary cancer thought to be resectable based on preoperative three-dimensional CT, the extent of local tumor burden involving the pancreas and peripancreatic tissues was accurately defined in 93% of the patients.[43] It was 95% accurate in determining cancer invasion of the superior mesenteric vessels and accurately predicted resectability and margin-negative resection in 98% and 86% of the patients, respectively. The ability of newer-generation CT scanners to predict margin-negative resectability is dependent on its enhanced ability to assess encasement of the portal or superior mesenteric vein and encasement of the superior mesenteric, celiac, or hepatic arteries.

In addition to local extent of disease, CT is effective in detecting liver metastases that are larger than 1 cm in size. CT scans in general are not highly accurate in assessing retroperitoneal lymphadenopathy or carcinomatosis without ascites or large metastatic lesions.[39] A CT scan of the chest is often performed at the same time as the staging CT to determine whether the patient has any lung metastases, but it is rare that a patient has metastatic lung disease without evidence of metastatic disease in the peritoneal cavity.

In some centers, EUS is used to help stage patients with periampullary tumors. It is very accurate in assessing the size of the primary lesion. The ability to predict vascular involvement is controversial, with some studies reporting high sensitivity and specificity and others reporting the opposite.[45,46] EUS is not very sensitive in determining lymph node involvement or distant metastatic disease unless the lesions are quite sizable. The accuracy of findings on EUS is very operator dependent.

The use of staging laparoscopy is also controversial. Some surgeons will always use staging laparoscopy in the belief that it will save a significant number of patients the morbidity and mortality of exploratory laparotomy only to determine that they have metastatic or locally unresectable disease.[47] In general, these same surgeons believe that if patients do not undergo resection for potential cure, they are best palliated by nonoperative means. Other surgeons will not routinely perform staging laparoscopy because current cross-sectional imaging studies are sensitive and specific enough that it does not make sense to subject all patients to laparoscopy to detect the few who have unresectable disease. Some argue that gastric outlet obstruction requiring surgical intervention will develop in as many as 20% of unresectable patients and that the ability to perform hepaticojejunostomy will more durably relieve obstructive jaundice.[48] Additionally, operative chemical splanchnicectomy may be performed at the same time. Yet other surgeons will use staging laparoscopy selectively by focusing on subgroups of patients at the highest risk of having unresectable disease.[49] Patients with adenocarcinoma involving the body or tail of the pancreas are more likely to have unresectable disease because these lesions do not cause obstructive jaundice and are generally larger and more advanced at the time of diagnosis. Patients with duodenal, ampullary, and distal common bile duct adenocarcinoma are much more likely to have resectable disease.

CLINICOPATHOLOGIC STAGING

Patients with cancer of the pancreas, ampulla, distal bile duct, and duodenum are staged according to the American Joint Committee on Cancer (AJCC) staging system. These staging criteria are based on the size and extent of the primary tumor (T), lymph node involvement (N), and the presence of distant metastases (M). Patients are stratified into stage groupings that guide prognosis and treatment. Pancreatic adenocarcinomas are staged with the AJCC exocrine pancreas guidelines, distal common bile duct cancers are staged with the AJCC extrahepatic bile duct guidelines, ampullary cancers are staged with the AJCC ampulla of Vater guidelines, and duodenal cancers are staged with the AJCC small intestine guidelines.

NONOPERATIVE PALLIATION

Approximately 80% to 85% of patients with pancreatic adenocarcinoma are found to have unresectable disease at diagnosis because of metastatic or locally invasive disease. For the majority of patients, palliation of symptoms and improvement in quality of life are the primary purposes of any intervention. The three main symptoms needing palliation are obstructive jaundice, gastric outlet obstruction, and pain. Patients with ampullary, distal bile duct, and duodenal adenocarcinoma are more likely to have resectable disease, but if they are initially found to have advanced disease, they will also require nonoperative palliation.

NONOPERATIVE PALLIATION OF OBSTRUCTIVE JAUNDICE

Nonoperative palliation of obstructive jaundice may be achieved either percutaneously (see Figure 93-6) or endoscopically during ERCP. Most centers will attempt endoscopic placement first and use percutaneous transhepatic approaches if required. Endoscopic placement is usually more comfortable for the patient and avoids trauma to the liver parenchyma and possible sequelae, including hemobilia and bile leakage. Endoscopic biliary stents may be made of plastic or metal. Plastic stents require periodic changing. Because of the size limitations of the accessory channel of endoscopes, the largest stent that can be placed is 12 French (12F). This relatively small diameter results in periodic occlusion necessitating periodic change. In an effort to decrease stent occlusion, self-expanding metallic stents that can reach a diameter of 30F have been developed. Metallic stents, however, eventually fail because of tumor ingrowth and, when they do fail, present a problem because they are not readily changeable. Additionally, they are more expensive than plastic stents. Covered stents are currently being developed and used and will, it is hoped, increase patency. Randomized controlled clinical trials comparing 10F or 11.5F plastic stents with 30F metallic stents have shown metallic stents to be associated with lower rates of cholangitis and stent replacement and fewer inpatient days.[50,51]

NONOPERATIVE PALLIATION OF DUODENAL OBSTRUCTION

Until recently, the standard method of nonoperative palliation of duodenal obstruction was the placement of a percutaneous endoscopic gastrostomy tube. The development of expandable metallic stents deployable in the duodenum has provided another nonoperative technique for controlling gastric outlet obstruction that allows the patient to eat. Gastroduodenal stenting can be successful in 80% to 90% of patients by providing adequate relief of obstruction.[52,53]

NONOPERATIVE PALLIATION OF PAIN

Standard management of pain has been based on opioids and nonsteroidal antiinflammatory agents. However, for patients to receive sufficient pain relief from narcotics, they often suffer many of the systemic side effects. US- and CT-guided celiac plexus nerve blocks have been used more recently in an attempt to specifically target the neurogenic pain caused by pancreatic and periampullary cancer. Several randomized controlled trials comparing standard oral narcotics with celiac plexus nerve blocks have demonstrated significant decreases in pain and narcotic use in patients undergoing these blocks.[54,55]

OPERATIVE PALLIATION

As discussed previously, current preoperative staging and imaging modalities allow resection in approximately 80% of patients explored for periampullary cancer. When a patient undergoes exploration and the cancer is found to be unresectable, a decision must be made regarding whether to operatively palliate the patient. Operative palliation is most beneficial in patients without widespread metastatic disease and with a life expectancy of more than several months. The potential morbidity and mortality associated with operative palliation should be weighed against the more durable palliation achieved with biliary bypass with or without gastrojejunostomy. Additionally, open chemical splanchnicectomy can be added to the operative palliative procedure.

OPERATIVE PALLIATION OF OBSTRUCTIVE JAUNDICE

The most effective operative procedure to relieve obstructive jaundice is hepaticojejunostomy.[56,57] Other less effective operative procedures include cholecystojejunostomy or simple drainage through a T-tube inserted above the site of obstruction. Cholecystojejunostomy is prone to reobstruction because the cystic duct insertion site into the common bile duct is often close to the site of original obstruction. T-tube drainage causes a high-output biliary fistula and results in major electrolyte abnormalities. The hepaticojejunostomy is performed by removing the gallbladder and circumferentially dissecting the common hepatic duct near the bifurcation and dividing it. The anastomosis can be performed to a loop of jejunum with a Braun jejunojejunostomy between the afferent and efferent limbs (Figure 93-8) or to a Roux-en-Y limb. In only a few patients palliated with a hepaticojejunostomy does recurrent jaundice develop before they die of their disease.[58]

OPERATIVE PALLIATION OF DUODENAL OBSTRUCTION

Periampullary cancers cause gastric outlet obstruction by compromising the lumen of the duodenum. Patients with gastric outlet obstruction who are not resection candidates and who do not have widely disseminated disease benefit from palliation, whether by operative or nonoperative stenting techniques. The role of prophylactic gastrojejunostomy is often debated. Much of the controversy stems from the discordant information on the exact percentage of patients with periampullary cancer in whom gastric outlet obstruction requiring surgical intervention eventually develops. This number ranges from 3% in some series[59] and approaches 20% in other series.[60] A prospective, randomized clinical trial was performed in 87 patients with unresectable periampullary cancer without gastric outlet obstruction in which they were randomized to undergo either retrocolic gastrojejunostomy or no bypass.[59] In none of the patients who underwent prophylactic gastrojejunostomy did gastric outlet

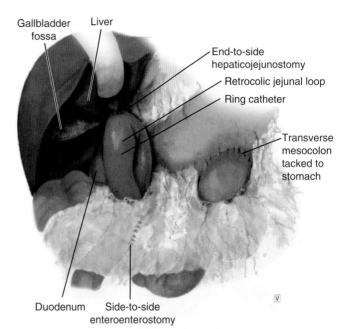

FIGURE 93-8 Anatomy after one method of palliative intervention. The biliary–enteric anastomosis is shown as a retrocolic end-to-side hepaticojejunostomy with a jejunal loop. A jejunojejunostomy was performed below the transverse mesocolon to divert the enteric stream away from the biliary–enteric anastomosis. Also shown is a retrocolic gastrojejunostomy. (From Cameron JL: *Atlas of surgery*, vol 1, Toronto, 1990, BC Decker, p 427.)

obstruction subsequently develop, whereas symptoms requiring intervention later developed in 19% of the patients who did not undergo gastric bypass. The addition of gastrojejunostomy did increase the operative time, but it had no effect on morbidity, mortality, or length of hospital stay. The gastrojejunostomies were retrocolic, to the left of the middle colic vessels, and isoperistaltic (see Figure 93-8). The gastrotomy was performed on the most dependent portion of the back wall of the stomach. Vagotomy is not routinely performed after operative palliation of gastric outlet obstruction.

OPERATIVE CHEMICAL SPLANCHNICECTOMY FOR PAIN

Operative chemical splanchnicectomy was first introduced in the 1960s in an attempt to relieve the neurogenic pain associated with unresectable pancreatic cancer.[61] A prospective randomized trial comparing intraoperative chemical splanchnicectomy with placebo in 137 patients with unresectable disease was performed by injecting 20 mL of 50% ethanol or saline through a spinal needle on either side of the aorta at the level of the celiac plexus (Figure 93-9).[62] There were no significant differences in morbidity, mortality, or length of hospital stay. The group randomized to alcohol had significantly lower pain scores at 2, 4, and 6 months. Even the patients who did not report pain preoperatively were shown to derive a benefit from chemical splanchnicectomy postoperatively as their disease progressed.

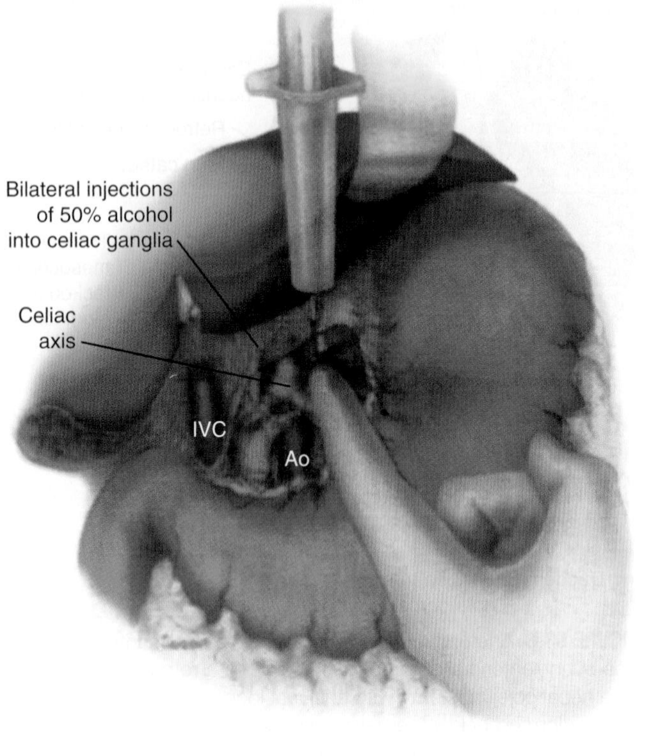

FIGURE 93-9 Technique of alcohol celiac nerve block in which 20 mL of 50% alcohol is injected on each side of the aorta (Ao) at the level of the celiac axis. *IVC,* Inferior vena cava. (From Lillemoe KD, Cameron JL, Kaufman HS, et al: Chemical splanchnicectomy in patients with unresectable pancreatic cancer: A prospective, randomized trial. *Ann Surg* 217:447, discussion 456, 1993.)

Labels in figure: Bilateral injections of 50% alcohol into celiac ganglia; Celiac axis; IVC; Ao

RESECTION OF PANCREATIC AND PERIAMPULLARY CARCINOMA

OPERATIVE TECHNIQUE OF PANCREATICODUODENECTOMY

The first successful resection of a periampullary tumor was performed by Halsted in 1898 at the Johns Hopkins Hospital. He described a local ampullary resection with reanastomosis of the pancreatic and bile ducts into the duodenum in a woman with obstructive jaundice.[63] Codivilla performed the first en bloc resection of the head of the pancreas and duodenum for periampullary carcinoma, but the patient did not survive beyond the postoperative period.[63] The first successful two-stage pancreaticoduodenectomy was performed by Kausch in 1909.[64] This patient survived to about 9 months but died of cholangitis. In 1914, Hirschel reported the first successful one-stage pancreaticoduodenectomy.[65] In the first part of the 20th century, most periampullary cancers were managed by a transduodenal approach similar to that first reported by Halsted.

Whipple et al in 1935 reported three successful two-stage en bloc resections of the head of the pancreas and the duodenum.[66] Over the next decade, modifications and technical refinements were made in the procedure, including the first one-stage pancreaticoduodenectomy in the United States by Trimble in 1941. The procedure

was infrequently performed until the 1980s despite technical advances because of the formidable operative morbidity, mortality, and poor prognosis associated with periampullary cancer. Beginning in the 1980s, Cameron perfected technical aspects and the postoperative management of the pancreaticoduodenectomy that greatly reduced the mortality of this procedure to the 1% to 3% range where it currently stands today. The reduction in mortality is at least in part due to the improved management of complications such as postoperative pancreatic fistulas, thus limiting their impact on outcome. Perhaps more importantly he trained a generation of surgeons to perform this operation with good outcomes resulting in the exponential increase in the use of this operation over the past 3 decades.

Exposure for a pancreaticoduodenectomy is obtained through a vertical midline incision from the xiphoid process to several centimeters below the umbilicus. Alternatively, a bilateral subcostal incision can be used. Exposure is greatly enhanced with the use of a mechanical retracting device.

The first portion of the operation focuses on assessing the extent of disease and resectability. The benefits and disadvantages of staging laparoscopy were discussed in the previous section. At open exploration, the entire liver is inspected and palpated to assess for the presence of metastases. The celiac axis is inspected for lymph node involvement. Tumor-bearing nodes within the resection zone do not contraindicate resection because long-term survival can be achieved with peripancreatic nodal involvement. The parietal and visceral peritoneal surfaces, the omentum, the ligament of Treitz, and the entire small and intraabdominal large intestine are carefully examined for the presence of metastatic disease. Drop metastases in the pelvis are also evaluated. A Kocher maneuver is performed by elevating the duodenum and head of the pancreas out of the retroperitoneum and into the midline. The gallbladder is mobilized and the porta hepatis is assessed. The common hepatic artery and proper hepatic artery should also be assessed to confirm resectability.

The distal common hepatic duct is divided close to the level of the cystic duct entry site early during the operation. For distal common bile duct cancers or pancreatic cancers near this area, more margin on the bile duct into the hilus of the liver may be required. The bile duct is retracted caudally, and a dissection plane is opened on the anterior surface of the portal vein. During these maneuvers, the portal structures should be assessed for a replaced right hepatic artery originating from the superior mesenteric artery. If found, this vessel should be dissected and protected from injury. If the patient appears to have an accessory right hepatic artery and a significant native right hepatic artery, the accessory vessel can often be taken. The gastroduodenal artery is next identified and occluded atraumatically. This maneuver confirms that the hepatic artery is not being supplied solely retrograde through the superior mesenteric artery collaterals (in the setting of celiac axis stenosis or occlusion).

In a standard Whipple procedure, a 30% to 40% distal gastrectomy is performed by dividing the right gastric and right gastroepiploic arteries. The antrectomy is then completed with a linear stapling device. For a pylorus-preserving pancreaticoduodenectomy, the proximal portion of the gastrointestinal tract is divided 2 to 3 cm distal to the pylorus with a linear stapling device. The right gastric artery can often be spared, but it may be taken if it allows better mobilization of the duodenum for reconstruction. The gastrointestinal tract is divided distally at a point of mobile jejunum, typically 20 cm distal to the ligament of Treitz. The mesenteric vasculature to this initial portion of the jejunum is carefully dissected and divided. Once the proximal jejunum is separated from its mesentery, it can be delivered dorsal to the superior mesenteric vessels from the left to the right side.

The superior mesenteric vein caudal to the neck of the pancreas can be identified running anterior to the third portion of the duodenum and is frequently surrounded by adipose tissue as it receives tributaries from the uncinate process and neck of the pancreas, the greater curve of the stomach, and the transverse mesocolon. In this location, the superior mesenteric vein is identified by dissecting the fatty tissue of the transverse mesocolon away from the uncinate process of the pancreas. Division of the branches emptying into the anterior surface of the superior mesenteric vein allows continued cephalad dissection. Often, a vein retractor to lift the inferior edge of the neck of the pancreas is useful for visualization (Figure 93-10). The plane anterior to the superior mesenteric vein is developed under direct vision while avoiding branches and tumor involvement. After the plane anterior to the portal vein and superior mesenteric vein is complete, a Penrose drain can be looped under the neck of the pancreas.

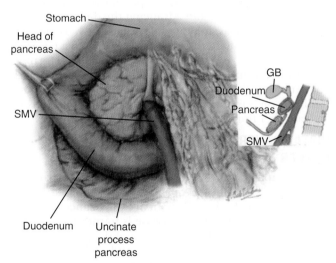

FIGURE 93-10 The superior mesenteric vein (SMV) can be visualized by performing an extended Kocher maneuver. At the level of the third portion of the duodenum (working laterally to medially), the SMV is the first and largest vascular structure running anterior to the duodenum. The inset shows the gallbladder (GB). (From Cameron JL: Rapid exposure of the portal and superior mesenteric veins. *Surg Gynecol Obstet* [now J Am Coll Surg] 176:395, 1993.)

Stay sutures are placed superiorly and inferiorly on the pancreatic remnant to reduce bleeding from the segmental pancreatic arteries. The pancreatic neck is then divided sharply after confirming a free plane anterior to the portal and superior mesenteric veins. The Penrose drain previously placed under the neck of the pancreas is used to elevate the pancreatic tissue to be divided and protect the underlying major veins. The main pancreatic duct should be noted so that it can be incorporated into the subsequent reconstruction.

The specimen now remains connected by the uncinate process of the pancreas. This structure is separated from the portal vein, superior mesenteric vein, and superior mesenteric artery by serially clamping, dividing, and tying the smaller branches off the portal and superior mesenteric vessels. Dissection should be performed flush with these structures to remove all pancreatic and nodal tissue in these areas but without injuring the superior mesenteric artery and vein at this level. The specimen can then be removed, and the pancreatic neck margin, uncinate margin, and common hepatic duct margins are marked for pathologic examination. To speed up analysis of these frozen-section margins, the common hepatic duct margin and the pancreatic neck margin should be sampled earlier and sent for pathologic examination while the main specimen is still being removed.

Multiple options for reconstruction after pancreaticoduodenectomy are available. The issues and controversies surrounding the pancreatic, biliary, and gastrointestinal reconstructions are outlined by multiple papers specifically addressing these issues.

The most common reconstruction involves placing the end of the divided jejunum through a defect in the right transverse mesocolon to create a pancreaticojejunostomy, followed by hepaticojejunostomy and then duodenojejunostomy (Figure 93-11). Some groups prefer to use a Roux limb for the pancreaticojejunostomy.

The pancreatic reconnection is the most problematic anastomosis and is responsible for the majority of the morbidity and mortality associated with the procedure. Controversy continues regarding the best type of pancreaticojejunostomy, the importance of duct-to-mucosa sutures, and the use of pancreatic duct stents. The pancreatic reconstruction can be performed with either a duct-to-mucosa anastomosis or an invagination technique. With either technique, the proximal jejunal stump is brought through a defect in the mesocolon to the right of the middle colic artery. The duct-to-mucosa anastomosis is constructed in an end-to-side fashion in which the outer back row is placed with interrupted 3-0 silk sutures that incorporate the capsule of the transected pancreas and seromuscular bites of the jejunum. A small defect is then made in the jejunum to which a duct-to-mucosa anastomosis is performed that incorporates the pancreatic duct and the full thickness of the jejunum with interrupted 5-0 Maxon suture. Some surgeons prefer to stent this anastomosis with a 6-cm stent cut from a 5F or 8F pediatric feeding tube. Three centimeters of the stent is placed in the pancreatic duct, and the other half is placed in the jejunum. The stent is held in place with one of the Maxon sutures from the back row. This stent typically

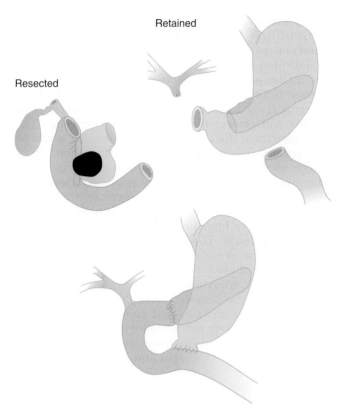

Retained

Resected

FIGURE 93-11 Pylorus-preserving pancreaticoduodenectomy. *Top left*, Structures resected include the duodenum (except for the initial 1 to 2 cm beyond the pylorus); the head, neck, and uncinate process of the pancreas, with tumor *(black)*; the gallbladder; and the distal extrahepatic biliary tree. *Top right*, Structures retained include the entire stomach, pylorus, proximal 1 to 2 cm of the duodenum, body and tail of the pancreas, proximal biliary tree, and jejunum distal to the ligament of Treitz. *Bottom*, The reconstruction is shown as a proximal end-to-end pancreaticojejunostomy, a hepaticojejunostomy decompressed with a percutaneous transhepatic catheter, and a distal duodenojejunostomy. (From Yeo CJ, Cameron JL: The pancreas. In Hardy JD, editor: *Hardy's textbook of surgery*, ed 2. Philadelphia, 1988, JB Lippincott, p 718.)

passes through the intestinal tract and into the stool within a couple of weeks.

The invagination technique is performed with an end-to-end or end-to-side pancreaticojejunostomy. The pancreatic remnant is circumferentially cleared and mobilized for 2 to 3 cm to allow for an optimal anastomosis. The pancreaticojejunostomy is performed in two layers, with the outer layer consisting of interrupted 3-0 silk suture that incorporates the capsule of the pancreas and the seromuscular layers of the jejunum. The inner layer consists of running 3-0 absorbable suture that incorporates the capsule and a portion of the cut edge of the pancreas and the full thickness of the jejunum. An attempt should be made to incorporate the pancreatic duct into the inner layer for several bites to splay it open. When completed, this anastomosis invaginates the cut surface of the pancreatic neck into the jejunal lumen for several centimeters.

If the stomach is used to reconnect the pancreas, it is invaginated into the back wall of the stomach as described

previously for the jejunum. In a prospective randomized trial comparing pancreaticogastrostomy with pancreaticojejunostomy, there was no difference in the leak or fistula rate between the two types of anastomoses.[67]

The biliary anastomosis is next performed with an end-to-side hepaticojejunostomy approximately 5 to 10 cm distal to the pancreaticojejunostomy. This anastomosis is performed with a single layer of interrupted absorbable suture such as 4-0 Maxon. If the patient has a percutaneous biliary stent, it is repositioned into the anastomosis. Preoperative biliary stenting remains controversial. Most groups believe that routine preoperative biliary stenting is of no benefit and carries potential risk, including an increased risk for wound or infectious complications, as well as an increased risk for pancreatic fistula formation.[68-70] Stenting can be considered in patients with obstructive jaundice who will have a substantial delay between initial evaluation and definitive surgery and in patients with cholangitis.

The third anastomosis performed is the duodenojejunostomy or gastrojejunostomy, depending on whether the pylorus has been preserved. This anastomosis can be performed 10 to 15 cm distal to the hepaticojejunostomy, proximal to the portion of jejunum traversing the defect in the mesocolon. Alternatively, it can be performed in antecolic fashion more distally on the jejunal limb, distal to where it traverses the mesocolic defect.

After the reconstruction is completed, closed suction drains are left in place near the pancreatic and biliary anastomoses. Some groups prefer not to drain and accept that if a fluid collection becomes clinically evident postoperatively, percutaneous drainage by interventional radiology may be required. They are also of the belief that closed-suction drains may contribute to the development of pancreatic leak and fistula.

Postoperative management after pancreaticoduodenectomy consists of keeping the patient with nothing by mouth for 1 or 2 days and advancing the diet with liquids and then solids as tolerated. The stomach is decompressed overnight after the day of surgery with a nasogastric tube, which is usually removed the next morning unless the output is high. The drains around the pancreatic anastomosis are typically removed once the patient has been on a regular diet and if significant amounts of amylase-rich fluid or bile are not draining.

DISTAL PANCREATECTOMY FOR PANCREATIC CANCER IN THE BODY OR TAIL

Staging laparoscopy should be considered in patients with distal pancreatic cancer because carcinomatosis is a more common finding in patients with cancers of the body and tail. If metastatic disease is found, pancreatectomy is unlikely to help in palliation of the patient. Exposure for distal pancreatectomy and splenectomy is obtained through a vertical midline incision from the xiphoid process to several centimeters below the umbilicus. Alternatively, a bilateral subcostal incision can be used. Exposure is greatly enhanced with the use of a mechanical retracting device. Folded sheets placed behind the patient underlying the spleen can also enhance exposure, especially in patients with a deep body habitus.

The lesser sac should be entered by elevating the greater omentum off the transverse colon. The splenic flexure of the colon should also be mobilized caudally and away from the spleen by dividing the lienocolic ligament. Splenectomy is usually performed with distal pancreatectomy in patients suspected of having carcinoma to obtain better margins, to remove the lymph nodes at the tip of the pancreas and the hilum of the spleen, and to avoid tedious dissection of the splenic artery and vein. The spleen is mobilized toward the midline by dividing the lienorenal ligament with the electrocautery device. The short gastric vessels in the lienogastric ligament are isolated and ligated. A plane is then developed behind the pancreatic tail and body to also mobilize the splenic artery and vein. This dissection is continued until an adequate margin is reached beyond the tumor. The splenic artery and vein are isolated at this level and suture-ligated. A row of overlapping "U" stitches of absorbable suture should then be placed. The electrocautery device is next used to transect the pancreatic parenchyma distal to this suture line (Figure 93-12). A frozen section should be performed on the pancreatic margin to confirm clearance of the lesion.

Postoperative management of patients after distal pancreatectomy is usually quite straightforward. Patients are advanced on a diet as tolerated. If an operative drain is left in place, it is monitored for signs of a pancreatic leak. Removing the spleen does place the patient theoretically at increased risk for postsplenectomy sepsis, and vaccines are given either preoperatively or after recovery for pneumococcus, *Neisseria meningitidis*, and *Haemophilus influenzae*.

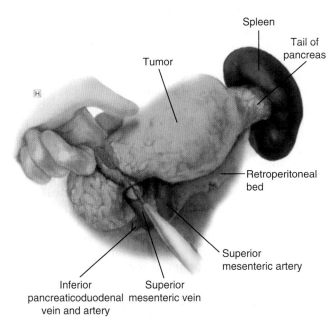

FIGURE 93-12 Near the completion of a distal pancreatectomy and splenectomy for a tumor in the body of the pancreas. The spleen and tail of the pancreas have been mobilized out of the retroperitoneum. The pancreatic parenchyma is being divided with the electrocautery device. (From Cameron JL: *Atlas of surgery*, vol 1. Toronto, 1990, BC Decker, p 27.)

MINIMALLY INVASIVE PANCREAS SURGERY

Laparoscopy, when applied appropriately to pancreatic tumors, can decrease surgical risks, postoperative pain, wound complications, and length of stay compared to the traditional open operation. The majority of the time when these techniques are being used it is for cystic neoplasms or neuroendocrine tumors. There are no prospective randomized trials to see whether laparoscopic pancreas surgery is appropriate for adenocarcinoma; however, different groups have shown that parameters of an oncologic resection such as lymph node harvest and margin status are equivalent to the traditional technique described earlier.

Laparoscopic Distal Pancreatectomy with Spleen Preservation

The operation begins with an infraumbilical port placed with a direct Hassan cut-down technique. Two ports are placed in the upper midline (or right of midline) and one left-lower quadrant port is inserted under direct visualization. The precise location for these ports depends on the location of the tumor, the intention to preserve the spleen, and the patient's body habitus. Once local landmarks are identified, the gastrocolic omentum and short gastric vessels are divided followed by take-down of the splenic flexure of the colon to achieve wide visualization of the lesser sac.

Mobilization of the pancreas is easiest from the inferior border of the gland. Thus, beginning with the inferior approach facilitates dissection of the posterior aspect of the gland from the retroperitoneal bed. The splenic artery and vein branches can be visualized from underneath the pancreas and one can alternate dissection of the splenic vessels from above and below the gland as the exposure best offers visualization. At all times, an endo GIA 2.5-mm stapler (white vascular load) is open, loaded, and ready to use in case of injury to the splenic vessels. Clips are avoided because stapling devices cannot engage on a clip. As a precaution, always keep a fresh No. 10-blade scalpel and a curved heavy Mayo scissor ready at all times in case a rapid conversion to an open operation is needed to control bleeding. Unlike other laparoscopic procedures, laparoscopic pancreas surgery may require expeditious conversion to an open approach given the intimate proximity of the large vessels in the region.

Once the pancreas is clear from the splenic vessels to allow for division of the gland, attempt to dissect as much of the tail as possible, freeing the entire tail when feasible. The gland is divided with an endo GIA 2.5-mm or 3.5-mm stapler (white vascular load or blue G.I. load) depending on pancreas thickness. The reticulating stapler is reinforced with a bioabsorbable staple line material (GORE Seamguard). Or, alternatively, energy devices or sewing the pancreatic stump can be used. The specimen is removed with an Endo Catch bag and a surgical drain is placed at the cut end of the pancreas.

When there is a suspicion of malignancy, or a technical reason that necessitates removal of the spleen, mobilization of the spleen is required after individual division of the splenic artery, vein, and organ? This allows resection of the distal pancreas and spleen en bloc. The inferior border of the pancreas is mobilized as previously described. The tail is suspended up by an instrument or umbilical tape used for upward traction, facilitating visualization of the splenic vessels. Dissection of the splenic artery toward the spleen or the celiac artery is sometimes required to ensure that the splenic artery is not mistaken for the hepatic artery. The splenic artery and the vein, respectively, are each ligated in turn with a vascular stapler, sometimes approaching these vessels from the posterior aspect of the spleen. On occasion, bleeding from branches of the splenic vein can be troublesome but these usually can be controlled with meticulous dissection and standard laparoscopic hemostatic techniques. The spleen is mobilized from its attachments as the last step of the operation. The specimen is removed en bloc in an Endo Catch bag requiring a small extension of one of the 12-mm port sites. A frozen-section analysis is performed intraoperatively to confirm a negative and adequate margin of resection before completing the operation.

Laparoscopic Pancreaticoduodenectomy

Laparoscopic pancreaticoduodenectomy is currently being done at select centers around the world. The steps involved are different from the traditional open approach described earlier. Typically six ports are used in a semicircle around the pancreas from the left upper quadrant (LUQ) to the RUQ. These 10-mm ports are placed evenly to give access from all directions. After evaluating the abdomen for metastasis, the lesser sac is entered standing on the patient's right side. The first portion of the duodenum and antrum is then lifted with a retractor. The hepatic artery is identified and dissected with the hook cautery to find the takeoff of the gastroduodenal artery, which is a landmark for the portal vein below. The gastroduodenal is dissected and ligated. The first portion of the duodenum is dissected until 1 to 2 cm beyond the pylorus and divided with a stapler. At this point, the inferior portion of the pancreas is dissected looking for the superior mesenteric vein. Earlier identification of the portal vein helps with superior mesenteric vein identification. Once found, the tunnel is created under the neck of the pancreas with gentle blunt dissection and encircled with an umbilical tape.

After the pancreas neck is completed, the gallbladder is mobilized and used to find the common bile duct, which is encircled with the distal end tied prior to transection. The tied end of the common bile duct can be used as an anchor to identify the portal vein below. Following the resection of the common bile duct, the kocher maneuver can be started by mobilizing the duodenum staying close to the bowel. After the extended Kocherization is complete, the distal jejunum is identified 10 cm distal to the ligament of Treitz and transected with a stapler. The stapled ends of the jejunum are sewn to each other with a 25-cm silk stitch with a large gap to facilitate pulling the distal jejunum through the ligament of Treitz for future anastomosis. Finally, the colon is lifted and the ligament of Treitz is freed with a hook cautery.

The final point of transection is the pancreas. The neck is transected with an energy device leaving behind

the uncinate, which is taken off the superior mesenteric vein and artery with an energy device. Larger branches may require ligation with clips or suture. The specimen is now free for removal with a bag to prevent contamination. As the specimen is pulled to the RUQ, the previously sewn jejunal limb will be pulled through the ligament of Treitz defect into proper place for pancreatic and biliary anastomosis. The jejunal suture can be cut at this point to remove the specimen.

Finally, the three anastomoses can be done with the jejunum already in proper position. These are anastomoses done similar to the open technique requiring intracorporal stitches. The pancreatic anastomosis can be done either from the duct to the mucosa or using the invagination technique. The hepaticojejunostomy is done with interrupted suture with the assistant holding the bowel up to facilitate this step. The final gastro/duodenal jejunal anastomosis can be done in a two-layered intracorporal sewn fashion or stapled. With everything being complete, the drains are placed around the anastomosis.

Laparoscopic pancreas surgery is a technically demanding operation. It requires the expertise of a pancreatic surgeon who also has advanced laparoscopic skills. This field is continuing to evolve and is currently available at high-volume centers.

COMPLICATIONS AFTER PANCREATICODUODENECTOMY AND DISTAL PANCREATECTOMY

The mortality rate after pancreaticoduodenectomy at centers specializing in pancreatic surgery is in the 2% to 3% range. Despite the low mortality rates, especially when compared with those reported before the 1980s, the rate of postoperative complications remains high. In a series of 564 pancreaticoduodenectomies performed for adenocarcinoma, the mortality rate was 2.3% with an overall complication rate of 31%.[69] In this series, the three most common complications were delayed gastric emptying in 14%, wound infection in 7%, and pancreatic fistula in 5% (Table 93-2). Delayed gastric emptying is not life-threatening and is almost always self-limited, but it can increase the length of stay and hospital costs significantly. The great majority of patients respond to nasogastric decompression and nutritional support. Erythromycin is sometimes used to increase gastrointestinal motility.[71]

Pancreatic fistulas are not uncommon after pancreaticoduodenectomy and can lead to very severe problems, including intraabdominal abscess and bleeding as a result of a pseudoaneurysm, if not properly controlled. In the majority of patients, a pancreatic leak will seal with conservative management. If closed-suction drains are in place and a CT scan confirms the absence of undrained abscesses, often no other major intervention is necessary. If a CT scan demonstrates an intraabdominal abscess, interventional radiologic techniques are usually successful at controlling the infection. If a patient is relatively asymptomatic with a controlled pancreatic leak and is on a regular diet, consideration can be given to sending the

TABLE 93-2 Mortality and Morbidity After Pancreaticoduodenectomy and Distal Pancreatectomy in 616 Patients

	Overall (*n* = 616)	Pancreaticoduodenectomy/ Pancreatectomy (*n* = 564)	Distal Pancreatectomy (*n* = 52)	*P* Value
Perioperative mortality	2.3%	2.3%	1.9%	NS
Overall complications	30%	31%	25%	NS
SPECIFIC COMPLICATIONS				
Reoperation	3%	3%	4%	NS
Delayed gastric emptying	—	14%	—	—
Cholangitis	—	3%	—	—
Bile leak	—	2%	—	—
Wound infection	7%	7%	5%	NS
Pancreatic fistula	5%	5%	8%	NS
Intraabdominal abscess	3%	3%	4%	NS
Pneumonia	1%	1%	0%	NS
Pancreatitis	1%	1%	0%	NS
POSTOPERATIVE LENGTH OF STAY				
Mean ± SE	13.7 ± 0.4 d	14.0 ± 0.4 d	11.5 ± 2.2 d	0.08
Median	11 d	11 d	7 d	

From Sohn TA, Yeo CJ, Cameron JL, et al: Resected adenocarcinoma of the pancreas—616 patients: Results, outcomes, and prognostic indicators. *J Gastrointest Surg* 4:567, 2000.
SE, Standard equivalent.

patient home with outpatient drain management. In most cases, the fistula will improve and cease within a couple of weeks. If the patient is symptomatic from the fistula or it has high output (>200 mL/day), consideration should be given to restricting the patient's diet and using parenteral nutrition.

In a series of 52 patients undergoing distal pancreatectomy for pancreatic adenocarcinoma of the body or tail, the mortality rate was 1.9% with an overall morbidity rate of 25%. The three most common complications were pancreatic fistula in 8%, wound infection in 5%, and intraabdominal abscess in 4% (see Table 93-2).

LONG-TERM SURVIVAL AFTER RESECTION OF PERIAMPULLARY CANCER

Survival of patients after resection of pancreatic and periampullary cancer is dependent on many factors, including the site of the primary cancer and the stage of the disease. In a series of 616 patients who underwent resection of pancreatic cancer, pancreaticoduodenectomy was performed in 85%, distal pancreatectomy in 9%, and total pancreatectomy in 6%.[72] The overall survival rate of the entire cohort was 63% and 17% at 1 and 5 years, respectively, with a median survival of 17 months. For right-sided lesions requiring pancreaticoduodenectomy, the survival rates were 64% and 17% versus 50% and 15% for left-sided lesions at 1 and 5 years, respectively (Figure 93-13). Factors that had favorable prognostic significance by univariate analysis were negative resection margins, tumor smaller than 3 cm, negative lymph nodes, blood loss less than 750 mL, absence of blood transfusions, well or moderate tumor differentiation, and postoperative chemoradiation.

An analysis was performed of 58 actual 5-year survivors from 242 consecutive patients with resected

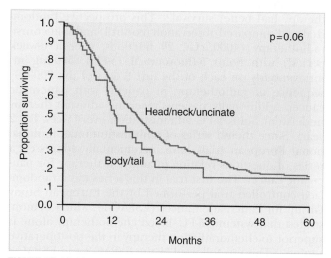

FIGURE 93-13 Kaplan–Meier actuarial survival curves comparing patients with head, neck, and uncinate lesions (right-sided, *n* = 563) with those who had body and tail lesions (left-sided, *n* = 49). (From Sohn TA, Yeo CJ, Cameron JL, et al: Resected adenocarcinoma of the pancreas—616 patients: Results, outcomes, and prognostic indicators. *J Gastrointest Surg* 4:567, 2000.)

periampullary adenocarcinoma; 62% had pancreatic adenocarcinoma, 19% had ampullary adenocarcinoma, 12% had distal bile duct adenocarcinoma, and 7% had duodenal adenocarcinoma.[72] The actual 5-year tumor-specific survival rates were 15% for pancreas, 39% for ampullary, 27% for distal bile duct, and 59% for duodenal adenocarcinoma. The 5-year survivors had a significantly higher rate of well-differentiated tumors, negative resection margins, and negative lymph nodes.

Some groups have advocated that patients with node-positive cancer have better survival after extended lymphadenectomy.[73] A trial was performed in which 299 patients with periampullary adenocarcinoma were randomized to standard pancreaticoduodenectomy or radical surgery in which the retroperitoneal lymph nodes were removed. For all periampullary cancer patients, those who underwent standard resection had 1- and 5-year survival rates of 78% and 25%, respectively, as compared with 76% and 31% ($P = .57$) for patients in the radical surgery group. For pancreatic adenocarcinoma patients, 1- and 5-year survival rates in the standard group were 75% and 13%, respectively, versus 73% and 29% in the radical surgery group ($P = .13$).[74]

ADJUVANT THERAPY

Several relatively large prospective randomized trials that assess the efficacy and safety of various adjuvant therapy regimens have been conducted. Early studies included all periampullary cancers, but based on the known differences in biology, contemporary trials more appropriately have been focused more on the particular cancers. The best studied periampullary cancer is pancreatic adenocarcinoma. The earliest trial on this disease was the 1985 Gastrointestinal Tumor Study Group (GITSG) trial and demonstrated that patients undergoing resection for pancreatic cancer who received adjuvant chemoradiotherapy had better survival.[75] This prospective randomized trial compared observation (control) and split-course radiotherapy (4000 cGy, 20 fractions, over a 6-week period) with bolus 5-fluorouracil (5-FU), 500 mg/m^2 intravenously on each of the first 3 days of the 200-cGy sequence of radiotherapy, in patients with pancreatic cancer. Additionally, patients receiving adjuvant therapy underwent bolus 5-FU administration every week for 2 years. Since then a series of multiinstitutional, multinational European trials have incrementally addressed a series of questions relating to adjuvant therapy for pancreatic cancer. The first trial in this series was a randomized controlled trial performed by the European Study Group for Pancreatic Cancer (ESPAC-1), which demonstrated that systemic 5-FU–based chemotherapy alone is superior to chemoradiation therapy in the postoperative setting.[76] This was followed by the ESPAC-2 and ESPAC-3 trials that were designed with the premise that chemoradiotherapy was inferior to chemotherapy alone and thus only assessed the latter. The ESPAC-3 trial compared 5-FU/leucovorin to gemcitabine in a two-armed trial and found no difference in survival.[77] However, the toxicity profile slightly favored gemcitabine as a result of reduced rates of stomatitis and diarrhea in that treatment arm. Taken together with the results of the CONKO-001 trial that demonstrated a significant survival advantage for adjuvant gemcitabine over observation, it is likely that gemcitabine-based regimens will be the standard in the near future.[78] It should be noted that the inferior outcomes for chemoradiotherapy in comparison to chemotherapy alone, and perhaps even observation, that was found in the ESPAC-1 trial is controversial. Other smaller prospective trials have suggested a potential benefit of chemoradiotherapy in particular in the battle against local recurrence.

The role of adjuvant chemoradiotherapy in the treatment of distal bile duct, ampullary, and duodenal cancer is less well understood than for pancreatic cancer because of the relative infrequency of these diseases.

NEOADJUVANT THERAPY

Neoadjuvant therapy has several theoretical advantages. It allows more timely administration of chemotherapy or chemoradiotherapy to patients who are at a high risk for failure after surgical resection. It has the potential to shrink the tumor and can theoretically decrease the extent of local disease. Patients in whom disseminated disease develops during neoadjuvant treatment are unlikely to have benefited from initial resection and are spared the time commitment, morbidity, and potential mortality from resection. It may allow better selection of patients who are most likely to benefit from surgical resection.

A series of 193 patients with biopsy-proven pancreatic adenocarcinoma who completed neoadjuvant chemoradiotherapy and 70 patients who underwent resection without neoadjuvant therapy has been reported. The exact treatment regimens varied, but 183 patients (95%) received 5-FU–based chemotherapy delivered concurrently with daily external-beam radiotherapy for a planned total dose of 4500 cGy at 180 cGy per fraction over a period of 5 weeks plus a 540-cGy boost to the tumor. Complete histologic responses were found in 6% of patients. Patients who underwent resection with minimal residual disease and those whose tumor specimens had significant tumor necrosis had significantly better survival.

The MD Anderson Cancer Center experience with neoadjuvant chemoradiotherapy for resectable pancreatic cancer was recently summarized.[79] Since 1988, four prospective neoadjuvant trials have been completed at that institution in patients with adenocarcinoma of the pancreatic head. The trials have evolved, with the first two using 5-FU as the chemotherapy component, the third using paclitaxel, and the fourth using gemcitabine. A total of 86 patients were enrolled in the most recent trial, with 58% of the resected surgical specimens showing at least 50% tumor cell kill and two with a complete pathologic response. With a median followup now extending more than 3 years, the median survival of resected patients was approximately 36 months.

PALLIATIVE CHEMOTHERAPY

5-FU was considered the standard therapy for advanced pancreatic cancer before approval of gemcitabine by the Food and Drug Administration (FDA). Although response rates greater than 20% were reported for treatment with 5-FU, most of these reports predated the era of CT imaging and were based primarily on clinical tumor evaluation. Modern phase II trials have reported response rates of less than 10% for 5-FU alone or with leucovorin.[80]

Gemcitabine was approved by the FDA because of its ability to alleviate tumor-related symptoms. A pivotal phase III trial was completed to quantify this effect in patients with metastatic, symptomatic pancreatic cancer. One hundred twenty-six patients who had not received previous chemotherapy for metastatic disease were randomized to weekly gemcitabine ($n = 63$) or weekly bolus 5-FU ($n = 63$). Overall survival in patients treated with gemcitabine was significantly improved over those treated with 5-FU (median survival, 5.7 vs. 4.4 months, respectively; $P < 0.0025$). One-year survival rates were 18% for patients treated with gemcitabine versus 2% for patients treated with 5-FU.

Trials are currently ongoing in which gemcitabine is combined with other chemotherapeutic agents such as topoisomerase I inhibitors, platinums, and taxanes. Additionally, gemcitabine is being combined with molecularly targeted agents such as antiangiogenic and epidermal growth factor receptor agents.[81]

IMMUNOTHERAPY

Immune-based therapies can exploit either the cellular or the humoral components of the immune system (or both). Strategies aimed at the cellular components recruit and activate T cells that recognize tumor-specific antigens. One approach is to transduce tumor cell lines from primary pancreatic tumor specimens to secrete cytokine-like granulocyte-macrophage colony-stimulating factor (GM-CSF) through gene transfer creating a tumor cell vaccine. GM-CSF tumor cell vaccines have been shown to have potent and lasting specific antitumor immunity by CD4 and CD8 pathways in several clinical trials. In a phase I trial of patients with surgically resected adenocarcinoma of the pancreas, 14 patients were treated with an allogeneic tumor cell vaccine transduced to secrete GM-CSF.[82] No dose-limiting toxicities were encountered. This vaccine approach induced dose-dependent systemic antitumor immunity as measured by increased postvaccination delayed-type hypersensitivity responses against autologous tumors. Moreover, the three long-term survivors had stage III disease but also had the strongest postvaccination responses. This strategy is currently being evaluated in a phase II trial at Johns Hopkins. Immune therapy is evolving in combining vaccine platforms as described with immune checkpoint regulation. This can involve enhancing the costimulatory receptors on T cells or blocking inhibitory receptors. In addition, clinical trials are ongoing looking at the role of vaccine and blockage of the immune inhibitory effects of FoxP3$^+$ T$_{reg}$ cells. The field of immunotherapy in pancreatic cancer is novel and continuing to grow, particularly in the area of combinatorial therapy with a vaccine and immune modulators. Recent trials have shown promise and continuing trials are underway evaluating the effectiveness.

CONCLUSION

Patients with pancreatic and periampullary cancer represent a difficult and challenging group to treat. It is clear that there is currently no single modality that can uniformly cure these patients; however, surgical resection should be attempted when appropriate because resection gives the only chance of long-term survival. Traditionally, these patients have had a poor prognosis, but with proper staging and patient selection, results are slowly improving. Resection should be performed by experienced surgeons to minimize morbidity and mortality. It is clear that there are many more developments that need to be made to improve the survival and well-being of these patients.

REFERENCES

1. American Cancer Society: *Facts and figures, 2005*. Atlanta, 2005, American Cancer Society.
2. Michaud DS: Epidemiology of pancreas cancer. *Minerva Chir* 59:99, 2004.
3. Neoptolemos JP, Talbot IC, Carr-Locke DL, et al: Treatment and outcome in 52 consecutive cases of ampullary carcinoma. *Br J Surg* 74:957, 1987.
4. Howe JR, Klimstra DS, Moccia RD, et al: Factors predictive of survival in ampullary carcinoma. *Ann Surg* 228:87, 1998.
5. Nakase A, Matsumoto Y, Uchida K, et al: Surgical treatment of cancer of the pancreas and the periampullary region: Cumulative results in 57 institutions in Japan. *Ann Surg* 185:52, 1977.
6. Yeo CJ: The Whipple procedure in the 1990s. *Adv Surg* 32:271, 1999.
7. Bettschart V, Rahman MQ, Engelken FJ, et al: Presentation, treatment and outcome in patients with ampullary tumours. *Br J Surg* 91:1600, 2004.
8. Matsumoto T, Hirano S, Yada K, et al: Malignant serous cystic neoplasm of the pancreas: Report of a case and review of the literature. *J Clin Gastroenterol* 39:253, 2005.
9. Sohn TA, Yeo CJ, Cameron JL, et al: Intraductal papillary mucinous neoplasms of the pancreas: An updated experience. *Ann Surg* 239:788, discussion 797, 2004.
10. Sanborn RE, Blanke CD: Gastrointestinal stromal tumors and the evolution of targeted therapy. *Clin Adv Hematol Oncol* 3:647, 2005.
11. Gold EB, Goldin SB: Epidemiology of and risk factors for pancreatic cancer. *Surg Oncol Clin N Am* 7:67, 1998.
12. Lowenfels AB, Maisonneuve P: Risk factors for pancreatic cancer. *J Cell Biochem* 95:649, 2005.
13. Boyle P, Maisonneuve P, Bueno DM, et al: Cigarette smoking and pancreas cancer: A case control study of the search programme of the IARC. *Int J Cancer* 67:63, 1996.
14. Engeland A, Andersen A, Haldorsen T, et al: Smoking habits and risk of cancers other than lung cancer: 28 years' follow-up of 26,000 Norwegian men and women. *Cancer Causes Control* 7:497, 1996.
15. Doll R, Peto R, Boreham J, Sutherland I: Mortality from cancer in relation to smoking: 50 years' observations on British doctors. *Br J Cancer* 92:426, 2005.
16. Kishi K, Nakamura K, Yoshimori M, et al: Morphology and pathological significance of focal acinar cell dysplasia of the human pancreas. *Pancreas* 7:177, 1992.
17. Gold EB: Epidemiology of and risk factors for pancreatic cancer. *Surg Clin North Am* 75:819, 1995.
18. Howe GR, Burch JD: Nutrition and pancreatic cancer. *Cancer Causes Control* 7:69, 1996.
19. Go VL, Gukovskaya A, Pandol SJ: Alcohol and pancreatic cancer. *Alcohol* 35:205, 2005.
20. MacMahon B, Yen S, Trichopoulos D, et al: Coffee and cancer of the pancreas. *N Engl J Med* 304:630, 1981.
21. Hseih C-C, MacMahon B, Yen S, et al: Coffee and pancreatic cancer (Chapter 2). *N Engl J Med* 315:587, 1986.
22. Angevine DM, Jablon S: Late radiation effects of neoplasia and other diseases in Japan. *Ann N Y Acad Sci* 114:823, 1964.
23. Thompson DE, Mabuchi K, Ron E, et al: Cancer incidence in atomic bomb survivors. Part II: Solid tumors, 1958-1987. *Radiat Res* 137:S17, 1994.
24. Hruban RH, Peterson GM, Ha PK, Kern SE: Genetics of pancreatic cancer: From genes to families. *Surg Oncol Clin N Am* 7:1, 1998.
25. Lowenfels AB, Maisonneuve P, Cavallini G, et al: Pancreatitis and the risk of pancreatic cancer: International Pancreatitis Study Group. *N Engl J Med* 328:1433, 1993.
26. Bansal P, Sonnenberg A: Pancreatitis is a risk factor for pancreatic cancer. *Gastroenterology* 109:247, 1995.
27. Fernandez E, LaVecchia C, Porta M, et al: Pancreatitis and the risk of pancreatic cancer. *Pancreas* 11:185, 1995.

28. Chow H-W, Gridley G, Nyren O, et al: Risk of pancreatic cancer following diabetes mellitus: A nationwide cohort study in Sweden. *J Natl Cancer Inst* 87:930, 1995.

29. LaVecchia C, Negri E, D'Avanzo B, et al: Medical history, diet and pancreatic cancer. *Oncology* 47:463, 1990.

30. Jones S, Zhang X, Parsons D, et al: Core signaling pathways in human pancreatic cancers revealed by global genomic analyses. *Science* 321:1801, 2008.

31. Jiao Y, Shi C, Edil BH: DAXX/ATRX, MEN1 and mTOR pathway genes are frequently altered in pancreatic neuroendocrine tumors. *Science* 331:1191, 2011.

32. Rozenblum E, Schutte M, Goggins M, et al: Tumor-suppressive pathways in pancreatic carcinoma. *Cancer Res* 57:1731, 1997.

33. Yeo CJ, Sohn TA, Cameron JL, et al: Periampullary adenocarcinoma: Analysis of 5-year survivors. *Ann Surg* 227:821, 1998.

34. Goggins M, Offerhaus GJA, Hilgers W, et al: Pancreatic adenocarcinomas with DNA replication errors (RER+) are associated with wild-type k-ras and characteristic histopathology: Poor differentiation, a syncytial growth pattern, and pushing borders suggest RER+. *Am J Pathol* 152:1501, 1998.

35. Shaib Y, El-Serag HB: The epidemiology of cholangiocarcinoma. *Semin Liver Dis* 24:115, 2004.

36. Wilentz RE, Chung CH, Sturm PDJ, et al: K-ras mutations in duodenal fluid of patients with pancreas carcinoma. *Cancer* 82:96, 1998.

37. Berthelemy P, Bouisson M, Escourrou J, et al: Identification of k-ras mutations in pancreatic juice early in the diagnosis of pancreatic cancer. *Ann Intern Med* 123:188, 1995.

38. Caldas C, Hahn SA, Hruban RH, et al: Detection of k-ras mutations in the stool of patients with pancreatic adenocarcinoma and pancreatic ductal mucinous cell hyperplasia. *Cancer Res* 54:3568, 1994.

39. Povoski SP, Karpeh MS Jr, Conlon KC, et al: Association of preoperative biliary drainage with postoperative outcome following pancreaticoduodenectomy. *Ann Surg* 230:131, 1999.

40. Sohn TA, Yeo CJ, Cameron JL, et al: Do preoperative biliary stents increase postpancreaticoduodenectomy complications? *J Gastrointest Surg* 4:258, 2000.

41. Bluemke DA, Fishman EK: CT and MR evaluation of pancreatic cancer. *Surg Oncol Clin N Am* 7:103, 1998.

42. House MG, Yeo CJ, Cameron JL, et al: Predicting resectability of periampullary cancer with three-dimensional computed tomography. *J Gastrointest Surg* 8:280, 2004.

43. Gambhir SS, Czernin J, Schimmer J, et al: A tabulated review of the literature. *J Nucl Med* 42:9S, 2001.

44. Delbeke D, Pinson CW: Pancreatic tumors: Role of imaging in the diagnosis, staging, and treatment. *J Hepatobiliary Pancreat Surg* 11:4, 2004.

45. Long EE, Van Dam J, Weinstein S, et al: Computed tomography, endoscopic, laparoscopic, and intra-operative sonography for assessing resectability of pancreatic cancer. *Surg Oncol* 14:105, 2005.

46. Aslanian H, Salem R, Lee J, et al: EUS diagnosis of vascular invasion in pancreatic cancer: Surgical and histologic correlates. *Am J Gastroenterol* 100:1381, 2005.

47. Conlon KC, Dougherty E, Klimstra DS, et al: The value of minimal access surgery in the staging of patients with potentially resectable peripancreatic malignancy. *Ann Surg* 223:134, 1996.

48. Lillemoe KD: Palliative therapy for pancreatic cancer. *Surg Oncol Clin N Am* 7:199, 1998.

49. Vollmer CM, Drebin JA, Middleton WD, et al: Utility of staging laparoscopy in subsets of peripancreatic and biliary malignancies. *Ann Surg* 235:1, 2002.

50. Knyrim K, Wagner HJ, Bethge N, et al: A controlled trial of an expansile metal stent for palliation of esophageal obstruction due to inoperable cancer. *N Engl J Med* 329:1302, 1993.

51. Davids PH, Groen AK, Rauws EA, et al: Randomised trial of self-expanding metal stents versus polyethylene stents for distal malignant biliary obstruction. *Lancet* 340:1488, 1992.

52. Kaw M, Singh S, Gagneja H: Clinical outcome of simultaneous self-expandable metal stents for palliation of malignant biliary and duodenal obstruction. *Surg Endosc* 17:457, 2003.

53. Maetani I, Tada T, Ukita T, et al: Comparison of duodenal stent placement with surgical gastrojejunostomy for palliation in patients with duodenal obstructions caused by pancreaticobiliary malignancies. *Endoscopy* 36:73, 2004.

54. Polati E, Finco G, Gottin L, et al: Prospective randomized double-blind trial of neurolytic coeliac plexus block in patients with pancreatic cancer. *Br J Surg* 85:199, 1998.

55. Bakkevold KE, Kambestad B: Palliation of pancreatic cancer. A prospective multicentre study. *Eur J Surg Oncol* 21:176, 1995.

56. Sarr MG, Cameron JL: Surgical management of unresectable carcinoma of the pancreas. *Surgery* 91:123, 1982.

57. Watanapa P, Williamson RCN: Surgical palliation for pancreatic cancer. Developments during the past two decades. *Br J Surg* 79:8, 1992.

58. Sohn TA, Lillemoe KD, Cameron JL, et al: Surgical palliation of unresectable periampullary adenocarcinoma in the 1990s. *J Am Coll Surg* 188:658, discussion 666, 1999.

59. Espat NJ, Brennan MF, Conlon KC: Patients with laparoscopically staged unresectable pancreatic adenocarcinoma do not require subsequent surgical biliary or gastric bypass. *J Am Coll Surg* 188:649, 1999.

60. Lillemoe KD, Cameron JL, Hardacre JM, et al: Is prophylactic gastrojejunostomy indicated for unresectable periampullary cancer? A prospective randomized trial. *Ann Surg* 230:322, 1999.

61. Lillemoe KD, Sauter PK, Pitt HA, et al: Current status of surgical palliation of periampullary carcinoma. *Surg Gynecol Obstet* 176:1, 1993.

62. Lillemoe KD, Cameron JL, Kaufman HS, et al: Chemical splanchnicectomy in patients with unresectable pancreatic cancer. A prospective randomized trial. *Ann Surg* 217:447, 1993.

63. Halsted WS: Contributions to the surgery of the bile passages, especially of the common bile duct. *Boston Med Surg J* 141:645, 1899.

64. Kausch W: Das Carcinoma der Papilla Duodeni und seine radikale Entfeinung. *Beitr Z Clin Chir* 78:439, 1912.

65. Hirschel G: Die Resection des Duodenums mit der Papille wegen Karzinoims. *Munchen Med Wochenschr* 61:1728, 1914.

66. Whipple AO, Parsons WB, Mullins CR: Treatment of carcinoma of the ampulla of Vater. *Ann Surg* 102:763, 1935.

67. Yeo CJ, Cameron JL, Maher MM, et al: A prospective randomized trial of pancreaticogastrostomy versus pancreaticojejunostomy after pancreaticoduodenectomy. *Ann Surg* 222:580, 1995.

68. Heslin MJ, Brooks AD, Hochwald SN, et al: A preoperative biliary stent is associated with increased complications after pancreaticoduodenectomy. *Arch Surg* 133:149, 1998.

69. Povoski SP, Karpeh MS, Conlon KC, et al: Association of preoperative biliary drainage with postoperative outcome following pancreaticoduodenectomy. *Ann Surg* 230:131, 1999.

70. Sohn TA, Yeo CJ, Cameron JL, et al: Preoperative biliary stents in patients undergoing pancreaticoduodenectomy: Increased risk of postoperative complications? *J Gastrointest Surg* 4:258, discussion 267, 2000.

71. Yeo CJ, Barry MK, Sauter PK, et al: Erythromycin accelerates gastric emptying following pancreaticoduodenectomy: A prospective, randomized placebo controlled trial. *Ann Surg* 218:229, discussion 237, 1993.

72. Sohn TA, Yeo CJ, Cameron JL, et al: Resected adenocarcinoma of the pancreas—616 patients: Results, outcomes, and prognostic indicators. *J Gastrointest Surg* 4:567, 2000.

73. Pedrazzoli S, DiCarlo V, Dionigi R, et al: Standard versus extended lymphadenectomy associated with pancreaticoduodenectomy in the surgical treatment of adenocarcinoma of the head of the pancreas: A multicenter, prospective, randomized study. Lymphadenectomy Study Group. *Ann Surg* 228:508, 1998.

74. Riall TS, Cameron JL, Lillemoe KD, et al: Pancreaticoduodenectomy with or without distal gastrectomy and extended retroperitoneal lymphadenectomy for periampullary adenocarcinoma—Part 3: Update on 5-year survival. *J Gastrointest Surg* 9:1191, 2005.

75. Kalser MH, Ellenberg SS: Pancreatic cancer—adjuvant combined radiation and chemotherapy following curative resection. *Arch Surg* 120:899, 1985.

76. Neoptolemos JP, Dunn JA, Stocken DD, et al: European Study Group for Pancreatic Cancer. Adjuvant chemoradiotherapy and chemotherapy in resectable pancreatic cancer: A randomised controlled trial. *Lancet* 358:1576, 2001.

77. Neoptolemos JP, Stocken DD, Bassi C, et al: Adjuvant chemotherapy with fluorouracil plus folinic acid vs gemcitabine following pancreatic cancer resection: A randomized controlled trial. *JAMA* 304:1073, 2010.

78. Oettle H, Post S, Neuhaus P, et al: Adjuvant chemotherapy with gemcitabine vs observation in patients undergoing curative-intent resection of pancreatic cancer: A randomized controlled trial. *JAMA* 297:267, 2007.

79. Raut CP, Evans DB, Crane CH, et al: Neoadjuvant therapy for resectable pancreatic cancer. *Surg Oncol Clin N Am* 13:639, 2004.

80. DeCaprio JA, Mayer RJ, Gonin R, et al: Fluorouracil and high-dose leucovorin in previously untreated patients with advanced adenocarcinoma of the pancreas: Results of a phase II trial. *J Clin Oncol* 9:2128, 1991.

81. Lockhart AC, Rothenberg ML, Berlin JD: Treatment for pancreatic cancer: Current therapy and continued progress. *Gastroenterology* 128:1642, 2005.

82. Jaffee EM, Hruban RH, Biedrzycki B, et al: Novel allogeneic granulocyte-macrophage colony-stimulating factor-secreting tumor vaccine for pancreatic cancer: A phase I trial of safety and immune activation. *J Clin Oncol* 19:145, 2001.

Neuroendocrine Tumors of the Pancreas

Daniela Ladner | Jeffrey A. Norton

The overall prevalence and incidence of functional pancreatic endocrine tumors are low, approximately 1 to 6 per million.[1] However, both the incidence and prevalence are increasing.[2] Gastrinoma and insulinoma are the two most common functional neuroendocrine tumors (NETs) and account for approximately 70% to 90%. Functional tumors all produce a surplus of hormone, leading to a specific syndrome with a characteristic symptom complex. The symptoms and presentation of NET may occasionally be life-threatening (e.g., perforated peptic ulcer or hypoglycemic seizures), an important reason to identify and remove the tumor. Most pancreatic endocrine tumors are malignant, although insulinomas are generally benign. However, malignancy is often not diagnosed until tumors are metastatic, although even malignant tumors tend to be slow growing and slowly progressive and may thus take a "benign" course. Obviously, in benign or malignant NET, resection of tumor leads to resolution of the characteristic syndrome. However, in many individuals, the extent of the disease limits the effectiveness of surgery. In patients whose tumor cannot be completely extirpated, effective medical treatments for controlling symptoms may be available and should be considered.

Beyond insulinoma, other pancreatic NETs include somatostatinoma, glucagonoma, pancreatic polypeptide–producing tumor (PPoma), vasoactive intestinal polypeptide–producing tumor (VIPoma), growth hormone–releasing factor–producing tumors (GRFomas), adrenocorticotropic hormone–producing tumors (ACTHomas), parathyroid hormone–related protein–producing tumors (PTHrpomas), neurotensinomas, and nonfunctional neuroendocrine tumors. Pancreatic endocrine tumors may contain ductular structures; may produce hormones that are not produced by the normal pancreas, including gastrin and VIP; and may produce more than one hormone.[3-5] These findings suggest that pancreatic endocrine tumors originate from dedifferentiation of an immature pancreatic stem cell.[5]

It has also been proposed that pancreatic endocrine tumors originate from cells that are part of the diffuse neuroendocrine system: amine precursor uptake and decarboxylation tumors (APUDomas).[6-8] These tumor cells contain dense secretory granules; may produce multiple peptides; and usually stain positive for neuron-specific enolase, chromogranin A, and synaptophysin.[3,4,9] APUDomas comprise many neuroendocrine tumors, including carcinoids, medullary thyroid carcinoma, and pheochromocytomas.[6-8]

Microscopically, pancreatic endocrine tumors are composed of sheets of small, round cells with uniform nuclei and cytoplasm (Figure 94-1). Mitotic figures are rare, and the precise determination of malignancy cannot be made by histologic appearance.[10,11]

Recent studies suggest that pancreatic neuroendocrine tumors can be grouped according to aggressive or nonaggressive behaviors. The aggressive forms include glucagonoma, VIPoma, somatostatinoma, and most nonfunctional tumors. Aggressive tumors are characterized by short disease duration, large size, liver metastases, and a reduced long-term survival rate. Studies have shown a number of clinical and tumoral factors that are predictors of aggressive growth. These include liver metastases, lymph node metastasis, local invasion, large primary tumor size, nonfunctional tumor, and incomplete tumor resection. The further definition of other factors will likely have a significant impact on the surgical management of pancreatic neuroendocrine tumors; that is, aggressive tumors may require more aggressive operation.

The molecular pathogenesis of pancreatic neuroendocrine tumors is just beginning to be elucidated. Recent studies demonstrate that alterations in the tumor suppressor gene DPC4 located on 18q21 may be involved in tumorigenesis. The specific role for the MEN 1 tumor suppressor gene product menin is unknown, although its diverse interactions suggest possible pivotal roles in transcriptional regulation, DNA processing and repair, and cytoskeletal integrity.[12] At present, no gene alteration sufficiently predicts aggressive behavior well enough to select for a more aggressive treatment strategy.

Pancreatic endocrine tumors are classified according to the functional syndrome they produce. All types of pancreatic endocrine tumor may be associated with MEN 1, and it is important to recognize this association because these patients generally have multiple tumors and a more indolent natural history.[13] Several studies suggest that, in addition to MEN 1, pancreatic neuroendocrine tumors are found in higher frequency in patients with von Recklinghausen disease,[14-16] von Hippel–Lindau disease,[17] and tuberous sclerosis.[18] In patients with von Recklinghausen disease, duodenal somatostatinoma and gastrinoma have been reported.[14-16] Of patients with von Hippel–Lindau disease, 17% had pancreatic endocrine tumors, including both adenomas and carcinomas. However, it is unusual for these tumors to be functional, and few patients have a clinical hormonal syndrome. Patients with tuberous sclerosis may have a higher incidence of insulinoma and nonfunctional pancreatic neuroendocrine tumors.

INSULINOMA

Insulinoma is a tumor of pancreatic beta cells that secrete insulin, leading to hypoglycemia. Insulinomas occur approximately in 1 per million population per year.[19]

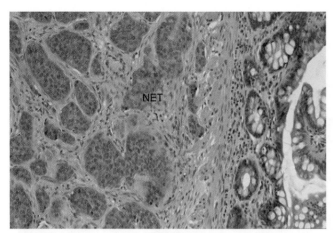

FIGURE 94-1 Neuroendocrine tumor (NET) within the wall of duodenum. This tumor was found to be a somatostatinoma.

Unlike other neuroendocrine tumors of the pancreas, these tumors are generally benign (90%) and are only occasionally malignant (10%). They are found uniformly distributed throughout the pancreas.[20] They present as sporadic cases (80%) or as part of a familial syndrome (MEN 1). In the sporadic form, the tumors are solitary and small (<2 cm in diameter), making localization difficult.[21] Tumors in the familial form are typically larger (>3 cm) and often multiple.

SYMPTOMS AND DIAGNOSIS

Diagnosis of insulinoma may be suggested by the presence of Whipple triad: neuroglycopenic symptoms, low blood glucose levels (<3 mmol/L), and relief of symptoms with glucose administration. Acute neuroglycopenic symptoms include anxiety, dizziness, obtundation, confusion, unconsciousness, personality changes, and seizures.[21,22] Symptoms are typically worse following exercise or fasting. Eighty percent of patients gain weight.[23] The majority (60% to 75%) of patients are female, and many have undergone extensive psychiatric evaluation. Many have been diagnosed with a neurologic condition such as seizure disorder, cerebrovascular accident, or transient ischemic attack.[23] In a review of 59 patients with insulinoma, the interval from the onset of symptoms to the time of diagnosis ranged from 1 month to 30 years, with the median time to diagnosis being 2 years.[23] Approximately 5% to 10% of patients with insulinoma also have MEN 1, which should be excluded or included based on history, symptoms, physical examination, and biochemical findings.

Patients with suspected insulinoma should undergo a 72-hour diagnostic fast. Factitious hypoglycemia, in which exogenous insulin or oral hypoglycemic drugs are administered clandestinely, may present exactly the same symptoms as an insulinoma and must be excluded.[24] Factitious hypoglycemia is seen more commonly in women than in men and may be suspected in individuals with access to insulin or oral hypoglycemic agents. Urinary sulfonylurea concentration should be measured by gas chromatography–mass spectroscopy to detect abuse of oral hypoglycemic drugs. Antiinsulin antibodies should not be detectable in patients with insulinoma.[25] An increased serum concentration of proinsulin or C-peptides during hypoglycemia effectively excludes the diagnosis of factitious hypoglycemia because exogenously administered insulin does not contain these proteins and actually suppresses their endogenous production. The diagnosis of insulinoma is difficult in patients with chronic renal failure because hypoglycemia may develop for other reasons.[26]

Any patient with a history of neuroglycopenic symptoms and hypoglycemia should undergo a diagnostic 72-hour fast in the inpatient hospital setting under close supervision. During the fast, the patient may only drink water or noncaloric beverages. The study is designed to induce symptoms of hypoglycemia in a controlled setting so that serum levels of glucose and insulin can be measured during symptoms. Blood is tested for serum glucose and immunoreactive insulin concentration every 6 hours and when symptoms develop. If the patient develops neuroglycopenic symptoms such as confusion, altered mental status, dizziness or seizure, serum levels of glucose, insulin, C-peptide, and proinsulin are drawn and the fast is terminated. Dextrose is administered to relieve the symptoms of hypoglycemia.

The diagnosis of insulinoma is made if the patient develops neuroglycopenic symptoms, the serum glucose level is lower than 45 mg/dL, and the concomitant serum level of insulin is higher than 5 µU/L. The symptoms should be ameliorated with the administration of glucose. Elevated serum levels of C-peptide (>0.7 ng/mL) and proinsulin are confirmatory and exclude factitious hypoglycemia.[21,25] Sixty percent of patients with insulinoma develop symptoms within 24 hours after fasting, and almost all patients develop symptoms within 72 hours.[25]

PREOPERATIVE LOCALIZATION

Sporadic nonfamilial insulinomas may be difficult to localize precisely preoperatively.[27] For this reason, the diagnosis must be unequivocal before contemplating an operation. Ultrasonography is an initial study to try to localize the insulinoma. The tumor appears sonolucent compared with the more echo-dense pancreas. However, ultrasound images only approximately 20% of insulinomas.[28,29] It is especially limited by overlying bowel gas and obesity.

Thin-cut pancreatic protocol CT with intravenous contrast and serial sections at small intervals through the pancreas (Figure 94-2) is the noninvasive study of choice.[22] Tumors are hypervascular compared to the surrounding pancreatic parenchyma. CT can demonstrate at least 80% of insulinomas[22,30,31] and may be useful for demonstrating liver metastases. Magnetic resonance (MR) is a newer but similarly sensitive modality for imaging insulinomas. Insulinomas appear bright on T2-weighted images. The sensitivity of MR is equivalent to that of CT[28,29] and increases with tumor size.

Somatostatin receptor scintigraphy (SRS) or Octreoscan has become an important imaging modality for neuroendocrine tumors of the pancreas. It images tumors based on the density of type 2 somatostatin receptors. Radiolabeled octreotide binds to tumors with somatostatin receptors, causing the tumor to appear as a "hot

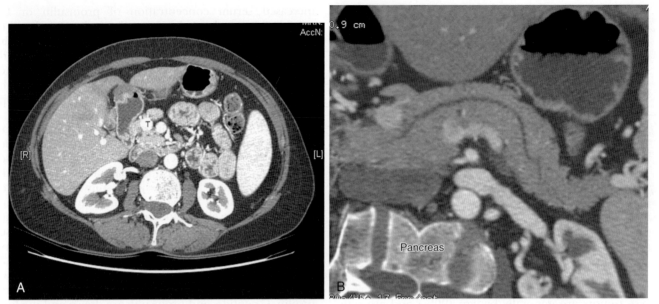

FIGURE 94-2 **A,** CT of a small insulinoma (T) within the head of the pancreas. **B,** Three-dimensional reconstruction of the same CT, which shows the small hypervascular insulinoma within the head of the pancreas.

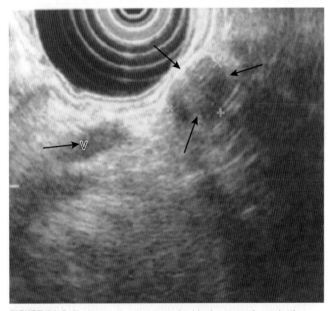

FIGURE 94-3 Endoscopic ultrasound with the transducer in the stomach. It demonstrates a small hypodense mass (insulinoma) within the tail of the pancreas *(arrows)*. The relationship to the splenic vein (V) is also seen.

spot" on whole-body gamma camera scintigraphy.[32] Although SRS correctly identifies 90% of NET and carcinoid tumors, small insulinomas often are not visible on SRS,[33] although combined with endoscopic ultrasound (EUS) the sensitivity for the diagnosis of insulinoma is reported to be higher than 90%.[34]

INVASIVE LOCALIZATION STUDIES

Approximately 50% of patients have small (<2 cm) insulinomas that are not detected by noninvasive imaging tests. EUS (Figure 94-3) is an important study that can identify tumors as small as 2 to 3 mm.[35-37] Sensitivity for EUS ranges from 70% to 90%, and specificity is near 100%.[38-40] It is more accurate in the head of the pancreas than in the body and the tail. Despite the tremendous potential, there are some limitations, including false-positive findings, such as accessory spleens and intrapancreatic lymph nodes. CT is a useful adjunct to EUS to image the liver and rule out disseminated malignancy.[41]

Differential insulin levels measured by portal venous sampling may correctly identify the insulinoma-bearing region of the pancreas in about 80% of patients with few false-positive results.[19,29] However, portal venous sampling is invasive and has largely been replaced by calcium angiography[28,42] which is preferred for patients with presumed insulinoma and negative imaging studies. Calcium gluconate (0.025 mEq/kg body weight) is injected selectively into arteries that perfuse the head (gastroduodenal artery, superior mesenteric artery), body, and tail (splenic artery) of the pancreas. Calcium stimulates a marked increase in insulin secretion from the insulinoma. Insulin concentration is measured in the hepatic vein. When the artery that perfuses the insulinoma is injected, the insulin level in the hepatic vein rises, localizing the tumor to that region of the pancreas. Sensitivity for calcium stimulation is approximately 90%, and few false-positive results occur.[43,44] Additionally, injection of contrast material may reveal a tumor blush confirming the location of the insulinoma by imaging the tumor.

A small portion of insulinomas remain unlocalizable despite extensive studies and are therefore considered occult. When the diagnosis is certain based on the result of a 72-hour fast, surgical exploration with careful inspection, palpation, and intraoperative ultrasound (IOUS) is indicated. Studies have shown that the combination of surgical exploration with IOUS identifies almost all insulinomas.[27,45-47]

THERAPY

Medical treatment should prevent hypoglycemia. Acute hypoglycemia is initially normalized with intravenous glucose infusion. Hypoglycemia can be prevented while establishing the diagnosis and tumor localization by giving frequent feeds of high-carbohydrate diet, including a night meal. Cornstarch added to the diet may prolong and slow down absorption. For patients who continue to become hypoglycemic between feedings, diazoxide may be added to the treatment regimen at a dose of 400 to 600 mg orally each day. Diazoxide inhibits insulin release in approximately 50% of patients with insulinoma.[48] In some patients, calcium channel blockers or phenytoin may suppress insulin production. Octreotide binds to and activates somatostatin receptors on cells expressing them. Its usefulness to inhibit insulin release, though, has been disappointing and unpredictable.[49-51]

Long-term medical management of hypoglycemia in patients with insulinomas is generally reserved for the few patients (<5%) with unlocalized, unresected tumors after thorough preoperative testing and exploratory laparotomy and for patients with metastatic, unresectable malignant insulinoma.[49] Patients with malignant insulinomas and refractory hypoglycemia may even require the placement of implantable glucose pumps for continuous glucose infusion.[48]

Surgery is the only curative therapy for insulinoma. Because most insulinomas are benign and small, the goal of surgery is to precisely localize the tumor and remove it with minimal morbidity. The major breakthrough in surgery for insulinoma has been IOUS.[46,52] It is the single best intraoperative method to localize insulinomas although in most cases the tumor is localized by other techniques preoperatively, or is visualized or palpated by the surgeon.

Midline or bilateral subcostal incisions allow for good exposure. Because virtually all insulinomas are located within the pancreas, an extended Kocher maneuver is performed and the lesser sac is opened, such that the entire pancreas can be examined. The tumor feels like a firm, nodular, and discrete mass. It may appear brownish-red purple, like a cherry. IOUS should be performed with a high-resolution near-field transducer (10 to 15 MHz). The tumor is sonolucent compared with the more echodense pancreas (Figure 94-4). The tumor should be imaged in two directions to identify it as a real structure. A recent study of 37 consecutive patients showed that IOUS identified tumors in 35 (95%), and the 2 that were missed were in the pancreatic tail.[52] The liver is examined, and suspicious lesions are biopsied or excised.

Patients who have clearcut preoperative localization including CT may be candidates for laparoscopic resection. This has been done with good results in these patients using laparoscopic ultrasound to image the tumor and guide the resection. Patients who undergo laparoscopic resection of insulinomas have less postoperative pain, shorter hospitalization, and faster return to work.[53,54]

Insulinomas presenting during pregnancy have been reported and are usually managed medically until the fetus can be delivered or the pregnancy is terminated.[55]

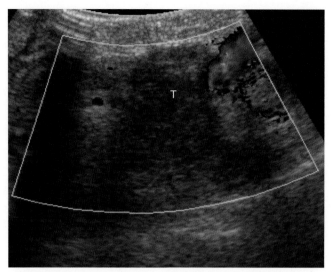

FIGURE 94-4 Intraoperative ultrasound (IOUS) that demonstrates a small, hypodense sonolucent tumor (T) within the head of the pancreas to the right of the superior mesenteric vein *(blue)* and artery *(red)*. This tumor was an insulinoma and IOUS facilitated the enucleation.

MULTIPLE ENDOCRINE NEOPLASIA 1

MEN 1 is an inherited autosomal dominant disease in which tumors develop in multiple endocrine organs. Patients classically have primary hyperparathyroidism secondary to four-gland parathyroid hyperplasia (94%), pituitary adenoma (35%) (most commonly prolactinoma), and multiple pancreatic neuroendocrine tumors that may be malignant (75%).[13] Gastrinoma and insulinoma are the most common functional neuroendocrine pancreatic tumors in MEN 1 patients, accounting for approximately 50% and 20% of the neuroendocrine tumor syndromes, respectively.[19,56] Nonfunctional pancreatic endocrine tumor and PPomas may be the most common pancreatic neuroendocrine tumors in MEN 1 patients because these tumors are almost always identified on careful histologic studies of the pancreas.[57,58] Patients may also have lipomas, thyroid adenomas, adrenal cortical adenomas or carcinomas, and carcinoid tumors of the entire neuroendocrine system.[13]

Of the rare pancreatic neuroendocrine tumors, MEN 1 is present in approximately 3% of patients with glucagonoma, 1% of patients with VIPoma, 33% of patients with tumors that secrete GRF (GRFomas), and 5% of patients with somatostatinoma.[13]

The genetic defect in patients with MEN 1 has been localized to the long arm of chromosome 11 and linked to the skeletal muscle glycogen phosphorylase gene.[59,60] Evidence from these studies suggests that the development of endocrine tumors in MEN 1 patients conforms to Knudson's two-hit model of neoplasm formation with an inherited mutation in one chromosome unmasked by a somatic deletion or mutation of the other normal chromosome, thereby removing the suppressor effects of the normal gene.[61] In contrast, in sporadic patients with pancreatic neuroendocrine tumors, tumors do not appear to develop by homozygous inactivation of the same gene.[59]

Growth factors have been identified in the plasma of patients with MEN 1. A circulating blood factor that was mitogenic for parathyroid cells in tissue culture has been identified,[62] and a subsequent study demonstrated that the factor was similar to fibroblast growth factor.[63]

DIAGNOSIS

The possibility of MEN 1 should be considered during the evaluation of all patients presenting with pancreatic NET. A careful family history of first-degree relatives should be taken, and suspicious comorbidities such as kidney stones, hyperparathyroidism, hypoglycemia, peptic ulcer disease, diarrhea, Cushing syndrome, and prolactinoma should be queried. All patients younger than age 40 years presenting with primary hyperparathyroidism due to hyperplasia should be screened for pancreatic endocrine tumors even if their family history is negative for MEN syndromes.[64] Physical examination should rule out lipomas. Screening of other family members is indicated, if suspicion of MEN 1 exists.[65] Evaluation should include serum calcium, gastrin, glucose, PP, chromogranin A, and prolactin levels.

Each patient with biochemical evidence of a neuroendocrine tumor should undergo complete radiologic assessment of disease to determine the feasibility of surgery. During the radiologic evaluation, medical management should be used to ameliorate symptoms secondary to excessive hormone secretion. It is clear that in some patients with neuroendocrine tumors (e.g., VIPoma) advances in medical control of the hormone production have improved the surgical outcome and reduced the operative complication rate.[19]

THERAPY

In MEN 1 patients with primary hyperparathyroidism and Zollinger–Ellison syndrome, surgery to correct the primary hyperparathyroidism ($3\frac{1}{2}$ gland parathyroidectomy) should be performed prior to pancreatic surgery because correction of the hypercalcemia will greatly ameliorate the signs and symptoms of Zollinger-Ellison syndrome. If MEN 1 is present, the pathologist will identify multiple neuroendocrine tumors within the pancreas,[57,58] so patients are seldom cured by surgery but most experts recommend that patients with neuroendocrine tumors greater than 2 cm undergo surgery because these tumors have a high probability of being malignant.[19,66-71] Medical management can only control the signs and symptoms, and tumor resection is the only potentially curative treatment for malignant NET. Resection is better in MEN 1 patients because of multiple tumors. Therefore, in patients with localized, potentially resectable, imageable (2 cm or larger) tumor, pancreatic resection by either a Whipple procedure (for pancreatic head tumors) or distal pancreatectomy (for pancreatic body and tail tumors) is indicated.

PROGNOSIS

Many variables associated with an individual patient have an impact on the surgical outcome. These include the extent of disease on preoperative imaging studies, whether the primary tumor is within the pancreas or duodenum, the exact area of the pancreas involved (head, body, or tail), the presence of liver or other distant metastases and whether they are resectable, the occurrence of the neuroendocrine tumor in a familial or a sporadic setting, and the simultaneous occurrence of other medical conditions that may limit the ability of a patient to undergo major surgery. The definition of success need not be equated with cure, as decreased medication requirement, decreased symptoms, and increased length of survival may be of considerable clinical value. In each patient, it is clear that neuroendocrine tumors may be malignant, that surgery is an effective way of accurately staging the true extent of disease, and that surgery may be curative, even in the patients with metastatic neuroendocrine tumor.[19,72-75]

Genetic counseling and screening should be provided to families at high risk of developing MEN 1. These patients should enter a clinical screening program, which can enable earlier detection and treatment of MEN 1–associated tumors and prompt treatment of hyperparathyroidism.[65,76]

SOMATOSTATINOMA

Somatostatinoma is a rare endocrine tumor of the pancreatic islet D cells or duodenum that secretes excessive amounts of somatostatin. Somatostatin excess causes a syndrome characterized by steatorrhea, mild diabetes, and cholelithiasis. Somatostatin is an inhibitory hormone originally discovered in the hypothalamus in 1973. It was discovered by its ability to inhibit growth hormone and thus was called somatotropin release–inhibiting hormone. In 1977, Ganda et al[77] and Larsson et al[78] reported the first two cases of somatostatinoma. Initially, the somatostatinoma syndrome included diabetes, cholelithiasis, weight loss, and anemia. Subsequently, diarrhea, steatorrhea, and hypochlorhydria were added.[79] Somatostatin inhibits the release of most other gastrointestinal hormones. It decreases many gastrointestinal functions, including acid secretion, pancreatic enzyme secretion, and intestinal absorption. It reduces gut motility and transit time. Contrary to their duodenal counterparts, pancreatic somatostatinomas are not associated with von Recklinghausen syndrome.[80]

PRESENTATION

Patients with pancreatic or intestinal somatostatinoma are typically in the sixth decade of life, with an equal proportion of men and women. Initial symptoms are diabetes, gallbladder disease, and steatorrhea. Diabetes mellitus and glucose intolerance are reported to occur in 60% of patients with pancreatic somatostatinomas; gallstones occur in 70%; diarrhea and steatorrhea are reported in 30% to 68%; and hypochlorhydria presents in 86%. The weight loss may be secondary to diarrhea and malabsorption.

DIAGNOSIS

In most instances, somatostatinomas are found incidentally at the time of cholecystectomy or during routine imaging studies.[10] In 75% of cases, they are metastatic and larger than 5 cm at the time of diagnosis.[81] Most somatostatinomas are located in the pancreas. Despite equal distribution of islet D cells throughout the pancreas, two-thirds of the tumors are located in the head of the pancreas, with the remainder found in the duodenum, at the ampulla, or small intestine.

Diagnosis of somatostatinoma requires the demonstration of elevated tissue concentration of somatostatin or by the documentation of increased fasting plasma somatostatin levels. A level greater than 14 pmol/L is suggestive of the diagnosis of somatostatinoma.[82] CT is a sensitive imaging study, given that the tumor is usually large at the time of diagnosis. Alternatively, MR imaging and EUS with biopsy and cytology or somatostatin scintigraphy can be helpful in obtaining the diagnosis.[83,84] The early diagnosis of somatostatinoma may be possible with greater awareness of its existence and reliable assays for the determination of somatostatin in the blood.

THERAPY

Most somatostatinomas are solitary and located within the pancreatic head or duodenum. A high proportion of these tumors are malignant. If the tumor is localized and not widely metastatic, surgical resection is the treatment of choice and the only chance for cure. In some, the severity of diarrhea and steatorrhea correlates with the size and degree of metastatic spread of the tumor, and it improves with tumor resection.[85] Therefore, surgical debulking of metastatic disease has been advocated, but patients are few and clear benefits have not been demonstrated. Five-year survival rates of patients with duodenal and pancreatic somatostatinomas are 30% and 15%, respectively.[86]

VIPoma

VIPomas are generally located within the pancreas. Most VIPomas have been found in the body and the tail of the pancreas.[87] The initial characterization of what was later recognized to be VIPoma was called the *Verner–Morrison syndrome*[88] and consisted of large-volume diarrhea, severe hypokalemia with muscle weakness, hypercalcemia, and hypochlorhydria. VIPoma typically occurs in adults. Approximately half the VIPomas are benign.[89]

PRESENTATION

Typically, the diarrhea is large in volume (>5 L/day), and it occurs in 70% of patients.[90] It is a secretory diarrhea and thus persists during a fast.[91] Hypokalemia is present in nearly every patient and is caused by excessive potassium losses in the diarrheal fluid, leading to severe muscle weakness and debilitation. Hypochlorhydria is found in 75% of patients with VIPoma and is due to inhibition of gastric acid secretion by VIP. The vasodilatory action of VIP leads to flushing in a minority of patients. Hyperglycemia occurs in 25% to 50% of patients and is caused by the glycogenolytic action of VIP. Hypercalcemia is present in a significant proportion of patients.

DIAGNOSIS

In patients with secretory diarrhea and hypokalemia suspected of having a VIPoma, a fasting plasma VIP level should be measured. Given that symptomatic tumors are usually larger than 1 cm, CT is a sensitive imaging study. MR imaging and ultrasound may also be helpful. SRS may also be useful for tumor localization.

TREATMENT

The first step in treating VIPoma includes the correction of the metabolic imbalance. Electrolyte losses from long-standing diarrhea should be aggressively corrected. Long-acting somatostatin analogue can decrease the diarrhea and help correct hypokalemia and the other metabolic derangements.[74] Surgical resection is the only chance for cure. IOUS may be considered for intraoperative identification. If complete surgical resection cannot be achieved, surgical debulking can be helpful, and postoperative medical treatment of the residual disease with octreotide is recommended.[92]

GLUCAGONOMA

Glucagonoma is an endocrine tumor of the pancreas that secretes excessive amounts of glucagon. This results in a characteristic syndrome that includes a rash called necrolytic migratory erythema, type 2 diabetes mellitus, weight loss, anemia, stomatitis, glossitis, thromboembolism, and other gastrointestinal and neuropsychiatric symptoms.[93] Liver disease and zinc deficiency may also add to the symptomatology.[69] Unlike other islet cell tumors, glucagonomas are almost always malignant and usually not resectable for cure. Tumor-related deaths occur in most patients after about 5 years of followup. Surgery is the only option for cure.[69] Surgical resection leads to complete resolution of all signs and symptoms in many patients.[69,94]

Patients with glucagonoma typically present between 50 and 60 years of age. The rash is migratory, red, and scaling and is associated with intense pruritus. It commonly occurs in the groin and lower extremities. The rash is pathognomonic of the tumor.[95,96] The rash is related to markedly disrupted plasma levels of amino acids, and can be completely reversed with total parenteral nutrition.[97] Others have also reported that infusion of peripheral amino acids did resolve the rash but it did not reverse hypoaminoacidemia.[75] Diabetes mellitus and glucose intolerance are among the most frequent findings in patients. However, about 20% of patients do not present with hyperglycemia.[98]

Weight loss and cachexia are common and may be profound. Thromboembolic symptoms occur more commonly in patients with glucagonoma. Both deep venous thrombosis and pulmonary emboli may ultimately cause death.

DIAGNOSIS

Diagnosis is established by the measurement of elevated plasma levels of glucagon. In all patients with glucagonoma, plasma glucagon concentration is elevated (>150 pg/mL). Plasma levels greater than 1000 pg/mL are diagnostic of glucagonoma. CT identifies the location of the tumor, which is usually larger than 4 cm (Figure 94-5, *A*). Glucagonomas are almost always found within the body and tail of the pancreas and only rarely

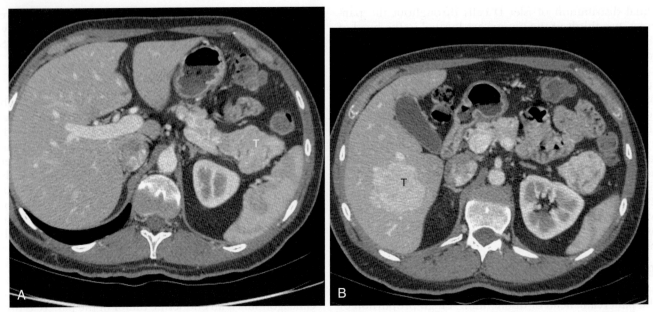

FIGURE 94-5 A, Glucagonoma (T) in the tail of the pancreas is demonstrated on CT scan. The patient presented with a rash known as necrolytic migratory erythema. **B,** The patient also had a large metastasis in the right lobe of the liver (T). He underwent a subtotal pancreatectomy/splenectomy and concomitant right hepatic lobectomy and recovered well. The rash resolved, and he has remained without imageable tumor for 2 years.

in the head. Seventy percent of patients present with liver metastasis at the time of the diagnosis.

THERAPY

Preoperative preparation involves control of diabetes, treatment of complications such as venous thrombosis, and nutritional support.[99] Resection of the primary tumor usually requires subtotal pancreatectomy with splenectomy. If the primary lesion is not fully resectable, debulking and resection of liver metastases may improve symptoms. Metastatic disease tends to progress slowly (Figure 94-5, *B*).[72] Other options include hepatic artery embolization, chemotherapy with bevacizumab (Avastin), 5-fluorouracil, and oxaliplatin or everolimus, long-term octreotide (Sandostatin LAR) for symptoms,[100,101] and transplantation of the liver and pancreas.

GRFoma

The GRFoma is a neuroendocrine tumor that secretes excessive amounts of growth hormone–releasing factor (GRF). GRFomas occur most frequently in the lung (bronchus), followed by pancreas, jejunum, adrenal glands, and retroperitoneum.[102] Pancreatic GRFomas are typically large (>6 cm). One-third will have metastasized at the time of diagnosis. Approximately 50% of patients with GRFomas also have Zollinger–Ellison syndrome and 33% have MEN 1. Patients present with acromegaly and a pancreatic mass. If liver metastasis or peptic ulcer disease is present, the diagnosis of GRFoma should also be considered.[100,101] The diagnosis of GRFoma is established using a plasma assay for GRF. Given that the tumor is usually large at the time of diagnosis, CT scan is a sensitive modality for localization. Surgical resection should

be attempted in these patients because complete resection may be curative, and debulking may decrease symptoms and prolong survival. Octreotide therapy can relieve the symptoms of acromegaly.

CORTICOTROPIN-PRODUCING TUMOR

Malignant NETs commonly secrete more than one peptide. When they produce corticotropin, patients present with Cushing syndrome. Excessive production of corticotropin by a pituitary tumor may occur in patients with MEN but is usually mild and clinically insignificant.[103] In 5% of patients with Zollinger–Ellison syndrome, Cushing syndrome has been reported.[103] In contrast, these patients have severe Cushing syndrome because of ectopic production of corticotropin by the neuroendocrine tumor.[104] Elevated blood levels of cortisol are diagnostic, and CT is used for localization. Corticotropin-producing pancreatic neuroendocrine tumors are usually not resectable. Therefore, either debulking or bilateral adrenalectomy may be indicated to control the severe signs and symptoms of hypercortisolism, given that medical management of the hypercortisolism in these patients is usually inadequate.[104]

TUMOR RELEASING PARATHYROID HORMONE–RELATED PROTEIN

Severe hypercalcemia has been reported to be due to a pancreatic neuroendocrine tumor releasing parathyroid hormone–related protein (PTHrP).[105,106] Hypercalcemia associated with pancreatic neuroendocrine tumors has also been reported to be due to the release of other substances such as VIP. In most cases, the pancreatic tumor is malignant and has spread to the liver by the time of diagnosis.

NEUROTENSINOMA

There have been reports of neuroendocrine tumors that secrete neurotensin. Neurotensin is a peptide that is found in the brain and the gastrointestinal tract. It can cause hypotension, tachycardia, cyanosis, pancreatic secretion, intestinal motility, and small intestinal secretion. Patients with neurotensinomas present with diarrhea and hypokalemia, weight loss, diabetes, cyanosis, hypotension, and flushing. Patients may be cured by resection of the tumor; others have responded to chemotherapy.[107,108] Some have questioned whether a separate neurotensinoma exists. Patients with VIPoma and gastrinoma have been found to have elevated plasma levels of neurotensin. At present, it is unclear whether a separate syndrome exists.

GHRELINOMA

Ghrelin is a novel gastrointestinal hormone that exerts a wide range of metabolic functions. It promotes growth hormone release and is an important regulator of energy balance. It has been demonstrated to increase appetite and food intake and modulate insulin secretion. It has significant homology with motilin, and it stimulates gastric contractility and acid secretion. A recent study suggested that a patient had a neuroendocrine tumor of the pancreas excreting the hormone ghrelin, a so-called ghrelinoma. This hormone had not been found in any other neuroendocrine tumor of the pancreas.[109]

PPoma AND NONFUNCTIONING NEUROENDOCRINE TUMOR

Neuroendocrine tumors that are not associated with a syndrome related to hormonal hypersecretion are referred to as nonfunctional. For example, PPomas secrete PP, but this hormone does not appear to cause symptoms; therefore, this tumor is considered nonfunctional. It is estimated that 10% to 25% of all neuroendocrine pancreatic tumors are nonfunctional.[3,110] They are therefore estimated to be among the most frequent neuroendocrine tumors of the pancreas.

PRESENTATION

Typically these tumors are large when diagnosed (>5 cm), and almost all (80%) are malignant and metastatic (Figure 94-6).[111,112] The incidence of malignancy is clearly higher than among the functioning pancreatic neuroendocrine tumors.[113] Symptoms occur secondary to mass effect. Cachexia, abdominal pain, intestinal bleeding, blockage, or hepatomegaly are common symptoms.[110] Some patients present with pancreatitis.[114]

DIAGNOSIS

Tumors are often found incidentally during surgery.[115] Given that these tumors are usually large by the time the patient is symptomatic, CT and MR imaging are good diagnostic imaging studies. PP and chromogranin A are presently the best serum markers to identify PPomas. Nonfunctioning pancreatic endocrine tumors are differentiated from PPomas on the basis of results of the serum PP assay. Adenocarcinoma of the pancreas can be distinguished from neuroendocrine tumors by immunohistochemical staining with chromogranin A.

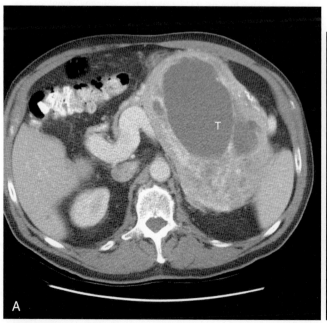
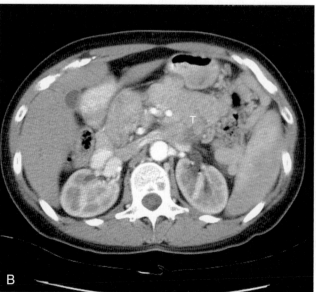

FIGURE 94-6 **A,** Large nonfunctional neuroendocrine tumor within the tail of the pancreas (T). This patient presented with stomach bleeding because the tumor had eroded into the posterior wall of the stomach. **B,** This patient presented with back pain. She was found to have a localized large nonfunctional neuroendocrine tumor within the body of the pancreas (T). Removal of this tumor required a total pancreatectomy/splenectomy. She has done well except that she developed small liver metastases at the 5-year followup.

THERAPY

Therapy includes resection of the tumor and chemotherapy. Most nonfunctioning islet cell tumors are in the head of the pancreas and require a pancreaticoduodenectomy. Debulking of hepatic tumor mass can be replaced by hepatic embolization.[116-118] Dopamine agonists have been shown to decrease circulating levels of PP and chromogranin A in patients with large unresectable islet cell tumors.[119] PPomas and nonfunctioning neuroendocrine tumors of the pancreas do not seem to differ in their biologic behavior[120,121]; however, PP and chromogranin levels may be used to monitor the result of therapy.

PROGNOSIS

Controversy exists concerning the 5-year survival of nonfunctioning versus functioning neuroendocrine pancreatic tumors.[122] Discrepancy in studies may be due to the small number of patients with this disease. Most likely there is no significant difference in behavior of functioning versus nonfunctioning tumors.

REFERENCES

1. Phan AT, Oberg K, Choi J, et al: NANETS consensus guideline for the diagnosis and management of neuroendocrine tumors: Well differentiated neuroendocrine tumors of the thorax (includes lung and thymus). *Pancreas* 39:784, 2010.
2. Yao JC, Hassan M, Phan A, et al: One hundred years after "carcinoid": Epidemiology of and prognostic factors for neuroendocrine tumors in 35,825 cases in the United States. *J Clin Oncol* 26:3063, 2008.
3. Kloppel G, Heitz PU: Pancreatic endocrine tumors. *Pathol Res Pract* 183:155, 1988.
4. Heitz PU, Kasper M, Polak JM, et al: Pancreatic endocrine tumors: Immunocytochemical analysis of 125 tumors. *Hum Pathol* 13:263, 1982.
5. Creutzfeldt W, Arnold R, Creutzfeld C: Pathomorphologic, biochemical, and diagnostic aspects of gastrinomas (Zollinger-Ellison syndrome). *Hum Pathol* 6:47, 1975.
6. Benish BM: The neurocristopathies: A unifying concept of disease arising in neural crest development [Letter]. *Hum Pathol* 6:128, 1975.
7. Pearse AG, Takor T: Embryology of the diffuse neuroendocrine system and its relationship to the common peptides. *Fed Proc* 38:2288, 1979.
8. Pearse AG: The APUD concept and hormone production. *Clin Endocrinol Metab* 9:211, 1980.
9. Lloyd RV, Mervak T, Schmidt K, et al: Immunohistochemical detection of chromogranin and neuron-specific enolase in pancreatic endocrine neoplasms. *Am J Surg Pathol* 8:607, 1984.
10. Jensen RT, Norton JA: Endocrine tumors of the pancreas in gastrointestinal disease. In Sleisenger MH, Fordtran JS, Scharschmidt BR, et al, editors: *Gastrointestinal Disease: Pathophysiology, Diagnosis, and Management,* ed 5, Philadelphia, 1993, WB Saunders, p 1695.
11. Norton JA, Levin B, Jensen RT: Cancer of the endocrine system. In Devita VT, Hellman S, Rosenberg SA, editors: *Cancer: Principles and Practice of Oncology,* ed 4, Philadelphia, 1993, JB Lippincott, p 1269.
12. Lairmore TC, Chen H: Role of menin in neuroendocrine tumorigenesis. *Adv Exp Med Biol* 668:87, 2009.
13. Modlin IM, Gustafsson BI, Moss SF, et al: Chromogranin A—biological function and clinical utility in neuroendocrine tumor disease. *Ann Surg Oncol* 17:2427, 2010.
14. Burke AP, Sobin L, Federspiel BH, et al: Carcinoid tumors of the duodenum: A clinicopathologic study of 99 cases. *Arch Pathol Lab Med* 114:700, 1990.
15. Burke AP, Sobin LH, Shekitka KM, et al: Somatostatin-producing duodenal carcinoids in patients with von Recklinghausen's neurofibromatosis: A predilection for black patients. *Cancer* 65:1591, 1990.
16. Chagnon JP, Barge J, Henin D, et al: Recklinghausen's disease with digestive localizations associated with gastric acid hypersecretion suggesting Zollinger-Ellison syndrome. *Gastroenterol Clin Biol* 9:65, 1985.
17. Binkovitz LA, Johnson CD, Stephens DH: Islet cell tumors in von Hippel-Lindau disease: Increased prevalence and relationship to the multiple endocrine neoplasias. *AJR Am J Roentgenol* 155:501, 1990.
18. Davoren PM, Epstein MT: Insulinoma complicating tuberous sclerosis. *J Neurol Neurosurg Psychiatry* 55:1209, 1992.
19. Norton JA: Neuroendocrine tumors of the pancreas and duodenum. *Curr Probl Surg* 31:77, 1994.
20. Peplinski GR, Norton JA: Gastrointestinal endocrine cancers and nodal metastases: Biological significance and therapeutic implications. *Surg Oncol Clin North Am* 5:159, 1996.
21. Doherty GM, Doppman JL, Shawker TH, et al: Results of a prospective strategy to diagnose, localize, and resect insulinomas. *Surgery* 110:989, 1991.
22. Fraker DL, Norton JA: Localization and resection of insulinomas and gastrinomas. *JAMA* 259:3601, 1988.
23. Dizon AM, Kowalyk S, Hoogwerf BJ: Neuroglycopenic and other symptoms in patients with insulinomas. *Am J Med* 106:307, 1999.
24. Grunberger G, Weiner JL, Silverman R: Factitious hypoglycemia due to surreptitious administration of insulin: Diagnosis, treatment, and long-term follow-up. *Ann Intern Med* 108:252, 1988.
25. Gorden P, Skarulis M, Roach P, et al: Plasma proinsulin-like component in insulinoma: A 25-year experience. *J Clin Endocrinol Metab* 80:2884, 1995.
26. Basu A, Sheehan MT, Thompson GB, et al: Insulinoma in chronic renal failure. *J Clin Endocrinol Metab* 87:4889, 2002.
27. Boukhman MP, Karam JM, Shaver J, et al: Localization of insulinomas. *Arch Surg* 134:818, 1999.
28. Doppman JL, Chang R, Fraker DL, et al: Localization of insulinomas to regions of the pancreas by intra-arterial stimulation with calcium. *Ann Intern Med* 123:269, 1995.
29. Vinik AI, Delbridge L, Moattari R, et al: Transhepatic portal vein catheterization for localization of insulinomas: A ten-year experience. *Surgery* 109:1, 1991.
30. Grant CS, van Heerden JA, Charboneau JW: Insulinoma: The value of intraoperative ultrasound. *Arch Surg* 123:843, 1988.
31. Rodallec M, Vilgrain V, Zins M, et al: Helical CT of pancreatic endocrine tumors. *J Comp Assist Tomogr* 26:728, 2002.
32. Lamberts SW, Bakker WH, Reubi JC, et al: Somatostatin receptor imaging in the localization of endocrine tumors. *N Engl J Med* 323:1246, 1990.
33. Lamberts SW, Hofland LJ, Van Koetsveld PM, et al: Parallel in vivo and in vitro detection of functional somatostatin receptors in human endocrine pancreatic tumors: Consequences with regard to diagnosis, localization, and therapy. *J Clin Endocrinol Metab* 71:566, 1990.
34. Proye C, Malvaux P, Pattou F, et al: Noninvasive imaging of insulinomas and gastrinomas with endoscopic ultrasonography and somatostatin receptor scintigraphy. *Surgery* 124:1134, 1998.
35. Owens LV, Huth JF, Cance WG: Insulinoma: Pitfalls in preoperative localization. *Eur J Surg Oncol* 32:326, 1995.
36. Thompson NW, Czako PF, Fritts LL: Role of endoscopic ultrasonography in the localization of insulinomas and gastrinomas. *Surgery* 116:1131, 1994.
37. Bottger TC, Junginger T: Is preoperative radiographic localization of islet cell tumors in patients with insulinoma necessary? *World J Surg* 17:427, 1993.
38. Heyder N: Localization of an insulinoma by ultrasonic endoscopy. *N Engl J Med* 312:860, 1985.
39. Glover JR, Shorvon PJ, Lees WR: Endoscopic ultrasound for localization of islet cell tumors. *Gut* 33:108, 1992.
40. Rosch T, Lightdale CJ, Botet JF, et al: Localization of pancreatic endocrine tumors by endoscopic ultrasonography. *N Engl J Med* 326:1721, 1992.
41. Richards M, Gauger PG, Thompson NW, et al: Pitfalls in the surgical treatment of insulinoma. *Surgery* 132:1040, 2002.
42. Doppman JL, Miller DL, Chang R, et al: Insulinomas: Localization with selective intraarterial injection of calcium. *Radiology* 178:237, 1991.

43. Cohen MS, Picus D, Lairmore TC, et al: Prospective study of provocative angiograms to localize functional islet cell tumors of the pancreas. *Surgery* 122:1091, 1997.

44. Brown CK, Bartlett DL, Doppman JL, et al: Intraarterial calcium stimulation and intraoperative ultrasonography in the localization and resection of insulinomas. *Surgery* 122:1189, 1997.

45. Norton JA: Intraoperative methods to stage and localize pancreatic and duodenal tumors. *Ann Oncol* 10:182, 1999.

46. Huai JC, Zhang W, Niu HO, et al: Localization and surgical treatment of pancreatic insulinomas guided by intraoperative ultrasound. *Am J Surg* 175:18, 1998.

47. Lo CY, Lam KY, Kung AWC: Pancreatic insulinomas: A fifteen-year experience. *Arch Surg* 132:926, 1997.

48. Grant CS: Insulinoma. *Surg Oncol Clin North Am* 7:819, 1998.

49. von Eyben FE, Grodum E, Gjessing HJ, et al: Metabolic remission with octreotide in patients with insulinoma. *J Intern Med* 235:245, 1994.

50. Arnold R, Neuhaus C, Benning R, et al: Somatostatin analog Sandostatin and inhibition of tumor growth in patients with metastatic endocrine gastroenteropancreatic tumors. *World J Surg* 17:511, 1993.

51. Arnold R, Frank M, Kajdan U: Management of gastroenteropancreatic endocrine tumors: The place of somatostatin analogues. *Digestion* 55:107, 1994.

52. Hiramoto JS, Feldstein VA, LaBerge JM, et al: Intraoperative ultrasound and preoperative localization detects all occult insulinomas. *Arch Surg* 136:1020, 2001.

53. Park AE, Heniford BT: Therapeutic laparoscopy of the pancreas. *Ann Surg* 236:149, 2002.

54. Iihara M, Kanbe M, Okamoto T, et al: Laparoscopic ultrasonography for resection of insulinomas. *Surgery* 130:1086, 2001.

55. Takacs CA, Krivak TC, Napolitano PG: Insulinoma in pregnancy: A case report and review of the literature. *Obstet Gynecol Surg* 57:229, 2002.

56. Sheppard BC, Norton JA, Doppman JL, et al: Management of islet cell tumors in patients with multiple endocrine neoplasia: A prospective study. *Surgery* 106:1108, 1989.

57. Thompson NW, Lloyd RV, Nishiyama RH, et al: MEN I pancreas: A histological and immunohistochemical study. *World J Surg* 8:561, 1984.

58. Kloppel G, Willemer S, Stamm B, et al: Pancreatic lesions and hormonal profile of pancreatic tumors in multiple endocrine neoplasia type I: An immunocytochemical study of nine patients. *Cancer* 57:1824, 1986.

59. Bale AE, Norton JA, Wong EL, et al: Allelic loss on chromosome 11 in hereditary and sporadic tumors related to familial multiple endocrine neoplasia type 1. *Cancer Res* 51:1154, 1991.

60. Oberg K, Skagseid B, Eriksson B: Multiple endocrine neoplasia type 1 (MEN-1): Clinical, biochemical, and genetic investigations. *Acta Oncol* 28:383, 1989.

61. Knudson AG Jr: Mutation and cancer: Statistical study of retinoblastoma. *Proc Natl Acad Sci U S A* 68:820, 1971.

62. Brandi ML, Aurbach G, Fitzpatrick LA, et al: Parathyroid mitogenic activity in plasma from patients with familial multiple endocrine neoplasia type 1. *N Engl J Med* 314:1287, 1986.

63. Zimering MB, Brandi M, deGrange DA, et al: Circulating fibroblast growth factor-like substance in familial multiple endocrine neoplasia type 1. *J Clin Endocrinol Metab* 70:149, 1990.

64. Langer P, Wild A, Hall A, et al: Prevalence of multiple endocrine neoplasia type 1 in young patients with apparently sporadic primary hyperparathyroidism or pancreaticoduodenal endocrine tumors. *Br J Surg* 90:1599, 2003.

65. Bartsch D, Kopp I, Bergenfelz A: MEN 1 gene mutations in 12 MEN1 families and their associated tumors. *Eur J Endocrinol* 139:416, 1998.

66. Legaspi A, Brennan M: Management of islet cell carcinoma. *Surgery* 104:1018, 1988.

67. Harris GJ, Tio F, Cruz AB Jr: Somatostatinoma: A case report and review of the literature. *J Surg Oncol* 36:8, 1987.

68. Higgins GA, Recant L, Fischman AB: The glucagonoma syndrome: Surgically curable diabetes. *Am J Surg* 137:142, 1979.

69. Chastain MA: The glucagonoma syndrome: A review of its features and discussion of new perspectives. *Am J Med* 321:306, 2001.

70. Mozell E, Stenzel P, Woltering EA, et al: Functional endocrine tumors of the pancreas: Clinical presentation, diagnosis, and treatment. *Curr Probl Surg* 27:301, 1990.

71. Wermers RA, Fatourechi V, Wynne AG, et al: The glucagonoma syndrome: Clinical and pathologic features in 21 patients. *Medicine (Baltimore)* 75:53, 1996.

72. Carty SE, Jensen RT, Norton JA: Prospective study of aggressive resection of metastatic pancreatic endocrine tumors. *Surgery* 112:1024, 1992.

73. Fraker DL, Norton JA: The role of surgery in the management of islet cell tumors. *Gastroenterol Clin North Am* 18:805, 1989.

74. Maton PN, Gardner JD, Jensen RT: Use of long-acting somatostatin analog SMS 201-995 in patients with pancreatic islet cell tumors. *Dig Dis Sci* 34:28S, 1989.

75. Alexander EK, Robinson M, Staniec M, et al: Peripheral amino acid and fatty acid infusion for the treatment of necrolytic migratory erythema in the glucagonoma syndrome. *Clin Endocrinol (Oxf)* 57:827, 2002.

76. Langer P, Wild A, Celik L, et al: Prospective controlled trial of a standardized meal stimulation test in the detection of pancreaticoduodenal endocrine tumors in patients with multiple endocrine neoplasia type 1. *Br J Surg* 88:1403, 2001.

77. Ganda OP, Soeldner JS: "Somatostatinoma": Follow-up studies. *N Engl J Med* 297:1352, 1977.

78. Larsson LI, Hirsch MA, Holst JJ, et al: Pancreatic somatostatinoma: Clinical features and physiological implications. *Lancet* 1:666, 1977.

79. Krejs GJ, Orci L, Conlon JM, et al: Somatostatinoma syndrome: Biochemical, morphologic, and clinical features. *N Engl J Med* 301:285, 1979.

80. Soga J, Yakuwa Y: Somatostatinoma/inhibitory syndrome: A statistical evaluation of 173 reported cases as compared to other pancreatic endocrinomas. *J Exp Clin Cancer Res* 18:13, 1999.

81. Snow N, Lauriaux R: Neuroendocrine tumors. In Rusygi A, editor: *Gastrointestinal cancers: Biology, diagnosis, and therapy*, Philadelphia, 1995, Lippincott-Raven, p 585.

82. Sakamoto T, Miyata M, Izukura M, et al: Role of endogenous somatostatin in postprandial hypersecretion of neurotensin in patients after gastrectomy. *Ann Surg* 225:377, 1997.

83. Stelow EB, Woon C, Pambuccian SE, et al: Fine-needle aspiration cytology of pancreatic somatostatinoma: The importance of immunohistochemistry for the cytologic diagnosis of pancreatic endocrine neoplasms. *Diagn Cytopathol* 33:100, 2005.

84. Angeletti S, Corleto VD, Schillaci O, et al: Use of the somatostatin analogue octreotide to localise and manage somatostatin-producing tumours. *Gut* 42:792, 1998.

85. Anene C, Thompson JS, Saigh J, et al: Somatostatinoma: Atypical presentation of a rare pancreatic tumor. *Am J Gastroenterol* 90:819, 1995.

86. O'Brien TD, Chejfec G, Prinz RA: Clinical features of duodenal somatostatinomas. *Surgery* 114:1144, 1993.

87. Virgolini I, Kurtaran A, Leimer M, et al: Location of a VIPoma by iodine 123-vasoactive intestinal peptide scintigraphy. *J Nucl Med* 39:1575, 1998.

88. Verner JV, Morrison AB: Islet cell tumor and a syndrome of refractory watery diarrhea and hypokalemia. *Am J Med* 29:529, 1958.

89. O'Dorisio TM, Mekhjian HS, Gaginella TS: Medical therapy of VIPomas. *Endocrinol Metab Clin North Am* 18:545, 1989.

90. Mekhjian HS, O'Dorisio TM: VIPoma syndrome. *Semin Oncol* 14:282, 1987.

91. O'Dorisio TM, Mekhjian HS: VIPoma syndrome. In Cohen S, Soloway RD, editors: *Hormone-producing tumors of the pancreas*. New York, 1985, Churchill-Livingstone, p 101.

92. Nagorney DM, Bloom SR, Polak JM, et al: Resolution of recurrent Verner-Morrison syndrome by resection of metastatic VIPoma. *Surgery* 93:348, 1983.

93. Mallinson CN, Bloom SR, Warin AP: A glucagonoma syndrome. *Lancet* 2:1, 1974.

94. Bornman PC, Beckingham IJ: ABC of diseases of liver, pancreas, and biliary system: Chronic pancreatitis. *BMJ* 322:595, 2001.

95. Kahan RS, Perez-Figaredo RA, Neimanis A: Necrolytic migratory erythema: Distinctive dermatosis of the glucagonoma syndrome. *Arch Dermatol* 113:792, 1977.

96. Vinik AI, Moattari AR: Treatment of endocrine tumors of the pancreas. *Endocrinol Metab Clin North Am* 18:483, 1989.

97. Wilkinson DS: Necrolytic migratory erythema with carcinoma of the pancreas. *Trans St. Johns Hosp Dermatol Soc* 59:244, 1973.

98. Stacpoole PW: The glucagonoma syndrome: Clinical features, diagnosis, and treatment. *Endocr Rev* 2:347, 1981.

99. Maton PN, Gardner JD, Densen RT: The incidence and etiology of Cushing's syndrome in patients with the Zollinger-Ellison syndrome. *N Engl J Med* 315:1, 1986.

100. Yao JC, Lombard-Bohas C, Baudin E, et al: Daily Oral Everolimus Activity in Patients With Metastatic Pancreatic Neuroendocrine Tumors After Failure of Cytotoxic Chemotherapy: A Phase II Trial. *J Clin Oncol* 28:69, 2009.

101. Rougier P, Mitry E: Chemotherapy in the treatment of neuroendocrine malignant tumors. *Digestion* 62:73, 2000.

102. Sano T, Asa SL, Kovacs K: Growth hormone–releasing hormone-producing tumors: Clinical, biochemical, and morphological manifestations. *Endocr Rev* 9:357, 1988.

103. Schoevaerdts D, Favet L, Zekry D, et al: VIPoma: Effective treatment with octreotide in the oldest old. *J Am Geriatr Soc* 49:496, 2001.

104. Zeiger MA, Pass HI, Doppman JD, et al: Surgical strategy in the management of non–small cell ectopic adrenocorticotropic hormone syndrome. *Surgery* 112:994, 1992.

105. Bresler L, Boissel P, Conroy T, et al: Pancreatic islet cell carcinoma with hypercalcemia: Complete remission 5 years after surgical excision and chemotherapy. *Am J Gastroenterol* 86:635, 1991.

106. Arps H, Dietel M, Schulz A, et al: Pancreatic endocrine carcinoma with ectopic PTH production and paraneoplasia hypercalcemia. *Virchows Arch A Pathol Anat Histopathol* 408:497, 1986.

107. Blackburn AM, Bryant MG, Adraian TE, et al: Pancreatic tumors produce neurotensin. *J Clin Endocrinol Metab* 52:820, 1981.

108. Shulkes A, Boden R, Cook I, et al: Characterization of a pancreatic tumor containing vasoactive intestinal peptide, neurotensin, and pancreatic polypeptide. *J Clin Endocrinol Metab* 58:41, 1984.

109. Corbetta S, Peracchi M, Cappiello V, et al: Circulating ghrelin levels in patients with pancreatic and gastrointestinal neuroendocrine tumors: Identification of one pancreatic ghrelinoma. *J Clin Endocrinol Metab* 88:3117, 2003.

110. Phan GQ, Yeo CJ, Hruban RH, et al: Surgical experience with pancreatic and peripancreatic neuroendocrine tumors: Review of 125 patients. *J Gastrointest Surg* 2:472, 1998.

111. Eckhauser FE, Cheung PS, Vinik AI: Nonfunctioning malignant neuroendocrine tumors of the pancreas. *Surgery* 100:978, 1986.

112. Lo CY, van Heerden JA, Thompson GB, et al: Islet cell carcinoma of the pancreas. *World J Surg* 20:878, 1996.

113. Schindl M, Kaczirek K, Kaserer K, et al: Is the new classification of neuroendocrine pancreatic tumors of clinical help? *World J Surg* 24:1312, 2000.

114. Grino P, Martinez J, Grino E, et al: Acute pancreatitis secondary to pancreatic neuroendocrine tumors. *JOP* 4:104, 2003.

115. Kent RB III, van Heerden JA, Weiland LH: Nonfunctioning islet cell tumors. *Ann Surg* 193:185, 1981.

116. Brown KT, Koh BY, Brody LA, et al: Particle embolization of hepatic neuroendocrine metastases for control of pain and hormonal symptoms. *J Vasc Interv Radiol* 10:397, 1999.

117. Delcore R, Friessen SR: Gastrointestinal neuroendocrine tumors. *J Am Coll Surg* 178:187, 1994.

118. McEntee GP, Nagorney DM, Kvols LK, et al: Cytoreductive hepatic surgery for neuroendocrine tumors. *Surgery* 108:1091, 1990.

119. Pathak RD, Tran TH, Burshell AL: A case of dopamine agonists inhibiting pancreatic polypeptide secretion from an islet cell tumor. *J Clin Endocrinol Metab* 89:581, 2004.

120. Venkatesh S, Ordonez NG, Ajani J, et al: Islet cell carcinoma of the pancreas: A study of 98 patients. *Cancer* 65:354, 1990.

121. Liu TH, Zhu Y, Cui QC, et al: Nonfunctioning pancreatic endocrine tumors: An immunohistochemical and electron microscopic analysis of 26 cases. *Pathol Res Pract* 188:191, 1992.

122. Broughan TA, Leslie JD, Soto JM, et al: Pancreatic islet cell tumors. *Surgery* 99:671, 1986.

Primary Pancreatic Cystic Neoplasms

George H. Sakorafas | Thomas Schnelldorfer | Michael G. Sarr

Primary pancreatic cystic neoplasms (PPCNs) are relatively rare neoplasms, but they are appreciated and recognized with increasing prevalence along with current increased access to and improvements in cross-sectional imaging. In 1978, Compagno and Oertel made the first important distinction between serous and mucinous cystic neoplasms of the pancreas and outlined the importance of identifying the mucinous neoplasms because of their overt or latent malignant potential.[1,2] In 1982, Ohashi et al in Japan[3] reported a seemingly new type of cystic neoplasm of the pancreas, which they termed *mucinous secreting cancer of the pancreas*. As our knowledge of this neoplasm has increased, the term *intraductal papillary mucinous neoplasm* (IPMN) has been accepted more widely to better describe this specific type of PPCN.[4] Since that time, there has been tremendous interest in further classifying these cystic lesions both histologically and clinically, and many groups throughout the world have refined the classification, diagnosis, differentiation, and appropriate management of PPCNs. Currently, PPCNs are increasingly important in clinical practice because of their increasing detection in asymptomatic patients. This presentation is a result of the widespread availability and use of modern, state-of-the-art imaging techniques for other reasons or for the investigation of patients with abdominal (often unrelated and nonspecific) complaints. The detection of presumed PPCNs may represent a particularly difficult dilemma for the practicing clinician because the biologic behavior of PPCNs ranges widely, not only between serous and mucinous neoplasms, but also between various subgroups of mucinous neoplasms. Moreover, the preoperative diagnosis of malignancy with certainty may be impossible, and these patients are often asymptomatic. This chapter focuses on these aspects of these neoplasms.

INCIDENCE AND EPIDEMIOLOGY

Pancreatic cystic lesions are surprisingly common. In an autopsy study,[5] 186 neoplastic cystic lesions were found in 73 of 300 autopsy cases (approximately 25%), equally distributed throughout the pancreas. The incidence of cystic lesions, however, did increase with age. Similar results have been reported by others.[6] One group of investigators in the United States tried to estimate the prevalence of pancreatic cysts in patients undergoing MRI for nonpancreatic diseases.[7] Nearly 20% of 1444 patients had at least one pancreatic cystic lesion. Therefore, it is not surprising that because of the increasing use of high-resolution abdominal imaging techniques, PPCNs are being identified increasingly, often as incidental findings.

Cystic lesions comprise approximately 15% of all pancreatic neoplasms.[8] Serous cystic neoplasms (SCNs), mucinous cystic neoplasms (MCNs), and IPMNs are the three most common types of PPCNs and represent approximately 90% of all PPCNs.[6] MCNs and IPMNs are the most prevalent and, importantly, have malignant potential, thus the clinical importance of differentiating these mucinous neoplasms from the SCN (or nonmucinous cystic neoplasms), which are almost always benign. SCNs are observed more commonly in women (75%), with an average age at diagnosis of 62 years.[9] Most SCNs are located in the head of the pancreas. MCNs are observed almost exclusively (>95%) in women, with a mean age at diagnosis of 53 years.[4,10] Unlike SCNs, MCNs are located most commonly in the body and tail of the pancreas (>75%). IPMNs represent approximately 25% of all cystic neoplasms.[4,6,10] In contrast to SCNs and MCNs, IPMNs are a bit more common in men and are encountered typically in older patients (usually in the sixth to seventh decades of life).[4,10] Most IPMNs arise in the pancreatic head but can be seen in any location and can occasionally involve the entire ductal system.[10] Unlike MCNs and SCNs, multifocal disease can occur in IPMNs. Overall, approximately two-thirds of all PPCNs are potentially premalignant or malignant lesions (see later).[11]

PATHOLOGY AND BIOLOGIC BEHAVIOR

Currently, the spectrum of PPCNs includes the following four groups: (1) SCNs, (2) MCNs, (3) IPMNs, and (4) unusual cystic neoplasms; the latter PPCNs will not be discussed in detail in this chapter but are outlined in Box 95-1. As noted earlier, there are substantive differences between these three subgroups of PPCNs; as a consequence, a selective management approach is necessary and required.

SEROUS CYSTIC NEOPLASM

SCNs, previously known as *microcystic adenomas*, form a well-demarcated mass (cluster) of individual small cysts (honeycomb-like appearance). Each cyst is almost always less than 2 cm, filled with a clear, watery fluid but distinctly without containing mucin (Figure 95-1). The overall size of the SCN tumor varies from a few centimeters to as large as 25 cm (usually, 6 to 10 cm). SCNs have a thin, almost translucent wall that usually separates easily from surrounding structures without the inflammatory or fibrous adherence seen in postinflammatory pancreatic pseudocysts. The cysts are lined by a single, uniform layer of cuboidal, glycogen-rich serous cells,[12] with round nuclei and abundant clear cytoplasm but notably without cellular characteristics of atypia or dysplasia. The stroma separating these microcystic areas is

---

BOX 95-1 Cystic Lesions of the Pancreas

CYSTIC NEOPLASMS
Serous cystic neoplasm
Mucinous cystic neoplasm
Intraductal papillary mucinous neoplasm
Other rare cystic neoplasms
  Solid pseudopapillary neoplasms of the pancreas
  Cystic islet cell neoplasms
  Cystic choriocarcinomas
  Cystic teratomas
  Angiomatous neoplasm (angioma, lymphangioma,
    hemangiothelioma)

ACQUIRED CYSTS
Parasitic cysts
  Echinococcal (hydatid) cyst
  Taenia solium cyst

Postinflammatory cystic fluid collection
  Pancreatic pseudocyst
  Pancreatic pseudopseudocyst (inflammatory exudative
    collection)
  Pancreatic sequestrum (postnecrotic fluid collection)

CONGENITAL TRUE CYSTS
Simple cysts
  Isolated pancreatic cyst
  Pancreatic cysts associated with polycystic disease of the
    kidneys
  Polycystic disease of the pancreas without related
    anomalies
  Pancreatic macrocysts associated with cystic fibrosis
  Polycystic disease of the pancreas associated with von
    Hippel-Lindau disease
Dermoid cysts

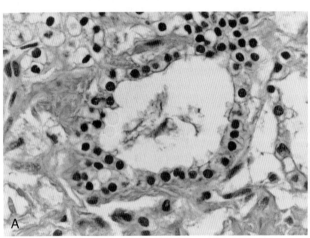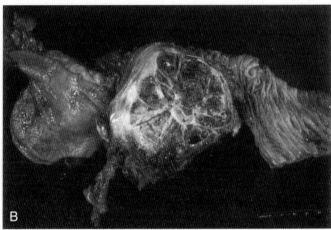

FIGURE 95-1 Serous cystadenoma of the pancreas (serous cystic neoplasm). **A,** Simple serous cuboidal cells without dysplasia. **B,** Gross appearance with multiple small cysts. (Reproduced with permission from Pyke CM, van Heerden JA, Colby TV, et al: The spectrum of serous cystadenoma of the pancreas: Clinical, pathological, and surgical aspects. *Ann Surg* 215:132, 1992.)

composed of a fibrous connective tissue that is quite vascular and is often calcified; indeed, this unique central calcification gives rise to a characteristic central sunburst, radial, or stellate scar pattern on computed tomography (CT) in approximately 30% of patients (see later). The much less common serous *oligocystic* (or *macrocystic*) SCN has fewer (sometimes only one) cystic spaces (>2 cm), but the histopathologic appearance is similar to that of the microcystic SCNs.[13] The cell of origin of SCNs appears to be the centroacinar cell, possibly explaining the peripheral anatomic location of these neoplasms within the pancreatic parenchyma.

Malignant SCNs (*serous cystadenocarcinomas*) have been reported in the literature as case reports[14] but are extremely rare, and, therefore, SCNs of the pancreas should be considered (and managed as) benign neoplasms.[4] The benign biologic behavior of SCNs has been confirmed in a recent series of 158 patients undergoing resection, with only two malignancies, one diagnosed initially, the other one on followup because of metastases

after an initial benign diagnosis from the resection specimen.[15] In the series by Bassi et al,[16] 50 patients with SCNs who were managed nonoperatively had no evidence of a "significant increase in the diameter of the lesion" after a median followup of 69 months. Tseng et al[9] from the Massachusetts General Hospital reported that 24 patients with SCNs experienced SCN rates of growth of 0.6 cm/yr. Growth rate was correlated with tumor size (0.1 cm/yr in tumors <4 cm in size [$n = 15$ patients] vs. 2 cm/yr in tumors ≥4 cm [$n = 9$ patients]). This observation served as the basis for their recommendation for resection of SCNs with a diameter of greater than or equal to 4 cm. Obviously, this information regarding natural history of untreated SCNs has great clinical importance.

MUCINOUS CYSTIC NEOPLASM

The gross appearance of MCNs, formerly known inappropriately as *macrocystic adenomas*, is different from that of SCNs. The individual cysts making up the mass are

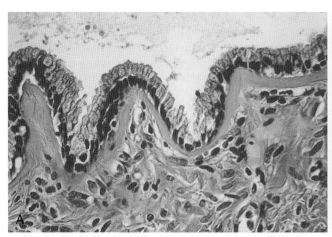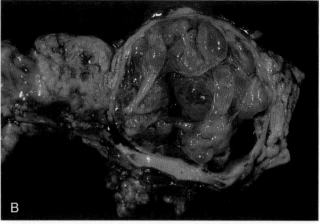

FIGURE 95-2 Mucinous cystic neoplasm (MCN) of the pancreas. **A,** Columnar mucinous cells line the cyst wall. **B,** Gross appearance of macrocysts with thin walls and mucinous cystic fluid. (Reproduced with permission from Sarr MG, Carpenter HA, Prabhakar LP, et al: Clinical and pathologic correlation of 84 mucinous cystic neoplasms of the pancreas: Can one reliably differentiate benign from malignant (or premalignant) neoplasms? *Ann Surg* 231:205, 2000.)

larger, typically greater than 2 cm, and the tumor mass can be as large as 25 cm (usually, 8 to 10 cm).[4] MCNs generally contain fewer than six separate cysts, do not communicate with the pancreatic ductal system (Figure 95-2), and usually are spherical (and not grape-like clusters as with branch-duct IPMNs). Rarely, the neoplasm has just one macrocyst. Often, the cysts are not unilocular but have septa within them and may have a solid, eccentric component.[4,10] As with SCNs, the surrounding tissues usually lack an inflammatory, pericystic reaction except when malignant transformation and tissue invasion have occurred. MCNs are almost always located in the body or tail of the pancreas (>95%).[4] Peripheral, eccentric (eggshell-like) calcifications occur in approximately 15% of MCNs and are considered almost pathognomonic of MCNs.[10]

MCNs contain a mucinous, columnar epithelium. The characteristics of this mucinous epithelium may vary widely throughout the neoplasm, with areas of a single layer of benign-appearing, mucin-secreting columnar epithelium resembling the mucinous cells of an ovarian mucous cystadenoma as well as the ovarian stroma that accompanies these neoplasms. In addition, the mucinous epithelial lining contains areas with papillary projections or invaginations and will often have atypia, dysplasia, carcinoma in situ, and even areas of tissue invasion (invasive carcinoma).[17] A spectrum of all these changes of epithelium may be found within the same neoplasm (Figure 95-3). The neoplasm is classified based on the greatest rather than the average degree of atypia. Foci of invasive carcinoma or carcinoma in situ can be patchy or very focal, not visible grossly, and often with an abrupt transition between histologically bland epithelium and epithelium with severe atypia. Therefore, numerous sections by the pathologist may be required to evaluate this neoplasm completely. Grossly papillary or nodular areas should be sampled first, because these areas are most likely to harbor the malignant component. Sometimes, mucin accumulating within neoplastic lobules causes pressure necrosis of the lining epithelium, causing the discontinuous nature of the epithelial lining.

Incomplete, denuded epithelium may be found in up to 70% of mucinous cystadenomas and cystadenocarcinomas, with a mean of 40% (but as great as 98%) of the cystic wall being devoid of an epithelial lining.[4,18] The intracystic fluid in MCNs is thicker and more viscous than in SCNs, because it contains mucus.

The presence of ovarian stroma is a particular and necessary characteristic of MCNs. Most pancreatologists agree that the presence of ovarian stroma is required for the diagnosis of MCN.[19] Because of this requirement, virtually all MCNs occur in women (>95%). The occurrence of MCNs with ovarian stroma in males is extremely unusual, and only a few definitive cases have been reported in the English literature.[19] The presence of ovarian stroma has been proposed as one of the differential findings to distinguish MCNs from IPMNs (mainly branch-duct type) in difficult cases (see later); indeed, in the past, many of the reported series of MCNs had a greater percentage of male patients who, now in retrospect, undoubtedly had branch-duct IPMNs.[17]

In contrast to SCNs, MCNs represent a more diverse, broader, heterogeneous spectrum. These neoplasms should be considered potentially premalignant. Malignant degeneration of a MCN can undoubtedly occur and has been described often after a long period,[17] but the incidence of malignant (invasive) degeneration is probably not as common as once thought because of the unknowing inclusion of patients with IPMNs in the older series of MCNs. The incidence of carcinoma within a MCN increases with the size and complexity of the lesion.[20] Foci of invasion may be found in up to a third of MCNs containing carcinoma in situ and, hence, extensive sampling of the entire tumor specimen is recommended (see earlier).[21] In an attempt to differentiate invasive MCNs from both the benign MCNs and the MCNs that show dysplastic changes limited to the surface epithelium (but not tissue invasion), a classification system has been proposed by investigators from the Mayo Clinic, which reliably separates the spectrum of MCNs into the following three subgroups[17]: (1) *mucinous cystadenomas* (~65% of MCNs), which contain a uniform,

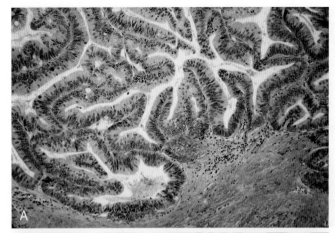

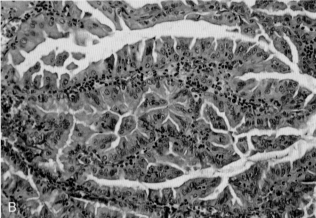

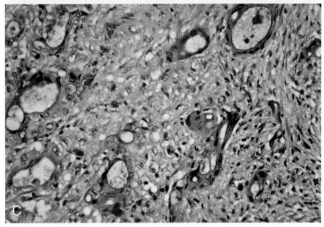

FIGURE 95-3 Spectrum of mucinous cystic neoplasm of the pancreas. **A,** Proliferative changes in epithelium with papillary fronds and low-grade dysplasia. **B,** High-grade dysplasia with papillary polypoid intracystic growth. **C,** Mucinous cystadenocarcinoma with tissue invasion and desmoplastic response. (Reproduced with permission from Sarr MG, Carpenter HA, Prabhakar LP, et al: Clinical and pathologic correlation of 84 mucinous cystic neoplasms of the pancreas: Can one reliably differentiate benign from malignant [or premalignant] neoplasms? *Ann Surg* 231:205, 2000.)

single layer of benign, columnar mucinous cells; (2) *noninvasive proliferative MCNs* (~30% of MCNs), composed of a varying degree of atypia, dysplasia, papillary endothelial infolding, and even changes of carcinoma in situ in the epithelial lining, but without any tissue

invasion; and (3) *mucinous cystadenocarcinomas*, which may have features throughout the neoplasm of the first two groups but also contain areas of overt stromal (tissue) invasion beyond the epithelium (i.e., true invasive cancer). Although the reported incidence of cancer in MCNs has ranged from 29% to 36%, the experience of the Mayo Clinic and of others is different with less than one-fifth of all MCNs (6% to 20%) actually having invasive carcinoma (8% in the Mayo Clinic experience).[4,10,20,22] This dichotomy stems from the tendency of some groups to call MCNs with areas of carcinoma in situ as cancers. In a recent case series report of 163 resected MCNs from both the University of Verona and the Massachusetts General Hospital, 118 patients (72%) had adenoma, 17 (11%) borderline neoplasms, 9 (6%) in situ carcinoma, and 19 (only 12%) invasive carcinoma.[23] Mutation of the *K-ras*2 oncogene located on chromosome 12 p is one of the earliest genetic changes seen within MCNs, and these mutations are detected in up to 20% of the mucinous cystadenomas and 90% of the MCNs with carcinoma in situ.[21]

Risk factors for the presence of underlying malignancy within a MCN are the following[19,23,24]:

1. **Large tumor size.** In the study by Goh et al, none of the 40 malignant MCNs (carcinoma in situ or invasive) were less than 3 cm, and only 1 was less than 4.5 cm (3 cm).[19] In the study by Crippa et al, of 163 resected MCNs, all neoplasms with cancer were 4 cm or larger, and malignant MCNs (both in situ and invasive carcinoma) were significantly larger than benign ones (80 vs. 45 mm).[23]

2. **Associated mass, mural nodules, asymmetrically thickened wall.**[10,23] Malignant MCNs (both in situ and invasive carcinoma) were 16 times more likely to harbor nodules (64 vs. 4%).[23] Extrinsic masses associated with the MCN are very worrisome for cystadenocarcinoma.

3. **Eggshell calcification.** This type of calcification differs from the centrally located radial, starburst-type calcification of SCNs.

4. **Age.** Patients with invasive carcinoma tend to be substantially older (>11 years old) than those with noninvasive MCNs, further justifying the concept of malignant degeneration.

5. **Symptomatology.** Many if not most benign MCNs are relatively asymptomatic. Concern about invasive malignancy should be emphasized if the patient has clinically relevant abdominal pain, weight loss, jaundice, or mechanical duodenal obstruction.

6. **Splenic vein obstruction.** Most MCNs are "pushers" rather than "invaders." The presence of splenic vein thrombosis in the absence of prior pancreatitis also should heighten the concern of invasive malignancy.

INTRADUCTAL PAPILLARY MUCINOUS NEOPLASM

IPMN is characterized by intraductal proliferation of neoplastic mucinous cells, which form micro- and macropapillae and lead to cystic dilation of the main pancreatic duct and/or secondary branches (branch ducts). These dilated, neoplastic ducts often contain globules of mucus that may appear as masses on imaging, most commonly in the pancreatic head and usually in older men (>60 years old).[25] The dysplastic lesions within the IPMN are usually contiguous but on rare occasions can be multicentric. These neoplasms often produce copious mucin. In approximately one-third of patients (~30%), mucus can be seen exuding from a bulging papilla at the ampulla of Vater at endoscopy when the main pancreatic duct is involved. IPMNs are characterized by the distinct lack of ovarian stroma, which differentiates IPMNs from MCNs.[4,10,25]

Depending on the morphology of changes of the ductal system, IPMNs have been classified into the following three variations[3,18,26]:

1. **Main-duct IPMN**, characterized by dilation of the main pancreatic duct. Duct dilation may be either diffuse (generalized) or segmental (usually involving the body and tail of the pancreas). A rare subtype of diffuse, main pancreatic duct ectasia is caused by complete filling of the dilated main pancreatic duct by papillary neoplasm.
2. **Branch-duct IPMN**, appearing as a cystic dilation of one or, on occasion, multiple side branches of the main pancreatic ductal system, communicating with the pancreatic ductal system, usually in the head or uncinate process of the pancreas.
3. **Mixed-type IPMN**, involving both the main pancreatic duct and the side branches.

Each variation has important implications regarding the probability of underlying malignancy (especially invasive malignancy) and the extent of resection potentially needed. The morphologic pattern of duct dilation is dependent on tumor location, mucus production, and the presence of proximal duct obstruction. Branch-duct IPMNs tend to be larger with evident intraductal, papillary projections. Side-branch IPMNs are frequently smaller, may not have a readily identifiable proliferative epithelial lining, and the communication with the main pancreatic duct may on occasion be difficult to visualize. In approximately 30% of branch-duct IPMNs, the disease is multifocal and characterized by the presence of multiple, cystic dilations of small branches of the pancreatic ductal system in two or more areas within the pancreatic parenchyma.[27] Interestingly, after resection of pancreatic parenchyma for presumably side-branch IPMN, in a substantial proportion of patients (up to 25%), histology shows concurrent histologic changes also within the main pancreatic duct; therefore, in these patients, the correct diagnosis is IPMN of the mixed type.[27]

Histologically and according to the World Health Organization, IPMNs can be subdivided into the following three subgroups: (1) benign (adenoma without dysplasia), (2) borderline (adenoma with mild to moderate dysplasia), and (3) carcinoma (noninvasive or invasive) (Box 95-2).[28] Note that this classification combines IPMN with carcinoma in situ and invasive IPMN; therefore, when reading the literature, one must be careful to remember this point. The hyperplastic or dysplastic epithelium may be flat, micropapillary, or grossly papillary (Figure 95-4).[4] Frequently, a wide spectrum of changes of the epithelium is recognized, including normal, hyperplasia, dysplasia, and carcinoma often within the same pancreas and similar in principle to MCNs.[11,25,27] This

---

BOX 95-2 World Health Organization Classification of Cystic Neoplasms of the Pancreas

Serous microcystic adenoma
Serous oligocystic adenoma
Serous cystadenocarcinoma
Mucinous cystadenoma
Mucinous cystic neoplasm–borderline
Mucinous cystadenocarcinoma
   Noninvasive
   Invasive
Intraductal papillary mucinous adenoma
Intraductal papillary mucinous neoplasm–borderline
Intraductal papillary mucinous carcinoma
   Noninvasive
   Invasive

---

histologic continuum implies a clonal progression within IPMN, similar to the adenoma-to-carcinoma sequence of colorectal neoplasms.[29] IPMN also exhibits several different patterns of histologic morphology of the papillary changes: gastric, intestinal, pancreatobiliary, oncocytic, and null types.[25] The prognosis of these subtypes appears to differ substantially and may be a clue to their natural biology. Most intestinal-type IPMNs are believed to progress to invasive colloid carcinomas that have a good prognosis, whereas most pancreatobiliary IPMNs are believed to progress to invasive ductal or tubular adenocarcinomas and portend a poor prognosis.[25] Gastric-type epithelium is often found at the periphery of other types of IPMNs.

Recent research has shown that IPMN is associated with frequent (50% to 80%) K-*ras* point mutations, thereby establishing these mutations as a potential genetic marker for IPMN as with typical pancreatic ductal adenocarcinoma. Other molecular alterations associated with IPMNs are loss of heterozygosity in 9p21 (p16) and 17p13 (p53), increased expression of cyclooxygenase-2, upregulation of several genes (such as claudin and mesothelin), increased expression of matrix metalloproteinase-7, proliferating-cell nuclear antigen, and vascular endothelial growth factor, and increased telomerase activity.[30] Telomerase is in part responsible for cell immortality and is activated in most human malignancies; therefore, telomerase may be a useful diagnostic tool in the distinction between adenoma and intraductal carcinoma.[30] The real question is whether any of these acquired genomic mutations are involved directly in the malignant transformation or rather are just markers of a more global genomic instability.

Unlike SCNs and MCNs, IPMNs are a more aggressive neoplasm; approximately 40% of patients at the time of diagnosis of main-duct IPMN already have an established invasive malignancy (see later).[31] Moreover most, if not all, benign main-duct IPMNs are believed to be at very high risk of progressing into invasive cancer.[27] Risk factors for the presence of underlying malignancy include the following[10,32]:

1. **Main-duct disease.** Patients with main-duct IPMNs or mixed-type IPMNs have a risk of malignancy (carcinoma in situ and invasive cancer) of approximately 50% but it may be as great as 90%.[20,24] *Invasive* malignancy is also common in these lesions and

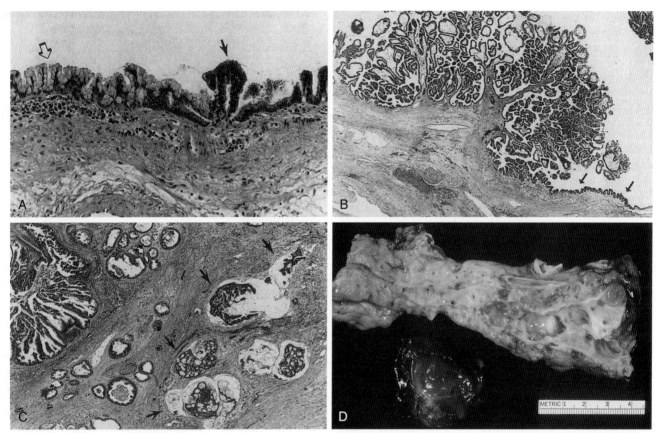

FIGURE 95-4 Intraductal papillary mucinous neoplasm. **A,** Ductal epithelium containing nondysplastic, micropapillary mucinous hyperplasia *(open arrow)* and micropapillary dysplasia *(solid arrow)*. **B,** Gross papillomatous changes with changes of flat micropapillary dysplasia *(arrows)*. **C,** Invasive adenocarcinoma *(arrows)*. **D,** Gross findings; main pancreatic duct dilation with copious intraductal mucin and ductal adenomas. (Reproduced with permission from Loftus EV Jr, Olivares-Pakzad BA, Batts KP, et al; members of the Pancreas Clinic and Pancreatic Surgeons of Mayo Clinic: Intraductal papillary-mucinous tumors of the pancreas: Clinicopathologic features, outcome, and nomenclature. *Gastroenterology* 110:1909, 1996.)

approaches 40% to 50%.[22,27] The risk of malignancy increases when the main pancreatic duct is dilated more than 1 cm and when mural nodules (>1 cm) are present[30]; the latter finding is extremely worrisome for invasive degeneration. In contrast, the risk of malignancy in patients with branch-duct IPMNs is much less (range, 6% to 46%; mean, 25%),[24,32] and the risk of *invasive* carcinoma in branch-duct IPMNs is even less (<15%).[22] Factors correlating with malignancy in branch-duct IPMNs include the presence of clinical symptoms, mural nodules (especially when >2 mm), cyst size larger than 3 cm, and coexistence of main-duct obstruction (dilation >10 mm).[27,32]

2. **Branch-duct dilation more than 3 cm** in size.
3. **Presence of a mural nodule(s).**
4. **Advanced age** (older than 70 years old).
5. **Presence of symptoms.** The majority of patients with invasive IPMNs have symptoms of pain (often a result of pancreatitis), weight loss, fatigue, and/or jaundice, but 30% of patients with malignant IPMNs are asymptomatic. Therefore, the absence of symptoms does not guarantee the absence of malignancy.[27]
6. **Increased telomerase activity in pancreatic juice.**[32]

Unlike typical ductal adenocarcinoma of the pancreas, histologic changes (atypia, dysplasia, or frank carcinoma in situ) may on occasion be found in discontinuous areas throughout the gland, raising the question of whether IPMN represents a generalized global disorder of the epithelium of the pancreatic duct or rather a more localized field defect. True multicentricity of main-duct IPMNs is not common (<10%), but in side-branch IPMNs, multicentricity has been recognized more frequently. IPMNs should be distinguished from pancreatic intraepithelial neoplasia (PanIN), the precursor lesion of ductal adenocarcinoma; indeed, IPMNs are radiographically detectable and grossly visible, while PanINs are detected microscopically and incidentally.[20] Moreover, IPMN is associated with invasive, colloid (mucinous noncystic) carcinoma in approximately 50% of cases, as opposed to the more traditional tubular adenocarcinomas, with which PanIN is typically associated.[10] There does appear, however, to be an increased incidence of extrapancreatic neoplasms in patients with IPMNs, especially colonic neoplasms[33] and also typical ductal carcinoma of the pancreas, raising the question of either a systemic predisposition or sharing of a local predisposition to malignant degeneration.

DIAGNOSTIC EVALUATION

Because of the markedly different biologic behavior of PPCNs, management of each type of neoplasm differs, and therefore an accurate preoperative diagnosis of the different types of PPCNs is crucial in making the correct therapeutic choices. After discovery of a cystic lesion in the pancreatic region, the three necessary diagnostic steps include the following: (1) confirm the pancreatic origin of the cystic lesion, (2) exclude the diagnosis of a pancreatic pseudocyst, and (3) identify those cystic neoplasms that should be resected because of overt or potential malignancy.[4]

CLINICAL PRESENTATION

PPCNs are usually discovered incidentally during diagnostic evaluation for other (often unrelated) symptoms or other indications. Clinical symptomatology may exist; when present, symptoms are usually not specific.

SCNs are typically asymptomatic. Clinical symptomatology is observed more commonly in large (>4 cm) compared to small (<4 cm) SCNs (72% vs. 22%); symptoms may include abdominal pain (25%), fullness or mass (10%), and rarely jaundice (7%).[9] MCNs are more commonly symptomatic compared to SCNs, probably because of their larger size. In patients with MCNs, the presence of clinical symptomatology should raise the suspicion for underlying malignancy. As with SCNs, symptoms are often nonspecific.[23] In patients with IPMN (mainly of the main-duct variant), recurrent episodes of pancreatitis or a scenario of idiopathic chronic pancreatitis may be observed; episodes of acute pancreatitis or development of chronic pancreatitis appear to be secondary to the presence of mucous or papillary projections within the pancreatic duct causing stenosis or obstruction of the ductal system. Branch-duct IPMNs are often asymptomatic, especially when "cyst" size is less than 3 cm. Clinical symptomatology typical of pancreatic

adenocarcinoma (i.e., painless jaundice, weight loss, etc.) may be observed in malignant IPMNs. Routine laboratory blood tests, including liver function tests, and amylase and lipase activities, should be obtained but are usually within normal limits or show nonspecific changes. The role of tumor markers, such as cancer antigen (CA) 19-9, carcinoembryonic antigen (CEA), and CA 125, are not completely established but appear to have limited value for diagnostic purposes.

CROSS-SECTIONAL IMAGING (ULTRASONOGRAPHY, COMPUTED TOMOGRAPHY, MAGNETIC RESONANCE IMAGING)

The suspicion of a PPCN is almost always evident first after a noninvasive imaging procedure (ultrasonography, CT, or MRI), often at the time of evaluation for unrelated reasons, for example, during followup for another indication or for vague abdominal complaints not correlated necessarily with PPCNs. Because of the known limitations of transabdominal ultrasonography in the evaluation of pancreatic lesions, CT (or alternatively magnetic resonane imaging [MRI]) should be considered the gold standard in the evaluation of PPCNs. Imaging should include the entire thorax, abdomen, and pelvis for appropriate staging, with special focus on the liver and lung as the most common sites for metastases for invasive PPCNs.

1. **SCN.** SCNs have three morphologic patterns on imaging: polycystic, oligocystic, and honeycomb. The polycystic pattern is the most common (70%) (Figure 95-5) and is characterized by a bosselated collection of multiple (usually more than six) small cysts, each of which are usually smaller than 2 cm.[4] A central, fibrous scar with a characteristic radial calcification manifested as a central starburst calcification on imaging occurs in up to 30% of these neoplasms and, when present, is considered virtually pathognomonic of SCNs. The honeycomb

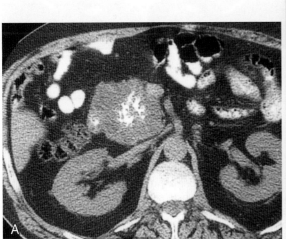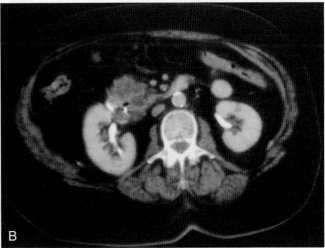

FIGURE 95-5 CT of serous cystic neoplasm. **A,** Solid-appearing lesion with central starburst calcification. **B,** "Microcystic" mass in head of pancreas. (**A** reproduced with permission from Pyke CM, van Heerden JA, Colby TV, et al: The spectrum of serous cystadenoma of the pancreas: Clinical, pathological, and surgical aspects. *Ann Surg* 215:132, 1992; **B** reproduced with permission from Sarr MG, Murr M, Smyrk TC, et al: Primary cystic neoplasms of the pancreas: Neoplastic disorders of emerging importance—current state-of-the-art and unanswered questions. *J Gastrointest Surg* 7:417, 2003.)

pattern (~20%) is characterized by numerous, sub-centimeter cysts that often cannot be well depicted as individual cysts by cross-sectional imaging; indeed, these lesions may appear as a solid mass on CT but will be hypoechoic on ultrasound imaging, of low attenuation on CT, and have a high signal intensity on T2-weighted MRI. The oligocystic or macrocystic pattern is the least common (<2%). These characteristic findings on imaging (predominance of small cystic areas with stromal hypervascularity) combined with an indolent course, lack of metastases or local invasion, and an appropriate clinical setting, permits the diagnosis of SCN to be made with an accuracy approaching 90% to 95%.[34]

2. **MCN.** MCNs are predominantly macrocystic and unilocular (80%); rarely, they can be multilocular (20%). Generally they are spherical in shape but may have several adjacent cysts (Figure 95-6).[4,34] MCNs do not communicate with the pancreatic ductal system but may cause partial pancreatic ductal obstruction because of extrinsic pressure on the pancreatic ductal system. The cysts have thicker, irregular walls, often with papillary excrescences extending into the lumen of the cystic lesion. The complex, internal architecture of the cysts often allows differentiation from SCNs. Although MCNs have often been misdiagnosed as pancreatic pseudocysts in the past, MCNs usually lack the prominent extracystic inflammatory component so characteristic of pancreatic pseudocysts. Calcifications are uncommon, but, when present (<20%), tend to be located in an eggshell distribution within the peripheral cyst walls. The presence of calcifications, an eccentrically located mass within a cystic area, multiple papillary invaginations (intracystic mural nodules), wall or septal enhancement, a recognizable pericystic mass or reaction, local invasion of adjacent vascular structures, extrahepatic biliary obstruction, associated metastatic lesions (usually in the liver), or ascites are imaging findings indicating the possibility of invasive carcinoma within the MCN (mucinous cystadenocarcinoma).[35] The size of mural nodules or papillary invaginations correlates with the probability of malignant degeneration[4,34]; however, in the absence of these imaging features, accurate preoperative differentiation of benign MCNs versus noninvasive proliferative MCNs (containing severe dysplasia or carcinoma in situ) versus malignant (invasive) MCNs is not possible.

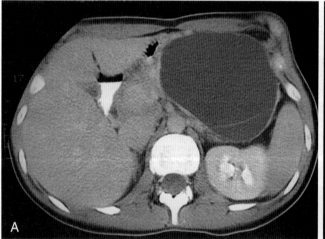
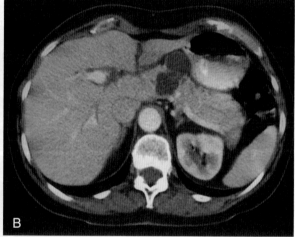
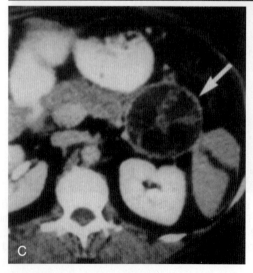

FIGURE 95-6 CT characteristics of primary mucinous cystic neoplasms of the pancreas. **A,** Macrocystic form: note septum and lack of surrounding inflammatory reaction. **B,** Several macrocystic areas (>2 cm) in midbody of pancreas. **C,** Complex cystic mass with solid intracystic component—invasive mucinous cystadenocarcinoma. (**A** and **B** reproduced with permission from Yeo CJ, Sarr MG: Cystic and pseudocystic diseases of the pancreas. *Current Probl Surg* 31:165, 1994; **C** reprinted with permission from Johnson CD, Stephens DH, Charboneau JW, et al: Cystic pancreatic tumors: CT and sonographic assessment. *Am J Roentgenol* 15:1133, 1988.)

3. **IPMN.** The characteristic feature of IPMNs on imaging is cystic dilation of either the main pancreatic duct (main-duct IPMN) or of a primary, segmental, side-branch of the main duct (branch-duct IPMN), most often in the uncinate lobe (Figure 95-7). Serial sections of the entire pancreatic specimen and three-dimensional reconstruction are extremely useful in determining the full extent of IPMNs. The mucinous globules or the areas of malignant transformation may appear as filling defects within the ductal system. CT (and alternatively MRI) can detect the location and degree of pancreatic duct dilation and can often differentiate IPMNs from other causes of duct dilation, such as chronic pancreatitis or obstructing neoplasms. Improved imaging techniques (e.g., MRI, see later) allow the detection of small cystic dilation of branch ducts with no or only mild dilation of the main pancreatic duct.[34,35] Main-duct IPMN (in contrast to branch-duct IPMN), especially when associated with a markedly dilated main pancreatic duct (>10 mm), the presence of mural nodules, and dilation of the biliary tree are imaging findings associated with a greater probability of underlying malignancy[20,25,27,35]; however, accurate preoperative discrimination of benign from malignant IPMNs is practically impossible; the implications of this problem has obvious clinical implications.

ENDOSCOPIC RETROGRADE CHOLANGIOPANCREATOGRAPHY

Endoscopic retrograde cholangiopancreatography (ERCP) is a very sensitive diagnostic modality used to identify a direct communication between the pancreatic duct and one of these cystic lesions.[4,8,34] ERCP may be helpful in the differentiation between pancreatic pseudocysts and cystic neoplasms, but ERCP has little to offer in the evaluation of SCNs or MCNs, because these neoplasms do not communicate with the pancreatic ductal system. In contrast, in IPMNs, ERCP may be important for several reasons. First, ERCP can depict the communication between the cystic dilation (or side-branch dilation) and the main pancreatic duct, and, second, ERCP can reveal a markedly dilated main pancreatic duct that may contain filling defects related to either mucinous concretions, papillary growths (intraductal papillomas), or areas of frank malignant degeneration/invasion (Figure 95-8).[4,17,34] Often, however, the intraductal mural nodules (adenomas or carcinomas) are obscured by the mucin and, sometimes, the mucin can be misinterpreted as a nodule. In approximately 30% of patients, copious egress of mucin noted from a bulging papilla on ERCP is considered as a virtually pathognomonic endoscopic finding.[34] ERCP may be particularly helpful in the differential diagnosis between branch-duct IPMN and MCN, which on occasion can be difficult on noninvasive imaging.[8,35] The presence of biliary or pancreatic duct dilation without an associated mass lesion on cross-sectional imaging is a particular indication for ERCP.[8] ERCP may also have a therapeutic role, allowing placement of a temporary, preoperative biliary endoprosthesis for decompression in jaundiced patients. Overall, the clinical role of ERCP, especially in diagnosis, is declining because of the improvements in quality of noninvasive cross-sectional imaging.

MAGNETIC RESONANCE CHOLANGIOPANCREATOGRAPHY

Magnetic resonance cholangiopancreatography (MRCP) is a noninvasive, diagnostic method with fewer procedure-related risks (compared to ERCP). On occasion, MRCP may be more specific than ERCP in imaging pancreatic duct anatomy (i.e., presence of communication of a cystic lesion with the ductal system), because filling of side-branch ducts at the time of ERCP may be obscured

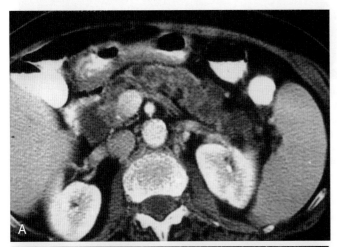
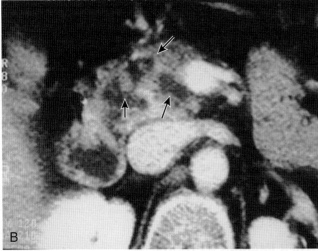

FIGURE 95-7 CT findings of intraductal papillary mucinous neoplasms (IPMNs) of the pancreas. **A,** Main-duct disease. Note dilation of main pancreatic duct and atrophy of the parenchyma. **B,** Branch-duct IPMN dilation of secondary branches of the ductal system. (**A** reproduced with permission from Loftus EV Jr, Olivares-Pakzad BA, Batts KP, et al; members of the Pancreas Clinic and Pancreatic Surgeons of Mayo Clinic: Intraductal papillary-mucinous tumors of the pancreas: Clinicopathologic features, outcome, and nomenclature. *Gastroenterology* 110:1909, 1996; **B** reproduced with permission from Sarr MG, Murr M, Smyrk TC, et al: Primary cystic neoplasms of the pancreas: Neoplastic disorders of emerging importance—current state-of-the-art and unanswered questions. *J Gastrointest Surg* 7:417, 2003.)

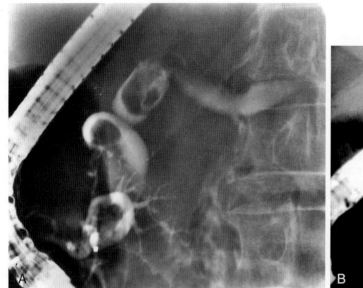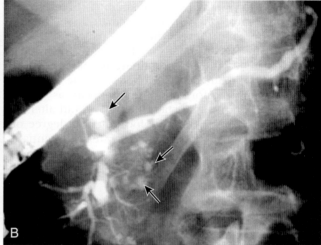

FIGURE 95-8 Endoscopic retrograde pancreatography of intraductal papillary mucinous neoplasms. **A,** Main-duct disease. Note intraductal filling defects secondary to mucin globules. **B,** Branch-duct disease. Note continuity with normal-sized main pancreatic duct. (**A** reproduced with permission from Loftus EV Jr, Olivares-Pakzad BA, Batts KP, et al; members of the Pancreas Clinic and Pancreatic Surgeons of Mayo Clinic: Intraductal papillary-mucinous tumors of the pancreas: Clinicopathologic features, outcome, and nomenclature. *Gastroenterology* 110:1909, 1996; **B** reproduced with permission from Sarr MG, Murr M, Smyrk TC, et al: Primary cystic neoplasms of the pancreas: Neoplastic disorders of emerging importance—current state-of-the-art and unanswered questions. *J Gastrointest Surg* 7:417, 2003.)

by intraductal plugs of mucin[34,36]; moreover, MRCP will image fluid collections that do not communicate with the pancreatic ductal system. Mural nodules or excrescences, main-duct IPMNs especially with main pancreatic duct dilation (>10 mm), and common bile duct dilation are findings on MRCP that suggest malignancy. As noted earlier, however, the absence of these findings does not guarantee that the neoplasm is benign.[36] MRCP is particularly helpful in delineating branch-duct lesions of IPMNs because of their characteristic appearance as a bunch of grapes.

ENDOSCOPIC ULTRASONOGRAPHY

Endoscopic ultrasonography (EUS) has emerged recently as a valuable diagnostic technique. By allowing high-frequency, high-resolution imaging of the pancreas and the cystic lesion, coupled with close proximity of the probe with the target lesion (imaging through the lumen of the stomach or duodenum), EUS allows a detailed imaging of the cyst morphology. Image-guided acquisition of tissue and fluid by fine-needle aspiration (FNA) is also possible during EUS (see later). EUS can often detect a communication between the main pancreatic duct and a cystic lesion.[4,10,35] Enthusiastic publications have suggested an accuracy of 40% to 90% in differentiating benign neoplasms from malignant neoplasms and from nonneoplastic cysts.[37] EUS criteria for malignant, mucinous neoplasms include size larger than 2 cm, main pancreatic duct dilation, presence of wall calcification, and perhaps more importantly, the presence of a frank mass or mural nodule.[22] Other investigators, however, remain more skeptical and emphasize that EUS is not sufficiently accurate in differentiating benign from malignant lesions reliably, reporting a wide range of diagnostic accuracy for EUS imaging (from 40% to 96%).[38,39] A recent, single-center, prospective study achieved a diagnostic accuracy of approximately 51% in differentiating mucinous from nonmucinous lesions.[38] Typically on EUS, SCNs are imaged as numerous small cysts with thin-walled septa and possibly calcification of the central septa. MCNs may be uni- or multilocular and may have macrocystic septations and/or an adjacent mass. Findings of IPMN on EUS include dilation of the main pancreatic duct (or branches) with or without mural ductal nodules.[39]

Problems with EUS include the relatively low availability in clinical practice (often limited to a small number of larger, tertiary centers) and the well-known fact that EUS is highly operator-dependent. Moreover, as with the other imaging methods, EUS is unreliable in distinguishing accurately between benign from malignant lesions, as suggested recently by the American Society for Gastrointestinal Endoscopy.[35,40]

OTHER IMAGING METHODS

Positron emission tomography–CT scan has been proposed as a new, useful imaging modality for the diagnosis of malignant lesions. Prospective case series have claimed sensitivities and specificities as great as 92% and 95%, respectively.[41] Its role in the evaluation of patients with pancreatic cystic lesions, however, has not been established precisely. *Intraductal pancreatoscopy* and *intraductal ultrasonography* have been used recently by some investigators with promising results in the diagnosis and differential diagnosis of pancreatic cystic neoplasms (Figures 95-9 and 95-10)[27]; however, experience with these newer diagnostic techniques remains limited to only a few centers with the interest and access to this technology.

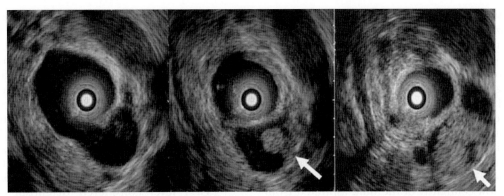

FIGURE 95-9 Intraductal ultrasonography showing branch-duct intraductal papillary mucinous neoplasm located in the pancreatic head with a mural nodule *(arrows)*. (Reprinted with permission from Tanaka M, Chari S, Volkan Adsay N, et al: Management of intraductal papillary mucinous neoplasms and mucinous cystic neoplasms of the pancreas. *Pancreatology* 6:20 [figure 6], 2006.)

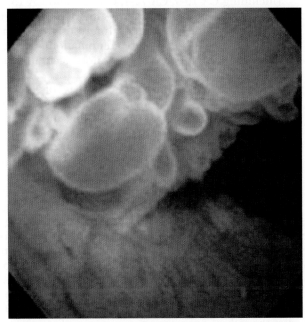

FIGURE 95-10 Intraductal pancreatoscopy in main-duct intraductal papillary mucinous neoplasm (fish-egg-like appearance). (Reprinted with permission from Tanaka M, Chari S, Volkan Adsay N, et al: Management of intraductal papillary mucinous neoplasms and mucinous cystic neoplasms of the pancreas. *Pancreatology* 6:22 [figure 7], 2006.)

FINE-NEEDLE ASPIRATION

Because imaging alone has limitations regarding definitive diagnosis, FNA and examination of the content of the cyst fluid has been studied extensively and has demonstrated some clinical usefulness. FNA is performed under image guidance, either endoscopically (EUS-guided) or percutaneously (CT-guided). EUS is preferred for guidance, because its imaging resolution is greater, and the endoscopic approach has fewer potential complications. Some reports are very enthusiastic about the value of the combination of EUS and FNA in predicting whether the cystic lesion requires resection, claiming sensitivities and specificities of 97% and 100%, respectively.[42] In contrast, other studies have reported

less convincing and more realistic results. EUS-guided FNA is well tolerated and safe in the hands of an experienced operator. Complications include bleeding (clinically serious bleeding, <1%; self-limiting intracystic hemorrhage, ~6%), pancreatitis (~1% to 2%), infection (<1%), and at least theoretically, the seeding of malignant cells along the tract of the needle.[10,37] Periprocedural antibiotics are used commonly to decrease the risk of cyst infection; most endoscopists tend to remove as much fluid as possible in an attempt to decrease the risk of bacterial inoculation of the fluid, despite the lack of evidence for this practice. Consideration should be given to the size of the lesion, because the volume of the aspirate may be very limited for small lesions and may be a problem for appropriate analysis and cytology. Small volume (<1 mL) aspirates may also be related to the high viscosity of the aspirated fluid (because of the presence of mucin) in MCNs and IPMNs.[22,37] EUS-guided FNA for cytology and/or other analysis of the cyst fluid remains limited to a few, large, tertiary centers with extensive experience in EUS and may be a limitation of this diagnostic approach (see earlier); moreover, analysis of the cystic fluid is often subject to local cytologic and laboratory expertise.

Endoscopic Ultrasound–Guided Fine-Needle Aspiration Cytology

When positive, the characteristic cytology of SCNs is that of cellular sheets of glycogen-containing, low-cuboidal cells, clear cytoplasm without vacuoles, and intracellular cytoplasmic inclusions.[34,35,37] Notably, the lack of appropriate cellular material is very common and limits the diagnostic accuracy in SCNs. In contrast, low-grade MCNs are characterized by honeycomb sheets and clusters of mucin-containing columnar cells with, rarely, small papillary sheets.[42,43] In addition, MCNs have abundant mucin in their background, which is not a feature of SCNs. Because of the heterogeneity of the epithelial lining of MCNs, there may be marked discrepancies between the cytologic typing and subsequent histologic diagnosis of these neoplasms, and thus cytologic findings should be used only to differentiate mucinous from serous neoplasms; again, lack of adequate cellular material should be considered as a nondiagnostic result and not as diagnostic of the lack of a mucinous neoplasm. IPMNs are characterized by the presence of papillary clusters lined by mucin-containing columnar cells, usually with some degree of atypia.[43] The degree of cytologic atypia has been shown to be predictive of malignancy.[10] Although low-grade MCNs may demonstrate a few papillary clusters, they are not usually as tall, abundant, and striking as the clusters observed in IPMNs. When pancreatic pseudocysts are aspirated, smears may show "dirty" material with macrophages and other inflammatory cells with proteinaceous precipitate and calcified debris.

As mentioned earlier, one major limitation of FNA cytology is the low cellularity of the fluid aspirated from the pancreatic cyst, resulting in a low sensitivity (~30%), especially for SCNs.[35] As a result, cytologic examination of the cyst fluid is often nondiagnostic, and FNA cytology has a diagnostic value only when it reveals obvious mucinous or malignant cells (specificity ~80%).[38] The ability to obtain image-guided mini-biopsies from the solid component of a cystic neoplasm or from the wall of the cyst increases the ability to make a differential diagnosis, but sampling error is a prominent limitation of this diagnostic method. "Contamination" of the aspirates from the normal (mucus-producing) gastrointestinal tract epithelium (during the passage of the needle) may be another problem in interpreting the results of FNA cytology.

Analysis of the Cystic Fluid

Biochemical analysis of the cystic fluid obtained by FNA may also be of diagnostic value. A typical analysis would include biochemical testing for mucin, CEA, and amylase levels.

1. **Mucin.** Fluid obtained from SCNs is characterized by the absence of mucin and, when adequate cellular material is present, positive immunostaining for the cytokeratins AE1 and AE3, or positive periodic acid–Schiff reaction.[4] In contrast, a positive mucin stain or a high viscosity (mucin) is highly specific for the mucinous (premalignant or overly malignant) neoplasms (MCN and IPMN) and can be used for their differential diagnosis from SCN and usually from pseudocysts as well.[8] Easily used and reliable assays for mucin are not, however, readily available; some groups no longer use mucin stains. Thick, viscid mucus may be appreciated grossly in the endoscopy suite, when smears are made.

2. **CEA.** Likewise, high intracystic levels of CEA differentiate a mucinous from a serous neoplasm with reasonable reliability. Currently, no standardized cutoff level for CEA exists, but many centers, particularly in the United States, use a CEA level of 192 ng/mL (as established by Brugge et al) as diagnostically sensitive (75%) and specific (84%) for differentiating mucinous from nonmucinous neoplasms (overall diagnostic accuracy, 79% for mucinous lesions).[22,38] The cutoff values, however, may vary from lab to lab depending on the assay used. As expected, by increasing the cutoff value of the CEA level considered diagnostic for mucinous lesions, the specificity of the test increases but at the expense of decreased sensitivity.[22] CEA levels of less than 5 ng/mL is quite sensitive for excluding a mucinous neoplasm.[4,34] Other tumor markers (including CA 19-9, CA 72-4, CA 125, and CA 15.3) may be present in greater levels in MCNs, but their diagnostic value is limited. Interestingly, in the study by Brugge et al, no combination of tests, including EUS appearance, was more accurate than CEA alone.[38]

3. **Amylase activity.** Amylase activity is of limited diagnostic value[37]; although a high amylase activity (>5 times serum activity) suggests that the cyst is a pancreatic pseudocyst, an important exception is IPMN, in which the neoplasm involves the epithelial cellular lining of the ductal system and is thus in contact with pancreatic juice (Table 95-1).

More recently, analysis of the fluid for telomerase activity, DNA quality, and a panel of mutations have suggested promising results in differentiation of benign versus malignant lesions.[44] Only a few drops of fluid are required, thus this molecular analysis can be applied to most cyst aspirates. K-*ras* mutations were found to be more prevalent in malignant lesions; however, these mutations are also found in normal and inflammatory pancreatic ducts.[45] The value of this expensive test to predict the risk of progression requires confirmation in prospective trials.

TREATMENT

Because of the substantial, clinically important differences regarding biologic behavior of PPCNs, treatment varies markedly with the type of cystic neoplasm of the pancreas. Each is discussed separately.

TABLE 95-1 Differential Diagnosis of Pancreatic Cystic Lesions Based on Analysis of Intracystic Fluid

Cystic Lesion	Amylase Activity	CEA Levels	Viscosity	Mucin Stain	Cytology
SCN	↓	↓	↓	−	Glycogen-rich cells
MCN	↓	↑↑↑	↑	+	Mucinous cells
IPMN	↑↑	↑↑	↑	+	Mucinous cells, papillary clusters
Pseudocyst	↑↑↑	↓	↓	−	Inflammatory cells

CEA, Carcinoembryonic antigen; *IPMN,* intraductal papillary mucinous neoplasm; *MCN,* mucinous cystic neoplasm; *SCN,* serous cystic neoplasm.

SEROUS CYSTIC NEOPLASM

The generally benign nature of SCNs, combined with the morbidity and potential mortality of major pancreatic resectional procedures, led historically to a philosophy weighted toward observation.[46] The marked decease in perioperative mortality after major pancreatectomy achieved during the last two decades may, however, account for the change of treatment policy toward a more aggressive approach. Some groups recommend operative resection for most (or even all) cystic neoplasms involving the body or tail of the pancreas, because the diagnosis is not always clear, and because the risk of resection is low. Conservative management, however, should be considered in the presence of a small, asymptomatic lesion in the pancreatic head (<4 cm), especially in the frail or elderly patient. Confirming these lesions as SCN (vs. MCNs) would allow a policy of observation (serial, noninvasive imaging annually or even every 2 or 3 years), given the very slow progression of these lesions over many years.[4,34] Currently, indications for operative therapy include (1) the presence of symptoms, (2) size larger than 4 cm (large SCNs probably will become symptomatic, even when diagnosed in asymptomatic patients; see earlier), and (3) uncertainty about the true nature of the cystic neoplasm (i.e., when differentiation from a MCN cannot be made confidently).[27,34] Anatomic pancreatectomy (i.e., pancreatoduodenectomy, preferentially with pylorus preservation or distal pancreatectomy with splenectomy, depending on the location of the neoplasm) is the procedure of choice, but other tissue-preserving procedures, such as segmental *central* pancreatectomy or spleen-preserving distal pancreatectomy, are acceptable alternatives. Enucleation has been reported, but in some studies, this approach was associated with a high morbidity (up to 35%), mainly because of the occurrence of postoperative pancreatic fistula.[46] Often, however, because of the large size of the neoplasm, enucleation is not a realistic possibility. In contrast, for a peripherally located neoplasm, enucleation would be an acceptable alternative. There is no role for lymphadenectomy or any type of *extended* resection in the management of SCNs.

There have been a few, very rare case reports of serous cystadenocarcinomas.[44,47] The true malignant nature of these extremely unusual cystadenocarcinomas was evident by the presence of distant metastases to liver. The appropriate treatment for these variant serous pancreatic cystic neoplasms is unknown, because the natural history is undefined.

MUCINOUS CYSTIC NEOPLASM

The unpredictable spectrum of multicentric metaplasia, dysplasia, carcinoma in situ, and tissue invasion implies that the majority, if not all of these neoplasms, can, in theory, evolve into invasive malignancy if left untreated.[17,48] Therefore, it is generally accepted that virtually all MCNs, whether in the proximal or in the distal pancreas, should be removed ideally, regardless of their size. For MCNs in the pancreatic head (a less common occurrence), a formal pancreatoduodenectomy (preferentially of the pylorus-preserving type) is usually indicated. Because,

however, MCNs are almost always located in the body and tail of the pancreas, standard distal pancreatectomy with splenectomy is the procedure of choice for most patients. For MCNs without any suggestion of malignancy, a spleen-preserving technique can be considered,[48] but if frozen-section analysis reveals evidence of invasion, a completion splenectomy with the splenic vessels and lymph nodes should be undertaken. A laparoscopic approach is the accepted approach for small or even medium-sized MCNs located in the tail of the pancreas,[49] but it is very important not to rupture the cyst during the procedure; spillage of its contents could potentially lead to tumor spread. Moreover, the cyst should be removed intact (i.e., not morcellized) so the pathologist can do an appropriate examination. Less extensive resections such as segmental central pancreatectomy could be considered, when there are no indications that the neoplasm has an invasive component[50]; yet, this decision is taken with a small calculated risk (<10%) of treating an invasive malignancy without appropriate margins of resection.[17] Lesser, nonanatomic resections, such as enucleation or duodenum-preserving subtotal resection of the pancreatic head—although theoretically feasible—are suboptimal procedures, given the limitations in preoperative and intraoperative diagnosis of invasive carcinoma. Excision of lymph nodes beyond those immediately adjacent to the pancreas is not necessary or beneficial, even when there is a high suspicion of malignancy, because the incidence of lymph node metastases is low in malignant MCNs.[23,48] Rarely, resection of involved adjacent structures or organs (including portal vein) may be required; however, unlike pancreatic adenocarcinomas, malignant MCNs tend to be "pushers" rather than "invaders."[17]

Frozen-section analysis is not usually required during operation for MCNs because cyst boundaries are easily discernible. Moreover, results of frozen-section analysis may be misleading, because a large part of the cyst wall may lack its epithelium (see earlier), and a diagnosis of benign cystadenoma may be inaccurate. Frozen sections should be obtained to exclude invasive malignancy if a dubious firmness is appreciated close to the resection margin. If invasive carcinoma is detected at the margin, it should be treated as any other invasive carcinoma of the pancreas.[27]

Of note, recently, some groups have undertaken a conservative approach in patients with small cystic lesions suspected of being MCNs or with low-risk MCNs for underlying malignancy, such as in asymptomatic MCN, smaller than 3 cm, without mural nodule(s), and without pancreatic or common bile duct dilation or peripancreatic adenopathy.[8,27] This approach (watchful waiting) represents a tradeoff between the morbidity and potential mortality of pancreatectomy when the lesion is still a benign neoplasm and the risk of enlargement and malignant degeneration in the future. The observational approach involves regular surveillance imaging to follow cyst size as well as to survey for development of mural nodules.[37] Long-term results of this approach are unknown currently. Similarly, the modality, frequency, and duration of surveillance imaging are undefined. If and when this strategy is adopted, both the patient and the surgeon should accept the risk, albeit low, of undertreating a potentially malignant and curable neoplasm. Therefore, it should be emphasized that current consensus favors resection in most patients with MCNs larger than 3 cm and, in some centers, regardless of their size.

INTRADUCTAL PAPILLARY MUCINOUS NEOPLASM

Because of the overt or latent malignant potential of IPMNs, operative resection is indicated in all but the poor-risk patient with main-duct IPMN. The aim of operative resection is to remove all adenomatous or malignant ductal epithelium and to minimize the probability of recurrence in the pancreatic remnant. The basic, and as yet not fully answered, question is whether or not IPMN represents a localized field defect limited to a segment of the pancreas or a more global abnormality with the potential to affect all the pancreatic ductal epithelium. If we knew IPMN was a localized process, as with typical ductal cancer of the pancreas, then a focused resection of the involved anatomic region of the gland would be all that is indicated. In contrast, if IPMN is a global disorder of all the pancreatic ductal epithelium, probably then all the pancreatic duct epithelium is at risk of malignant transformation, and therefore, in selected individuals, a total pancreatectomy should at least be entertained.[4] Total pancreatectomy with its obligate apancreatic state has its own potential problems (brittle diabetes, exocrine insufficiency) and may not be appropriate for many patients, especially the elderly or the medically unsophisticated patient.

The operative approach to IPMN is determined based on the type of ductal distribution (main or mixed-duct IPMN vs. branch-duct IPMN). In localized, branch-duct IPMN, a localized but formal anatomic, oncologic pancreatectomy is the favored procedure (i.e., pancreatoduodenectomy, preferentially of the pylorus-preserving type for neoplasms located in the pancreatic head and uncinate process or distal pancreatectomy for body and tail lesions).[32,34] Recently, a consensus policy toward a more conservative management of selected patients with branch-duct IPMN has been proposed.[10,27] This strategy could be considered for asymptomatic patients with branch-duct IPMN with a cyst size of less than 3 cm and without mural nodules.[10,21,27,51,52] This approach is based on the low incidence of malignancy (~2%) in these patients, which approximates the mortality risk from major surgical resection.[51] In multifocal branch-duct IPMN, which is observed in 20% to 30% of patients with branch-duct IPMN when really searched for with high-resolution, multislice CT or MRI,[21,32] total pancreatectomy would be the ideal procedure theoretically, but the formidable and obligate long-term morbidity of this operation should be considered seriously. A more conservative approach in this situation would be an anatomic pancreatic resection removing the most suspicious (or dominant) lesion(s) and surveillance observation of the remnant gland/lesions until these cystic lesions enlarge or develop findings suggestive of malignancy.[27]

Management of main-duct IPMNs is less controversial. Because of the high incidence of overt or latent malignancy, resection is warranted.[3,4,27] When main-duct IPMN is localized in the pancreatic body and tail (10% to 25%

of patients), distal pancreatectomy and splenectomy with frozen-section analysis of the proximal pancreatic margin is the procedure of choice.[32,34] If the frozen section is negative for true adenomatous changes (not reactive ductal hyperplasia) in the ductal epithelium, total pancreatectomy is not indicated in the absence of objective evidence that the proximal duct is involved. In contrast, when the margin is positive for invasive or noninvasive malignant IPMN, most surgeons would advocate a further pancreatic resection; if a tumor-free margin is not attainable after two further "creeping" resections, most surgeons would proceed with total pancreatectomy, provided the patient is an appropriate candidate and has been consented appropriately[4,32,34]; obviously this discussion would have occurred preoperatively between patient and surgeon. When the entire pancreatic duct is diffusely dilated, the assumption is that the disease is the pancreatic head causing obstruction by growth of the neoplasm or by mucus production. Based on this assumption and provided no intraluminal or extraluminal solid mass is evident elsewhere in the duct outside the boundaries of a pancreatic head resection, a pancreatoduodenectomy is undertaken with immediate frozen-section analysis of the distal margin. A positive margin for adenomatous changes necessitates a further "creeping" resection, keeping in mind that IPMNs may involve the pancreatic duct diffusely. If the frozen section remains positive after two attempts for further resection, total pancreatectomy should be entertained (in up to 10% to 20% of patients).[21,27,32,34] The concept of prophylactic total pancreatectomy is considered by most pancreatic surgeons as an unacceptable option.[21] In evaluating the results of frozen sections, it should be emphasized that the surgeon should keep in mind that even a negative margin does not ensure the absence of neoplastic cells in the remaining pancreas (multifocal disease with *skip* lesions indicating a generalized instability of the epithelium).[27] Intraoperative pancreatic ductoscopy to evaluate the pancreatic remnant has been tried with limited success. Certainly, one should make every effort to evaluate both the pancreatic duct and the parenchyma of any pancreatic tissue being left in-site when performing a resection for an IPMN.

OTHER CONSIDERATIONS

All symptomatic PPCNs, regardless of etiology, should be treated surgically. In contrast, management of incidentally discovered PPCNs is more complicated. Recent improvements in clinical diagnosis and in the understanding of clinicopathologic factors that predict the presence or absence of malignancy now provide an opportunity for selective use of resection targeted at those patients most likely to benefit from pancreatic resection and to avoid the morbidity and potential mortality of resection in selected patients with PPCNs that may never require resection.[24] The goal of this approach is to identify preoperatively those patients with premalignant or malignant disease.[24]

The general medical performance status of the patient is an important factor that should be taken into consideration when deciding to resect a pancreatic cystic lesion.

Indeed, the risk of resection should be weighed against and not exceed the risk of malignancy. High-risk patients, such as those with severe comorbidities or advanced age, may best be followed with periodic, noninvasive imaging; aggressive evaluation (including EUS with FNA cytology and analysis of cyst fluid) might not be worthwhile in these patients. This conservative approach appears to be safe, especially when the cystic lesion is small (<2 cm) and lacks any worrisome findings on imaging suggestive of malignancy.[8,23,52,53] Direct injection of ablative agents (such as alcohol, paclitaxel [Taxol], etc.) has been proposed recently for the management of these high-risk patients who are poor candidates for operation. Early trials have been published showing a low complication rate with EUS-guided ethanol ablation of SCNs, MCNs, and IPMNs[54]; however, the followup is too short to make conclusions on its efficacy, and endoscopic treatment should therefore still be considered experimental. Success of these new treatments awaits outcome data.

Diagnostic evaluation should proceed on a practical, cost-effective basis. If resection is otherwise indicated (based on the results of cross-sectional imaging or because the patient is symptomatic), then expensive and invasive diagnostic procedures (such as EUS combined with FNA cytology and analysis of the aspirated fluid) are not indicated. In a substantial number of patients, however, modern diagnostic methods will fail to differentiate reliably the premalignant and malignant cystic lesions from benign ones, and therefore, when a definitive preoperative diagnosis cannot be established, resection should be favored based on the results of diagnostic workup.[24]

As expected, the greatest risk of resection is when the PPCN is located in the pancreatic head. Because most MCNs are located in the body and tail of the pancreas, the decision to proceed to operative resection (distal pancreatectomy or even segmental central pancreatectomy) is easier compared to lesions of the head of the gland, which would require pancreatoduodenectomy. In this case, if a SCN is diagnosed with confidence, a conservative observational approach should be followed, especially in high-risk patients. From a technical point of view, pylorus preservation should probably be favored over classic pancreatoduodenectomy in patients with cystic neoplasms. Pancreatoduodenectomy in the setting of a PPCN, in contrast to pancreatic ductal adenocarcinoma, can be complicated frequently by the presence of a soft pancreatic parenchyma and nondilated pancreatic and biliary ducts. Segmental central pancreatectomy preserves islet cell mass, and the risk for development of insulin-dependent diabetes can be minimized.

ADJUVANT AND NEOADJUVANT THERAPY

Historically, the experience with adjuvant treatment of pancreatic ductal adenocarcinoma has been extrapolated to the treatment of invasive PPCNs. If tissue invasion is present, some form of adjuvant therapy probably should be considered, despite a "curative" resection, even if there are no nodal metastases.[4,17,34] Because of the absence of any randomized clinical trials, the type of treatment used is similar to that of ductal adenocarcinoma, that is, gemcitabine-based chemotherapy with radiation. In a recent study from the Johns Hopkins Hospital, 70 patients with malignant (invasive) IPMN received postoperative (adjuvant) chemoradiotherapy, which appeared to confer a 57% decrease in the relative risk of mortality; patients with lymph node metastases or positive margins appeared to benefit particularly from chemoradiation therapy after a curative resection.[55] Other studies, however, have not shown such a dramatic benefit.[47,56]

Concerning neoadjuvant therapy, although there is anecdotal evidence that apparently unresectable neoplasm with no metastases can become resectable after combined chemoradiation therapy, the experience is limited, thereby precluding definite recommendations.

PROGNOSIS AND FOLLOWUP

Complete operative resection of SCNs and MCNs lacking an invasive component (i.e., benign MCNs and, more important, noninvasive proliferative MCNs) ensures cure. These neoplasms are generally solitary, not multicentric, and do not recur either locally or distally after complete operative resection.[4,17] Therefore, a regular followup program with surveillance (using mainly imaging tests) is probably not necessary, thereby saving money and eliminating patient worry.[17,27] More controversial is the long-term survival of patients undergoing complete resection for MCN with tissue invasion. In the past, numerous articles claimed 5-year survival rates greater than 50% and up to 70% for "mucinous cystadenocarcinomas"[4,48]; however, now in retrospect, we know that these series lumped together MCN containing a proliferative epithelium (but without tissue invasion) with the true cystadenocarcinomas and probably a substantial portion of branch-duct IPMNs. In contrast, after a careful evaluation of MCN containing true invasive carcinoma, 5-year survival rates appear to be much less (15% to 35%) but still better than those for typical ductal cancer of the pancreas.[17] Patients with resected malignant MCNs should be followed closely, possibly with imaging every 6 months for the first 2 years regarding local recurrence and distant metastases (mainly hematogenous) using either CT or MRI.[27] The prognosis for nonresectable, malignant MCN appears to be as poor as that for nonresectable pancreatic adenocarcinoma.[4,17]

In IPMNs, the dysplastic component may remain in situ for many years. For single, branch-duct IPMNs, several studies suggest strongly that a local anatomic resection is essentially curative. In contrast, for noninvasive, main-duct IPMNs, occurrence in the remnant gland has been found with variable rates (0% to 10%), provided that the frozen-section margin was negative for adenomatous changes and the resected specimen lacked invasive IPMN.[4,17,27] Under these conditions, recurrence in the remnant may be caused by the presence of multifocal disease.[21] The 5-year survival after resection of IPMN without invasive cancer is greater than 70% in most series.[21] Some reports have even suggested a 5-year survival in excess of 90% after resection. In distinct contrast, when the resection specimen contains invasive disease, even if the margins are negative, recurrent IPMN either in the pancreatic remnant or more commonly in extra-pancreatic sites occurs in 50% to 90% of patients, thereby decreasing the 5-year survival to 30% to 50%.[10,31,47] Features predicting a decreased survival when invasive cancer is present include lymph node metastases, vascular invasion, and positive resection margins.[21,47] Invasive IPMN should be managed as an aggressive malignancy that behaves, in many respects, similar to ductal cancer of the pancreas. Overall survival appears to be better with invasive IPMN compared to pancreatic ductal cancer, but whether this ostensible survival advantage is because of a phase shift with earlier diagnosis of IPMN (as shown in some studies[47]) or because of a truly less aggressive tumor biology remains controversial. Routine followup surveillance with noninvasive imaging is indicated in all patients with IPMN, because if recurrence occurs, these patients may benefit from further resection or other treatments.[27] There are no established guidelines regarding the frequency or type of surveillance imaging to detect potential recurrence. A reasonable strategy would be to get yearly followup with CT or MRI, and then increase the interval between imaging if no changes have occurred over several years. Because patients with invasive IPMNs have a significantly greater risk of recurrence, this population probably should be evaluated every 6 months.[27] Serum levels of CEA and CA 19-9 have no definitive value in the followup of these patients. The discovery of a pancreatic cyst or mass lesion after operative resection may be related to the presence of a postoperative pseudocyst or contained leak, a recurrence of IPMN linked to incomplete resection, a new site of IPMN, or rarely a cystadenocarcinoma after inadequate, histopathologic examination.[4]

As has become well known (see earlier), IPMN is associated with a high incidence (~25% to 30%) of synchronous or metachronous extrapancreatic neoplasms in other organs (including colon, rectum, stomach, lung, breast, liver, etc.), but also of pancreatic cancer of the ordinary ductal type.[27] Whether this association is because of increased use of imaging studies in this population or represents a true genetic instability is unknown. Nevertheless, this important information should be taken into consideration when scheduling both the initial evaluation and followup plan of patients with IPMN; screening colonoscopy may be warranted in these patients because of the increased frequency of colonic neoplasms.[53]

REFERENCES

1. Compagno J, Oertel JE: Mucinous cystic neoplasms of the pancreas with overt and latent malignancy (cystadenocarcinomas and cystadenomas): A clinicopathologic study of 41 cases. *Am J Clin Pathol* 69:573, 1978.
2. Compagno J, Oertel JE: Microcystic adenomas of the pancreas (glycogen-rich cystadenomas): A clinicopathologic study of 34 cases. *Am J Clin Pathol* 69:289, 1978.
3. Ohashi K, Murakami Y, Takekoshi T, et al: Four cases of mucin producing cancer of the pancreas on specific findings of the papilla of Vater. *Prog Dig Endosc* 20:348, 1982.
4. Sarr MG, Murr M, Smyrk TC, et al: Primary cystic neoplasms of the pancreas: Neoplastic disorders of emerging importance—current state-of-the-art and unanswered questions. *J Gastrointest Surg* 7:417, 2003.
5. Kimura W, Nagai H, Kuroda A, et al: Analysis of small cystic lesions of the pancreas. *Int J Pancreatol* 18:197, 1995.
6. Kosmahl M, Pauser U, Peters K, et al: Cystic neoplasms of the pancreas and tumor-like lesions with cystic features: A review of 418 cases and a classification proposal. *Virchows Arch* 445:168, 2004.
7. Zhang XM, Mitchell DG, Dohke M, et al: Pancreatic cysts: Depiction on single-shot fast spin-echo MR images. *Radiology* 223:547, 2002.
8. Ceppa EP, De la Fuente S, Reddy SK, et al: Defining criteria for selective operative management of pancreatic cystic lesions: Does size really matter? *J Gastrointest Surg* 14:236, 2010.
9. Tseng JF, Warshaw AL, Sahani DV, et al: Serous cystadenoma of the pancreas: Tumor growth rates and recommendations for treatment. *Ann Surg* 242:413, 2005.
10. Fasanella KE, McGrath K: Cystic lesions and intraductal neoplasms of the pancreas. *Best Pract Res Clin Gastroenterol* 23:35, 2009.
11. Fernandez-del Castillo C, Warshaw AL: Cystic neoplasms of the pancreas. *Pancreatology* 1:641, 2001.
12. Belsley NA, Pitman MB, Lauwers GY, et al: Serous cystadenoma of the pancreas. *Cancer (Cancer Cytopathol)* 114:102, 2008.
13. Chatelain D, Hammel P, O'Toole D, et al: Macrocystic form of serous pancreatic cystadenoma. *Am J Gastroenterol* 97:2566, 2002.
14. Strobel O, Z'Graggen K, Schmitz-Winnenthal FH, et al: Risk of malignancy in serous cystic neoplasms of the pancreas. *Digestion* 68:24, 2003.
15. Galanis C, Zamani A, Cameron JL, et al: Resected serous cystic neoplasms of the pancreas: A review of 158 patients with recommendations for treatment. *J Gastrointest Surg* 11:820, 2007.
16. Bassi C, Salvia R, Molinari E, et al: Management of 100 consecutive cases of pancreatic serous cystadenoma: Wait for symptoms and see at imaging or vice versa? *World J Surg* 27:319, 2003.
17. Sarr MG, Carpenter HA, Prabhakar LP, et al: Clinical and pathologic correlation of 84 mucinous cystic neoplasms of the pancreas: Can one reliably differentiate benign from malignant (or premalignant) neoplasms? *Ann Surg* 231:205, 2000.
18. Warshaw AL, Compton CC, Lewandrowski K, et al: Cystic tumors of the pancreas: New clinical, radiologic, and pathologic observations in 67 patients. *Ann Surg* 212:432, 1990.
19. Goh BK, Yu-Meng Tan J, Chung YFA, et al: A review of mucinous cystic neoplasms of the pancreas defined by ovarian-type stroma: Clinicopathological features of 344 patients. *World J Surg* 30:2236, 2006.
20. Basturk O, Coban I, Adsay VN: Pancreatic cysts. Pathologic classification, differential diagnosis, and clinical implications. *Arch Pathol Lab Med* 133:423, 2009.
21. Garcea G, Ong SL, Rajesh A, et al: Cystic lesions of the pancreas. *Pancreatology* 8:236, 2008.
22. Hutchins GF, Draganov PV: Cystic neoplasms of the pancreas: A diagnostic challenge. *World J Gastroenterol* 15:48, 2009.
23. Crippa S, Salvia R, Warshaw AL, et al: Mucinous cystic neoplasm of the pancreas is not an aggressive entity: Lessons from 163 resected patients. *Ann Surg* 247:571, 2008.
24. Katz MHG, Mortenson MM, Wang H, et al: Diagnosis and management of cystic neoplasms of the pancreas: An evidence based approach. *J Am Coll Surg* 207:106, 2008.
25. Volkan Adsay N, Merati K, Basturk O, et al: Pathologically and biologically distinct types of epithelium in intraductal papillary mucinous neoplasms. *Am J Surg Pathol* 28:839, 2004.
26. Hruban RH, Takaori K, Klimstra DS, et al: An illustrated consensus on the classification of pancreatic intraepithelial neoplasia and intraductal papillary mucinous neoplasms. *Am J Surg Pathol* 28:977, 2004.
27. Tanaka M, Chari S, Volkan Adsay N, et al: International consensus guidelines for management of intraductal papillary mucinous neoplasms and mucinous cystic neoplasms of the pancreas. *Pancreatology* 6:17, 2006.
28. Longnecker DS, Adler G, Hruban RH, et al: Intraductal papillary-mucinous neoplasms of the pancreas. In Hamilton SR, Aaltonen LA, editors: *World Health Organization classification of tumors. Pathology and genetics of tumors of the digestive system.* Lyon, 2000, IARC Press, p 237.
29. Wada K, Takada T, Yasuda H, et al: Does 'clonal progression' relate to the development of IPMT of the pancreas? *J Gastrointest Surg* 8:289, 2004.
30. Jeurnink SM, Vleggaar FP, Siersema PD: Overview of the clinical problem: Facts and current issues of mucinous cystic neoplasms of the pancreas. *Dig Liver Dis* 40:837, 2008.

31. Adsay NV, Conlon KC, Zee SY, et al: Intraductal papillary mucinous neoplasms of the pancreas: An analysis of in situ and invasive carcinomas in 28 patients. *Cancer* 94:62, 2002.

32. Farnell MB: Surgical management of intraductal papillary mucinous neoplasm (IPMN) of the pancreas. *J Gastrointest Surg* 12:414, 2008.

33. Reid-Lombardo KM, Mathis KL, Wood CM, et al: Frequency of extrapancreatic neoplasms in intraductal papillary mucinous neoplasm of the pancreas: Implications for management. *Ann Surg* 251:64, 2010.

34. Sarr MG, Kendrick ML, Nagorney DM, et al: Cystic neoplasms of the pancreas. *Surg Clin North Am* 81:497, 2001.

35. Ng DZW, Goh BKP, Tham EHW, et al: Cystic neoplasms of the pancreas: Current diagnostic modalities and management. *Ann Acad Med Singapore* 38:251, 2009.

36. Arakawa A, Yamashita Y, Namimoto T, et al: Intraductal papillary tumors of the pancreas: Histopathologic correlation of MR cholangiopancreatography findings. *Acta Radiol* 41:343, 2000.

37. Scheiman JM: Management of cystic lesions of the pancreas. *J Gastrointest Surg* 12:405, 2008.

38. Brugge WR, Lewandrowski K, Lee-Lewandrowski E, et al: Diagnosis of pancreatic cystic neoplasms: A report of the cooperative pancreatic cyst study. *Gastroenterology* 126:1330, 2004.

39. Papanikolaou IS, Adler A, Neumann U, et al: Endoscopic ultrasound in pancreatic disease—its influence on surgical decision-making. *Pancreatology* 9:55, 2009.

40. American Society of Gastrointestinal Endoscopy Guidelines: The role of endoscopy in the diagnosis and management of cystic lesions and inflammatory fluid collection of the pancreas. *Gastrointest Endosc* 61:363, 2005.

41. Sperti C, Bissoli S, Pasquali C, et al: 18-Fluorodeoxyglucose positron emission tomography enhances computed tomography diagnosis of malignant intraductal papillary mucinous neoplasms of the pancreas. *Ann Surg* 246:932, 2007.

42. Frossard JL, Amouyal P, Amouyal G, et al: Performance of endoscopically guided fine needle aspiration and biopsy in the diagnosis of pancreatic cystic lesions. *Am J Gastroenterol* 98:1516, 2003.

43. Recine M, Kaw M, Evans DB: Fine-needle aspiration cytology of mucinous tumors of the pancreas. *Cancer* 102:92, 2004.

44. Khalid A, McGrath KM, Zahid M, et al: The role of pancreatic cyst fluid molecular analysis in predicting cyst pathology. *Clin Gastroenterol Hepatol* 3:967, 2005.

45. Schoedel KE, Finkelstein SD, Ohori NP: K-ras and microsatellite marker analysis of fine-needle aspirates from intraductal papillary mucinous neoplasms of the pancreas. *Diagn Cytopathol* 34:605, 2006.

46. Pyke CM, van Heerden JA, Colby TV, et al: The spectrum of serous cystadenoma of the pancreas. *Ann Surg* 215:132, 1992.

47. Schnelldorfer T, Sarr MG, Nagorney DM, et al: Experience with 208 resections for intraductal papillary mucinous neoplasm of the pancreas. *Arch Surg* 143:639, 2008.

48. Fernandez-del Castillo C: Mucinous cystic neoplasms. *J Gastrointest Surg* 12:411, 2008.

49. Melotti G, Butturini G, Piccoli M, et al: Laparoscopic distal pancreatectomy: Results on a consecutive series of 58 patients. *Ann Surg* 246:77, 2007.

50. Crippa S, Bassi C, Warshaw AL, et al: Middle pancreatectomy: Indications, short- and long-term operative outcomes. *Ann Surg* 246:69, 2007.

51. Woo SM, Ryu JK, Lee SH, et al: Branch duct IPMNs in a retrospective series of 190 patients. *Br J Surg* 96:405, 2009.

52. Rodriguez JR, Salvia R, Crippa S, et al: Branch-duct IPMNs: Observations in 145 patients who underwent resection. *Gastroenterology* 133:72, 2007.

53. Handrich SJ, Hough DM, Fletcher JG, et al: The natural history of the incidentally discovered small simple pancreatic cyst: Long-term follow-up and clinical implications. *AJR Am J Roentgenol* 184:20, 2005.

54. DeWitt J, McGreevy K, Schmidt CM, et al: EUS-guided ethanol versus saline solution lavage for pancreatic cysts: A randomized, double-blind study. *Gastrointest Endosc* 70:710, 2009.

55. Swartz MJ, Hsu CC, Pawlik TM, et al: Adjuvant chemoradiotherapy after pancreatic resection for invasive carcinoma associated with intraductal papillary mucinous neoplasm of the pancreas. *Int J Radiat Oncol Biol Phys* 76:839, 2010.

56. Turrini O, Waters JA, Schnelldorfer T, et al: Invasive intraductal papillary mucinous neoplasm: Predictors of survival and role of adjuvant therapy. *HPB (Oxford)* 12:447, 2010.

Pancreatic Trauma

Amy P. Rushing | Edward E. Cornwell, III | Elliott R. Haut

Among all types of intraabdominal trauma, pancreatic injuries remain some of the most challenging. Even in the hands of experienced trauma surgeons, pancreatic injuries carry a high rate of morbidity and mortality primarily because of the concomitant vascular and visceral trauma. Pancreatic injuries account for 5% of significant blunt abdominal trauma, and only a slightly higher percentage of abdominal gunshot and stab wounds.[1] More than 70% of pancreatic injuries occur as a result of penetrating trauma, with a mortality rate approaching 25%. The majority of deaths result from early massive hemorrhage. Systemic inflammatory response syndrome (SIRS), sepsis, and multisystem organ failure (MSOF) account for the majority of delayed deaths. As for the patients with major pancreatic injury who survive the initial insult, nearly half will have a complication of their pancreatic wound such as abscess, fistula, pseudocyst, false aneurysm, or anastomotic leak.[2]

Patients with penetrating trauma to the pancreas experience injuries with equal frequency along the head, body, and tail of the organ.[2,3] In victims of blunt trauma, the deceleration and direct compression of the pancreas against the spine most frequently results in significant injury to the neck of the pancreas. This is commonly seen in collisions involving seatbelts, steering wheels, or handlebars.[4] Not only is the surgical treatment of pancreatic injury complicated by the gland's complex anatomic relationship to multiple vital structures, its overall management is challenging given its often delayed clinical presentation and lack of specific diagnostic modalities. Thus, it is essential that the trauma surgeon maintains a high index of suspicion for pancreatic injury and, once the injury is identified, timely treatment is carried out. The use of computed tomographic (CT) scans and endoscopic retrograde cholangiopancreatography (ERCP) has fostered the nonoperative management of pancreatic trauma, yet there remains a role for definitive operative therapy in the setting of hemorrhage and main pancreatic duct disruption. This chapter will outline the clinical presentation of pancreatic injuries, address critical points regarding technical surgical approaches, and review the common complications related to these difficult injuries.

DIAGNOSIS

Patients who exhibit signs of intraabdominal hemorrhage or peritonitis should undergo prompt evaluation for pancreatic injury via emergency surgical exploration. For patients who are hemodynamically stable, a thorough diagnostic evaluation is warranted. There are several challenges that accompany timely diagnosis of pancreatic injuries. First, the patient's clinical presentation is not specific for pancreatic injury alone as there are no specific physical examination findings or laboratory tests that can confirm or exclude pancreatic injury. Second, modern imaging modalities have yet to achieve the same level of sensitivity and specificity for pancreatic injury when compared to injuries of the liver and spleen. Third, the natural history of pancreatic injuries has demonstrated a more gradual progression of signs and symptoms because of the secondary inflammatory process that occurs with pancreatic parenchymal damage.

Physical examination and evaluation of hemodynamic status remain the key factors in the diagnostic algorithm of abdominal trauma. A hypotensive patient with abdominal trauma should proceed to the operating room without delay. For the clinically stable patient, selective management can be successful as long as careful attention is given to clinical progress or deterioration. Pancreatic injuries are no exception. The initial evaluation following the primary survey should include a focused abdominal physical examination as well as focused abdominal sonography for trauma (FAST) to assess for free fluid in the peritoneal cavity. Additionally, a full laboratory panel should be collected including serum amylase and lipase levels. For decades, surgeons have evaluated the value of serum amylase in the diagnosis of pancreatic injuries. In 1985, Jones reported on the 35-year experience of managing pancreatic injuries at Parkland Memorial Hospital. His work demonstrated that among the 270 patients who had preoperative serum amylase levels, only 16% of patients with penetrating pancreatic injuries and 61% of patients with blunt injuries had elevated amylase levels. It was also noted that among patients with complete transection of the pancreas, a mere 65% had elevated serum amylase levels.[5] In contrast, Takishima et al reported that serum amylase levels were elevated in all patients with pancreatic injuries when the level was drawn at least 3 hours after the injury occurred.[6] Amylase levels have not consistently been shown to predict pancreatic injury; however, they may serve as a useful adjunct in the serial monitoring of a patient with a known pancreatic injury who is being managed nonoperatively.[1]

Following the initial physical examination, the hemodynamically stable patient should undergo a CT scan of the abdomen and pelvis (with intravenous contrast) to elucidate the presence of any visceral injuries. A pancreatic injury can be challenging to assess given some injuries may not be obvious without significant inflammatory changes. Such findings may not be apparent in the initial

24 hours postinjury.[7] In 2009, the American Association for the Surgery of Trauma (AAST) published a multicenter study examining the use of CT scan in the evaluation of pancreatic injuries. They enrolled 206 patients with confirmed pancreatic injuries on operative exploration and determined the following radiographic characteristics were "hard signs" of a pancreatic injury:

Active bleeding
Pancreatic hematoma or laceration
Diffuse enlargement or edema of pancreas
Low pancreatic attenuation

Additionally, the study suggested that lacerations greater than 50% of the gland thickness on CT scan should raise concern for a pancreatic ductal injury.[8]

Although CT scan has become integral to the diagnostic algorithm of abdominal trauma, it is far from the criterion standard in detecting pancreatic injuries. According to a single-institution study reported by Ilahi et al in 2002, spiral CT imaging was only 68% sensitive in detecting pancreatic injuries.[9] In 2009, Velmahos et al reported an overall sensitivity of 76% in a multicenter study that included 230 patients diagnosed with blunt pancreaticoduodenal injuries. This study combined old- and new-generation scanners and found that the newer 16-slice or 64-slice CT scanners offered 83% sensitivity compared to the older 4-slice CT scanner, which detected a pancreatic injury with only a sensitivity of 67%.[10] The AAST multicenter study reported lower sensitivities of 60% and 47% for the 16-slice and 64-slice multidetector CT scanners, respectively. However, the AAST study reported that the scanners were highly specific for pancreatic ductal injuries with specificities of 95% and 90%, respectively. Interestingly, the 16-slice scanner yielded better results than the 64-slice modality, which perhaps further demonstrates that CT scan alone is not a reliable workup for this injury.[8] The current literature suggests maintaining a high index of suspicion for pancreatic injury and, if there is persistent concern, serial CT scan imaging may be warranted.[10]

Other options that should be considered when a CT scan suggests pancreatic injury are magnetic resonance cholangiopancreatography (MRCP) and/or ERCP. MRCP has not been evaluated specifically in large numbers of trauma patients, but its use has been extrapolated from other uses in nontraumatic issues related to the pancreas and biliary tree. Its potential benefits include its noninvasive nature and the fact it can be performed even after anatomy-altering surgery has made ERCP impossible (i.e., pyloric exclusion). However, it does have potential downsides, including the need to send a patient to a remote location and the fact that it is only diagnostic without any therapeutic option. Alternatively, ERCP has proven itself useful in both the diagnosis and therapeutic intervention for pancreatic ductal injuries. ERCP will clearly delineate the anatomy of the pancreatic duct and identify an injury by demonstrating a complete cutoff or extravasation of contrast (Figure 96-1). In 2010, Rogers examined 26 patients with pancreatic injuries who underwent ERCP. Eighteen patients had significant ductal injuries ranging from partial transection of secondary ducts to high-grade stenosis and complete disruption of the main pancreatic

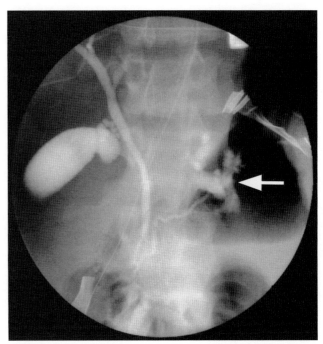

FIGURE 96-1 Endoscopic retrograde cholangiopancreatography performed after original damage control surgery for gunshot wound to the abdomen and before reexploration.

duct. Overall, 11 patients were able to receive endoscopic treatment that either eliminated or relegated further surgical intervention.[7]

INTRAOPERATIVE EVALUATION

In most cases, pancreatic injuries are diagnosed at the time of exploration. Evaluation of pancreatic trauma requires several surgical maneuvers to ensure proper exposure. A Kocher maneuver involves incising the lateral peritoneal attachments to the second and third portions of the duodenum in order to mobilize the duodenum and head of the pancreas to the patient's left side. This proceeds along the avascular plane to the superior mesenteric vein. Occasionally, a replaced right hepatic artery is encountered as a branch of the superior mesenteric artery and care must be taken to avoid its injury during the dissection. The maneuver facilitates inspection of the posterior aspect of the pancreatic head as well as the duodenum and provides a view of the suprarenal inferior vena cava.

The anterior aspect of the entire pancreas is evaluated by entering the lesser sac through the gastrocolic omentum. With a wide incision through the omentum and retraction of the stomach superiorly and the transverse colon inferiorly, thorough evaluation of a parenchymal or ductal injury is possible (Figure 96-2). Occasionally, a patient may present with severe injury to the posterior aspect of the pancreas with the anterior capsule intact. This is seen most commonly in patients with blunt mechanisms of injury. Any hematoma or contusion should raise suspicion for an injury involving the posterior aspect of the gland, and prompt exploration via an incision in the peritoneum and areolar tissue

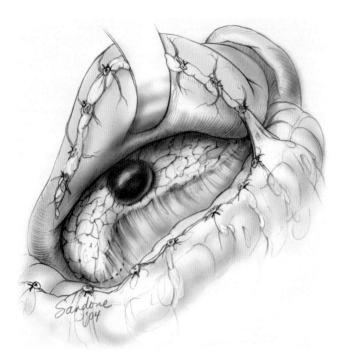

FIGURE 96-2 Any hematoma overlying the pancreas must be "unroofed."

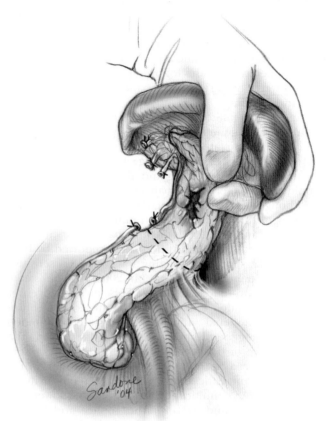

FIGURE 96-4 The Aird maneuver is employed to mobilize the spleen and tail of the pancreas.

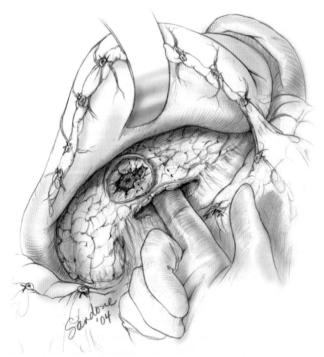

FIGURE 96-3 With the peritoneum along the inferior border of the pancreas divided, the surgeon's finger is slipped behind the pancreas to evaluate for palpable parenchymal defects.

along the inferior aspect of the pancreas needs to be performed. Most injuries will reside in the prevertebral region of the pancreas. After division of the peritoneum along the inferior border of the pancreas, the surgeon's finger is slipped behind the gland to evaluate for palpable parenchymal defects (Figure 96-3).

Full evaluation of the pancreatic tail is facilitated by the Aird maneuver.[11] Originally described in 1955 for adrenalectomy, this technique involves division of the avascular splenic ligaments—splenorenal, spleno-colic, and splenophrenic—followed by mobilization of the spleen and tail of the pancreas from the patient's left to right (Figure 96-4). Ultimately, one should be able to visualize the anterior and posterior aspects of the distal body and tail of the pancreas. In addition, this provides good exposure to zone I and zone II of the retroperitoneum.

OPERATIVE INTERVENTION

The indications for and extent of the initial operative intervention of pancreatic injuries are determined by several factors: the anatomy of the pancreatic injury, associated injuries, and the patient's overall hemodynamic status.[12] Treatment can range from simple drainage to total pancreatectomy or pancreaticoduodenectomy (Whipple procedure). The key steps in management decisions include recognizing not only the appropriate intervention but the correct timing as the patient's overall status may preclude definitive operative therapy at the initial operation.

The AAST devised a pancreatic organ injury scale grading injuries from one through five (Table 96-1).

TABLE 96-1 AAST Organ Injury Scale

Grade I	Type of Injury
Hematoma	Minor contusion without duct injury
Laceration	Superficial laceration without duct injury
Grade II	
Hematoma	Major contusion without duct injury or tissue loss
Laceration	Major laceration without duct injury or tissue loss
Grade III	
Hematoma	Distal transection or parenchymal injury with duct injury
Grade IV	
Laceration	Proximal transection or parenchymal injury involving ampulla
Grade V	
Laceration	Massive disruption of pancreatic head

AAST, American Association for the Surgery of Trauma.

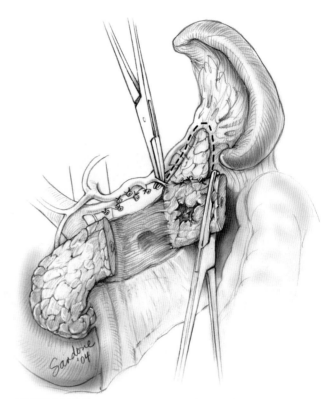

FIGURE 96-5 Distal pancreatectomy with splenic preservation.

The scale classifies pancreatic injuries in order to standardize operative findings and help guide therapeutic interventions. Grade I and II injuries are usually managed with debridement and drainage alone. Integrity of the main pancreatic duct differentiates low-grade versus high-grade injury and determines subsequent operative management. Suspicion of ductal involvement is raised by the anatomic location of the injury and the amount of local pancreatic tissue disruption. At times, pancreatic secretions can be identified at the open ends of a duct. Major ductal injury prompts definitive therapy. However, the therapy may be provided as a staged procedure if the patient's physiology is unfavorable as in the case of patients with the lethal triad (acidosis, coagulopathy, and hypothermia) who are managed with damage control techniques.

Once a main pancreatic duct injury is identified, the location of the injury will determine the appropriate treatment. Ductal injuries are classified as proximal or distal based on their relationship to the superior mesenteric vessels. Those to the right of the vessels are recognized as proximal injuries (AAST grade IV or V), whereas those to the left are distal injuries (AAST grade III). Distal pancreatic injuries are more amenable to definitive operative intervention, as a distal pancreatectomy is less morbid and has fewer complications than surgery for more proximal injuries. In the case of ongoing intraabdominal hemorrhage, distal pancreatectomy should be accompanied by a splenectomy to ensure prompt hemostasis with minimal dissection. In this situation, the spleen and pancreatic tail are easily mobilized, leaving only the division of the pancreas, the short gastric arteries, splenic artery, and splenic vein. The pancreas is transected using one of several techniques, including stapling, suture ligation, or electrocautery. The transected pancreatic duct should be identified and closed using a figure-of-8 suture or U-stitch. Additionally, an omental patch or fibrin glue may be utilized to further control drainage

from the duct and prevent fistula formation. Following dissection and specimen removal, the surgical field should be widely drained in anticipation of a potential postoperative pancreatic leak. There is ongoing controversy regarding use of spleen-preserving distal pancreatectomy in trauma. This operation takes significantly longer and may be associated with higher early complications and therefore should only be performed in highly selected cases (Figure 96-5).

An extended distal pancreatectomy can be performed if the laceration resides to the right of the superior mesenteric vessels and may be an option that potentially avoids a Whipple procedure. Another alternative is a central pancreatectomy, which can be considered in the setting of a proximal ductal transection with otherwise normal distal pancreatic parenchyma. The procedure involves resecting the central portion of the gland and debriding back to viable tissue in order to properly close the end of the proximal duct. The distal pancreatic remnant is then drained by creating a Roux-en-Y pancreaticojejunostomy. Again, wide drainage should be performed to control a postoperative fistula.

In the case of a grade IV or V pancreatic injury, one must consider not only the associated duodenal injury but the patient's overall hemodynamic status at the time of initial laparotomy. These injuries may require extensive interventions that may best be performed as staged procedures as described by Seamon et al in their series of patients who underwent damage control laparotomy with concomitant pancreatic injuries. Of the 42 patients, three underwent pancreaticoduodenectomy for grade IV injuries. One patient underwent resection with delayed reconstruction following appropriate resuscitation while

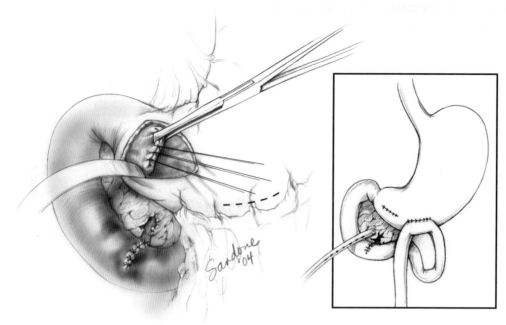

FIGURE 96-6 Pyloric exclusion.

the remaining two patients underwent definitive resection and reconstruction at subsequent operations. All patients survived. This serves as an example of how a staged procedure and the principles of damage control surgery may be the safest alternative in a physiologically labile patient who requires an extensive operation for a complex injury.[12]

When the patient is deemed suitable for a prolonged procedure, there are several techniques that can be applied depending on the associated duodenal injury. Thirty years ago, the classic duodenal diverticulization was used to protect the healing duodenal repair and consisted of a vagotomy, antrectomy, and Billroth II gastrojejunostomy.[13] This has since been replaced by the pyloric exclusion technique that entails closing the pylorus to divert gastric contents from entering the duodenum. The pylorus can be sewn closed from the inside of the stomach through an anterior gastrotomy or stapled across externally with a TA stapler. This is followed by closure of the gastrotomy and creation of a gastrojejunostomy through a separate gastric incision (Figure 96-6). Finally, the surgical field should be widely drained both with external drains and intraluminal decompression (i.e., nasogastric tube). Gastroduodenal continuity is restored from either approach by at most 4 to 6 weeks when the pylorus reopens.[14] This procedure should be performed in conjunction with wide drainage for the patient with a pancreatic head injury.

In the setting of complete disruption of the pancreatic head and duodenum (AAST grade V), a Whipple procedure may be the only course of action to restore continuity between the pancreatic duct, biliary tree, and intestinal tract. A staged Whipple may be the safest option for the patient after hemorrhage and enteric contamination are controlled, as peripancreatic packing and drainage are safe and effective temporary measures until the patient's

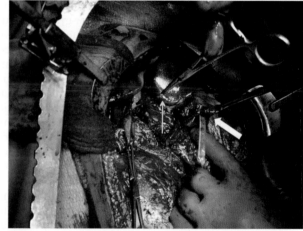

FIGURE 96-7 Intraoperative photo following pancreaticoduodenectomy for blunt trauma. The *yellow arrow* denotes the common bile duct and the *white arrow* denotes the proximal duodenum as the pylorus is spared. (Courtesy Gregory D. Rushing, MD.)

physiology is restored.[12] Often, the nature of the initial injury has provided a large amount of dissection for the surgeon and one may only have to find the avascular plane between the neck of the pancreas and the superior mesenteric vein to finish mobilization of the gland. This is often performed at the index laparotomy in addition to debridement of necrotic tissue and ligation of the common bile duct (Figure 96-7). Ligation of the common bile duct will result in its dilation, which will facilitate a technically easier choledochojejunostomy during the delayed reconstruction.[15] The specific surgical approach depends on the patient's overall physiology and one must

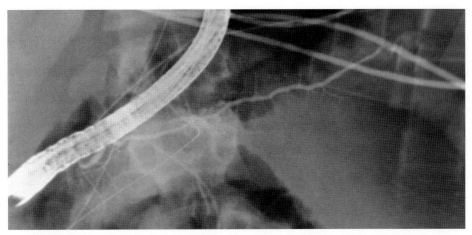

FIGURE 96-8 Same patient as in Figure 96-1 following placement of a pancreatic stent.

be willing to plan on a series of operations to perform a safe and technically adequate procedure.

POSTOPERATIVE CONSIDERATIONS

Following operative intervention for pancreatic trauma, there are several factors to consider, as the complication rate approaches 50% in some series.[16] Pancreatic fistulas, pseudocysts, posttraumatic pancreatitis, and intraabdominal abscesses represent the most common complications. Up to one-third of patients with major pancreatic injuries will develop pancreatic fistulas. Most will resolve spontaneously with adequate drainage. There is some evidence that somatostatin may reduce fistula output and promote healing; however, the medication's high cost must be considered.[17,18] Rarely, a pancreatic fistula may persist after weeks of nonoperative management leading to pseudocyst formation and necessitating internal drainage via a Roux-en-Y jejunal limb or possibly internal drainage to the stomach via advanced endoscopic techniques. ERCP with pancreatic duct stenting may also be used to divert pancreatic secretions from a fistula tract (Figure 96-8). Postoperative pancreatic abscess may frequently develop and is most often managed with CT-guided percutaneous drainage as the first-line approach, with open debridement and wide drainage as the backup technique. When looking at risk factors for postoperative complications, recent literature has shown that injury location, injury grade, and associated vascular injuries are predictors of morbidity. Recinos et al demonstrated that pseudocyst formation was associated with wide drainage alone versus pancreatic resection.[16] Regardless of the surgical approach, close postoperative observation is warranted to ensure that prompt action is taken when a complication arises.

CONCLUSION

Pancreatic injuries continue to be some of the most complex injuries a trauma surgeon will encounter. They are associated with a high incidence of vascular and other major visceral injuries. Therefore, treating other injuries and stabilizing the patient may be necessary before definitive operative management of the pancreatic injury can occur. Prompt diagnosis, appropriate resuscitation, and careful surgical technique are paramount in the proper treatment of pancreatic trauma. In spite of evolving technology, no noninvasive test definitively diagnoses pancreatic injury with absolute sensitivity and specificity. Therefore, a high index of suspicion should remain when a patient presents with a significant trauma mechanism and/or abdominal pain. During operative intervention, the integrity of the pancreatic duct will determine the role of simple drainage versus major pancreatic resection, which may have to occur in stages given the patient's hemodynamic status. Finally, complications are likely to occur, so close observation and early interventions are key to ensure that patients with pancreatic trauma can recover given proper and meticulous care.

REFERENCES

1. Subramanian A, Dente CJ, Feliciano DV: The management of pancreatic trauma in the modern era. *Surg Clin N Am* 87:1515, 2007.
2. Ivatury R, Nallathambi M, Ran P, et al: Penetrating pancreatic injuries: Analysis of 103 consecutive cases. *Am J Surg* 56:90, 1990.
3. Young PR Jr, Meredith JW, Baker CC, et al: Pancreatic injuries resulting from penetrating trauma: A multi-institution review. *Am J Surg* 64:838, 1998.
4. Ahmed N, Vernick JJ: Pancreatic injury. *South Med J* 102:1253, 2009.
5. Jones RC: Management of pancreatic trauma. *Am J Surg* 150:698, 1985.
6. Takishima T, Sugimoto K, Hirata M, et al: Serum amylase on admission in the diagnosis of blunt injury to the pancreas: Its significance and limitations. *Ann Surg* 226:70, 1997.
7. Rogers SJ, Cello JP, Schecter WP: Endoscopic retrograde cholangiopancreatography in patients with pancreatic trauma. *J Trauma* 68:538, 2010.
8. Phelan HA, Velmahos GC, Jurkovich GJ, et al: An evaluation of multidetector computed tomography in detecting pancreatic injury: Results of a multicenter AAST study. *J Trauma* 66:641, 2009.
9. Ilahi O, Bochicchio GV, Scalea TM: Efficacy of computed tomography in the diagnosis of pancreatic injury in adult blunt trauma patients. A single-institutional study. *Am Surg* 68:704, 2002.
10. Velmahos GC, Tabbara M, Gross R, et al: Blunt pancreatoduodenal injury: A multicenter study of the research consortium of New England Centers for Trauma (ReCONECT). *Arch Surg* 144:413, 2009.

11. Aird I, Helman P: Bilateral anterior transabdominal adrenalectomy. *Br Med J* 2:708, 1955.

12. Seamon MJ, Kim PK, Stawicki SP, et al: Pancreatic injury in damage control laparotomies: Is pancreatic resection safe during the initial laparotomy? *Injury* 40:61, 2009.

13. Levison MA, Petersen SR, Sheldon GF, et al: Duodenal trauma: Experience of a trauma center. *J Trauma* 24:475, 1984.

14. Vaugham G, Grazier O, Graham D, et al: The use of pyloric exclusion in the management of severe duodenal injuries. *Am J Surg* 134:785, 1977.

15. Gross RI, Jacobs LM, Luk S: *Advanced trauma operative management.* Woodbury, Conn, 2004, Cine-Med.

16. Recinos G, Dubose JJ, Teixeira P, et al: Local complications following pancreatic trauma. *Injury* 40:516, 2009.

17. Amirata E, Livingston DH, Elcavage J: Octreotide acetate decreases pancreatic complications after pancreatic trauma. *Am J Surg* 168:345, 1994.

18. Nwariaku FE, Terracina A, Mileski WJ, et al: Is octreotide beneficial following pancreatic injury? *Am J Surg* 170:582, 1995.

Pancreatic Problems in Infants and Children

David A. Rodeberg | Charles N. Paidas

There is much about the pediatric pancreas that can be informative to the adult surgical specialist. Problems that are commonly seen in infants and children, such as annular pancreas, may remain occult until adulthood. Pediatric management strategies, such as the nonoperative management of pancreatic trauma, have been found to be effective in this patient population, and the adult clinician must make an informed decision whether to extend these approaches to adult patients.

This chapter discusses surgical pancreatic conditions commonly seen in infancy, childhood, and adolescence. We review annular pancreas and its relation to duodenal atresia; hyperinsulinism (HI) of infancy; pancreas divisum; and the pediatric surgical strategies for chronic pancreatitis, tumors, and trauma. The safety and efficacy of endoscopic retrograde cholangiopancreatography (ERCP) in children are also discussed.

ANNULAR PANCREAS

In the fetus, the caudal portion of the developing foregut develops into the proximal duodenum as well as the dorsal and ventral pancreatic buds. At 5 weeks of gestation, rightward rotation begins to bring the ventral pancreatic bud to the right of the duodenum, where it comes to join the dorsal pancreatic bud to give rise to the head of the pancreas (Figure 97-1). The lumen of the duodenum becomes transiently obliterated with proliferation of the lining cells during the same period of development. By the eighth week of gestation, rotation of the pancreas is complete and recanalization of the duodenum has occurred.[1] Thus, it is easy to understand that any perturbation influencing the rotation of pancreatic tissue may also impact recanalization of the duodenum. Therefore, annular pancreas is occasionally associated with various degrees of intrinsic duodenal stenosis and atresia. However, in most cases, annular pancreas is associated with external compression of the duodenum resulting in partial or complete obstruction.

Annular pancreas generally presents in the newborn period, with 75% of cases presenting in the first week of life, but it has been reported in an 11-year-old and may be encountered incidentally in adults.[2,3] It has been suggested that a large percentage of patients with annular pancreas remain asymptomatic; however, it is impossible to know because the denominator is unknown.[4] Prenatal ultrasound may detect polyhydramnios or may diagnose duodenal obstruction directly in 30% of patients (Figure 97-2).[3] At birth, infants have a scaphoid abdomen. Radiographs showing the "double bubble" sign, classically attributed to duodenal atresia, may be seen in more than 88% of patients (Figure 97-3).[3,5] Emesis may be bilious (up to 50%) or more commonly nonbilious (>90%) depending on whether the obstruction is above or below the ampulla of Vater.[2,3,6]

Associated congenital anomalies occur in approximately 70% of patients (32% chromosomal and 38% other malformations) and should be looked for prior to, and during, operation for annular pancreas.[7] These may include nonsurgical anomalies such as Down syndrome and operative conditions including esophageal atresia, malrotation, Meckel diverticulum, and imperforate anus. In addition, 4% of patients with annular pancreas may have a second duodenal obstruction related to stenosis or web usually noticed intraoperatively as a dilated duodenum distal to the annular pancreas.[8] Congenital cardiac defects must be assessed with preoperative echocardiogram.

At operation, a transverse right upper quadrant skin incision is used. In the newborn, the proximal, obstructed, duodenal bulb may be markedly dilated, with the rim of annular pancreas visible just caudal to it. Repair is by duodenoduodenostomy, done in diamond-shaped fashion by making a transverse incision in the proximal duodenum and a perpendicular longitudinal incision in the distal duodenum (Figure 97-4). The two ends may then be "fish mouthed" or "diamond shaped" together using a single layer of interrupted, absorbable, monofilament suture. If duodenoduodenostomy is precluded by excess tension or a poorly developed distal duodenum, then duodenojejunostomy should be performed.

Nasogastric or orogastric decompression is used postoperatively. Enteral feeding may be initiated approximately 1 week after operation. Thus, annular pancreas, which Merrill and Raffensperger in 1976 deemed an "eminently curable lesion," is cured without ever touching the pancreas itself.

Occasionally after correction for annular pancreas a patient may experience recurrent abdominal pain that may be related to biliary anomalies such as pancreatic divisum or pancreaticobiliary maljunction.[9] These anomalies can be detected by ERCP or MRCP and may require surgical intervention for recurrent or chronic pancreatitis.

HYPERINSULINISM

HI is characterized by dysregulated insulin secretion that results in persistent mild to severe hypoglycemia. The various forms of HI represent a group of clinically, genetically, and morphologically heterogeneous disorders.[10,11] HI occurs at a frequency of 1 in 30,000 to 50,000 live births.[6] There has been significant ambiguity surrounding the pathophysiology of congenital HI. Early recognition of congenital HI is critical because, if untreated,

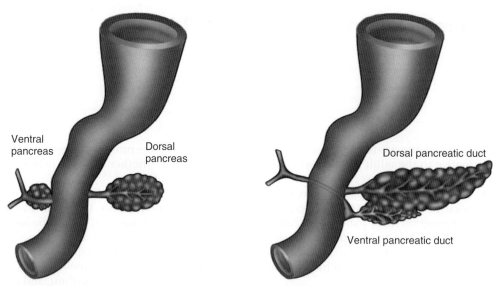

FIGURE 97-1 Embryology of the pancreas at 5 weeks' gestational age. The caudal portion of the foregut gives rise to a ventral and dorsal pancreatic bud. Rotation of the ventral bud to the right allows fusion with the dorsal component. The ventral portion gives rise to the head of the pancreas and the body and tail are formed from the dorsal bud. (From Goldin S: The pancreas. In Lawrence PF, Bell RM, Dayton MT, editors: *Essentials of general surgery*, ed 5. Philadelphia, 2011, Lippincott Williams & Wilkins.)

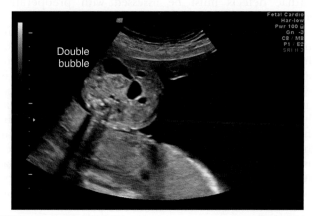

FIGURE 97-2 Antenatal ultrasound showing a double bubble and polyhydramnios indicative of duodenal obstruction or atresia. The double bubble consists of dilated stomach and proximal duodenal obstruction. Polyhydramnios is the result of an inability for the fetus to pass meconium beyond the duodenal obstruction. (Courtesy Victoria Belogolvkin MD, Assistant Professor, Division of Maternal Fetal Medicine, Department of Obstetrics and Gynecology, University of South Florida College of Medicine, Tampa, Fla.)

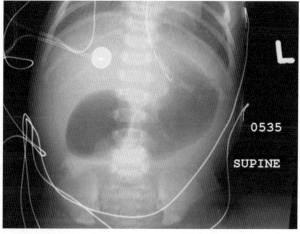

FIGURE 97-3 Postpartum plain abdominal film showing the classic double bubble.

profound hypoglycemia may lead to brain damage. The clinical manifestations of congenital HI include babies that are jittery, floppy, or lethargic; seizures are common, and near-death events may occur.[12,13] Diagnosis requires the presence of inappropriately elevated insulin in the setting of hypoglycemia, along with the need for continuous glucose infusion (>15 mg/kg/min) to maintain normoglycemia. The presence of low ketone bodies and an increase in blood glucose after glucagon administration may additionally be used as diagnostic criteria.[12]

Mutations in six genes have been associated with HI: the sulfonylurea receptor 1 (SUR-1; encoded by *ABCC8*)[14]; potassium inward rectifying channel (Kir6.2; encoded by *KCNJ11*)[15]; glucokinase (GK; encoded by *GCK*)[16]; glutamate dehydrogenase (GDH; encoded by *GLUD-1*)[17]; short-chain 3-hydroxyacyl-CoA dehydrogenase (SCHAD; encoded by *HADH*)[18]; and ectopic expression on β-cell plasma membrane of *SLC16A1* (encodes monocarboxylate transporter 1 [MCT1]).[19] Genetic testing is available through commercial laboratories for four of the six genes known to be associated with HI (*ABCC8, KCNJ11, GCK, GLUD-1*).

SUR-1 and Kir6.2 combine to form the β-cell plasma membrane K_{ATP} channel. Inactivating mutations in the K_{ATP} channel result in membrane depolarization and calcium influx into the β cell, resulting in constitutive insulin secretion. This is the most common and severe form of HI. There are two distinct histologic forms of K_{ATP}-HI, diffuse HI and focal HI.

Glutamate dehydrogenase HI is the second most common form of HI. It is also known as the hyperinsulinism and hyperammonemia (HI/HA) syndrome. GDH-HI presents with recurrent episodes of hypoglycemia that

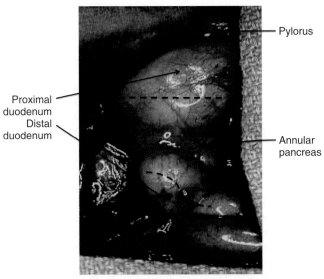

FIGURE 97-4 Reconstruction of annular pancreas. The absence of ventral and dorsal bud fusion results in an obstructing ring or annulus around the duodenum. Shown in the operative photo is pylorus, annular pancreas, and proximal and distal duodenum. The *dotted lines* represent duodenal incisions for fish-mouth or diamond-shaped duodenoduodenal anastomosis. (Adapted from Eckholdt-Wolke F, Hesse A, Krishnaswami S: Duodenal atresia and stenosis. In *Pediatric surgery: A comprehensive text for Africa*, chap 62, www.global-help.org/publications/books/help_pedsurgeryafrica62.pdf.)

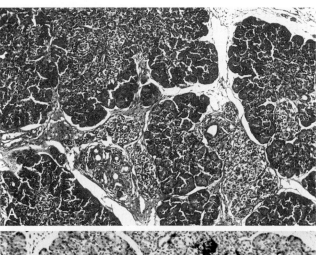

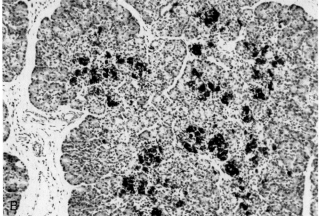

FIGURE 97-5 Diffuse hyperinsulinism from a 95% pancreatectomy specimen of a 1-month-old infant. **A,** In the diffuse form of HI, islet cell tissue is increased both at the center of the pancreatic acinus and in connective tissue between the lobules. **B,** Pancreas stained by immunocytochemistry using antiinsulin antibody. Numerous small packets of islets scattered throughout the parenchyma and multiple larger islets consistent with the diffuse form of HI. (From Gilbert-Barness E, editor: *Potter's pathology of the fetus, infant and child*, ed 2. New York, 2007, Elsevier, chap 25.)

are less severe than in K_{ATP}-HI, and can be precipitated by a protein-rich meal.[20] These patients do not typically present with hypoglycemia at birth, but are frequently diagnosed after several months of age. The hypoglycemia in patients with GDH-HI is easily controlled with diazoxide.

HI can also occur in the setting of perinatal stress resulting in prolonged neonatal hypoglycemia. Unlike the transient HI seen in the infants of diabetic mothers, perinatal stress–induced HI can persist for several days to a year.[21] The mechanism is unknown. These infants usually respond well to diazoxide. Mimickers of HI include neonatal panhypopituitarism, drug-induced hypoglycemia, insulinoma, antiinsulin and insulin-receptor stimulating antibodies, Beckwith-Wiedemann syndrome, and congenital disorders of glycosylation.

The ability to distinguish focal and diffuse HI is of paramount importance, in that focal HI is curable by partial pancreatectomy. Interventional radiology studies, such as transhepatic portal venous insulin sampling[22] and selective pancreatic arterial calcium stimulationm[23] have been used to localize focal lesions. More recently, positron emission tomography (PET) scans with ^{18}F-dihydroxyphenylalanine (DOPA) have been shown to accurately discriminate focal HI from diffuse HI.[24-26] PET-CT may offer even better localization.[27] Supplemental imaging modalities such as computed tomography (CT), ultrasound, and intraoperative ultrasound have not yet been validated in the literature for this problem in infancy; however, PET-MRI appears promising.[28] In diffuse HI, β cells throughout the pancreas are functionally abnormal and have characteristic enlarged nuclei in about 2% to 5% of cells (Figure 97-5). Focal HI lesions

are usually less than 1 cm in diameter and are characterized by the presence of a confluent proliferation of islet-cell clusters (focal adenomatosis).[12]

The goal of treatment in infants with HI is to prevent brain damage from hypoglycemia by maintaining plasma glucose levels above 700 mg/L (70 mg/dL). First-line pharmacologic therapy in patients with HI is diazoxide, a K_{ATP} channel agonist. Because a functional K_{ATP} channel is required for diazoxide to exert an effect, patients with recessive focal or diffuse K_{ATP}-HI do not respond to therapy with diazoxide. Patients with GDH-HI, SCHAD-HI, and perinatal stress–induced HI typically respond well to diazoxide. Second-line medical therapy for infants unresponsive to diazoxide is octreotide.

The decision to operate is based on a laboratory evaluation consistent with HI, medical responsiveness, genetic testing, and imaging. Operation is necessary in more than two-thirds of cases.[28] The decision to operate should hinge on the demonstration of focality or, in the case of diffuse disease, on the failure of medical management. Treatment of the focal form of congenital HI is by partial pancreatectomy. Cretolle et al have reported cure in 44 of 45 patients undergoing partial pancreatectomy following localization, and most, although not all, were found to appropriately correlate with preoperative venous localization. The authors approached lesions of the midportion of the pancreas by means of middle pancreatectomy with preservation of the head, along with Roux-en-Y jejunal loop to the transected portion of the pancreatic tail. Forty-four patients in the series had normal postoperative glucose and glucose tolerance tests as well as hemoglobin A_{1c}, and all patients were without exocrine dysfunction, with a reported mean followup of 3.7 years.[19] Curative laparoscopic enucleation of focal lesions has been reported by others.[29]

Infants with diffuse disease will normally require a near-total pancreatectomy (95% to 98%) to control the HI and might require additional therapy with diazoxide, octreotide, and/or frequent feedings to maintain euglycemia. In the diffuse form of congenital HI, there is diffuse hyperfunction of pancreatic β cells with enlargement of their nuclei, but neither the β-cell proliferation rate nor the overall β-cell mass is increased.[14,15] Diagnosis may also be made by pancreatic venous sampling or by the observation on frozen section of diffuse enlargement of nuclei seen in all specimens. In this case, near-total pancreatectomy is required. Classic anatomic benchmarks, such as removing all pancreatic tissue up to the superior mesenteric vein, should be taken with caution in light of a pediatric autopsy study by Reyes et al, who demonstrated that distal pancreatectomy taken past the mesenteric vessels, up to the left border of the pancreaticoduodenal vessels in the head of the pancreas, only accounted for removal of an average of 71.3% of the pancreas by weight, with a highly variable range of 43.5% to 95.8%.[30] The approach of Fékété et al is to perform near-total pancreatectomy, leaving only a "small lump of pancreatic tissue in the concavity of the duodenal genu superius, with choledochal dissection."[28] Long-term complications reported following near-total pancreatectomy have included growth disturbance, glucose intolerance or overt diabetes, and variceal bleeding due to splenic vein thrombosis, the latter presenting as late as 18 years postoperatively.[31-33] Reports of long-term pancreatic exocrine deficiency are hard to find. Regeneration of the pancreas following near-total pancreatectomy in infancy has been documented.[12,13] Patients with HI requiring surgical therapy have a higher incidence of neurodevelopmental problems compared to patients responsive to medical therapy.[34] The risk of developing diabetes has been attributed to pancreatectomy[35]; however, it has also been observed in patients who did not have surgery. In a series of 114 patients with HI, the incidence of diabetes was as high as 27% after pancreatectomy, and 71% in patients requiring multiple surgical resections.[36]

PANCREAS DIVISUM

Pancreas divisum is a congenital anomaly, but it may or may not manifest itself at any time during life. During fetal development, as the pancreas forms from the rotation and fusion of the ventral pancreatic anlage and the dorsal pancreatic anlage, the ventral duct of Wirsung and the dorsal duct of Santorini ordinarily join. Failure of fusion of the two ducts results in a spectrum of anomalies known as pancreas divisum (Figure 97-6). In the most common variant, the duct of Wirsung drains the uncinate process and variable amounts of the head of the pancreas through the major papilla, while the smaller duct of Santorini drains the majority of the pancreas through a more cephalad accessory papilla. Stenosis of one or both ducts may contribute to the development of pancreatitis.

Pancreas divisum is associated with 25% of patients with recurrent pancreatitis.[37] In contrast, a group of patients with primary biliary disease who had ERCP manifested a 3.6% incidence of pancreas divisum. Necropsy series show a 5% to 10% incidence in the general population. A more recent pediatric study corroborates that of 52 children with relapsing or chronic pancreatitis, 10 of whom had variants of pancreas divisum.[20] The etiology of chronic or recurrent pancreatitis is multifactorial; however, an association with pancreas divisum has not been disproved, and it may have a contributory role in some individuals.

A concept for the surgical treatment of recurrent pancreatitis in the setting of pancreas divisum with ductal stenosis has been advocated.[20,38,39] This includes transduodenal sphincteroplasty of the minor papilla draining the stenotic accessory duct of Santorini, as well as sphincteroplasty of the major papilla. The sphincteroplasties are done by insinuating a probe into the papilla and sharply dividing anterior to the probe, in gradual fashion. During the course of this sharp division, which serves to splay open the sphincter, interrupted 6-0 or 7-0 synthetic, monofilament, absorbable sutures are sequentially placed from ductal mucosa to surrounding duodenal mucosa. No stent is left. The duodenotomy, opened longitudinally, is closed transversely. Secretin (1 U/kg) given during the operation may assist in the localization of the papilla.

However, this treatment does not ensure resolution of the patient's symptoms. In one study of six patients, all patients had preoperative evidence of pancreas divisum with ductal obstruction by ERCP.[20] Of the six, just one had a long-term excellent result. Another required ERCP and stenting 3 years later. Two of the six patients continued to have attacks of abdominal pain. Two others went on to have Puestow procedures, with achievement of long-term improvement. Clearly, for some patients with recurrent or chronic pancreatitis and pancreas divisum, sphincteroplasty alone may not address the whole problem, and pancreaticoenteric anastomosis may be required.

PANCREATICOENTERIC PROCEDURES FOR CHRONIC PANCREATITIS

The most frequent symptoms of pancreatitis in children are pain followed by emesis and ileus.[40] Approximately a third of pancreatitis episodes represent recurrent pancreatitis. In stark contrast with cases of pancreatitis in adults, where the most frequent causes are alcohol and gallstones, in children the etiology is much more diverse

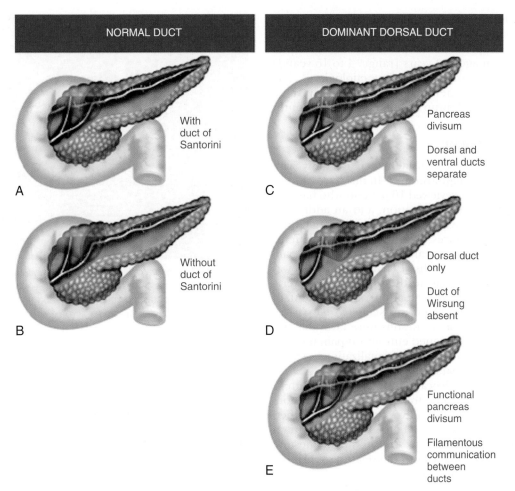

NORMAL DUCT	DOMINANT DORSAL DUCT

A — With duct of Santorini

B — Without duct of Santorini

C — Pancreas divisum / Dorsal and ventral ducts separate

D — Dorsal duct only / Duct of Wirsung absent

E — Functional pancreas divisum / Filamentous communication between ducts

FIGURE 97-6 The spectrum of pancreas divisum. The most common variant is shown in **C.** In this case the duct of Wirsung drains the uncinate process and head of the pancreas into the major papilla. Through a more cephalad accessory papilla, the duct of Santorini drains the majority of the head of the pancreas. (From Goldin S: The pancreas. In Lawrence PF, Bell RM, Dayton MT, editors: *Essentials of general surgery*, ed 5. Philadelphia, 2011, Lippincott Williams & Wilkins.)

and includes biliary stones, familial, drug ingestion, hypercalcemia, trauma, hypertriglyceridemia, and pancreatic anomalies such as divisum.[40,41]

Medical management of chronic pancreatitis revolves around the use of total parenteral nutrition (TPN), somatostatin, pain management, pancreatic enzyme replacement, and endoscopic sphincterotomy and stenting. When these fail, surgical therapy is indicated. There are three pancreaticoenteric procedures described for the surgical management of chronic pancreatitis in children: (1) the Frey procedure, (2) the modified Puestow procedure, and (3) the Duval procedure.

THE FREY PROCEDURE

The Frey procedure is designed to drain the head as well as the body and tail of the pancreas. The Frey procedure involves opening the main pancreatic duct throughout its length in the neck, body, and tail of the gland, after which the head is "cored out" in continuity with the opened duct.[42] A longitudinal anastomosis is then constructed between the gland and a Roux-en-Y limb of intestine. This retrospective study by Rollins and Meyers in 2004 included nine patients who underwent the Frey procedure. Improvements in symptoms and in quality of

life were found in seven of the nine. Notably, the average patient age was 12.8 years at the time of operation. One patient was successfully operated on in the setting of a previous, failed Puestow procedure. There were multiple causes of pancreatitis in this cohort, and only one of those undergoing the Frey procedure had hereditary pancreatitis.

THE MODIFIED PUESTOW PROCEDURE

The modified Puestow procedure may also be successfully employed in children. DuBay et al described its applicability in 12 cases of hereditary pancreatitis.[43] The patients were a mean of 9.3 years old (range, 2 to 16 years) and all had dilated ducts, with symptoms including either intractable pain or failure to thrive with recurrent pancreatitis. They used a two-layer, side-to-side anastomosis between the opened pancreatic duct and a retrocolic, Roux-en-Y jejunal limb. These authors found significantly decreased rates of hospitalizations after 1 and 3 years and a significant gain in percentage of ideal body weight after 3 years. All but 1 of the 12 patients rated their own outcome as good or excellent. One patient developed pancreatic stones postoperatively and underwent ERCP with sphincterotomy and extraction.

Crombleholme et al also reported favorable results using the Puestow (with splenectomy) or the modified Puestow (without splenectomy) procedure in a group of 10 children (mean age, 9.4 years [range, 4 to 16 years]) with chronic pancreatitis of varying etiologies.[44] The authors found improvement or resolution of pain in all patients with a mean followup of 4 years (range, 7 months to 19.75 years).

THE DUVAL PROCEDURE

The Duval procedure is a distal pancreatectomy with Roux-en-Y pancreaticojejunostomy.[45] In this retrospective study Weber and Keller reviewed 16 patients who had this procedure as the primary operation, and an additional 2 patients who were converted to Duvals following failure of prior Puestow procedures. Mean age for the 18 patients was 8 years (range, 3 to 13 years). Half had familial pancreatitis. The extent of distal pancreatectomy was described as going generally to the superior mesenteric vessels, but intraoperative evaluation of the extent of pancreatitis in the distal gland was stated to be part of the decision-making process. Results were favorable. Of the 18 patients, 13 were weaned entirely off pain medications and required no further hospitalizations, with a mean followup of 7.5 years.

Among these series, advocates of the Duval procedure point out that two failed Puestows were successfully converted to Duvals. In contrast, advocates of the modified Puestow included a patient who failed to improve after a Duval and so was converted to the modified Puestow. Thus, no claim can be made as to the relative superiority of one approach over the other.

TUMORS

Pancreatic tumors are very rare in children and have better outcomes as compared to adult pancreatic tumors. As a general principle, pancreatic tumors in children are well demarcated rather than infiltrative. Several pancreatic tumors are unique to pediatric patients. Patients are usually asymptomatic; however, presenting signs and symptoms in pediatric patients may include a mass, pain, weight loss, or hypoglycemia, but jaundice is a much less common presentation than is experienced with adults. Surgery figures prominently in the treatment of each of these conditions.

Pediatric pancreatic tumors include pancreatoblastoma, solid-pseudopapillary tumors, and primitive neuroectodermal tumors (PNETs). Lymphoid malignancies and metastatic disease may also affect the pancreas. Other pancreatic masses and cysts such as neuroendocrine tumors, serous cystadenomas, and hydatid cysts can occur in children, and their management parallels that of the same conditions in adults.[46-48]

PANCREATOBLASTOMA

Pancreatoblastoma usually presents in the first decade of life. Originally termed *infantile pancreatic carcinoma*, these tumors comprise both epithelial and stromal components. Pathologists look for characteristic squamoid corpuscles, which are nests of squamous-appearing spindle cells that may have keratinization (Figure 97-7). Tumors

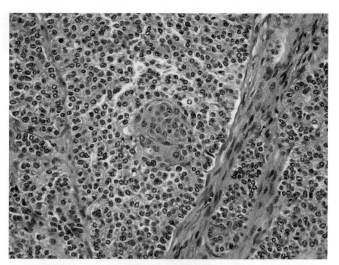

FIGURE 97-7 Pancreatoblastoma. This adenocarcinoma of infancy consists of corpuscles of centrally localized squamous cells, an intermediate dark-staining zone of cells, and finally a peripheral rim of duct like tubular structures. (From Gilbert-Barness E, editor: *Potter's pathology of the fetus, infant and child,* ed 2. New York, 2007, Elsevier, chap 25.)

are distributed similarly between males and females. There is no predilection for the head versus the tail of the pancreas; however, it has been noted in one study that four of six patients with tumors in the head of the pancreas died, whereas five of five with tumors in the body or tail survived.[49]

Wide local excision carries an important role in pancreatoblastoma, so the pediatric surgeon must be prepared for whatever resection is required, whether distal pancreatectomy or pancreaticoduodenectomy, even if in an infant.[50] Involvement of adjacent organs, regional nodes, and vessels is common; many patients present with metastases. Neoadjuvant and adjuvant therapy have been used with variable success. Initial diagnosis may be made by fine-needle aspiration.[36] Recurrences are common and therefore long term followup is critical.[51]

PRIMITIVE NEUROECTODERMAL TUMOR

PNETs are members of the Ewing sarcoma family of tumors. Primary pancreatic PNETs, of which only 13 cases have been reported in the literature,[52-57] are aggressive tumors that typically affect patients in the second or third decades of life. The overwhelming preponderance has occurred in the head of the pancreas, which may explain why patients with pancreatic PNET, unlike those with the other pediatric histologies described here, frequently present with jaundice.

Histologically, PNETs are small round cell tumors. They share the characteristic t(19;37)(q24;q12) chromosomal translocation of Ewing sarcoma, and this results in the *EWS-FLI1* fusion gene. Histologic diagnosis may not be straightforward, and thus obtaining enough tissue to perform molecular diagnostic studies may be critical.

All reported patients have undergone either biopsy or resection. Infiltration into surrounding organs and lymph nodes has been described. Given the similarities with Ewing sarcoma and PNETs at other locations, chemotherapy is indicated; the only survivors reported in the

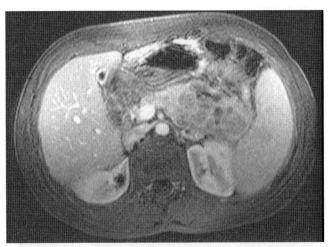

FIGURE 97-8 MRI showing neuroblastoma metastatic to the tail of the pancreas in a 16-year-old girl, appearing as a heterogeneous, multilobulated mass.

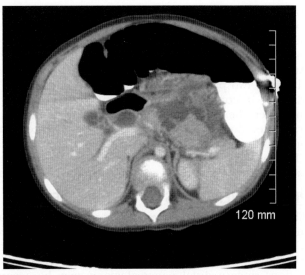

120 mm

FIGURE 97-9 Midbody pancreas injury following blunt trauma to abdomen in a 5-year-old girl. Note incidental finding of choledochal cyst.

literature have been those who have complied with this. Radiation therapy has been used as well.

SOLID-PSEUDOPAPILLARY TUMOR

In the past, solid-pseudopapillary tumors have also been termed *papillary cystic neoplasm, Hamoudi tumor,* or *Frantz tumor.* It is an epithelial tumor of low-grade malignant potential, occurring more frequently in females of reproductive age that usually presents as an asymptomatic large mass or with pain.[58-60] Radiographically and grossly, solid-pseudopapillary tumors have cystic and solid elements. Diagnosis may be made by fine-needle aspirate, which may be accomplished at the time of endoscopic ultrasound in an adolescent patient.[61]

Solid-pseudopapillary tumors occur in all regions of the pancreas with equal frequency. They do not tend to invade adjacent organs. Depending on location, pancreaticoduodenectomy, central pancreatectomy with anastomosis of the distal portion to a Roux-en-Y jejunal loop, and distal pancreatectomy have each been applied.[59,61-64] Treatment is by complete excision and if completely excised has an excellent prognosis. There is no established role for chemotherapy or radiation therapy.

OTHER TUMORS

Lymphomas may arise in the pancreas. The pancreas also may be the site of metastatic spread of other pediatric malignancies, such as neuroblastoma (Figure 97-8).

TRAUMA

Pancreatic trauma is uncommon and is frequently missed during initial evaluation. Blunt injury to the pancreas in children typically occurs in the setting of three characteristic mechanisms. These include handlebar injuries, blows to the abdomen, or motor vehicle crashes. Ordinarily, mechanism, symptoms, or a "seat-belt" sign will lead to the performance of a CT scan. The administration of intravenous contrast is essential to suitably visualize solid organ injury, but the utility of oral or intragastric contrast is debatable. Most patients will have grade 3 or 4 injuries usually in the body of the pancreas

(Figure 97-9).[65] The accuracy of CT to detect pancreatic injury increases from 70% at time of injury to 90% after 3 days. Hemodynamic instability after volume resuscitation of 40 mL/kg (20 mL/kg × 2) of crystalloid should prompt celiotomy, but this scenario is unusual.

Successful surgeon-directed nonoperative management of pancreatic injuries has been reported in multiple case series since the 1990s. In 1994 the Johns Hopkins group found that of 2900 children admitted for blunt trauma to a pediatric trauma center, 7 had CT-proven lacerations of the pancreas. Four of these 7 patients recovered without intervention. The remaining 3 required partial resection or operative treatment of a pseudocyst.[66] A subsequent review of the National Pediatric Trauma Registry stratified 154 pediatric pancreatic injuries by severity and found that 79% of the children without major ductal injury, and 48% of the children with major ductal injury, evaded celiotomy.[67] Although encouraging, these data must be counterbalanced by a consideration of the morbidity associated with nonoperative management. Nonoperative management has shown complication rates up to 78%.[65] However, even with the higher complication rate for nonoperative therapy, when compared to operative treatment, the patients had similar lengths of stay and rates of readmission.[68,69] In another review of 19 Japanese children reported in a 1999 series, nonoperative management had complications, including two pseudocyst ruptures secondary to patient motion and one death from TPN-associated complications.[23]

The data on nonoperative management highlight the observation that in some cases, even after complete transection, the pancreatic duct may seal. The resiliency of the duct is illustrated by a case of an 8-year-old who sustained a complete, ERCP-proven transection of the proximal duct. Surgical debridement and placement of two Jackson-Pratt drains—but no pancreatic resection or enteric anastomosis—were performed, and in 3 months' time complete reconstruction of the duct was demonstrated.[70] Similarly, a review of nine children with complete pancreatic transection who were treated nonoperatively showed that percutaneous pseudocyst drainage was later required in three of the nine patients. Atrophy of the body and tail were observed in some cases. However, two patients reconstituted completely normal glands.[71] In contrast, other investigators have suggested that given the high complication rate in patients with a transected duct, those are the patients best treated with operative resection.[68] This study also suggested that ERCP was the tool best employed to determine which patients had ductal injury and would require resection.

PROXIMAL VERSUS DISTAL DUCT INJURIES

The decision to render operative or nonoperative treatment to a child with a ductal injury revolves, in part, on whether the injury is in the proximal duct or distal duct. The distal duct presents more straightforward surgical options since a distal pancreatectomy may be accomplished by standard suture or staple closure of the pancreatic remnant without the requirement for an enteric anastomosis. This distal resection could even be performed laparoscopically.[72] Therefore, groups at several children's hospitals have advocated early operation for distal duct transections, citing earlier return to health and obviation of the need for TPN.[22,24]

Proximal duct injuries, however, have prompted wide-ranging solutions including Whipple procedure[24] and onlay of a Roux limb of jejunum.[25] The track record of nonoperative management makes observation a more attractive alternative than complex operations for proximal ductal transection. All that may be required is interval drainage of the potentially resulting pseudocyst.[26,73]

Alternatively, Canty and Weinman treated their patients with ductal injury by ERCP and transampullary stenting of the pancreatic duct.[74] In this study, both patients healed without pseudocyst formation. Ductal disruption occurred in the midbody in one and in the distal duct in the other, and in one case the stent did not even traverse the injury. Thus, the healing of the ductal injury is attributed to decompression of the pancreatic duct as a whole. The investigators pointed out that these cases involved ductal extravasation but not full-scale ductal transection.

OPTIONS FOR PSEUDOCYST DRAINAGE

If a pseudocyst develops (Figure 97-10), it may be dealt with by standard cystogastrostomy or cystojejunostomy. Percutaneous drainage and internal, endoscopic drainage using a double-pigtail stent into the stomach have also been reported in children as young as 2 years old (Figure 97-11). Like open operative techniques, these methods rely on the development of a rind around the pseudocyst cavity.[75,76]

ENDOSCOPIC RETROGRADE CHOLANGIOPANCREATOGRAPHY IN CHILDREN

The assumption that ERCP is more dangerous in children than in adults has not been substantiated by the

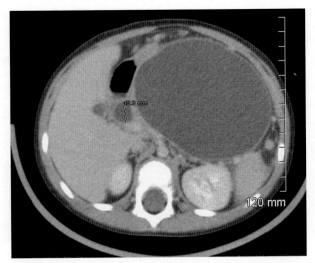

FIGURE 97-10 Posttraumatic pseudocyst in a 4-year-old girl following blunt injury to the abdomen. Extrinsic compression of the common bile duct (18.3 mm).

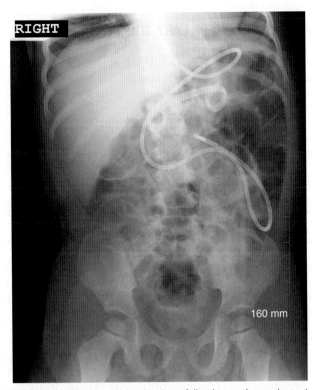

FIGURE 97-11 Pigtail catheter in place following endoscopic cyst gastrostomy for management of posttraumatic pseudocyst in 4-year-old shown in Figure 97-10. Nasoduodenal feeding tube remains in place.

bulk of data in the literature. Some concerns center on a 2001 study from Montreal Children's Hospital, delineating 21 ERCP procedures performed in children (mean age, 11.3 years [range, 4 to 17 years]). Although the success rate was more than 90%, the authors reported a high complication rate of 33%. Pancreatitis occurred in four patients who underwent sphincterotomy, in one who had a strictly diagnostic ERCP, and in one in whom the ampulla could not be cannulated at all. Another patient had bleeding following sphincterotomy, requiring transfusion.[77]

However, these findings are counterbalanced by data from other centers. Allendorph et al reported four complications among 39 diagnostic and/or therapeutic ERCPs in children (mean age, 12.5 years [range, 6 months to 18 years]); all four complications were mild cases of pancreatitis.[78] Guelrud has reported 95% cannulation success in a series of 155 neonates and infants and 98% success among 125 children older than 1 year, with major complications (cholangitis and pancreatitis) occurring in only 2 patients.[34] Therapeutic ERCP may be useful for children with chronic pancreatitis, enabling papillotomy, stone extraction, and stenting with an acceptable short-term complication rate.[35]

However, for patients requiring purely diagnostic studies, the use of magnetic resonance cholangiopancreatography (MRCP) to study the pancreatic ducts has been retrospectively validated in a small pediatric series by Arcement et al, who compared findings with those of ERCPs performed on the same children.[36] Given that the only complications of MRCP seem to be those of general anesthesia, MRCP is beginning to supplant ERCP when a diagnostic, not therapeutic, study is needed. For premature infants or children with respiratory concerns, overnight observation in the hospital may still be needed after anesthesia for MRCP.

REFERENCES

1. Moore KM: *The developing human: Clinically oriented embryology*, ed 4. Philadelphia, 1988, WB Saunders.
2. Merrill JR, Raffensperger JG: Pediatric annular pancreas: Twenty years' experience. *J Pediatr Surg* 11:921, 1976.
3. Jimenez JC, Emil S, Podnos Y, et al: Annular pancreas in children: A recent decade's experience. *J Pediatr Surg* 39:1654, 2004.
4. Lainakis N, Antypas S, Panagidis A, et al: Annular pancreas in two consecutive siblings: An extremely rare case. *Eur J Pediatr Surg* 15:364, 2005.
5. Sencan A, Mir E, Gunsar C, et al: Symptomatic annular pancreas in newborns. *Med Sci Monit* 8:CR434, 2002.
6. Lin Y-T, Chang M-H, Hsu H-Y, et al: A follow-up study of annular pancreas in infants and children. *Zhongua Min Guo Xiao Er Ke Yi Xue Hui Za Zhi* 39:89, 1998.
7. Scheida N, Wales PW, Krishnamurthy G, et al: Ectopic drainage of the common bile duct into the lesser curvature of the gastric antrum in a newborn with pyloric atresia, annular pancreas and congenital short bowel syndrome. *Pediatr Radiol* 39:66, 2009.
8. Papandreou E, Baltogiannia N, Cigliano B, et al: Annular pancreas combined with distal stenosis. A report of four cases and review of the literature. *Pediatr Med Chir* 26:256, 2004.
9. Urushihara N, Fukumoto K, Fukuzawa H, et al: Recurrent pancreatitis caused by pancreatobiliary anomalies in children with annular pancreas. *J Pediatr Surg* 45:741, 2010.
10. Palladino A, Bennett MJ, Santley CA: Hyperinsulinism in infancy and childhood: When an insulin level is not always enough. *Clin Chem* 4:256, 2008.
11. Darendeliler F, Bas F: Hyperinsulinism in infancy—genetic aspects. *Pediatr Endocrinal Rev* 3:521, 2006.
12. Aynsley-Green A, Polak JM, Bloom SR, et al: Nesidioblastosis of the pancreas: Definition of the syndrome and the management of the severe neonatal hyperinsulinaemic hypoglycaemia. *Arch Dis Child* 56:496, 1981.
13. Schonau E, Deeg KH, Huemmer HP, et al: Pancreatic growth and function following surgical treatment of nesidioblastosis in infancy. *Eur J Pediatr* 150:550, 1991.
14. Sempoux C, Poggi F, Brunelle F, et al: Nesidioblastosis and persistent neonatal hyperinsulinism. *Diabete Metab (Paris)* 21:402, 1995.
15. Rahier J, Guiot Y, Sempoux C: Persistent hyperinsulinaemic hypoglycemia of infancy: A heterogeneous syndrome unrelated to nesidioblastosis. *Arch Dis Child Fetal Neonatal Ed* 82:F108, 2000.
16. Verkarre V, Fournet J-C, de Lonlay P, et al: Paternal mutation of the sulfonylurea receptor (*SUR1*) gene and maternal loss of 11p15 imprinted genes lead to persistent hyperinsulinism in focal adenomatous hyperplasia. *J Clin Invest* 102:1286, 1998.
17. Dubois J, Brunelle F, Touati G, et al: Hyperinsulinism in children: Diagnostic value of pancreatic venous sampling correlated with clinical, pathological, and surgical outcome in 25 cases. *Pediatr Radiol* 25:512, 1995.
18. Brunelle F, Negre V, Barth MO, et al: Pancreatic venous samplings in infants and children with primary hyperinsulinism. *Pediatr Radiol* 19:100, 1989.
19. Cretolle C, Fékété CN, Jan D, et al: Partial elective pancreatectomy is curative in focal form of permanent hyperinsulinemic hypoglycemia in infancy: A report of 45 cases from 1983 to 2000. *J Pediatr Surg* 37:155, 2002.
20. Neblett WW, O'Neill JA: Surgical management of recurrent pancreatitis in children with pancreas divisum. *Ann Surg* 231:899, 2000.
21. Silverman JF, Holbrook CT, Pories WJ, et al: Fine-needle aspiration cytology of pancreatoblastoma with immunocytochemical and ultrastructural studies. *Acta Cytol* 34:632, 1990.
22. Jobst MA, Canty TG, Lynch FP: Management of pancreatic injury in pediatric blunt abdominal trauma. *J Pediatr Surg* 34:818, 1999.
23. Kouchi K, Tanabe M, Yoshida H, et al: Nonoperative management of blunt pancreatic injury in childhood. *J Pediatr Surg* 34:1736, 1999.
24. Meier DE, Coln CD, Hicks BA, et al: Early operation in children with pancreas transection. *J Pediatr Surg* 36:341, 2001.
25. Mboyo A, Flurin V, Allamand P, et al: Internal drainage into an onlay-Roux-en-Y jejunal loop in isolated pancreatic injury with ductal transection: Short-term and long-term follow-up in two pediatric cases. *Eur J Pediatr Surg* 10:398, 2000.
26. Ohno Y, Ohgami H, Nagasaki A, et al: Complete disruption of the main pancreatic duct: A case successfully managed by percutaneous drainage. *J Pediatr Surg* 30:1741, 1995.
27. Cherubini V, Bagalini LS, Ianilli A, et al: Rapid genetic analysis, imaging with ^{18}F-DOPA-PET/CT scan and laparoscopic surgery in congenital hyperinsulinism. *J Pediatr Endocrinol Metab* 23:171, 2010.
28. Fékété CN, de Lonlay P, Jaubert F, et al: The surgical management of congenital hyperinsulinemic hypoglycaemia in infancy. *J Pediatr Surg* 39:267, 2004.
29. De Vroede M, Bax NMA, Brusgaard K, et al: Laparoscopic diagnosis and cure of hyperinsulinism in two cases of focal adenomatous hyperplasia in infancy. *Pediatrics* 114:e520, 2004.
30. Reyes GA, Fowler CL, Pokorny WJ: Pancreatic anatomy in children: Emphasis on its importance to pancreatectomy. *J Pediatr Surg* 28:712, 1993.
31. Soliman AT, Alsalmi I, Darwish A, et al: Growth and endocrine function after near total pancreatectomy for hyperinsulinaemic hypoglycaemia. *Arch Dis Child* 74:379, 1996.
32. Chevalier SG: Long-term complication following subtotal pancreatectomy for nesidioblastosis: A case report. *Conn Med* 60:335, 1996.
33. Maier JP, Weiss WM: Variceal hemorrhage 18 years after pancreatectomy for nesidioblastosis: A case report and discussion. *J Pediatr Surg* 38:1102, 2003.
34. Guelrud M: Endoscopic retrograde cholangiopancreatography in children. *Gastroenterologist* 4:81, 1996.
35. Kozarek RA, Christie D, Barclay G: Endoscopic therapy of pancreatitis in the pediatric population. *Gastrointest Endosc* 39:665, 1993.
36. Arcement CM, Meza MP, Arumanla S, et al: MRCP in the evaluation of pancreaticobiliary disease in children. *Pediatr Radiol* 31:92, 2001.
37. Cotton PB: Congenital anomaly of pancreas divisum as cause of obstructive pain and pancreatitis. *Gut* 21:105, 1980.
38. Adzick NS, Shamberger RC, Winter HS, et al: Surgical treatment of pancreas divisum causing pancreatitis in children. *J Pediatr Surg* 24:54, 1989.
39. O'Rourke RW, Harrison MR: Pancreas divisum and stenosis of the major and minor papillae in an eight-year-old girl: Treatment by dual sphincteroplasty. *J Pediatr Surg* 33:789, 1998.
40. Sanchez-Ramirez CA, Larosa-Haro A, Flores-Martinez S, et al: Acute and recurrent pancreatitis in children: Etiological factors. *Acta Paeditr* 96:534, 2007.

41. Stringer MD, Davison DM, McClean P, et al: Multidisciplinary management of surgical disorders of the pancreas in childhood. *J Pediatr Gastroenterol Nutr* 40:363, 2005.

42. Rollins MD, Meyers RL: Frey procedure for surgical management of chronic pancreatitis in children. *J Pediatr Surg* 39:817, 2004.

43. DuBay D, Sandler A, Kimura K, et al: The modified Puestow procedure for complicated hereditary pancreatitis in children. *J Pediatr Surg* 35:343, 2000.

44. Crombleholme TM, deLorimier AA, Way LW, et al: The modified Puestow procedure for chronic relapsing pancreatitis in children. *J Pediatr Surg* 25:749, 1990.

45. Weber TR, Keller MS: Operative management of chronic pancreatitis in children. *Arch Surg* 136:550, 2001.

46. Beccaria L, Bosio L, Burgio G, et al: Multiple insulinomas of the pancreas: A patient report. *J Pediatr Endocrinol Metab* 10:309, 1997.

47. Montero M, Vazques JL, Rihuete MA, et al: Serous cystadenoma of the pancreas in a child. *J Pediatr Surg* 38:E36, 2003.

48. Arikan A, Sayan A, Erikci VS: Hydatid cyst of the pancreas: A case report with five years' follow-up. *Pediatr Surg Int* 15:579, 1999.

49. Klimstra DS, Wenig BM, Adair CF, et al: Pancreatoblastoma: A clinicopathologic study and review of the literature. *Am J Surg Pathol* 19:1371, 1995.

50. Jaksic T, Yaman M, Thorner P, et al: A twenty-year review of pediatric pancreatic tumors. *J Pediatr Surg* 27:1315, 1992.

51. Lee YJ, Hah JO: Long-term survival of pancreatoblastoma in children. *J Pediatr Hematol Oncol* 29:845, 2007.

52. Danner DB, Hruban RH, Pitt HA, et al: Primitive neuroectodermal tumor arising in the pancreas. *Mod Pathol* 7:200, 1994.

53. Luttges J, Pierre E, Zamboni G, et al: Maligne nichtepthliale tumoren des pancreas. *Pathologe* 18:233, 1997.

54. Bulchmann G, Schuster T, Haas RJ, et al: Primitive neuroectodermal tumor of the pancreas: An extremely rare tumor. *Klin Padiatr* 212:185, 2000.

55. Movahedi-Lankarani S, Hruban RH, Westra WH, et al: Primitive neuroectodermal tumors of the pancreas: A report of seven cases of a rare neoplasm. *Am J Surg Pathol* 26:1040, 2002.

56. Shorter NA, Glick RD, Klimstra DS, et al: Malignant pancreatic tumors in childhood and adolescence: The Memorial Sloan-Kettering experience, 1967 to present. *J Pediatr Surg* 37:887, 2002.

57. Perek S, Perek A, Sarman K, et al: Primitive neuroectodermal tumor of the pancreas: A case report of an extremely rare tumor. *Pancreatology* 3:352, 2003.

58. Martin RCG, Klimstra DS, Brennan MF, et al: Solid-pseudopapillary tumor of the pancreas: A surgical enigma? *Ann Surg Oncol* 9:35, 2002.

59. Raffel A, Cupisti K, Krausch M, et al: Therapeutic strategy of papillary cystic and solid neoplasm (PCSN): A rare non-endocrine tumor of the pancreas in children. *Surg Oncol* 13:1, 2004.

60. Lee YJ, Jang JY, Hwang DW, et al: Clinical features and outcome of solid pseudopapillary neoplasm. *Arch Surg* 143:218, 2008.

61. Nadler EP, Novikov A, Landzberg BR, et al: The use of endoscopic ultrasound in the diagnosis of solid pseudopapillary tumors of the pancreas in children. *J Pediatr Surg* 37:1370, 2002.

62. Wunsch LP, Flemming P, Werner U, et al: Diagnosis and treatment of papillary cystic tumor of the pancreas in children. *Eur J Pediatr Surg* 7:45, 1997.

63. Ward HC, Leake J, Spitz L: Papillary cystic cancer of the pancreas: Diagnostic difficulties. *J Pediatr Surg* 28:89, 1993.

64. Casanova M, Collini P, Ferrari A, et al: Solid-pseudopapillary tumor of the pancreas (Frantz tumor) in children. *Med Pediatr Oncol* 41:74, 2003.

65. Thomas H, Madanur M, Bartlett A, et al: Pancreatic trauma: 12-year experience from a tertiary center. *Pancreas* 38:113, 2009.

66. Haller JA, Papa P, Drugas G, et al: Nonoperative management of solid organ injuries in children: Is it safe? *Ann Surg* 219:625, 1994.

67. Keller MS, Stafford PW, Vane DW: Conservative management of pancreatic trauma in children. *J Trauma* 42:1097, 1997.

68. Wood JH, Partrick DA, Bruny JL, et al: Operative vs nonoperative management of blunt pancreatic trauma in children. *J Pediatr Surg* 45:401, 2010.

69. de Blaauw I, Winkelhorst JT, Rieu PN, et al: Pancreatic injury in children: Good outcome of nonoperative treatment. *J Pediatr Surg* 43:1640, 2008.

70. Arkovitz MS, Garcia VF: Spontaneous recanalization of the pancreatic duct: Case report and review. *J Trauma* 40:1014, 1996.

71. Wales PW, Shuckett B, Kim PCW: Long-term outcome after nonoperative management of complete traumatic pancreatic transection in children. *J Pediatr Surg* 36:823, 2001.

72. Yoder SM, Rothenberg S, Tsao K, et al: Laparoscopic treatment of pancreatic pseudocysts in children. *J Laparoendosc Adv Surg Tech A* 19:S37, 2009.

73. Canty TG, Weinman D: Management of major pancreatic duct injuries in children. *J Trauma* 50:1001, 2001.

74. Canty TG, Weinman D: Treatment of pancreatic duct disruption in children by an endoscopically placed stent. *J Pediatr Surg* 36:345, 2001.

75. Kimble RM, Cohen R, Williams S: Successful endoscopic drainage of a posttraumatic pancreatic pseudocyst in a child. *J Pediatr Surg* 34:1518, 1999.

76. Patty I, Kalaoui M, Al-Shamali M, et al: Endoscopic drainage for pancreatic pseudocyst in children. *J Pediatr Surg* 36:503, 2001.

77. Prasil P, Laberge J-M, Barkun A, et al: Endoscopic retrograde cholangiopancreatography in children: A surgeon's perspective. *J Pediatr Surg* 36:733, 2001.

78. Allendorph M, Werlin SL, Geenen JE, et al: Endoscopic retrograde cholangiopancreatography in children. *J Pediatr* 110:206, 1987.

Pancreas and Islet Allotransplantation

Piotr Witkowski | Ryosuke Misawa | J. Michael Millis

CHAPTER

98

I n 1993, the Diabetes Control and Complications Trial Research Group reported that patients with insulin-dependent diabetes mellitus (IDDM) treated with intensive insulin therapy showed a reduced risk of developing retinopathy, albuminuria or microalbuminuria, and clinical neuropathy, when compared to patients who received conventional insulin therapy.[1] In this trial, the intensive therapy group was shown to have achieved sustained lowered blood glucose concentrations over time as reflected by significantly lower hemoglobin (Hb) A_{1c} values compared to those of the conventional insulin therapy group. Although the intensive therapy group benefited from reduced long-term complications, the risk of severe hypoglycemia, which compromised life quality associated with tight glycemic control, was three times greater than in the conventional therapy group. Successful β-cell replacement therapy in the form of pancreas or islet transplantation offers the advantages of attaining normal or near-normal blood glucose control without the risks of severe hypoglycemia associated with intensive insulin therapy. Thus, the goal of pancreas and islet transplantation is to restore normal glycemic control and thereby reduce the complications of IDDM by providing sufficient β-cell mass.[2] Although pancreas transplantation remains the gold standard, as β-cell replacement therapy, an alternative approach, that is, pancreatic islet transplantation, is a developing procedure, and recent results indicate it may be as effective as solitary pancreas transplantation.[3] Islet cell allotransplantation has become an approved and reimbursed procedure in Canada, Europe, and Australia in selected patients. In the United States, it should achieve the same status in a few years, once the National Institutes of Health (NIH)-sponsored multicenter trial is completed.[4] Therefore, as pancreatic islet allotransplantation has become a clinical reality and an option in the treatment of IDDM, we have elected to present it with pancreas transplantation.

HISTORY OF PANCREAS TRANSPLANTATION

The first pancreas transplants were performed in combination with a kidney in uremic type 1 diabetic patients in 1966 at the University of Minnesota. They proved that pancreas transplantation could obtain a euglycemic state without the need for exogenous insulin.[5] However, early procedures were complicated by a high rate of morbidity, early graft failure, and poor patient survival, so few transplants were performed.[5] Improvements in transplantation techniques, immunosuppressive therapies, and posttransplantation monitoring of graft function and rejection have resulted in a dramatic improvement in patient morbidity and graft survival. According to the

International Pancreas Transplant Registry (IPTR), from 1966 to 2008 more than 30,000 pancreases have been transplanted worldwide (22,000 in the United States and 9000 in Europe), and more than 1200 procedures are performed annually in the United States.[4-6] Nevertheless, since 2004, the number of all types of pancreas transplants declined. Currently, simultaneous pancreas-kidney (SPK) transplantation accounts for 73% of pancreas transplants, pancreas after kidney (PAK) transplantation accounts for 19%, and pancreas transplantation alone (PTA) accounts for 8% (Figure 98-1).[6]

HISTORY OF PANCREATIC ISLET TRANSPLANTATION

In 1965, Moskalewski first isolated pancreatic islets from the guinea pig, but in 1967 Lacy's group described a novel collagenase-based method to isolate rat islets, thus paving the way for islet transplantation.[7,8] Subsequent studies showed that transplanted islets could reverse diabetes not only in rodents but also in nonhuman primates.[9] However, early efforts to treat type 1 diabetics with pancreatic islet transplantation were mostly unsuccessful. Although the first human pancreatic islet allografts were performed in 1977,[10] it was not until 1990 that a pancreatic islet transplant recipient achieved sustained euglycemia off insulin (for 1 year).[11] The Pittsburgh group reported the first successful series of human islet allografts when transplanted together with the liver from the same donor. Although they did not address the added issue of autoimmunity in type 1 diabetes (none of their patients were type 1 diabetics), this study provided the first evidence of long-term reversal of diabetes after islet allotransplantation, with more than 50% of recipients having sustained insulin independence, lasting in one case up to 5 years.

EDMONTON PROTOCOL

Of the patients receiving islet transplants in the 1990s, only 7% of patients remained insulin free 1 year after islet transplantation. In 2000, the Edmonton group reported seven consecutive islet transplant recipients, all of whom achieved insulin independence at the end of 1 year without major complications.[12] All recipients received islets from at least two donors and were maintained on a glucocorticoid-free immunosuppression protocol using rapamycin and low-dose tacrolimus.[12] The success of the Edmonton program has led to a general acceptance that islet transplantation is a clinically feasible therapy, which may be considered for the treatment of patients with type 1 diabetes, especially when accompanied by severe hypoglycemia. Since the report of

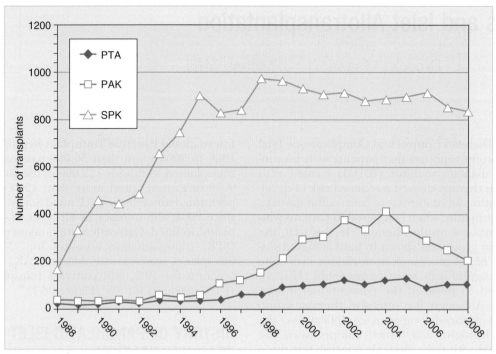

FIGURE 98-1 Annual number of pancreas transplants in the United States, 1988-2008. *PAK,* Pancreas after kidney; *PTA,* pancreas transplant alone; *SPK,* simultaneous pancreas–kidney. (From Gruessner AC, Sutherland DE, Gruessner RW: Pancreas transplantation in the United States: A review. *Curr Opin Organ Transplant* 15:93, 2010.)

success from Edmonton, interest has grown in islet transplantation, and more than 46 centers worldwide have performed this procedure. According to the Collaborative Islet Transplant Registry (CITR), from 1999 to 2008, a total of 828 islet transplantations in 412 recipients were reported.[13]

CANDIDATES FOR PANCREAS OR ISLET ALLOTRANSPLANTATION

Neither pancreas nor islet transplantation is a life-saving procedure. The aim for both procedures is to improve quality of life and prevent secondary complications. Therefore, patient selection criteria are stricter than for other organ transplant procedures in order to protect patient safety and identify candidates who will benefit from the procedures.

Guidelines of the American Diabetes Association for indication for pancreas transplantation include patients with IDDM, with undetected C-peptide who suffer from end-stage renal disease or symptoms of hypoglycemic unawareness with progressive secondary diabetic complications such as (1) history of frequent, acute, and severe metabolic complications (hypoglycemia, hyperglycemia, ketoacidosis) requiring medical attention; (2) clinical and emotional problems with exogenous insulin therapy that are so severe as to be incapacitating; or (3) consistent failure of insulin-based management to prevent acute complications.[14]

Currently, general indications for islet allotransplantation in most of the clinical studies are the same as described earlier for pancreas transplantation. For example, the NIH-funded, Food and Drug Administration (FDA)–regulated, multicenter Clinical Islet Transplantation trial

targets patients who failed intensive insulin treatment defined as intensive insulin therapy with target HbA_{1c} levels of lower than 6.5% as suggested by the American Association of Clinical Endocrinologists/American College of Endocrinology (AACE/ACE) consensus panel statement on type 2 diabetes mellitus and glycemic control. Following a period of longer than 4 months on this therapy, only patients who evidence continued inadequate glucose control characterized by either HbA_{1c} level higher than 7.5% or HbA_{1c} level lower than 7.5% but with severe hypoglycemic episodes are included.[4]

Currently, one limitation of islet allotransplantation is the insufficient number of islets isolated from a single organ to restore normoglycemia in each type 1 diabetic patient. Even with two or three sequential infusions, success cannot be achieved in patients with high insulin demand. Most studies limit recipients to body mass index (BMI) less than 30 kg/m^2 and body weight less than 90 kg and daily insulin requirements below 1 unit/kg.[4]

It is worth emphasizing that 5.9% of pancreas transplants are performed in selected type 2 diabetics.[5] Additionally, 4% of pancreas allografts are implanted in nondiabetic patients after extended intraabdominal resection as part of multiorgan transplantation (including liver, intestine, and/or kidney transplants).[6] Islet transplantation is also an option in such cases with good results, in cases where the patient is not suitable for whole pancreas transplantation.[11]

DONOR CHARACTERISTICS

Most pancreas allografts (95%) come from deceased heart-beating donors. The remainder are from highly selected non-heart-beating donors or from living donors.[2]

To improve results, optimal parameters of donors are as follows: age 14 to 45 years; BMI less than 28 kg/m^2; head trauma as the preferred cause of death; organ procured by a local organ procurement organization to minimize cold ischemic time, preferably less than 12 hours. Pancreas donors are excluded based on presence of diabetes, pancreatitis, sepsis, malignancy, and positive markers for viral infection such as hepatitis B or C, HIV, or human T-lymphocyte virus. Undesired conditions include BMI greater than 30 kg/m^2, Center for Disease Control (CDC) high risk, downtime, disseminated intravascular coagulopathy (DIC), need for pressors, and pancreas injury, fibrosis, or steatosis. Hyperglycemia or need for insulin therapy in the donor at the time of organ procurement is not a contraindication, but it is a minor risk factor for long-term graft loss.[2] Hyperamylasemia can be of salivary origin, and it is not itself a contraindication for donation. Some centers have exclusion criteria for the pancreas based on age (younger than 8 years), body weight (<30 kg), or diameter of the splenic artery (<2 mm).[14] Donors with BMI greater than 35 kg/m^2 or who are older than 55 years of age are used very rarely; only 6% of donors are younger than 14 years of age, and 6% are older than 45 years of age.[2]

Exclusion donor criteria for the purpose of islets are the same as for pancreas transplantation in order to prevent transmission of disease to the recipient. However, donor and organ quality criteria are much less selective. Desired age is older than 18 years without an upper limit and BMI is unrestricted as long as the patient is not diabetic (HbA$_{1c}$ < 6%). The main limiting factor regarding the effectiveness of the islet isolation is cold ischemia time; less than 8 hours is preferable. In the United States and United Kingdom, preferential pancreas allocation to islet transplant recipients was established for donors older than 50 years of age or with a BMI greater than 30 kg/m^2.[2] The goal is to limit cold ischemia time and enhance availability of the organ and improve isolation results. Otherwise, the current organ allocation system promotes pancreas transplantation over islet transplantation. Therefore, each pancreas is offered first to potential whole-organ recipients, and then if rejected, is considered for islet transplant patients. In this way, only lower quality organs are used for islet isolation. This allocation schema may be changed in the future, once islet transplantation achieves the same effectiveness and status as whole-organ pancreas transplantation.

PANCREAS PROCUREMENT TECHNIQUES

PANCREAS PROCUREMENT FOR WHOLE-ORGAN TRANSPLANTATION

Cadaveric-donor pancreatectomy is performed as part of a multiorgan procurement through a midline incision. The gastrocolic ligament is divided to enter the lesser sac and expose the anterior aspect of the pancreas. At this point, the pancreas is evaluated for signs of fat infiltration, edema, injury, hematoma, calcification, and tumor. If the organ is still suitable, a Kocher maneuver is performed to expose the inferior vena cava and aorta. The gastroduodenal artery is ligated and divided. If a replaced (accessory) right hepatic artery is present, it may be divided at its origin. If liver is procured at the same time, usually the liver surgeon decides whether to include the superior mesenteric artery (SMA) with the right replaced hepatic artery or not, allowing for easier arterial reconstruction of pancreas vasculature and transplantation. Next, the spleen and tail of the pancreas are mobilized to allow for placement of the ice-slush posterior to the gland during perfusion. After the thoracic aorta is cross-clamped, cold preservation solution (most commonly University of Wisconsin [UW] or histidine-tryptophan-ketoglutarate [HTK]) is introduced through cannulas in the inferior mesenteric vein and distal aorta. On completion of organ perfusion, the splenic artery is divided from the celiac trunk; the aorta is divided above and below the origin of the celiac trunk, and the portal vein is divided usually 2.5 cm above the superior border of the pancreas. The SMA is harvested with an aortic Carrel patch and distal to the origin of interior pancreaticoduodenal artery. The duodenum is divided by GIA stapler at the level of pylorus and ligament of Treitz after flushing the lumen with an antiseptic solution. The spleen remains attached to the pancreas to protect the tail during the procurement. Iliac venous and arterial grafts are obtained from the donor for the reconstruction of the pancreas vasculature.[14] When the small bowel is procured for transplantation at the same time, it is essential to ensure that the inferior pancreaticoduodenal artery is not divided during dissection of the root of the small bowel. Next the pancreas with spleen and duodenum in continuity are placed in a container with preservation solution and placed on ice during transportation.

PANCREAS PROCUREMENT FOR THE ISLET ALLOTRANSPLANTATION

Basically, the pancreas for the islet isolation is procured in the same way. However, different elements of the procurements are more crucial. First, the pancreas for islet procurement is more sensitive to warm injury; therefore the organ should be well flushed with the preservation solution to eliminate blood. Then, the organ should be constantly kept surrounded by ice, even during dissection. Next, because no blood vessels are necessary for the isolation, the presence of a right hepatic artery does not preclude pancreas procurement. Instead, it is extremely important during the dissection not to cut or open the pancreas capsule because it compromises enzyme distention, organ digestion, and eventually the yield of the isolation. Because results of the islet isolation depend strongly on proper pancreas preservation, it is hard to overemphasize the importance of the pancreas procurement technique for the success of the islet isolation and then transplantation. In multivariable analysis, the procuring team from the islet isolation center is the strongest independent factor (odds ratio [OR] = 10.9) regarding the success of the isolation.[15]

BACK-TABLE PREPARATION FOR WHOLE PANCREAS TRANSPLANTATION

Before implantation, the pancreas needs to be prepared for transplantation while still on ice at the back-table. During this important procedure, the pancreas vasculature is restored, excess surrounding fat, connective tissue, and the spleen are removed, followed by meticulous ligation of the surrounding blood vessels. This is all done to minimize unnecessary ischemic or bleeding injury, improving the results of pancreas transplantation. Because the celiac trunk and hepatic artery are allotted to the liver, the splenic artery and SMA are maintained with the pancreas. To make a single arterial pedicle, the donor iliac artery is used as a Y graft to suture onto the donor SMA and splenic artery. The portal vein is available for anastomosis and usually does not require elongation. The standard pancreas graft includes the entire pancreas and the second portion of the duodenum. Some authors recommend reconstruction of the gastroduodenal artery as well with an arterial conduit in order to improve blood supply to the head and duodenum and decrease risk for complications; however, the advantage of such a maneuver has not been confirmed in comparative studies.[16]

LIVING-DONOR PANCREAS TRANSPLANTATION

Since 1978, when for the first time living-donor pancreas transplantation was performed at the University of Minnesota, there have been 72 such procedures reported to the IPTR, and currently only three American centers are involved.[17] Improved graft survival was the main goal of the procedure when azathioprine and cyclosporine were the main immunosuppressive agents, despite the magnitude and potential complications of the donor operation. However, with the introduction of tacrolimus, mycophenolate mofetil (MMF) and antibodies used for induction therapy, graft survival improved dramatically for living-donor and cadaveric-donor pancreas transplants. As a result, the immunologic advantage of pancreas transplantation with living-donor transplants in the recent era is no longer as critical as it was before. Moreover, cadaver donors for pancreas transplantation are more available than for other organ transplants. Thus, living donors for solitary pancreas transplants are only considered in limited cases such as (1) a highly sensitized recipient (panel-reactive antibody >80%), (2) to avoid high doses of immunosuppression, or (3) a nondiabetic identical twin or a 6-antigen matched sibling.[2]

In the living-donor pancreas recovery procedure, the short gastric artery arcade should be preserved so that the spleen can be safely left in place. The splenic artery is divided just distal to its origin, and the splenic vein is divided proximal to its confluence with the superior mesenteric vein. The splenic arterial anastomosis is to the recipient common iliac artery, whereas venous drainage is to the common iliac vein. The pancreatic drainage is accomplished by pancreaticojejunostomy or pancreaticocystostomy.[2]

PANCREAS TRANSPLANTATION

The pancreas may be transplanted as the only organ in PTA or as a PAK transplantattion. Most commonly, however, it is transplanted from the same donor with the kidney as an SPK transplantation. In this situation, during the same procedure, the pancreas may be transplanted first since it has a shorter "shelf life" (optimal cold storage time is <12 hours vs. 24 to 48 hours for kidney), so to reduce preservation injury and the risk of complication.[2] Alternatively, the kidney may be grafted first to reduce the incidence of acute tubular necrosis and to avoid pancreas manipulation during kidney transplantation. The pancreas is usually placed in the right pelvis, as in kidney transplantation, with the arterial anastomosis performed on the recipient common iliac artery. Venous drainage can be connected to the lower cava or the common iliac vein (systemic drainage) or superior mesenteric vein (portal drainage). The standard pancreas graft includes the entire pancreas and a portion of the duodenum. The donor duodenum is anastomosed to the recipient's small bowel or urinary bladder allowing drainage of the exocrine pancreas secretions. Each alternative procedure has its own pros and cons.

PORTAL VERSUS SYSTEMIC VENOUS DRAINAGE

Portal venous drainage directs the insulin released by the pancreas transplant initially to the liver, in a fashion similar to normal physiologic conditions allowing for 50% first-pass metabolism. It also lowers the concentration of low-density lipoprotein and apolipoprotein B, free cholesterol, as well as very-low-density lipoprotein. It was postulated based on experimental models that portal venous drainage decreases immunologic response to the graft; however, this was not confirmed clinically.[16] Systemic drainage, on the other hand, omitting first passage through the liver leads to hyperinsulinemia and increased level of low-density lipoprotein. However, clinically, the advantages of the portal over systemic drainage in maintaining normal glucose homeostasis or lipid metabolism have never been shown.[16] Similarly, carbohydrate metabolism does not differ in recipients having SPK transplantation compared with nondiabetic recipients after kidney transplantation only, when similar immunosuppression is used.[2] Therefore, currently, portal drainage is used in only 20% of patients as it is more challenging, requires more experience, and has a somewhat higher risk of graft thrombosis.[18]

ENTERIC DRAINAGE VERSUS BLADDER DRAINAGE

Historically, restoration of pancreatic exocrine secretion drainage was challenging. After the failure of attempts at pancreatic duct ligation and obliteration, the urinary bladder with pancreas-duodenum anastomosis was developed. The advantage of this approach is that amylase concentration in urine allows for monitoring of graft function, enabling early detection of rejection. It is especially useful in PTA and PAK transplantation. However, the major disadvantage is metabolic acidosis because of loss of bicarbonate with the relatively large amount of pancreas juice, frequent reflux pancreatitis (50%), cystitis, urinary tract infection, and perineal irritation.[14] Therefore, once more potent immunosuppression was introduced including induction therapy and the need for pancreas monitoring was diminished, enteric drainage was more widely adopted, improving postoperative course and patient satisfaction. Additionally, pancreas rejection is usually associated with kidney graft dysfunction in SPK transplantation, which allows additional monitoring of the pancreas graft state. Therefore, currently 80% of patients undergo enteric drainage. There are many different methods for enteric drainage in use: The duodenum may be connected with a loop of jejunum, ileum, or even recipient duodenum. It is usually a side-to-side configuration with the loop or Roux-en-Y limb of the bowel, either a hand-sewn double layer or a stapled anastomosis. However, in the latter approach, there is a higher risk of postoperative mucosal bleeding. It seems that enteric drainage has a slightly higher incidence of graft thrombosis than bladder anastomosis: 5.5% to 11.6% versus 5% to 7.2%, respectively.[2] Postoperative enteric leak usually requires reoperation for repair with Roux-en-Y conversion of the bowel loop. In cases of a leak from a bladder anastomosis, drainage with a Foley urinary catheter is usually sufficient.[16] Although enteric drainage dominates in SPK patients now (80%), bladder anastomosis is still in use for solitary pancreas transplant. Based on considerable data from both registries and various retrospective and prospective trials, neither of those two drainage techniques has a clear advantage as regards overall patient or pancreas graft survival.[18]

COMPLICATIONS

The hypoxic injury inherent in cadaveric organ procurement accounts for some of the complications related to the pancreatic allograft. During the 1980s, 25% of all pancreata were lost because of surgical technical failure. According to the IPTR, from 2004 through 2008, the incidence was reduced to an 8% average in all three categories (SPK, PTA, and PAK recipients). Nonetheless, surgical complications, such as pancreas graft thrombosis, leakage, graft pancreatitis, and bleeding, remain high concerns because the rate of the relaparotomy is as high as 35%.[19]

Pancreas Graft Thrombosis

Pancreas graft thrombosis remains, by far, the most frequent and serious surgical complication (incidence ranges from 3% to 10%).[19] With rare exceptions, it results in graft loss and the need for transplant pancreatectomy. Anticoagulation is often used, and tight postoperative management and monitoring with ultrasound, contrast-enhanced computed tomography (CT), or magnetic resonance imaging (MRI) is required.[20] Ultrasound is less useful in patients with enteric drainage, where bowel gas obscures the window.

Leakage

Leakage remains a clinically significant entity, as it typically causes intraabdominal infection. In the case of enteric drainage, intestinal contents leak and cause peritonitis and sepsis. This complication usually requires graft duodenal diversion with a Roux-en-Y limb. From this perspective, bladder drainage has a lower incidence of leakage, but also if it occurs, can be managed conservatively.

Graft Pancreatitis

Although only the endocrine part of the pancreas is needed to control normoglycemia, whole pancreas grafts have both islets and exocrine tissue. Postoperative graft pancreatitis occurs more frequent in PAK and PTA

recipients with bladder drainage (1.7% and 2.0%, respectively). Postoperative pancreatitis may be treated conservatively, but severe cases may require relaparotomy with debridement or occasionally graft pancreatectomy. Also, repetitive episodes of reflux pancreatitis in bladder-drained recipients are an indication for conversion from bladder to enteric drainage.

Hemorrhage

Significant intraabdominal bleeding after pancreas transplantation frequently requires relaparotomy, however, currently, less than 0.3% of all pancreas grafts are lost because of bleeding. Gastrointestinal (GI) bleeding may occur in the early postoperative period, most often from mucosal bleeding at the duodenoenteric anastomosis, and especially when the stapler was applied. Further, late GI bleeding may be a sign of chronic graft rejection.[2]

Rejection and Immunosuppression

Pancreas transplantation is associated with graft loss by rejection as a result of alloimmunity or autoimmune recurrence. Even transplants between identical twins need immunosuppression to prevent autoimmune recurrence.[2] Although the introduction of cyclosporine improved overall results of organ transplantation, the pancreas graft rejection rate was still as high as 78% (for PTA), with up to a third of patients experiencing recurrent rejections. Currently, tacrolimus and MMF with low-dose steroids in combination with different induction therapies are most commonly used as the maintenance immunosuppressive regimen. Such combinations lead to rejection rates at the level of 5% to 25%.[2] Anti-T-cell antibody induction with a combination of maintenance treatment is used in 80% of all pancreas transplant recipients.[18] Antihuman thymocyte antibody (thymoglobulin), anti-interleukin-2 (IL-2) receptor antibody (basiliximab), or anti-CD52 antibody (alemtuzumab) are most commonly used for induction.

Because acute rejection is a strong predictor of chronic rejection (relative risk [RR], 4.4), which is the second most common cause of graft loss (after technical failure), there is a hope that reduction of the number and severity of acute graft rejection episodes will improve long-term results.[14] However, so far clinically, it has not been proved that reduced graft rejection rate (diagnosed with biopsy) prolongs pancreas graft or patient survival.[2] Side effects of the immunosuppression compromise overall health and function of the other organs, for example, steroids lead to insulin resistance, dyslipidemia, bone loss, and impaired wound healing; tacrolimus causes nephrotoxicity. Recent large trials tested a steroid-free regimen or minimization of calcineurin inhibitors, showing a slightly increased rejection rate of 20% to 30% without the hoped-for improvement in long-term results.[2]

OUTCOME OF PANCREAS TRANSPLANTATION

Although pancreas transplantation is not a life-saving procedure but aims to improve quality of life and prevent secondary complications, the benefits of the pancreas transplantation may be only considered in patients with functioning grafts; therefore, we primarily assess both graft and patient survival.

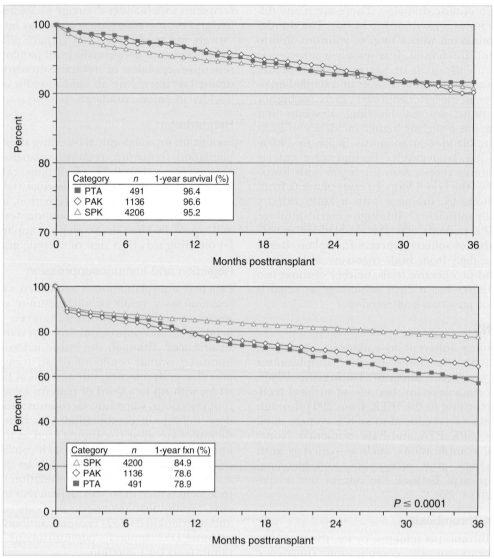

FIGURE 98-2 Three-year patient and pancreas graft survival, based on the International Pancreas Transplant Registry. *PAK,* Pancreas after kidney; *PTA,* pancreas transplant alone; *SPK,* simultaneous pancreas–kidney. (From Gruessner AC, Sutherland DE, Gruessner RW: Pancreas transplantation in the United States: A review. *Curr Opin Organ Transplant* 15:93, 2010.)

Patient Survival

According to the IPTR, the patient survival rate for primary deceased-donor pancreas transplants has constantly improved over the last several years. The 1-year survival rate increased from 67% in 1980 to more than 95% currently.[2,4,5] The 3-year survival rate reached more than 90% in all three transplantation categories (Figure 98-2).[18] Fifteen-year actuarial patient survival is 56% in SPK transplants, 42% for PAK transplants, and 59% after PTA.[2]

Interestingly, there was a substantial increase in survival in age-matched diabetics 10 years after SPK transplantation compared to deceased-donor kidney transplantation.[21] Reddy et al found similar benefits 5 and 8 years after the procedures.[22] SPK recipients have a 10-year longer expected survival time than do kidney transplantation alone (KTA) recipients (23 vs. 13 years); however, the difference is not obvious for patients older than 50 years of age before transplantation.[23] The presence of a

functioning graft increases survival by almost 20% at 8-year followup.

Despite that, there has been a debate recently whether the benefits of pancreas transplantation translate into patient survival. It turned out that overall patient survival was similar in SPK recipients when compared to living-donor kidney transplantation (LDKT) recipients.[21-23] The adjusted survival rate was 67% for SPK recipients, 65% for LDKT, and 46% for deceased-donor kidney transplantation.[23] Additionally, it was also reported that patients with preserved renal function after receiving solitary pancreas transplantation had worse survival rates than those diabetics who were treated with conventional therapy (insulin) while waiting to be transplanted.[24] The relative risk of dying was 2.7 (CI, 0.84-6.13) for PTA and 2.89 (CI, 1.67-5.00) for PAK transplantation within 90 days after the procedure. For SPK transplantation, the risk was lower (RR, 1.7; 95% CI, 0.97-2.98), but reversed as late as 4 years after transplantation. Other authors, however, reanalyzed the same United Network for Organ Sharing data and found several factors that could bias the previous results. Several patients were listed for many procedures at the same time, and the mortality rate of the patients on the waiting list was underestimated.[25] The current conclusion is that the benefit in patient survival starts 3 months after surgery for SPK patients, and 1 year after PTA and PAK transplantation compared to patients on the waiting list.[25] Overall mortality after pancreas transplantation is not higher than mortality on the waiting list and for SPK transplantation is even decreased (hazard ratio [HR], 0.29; CI 0.27-0.33). At least 40% of patients die within the first 4 years waiting for SPK transplants, whereas only 10% die after the transplantation.[25] For PTA and PAK transplantation, 4-year survival is comparable to survival on the waiting list. The most important factor for long-term patient survival is preservation of the pancreas graft (RR around 3 [for mortality]). However for SPK and PAK patients, kidney graft failure has a much stronger influence on mortality than pancreas graft loss (RR, 11 vs. 2.65 and 8 vs. 3, respectively).[6]

The main causes of death after pancreas transplantation remain cardiac or cerebrovascular incidents and infection. Infection peaks between 3 and 12 months after the transplantation.[6]

Graft Survival

Pancreas graft survival defined by insulin independence is the best for SPK transplants and reaches 80% at 3 years after the procedure. Graft survival for PAK transplants is better than for PTA (see Figure 98-2).[18] Early technical failure rates are similar for all types of pancreas transplantation, and approach 8%. Differences in long-term graft survival between SPK and PTA/PAK recipients are mainly caused by immunologic graft loss (acute or chronic rejection). The second leading cause of graft failure in SPK patients is death with a functioning graft. Loss because of chronic rejection increases with time. In multifactorial analyses of registry data, deceased-donor factors and preservation time impacted outcomes the most. Grafts from younger trauma victims, with shorter preservation time, recipients on tacrolimus and MMF immunosuppression, and those operated on in high-volume centers had better graft survival. Interestingly, young recipients (<30 years old) had worse outcomes than older patients (RR, 1.25 to 2).[6] Bladder versus enteric drainage had no influence on graft survival.

Impact on the Health Status and Quality of Life of Patients

The effect of pancreas transplantation on diabetic complications and quality of life is often difficult to assess because complications are often too advanced to reverse. Also SPK patients are usually younger and in better general health than KTA recipients. Additionally, conclusions are not drawn from the 5% of SPK patients who die within the first year.[2] There are clear data that the quality of life improves when the patient has an uncomplicated postoperative course and good pancreas graft function. Cessation of insulin injections, removal of dietary constraints, and most importantly the fear about hypoglycemic episodes improves the quality of life in

SPK patients and, to a lesser degree, in KTA recipients. However, diabetic patients have also improved quality of life once they have a kidney transplant working, irrespective if they received a pancreas graft as well. Nevertheless, successful PTA recipients also report improved quality of life despite surgery and the side effects of immunosuppression.[25] These improvements disappear once the patient develops a pancreas graft failure, serious complication, or serious side effects of immunosuppression.[26]

Glycemic Control

Successful pancreas transplantation restores a normoglycemic state in the majority of the patients immediately after pancreas implantation. Delayed onset of normoglycemia may occur because of organ injury caused by the donor's condition, preservation, extended preservation time, in transplants of a small pancreas into a large adult, or with insulin resistance. Abnormal glucose control may be caused also by complications (arterial or venous thrombosis of the graft, pancreatitis, or rejection). Therefore, blood glucose levels and insulin requirements should be closely observed in the postoperative period. Once the pancreas recovers from perioperative stress, patients typically experience normal fasting and postprandial blood glucose concentrations. Results after glucose challenge are also similar to those who are nondiabetic.[27] However, the most important and long-term benefit is that pancreas transplantations fully protect the patient from disabling and life-threatening severe hypoglycemia unawareness episodes so that the patients can fearlessly resume normal life activities.

Retinopathy

Retinopathy can deteriorate in 10% to 35% of patients with unstable eye disease immediately after pancreas transplantation.[2] Because proper pretransplantation screening and treatment is applied, such complications are preventable. Most of the patients have already developed advanced retinopathy or blindness at the time of transplantation. The long-term effects of pancreas transplantation on diabetic retinopathy have been conflicting. Many early reports showed clear improvement, some found progression of retinal lesions,[28] others reported slower progression of vascular proliferation, improvement of retinal arterial flow velocities, and less need for laser therapy in SPK and PTA recipients.[29] Additionally, post–pancreas grafting cataracts may develop or worsen because of calcineurin inhibitors and steroids.[2]

Nephropathy

In general, normoglycemia can stop the progression of diabetic nephropathy in kidneys and even partially reverse histologic changes secondary to diabetes in native kidneys, but the effect is only observed after a long time. The time frame for this improvement is 5 to 10 years after pancreas engraftment, and many patients may never reach that time point and obtain this benefit.[30] Whether native renal function benefits from PTA is uncertain, as the nephrotoxic effect of calcineurin-inhibitor–based immunosuppression therapy must be considered. Despite the morphologic improvement and reduced urinary protein excretion, creatinine clearance usually gradually deteriorates. According to IPTR data, 2% to 8% of PTA recipients develop end-stage renal failure and require a kidney transplant within the first year after transplantation.[18]

Neuropathy

Polyneuropathy is a common complication of both IDDM and end-stage renal failure, and advanced motor, sensory, and autonomic neuropathies are frequently seen in patients undergoing whole pancreas transplantation. Early reports demonstrated that the motor and sensory nerve conduction indices increased significantly at all intervals after pancreas transplantation; however, the clinical examination and autonomic tests improved only slightly.[31] The impact of restored normoglycemia probably depends on the degree of degeneration before transplantation. In more advanced neuropathy, prevention from progression is observed. In those with mild neuropathy before transplantation, some degree of improvement may be observed.

Vascular Disease

Macrovascular disease naturally progresses with age, and it is difficult to observe any beneficial influence following pancreas transplantation. However, coronary atherosclerosis can regress in nearly 40% of patients with functioning pancreas grafts.[32] Diastolic dysfunction can return to normal after 4 years.[33]

Stabilization and improvement of cardiac autonomic function have also been noted. Peripheral vascular disease is usually too advanced to see substantive improvement after pancreas transplant.

ISLET ALLOTRANSPLANTATION

Once the pancreas is procured, it should be immediately shipped to the islet isolation laboratory (good manufacture practice [GMP] facility) in order to limit cold ischemia time and improve outcome.

ISLET ISOLATION

The pancreas is trimmed from surrounding tissue and blood vessels and then distended with cold enzyme (collagenase) through the pancreatic duct. An intact capsule of the pancreas allows for full distention of the organ and effective digestion in the next step. During enzymatic digestion, the pancreas dissociates into acinar (exocrine tissue) and islets. In the next step, the enzymes are washed out of the collected tissue. The digested tissue is then purified to separate islets from acinar tissue. The final product, purified islets, are tested for bacterial contamination, level of endotoxin, and mycoplasma. Quality tests include purity (>40%), viability (intracellular staining assessed under microscope instantly), and stimulation index (an in vitro functional test assessing the response of the islets to high and low glucose concentration). The final criterion is a sufficient amount of islets after the isolation, so as to benefit the patient. The minimal amount based on previous experience is 5000 IEQ/kg body mass.[12] Islets may be infused fresh (just after the isolation) or after in vitro culture, usually up to 72 hours.

ISLET INFUSION INTO LIVER

Pancreatic islet allotransplantation, in contrast to whole-organ pancreas transplantation, is a minor procedure usually performed under local anesthesia in a radiology suite. The interventional radiologist first inserts a small (7 French) catheter under ultrasound and fluoroscopy guidance into the main portal vein through a percutaneous, transhepatic approach. Islets (usually 2 to 5 mL; up to 10-mL tissue pellet) are suspended in 200 to 400 mL solution (transplant media) with heparin and human albumin contained in a plastic infusion bag. The procedure starts with portal pressure measurements to ensure absence of portal hypertension. Next, islets are dripped slowly through the intravenous line connecting the harvested islet bag with the portal catheter. Portal pressure is measured at the midpoint and the conclusion of the infusion. Typically, the infusion, performed slowly, takes 30 to 45 minutes. Alternatively, it can be done under general anesthesia and in the operating room during a minilaparotomy with infusion through the mesocolonic vein if percutaneous access via the portal vein fails. Postoperatively, subcutaneous heparin and insulin are administered for at least 2 weeks to promote islet engraftment.

COLLABORATIVE ISLETS TRANSPLANT REGISTRY

CITR was established by NIH in 2001, to collect, record, and analyze and report data about islet transplantation. To maintain integrity of the data, it is collected only from accredited centers, which meet all requirements and pass CITR audit. Currently, 32 centers in the United States report their own data to the CITR, as well as 3 centers from Europe, and another 3 from Australia. Yearly reports summarize the updated results.[13]

INFUSION-RELATED COMPLICATIONS

Infusion of islets into the portal vein usually causes transient transaminase elevation (2 to 5 times), but native liver or liver graft (in the case of simultaneous liver and islet transplantation) long-term dysfunction has not been reported.[13] Postinfusion portal-vein thrombosis has been reported based on routine Doppler screening without clinical symptoms in 4% of cases. However, it has always resolved without any treatment.[34] Since the process of purification has been optimized, less tissue is infused, and currently, the risk for thrombosis is even lower. Intraabdominal bleeding was reported initially in 10% of patients.[34] However, when the access technique was optimized (smaller catheters, obliteration of the puncture track), the risk for such a complication has been much decreased (1% to 2%).

Immunosuppression

Since 2000, when the Edmonton group reported success of the corticosteroid-free immunosuppressive regimen, more than 90% of islet programs have followed the same protocol.[12] It consists of rapamycin-based therapy, with low doses of tacrolimus and anti-IL-2 receptor antibody (daclizumab) as induction therapy. Because islets were used in "brittle" type 1 diabetics with preserved kidney function, the main rationale was to improve islet survival and function (thus a steroid-free approach) and protect kidney function (calcineurin inhibitors were minimized). After 5 years of disappointing experience with this approach, many different protocols were developed. The most successful were those involving stronger immunosuppression, involving T-cell depletion induction therapy in the form of thymoglobulin, anti-CD52 antibody (alemtuzumab), or anti-CD3 humanized antibody. Recently, tacrolimus, as well as cyclosporine, MMF, and even steroids, has been used for maintenance. Because the immunosuppression for islet transplant currently does not differ from that routinely used for other organ grafts, the side effects are also the same and not unexpected.

Allosensitization

Because pancreatic islet allotransplantation usually requires two or three islet infusions from the same number of different donors, there is theoretically an increased risk for allosensitization. Clinical observation confirmed that when patients stop immunosuppression because of islet graft failure or side effects, as many as 70% of them develop donor-specific antibody and high panel-reactive antibody (PRA) (>50%).[35-37] However, recent reports show that as long as patients remain on adequate immunosuppression, the risk for donor-specific antibody and high PRA is small even after their fourth and fifth islet infusion.[36,38]

OUTCOME OF PANCREATIC ISLET ALLOTRANSPLANTATION

Insulin Dependence and Graft Function

Islet allotransplantation is an attractive alternative for pancreas transplantation as β-cell replacement therapy because it is a mini-invasive procedure and does not deal with the exocrine part of the pancreas, limiting the risk for complications. Because the number of patients is still limited in each study, cumulative results are reported by the CITR, which helps to analyze the data.[13] There were 412 recipients of 828 islet transplants in the last 10 years (1999 through 2008), including 65 patients receiving islets after kidney allografts.

Overall, as expected for a new and sophisticated procedure, results in the experienced centers are superior as compared to others. Overall, approximately 70% to 90% of all islet recipients are estimated to have achieved insulin independence at some point. The median time to achievement of insulin independence was 6 to 7 months after the first transplant; however, there are centers that reported such success after only one islet infusion.[39] As mentioned before, immunosuppression based on the Edmonton protocol did not protect islets sufficiently, so the number of insulin-free patients gradually decreased from 70% after the first year, to only 9% at 5 years posttransplant.[34] These results were disappointing compared to whole pancreas transplantation. However, even those patients who had only partial islet graft function (required some insulin, but much less than before the transplantation) were protected from hypoglycemic episodes. Overall, 70% to 80% of patients 5 years after the transplantation had full or partial islet graft function (C-peptide positive) protecting them from

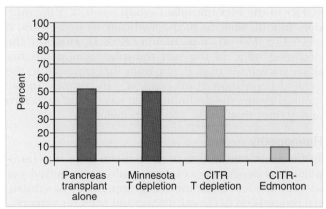

FIGURE 98-3 Results of islet transplant alone (ITA) depending on induction therapy, in comparison to pancreas transplant alone, based on data from the Collaborative Islet Transplant Registry (CITR). Rate of insulin-free patients 5 years after transplant: pancreas transplant alone (PTA), N = 132; University of Minnesota, N = 21; CITR T-cell depletion, N = 73; CITR Edmonton protocol, N = 221. When T-cell depletion induction therapy was applied in ITA, 5-year results were comparable with PTA. (Data from Hering B, Bellin M, Barton F: Induction immunosuppression with T-cell depleting antibodies facilitates long-term insulin independence after islet allotransplantation in type I diabetes. *Am J Transplant* 10:141, 2010.)

hypoglycemia. Those patients had improved blood glucose control and had much lower levels of HbA$_{1c}$ when compared to their pre–islet transplant status.[34]

For the last 5 years, different protocols have been tested with some improvement. Recent data from the CITR indicate that when T-cell depletion induction is applied, 5-year insulin independence might improve to 40% to 50% of patients, which is comparable to that with PTA (Figure 98-3).[3] Those results are preliminary, based on 73 patients, already presented during major international conferences.[3] The results indicate a positive trend that islet transplantation may be as effective as whole pancreas grafts, with the advantage of harboring a lesser risk of complications. Recent results from the Edmonton group confirm this observation. The Edmonton group also has data indicating that supplemental fourth and fifth islet infusions performed a few years after the initial one may be an effective option for patients, without an additional risk of portal-vein thrombosis or development of PRA.[38]

Patient Survival

The recent CITR report notes 9 deaths among 412 recipients of the 828 islet transplant alone (ITA) in the last 10 years (1999 to 2008). Only one death might have possibly been related to immunosuppression—viral meningitis 3 years after islet transplant.[13]

Kidney Function

The same report indicates that serum creatinine increased more then 0.5 mg/dL above baseline in only 42 (16%) of ITA recipients; however, it includes all patients independent of islet graft status. Three years after the transplantation, the decline in glomerular filtration rate

(GFR) in the islet transplant group was 0.12 ± 0.7 mL/min/month, whereas in the medically treated group, it was 0.45 ± 0.77 mL/min/month ($P = 0.1$). However, the declining value in the islet transplant group did not differ statistically from 0, nor from that expected in the general population (1 mL/min/yr). In contrast, in the medical group, the declining value was greater than zero and greater than in the general population.[40]

Retinopathy

In the same study, none of the patients after islet transplant had progression of retinopathy, or required eye surgery, whereas in the medical group, there was substantial progression of the eye disease and need for surgery.[40] Similar observation with stabilization of the retinal disease and occasional improvement can be found in other reports.[13,41]

Neuropathy

Improved glycemic control after islet transplantation leads to improvement or stabilization of neuropathy in more than 50% of patients.[41] These observations are exciting, as they were made after only a 2-year followup.

PATIENT SELECTION

Results of pancreas, as well as islet, transplantation constantly evolve, so algorithms for β-cell replacement therapy should be constantly updated. Nevertheless, medical indications for pancreas and islet transplantation remain the same.

Pancreas transplant candidates must be in good medical condition to safely survive major surgery. There is no age limit for pancreas transplantation. Younger patients have higher rates of rejection, but those older than 50 years of age have higher postoperative complication rates.

The most appropriate type of pancreas transplant depends on patient comorbidity, renal function, and availability of living or cadaveric donor. Patients with hypoglycemic unawareness and stable kidney function (GFR, 80-100 mL/min/1.73 m^2) may be candidates for PTA or ITA, depending on whether the patient can tolerate major surgery. However, 30% of those patients will require a kidney transplant in 9 to 10 years because of calcineurin-inhibitor nephrotoxicity, which is an independent risk factor for progression of kidney failure.[2] If a patient has a GFR less than 80 mL/min/1.73 m^2, they will most likely require a kidney graft in the future. Patients with a GFR of less than 50 to 60 mL/min/1.73 m^2 will likely need a kidney graft before, with, or soon after the pancreas. Of course, preemptive LDKT would be the best option for these patients.

SPK transplantation would be the best option for uremic type 1 diabetics because long-term results are the best for combined kidney and pancreas grafts. However, because of the shortage of deceased-donor organs, instead of waiting long on dialysis for proper organs and developing complications, a better option is to have a preemptive LDKT followed by deceased-donor pancreas transplant. Immediate results of PAK transplantation in such situations are good, because the patient has never been uremic. Patient survival for LDKT and SPK transplantation are comparable.[2]

REFERENCES

1. The Diabetes Control and Complications Trial Research Group: The effect of intensive treatment of diabetes on the development and progression of long-term complications in insulin-dependent diabetes mellitus. *N Engl J Med* 329:977, 1993.
2. White SA, Shaw JA, Sutherland DE: Pancreas transplantation. *Lancet* 373:1808, 2009.
3. Hering B, Bellin M, Barton F: Induction immunosuppression with T-cell depleting antibodies facilitates long-term insulin independence after islet allotransplantation in type I diabetes. *Am J Transplant* 10:141, 2010.
4. Clinical Islet Transplantation Consortium: Clinical islet transplantation study. Available at http://www.isletstudy.org/
5. Kelly WD, Lillehei RC, Merkel FK, et al: Allotransplantation of the pancreas and duodenum along with the kidney in diabetic nephropathy. *Surgery* 61:827, 1967.
6. Gruessner AC, Sutherland DE, Gruessner RW: Pancreas transplantation in the United States: A review. *Curr Opin Organ Transplant* 15:93, 2010.
7. Moskalewski S: Isolation and culture of the islets of Langerhans of the guinea pig. *Gen Comp Endocrinol* 44:342, 1965.
8. Lacy PE, Kostianovsky M: Method for the isolation of intact islets of Langerhans from the rat pancreas. *Diabetes* 16:35, 1967.
9. Scharp DW, Murphy JJ, Newton WT, et al: Transplantation of islets of Langerhans in diabetic rhesus monkeys. *Surgery* 77:100, 1975.
10. Najarian JS, Sutherland DE, Matas AJ, et al: Human islet transplantation: A preliminary report. *Transplant Proc* 9:233, 1977.
11. Tzakis AG, Ricordi C, Alejandro R, et al: Pancreatic islet transplantation after upper abdominal exenteration and liver replacement. *Lancet* 336:402, 1990.
12. Shapiro AM, Lakey JR, Ryan EA, et al: Islet transplantation in seven patients with type 1 diabetes mellitus using a glucocorticoid-free immunosuppressive regimen. *N Engl J Med* 343:230, 2000.
13. Collaborative Islet Transplant Registry (CITR): Website http://www.citregistry.org/.
14. Leeser DB, Bartlett ST: Pancreas transplantation. In Yeo CJ, Dempsey DT, Klein AS, et al, editors: *Shackelford's surgery of the alimentary tract*, ed 6. Philadelphia, 2005, Saunders, p 1415.
15. O'Gorman D, Kin T, Murdoch T, et al: The standardization of pancreatic donors for islet isolations. *Transplantation* 80:801, 2005.
16. Boggi U, Amorese G, Marchetti P: Surgical techniques for pancreas transplantation. *Curr Opin Organ Transplant* 15:102, 2010.
17. Sutherland DE, Goetz FC, Najarian JS: Living-related donor segmental pancreatectomy for transplantation. *Transplant Proc* 12:19, 1980.
18. University of Minnesota: International Pancreas Transplant Registry (IPTR). Available at http://www.iptr.umn.edu/.
19. Troppmann C: Complications after pancreas transplantation. *Curr Opin Organ Transplant* 15:112, 2010.
20. Chandra J, Phillips RR, Boardman P, et al: Pancreas transplants. *Clin Radiol* 64:714, 2009.
21. Tyden G, Bolinder J, Solders G, et al: Improved survival in patients with insulin-dependent diabetes mellitus and end-stage diabetic nephropathy 10 years after combined pancreas and kidney transplantation. *Transplantation* 67:645, 1999.
22. Reddy KS, Stablein D, Taranto S, et al: Long-term survival following simultaneous kidney-pancreas transplantation versus kidney transplantation alone in patients with type 1 diabetes mellitus and renal failure. *Am J Kidney Dis* 41:464, 2003.
23. Ojo AO, Meier-Kriesche HU, Hanson JA, et al: The impact of simultaneous pancreas-kidney transplantation on long-term patient survival. *Transplantation* 71:82, 2001.
24. Venstrom JM, McBride MA, Rother KI, et al: Survival after pancreas transplantation in patients with diabetes and preserved kidney function. *JAMA* 290:2817, 2003.
25. Gruessner RW, Sutherland DE, Gruessner AC: Mortality assessment for pancreas transplants. *Am J Transplant* 4:2018, 2004.
26. Sutherland DE, Gruessner RW, Dunn DL, et al: Lessons learned from more than 1,000 pancreas transplants at a single institution. *Ann Surg* 233:463, 2001.

27. Larsen JL: Pancreas transplantation: Indications and consequences. *Endocr Rev* 25:919, 2004.
28. Ramsay RC, Goetz FC, Sutherland DE, et al: Progression of diabetic retinopathy after pancreas transplantation for insulin-dependent diabetes mellitus. *N Engl J Med* 318:208, 1988.
29. Dean PG, Kudva YC, Stegall MD: Long-term benefits of pancreas transplantation. *Curr Opin Organ Transplant* 13:85, 2008.
30. Fioretto P, Steffes MW, Sutherland DE, et al: Reversal of lesions of diabetic nephropathy after pancreas transplantation. *N Engl J Med* 339:69, 1998.
31. Navarro X, Sutherland DE, Kennedy WR: Long-term effects of pancreatic transplantation on diabetic neuropathy. *Ann Neurol* 42:727, 1997.
32. Stratta RJ: Mortality after vascularized pancreas transplantation. *Surgery* 124:823, 1998.
33. La Rocca E, Fiorina P, di Carlo V, et al: Cardiovascular outcomes after kidney-pancreas and kidney-alone transplantation. *Kidney Int* 60:1964, 2001.
34. Ryan EA, Paty BW, Senior PA, et al: Five-year follow-up after clinical islet transplantation. *Diabetes* 54:2060, 2005.
35. Rickels MR, Kearns J, Markmann E, et al: HLA sensitization in islet transplantation. *Clin Transpl* 413, 2006.
36. Cardani R, Pileggi A, Ricordi C, Gomez C, et al: Allosensitization of islet allograft recipients. *Transplantation* 84:1413, 2007.
37. Campbell PM, Senior PA, Salam A, et al: High risk of sensitization after failed islet transplantation. *Am J Transplant* 7:2311, 2007.
38. Koh A, Imes S, Kin T, et al: Supplemental islet infusions restore insulin independence after graft dysfunction in islet transplant recipients. *Transplantation* 89:361, 2010.
39. Hering BJ, Kandaswamy R, Ansite JD, et al: Single-donor, marginal-dose islet transplantation in patients with type 1 diabetes. *JAMA* 293:830, 2005.
40. Warnock GL, Thompson DM, Meloche RM, et al: A multi-year analysis of islet transplantation compared with intensive medical therapy on progression of complications in type 1 diabetes. *Transplantation* 86:1762, 2008.
41. Lee TC, Barshes NR, O'Mahony CA, et al: The effect of pancreatic islet transplantation on progression of diabetic retinopathy and neuropathy. *Transplant Proc* 37:2263, 2005.

Autologous Islet Cell Transplantation

John D. Christein | Christopher W. Snyder

Autologous pancreatic islet cell transplantation, or islet autotransplantation (IAT), is an adjunct to pancreatic resection that aims to preserve endocrine function without a need for immunosuppression. The purpose of this chapter is to provide an overview of IAT indications, preoperative workup, techniques, and published outcomes.

ISLET CELL PHYSIOLOGY AND BRITTLE DIABETES

The average adult pancreas weighs 70 g and contains 1 to 2 million endocrine islets of Langerhans, which constitute only 0.8% to 3.8% of the total gland mass.[1] The islets are scattered throughout the gland but are most highly concentrated in the tail. Each islet measures approximately 76 by 175 μm and consists of an ovoid collection of multiple endocrine cells.[2] Each islet cell type produces a unique profile of important gastrointestinal hormones (Table 99-1), which contribute to a complex milieu of regulation and counterregulation to achieve glycemic homeostasis.

The predominant islet cell type is the insulin-producing B cell. Insulin has multiple complex physiologic effects, but is best known for its rapid hypoglycemic effect, which is produced by increased transport of glucose into insulin receptor–bearing cells. The net effect of this "hormone of abundance" is storage of fat, protein, and carbohydrate.

Glucagon is secreted by the A islet cells and generates glycogenolytic, gluconeogenic, lipolytic, and ketogenic effects, thus acting as the primary counterregulatory hormone for insulin. The F cells produce pancreatic polypeptide, which is believed to regulate the rate of food absorption. Somatostatin is produced by the D islet cell type and inhibits the secretion of insulin, glucagon, and pancreatic polypeptide. The islet cell types are spatially arranged within each islet in such a way that they regulate one another; each islet is believed to function as a secretory unit. However, these secretory units are not all identical. At least two types of islets—glucagon-rich and pancreatic polypeptide-rich—have been described, but their relationship and physiologic significance are poorly understood.

When a critical mass of islet cells is lost, as occurs in end-stage chronic pancreatitis or after extensive pancreatic resection, "pancreatogenic diabetes" or "brittle diabetes" ensues. Because of the loss of both insulin and counterregulatory hormones, patients with this condition have great difficulty achieving glycemic homeostasis and are prone to both hypoglycemia and hyperglycemia. Hypoglycemic unawareness is a particularly concerning feature of brittle diabetes; in this condition, hypoglycemia produces cerebral dysfunction (e.g., syncope) without the usual early warning symptoms of tremor, diaphoresis, and anxiety. Brittle diabetes has been associated with increased rates of diabetic complications, decreased quality of life, and higher mortality relative to stable diabetics.[3]

CHRONIC PANCREATITIS

Chronic pancreatitis (CP) is characterized by persistent inflammation and fibrosis of the pancreas, resulting in damage to the ductal system, exocrine acinar cells, and endocrine islets of Langerhans. The prevalence of CP in a recent population-based study was 12 per 100,000 women and 45 per 100,0000 men.[4] Although several studies suggest that the incidence and prevalence of CP are rising, it is unclear whether these findings are attributable to more frequent abdominal imaging and more inclusive diagnostic criteria.[5] In the United States, long-term alcohol use is the most common cause of CP, comprising approximately 70% of cases. However, CP can arise from multiple causes, including other toxins, autoimmune and genetic factors, obstruction, recurrent severe acute pancreatitis, and idiopathic causes.[6]

CP manifests clinically as abdominal pain and progressive loss of pancreatic function. Pain varies considerably from patient to patient, but is often severe, chronic, and disabling. Exocrine insufficiency occurs early, with variable degrees of malabsorption and steatorrhea. Islet cells are often preserved for a prolonged period despite extensive fibrosis (Figure 99-1), but eventually endocrine insufficiency occurs and diabetes ensues. The prevalence of impaired glucose tolerance among patients with long-term CP is 60% to 80%. Of CP patients, 30% to 35% require insulin, and the prevalence of diabetes increases with longer duration of disease.[7-9] CP is also an established risk factor for pancreatic carcinoma, carrying a cumulative risk of 1.8% and 4% at 10 and 20 years after diagnosis, respectively.[10-13]

DIAGNOSIS AND TREATMENT OF CHRONIC PANCREATITIS

Because biopsies of the pancreas for histologic analysis are difficult to obtain, the diagnosis of CP depends on radiologic evidence of pancreatic inflammation and fibrosis, along with concordant clinical manifestations.[14,15] At our institution, diagnostic workup of CP begins with a complete history and physical examination and a contrast-enhanced computed tomography (CT) scan of the abdomen. CT findings consistent with CP include

TABLE 99-1 Islet Cell Content

Cell Type	Percent	Hormonal Content
B (β)	50-80	Insulin
A (α)	15-20	Glucagon
F	15-20	Pancreatic polypeptide
D (δ)	5-10	Somatostatin
D1	<1	VIP
EC	<1	Substance P
G	<1	Gastrin

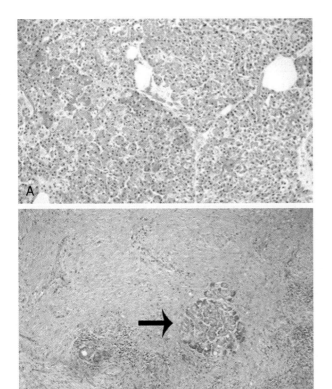

FIGURE 99-1 Preservation of islet cells in setting of chronic pancreatitis: **A,** Normal pancreatic architecture. **B,** Extensive fibrosis with preserved islets *(arrow).*

ductal calcifications, ductal stricturing, and other ductal abnormalities.

Treatment of CP focuses on relieving pain and replacing pancreatic function. Initial conservative treatment measures include avoidance of precipitating factors such as alcohol, appropriate pain control, and supplementation. Many patients are already narcotic-dependent at the time of presentation. Malabsorption and malnutrition from compromised exocrine function are treated with pancreatic enzymes and nutritional supplements. Diabetes from advanced CP with endocrine insufficiency is treated with insulin replacement. Chronic pancreatitis is a multifaceted disease, and the importance of a multidisciplinary approach cannot be overemphasized. A multidisciplinary team that includes gastroenterology, interventional endoscopy, diagnostic and interventional radiology, gastrointestinal surgery, and endocrinology is necessary for the optimal management of the patient.

Endoscopic retrograde cholangiopancreatography (ERCP) and endoscopic ultrasound (EUS) are useful modalities for both diagnosis and treatment. Diagnostic criteria for CP based on EUS features have been described.[16] EUS and ERCP define ductal anatomy and complications of CP, such as pancreatic duct strictures and stones. With ERCP, strictures can be dilated and/or stented, and stones can be treated with sphincterotomy, dilation, or lithotripsy. Unfortunately, such measures are highly endoscopist-dependent and only about 50% effective.[17,18]

Goals of surgical treatment are to provide durable relief from pain and obstruction, and to rule out malignancy in suspicious-appearing lesions.[19] The key to successful surgical treatment is adequate radiologic and endoscopic workup and proper patient selection. Operative treatments fall into two main categories: resection and drainage. Resection options include pancreaticoduodenectomy (Whipple procedure), distal pancreatectomy, and total pancreatectomy with or without islet cell autotransplantation. Drainage options include lateral pancreaticojejunostomy (Puestow procedure) and the Frey procedure. Patients with a dilated pancreatic duct (PD) on imaging studies, or large-duct disease, may be candidates for a drainage procedure.[20] Patients with a normal-caliber PD, or small-duct disease, may be candidates for resection. Figure 99-2 shows the current algorithm for management of chronic pancreatitis used at our institution.

RATIONALE AND HISTORY OF ISLET CELL AUTOTRANSPLANTATION

Although surgical resection provides durable relief of pain in a majority of patients with chronic pancreatitis, the removal of endocrine pancreatic tissue often results in diabetes. Pancreaticoduodenectomy results in diabetes in up to 40% of patients.[21] In addition, up to 30% of patients who undergo partial pancreatic resection procedures may eventually require completion pancreatectomy.[22-24] Total pancreatectomy provides effective pain relief in 58% to 70% of patients but places the patient in an apancreatic state, with accompanying brittle diabetes that may severely compromise quality of life.[25]

IAT was conceived as a means to avoid the morbidity of brittle diabetes induced by extensive pancreatic resection. Because islets are preserved until late in the course of the disease, viable islets often remain despite severe fibrosis and exocrine insufficiency. IAT seeks to give these viable islets back to the patient, allowing autologous endocrine pancreatic function to be maintained. The relatively small islet mass must be separated from the surrounding exocrine tissue and purified in such a way that the islets remain viable. The resulting islet cell preparation must then be reinfused safely into an anatomic site where the islets can engraft and maintain long-term viability and function.

Islet isolation was first attempted for the purpose of allogeneic transplantation and was successfully

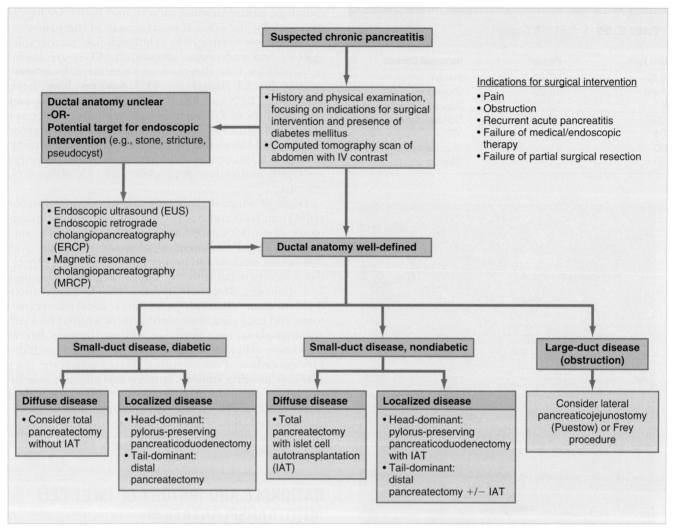

FIGURE 99-2 Treatment algorithm for chronic pancreatitis, with incorporation of islet autotransplantation. *IV,* Intravenous.

performed in rats in 1967.[1] In 1972 at Washington University, Dr. Paul E. Lacy and colleagues successfully reversed chemically induced diabetes mellitus in rats with allogeneic islet transplantation. Subsequently, the fields of human allogeneic and autologous islet transplantation have developed in parallel. Many of the challenges of the field are common to both procedures, including the development of isolation techniques to maximize purity and viability and choosing an anatomic site for safe infusion and engraftment. Both approaches have achieved good islet function initially, but must contend with diminishing islet function over time. IAT does have an advantage over allogeneic transplantation in that it involves autologous tissue, thereby avoiding the problems of tissue rejection and immunosuppression.

In 1977, Dr. David Sutherland and colleagues at the University of Minnesota (UMN) performed the first IAT. UMN has the largest experience with IAT, having performed more than 200 procedures as of 2007. IAT requires significant multidisciplinary resources and expertise and is consequently performed at only a few specialized centers. Centers with published results include UMN, the University of Cincinnati (UC), Leicester General Hospital (LGH), the University of Alabama

at Birmingham (UAB), the University of Geneva (U Geneva), the Medical University of South Carolina (MUSC), and Baylor University Medical Center (Baylor). Other institutions performing this procedure in the United States include the Mayo Clinic, Weill Cornell Medical College, the University of Pittsburgh, the University of Chicago, and the University of Arizona. Table 99-2 provides a review of current published institutional series of IAT. Some centers also rarely perform IAT after pancreatic resection for benign tumors or trauma[26]; these cases are not included in this review.

TECHNIQUE

The surgical procedure follows standard techniques for total pancreatectomy with splenectomy and reconstruction described elsewhere. However, special attention is given to preserving the arterial supply to the pancreas for as long as possible to minimize islet warm ischemia time. To accomplish this, the splenic artery is divided first, followed by the gastroduodenal artery. The pancreaticoduodenal artery is divided at the last possible moment and the specimen is handed off the field for processing.

A separate table is set up in the operating room to receive the resected pancreas and prepare it for islet isolation. The pancreas is immediately submerged in University of Wisconsin (UW) solution (Viaspan) at 4° C, where the peripancreatic fat is removed and the pancreatic duct cannulated with a small angiocatheter if patent. To rule out cancer, multiple biopsies are taken from the head, body, and tail of the pancreas and sent for frozen-section analysis.

The skeletonized pancreas is then transported in fresh, cold UW solution to the processing facility, where it is intraductally perfused or interstitially injected with a solution containing collagenase NB1 and neutral protease. The distended pancreas is divided in several pieces and placed into a 500-mL metallic chamber containing metallic marbles and a 500-μm-pore-sized steel mesh screen. The tissue is mechanically and enzymatically dissociated using a semiautomated technique described by Ricordi et al. Digested samples are collected at regular intervals to monitor the dissociation of islets from exocrine tissue following dithizone staining. When the digestion is judged to be complete, the process is terminated by adding human albumin, diluting the islet-containing solution, and lowering the temperature of the system (7° to 20° C).

To maximize islet yields, islet preparations with packed cell volume less than 15 mL are not purified. If required, islet purification is performed in a COBE 2991 Cell Processor using discontinuous density gradients. Aliquots of the final product are taken for determination of islet counts, purity, viability, sterility, and endotoxin content. To prepare the final islet infusion, islets are resuspended in 200 mL of Transplant Media (CMRL 1066-based) supplemented with 20% human albumin, HEPES 1 M, ciprofloxacin 1%, and heparin (35 to 70 units/kg recipient body weight) and returned to the operating room. Islets were infused into the liver via portal vein injection or through the middle colic vein by gravity using a closed-bag system.

OUTCOMES AND COMPLICATIONS

A summary of published institutional series of IAT is provided in Table 99-2. Reported complications specific to IAT are usually related to islet infusion and include portal vein thrombosis, portal hypertension, disseminated intravascular coagulation, hepatic infarction, and liver failure. However, these complications occurred in the early 1980s before the introduction of semiautomated processing techniques and routine use of heparinization.

METABOLIC OUTCOMES

Islet yields are measured in islet equivalents (IEQ). A summary of islet yields and metabolic outcomes from published institutional series is provided in Table 99-3.

Islet yield has been shown to be affected by multiple factors and maximizing yield remains a

TABLE 99-2 Published Institutional Series of Islet Cell Autotransplantation After Resection for Chronic Pancreatitis

Institution	Number of Patients	Age (Mean)	Etiology	Followup Time	Mean Operative Time	30-Day Mortality	Complication Rate, n (%)	Mean Length of Hospital Stay
UMN[13,24,27]	N = 136 (93% total*, 7% partial)	36 yr	43% idiopathic	4 mo-22 yr	10 hr	1/48 (2%) 1977-1995	12/48 (25%) 1977-1995	22 d
UC[22]	N = 45 (91% total, 9% partial)	39 yr	87% idiopathic	Median, 18 mo (range, 1-46 mo)	8.9 hr	1/45 (2%)	19/45 (42%)	11 d (insulin dependent), 15 d (insulin independent)
LGH[28,29]	N = 46	43 yr	50% idiopathic	3 mo-10 yr	NR	1/46 (2%)	9/24 (38%), 1994-1999	21 d
UAB[23]	N = 27 (77% total, 23% partial)	44 yr	35% alcoholic	Mean, 6.5 mo	6.9 hr	0/27 (0%)	16/27 (59%)	10 d
U Geneva[26]	N = 7 (86% total, 14% partial)	NR	NR	Median, 51 mo (range, 22-72 mo)	NR	0/7 (0%)	NR	NR
MUSC[30]	N = 7	16-50 yr	57% sphincter of Oddi dysfunction	NR	NR	0/7 (0%)	NR	NR
Baylor[31]	N = 17	40 yr	53% idiopathic	Mean, 7.3 mo	NR	NR	NR	NR

NR, Not reported.
*Includes completion and near-total (≥95%) pancreatectomies.

TABLE 99-3 Islet Yield and Metabolic Outcomes After Islet Cell Autotransplantation

Institution	Total Islet Equivalents (IEQ), Mean	IEQ Per Kilogram Body Weight	Discharge Insulin Requirement (units/day)	No. (%) of Patients Insulin Independent
UMN[13,24,27]	238,010 (1977-1995)	3996 if no pancreatic surgery, 3687 if previous resection, 1531 if previous Puestow (1977-2004)	NR	20/39 (51%) at 1 yr, 34% at 2 yr (1977-1995); if >2500 IEQ/kg received, 72% complete independence, 14% partial independence (1995-2004)
UC[22]	297,889 (dependent), 413,542 (independent)	3749 dependent, 6635 independent	18.9 dependent, 5.7 independent	18/45 (40%)
LGH[28,29]	130,108 (range, 24,332-1,165,538)	2605	NR	10/24 (42%) transient independence, 7/9 (78%) if >2500 IEQ/kg received
UAB[23]	82,094	1331 (3145 total, 1317 partial)	10.7 (11.0 total, 5.0 partial)	4/26 (18%)
U Geneva[26]	129,101	2167	NR	5/7 (71%) transiently independent for 8-54 mo (median, 36 mo)
MUSC[30]	NR	NR	NR	1/5 (20%)
Baylor[31]	168,000 (low-yield), 573,000 (high-yield)	2717 (low-yield), 7556 (high-yield)	NR	8/17 (47%)

NR, Not reported.

challenge. Gruessner et al demonstrated that the type and extent of previous pancreatic surgery affects islet yield.[24] Patients with a previous Puestow procedure had median yields of 1052 IEQ/kg body weight, whereas those with distal pancreatectomy, Whipple, or no surgery had median yields of 2112, 4719, and 3249 IEQ/kg, respectively. Takita et al found that higher degrees of preoperative radiographic pancreatic inflammation, as measured by CT, EUS, or ERCP, were predictive of lower islet yield (<5000 IEQ/kg).[31]

Clear prognostic factors for insulin independence after IAT have proven elusive. It is intuitive that patients receiving greater numbers of IEQ per kilogram body weight would have a greater likelihood of remaining insulin independent. The UMN series demonstrated a strong correlation between insulin independence and the number of islet equivalents transplanted,[27] leading this group to report that a minimum of 2000 to 2500 IEQ/kg are required for insulin independence. However, other groups have found no correlation between long-term insulin requirements and number of islets transplanted. In the LGH series, several patients receiving <2000 IEQ/kg had low or no insulin requirements at 1 year.[28] Clear conclusions regarding insulin independence after IAT are limited by varying definitions (i.e., partial vs. complete independence) as well as various reporting time points (discharge, 1 year, 5 years, etc.) in the published literature. Initial complete insulin independence has been achieved in 18% to 72% of patients in the current series, but in most cases this independence is transient and some insulin supplementation is eventually required. However, transplanted islet cells do maintain long-term function, as evidenced by persistent C-peptide levels, which may be sufficient to prevent the development of brittle diabetes. Insulin requirements after IAT are likely dependent on multiple factors, and complete independence from insulin may not be a consistently achievable goal. Diabetes that is well controlled with moderate doses of insulin may be a more reasonable goal and provide similar quality of life. Several series have demonstrated no complications of brittle diabetes after IAT.[23]

PATIENT-ORIENTED OUTCOMES

Chronic pain is usually the most disabling manifestation of CP and the primary indication for surgical resection. Table 99-4 provides a summary of patient-oriented outcomes in published IAT series. As with metabolic outcomes, conclusions are limited by various nonstandardized measures of pain control and quality of life in the published literature. However, a majority of patients do report decreased pain after pancreatic resection. UAB found significant reduction in pain scores at 6 months and 1 year after pancreatic resection with IAT using the validated McGill Pain Questionnaire. Significant increases in health-related quality of life by the Short Form 36 (SF-36) questionnaire at 1 year were also observed.

CONCLUSION

Islet cell autotransplantation has been shown to be effective in preventing or lessening the metabolic impact of pancreatogenic diabetes after resection. Current surgical treatment for chronic pancreatitis consists of drainage procedures for large-duct disease and resection for small-duct disease in appropriate operative candidates. This current criterion standard is well established and should not be abandoned. IAT should be considered as an adjunctive procedure as part of a multidisciplinary approach at specialized centers.

TABLE 99-4 Patient-Oriented Outcomes After Islet Cell Autotransplantation

Institution	Pain	Quality of Life
UMN[13,24,27]	90% pain resolved or improved, 50% narcotic independent*	NR
UC[22]	26/45 (58%) narcotic independent; overall mean daily morphine equivalents decreased from 206 to 90.	22-patient subset (2000-2003) had improved scores on SF-36 at 19-mo followup
LGH[28,29]	16/21 (76%) narcotic independent, 4/21 (19%) persistent but decreased narcotic use	NR
UAB[23]	2/14 (14%) and 3/5 (60%) narcotic independent at 3 and 6 mo; decreased pain on McGill Pain Scale (56%-20% of maximum total score) and Visual Analogue Scale (63%-24% of maximum)*	Significant improvements in SF-36 Physical and Mental Component Scores at 6 mo and 1 year*
MUSC[30]	0/5 (0%) narcotic independent	Decreased hospitalizations (2.8-1.0) and clinic visits (16.6-7.2) per year
Baylor[31]	6/17 (35%) narcotic independent, significant decrease in mean daily morphine equivalents	NR

NR, Not reported.
*Unpublished data.

REFERENCES

1. Truong W, Shapiro AMJ: Islet transplantation. In Yeo C, et al, editors: *Shackelford's surgery of the alimentary tract*, Philadelphia, 2006, Saunders, p 1422.
2. Ganong WF: *Review of medical physiology*, ed 22. New York, 2005, McGraw-Hill.
3. Kent LA, Gill GV, Williams G: Mortality and outcome of patients with brittle diabetes and recurrent ketoacidosis. *Lancet* 344:778, 1994.
4. Lin Y, Tamakoshi A, Matsuno S, et al: Nationwide epidemiological survey of chronic pancreatitis in Japan. *J Gastroenterol* 35:136, 2000.
5. Nair RJ, Lawler L, Miller MR: Chronic pancreatitis. *Am Fam Physician* 76:1679, 2007.
6. Etemad B, Whitcomb DC: Chronic pancreatitis: Diagnosis, classification, and new genetic developments. *Gastroenterology* 120:682, 2001.
7. Bank S, Marks IN, Vinik AI: Clinical and hormonal aspects of pancreatic diabetes. *Am J Gastroenterol* 64:13, 1975.
8. Angelopoulos N, Dervenis C, Goula A, et al: Endocrine pancreatic insufficiency in chronic pancreatitis. *Pancreatology* 5:122, 2005.
9. Larsen S, Hilsted J, Tronier B, et al: Metabolic control and B cell function in patients with insulin-dependent diabetes mellitus secondary to chronic pancreatitis. *Metabolism* 36:964, 1987.
10. Warshaw AL, Banks PA, Fernandez-Del Castillo C: AGA technical review: Treatment of pain in chronic pancreatitis. *Gastroenterology* 115:765, 1998.
11. Lowenfels AB, Maisonneuve P, Cavallini G, et al: Pancreatitis and the risk of pancreatic cancer. International Pancreatitis Study Group. *N Engl J Med* 328:1433, 1993.
12. Lankisch PG: Natural course of chronic pancreatitis. *Pancreatology* 1:3, 2001.
13. Blondet JJ, Carlson AM, Kobayashi T, et al: The role of total pancreatectomy and islet autotransplantation for chronic pancreatitis. *Surg Clin North Am* 87:1477, 2007.
14. Sarner M, Cotton PB: Classification of pancreatitis. *Gut* 25:756, 1984.
15. Homma T, Harada H, Koizumi M: Diagnostic criteria for chronic pancreatitis by the Japan Pancreas Society. *Pancreas* 15:14, 1997.
16. Raimondo M, Wallace MB: Diagnosis of early chronic pancreatitis by endoscopic ultrasound. Are we there yet? *JOP* 5:1, 2004.
17. Topazian M, Aslanian H, Andersen D: Outcome following endoscopic stenting of pancreatic duct strictures in chronic pancreatitis. *J Clin Gastroenterol* 39:908, 2005.
18. Guda NM, Freeman ML, Smith C: Role of extracorporeal shock wave lithotripsy in the treatment of pancreatic stones. *Rev Gastroenterol Disord* 5:73, 2005.
19. Sakorafas GH, Farnell MB, Nagorney DM, et al: Surgical management of chronic pancreatitis at the Mayo Clinic. *Surg Clin North Am* 81:457, 2001.
20. Prinz RA, Greenlee HB: Pancreatic duct drainage in 100 patients with chronic pancreatitis. *Ann Surg* 194:313, 1981.
21. Sakorafas GH, Farnell MB, Nagorney DM, et al: Pancreatoduodenectomy for chronic pancreatitis: Long-term results in 105 patients. *Arch Surg* 135:517; discussion 523, 2000.
22. Ahmad SA, Lowy AM, Wray CJ, et al: Factors associated with insulin and narcotic independence after islet autotransplantation in patients with severe chronic pancreatitis. *J Am Coll Surg* 201:680, 2005.
23. Argo JL, Contreras JL, Wesley MM, et al: Pancreatic resection with islet cell autotransplant for the treatment of severe chronic pancreatitis. *Am Surg* 74:530; discussion 536, 2008.
24. Gruessner RW, Sutherland DE, Dunn DL, et al: Transplant options for patients undergoing total pancreatectomy for chronic pancreatitis. *J Am Coll Surg* 198:559; discussion 568, 2004.
25. Petrin P, Andreoli A, Antoniutti M, et al: Surgery for chronic pancreatitis: What quality of life ahead? *World J Surg* 19:398, 1995.
26. Oberholzer J, Triponez F, Mage R, et al: Human islet transplantation: Lessons from 13 autologous and 13 allogeneic transplantations. *Transplantation* 69:1115, 2000.
27. Wahoff DC, Papalois BE, Najarian JS, et al: Autologous islet transplantation to prevent diabetes after pancreatic resection. *Ann Surg* 222:562; discussion 575, 1995.
28. Webb MA, Illouz SC, Pollard CA, et al: Islet auto transplantation following total pancreatectomy: A long-term assessment of graft function. *Pancreas* 37:282, 2008.
29. Clayton HA, Davies JE, Pollard CA, et al: Pancreatectomy with islet autotransplantation for the treatment of severe chronic pancreatitis: The first 40 patients at the Leicester General Hospital. *Transplantation* 76:92, 2003.
30. Dixon J, DeLegge M, Morgan KA, et al: Impact of total pancreatectomy with islet cell transplant on chronic pancreatitis management at a disease-based center. *Am Surg* 74:735, 2008.
31. Takita M, Naziruddin B, Matsumoto S, et al: Variables associated with islet yield in autologous islet cell transplantation for chronic pancreatitis. *Proc (Bayl Univ Med Cent)* 23:115, 2010.

Unusual Pancreatic Tumors

Susan Tsai | Melinda M. Mortenson | Huamin Wang |

Eric P. Tamm | Douglas B. Evans

Pancreatic ductal adenocarcinoma and cystic neo-plasms of the pancreas account for the majority of all pancreatic neoplasms. However, there is a subset of rare and unusual conditions of the pancreas that have been increasingly identified over the last two decades, in part by increased use of computed tomography (CT). These conditions can often be challenging to clinicians, as the presentation and diagnostic findings can often mimic pancreatic ductal adenocarcinoma. This chapter will focus on these less appreciated lesions and will discuss the optimal diagnostic and therapeutic approaches to their management.

SOLID PSEUDOPAPILLARY TUMOR

Solid pseudopapillary tumors (SPTs) of the pancreas are rare neoplasms with low malignant potential that were first described in 1959.[1] Historically, several other names have been associated with this tumor, including Franz tumors, Hamoudi tumors, and papillary cystic neoplasm. In 1996, the World Health Organization (WHO) classified these tumors as SPTs and further defined malignant SPTs as those tumors with histologic characteristics of angioinvasion, perineural invasion, or extension into the surrounding pancreatic parenchyma.[2] It is estimated that SPTs represent approximately 2% of all pancreatic tumors and 9% of pancreatic cystic neoplasms.[3] The largest review of the literature included 718 patients over a 70-year time period.[4] The authors observed that the prevalence of SPT is 10-fold higher in women than in men and affected predominantly younger individuals (mean age, 22 years; range, 2 to 85 years).

CLINICOPATHOLOGIC FEATURES

More than 80% of patients with SPT present with symptoms, the most common being pain (45%) and/or an abdominal mass (34%).[4] In the asymptomatic patient, the tumors may also be discovered as a palpable mass on routine physical examination or as an incidental finding on imaging for an unrelated complaint. Although SPT can occur throughout the pancreas, they are slightly more common in the pancreatic tail and, when discovered, are generally large in size (mean diameter, 6 cm; range, 0.5 to 34.5 cm). On CT imaging, SPTs are characteristically large, heterogeneously enhancing lesions with solid and cystic components, and they frequently demonstrate peripheral enhancement and variable calcification (Figure 100-1). Although SPTs are often categorized as cystic lesions, they do not form true cysts; rather the cystic appearance is secondary to necrotic degeneration of the primary cytoarchitecture. The solid papillary

vascular stalks within the tumor slough and hemorrhage as the tumor increases in size, resulting in cystic degeneration. The differential diagnosis of a predominantly cystic SPT should include other cystic neoplasms including mucinous or serous cystadenomas and intraductal papillary mucinous neoplasms, as well as cystic degeneration of a typically solid neoplasm, such as a pancreatic neuroendocrine tumor or acinar cell cancer.

Fine-needle aspiration (FNA) biopsy may be useful when routine imaging is inconclusive and diagnostic uncertainty exists; however, because of the tumor's largely necrotic composition, FNA biopsy can be nondiagnostic. Characteristic cytologic features of SPTs include branching papillary fronds with sheets and cords of cells arranged around a fibrovascular septa. The cells contain eosinophilic granules rich in α_1-antitrypsin and the nuclei are typically grooved. The immunophenotype is nonspecific with positive staining for vimentin, α_1-antitrypsin, neuron-specific enolase, CD10, and CD56.[5] Keratins, chromogranin, synaptophysin, and endocrine and pancreatic enzymes are generally not expressed. In addition, SPTs often stain positive for progesterone receptors, while estrogen receptor positivity is more variable.[6]

The molecular changes associated with the development of SPT have been well described and are distinct from the pattern of mutations seen in pancreatic ductal adenocarcinoma. In particular, the genetic profile associated with SPT is different from PDAC, most notably for an absence of KRAS and DPC4 mutations. SPTs are characterized by the presence of an activating β-catenin gene mutation that interferes with protein phosphorylation.[7] This results in the accumulation of β-catenin within the cytoplasm and the subsequent translocation of β-catenin into the nucleus, where it functions as a transcriptional regulator of the cyclin D1 and c-myc genes.

TREATMENT

Given the unpredictable but real metastatic potential of these tumors, surgical resection is recommended for SPT. Although these tumors may be extremely large and can invade critical vasculature, most lesions are usually amenable to complete resection. Pancreaticoduodenectomy or distal pancreatectomy is performed most commonly, with en bloc resection of involved adjacent organs when indicated. Complete margin-negative resection (R0) is associated with long-term disease-free survival; the impact of a microscopically positive margin of resection (R1) is not known. In a single-institution series of 24 patients, 17 of 19 patients underwent complete R0 resection. At a median followup of 8 years, no evidence of recurrent disease was present in all patients who received an R0 resection.[8] Multiple groups have reported that 10% to 15% of patients with SPT have metastases at the time of diagnosis or develop metastases at some point in the future.[8,9] The most common sites of metastases include liver, mesentery, and peritoneum. Several series have reported long-term survival following metastasectomy. Martin et al[8] have reported 4 patients who presented with synchronous liver metastases and underwent concurrent liver and pancreas resection. Although two patients recurred, three of the four patients were still alive at 6 months, 6 years, and 11 years of followup.

The 5-year survival rate for patients with resectable SPT is 95%. Tumor size, as well as vascular, lymphatic, or perineural invasion have not been useful in predicting recurrence. However, the presence of nuclear atypia and high mitotic rate may suggest an aggressive subtype.[10] Given the excellent survival rates following surgical resection alone, adjuvant systemic therapy is not routinely utilized. When metastatic disease develops, small series have reported excellent survival after complete metastasectomy. For unresectable metastatic disease, there are anecdotal case reports of success with regimens including cisplatin, 5-fluorouracil, or gemcitabine.[11,12] In addition, at least one series has suggested that SPT may be radiosensitive, with a report of one patient with an unresectable tumor treated with 40 Gy of external beam radiation therapy who demonstrated tumor response and symptom control at 3 years.[2]

ACINAR CELL CARCINOMA

Acinar cell carcinoma (ACC) is a rare tumor accounting for less than 1% of pancreatic cancers. It has a unique clinical presentation initially characterized by Berner in 1908. ACC mimics the growth pattern of normal pancreatic acini and often produces digestive enzymes such as trypsin, chymotrypsin, lipase, and amylase. In addition, ACC has been associated with lipase hypersecretion syndrome, a paraneoplastic syndrome that includes subcutaneous fat necrosis, polyarthralgia, and eosinophilia associated with elevated serum lipase related to ACC, but occurs in less than 10% of patients.[13] In contrast to SPT, ACC occurs more commonly in men than women (2:1) and primarily affects individuals in the sixth and seventh decades of life.

CLINICOPATHOLOGIC FEATURES

Patients with ACC may be asymptomatic or may present with nonspecific symptoms, such as abdominal pain, weight loss, and change in bowel function.[13,14] The most common signs at presentation are a palpable abdominal mass, jaundice, and elevated liver enzymes. ACCs tend to be large (ranging from 5 to 10 cm), unifocal lesions that are slightly more likely to occur in the head of pancreas. There are no specific laboratory studies that are highly sensitive for ACC, but serum lipase levels can be elevated in up to 25% of patients.[13] Serum tumor markers such as CA 19-9, AFP, and CEA are variably expressed.[15] Diagnostic imaging with either CT or magnetic resonance imaging (MRI) generally reveals an exophytic, well-circumscribed mass (Figure 100-2, A). The tumor may be solid or cystic in appearance with homogenous enhancement of the solid components, of variable nature when

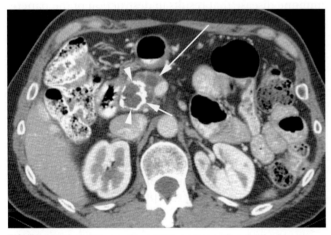

FIGURE 100-1 Solid pseudopapillary tumor with solid and cystic characteristics and coarse calcification.

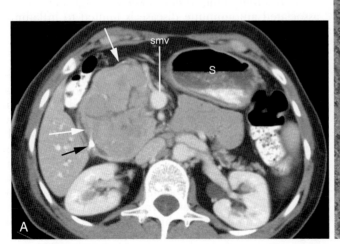
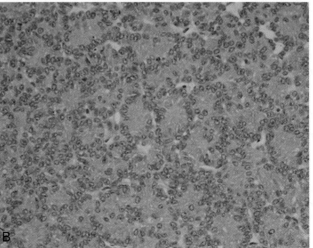

FIGURE 100-2 A, Large acinar cell carcinoma with local compression of the duodenum. **B,** Periodic acid–Schiff positivity.

compared with the surrounding normal pancreas. ACC may also demonstrate radiographic features that can be used to distinguish it from pancreatic ductal adenocarcinoma including a central hypodense area and internal foci of calcifications.[15] Mass effect may also be demonstrated with either biliary or pancreatic ductal dilation or duodenal invasion.[16] The differential diagnosis of ACC includes pancreatic ductal adenocarcinoma, pancreatic neuroendocrine tumor, SPT, pancreatoblastoma, and mucinous cystic neoplasm.

On histopathologic examination, pure ACCs have two predominant cellular patterns of growth: an acinar pattern consisting of cells growing in well-formed acini and a solid pattern characterized by sheets of cells in a fibrovascular stroma.[17] ACCs often stain positive for periodic acid–Schiff (PAS), corresponding to zymogen granules (Figure 100-2, *B*).[13] Mucin stains are typically negative. ACC displays an immunochemical staining pattern that is strongly positive for digestive enzymes, including trypsin, chymotrypsin, lipase, and phospholipase A_2.[13] In contrast to the staining pattern of pancreatic ductal adenocarcinoma, ACCs generally stain negative, for CEA, and mucicarmine. Although FNA biopsy can usually differentiate pancreatic ductal adenocarcinoma from ACC, the greater diagnostic dilemma is distinguishing between ACC and a well-differentiated pancreatic endocrine neoplasm and pancreatoblastoma. Because ACCs can be focally positive for endocrine markers, it may be difficult to distinguish between ACCs and endocrine neoplasms by cytology alone. Tumors that display both acinar and endocrine features that constitute more than 25% of cells have been termed "mixed acinar-endocrine carcinomas." On gross examination, the tumors are large, well–circumscribed lesions with scattered areas of hemorrhage and necrosis, and unlike pancreatic endocrine neoplasms, lack a desmoplastic stroma.

Although the molecular characterization of ACC has not been well established, ACCs generally do not exhibit the characteristic mutations observed in pancreatic ductal adenocarcinoma, such as KRAS, p53, p16, or DPC4. In addition, loss of heterozygosity at 3q and 16p are the most common alterations in pancreatic endocrine tumors, but these are relatively infrequent mutations in ACC and may be helpful in distinguishing between these two entities.[18] Finally, pancreatoblastoma frequently involves abnormalities of chromosome 1 (deletion), 6p, 13q, and 22q, which are uncommon in pancreatic ductal adenocarcinoma.[19] Abraham et al[20] evaluated 21 cases of ACC and observed allelic loss of 11p in 6 of 12 patients and molecular alterations in the APC/β-catenin pathway in 4 of 17 patients.

TREATMENT

Operative resection is the treatment of choice for patients with ACC. Although ACCs are generally large, they tend to be well circumscribed and are often amenable to complete surgical resection. Initially, the survival after resection of ACC was considered to be similar to that of pancreatic ductal adenocarcinoma. However, recent series have supported a slightly more favorable prognosis of ACC over pancreatic ductal adenocarcinoma. A recent

report from Memorial Sloan Kettering Cancer Center included 39 patients with resected ACC who had a median disease-free survival of 14 months and median actuarial survival of 36 months.[13] These data were supported by a series of 14 patients reported from the Johns Hopkins University in which the median and disease-free survival were 33 and 25 months, respectively.[14] Furthermore, in a recent review of the National Cancer Database, the 5-year survival rate of 865 patients who underwent resection for ACC was 36.2%.[21] Adjuvant gemcitabine is often administered after surgical resection; however, ACCs are generally less responsive to systemic chemotherapies than are pancreatic ductal adenocarcinoma.[21]

AUTOIMMUNE PANCREATITIS

Autoimmune pancreatitis (AIP) is a chronic inflammatory disease of the pancreas that was first recognized by Sarles et al[22] in 1961, and can mimic a pancreatic tumor. The true incidence of AIP is unknown because most reported series describe the incidence of AIP in the context of resected specimens, in which AIP accounts for 2% to 3% of such surgical specimens.[23,24] AIP is an autoimmune disease that results in destruction of the pancreatic parenchyma mediated by both humoral and cellular components. Histopathologic characteristics include diffuse lymphoplasmacytic infiltration, marked interstitial fibrosis, and acinar atrophy. More recently, the worldwide experience with AIP has suggested that there may be two subtypes with unique histopathologic and clinical characteristics.[25] In general, AIP in the Asian experience is more commonly described as having histopathologic features of lymphoplasmacytic sclerosing pancreatitis (type 1), as opposed to the experience in Europe and the Americas, which have additionally described a second subtype with characteristics of idiopathic duct-centric pancreatitis (type 2). The acceptance of the latter subtype remains controversial. Interestingly, these subtypes are associated with distinct clinical profiles. Type 1 patients are typically older men, who often have associated increases in serum IgG4 levels and radiographic evidence of extrapancreatic involvement. In contrast, type 2 AIP is seen with equal frequency in younger patients of both genders, often in the absence of elevated IgG4 levels, and associated autoimmune disease is limited to inflammatory bowel disease.[26]

CLINICOPATHOLOGIC FEATURES

AIP can have a variable presentation; however, jaundice, weight loss, and abdominal pain are common symptoms. The abdominal pain tends to be mild and variable in duration, lasting weeks to months. Jaundice has been reported in up to 70% to 80% of patients and is likely due to inflammation and narrowing of the distal common bile duct.[27] Up to 60% of patients are diabetic, the majority of whom have type 2 diabetes with impaired glucose tolerance. AIP can be associated with other autoimmune diseases; type 1 AIP has been associated with Sjögren syndrome, rheumatoid arthritis, primary sclerosing cholangitis, orbital pseudotumor, and inflammatory bowel disease.[28-32] Extrapancreatic organ involvement can occur prior to, synchronous with, or after the diagnosis of AIP; however, swelling of salivary and lacrimal glands tends to precede the onset of AIP.[33] Affected extrapancreatic organs demonstrate the characteristic lymphoplasmacytic infiltrate rich in immunoglobulin G4 (IgG4)–positive cells and can be helpful additional sites for biopsy to establish the correct diagnosis. In contrast to type 1 AIP, the only known association of an autoimmune disease with type 2 AIP is inflammatory bowel disease, which is prevalent in 30% of patients.[26]

The classic radiographic feature of AIP is a diffusely enlarged, sausage-shaped pancreas with homogeneous attenuation and moderate enhancement. In contrast to alcoholic pancreatitis, AIP often lacks the radiographic features of ductal dilation, calculi, and pseudocyst formation. The pancreatic duct may have a long narrow stricture with lack of upstream dilation or multiple noncontiguous strictures.[34] In addition, AIP may also present as a focal mass-forming lesion in the pancreas that can be easily confused with pancreatic ductal adenocarcinoma.[35] In such cases, serologic studies may aid in the diagnosis of AIP, and serum levels of IgG4 remain the main antibody of choice to support the diagnosis of AIP. However, the sensitivity and specificity of the serologic diagnosis of AIP may vary according to histologic subtype, with 80% of type 1 AIP demonstrating elevated serum IgG4 levels as opposed to only 17% of type 2 AIP.[36] Nevertheless, elevation of serum IgG above twice the upper limit of normal remains highly suggestive of AIP.[37] Recently, Frulloni et al[35] identified an antiplasminogen-binding peptide antibody that was elevated in 94% of AIP patients, with 100% sensitivity in the IgG4-negative cohort. Unfortunately, the antibody was positive in 5% of patients with pancreatic ductal adenocarcinoma, and therefore will not be of value in distinguishing cancer from AIP (see Table 100-1).

Cytopathology is useful in the diagnosis of AIP; however, there exists some controversy as to the classification of type 1 and 2 histologies. A consensus conference of experts from Japan, Korea, Europe, and the United States was convened in Honolulu in 2009 to establish histologic criteria for AIP (Table 100-1). Type 1 AIP has

three essential features: (1) lymphoplasmacytic infiltrate surrounding small-sized interlobular pancreatic ducts that spare the pancreatic ductal epithelium; (2) fibrosis centered around ducts and veins affecting predominantly the peripancreatic adipose tissue; (3) obliterative phlebitis affecting the pancreatic veins. Immunostaining often demonstrates abundant (>10 cell/high-power field) IgG4-positive cells (Figure 100-3). Type 2 AIP differs from type 1 by less prominent fibrosis and phlebitis and lack of IgG4 positivity.[38] In type 2 AIP, lymphoplasmacytic infiltrates may result in obliteration of the duct lumen, in contrast to type 1 AIP, in which the ductal epithelium is generally spared.

The diagnosis of AIP can be clinically challenging and no single diagnostic test is sufficient. Diagnostic criteria rely on a combination of histology, cross-sectional and endoscopic imaging, serologic findings, and a detailed clinical history. Furthermore, diagnostic criteria can vary by region, for example, by the Japanese criteria (Box 100-1), endoscopic retrograde pancreatogram is mandated to diagnose AIP, whereas it is not essential to the American HISORt criteria (Box 100-2). In general, the diagnosis of AIP requires a multidisciplinary team consisting of a radiologist, pathologist, and gastroenterologist all familiar with the disease.

TREATMENT

Treatment of AIP consists of corticosteroid therapy. Although AIP can resolve spontaneously, treatment with corticosteroids has been associated with an increased remission of AIP when compared to no treatment (98% vs. 75%, $P < 0.001$).[39] Several studies have demonstrated a reversal of jaundice, diabetes, and exocrine dysfunction after treatment. However, there is no consensus regarding the corticosteroid dose or duration of the initial treatment or the need for maintenance therapy. A common practice pattern utilizes 40 mg of prednisone/day for 4 weeks. With clinical and radiologic improvement, the prednisone can be tapered by 5 mg/week. Because clinical relapse can occur in up to 30% of patients[40] some investigators advocate administering a low-dose maintenance dose of prednisone. In Japan, prednisone (2.5 to

TABLE 100-1 Comparison of Histologic Descriptions of Type 1 and 2 Autoimmune Pancreatitis

	Type 1	Type 2
General description	Fibroinflammatory process involving pancreatic ducts, lobules, veins, and common bile duct	Fibroinflammatory process involving mainly pancreatic ducts and intrapancreatic common bile duct but less marked in lobules and veins
Infiltrate	Lymphoplasmacytic, often with eosinophils and rare neutrophils	Lymphoplasmacytic with neutrophilic infiltration of medium-sized and small ducts and acini
Pancreatic ducts	Dense periductal inflammation without epithelial damage	Periductal infiltration with destruction of duct epithelium by neutrophilic granulocytes. (Granulocytic epithelial lesion, GEL)
Lobules	Lymphoplasmacytic invasion with replacement of acinar tissue	Patchy lymphoplasmacytic invasion
Veins	Obliterative phlebitis	Rare venous obliteration
Peripancreatic fat	Fibroinflammatory process extends to peripancreatic region	Inflammation usually limited to the pancreas
IgG4 positivity	Abundant (>10 cell/hpf)	Scant to absent

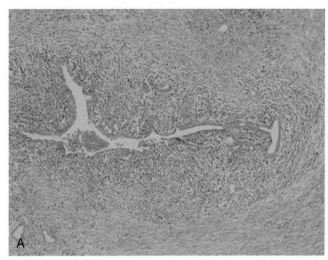 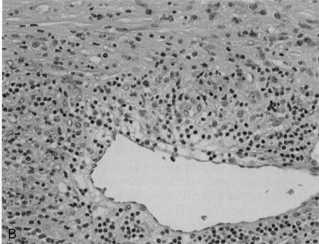

FIGURE 100-3 Histologic changes associated with type 1 autoimmune pancreatitis including **(A)** periductal lymphoplasmacytic infiltrates and preductal fibrosis and **(B)** focal venulitis.

BOX 100-1 Clinical Diagnostic Criteria for Autoimmune Pancreatitis, 2006

1. Diffuse or segmental narrowing of the main pancreatic duct with irregular wall or diffuse or localized enlargement of the pancreas by imaging studies
2. High serum γ-globulin, IgG or IgG4, or the presence of autoantibodies such as antinuclear antibodies and rheumatoid factor
3. Marked intralobular fibrosis and prominent infiltration of lymphocytes and plasma cells in the periductal area, occasionally with lymphoid follicles in the pancreas
   Diagnosis of AIP is established when criteria 1 and 2 and/or 3 are fulfilled

---

BOX 100-2 HISORt Criteria of Autoimmune Pancreatitis

HISTOLOGY
1. Diagnostic
   a. Pancreatic lymphoplasmacytic infiltrate with obliterative phlebitis
   b. Pancreatic lymphoplasmacytic infiltrate with (>10/hpf) IgG4-positive cells
2. Suggestive
   a. Lymphoplasmacytic infiltrate with (>10/hpf) IgG4-positive cells from an extrapancreatic organ
   b. Lymphoplasmacytic infiltrate with fibrosis in the pancreas

IMAGING
Typical imaging features
1. CT/MR: diffusely enlarged gland with delayed rim enhancement
2. ERCP: diffusely irregular attenuated main pancreatic duct

SEROLOGY
Elevated serum IgG4 levels (normal 8-140 mg/dL)

OTHER ORGAN INVOLVEMENT
Hilar/intrahepatic biliary strictures, persistent distal biliary stricture, parotid/lacrimal gland involvement, mediastinal lymphadenopathy, retroperitoneal fibrosis

RESPONSE TO STEROID THERAPY
Resolution or improvement of pancreatic extrapancreatic manifestation with steroid therapy

CT, Computed tomography; *ERCP,* endoscopic retrograde cholangiopancreatography; *MR,* magnetic resonance imaging.

---

5 mg/day) is administered for up to 3 years, which has demonstrated lower relapse rates (23% vs. 24%, P< 0.05) in a retrospective analysis of more than 500 patients managed with this strategy.[39] Ongoing interest in other immunologic therapies, such as rituximab, for the induction and maintenance of remission has been encouraging. In a report of four patients, the addition of rituximab was associated with a 65% decline in IgG4 levels and rapid tapering of corticosteroids in all patients in less than 2 months.[41]

PRIMARY PANCREATIC LYMPHOMA

Primary pancreatic lymphoma (PPL) accounts for less than 0.5% of all pancreatic tumors.[42] The Behrns criteria are often used to establish the diagnosis of PPL and includes a pancreatic mass with grossly involved lymph nodes confined to the peripancreatic region, in the absence of superficial or mediastinal lymphadenopathy, no splenic or hepatic involvement, and a normal leukocyte count. In a review of over 100 case reports, the majority of PPLs are diffuse, large cell high-grade lymphomas (45%), low-grade B-cell lymphomas (15%), and other B-cell lymphomas (34%).[43] The disease occurs more often in men than women and usually presents in the fifth to sixth decade of life.[44]

CLINICOPATHOLOGIC FEATURES

Patients often present with nonspecific symptoms, including weight loss, abdominal pain, nausea, and vomiting. Symptoms of PPL are distinguished from that of pancreatic ductal adenocarcinoma in that the abdominal pain

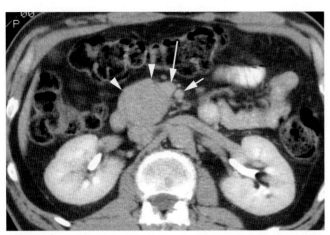

FIGURE 100-4 Primary pancreatic lymphoma of the head of pancreas with possible adherence to the superior mesenteric vein.

rarely radiates to the back and jaundice is an infrequent sign. Unlike secondary non-Hodgkin lymphoma, only 2% of patients present with classic B symptoms of fevers and night sweats.[45] These symptoms usually prompt additional body imaging, which identifies a bulky pancreatic head lesion with considerable multifocal regional lymphadenopathy and the absence of pancreatic ductal dilation. Tumors may have a significant extrapancreatic component, with encroachment upon adjacent mesenteric vessels (Figure 100-4). Less commonly, there may be a mass in the body or tail of the pancreas.[46] By endoscopic ultrasound (EUS), the mass may be hypoechoic with cystic and solid components and a central stellate fibrous band.[47] No specific biochemical markers have been identified for PPL, although serum lactic dehydrogenase (LDH) may be elevated in up to 50% of cases. An elevated serum level of CA19-9 may also occasionally be associated with PPL.[43,48]

On histopathologic examination, PPL may be difficult to distinguish from pancreatic endocrine neoplasms and acinar cell carcinomas. However, key immunohistochemical stains which are positive in pancreatic endocrine neoplasms, such as synaptophysin, are generally negative in PPL. Histologically, PPL often exhibits characteristic large, malignant lymphocytic nuclei, and abundant karyorrhexis. Immunohistochemical stains are usually positive for leukocyte common antigen and CD20 and are negative for CD34 and CD68.[49] Unfortunately, biopsy samples of tumor tissues are often necrotic and nondiagnostic. The addition of flow cytometry has also been reported to have high diagnostic value in PPL, with a 84% sensitivity and 100% specificity.[50] However, the samples must be of adequate cellularity for this diagnostic procedure. A combination of imaging and histologic findings should allow differentiation of PPL from secondary lymphomas, pancreatic endocrine neoplasms, and acinar cell carcinomas.

TREATMENT

Although surgical resection was previously considered a primary treatment option for PPL, significant improvements in chemotherapy have limited the role of surgery to circumstances in which the diagnosis is uncertain or

in the setting of failed chemotherapy or chemoradiation. PPL is most commonly treated with a multidrug regimen such as cyclophosphamide, doxorubicin, vincristine, and prednisone (CHOP). Complete remission can be expected with multidrug therapy in 63% to 77% of patients with large B-cell lymphoma.[51] However recurrence is common in patients older than age 60. In a recent literature review of 105 cases of PPL, radiotherapy was administered with chemotherapy in one-third of cases but did not appear to be associated with an increase in overall survival.[43] The use of an anti-CD20 antibody, rituximab, to CHOP has been associated with improved response rates of up to 85% in diffuse large B-cell lymphoma. Given the rarity of PPL, the addition of rituximab to chemotherapy has been reported in only two cases with variable benefit.

METASTATIC RENAL CELL CANCER

Metastases from renal cell carcinoma (RCC) are frequently found at unusual sites, such as thyroid, skeletal muscle, and pancreas. Although most cancers rarely metastasize to the pancreas and account for only 2% of all pancreatic malignancies, approximately 40% of metastatic lesions to the pancreas are found to be RCC. Synchronous metastases can occur in up to 25% to 30% of patients, and metachronous metastases occur in approximately 40% of all patients with RCC.[52,53] A recent systematic review of pancreatic surgery for metastatic RCC identified 311 cases of surgically resected RCC in the published literature.[54] The mean age of diagnosis was 63 years, with a mean disease-free interval of approximately 10 years (range, 1 to 25 years) after the primary RCC was surgically excised. Men and women were equally affected and there were no differences in the laterality of the primary and the location of the metastases. The majority of patients had solitary metastases, although 34% of patients had multiple pancreatic metastases.

CLINICOPATHOLOGIC FEATURES

The majority of patients with metastatic RCC are asymptomatic.[54] Among symptomatic patients, the most frequent symptoms included abdominal or back pain, gastrointestinal bleeding, weight loss, and jaundice. On cross-sectional imaging, the metastatic RCC often appears as a large hypervascular spherical mass with well-defined margins with a central area of low attenuation on the arterial phase (Figure 100-5). The hypervascularity of the lesion is inconsistent with pancreatic ductal adenocarcinoma; however, pancreatic endocrine neoplasm remains in the differential. A tissue biopsy is helpful if the diagnosis is uncertain, the patient has a history of a non-RCC malignancy, or a nonoperative approach is planned. However, in the majority of patients with a history of RCC, the CT findings are characteristic and there is no need for a preoperative biopsy.

Histologically, RCC forms solid sheets of tumor cells that are separated into solid acini by vascular septae, which can be distinguished from pancreatic endocrine neoplasms (see Figure 100-5, *B*). Metastatic RCC may appear histologically different from the primary RCC because of alterations in differentiation and expression

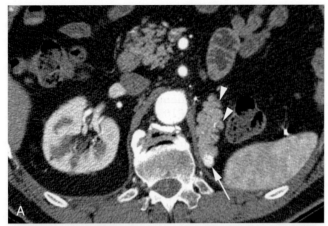

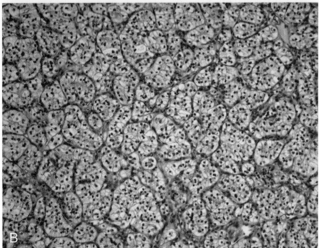

FIGURE 100-5 Metastatic renal cell carcinoma to the pancreas with **(A)** enhancement on arterial phase imaging and **(B)** solid growth of clear cell RCC with acini formation.

proteins. Multiple studies have compared the markers in metastatic and primary RCC. The tumor-type–specific profiles for primary RCC are largely retained in their metastases but significant attenuation of staining frequency has been observed.[55] Immunohistochemistry can be helpful in diagnosing metastatic RCC. In particular PAX2, a nuclear transcription factor essential for fetal kidney development, is the most useful marker for metastatic RCC with a frequency and extent of staining of up to 74% of cases. Furthermore, depending on the histology of the primary, several stains have 100% positivity: CD10 for clear cell RCC and α-methylacyl coenzyme A racemase for papillary RCC.[55]

TREATMENT

Approximately 22% of patients with metastatic RCC will have extrapancreatic disease. Tanis et al[54] have identified extrapancreatic disease as the only adverse risk factor for disease-free survival following pancreatic resection. Therefore, a thorough staging evaluation should be performed in patients with suspected or biopsy-proven metastatic disease to the pancreas. In a systematic review, the in-hospital mortality rate after pancreatic surgery was 2.8%, similar to mortality rates associated with pancreatic surgery for primary pancreatic neoplasms at high-volume

centers. Metachronous pancreatic recurrences were reported in 4% of patients and extrapancreatic recurrences in 17%, of which 45% were amenable to resection. In patients with isolated RCC metastases, surgical resection may offer significant survival benefit. Following resection, disease-free survival and overall survival are 57% and 72% at 5 years, respectively.[54] In recent years, phase III trials of sunitinib, sorafenib, temsirolimus, and bevacizumab have demonstrated promising results in patients with metastatic RCC (excluding those with brain metastases). These agents can also be used sequentially or in association with surgery in a multimodal approach.

CONCLUSION

Although the majority of pancreatic neoplasms are pancreatic ductal adenocarcinoma, a thorough understanding of rare and unusual pancreatic neoplasms is important as some of these lesions are best managed with medical therapy. An accurate pretreatment diagnosis is critical to developing the optimal treatment strategy. This is best achieved by a coordinated approach involving a multidisciplinary team of physicians: gastroenterologist, pathologist, radiologist, and surgeon. Although cross-sectional imaging can be diagnostic, in many cases a cytopathologic diagnosis may be necessary. Surgery is the cornerstone of therapy for SPT, ACC, and RCC metastases; however, medical therapy is more appropriate for AIP and PPL.

REFERENCES

1. Franz VK: *Tumors of the pancreas.* In Atlas of tumor pathology, Section 7, Fascicles 27 and 28. Washington, D.C. 1959.
2. Kloppel G, Solcia E, Longnecker DS, et al: *Histological typing of tumors of the exocrine pancreas: World Health Organization international histological classification of tumors,* ed 2. New York, 1996, Springer-Verlag.
3. Casadei R, Santini D, Calculli L, et al: Pancreatic solid-cystic papillary tumor: Clinical features, imaging findings and operative management. *JOP* 7:137, 2006.
4. Papavramidis T, Papavramidis S: Solid pseudopapillary tumors of the pancreas: Review of 718 patients reported in English literature. *J Am Coll Surg* 200:965, 2005.
5. Klimstra DS, Wenig BM, Heffess CS: Solid-pseudopapillary tumor of the pancreas: A typically cystic carcinoma of low malignant potential. *Semin Diagn Pathol* 17:66, 2000.
6. Santini D, Poli F, Lega S: Solid-papillary tumors of the pancreas: Histopathology. *JOP* 7:131, 2006.
7. Abraham SC, Klimstra DS, Wilentz RE, et al: Solid-pseudopapillary tumors of the pancreas are genetically distinct from pancreatic ductal adenocarcinomas and almost always harbor beta-catenin mutations. *Am J Pathol* 160:1361, 2002.
8. Martin RC, Klimstra DS, Brennan MF, et al: Solid-pseudopapillary tumor of the pancreas: A surgical enigma? *Ann Surg Oncol* 9:35, 2002.
9. Kang CM, Kim KS, Choi JS, et al: Solid pseudopapillary tumor of the pancreas suggesting malignant potential. *Pancreas* 32:276, 2006.
10. Tang LH, Aydin H, Brennan MF, et al: Clinically aggressive solid pseudopapillary tumors of the pancreas: A report of two cases with components of undifferentiated carcinoma and a comparative clinicopathologic analysis of 34 conventional cases. *Am J Surg Pathol* 29:512, 2005.
11. Strauss JF, Hirsch VJ, Rubey CN, et al: Resection of a solid and papillary epithelial neoplasm of the pancreas following treatment with cis-platinum and 5-fluorouracil: A case report. *Med Pediatr Oncol* 21:365, 1993.

12. Maffuz A, Bustamante Fde T, Silva JA, et al: Preoperative gemcitabine for unresectable, solid pseudopapillary tumour of the pancreas. *Lancet Oncol* 6:185, 2005.

13. Holen KD, Klimstra DS, Hummer A, et al: Clinical characteristics and outcomes from an institutional series of acinar cell carcinoma of the pancreas and related tumors. *J Clin Oncol* 20:4673, 2002.

14. Seth AK, Argani P, Campbell KA, et al: Acinar cell carcinoma of the pancreas: An institutional series of resected patients and review of the current literature. *J Gastrointest Surg* 12:1061, 2008.

15. Chiou YY, Chiang JH, Hwang JI, et al: Acinar cell carcinoma of the pancreas: Clinical and computed tomography manifestations. *J Comput Assist Tomogr* 28:180, 2004.

16. Tatli S, Mortele KJ, Levy AD, et al: CT and MRI features of pure acinar cell carcinoma of the pancreas in adults. *AJR Am J Roentgenol* 184:511, 2005.

17. Klimstra DS, Heffess CS, Oertel JE, et al: Acinar cell carcinoma of the pancreas. A clinicopathologic study of 28 cases. *Am J Surg Pathol* 16:815, 1992.

18. Chung DC, Brown SB, Graeme-Cook F, et al: Localization of putative tumor suppressor loci by genome-wide allelotyping in human pancreatic endocrine tumors. *Cancer Res* 58:3706, 1998.

19. Henke AC, Kelley CM, Jensen CS, et al: Fine-needle aspiration cytology of pancreatoblastoma. *Diagn Cytopathol* 25:118, 2001.

20. Abraham SC, Wu TT, Klimstra DS, et al: Distinctive molecular genetic alterations in sporadic and familial adenomatous polyposis-associated pancreatoblastomas : Frequent alterations in the APC/beta-catenin pathway and chromosome 11p. *Am J Pathol* 159:1619, 2001.

21. Schmidt CM, Matos JM, Bentrem DJ, et al: Acinar cell carcinoma of the pancreas in the United States: Prognostic factors and comparison to ductal adenocarcinoma. *J Gastrointest Surg* 12:2078, 2008.

22. Sarles H, Sarles JC, Muratore R, et al: Chronic inflammatory sclerosis of the pancreas—an autonomous pancreatic disease? *Am J Dig Dis* 6:688, 1961.

23. de Castro SM, de Nes LC, Nio CY, et al: Incidence and characteristics of chronic and lymphoplasmacytic sclerosing pancreatitis in patients scheduled to undergo a pancreatoduodenectomy. *HPB (Oxford)* 12:15, 2010.

24. Hardacre JM, Iacobuzio-Donahue CA, Sohn TA, et al: Results of pancreaticoduodenectomy for lymphoplasmacytic sclerosing pancreatitis. *Ann Surg* 237:853; discussion 858, 2003.

25. Weber SM, Cubukcu-Dimopulo O, Palesty JA, et al: Lymphoplasmacytic sclerosing pancreatitis: Inflammatory mimic of pancreatic carcinoma. *J Gastrointest Surg* 7:129; discussion 137, 2003.

26. Chari ST, Longnecker DS, Kloppel G: The diagnosis of autoimmune pancreatitis: A Western perspective. *Pancreas* 38:846, 2009.

27. Okazaki K, Uchida K, Chiba T: Recent concept of autoimmune-related pancreatitis. *J Gastroenterol* 36:293, 2001.

28. Kamisawa T, Tu Y, Egawa N, et al: Salivary gland involvement in chronic pancreatitis of various etiologies. *Am J Gastroenterol* 98:323, 2003.

29. Kulling D, Tresch S, Renner E: Triad of sclerosing cholangitis, chronic pancreatitis, and Sjogren's syndrome: Case report and review. *Gastrointest Endosc* 57:118, 2003.

30. Uchida K, Okazaki K, Asada M, et al: Case of chronic pancreatitis involving an autoimmune mechanism that extended to retroperitoneal fibrosis. *Pancreas* 26:92, 2003.

31. Webster GJ, Pereira SP, Chapman RW: Autoimmune pancreatitis/IgG4-associated cholangitis and primary sclerosing cholangitis—overlapping or separate diseases? *J Hepatol* 51:398, 2009.

32. Ravi K, Chari ST, Vege SS, et al: Inflammatory bowel disease in the setting of autoimmune pancreatitis. *Inflamm Bowel Dis* 15:1326, 2009.

33. Takuma K, Kamisawa T, Anjiki H, et al: Metachronous extrapancreatic lesions in autoimmune pancreatitis. *Intern Med* 49:529, 2010.

34. Kamisawa T, Imai M, Yui Chen P, et al: Strategy for differentiating autoimmune pancreatitis from pancreatic cancer. *Pancreas* 37:e62, 2008.

35. Frulloni L, Scattolini C, Falconi M, et al: Autoimmune pancreatitis: Differences between the focal and diffuse forms in 87 patients. *Am J Gastroenterol* 104:2288, 2009.

36. Sah RP, Chari ST, Pannala R, et al: Differences in clinical profile and relapse rate of type 1 versus type 2 autoimmune pancreatitis. *Gastroenterology* 139:140, 2010.

37. Ghazale A, Chari ST, Zhang L, et al: Immunoglobulin G4-associated cholangitis: Clinical profile and response to therapy. *Gastroenterology* 134:706, 2008.

38. Chari ST, Kloeppel G, Zhang L, et al: Histopathologic and clinical subtypes of autoimmune pancreatitis: The Honolulu consensus document. *Pancreas* 39:549, 2010.

39. Kamisawa T, Shimosegawa T, Okazaki K, et al: Standard steroid treatment for autoimmune pancreatitis. *Gut* 58:1504, 2009.

40. Gardner TB, Chari ST: Autoimmune pancreatitis. *Gastroenterol Clin North Am* 37:439, 2008.

41. Khosroshahi A, Bloch DB, Deshpande V, et al: Rituximab therapy leads to rapid decline of serum IgG4 levels and prompt clinical improvement in IgG4-related systemic disease. *Arthritis Rheum* 62:1755, 2010.

42. Baylor SM, Berg JW: Cross-classification and survival characteristics of 5,000 cases of cancer of the pancreas. *J Surg Oncol* 5:335, 1973.

43. Grimison PS, Chin MT, Harrison ML, et al: Primary pancreatic lymphoma—pancreatic tumours that are potentially curable without resection, a retrospective review of four cases. *BMC Cancer* 6:117, 2006.

44. Koniaris LG, Lillemoe KD, Yeo CJ, et al: Is there a role for surgical resection in the treatment of early-stage pancreatic lymphoma? *J Am Coll Surg* 190:319, 2000.

45. Battula N, Srinivasan P, Prachalias A, et al: Primary pancreatic lymphoma: Diagnostic and therapeutic dilemma. *Pancreas* 33:192, 2006.

46. Behrns KE, Sarr MG, Strickler JG: Pancreatic lymphoma: Is it a surgical disease? *Pancreas* 9:662, 1994.

47. McCauley AM, Gottlieb KT: Primary pancreatic lymphoma coexisting with chronic lymphocytic leukemia: EUS findings. *Gastrointest Endosc* 68:188, 2008.

48. Lin H, Li SD, Hu XG, et al: Primary pancreatic lymphoma: Report of six cases. *World J Gastroenterol* 12:5064, 2006.

49. Naito Y, Okabe Y, Kawahara A, et al: Guide to diagnosing primary pancreatic lymphoma, B-cell type: Immunocytochemistry improves the diagnostic accuracy of endoscopic ultrasonography-guided fine needle aspiration cytology. *Diagn Cytopathol* Mar 17 2011.

50. Khashab M, Mokadem M, DeWitt J, et al: Endoscopic ultrasound-guided fine-needle aspiration with or without flow cytometry for the diagnosis of primary pancreatic lymphoma—a case series. *Endoscopy* 42:228, 2010.

51. Coiffier B: Monoclonal antibody as therapy for malignant lymphomas. *C R Biol* 329:241, 2006.

52. Motzer RJ, Bander NH, Nanus DM: Renal-cell carcinoma. *N Engl J Med* 335:865, 1996.

53. Zweizig SL: Cancer of the kidney. *Clin Obstet Gynecol* 45:884, 2002.

54. Tanis PJ, van der Gaag NA, Busch OR, et al: Systematic review of pancreatic surgery for metastatic renal cell carcinoma. *Br J Surg* 96:579, 2009.

55. Truong LD, Shen SS: Immunohistochemical diagnosis of renal neoplasms. *Arch Pathol Lab Med* 135:92, 2011.

Prevention and Management of Complications of Pancreatic Surgery

Mark P. Callery | Tara Kent

Mortality after pancreatic resection has greatly decreased in comparison with historical series, from 33% following Whipple's initial reports, to currently less than 5% in most high-volume centers,[1] resulting in the recognition that assessment of surgical quality for these high-acuity patients warrants further refinement.[2] Birkmeyer et al have demonstrated the impact of hospital volume on actual operative mortality for pancreatic cancer resections, among other high-acuity operations,[3] but these two measures accounted for only half of the hospital-level variation in mortality. In the highest-volume centers, mortality no longer correlates well with volume,[2] yet overall morbidity remains high for pancreatic resections, in the range of 35% to 50%.[2,4] Previously published outcomes after pancreatic resection in a high-volume institution are demonstrated in Table 101-1; the three most common complications were delayed gastric emptying in 14%, wound infection in 7%, and pancreatic fistula in 5%.[5] This chapter will also discuss postpancreatectomy hemorrhage.

Initial efforts to better understand perioperative mortality after pancreatic resection demonstrated the importance of hospital volume on outcome, with a three- to fourfold greater operative mortality at low-volume hospitals versus high-volume hospitals.[6-8] Fong et al also demonstrate an ongoing survival benefit (6% at 2 years) for patients undergoing pancreatic cancer resection at a high-volume institution.[8] A recent single-institution study of similar issues reports that higher surgeon volume is associated with shorter operative time, less intraoperative blood loss, and higher lymph node harvest (for cancer cases).[9] However, surgeon experience mitigated these differences, with experienced surgeons (>50 pancreaticoduodenectomies) having significantly lower morbidity compared to less experienced surgeons, and in particular, less blood loss, shorter operative time, and a lower postoperative pancreatic fistula (POPF) rate.[9] Twenty pancreaticoduodenectomies (PDs) were required to equalize the experienced and inexperienced surgeons. However, adequacy of oncologic resection did not differ.

This chapter will focus on technical and clinical means of preventing and managing pancreatic surgical complications, but the import of surgeon and hospital volume, as well as experience, on complications and overall outcome after pancreatic resection should not be lost on the reader. Schmidt et al also emphasize the importance of the institution's systems support for the diagnosis and management of postoperative complications, that is, interventional radiology and gastroenterology, intensive care, and surgical team members.[9]

POSTPANCREATECTOMY HEMORRHAGE

Hemorrhage associated with pancreatic resection (PPH) occurs in up to 8% of cases, but may account for 11% to 38% of mortality.[10-13] Because of the potential consequences of this problem, a consensus definition was developed by the International Study Group of Pancreatic Surgery (ISGPS) in 2007[14] and is seen in Table 101-2. It may occur intraoperatively, early in the postoperative period, or late (more than 24 hours postoperatively). Intraoperative hemorrhage may be more likely to occur in the event of aberrant vasculature particularly when not preoperatively identified.[15] Figure 101-1 demonstrates normal peripancreatic vasculature as seen on CT angiography.[15] The common variations include a replaced right hepatic artery (11% to 21%), replaced left hepatic artery (4% to 10%), accessory right or left hepatic artery (<1% to 8%), and celiac artery stenosis (2% to 8%).[15]

Intraoperative vascular complications are known to adversely affect ultimate outcome,[16] including the mortality rate; thus, efforts to delineate vasculature preoperatively by means of a pancreatic protocol computed tomography (CT) including arterial, venous, and portal venous phases,[15] should allow the surgeon to be better prepared intraoperatively and limit the occurrence of intraoperative hemorrhage related to an unexpected encounter with abnormal vascular anatomy. These efforts should continue intraoperatively by inspection and palpation of the operative field to further define the vascular anatomy. For example, a replaced right hepatic artery may be appreciated by palpation of a pulse posterior and lateral to the bile duct and portal vein. Intraoperative hemorrhage may also occur in the setting of tumor infiltration that involves the relevant vasculature.

To obtain intraoperative control of hemorrhage, direct pressure should be applied initially to allow for mobilization of appropriate anesthetic and surgical resources such as blood products, vascular sutures and clamps, and appropriate surgical assistance. Aberrant vasculature such as a replaced right hepatic artery may need to be reconstructed or anastomosed to an alternate vessel in order to preserve hepatic arterial blood flow. Doppler ultrasonography may be useful to determine whether there is already alternate arterial flow. Venous injuries may be able to be addressed with venorrhaphy or with patch venoplasty. In exsanguinating, uncontrolled hemorrhage, portal vein ligation has been described, with a potential for survival, when accompanied by a "second-look" laparotomy in 24 hours to evaluate for signs of ischemia.[17] A more recent paper reports on a small series

TABLE 101-1 Mortality and Morbidity after Pancreaticoduodenectomy and Distal Pancreatectomy in 616 Patients

	Overall (*N* = 616)	Pancreaticoduodenectomy/Total Pancreatectomy (*n* = 564)	Distal Pancreatectomy (*n* = 52)	*P* value
Perioperative mortality	2.3%	2.3%	1.9%	NS
Overall complications	30%	31%	25%	NS
SPECIFIC COMPLICATIONS				
Reoperation	3%	3%	4%	NS
Delayed gastric emptying	—	14%	—	—
Cholangitis	—	3%	—	—
Bile leak	—	2%	—	—
Wound infection	7%	7%	5%	NS
Pancreatic fistula	5%	5%	8%	NS
Intraabdominal abscess	3%	3%	4%	NS
Pneumonia	1%	1%	0%	NS
Pancreatitis	1%	1%	0%	NS
POSTOPERATIVE LENGTH OF STAY				
Mean ± SE	13.7 ± 0.4 d	14.0 ± 0.4 d	11.5 ± 2.2 d	.08
Median	11 d	11 d	7 d	

From Sohn TA, Yeo CJ, Cameron JL, et al: Resected adenocarcinoma of the pancreas—616 patients: Results, outcomes, and prognostic indicators. *J Gastrointest Surg* 4:567, 2000.

TABLE 101-2 Classification of PPH: Clinical Condition and Diagnostic and Therapeutic Consequences

Grade	Time of Onset, Location, Severity and Clinical Impact of Bleeding		Clinical Condition	Diagnostic Consequence	Therapeutic Consequence
A	Early, intra- or extraluminal, mild		Well	Observation, blood count, ultrasonography and, if necessary, computed tomography	No
B	Early, intra- or extraluminal, severe	Late, intra- or extraluminal, mild*	Often well/intermediate, very rarely life-threatening	Observation, blood count, ultrasonography, computed tomography, angiography, endoscopy[†]	Transfusion of fluid/blood, intermediate care unit (or ICU), therapeutic endoscopy,[†] embolization, relaparotomy for early PPH
C		Late, intra- or extraluminal, severe	Severely impaired, life-threatening	Angiography, computed tomography, endoscopy[†]	Localization of bleeding, angiography and embolization (endoscopy[†]), *or* relaparotomy, ICU

From Wente MN, Veit JA, Bassi C, et al: Postpancreatectomy hemorrhage (PPH)—an International Study Group of Pancreatic Surgery definition. *Surgery* 142:20, 2007.
ICU, Intensive care unit; *PPH*, postpancreatectomy hemorrhage.
*Late, intra- or extraluminal, mild bleeding may not be immediately life-threatening to patient but may be a warning sign for later severe hemorrhage ("sentinel bleed") and is therefore grade B.
[†]Endoscopy should be performed when signs of intraluminal bleeding are present (melena, hematemesis, or blood loss via nasogastric tube).

of patients undergoing damage control laparotomy (DCL) for pancreatic surgery,[18] primarily for portal vein injury, with the goal of allowing intensive care unit (ICU) resuscitation to reverse the accompanying hypothermia, acidosis, and coagulopathy. They describe initial venous compression to allow for identification/visualization of the site of injury as well as for preparation of the surgical and anesthetic teams. Useful maneuvers for compression included the Kocher maneuver and sponge sticks. The pancreas was then divided and the specimen quickly extirpated when possible. Other techniques used to shorten operating time included external drainage,

packing, stapled bowel closure, and rapid abdominal closure.[18] The authors emphasize that there was significant resource utilization but no mortality.

Management of early and late PPH is addressed by the ISGPS classification schema.[14] Early PPH is most often a result of technical failure to achieve appropriate hemostasis at the index operation, or else secondary to underlying coagulopathy. When significant, and thought to be technical failure, prompt relaparotomy is mandated.[19] PPH occurring later than the first postoperative day and up to several weeks postoperatively is often a result of other postoperative complications such as fistula,

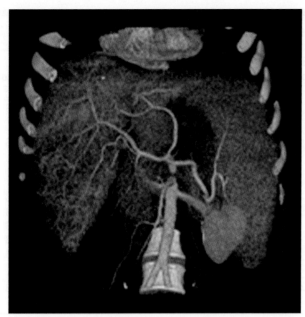

FIGURE 101-1 CT angiography of normal peripancreatic arterial anatomy. (From Shukla PJ, Barreto SG, Kulkarni A, et al: Vascular anomalies encountered during pancreatoduodenectomy: Do they influence outcomes? *Ann Surg Oncol* 17:186, 2010.)

anastomotic ulceration, or pseudoaneurysm.[11,14,20] PPH may represent bleeding from intra- or extraluminal sources: unsecured vessels, vessels with pseudoaneurysm, anastomotic suture lines or ulceration, resection cut surfaces, or hemobilia. Named vascular structures that may be the source of bleeding are the gastroduodenal, hepatic, or splenic artery, branches of the superior mesenteric artery, or the splenic vein stump.[13,14] The classification system for PPH is described in Table 101-2.

Once PPH becomes apparent, evaluation must occur in a timely fashion, and may include a variety of modalities depending on the hemodynamic status of the patient and apparent location of the bleeding (intra- or extraluminal): endoscopy, angiography, CT scan, or reoperation.[14] Early extraluminal PPH requires reexploration. Intraluminal bleeding may manifest as extraluminal if there is associated anastomotic breakdown,[13] and this may be amenable to angiographic intervention when involving the pancreaticojejunostomy. Bleeding from the gastro- or duodenojejunostomy may first be excluded by endoscopy. Over time, conservative management has become more successful for late PPH but surgical intervention has continued to be the mainstay of treatment. Mortality in patients with late PPH is much higher than for the routine pancreatic resection, with rates of 16% to 27%[13-21] but is strongly associated with a bleed in the setting of a septic complication such as pancreatic fistula. Patients present with septic complications and/or a sentinel bleed. Radiographic embolization has become a more successful modality, with up to 80% success,[13] but is limited by the initially intermittent nature of the bleeding.[21] Reexploration is indicated when angiographic intervention is not technically feasible or successful, or when the site is not visualized on angiography and the patient is hemodynamically unstable.[13]

PANCREATIC FISTULA

POPF continues to be the nemesis of pancreatic resection. Occurring in up to 30% of cases even in the setting of vast improvements in the safety and efficacy of pancreatic surgery overall as mentioned earlier, fistula rates have failed to decrease significantly.[22-24] One must first recall the definition of *fistula* as "an abnormal communication from one epithelialized surface to another" compared to that of *leakage*, referring to "an abnormal escape of fluid through an orifice or opening."[23]

In addition, POPF occurs with the leakage of amylase-rich fluid from the transection margin of the gland and/or from the pancreatic-enteric anastomosis. Although many literature reports have been devoted to studying the diagnosis, management, and effect of POPF on patient outcome, comparison of these studies has been difficult because there was no uniform definition available. To better understand POPF, the ISGPF developed a classification scheme that is presented in Table 101-3.[25] POPF was defined as inclusive of all peripancreatic fluid collections, abscesses, leaks, or fistulas, and diagnosed by virtue of drain amylase, output, imaging, and clinical picture (well, septic).[25] According to the classification scheme, grade A fistulas are biochemical only and not clinically relevant, whereas grades B and C fistulas are clinically relevant, requiring further evaluation and management, such as antibiotics, nutritional support, octreotide, and percutaneous drainage (grade B) or surgical exploration (grade C) in the setting of sepsis.[25] Subsequent efforts to validate this classification scheme demonstrate that grade A fistulas comprise nearly half of all POPF, yet have no apparent significant effect on outcome. However, grade B/C fistulas occur less often (40% and 11%, respectively) but are associated with higher resource utilization (ICU stay, nursing services postdischarge, readmission rate), longer hospital stay, more complications, and accordingly, increase in cost, grade for grade.[24]

RISK STRATIFICATION

Prevention of POPF relates to appropriate risk stratification[26] according to disease-related, patient-related, and operative risk factors. A soft gland or diagnoses of ampullary, duodenal, cystic, or islet cell pathologies increases the risk of POPF development by up to 10-fold.[26,27] Pancreatic duct size is also crucial, with small ducts up to 3 mm in diameter conferring increased risk of POPF[26,28] with an odds ratio greater than 3. As for patient-related risk factors, conflicting information exists in the literature. Some investigators have identified older age, male gender, coronary artery disease, jaundice, and low creatinine clearance as predictors of POPF.[27,29,30] However, other studies fail to find any impact of gender in multivariate analysis.[28] Interestingly, neoadjuvant therapy appears to reduce the risk of fistula.[31] Operative risk factors include blood loss higher than 1000 mL and longer operative time.[26,28,29] Importantly, there appears to be an additive effect of these risk factors, whereby the percentage of patients developing a POPF increases sequentially as the number of risk factors increases,[26] as seen in Table 101-4, and is associated with increased cost and hospital stay.

TABLE 101-3 Criteria for Grading Pancreatic Fistula (ISGPF Classification Scheme)

Criteria	No Fistula	Grade A Fistula	Grade B Fistula	Grade C Fistula
Drain amylase	<3 times normal serum amylase	>3 times normal serum amylase	>3 times normal serum amylase	>3 times normal serum amylase
Clinical conditions	Well	Well	Often well	Ill appearing/bad
Specific treatment	No	No	Yes/no	Yes
Ultrasonography/CT (if obtained)	Negative	Negative	Negative/positive	Positive
Persistent drainage (>3 wk)	No	No	Usually yes	Yes
Signs of infection	No	No	Yes	Yes
Readmission	No	No	Yes/no	Yes/no
Sepsis	No	No	No	Yes
Reoperation	No	No	No	Yes
Death related to fistula	No	No	No	Yes

Adapted from Bassi C, Dervenis C, Butturini G, et al: Postoperative pancreatic fistula: An international study group definition. *Surgery* 138:8, 2005.
Note: Signs of infection include elevated body temperature >38° C, leukocytosis, and localized erythema, induration, or purulent drainage. Readmission is any hospital admission within 30 days following hospital discharge from the initial operation. Sepsis is the presence of localized infection and positive culture with evidence of bacteremia (i.e., chills, rigors, elevated WBC count) requiring IV antibiotic treatment, or hemodynamic compromise as demonstrated by high cardiac output and low systemic vascular resistance within 24 hour of body temperature >38° C.

TABLE 101-4 The Impact of Increasing Number of Risk Factors for Pancreatic Fistulas

Outcomes	No Risk Factors ($n = 63$)	1 Risk Factor ($n = 88$)	2 Risk Factors ($n = 66$)	3 Risk Factors ($n = 13$)	4 Risk Factors ($n = 3$)	P value
Clinically relevant fistulas (%)	1 (2)	7 (8)	16 (24)	4 (31)	3 (100)	<.001
Nonfistulous complications (%)	22 (35)	38 (43)	38 (58)	6 (42)	2 (67)	0.113
Hospital duration (median, days)	8	8	8	9	19	0.001
Total hospital costs (median)	$16,969	$17,797	$20,179	26,776	$40,517	0.002
Total cost increase (beyond no risk factors)	—	$828	$3210	$9807	$23,548	—

Adapted from Pratt WB, Callery MP, Vollmer CM Jr: Risk prediction for development of pancreatic fistula using the International Study Group of Pancreatic Surgery classification scheme. *World J Surg* 32:419, 2007.
Risk factors for pancreatic fistulas consist of (1) small pancreatic duct size (<3 mm); (2) pancreatic parenchyma of soft texture; (3) ampullary, duodenal, cystic, or islet cell pathology; and (4) increased intraoperative blood loss (>1000 mL).

Although the incidence of POPF seems to be similar after distal and central pancreatectomy versus proximal pancreatectomy, the clinical course in the setting of a distal resection is milder.[32] However, risk factors particular to distal resections remain poorly understood. Again, a soft gland is predictive of POPF, as well as primary pancreatic pathology, splenic preservation, and failure to use somatostatin (Editors' note: this latter point is debatable).[33] Division of the pancreas at the body rather than the neck, and failure to ligate the main pancreatic duct were also identified as predictors of POPF after distal pancreatectomy.[34] Furthermore, there was no difference in fistula rate for stump closure with suture versus stapler, nor for any demographic measures.[33]

PREVENTIVE MEASURES

Many technical variations have been studied with the hope of decreasing the incidence of POPF. For pancreaticoduodenectomy, both the type of anastomosis and the technique utilized have been evaluated. The pancreatic-enteric anastomosis may be to the jejunum or to the stomach. For the more typical pancreaticojejunal anastomosis, a duct-to-mucosa or invagination technique may be employed, as demonstrated in Figures 101-2 and 101-3, respectively.[35] Most groups have found the

duct-to-mucosa technique to be superior in terms of fistula rates, according to a large metaanalysis by Poon et al published in 2002 and reflecting the studies of the 1990s.[36] Additional variations include the use of a single- or double-layer anastomosis as well as the choice between continuous and interrupted suture. The binding pancreaticojejunostomy, in which invagination is used with ablation of the overlapping jejunal mucosa, has recently been shown to have equivalent fistula rates versus duct-to-mucosa, but increased incidence of PPH.[37] There is one recent report of superiority of the invagination technique over the duct-to-mucosa technique in terms of fistula rate[38] but the usual practice of the surgeons involved is taken into account; thus, the results are difficult to interpret, and at this point, duct-to-mucosa continues to be the preferred technique.

Pancreaticogastrostomy has been postulated to be advantageous with respect to POPF occurrence, because of the thickness and blood supply of the gastric wall, its proximity to the pancreas, and incomplete activation of pancreatic enzymes in the presence of gastric acid.[23,32] Yeo et al[39] completed a prospective, randomized trial comparing pancreaticojejunostomy to pancreaticogastrostomy (Figure 101-4), which failed to demonstrate any benefit to either technique, as the

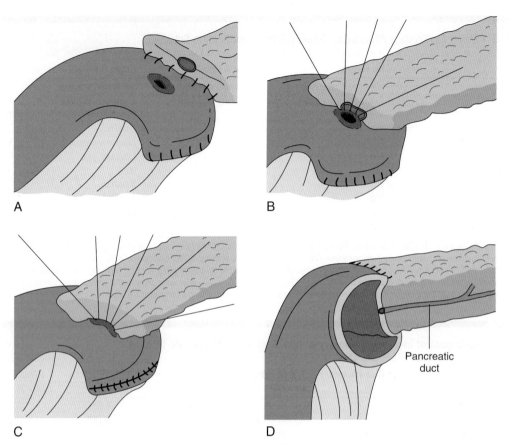

FIGURE 101-2 Duct-to-mucosa pancreaticojejunostomy. **A,** Posterior outer row of interrupted silk sutures. **B,** Posterior inner layer of duct-to-mucosa sutures. **C,** Anterior inner layer of duct to mucosa interrupted sutures have been placed and tied. **D,** Side view of completed anastomosis. Note in this trial, in-dwelling stents were not used. (Redrawn from Cameron JL, Sandone C: *Atlas of gastrointestinal surgery*, vol 1, ed 2. Hamilton, Ontario, 2007, Decker, p 296, Figs 26, 27, 30, and 31.)

fistula rate was approximately 12% in both groups, which were similar in terms of gland texture and operative characteristics. Of note, surgeon volume did affect fistula rate.[38] There have been several nonrandomized similar studies that have concluded that pancreaticogastrostomy does in fact have a lower fistula rate and in one case, a lower associated mortality,[36] but because of study design, the true value is difficult to assess. Furthermore, long-term patency and functional results may be problematic with this variation, as described in smaller case series.[36] Thus, pancreaticojejunostomy continues as the mainstay of the reconstruction, although there may be some merit to performing the invagination technique or pancreaticogastrostomy when the duct is very small and/or difficult to delineate, and other high-risk factors are present, or when the surgeon is more practiced with those techniques.

In summary and at a most fundamental level, a successful pancreaticoenteric anastomosis requires a tension-free anastomosis with properly placed and tied sutures, preserved blood supply to the pancreatic remnant and jejunum, and unobstructed flow from the pancreas into the gastrointestinal tract, whatever the chosen technique may be.

Neither internal stenting nor creation of an isolated Roux loop has been found to positively affect fistula rate.[40] There is, however, one prospective randomized trial that demonstrates a significantly lower rate of POPF formation with external stenting compared to no stent.[41] In theory, such external drainage might be advantageous because it should completely divert the pancreatic secretions away from the anastomosis.[40]

After distal pancreatectomy, fistula rates have been studied to compare stapled versus sutured pancreatic remnant[33] without clear demonstration of benefit with one technique over another evaluating the various papers in the literature[33,34]; thus, either approach is acceptable. Investigation of the success of fibrin glue for preventing POPF has been marred by bias, and thus no conclusion has been reached as regards its utility.[23]

Octreotide, a long-lasting analogue of somatostatin, inactivates gastric and pancreatic exocrine secretion, and may thus support a fragile pancreaticojejunostomy[23] or soft remnant after distal pancreatectomy. Studies of the utility of octreotide for decreasing POPF have been conflicting.[23,33,34] Some authors have found octreotide to be effective for distal[33] or local resection but not helpful in pancreaticoduodenectomy.[36] However, the benefit is clearer for high-risk glands[36,42] after pancreaticoduodenectomy. Prophylactic octreotide was efficacious and cost-efficient when given to patients at high risk for POPF, with the criteria as listed previously,[26] and thus may be used selectively for those patients. No benefit was found for low-risk patients.

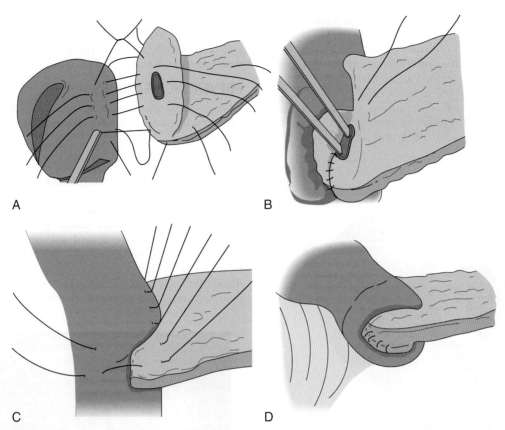

FIGURE 101-3 Invagination pancreaticojejunostomy. **A,** Posterior outer row of silk interrupted sutures. **B,** Inner continuous suture. **C,** Outer layer of interrupted silk sutures. **D,** Completed anastomosis demonstrating the "dunking" of the pancreatic remnant. (Redrawn from Cameron JL, Sandone C: *Atlas of gastrointestinal surgery,* vol 1, ed 2, Hamilton, Ontario, 2007, Decker, p 294, Figs 21, 23, 24, and 25.)

MANAGEMENT

Management of clinically relevant pancreatic fistulas hinges on timely diagnosis. Especially because latent leaks or fistulas may develop[43] and the patient may be home already, with the operative drain out, it is critical to acknowledge and respond to patient reports of worsening abdominal pain, fever, failure to thrive, or inability to tolerate a diet. According to the ISGPF classification, diagnosis requires drain amylase measurement, as well as clinical and imaging data. Furthermore, a sinister character of drain effluent, or output greater than 200 mL/day after postoperative day 5 may be associated with clinically relevant POPF.[23] Grade A fistulas are not of clinical consequence.[24] Patients having had a proximal or central pancreatectomy are more likely to require aggressive resuscitation and/or intervention than are patients after distal pancreatectomy.[32]

Much of the treatment of clinically relevant POPF is empiric. Initial management often includes hydration, being "nil per os" (NPO), supplemental nutrition, and antibiotics when patients present with signs and symptoms of infection (i.e., fever, leukocytosis). Octreotide may be given for high-output fistulas. Patients with amenable collections may undergo radiology-guided drainage, particularly if the operative drain has already been removed or if it is not adequately draining the site of the collection.

Reexploration is rarely required but may be necessary in the setting of clinical decline, undrainable fistula/abscess, or for the suspicion of pancreaticojejunal anastomotic dehiscence (Figure 101-5). Options include wide drainage, anastomotic revision or conversion to alternate pancreatic duct drainage site, completion pancreatectomy, or use of a bridge-stent technique[44] as depicted in Figure 101-6. Pancreaticojejunal anastomotic dehiscence following pancreaticoduodenectomy is a rare but difficult problem to manage. The above-mentioned traditional surgical options are associated with significant morbidity and mortality. With a patient who is already compromised physiologically, the goal is a safe, efficient reoperation. The bridge-stent technique allowed a small group of patients to recover to hospital discharge with limited long-term sequelae[44] and is another option in the armamentarium to deal with this complex problem.

Patients with clinically relevant POPF are known to have longer hospital stays, more additional complications, ICU requirements, transfusion requirements, and need for services or rehabilitation placement on discharge.[24] Accordingly, total costs increase significantly as the grade of fistula increases.[24]

DELAYED GASTRIC EMPTYING

Although delayed gastric emptying (DGE) is rarely life-threatening and typically is self-limited, it can increase the length of hospital stay, likelihood of readmission, other complications, and ultimately cost.[45,46] Until 2007, there was no standard definition of DGE and, thus, it was difficult to compare the multitude of literature reports on the topic, which described an incidence after pancreaticoduodenectomy of 6% to more than 50%.[5,45,47-49] The ISGPS has now created a definition (Table 101-5) of DGE, dividing it into grades of severity. Similar to the consensus definitions for PPH and POPF, this effort resulted in a standardized classification scheme based on duration of NGT decompression required, time until solid food is tolerated, the presence of vomiting or gastric distention, and the use of prokinetics.[45,49]

PREVENTIVE MEASURES

DGE is likely multifactorial but may be related to the decrease in plasma motilin that occurs following duodenal resection, vagal innervation to the pylorus and antrum with gastric atony, and/or relative devascularization of the pylorus.[45] Thus, attempts to prevent DGE have centered on technical modifications to modulate the above-mentioned factors.

Some groups have found a decreased rate of DGE with pylorus-preserving versus classic pancreaticoduodenectomy, but others have found the opposite, leaving no clearly better technique at this point in time.[45,46,50] Still other surgeons advocate pylorus-preserving pancreaticoduodenectomy with the addition of a pyloric dilation or pyloromyotomy to decrease the incidence of DGE.[4,45,51]

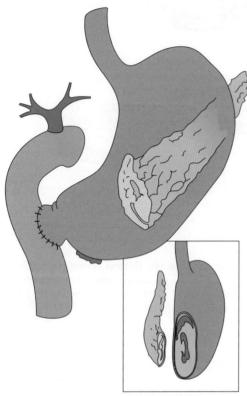

FIGURE 101-4 Pancreaticogastrostomy illustration, with anastomosis of the pancreas to the posterior gastric wall. (Redrawn from Yeo CJ, Cameron JL, Maher MA, et al: A prospective randomized trial of pancreaticogastrostomy versus pancreaticojejunostomy after pancreaticoduodenectomy. *Ann Surg* 222:580, 1995.)

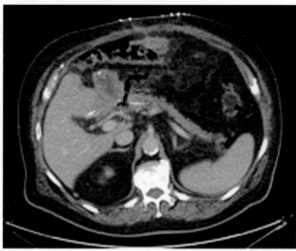

FIGURE 101-5 *Arrows* demonstrate gap between the pancreas and the jejunum, with associated peripancreatic gas. (From Kent TS, Callery MP, Vollmer CM: The bridge-stent technique for salvage of pancreatico-jejunal anastomotic dehiscence. *HPB [Oxford]* 12:577, 2010.)

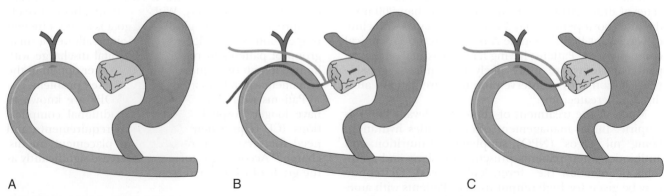

A   B   C

FIGURE 101-6 **A,** Dehiscence of the pancreaticojejunal anastomosis is illustrated, with a gap between the pancreatic remnant and jejunum. **B,** Bridge-stent technique with externalized stent plus external drain. **C,** Bridge-stent technique with internal stent and external drain adjacent to gap. (From Kent TS, Callery MP, Vollmer CM: The bridge-stent technique for salvage of pancreatico-jejunal anastomotic dehiscence. *HPB [Oxford]* 12:577, 2010.)

TABLE 101-5 Consensus Definition of DGE After Pancreatic Surgery

DGE Grade	NGT Required	Unable to Tolerate Solid Oral Intake by POD	Vomiting/Gastric Distention	Use of Prokinetics
A	4-7 d or reinsertion > POD 3	7	±	±
B	8-14 d or reinsertion > POD 7	14	+	+
C	>14 d or reinsertion > POD 14	21	+	+

From Wente MN, Bassi C, Dervenis C, et al: Delayed gastric emptying after pancreatic surgery: A suggested definition by the International Study Group of Pancreatic Surgery. *Surgery* 142:761, 2007.
DGE, Delayed gastric emptying; *NGT*, nasogastric tube; *POD*, postoperative day.
Note: To exclude mechanical causes of abnormal gastric emptying, the patency of either the gastrojejunostomy or the duodenojejunostomy should be confirmed by endoscopy or upper gastrointestinal gastrograph in series.

These studies have been difficult to interpret in light of variable DGE definitions and variation in the diagnoses of included cases, and recent reviews conclude equivalency.[52,53] Another decision point is the location (retro- or antecolic) of the gastro or duodenojejunostomy. Nikfarjam et al found a significant decrease in the rate of DGE when they switched from retrocolic to antecolic gastro- or duodenojejunostomy.[54] This finding was confirmed by a small, but prospective, randomized trial in which DGE was 5% for antecolic duodenojejunostomy versus 50% for the retrocolic approach.[55]

Promotility agents have also been evaluated as to their efficacy at decreasing the incidence of DGE after pancreatic resection. A prospective study in 1993 found that erythromycin, a motilin agonist, was associated with a 37% reduction in the incidence of DGE, and with a significant reduction in the percentage liquid retention in gastric emptying studies.[56] Another similar study supported this finding.[57] Metoclopramide is often used instead of, or in addition to erythromycin, but is not well studied in this patient population. Octreotide also may have an adjunctive role in decreasing DGE in terms of its ability to limit POPF.

MANAGEMENT

Nearly all patients with DGE resolve with conservative management, consisting of nasogastric tube decompression and nutritional support, either with a feeding jejunostomy tube or with total parenteral nutrition (TPN) until symptoms resolve and a regular diet can be tolerated. Additionally, management of the primary associated problem, that is, pancreatic fistula, is crucial.

In summary, many technical modifications have been investigated with respect to limiting DGE. Again, the ability to draw meaningful conclusions from most of these published reports is limited by the lack of uniform definition and by, in general, longer time to remove the nasogastric tube or initiate diet in the older studies. Furthermore, when one technical aspect was compared, many other factors varied, again limiting comparison. However, the use of an antecolic duodenojejunostomy does seem to be consistently associated with decreased DGE rates.[53,55] Most important in the prevention of DGE is the avoidance of other complications, namely POPF, as discussed earlier, since such complications are clearly associated with a secondary DGE.[45,47,58,59]

INFECTIOUS COMPLICATIONS

Infectious complications occur frequently following pancreatectomy. In a recent review of our own data, infections occurred in nearly one-third of patients, including both proximal and distal resections, and accounted for a nearly 40% increase in total cost as well as one extra hospital day. Among major infections, infected pancreatic fistula was responsible for 28%, followed by wound infection at 24%. Other major infections included pneumonia (17%), abscess (15%), urinary tract infection (10%), and sepsis (6%). Many patients with at least one infection incurred multiple infections. Thus, infectious complications, of both minor and major significance, occur frequently following pancreatic resections and are most commonly wound infections and infected pancreatic fistulas. These are responsible for a significant burden to patients, practitioners, and systems alike. Their common occurrence in the setting of excellent adherence to infection control regulations emphasizes the need to discover better process improvements to decrease the incidence of infectious complications, including reevaluating the effectiveness of chosen antimicrobial prophylaxis regimens and adjusting the regimens according to various risk profiles.

SUMMARY

Pancreatic resection remains a high-acuity operation that can be safely performed by appropriately trained and experienced surgeons, in adequately equipped facilities. Although mortality has declined, morbidity remains high. Major potential complications as discussed here include postoperative pancreatic fistula, postpancreatectomy hemorrhage, and delayed gastric emptying. Other, more generic, complications remain prevalent as well, particularly wound infections, which have been reported at 7% to 15%, and in association with fistulas.[5,39,54]

Aside from efforts to prevent and appropriately manage individual complications, the system of care delivery for pancreatic surgical patients plays a crucial role in improving outcomes overall. Adequate system-wide support for the diagnosis and management of complications must be sufficient to provide the appropriate level of care.[9] For example, services available should include ICU level of care, adequate blood bank, interventional radiology and gastroenterology, nurses accustomed to managing complex postoperative care and drains, and case management. Standardized care plans have been developed to care for postpancreatectomy patients. "Critical" or "clinical" pathways have been defined as "structured multidisciplinary care plans that detail essential steps (process measures) in the care of patients with specific problems."[60] Such structured plans have been shown to positively impact outcomes for these patients. Initial results included a decrease in resource utilization and cost.[61,62] Further investigation confirmed the decreased resource utilization, readmission, and cost, and increased bed/operation theater availability,[61,63,64] and also demonstrated fewer deviations from the expected postoperative course after initiation of the clinical pathway.[23,63] As a result of these data, it has been suggested that development and maintenance of such pathways should be a requirement for institutions to serve as referral centers.[60]

REFERENCES

1. Howard JM: Development and progress in resective surgery for pancreatic cancer. *World J Surg* 23:901, 1999.
2. Vollmer CM, Pratt W, Vanounou T, et al: Quality assessment in high acuity surgery: Volume and mortality are not enough. *Arch Surg* 2:371, 2007.
3. Birkmeyer JD, Dimick JB, Staiger DO, et al: Operative mortality and procedure volume as predictors of subsequent hospital performance. *Ann Surg* 243:411, 2006.
4. Bassi C, Falconi M, Salvia R, et al: Management of complications after pancreaticoduodenectomy in a high volume center: Results on 150 consecutive patients. *Dig Surg* 18:453, 2001.
5. Sohn TA, Yeo CJ, Cameron JL, et al: Resected adenocarcinoma of the pancreas—616 patients: Results, outcomes, and prognostic indicators. *J Gastrointest Surg* 4:567, 2000.
6. Birkmeyer JD, Finlayson SR, Tosteson AN, et al: Effect of hospital volume on in-hospital mortality with pancreaticoduodenectomy. *Surgery* 125:250. Comment in *Surgery* 1999;127: 238, 1999.
7. Finlayson EV, Goodney PP, Birkmeyer JD: Hospital volume and operative mortality in cancer surgery. *Arch Surg* 138:721, 2003.
8. Fong Y, Gonen M, Rubin D, et al: Long-term survival is superior after resection for cancer in high-volume centers. *Ann Surg* 242:540; discussion 544, 2005.
9. Schmidt CM, Turrini O, Parikh P, et al: Effect of hospital volume, surgeon experience, and surgeon volume on patient outcomes after pancreaticoduodenectomy: A single-institution experience. *Arch Surg* 145:634, 2010.
10. van Berge Henegouwen MI, Allema JH, van Gulik TM, et al: Delayed massive haemorrhage after pancreatic and biliary surgery. *Br J Surg* 82:1527, 1995.
11. Tien YW, Lee PH, Yang CY, et al: Risk factors of massive bleeding related to pancreatic leak after pancreaticoduodenectomy. *J Am Coll Surg* 201:554, 2005.
12. Trede M, Schwall G: The complications of pancreatectomy. *Ann Surg* 207:39, 1998.
13. Yekebas EF, Wolfram L, Cataldegirmen G, et al: Postpancreatectomy hemorrhage: Diagnosis and treatment: An analysis in 1669 consecutive pancreatic resections. *Ann Surg* 246:269, 2007.
14. Wente MN, Veit JA, Bassi C, et al: Postpancreatectomy hemorrhage (PPH)—an International Study Group of Pancreatic Surgery (ISGPS) definition. *Surgery* 142:20, 2007.
15. Shukla PJ, Barreto SG, Kulkarni A, et al: Vascular anomalies encountered during pancreatoduodenectomy: Do they influence outcomes? *Ann Surg Oncol* 17:186, 2010.
16. Kim AW, McCarthy WJ 3rd, Maxhimer JB, et al: Vascular complications associated with pancreaticoduodenectomy adversely affect clinical outcome. *Surgery* 132:738, 2002.
17. Pachter HL, Drager S, Godfrey N, et al: Traumatic injuries of the portal vein. *Ann Surg* 189:383, 1979.
18. Morgan K, Mansker D, Adams DB: Not just for trauma patients: Damage control laparotomy in pancreatic surgery. *J Gastrointest Surg* 14:768, 2010.
19. Standop J, Glowka T, Schmitz V, et al: Operative re-intervention following pancreatic head resection: Indications and outcome. *J Gastrointest Surg* 13:1503, 2009.
20. Choi SH, Moon HJ, Heo JS, et al: Delayed hemorrhage after pancreaticoduodenectomy. *J Am Coll Surg* 199:186, 2004.
21. De Castro SM, Kuhlmann KF, Busch OR, et al: Delayed massive hemorrhage after pancreatic and biliary surgery. *Ann Surg* 241:85, 2005.
22. Reid-Lombardo KM, Farnell MB, Crippa S, et al: Pancreatic Anastomotic Leak Study Group. Pancreatic anastomotic leakage after pancreaticoduodenectomy in 1,507 patients: A report from the Pancreatic Anastomotic Leak Study Group. *J Gastrointest Surg* 11:1451, 2007.
23. Callery MP, Pratt WB, Vollmer CM: Prevention and management of pancreatic fistula. *J Gastrointest Surg* 13:163, 2009.
24. Pratt WB, Maithel SK, Vanounou T, et al: Clinical and economic validation of the International Study Group of Pancreatic Fistula (ISGPF) classification scheme. *Ann Surg* 245:443, 2007.
25. Bassi C, Dervenis C, Butturini G, et al: Postoperative pancreatic fistula: An international study group (ISGPF) definition. *Surgery* 138:8, 2005.
26. Pratt WB, Callery MP, Vollmer CM: Risk prediction for development of pancreatic fistula utilizing the ISGPF classification scheme. *World J Surg* 32:419, 2007.
27. Lin JW, Cameron JL, Yeo CJ, et al: Risk factors and outcomes in postpancreaticoduodenectomy pancreaticocutaneous fistula. *J Gastrointest Surg* 8:951, 2004.
28. de Castro SM, Busch OR, van Gulik TM, et al: Incidence and management of pancreatic leakage after pancreatoduodenectomy. *Br J Surg* 92:1117, 2005.
29. Yeh TS, Jan YY, Jeng LB, et al: Pancreaticojejunal anastomotic leak after pancreaticoduodenectomy—multivariate analysis of perioperative risk factors. *J Surg Res* 67:119, 1997.
30. Matsusue S, Takeda H, Nakamura Y, et al: A prospective analysis of the factors influencing pancreaticojejunostomy performed using a single method, in 100 consecutive pancreaticoduodenectomies. *Surg Today* 28:719, 1998.
31. Cheng TY, Sheth K, White RR, et al: Effect of neoadjuvant chemoradiation on operative mortality and morbidity for pancreaticoduodenectomy. *Ann Surg Oncol* 13:66, 2006.
32. Pratt W, Maithel SK, Vanounou T, et al: Postoperative pancreatic fistulas are not equivalent after proximal, distal, and central pancreatectomy. *J Gastrointest Surg* 10:1264, 2006.
33. Ridolfini MP, Alfieri S, Gourguitis S, et al: Risk factors associated with pancreatic fistula after distal pancreatectomy: Which technique of pancreatic stump closure is more beneficial? *World J Gastroenterol* 13:5096, 2007.
34. Pannegeon V, Pessaux P, Sauvanet A, et al: Pancreatic fistula after distal pancreatectomy: Predictive risk factors and value of conservative treatment. *Arch Surg* 141:1071, 2006.
35. Cameron JL, Sandone C: *Atlas of gastrointestinal surgery*, Vol. 1, ed 2. Hamilton, Ontario, 2007, Decker, p 294.
36. Poon RT, Lo SH, Fong D, et al: Prevention of pancreatic anastomotic leakage after pancreaticoduodenectomy. *Am J Surg* 183:42, 2002.
37. Maggiori L, Sauvanet A, Nagarajan G, et al: Binding versus conventional pancreaticojejunostomy after pancreaticoduodenectomy: A case-matched study. *J Gastrointest Surg* 14:1395, 2010.
38. Berger AC, Howard TJ, Kennedy EP, et al: Does type of pancreaticojejunostomy after pancreaticoduodenectomy decrease rate of pancreatic fistula? A randomized, prospective, dual-institution trial. *J Am Coll Surg* 208:738, 2009.
39. Yeo CJ, Cameron JL, Maher MA, et al: A prospective randomized trial of pancreaticogastrostomy versus pancreaticojejunostomy after pancreaticoduodenectomy. *Ann Surg* 222:580, 1995.
40. Lai EC, Lau SH, Lau WY: Measures to prevent pancreatic fistula after pancreaticoduodenectomy: A comprehensive review. *Arch Surg* 144:1074, 2009.
41. Poon RT, Fan ST, Lo CM, et al: External drainage of pancreatic duct with a stent to reduce leakage rate of pancreaticojejunostomy after pancreaticoduodenectomy: A prospective randomized trial. *Ann Surg* 246:425, 2007.
42. Vanounou T, Pratt WB, Callery MP, et al: Selective administration of prophylactic octreotide during pancreaticoduodenectomy: A clinical and cost-benefit analysis in low- and high-risk glands. *J Am Coll Surg* 205:546, 2007.
43. Pratt WB, Callery MP, Vollmer CM Jr: The latent presentation of pancreatic fistulas. *Br J Surg* 96:641, 2009.
44. Kent TS, Callery MP, Vollmer CM: The bridge-stent technique for salvage of pancreatico-jejunal anastomotic dehiscence. *HPB (Oxford)* 12:577, 2010.

45. Wente MN, Bassi C, Dervenis C, et al: Delayed gastric emptying (DGE) after pancreatic surgery: A suggested definition by the International Study Group of Pancreatic Surgery (ISGPS). *Surgery* 142:761, 2007.

46. van Berge Henegouwen MI, van Gulik TM, DeWitt LT, et al: Delayed gastric emptying after standard pancreaticoduodenectomy versus pylorus-preserving pancreaticoduodenectomy: An analysis of 200 consecutive patients. *J Am Coll Surg* 185:373, 1997.

47. Miedema BW, Sarr MG, van Heerden JA, et al: Complications following pancreaticoduodenectomy. Current management. *Arch Surg* 127:945, 1992.

48. Richter A, Niedergethmann M, Sturm JW, et al: Long-term results of partial pancreaticoduodenectomy for ductal adenocarcinoma of the pancreatic head: 25-year experience. *World J Surg* 27:324, 2003.

49. Welsch T, Borm M, Degrate L, et al: Evaluation of the International Study Group of Pancreatic Surgery definition of delayed gastric emptying after pancreaticoduodenectomy in a high-volume centre. *Br J Surg* 97:1043, 2010.

50. Witzigmann H, Max D, Uhlmann D, et al: Outcome after duodenum-preserving pancreatic head resection is improved compared with classic Whipple procedure in the treatment of chronic pancreatitis. *Surgery* 134:53, 2003.

51. Kim DK, Hindenburg AA, Sharma SK, et al: Is pylorospasm a cause of delayed gastric emptying after pylorus-preserving pancreaticoduodenectomy? *Ann Surg Oncol* 12:222, 2005.

52. Lytras D, Paraskevas KI, Avgerinos C, et al: Therapeutic strategies for the management of delayed gastric emptying after pancreatic resection. *Langenbecks Arch Surg* 392:1, 2007.

53. Paraskevas K, Avgerinos C, Manes C, et al: Delayed gastric emptying is associated with pylorus-preserving but not classical Whipple pancreaticoduodenectomy: A review of the literature and critical reappraisal of the implicated pathomechanism. *World J Gastroenterol* 12:5951, 2006.

54. Nikfarjam M, Kimchi ET, Gusani NJ, et al: A reduction in delayed gastric emptying by classic pancreaticoduodenectomy with an antecolic gastrojejunal anastomosis and a retrogastric omental patch. *J Gastrointest Surg* 13:1674, 2009.

55. Tani M, Terasawa H, Kawai M, et al: Improvement of delayed gastric emptying in pylorus-preserving pancreaticoduodenectomy: Results of a prospective, randomized, controlled trial. *Ann Surg* 243:316, 2006.

56. Yeo CJ, Barry MK, Sauter PK, et al: Erythromycin accelerates gastric emptying following pancreaticoduodenectomy: A prospective, randomized placebo controlled trial. *Ann Surg* 218:229, 1993.

57. Ohwada S, Satoh Y, Kawate S, et al: Low-dose erythromycin reduces delayed gastric emptying and improves gastric motility after Billroth I pylorus-preserving pancreaticoduodenectomy. *Ann Surg* 234:668, 2001.

58. Park YC, Kim SW, Jang JY, et al: Factors influencing delayed gastric emptying after pylorus-preserving pancreatoduodenectomy. *J Am Coll Surg* 196:859, 2003.

59. Sauvanet A: Complications chirurgicales des pancréatectomies. *J Chir* 145:103, 2008.

60. Riall TS, Nealon WH, Goodwin JS, et al: Outcomes following pancreatic resection: Variability among high-volume providers. *Surgery* 144:133, 2008.

61. Porter GA, Pisters PW, Mansyur C, et al: Cost and utilization impact of a clinical pathway for patients undergoing pancreaticoduodenectomy. *Ann Surg Oncol* 7:484, 2000.

62. Kennedy EP, Rosato EL, Sauter PK, et al: Initiation of a critical pathway for pancreaticoduodenectomy at an academic institution— the first step in multidisciplinary team building. *J Am Coll Surg* 204:917, 2007.

63. Vanounou T, Pratt W, Fischer JE, et al: Deviation-based cost modeling: A novel model to evaluate the clinical and economic impact of clinical pathways. *J Am Coll Surg* 204:570, 2007.

64. Kennedy EP, Grenda TR, Sauter PK, et al: Implementation of a critical pathway for distal pancreatectomy at an academic institution. *J Gastrointest Surg* 13:938, 2009.

PART TWO

Biliary Tract

Anatomy, Embryology, Anomalies, and Physiology

Henry A. Pitt | Thomas R. Gadacz

The anatomy of the biliary tract is intimately associated with both the liver and the pancreas. Thus, an understanding of biliary anatomy must include these adjacent organs as well as their embryology. Similarly, anomalies of the biliary tract and the associated vasculature are common and result from arrested or abnormal development during embryonic growth. Biliary physiology also is closely associated with the liver where bile is formed, as well as with the pancreas, because the sphincter of Oddi regulates the flow of both bile and pancreatic juice. Thus, for a complete picture of the anatomy, embryology, and physiology of the biliary tract, the reader is referred to corresponding chapters in the sections on the liver and the pancreas.

ANATOMY AND EMBRYOLOGY

The first step in understanding the anatomy of the biliary tract is a review of the embryology of the liver, biliary tract, and pancreas. At the fourth week in the development of the human embryo, a projection appears in the ventral wall of the primitive midgut. At this 3-mm stage, three buds can be recognized. The cranial bud develops into two lobes of the liver, whereas the caudal bud becomes the gallbladder and extrahepatic biliary tree (Figure 102-1). The ventral pancreas, which eventually becomes the pancreatic head and uncinate process, also develops from the caudal bud. The third primitive bud develops from the dorsal surface of the midgut to become the anlage of the remainder of the pancreatic head as well as the neck, body, and tail of the pancreas.[1] At the 5-mm stage, the primitive gallbladder and common bile duct have appeared.

At the 7-mm stage (see Figure 102-1), the liver and hepatic ducts have formed, and the gallbladder, the cystic duct, and the ventral pancreas have arisen from the common duct. At this stage, the stomach has begun to form, and the ventral pancreas has developed from the dorsal mesogastrium. By the 12-mm stage, the ventral pancreatic bud has rotated 180 degrees clockwise around the duodenum. This rotation causes fusion of the ventral

and dorsal buds to form the complete pancreas by the sixth or seventh week of gestation. Within another week, a completely open lumen has formed in the gallbladder, bile ducts, and pancreatic ducts. By the twelfth week of fetal life, the liver begins to secrete bile, and the pancreas secretes fluid that flows through the extrahepatic biliary tree and pancreatic ducts, respectively, into the duodenum.

INTRAHEPATIC DUCTS

The anatomy of the biliary tract can be divided into various segments, including the intrahepatic ducts, the extrahepatic ducts, the gallbladder and cystic duct, and the sphincter of Oddi. The anatomy of the intrahepatic ducts is intimately associated with the anatomy of the liver. The lobar and segmental anatomy of the liver is determined by the sequential branching of the portal vein, hepatic artery, and biliary tree as they enter the parenchyma at the hilum. All three of these structures follow roughly parallel courses and bifurcate just before entering the liver. This major bifurcation divides the liver into left and right lobes. According to Couinaud's classification, the caudate lobe is segment I; segments II to IV are on the left; and segments V to VIII are on the right (Figure 102-2).

The biliary drainage of the right and left liver is into the right and left hepatic ducts, respectively. The left hepatic duct is formed within the umbilical fissure from the union of the three segmental ducts draining the left side of the liver (segments II through IV). The left hepatic duct crosses the base of segment IV (medial segment of the left lobe) in a horizontal direction to join the right hepatic duct and form the common hepatic duct. The right hepatic duct drains segments V through VIII and is formed from the union of the right posterior and right anterior segmental ducts. The right posterior segmental duct is formed by the confluence of ducts draining segments VI and VII. The posterior segmental duct initially courses in a nearly horizontal direction before descending in a more vertical direction to join the anterior segmental duct. The right anterior segmental

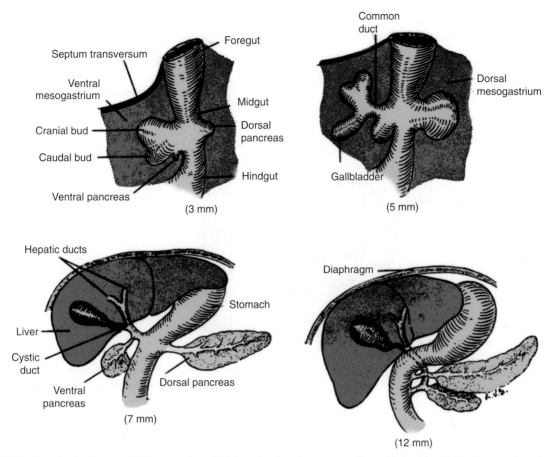

FIGURE 102-1 Embryonic development of the extrahepatic biliary tract and pancreas. (From Linder HH: Embryology and anatomy of the biliary tree. In Way LW, Pellegrini CA, editors: *Surgery of the gallbladder and bile ducts*. Philadelphia, 1987, Saunders, p 4.)

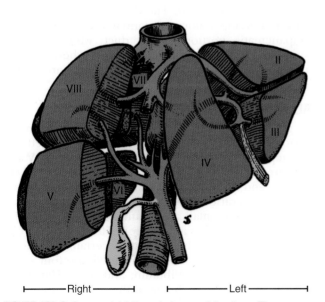

FIGURE 102-2 Segmental biliary drainage of the liver. (From Smadja C, Blumgart LH: The biliary tract and the anatomy of biliary exposure. In Blumgart LH, editor: *Surgery of the liver and biliary tract*. Edinburgh, 1988, Churchill Livingstone, p 11.)

duct is formed by the union of the ducts draining segments V and VIII. In approximately 15% to 20% of cases, the right posterior duct drains into the left hepatic duct.[2] The biliary drainage of the caudate lobe (segment I) is variable.[3] In approximately 80% of the individuals, the caudate lobe drains into both the right and left hepatic ducts. In 15% of cases, the caudate lobe drains only into the left hepatic duct, and in the remaining 5% of cases, the caudate is drained exclusively by the right hepatic duct.[4]

EXTRAHEPATIC DUCTS

Most patients have a bifurcation where the right and left hepatic ducts join to form the common hepatic duct. This junction may occur as a wide or an acute angle, or the two hepatic ducts may run parallel to each other before joining. In some patients, three hepatic ducts join to form the common hepatic duct. Usually, the hepatic ducts meet just outside of the liver parenchyma, with the cystic duct entering 2 to 3 cm distally. Occasionally, the two hepatic ducts do not unite until after the cystic duct has joined the right hepatic duct. The common hepatic duct extends for a variable length from the junction of the right and left hepatic ducts to the entrance of the cystic duct into the gallbladder (Figure 102-3).

The common bile duct is formed by the union of the cystic and common hepatic ducts. The common bile duct is approximately 8 cm in length, but, like the hepatic

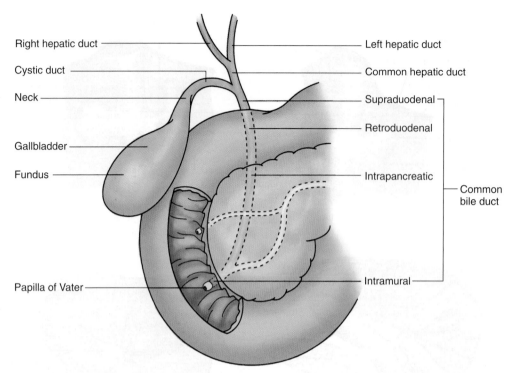

FIGURE 102-3 Anatomic divisions of the gallbladder and extrahepatic biliary tree. (From Gadacz TR: Biliary anatomy and physiology. In Greenfield LJ, Mulholland MW, Oldham KT, editors: *Surgery: Scientific principles and practice.* Philadelphia, 1993, Lippincott, p 931.)

duct, it varies in length according to the point of union of the cystic duct and the common hepatic duct. The normal diameter of the common bile duct ranges from 4 to 9 mm. The common bile duct is considered enlarged if the duct diameter exceeds 10 mm. The upper third, or supraduodenal portion, of the common bile duct courses downward in the free edge of the lesser omentum, anterior to the portal vein and to the right of the proper hepatic artery. The middle third, or retroduodenal portion, of the common bile duct passes behind the first portion of the duodenum, lateral to the portal vein and anterior to the inferior vena cava. The lower third, or intrapancreatic portion, of the common bile duct traverses the posterior aspect of the pancreas in a tunnel or groove to enter the second portion of the duodenum, where it is usually joined by the pancreatic duct. The intramural or intraduodenal portion of the common bile duct passes obliquely through the duodenal wall to enter the duodenum at the papilla of Vater.

The relationship between the lower common bile duct and pancreatic duct is variable: (1) the two structures may rarely unite outside the duodenal wall to form a long common channel; (2) the bile duct and pancreatic duct usually join within the duodenal wall to form a short common channel; or (3) the two structures may rarely enter the duodenum independently through separate orifices. The lower portion of the common bile duct and the terminal portion of the pancreatic duct are enveloped and regulated by a complex sphincter, the sphincter of Oddi. In 5% to 10% of patients who have pancreas divisum, the dorsal pancreatic duct enters the duodenum through an accessory sphincter, whereas the ventral pancreatic duct joins the common bile duct at the sphincter of Oddi.

The extrahepatic bile ducts contain a columnar mucosa surrounded by a connective tissue layer. The surface is relatively flat, with basal nuclei and an absent or small nucleolus. The lamina propria consists of collagen, elastic fibers, and vessels. Occasional lymphocytes are found, and pancreatic acini and ducts may be seen in the wall of the intrapancreatic portion of the distal common bile duct. Muscle fibers in the bile duct are sparse and discontinuous. The muscle fibers that are present are usually longitudinal, although occasional circular fibers are observed. The distal common bile duct begins to develop a more substantial muscle layer in the intrapancreatic portion of the duct, which becomes prominent at the sphincter of Oddi, where distinct bundles of longitudinal and circular fibers are clearly identified.

GALLBLADDER AND CYSTIC DUCT

The gallbladder is a pear-shaped organ that lies on the inferior surface of the liver at the junction of the left and right hepatic lobes between Couinaud's segments IV and V (Figure 102-4).[5] The gallbladder varies from 7 to 10 cm in length and from 2.5 to 3.5 cm in width. The gallbladder's volume varies considerably, being large during fasting states and small after eating. A moderately distended gallbladder has a capacity of 50 to 60 mL of bile but may become much larger with certain pathologic states. The gallbladder has been divided into four areas: the fundus, body, infundibulum, and neck. Hartmann pouch is an asymmetric bulge of the infundibulum that lies close to the gallbladder's neck. The neck points in a cephalad and dorsal direction to join the cystic duct.

The gallbladder wall consists of five layers. The innermost layer is the epithelium, and the other layers are the

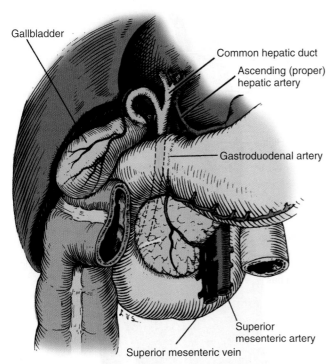

FIGURE 102-4 Anatomic relationships of the gallbladder. (From Linder HH: Embryology and anatomy of the biliary tree. In Way LW, Pellegrini CA, editors: *Surgery of the gallbladder and bile ducts*. Philadelphia, 1987, Saunders, p 8.)

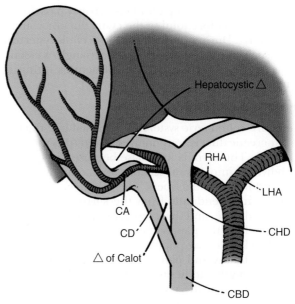

FIGURE 102-5 The triangle (Δ) of Calot and the hepatocystic triangle. The two triangles differ in their upper boundaries. The upper boundary of Calot triangle is the cystic artery *(CA)*, whereas that of the hepatocystic triangle is the inferior margin of the liver. *CBD,* Common bile duct; *CD,* cystic duct; *CHD,* common hepatic duct; *LHA,* left hepatic artery; *RHA,* right hepatic artery. (From Skandalakis JE, Gray SW, Rowe JS Jr: Biliary tract. In Skandalakis JE, Gray SW, editors: *Anatomical complications in general surgery.* New York, 1983, McGraw-Hill, p 31.)

lamina propria, smooth muscle, perimuscular subserosal connective tissue, and serosa. The gallbladder has no muscularis mucosae or submucosa. Most cells in the mucosa are columnar cells, and their main function is absorption, but they also are capable of active secretion.[6] These cells are aligned in a single row, with slightly eosinophilic cytoplasm, apical vacuoles, and basal or central nuclei.

The lamina propria contains nerve fibers, vessels, lymphatics, elastic fibers, loose connective tissue, and occasional mast cells and macrophages. The muscle layer is a loose arrangement of circular, longitudinal, and oblique fibers without well-developed layers. Ganglia are found between smooth muscle bundles. The subserosa is composed of a loose arrangement of fibroblasts, elastic and collagen fibers, vessels, nerves, lymphatics, and adipocytes.

Rokitansky-Aschoff sinuses are invaginations of epithelium into the lamina propria, muscle, and subserosal connective tissue. These sinuses are present in approximately 40% of normal gallbladders and are present in abundance in almost all inflamed gallbladders. The ducts of Luschka are tiny bile ducts found around the muscle layer on the hepatic side of the gallbladder. They are found in approximately 10% of normal gallbladders and have no relation to the Rokitansky-Aschoff sinuses or to cholecystitis.

The cystic duct arises from the gallbladder and joins the common hepatic duct to form the common bile duct (see Figure 102-3). The length of the cystic duct is variable, averaging between 2 and 4 cm. The cystic duct usually courses downward in the hepatoduodenal ligament to join the lateral aspect of the supraduodenal portion of the common hepatic duct at an acute angle.[2] Occasionally, the cystic duct may join the right hepatic duct, or it may extend downward to join the retroduodenal duct. In addition, the cystic duct may join the common hepatic duct at a right angle, may run parallel to the common hepatic duct, or may enter the common hepatic duct dorsally, on its left side, behind the duodenum, or, rarely, may enter the duodenum directly. The cystic duct contains a variable number of mucosal folds, similar to those found in the neck of the gallbladder. Although referred to as valves of Heister, these spiral folds do not have a valvular function. Variations in the length and course of the cystic duct and its point of union with the common hepatic duct are common.

In 1891, Calot described a triangular anatomic region formed by the common hepatic duct medially, the cystic duct laterally, and the cystic artery superiorly.[7] Calot triangle is considered by most to comprise the triangular area with an upper boundary formed by the inferior margin of the right lobe of the liver, rather than the cystic artery (Figure 102-5).[8,9] A thorough appreciation of the anatomy of Calot triangle is essential during performance of a cholecystectomy because numerous important structures pass through this area. In most instances, the cystic artery arises as a branch of the right hepatic artery within the hepatocystic triangle. A replaced or aberrant right hepatic artery arising from the superior mesenteric artery usually courses through the medial aspect of the triangle, posterior to the cystic duct.

Aberrant or accessory hepatic ducts also may pass through Calot triangle before joining the cystic duct or common hepatic duct. During performance of a cholecystectomy, clear visualization of the hepatocystic triangle is essential with accurate identification of all structures within this triangle.

SPHINCTER OF ODDI

The entire sphincteric system of the distal bile duct and the pancreatic duct is commonly referred to as the *sphincter of Oddi*. This term is imprecise because the sphincter is subdivided into several sections and contains both circular and longitudinal fibers. The sphincter mechanism functions independently from the surrounding duodenal musculature and has separate sphincters for the distal bile duct, the pancreatic duct, and the ampulla. In more than 90% of the population, the common channel, where the biliary and pancreatic ducts join, is less than 1.0 cm in length and lies within the ampulla. In the rare situation in which the common channel is longer than 1.0 cm or the biliary and pancreatic ducts open separately into the duodenum, pathologic biliary or pancreatic problems are likely to develop. The entire sphincter mechanism is actually composed of four sphincters containing both circular and longitudinal smooth muscle fibers (Figure 102-6). The four sphincters are the superior and inferior sphincter choledochus, the sphincter pancreaticus, and the sphincter of the ampulla.[10]

VASCULAR

The blood supply to the right and left hepatic ducts and upper portion of the common hepatic duct is from the cystic artery and the right and left hepatic arteries. The supraduodenal bile duct is supplied by arterial branches from the right hepatic, cystic, posterior superior pancreaticoduodenal, and retroduodenal arteries. The axial blood supply of the supraduodenal bile duct has been emphasized by Terblanche and colleagues (Figure 102-7).[11] The most important arteries to the supraduodenal bile duct run parallel to the duct at the 3- and 9-o'clock positions. Approximately 60% of the blood supply to the supraduodenal bile duct originates inferiorly from the pancreaticoduodenal and retroduodenal arteries, whereas 38% of the blood supply originates superiorly from the right hepatic artery and cystic duct artery. Injury to this important axial blood supply may result in the formation of an ischemic ductal stricture. Only 2% of the arterial blood supply to the supraduodenal bile duct is segmental (nonaxial). These small segmental arterial branches arise directly from the proper hepatic artery as it ascends in the hepatoduodenal ligament, adjacent to the common bile duct. The blood supply to the retroduodenal and intrapancreatic bile duct is from the retroduodenal and pancreaticoduodenal arteries.

The cystic artery usually arises as a single branch from the right hepatic artery within Calot triangle (Figure 102-8).[12,13] Infrequently, the cystic artery may arise from the left hepatic, common hepatic, gastroduodenal, or superior mesenteric artery.[14] When the cystic artery arises from the right hepatic artery, it usually courses parallel, adjacent, and medial to the cystic duct. This relation is

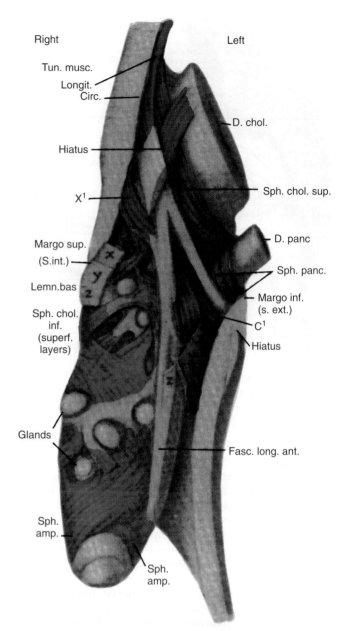

FIGURE 102-6 Human choledochoduodenal junction at the terminal portion of the common bile duct and pancreatic ducts. (From Boyden EA: The anatomy of the choledochoduodenal junction in man. *Surg Gynecol Obstet* 104:646, 1957.)

far from constant, however; and if the artery arises from the proximal right hepatic artery or from the common hepatic artery, it may lie close to the hepatic duct, which may be injured when the artery is ligated.

As it crosses Calot triangle, the cystic artery often supplies the cystic duct with one or more small arterial branches. Near the gallbladder, the cystic artery usually divides into a superficial branch and a deep branch. The superficial branch of the cystic artery courses along the anterior surface of the gallbladder, whereas the deep branch passes between the gallbladder and liver within the cystic fossa.

The right hepatic artery passes posterior to the common hepatic duct as it ascends to the liver in 85% of

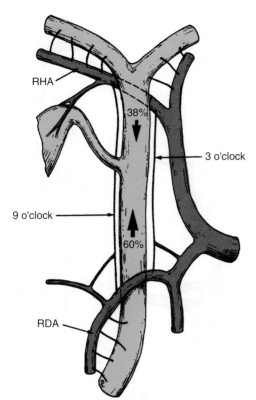

FIGURE 102-7 Arterial blood supply of the extrahepatic biliary tree. The proximal or hilar ducts and the retropancreatic bile duct receive a rich blood supply. The supraduodenal bile duct supply is axial and tenuous, with 60% from below and 38% from above. The small axial vessels (3 o'clock and 9 o'clock arteries) are vulnerable and easily damaged. *RDA,* Retroduodenal artery; *RHA,* right hepatic artery. (From Terblanche J, Allison HF, Northover JMA: An ischemic basis for biliary strictures. *Surgery* 94:56, 1983.)

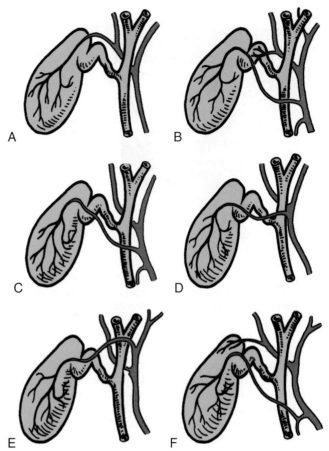

FIGURE 102-8 Cystic artery and its variations. **A,** Usual origin and course of the cystic artery. **B,** Double cystic artery. **C,** Cystic artery crossing anterior to main bile duct. **D,** Cystic artery originating from the right branch of the hepatic artery and crossing the common hepatic duct anteriorly. **E,** Cystic artery originating from the left branch of the hepatic artery. **F,** Cystic artery originating from the gastroduodenal artery. (From Smadja C, Blumgart LH: The biliary tract and the anatomy of biliary exposure. In Blumgart LH, editor: *Surgery of the liver and biliary tract,* Edinburgh, 1988, Churchill Livingstone, p 16.)

individuals and anterior to the common hepatic duct in the remaining 15%. In approximately 15% of individuals, a replaced or aberrant right hepatic artery originates from the superior mesenteric artery and courses through the medial aspect of Calot triangle, posterior to the cystic duct.

The venous drainage from the hepatic ducts and hepatic surface of the gallbladder is through small vessels that empty into branches of the hepatic veins within the liver. A small venous trunk ascending parallel to the portal vein receives veins draining the gallbladder and bile duct before entering the liver, separate from the portal vein.[4] Venous drainage of the lower portion of the bile duct is directly into the portal vein.

LYMPHATIC DRAINAGE

Lymphatic vessels from the hepatic ducts and upper common bile duct drain into the hepatic lymph nodes, a chain of lymph nodes that follows the course of the hepatic artery to drain into the celiac lymph nodes. Lymph from the lower bile duct drains into the lower hepatic nodes as well as the upper pancreatic lymph nodes. Lymphatic vessels from the gallbladder and cystic duct drain primarily into the hepatic nodes by way of the cystic duct node, a constant lymph node located at the junction of the cystic duct and common hepatic duct. Lymphatic vessels from the hepatic surface of the gallbladder may also communicate with lymphatic vessels within the liver.

NEURAL INNERVATION

The gallbladder and biliary tree receive sympathetic and parasympathetic nerve fibers that are derived from the celiac plexus and course along the hepatic artery (Figure 102-9). The left (anterior) vagal trunk branches into hepatic and gastric components. The hepatic branch supplies fibers to the gallbladder, bile duct, and liver. Sympathetic fibers originating from the fifth to the ninth thoracic segments pass through the greater splanchnic nerves to the celiac ganglion. Postganglionic sympathetic fibers travel along the hepatic artery to innervate the gallbladder, bile duct, and liver. Visceral afferent nerve fibers from the liver, gallbladder, and bile duct travel with sympathetic afferent fibers through the greater splanchnic nerves to enter the dorsal roots of the fifth through

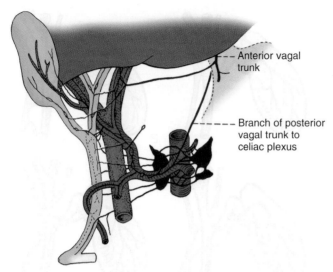

FIGURE 102-9 Nerve supply to the extrahepatic bile tree. (From Linder HH: Embryology and anatomy of the biliary tree. In Way LW, Pellegrini CA, editors: *Surgery of the gallbladder and bile ducts.* Philadelphia, 1987, Saunders, p 21.)

ninth thoracic segments. Sensory fibers from the right phrenic nerve also innervate the gallbladder, presumably through the communications between the phrenic plexus and the celiac plexus. This innervation may explain the phenomenon of referred shoulder pain in patients with gallbladder disease.

ANOMALIES

BILIARY DUCTS

The anatomy of the extrahepatic biliary tree is highly variable. A thorough knowledge of this variable anatomy is important because failure to recognize the frequent anatomic variations may result in significant ductal injury. Anomalies of the extrahepatic biliary tree may involve the hepatic ducts, common bile duct, or cystic duct.

Hepatic Ducts

In 57% to 68% of patients, the right anterior and right posterior intrahepatic ducts join, and the right hepatic duct unites with the left hepatic duct to form the common hepatic duct (Figure 102-10).[3,15,16] Three other common variations are recognized. In 12% to 18% of patients, the right anterior, right posterior, and left hepatic ducts unite to form the common hepatic duct. In 8% to 20% of patients, the right posterior and left hepatic ducts join to form the common hepatic duct, and the right anterior duct joins below the union. In 4% to 7% of patients, the right posterior duct joins the common hepatic duct below the union of the right anterior and the left hepatic ducts. In 1.5% to 3% of patients, the cystic duct joins at the union of all the ducts or with one of the right hepatic ducts.

Accessory hepatic ducts may emerge from the liver to join the right hepatic duct, common hepatic duct, cystic duct, common bile duct, or gallbladder (Figure 102-11). These ducts are present in approximately 10% of

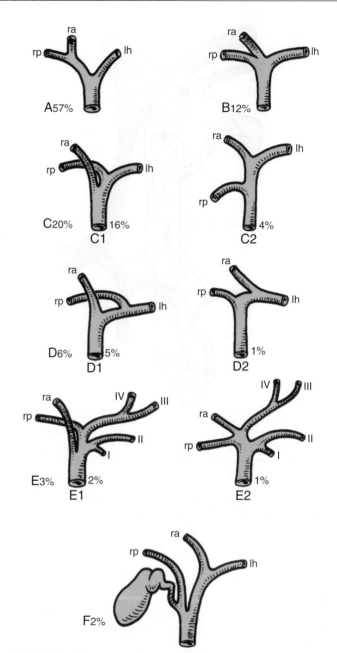

FIGURE 102-10 A to **F,** Variations in hepatic ducts and hepatic duct bifurcation. *lh,* Left hepatic duct; *ra,* right anterior segmental duct; *rp,* right posterior segmental duct. The Roman numerals *I* to *IV* refer to hepatic segmental ducts. (From Smadja C, Blumgart LH: The biliary tract and the anatomy of biliary exposure. In Blumgart LH, editor: *Surgery of the liver and biliary tract.* Edinburgh, 1988, Churchill Livingstone, p 17.)

individuals. Although accessory hepatic ducts may approach the size of a normal cystic duct, they are often delicate, thin structures that may easily be overlooked. Accessory hepatic ducts often course through Calot triangle and may be injured during dissection in this area. Cholecystohepatic ducts are small biliary ducts that emerge from the liver to enter the hepatic surface of the gallbladder directly.[17] If a cholecystohepatic duct is discovered during dissection of the gallbladder from the cystic fossa, it should be ligated to avoid a postoperative bile leak.

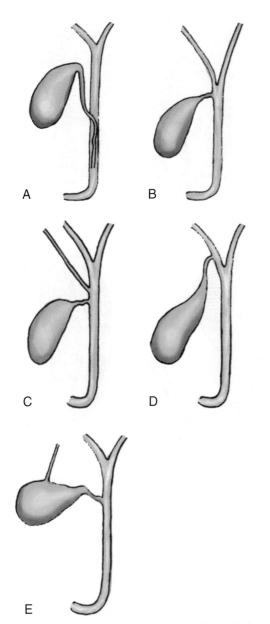

FIGURE 102-11 Duct anomalies. **A,** Long cystic duct with low fusion with common hepatic duct. **B,** Abnormally high fusion of cystic duct with common hepatic duct (trifurcation). **C,** Accessory hepatic duct. **D,** Cystic duct entering right hepatic duct. **E,** Cholecystohepatic duct. (From Benson EA, Page RE: A practical reappraisal of the anatomy of the extrahepatic bile ducts and arteries. *Br J Surg* 63:854, 1976.)

Common Bile Duct

Malpositions or duplications of the common bile duct are rare anomalies. However, recognition of their presence is extremely important to prevent serious injury to the common bile duct during operations on the biliary tract or stomach. Several variations of common bile duct malposition and duplication have been described: (1) a single duct opening into the pylorus or antrum; (2) a single duct opening into the gastric fundus; (3) a single duct entering the duodenum independently of the pancreatic duct; (4) two separate ducts entering the duodenum; (5) a bifurcating duct, with one branch entering

the duodenum and the other branch entering the stomach; (6) a bifurcating duct with both branches entering the duodenum; and (7) a septate common bile duct, with two openings of the single duct into the duodenum. The mere presence of these anomalies does not produce symptoms, and their clinical importance rests solely on their recognition and on the avoidance of injury during an operation.

Cystic Duct

In 1976, Benson and Page described five ductal anomalies of clinical significance to the surgeon during performance of a cholecystectomy.[12] Of these five anomalies, three involve abnormalities in the length, course, or insertion of the cystic duct into the common hepatic duct (see Figure 102-11). The cystic duct may run parallel to the common hepatic duct for a variable distance, or it may spiral anterior or posterior to the common hepatic duct to form a left-sided union. Parallel cystic ducts occur in 15% of individuals, whereas spiral cystic ducts are found in approximately 8%. The parallel or spiral cystic duct may be normal in length or may course downward in the hepatoduodenal ligament for a considerable distance before forming a low union with the common hepatic duct. In both situations, the cystic duct is usually closely adhered to the common hepatic duct by a sheath of connective tissue.

The cystic duct may join the right hepatic duct or a right segmental duct. Less often, the cystic duct, right hepatic duct, and left hepatic duct may join at the same level to form a trifurcation. In these situations, the right hepatic duct may easily be mistaken for the cystic duct and may be inadvertently ligated and divided. Occasionally, the gallbladder may join the common hepatic duct with a short or virtually nonexistent cystic duct. During ligation of a short cystic duct, care must be taken not to compromise the lumen of the common bile duct.

GALLBLADDER

Some apparent anomalies are acquired, but most result from arrested or abnormal development at some stage of embryonic growth. These anomalies vary in their clinical significance: Some are only medical curiosities and require no attempt at correction, whereas others require surgical intervention. The gallbladder anomalies may be divided into three groups based on formation, number, and position (Box 102-1).

Phrygian Cap

This anomaly of formation is the most common of the gallbladder (Figure 102-12, *A*). Phrygian cap occurs in individuals of all ages and more commonly in women. Boyden found that this anomaly was present as confirmed by oral cholecystography in 18% of patients with a functioning gallbladder.[18] The phrygian cap deformity is created by an infolding of a septum between the body and the fundus. The gallbladder functions normally, and this anomaly is not an indication for cholecystectomy.

Bilobed Gallbladder

This rare anomaly of formation consists of a completely divided gallbladder drained by a common cystic duct

> ### BOX 102-1 Anomalies of the Gallbladder
>
> **FORMATION**
>   Phrygian cap
>   Bilobed gallbladder
>   Hourglass gallbladder
>   Diverticulum of the gallbladder
>   Rudimentary gallbladder
>
> **NUMBER**
>   Absence of the gallbladder (agenesis)
>   Duplication of the gallbladder
>
> **POSITION**
>   Floating gallbladder
>   Intrahepatic gallbladder
>   Left-sided gallbladder
>   Transverse gallbladder
>   Retrodisplaced gallbladder

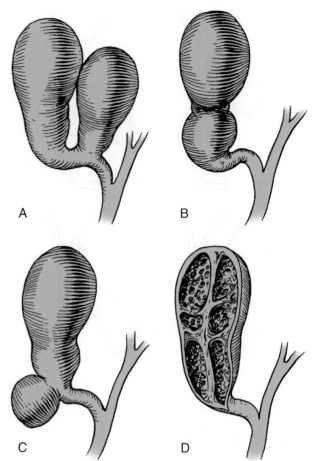

FIGURE 102-13 Anomalies of the gallbladder. **A,** Bilobed gallbladder. **B,** Hourglass gallbladder. **C,** Congenital diverticulum of the infundibulum. **D,** Septate gallbladder. (From Linder HH: Embryology and anatomy of the biliary tree. In Way LW, Pellegrini CA, editors: *Surgery of the gallbladder and bile ducts.* Philadelphia, 1987, Saunders, p 5.)

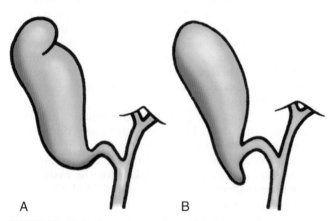

FIGURE 102-12 Deformations of the gallbladder. **A,** Phrygian cap deformity. **B,** Hartmann pouch of the infundibulum. (From Gray SW, Skandalakis JE: *Embryology for surgeons.* Philadelphia, 1972, Saunders, p 254.)

(Figure 102-13, *A*). Bilobed gallbladder occurs in two forms: (1) a type that has the outward appearance of a single gallbladder but is divided internally by a longitudinal fibrous septum; and (2) a type that has the outward appearance of two separate gallbladders that are fused at the neck. A bilobed gallbladder has no clinical significance and does not require excision unless it becomes symptomatic.

Hourglass Gallbladder

Alterations in the contour of the gallbladder may result in a dumbbell or hourglass form (Figure 102-13, *B*). These anomalies are not rare and can be congenital or acquired. In children, this anomaly is congenital and does not require removal. In adults, this abnormality usually results from chronic cholecystitis and should be removed in patients with appropriate biliary symptoms.

Diverticulum of the Gallbladder

Congenital diverticula of the gallbladder are rare, being found in only 25 of 29,701 gallbladders removed surgically at the Mayo Clinic (Figure 102-13, *C*).[19]

Diverticula may occur in any part of the gallbladder and may vary greatly in size from 0.5 to 9 cm in diameter. These diverticula are clinically insignificant unless they become the site of disease, in which case they may contain stones, become acutely inflamed, or even perforate. Hartmann pouch is an acquired diverticulum of the infundibulum or neck of the gallbladder (Figure 102-12, *B*). This pouch projects from the convexity of the gallbladder neck and may be closely adherent to the common bile duct. Hartmann pouch is associated with pathologic conditions of the gallbladder, especially those involving prolonged obstruction to gallbladder emptying.[20]

Rudimentary Gallbladder

This condition consists of a small nubbin at the end of the cystic duct. When found in infants and children, a rudimentary gallbladder is believed to be caused by congenital hypoplasia and usually requires no treatment. In an elderly person, this situation may be the result of fibrosis from cholecystitis and may require removal if causing biliary symptoms.

Absence of the Gallbladder (Agenesis)

More than 200 cases of absence of the gallbladder have been reported. Most cases are associated with other biliary abnormalities, and most of the patients died before 6 months of age. One publication reviewed 185 cases of gallbladder agenesis. In this series, 70 (38%) were completely absent, 60 (32%) were rudimentary, and 55 (30%) were a fibrous structure.[21]

Duplication

This anomaly occurs in approximately 1 in 4000 persons. A true duplicated gallbladder has two separate cavities, each drained by its own cystic duct and sometimes supplied by its own cystic artery (Figure 102-14). Duplication

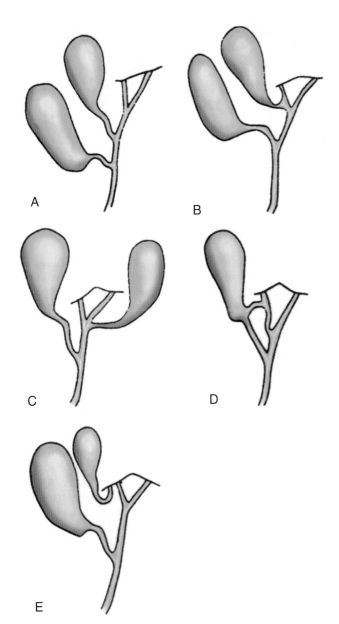

FIGURE 102-14 A to **E,** Duplication of the gallbladder. (From Glassman JA: A short practical review of surgical anatomy of the biliary tract. In Glassman JA, editor: *Biliary tract surgery: Tactics and techniques*. New York, 1989, Macmillan, p 18.)

occurs as one of two varieties: (1) the more common ductular type, in which each gallbladder has its own cystic duct that empties independently into the same or different parts of the extrahepatic biliary tree; and (2) a type in which the two ducts gradually merge into a common cystic duct before emptying into the common bile duct. The gallbladder itself may be seen as two distinct organs at variable distances apart or may outwardly have the appearance of a single organ. Each cavity may function normally or become diseased independently of the other. Duplication of the gallbladder is clinically unimportant and generally requires no treatment.

Rarely, a gallbladder may be found in an abnormal location. This type of gallbladder requires no treatment unless it causes symptoms. Five different conditions are recognized: floating, intrahepatic, left-sided, transverse, and retrodisplaced.

Floating Gallbladder

A floating gallbladder has been reported to occur in approximately 5% of persons. In this condition, the gallbladder is completely surrounded by peritoneum and is attached to the undersurface of the cystic fossa by the peritoneal reflection from the liver. This attachment may extend the entire length of the gallbladder, or it may include only the cystic duct, thus leaving the gallbladder unsupported and ptosed (Figure 102-15, *A* and *B*). This condition usually occurs in women older than 60 years of age. Such a gallbladder not only is subject to the same pathologic changes as a normally placed gallbladder but also may undergo torsion around its pedicle. Torsion of the gallbladder usually occurs in persons 60 to 80 years of age, but it also has been reported to occur in young children. When torsion of the gallbladder occurs, an abrupt onset of symptoms may include acute right upper quadrant abdominal pain, nausea, and vomiting. Torsion of the gallbladder requires operative detorsion and removal of the gallbladder, which may be infarcted as a result of occlusion of its blood vessels.

Intrahepatic Gallbladder

The gallbladder is usually intrahepatic during its embryologic period and becomes extrahepatic later in its development. An intrahepatic gallbladder is one that is partially or completely embedded within the substance of the liver (Figure 102-15, *C*). The condition may be suspected if the cholecystogram or ultrasound reveals a gallbladder in an unusually high location. In adults, approximately 60% of intrahepatic gallbladders are associated with gallstones. Most intrahepatic gallbladders are only partially embedded within the hepatic parenchyma, and they can usually be easily identified at the time of cholecystectomy. Those that are completely buried within the liver may be a challenge to remove. A completely embedded gallbladder is best approached by first identifying the cystic duct where it joins the common hepatic duct and then following the cystic duct back to the gallbladder.

Left-Sided Gallbladder

The two types of left-sided gallbladders are (1) left-sided gallbladder associated with situs inversus, in which the

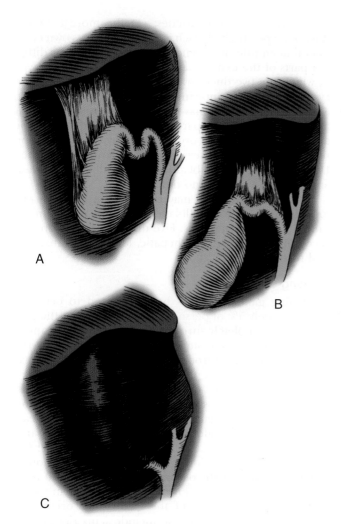

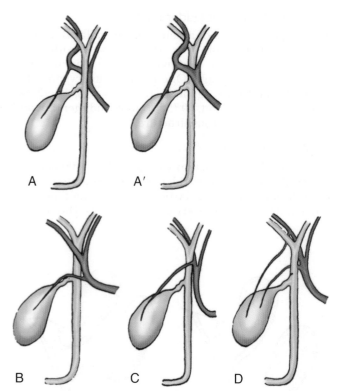

FIGURE 102-15 Anomalies of gallbladder position. **A,** Floating gallbladder with mesentery. **B,** Cystic duct with mesentery. **C,** Intrahepatic gallbladder. (From Linder HH: Embryology and anatomy of the biliary tree. In Way LW, Pellegrini CA, editors: *Surgery of the gallbladder and bile ducts.* Philadelphia, 1987, Saunders, p 5.)

FIGURE 102-16 Vascular anomalies. **A, A′,** "Caterpillar hump" right hepatic artery. **B,** Right hepatic artery anterior to common hepatic (or common bile) duct. **C,** Cystic artery anterior to common hepatic (or common bile) duct. **D,** Accessory cystic artery. (From Benson EA, Page RE: A practical reappraisal of the anatomy of the extrahepatic bile ducts and arteries. *Br J Surg* 63:854, 1976.)

heart and abdominal viscera are transposed from their usual position; and (2) the type in which the gallbladder alone is transposed. Both types of left-sided gallbladders are rare. The malpositioned gallbladder is usually located on the undersurface of the left lobe of the liver. In most instances, the cystic duct joins the common hepatic duct in the usual location, but it may occasionally join the left hepatic duct.

Transverse Gallbladder

In this rare anomaly, the gallbladder is positioned horizontally in the transverse fissure of the liver. In these cases, the gallbladder is usually deeply embedded within the liver parenchyma.

Retrodisplaced Gallbladder

Retrodisplacement of the gallbladder is a condition in which the organ is not situated in the gallbladder fossa but is bound to another portion of the liver or freely suspended from the liver with the fundus extending posteriorly. The retrodisplaced gallbladder may be partially or completely located within the retroperitoneum. This type of gallbladder may be difficult to expose and excise. If the gallbladder is located retroperitoneally, dividing the peritoneum overlying it will facilitate its removal.

VASCULAR

Variations in the arterial supply of the extrahepatic biliary tree are more common than variations in the ductal anatomy. Anatomic variations of the hepatic and cystic arteries are present in approximately 50% of individuals.[4,12,22] Based on their anatomic dissections, Benson and Page described three surgically important variations in the arterial anatomy (Figure 102-16).[12] An accessory or double cystic artery occurs in approximately 15% to 20% of individuals.[12,23] These arteries usually arise from the right hepatic artery within Calot triangle. Triple cystic arteries are unusual and occur in less than 1% of individuals. During dissection of Calot triangle, care should be taken to exclude the presence of an accessory cystic artery.

In 5% to 15% of individuals, the right hepatic artery courses through Calot triangle in close proximity to the cystic duct before turning upward to enter the hilum of the liver.[12,22] In this location, the cystic artery arises from the convex aspect of the angled or humped portion of the hepatic artery. This "caterpillar hump" right hepatic artery may easily be mistaken for the cystic artery and may be inadvertently ligated during performance of a cholecystectomy. The cystic artery that arises from the caterpillar hump is typically short and may easily be avulsed from the hepatic artery if excessive traction is applied to the gallbladder.[12]

The cystic artery may occasionally pass anterior to the common bile duct or common hepatic duct.[13] In this location, the cystic artery, rather than the cystic duct, is usually the first structure encountered during dissection of the lower border of Calot triangle.[23,24] These arteries usually require ligation and division early in the dissection during a cholecystectomy, to provide adequate exposure of the cystic duct.

PHYSIOLOGY

BILE PRODUCTION

Bile Formation

The formation of bile by the hepatocyte serves two purposes. Bile represents the route of excretion for certain organic solutes, such as bilirubin and cholesterol, and it facilitates intestinal absorption of lipids and fat-soluble vitamins. Bile secretion results from the active transport of solutes into the canaliculus followed by the passive flow of water. Water constitutes approximately 85% of the volume of bile.

The major organic solutes in bile are bilirubin, bile salts, phospholipids, and cholesterol. Bilirubin, the breakdown product of spent red blood cells, is conjugated with glucuronic acid by the hepatic enzyme glucuronyl transferase and is excreted actively into the adjacent canaliculus. Normally, a large reserve exists to handle excess bilirubin production, which might exist in hemolytic states. Bile salts are steroid molecules synthesized by the hepatocyte. The primary bile salts in humans, cholic and chenodeoxycholic acid, account for more than 80% of those produced. The primary bile salts, which are then conjugated with either taurine or glycine, can undergo bacterial alteration in the intestine to form the secondary bile salts, deoxycholate and lithocholate. The purpose of bile salts is to solubilize lipids and facilitate their absorption. Phospholipids are synthesized in the liver in conjunction with bile salt synthesis. Lecithin is the primary phospholipid in human bile, constituting more than 95% of its total. The final major solute of bile is cholesterol, which also is produced primarily by the liver with little contribution from dietary sources.

The normal volume of bile secreted daily by the liver is 750 to 1000 mL. Bile flow depends on neurogenic, humoral, and chemical control. Vagal stimulation increases bile secretion. Splanchnic stimulation causes vasoconstriction with decreased hepatic blood flow and, thus, diminished bile secretion. Gastrointestinal hormones including secretin, cholecystokinin, gastrin, and glucagon all increase bile flow, primarily by increasing water and electrolyte secretion. This action probably occurs at a site distal to the hepatocyte. Finally, the most important factor in regulating the volume of bile flow is the rate of bile salt synthesis by the hepatocyte. This rate is regulated by the return of bile salts to the liver by the enterohepatic circulation.

Bile Salt Secretion

Bile is secreted from the hepatocyte into canaliculi that drain their contents into small bile ducts. Secretion of bile salts is the major osmotic force for the generation of bile flow. Bile acids are formed at a rate of 500 to 600 mg per day. The majority of the bile salt pool is maintained in the gallbladder followed by the liver, the small intestine, and the extrahepatic bile ducts. Bile acids are synthesized from cholesterol via (1) a classic pathway that leads to the formation of cholic acid and (2) an alternate pathway that results in the synthesis of chenodeoxycholic acid which occurs less commonly in human bile.[25]

In plasma, bile acids circulate in a bound state either to albumin or lipoproteins. In the space of Disse in the liver, bile salt uptake into the hepatocytes is very efficient. This process is mediated by sodium-dependent and sodium-independent mechanisms. The sodium-dependent pathway accounts for more than 80% of taurocholate uptake but less than 50% of cholate uptake.[26] In recent years, a number of transport proteins have been identified that play a key role in this process. The bile salt transporter, sodium-taurocholate cotransporting polypeptide (NTCP), is exclusively expressed in the liver and is located in the basolateral membrane of the hepatocyte. Sodium-independent hepatic uptake of bile acids is mediated primarily by a family of transporters termed the *organic anion-transporting polypeptides* (OATPs). In contrast to NTCP, these transporters have a broader substrate affinity and transport a variety of organic anions including the bile salts. OATP-C is the major sodium-independent bile salt uptake system. OATP-A also uptakes bile acids, and OATP8 mediates taurocholate uptake.

Intracellular bile acid transport occurs within a matter of seconds. Two mechanisms may be responsible for bile acid transcellular movement. One involves transfer of bile acids from the basolateral membrane to the canalicular membrane via bile-acid binding proteins.[27] The other proposed mechanism for intracellular bile salt movement is through vesicular transport. In contrast, the transport of bile salts across the canalicular membrane of hepatocytes represents the rate-limiting step in the overall secretion of bile salts from the blood into bile.

Bile salt concentrations are 1000-fold greater within the canaliculi than in the hepatocyte. This gradient necessitates an active transport mechanism which is an adenosine triphosphate (ATP)-dependent process. This bile salt export pump (BSEP) is closely related to the proteins encoded by the multidrug resistance (MDR) gene family of ATP-binding cassette (ABC) transporters.[25] The ABC transporters mediate the transport of metabolites, peptides, fatty acids, cholesterol, and lipids in the liver, intestine, pancreas, lungs, kidneys, brain, and in macrophages. Although BSEP is the major transporter for monovalent bile salts into the canaliculus, MRP2, a member of the multidrug resistance protein family, also transports sulfated and glucuronidated bile salts into the canaliculus. MRP2 also mediates the export of multiple other organic anions, including conjugated bilirubin, leukotrienes, glutathione disulfide, chemotherapeutic agents, uricosurics, antibiotics, toxins, and heavy metals.[28]

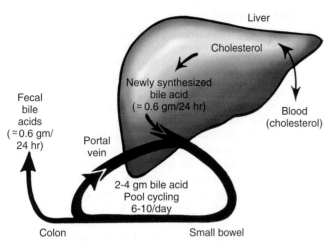

FIGURE 102-17 Enterohepatic circulation of bile salts. Cholesterol is taken up from plasma by the liver. Bile acids are synthesized at a rate of 0.6 g/24 hours and are excreted through the biliary system into the small bowel. Most of the bile salts are reabsorbed in the terminal ileum and are returned to the liver to be extracted and reextracted. (Modified from Dietschy JM: The biology of bile acids. *Arch Intern Med* 130:472, 1972.)

Enterohepatic Circulation

Bile salts are synthesized and conjugated in the liver, secreted into bile, stored temporarily in the gallbladder, passed from the gallbladder into the duodenum, absorbed throughout the small intestine but especially in the ileum, and returned to the liver via the portal vein. This cycling of bile acids between the liver and the intestine is referred to as the *enterohepatic circulation* (Figure 102-17). The total amount of bile acids in the enterohepatic circulation is defined as the circulating bile pool. In this highly efficient system, nearly 95% of bile salts are reabsorbed. Thus, of the total bile salt pool of 2 to 4 g, which recycles through the enterohepatic cycle 6 to 10 times daily, only approximately 600 mg of bile salt is actually excreted into the colon. Bacterial action in the colon on the two primary bile salts, cholate and chenodeoxycholate, results in the formation of the secondary bile salts, deoxycholate and lithocholate. Although some deoxycholate is reabsorbed passively by the colon, the remainder is lost in fecal waste.

The enterohepatic circulation provides an important negative feedback system on bile salt synthesis. Should the recirculation be interrupted by resection of the terminal ileum, or by primary ileal disease, abnormally large losses of bile salts can occur. This situation increases bile salt production to maintain a normal bile salt pool. Similarly, if bile salts are lost by an external biliary fistula, increased bile salt synthesis is necessary. However, except for those unusual circumstances in which excessive losses occur, bile salt synthesis matches losses, maintaining a constant bile salt pool size. During fasting, approximately 90% of the bile acid pool is sequestered in the gallbladder.

Cholesterol Saturation

Cholesterol is highly nonpolar and insoluble in water; thus, it is insoluble in bile. The key to maintaining cholesterol in solution is the formation of micelles, a bile salt–phospholipid-cholesterol complex. Bile salts are amphipathic compounds containing both a hydrophilic and hydrophobic portion. In aqueous solutions, bile salts are oriented with the hydrophilic portion outward. Phospholipids are incorporated into the micellar structure, allowing cholesterol to be added to the hydrophobic central portion of the micelle. In this way, cholesterol can be maintained in solution in an aqueous medium. The concept of mixed micelles as the only cholesterol carrier has been challenged by the demonstration that much of the biliary cholesterol exists in a vesicular form. Structurally, these vesicles are made up of lipid bilayers of cholesterol and phospholipids. In their simplest and smallest form, the vesicles are unilamellar, but an aggregation may take place, leading to multilamellar vesicles. Present theory suggests that in states of excess cholesterol production, these large vesicles may also exceed their capability to transport cholesterol, and crystal precipitation may occur (Figure 102-18).

Cholesterol solubility depends on the relative concentration of cholesterol, bile salts, and phospholipids.[29] By plotting the percentages of each component on triangular coordinates, the micellar zone in which cholesterol is completely soluble can be demonstrated (Figure 102-19). In a solution composed of 10% solutes similar to bile, the area under the curve represents the concentration at which cholesterol is maintained in solution. In the area above the curve, bile is supersaturated with cholesterol, and precipitation of cholesterol crystals can occur.

A mathematical model of cholesterol solubility has been developed and is influenced by the relative concentrations of lipid components and the total lipid composition.[30] A numerical value, known as the *cholesterol saturation* (or lithogenic) *index,* is derived that expresses the relative degrees of cholesterol saturation. When the cholesterol saturation index is greater than 1.0, the solution is supersaturated with cholesterol. Changes in the relative concentrations of bile salts, cholesterol, or phospholipids alter the capacity of micelles, thus changing the solution's cholesterol saturation index.

Bilirubin Metabolism

Heme, released at the time of degradation of senescent erythrocytes by the reticuloendothelial system, is the source of approximately 80% to 85% of the bilirubin produced daily. The remaining 15% to 20% is derived largely from the breakdown of hepatic hemoproteins.[31] Both enzymatic and nonenzymatic pathways for the formation of bilirubin have been proposed. Although both may be important physiologically, the microsomal enzyme heme oxygenase, found in high concentration throughout the liver, spleen, and bone marrow, plays a major role in the initial conversion of heme to biliverdin. Biliverdin is then reduced to bilirubin by the cytosolic enzyme biliverdin reductase in a nicotinamide adenine dinucleotide (NADH)-dependent reaction before being released into the circulation. In this "unconjugated" form, bilirubin has a very low solubility. Bilirubin is bound avidly to plasma proteins, primarily albumin, before uptake and further processing by the liver. The liver is the sole organ capable of removing the albumin-bilirubin complex from the circulation and esterifying the potentially toxic

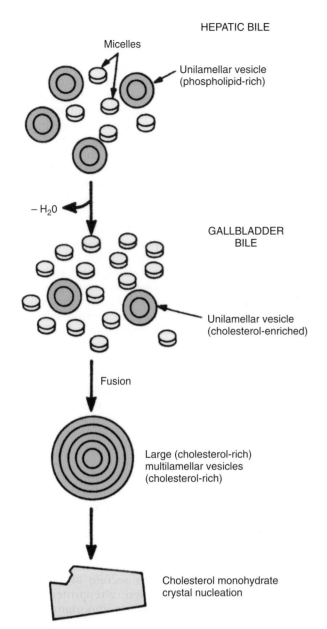

FIGURE 102-18 Concentration of bile leads to net transfer of phospholipids and cholesterol from vesicles to micelles. Phospholipids are transferred more efficiently than cholesterol, leading to cholesterol enrichment of the remaining (remodeled) vesicles. Aggregation of these cholesterol-rich vesicles forms multilamellar liquid crystals of cholesterol monohydrate. (From Vessey DA: Metabolism of drugs and toxins by the human liver. In Zakin D, Boyer TD, editors: *Hepatology: A textbook of liver disease*, ed 2. Philadelphia, 1990, Saunders, p 1492.)

bilirubin to water-soluble, nontoxic monoconjugated and deconjugated derivatives. Conjugated bilirubin is then excreted into the duodenum.

BILE FLOW

The bile ducts, gallbladder, and sphincter of Oddi act in concert to modify, store, and regulate the flow of bile. Approximately 750 to 100 mL of bile is produced daily. During its passage through the bile ductules, canalicular bile is modified by the absorption and secretion

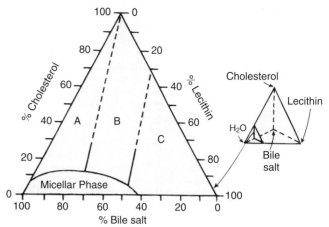

FIGURE 102-19 Interrelationships of bile salts, lecithin, and cholesterol. The graph is a plan taken from a tetrahedron at 90% water concentration. The tetrahedral plot is used to record the relationships of the four major constituents of bile: water, bile salts, lecithin, and cholesterol. The triangular coordinates can be divided into four zones, representing the physical state of the solutes in bile: crystals of cholesterol plus liquid (A); cholesterol crystals plus cholesterol liquid crystals plus liquid (B); liquid crystals plus liquid (C); and the micellar zone in which cholesterol is in water solution through the formation of cholesterol-lecithin-bile salt micelles (D). The *solid line* is the 10% solute line. (From Admirand WH, Small DM: The physicochemical basis of cholesterol gallstone formation in man. *J Clin Invest* 47:1043, 1968.)

of electrolytes and water. The gastrointestinal hormone secretin increases bile flow primarily by increasing the active secretion of chloride-rich fluid by the bile ducts. Bile ductular secretion also is stimulated by other hormones such as cholecystokinin and gastrin. The bile duct epithelium also is capable of water and electrolyte absorption, which may be of primary importance in the storage of bile during fasting in patients who have previously undergone cholecystectomy. The main functions of the gallbladder are to concentrate and store hepatic bile during the fasting state and deliver bile into the duodenum in response to a meal. The usual capacity of the human gallbladder is about 40 to 50 mL. Only a small fraction of the 750 to 100 mL of bile produced each day would be stored were it not for its remarkable absorptive capacity. The gallbladder mucosa has the greatest absorptive capacity per unit of any structure in the body.

BILE COMPOSITION

Bile is usually concentrated 5-fold to 10-fold by the absorption of water and electrolytes leading to a marked change in bile composition (Table 102-1).[32,33] Active sodium chloride transport by the gallbladder epithelium is the driving force for the concentration of bile. Water is passively absorbed in response to the osmotic force generated by solute absorption. The concentration of bile may affect the solubilities of two important components of gallstones: cholesterol and calcium. Although the gallbladder mucosa does absorb calcium, this process is not nearly as efficient as for sodium or water, leading to a greater relative increase in calcium concentration.[34] As the gallbladder bile becomes concentrated, several

TABLE 102-1 Composition of Hepatic and Gallbladder Bile

Characteristics*	Hepatic Bile	Gallbladder Bile
Na	160	270
K	5	10
Cl	90	15
HCO₃	45	10
Ca	4	25
Mg	2	4
Bilirubin	1.5	15
Protein	150	200
Bile acids	50	150
Phospholipids	8	40
Cholesterol	4	18
Total solids	—	125
pH	7.8	7.2

*All determinations are milliequivalents per liter; except for pH. Significant ranges of all elements may occur.

changes occur in the capacity of bile to solubilize cholesterol. The solubility in the micellar fraction is increased, but the stability of phospholipids-cholesterol vesicles is greatly decreased. Because cholesterol crystal precipitation occurs preferentially by vesicular rather than micellar mechanisms, the net effect of concentrating bile is an increased tendency to form cholesterol crystals.[32]

GALLBLADDER FUNCTION

The main function of the gallbladder is to concentrate and store hepatic bile during the fasting state, thus allowing for its coordinated release in response to a meal. To serve this overall function, the gallbladder has absorptive, secretory, and motor capabilities. Absorption of water results from an active process via the sodium-hydrogen exchanger. As a result, the gallbladder stores concentrated bile that reenters the distal bile duct and is secreted into the duodenum in response to a meal. In addition to absorption and concentration, the gallbladder's mucosa actively secretes glycoproteins and hydrogen ions. Secretion of mucus glycoproteins occurs primarily from the glands of the gallbladder neck and cystic duct. The resultant mucin gel is believed to constitute an important part of the unstirred layer (diffusion-resistant barrier) that separates the gallbladder cell membrane from the luminal bile.[35,36] This mucus barrier may be very important in protecting the gallbladder epithelium from the strong detergent effect of the highly concentrated bile salts found in the gallbladder. However, considerable evidence also suggests that mucin glycoproteins play a role as pronucleating agents for cholesterol crystallization.[37] The transport of hydrogen ions by the gallbladder epithelium leads to a decrease in gallbladder bile pH through a sodium-exchange mechanism. Acidification of bile promotes calcium solubility, thereby preventing its precipitation as calcium salts. The gallbladder's normal acidification process lowers the pH of entering hepatic bile from 7.5 to 7.8 down to 7.1 to 7.3.[32,33]

Absorption

The gallbladder's mucosa has the greatest absorptive capacity per unit of any structure in the body. Bile is usually concentrated fivefold by the absorption of water and electrolytes. Active Na-Cl transport by the gallbladder epithelium is the driving force for the concentration of bile (Figure 102-20). Water is passively absorbed in response to the osmotic force generated by solute absorption. The concentration of bile may affect both calcium and cholesterol solubilities. The concentration of calcium in gallbladder bile, which is an important factor in gallstone pathogenesis, is influenced by serum calcium, hepatic bile calcium, gallbladder water absorption, and the concentration of organic substances such as bile salts in gallbladder bile.[34] Although the gallbladder mucosa does absorb calcium, this process is not nearly as efficient as for sodium or water.

As the gallbladder bile becomes concentrated, several changes occur in the bile's capacity to solubilize cholesterol. The solubility in the micellar fraction is increased, but the stability of phospholipids-cholesterol vesicles is greatly decreased. Because cholesterol crystal precipitation occurs preferentially by vesicular rather than micellar mechanisms, the net effect of concentrating bile is an increased tendency to nucleate cholesterol.[37] Absorption of organic compounds also occurs; lipid solubility is the major determinant of movement across the gallbladder mucosa. However, the absorption of bilirubin, cholesterol, phospholipids, and bile salts is minimal compared with that of water. Thus, these organic compounds are significantly concentrated by the normal absorptive process that occurs in the gallbladder. Unconjugated bile salts are absorbed more readily than conjugated bile salts and may actually damage the gallbladder's mucosa, causing a nonselective increase in absorption of other solutes. Thus, increased absorption of unconjugated bile salts, caused by bacterial deconjugation or mucosal inflammation, may impair cholesterol solubility and therefore promote cholesterol gallstone formation.

Secretion

The gallbladder's epithelial cells secrete at least two important products into its lumen: glycoproteins and hydrogen ions. Prostaglandins play an important role as stimulants of gallbladder mucin secretion. Furthermore, mucin glycoproteins are key pronucleating agents for cholesterol crystallization.

The acidification of bile occurs by the transport of hydrogen ions by the gallbladder epithelium, through a sodium-exchange mechanism. Acidification of bile promotes calcium solubility, thereby preventing its precipitation as calcium salts. The gallbladder's normal acidification process lowers the pH of gallbladder bile, which normally varies from approximately 7.1 to 7.3. Compared with gallbladder bile, the bile secreted by the liver is slightly alkaline, pH 7.5 to 7.8, so that excess losses of hepatic bile may cause metabolic acidosis.

Motility

Gallbladder filling is facilitated by tonic contraction of the ampullary sphincter, which maintains a constant pressure in the common bile duct (10 to 15 mm Hg). However, the gallbladder does not simply fill passively and continuously during fasting. Rather, periods of filling are punctuated by brief periods of partial emptying (10%

Lumen   Connective tissue

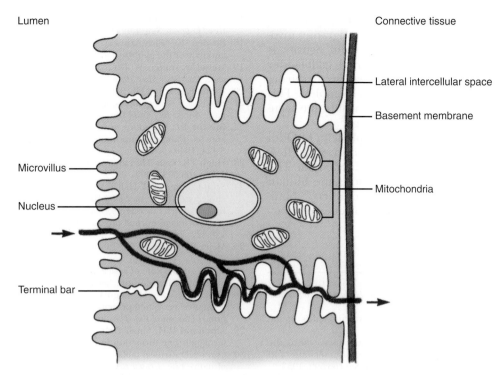

FIGURE 102-20 Cellular mechanisms of gallbladder mucosal absorption. The *arrows* indicate the route of water flow across the cell membrane and into the intercellular spaces. Sodium chloride is pumped into the intercellular space, and the result is a hypertonic environment. As water is transported into the space, the space distends, and an isotonic solution enters the connective tissue space. (From Gadacz TR: Biliary anatomy and physiology. In Greenfield LJ, Mulholland MW, Oldham KT, editors: *Surgery: Scientific principles and practice*. Philadelphia, 1993, Lippincott, p 935.)

to 15% of its volume) of concentrated gallbladder bile, which are coordinated with each passage through the duodenum of phase III of the migrating myoelectric complex. This process is mediated, at least in part, by the hormone motilin.[38-40] Following a meal, the release of stored bile from the gallbladder requires a coordinated motor response of gallbladder contraction and sphincter of Oddi relaxation. One of the main stimuli to gallbladder emptying is the hormone cholecystokinin, which is released from the duodenal mucosa in response to a meal. When stimulated by eating, the gallbladder empties 50% to 70% of its contents within 30 to 40 minutes. Gallbladder refilling then occurs gradually over the next 60 to 90 minutes. Many other hormonal and neural pathways are also necessary for the coordinated action of the gallbladder and sphincter of Oddi. Defects in gallbladder motility, which increase the residence time of bile in the gallbladder, play a central role in the pathogenesis of gallstones.[32]

SPHINCTER OF ODDI

The human sphincter of Oddi is a complex structure that is functionally independent from the duodenal musculature. Endoscopic manometric studies have demonstrated that the human sphincter of Oddi creates a high-pressure zone between the bile duct and the duodenum (Figure 102-21). The sphincter regulates the flow of bile and pancreatic juice into the duodenum and also prevents the regurgitation of duodenal contents into the biliary tract. These functions are achieved by keeping pressure within the bile and pancreatic ducts higher than

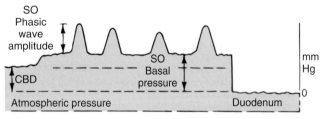

FIGURE 102-21 Sphincter of Oddi *(SO)* manometric pressure profile obtained by catheter pull-through from the common bile duct *(CBD)* into the duodenum. The CBD pressure and SO basal pressure are both referenced to duodenal pressure. SO phasic-wave amplitude was measured from basal SO pressure. The CBD-to-duodenal pressure gradient is indicated by the *parallel broken lines*. (From Geenen JE, Toouli J, Hogan WJ, et al: Endoscopic sphincterotomy: Follow-up evaluation of effects on the sphincter of Oddi. *Gastroenterology* 87:754, 1984.)

duodenal pressure.[41] The sphincter of Oddi also has high-pressure phasic contractions, which may play a role in preventing the regurgitation of duodenal contents into the biliary tract.

Both neural and hormonal factors influence the sphincter of Oddi. In humans, sphincter of Oddi pressure and phasic wave activity diminish in response to cholecystokinin. Thus, sphincter pressure relaxes after a meal, allowing the passive flow of bile into the duodenum. During fasting, high-pressure phasic contractions of the sphincter of Oddi persist through all phases of the migrating myoelectric complex. However, recent animal studies suggest that sphincter of Oddi phasic waves do vary to some degree in concert with the migrating myoelectric complex. Thus, sphincter of Oddi activity is undoubtedly coordinated with the partial gallbladder emptying and increases in bile flow that occur during phase III of the migrating myoelectric complex. This activity may be a preventive mechanism against the accumulation of biliary crystals during fasting.[32]

Neurally mediated reflexes link the sphincter of Oddi with the gallbladder and stomach to coordinate the flow of bile and pancreatic juice into the duodenum. The cholecysto–sphincter of Oddi reflex allows the human sphincter to relax as the gallbladder contracts.[42] Similarly, antral distention causes both gallbladder contraction and sphincter relaxation.[43]

REFERENCES

1. Linder HH: Embryology and anatomy of the biliary tree. In Way LW, Pellegrini CA, editors: *Surgery of the gallbladder and bile ducts.* Philadelphia, 1987, Saunders, p 3.
2. Moorman DA: The surgical significance of six anomalies of the biliary duct system. *Surg Gynecol Obstet* 131:665, 1970.
3. Healey JE, Schroy PC: Anatomy of the biliary ducts within the human liver: Analysis of the prevailing pattern of branchings and the major variations of the biliary ducts. *Arch Surg* 66:599, 1953.
4. Johnson EV, Anson BJ: Variations in the formation and vascular relationships of the bile ducts. *Surg Gynecol Obstet* 94:669, 1952.
5. Frierson H Jr: The gross anatomy and histology of the gallbladder, extrahepatic bile ducts, vaterian system, and minor papilla. *Am J Surg Pathol* 13:146, 1989.
6. Swartz-Basile DA, Lu D, Basile DP, et al: Leptin regulates gallbladder genes related to absorption and secretion. *Am J Physiol* 293:84, 2007.
7. Rock J, Swan KG, Diego J: Calot's triangle revisited. *Surg Gynecol Obstet* 153:410, 1981.
8. Skandalakis JE, Gray SW, Rowe JS Jr: Biliary tract. In Skandalakis JE, Gray SW, editors: *Anatomical complications in general surgery.* New York, 1983, McGraw-Hill, p 31.
9. Specht MJ: Calot's triangle [letter]. *JAMA* 200:1186, 1967.
10. Boyden EA: The anatomy of the choledochoduodenal junction in man. *Surg Gynecol Obstet* 104:646, 1957.
11. Terblanche J, Allison HF, Northover JMA: An ischemic basis for biliary strictures. *Surgery* 94:52, 1983.
12. Benson E, Page RE: A practical reappraisal of the anatomy of the extrahepatic bile ducts and arteries. *Br J Surg* 63:853, 1976.
13. Michels NA: The hepatic, cystic, and retroduodenal arteries and their relations to the biliary ducts with samples of the entire celiacal blood supply. *Ann Surg* 133:503, 1951.
14. Daseler EH, Anson BJ, Hambley WD, et al: The cystic artery and constituents of the hepatic pedicle: A study of 500 specimens. *Surg Gynecol Obstet* 85:47, 1947.
15. Couinaud C: Cited in Smadja C, Blumgart LH: The biliary tract and the anatomy of biliary exposure. In Blumgart LH, editor: *Surgery of the liver and biliary tract.* Edinburgh, 1988, Churchill Livingstone, p 16.
16. Yoshida J, Chijiiwa K, Yamaguchi K, et al: Practical classification of the branching types of the biliary tree: An analysis of 1,094 consecutive direct cholangiograms. *J Am Coll Surg* 182:37, 1996.
17. Bockman DE, Freeny PC: Anatomy and anomalies of the biliary tree. *Laparosc Surg* 1:92, 1992.
18. Boyden E: "Phrygian cap" in cholecystography: A congenital anomaly of the gallbladder. *AJR Am J Roentgenol* 33:589, 1935.
19. Weisel W, Walters W: Diverticulosis of the gallbladder: Report of a case. *Proc Staff Meet Mayo Clin* 16:753, 1941.
20. Davies F, Harding HE: The pouch of Hartmann. *Lancet* 1:193, 1942.
21. Stoklind E: Congenital abnormalities of gallbladder and extrahepatic ducts. *Br J Child Dis* 36:115, 1939.
22. Browne EZ: Variations in origin and course of the hepatic artery and its branches: Importance from a surgical viewpoint. *Surgery* 8:424, 1940.
23. Hugh TB, Kelly TB: Laparoscopic anatomy of the cystic artery. *Am J Surg* 163:593, 1992.
24. Scott-Conner CEH, Hall T: Variant arterial anatomy in laparoscopic cholecystectomy. *Am J Surg* 163:590, 1992.
25. Kullak-Ublick GA, Stieger B, Meier PJ, et al: Enterohepatic bile salt transporters in normal physiology and liver disease. *Gastroenterology* 126:322, 2004.
26. Meier PJ, Stieger B: Bile salt transporters. *Annu Rev Physiol.* 64:635, 2002.
27. Crawford JM: Role of vesicle-mediated transport pathways in hepatocellular bile secretion. *Semin Liver Dis* 16:169, 1996.
28. Gerk PM, Vore M: Regulation of expression of the multidrug resistance-associated protein 2 (MRP2) and its role in drug disposition. *J Pharmacol Exp Ther* 302:407, 2002.
29. Admirand WH, Small DM: The physicochemical basis of cholesterol gallstone formation in man. *J Clin Invest* 47:1043, 1968.
30. Carey MD: Critical tables for calculating the cholesterol saturation of native bile. *J Lipid Res* 19:945, 1978.
31. Blanckaert N, Schmid R: Physiology and pathophysiology of bilirubin metabolism. In Zakmin D, Boyer TD, editors: *Hepatology: A textbook of liver disease,* ed 2. Philadelphia, 1990, Saunders, p 246.
32. Klein A, Lillemoe K, Yeo C, et al: Liver, biliary tract, and pancreas. In O'Leary J, editor: *Physiologic basis of surgery.* Baltimore, 1996, Wilkins & Wilkins, p 441.
33. Gadacz TR: Biliary anatomy and physiology. In Greenfield LJ, Mulholland MW, Oldham KT, editors: *Surgery: scientific principles and practice.* Philadelphia, 1993, Lippincott, p 925.
34. Moore EW: Biliary calcium and gallstone formation. *Hepatology* 12:206S, 1990.
35. Smithson KW, Miller DB, Jacobs LR, et al: Intestinal diffusion barrier: Unstirred water layer or membrane surface mucous coat? *Science* 214:1241, 1981.
36. Glickerman DJ, Kim MH, Malik R, et al: The gallbladder also secretes. *Dig Dis Sci* 42:489, 1997.
37. Holzbach RT: Recent progress in understanding cholesterol crystal nucleation as a precursor to human gallstone formation. *Hepatology* 6:1403, 1986.
38. Itoh A, Takahasi I: Periodic contractions of the canine gallbladder during interdigestive state. *Am J Physiol* 240:G183, 1981.
39. Niebergall-Roth E, Teyssen S, Singer MV: Neurohormonal control of gallbladder motility. *Scand J Gastroenterol* 32:737, 1997.
40. Svenberg T, Christofides ND, Fitzpatrick ML, et al: Interdigestive biliary output in man: Relationship to fluctuations in plasma motilin and effect of atropine. *Gut* 23:1024, 1982.
41. Geenen JE, Hoagan WJ, Dodds WJ, et al: Intraluminal pressure recording from the human sphincter of Oddi. *Gastroenterology* 78:317, 1980.
42. Muller EL, Lewinski MA, Pitt HA: The cholecysto-sphincter of Oddi reflex. *J Surg Res* 36:377, 1984.
43. Webb TH, Lillemoe KD, Pitt HA: The gastro-sphincter of Oddi reflex. *Am J Surg* 155:193, 1988.

Imaging and Intervention in the Biliary System

Anthony C. Venbrux | Merissa N. Zeman | Nadia J. Khati

Bhupender Yadav | Albert K. Chun | Andrew S. Akman

Amy P. Harper | Shawn N. Sarin | Emily T. Jackson

This chapter provides a broad overview of imaging and percutaneous intervention in the biliary system. Optimal management of these complex patients requires a multidisciplinary approach involving the primary care physician, internist, surgeon, gastroenterologist, and interventional radiologist. The evaluation of a patient with obstructive jaundice includes a detailed medical history, physical examination, and review of laboratory data and radiologic studies. Additionally, noninvasive imaging is an integral part of preplanning for either percutaneous interventions or surgery. Should the patient be deemed a surgical candidate, percutaneous interventions may play a role in "setting the stage" for subsequent corrective surgical procedures. In certain patients, percutaneous interventions may prove to be both diagnostic and therapeutic. The objectives of this chapter are as follows: (1) examine the noninvasive imaging techniques used in the management of patients with biliary disease and (2) examine the minimally invasive percutaneous techniques used to treat patients with benign or malignant biliary obstruction or injury.

The authors in this chapter provide an overview of the role of imaging in patients with biliary disease to include the use of ultrasound (US), computed tomography (CT), magnetic resonance imaging (MRI), and nuclear medicine.

As to percutaneous interventions, percutaneous transhepatic cholangiography (PTC) and percutaneous biliary drainage (PBD) are reviewed. Additional therapeutic interventions that are discussed include percutaneous biliary stricture dilation, biopsy, use of drainage catheters, and biliary endoprosthesis. Appropriate patient selection for application of such minimally invasive techniques is discussed (i.e., use in benign or malignant disease). Newer modalities for treatment of biliary malignancy are covered to include use of yttrium-90 therapy for unresectable intrahepatic cholangiocarcinoma. Also included is a brief section on the percutaneous management of iatrogenic injuries.

We hope that this chapter will allow the reader to acquire a broad understanding of the role of imaging and image-guided interventions in the management of patients with complex biliary disease.

A patient presenting with signs and symptoms of obstructive jaundice undergoes clinical evaluation and a diagnostic workup. Included in the latter are laboratory data (i.e., blood work) and imaging. The goals of imaging include

1. Confirm the presence of obstructive jaundice using cross-sectional imaging (i.e., US, CT, or MRI).
2. Precisely define biliary anatomy to determine the severity and the level of obstruction using the following techniques:
   a. Magnetic resonance cholangiopancreatography (MRCP) (noninvasive)
   b. Percutaneous transhepatic cholangiography (PTC or PTHC)
   c. PBD or percutaneous transhepatic biliary drainage (PTBD) (invasive)
   d. Endoscopic retrograde cholangiopancreatography (ERCP) (invasive)
3. Staging malignant disease with image-based assistance.
4. Guiding possible nonsurgical therapy with image-based assistance.

IMAGING MODALITIES FOR THE BILIARY SYSTEM

ULTRASOUND

US is a relatively inexpensive, noninvasive imaging modality used to confirm the presence of biliary ductal dilation (Figure 103-1). When performed correctly, US may provide considerable information to assist the physician in the management of patients with hepatobiliary disease. Although operator dependent, US is generally readily available in most medical institutions and should be the first imaging modality used when assessing patients with suspected biliary disease. The normal gallbladder is an anechoic (fluid-filled) oval structure.[1] The position of the gallbladder fundus is variable; however, the gallbladder neck has a fixed relationship with the interlobar fissure of the liver. The wall of the gallbladder is a thin, smooth, echogenic line that should not exceed 3 mm in thickness. The gallbladder will be contracted in the nonfasting state, and the wall may appear abnormally thickened. Pathologic gallbladder wall thickening may be secondary to acute or chronic cholecystitis, cholangitis,

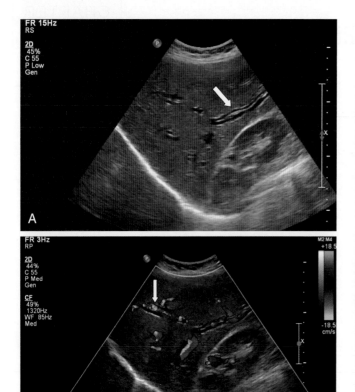

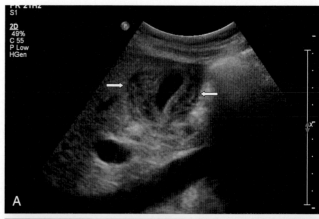

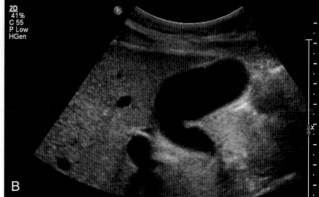

FIGURE 103-1 Gray scale **(A)** and color Doppler **(B)** transabdominal sagittal right upper quadrant ultrasound images showing the "parallel channels" sign consistent with intrahepatic biliary ductal dilation *(arrow)*. The color Doppler scan **(B)** depicts prominent intrahepatic bile ducts adjacent to blood vessels *(arrow)*. This patient presented with painless jaundice and weight loss.

FIGURE 103-2 Sagittal transabdominal ultrasound images of the gallbladder **(A)** in a patient with hypoalbuminemia showing marked gallbladder wall thickening with stratification *(arrows)*. **B,** One-week followup in the same patient after correction of the albumin level, showing a normal-appearing gallbladder wall (thickness <3 mm).

hepatitis, hepatic failure, cirrhosis, pancreatitis, congestive heart failure, renal failure, hypoalbuminemia (Figure 103-2), neoplasm, or human immunodeficiency virus (HIV).

The common hepatic duct is easily visualized in the porta hepatis as it crosses the undivided right portal vein. In most cases, the hepatic artery passes between the common hepatic duct and portal vein; however, in 10% to 15% of patients, the hepatic artery is located anterior to the common hepatic duct. The joining of the cystic duct with the common hepatic duct forms the common bile duct. The cystic duct is generally located posterior to the common hepatic duct and may travel a variable distance before joining the common hepatic duct. Within the hepatoduodenal ligament, the common bile duct is anterior and lateral to the portal vein and to the right of the hepatic artery. As the common bile duct travels caudally to the second portion of the duodenum, it assumes a more posterior position.[1,2] On US, the normal diameter of the extrahepatic bile ducts can range from 4 to 8 mm.[3] The size of the extrahepatic bile ducts can increase slightly with increasing patient age, after cholecystectomy or bile duct surgery, or after endoscopic manipulation of the duct. The maximum upper limit of normal in the extrahepatic biliary tree after cholecystectomy is 10 mm.

However, it is generally accepted that a duct that measures 6 mm or greater in symptomatic patients warrants further investigation.[4]

Intrahepatic bile ducts can be considered normal if they are less than 40% of the diameter of the accompanying portal vein, or if they are 2 mm or smaller in diameter.[2] Intrahepatic biliary dilation may appear as an alteration in the normal anatomic relationships in the portal triads and a confluence of tubular structures near the hilum of the liver. The appearance of peripheral intrahepatic duct dilation has been called the *parallel-channel* sign.[5] Color Doppler US is useful in this setting to confirm the presence of biliary dilation. Using color Doppler US, one may differentiate between vessels and dilated biliary ducts (see Figure 103-1). US accurately predicts the level of biliary obstruction in the majority of cases (92%), but it is less accurate in suggesting the correct cause (71%).[6] The use of US guidance in the critically ill patient at bedside has provided the interventionalist with portable, inexpensive, easy-to-use technology for drainage of structures such as the gallbladder in a patient with acute cholecystitis.

There are many causes of biliary obstruction. These include (1) stones, (2) neoplasms, (3) inflammatory disease, (4) congenital causes (rare), and (5) extrinsic compression (e.g., Mirizzi syndrome). The use of higher frequency transducers and newer noninvasive techniques, such as harmonic imaging, allow for better resolution and improved visualization of the bile ducts by increasing the contrast-to-noise ratio.[7] US coupled with the use of CT or MRCP to determine extent of disease assists the interventional radiologist, gastroenterologist, or surgeon in planning therapy.

COMPUTED TOMOGRAPHY

In many institutions, the initial noninvasive imaging modality of choice for patients with suspected biliary obstruction is CT, specifically, helical CT scanning (Figure 103-3). With the advent of multidetector CT scanners, imaging of the entire biliary tract can be performed in a single breath hold allowing for shorter scan durations and the acquisition of volumetric data, which can subsequently be reconstructed at very thin sections. This is especially helpful when scanning pediatric or critically ill

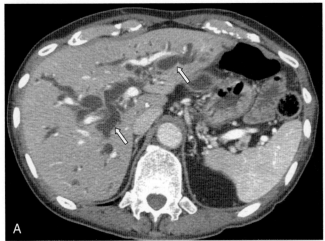

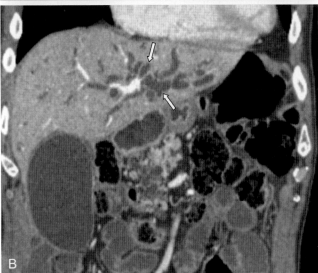

FIGURE 103-3 Axial **(A)** and reconstructed coronal **(B)** contrast-enhanced computed tomography scans through the liver and biliary tree in a patient with painless jaundice and weight loss. There is marked, diffuse intrahepatic biliary ductal dilation *(arrows)*. The patient had a pancreatic head mass causing distal obstruction of the common bile duct.

patients. The disadvantages include (1) the requirement for intravenous contrast administration (not always possible in patients with renal dysfunction), (2) use of ionizing radiation, and (3) additional cost as compared to US.

CT is less "operator dependent" than US. Thus, it is reproducible, and studies are easily compared. It is therefore important for followup after biliary surgical or interventional procedures. When correctly performed, CT provides valuable information not only of the intra- and extrahepatic bile ducts but also of structures outside the biliary system (e.g., liver parenchyma, adjacent lymph nodes, the presence of choledocholithiasis, neoplasms, etc.).

To optimize biliary tract imaging with multidetector helical CT, a noncontrast scan followed by a contrast-enhanced CT scan through the liver, biliary tree, and pancreas should be performed. Thin-section (1 to 2.5 mm) images should be performed from the porta hepatis through the pancreatic head following the injection of contrast using a multiphase scan that includes late arterial and portal venous phases (45- to 50-second delay and a 70-second delay, respectively) when a neoplastic process is suspected. A 10-minute-delayed scan can be added if there is suspicion for cholangiocarcinoma as the cause of biliary tract dilation.[8] With the volumetric acquisition of thin-section scans, multiplanar reconstruction images can be obtained in the coronal or coronal oblique planes. Reformatted curved planar images can also be acquired allowing for improved evaluation of the biliary tract. Similarly, image reconstruction can be performed for CT angiography and CT cholangiography.

The extrahepatic bile duct is typically visualized throughout its entire course in the hepatoduodenal ligament as a water-density tubular structure. At the level of the pancreatic head, the distal common bile duct has a round or oval configuration. Although normal intrahepatic bile ducts can occasionally be seen with current CT technology, it usually is not difficult to differentiate normal intrahepatic bile ducts from true dilated ducts. Normal intrahepatic ducts should be less than 2 mm and not confluent.[8]

The use of CT guidance with real-time imaging (fluoro-CT) allows the operator to rapidly access specific biliary structures. Examples might be the requirement for percutaneous biopsy of a lesion in the liver adjacent to bile ducts, percutaneous drainage of a biloma located near vital structures (e.g. aorta), and so forth. Thus image acquisition coupled with rapid feedback facilitates interventions that would otherwise require potentially lengthy procedures in a patient with complex biliary disease.

MAGNETIC RESONANCE IMAGING

Perhaps the most significant contribution in the use of noninvasive imaging for management of patients with suspected biliary disease is MRI. MRCP has played an increasing role in the evaluation of such patients (Figure 103-4). In fact, accurately performed MRCP has, in many institutions, replaced conventional ERCP and PTC.

Although more expensive than US or CT, MRCP is considered an accurate, noninvasive technique for

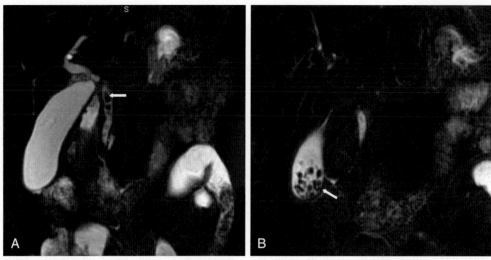

FIGURE 103-4 Coronal images from a magnetic resonance cholangiopancreatography scan in a patient with known gallstones and elevated bilirubin levels. **A,** Multiple hypointense well-defined foci are shown in the common bile duct *(arrow)* consistent with stones. The common bile duct is dilated. **B,** The remaining stones in the gallbladder *(arrow)* are shown.

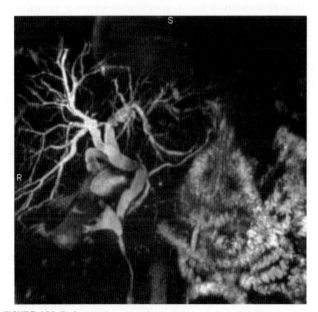

FIGURE 103-5 Coronal magnetic resonance cholangio-pancreatography (MRCP) scan through the intrahepatic and extrahepatic biliary ductal system. There is marked diffuse intrahepatic and common bile duct dilation. MRCP uses heavily T2-weighted sequences and provides a noninvasive means of defining biliary anatomy. This patient had a stone impacted distally in the common bile duct (not shown).

evaluation of the biliary tract. MRCP uses heavily T2-weighted sequences to show bile ducts as high signal intensity structures (Figure 103-5). Many MRI techniques (i.e., pulse sequences) have been described to generate high-resolution images.[9-14] More recently, MRCP is performed using two-dimensional and three-dimensional heavily T2-weighted sequences. Decreased imaging time and decreased respiratory motion artifacts can both be achieved with newer technical advances in MRI.[8] This is especially helpful when imaging critically ill patients who might have difficulty holding their breath for long

periods of time. MRCP has a high sensitivity and specificity in demonstrating biliary tract stone disease, allowing visualization of stones as small as 2 mm in size.[8] MRCP is also useful in the evaluation of congenital disorders, benign and malignant biliary strictures, and for patients with failed or incomplete ERCP or PTC.[13,15,16] This is a valuable noninvasive means to visualize the biliary tree before therapeutic intervention or surgery.[1]

NUCLEAR MEDICINE

A suspected traumatic injury to the biliary system may be confirmed using nuclear medicine scintigraphy (e.g., technetium-99m diisopropyl iminodiacetic acid [DISIDA] scan). Confirmation of the presence of a biliary leak will mobilize the multidisciplinary team to rapidly manage the patient (Figure 103-6). In addition to confirming the presence of bile duct injury (i.e., leak), the technique may also prove useful in confirming the presence of gallbladder disease, biliary obstruction, and so forth.

BILIARY INTERVENTIONS

THE ROLE OF THE INTERVENTIONAL RADIOLOGIST

As mentioned earlier, the interventional radiologist is frequently involved at multiple levels in the workup of patients with biliary disease including the following:

1. Precisely defining biliary anatomy to determine the severity and level of obstruction using percutaneous techniques (i.e., PTC).
2. Draining obstructed bile ducts (i.e., PTBD) (Figure 103-7).
3. Obtaining tissue and/or bile to confirm a suspected diagnosis (i.e., percutaneous biopsy and/or bile sampling for cytopathology).
4. Percutaneous management of benign biliary strictures in those patients who are not good surgical candidates because of other comorbid diseases (e.g., advanced cardiopulmonary disease).

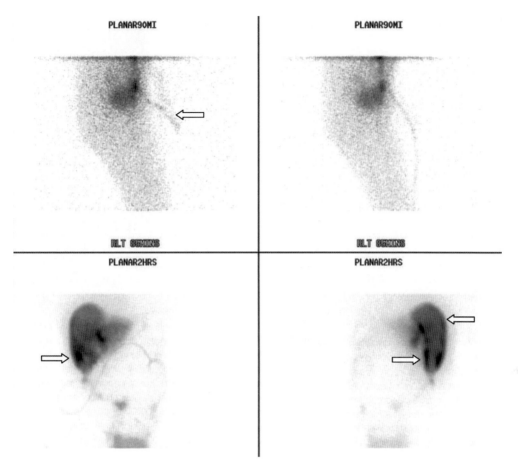

PLANAR90MI

RLT 95MINS

PLANAR2HRS

PLANAR90MI

RLT 95MINS

PLANAR2HRS

FIGURE 103-6 Nuclear medicine scintigraphy 90-minute– and 2-hour–delayed (DISIDA scan) showing extravasation of radiotracer into the inferior percutaneous drain and surrounding the right surface of the liver, extending superiorly consistent with a bile leak *(arrows)*. This patient was status post cholecystectomy and was found to have fusiform dilation of the common bile duct, consistent with a type I choledochal cyst.

5. Percutaneous management of patients with retained intrahepatic or extrahepatic biliary stones in those patients who cannot undergo ERCP (e.g., patients who have undergone biliary reconstructive surgery such as a Roux-en-Y loop or have stones located beyond the reach of the endoscope) (Figures 103-8 through 103-10).
6. Palliative measures for patients with biliary malignancy including deployment of biliary endoprostheses (Figures 103-11 and 103-12).
7. Confirming the presence of a biliary leak or gallbladder obstruction using radionuclide hepatobiliary scintigraphy.
8. Diversion of bile in the setting of major bile duct injury.
9. Newer techniques such as transhepatic arterial radioembolization using yttrium-90 to treat intrahepatic lesions such as cholangiocarcinoma.

In many institutions, after initial clinical, laboratory, and imaging evaluations, ERCP is generally the first minimally invasive procedure performed in patients with known biliary disease. This is especially true for patients with nondilated biliary ducts (e.g., patients with a suspected bile duct injury, such as a leak after surgery, or with sclerosing cholangitis, etc.)

In general, ERCP should be used in patients when
1. Intrahepatic bile ducts are nondilated.
2. The patient has an absolute contraindication to PTC/PBD (i.e., a coagulopathy that cannot be corrected).
3. The patient has a relative contraindication to PTC/PBD (i.e. ascites, polycystic liver disease, etc.).
PTC (often followed by PBD) should be performed:
1. When ERCP fails, and the patient is symptomatic (e.g., obstruction with sepsis, etc.).
2. When the patient has had a prior biliary-enteric anastomosis. Such surgical biliary reconstruction frequently prevents successful cannulation of the ampulla during attempted ERCP.
3. If surgical resection of a tumor at the biliary confluence is planned, PBD (often bilateral) is performed to relieve symptoms (i.e., to drain obstructed and potentially infected bile). In some centers, it is felt that the presurgical placement of percutaneously placed biliary drainage catheter(s) facilitates intraoperative biliary reconstruction and aids in the surgical creation of a biliary-enteric anastomosis(es).
4. In those patients who are not surgical candidates and who have known malignant tumors at the biliary confluence, bilateral PTC/PBD will allow

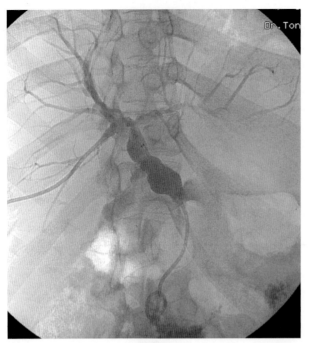

FIGURE 103-7 Right anterior oblique digital spot film after right midaxillary percutaneous transhepatic biliary drainage. This elderly female presented with a clinical picture of obstructive jaundice and was found to have unresectable pancreatic carcinoma. This cholangiogram documents placement of a multisidehole biliary drainage catheter, which is seen coursing from the peripheral right biliary ducts (intrahepatic ducts) to the duodenum.

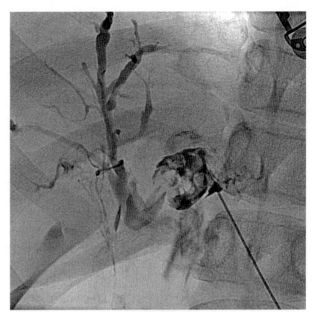

FIGURE 103-8 Digital spot film obtained during initial left percutaneous transhepatic cholangiogram (subxiphoid approach). The skinny needle (21-gauge trocar needle) partially opacifies a markedly dilated left biliary system that is filled with numerous stones. There is reflux of contrast into the right-sided bile ducts. These ducts are irregular in caliber and "pruned" (i.e., demonstrate a reduced branching pattern). Such findings are consistent with sclerosing cholangitis, in this case because of numerous episodes of sepsis (cholangitis) associated with the intrahepatic stones.

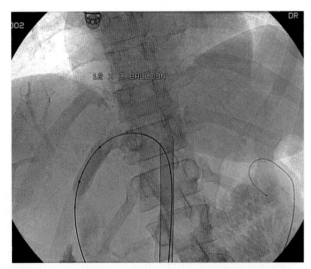

FIGURE 103-9 Digital spot film obtained during fluoroscopically guided left biliary duct stone removal (same patient as in Figure 103-8). After outpatient sequential left biliary drainage catheter upsizings, a large sheath has been placed into the left biliary system to facilitate placement of stone baskets and to remove stone fragments. A 12-mm-diameter balloon has been inflated to dilate a left central (hilar) stricture. This stricture was biopsied and found to be benign on pathologic analysis. The stricture was felt to contribute to left biliary duct stone formation. This patient had a remote history of a cholecystectomy.

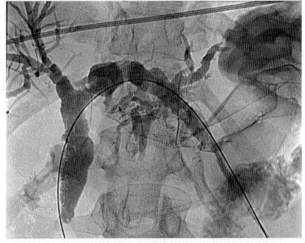

FIGURE 103-10 Completion cholangiogram after outpatient left biliary stone extraction procedures (same patient as in Figures 103-8 and 103-9). Using both fluoroscopic and endoscopic guidance, the patient's left biliary system was rendered stone free. The left central hilar biliary stricture (benign) was dilated (see Figure 103-9) and stented with a large-caliber 16-French Silastic external/internal biliary drainage catheter (not shown). This final "over the wire" cholangiogram was performed after stenting the stricture for 3 months. Contrast rapidly flowed across the previously dilated and stented central left biliary stricture and opacified the right biliary system, common hepatic, and common bile ducts. The duodenum is also opacified, indicating no ampullary obstruction. This patient's tube was removed, and the patient remains asymptomatic at 3-year followup.

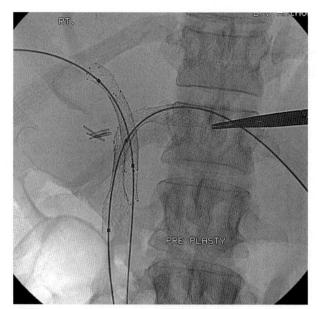

FIGURE 103-11 Digital spot film in a 65-year-old woman with unresectable biliary malignancy (end-stage hilar cholangiocarcinoma). Overlapping bilateral self-expanding bare metal stents (biliary endoprostheses) have been placed from the right and left percutaneous biliary access sites (Zilver stents). This image was obtained before gentle balloon dilation of the stents and bilateral guidewire removals. Use of biliary endoprostheses for palliation frees a patient from the encumbrance of external/internal biliary drainage catheters.

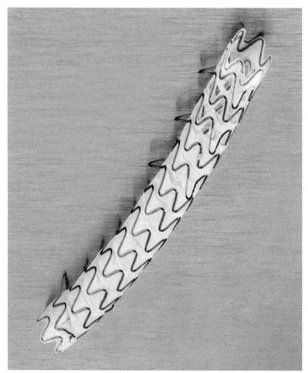

FIGURE 103-12 Photograph of a self-expanding covered biliary endoprosthesis (Viabil). (Courtesy W. L. Gore and Associates, Flagstaff, Ariz.)

palliative endoprosthesis placement.[17-31] The endoscopist may not be able to successfully relieve obstruction from malignant tumors located at the biliary confluence. An endoprosthesis placed during endoscopy is frequently deployed into either the right or the left biliary duct. If both sides are not stented, this may result in inadequate biliary drainage. (See also Percutaneous Image-Guided Therapy of Malignant Biliary Tract Disease later in this chapter.)

Percutaneous techniques are especially well suited for patients with biliary bifurcation (i.e., hilar) or intrahepatic lesions and in those patients with prior surgical failures (e.g., anastomotic strictures at the site of a prior biliary-enteric surgical reconstruction). As mentioned earlier, ERCP may prove inadequate when biliary strictures are located in the hilum. In fact, ERCP may lead to emergency PTC/PBD because of "instrumentation" in the clinical setting of inadequate biliary drainage. This is because of the inability of the endoscopic stent to reach the upper level of the biliary obstruction. Such patients, with high-grade obstruction and subsequent unsuccessful bile duct manipulation, may require emergent percutaneous transhepatic drainage or surgery because of sepsis.

TECHNIQUE OF PERCUTANEOUS TRANSHEPATIC CHOLANGIOGRAPHY, PERCUTANEOUS BILIARY DRAINAGE, AND DILATION OF BENIGN BILIARY STRICTURES

The techniques of PTC and PBD are well described.[32-34] Access to the biliary system may be achieved under cross-sectional imaging or fluoroscopic guidance. The authors prefer fluoroscopy. Briefly, after informed consent, conscious sedation, and intravenous antibiotics, biliary anatomy is defined from either a right (midaxillary) or a left (subxiphoid) approach (see Figure 103-7). A second needle may be used to select the appropriate peripheral duct for percutaneous biliary drainage. Generally an 8- to 10-French (8 to 10F) locked multisidehole catheter is placed at the initial biliary drainage procedure. Depending on the location and nature of the biliary lesion (e.g., benign hilar stricture), the patient is brought back to the interventional suite, and balloon cholangioplasty is performed. In general, cholangioplasty of the distal common bile duct is achieved with a 10- to 12-mm-diameter balloon; a hilar stricture with an 8- to 10-mm-diameter balloon. Similar sized balloons (e.g., 10-mm diameter) are used for a benign stricture at a biliary-enteric anastomosis (e.g., a Roux-en-Y choledochoenterostomy anastomosis). Following balloon dilation, upsizing to a larger caliber external/internal biliary drainage catheter is generally felt to be the most appropriate therapy. At the authors' institution, soft Silastic biliary tubes (e.g., 16F) are often used after sequential tube upsizing. The drainage catheters are sutured to the skin entry site. Patients flush their tubes with 10 mL of normal saline once or twice daily. When internal/external biliary drainage has been achieved, it is important to instruct the patient as to the correct technique for biliary catheter flushing. A patient should be instructed to gently flush saline into the tube but not to aspirate, as there is a risk of colonizing the biliary system with gastrointestinal flora.

Should intrahepatic strictures be found, the appropriate duct must be chosen for percutaneous access such that the stricture is negotiated (i.e., crossed), and balloon dilation is performed (see Figure 103-9) followed by external/internal biliary stenting. Should a patient fail a course of balloon dilation and stenting (i.e., failure of a clinical trial in which the biliary drainage catheter is pulled above the stricture), or should the patient fail a graduated infusion "stress" test across the stricture (i.e., a biliary manometric perfusion test), a retrial of balloon dilation and stenting is an option. Dialogue with the patient, gastroenterologist, and surgeon is critical to formulate an appropriate treatment plan. Should the patient be deemed a poor surgical candidate, the patient may have to be maintained with permanent internal/external biliary drainage catheters changed every 2 to 3 months on an outpatient basis.

Recent data suggest that benign biliary strictures that are extremely fibrotic may be treated with cutting balloons (i.e., a balloon with cutting blades mounted on the device). Data on use of cutting balloons are limited, and only case reports indicate potential improved outcomes in patients who have no surgical or interventional alternatives aside from the placement of long-term internal/external biliary drainage catheters (i.e., permanent internal/external catheters).

For benign biliary strictures, noncovered metallic stents should not be used because (1) such devices generally will occlude in 6 to 12 months; (2) the metallic struts of the stent become incorporated into the bile duct epithelium; and (3) should future surgery be required, additional nondiseased bile duct may be sacrificed, complicating the originally planned biliary reconstructive surgery. At the authors' institution, external/internal biliary stenting is the norm for percutaneous management of patients with benign biliary strictures. As mentioned earlier, catheters are routinely changed on an outpatient basis at 2- to 3-month intervals. In general, bile duct injury requires a lengthy healing process. Although controversial, it is not unusual for patients, after biliary enteric reconstructive surgery, to be stented for 6 months to a year with large-caliber Silastic stents (generally 16F). On completion of the stenting interval, successful completion of a clinical trial and/or biliary manometric perfusion test is required before stent removal.

Rarely, benign biliary strictures may be treated with covered stents. Recent data suggest that covered metallic biliary stents may be used in the setting of benign biliary strictures and removed once "healing" and stricture "remodeling" has occurred.[35] The use of such a covered stent might be in the setting of (1) a patient who cannot psychologically tolerate an internal/external biliary drainage catheter, (2) in a patient with a short life expectancy because of other comorbid conditions despite benign biliary disease, and (3) the occasional patient who cannot undergo surgery. For example, a patient with a liver transplant and a focal stricture at a choledocho-choledochostomy anastomosis might, if no surgical

option exists, be a candidate for a short-segment covered metallic biliary stent (i.e., endoprosthesis).

PERCUTANEOUS MANAGEMENT OF BILIARY STONES

In general, biliary stones are associated with infected bile. Thus, complete removal of stones is essential in order to render the patient "stone free" and to prevent further episodes of cholangitis. Often, biliary stones are associated with underlying biliary strictures. Extrahepatic biliary stones may be treated by the endoscopist. Treatment may consist of a sphincterotomy followed by endoscopic stone removal using baskets, balloons, and so forth. Intrahepatic stones present a particular challenge to the endoscopist, surgeon, and interventional radiologist. The multidisciplinary approach is necessary for optimal patient management. This may consist of an ERCP with sphincterotomy and removal of distal common bile and common hepatic duct stones. Following this, percutaneous access may be necessary from the right (midaxillary), left (subxiphoid), or both approaches. With appropriate biliary drainage catheter upsizing, fluoroscopically directed interventions may be performed to remove intrahepatic stones. These include balloon dilation of strictures and removal of stones with stone baskets and grasping forceps. Additional techniques include the use of compliant latex occlusion balloons that may be inflated and used to push stones forward into duodenum. Before this maneuver, balloon cholangioplasty of the sphincter is required as stones may otherwise become impacted in the distal common bile ducts. Following removal of stones, stenting with an internal/external biliary drainage catheter is required. Stone removal procedures are repeated until the patient is stone free. Such procedures may be performed on an outpatient basis (see Figures 103-8 through 103-10).

The increase in use of fiberoptic transhepatic or trans-T-tube cholangioscopy by interventional radiologists has changed management of patients with retained intrahepatic biliary stones.[36,37] Such a technique generally necessitates the use of larger cholangioscopes (e.g., 15 to 16F) and requires tube upsizing to 18 to 20F before stone removal.

The advantages of percutaneous cholangioscopy include (1) the use of electrohydraulic or laser lithotripsy under direct vision to fragment large stones, (2) the ability to negotiate eccentric biliary strictures under direct vision when fluoroscopically guided attempts have failed, (3) the ability to biopsy suspicious lesions seen during biliary interventions (i.e., to biopsy suspected malignant biliary lesions), (4) a reduction in radiation both to the patient and healthcare personnel in the interventional suite, and (5) the procedure (i.e., percutaneous cholangioscopy) may be performed generally on an outpatient basis.

Disadvantages of cholangioscopy include (1) the general lack of familiarity of radiologists with the use of a fiberoptic scope, (2) considerable cost for initial purchase of equipment (unless it can be borrowed from other services such as urology, etc.), (3) the need for a different type of recording system other than that found in a conventional interventional suite (i.e., digital endoscopic images, etc.), and (4) a requirement for purchase or loan of an energy source for laser or electrohydraulic lithotripsy. The equipment cost and lack of training are generally reasons why the use of cholangioscopy for biliary interventions has not received widespread acceptance in the interventional radiology community.

When using fluoroscopy, biliary calculi, once captured in a stone basket, are generally "swept" forward into the bowel. Theoretical risks of pulling stones through a transhepatic tract include tract trauma and the potential risk of stone fragments being "lost" and becoming a nidus of infection in the transhepatic tract. The use of a large percutaneously placed transhepatic sheath may facilitate stone removal by this route (see Figure 103-9).

At the authors' institution, the preference is to perform percutaneous cholangioscopy with electric hydraulic lithotripsy or holmium laser stone fragmentation followed by the use of a soft latex occlusion balloon to "sweep" stone fragments into the bowel. As mentioned earlier, before pushing stones into the bowel, cholangioplasty is performed using a 10- to 12-mm-diameter balloon to facilitate passage of stone fragments through the ampulla and into the bowel without stone impaction.

PERCUTANEOUS IMAGE-GUIDED THERAPY OF MALIGNANT BILIARY TRACT DISEASE

Patients with malignant biliary obstruction may benefit from the use of either (1) plastic, (2) open mesh (i.e., bare metal or uncovered) (see Figure 103-11), or (3) covered biliary endoprostheses (see Figure 103-12). As compared to plastic endoprostheses, the bare metal or covered metallic endoprostheses have gained in popularity because of their simplicity and, once deployed, the large caliber of the lumen. Recent data have suggested that covered biliary stents (i.e., a metallic "skeleton or scaffold" covered with fabric) have an increased long-term patency rate. Most investigators feel that metallic biliary endoprostheses (covered or uncovered) are advantageous for the following reasons:

1. There is controversy in the medical literature, but it is generally agreed that bare metal or covered biliary endoprostheses have better long-term patency than plastic endoprostheses.
2. The bare metal biliary stents (endoprostheses) used for palliation of malignant biliary obstruction are generally placed through a smaller percutaneous transhepatic tract than a plastic endoprosthesis.
3. Bare metal endoprostheses may be placed in a single-step procedure (i.e., PTC followed by PBD and endoprostheses placement) in those patients deemed nonsurgical candidates.

Disadvantages of bare metal or covered endoprostheses include

1. Their cost is considerable (at least 10 to 20 times that of plastic endoprostheses).
2. The uncovered bare metal stent generally cannot be removed except through a significant endoscopic procedure or surgical resection. In contrast, covered stents may be removed percutaneously or with endoscopy.

3. Bare metal uncovered endoprostheses may occlude, necessitating repeat percutaneous or endoscopic drainage.

Below is a partial listing of metallic endoprostheses commercially available in the United States and approved for palliation of malignant biliary obstruction by the Food and Drug Administration (FDA):

1. Self-expanding bare metal (open mesh or uncovered) stents, for example:
   a. Smart Stent
   b. Wallstent
   c. Zilver Stent
2. Balloon-expandable bare metal (open mesh or uncovered) stents, for example:
   a. Express Biliary LD
   b. Palmaz and Palmaz Genesis
3. Self-expanding covered biliary stent, for example:
   a. Viabil (see Figure 103-12)

In general, open mesh (i.e., uncovered biliary endoprostheses) require a 7 to 9F percutaneous transhepatic access, whereas the less expensive but larger caliber plastic endoprostheses generally require a 10 to 14F transhepatic tract. In the case of placement of a plastic endoprosthesis, tract dilation may be associated with considerable patient discomfort and risk of hemobilia. For patients requiring palliation for malignant biliary obstruction, using a covered biliary endoprosthesis (e.g., Viabil) with 11F transhepatic access is required.

If no hemobilia is noted after PTC/PBD, the metallic covered or uncovered endoprosthesis may be placed in a single step, thus offsetting the increased cost of the device. In contrast, plastic endoprosthesis placement from a percutaneous transhepatic approach often includes multiple steps (i.e., PTC/PBD), tube tract maturation, tract dilation, and plastic endoprosthesis placement. Multiple steps add to the overall cost and to the potential patient discomfort and risk.

Given the limitations of uncovered bare metal and plastic endoprostheses in patients with malignant obstruction of the biliary system, the application of covered stents for improving long-term patency continues to be actively studied in clinical trials (see Figure 103-12). Such stents are self-expanding, covered with prosthetic material, and have both anchoring "fins" and holes, the latter placed to prevent obstruction of the cystic duct or major branch ducts. As mentioned, such devices require a larger transhepatic tract and are considerably more expensive than uncovered metallic stents.

In a multicenter study by Schoder et al,[30] 42 patients with malignant biliary obstruction were treated by using an expanded polytetrafluoroethylene and fluorinated ethylene-propylene (ePTFE/FEP)-covered biliary endoprosthesis. In this series, patients had obstruction of the common bile duct, common hepatic duct, and hilar confluence. Unilateral ($n = 38$) or bilateral ($n = 4$) drainage was accomplished using covered endoprostheses with anchoring fins. To avoid branch duct blockage, endoprostheses with drainage holes at the proximal end were available. Procedure- and device-related complications were recorded. Successful deployment, correct positioning, and patency of the device were achieved in all patients. Procedure-related complications occurred in two (5%) patients. Thirty-day mortality rate was 20% (8 of 41 patients), and median survival time was 146 days. Laboratory values decreased significantly after the procedure ($P < 0.001$). Recurrent obstructive jaundice occurred in six (15%) patients. Primary patency rates at 3, 6, and 12 months were 90%, 76%, and 76%, respectively. Calculation of the composite endpoint of death or obstruction revealed a median patency duration of 138 days. No endoprosthesis migration was observed. Branch-duct obstruction was observed in four (10%) patients. Postmortem examination of one stent revealed a widely patent endoprosthesis with intact covering.

In another clinical study by Miyayama et al,[31] 62 patients with malignant biliary obstruction distal to the hilar confluence were treated with a covered stent (group 1, $n = 22$), a bare metal stent with large interstices (i.e., Z stent) (group 2, $n = 19$), and a bare metal stent with smaller interstices (i.e., mesh) (group 3, $n = 21$). Patency rates of each group were compared. Early stent revision was required after 3 days in 18% (4/22) of group 1, 26% (5/19) of group 2, and 0% (0/21) of group 3. The 10-, 20-, and 40-week primary patency rates were 77%, 77%, and 59% (group 1); 42%, 25%, and 8% (group 2); and 76%, 71%, and 55% (group 3), respectively. Primary patency rates of groups 1 and 3 were significantly higher than those of group 2 ($P < 0.05$), and there was no statistically significant difference between those of group 1 and group 3. The 10-, 20-, and 40-week assisted primary (secondary) patency rates were 96%, 96%, and 96% (group 1); 68%, 49%, and 39% (group 2); and 86%, 74%, and 58% (group 3), respectively. Assisted primary patency (secondary) rates of group 1 were significantly higher than those of groups 2 and 3 ($P < 0.01$ and $P < 0.05$, respectively). The authors concluded that their study suggests the primary patency rate of the covered stents is equal to that of mesh stents, and that covered stent patency may be improved further to possibly avoid the need for early revision.[31]

The advantages of palliative percutaneous placement of an endoprosthesis in the setting of unresectable malignant distal biliary obstruction include (1) restoration of bile flow into the duodenum with its associated improved physiologic and metabolic effects, and (2) conversion of an external/internal biliary drainage catheter (stent) into a "self contained" intraductal device eliminating the external component of the tube and the daily care required for an external/internal biliary drainage catheter. The endoprosthesis offers the patient the advantage of enhanced quality of life (i.e., the patient is no longer burdened with a catheter that requires maintenance such as dressing changes, flushing of the tube once or twice daily, elimination of potential bile leakage and infection at the catheter skin entry site, and routine periodic catheter exchanges).

The disadvantages of an endoprosthesis (plastic or bare metal) for palliation include (1) premature endoprosthesis occlusion with the associated complications (e.g., recurrent jaundice, possible sepsis, etc.), (2) possible dislodgement of the device, and (3) increased cost of the metallic device (offset by a reduced hospitalization time). A bare metal uncovered biliary endoprosthesis (stent) in place for weeks or months cannot be exchanged

either endoscopically or transhepatically. Should premature occlusion occur or should the patient outlive the patency of the stent, a repeat percutaneous biliary drainage is necessary either with placement of a new endoprosthesis inside the old one, or an external/internal biliary drainage catheter. A second option is attempted endoscopic placement of an endoprosthesis through the occluded metallic stent. If tumor "overgrowth" has occurred, the site of obstruction may be beyond the "reach" of the endoscopic cannula.

There is recent experimental work on other novel biliary endoprosthesis designs. One is a flexible, open mesh (uncovered) coil-like stent; it is a potentially removable device for use in patients with benign biliary disease (e.g., strictures). However, extensive clinical data on its use in humans are lacking.

BENIGN BILIARY DISEASE: IATROGENIC OR TRAUMATIC INJURIES OF THE BILIARY SYSTEM

The clinical results of percutaneous (nonsurgical) management of patients with biliary tract injuries have also received considerable attention in the medical literature.[38-40] Bile duct injuries occur in 0.3% to 0.6% and 0.06% to 0.21% of laparoscopic and conventional cholecystectomy procedures, respectively. In general, the role of the interventional radiologist in the management of patients with biliary leaks includes (1) defining biliary anatomy before definitive surgical biliary reconstruction, (2) diverting bile externally in those patients with complete obstruction of the extrahepatic biliary system (e.g., because of inadvertent clipping of the common hepatic or common bile duct), or in those patients who have sustained complete duct transection with free spillage of bile into the subhepatic space. In the clinical setting where there is free spillage of bile into the abdomen, external diversion coupled with percutaneous biloma drainage may set the stage for surgical reconstruction and allow clinical stabilization of the patient. In the setting of iatrogenic or posttraumatic ductal injury, a focal stricture may be treated solely with percutaneous methods. However, the role of the interventional radiologist is generally to prepare the patient for eventual biliary reconstructive surgery. Trerotola et al reported a series of 13 patients who had undergone laparoscopic cholecystectomy and had experienced a ductal injury.[38] Six patients (46%) had postoperative bilomas or bile leaks. Of these, two (33%) were managed by percutaneous means alone thus avoiding a second operation. Van Sonnenberg et al reported on management of 21 patients with laparoscopic cholecystectomy injuries, 11 of which consisted of bilomas or bile leaks. Seven of these patients were treated percutaneously and without further surgical intervention.[39]

COMPLICATIONS OF PERCUTANEOUS TRANSHEPATIC CHOLANGIOGRAPHY, PERCUTANEOUS BILIARY DRAINAGE, AND BILIARY INTERVENTIONS

The incidence of major complications associated with percutaneous biliary drainage varies from 4.6% to 25%, and the incidence of procedure-related deaths is 0% to

5.6%.[25-29] Major complications include hemobilia requiring blood transfusion and cholangitis associated with hypotension. Hemobilia, a recognized complication of PTC/PBD, occurs in 2.6% to 9.6% of cases.[29,32] Although bleeding is the most common cause of serious procedure-related morbidity, it is rarely a cause of death in patients undergoing percutaneous transhepatic biliary interventions. Should a patient develop hemobilia, a cholangiogram is initially performed to assess whether or not the vascular system opacifies. During cholangiography, should injected contrast opacify only the venous system (e.g., hepatic vein or portal vein), tube repositioning or upsizing is generally all that is required to tamponade the bleeding site. It is important to first check that the proximal most (i.e., most peripheral) sidehole is intraductal (i.e., not outside and in the transhepatic tube tract). If the proximal sidehole is outside the biliary system, the last sidehole may serve as a site of egress for venous blood should a vein have been inadvertently transgressed during initial placement of the tube. Biliary drainage catheter upsizing may be tried next if venous bleeding (oozing) persists despite catheter sidehole repositioning.

Infrequently, should a major central portal venous branch be injured, repeat biliary drainage at a different site with embolization of the original transhepatic tube tract using embolic spring coils, Gelfoam, or both may be necessary.

If, during a biliary catheter exchange, pulsatile bright red blood is seen, an arterial injury must be suspected. The nonsurgical treatment of patients with arterial hemobilia is transcatheter embolotherapy of the injured hepatic arterial branch. Such arterial injuries may occasionally be life threatening. Patients are consented for an emergency hepatic arteriogram and embolization. If the hepatic artery injury is not seen on the initial arteriogram (i.e., with the biliary drainage catheter in place), the arteriogram must be repeated with the biliary drainage catheter briefly pulled out over a guidewire. This is performed to maximize the chance of identifying the injured vessel. Once the site of bleeding is identified (e.g., pseudoaneurysm of the hepatic artery, fistula between hepatic artery and a bile duct, etc.), the arterial catheter is advanced distal to the site of injury, and spring coils or other suitable embolic material are deployed in the hepatic artery branch to occlude the segment of artery injured during PBD. It is important to begin embolization distal (i.e., peripheral) to the site of injury and then to continue embolization proximal to the site. This technique "bridges," "isolates," or "traps" the segment of injured vessel, preventing recurrent bleeding caused by collateral hepatic arterial blood flow. The injured arterial branch is functionally "double ligated."

Another complication of PTC/PBD is biliary infection. Fevers and chills may occur in 5% to 26% of patients undergoing biliary drainage. Four percent to 12% of patients develop frank biliary septicemia. Cholangitis with long-term drainage may occur in as many as 50% of patients.[27,30] Occasionally, complications of PTC/PBD will include inadvertent puncture of other structures such as the transverse colon, especially in subxiphoid or left biliary drainage procedures. With adequate review of previously obtained cross-sectional imaging studies and appropriate use of US and fluoroscopic monitoring during PBD, such injuries can generally be avoided during left-sided percutaneous biliary drainage procedures.

Of the patients undergoing biliary drainage procedures reported in the literature, the presence of malignant biliary obstruction and the high complication rate is generally attributed to the fact that these patients are more debilitated than those presenting with biliary obstruction caused by benign biliary strictures. A review by Yee and Ho combine the results of six groups of investigators (702 patients) and report major complication rates of 8% and death in 2%. In this retrospective review, 609 of the 702 patients (87%) had malignant biliary obstruction.[29]

NEW DEVELOPMENTS

As mentioned, one new development includes reports of the use of transcatheter radioembolization using yttrium-90 therapy for treatment of nonresectable intrahepatic cholangiocarcinoma. Data are limited, and clinical studies are ongoing.

CONCLUSION AND SUMMARY

Imaging and interventional procedures used in the management of patients with biliary obstruction have evolved rapidly. The interventional radiologist provides minimally invasive, image-guided therapeutic options for management of patients with benign or malignant biliary disease. Percutaneous biliary interventions performed for malignant biliary disease may be palliative, or if the patient's malignant disease is deemed resectable, may set the stage for surgery. Similarly, for benign biliary disease, such percutaneous interventions may be definitive treatment or prepare the patient for surgical reconstruction with creation of a Roux-en-Y loop. Percutaneous biliary access provides a means for adjunctive biliary interventions whether that be stricture dilation, stone removal, access for bile cytology or biopsy, intraductal brachytherapy, or placement of an endoprosthesis.[41-45] The use of plastic or metallic biliary endoprostheses for patients with malignant biliary obstruction is a technique that eliminates the physical and psychological encumbrances of an external appliance needing daily maintenance. In patients with benign disease (e.g., a biliary stricture), percutaneous biliary interventions provide a minimally invasive therapeutic option. However, long-term success is not as good as that reported in the surgical literature. Of benign biliary strictures managed percutaneously, the best results are generally felt to be in the clinical setting where balloon dilation is performed at a biliary-enteric anastomosis. Such anastomotic strictures may occur after biliary reconstructive surgery. Long-term patency in such patients ranges between 60% and 70% as compared to 80% and 90% in the surgical literature.[46] Use of covered biliary stents for improving long-term endoprosthesis patency is a relatively recent development in patient management.[17] Radioembolization (i.e., yttrium-90) for intrahepatic cholangiocarcinoma is an area of ongoing clinical research.[47]

It is hoped that the information covered in this chapter provides the multidisciplinary health team caring for such patients with a comprehensive overview of imaging and percutaneous interventional options available to patients with biliary disease.

ACKNOWLEDGMENT

The authors wish to express their thanks to Ms. Shundra Dinkins for her expertise in the preparation of this manuscript.

REFERENCES

1. Levy AD: Noninvasive imaging approach to patients with suspected hepatobiliary disease. *Tech Vasc Interv Radiol* 4:132, 2001.
2. Khalili K, Wilson SR: The biliary tree and gallbladder. In Rumack CM, Wilson SR, Charboneau JW, et al, editors: *Diagnostic ultrasound*, vol 1, ed 3. St. Louis, 2005, Mosby, p 171.
3. Niederau C, Muller J, Sonnenberg A, et al: Extrahepatic bile ducts in healthy subjects, in patients with cholelithiasis, and in postcholecystectomy patients: A prospective ultrasonic study. *J Clin Ultrasound* 11:23, 1983.
4. Graham MF, Cooperberg PL, Cohen MM, et al: The size of the normal common hepatic duct following cholecystectomy: An ultrasonographic study. *Radiology* 135:137, 1980.
5. Conrad MR: Sonographic "parallel channel" sign in obstructive jaundice. *AJR Am J Roentgenol* 146:645, 1986.
6. Laing FC, Jeffrey RB Jr, Wing VW, et al: Biliary dilatation: Defining the level and cause by real-time US. *Radiology* 160:39, 1986.
7. Ortega D, Burns PN, Hope SD, et al: Tissue harmonic imaging: Is it a benefit for bile duct sonography? *AJR Am J Roentgenol* 176:653, 2001.
8. Yeh BM, Liu PS, Soto JA, et al: MR imaging and CT of the biliary tract. *Radiographics* 29:1669, 2009.
9. Sodickson A, Mortele K, Barish M, et al: Three-dimensional fast-recovery fast spin-echo MRCP: Comparison with two-dimensional single-shot fast spin-echo techniques. *Radiology* 238:549, 2006.
10. Kondo H, Kanematsu M, Shiratori Y, et al: MR cholangiography with volume rendering: Recover operating characteristic curve analysis in patients with choledocholithiasis. *AJR Am J Roentgenol* 176:1183, 2001.
11. Fayad LM, Kamel I, Mitchell D, et al: Functional MR cholangiography: Diagnosis of functional abnormalities of the gallbladder and biliary tree. *AJR Am J Roentgenol* 184:1563, 2005.
12. Fulcher AS, Turner MA, Capps GW, et al: Half-Fourier RARE MR cholangiopancreatography: Experience in 300 subjects. *Radiology* 207:21, 1998.
13. Fulcher AS, Turner MA, Capps GW: MR cholangiography: Technical advances and clinical applications. *Radiographics* 19:25, 1999.
14. Merkle EM, Haugan PA, Thomas J, et al: 3.0-versus 1.5–T MR cholangiography: A pilot study. *AJR Am J Roentgenol* 186:516, 2006.
15. Fulcher AS, Turner MA: Benign diseases of the biliary tract: Evaluation with MR cholangiography. *Semin Ultrasound CT MR* 20:294, 1999.
16. Hekimoglu K, Ustundag Y, Dusak A, et al: MRCP vs ERCP in the evaluation of biliary pathologies: Review of current literature. *J Dig Dis* 9:162, 2008.
17. Bezzi M, Zolovkins A, Cantisani V, et al: New ePTFE/FEP-covered stent in the palliative treatment of malignant biliary obstruction. *J Vasc Interv Radiol* 13:581, 2002.
18. McLean GK, Burke DR: Role of endoprostheses in the management of malignant biliary obstruction. *Radiology* 170:961, 1989.
19. Lammer J, Neumayer K: Biliary drainage endoprostheses: Experience with 201 placements. *Radiology* 159:625, 1986.
20. Lammer J: Biliary endoprostheses: Plastic versus metal stents. *Radiol Clin North Am* 28:1211, 1990.
21. Mueller PR, Ferrucci JT Jr, Teplick SK, et al: Biliary stent endoprosthesis: Analysis of complications in 113 patients. *Radiology* 156:637, 1985.
22. Becker CD, Glattli A, Maibach R, et al: Percutaneous palliation of malignant obstructive jaundice with the Wallstent endoprosthesis: Follow-up and reintervention in patients with hilar and non-hilar obstructions. *J Vasc Interv Radiol* 4:597, 1993.
23. Gordon RL, Ring EJ, LaBerge JM, et al: Malignant biliary obstruction: Treatment with expandable metallic stents—follow-up of 50 consecutive patients. *Radiology* 182:697, 1992.
24. Salomonowitz EK, Adam A, Antonucci F, et al: Malignant biliary obstruction: Treatment with self-expandable stainless steel endoprosthesis. *Cardiovasc Intervent Radiol* 15:351, 1992.
25. Mueller PR, van Sonnenberg E, Ferrucci JT Jr: Percutaneous biliary drainage: Technical and catheter related problems in 200 procedures. *AJR Am J Roentgenol* 138:17, 1982.
26. Carrasco CH, Zounoza J, Bechtel WJ: Malignant biliary obstruction: Complications of percutaneous biliary drainage. *Radiology* 152:343, 1984.
27. Hamlin JA, Friedman M, Stein MG, et al: Percutaneous biliary drainage: Complications of 118 consecutive catheterizations. *Radiology* 158:199, 1986.
28. Nakayama T, Ikeda A, Okuda K: Percutaneous drainage of the biliary tract: Technique and results in 104 cases. *Gastroenterology* 2:305, 1980.
29. Yee CAN, Ho CS: Complications of percutaneous biliary drainage: Benign vs malignant diseases. *AJR Am J Roentgenol* 148:1207, 1987.
30. Schoder M, Rossi P, Uflacker R, et al: Malignant biliary obstruction: Treatment with ePTFE-FEP-covered endoprostheses initial technical and clinical experience in a multicenter trial. *Radiology* 225:35, 2002.
31. Miyayama S, Matsui O, Akakura Y, et al: Efficacy of covered metallic stents in the treatment of unresectable malignant biliary obstruction. *Cardiovasc Intervent Radiol* 27:349, 2004.
32. Osterman FA Jr, Venbrux AC: Obstructive jaundice: Percutaneous transhepatic interventions. In Cameron JL, editor: *Current surgical therapy*. St. Louis, 1995, Mosby-Year Book, p 394.
33. Venbrux AC, Osterman FA Jr: Malignant obstruction of the hepatobiliary system. In Baum S, Pentecost MJ, editors: *Abrams' angiography. Interventional radiology*, Vol III. Boston, 1997, Little, Brown and Co., p 472.
34. Savader SJ, Venbrux AC, Osterman FA: Interventional radiology in cancer diagnosis and management. In Niederhuber JE, editor: *Current therapy in oncology*, Philadelphia, 1993, Mosby-Year Book, p 98.
35. Personal communication, Renan P. Uflacker, M.D., December 2004.
36. Venbrux AC, Robbins KV, Savader SJ, et al: Endoscopy as an adjuvant to biliary radiologic intervention. *Radiology* 180:355; 1991.
37. Venbrux AC, Osterman FA: Percutaneous transhepatic cholangiography and percutaneous biliary drainage: Step-by-step. In Society of Cardiovascular and Interventional Radiology, editor: *SCVIR syllabus: volume 2: Biliary interventions*. Philadelphia, 1995, Lippincott Williams & Wilkins, p 129.
38. Trerotola SO, Savader SJ, Lund GB, et al: Biliary tract complications following laparoscopic cholecystectomy: Imaging and intervention. *Radiology* 184:195, 1992.
39. van Sonnenberg E, Casola G, Wittich GR, et al: The role of interventional radiology for complications of cholecystectomy. *Surgery* 107:632. 1990.
40. Mirsa S, Melton GB, Geschwind JF, et al: Percutaneous management of bile duct strictures and injuries associated with laparoscopic cholecystectomy: A decade of experience. *J Am Coll Surg* 198:218, 2004.
41. Venbrux AC, McCormick CD: Percutaneous endoscopy for biliary radiological interventions. *Tech Vasc Interv Radiol* 4:186, 2001.
42. Teplick SK, Haskin PH, Kline TS, et al: Percutaneous pancreaticobiliary biopsies in 173 patients using primarily ultrasound or fluoroscopic guidance. *Cardiovasc Intervent Radiol* 11:26, 1988.
43. Muro A, Mueller JPR, Ferrucci JT, et al: Bile cytology: A routine addition to percutaneous biliary drainage. *Radiology* 149:846, 1983.
44. Nunnerly HB, Karani JB: Intraductal radiation in interventional radiology of the biliary tract. *Radial Clin North Am* 28:1237, 1990.
45. Lammer J, Deu E: Percutaneous management of benign biliary strictures. In Kadir S, editor: *Current practice of interventional radiology*, Philadelphia, 1991, Decker, p 550.
46. Pitt HA, Cameron JL, Postier RG, et al: Factors affecting mortality in biliary tract surgery. *Am J Surg* 141:66, 1981.
47. Saxena A, Bester L, Chua TC, et al: Yttrium-90 radiotherapy for unresectable intrahepatic cholangiocarcinoma: A preliminary assessment of this novel treatment option. *Ann Surg Oncol* 17:484, 2010.

Operative Management of Cholecystitis and Cholelithiasis

Leonardo Villegas | Theodore N. Pappas

Cholelithiasis is a disease prevalent worldwide because of an imbalance of bile salt and cholesterol concentrations that leads to precipitation inside the gallbladder. About 15% of the adult Western population will develop gallstones; only between 1% and 4% a year will develop symptoms.[1] In both sexes, the prevalence increases with age; however, overall gallstones are nearly twice as common in females as in males. Obesity and family history are also significant risk factors.

Symptomatic gallstone disease consists mostly of biliary colic, followed by acute cholecystitis in up to 20% of the patients eventually if left untreated. Younger patients do have a higher chance for complications over a lifetime, with small stones associated with a higher risk for pancreatitis.[2] Complications of cholelithiasis include cholecystitis, common bile duct obstruction/impingement (Mirrizzi syndrome), pancreatitis, cholangitis, and rarely gallbladder cancer. Approximately 65% of patients with acute cholecystitis have some element of chronic cholecystitis, which is characterized by fibrosis and inflammatory infiltrate of the gallbladder wall.[3] Regardless of the cause, almost all cases of symptomatic or complicated cholelithiasis are treated by cholecystectomy.

Gallstone disease management has evolved considerably over the past 2 decades after the development of laparoscopic cholecystectomy. The surgical approach has evolved from same-day elective laparoscopic cholecystectomy and early cholecystectomy for cholecystitis to single-port laparoscopic cholecystectomy and even robotic procedures.

Initial review of laparoscopic cholecystectomy complications showed a higher incidence of bile duct injuries (0.2% to 0.8%) compared to open cholecystectomy (0.1% to 0.25%).[4-9] Previous abdominal operations may create technical difficulties with trocar placement, exposure, and visualization during laparoscopy. Furthermore, conversion to open cholecystectomy should not be considered a complication, but rather, a reflection of sound surgical judgment in difficult cases. The rate of conversion in the United States is 5% to 10%.[10-13] Cholecystectomy and related procedures are discussed in detail in this chapter; the focus is on the indications for operative management for cholelithiasis and cholecystitis and the open technique for cholecystectomy. The indications for an open cholecystectomy are shown in Box 104-1.

ASYMPTOMATIC CHOLELITHIASIS

The large number of asymptomatic individuals who harbor gallstones but do not require a cholecystectomy makes the management of cholelithiasis challenging.

Although cholecystectomy for symptomatic cholelithiasis is standard practice, the natural history of asymptomatic gallstones is not well defined and therefore a standard treatment path does not exist. At present, prophylactic cholecystectomy is not recommended for most cases of asymptomatic cholelithiasis. However, there are certain instances when a prophylactic cholecystectomy for silent gallstones may be warranted (Box 104-2). Certain transplant recipients or immunocompromised patients may benefit from early intervention. It has been shown that heart and lung transplant recipients develop gallbladder-related disease at a higher rate than the general population and may require an emergency operation associated with a significantly higher mortality rate than the general population.[14,15] In contrast, renal transplant recipients do not appear to have a higher rate of gallstone formation and associated complications.[16] It is not clear why this relationship exists, but one possible explanation may have to do with the duration of cyclosporine use in heart/lung transplant patients and its effects on bile formation. Many heart/lung transplant recipients continue to use cyclosporine as maintenance immunotherapy for 2 years or more. Long-term cyclosporine use (>2 years) has been associated with the prevalence of gallstones. In contrast, maintenance immunosuppressive regimens for renal transplant recipients have transitioned away from nephrotoxic calcineurin inhibitors such as cyclosporine in favor of newer less nephrotoxic agents such as sirolimus. Thus, prospective heart and lung transplant recipients may benefit from prophylactic cholecystectomy before their transplant.

Another subset of patients who may benefit from prophylactic cholecystectomy are those requiring long-term total parenteral nutrition (TPN). Prolonged TPN use and gallbladder stone and sludge formation has been established, and the number of these patients who progress to symptoms and require a cholecystectomy is higher than those in the general population who have asymptomatic gallstones.[17]

Other cases in which a prophylactic cholecystectomy may be prudent is in patients who have certain hemoglobinopathies, such as hereditary spherocytosis, thalassemia, and sickle cell disease. Patients who have a family history of gallbladder cancer or calcification of the gallbladder wall should also undergo a cholecystectomy for asymptomatic cholelithiasis.

CHOLECYSTITIS

Acute cholecystitis results from obstruction of the cystic duct, usually secondary to a gallstone. Local inflammatory responses may also result in edema and

---

BOX 104-1 Indications and Relative Indications for an Open Cholecystectomy

Severe cholecystitis (relative)
Inability to delineate anatomy during laparoscopic cholecystectomy
Emphysematous gallbladder (relative)
Suspicion for gallbladder cancer
Perforation of gallbladder/abscess (relative)
Fistulization of gallbladder and gallstone ileus (relative)
Cholangitis (relative)
Multiple past abdominal procedures (relative)
Cirrhosis/portal hypertension (relative)
Blood dyscrasias (relative)
Contraindication for laparoscopy

BOX 104-2 Relative Indications for Prophylactic Cholecystectomy

Chronic total parenteral nutrition requirement
Family history of gallbladder cancer and asymptomatic stones
Children with hemoglobinopathy (sickle cell, thalassemia, spherocytosis)

---

inflammation of the gallbladder. Nearly 90% to 95% of cases of cholecystitis are calculous in origin. Acalculous cholecystitis accounts for the remaining 5% to 10% of the cases and is more common in critically ill trauma, burn, and sepsis patients and individuals with cardiac, diabetic, and acquired immunodeficiency syndrome conditions. Patients who are on TPN, postpartum, taking steroids or narcotics, or have received transfusions are also more likely to have the acalculous variant. Acalculous cholecystitis has a higher incidence of gangrene, emphysematous infection, perforation, and mortality. These patients usually require an emergent intervention, either a percutaneous cholecystostomy tube to decompress the gallbladder or cholecystectomy.

It was once thought that stagnation of bile and resultant infection from an impacted gallstone was the main pathophysiology in the development of cholecystitis. However, studies investigating bile cultures have shown that only 15% to 30% of patients undergoing cholecystectomy for cholecystitis have positive bile cultures.[18] This indicates that inflammation of the gallbladder is not simply an infectious process but rather a multifactorial series of events that are initiated by gallstone obstruction of the cystic duct. A well-described "ball-valve" mechanism has been attributed to the characteristic pain. Initially, a gallstone is impacted at the neck of the gallbladder leading to obstruction and wall edema. This leads to the formation of lysolecithin, a mucosal toxin. Prostaglandin synthesis increases and amplifies the inflammatory response. The edema and inflammation can then result in the lifting of the gallbladder wall away from the stone, thereby disimpacting the stone and effecting drainage through the cystic duct. In most patients, this series of events plays through and conservative management is effective. In some patients, however, disimpaction does

not occur, and this results in continued cystic duct obstruction leading to venous congestion, gallbladder ischemia, biliary stasis, and a systemic inflammatory response that necessitates operative intervention.

The present recommendations for antibiotic for cholecystitis are second-generation cephalosporin or a combination of a fluoroquinolone and metronidazole to cover microorganisms in the Enterobacteriaceae family; activity against enterococci is not required.

The timing of cholecystectomy during acute cholecystitis has been debated.[19-21] To compare early (<1 week) versus late (>6 weeks) cholecystectomy for acute cholecystitis, the Cochrane review evaluated 451 randomized patients and found no difference in bile duct injury or conversion to open cholecystectomy, with a shorter hospital stay in the early group.[22] Another study demonstrated a 28% readmission for the late group.[23] Early cholecystectomy is considered the treatment of choice today.

In 2007, an International Consensus group established the Tokyo Guidelines for diagnosis and management of acute cholecystitis.[24] Diagnosis was made with one local sign (Murphy sign, right upper quadrant pain or mass) and one systemic sign (fever, leukocytosis, or elevated C-protein level) with a confirmatory imaging test (ultrasound or hepatobiliary scintigraphy). Ultrasound confirmation was established with thickened gallbladder wall (>4 mm; if the patient does not have chronic liver disease and/or ascites or right heart failure), enlarged gallbladder (long axis diameter >8 cm, short axis diameter >4 cm), incarcerated gallstone, debris echo, pericholecystic fluid collection, sonolucent layer in the gallbladder wall, striated intramural, lucencies, and Doppler signals. They also defined the severity in mild, moderate (symptoms >72 hours, white blood cell count >18,000) and severe (organ failure) to guide treatment options.

The present recommendations in the management for acute cholecystitis are early cholecystectomy for mild and moderate acute cholecystitis, with low threshold of conversion to open cholecystectomy for moderate cholecystitis if the anatomy is not clear in order to avoid biliary injury. The single factors that influence conversion are males, older, obese, cirrhosis, and previous laparotomies. For the severe form of acute cholecystitis, a conservative management with antibiotics and cholecystostomy tube as needed is recommended, leaving surgical treatment when conservative treatments fail.

ANATOMIC CONSIDERATIONS FOR CHOLECYSTECTOMY

Successful surgical removal of the gallbladder requires knowledge of normal anatomy as well as the anatomic variants associated with the liver, gallbladder, bile duct, and the arterial supply to them. Iatrogenic injuries often result from unidentified anatomic anomalies. All important structures must be identified before dividing or ligating any structure (Figure 104–1). Vital structures include the hepatoduodenal ligament and its contents, cystic duct, common hepatic duct, common bile duct, cystic artery, and right hepatic artery. The cholecystectomy

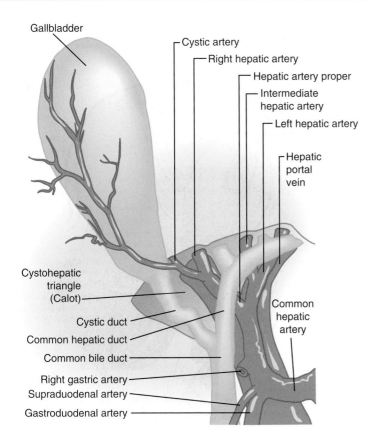

Gallbladder

Cystic artery

Right hepatic artery

Hepatic artery proper

Intermediate hepatic artery

Left hepatic artery

Hepatic portal vein

Cystohepatic triangle (Calot)

Cystic duct

Common hepatic duct

Common bile duct

Right gastric artery

Supraduodenal artery

Gastroduodenal artery

Common hepatic artery

FIGURE 104-1 The most common anatomy of the gallbladder and relevant adjacent structures. The surgeon must also be familiar with the variations in ductal and arterial anatomy that can be encountered during a cholecystectomy.

triangle, also known as *Calot triangle,* is formed by cystic duct, common hepatic duct, and the inferior edge of the liver. It is important to identify this triangle and its related structures during any cholecystectomy (open or laparoscopic). Commonly, the right hepatic artery is located posterior to the common hepatic duct, and the origination of the cystic artery from the right hepatic artery is within the triangle of Calot. Occasionally the cystic artery may arise from the gastroduodenal artery. The cystic duct and common duct junction is variable. The cystic duct may be long, short, or nearly nonexistent. It may run adherent to the common bile duct in a parallel course. The cystic duct may join the right or left side of the common bile duct, or it may connect to the right hepatic duct. In inflammatory states such as Mirizzi syndrome, the cystic duct may be unrecognizably contracted.

In difficult cases where the ductal anatomy is not certain, the use of an intraoperative cholangiogram is often helpful. Routine versus selective intraoperative cholangiography is still a matter of debate, especially in laparoscopic approaches. An intraoperative cholangiogram can provide ductal anatomy, demonstrate unidentified stones in the biliary system, and identify disease in the intrahepatic or extrahepatic biliary tree. Although intraoperative cholangiography does not prevent bile duct injury, it can help to limit the severity of injury by early identification and influence the success of repair and outcomes.[25-27] In some instances, the biliary injury can be repaired at the initial operative setting. Hence, the intraoperative cholangiogram can be an important adjunct to cholecystectomy.

LAPAROSCOPIC CHOLECYSTECTOMY

The laparoscopic approach has become the standard for the cholecystectomy; it reproduces the open cholecystectomy technique with the neck-toward-fundus approach as described later. With the patient in a supine position, general endotracheal anesthesia is induced, preoperative antibiotics are administered, and bilateral lower extremity sequential compression devices are placed. The abdomen is widely prepped and draped in the usual sterile fashion. In general, the abdomen is accessed with an open-technique Hasson port placement at the umbilicus and the pneumoperitoneum established. Alternatively, a Veress needle could be used to access the abdominal cavity. The intraperitoneal placement of the needle is confirmed with a saline drop test. Using the Veress technique, the Veress needle is exchanged for a 5-mm port and the pneumoperitoneum is initiated. A laparoscope is introduced through the Hasson port or the 5-mm port used for access, and diagnostic laparoscopy is used to confirm there was no injury to intraabdominal contents during the access placement. Under direct vision, three additional 5-mm ports are introduced in the abdominal cavity, two in the right upper quadrant and right flank and one port in the subxiphoid region. If the Veress technique was used and a 5-mm port placed at the umbilicus, a 10-mm port is placed in the subxiphoid region along with the other two lateral ports. The patient is then positioned with the head up and left side down, and attention is given to the right upper quadrant.

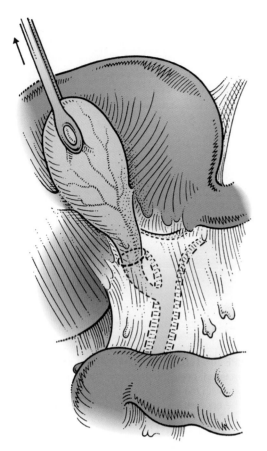

FIGURE 104-2 Cholecystectomy commences with adequate exposure of the gallbladder, grasping the fundus with a clamp to provide traction.

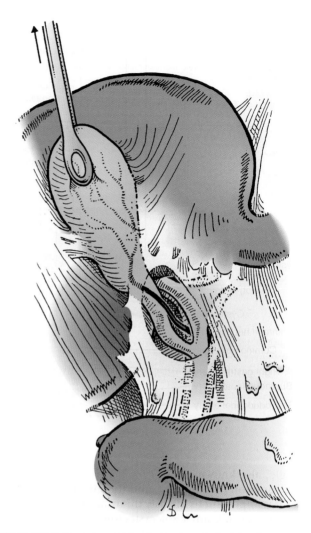

FIGURE 104-3 Neck-toward-fundus approach. Incising the peritoneum overlying the hepatoduodenal ligament will expose the Calot triangle.

NECK-TOWARD-FUNDUS APPROACH

With one of the lateral ports, a gallbladder grasper is used to retract the fundus cephalad above the liver by the assistant surgeon. Another grasper may be used to retract the infundibulum of the gallbladder and lateral and anterior traction is applied to straighten the cystic duct away from the common bile duct. The operation commences with an incision to the peritoneal undersurface of the gallbladder with the hook electrocautery and extends to the anterior aspect of the hepatoduodenal ligament (Figures 104-2 and 104-3). Too much traction may cause tenting of the common bile duct, which can lead the surgeon to misidentify it as the junction of the common bile duct and the cystic duct. Blunt dissection of the triangle is performed to identify the cystic duct and its junction with the gallbladder and the common bile duct. A grasper can be used to palpate the duct and identify stones and milk them back up into the gallbladder as performed in the open surgery (Figure 104-4). At this point, an intraoperative cholangiogram may be performed if there is suspicion for a common bile duct stone (Figure 104-5). The common bile duct may be opened and explored if a stone is palpable or detected on cholangiogram. The cystic duct and the cystic artery are dissected in the Calot triangle.

Next, the "critical view of safety" technique is performed. This technique requires three elements: the triangle of Calot must be dissected free of fat (without exposing the common bile duct), the base of the gallbladder must be dissected off the liver bed (or cystic plate), two structures (and only two, the cystic duct and artery) enter the gallbladder and these can be seen circumferentially (360-degree view). This creates two windows, one between the cystic duct and the artery and the other between the artery and the liver bed. Once this technique is completed, the cystic structures are safely divided. When exposing these windows, enough of the gallbladder should be taken off the liver bed (similar to the technique used in open cholecystectomy on the fundus-down approach and more in acute cholecystitis), so that it is obvious that the only remaining step is the division of the structures.

Once the anatomy is fully recognized, the cystic duct is clipped and transected as close to the gallbladder as feasible to prevent injury to the common bile duct. The length of the cystic duct stump, once thought to be related to postcholecystectomy syndrome, is not critical.

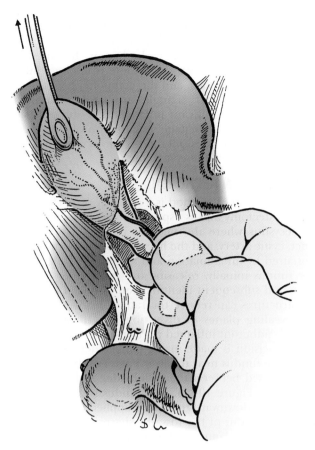

FIGURE 104-4 Digital palpation of the portal structures can identify stones in the cystic duct. The stones are gently milked back into the gallbladder.

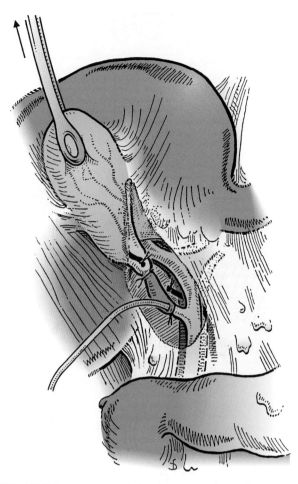

FIGURE 104-5 Intraoperative cholangiogram can be performed to identify anatomy or if a common bile duct stone is suspected. (Optionally, the cystic artery may be divided prior to cholangiogram if it has been identified.)

It is far more important not to injure the common bile duct. Once the cystic artery has been isolated and distinguished from a right hepatic artery, it is sharply divided between clips and transected.

Once the cystic artery and cystic duct have been divided, the neck of the gallbladder should be free and dissecting the gallbladder from its hepatic fossa begins. Continuous upward traction on the neck of the gallbladder facilitates exposure of the investing peritoneum around the gallbladder and the alveolar tissue between the gallbladder and the liver. The gallbladder is freed from its fossa by a combination of electrocautery and blunt dissection. This continues all the way up to the fundus until the gallbladder is free (Figure 104-6). Occasionally, there may be aberrant bile duct branches from the right hepatic or common hepatic ducts communicating directly with the cystic fossa, the so-called ducts of Luschka. These may be clipped and divided. In case of a postoperative bile leak, these ducts often cease draining spontaneously.[28,29] The gallbladder bed and cystic artery are inspected for hemostasis.

There have been valuable lessons learned from complications of laparoscopic cholecystectomy, such as developing techniques to minimize these complications. One potential fatal complication is the injury of the common bile duct. This usually happens because of anatomy misidentification, such as when the common bile duct is mistaken for the cystic duct. The "critical view of safety" technique described previously, published by Strasberg in 1995[30,31] has been used to minimize biliary injuries in the era of laparoscopy and has become a very important safety maneuver.

OPEN CHOLECYSTECTOMY TECHNIQUE

The location of the gallbladder on the posterior surface of the liver combined with the liver's residence beneath the ribs makes exposure a key aspect in the successful performance of a cholecystectomy. The right subcostal incision (8 to 12 cm) provides good, direct access to the liver, gallbladder, and the extrahepatic biliary tree and is the standard incision. The limitation of this incision is in providing exposure to lower abdominal organs. In cases where the costal angle is narrow or access to the entire abdominal cavity is preferred, a midline incision may offer better exposure as it can be easily extended superiorly or inferiorly.

Retraction of the right costal margin is best accomplished with the aid of a retraction system that is fixed to the operating table. This provides steady retraction, spares a hand, and limits the need for additional

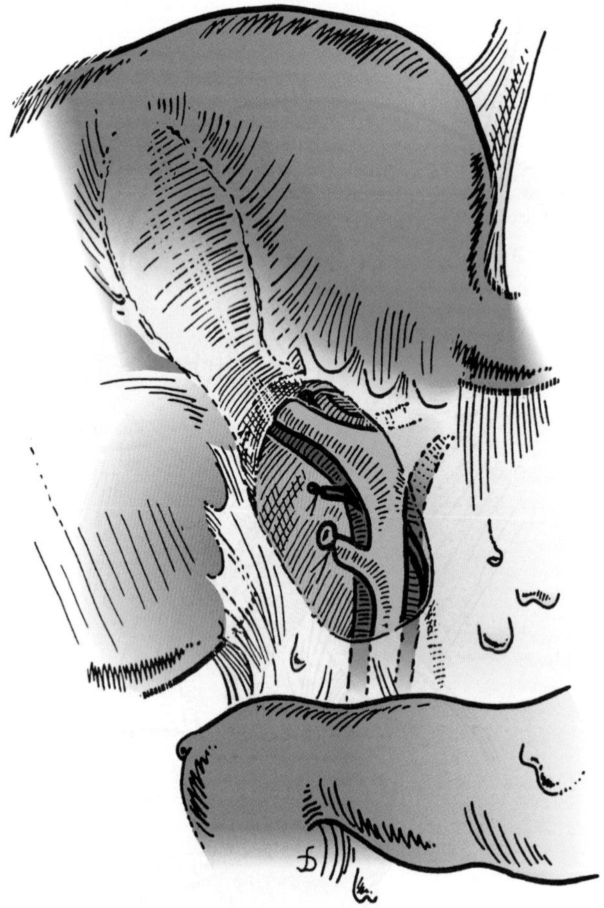

FIGURE 104-6 View of the gallbladder fossa on completion of the cholecystectomy with intact cystic artery and cystic duct stumps.

assistants. The patient is placed in a reverse Trendelenburg position to help bring the liver down from under the costal margin and moist gauze packs may be placed behind the right hepatic lobe to bring the liver forward. Division of the falciform ligament, and using it as a handle to lift the liver up, provides additional exposure. Alternatively, a retractor to lift the inferior aspect of the liver up may be used taking care not to tear the liver capsule. Moist packs are used to pack away adjacent structures and a wide hand-held or fixed retractor can be used to hold them in place. An orogastric or nasogastric tube is used for decompressing the stomach and enhancing exposure. Dense inflammatory adhesions to the colon or duodenum are often encountered and must be dissected free. Dissection in all instances should be performed close to the gallbladder wall. The presence of cholecystenteric fistulas must also be kept in mind.

The gallbladder fundus is grasped with a clamp for traction. A distended gallbladder may be difficult to grasp and may be aspirated to facilitate manipulation. During states of inflammation caused by cystic duct obstruction, the absorptive capacity of the gallbladder mucosa is impaired by the mucosal toxin lysolecithin. As a result, there is net secretion into the gallbladder with no outlet. This produces hydrops of the gallbladder and its characteristic whitish/clear gallbladder aspirate.

At this stage of the operation, the surgeon has two methods available to remove the gallbladder. Cholecystectomy from the neck toward the fundus (see Laparoscopic Cholecystectomy, earlier) can be used for straightforward cases in which there is minimal inflammation and adhesions, and the components of the cholecystectomy (Calot) triangle are easily identifiable. When there is significant inflammation and adhesions that impede safe, adequate visualization of the triangle components, the safest method is cholecystectomy from the fundus toward the cystic duct.

FUNDUS-DOWN APPROACH

The fundus-down method is a safe way of performing a cholecystectomy and is especially useful in the cases of cholecystitis where the neck of the gallbladder, cystic duct, cystic artery, and the hepatoduodenal ligament are obscured by inflammation and adhesions. Dissection of the fundus initially, releasing the gallbladder from the liver, and subsequent identification of ductal and vascular structures can reduce the rate of inadvertent injury by revealing planes of dissection away from the most densely adherent inflamed portions.

An incision is made in the gallbladder serosa at the tip of the fundus near the liver edge. A subserosal plane is developed between the gallbladder and the liver on each side (Figure 104-7). The fundus is grasped with a clamp, and downward traction is applied as the gallbladder is taken out of the fossa by sharp and blunt dissection. Another clamp on the gallbladder can be used to manipulate the gallbladder laterally and medially during the dissection (Figure 104-8). With inflammation and edema, this plane is easily dissected sharply.

It is best not to aspirate the contents of the gallbladder because it is easier to identify the wall of the gallbladder when it is full and helps define the plane of dissection. However, if it interferes with grasping or visualization, it may be aspirated as described earlier. A useful maneuver in dissecting a collapsed gallbladder is to place a finger inside the gallbladder and use it as a guide for the gallbladder wall.

When the infundibulum and neck is reached, the cystic artery will be encountered entering the gallbladder wall (Figure 104-9). The cystic artery is sharply divided between clamps and ligated close to the gallbladder. Light traction on the gallbladder and skeletonization of the infundibulum will reveal the cystic duct. The cystic duct, common bile duct, and common hepatic duct should be identified. The cystic duct is then clamped close to the gallbladder and then sharply divided between two clamps and ligated. The gallbladder is removed from the field. The cystic duct stump may further be suture ligated or reinforced with clip. The gallbladder fossa and cystic artery stump are inspected for hemostasis.

The use of a closed suction drain is only indicated if the surgeon is concerned about identifying or controlling a bile leak. The drain is placed in the gallbladder fossa and brought out through a separate lateral stab incision. The drain is removed when the output is low and nonbilious. The abdominal incision is closed in one or two layers using a monofilament absorbable suture.

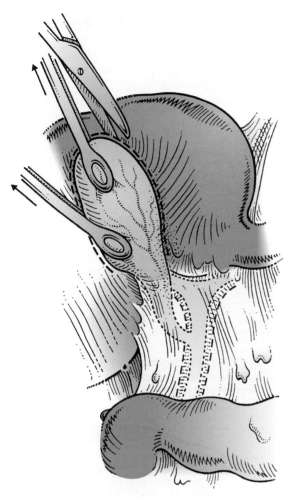

FIGURE 104-7 Fundus-toward-neck approach. The peritoneum over the gallbladder, close to the liver edge at the tip of the fundus, is incised.

The skin can almost always be closed primarily except in cases of the most infected gallbladder fossa.

MINICHOLECYSTECTOMY

Minicholecystectomy was first described by Dubois and Barthelot in 1982. It was initially applied to compare its effectiveness with the then rapidly advancing laparoscopic cholecystectomy. With the patient in reverse Trendelenburg position, a transverse 5-cm incision is made just lateral to the midline in the right upper quadrant and extended as necessary. The cholecystectomy is performed in a fundus-to-neck fashion. This is in comparison to the 8- to 12-cm incision that cuts the majority of the rectus muscle in the traditional open cholecystectomy.

This technique was modified by Tyagi in 1994 and results compared later to laparoscopic cholecystectomy. The technique by Tyagi described a 3-cm transverse incision performed just lateral to the linea alba at the "minimal stress triangle" in the subxiphoid area until the plane joining the eighth costochondral cartilages.[32] Once the anterior rectus sheath was visualized, a 5-cm vertical incision was made 1 cm lateral to the linea alba for the

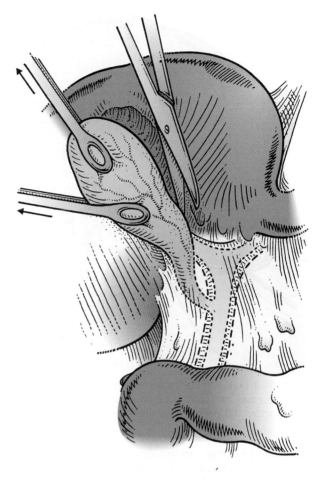

FIGURE 104-8 A plane is developed between the liver and the gallbladder wall. The second clamp can facilitate maneuvering of the gallbladder laterally and medially. In cases of acute inflammation, the surgeon can take advantage of the edema commonly found in this plane. The plane is most easily created by sharp dissection, but electrocautery may also be used.

anterior and posterior rectus sheath, retracting laterally the rectus muscle. This gives a vertical projection to the Calot triangle.

The minicholecystectomy (defined as an incision <8 cm long) was evaluated in a Cochrane review and other reports and compared with standard laparoscopy.[33-35] No differences were found in mortality, complications, and postoperative recovery, but minicholecystectomy had a shorter operative time. Although this technique does not offer much advantage relative to laparoscopic cholecystectomy, it should be a tool that every surgeon should be familiar with and utilize when the laparoscopic approach is not possible, namely, due to multiple adhesions from previous laparotomies, poor tolerance to the pneumoperitoneum, or the lack of laparoscopic equipment.

PARTIAL CHOLECYSTECTOMY

In rare emergent situations, a cholecystectomy may become hazardous because of the inability to identify most of the gallbladder and the triangle of Calot, excessive bleeding (portal hypertension, cirrhosis), or patient

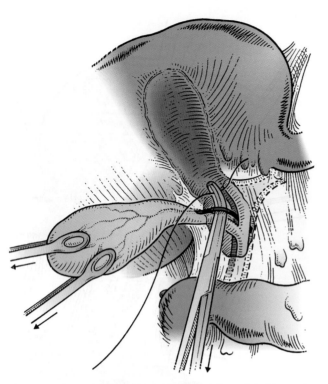

FIGURE 104-9 During this dissection toward the gallbladder neck, the first structure encountered will be the cystic artery as it enters the gallbladder. It is appropriately ligated and divided.

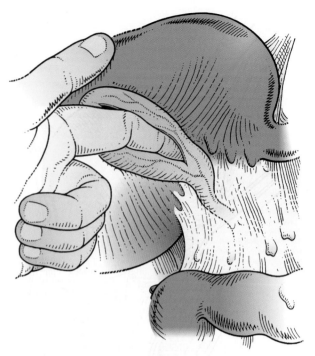

FIGURE 104-10 Partial cholecystectomy. The gallbladder has been opened and its contents evacuated. A finger may be used to inspect the cystic duct origination.

instability. In these circumstances, partial cholecystectomy may be indicated. The fundus of the gallbladder is opened and the contents evacuated. The surgeon places a finger in the cavity and uses it as a guide to remove the entire anterior wall of the gallbladder above the cystic duct (Figure 104-10). Impacted stones in the cystic duct should be removed. The posterior wall of the gallbladder that is in contact with the liver is left in place and its mucosa is removed with a curette or scoured with electrocautery (Figure 104-11). The cystic duct is ligated only if it is clearly identified. Blind stitching of possible cystic duct orifice can result in common bile duct injury. Alternatively, the cystic duct is left without further intervention and will seal, provided there is no distal common bile duct obstruction. An endoscopically placed stent across the cystic orifice may also be placed after patient stabilization. The area is drained using a closed suction device. Drainage of bile usually ceases spontaneously. If drainage persists, a reoperation may be necessary, although this is quite uncommon.

CHOLECYSTOSTOMY

In high-risk surgical patients with acute cholecystitis, such as those in the intensive care unit or with extensive cardiopulmonary disease, the mortality rates for an emergent operation can be as high as 46%.[36-40] High-risk surgical patients with severe acute cholecystitis (Tokyo Guidelines) may be managed with a percutaneous cholecystostomy tube, where biliary decompression can be obtained in 98% of the patients, and allows them to recover and leave the hospital.[36] Cholecystostomy can be

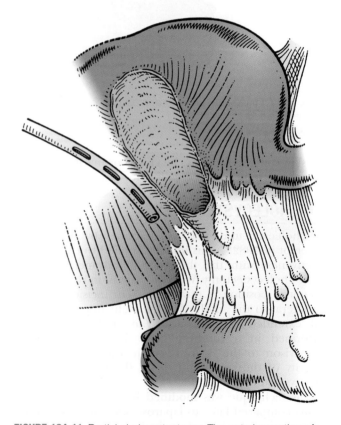

FIGURE 104-11 Partial cholecystectomy. The anterior portion of the gallbladder is excised, leaving the posterior wall intact within the cystic plate and the infundibulum. The cystic duct, if clearly identifiable, may be closed by suture ligation being mindful of the common bile duct. The gallbladder mucosa is removed with a curette or cauterized. A closed suction drain is placed.

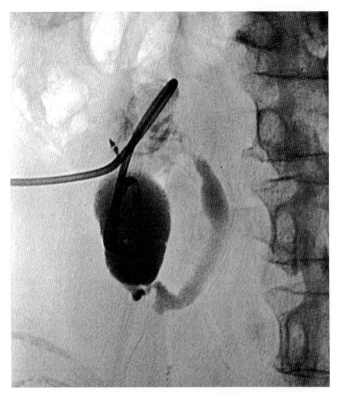

FIGURE 104-12 Percutaneous cholecystostomy tube is placed under fluoroscopy for acute cholecystitis. Note that there is a large intraluminal filling defect in the common bile duct, consistent with a calculus.

followed by delayed cholecystectomy or percutaneous stone extraction in poor surgical candidates.

A cholecystostomy can be accomplished either percutaneously or via a small subcostal incision under local anesthesia. It allows immediate decompression of the inflamed gallbladder and can serve as a temporizing measure or as a definitive treatment (Figure 104-12). Percutaneous transhepatic cholecystostomy is the preferred route and can even be done under ultrasound guidance in patients who are not stable to travel out of the intensive care setting. If the percutaneous method is not readily available, a small right subcostal incision permitting visualization of the fundus is made. The gallbladder is emptied as much as possible, a Malecot-type or similar catheter is placed in the gallbladder secured with a purse-string suture and exteriorized. Cholecystography is performed through the tube after resolution of cholecystitis. If there is free flow of contrast into the duodenum via a patent cystic duct and common duct, and there are no stones, the tube may be removed and cholecystectomy is not necessarily needed. Patients with gallstones who recover from their acute illness and are fit for surgery should undergo an elective cholecystectomy. In a retrospective analysis from our institution, 36 of 45 patients who underwent percutaneous cholecystostomy improved clinically within 5 days. Nine patients died within 30 days of the procedure, and only one death was attributable to gallbladder sepsis.[40] Thus, cholecystostomy is an easy, safe option with a low complication and high success rate for high-risk patients with acute cholecystitis.

SINGLE-INCISION LAPAROSCOPIC SURGERY

Single-incision laparoscopic surgery (SILS) was developed to reduce the number of incisions required to perform a procedure. SILS was developed in 1992 by Pelosi for single-puncture laparoscopic appendectomy and in 1997 Navarra described the first SILS cholecystectomy via transumbilical trocars and transabdominal stay sutures. One of the concerns with this technique is the difficulty in obtaining the "critical view of safety" while performing the cholecystectomy. This is particularly difficult because of the lack of triangulation, making the exposure of the Calot triangle more challenging, and the dissection of the cystic duct is on top of the common bile duct instead of being lateral to it. Navarra et al reported 30 cases of SILS cholecystectomy[41]; his enthusiasm decreased later when he randomized this technique (unpublished) with standard four-trocar laparoscopic cholecystectomy. He did not notice a difference in cosmetics or pain, but did notice that the operative time was longer with SILS. Recent reports evaluating these two techniques defined similar safety and efficacy. This is an interesting and novel technique, but the critical view of safety technique should be preserved to avoid biliary injuries.

MORBIDITY AND MORTALITY

The morbidity rate for an open cholecystectomy ranges from 5% to 20% when all complications are reported, including problems associated with any operation such as ileus, electrolyte abnormalities, atelectasis/pneumonia, and urinary retention. The overall mortality rate from an open cholecystectomy is 0.1% to 0.5%.[42-44]

Aside from the usual complications associated with any surgical procedure, the most significant complication from a cholecystectomy is a bile duct injury. The incidence of bile duct injury in open cholecystectomy is between 0.1% and 0.2%.[42,45,46]

The anatomic variations of the cystic and hepatic ducts and arteries are common enough to warrant no clamping, transection, or ligation until all critical structures have been properly identified. Injury to the hepatic duct or common bile duct often results by mistaking them for the cystic duct. Excessive traction can result in clamping of the hepatic or common duct (Figure 104-13). If identification of the ductal anatomy is difficult, a cholangiogram should be performed to identify the relationships of the ducts. If an injury has occurred, repair is best if it can be done safely at the time of the original operation. Primary repair can be performed over a T-tube if the defect is small (<1 cm) and there is no crush or burn injury or, alternatively, a Roux-en-Y reconstruction can be performed for larger defects.

Vascular injury to the right hepatic artery occurs when it is mistaken for the cystic artery. This can lead to future biliary strictures, cholangitis, and significant morbidity. In rare instances inadvertent ligation of the right hepatic artery has been fatal. The variations of the hepatic artery and cystic artery confluences and the possibility of accessory arteries mandate proper identification prior to clamping.

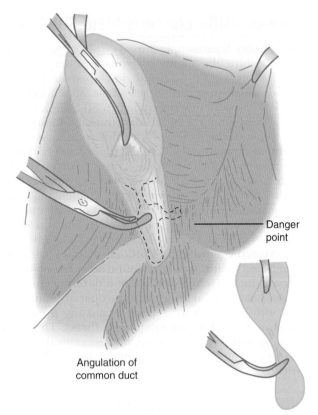

Danger point

Angulation of common duct

FIGURE 104-13 A common cause for common bile duct injury. Excessive traction on the gallbladder results in tenting of the common bile duct. This can lead to angulation of the cystic duct–common bile duct junction and erroneous clamping.

Bile leaks occur in less than 1% of the cases and are most commonly from the cystic duct stump, accessory duct, or intrahepatic bile duct. They are usually self-limiting and cease drainage in 1 to 2 weeks. If there is failure to close in a reasonable period, a contrast study via a percutaneous cholangiogram or endoscopic retrograde cholangiogram may be diagnostic and therapeutic.[47] During endoscopic retrograde cholangiopancreatography (ERCP), a stent or sphincterotomy may sufficiently relieve the elevated bile duct pressure that is maintaining patency of the leak or fistula and allow for sealing.

In a small subset of patients, new abdominal complaints arise after cholecystectomies that are of an unclear cause despite an extensive workup. This has been commonly referred to as the *postcholecystectomy syndrome*. Proposed etiologies for this syndrome include papillary stenosis and sphincter of Oddi dysfunction. Biliary manometry, magnetic resonance cholangiopancreatography, ERCP, and ultrasonography may help establish the diagnosis.

Length of stay for an open cholecystectomy is on average 2 to 3 days for an uncomplicated case. A few randomized studies had tried to evaluate if it is safe to do a laparoscopic cholecystectomy as an outpatient or if they should stay overnight. A Swedish randomized clinical trial compared day case cholecystectomy with "overnight stay." The average stay for the day case group was between 4 and 8 hours. The results found no difference in complication, readmission rate (8%), and patient

acceptance, but day-case surgery costs less.[48] The majority of the readmissions were due to patient's nausea or suboptimal pain control. Patient acceptance and anxiety play a significant role as well. Another study demonstrated a less than 2% readmission rate.[49]

Although laparoscopic cholecystectomy has largely supplanted the open variant, there will always remain a role for the open cholecystectomy and its usefulness should not be overlooked.

NATURAL ORIFICE TRANSLUMINAL ENDOSCOPIC SURGERY (NOTES) CHOLECYSTECTOMY

Natural orifice transluminal endoscopic surgery (NOTES), which uses natural orifices (transgastric, colonic, urethral, vagina) to introduce an endoscope, has been reported since early 2000 as a less invasive approach to laparoscopy. The growing interest in this technique motivated a working group of surgeons from the Society of American Gastrointestinal and Endoscopic Surgeons (SAGES) and gastroenterologists to form the Natural Orifice Surgery Consortium for Assessment and Research (NOSCAR), which oversees IRB approvals for human investigations. Today, almost 617 human patients have undergone NOTES procedures; most are transvaginal cholecystectomy or appendectomies and transgastric cholecystectomy.[49] The transvaginal access has a long history of interventions by gynecologists dating back to early 1800. The first human NOTES transvaginal cholecystectomy was reported in 2007, and later the report of a hybrid combination of flexible scope by a transvaginal approach in combination with an umbilical needle or port for laparoscopic instruments for retraction, dissection, or clips application. This hybrid technique allowed for a quicker and safer procedure; the present deficiency is in the proper endoscopic instrumentation. The first totally NOTES (T-NOTES) cholecystectomy was reported in 2009. For the transvaginal approach, a Foley catheter is placed, a dissection is performed in the posterior vaginal cul-de-sac to allow a port placement, and when the case is over, the closure is easier than a transgastric or transcolonic approach, which continues to be an issue. NOTES technique is evolving; the development of new instruments and randomization data could define the future application of this tool.

SUGGESTED READINGS

Bingener-Casey J, Richards ML, Strodel WE, et al: Reasons for conversion from laparoscopic to open cholecystectomy: A 10-year review. *J Gastrointest Surg* 6:800, 2002.

Flum DR, Cheadle A, Prela C, et al: Bile duct injury during cholecystectomy and survival in Medicare beneficiaries. *JAMA* 290:2168, 2003.

Hirota M, Takada T, Kawarada Y, et al: Diagnostic criteria and severity assessment of acute cholecystitis: Tokyo guidelines. *J Hepatobiliary Pancreat Surg* 14:78, 2007.

Lo CM, Liu CL, Lai EC, et al: Prospective randomized study of early versus delayed laparoscopic cholecystectomy for acute cholecystitis. *Ann Surg* 227:461, 1998.

Roslyn JJ, Binns GS, Hughes EX, et al: Open cholecystectomy: A contemporary analysis of 42,474 patients. *Ann Surg* 218:219, 1993.

Strasberg SM, Brunt LM: Rationale and use of the critical view of safety in laparoscopic cholecystectomy. *J Am Coll Surg* 211:132, 2010.

REFERENCES

1. Halldestam I, Enell EL, Kullman E, et al: Development of symptoms and complications in individuals with asymptomatic gallstones. *Br J Surg* 91:734, 2004.
2. Venneman NG, Buskens E, Besselink MG, et al: Small gallstones are associated with increased risk of acute pancreatitis: Potential benefits of prophylactic cholecystectomy? *Am J Gastroenterol* 100:2540, 2005.
3. Pappas TN, Posther KE: Acute cholecystitis. In Cameron JL, editor: *Current surgical therapy*, ed 8. Philadelphia, 2004, Mosby, p 385.
4. Shamiyeh A, Wayand W: Laparoscopic cholecystectomy: Early and late complications and their treatment. *Langenbecks Arch Surg* 389:164, 2004.
5. Z'graggen K, Wehrli H, Metzger A, et al: Complications of laparoscopic cholecystectomy. *Surg Endosc* 12:1303, 1998.
6. Regoly-Merei J, Ihasz M, Szeberin Z, et al: Biliary tract complications in laparoscopic cholecystectomy. *Surg Endosc* 12:294, 1998.
7. Macfayden BV Jr, Vecchio R, Ricardo AE, et al: Bile duct injury after laparoscopic cholecystectomy. *Surg Endosc* 12:315, 1998.
8. Mahatharadol V: Bile duct injuries during laparoscopic cholecystectomy: An audit of 1522 cases. *Hepatogastroenterology* 51:12, 2004.
9. Schmidt SC, Settmacher U, Langrehr JM, et al: Management and outcome of patients with combined bile duct and hepatic arterial injuries after laparoscopic cholecystectomy. *Surgery* 135:613, 2004.
10. Livingston EH, Rege RV: A nationwide study of conversion from laparoscopic to open cholecystectomy. *Am J Surg* 188:205, 2004.
11. Feldman LS, Medeiros LE, Hanley J, et al: Does a special interest in laparoscopy affect the treatment of acute cholecystitis? *Surg Endosc Intervent Tech* 16:1697, 2002.
12. Bender JS, Duncan MD, Freeswick PD, et al: Increased laparoscopic experience does not lead to improved results with acute cholecystitis. *Am J Surg* 184:591, 2002.
13. Rosen M, Brody F, Ponsky J: Predictive factors for conversion of laparoscopic cholecystectomy. *Am J Surg* 184:254, 2002.
14. Gupta D: Management of biliary tract disease in heart and lung transplant patients. *Surgery* 128:641, 2000.
15. Peterseim DS, Pappas TN, Meyers CH, et al: Management of biliary complications after heart transplantation. *J Heart Lung Transplant* 14:623, 1995.
16. Greenstein SM, Katz S, Sun S, et al: Prevalence of asymptomatic cholelithiasis and risk of acute cholecystitis after kidney transplantation. *Transplantation* 63:1030, 1997.
17. Roslyn JJ, Pitt HA, Mann L: Parenteral nutrition-induced gallbladder disease: A reason for early cholecystectomy. *Am J Surg* 148:58, 1994.
18. Den-Hoed PT, Boelhouwer RU, Veen HF, et al: Infections and bacteriologic data after laparoscopic and open gallbladder surgery. *J Hosp Infection* 39:27, 1999.
19. Lo CM, Liu CL, Lai EC, et al: Prospective randomized study of early versus delayed laparoscopic cholecystectomy for acute cholecystitis. *Ann Surg* 227:461, 1998.
20. Rutledge D, Jones D, Rege R, et al: Consequences of delay in surgical treatment of biliary disease. *Am J Surg* 180:466, 2000.
21. Uchiyama K, Onishi H, Tani M, et al: Timing of cholecystectomy for acute cholecystitis with cholecystolithiasis. *Hepatogastroenterology* 51:346, 2004.
22. Gurusamy KS, Samraj K: Early versus delayed laparoscopic cholecystectomy for acute cholecystitis. *Cochrane Database Syst Rev* CD005440, 2006.
23. Cheruvu CV, Eyre-Brook IA: Consequences of prolonged wait before gallbladder surgery. *Ann R Coll Surg Engl* 84:20, 2002.
24. Hirota M, Takada T, Kawarada Y, et al: Diagnostic criteria and severity assessment of acute cholecystitis: Tokyo guidelines. *J Hepatobiliary Pancreat Surg* 14:78, 2007.
25. Metcalfe MS, Ong T, Bruening MH, et al: Is intraoperative cholangiogram a matter of routine? *Am J Surg* 187:475, 2004.
26. Fletcher DR, Hobbs MS, Tan P, et al: Complications of cholecystectomy: Risks of the laparoscopic approach and protective effects of operative cholangiography—a population-based study. *Ann Surg* 229:449, 1999.
27. Ludwig K, Bernhardt J, Steffen H, et al: Contribution of intraoperative cholangiography to incidence and outcome of common bile duct injuries during laparoscopic cholecystectomy. *Surg Endosc* 16:1098, 2002.
28. Sharif K, de Goyet J: Bile duct of Luschka leading to bile leak after cholecystectomy: Revisiting the biliary anatomy. *J Pediatr Surg* 38:21, 2003.
29. Suhocki PV, Meyers WC: Injury to aberrant bile ducts during cholecystectomy: A common cause of diagnostic error and treatment delay. *AJR Am J Roentgenol* 172:955, 1999.
30. Strasberg SM, Hertl M, Soper NJ: An analysis of the problem of biliary injury during laparoscopic cholecystectomy. *J Am Coll Surg* 180:101, 1995.
31. Strasberg SM, Brunt LM: Rationale and use of the critical view of safety in laparoscopic cholecystectomy. *J Am Coll Surg* 211:132, 2010.
32. Tyagi NS, Meredith MC, Lumb JC, et al: A new minimal invasive technique for cholecystectomy: Subxiphoid "minimal stress triangle" microceliotomy. *Ann Surg* 220:617, 1994.
33. Harju J, Juvonen P, Eskelinen M, et al: Minilaparotomy cholecystectomy versus laparoscopic cholecystectomy: A randomized study with special reference to obesity. *Surg Endosc* 20:583, 2006.
34. Ros A, Nilsson E: Abdominal pain and patient overall and cosmetic satisfaction one year after cholecystectomy: Outcome of a randomized trial comparing laparoscopic and minilaparotomy cholecystectomy. *Scand J Gastroenterol* 39:773, 2004.
35. Keus F, de Jong JA, Gooszen HG, et al: Laparoscopic versus small-incision cholecystectomy for patients with symptomatic cholecystolithiasis. *Cochrane Database Syst Rev* (13): CD006229, 2006.
36. Spira RM, Nissan A, Zamir O, et al: Percutaneous transhepatic cholecystostomy and delayed laparoscopic cholecystectomy in critically ill patients with acute calculus cholecystitis. *Am J Surg* 183:62, 2002.
37. Chang L, Moonka R, Stelzner M, et al: Percutaneous cholecystostomy for acute cholecystitis in veteran patients. *Am J Surg* 180:198, 2000.
38. Patel M, Miedema BW, James MA, et al: Percutaneous cholecystostomy is an effective treatment for high-risk patients with acute cholecystitis. *Am Surg* 66:33, 2000.
39. Barie PS, Eachempati SR: Acute acalculous cholecystitis. *Curr Gastroenterol Rep* 5:302, 2003.
40. Byrne MF, Suhocki P, Mitchell RM, et al: Percutaneous cholecystostomy in patients with acute cholecystitis: Experience of 45 patients at a U.S. referral center. *J Am Coll Surg* 197:206, 2003.
41. Navarra G, La Malfa G, Bartolotta G, et al: The invisible cholecystectomy: A different way. *Surg Endosc* 22:2103, 2008.
42. Morgenstern L, Wong L, Berci G: Twelve hundred open cholecystectomies before the laparoscopic era: A standard for comparison *Arch Surg* 127:400, 1992.
43. Chen AY, Daley J, Pappas TN, et al: Growing use of laparoscopic cholecystectomy in the national Veterans Affairs Surgical Risk Study: Effect on volume, patient selection, and selected outcomes. *Ann Surg* 227:12, 1998.
44. Lillemoe KD, Melton GB, Cameron JL, et al: Postoperative bile duct strictures: Management and outcome in the 1990s. *Ann Surg* 232:430, 2000.
45. Blumgart LH, Kelly CJ, Benjamin IS: Benign bile duct stricture following cholecystectomy: Critical factors in management. *Br J Surg* 71:836, 1984.
46. Sandha GS, Bourke MJ, Haber GB, et al: Endoscopic therapy for bile leak based on new classification: Results in 207 patients. *Gastrointest Endosc* 60:567, 2004.
47. Johansson M, Thune A, Nelvin L, et al: Randomized clinical trial of day-care versus overnight-stay laparoscopic cholecystectomy. *Br J Surg* 93:40, 2006.
48. Leeder PC, Matthews T, Krzeminska K, et al: Routine day-case laparoscopic cholecystectomy. *Br J Surg* 91:312, 2004.
49. Chukwumah C, Zorron R, Marks JM, et al: Current status of natural orifice translumenal endoscopic surgery (NOTES). *Curr Probl Surg* 47:630, 2010.

Management of Common Bile Duct Stones

Eric S. Hungness | Nathaniel J. Soper

The optimal treatment of choledocholithiasis is controversial and mainly depends on the patient's condition and the relative local expertise in laparoscopy, endoscopy, and interventional radiology. Before the age of laparoscopy, patients with choledocholithiasis required a laparotomy with common bile duct (CBD) exploration and T-tube placement. Laparoscopic CBD exploration (LCBDE) has largely replaced the open approach with both transcystic and transcholedochal techniques available. Endoscopic retrograde cholangiography (ERC) with or without endoscopic sphincterotomy (ES) is commonly performed by endoscopists. In addition, interventional radiologists may dislodge or disintegrate stones by percutaneous transhepatic cholangiography techniques. One of the main determining factors of who performs these procedures is if choledocholithiasis is detected before, during, or after cholecystectomy, and if altered anatomy is present (Roux-en-Y gastrojejunostomy). In this chapter, we review the various techniques available to clear the CBD of stones, focusing on LCBDE. We propose an algorithm that assumes an advanced laparoscopic surgeon with excellent endoscopic and radiologic support (Figure 105-1) and that takes into account the ability to clear the CBD in the safest and most cost-effective manner.

DETECTION OF COMMON DUCT STONES

The most common clinical presentations for patients with choledocholithiasis are cholecystitis, pancreatitis, biliary colic, cholangitis, and jaundice. Cholangitis is most predictive, with some studies showing 100% specificity.[1] However, none of the other more common clinical presentations are predictive. A recent study by Tranter and Thompson[1] demonstrated a 14.2% incidence of choledocholithiasis in 1000 consecutive laparoscopic cholecystectomies (LCs) with routine intraoperative cholangiogram. Patients presenting with cholecystitis, biliary colic, pancreatitis, and jaundice were found to have common duct stones 7%, 16%, 20%, and 45% of the time, respectively.

Transabdominal ultrasound is the most common imaging modality used in evaluating patients with biliary symptoms. Compared to its high accuracy in diagnosing cholelithiasis and cholecystitis, transabdominal ultrasound only has 50% to 80% sensitivity in detecting common duct stones, depending mostly on the presence of CBD dilation.[2,3] Some studies have shown that if sonographic CBD dilation is combined with age older than 55 years and abnormal liver enzymes, choledocholithiasis can be predicted up to 95% of the time.[4]

For those patients in which choledocholithiasis is suspected, more definite tests may be performed. ERC is

highly specific in diagnosing common duct stones and may be therapeutic with sphincterotomy and duct clearance. However, this procedure is invasive and associated with significant morbidity. A recent prospective study of 1177 consecutive ERCs demonstrated a 30-day morbidity rate of 15.9% with procedure-related mortality at 1%.[5] Also, up to 61% of patients undergoing ERC will be found not to have common duct stones and will have undergone an unnecessary invasive test.[6,7]

Recently, endoscopic ultrasound (EUS) and magnetic resonance technology have been used to diagnose choledocholithiasis. To decrease unnecessary ERC/ES, some centers now routinely perform EUS before ERC. A recent study showed the sensitivity and specificity of EUS to be 98% and 99%, respectively.[8] In light of these findings and the decreased risk of pancreatitis, two recently published clinical guidelines advocate EUS in symptomatic patients with indeterminate risk of choledocholithiasis.[9,10] Additionally, magnetic resonance imaging has shown promise as a noninvasive alternative to diagnose choledocholithiasis, with a recent study showing a positive predictive value of 95%.[11] Magnetic resonance cholangiopancreatography (MRCP) is quite expensive, however, and does not have the therapeutic possibilities of ERC. MRCP is also useful in patients who have had a prior Billroth II or Roux-en-Y gastrojejunostomy, particularly for the hundreds of thousands of patients having undergone a gastric bypass operation for the treatment of morbid obesity.

PREOPERATIVE ENDOSCOPIC THERAPY

ERC plays an important role in the early treatment of common duct stones for elderly or debilitated patients and in patients who present with jaundice, cholangitis, or severe pancreatitis. For patients who may not tolerate an operation, performing ERC/ES and leaving the gallbladder in situ is a good alternative to cholecystectomy, because recent studies have demonstrated that 75% to 84% of patients remain symptom free with up to 70-month followup.[12,13] Other studies have demonstrated a decreased mortality for patients undergoing ERC versus surgical drainage for cholangitis and severe pancreatitis.[14-16] The use of routine preoperative ERC for suspected choledocholithiasis, however, is not warranted because recent studies demonstrate that up to 61% of patients with suspected common duct stones undergo an unnecessary ERC with its associated morbidity.[6] If a patient with choledocholithiasis does undergo successful preoperative ERC, early laparoscopic cholecystectomy should be considered, as a recent randomized trial showed 36% recurrent biliary events within 6 to 8 weeks.[17] Additionally, two prospective randomized trials comparing two-stage versus single-stage management

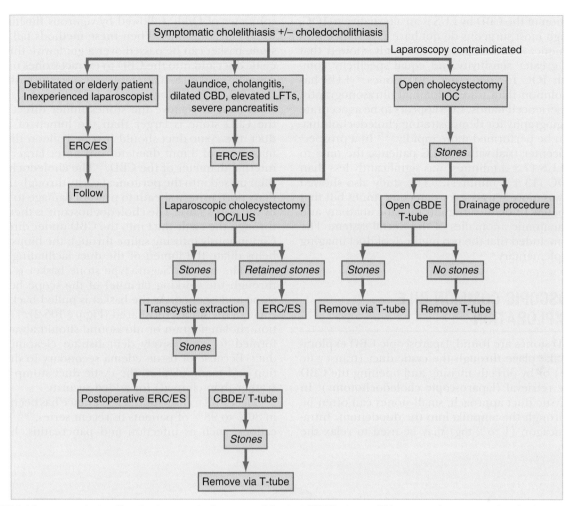

FIGURE 105-1 Management algorithm for treatment of common bile duct (CBD) stones. This approach assumes that the laparoscopist is experienced in transcystic techniques and that endoscopic retrograde cholangiography and endoscopic sphincterotomy is at least 90% successful at CBD stone clearance. *CBDE,* Common bile duct exploration; *ERC,* endoscopic retrograde cholangiography; *ES,* endoscopic sphincterotomy; *LFT,* liver function test; *IOC,* intraoperative cholangiography; *LUS,* laparoscopic ultrasonography. (From Jones DB, Soper NJ: The current management of common bile duct stones. *Adv Surg* 29:271, 1996.)

demonstrate equivalent success rates for LCBDE versus preoperative ERC/ES followed by LC.[18,19] One-stage LCBDE has also been shown to significantly reduce hospital stays and hospital costs.[19,20] Tai et al showed that LCBDE had a 100% success rate in salvaging failed preoperative ERC/ES.[21]

Much of the morbidity associated with ERC/ES is associated with the sphincterotomy. Endoscopic papillary dilation has been suggested as an alternative; however, a recent multicenter, controlled, randomized study demonstrated that endoscopic balloon dilation resulted in a higher rate of pancreatitis compared with sphincterotomy and recommended that it should be avoided in routine practice.[22] A recent metaanalysis suggested that dilation should be the preferred method for endoscopic removal of common duct stones in patients with coagulopathy.[23]

INTRAOPERATIVE DIAGNOSIS

For patients undergoing LC, the CBD should be imaged if choledocholithiasis is suspected (past or present

elevation of liver function tests, gallstone pancreatitis, CBD dilation or choledocholithiasis on preoperative ultrasound) or if the biliary anatomy is unclear.[24] This can be achieved by intraoperative cholangiography (IOC) or laparoscopic ultrasonography (LUS). Before either procedure, a clip is applied high on the cystic duct at its junction with the gallbladder to prevent stones migrating down the duct. To perform IOC, the cystic duct is partially transected and "milked," moving stones away from the CBD and out the ductotomy. A cholangiography catheter is inserted into the cystic duct and secured in place with a clip, grasping jaws, or balloon fixation. Cholangiography is now routinely performed with real-time fluoroscopy while injecting 5 to 10 mL of water-soluble contrast medium diluted 1:1 with normal saline. The following characteristics should be ascertained: (1) the length of cystic duct and location of its junction with the CBD, (2) the size of the CBD, (3) the presence of intraluminal filling defects, (4) the free flow of contrast into the duodenum, and (5) the anatomy of the extrahepatic and intrahepatic biliary tree.

Evaluation of the CBD by LUS is an alternative to IOC, even though most surgeons do not have experience with this technique. A recent prospective study showed that LUS had greater sensitivity and equal specificity compared with IOC for detecting CBD stones.[25] LUS has better resolution than transabdominal ultrasonography, and in experienced hands, LUS appears to be as accurate as cholangiography for demonstrating choledocholithiasis and can be performed more rapidly.[26,27] In a prospective, multicenter trial with 209 LC patients, the time to perform LUS (7 ± 3 minutes) was significantly less than that of IOC (13 ± 6 minutes).[26] The study also showed that LUS was more sensitive for detecting stones but that IOC was better in delineating intrahepatic anatomy and defining anatomic anomalies of the ductal system. The authors concluded that the two methods of duct imaging were complementary.

LAPAROSCOPIC COMMON BILE DUCT EXPLORATION

When CBD stones are found, laparoscopic CBD exploration can take place through the cystic duct (transcystic technique) or by directly incising and opening the CBD with stone retrieval (laparoscopic choledochotomy). In the transcystic duct approach, small stones can often be flushed through the ampulla into the duodenum. Intravenous glucagon (1 to 2 mg) may be used to relax the sphincter of Oddi, followed by vigorous flushing of 100 to 200 mL of saline. When these methods fail, a helical stone basket can be passed over a guidewire through the cystic duct and into the CBD to extract stones under fluoroscopic guidance. If attempts at transcystic basket extraction fail, a choledochoscope (≤10 French) should be tried next to remove the stones under direct vision. If the CBD stone is larger than the lumen of the cystic duct, the cystic duct should first be balloon dilated to a maximum of 8 mm diameter but never larger than the internal diameter of the CBD.[28] The choledochoscope is then passed into the peritoneal cavity through the midaxillary port, using a sheath to prevent damage to the scope by the port's valve. The choledochoscope is then inserted through the cystic duct into the CBD under direct vision. Continuously infusing saline through the biopsy channel helps dilate the lumen of the duct facilitating visualization. The tip of a Segura-type stone basket is advanced through the working channel of the scope beyond the stone and opened. As the basket is pulled backward and rotated, the stone is ensnared (Figure 105-2).[29] A completion cholangiogram or ultrasound should always be performed to conclusively demonstrate clearance of the duct. Because of tissue edema secondary to ductal dilation and manipulation, the cystic duct stump is ligated (rather than clipped) for added security.

Successful transcystic duct clearance has been reported in 80% to 98% of patients in recent series.[18,30,31] Complications, such as infection and pancreatitis, have been

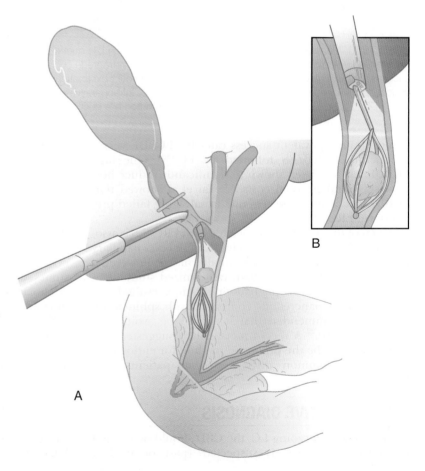

FIGURE 105-2 Transcystic choledochoscopy. **A,** The flexible choledochoscope is passed into the common bile duct through the cystic duct. Under direct vision the basket is advanced distal to the stone and opened. **B,** As the basket is withdrawn through the working channel of the choledochoscope, the stone is ensnared. The basket, stone, and choledochoscope are then removed as a unit. (From Jones DB, Soper NJ: The current management of common bile duct stones. *Adv Surg* 29:271, 1996.)

reported in 5% to 10% of patients with a mortality rate of 0 to 2%. The duration of hospitalization following an uncomplicated transcystic duct stone extraction is the same as that for LC alone, averaging 1 to 2 days. The main advantage of the transcystic approach is that it avoids choledochotomy. Poor candidates for transcystic extraction techniques are those with large or multiple CBD stones, those with stones in the proximal ductal system, and those with small or tortuous cystic ducts.[32]

Other novel transcystic approaches include balloon dilation of the sphincter of Oddi and antegrade sphincterotomy. Carroll et al reported successful clearance of CBD stones in 17 (85%) of 20 patients by balloon dilation; however, even in this small series, three patients (15%) experienced mild postoperative pancreatitis.[33] This method should be avoided in patients with preexisting pancreatitis, biliary dyskinesia, or anatomic sphincter anomalies. A sphincterotome may be inserted through the cystic duct and its tip placed just through the ampulla of Vater into the duodenum. A duodenoscope is passed transorally and used to allow proper positioning of the sphincterotome before applying current to perform a sphincterotomy. DePaula et al have reported the performance of transcystic antegrade sphincterotomy at the time of LC in 22 patients, and all had successful stone clearance without complications; the procedure added only 17 minutes to the operation.[34]

If the transcystic approach fails, we recommend laparoscopic choledochotomy. Indications for this procedure are multiple or large stones or those positioned within the proximal bile ducts in patients with a CBD diameter larger than 8 to 10 mm.[35,36] Stay sutures are usually placed on either side of the midline of the anterior CBD wall to allow anterior traction on the duct. A longitudinal choledochotomy is made on the distal CBD, of adequate length to allow easy placement of a choledochoscope and removal of the largest stone.

After the stones are removed under endoscopic visualization, the ductotomy is usually closed either primarily or over an appropriately sized T-tube. Some centers have used transcystic tubes (C-tubes) or antegrade stenting with choledochorrhaphy for CBD drainage.[37,38] Common duct closure is accomplished with fine absorbable sutures using intracorporeal suturing techniques, and if a T-tube or C-tube is used, it is exteriorized through the lateral port site. Recent studies have demonstrated comparable results regardless of the technique of duct closure.[39] Others have shown decreased complications with primary closure compared with T-tube use, including a recent metaanalysis, as well as a prospective, randomized trial that also suggested decreased operative time and hospital stay.[37,40,41] The patient is generally discharged 2 to 4 days postoperatively. If a T-tube is used, a final cholangiogram is performed 14 to 21 days postoperatively with removal of the tube if no abnormalities are noted. Retained stones demonstrated by T-tube cholangiography may be effectively removed percutaneously after allowing maturation of the T-tube tract. Percutaneous extraction is successful in more than 95% of patients with retained stones[42]; otherwise postoperative ERC will be required.

Overall, laparoscopic choledochotomy is successful in 84% to 94% of patients with a minor morbidity rate of 4% to 16% and a mortality rate of 0 to 2%.[18,30,31] Potential complications of this technique include CBD laceration, bile leak, sewn-in T-tubes, and stricture formation.[35] Many surgeons have not mastered laparoscopic suturing and feel uncomfortable closing the choledochotomy for fear of a resultant stricture; however, no biliary strictures were identified in two recently published studies of more than 500 patients undergoing LCBDE with a mean followup of more than 3 years.[43,44]

Recently, some centers have explored intraoperative ERC as an alternative to CBD exploration. Enochsson et al reported that the technique was safe with 93.5% duct clearance; however, it added 1 hour of operative time compared with LC alone.[45] In another study, intraoperative ERC was as effective as LCBDE in duct clearance (≈90%), but morbidity was doubled, and hospital costs were significantly increased.[46] Intraoperative ERC also relies on preoperative coordination with a skilled endoscopist if the surgeon is not trained in ERC. Positioning in the operating room also makes the technique more difficult than in the endoscopy suite.

The possibility of finding CBD stones at the time of LC and potential treatment plans must be discussed with the patient before the operation. Many surgeons routinely leave CBD stones in place during LC for planned postoperative endoscopic removal. Additionally, a recent prospective study reported that more than 50% of clinically silent CBD stones passed spontaneously within 6 weeks.[47] Neither the number of stones nor stone size was predictive of spontaneous stone passage. The authors suggested a short-term expectant management approach for patients with clinically silent choledocholithiasis.

POSTOPERATIVE ENDOSCOPIC THERAPY

Postoperative ERC/ES should be considered when (1) LCBDE fails to clear the duct; (2) the surgeon is inexperienced in LCBDE; (3) retained stones are discovered postoperatively; (4) a patient's comorbidities make a prolonged operation risky; and (5) the CBD is small and prone to postoperative stricture. Multiple studies have shown that the incidence of retained CBD stones after LC is approximately 2.5%.[44,48] Regardless of the reason, postoperative ERC/ES maintains the goals of minimally invasive surgery with a rapid return to full activity. However, relying on postoperative ERC/ES subjects the patient to an additional procedure with its associated morbidity and possibly a second operation if endoscopic stone extraction fails. In a recent study by Rhodes et al, 80 patients discovered to have choledocholithiasis at the time of LC were randomized to have LCBDE versus postoperative ERCP.[49] Clearance of the duct was 100% for LCBDE and 93% for ERC, with a significantly decreased hospital stay for patients undergoing LCBDE. Other studies have shown that even in experienced hands, endoscopic sphincterotomy has an overall failure rate for stone clearance of 4% to 18%.[50] Because of the uncertainty of postoperative ERC, it may be reasonable to insert a catheter through the cystic duct into the CBD at the time of LC when CBD stones are discovered. Leaving a transcystic catheter in the CBD may increase postoperative ERC success by allowing a guidewire to be passed into the duodenum, thereby ensuring cannulation of the duct.[51]

PATIENTS WITH ROUX-EN-Y GASTROJEJUNOSTOMY

Patients who have had a prior Roux-en-Y gastrojejunostomy, most commonly performed now during gastric bypass operation for the treatment of obesity, who present with choledocholithiasis pose certain challenges that must be considered (Figure 105-3). The typical anatomy consists of a small gastric pouch connected to a 75- to 150-cm Roux limb and a 40- to 50-cm biliopancreatic limb. If the patient presents with symptomatic cholelithiasis and/or suspected choledocholithiasis, an intraoperative cholangiogram with or without LCBDE should be routinely performed because postoperative ERC is very difficult, if not impossible, to perform. If the patient has already had a cholecystectomy and has suspected choledocholithiasis, MRCP should be performed. If choledocholithiasis is confirmed, attempts at ERC with the assistance of a single- or double-balloon enteroscope can be made. Recent studies have demonstrated 60% to 80% successful CBD clearance using either single- or double-balloon enteroscopes.[52] If this is not successful,

laparoscopic-assisted ERC has been described.[53] In this technique, after a laparoscopic gastrotomy is created in the remnant stomach, a 15-mm laparoscopic trocar is inserted directly into the stomach. The endoscope is then passed into the previously "bypassed" GI tract through this trocar, and ERC is performed. Laparoscopic choledochotomy is another alternative in this group of challenging patients.

OPEN COMMON BILE DUCT EXPLORATION

Open common bile duct exploration (OCBDE) should be considered the default position, not a "failure," if LCBDE and/or ERC are unsuccessful. The most common reason to convert to OCBDE is an impacted stone at the ampulla of Vater, and these cases require a transduodenal exploration. OCBDE should also be considered as the initial procedure of choice if patients present with dilated CBD or multiple CBD stones. This entails performing either a choledochoenterostomy or a sphincterotomy ("-plasty"). Studies have shown overall similar results with either of the two operations. Therefore, surgeon experience should dictate which one is performed.[54] Some authors, however, have suggested choledochoenterostomy for CBD greater than 2 cm in diameter to create a large opening between the bile duct and intestine.

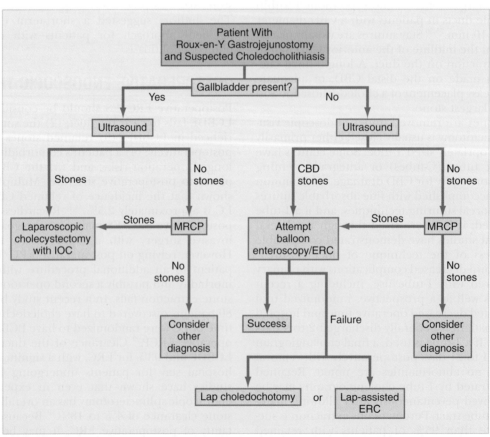

FIGURE 105-3 Treatment algorithm for patients with suspected choledocholithiasis and Roux-en-Y gastrojejunostomy. *CBD,* Common bile duct; *ERC,* endoscopic retrograde cholangiography; *IOC,* intraoperative cholangiography; *MRCP,* magnetic resonance cholangiopancreatography.

SPHINCTEROTOMY AND SPHINCTEROPLASTY

Sphincterotomy consists of incising the distal part of the sphincter musculature for a distance of approximately 1 cm. This incision should not extend beyond the outer wall of the duodenum. A sphincteroplasty requires complete division of the sphincter muscle. This creates a patulous, wide opening that is followed by suture approximation of the wall of the duodenum to the wall of the CBD.

After a choledochotomy is made as described earlier, a catheter or dilator is passed distally and left in place to serve as a guide. A generous Kocher maneuver is then performed, after which a longitudinal anterior duodenotomy is made at the level of the ampulla, which can be palpated. The dilator is then used to bring the ampulla into the operative field, being careful not to perforate the duct. For sphincterotomy, the ampulla is then incised sufficiently along the anterosuperior side (opposite the pancreatic duct orifice) to permit removal of the impacted calculus.

For sphincteroplasty, the ampulla and distal CBD are divided for a distance of 1.5 to 2 cm directed anteromedially. The sphincter is usually divided sequentially between small clamps, with sequential suture approximation of the duodenal and bile duct mucosa. This is done using fine interrupted absorbable suture. The duodenum is closed transversely, and the choledochotomy is managed as described earlier.

CHOLEDOCHOENTEROSTOMIES

The most common choledochoenterostomy is the side-to-side choledochoduodenostomy, usually in the setting of a dilated CBD with multiple stones. A generous Kocher maneuver is performed, and the distal CBD is exposed. A 2- to 3-cm longitudinal choledochotomy is made close to the lateral border of the duodenum along with a similar-sized longitudinal duodenotomy at the corresponding location. A "diamond-shaped" anastomosis is made with interrupted absorbable sutures. One potential complication from this is the "sump syndrome" caused by food or other debris becoming lodged and impacted in the distal CBD. This complication is rare ($\approx 1\%$) and can be managed with ERC/ES.[55,56] Other authors have suggested end-to-side choledochoduodenostomy as well as choledochojejunostomy as alternatives,[57] although endoscopic biliary access following these operations is technically challenging.

CONCLUSION

There are many ways to treat patients with choledocholithiasis. The algorithm proposed is only a guideline, and ultimate treatment will depend on physician experience and available resources.

SUGGESTED READINGS

Collins C, Maguire D, Ireland A, et al: A prospective study of common bile duct calculi in patients undergoing laparoscopic cholecystectomy: Natural history of choledocholithiasis. *Ann Surg* 239:28, 2004.

Cuschieri A, Lezoche E, Morino M, et al: E.A.E.S. multicenter prospective randomized trial comparing two-stage versus single-stage management of patients with gallstone disease and ductal calculi. *Surg Endosc* 13:952, 1999.

Hunter JG, Soper NJ: Laparoscopic management of common bile duct stones. *Surg Clin North Am* 72:1077, 1992.

Rhodes M, Sussman L, Cohen L, et al: Randomised trial of laparoscopic exploration of common bile duct versus postoperative endoscopic retrograde cholangiography for common bile duct stones. *Lancet* 351:159, 1998.

Williams EJ, Green J, Beckingham I, et al: Guidelines on the management of common bile duct stones (CBDS). *Gut* 57:1004, 2008.

REFERENCES

1. Tranter SE, Thompson MH: Spontaneous passage of bile duct stones: Frequency of occurrence and relation to clinical presentation. *Ann R Coll Surg Engl* 85:174, 2003.
2. Cronan JJ: US diagnosis of choledocholithiasis: A reappraisal. *Radiology* 161:133, 1986.
3. Gross BH, Harter LP, Laing FC, et al: Ultrasonic evaluation of common bile duct stones: Prospective comparison with endoscopic retrograde cholangiopancreatography. *Radiology* 146:471, 1983.
4. Barkun AN, Barkun JS, Fried GM, et al: Useful predictors of bile duct stones in patients undergoing laparoscopic cholecystectomy. *Ann Surg* 220:32, 1994.
5. Christensen M, Matzen P, Schulze S, et al: Complications of ERCP: A prospective study. *Gastrointest Endosc* 60:721, 2004.
6. Nataly Y, Merrie AE, Stewart ID: Selective use of preoperative endoscopic retrograde cholangiopancreatography in the era of laparoscopic cholecystectomy. *Austr N Z J Surg* 72:186, 2002.
7. Lakatos L, Mester G, Reti G, et al: Selection criteria for preoperative endoscopic retrograde cholangiopancreatography before laparoscopic cholecystectomy and endoscopic treatment of bile duct stones: Results of a retrospective, single-center study between 1996-2002. *World J Gastroenterol* 10:3495, 2004.
8. Buscarini E, Tansini P, Vallisa D, et al: EUS for suspected choledocholithiasis: Do benefits outweigh costs? A prospective, controlled study. *Gastrointest Endosc* 57:510, 2003.
9. Williams EJ, Green J, Beckingham I, et al: Guidelines on the management of common bile duct stones (CBDS). *Gut* 57:1004, 2008.
10. The Standards of Practice Committee: The role of endoscopy in the evaluation of suspected choledocholithiasis. *Gastrointest Endosc* 71:1, 2010.
11. Kejriwal R, Liang J, Anderson G, et al: Magnetic resonance imaging of the common bile duct to exclude choledocholithiasis. *Austr N Z J Surg* 74:619, 2004.
12. Vazquez-Inglesias JL, Gonzalez-Conde B, Lopez-Roses L, et al: Endoscopic sphincterotomy for prevention of the recurrence of acute biliary pancreatitis in patients with gallbladder in situ. *Surg Endosc* 18:1442, 2004.
13. Schreurs WH, Vles WJ, Stuifbergen WH, et al: Endoscopic management of common bile duct stones leaving the gallbladder in situ: A cohort study with long-term follow-up. *Dig Surg* 21:60, 2004.
14. Lai EC, Mok FP, Tan ES, et al: Endoscopic biliary drainage for severe acute cholangitis. *N Engl J Med* 326:1582, 1992.
15. Neoptolemos JP, Carr-Locke DL, London NJ, et al: Controlled trial of urgent ERCP versus conservative treatment for acute pancreatitis due to gallstones. *Lancet* 2:979, 1988.
16. Fan S, Lai EC, Mok FP, et al: Early treatment of acute biliary pancreatitis by endoscopic papillotomy. *N Engl J Med* 328:228, 1993.
17. Reinders JK, Goud A, Timmer R, et al: Early laparoscopic cholecystectomy improves outcomes after endoscopic sphincterotomy for choledochocystolithiasis. *Gastroenterology* 138:2315, 2010.
18. Cuschieri A, Lezoche E, Morino M, et al: E.A.E.S. multicenter prospective randomized trial comparing two-stage versus single-stage management of patients with gallstone disease and ductal calculi. *Surg Endosc* 13:952, 1999.
19. Rogers SJ, Cello JP, Horn JK, et al: Prospective randomized trial of LC + LCBDE vs ERCP/S + LC for common bile duct stone disease. *Arch Surg* 145:28, 2010.

20. Topol B, Vromman K, Aerts R, et al: Hospital cost categories of one-stage versus two-stage management of common bile duct stones. *Surg Endosc* 24:413, 2010.

21. Tai CK, Tang CN, Ha JP, et al: Laparoscopic exploration of common bile duct in difficult choledocholithiasis. *Surg Endosc* 18:910, 2004.

22. Disario JA, Freeman ML, Bjorkman DJ, et al: Endoscopic balloon dilation compared with sphincterotomy for extraction of bile duct stones. *Gastroenterology* 127:1291, 2004.

23. Baron TH, Harewood GC: Endoscopic balloon dilation of the biliary sphincter compared to endoscopic biliary sphincterotomy for removal of common duct stones during ERCP: A meta-analysis of randomized, controlled trials. *Am J Gastroenterol* 99:1455, 2004.

24. Horwood J, Akbar F, Davis K, et al: Prospective evaluation of a selective approach to cholangiography for suspected common bile duct stones. *Ann R Coll Surg Engl* 92:206, 2010.

25. Tranter SE, Thompson MH: A prospective single-blinded controlled study comparing laparoscopic ultrasound of the common bile duct with operative cholangiogram. *Surg Endosc* 17:216, 2003.

26. Stiegmann GV, McIntyre RC, Pearlman NW, et al: Laparoscopic intracorporeal ultrasound: An alternative to cholangiography? *Surg Endosc* 8:167, 1994.

27. Halpin VJ, Dunnegan D, Soper NJ: Laparoscopic intracorporeal ultrasound versus intraoperative cholangiography: After the learning curve. *Surg Endosc* 16:336, 2002.

28. Hunter JG, Soper NJ: Laparoscopic management of common bile duct stones. *Surg Clin North Am* 72:1077, 1992.

29. Jones DB, Soper NJ: The current management of common bile duct stones. *Adv Surg* 29:271, 1996.

30. Rojas-Ortega S, Arizpe-Bravo D, Marin Lopez ER, et al: Transcystic common bile duct exploration in the management of patients with choledocholithiasis. *J Gastrointest Surg* 7:492, 2003.

31. Thompson MH, Tranter SE: All-comers policy for laparoscopic exploration of the common bile duct. *Br J Surg* 89:1608, 2002.

32. Strömberg C, Nilsson M, Leijonmarck CE: Stone clearance and risk factors for failure in laparoscopic transcystic exploration of the common bile duct. *Surg Endosc* 22:1194, 2008.

33. Carroll BJ, Phillips EH, Chandra M, et al: Laparoscopic transcystic duct balloon dilatation of the sphincter of Oddi. *Surg Endosc* 7:514, 1993.

34. DePaula AL, Hashiba K, Bafutto M, et al: Laparoscopic antegrade sphincterotomy. *Semin Laparosc Surg* 4:42, 1997.

35. Dion YM, Ratelle R, Morin J, et al: Common bile duct exploration: The place of laparoscopic choledochotomy. *Surg Laparosc Endosc* 4:419, 1994.

36. Phillips EH: Laparoscopic transcystic duct common bile duct exploration. *Surg Endosc* 12:365, 1998.

37. Isla AM, Griniatsos J, Karvounis E, et al: Advantages of laparoscopic stented choledochorrhaphy over T-tube placement. *Br J Surg* 91:862, 2004.

38. Hotta T, Taniguchi K, Kobayashi Y, et al: Biliary drainage tube evaluation after common bile duct exploration for choledocholithiasis. *Hepatogastroenterology* 50:315, 2003.

39. Petelin JB: Laparoscopic common bile duct exploration. *Surg Endosc* 17:1705, 2003.

40. Zhu QD, Tao CL, Zhou MT, et al: Primary closure versus T-tube drainage after common bile duct exploration for choledocholithiasis. *Langenbecks Arch Surg* 396:53, 2011.

41. El-Geidie AA: Is the use of T-tube necessary after laparoscopic choledochotomy? *J Gastrointest Surg* 14:844, 2010.

42. Burhenne HJ: Garland lecture. Percutaneous extraction of retained biliary tract stones: 661 patients. *AJR Am J Roentgenol* 134:889, 1980.

43. Waage A, Strömberg C, Leijonmarck CE, et al: Long-term results from laparoscopic common bile duct exploration. *Surg Endosc* 17:1185, 2003.

44. Riciardi R, Islam S, Canete JJ, et al: Effectiveness and long-term results of laparoscopic common bile duct exploration. *Surg Endosc* 17:19, 2003.

45. Enochsson L, Lindberg B, Swahn F, et al: Intraoperative endoscopic retrograde cholangiopancreatography (ERCP) to remove common bile duct stones during routine laparoscopic cholecystectomy does not prolong hospitalization: A two-year experience. *Surg Endosc* 18:367, 2003.

46. Wei Q, Wang JG, Li LB, et al: Management of choledocholithiasis: Comparison between laparoscopic common bile duct exploration and intraoperative endoscopic sphincterotomy. *World J Gastroenterol* 9:2856, 2003.

47. Collins C, Maguire D, Ireland A, et al: A prospective study of common bile duct calculi in patients undergoing laparoscopic cholecystectomy: Natural history of choledocholithiasis. *Ann Surg* 239:28, 2004.

48. Anwar S, Rahim R, Agwunobi A, et al: The role of ERCP in management of retained bile duct stones after laparoscopic cholecystectomy. *N Z Med J* 117:U1102, 2004.

49. Rhodes M, Sussman L, Cohen L, et al: Randomised trial of laparoscopic exploration of common bile duct versus postoperative endoscopic retrograde cholangiography for common bile duct stones. *Lancet* 351:159, 1998.

50. Tranter SE, Thompson MH: Comparison of endoscopic sphincterotomy and laparoscopic exploration of the common bile duct. *Br J Surg* 89:1495, 2002.

51. Deslandres E, Gagner M, Pomp A: Intraoperative endoscopic sphincterotomy for common bile duct stones during laparoscopic cholecystectomy. *Gastrointest Endosc* 39:54, 1993.

52. Saleem A, Baron TH, Gostout CJ, et al: Endoscopic retrograde cholangiopancreatography using a single-balloon enteroscope in patients with altered Roux-en-Y anatomy. *Endoscopy* 42:656, 2010.

53. Lopes TL, Clements RH, Wilcox CM: Laparoscopic-assisted ERCP: Experience of a high-volume bariatric surgery center (with video). *Gastrointest Endosc* 70:1254, 2009.

54. Baker AR, Neoptolemos JP, Leese T, et al: Long-term follow-up of patients with side-to-side choledochoduodenostomy and transduodenal sphincteroplasty. *Ann R Coll Surg Engl* 68:253, 1987.

55. Escudero-Fabre A, Escallon A Jr, Sack J, et al: Choledochoduodenostomy: Analysis of 71 cases followed for 5 to 15 years. *Ann Surg* 213:635, 1991.

56. Caroli-Bosc FX, Demarquay JF, Peten EP, et al: Endoscopic management of sump syndrome after choledochoduodenostomy: Retrospective analysis of 30 cases. *Gastrointest Endosc* 51:180, 2000.

57. Cuschieri A: Common bile duct exploration. In Zinner MJ, Schwartz SI, Ellis H, editors: *Maingot's abdominal operations*, Norwalk, CT, 1997, Appleton & Lange, p 1875.

Biliary Dyskinesia and Sphincter of Oddi Dysfunction

Katherine A. Morgan | David B. Adams

Biliary dyskinesia and sphincter of Oddi dysfunction are functional disorders of the pancreas and biliary tract that challenge the practicing surgeon. Both disease entities are characterized by pancreatobiliary pain syndromes and are fraught with controversy over their definition, diagnosis, and management.

BILIARY DYSKINESIA

Acalculous gallbladder disease has been recognized by surgeons for almost a century. In 1924, Alfred Blalock described a series of greater than 100 patients who underwent cholecystectomy in the absence of gallstones with excellent results in pain relief (83% were improved). Allen Oldfather Whipple, in 1926, reported on 36 of 47 patients (76%) who were improved with cholecystectomy for acalculous biliary disease.

Biliary dyskinesia is a disease process characterized by right upper quadrant biliary-type pain in the absence of gallstones. Biliary dyskinesia is also referred to as *chronic acalculous cholecystitis* and *acalculous biliary pain*. Biliary dyskinesia is presumed to represent pain secondary to the abnormal motile function of the gallbladder. The frequency of acalculous biliary pain may be as high as 8% in men and 21% in women.

PHYSIOLOGY

The purpose of the gallbladder is to store and concentrate bile after production by the liver. Gallbladder emptying is achieved by contraction of the smooth muscle of the gallbladder wall, which occurs in coordination with sphincter of Oddi relaxation. In the fasting state, the gallbladder empties partially cyclically in conjunction with the migrating motor complex. In response to meal intake, contraction of the gallbladder occurs because of neural reflex stimuli as well as enterohormonal cues from the foregut, most notably cholecystokinin (CCK).

The pathophysiology of biliary dyskinesia is incompletely understood. In some cases, the cystic duct is implicated as problematic, with narrowing, possibly because of inflammation or fibrosis, and a resultant obstruction to gallbladder emptying. In other cases, an intrinsic functional motility disorder of the smooth muscle of the gallbladder wall or the cystic duct seems to be causative. Up to 43% of gallbladders on final pathology after cholecystectomy for presumed biliary dyskinesia show no histologic abnormalities.

Likely, biliary dyskinesia encompasses a diverse group of patients with variable factors contributing to poor gallbladder emptying.

CLINICAL PRESENTATION

Patients with biliary dyskinesia present with typical pancreatobiliary-type pain, as outlined by the Rome II diagnostic criteria, in the absence of gallstones (Box 106-1). The pain is located in the right upper quadrant or epigastrium, is colicky in nature, occurs postprandially, and is associated with nausea or bloating. The patient may have associated emesis or diarrhea. In addition, the patient may report anorexia and weight loss.

DIAGNOSIS

The essential component of the diagnostic evaluation of the patient with suspected biliary dyskinesia is a typical pain history. The physical examination may be remarkable for abdominal tenderness, particularly in the right upper quadrant, but often the abdominal examination is entirely benign. Liver biochemistries and pancreatic enzymes are within normal limits. A transabdominal ultrasound of the right upper quadrant should exclude the presence of gallstones (sensitivity >95%).

The differential diagnosis of upper abdominal pain in patients with an intact gallbladder but without gallstones is broad, including peptic ulcer disease, sphincter of Oddi dysfunction, microlithiasis, and generalized functional gut motility disorders. In addition, there is often overlap with these disorders, making diagnosis and management decisions challenging. In fact, some authors have reported residual or recurrent abdominal pain in patients treated with cholecystectomy for symptomatic cholelithiasis. Accordingly, these alternative or additional diagnoses should be sought with appropriate diagnostic studies where indicated by the clinical picture, including upper endoscopy.

CCK-stimulated hepatoiminodiacetic acid (CCK-HIDA) nuclear scintigraphy is considered the cornerstone diagnostic test for biliary dyskinesia. This study is useful in quantifying gallbladder ejection fraction (EF) as a marker for abnormal motility. In addition, the reproduction of pain with the infusion of CCK lends credence to the diagnosis of biliary dyskinesia. Most physicians define an abnormal gallbladder EF as less than 35%, based on the original descriptive study by Krishnamurthy et al in 1982. This group evaluated 7 subjects with a fast (1 to 3 minute) technique of CCK injection. In 1991, Yap et al evaluated 40 normal subjects with a slow (45 minute) CCK infusion technique, and found a mean EF of 75%. The authors therefore proposed an EF less than 40%, 3 standard deviations below the mean, as abnormal. In 1985, Fink-Bennett et al demonstrated a correlation between an abnormal preoperative CCK-HIDA and postoperative pain relief after cholecystectomy in 14 patients.

TREATMENT

Cholecystectomy is the treatment of choice for biliary dyskinesia. With the introduction of laparoscopic technology in the late 1980s, the number of patients undergoing cholecystectomy for this indication has at least

TABLE 106-1 Milwaukee Classification System

Type	Criteria
I	Pancreatobiliary pain **and** Elevated liver or pancreatic biochemistries* **and** Dilated bile or pancreatic duct† **and** [Delayed drainage of contrast on ERCP]‡
II	Pancreatobiliary pain **and** Elevated liver or pancreatic biochemistries* **or** Dilated bile or pancreatic duct† **or** [Delayed drainage of contrast on ERCP]‡
III	Pancreatobiliary pain **only**

From Hogan WJ, Geenen JE: Biliary dyskinesia. *Endoscopy* 20:179, 1988.
ERCP, Endoscopic retrograde cholangiopancreatography.
*Aspartate aminotransferase, alkaline phosphatase or amylase, lipase greater than twice normal on two occasions.
†Common bile duct greater than 12 mm or pancreatic duct greater than 5 mm.
‡Not generally included in the modern criteria.

tripled. Multiple retrospective studies have demonstrated benefit in terms of pain relief (79% to 100%) after cholecystectomy for biliary dyskinesia. One small, randomized, controlled trial of 21 patients has shown benefit as well.

Some authors have proposed that patients with a very low gallbladder EF by CCK stimulation (<15%) have a higher rate of pain relief after cholecystectomy, while others have not found this correlation.

Alternatively, some have suggested that a consistent history, more than results of objective testing with CCK-HIDA, is more predictive of a favorable outcome. These authors report excellent rates of pain relief in patients with typical symptoms regardless of the measured gallbladder EF (and notably even in patients with a normal gallbladder EF).

SPHINCTER OF ODDI DYSFUNCTION

Francis Glisson described circular muscle fibers surrounding the distal common bile duct in 1654. As a young medical student in 1887, Ruggero Oddi, elucidated the sphincter of the hepatopancreatic ampulla. He went on to become an acclaimed academician in Genoa, but his career was thwarted by a series of professional and financial indiscretions; he was therefore obligated to practice clinical medicine to make a living. Perhaps fittingly, since its description by this controversial man, the sphincter of Oddi, along with its associated disorders, has been viewed with skepticism. Patients with sphincter of Oddi dysfunction are often challenging in their fractious presentation, difficult diagnosis, and laborious management.

Sphincter of Oddi dysfunction (SOD) represents a benign, noncalculous obstruction to the flow of biliary or pancreatic secretions through the pancreaticobiliary junction. SOD is known by many names, including ampullary stenosis, papillary stenosis, papillitis, and postcholecystectomy syndrome. It is a disorder of the contractile function of the ampullary sphincter. It is a heterogeneous disorder, consisting of a fixed obstruction because of a stenotic ampulla in some patients and a functional obstruction because of abnormal motility in others.

SOD is an uncommon disorder, affecting most often middle-aged women. Approximately 10% of patients

develop pain postcholecystectomy, and 10% of those will have SOD. Depending on the group studied, 15% to 76% of patients with idiopathic recurrent pancreatitis will have SOD.

ANATOMY AND PHYSIOLOGY

The sphincter of Oddi is located at the terminal portions of the common bile duct and main pancreatic duct as they enter into the second portion of the duodenum. The sphincter consists of a common muscular complex, also known as the ampullary zone, as well as an intrapancreatic and an intrabiliary sphincteric mechanism.

The sphincter of Oddi exhibits a baseline zone of elevated pressure, with superimposed phasic contractions. It demonstrates a cyclical change in motor activity that is closely associated with the migrating motor complex. There is some neural influence on the sphincter through the parasympathetic and sympathetic systems. Hormonal factors, however, seem to play a significant role in the motility pattern. CCK is a potent inhibitor of the ampullary sphincter. Secretin acts to inhibit the pancreatic portion of the sphincter of Oddi.

SOD is marked by aberrations in the function of the sphincteric mechanism. It is most commonly defined by elevated intraductal pressures on manometric evaluation.

CLINICAL PRESENTATION

Patients with SOD are marked clinically by classic pancreatobiliary type pain, similar to the pain of biliary dyskinesia. This pain, as defined by the Rome II criteria (see Box 106-1), is episodic upper abdominal pain, typically postprandial in nature and associated with nausea. The physical examination is generally unremarkable. Patients may have transient elevation of their liver or pancreatic serum biochemical markers, or they may present with recurrent idiopathic pancreatitis.

Hogan and Geenen in Milwaukee developed a classification system for patients presenting with presumed SOD (Table 106-1). This system seems to effectively

TABLE 106-2 Milwaukee Classification System and Response to Therapy

SOD Type	Probability of Abnormal Manometry	Response to Treatment if Manometry Abnormal	Response to Treatment if Manometry Normal	Manometry Recommended?
I	75%-95%	90%-95%	90%-95%	No
II	55%-65%	85%	35%	Yes
III	25%-60%	55%-65%	<10%	Yes

Adapted from Sherman S, Lehman G: Sphincter of Oddi dysfunction: Diagnosis and treatment. *JOP* 2:382, 2001.
SOD, Sphincter of Oddi dysfunction.

predict diagnosis as well as management options and outcomes (Table 106-2). Type I patients have typical pancreatobiliary pain, elevated liver or pancreatic biochemistries, and a dilated biliary or pancreatic duct. Type II patients have typical pain, along with one other objective finding, and type III patients have pain alone.

DIAGNOSIS

The most important component of the diagnostic evaluation for SOD is a consistent history of pancreatobiliary type pain. Other more common etiologies of abdominal pain should be excluded with appropriate tests, including computed tomography (CT), esophagogastroduodenoscopy, and colonoscopy.

Historically, the Nardi test (morphine-prostigmin provocation test) was used as a diagnostic tool in the evaluation of the patient for SOD. In this test, the patient is administered morphine and neostigmine, and then evaluated for pain or elevated liver or pancreatic serum biochemistries. Biliary scintigraphy can evaluate for delayed hepatic hilum to duodenum transit time of the nuclear medicine tracer, correlating with ampullary obstruction. Ultrasound stimulation tests (transabdominal, endoscopic) have been used to evaluate the biliary or pancreatic duct diameter after administration of CCK or secretin, respectively. Sustained ductal enlargement from baseline suggests a relative obstruction caused by SOD. Similarly, secretin-stimulated magnetic resonance cholangiopancreatography (ssMRCP) can show a persistent increase in the pancreatic duct diameter after secretin administration. In general, these tests are of variable accuracy because of operator inconsistencies.

The standard for diagnosis of SOD in the modern era is endoscopic retrograde cholangiopancreatography (ERCP) with endoscopic sphincter of Oddi manometry (ESOM) (Figure 106-1). ESOM allows for the direct measurement of ductal pressures to assess for sphincteric hypertension. A smal-caliber (typically 5 French) multilumen perfusion catheter with an aspiration port is used for pressure monitoring. Sustained ductal pressures greater than 35 to 40 mm Hg above baseline are indicative of SOD. Abnormal pressures can be localized to the pancreatic duct, the bile duct, or may be present in both. ERCP with ESOM does carry some risk for morbidity, with pancreatitis reported in 4% to 31% of patients. A small percentage of these will be clinically significant. Pancreatitis is minimized by use of an aspiration port and by limiting perfusion time and pressure. In cases with equivocal manometry or where manometry is not available, endoscopic transpapillary stenting or endoscopic

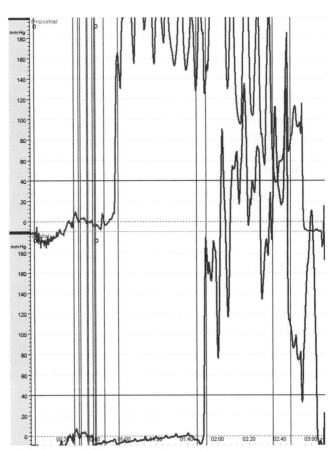

FIGURE 106-1 Endoscopic sphincter of Oddi manometry tracing shows abnormally high pressures (>40 mm Hg) measured in both the proximal and distal channels of the catheter.

intrasphincteric injection of botulinum toxin have been shown to be potentially predictive of response to endoscopic sphincterotomy (ES) therapy.

TREATMENT

The indications for intervention in patients with SOD are debilitating pain episodes or episodes of recurrent pancreatitis.

The medical approach to SOD has shown limited success. Smooth muscle–relaxing agents such as nitrates and calcium channel blockers have been used, although without data to show long-term improvement. Alternative strategies of pain management, including electroacupuncture, biofeedback, and use of transcutaneous electrical nerve stimulation have also been described.

TABLE 106-3 Randomized Controlled Trials of Endoscopic Sphincterotomy for Sphincter of Oddi Dysfunction

Study	N	Followup (Years)	Design	Response
Geenen et al, 1989	47	4	ES vs. Sham All SOM	+SOM ES, 90% +SOM Sham, 30% −SOM ES, 35% −SOM Sham, 35%
Sherman et al, 1994	23	3	ES vs. SSpx vs. ESham	ES, 83% SSpx, 80% ESham, 29%
Toouli et al, 2000	58	2	ES vs. Sham	+SOM ES, 85% +SOM Sham, 38% −SOM ES = Sham

From Geenen JE, Hogan WJ, Dodds WJ, et al: The efficacy of endoscopic sphincterotomy after cholecystectomy in patients with sphincter-of-Oddi dysfunction. *N Engl J Med* 320:82, 1989; Sherman S, Lehman GA, Jamidar P, et al: Efficacy of endoscopic sphincterotomy and surgical sphincteroplasty for patients with sphincter of Oddi dysfunction: Randomized, controlled study. *Gastrointest Endosc* 40:A125, 1994; and Toouli J, Roberts-Thomson IC, Kellow J, et al: Manometry based randomised trial of endoscopic sphincterotomy for sphincter of Oddi dysfunction. *Gut* 46:98, 2000.
ES, Endoscopic sphincterotomy; *Esham,* endoscopy without sphincterotomy; *Sham,* endoscopy without sphincterotomy; *SOM,* sphincter of Oddi manometry (+ abnormal; − normal); *SSpx,* surgical sphincteroplasty.

ENDOSCOPY

The current standard for management of SOD is ES. Successful pain relief is achieved in 55% to 95% of patients after this intervention, depending on patient selection. Three randomized, controlled trials have demonstrated the efficacy of ES in properly selected patients (Table 106-3). ES does carry a significant risk for postprocedure pancreatitis, 5% to 20%, although this is improved with use of prophylactic endoscopic stenting. Restenosis rates of 25% to 33% are reported.

SURGERY

Historically, before the modern endoscopic era, operative transduodenal sphincteroplasty with pancreatic septoplasty was the treatment of choice for patients with SOD, with good outcomes reported. With the success of endoscopic therapies, however, the surgical approach to SOD is relevant to two groups of patients currently: those patients who have failed prior endoscopic intervention (generally because of restenosis) and those patients who have undergone previous gastric surgery, particularly gastric bypass with Roux-en-Y reconstruction, where endoscopic access to the ampulla is difficult except with advanced techniques.

Transduodenal sphincteroplasty is undertaken through a midline laparotomy. A generous Kocher maneuver is employed to fully mobilize the duodenum and bring it up into the operative field. The duodenum and head of pancreas are assessed, noting signs of chronic pancreatitis, which may portend a poor prognosis for postoperative relief of symptoms. A fibrotic ampulla may be palpable through the duodenal wall and can help guide the location of the duodenotomy. An oblique duodenotomy is made overlying the estimated location of the ampulla using electrocautery. The ampulla is sought within the duodenum, with care taken not to traumatize the duodenal mucosa. A lacrimal duct probe is used to cannulate the distal common bile duct. The needle-tipped cautery is used to make a generous sphincterotomy, dividing the duodenal mucosa and sphincter on top of the lacrimal duct probe. The sphincterotomy is continued until there is easy flow of bile into the operative field.

The pancreatic duct is then sought and cannulated with a separate lacrimal duct probe. The septum between the bile duct and pancreatic duct is divided using electrocautery. The septotomy is continued until there is good flow of pancreatic secretions. Interrupted fine absorbable monofilament suture (such as 5-0 polydiaxanone) is used to approximate duodenal mucosa to bile duct mucosa and bile duct mucosa to pancreatic duct mucosa to complete the biliary sphincteroplasty and pancreatic septoplasty. The duodenotomy is closed obliquely with a running 3-0 absorbable monofilament suture.

In the modern era, pain relief rates in excess of 60% can be expected on long-term followup after operative transduodenal sphincteroplasty with pancreatic septoplasty. Younger patients and patients with chronic pancreatitis have poorer outcomes.

POST–GASTRIC SURGERY PATIENTS

In patients who have undergone prior gastric surgery, and are therefore not easily amenable to ESOM, the diagnosis of SOD can be difficult. In these patients, the most important component of the evaluation is a proper history. Laboratory evidence with abnormal biliary or pancreatic serum biochemistries, particularly during a pain exacerbation episode, is sought. Other more common diagnoses, such as ulcer disease, anastomotic stricture, internal hernia, or adhesions, are excluded with proper tests, including upper endoscopy and abdominal CT. ssMRCP can be used to evaluate for biliary or pancreatic ductal dilation at baseline or a persistently dilated pancreatic duct after secretin administration, both suggestive of SOD. ssMRCP seems to be specific but not very sensitive in the diagnosis of SOD. ssMRCP can help to exclude other pathology such as stones or neoplasm. Importantly, ssMRCP can also help to evaluate for chronic pancreatitis, as patients who have chronic pancreatitis tend to have a poor response to sphincteroplasty and may do better with an alternative procedure such as total pancreatectomy with islet autotransplantation.

These patients are well treated with operative transduodenal sphincteroplasty with pancreatic septoplasty. With proper patient selection, long-term pain relief is expected in 85% of patients.

Alternatively, in the patient who is post–gastric bypass, the excluded stomach can be accessed by radiographic or operative means. This site can then be used to allow endoscopic access for ERCP, ESOM, and ES. This approach has been favored by some authors. It does, however, require multiple procedures and carries morbidity.

SUMMARY

Biliary dyskinesia and sphincter of Oddi dysfunction, the functional disorders of the biliary tract and pancreas, are vexing in diagnosis and management. They are becoming increasingly recognized, and more objective means of evaluation have become available over the past two decades. However, significant controversy still remains regarding their ideal evaluation and therapy.

SUGGESTED READINGS

Adams DB, Tarnasky PR, Hawes RH, et al: Outcome after laparoscopic cholecystectomy for chronic acalculous cholecystitis. *Am Surg* 64:1, 1998.

Bingener J, Richards ML, Schwesinger WH, et al: Laparoscopic cholecystectomy for biliary dyskinesia: Correlation of preoperative cholecystokinin cholescintigraphy results with postoperative outcome. *Surg Endosc* 18:802, 2004.

Blalock A: A statistical study of eight hundred and eighty-eight cases of biliary tract disease. *Johns Hopkins Hosp Bull* 35:391, 1926.

Corriazziari E, Shaffer EA, Hogan WJ, et al: Functional disorders of the biliary tract and pancreas. *Gut* 45:1148, 1999.

Fink-Bennett D, DeRidder P, Kolozsi W, et al: Cholecystokinin cholescintigraphic findings in the cystic duct syndrome. *J Nucl Med* 26:1123, 1985.

Krishnamurthy GT, Bobba VR, Kingston E, et al: Measurement of gallbladder emptying sequentially using a single dose of 99mTc-labeled hepatobiliary agent. *Gastroenterology* 83:773, 1982.

Morgan KA, Glenn JB, Byrne TK, et al: Sphincter of Oddi dysfunction after Roux-en-Y gastric bypass. *Surg Obes Relat Dis* 5:571, 2009.

Morgan KA, Romagnuolo J, Adams DB: Transduodenal sphincteroplasty in the management of sphincter of Oddi dysfunction and pancreas divisum in the modern era. *J Am Coll Surg* 206:908, 2008.

Yap L, Wycherly AG, Morphett AD, et al: Acalculous biliary pain: Cholecystectomy alleviates symptoms in patients with abnormal cholescintigraphy. *Gastroenterology* 101:786, 1991.

Yost F, Margenthaler J, Presti M, et al: Cholecystectomy is an effective treatment for biliary dyskinesia. *Am J Surg* 178:462, 1999.

Whipple AO: Surgical criteria for cholecystectomy. *Am J Surg* 40:129, 1926.

CHAPTER

107

Endoscopic Retrograde Cholangiopancreatography in the Evaluation and Management of Hepatobiliary and Pancreatic Disease

James L. Watkins | Stuart Sherman | Lee McHenry, Jr. |

Evan L. Fogel | Kyo-Sang Yoo | Glen A. Lehman

Endoscopic cannulation of the major papilla with imaging of the pancreatic duct and biliary tree (endoscopic retrograde cholangiopancreatography [ERCP]) was first successfully accomplished with an end-viewing duodenoscope and reported in 1968. The subsequent development of side-viewing endoscopes with a catheter-deflecting elevator greatly facilitated the technique. Diagnostic studies were supplemented by the first endoscopic sphincterotomies in 1973. Techniques of biliary stone extraction, nasobiliary tube (NBT) placement, and biliary stent placement soon followed. These developments permitted less invasive diagnostic and therapeutic maneuvers in the pancreatic and bile duct that were previously limited to open surgical and percutaneous techniques. Although these procedures are more technically demanding than most other gastrointestinal endoscopic techniques, they are now being widely applied and are the method of choice for many clinical problems involving the pancreatic duct and the hepatobiliary system.

ENDOSCOPIC RETROGRADE CHOLANGIOPANCREATOGRAPHY

INDICATIONS

The role for diagnostic ERCP alone is diminishing as other less invasive/noninvasive imaging techniques (e.g., endoscopic ultrasound [EUS], magnetic resonance cholangiopancreatography [MRCP]) become more widely used. ERCP is indicated in clinical settings in which there is significant suspicion of an obstructing, inflammatory, or neoplastic pancreaticobiliary lesion that if detected or ruled out, would alter clinical management. A general classification of indications is listed in Box 107-1.

PREPARATION

Preparation for ERCP involves assembly of a skilled team that includes a physician or physicians, nursing personnel, and a radiology technician. A quality fluoroscopic unit is needed. A wide variety of catheters, guidewires, stone extraction balloons and baskets, sphincterotomes, stents, drainage catheters, lithotripters, and tissue-sampling devices should be available.

Patient preparation includes an updated history and physical examination and a recent complete blood count, serum liver chemistry panel, serum amylase or lipase (or both), coagulation studies, and noninvasive imaging of the upper part of the abdomen with abdominal ultrasonography, CT, or MRI/MRCP, depending on the clinical situation. Platelet count, prothrombin time, and partial thromboplastin times may be obtained if therapeutics are anticipated. However, a history of liver disease, renal disease, and bleeding are adequate to detect most patients with increased bleeding risk. Patients with a history of easy bruising, excessive bleeding after dental extraction, other postoperative bleeding, or a family history of coagulopathy are best evaluated with the help of hematology consultation. Special risk factors such as anticoagulant therapy, bleeding disorders, prosthetic heart valves, and allergies must be addressed. If possible, aspirin and nonsteroidal antiinflammatory drugs should be avoided for 7 days before the procedure. Iodine allergic patients are at very low risk of allergic reaction; nevertheless, some centers continue to use prednisone 30 to 40 mg orally 15 and 3 hours before the examination. Diphenhydramine (Benadryl) 25 mg intravenously may be added if serious past reactions have occurred. Iodine allergy appears to never be a reason to omit a needed examination but limiting volume of contrast media used is logical.

Informed consent for ERCP must be obtained. It is both legally and ethically necessary to apprise the patient and family of the risks, benefits, and alternatives of ERCP. Table 107-1 lists the potential complications of diagnostic and therapeutic ERCP and their relative frequency. Although legal standards continue to evolve, we recommend that patients not only be informed of the frequency of potential complications but also be told that a severe complication may possibly result in a prolonged hospital stay, intensive care unit (ICU) monitoring, or open surgery and may very rarely result in permanent disability or death. Complication rates vary according to patient and procedure risk factors, as well as the disease process being evaluated and treated. Patients with uncomplicated biliary stones, malignancy, or chronic pancreatitis have lower complication rates, whereas patients with recurrent pancreatitis and sphincter of Oddi dysfunction have twofold to threefold higher

---

BOX 107-1 Indications for Endoscopic Retrograde Cholangiopancreatography

SUSPECTED BILIARY DUCTAL DISORDER
Jaundice or cholestasis of suspected obstructive origin
Acute cholangitis
Gallstone pancreatitis
Clarification of biliary lesion seen on other imaging tests
Biliary fistula

SUSPECTED PANCREATIC DUCTAL DISORDER
Pancreatic cancer
Mucinous or cystic neoplasm
Unexplained recurrent pancreatitis
Chronic pancreatitis with unrelenting pain
Clarification of pancreatic lesion detected on other imaging tests
Ascites or pleural effusion of suspected pancreatic origin
Pancreatic pseudocyst or fistula

TO DIRECT ENDOSCOPIC THERAPY
Sphincterotomy
Biliary drainage
Pancreatic drainage

TO DIRECT ENDOSCOPIC TISSUE/FLUID SAMPLING
Biopsy, brush, fine-needle aspiration
Bile/pancreatic juice collection

PREOPERATIVE DUCTAL MAPPING
Malignant tumors
Benign strictures
Chronic pancreatitis
Pancreatic pseudocysts and ductal disruptions
Mucinous or cystic tumors of the pancreas

TO PERFORM MANOMETRY
Sphincter of Oddi
Ductal

TABLE 107-1 Approximate Frequencies of Complications After Endoscopic Retrograde Cholangiopancreatography and Sphincterotomy (%)

Complication	AVERAGE-RISK PATIENTS		HIGH-RISK PATIENTS*	
	ERCP	*Sphincterotomy*	*ERCP*	*Sphincterotomy*
Pancreatitis	3	5	8	12
Bleeding	0.2	1.5	0.4	3.5
Perforation	0.1	0.8	0.3	1.5
Infection	0.1	0.5	2	2
Sedation reaction or cardiopulmonary	0.5	0.5	2	2
Total[†]	3.9[‡]	8.3[‡]	12.7[‡]	21[‡]

*Certain patient characteristics and technical aspects of the procedure increase the risk for complications, including suspected sphincter of Oddi dysfunction, recurrent pancreatitis, difficult cannulation, precut sphincterotomy, coagulopathy, renal dialysis, cirrhosis, and advanced cardiopulmonary disease.
[†]Some patients have more than one complication.
[‡]Approximate severity of complications: mild, 70%; moderate, 20%; and severe, 10%.

---

complication rates. Procedure techniques associated with higher complication rates include repeated cannulation attempts, repeated pancreatic duct injections, pancreatic parenchymal acinarization, and precut sphincterotomy. Attention to details of the technique and patient selection can minimize but not eliminate complications. Early recognition plus treatment of complications help limit morbidity.

ERCP can be performed with fiberoptic or video chip instruments, which have similar performance characteristics. Video systems have the advantage of television monitor viewing by all persons in the endoscopy suite. Such systems offer better teaching capabilities and allow better coordination between the endoscopist and nursing assistants. Most ERCPs are done with air insufflation. Limited data show that CO_2 inflation reduces postprocedure abdominal distention. For Billroth II patients, we generally start with a standard side-viewing duodenoscope, but an end-viewing endoscope is occasionally needed. In patients with a long Roux-en-Y

gastroenterostomy, or choledochojejunostomy, a 160-cm pediatric colonoscope or a 220-cm enteroscope will reach the bile duct in greater than half of patients. Double balloon enteroscopy has facilitated Roux-limb traversal.[1] The lack of a catheter-deflecting elevator and limited compatible accessories make end-viewing endoscopy difficult in these settings.

TECHNIQUE

The patient is positioned in a prone to slightly left lateral decubitus position on a fluoroscopic table. Less often, the supine position is preferred as in difficult patients with recent abdominal incisions, multiple abdominal drain tubes, or Billroth II patients. Intravenous access and monitoring equipment for blood pressure, pulse, and pulse oximetry are needed. Electrocardiographic monitoring is desirable for patients with angina or a history of a cardiac arrhythmia. Sedation and analgesia are achieved by slow intravenous administration of common agents such as diazepam (10 to 40 mg), midazolam (1 to 5 mg), or meperidine (25 to 150 mg). Droperidol (2.5 to 5.0 mg) is a common supplement or alternative, particularly for alcoholics or persons taking narcotics or benzodiazepines. However, recent concerns about QT interval prolongation has limited the use of droperidol for conscious sedation. Although propofol may offer better procedure tolerance and a much shorter recovery time than standard sedation does, the complication rate when administered by endoscopists and not anesthesiologists has not been well studied. A topical pharyngeal anesthetic spray is desirable. An antiperistaltic drug (e.g., glucagon or atropine) to inhibit duodenal motility is commonly needed.

Initially, a brief endoscopic examination of the esophagus, stomach, duodenum, and major duodenal papilla is performed. The finding of a large ulcer or neoplasm may cancel the need for ERCP. Other findings such as varices, a pseudocyst pressing on the gut wall, or edema of the medial wall of the duodenum help quantitate or localize disease processes. The major papilla is usually located on the medial aspect of the mid-descending duodenum. Before attempts at cannulation, fluoroscopic visualization (or still image acquisition) of the field of interest should be performed to look for calcifications, masses, and old contrast material. The major papilla is then cannulated, usually with a 5F-diameter plastic catheter. Orientation of the catheter tip toward the 11- to 12-o'clock position will more likely permit entrance into the bile duct; orientation of the catheter toward the 3- to 5-o'clock position will more likely permit entrance into the pancreatic duct. Cannulation may be accomplished by gentle impaction of the catheter tip in the papillary orifice. There are increasing observations that initial use of a guidewire facilitates cannulation and decreases post-ERCP pancreatitis.[2] Deep cannulation (>1-cm penetration of the catheter into the duct) more securely establishes an intraductal position, which allows contrast injection, fluid aspiration, patient position changes, and endoscope position changes without loss of access to the duct.

Standard ionic contrast media (e.g., meglumine diatrizoate) at a 50% to 60% (full-strength) concentration is used for pancreatography, whereas a 25% to 30% (half-strength) concentration is recommended for cholangiography. Biliary stricture detail is better defined with full-strength contrast, however. Nonionic and lower-osmolality contrast media, which are more expensive, offer no safety advantage. Many manufacturers have abandoned marketing of inexpensive ionic agents, making use of nonionic agent necessary. Injection of contrast media is done with continuous fluoroscopic monitoring. The extent of ductal filling should be correlated with the clinical need to know the ductal anatomy. Complete pancreatography involves filling of the main duct and side branches to the tail. High-resolution fluoroscopy is needed to see such detail. In settings in which there is excess overlying gas or obesity, underfilling of the pancreatic duct is recommended to avoid acinarization (instillation of contrast media into the pancreatic parenchyma). For a very dilated duct, initial aspiration of fluid will allow better contrast visualization without overdistention of the duct. Complete cholangiography

requires filling of the peripheral intrahepatic radicles. The left lobe is more dependent in the prone position and fills preferentially. Right lobe filling may require tilting the patient's head down 15 to 20 degrees on the fluoroscopy table, more forceful injection (a balloon occlusion catheter is helpful), or turning the patient to the supine position. Contrast media mixes slowly with gallbladder bile, and final films are best taken in the supine position after withdrawal of the endoscope (and additional time for mixing with gallbladder contents). Occasionally, delayed gallbladder films taken 4 to 12 hours after completion of the procedure allow the passage of intraluminal gas and give better diagnostic film quality. In settings of tight biliary strictures, limited contrast filling upstream should be done until catheter access above the stricture is achieved. Similarly, limited pseudocyst filling should be done unless immediate drainage is certain. Several views of each ductal position are recommended in both the limited-filling and more completely filled state.

Sphincter of Oddi manometry (SOM) is usually performed at the time of ERCP, if indicated. All drugs that relax (e.g., anticholinergics, nitrates, calcium channel blockers, glucagon) or stimulate (e.g., certain narcotics, cholinergic agents) should be avoided for at least 8 to 12 hours before SOM and during the manometric session. SOM is performed with a low-compliance infusion pump system and a 5F catheter.

Endoscopic sphincterotomy (ES) of the bile duct is commonly performed before removing bile duct stones or placing a biliary stent. A pull-type (traction) sphincterotome is advanced into the bile duct and its position confirmed with fluoroscopy. The sphincterotome is pulled back until 5 to 7 mm of cutting wire is passed into the papillary orifice. The instrument is bowed to apply gentle tension in the 11- to 12-o'clock direction. Cautery current at 40 to 60 W is applied in bursts of less than 1 second to cut stepwise 80% to 90% of the intramural portion of the bile duct. Although blended current is most commonly used, pure cut current may be associated with a lower incidence of pancreatitis without increasing the rate of sphincterotomy-induced bleeding. Many endoscopists are now using a microprocessor-controlled electrosurgical generator (Endocut by Erbe). Adequacy of the sphincterotomy is judged by pulling a bowed sphincterotome through the incised sphincter. Small papillae and papillae associated with diverticula may require smaller cuts. Minor bleeding may occur but usually stops spontaneously. Bleeding that limits the endoscopic view should be controlled by hydrostatic balloon tamponade, bipolar cautery, or epinephrine injection. Pancreatic sphincterotomy is performed in a similar fashion as biliary sphincterotomy (once access to the pancreatic duct is obtained with the sphincterotome), except that the direction of the cut is usually made in the 1- to 2-o'clock position. Some authorities advocate performing pancreatic sphincterotomy after placing a 3- to 4F, 6- to 8-cm-long, unflanged polyethylene stent into the pancreatic duct and then cutting over the stent with a needle knife.

Precut sphincterotomy involves cutting the papilla to gain deep intraductal access to the biliary tree. This

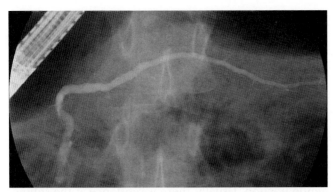

FIGURE 107-1 A normal pancreatogram obtained by placing a catheter in the duct of Wirsung. Note the gradual tapering of the main pancreatic duct and the delicate side branches.

technique should be limited to experienced endoscopists and used when there is high clinical suspicion of obstructive pathology (e.g., a jaundiced patient with a dilated bile duct on ultrasound) after standard techniques fail. Precutting can be achieved by impaction of a short-nosed, pull-type sphincterotome into the papillary orifice with sequential shallow cephalad cuts until the biliary orifice is identified. Similar sequential shallow cuts can be made with a needle knife. We prefer to place a 3- to 4F, 6- to 8-cm-long, unflanged polyethylene stent into the pancreatic duct first, if possible, and use the stent to guide needle knife cutting. Another way of gaining access is a suprapapillary fistulotomy using needle knife. Typically this is done by inserting the needle a few millimeters above the papillary orifice in the 11 o'clock orientation, and cutting in a downward motion toward the orifice to expose the bile duct.

RADIOLOGY

Figure 107-1 shows a normal pancreatogram. The contour of the main duct is typically S shaped, but numerous other configurations are common and normal. The upper limits of normal for main duct diameter are 5 mm in the head, 4 mm in the body, and 2 mm in the tail. Side branches are delicate with terminal branching. The accessory duct extends from the genu at the junction of the head and body of the main duct to the minor papilla. The minor papilla has a patent orifice in approximately 85% of patients. Pancreas divisum is discussed later.

A normal cholangiogram is shown in Figure 107-2. The upper limit of normal diameter for the common bile duct is 10 mm. The cystic duct commonly joins the common duct approximately halfway from the hilum to the papilla, but this junction may be quite variable. The intrahepatic radicles have a tree-like branch pattern with marked variation in distribution.

CANNULATION SUCCESS RATES

The papilla is readily identified by experienced endoscopists in nearly all patients with normal anatomy. Difficulty finding the papilla may arise in patients with large papillary tumors, duodenal stenosis, or edematous folds caused by acute pancreatitis, as well as in patients whose papilla is located inside a diverticulum. In patients with a Billroth II gastrojejunostomy, the success rate should

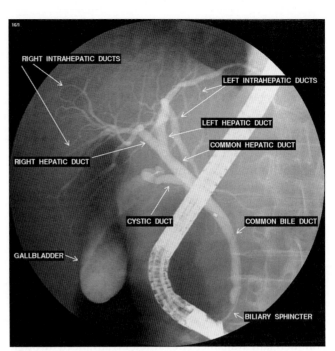

FIGURE 107-2 The normal common bile duct becomes the common hepatic duct proximal to the insertion of the cystic duct. The common hepatic duct bifurcates into the right and left hepatic ducts. The cystic duct has a spiral shape because of the valves of Heister and connects the gallbladder to the bile duct.

be greater than 80% when the procedure is performed by an expert. Initial cannulation success rates with ductography vary from 80% to 98%, depending on operator experience, anatomy, and disease state. Cannulation is easiest in patients with biliary stones but more difficult in patients with periampullary neoplasms, sphincter of Oddi dysfunction, and chronic pancreatitis with obstructing stones. In experienced centers, cannulation success rates exceed 95%, even in difficult cases when a previous attempt at cannulation failed. Such high success rates require supplemental use of precut sphincterotomy and minor papilla cannulation in 10% to 25% of cases.

COMPLICATIONS OF ENDOSCOPIC RETROGRADE CHOLANGIOPANCREATOGRAPHY/SPHINCTEROTOMY

Complications of ERCP/ES are undesirable outcomes related to some portion of the procedure or sedation required for the procedure. Unsuccessful cannulation, stent placement, or stone removal and making an incorrect diagnosis are failures of the procedure but are not generally included as complications. Table 107-1 lists the more common complications of diagnostic and therapeutic ERCP. Since 1991, a more uniform classification of ERCP complications and their severity has been developed.[3]

BILE DUCT STONES

The introduction of ES by Classen and Kawai in 1974 initiated a change in the management of bile duct stones. Before that time, laparotomy with common bile duct exploration was the main therapeutic recourse for patients with choledocholithiasis. With improvements in equipment and accessories, growth in number and skill of biliary endoscopists, and the introduction of laparoscopic cholecystectomy, the clinical settings in which endoscopic management is applied to common duct stones has been broadened considerably.

METHODS OF STONE EXTRACTION

Standard (Basket and Balloon Catheters)

After identification of a common duct stone, a sphincterotomy is usually performed. The length of the cut is dictated by the length of the endoscopically visible intramural bile duct and the size of the stone. Balloon catheters are most useful for extracting one or more relatively small stones (<10 mm) in a nondilated duct. They are not as effective for extracting larger stones or small stones in a markedly dilated bile duct because the balloon will often slide past the stone. A major advantage of a stone retrieval balloon (vs. a basket) is that it cannot become impacted, although the stone can.

Catheters with balloons that inflate to 8 to 18 mm are commercially available. The catheter is advanced through the sphincterotomy into the bile duct proximal to the stone under fluoroscopic guidance. The balloon is then inflated to the diameter of the duct, and gentle traction is applied to deliver the stone through the sphincterotomy (Figure 107-3). Passage of the balloon catheter over a guidewire is often helpful to allow frequent easy catheter passage through the sphincterotomy without trauma, to position the balloon proximal to the stone without pushing the stone proximally, and to avoid repeated cystic duct entry.

Stone retrieval baskets with different configurations, length/width, types of wire, and number of wires are commercially available. Settings in which a basket may be preferred over a balloon include larger stones (>10 mm), intrahepatic stones, smaller stones in a dilated duct, and stones that are larger than the downstream duct (e.g., stone proximal to a stricture). The basket is advanced through the sphincterotomy and partially or fully opened alongside or above the stone while taking care to not push the stone up the duct. The basket is then moved to and fro with the stone adjacent to the widest portion of the basket. Once captured, the stone is removed with gentle traction. Usually, there is resistance at the sphincterotomy orifice. By deflecting the scope tip down and applying extra force in the correct axis, stone removal is often successful. Vigorous pulling on the endoscope is sometimes necessary but has the potential to produce a duodenal tear.

In experienced centers, common duct stones can be successfully removed in 80% to 90% of patients after sphincterotomy with standard baskets and balloon catheters. Difficulty clearing or failure to clear the common duct of stones may occur for a variety of reasons. In most cases, stone size is the major determinant of success. In one series,[4] stones less than 10 mm in diameter ($n = 21$) were all removed successfully, whereas only 3 of 25 (12%) larger than 15 mm were cleared by extraction with balloons and baskets. Stones greater than 15 mm are generally considered to be large; equally important, however, are stone factors, such as number, consistency, shape, and location, and ductal factors, such as contour, diameter at the level of and distal to the stone, and the presence of coexisting pathology such as a stricture or tumor.

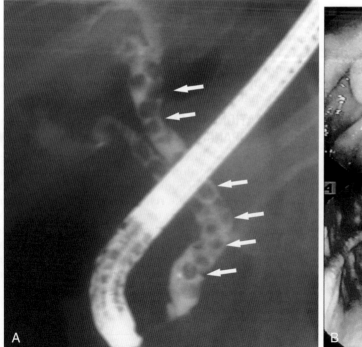
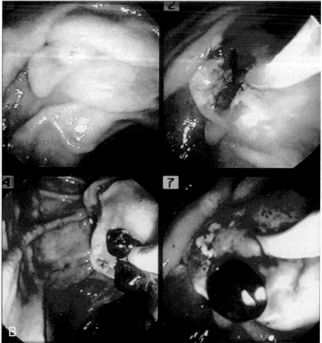

FIGURE 107-3 A, Numerous bile duct stones present in the entire common duct *(arrows)*. Note stones also in the cystic duct. **B,** Stones removed after biliary sphincterotomy. *Top left,* Normal papilla. *Top right,* Completed biliary sphincterotomy. *Bottom left* and *bottom right,* Stones being removed with a stone retrieval balloon.

Lithotripsy Techniques

A variety of lithotripsy techniques (mechanical, electrohydraulic, laser, and extracorporeal shock wave lithotripsy [ESWL]) and dissolution therapies have been used to facilitate the retrieval of stones not removable by standard methods.[5] The simplest endoscopic adjunct for the management of common duct stones that have failed to be removed by conventional baskets and balloons is the mechanical lithotripter or crushing basket. It is a safe, effective, low-cost procedure that can be performed at the time of the initial ERCP. With this technique, the stone is captured in a strong wire basket that has been advanced through a metal sheath. Longitudinal traction is then applied by turning a crank handle to withdraw the basket into the metal sheath, which results in stone fragmentation or wire breakage. In experienced centers, mechanical lithotripsy allows for the removal of more than 85% to 90% of difficult bile duct stones that are refractory to standard extraction techniques. Failure of mechanical lithotripsy is typically due to an inability to engage the stone within the basket and rarely to insufficient shearing power to fragment the stone.

Lithotripsy techniques using ESWL or intracorporeal (laser or electrohydraulic) modalities are acceptable adjuncts to standard endoscopic management when attempting bile duct clearance. The choice between these methods or surgery largely depends on availability because they are usually concentrated in tertiary centers. Intracorporeal lithotripsy can be achieved by producing a shock wave directly on the surface of the stone with either a flexible electrohydraulic probe or a flexible quartz fiber to deliver light from a laser. Both techniques require a fluid medium that is delivered coaxially along the probe or through an NBT. Because of the risk for bile duct injury (electrohydraulic methods have a greater risk for injury than the pulsed dye laser does), intracorporeal lithotripsy is usually performed under direct endoscopic control via the mother–baby endoscope system. In this technique, a small-caliber endoscope (baby scope) is advanced through the working channel of the duodenoscope (mother scope) into the bile duct. The laser fiber or electrohydraulic probe is advanced through the working channel of the baby scope, and apposition with the stone is ensured under direct vision. Laser lithotripsy has become possible under fluoroscopic guidance with the development of a device (smart laser) that can identify bile duct stones by analyzing backscattered light, with the pulse interrupted in the event of tissue contact. Complete duct clearance rates with intracorporeal lithotripsy techniques range from 80% to 90%. The main advantages of electrohydraulic lithotripsy over laser technology are its low cost and portability; however, the potential risk for bile duct injury is greater.

ESWL is used to treat bile duct stones in a fashion similar to renal and gallbladder applications. Most centers use machines that require fluoroscopy to target the stones and rely on injection of contrast material through an NBT, but some centers have reported good visualization of the stone in 90% of patients with ultrasound imaging. Complete stone clearance can be expected in approximately 80% of patients, but a number of ESWL and endoscopic sessions are generally required.[6]

Mother and Baby Choledochoscopy and Intraductal Lithotripsy

Intraductal electrohydraulic lithotripsy (EHL) or laser lithotripsy is best performed under direct visual control using the mother and baby scope system. Newer baby scopes are smaller, with a 3.2-mm diameter and a 1-mm instrument channel, than old ones. Such small-diameter scopes can be inserted through a standard therapeutic duodenoscope with a 4.2-mm instrument channel. Spyglass Spyscope (Boston Scientific, Natick, MA) is a new partially disposable, less-expensive, single-operator endoscope. It includes a baby scope, which is 10F in diameter, has four-way tip deflection, and a 1.2-mm working channel. EHL can be readily applied by this system.

Dissolution Therapy

Contact dissolution of biliary stones has been attempted by perfusing the bile duct with solvents administered via an indwelling NBT, percutaneous transhepatic catheter, cholecystostomy tube, or T-tube. The results with these agents (monooctanoin and methyl-*tert*-butyl ether) have been disappointing because of incomplete stone dissolution and the potential for complications from these solvents. As a result of their low efficacy and high morbidity, contact dissolution has not assumed an important role in patients with refractory bile duct stones.

Stents and Nasobiliary Tubes

When stone extraction is incomplete or has failed, biliary drainage should be established to prevent stone impaction and cholangitis. In most situations, this therapy serves as a temporizing measure that allows for improvement in the patient's clinical condition pending repeat attempts at stone removal. The stent (or NBT) is placed so that one limb is above the stone and the other is in the duodenum (in the case of an NBT, the end of the tube is brought out the patient's nose and connected to a drainage bag) (Figure 107-4). Most authorities recommend double-pigtail stents, although favorable experience is reported with straight 10F stents.[7] NBTs allow for repeat contrast injection without the need for another ERCP to visualize the biliary tree. However, they are often poorly tolerated and frequently dislodged by a confused/uncooperative patient, and out-of-hospital tube management is not optimal. Endoprostheses are better tolerated, but migration or occlusion may occur and lead to recurrent symptoms of biliary obstruction and cholangitis.

Biliary stenting not only serves to drain the bile duct but may also aid in mechanically fragmenting the stone and thereby facilitating subsequent attempts at endoscopic removal. The addition of oral dissolution therapy may also soften and reduce the size of the stone and thus aid endoscopic removal. In a study by Johnson et al,[8] 9 of 10 patients (90%) with nonextractable stones treated with ursodeoxycholic acid plus stenting had clearance of their bile duct after a mean of 2.7 followup procedures, in contrast to 0 of 12 patients (0%; $P < 0.01$) treated with stenting alone and a mean of 5.3 followup procedures.

Long-term internal stenting was believed to be a good palliative measure in elderly and high-risk patients with

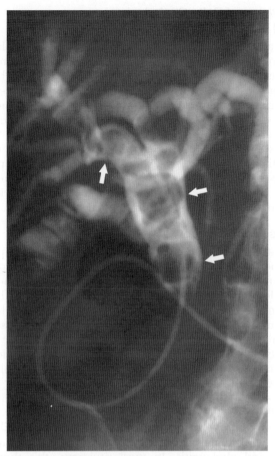

FIGURE 107-4 A nasobiliary tube has been placed to provide temporary biliary drainage in this patient with multiple large bile duct stones *(arrows)*.

nonextractable bile duct stones. In several reports, the rate of late complications (primarily cholangitis) was 12% to 15%. Enthusiasm for this approach has been tempered by the results of a study conducted by Bergman et al,[7] who reported 34 complications in 23 of 58 patients (40%) stented for a median of 36 months (range, 1 to 117 months). There were nine (16%) biliary-related deaths occurring at a median of 42 months. The rate of late complications was shown to increase proportionally with time (16% at 1 year and 50% at 4 years). They advised that permanent stenting be restricted to patients unfit for elective surgical, endoscopic, or percutaneous treatment and in patients with a short life expectancy. This recommendation was supported by the results of a randomized study of endoprosthesis insertion versus standard duct clearance techniques in a group of high-risk patients with symptomatic stones. DePalma and Catanzano[9] retrospectively compared the results of endoscopic biliary stenting ($n = 31$) with those of surgery ($n = 37$) in 68 patients older than 70 years with failed endoscopic bile duct clearance. Although early complications were significantly less frequent in the stented group (12.9% vs. 29.7%; $P < 0.0005$), complications (35.5% vs. 8.1%; $P < 0.001$) and biliary mortality (9.6% vs. 0%) during long-term followup were significantly more common in the stented group.

Endoscopic Balloon Dilation of the Biliary Sphincter for Stone Removal

Because of the significant risks and unknown long-term effects of sphincter ablation, some authorities have suggested that small common duct stones be removed after papillary balloon dilation. The main theoretical advantages of not cutting the sphincter are that acute complications might be less frequent and that by preserving sphincter function, long-term complications (a particular concern in younger patients undergoing laparoscopic cholecystectomy) may be avoided. Bergman et al[10] reported 36 biliary tract complications in 22 patients (among 93 patients) monitored for a mean of 15 years after sphincterotomy and stone removal. The same group[11] later found that after biliary sphincterotomy the function of the biliary sphincter was permanently lost, with associated bacterial colonization, the presence of cytotoxic components in the bile, and chronic inflammation of the biliary ductal mucosa. In contrast, manometric studies have suggested recovery of sphincter function within a few weeks of balloon dilation of the sphincter.

In this technique, the papilla is dilated with an 8- to 10-mm hydrostatic balloon. After dilation, the stones are removed via stone retrieval balloons, baskets, or mechanical lithotripsy. Initial reluctance to use this technique arose because of concern regarding a high risk for post-procedural pancreatitis and cholangitis. A metaanalysis of eight randomized trials that compared balloon dilation with ES showed that the initial success of duct clearance was higher with ES (80% vs. 70%) but that overall success did not differ significantly between the two groups (97% vs. 94%) because of rescue ES when balloon dilation failed.[12] Mechanical lithotripsy was used more frequently with balloon dilation (21% vs. 15%). Overall complications were similar in the two groups (10.5% vs. 10.3%). The bleeding rate was higher in the ES group (2% vs. 0%; $P = 0.001$), whereas pancreatitis occurred more frequently in the balloon dilation group (7.4% vs. 4.3%; $P = 0.05$). Results from a more recently published randomized trial, not included in the metaanalysis, demonstrated equivalent success rates for balloon dilation and ES (98% vs. 93%), but significantly higher 30-day morbidity (18% vs. 3.3%) for balloon dilation, including severe pancreatitis in 5.1% (vs. 0% after ES) and higher mortality (1.7% vs. 0%).[13] In another randomized study comparing the two techniques, the frequency of recurrent bile duct stones and cholecystitis at 1 year was similar.[14] Moreover, 1 year after balloon dilation, common bile duct pressure, sphincter of Oddi basal and peak pressure, and sphincter of Oddi contraction frequency were significantly lower than predilation values. These results suggest that balloon dilation should probably not be used routinely but should be reserved for patients at high risk for complications of sphincterotomy, such as those with uncorrectable coagulopathy and cirrhosis.

Supplemental Endoscopic Papillary Large Balloon Dilation

Use of large-diameter (12 to 20 mm) dilation balloons after near-maximal or limited ES has been introduced as an adjunctive tool to enlarge a papillary orifice for the removal of large or difficult bile duct stones.

Theoretically, risk of perforation or bleeding would be reduced by performing a less than maximal sphincterotomy and risk of pancreatitis from balloon dilation would be reduced by first separating the biliary and pancreatic orifices with biliary sphincterotomy. Data regarding supplemental endoscopic papillary large-balloon dilation are relatively limited. Details of the method not yet standardized include optimal size of balloon, duration of dilation, and extent of sphincterotomy. Recent studies have reported the results for large/difficult stones with complete stone removal rate at 95% to 100%, overall complication rate at 3.8% to 8.3%, and low incidence of pancreatitis.[15] This technique may be helpful in patients with difficult papillary anatomy, such as those with small papilla or intra- or peridiverticular papilla. Its role in patients with coagulopathy, however, or other risks of bleeding remain to be investigated.

INTERFACE OF ERCP AND LAPAROSCOPIC CHOLECYSTECTOMY

Laparoscopic cholecystectomy has become the standard, accepted, and preferred technique for the treatment of gallbladder stones because it is associated with less postoperative pain, reduced hospitalization time, shorter convalescence, and better cosmetic results than open cholecystectomy is. However, laparoscopic management of common duct stones is much more complex than cholecystectomy alone; advanced surgical skills and sophisticated instrumentation are required; and it is not widely available. Thus, ERCP plays an integral role in the treatment of common duct stones in the laparoscopic cholecystectomy era. The timing and need for ERCP in relation to laparoscopic cholecystectomy are dependent on the likelihood of stones being present (low, medium, and high), the skill of the endoscopist, and the ability of the laparoscopist to perform common duct exploration. There appears to be little value of routine ERCP before laparoscopic cholecystectomy in patients with a low likelihood of having bile duct stones. When comparing the low yield of detecting clinically important anatomic variants and unsuspected bile duct stones with the generally accepted 3% to 7% ERCP complication rate, the routine use of ERCP before cholecystectomy cannot be justified. Patients judged to have a high likelihood of harboring duct stones are likely to benefit from preoperative ERCP and stone extraction (if stones are present). Patients in the medium-risk group create a diagnostic and therapeutic dilemma whose resolution depends on the skills of the endoscopist and laparoscopist at each particular center. EUS, MRCP, and spiral CT cholangiography have high sensitivity and specificity for stone detection; however, these imaging modalities are operator dependent and not universally available (Figure 107-5). The value of these noninvasive and less invasive techniques in the evaluation of patients at medium risk for bile duct stones needs further study.

Ultimately, a laparoscopic procedure that treats both cholelithiasis and choledocholithiasis in a single setting would be the best approach in the majority of patients. This strategy appears to be cost-effective and associated with a shorter hospital stay than with a two-stage procedure (preoperative ERCP with sphincterotomy followed by laparoscopic cholecystectomy). When these laparoscopic skills become widely disseminated, the use of ERCP will be relegated to its well-established role in the open cholecystectomy era, specifically, the treatment of acute cholangitis, severe gallstone pancreatitis, retained common duct stones, and complications of biliary surgery.

ACUTE GALLSTONE PANCREATITIS

In Western countries, gallstone disease is a leading cause of acute pancreatitis and accounts for 34% to 54% of cases. Most patients with acute gallstone pancreatitis (AGP) have a mild attack and can be treated conservatively. However, the case fatality rate in severe pancreatitis remains unacceptably high, approaching 10%. In the open cholecystectomy era, urgent surgical intervention for severe AGP did not gain general acceptance because of the increased morbidity and mortality associated with this approach. Coincident with these surgical reports were uncontrolled endoscopic series reporting the efficacy and safety of ERCP and ES in the setting of AGP. Although the results were encouraging, the studies varied in their criteria for patient selection and timing of ES in relation to the acute attack (many were performed in the recovery phase, when surgery is also safe). These early series prompted the three randomized controlled trials[16-18] that now serve as the basis for the endoscopic treatment of AGP. The therapeutic principle for ES in AGP is simply removal of the obstructing calculus and reestablishment of bile and pancreatic juice flow.

In a randomized prospective controlled trial from the United Kingdom, 121 patients with AGP either received conventional therapy (i.e., gut rest, analgesics, intravenous fluids, and antibiotics) or underwent urgent (within 72 hours after admission) ERCP with ES and stone extraction (if stones were present in the common bile duct at the time of ERCP).[16] Patients were stratified by the predicted severity of their attacks with the modified Glasgow system. Choledocholithiasis was found in 25% of patients with predicted mild attacks and 63% with predicted severe attacks. The four important findings were that (1) ERCP could be safely performed in the setting of gallstone pancreatitis, (2) there was a significant reduction in major complications in patients who underwent urgent ERCP and ES, (3) the reduction in morbidity was apparent only in patients with predicted severe attacks (61% vs. 24%; $P = 0.007$), and (4) there was a significant reduction in hospital stay for those with severe attacks treated by urgent ERCP and ES (median of 9.5 vs. 17 days, $P = 0.03$). The mortality rate was improved, but the difference was not statistically significant.

A second randomized controlled study was performed by the department of surgery at the University of Hong Kong.[17] One hundred ninety-five patients with acute pancreatitis were randomized to early ERCP (within 24 hours of admission) or conservative therapy. Although the methodology, patient selection, and assessment of the severity of the acute pancreatitis used in this study differed from that in the United Kingdom study, the results in the subgroup of patients with gallstone pancreatitis ($n = 127$) were quite similar. Patients with mild

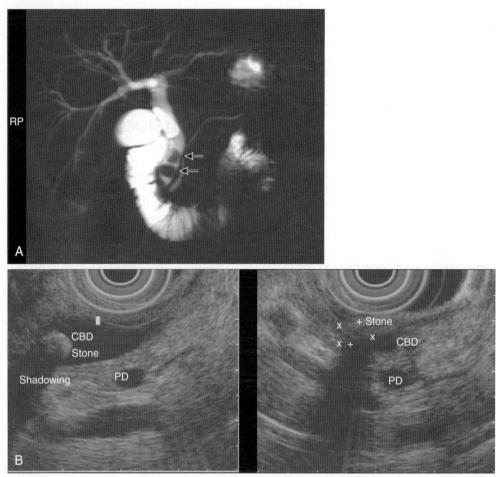

FIGURE 107-5 **A,** Magnetic resonance cholangiopancreatography demonstrating bile duct stones *(arrows)*. **B,** Endoscopic ultrasound showing bile duct stones with acoustic shadowing. *CBD*, Common bile duct; *PD*, pancreatic duct.

pancreatitis had similar morbidity and mortality regardless of the therapy. In contrast, patients with predicted severe attacks who underwent endoscopic therapy had a lower complication rate (54% vs. 13%; $P = 0.003$) and a lower mortality rate (18% vs. 3%; $P = 0.07$) than did patients treated conservatively.

The third study[18] was a prospective multicenter randomized controlled study from Germany in which 238 patients with AGP and no evidence of severe biliary obstruction (severe biliary obstruction defined as a bilirubin concentration >5 mg/dL) were randomized to ERCP with ES and stone extraction or conservative therapy within 72 hours of symptom onset. This study attempted to address the major criticism of the United Kingdom and Hong Kong studies: the need to exclude patients with concomitant cholangitis because these patients are known to benefit from ERCP. The two treatment groups did not differ significantly in mortality (11% vs. 6% overall mortality, 8% vs. 4% AGP mortality, ERCP vs. conservative therapy) or overall complications (46% vs. 51%, ERCP vs. conservative therapy) regardless of the predicted severity of the pancreatitis. However, respiratory failure was more frequent in the ERCP group (12% vs. 5%; $P = 0.03$), and jaundice was more frequent in patients who received conservative treatment (11% vs. 1%; $P = 0.02$).

Although all three studies concluded that there was no difference in outcomes for patients with mild pancreatitis treated conservatively or by ERCP, only the study from Germany suggested that early ERCP was of no benefit in patients with severe gallstone pancreatitis. Even though ERCP is clearly indicated in patients with AGP complicated by cholangitis or biliary obstruction, its role in the setting of severe AGP alone warrants further investigation. A metaanalysis[19] of these three published studies and an abstracted randomized study[20] revealed a statistically significant reduction in morbidity from 38% to 25% and mortality from 9% to 5% in the ERCP/ES group versus the conservatively treated group. A subgroup analysis based on the severity of pancreatitis was not reported in this metaanalysis. The role of EUS and MRCP in detecting bile duct stones and triaging patients with stones to ERCP is evolving. In one series of 100 AGP patients, EUS was found to be more sensitive than transcutaneous ultrasound in detecting cholelithiasis (100% vs. 84%; $P < 0.005$) and had a sensitivity, specificity, and accuracy of 97%, 98%, and 98%, respectively, for detecting choledocholithiasis.[21] In another series of 32 patients with gallstone pancreatitis, the sensitivity, specificity, and overall accuracy of MRCP detection of bile duct stones was 80%, 83%, and 81%, respectively. Stones missed by MRCP were smaller than 6 mm in diameter.[22] Because small stones commonly cause AGP, MRCP will probably have lower sensitivity in this setting than in the overall population of patients with bile duct stones.

Sphincterotomy has been shown to prevent recurrent episodes of AGP and is an alternative to surgery in high-risk patients. If sphincterotomy is not performed, early cholecystectomy is mandatory to prevent recurrent pancreatitis.

ACUTE CHOLANGITIS

Cholangitis is a potentially life-threatening disease that results from bacterial infection of obstructed bile. Systemic toxicity occurs when intraductal pressure is sufficiently elevated to cause reflux of bacteria or endotoxin into blood. Thus, obstruction plays a key role by both increasing intraductal pressure and promoting bacterial overgrowth as a result of bile stasis. The most common cause of acute cholangitis is choledocholithiasis, which occurs in approximately 80% to 90% of unselected cases. Therapy for cholangitis must be individualized because of the spectrum of severity of illness. Antibiotic therapy should be initiated promptly. Analysis of bile and stone cultures indicates that *Escherichia coli*, *Klebsiella* spp., *Enterobacter* spp., *Enterococcus* spp., and *Streptococcus* spp. are the most commonly isolated bacteria. The antibiotic selected should preferably penetrate an obstructed biliary tree. The majority of patients will respond to conservative management, thereby allowing for a more elective approach to biliary decompression.[23] Urgent decompression is indicated if improvement is not seen within a few hours of initial resuscitation. The latter group will invariably have a fatal outcome if conservative treatment is continued.

Options for bile duct decompression include surgical, percutaneous, and endoscopic methods. Endoscopic intervention is now accepted as definitive therapy for acute cholangitis. The advantages of ERCP are that it can delineate the cause of obstruction, facilitate sampling of bile for culture, and decompress the biliary tree in a relatively short time with low morbidity. Biliary decompression is the goal of therapy and can be complete (e.g., stone removal) or temporary (e.g., placement of a stent without stone removal), pending more definitive management (to allow stabilization of an unstable patient). The endoscopic procedure consists of sphincterotomy with stone extraction or biliary drainage with an NBT or endoprosthesis.

Ideally, the patient should be stabilized or made as stable as possible before performing ERCP. Patients with respiratory compromise can have their ERCP performed while on ventilatory assistance. Although the procedure is best performed in a dedicated fluoroscopy room, unstable patients can undergo ERCP in an ICU or operating room. A mobile fluoroscopy unit can be used, but reports indicate that ductal decompression can be performed without fluoroscopic assistance. Because intrabiliary pressure is increased in acute cholangitis, contrast injection should be limited to reduce further systemic seeding of bacteria. Enough contrast should be injected to define the anatomy and the cause of obstruction. Alternatively, the bile duct should be aspirated completely of infected bile before injection of contrast.

Aspirated bile should be cultured. In a stable patient, definitive therapy can be performed. In an unstable patient, the length of the procedure should be limited. In such cases a stent or NBT should be placed, and once the patient is stabilized, more definitive therapy can be performed.

The high morbidity and mortality associated with surgical and percutaneous therapy for acute cholangitis prompted evaluation of the safety and utility of endoscopic management. In a retrospective analysis, Leese et al[24] reported on 71 patients with stone-related cholangitis treated by early decompression either surgically ($n = 28$) or by ES ($n = 43$). Early surgery was associated with significantly higher 30-day mortality (21% vs. 5%) and morbidity (57% vs. 8%) than was sphincterotomy. The endoscopic group was significantly older than the surgical group and had more medical risk factors, but there were no significant differences in the severity of cholangitis. Leung et al[23] reported their experience in a retrospective analysis of 105 patients with acute calculous cholangitis who did not respond to conservative management and underwent urgent endoscopic decompression at a mean of 1.5 days after admission. Thirty-nine percent of patients had coexisting medical problems, 85% had Charcot triad, and 40% were in shock at the time of admission. Endoscopic drainage was successful in 102 patients (97%). Ninety-seven percent of patients responded with striking improvement in abdominal pain, and 93% had resolution of fever within 3 days. The overall 30-day mortality was 5%. Among those in shock, 2 of 4 drained after 72 hours died, as compared with 3 of 38 drained before 72 hours. There were no deaths in the group without shock, irrespective of the timing of drainage. The mortality of 5% compares favorably with that of urgent surgical intervention, in which mortality has been reported to be greater than 40% in some series. The ERCP complication rate was 5% and was limited to five postsphincterotomy bleeding episodes managed by endoscopic techniques. The safety and efficacy of endoscopic therapy were corroborated in a large retrospective study of 947 patients with cholangitis secondary to stones ($n = 898$) or stricture ($n = 49$).[25] In a randomized prospective study, Lai et al compared the safety and efficacy of biliary decompression by surgical and endoscopic techniques in 82 patients with severe cholangitis as a result of stones.[26] Patients treated with laparotomy and common bile duct exploration had significantly higher morbidity (64% vs. 34%) and mortality (32% vs. 10%) than those treated with endoscopic therapy. These and other studies clearly demonstrate the efficacy and safety of biliary decompression either as definitive therapy or as a temporizing measure pending more definitive intervention once the patient is stabilized.

BILIARY DRAINAGE PROCEDURES

BENIGN BILIARY STRICTURES
Postoperative

Postoperative strictures of the extrahepatic bile duct occur after 0.25% to 1% of cholecystectomies. Most such lesions are manifested as abnormal liver test results,

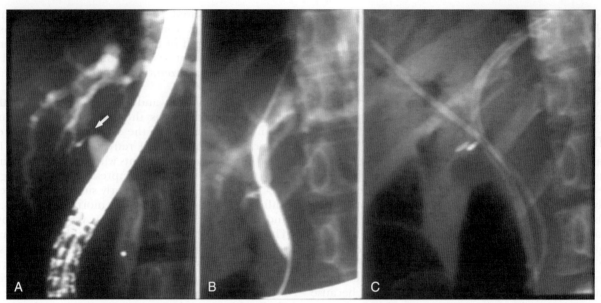

FIGURE 107-6 This patient was evaluated for obstructive jaundice 2 months after laparoscopic cholecystectomy. **A,** The cholangiogram shows a common duct stricture *(arrow)*. Note the clips in the region of the common duct. **B,** The stricture was then dilated with a balloon-dilating catheter. **C,** Two biliary stents were placed to bridge the stricture.

obstructive jaundice, and cholangitis within 2 to 3 months postoperatively, although a much more delayed response may occur. In contrast, when the common duct has been completely occluded with a clip, progressive jaundice will become obvious early in the postoperative period.

The cholangiogram commonly shows a short, smooth narrowing near the cystic duct stump and surgical clips with proximal duct dilation (Figure 107-6). Strictures greater than 2 cm in length, those with clips placed securely across the duct, or those associated with resected segments of duct require operative management. Irrespective of the site or pathogenesis of the stricture, the primary aim of endoscopy is to pass a guidewire through the stricture to permit passage of dilators (balloon or catheter) and stents. Sphincterotomy before stricture manipulation permits greater instrument maneuverability. The preferred treatment of short, simple strictures is balloon dilation to 6 to 10 mm with ultimate placement of two to three 10F plastic stents across the stricture and extending into the duodenum. The stricture is redilated and stents are exchanged at 3- to 4-month intervals for 8 to 12 months until the stricture profile is nearly as open as the downstream adjacent duct. The goals of treatment are to render the patient free of symptoms and to achieve sustained normalization of liver test results after the stents are permanently removed. Because strictures can recur many years after therapy, the long-term outcome after endoscopic intervention is of critical concern. In three uncontrolled endoscopic studies,[27-29] a good to excellent result was achieved in 70% to 80% of patients monitored for an average of 4 years. Assessment of good to excellent outcomes was based on resolution of symptoms and normalization or significant improvement in biochemical test results and radiographic findings. Two long-term followup studies of endoscopic stenting of biliary strictures were recently reported.[30,31] Bergman

et al[30] reported late complications (median followup of 9.1 years) in 34% of 44 patients undergoing biliary stenting with two 10F stents for a maximum of 1 year. Restenosis at the site of the original stricture occurred in 20% of patients. Costamagna et al[31] undertook a more aggressive endoscopic approach. Each patient received as many large-diameter stents as necessary (based on stricture tightness and bile duct diameter) to eliminate the stricture. Stents were exchanged electively at 3-month intervals and were removed after complete resolution of the stricture. There were no symptomatic recurrent biliary strictures in the 40 patients completing the stenting protocol during a 49-month followup period. In a nonrandomized study, Davids et al[32] compared the outcome of 35 patients treated surgically (biliary-enteric anastomosis) and 66 patients managed by endoscopic balloon dilation and stenting (stents changed every 3 months for 1 year). The mean followup interval for the surgically and endoscopically treated patients was 50 and 42 months, respectively. Eighty-three percent of patients in both groups attained good to excellent results. The total morbidity rates (surgery, 26%; endoscopy, 35%) and stricture recurrence rates (17% for both groups) were similar for the two groups. The long-term outcome after endoscopic biliary stenting of postoperative biliary strictures has been shown to be superior to that after stenting of biliary strictures in the setting of chronic pancreatitis. Collectively, these data support the use of endoscopic therapy in patients with postoperative biliary strictures. Surgically fit patients who fail initial endoscopic therapy or have recurrent strictures are best managed by a bilio-enteric bypass. Although metal expandable stents offer prolonged patency in comparison to plastic stents, their use for treating benign postoperative biliary strictures should be discouraged. Dumonceau et al[33] reported mucosal hyperplasia and Wallstent occlusion in all six patients who underwent this therapy.

Endoscopic techniques have been used to treat biliary strictures complicating orthotopic liver transplantation. Such strictures are often treated in a fashion similar to strictures occurring after other biliary tract surgeries. Anastomotic strictures appear to be more responsive to endoscopic therapy than do strictures occurring at non-anastomotic sites.

Distal Common Bile Duct Strictures Secondary to Chronic Pancreatitis

Intrapancreatic common bile duct strictures have been reported to occur in 3% to 46% of patients with chronic pancreatitis (Figure 107-7). Deviere et al[34] were the first to report the use of biliary stenting in patients with common bile duct obstruction and significant cholestasis (alkaline phosphatase >2 times the upper limits of normal) secondary to chronic pancreatitis. Nineteen of the 25 patients had jaundice, and 7 had cholangitis. The patients were treated with ES followed by insertion of one or two 10F biliary stents placed across the stricture. The stents were changed when clinical or ultrasonographic evidence of blockage was present. Cholestasis, hyperbilirubinemia, and cholangitis resolved in all patients after stent placement. The late followup (mean, 14 months; range, 4 to 72 months) on 22 patients was much less satisfactory. One patient died 1 month after treatment as a result of acute cholecystitis and postsurgical complications, whereas a second died 10 months after stenting as a result of sepsis that was believed to be caused by stent blockage or dislodgment. Stent migration occurred in 10 patients and stent blockage in 8 and resulted in cholestasis with or without jaundice ($n = 12$), cholangitis ($n = 4$), or no symptoms ($n = 2$). These patients were treated by stent replacement or surgery, or both ($n = 7$). Ten patients continued to have a stent in place (mean followup, 8 months) and remained asymptomatic. Only three patients required no further stents because of resolution of their biliary stricture. Other authors have also reported a low stricture resolution rate ranging from 11% to 32% (Table 107-2).[35-40] The salient point of these studies was that biliary drainage via a plastic biliary stent is an effective therapy for resolving cholangitis or jaundice in patients with chronic pancreatitis and a biliary stricture. However, the long-term efficacy of this treatment is much less satisfactory because stricture resolution rarely occurs. The results of nearly all studies stand in distinct contrast to those of Vitale et al,[38] who reported that 20 of 25 patients undergoing plastic biliary stenting for a median period of 13.3 months remained stent-free without stricture recurrence during a 32-month followup interval. Catalano et al[41] have demonstrated better outcomes for multiple stents than for a single stent.

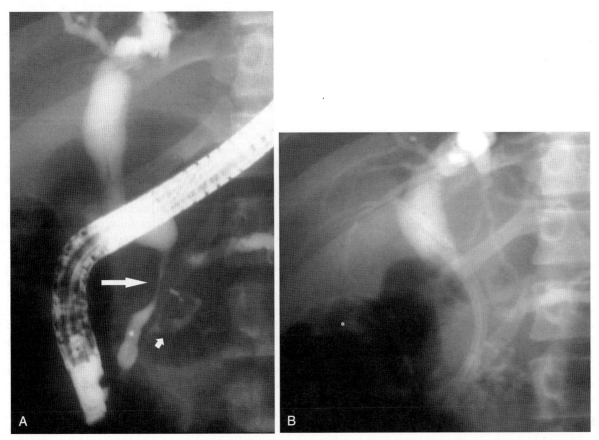

FIGURE 107-7 Chronic pancreatitis-induced common bile duct stricture. **A,** The cholangiogram shows a 2-cm common bile duct stricture *(large arrow)* with proximal dilation. Note the pancreatic duct stone *(small arrow)* and pancreatic stricture. **B,** Two biliary stents were placed.

TABLE 107-2 Summary of Selected Series Evaluating the Efficacy of Endoscopic Biliary Polyethylene Stent Insertion for the Treatment of Chronic Pancreatitis–Induced Common Bile Duct Strictures

Investigator	N	Technical Success (%)	Stricture Resolution (%)	STENT DYSFUNCTION (%)		Followup (mo)
				Clogging	Migration	
Deviere et al[34]	25	100	3 (12%)	32	40	14
Barthet et al[35]	19	100	2 (11%)	0	5	18
Smits et al[36]	58	100	16 (28%)	62	7	49
Kiehne et al[37]	14	100	2 (16%)	36	NM	NM
Vitale et al[38]	25	100	20 (80%)	12	8	32
Farnbacher et al[39]	31	100	10 (32%)	29	23	24
Eikhoff et al[40]	39	100	12 (31%)	33	10	58

NM, Not mentioned.

Because of the disappointing results with plastic stents and concern for the high morbidity associated with surgically performed biliary drainage procedures in alcoholic (frequently debilitated) patients, the group from Brussels evaluated the use of uncoated expandable metal stents for this indication.[42] Twenty patients were treated with a 34-mm-long metal stent that becomes 10 mm in diameter when fully expanded. The short length of the stent was chosen so that surgical bypass (e.g., choledochoduodenostomy) would still be possible if necessary. Cholestasis ($n = 20$), jaundice ($n = 7$), and cholangitis ($n = 3$) resolved in all patients. Eighteen patients had no further biliary problems during a followup period of 33 months (range, 24 to 42 months). Epithelial hyperplasia within the stent developed in two patients (10%) and resulted in recurrent cholestasis in one and jaundice in the other. These patients were treated endoscopically with standard plastic stents, with one of these patients ultimately requiring surgical drainage. The authors concluded that this therapy could be an effective alternative to surgical biliary diversion but that longer followup and controlled trials will be necessary to confirm these results. We suspect that all the metal stents would ultimately occlude. In a series of 14 patients treated with partially covered metal stents (0.5-cm-long uncovered metal meshes at both ends), stent dysfunction developed in 7 (50%) during a median followup of 22 months. Stent patency was 100% at 12 months, 40% at 24 months, and 37.5% at 30 months.[43]

The studies just presented and others indicate that plastic biliary stents are a useful alternative to surgery for short-term treatment of chronic pancreatitis–induced common bile duct strictures complicated by cholestasis, jaundice, and cholangitis. This therapy should also be considered for high-risk surgical patients. However, because the long-term efficacy of this treatment is much less satisfactory, operative intervention appears to be a better long-term solution for this problem in average-risk patients. More data on the long-term outcome, preferably in controlled trials, are necessary before expandable stents can be advocated for this indication.

PRIMARY SCLEROSING CHOLANGITIS

Cholangiographic imaging is the gold standard for diagnosing primary sclerosing cholangitis (PSC), although conditions that mimic PSC must be excluded. In a variant, small-duct PSC, the cholangiogram is normal. Both percutaneous transhepatic cholangiography (PTC) and ERCP can be used to show the characteristic changes associated with PSC. The choice between PTC and ERCP depends on local and regional expertise and availability. However, when available, ERCP is the preferred modality because (1) the often small fibrotic ducts of patients with PSC may be difficult to puncture via the percutaneous route; (2) ERCP has a better safety profile; and (3) the pancreatic duct and cystic duct, which may be involved in up to 20% of patients with PSC, can be examined at ERCP. PTC is reserved for ERCP failures and patients with altered anatomy. The role of MRCP and spiral CT cholangiography in the diagnosis of PSC awaits further study.

The classic cholangiographic features in PSC are diffuse multifocal strictures of the intrahepatic and extrahepatic bile ducts (Figure 107-8). These strictures are usually short, with intervening normal or dilated segments giving a beaded appearance. Other frequent findings on cholangiography include pseudodiverticula, mural irregularities, and biliary stones and sludge.

The rationale for endoscopic intervention is based on the hypothesis that progressive liver disease and deterioration of liver function may be aggravated or accelerated by backpressure from dominant strictures and stones or debris when present. It is further hypothesized that relief of obstruction may halt, delay, or even reverse progression to cirrhosis and liver failure. Because no medical therapy has definitively proved effective for PSC, a trial of endoscopic therapy in symptomatic patients seems reasonable. Indications for considering endoscopic management of PSC are treatment of jaundice or pruritus and symptomatic cholangitis, deteriorating serum hepatic chemical profile, and when concern for bile duct cancer is high, tissue sampling. The most favorable candidates for therapy are patients with a dominant extrahepatic stricture with or without stones and limited or no intrahepatic involvement. Such ideal anatomy is uncommon.

When performing ERCP in the setting of PSC, therapeutic skills are mandatory because of the serious risk for infection. Not uncommonly, contrast media will take the path of least resistance and enter the cystic duct and gallbladder; intrahepatic filling is therefore limited. Preferably, a balloon catheter is then manipulated above the

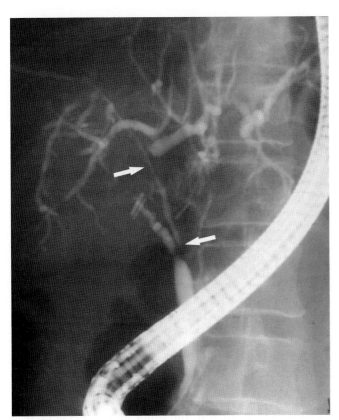

FIGURE 107-8 This patient has primary sclerosing cholangitis involving the extrahepatic and intrahepatic ducts. There is a long, high-grade stricture involving the common hepatic duct *(arrows)* and the right and left hepatic ducts, as well as narrowings/irregularities of the intrahepatic ducts.

cystic duct takeoff, and higher-pressure injection of the intrahepatic radicles is performed with the balloon inflated. Moreover, because the risk for post-ERCP cholangitis in patients with PSC may be as high as 20% to 30% after diagnostic and therapeutic procedures (particularly in those in whom obstructed segments are not decompressed), antibiotic prophylaxis has been advocated.

All therapeutic procedures aim at improving bile flow. Endoscopic techniques that may be used to achieve this goal are ES, stone/sludge removal, stricture dilation with balloons and catheters, placement of stents and NBTs (with or without instillation of corticosteroids and saline lavage), and combinations of therapy. Endoscopic stricture dilation and stenting have been reported in PSC patients since the early 1980s. The techniques have been standardized. The goals of endoscopic intervention in patients with PSC are to relieve jaundice and pruritus, treat cholangitis, and theoretically, delay the onset of biliary cirrhosis and thus buy time before liver transplantation. Interpretation of the reported results of endoscopic therapy is difficult because there are no randomized controlled trials, therapies are not uniform, treated patients have variable anatomy, the definition of success varies, studies are generally small, the course of untreated PSC is variable, and there is no long-term followup.

Johnson and associates[44] reported their results of endoscopic dilation in 35 symptomatic PSC patients (29

with cholangitis and 6 with jaundice alone). Patients were treated by dilation (balloon or catheter) with or without biliary stenting. During a mean followup period of 24 months, there was a significant reduction in the frequency of hospitalization for cholangitis, bilirubin, and stricture score. Cholangitis occurred shortly after treatment in six patients; five of the six had a biliary stent placed. As a result, these authors recommended avoiding biliary stents in patients with PSC.

Lee and associates[45] retrospectively reviewed the records of 85 PSC patients who underwent 175 ERCP procedures (75 diagnostic and 100 therapeutic). Endoscopic therapy was associated with a 15% major complication rate (7% pancreatitis and 8% cholangitis). Clinical followup (median of 31 months) was obtained in 50 of 53 patients who underwent 85 therapeutic procedures. Twenty-eight patients improved clinically, whereas 21 felt the same and 1 felt worse. Serum liver chemistry results obtained within 3 months of the endoscopic intervention were significantly improved in comparison to pretreatment values. Overall, 41 of 53 patients (77%) had improvement in their clinical symptoms, liver function test results, or cholangiograms.

Van Milligen de Wit et al[46] reported the results of stent therapy in 25 patients with PSC and dominant extrahepatic strictures. Stents were exchanged or removed electively at 2- to 3-month intervals or because of symptoms attributable to stent clogging. Endoscopic therapy was technically successful in 21 patients (84%). In these 21 patients, the results of all serum biochemical liver tests improved significantly within 6 months of stent therapy. During a median followup of 29 months (range, 2 to 120 months) after stent removal, 12 patients (57%) remained asymptomatic with stable biochemical liver test results and 4 (19%) had clinical and biochemical relapse of disease that responded favorably to repeat endoscopic therapy. Early procedure-related complications occurred in 14% of the procedures. The value of short-term endoscopic stenting (mean, 11 days; range, 1 to 23 days) for 32 patients with dominant strictures was reported by Ponsioen et al.[47] Cholestatic symptoms improved in 83%, and there were statistically significant reductions in abdominal pain, fatigue, and pruritus. Serum liver chemistry results were significantly improved. Eighty percent of patients were free of reinterventions at 1 year and 60% at 3 years. Procedure-related complications occurred in 15%, but there were no episodes of cholangitis. The authors advocated this technique because it was efficacious and overcame the complications associated with stent occlusion. Kaya et al[48] reported that stenting after balloon dilation (median stenting interval of about 4.5 months) of dominant strictures provides no additional benefit and is associated with more complications than balloon dilation alone is. Baluyut et al[49] found that repeated endoscopic treatment to maintain bile duct patency was associated with a significantly higher observed 5-year survival rate than predicted by the Mayo Clinic survival model.

Cholangiocarcinoma is a dreaded complication of PSC that occurs in 9% to 15% of patients. The risk appears to be greatest in patients with long-standing ulcerative colitis and cirrhosis. Surprisingly, recent studies suggest that there may be an inverse relationship between the duration of PSC and the risk for cholangiocarcinoma.[50] Sudden worsening of jaundice should raise the possibility of the development of cholangiocarcinoma. Cholangiographic findings that suggest malignant transformation include markedly dilated ducts of the ductal segments proximal to a stricture, the presence of a polypoid mass, and progressive stricture formation. Comparison with previous ERCP results is essential to signal the presence of complicating cholangiocarcinoma because with PSC uncomplicated by malignancy, the cholangiographic appearance frequently remains static for years. Unfortunately, early diagnosis of cancer is difficult because of the absence of a sensitive, specific serologic marker and the relative insensitivity of bile duct tissue sampling. However, tissue sampling of any suspicious lesion at ERCP is indicated.

Although the utility of ERCP in helping make the diagnosis of PSC is clear, its therapeutic efficacy in improving the course of the disease appears highly likely but has not definitively been established. Clearly, symptomatic patients with dominant extrahepatic strictures are the best candidates for therapy.

BILIARY FISTULAS

Biliary fistulas most commonly occur as a complication of cholecystectomy, common bile duct exploration, or inadvertent operative injury of the bile duct or as a consequence of a local infection. Rarely, biliary fistulas result from long-standing untreated biliary tract disease. With more widespread use of laparoscopic cholecystectomy, the incidence of bile duct injury, including biliary fistula, has increased. Bile leakage from the cystic duct remnant is among the most common injuries reported as a complication of laparoscopic cholecystectomy. The most common cause of cystic duct leaks involves imprecise application of clips on the duct or their subsequent dislodgment during the procedure. Biliary fistulas may also arise from the intrahepatic ducts and common duct. A duct of Luschka in the gallbladder bed, if present, is quite vulnerable to transection during cholecystectomy. Clearly, distal obstruction from a stone, stricture, or papillary stenosis increases ductal pressure proximally and may promote and maintain the biliary fistula.

Postoperative bile duct leaks are usually manifested within a week after surgery.[51] In a series of 62 patients with postcholecystectomy leaks, initial symptoms included abdominal pain in 89%, abdominal tenderness in 81%, fever in 74%, nausea and vomiting in 43%, and jaundice in 43%.[51] Only 2% had a clinically detectable mass or ascites. Biochemical testing is usually nonspecific with variable elevations in serum hepatic chemistry values and the white blood cell count.

A high index of suspicion for bile duct injuries after laparoscopic cholecystectomy should be maintained in any patient who fails to follow a smooth, uneventful postoperative course. Patients with suspected biliary fistulas often undergo abdominal ultrasonography or CT to look for evidence of a biloma, as well as a hepatobiliary iminodiacetic acid (HIDA) scan to diagnose the leak. However, direct cholangiography (most often by ERCP) is the most sensitive test to detect a biliary fistula.[51]

Treatment options for biliary leaks include percutaneously or endoscopically placed biliary drains or stents and surgical drainage and repair of the leak. Patients with large bilomas should undergo percutaneous drainage of the fluid collection (unless surgery is performed). Endoscopic therapy has been shown to be definitive therapy in this setting with low morbidity. Patients with leaks from the cystic duct, duct of Luschka, and T-tube tract are optimal candidates for endoscopic treatment. However, patients with injuries of the common bile duct, common hepatic duct, and intrahepatic ducts can also be managed by endoscopic techniques.

The primary goal of endoscopic therapy is to decrease the pressure gradient between the bile duct and duodenum and thereby allow drainage of bile along the path of least resistance and away from the site of leakage (to permit the defect to seal). This objective can be accomplished with biliary sphincterotomy alone, stenting alone, an NBT alone, or any combination thereof.[51-55] Kaffes et al[54] performed ES alone (n = 18), bile duct stenting alone (n = 40), or ES plus stenting (n = 31) in 89 patients, with leaks arising in 80 from the cystic duct stump (n = 48), duct of Luschka (n = 15), T-tube tract (n = 7), common duct (n = 5), an intrahepatic duct (n = 4), and an uncertain site (n = 1). The biliary fistula closure rate was 95%, and significantly more patients in the sphincterotomy-alone group required surgery to control leaks than in the other groups (22% vs. 0%; P = 0.001). Sandha et al[55] recommended a systematic approach to bile duct fistulas based on their experience in 207 patients. Low-grade leaks (leak identified only after intrahepatic opacification) resolved in 91% with sphincterotomy alone (along with bile duct stone removal when present), and 100% of high-grade leaks (leak observed before intrahepatic opacification) resolved with stenting with or without ES (and stone extraction when present). Patients with clinically evident leaks not identified on cholangiography usually have a disconnected duct. Kalacyi et al showed that MRCP may be helpful in identifying the upstream disconnected bile duct and the site of injury.[56] This occurs most frequently when there is low insertion of a right posterior sectoral duct which is clipped along with the cystic duct.

Experience with NBTs to treat biliary leaks is limited, but data available from several investigators have been favorable. Because most fistulas seal in a few days, NBT placement is a reasonable option. Advantages of an NBT include the ability to monitor closure of the leak with repeat cholangiography, the possibility of applying maximum decompression with suction, and easy removal of the tubes without the need for a second endoscopic procedure. However, the risk of infection when improperly cared for, poor patient acceptance and discomfort, and potential electrolyte disturbances from external drainage have been cited as potential disadvantages of this approach. Biliary stents are a very effective therapy for resolving biliary leaks. The observation from several uncontrolled studies that patients treated with stents alone experience equally good outcomes as patients treated with a combination of stents and sphincterotomy suggests that sphincterotomy can be avoided in patients with otherwise unobstructed ducts. Therapeutic efficacy for 7F stents has been high. However, Foutch et al[53] reported a 22% failure rate with 7F stents; these fistulas resolved by upsizing the stent to 10F. Larger-caliber stents are certainly preferred when a concomitant stricture is present. In most reported series, stents were inserted with the proximal end positioned above the leak site. It is assumed that the stent can partially mechanically occlude the leak site, thus favoring more rapid closure. However, Bjorkman et al[52] reported a 100% fistula closure rate in 15 patients after placing one short (2 to 3 cm) 10F stent with the stent tip distal to the leak site. The results of this study confirm the importance of eliminating the transpapillary pressure gradient. Most studies that monitor drain output or reassess the fistula by repeat cholangiography report rapid closure of the fistula in most cases with cessation of bile extravasation in 1 to 7 days. The precise time when the fistula site is permanently closed is difficult to determine from reported series, however.

The available data suggest that biliary fistulas are likely to heal regardless of the therapy used to decrease the pressure gradient in the direction of the duodenum. Randomized studies comparing sphincterotomy, internal stents, and NBTs will be necessary to determine which of these therapies is the safest, most reliable, and most cost-effective management option. Biliary fistulas associated with bile duct strictures will require long-term stenting, preferably with large-bore stents (10- and 11.5F stents).

MALIGNANT BILE DUCT OBSTRUCTION

A variety of palliative options can be offered to a patient with malignant obstructive jaundice, including surgical, percutaneous, endoscopic, and medical therapy (chemotherapy and radiation therapy). Certainly, a surgically fit patient with a resectable tumor after staging should be offered the option of surgical resection for cure. In a high-risk patient or one with an unresectable tumor, endoscopic placement of polyethylene stents has become a widely accepted method of management (Figure 107-9). Soehendra and Rejinders-Frederix[57] first described endoscopic biliary stenting in 1980. Since then, many advances in stent technology have been made. Despite these developments, stent patency remains a major problem, with 10F stents becoming occluded after 3 to 6 months. The problem with stent occlusion has been studied intensively, but attempts at altering bile composition with choleretic agents, reducing bacterial load with antimicrobial agents, changing the stent material, or influencing mucin production with aspirin have failed to prolong stent patency. Because deposition of sludge (leading to stent occlusion) may depend on the flow rate through the stent, a change in stent diameter may influence the process of stent clogging. Theoretically, a small increase in stent diameter may result in an appreciable increase in flow. The limiting factor for insertion of larger plastic biliary stents is the size of the instrumentation channel of the duodenoscope. With presently available endoscopes, plastic stents up to 12F can be placed. The question of whether bigger is better still cannot be definitively answered for plastic stents. In some studies, stent patency was significantly longer for large-diameter plastic stents than for small-diameter ones. Others have found no prolongation of stent patency and more complications when larger stents are used. The divergent results of these studies may be explained by study design, patient selection criteria, and sample size.

Preoperative biliary drainage for malignant bile duct obstruction has been debated and still now unclear. Studies to date have reported differing outcomes, and some have suggested that morbidity and mortality are greater in patients undergoing drainage than in those proceeding directly to surgery. Preoperative biliary drainage is unnecessary, except for patients with cholangitis or poor hepatic function, before pancreaticoduodenectomy or less invasive surgery. However, it should be recommended before extended hepatectomy for patients with hilar cholangiocarcinoma.[58] There is considerable debate about whether patients with strictures involving the confluence require ductal decompression of both the right and left intrahepatic systems. Advocates of a

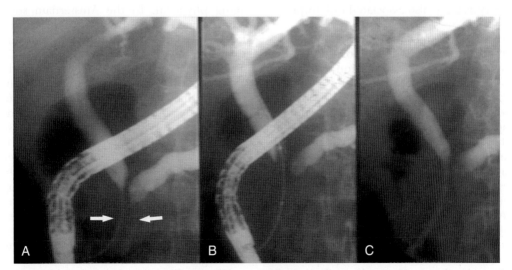

FIGURE 107-9 This patient has pancreas cancer. **A,** Endoscopic retrograde cholangiopancreatography demonstrates a classic double-duct sign with strictures of both the common bile duct *(left arrow)* and the pancreatic duct *(right arrow)* in the pancreas head with upstream ductal dilation. The stricture was then dilated **(B)** and a biliary stent was placed **(C).**

single stent argue that ductal decompression of one lobe improves symptoms of cholestasis and allows jaundice to resolve. Proponents of decompressing both sides of the liver point to the 30% to 40% incidence of cholangitis, increased mortality, and death from sepsis when only one lobe is drained. Our approach to hilar strictures is as follows: once a guidewire is advanced into an intrahepatic duct, bile is aspirated to limit systemic seeding of any resident bacteria when contrast is injected. Only enough contrast should be injected to define the stricture anatomy. If a good stentable duct is identified, that lobe is drained. When draining only one lobe of the liver, it is imperative to limit contrast injection to the lobe to be drained and avoid manipulation of the other lobe. The other lobe should be stented if cholangitis develops or symptoms of cholestasis persist. Two recent studies support this approach.[59,60] De Palma et al randomized 157 consecutive patients with malignant hilar obstruction to undergo unilateral or bilateral hepatic duct drainage.[60] In the intention-to-treat analysis, unilateral drainage was associated with significantly higher rates of successful drainage and lower early complication rates (primarily because of lower rates of cholangitis). Thirty-day mortality, late complications, and median survival were similar for the two groups. MRCP can help in selecting the liver lobe to be drained, thus avoiding injection of contrast medium into the contralateral lobe. Freeman and Overby used MRCP and CT to guide unilateral metal stent placement in 35 patients with no episodes of cholangitis.[61]

The success rate of plastic stent insertion is about 90%, and it is higher with distal than with proximal tumors. If endoscopic stent placement fails, percutaneous drainage or a combined endoscopic radiologic procedure (rendezvous procedure) can be performed. If contrast was injected into the biliary tree, such therapy should be performed urgently to prevent cholangitis. In a surgically fit patient, particularly if duodenal obstruction is present, surgical bypass is a reasonable option. Relief of symptoms can be expected in nearly all patients after successful deployment of a plastic stent. Stenting not only resolves jaundice and pruritus but is also associated with improvement in quality of life.

Early postprocedure complications, which have been reported in 10% to 20% of patients in most studies, are related to the sphincterotomy or to insertion of the stent itself. The most frequent early complication is cholangitis, which is reported to occur in as many as 10% to 15% of patients and is probably due to the introduction of bacteria during the procedure into the stagnant bile proximal to the stricture.[3] The risk for cholangitis is higher if incomplete drainage is achieved.

The main late complication of biliary stenting is cholangitis as a result of stent occlusion. Stents placed for hilar obstruction appear to occlude faster than stents placed for more distal obstructing lesions.[62] Patients with symptomatic stent occlusion will require stent change and possibly hospitalization for treatment of cholangitis. As a result, some authorities have advocated prophylactic stent changes in the hope of avoiding cholangitis. Sherman et al have demonstrated that nearly 50% of patients undergoing stenting with 10- or 11.5F plastic

biliary stents die before stent occlusion.[62] Thus, patients with a short life expectancy would be subjected to unnecessary procedures if prophylactic stent changes were performed. Using computer modeling, Tarnasky et al suggested that indicated stent exchanges are more cost-effective than prophylactic stent change at any interval.[63] Prat et al reported that symptom-free survival was longer in patients undergoing planned stent exchange every 3 months but that planned stent exchange offered no cost advantage over stent exchange for symptomatic occlusion.[64] The preliminary results of a randomized trial comparing scheduled stent change every 4 months with symptomatic stent change revealed no difference in the number of ERCP procedures per patient, number of stents per patient, mortality rate, need for metal stenting, frequency of surgery, mean stent survival, frequency of cholangitis, and time to death.[65]

One of the major advances in stent technology was development of the metal expandable stent. Expandable metal stents may offer improved biliary drainage with prolonged patency rates because of their large diameter and small surface area. Several types of expandable metal stents are available that are characterized by different insertion devices, methods of deployment, radial forces, and metal composition. To date, most experience has been gained with the Wallstent. This stent is easily inserted over a well-positioned guidewire and is successfully deployed in more than 95% of cases. The Wallstent is mounted on a 7.5F delivery device and shortens and expands to 8 to 10 mm as it is deployed. Five prospective, randomized trials[66-70] (four endoscopic and one percutaneous) have shown that a metal expandable biliary stent occludes less frequently and less rapidly than do conventional 10- and 11.5F plastic stents. This translated into a reduction in hospitalization requirements (for cholangitis and stent change) and an overall cost savings for the metal stents. Because metal stents are more costly initially and approximately half the patients in most plastic stent series will need a second stent, identification of patients who are likely to outlive their first plastic stent (and warrant a metal stent) is a major challenge for the managing physician. In the Amsterdam study,[66] the stent patency curves of Wallstents and plastic stents ran parallel during the first 3 months after stent insertion. After that time, the curves diverged in favor of the Wallstent. Therefore, based on data from this study, the authors recommended that only patients with a life expectancy of more than 3 months be potential candidates for the use of an expandable metal stent. An additional indication for the use of metal stents is in the small group of patients who suffer rapid and repeated obstruction of plastic stents. These patients have not been well studied and can, at present, not be identified at the initial stenting session. Studies comparing endoscopically placed metal stents with plastic stents for malignant hilar obstruction have not been performed. However, using MRCP and CT targeting, metal stents can be successfully placed with long patency rates and infrequent episodes of cholangitis.

When palliation is the goal of therapy for patients with malignant bile duct obstruction, how does endoscopic decompression compare with percutaneous and surgical drainage procedures? In a randomized study comparing percutaneous with endoscopic drainage,[71] endoscopic stenting was associated with more frequent successful drainage (81% vs. 61%; $P < 0.05$), a lower complication rate (19% vs. 67%; $P < 0.05$), and lower 30-day mortality (15% vs. 33%; $P < 0.05$). Median survival was similar for the two groups (23 vs. 16 weeks). Three prospective, randomized trials[72-74] have compared endoscopic and surgical drainage for malignant distal biliary obstruction. Endoscopic stenting and surgery were equally effective palliative treatments, with endoscopic treatment having a lower early complication rate and mortality, but a higher risk for late complications such as stent blockage and gastric outlet obstruction. None of these studies demonstrated a difference in survival rates between treatment groups.

Tissue Sampling at ERCP

ERCP frequently provides the first opportunity to obtain a histologic or cytologic specimen from an unexplained biliary or pancreatic stricture. A variety of tissue-sampling techniques are available to the endoscopist at the time of ERCP, including bile and pancreatic juice cytology, brush cytology, intraductal forceps biopsy, intraductal fine-needle aspiration, stent cytology, and juice and tissue evaluation for aneuploidy, tumor markers (e.g., carcinoembryonic antigen [CEA], CA 19-9), p53 immunoreactivity, and K-*ras* oncogene mutations.

Brush cytology is the most commonly applied method of tissue sampling and the most extensively studied. Although the technical success rate is high (90% to 95%), most studies demonstrate cancer detection rates in the 20% to 60% range.[75] The sensitivity of bile duct brush cytology is higher for cholangiocarcinoma than for pancreatic cancer.[100] Sawada et al[76] have shown that brushing the pancreatic duct may increase the diagnostic yield of brush cytology (vs. brushing the bile duct) in pancreatic cancer. However, pancreatic cancers often disrupt the duct and prevent passage of the brush through the tumor in more than 25% of patients. In an attempt to improve on the sensitivity of brush cytology, other methods have been used more recently. Howell et al[77] originated use of the ERCP endoscopic needle aspiration (ENA) technique and reported 62% sensitivity for detection of cancer from biliary samplings in patients with biliary strictures (including 53% in pancreatic cancer and 80% in cholangiocarcinoma). These impressive results for ENA were not found in subsequent reports,[78,101] where the sensitivity ranged from 26% to 30%.

Endobiliary forceps biopsy allows examination of tissue specimens below the bile duct epithelium. The results of six selected studies have shown improved cancer detection rates in comparison to cytologic techniques, with a cancer detection rate of 56% in 502 patients.[79]

Although it would be preferable to have one technique that would have a cancer detection rate similar to that seen with biopsy of upper gastrointestinal and colonic neoplasms, this goal has not been reached in the pancreaticobiliary tree. Investigators have therefore evaluated the added sensitivity of combining a number of tissue sampling techniques. Jailwala et al[75] reported their results of the cumulative sensitivity of triple tissue sampling at one ERCP session with brush cytology, fine-needle aspiration, and forceps biopsy in 104 patients with malignant bile duct obstruction. Tissue sampling sensitivity varied according to the type of cancer; the highest yield was seen in patients with ampullary cancer. The combination of techniques was superior to individual methods, with the addition of a second or third technique increasing cancer sensitivity rates in most instances.

It is clear that the cancer detection sensitivity of these standard techniques individually is suboptimal. Methods to improve this sensitivity are therefore being evaluated. Preliminary studies suggest that the yield may be increased by evaluating aspirated fluid and tissue for aneuploidy and tumor markers such as CEA and CA 19-9. Recent investigation has suggested that evaluation of tissue or fluid for K-*ras* mutations is more accurate than cytology in the diagnosis of pancreatic cancer. However, some authors have identified K-*ras* mutations in patients with chronic pancreatitis, thus reducing the specificity of this test. Further study is warranted to determine the role of these new techniques in the assessment of pancreatic and biliary strictures.

Other ancillary cytologic tests such as digital image analysis (DIA) and fluorescence in situ hybridization (FISH) have been also developed to improve the sensitivity of routine cytology. DIA and FISH use cells obtained from ERCP brushing specimens. DIA is used to assess for aneuploidy by determining the DNA content of cells. FISH is a technique that utilizes fluorescently labeled DNA probes to examine cells for chromosomal abnormalities. The detection of nondiploid (DIA) or chromosomally abnormal (FISH) cells generally correlates with the presence of tumor. Recent studies showed that FISH and DIA may enhance the accuracy of standard techniques in evaluation of indeterminate pancreatobiliary strictures.[80]

SUMP SYNDROME

Sump syndrome is an infrequent complication of the now rarely performed side-to-side choledochoduodenostomy. Some degree of stenosis of the surgical anastomosis is usually present. Cholangitis, pain, and pancreatitis may occur as food, stones, or other debris accumulates in the distal common bile duct in the bypassed segment caudal to the biliary–duodenal anastomosis. The reported median time interval between surgery and the appearance of symptoms was 5 years and between surgery and the diagnosis of sump syndrome was 6 years. ES with removal of the debris has been shown to be effective treatment. Although it may be possible to extract debris and stones via the choledochoduodenostomy, thereby obviating the need for sphincterotomy, this approach puts the patient at risk for recurrent symptoms.

CHOLEDOCHAL CYSTS AND ANOMALOUS PANCREATICOBILIARY UNION

Choledochal cysts are uncommon anomalies of the biliary tree that are manifested as cystic dilation of the intrahepatic or extrahepatic ducts (or both). These cysts are most often classified by the scheme proposed by

Todani et al. Type I cysts, which involve only the extrahepatic biliary tree, are the most common form and account for 80% to 90% of all choledochal cysts. In this form of the anomaly, the cystic duct generally enters the choledochal cyst, and the right and left hepatic ducts and the intrahepatic ducts are normal in size. Type II cysts are extrapancreatic bile duct diverticula and make up 2% of reported cases. Type III cysts, which account for 1.4% to 5% of cases, are choledochoceles and most often involve only the intraduodenal part of the common bile duct, but occasionally the intrapancreatic portion. Type IV cysts are subdivided into type IV A, or multiple intrahepatic and extrahepatic cysts, and type IV B, or multiple extrahepatic cysts. Type IV A cysts account for approximately 19% of reported cases, whereas type IV B cysts are much less common. Finally, a type V cyst, or Caroli disease, consists of either single or multiple solely intrahepatic cysts. This form of cystic disease within the liver communicates with the biliary system, as opposed to fibrocystic disease, in which cysts filled with bile do not.

An anomalous pancreaticobiliary union is an anomaly frequently combined with choledochal cysts that is more common in the Asian population. However, anomalous pancreaticobiliary union is not associated with choledochal cyst in 22% to 37%.[81] An anomalous pancreaticobiliary union is considered to be present when the common channel is longer than 15 mm. In this situation, the pancreatic duct and bile duct junction is outside the duodenal wall and proximal to the sphincter of Oddi, thus promoting reflux of pancreatic juice into the biliary tree. Japanese criteria emphasize the junction of the ducts outside the duodenal wall.[81] Reflux of pancreatic juice has been postulated to be involved in the pathogenesis of carcinoma, which occurs in 2.5% to 17% of patients with choledochal cysts.

Surgery is the recommended treatment for most patients with choledochal cysts (most notably types I and II). Cholangiography is the gold standard for diagnosing choledochal cysts. Although ERCP and PTC are invasive, they can thoroughly assess the cyst anatomy, site of biliary origin, extent of intrahepatic and extrahepatic disease, associated biliary tract anomalies, and complications (e.g., bile duct strictures, stones); in addition, they shed light on possible therapeutic intervention, either definitive or temporizing pending surgery. ERCP is often the preferred modality because it provides detailed evaluation of the pancreatic duct and the pancreaticobiliary union and is very useful in the diagnosis of type III choledochal cysts (choledochocele). MRCP can also delineate the anatomy noninvasively.

ERCP has become the procedure of choice to evaluate and treat most patients with type III choledochal cysts.[82] Patients with choledochoceles will commonly have biliary symptoms (biliary colic, cholestatic jaundice, jaundice) or unexplained pancreatitis prompting evaluation by ERCP. The endoscopic features of a choledochocele include the following: the intramural segment of the common bile duct protrudes into the duodenum in continuity with an enlarged papilla, the papilla is soft and smooth, ballooning of the papilla is noted with contrast injection, on contrast injection a cyst-filled structure is apparent on fluoroscopy and in continuity with the common bile duct, and no impacted stone is present. Several small series have reported the utility of endoscopic cyst unroofing and sphincterotomy for both pancreatic and biliary indications.[82,83] Ladas et al[82] identified 15 symptomatic choledochocele patients among 1019 (1.5%) referred for ERCP. Twelve patients were treated by endoscopic therapy. During long-term followup (mean, 26 months; range, 4 to 56 months), 10 of 12 patients were asymptomatic with normal liver test results. One patient had a mild episode of cholangitis, and carcinoma developed in the choledochocele in another. This unusually high frequency of choledochoceles may represent overdiagnosis because several of these patients appeared to have only bile duct and ampulla of Vater dilation associated with ductal stones (not true choledochoceles). Although the risk for cancer in these patients is uncertain, it appears appropriate to recommend long-term followup in patients treated by endoscopic therapy alone. How this followup should be pursued remains to be clarified. Elton et al[83] described a variant of a choledochocele that they called a dilated common channel syndrome. These patients have enlarged common pancreaticobiliary channels that were thought to have developed because of papillary stenosis. Among 77 patients treated by unroofing and sphincterotomy, 77% had complete and long-lasting resolution of symptoms.

Management of anomalous pancreaticobiliary union in the absence of a choledochal cyst is unclear. Because of the high risk for gallbladder cancer, prophylactic cholecystectomy has been recommended by some.[81] In one series of 15 patients with an anomalous pancreaticobiliary union (7 had choledochal cysts) and recurrent pancreatitis or abdominal pain (or both) treated by ES, 13 had resolution or a reduction in the frequency of pancreatitis and pain.[84] Ng et al[85] similarly reported resolution of pain and pancreatitis in 5 of 6 patients with a long common channel after endoscopic therapy. Whether patients with anomalous junctions without choledochal cysts treated by sphincterotomy need surveillance for cancer cannot be answered at the current time.

PANCREATIC DRAINAGE PROCEDURES

CHRONIC PANCREATITIS

Pancreatic duct pressure is generally increased in patients with chronic pancreatitis regardless of the etiology and whether the main pancreatic duct is dilated. The aim of endoscopic therapy (and decompressive surgical therapy) for patients with chronic pancreatitis and pain or clinical episodes of acute pancreatitis (or both) is to alleviate the obstruction to outflow of exocrine juice. Certain pathologic alterations of the pancreatic duct, bile duct, or sphincter lend themselves to endoscopic therapy. The techniques (e.g., sphincterotomy, dilation, stenting) and instruments (e.g., sphincterotome, dilating balloon, pancreatic stent) used to treat biliary tract disease have been adapted for use in the pancreatic duct.

Data in this area are often difficult to interpret because of heterogeneous populations with one or more pathologic processes being treated (e.g., pancreatic duct stones, strictures, pseudocysts) and because of the multiple therapies being performed in a given patient (e.g., stricture dilation, stone extraction, bile or pancreatic duct ES). No controlled studies have been reported to date.

Pancreatic Strictures

Benign strictures of the main pancreatic duct may be a complication of a previous embedded stone or a consequence of acute inflammatory changes around the main pancreatic duct.[86] In Cremer et al's large referral population, only 10% of patients had a stricture without associated calcified pancreatic stones.[86] Pancreatic duct strictures can be treated by stent therapy. If stents larger than 7F are to be used, patients often require both pancreatic and bile duct sphincterotomy followed by stricture dilation. For optimal results, the therapy must address both the pancreatic duct stricture and duct stones. The best candidates for stenting are those with a distal stricture (in the pancreatic head) and upstream dilation.

The technique for placing a stent in the pancreatic duct is similar to that used for inserting a biliary stent. A guidewire must be maneuvered upstream to the narrowing. Hydrophilic flexible-tip wires are especially helpful. The pancreatic stent is advanced over the wire through the stricture with a pusher tube. Most pancreatic stents are just standard biliary stents with extra side holes at approximately 1-cm intervals to permit better side branch juice flow. In general, the size of stent should not exceed the size of the normal downstream duct. Therefore, 4- to 7F stents are commonly used in small ducts, whereas 10- to 11.5F stents can be used in patients with advanced chronic pancreatitis and grossly dilated ducts. Pancreatic sphincterotomy (major or minor papilla, or both) is often performed before (or after) placing a pancreatic stent. This procedure is done with a standard pull-type sphincterotome or by using a needle knife to incise the sphincter over a previously placed stent. Some authorities favor performing biliary sphincterotomy before pancreatic sphincterotomy because of the high incidence of bile duct obstruction and cholangitis, as reported by one group, if this is not done.[87] Such complications were not found by others and have been infrequent in our experience. Performing biliary sphincterotomy first, however, can expose the pancreaticobiliary septum and allow the length of the cut to be gauged more accurately.

Wilcox summarized the results of pancreatic duct stent placement, usually with ancillary procedures.[86,88] Among the 1500 patients treated in 15 series, benefit was seen in 31% to 100% of patients during a followup interval of 8 to 72 months. The greatest benefit was achieved in patients with dominant strictures and dilated ducts. Like surgical decompressive procedures, it appears that the response attenuates over time. Quantification of the degree of improvement is often poorly defined. Partial or complete symptom improvement after stenting suggests that intraductal hypertension was an etiologic factor. Continued symptom relief after stent removal indicates adequate dilation of the narrowing. Differentiation of these two types of improvement is, unfortunately, not clarified in some reports. In the largest published study, 1018 patients with chronic pancreatitis were monitored prospectively for a mean of 4.9 years after endoscopic intervention.[89] At followup, 60% of patients had completed endotherapy, 16% were still undergoing endoscopic treatments, and 24% had undergone surgery. Complete (69%) or partial (19%) technical success of endoscopic therapy was achieved in 88%. All patients had pain initially, but only 34% had pain at followup ($P < 0.0001$); a significant reduction in pain (no or weak pain) was achieved in 85%. Rates of pain relief were similar in patients with dominant strictures in the head or body (or both), pancreatic stones in the head or body (or both), a combination of stones and strictures, and complex pathology. Dite et al[90] reported the results of a randomized study comparing surgical and endoscopic treatment in 72 patients with a dilated pancreatic duct and stones, strictures, or both. An additional 68 patients who refused randomization and opted for endoscopic therapy ($n = 28$) or surgery ($n = 40$) were included in the total results. At 1 year after the intervention, 92% of patients in each group had complete or partial pain relief. After 5 years, rates were 65% for endotherapy patients and 86% for surgical patients (complete resolution, 14% vs. 37%, respectively, $P = 0.002$; partial relief, 51% vs. 49%, $P = NS$). Weight gain was similarly common in the two groups at 1 year (66% vs. 60%, respectively), but significantly more patients had gained weight in the surgical group (52%) than in the endotherapy group (27%) by 5 years. Outcomes in the randomized group were similar to those in the total group. Despite the many methodologic problems associated with this study, the data suggest that surgical outcomes are more durable. In a long-term outcome study, 100 patients with severe chronic pancreatitis and pancreatic duct strictures were treated with plastic pancreatic stents (median duration of 23 months) and monitored for 69 months from study entry, including a median period of 27 months after stent removal.[91] The stents were exchanged when recurrent pain developed and removed when defined clinical and endoscopic parameters were met. After stent removal, 30 patients (30%) required restenting within the first year of followup, whereas in 70 (70%) patients, pain control was adequate during that period. By the end of the followup period, 38 patients required restenting and 4 ultimately underwent pancreaticojejunostomy. Pancreas divisum was the only factor significantly associated with a higher risk for restenting.

It appears that complete stricture resolution is not mandatory for improvement in symptoms, which implies that luminal patency was sufficient or other therapies performed along with the stenting contributed to the benefit. Because the stricture persists in many patients, Cremer et al evaluated the expandable metal stent (18F in diameter, 23 mm in length) in 29 patients.[92] After 6 months, mucosal hyperplasia resulted in stent occlusion in most patients.

Pancreatic Ductal Stones

It has been postulated that increased intraductal pressure proximal (upstream) to an obstructed focus within the pancreatic duct, as with pancreatic duct stones, is one of the potential mechanisms responsible for attacks of acute pancreatitis or exacerbations of chronic abdominal pain in patients with chronic pancreatitis. Reports indicating that endoscopic (with or without ESWL) or surgical removal of pancreatic calculi results in improvement in symptoms support this notion.[87,93] In one series,[93] 32 patients with pancreatic duct stones underwent attempted endoscopic removal. Of these patients, 72% had complete or partial stone removal and 68% improved after endoscopic therapy. Symptomatic improvement was most evident in the group of patients with chronic relapsing pancreatitis (vs. those with chronic continuous pain alone; 83% vs. 46%). Factors favoring complete stone removal included (1) three or fewer stones, (2) stones confined to the head or body of the pancreas (or both), (3) absence of a downstream stricture, (4) stone diameter less than 10 mm, and (5) absence of impacted stones. After successful stone removal, 25% of patients demonstrated regression of the ductographic changes of chronic pancreatitis and 42% had a decrease in diameter of the main pancreatic duct. The only complication from therapy was mild pancreatitis in 8%. These data suggest that removal of pancreatic duct stones may result in symptomatic improvement. Longer followup will be necessary to determine the stone recurrence rate and whether endoscopic success results in long-standing clinical improvement. It is apparent from this and other studies that the success rate for complete stone extraction from the pancreatic duct by endoscopic techniques alone is significantly inferior to that seen in the bile duct. The problem of delivering a large stone, an impacted stone, or a stone upstream to a stricture can be overcome by reducing the stone's size by either dissolution or fragmentation. No chemical agents have been found to effectively dissolve stones.

ESWL can be used to facilitate fragmentation and stone removal when endoscopic therapy alone fails or as a primary therapy.[87] Thus, this procedure is complementary to endoscopic techniques and improves the success of nonsurgical ductal decompression. This technique is a widely available alternative that has been performed since 1987 and for which substantial clinical experience has accumulated. There are more than 18 published reports totaling more than 700 patients who were treated with ESWL. Patients with obstructing prepapillary concrements and upstream ductal dilation appear to be the best candidates for ESWL. In the largest reported series,[87] 123 patients with main pancreatic duct stones and proximal dilation were treated with the electromagnetic lithotripter, usually before pancreatic duct sphincterotomy. Stones were successfully fragmented in 99% and resulted in a decrease in duct dilation in 90%. The main pancreatic duct was completely cleared of all stones in 59%. Eighty-five percent of patients noted improvement in pain during a mean followup of 14 months. However, 41% of patients had a clinical relapse as a result of stone migration into the main pancreatic duct, a progressive stricture, or stent occlusion. Complications in series using ESWL were mostly minor and primarily related to the endoscopic procedure. A metaanalysis of 16 studies published between 1989 and 2002 that included 588 patients showed that ESWL had a significant impact on reduction of pancreatic stone burden and improvement in pain.[94] Brand et al[95] showed that the global quality of life was improved in 68% of patients undergoing ESWL. Overall, the endoscopist is encouraged to remove pancreatic duct stones in symptomatic patients when the stones are located in the main duct (in the head or body, or both) and are thus readily accessible. The currently available data suggest that the clinical outcome after successful endoscopic removal is similar to the surgical outcome,[96] but with lower morbidity and mortality. Long-term followup studies have shown that ESWL combined with ERCP may avoid the need for surgery in approximately two-thirds of patients on an intention-to-treat basis. However, to date, no comparative trials have been conducted in patients with pancreatic stones alone.

Pancreatic Pseudocysts and Fistulas

Pancreatic pseudocysts are defined as encapsulated collections (without an epithelial lining) of pancreatic juice, either pure or containing necrotic debris or blood (or both), that are situated either outside or within the limits of the pancreas from which they arise. A pancreatic pseudocyst develops as a consequence of acute pancreatitis, chronic pancreatitis, or pancreatic trauma. The optimal pseudocyst candidate for endoscopic drainage has a single mature cyst without pancreatic necrosis, residual adjacent inflammation, or portal hypertension. More complex patients are generally best managed by a multidisciplinary approach with input from surgery, medicine, and interventional radiology.

Two endoscopic approaches can be used, depending on whether the cyst communicates with the pancreatic duct.[97-105] Cysts communicating with the ductal system can be drained by a transpapillary approach (Figure 107-10). The proximal tip of the prosthesis has generally been placed in the cystic cavity, but it can be placed upstream at the site of disruption. A pancreatic duct sphincterotomy may be required.

Noncommunicating pseudocysts can be treated by direct cystoenterostomy via the stomach (endoscopic cystogastrostomy) or duodenum (endoscopic cystoduodenostomy). The aim of therapy is to create a communication between the cystic cavity and the gastric or duodenal lumen. Two prerequisites should be fulfilled before attempting this treatment: bulging because of the cyst should be obvious during upper endoscopy, and the distance between the cyst and the lumen should not exceed 1 cm. This distance can usually be assessed by CT, ultrasound, or endosonography, but when the compression is visible, usually the distance from the cyst to the lumen is less than 1 cm. In addition, the cyst wall should be mature. A double- or triple-lumen, beveled-tip needle knife is used to burrow a hole (usually with blended current) into the cyst cavity. A cystoenterotome is commercially available. Many authorities advocate needle localization to identify a safe entry site before diathermic puncture. The complication rate of this procedure may also be reduced by using the Seldinger technique without electrocautery. A guidewire is advanced into the cyst and looped 360 degrees to secure positioning. Puncture should be performed perpendicular to the cyst wall, and thus a duodenoscope is preferred. The newly created tract is then balloon-dilated to 8 to 10 mm. Vigorous flow of pseudocyst fluid into the gut lumen generally occurs,

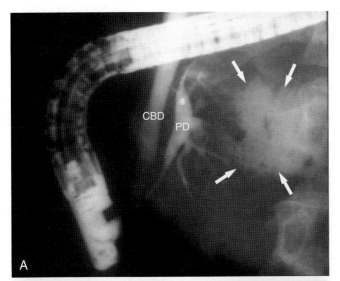

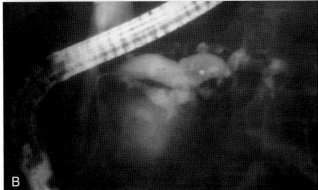

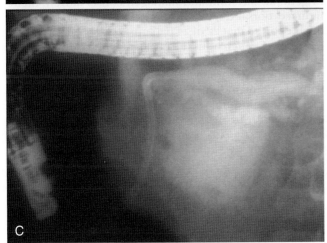

FIGURE 107-10 Chronic pancreatitis with a 5-cm communicating pseudocyst. **A,** The pancreatogram demonstrates a leak from the neck of the pancreatic duct that is filling a pseudocyst cavity *(arrows)*. *CBD,* Common bile duct; *PD,* pancreatic duct. **B,** The upstream duct is accessed and demonstrates marked dilation of the main duct and side branches. **C,** A pancreatic stent was placed to bridge the site of disruption.

and this fluid must be aspirated to maintain the endoscopic view. Two or more double-pigtail stents are then placed to bridge the cyst and the intestinal lumen. When significant debris or necrotic tissue is present, use of a nasocystic drain should be considered to allow for lavage of the cyst cavity. It is appropriate to maintain the patient

with nothing by mouth (NPO) and administer broad-spectrum antibiotics intravenously for 1 to 3 days if the cyst is larger than 6 cm or contains debris. Diabetics, patients with debris in the cyst, and immunosuppressed patients may need a longer NPO interval because oral intake permits food and a greater concentration of bacteria to enter the residual cyst. Pseudocyst size is monitored by ultrasonography or CT at 4- to 6-week intervals. After resolution (usually in 1 to 2 months), the stents are endoscopically removed and followup pancreatography is performed. Pseudocysts resolve after endotherapy in approximately 80% to 90% of patients, with the complication rate ranging from 4% to 20%. The pseudocyst recurs in 10% to 20% of endoscopically managed patients, especially those with duct cutoff on the pancreatogram. Table 107-3 shows the results of endoscopic management from large centers. EUS has been used increasingly for the evaluation and treatment of pancreatic fluid collections. This endoscopic procedure can (1) determine whether there is significant solid debris within a collection, (2) differentiate between a pseudocyst and other noninflammatory cystic lesions, (3) guide transmural drainage, and (4) be used to perform drainage of the pseudocyst. Because a visible luminal bulge is not required for direct EUS pseudocyst drainage, the number of potential patients available for endoscopic therapy has increased.

These excellent results certainly support the use of endoscopic therapy in appropriate candidates. When compared with other endoscopic techniques, this procedure has a relatively high bleeding and perforation rate. Bleeding complications are decreased by use of a hydrostatic balloon (not sphincterotome) to enlarge the tract orifice or by initial puncture with a needle catheter instead of the needle knife. Nevertheless, the overall complication rate probably compares favorably with surgical series. Coordination with the surgeon is necessary when performing this procedure.

Pancreatic duct disruptions or leaks occur as a result of acute or chronic pancreatitis, trauma, or surgical injury and can produce pancreatic ascites, pseudocyst formation, pleural effusions, and cutaneous fistulas. Pancreatic leaks and fistulas can be successfully treated with transpapillary stents. Telford et al[106] reported that 25 of 43 (58%) disruptions resolved with pancreatic stenting, with no recurrence during a 2-year followup interval. Bridging the disruption was found on multivariate analysis to be predictive of a successful outcome.[106] Endoscopic injection of tissue glue has also been used to close pancreatic fistulas.

Endoscopic therapy has been used to treat sterile organized necrosis in symptomatic patients.[104] The procedure is more technically difficult, carries a higher rate of complications, has a lower cure rate, and tends to be performed in more severely ill patients than those with pseudocysts.

PANCREAS DIVISUM

Pancreas divisum, the most common congenital variant of pancreatic ductal anatomy, occurs when the ductal systems of the dorsal and ventral pancreatic ducts fail to

TABLE 107-3 Results of Endoscopic Management of Pseudocysts

Author	Technical Success	METHOD OF PSEUDOCYST DECOMPRESSION			Complications	Death
		Transpapillary	Cystogastrostomy	Cystoduodenostomy		
Binmoeller[97]	47/53*	31	6	10	6	0
Catalano[98]	17/21	17	0	0	1	0
Cremer[99]	32/33	0	11	21	3	0
Kozarek[100]	12/14	12	0	0	5	0
Barthet[101]	58/67	26	1	31	9	1
Smits[102]	31/37*	16	8	7	6	0
Howell[103]	100/108	37	38	25	25	0
Baron[104]	82/95	NM	NM	NM	17	0
Grimm[105]	14/16	5	1	8	5	1
Total	393/444 (89%)	144†	65†	102†	77 (17%)	2 (0.5%)

NM, Not mentioned.
*Combination therapy in several patients.
†Does not include numbers from Baron et al.[104]

fuse during the second month of gestation. With non-union of the ducts, the major portion of pancreatic exocrine juice drains into the duodenum via the dorsal duct and minor papilla. It has been proposed that a relative obstruction to pancreatic exocrine juice flow through the minor papilla could result in pancreatic pain or acute pancreatitis (or both) in a subpopulation of patients with pancreas divisum. Endoscopic attempts to decompress the dorsal duct in symptomatic patients with pancreas divisum have been performed primarily by dilation, stent insertion, minor papilla sphincterotomy, or any combination of these techniques.[107-109] Lans et al[107] reported their results of a randomized controlled trial of long-term (12 months) stenting of the minor papilla in patients with recurrent pancreatitis ($n = 19$). Followup continued for at least 12 months after stent removal. Stented patients had fewer hospitalizations and episodes of pancreatitis ($P < 0.05$) and were more frequently judged to be improved (90% vs. 11% for controls, $P < 0.05$). Although the symptomatic improvement after this therapy has been encouraging, multiple stent changes are generally required and the risk for stent-related complications is considerable. Ertan[108] reported that stent-induced ductal changes developed in 21 of 25 patients (84%) with pancreas divisum after stenting periods of 6 to 9 months.

A more permanent enlargement of the minor papilla orifice is possible with sphincterotomy. Lehman et al[109] attempted to evaluate the efficacy of minor papilla ES for patients with pancreas divisum ($N = 52$) and disabling pancreatic-type pain ($n = 24$), idiopathic acute recurrent pancreatitis ($n = 17$), or chronic pancreatitis ($n = 11$). A short 4- to 7F stent was placed in the minor papilla and a 3- to 6-mm sphincterotomy was performed over the stent, with the stent used as a guide for cutting and a bridge to prevent edema-induced closure of the cut. The stent was then removed in approximately 2 weeks. The mean duration of preintervention symptoms was 5.1 years, and followup averaged 1.7 years, with all patients being observed for at least 6 months after therapy. Although 76.5% of the acute recurrent pancreatitis group improved after therapy, only 26% of the chronic pain group ($P = 0.002$) and 27% of the chronic

pancreatitis group ($P = 0.01$) benefited. Similarly, when compared with the chronic pain and chronic pancreatitis groups, the acute recurrent pancreatitis group had a significant reduction in mean pain score and number of hospital days per month required for severe pain or pancreatitis (or both). These discordant results in responsiveness to therapy for the acute recurrent pancreatitis group versus the chronic pancreatitis and chronic pain groups were noted in several surgical series evaluating dorsal duct decompression and other endoscopic series. Pancreatitis complicating therapy occurred in 13% but, in general, was mild and managed conservatively. Stent-induced dorsal duct changes occurred in 50%. Heyries et al reported that 22 of 24 patients (92%) had no further episodes of pancreatitis during a median followup period of 39 months (range, 24 to 105 months) after minor papilla sphincterotomy in 8 and dorsal duct stenting for a median time of 8 months in 16 patients.[110] When summarizing eight published studies that evaluated the efficacy of minor papilla therapy in 127 patients, no further attacks occurred in 81% monitored for a mean of 27 months after the intervention.[111] The results of these studies suggest that patients with pancreas divisum and acute recurrent pancreatitis are good candidates for endoscopic therapy, whereas patients with chronic pancreatitis or chronic pain alone (or both) do not appear to do as well.

REFERENCES

1. Haber GB: Double balloon endoscopy for pancreatic and biliary access in altered anatomy (with videos). *Gastrointest Endosc* 66:S47, 2007.
2. Cheung J, Tsoi KK, Quan WL, et al: Guidewire versus conventional contrast cannulation of the common bile duct for the prevention of post-ERCP pancreatitis: A systematic review and meta-analysis. *Gastrointest Endosc* 70:1211, 2009.
3. Cotton PB, Lehman GA, Vennes J, et al: Endoscopic sphincterotomy complications and their management: An attempt at consensus. *Gastrointest Endosc* 37:383, 1991.
4. Lauri A, Horton RC, Davidson BR, et al: Endoscopic extraction of bile duct stones: Management related to stone size. *Gut* 34:1718, 1993.
5. Yoo KS, Lehman GA: Endoscopic management of biliary ductal stones. *Gastroenterol Clin North Am* 39:209, 2010.

6. Tandan M, Reddy DN, Santosh D, et al: Extracorporeal shock wave lithotripsy of large difficult common bile duct stones: Efficacy and analysis of factors that favor stone fragmentation. *J Gastroenterol Hepatol* 24:1370, 2009.

7. Bergman JJ, Rauws EA, Tijssen JG, et al: Biliary endoprosthesis in elderly patients with endoscopically irretrievable common bile duct stones: Report on 117 patients. *Gastrointest Endosc* 42:195, 1995.

8. Johnson GK, Geenen JE, Venu RP, et al: Treatment of non-extractable common bile duct stones with combination ursode-oxycholic acid plus endoprostheses. *Gastrointest Endosc* 39:528, 1993.

9. DePalma GD, Catanzano C: Stenting or surgery for treatment of irretrievable common bile duct calculi in elderly patients. *Am J Surg* 178:390, 1999.

10. Bergman JJ, van der Mey S, Rauws EA, et al: Long-term follow-up after endoscopic sphincterotomy for bile duct stones in patients younger than 60 years of age. *Gastrointest Endosc* 44:643, 1996.

11. Bergman JJ, van Berkel AM, Groen AK, et al: Biliary manometry, bacterial characteristics, bile composition, and histologic changes fifteen to seventeen years after endoscopic sphincterotomy. *Gastrointest Endosc* 45:400, 1997.

12. Baron TH, Harewood GC: Endoscopic balloon dilation of the biliary sphincter compared to endoscopic biliary sphincterotomy for removal of common bile duct stones during ERCP: A meta-analysis of randomized, controlled trials. *Am J Gastroenterol* 99:1455, 2004.

13. DiSario JA, Freeman ML, Bjorkman DJ, et al: Endoscopic balloon dilation compared with sphincterotomy for extraction of bile duct stones. *Gastroenterology* 127:1291, 2004.

14. Yasuda I, Tomita E, Enya M, et al: Can endoscopic papillary balloon dilation really preserve sphincter of Oddi function? *Gut* 49:686, 2001.

15. Attasaranya S, Cheon YK, Vittal H, et al: Large-diameter biliary orifice balloon dilation to aid in endoscopic bile duct stone removal: A multicenter series. *Gastrointest Endosc* 67:1046, 2008.

16. Neoptolemos JP, London NJ, Carr-Locke DL, et al: Controlled trial of urgent endoscopic retrograde cholangiopancreatography and endoscopic sphincterotomy versus conservative treatment for acute pancreatitis due to gallstones. *Lancet* 2:979, 1988.

17. Fan S-T, Lai E, Mok F, et al: Early treatment of acute biliary pancreatitis by endoscopic papillotomy. *N Engl J Med* 328:228, 1993.

18. Fölsch UR, Nitsche R, Lüdtke R, et al: Early ERCP and papillotomy compared with conservative treatment for acute biliary pancreatitis. *N Engl J Med* 336:237, 1997.

19. Sharma VK, Howden CW: Metaanalysis of randomized controlled trials of endoscopic retrograde cholangiography and endoscopic sphincterotomy for the treatment of acute biliary pancreatitis. *Am J Gastroenterol* 94:3211, 1999.

20. Nowak A, Nowakowska-Dulawa E, Marek T, et al: Final results of the prospective, randomized, controlled study on endoscopic sphincterotomy versus conventional management in acute biliary pancreatitis. *Gastroenterology* 108:A380, 1995.

21. Liu CL, Lo CM, Chan JK, et al: Detection of choledocholithiasis by EUS in acute pancreatitis: A prospective evaluation in 100 consecutive patients. *Gastrointest Endosc* 54:325, 2001.

22. Moon JH, Cho JD, Cha SW, et al: The detection of bile duct stones in suspected biliary pancreatitis: Comparison of MRCP, ERCP, and intraductal US. *Am J Gastroenterol* 100:1051, 2005.

23. Leung JW, Chung SC, Sung JJ, et al: Urgent endoscopic drainage for acute suppurative cholangitis. *Lancet* 1:1307, 1989.

24. Leese T, Neoptolemos JP, Baker AR, et al: Management of acute cholangitis and the impact of endoscopic sphincterotomy. *Br J Surg* 73:988, 1986.

25. Siegel JH, Rodriquez R, Cohen SA, et al: Endoscopic management of cholangitis: Critical review of an alternative technique and report of a large series. *Am J Gastroenterol* 89:1142, 1994.

26. Lai EC, Mok FP, Tan ES, et al: Endoscopic biliary drainage for severe acute cholangitis. *N Engl J Med* 326:1582, 1992.

27. Davids PH, Rauws EA, Coene PP, et al: Endoscopic stenting for postoperative biliary strictures. *Gastrointest Endosc* 38:12, 1992.

28. Berkelhammer C, Kortan P, Haber GB: Endoscopic biliary prosthesis as treatment for benign postoperative bile duct strictures. *Gastrointest Endosc* 38:98, 1989.

29. Geenen DJ, Geenen JE, Hogan WJ, et al: Endoscopic therapy for benign bile duct strictures. *Gastrointest Endosc* 35:367, 1989.

30. Bergman JJ, Burgemeister L, Bruno MJ, et al: Long-term follow-up after biliary stent placement for postoperative bile duct stenosis. *Gastrointest Endosc* 54:154, 2001.

31. Costamagna G, Pandolfi M, Mutignani M, et al: Long-term results of endoscopic management of postoperative bile duct strictures with increasing numbers of stents. *Gastrointest Endosc* 54:162, 2001.

32. Davids PH, Tanka AK, Rauws EA, et al: Benign biliary strictures. Surgery or endoscopy? *Ann Surg* 217:237, 1993.

33. Dumonceau JM, Deviere J, Delhaye M, et al: Plastic and metal stents for postoperative benign bile duct strictures: The best and the worst. *Gastrointest Endosc* 47:8, 1998.

34. Deviere J, Devaere S, Baize M, et al: Endoscopic biliary drainage in chronic pancreatitis. *Gastrointest Endosc* 36:96, 1990.

35. Barthet M, Bernard JP, Duval JL, et al: Biliary stenting in benign biliary stenosis complicating chronic calcifying pancreatitis. *Endoscopy* 26:569, 1994.

36. Smits ME, Rauws EA, van Gulik TM, et al: Long-term results of endoscopic stenting and surgical drainage for biliary stricture due to chronic pancreatitis. *Br J Surg* 83:764, 1996.

37. Kiehne K, Fölsch UR, Nitsche R: High complication rate of bile duct stents in patients with chronic alcoholic pancreatitis due to noncompliance. *Endoscopy* 32:377, 2000.

38. Vitale GC, Reed DN, Nguyen CT, et al: Endoscopic treatment of distal bile duct stricture from chronic pancreatitis. *Surg Endosc* 14:227, 2000.

39. Farnbacher MJ, Rabenstein T, Ell C, et al: Is endoscopic drainage of common bile duct stenoses in chronic pancreatitis up-to-date. *Am J Gastroenterol* 95:1466, 2000.

40. Eickhoff A, Jakobs R, Leonhardt A, et al: Endoscopic stenting for common bile duct stenosis in chronic pancreatitis: Results and impact on long-term outcome. *Eur J Gastroenterol Hepatol* 13:1161, 2001.

41. Catalano MF, Linder JD, George S, et al: Treatment of symptomatic distal common bile duct stenosis secondary to chronic pancreatitis: Comparison of single vs. multiple simultaneous stents. *Gastrointest Endosc* 60:945, 2004.

42. Deviere J, Cremer M, Baize M, et al: Management of common bile duct strictures caused by chronic pancreatitis with metal mesh self-expandable stents. *Gut* 35:122, 1994.

43. Cantu P, Hookey LC, Morales A, et al: The treatment of patients with symptomatic common bile duct stenosis secondary to chronic pancreatitis using partially covered metal stents: A pilot study. *Endoscopy* 37:735, 2005.

44. Johnson GK, Geenen JE, Venu RP, et al: Endoscopic treatment of biliary tract strictures in sclerosing cholangitis: A larger series and recommendations for treatment. *Gastrointest Endosc* 37:38, 1991.

45. Lee JG, Schutz SM, England RE, et al: Endoscopic therapy of sclerosing cholangitis. *Hepatology* 21:661, 1995.

46. van Milligen de Wit AW, van Bracht J, Rauws EA, et al: Endoscopic stent therapy for dominant extrahepatic bile duct strictures in primary sclerosing cholangitis. *Gastrointest Endosc* 44:293, 1996.

47. Ponsioen CY, Lam K, Van Milligen de Wit AW, et al: Four years experience with short term stenting in primary sclerosing cholangitis. *Am J Gastroenterol* 94:2403, 1999.

48. Kaya M, Petersen BT, Angulo P, et al: Balloon dilation compared to stenting of dominant strictures in primary sclerosing cholangitis. *Am J Gastroenterol* 96:1059, 2001.

49. Baluyut AR, Sherman S, Lehman GA, et al: Impact of endoscopic therapy on the survival of patients with primary sclerosing cholangitis. *Gastrointest Endosc* 53:308, 2001.

50. Chalasani N, Baluyut A, Ismail A, et al: Cholangiocarcinoma in patients with primary sclerosing cholangitis: A multicenter case-control study. *Hepatology* 31:7, 2000.

51. Barkun AN, Rezieg M, Mehta SN, et al: Postcholecystectomy biliary leaks in the laparoscopic era: Risk factors, presentation, and management. *Gastrointest Endosc* 45:277, 1997.

52. Bjorkman DJ, Carr-Locke DL, Lichtenstein DR, et al: Postsurgical bile leaks: Endoscopic obliteration of the transpapillary pressure gradient is enough. *Am J Gastroenterol* 90:2128, 1995.

53. Foutch PG, Harlan JR, Hoefer M: Endoscopic therapy for patients with a post-operative biliary leak. *Gastrointest Endosc* 39:416, 1993.

54. Kaffes AJ, Hourigan L, De Luca N, et al: Impact of endoscopic intervention in 100 patients with suspected postcholecystectomy bile leak. *Gastrointest Endosc* 61:269, 2005.

55. Sandha GS, Bourke MJ, Haber GB, et al: Endoscopic therapy for bile leak based on a new classification: Results in 207 patients. *Gastrointest Endosc* 60:567, 2004.

56. Kalayci C, Aisen A, Canal D, et al: Magnetic resonance cholangio-pancreatography documents bile leak site after cholecystectomy in patients with aberrant right hepatic duct where ERCP fails. *Gastrointest Endosc* 52:277, 2000.

57. Soehendra N, Rejinders-Frederix V: Palliative bile duct drainage: A new endoscopic method of introducing a transpapillary drain. *Endoscopy* 12:8, 1980.

58. Nagino M, Takada T, Miyazaki M, et al: Preoperative biliary drainage for biliary tract and ampullary carcinomas. *J Hepatobiliary Pancreat Surg* 15:25, 2008.

59. Chang WH, Kortan P, Haber GB: Outcome in patients with bifurcation tumors who undergo unilateral versus bilateral hepatic duct drainage. *Gastrointest Endosc* 47:354, 1998.

60. De Palma GD, Galloro G, Siciliano S, et al: Unilateral versus bilateral endoscopic hepatic duct drainage in patients with malignant hilar biliary obstruction: Results of a prospective, randomized and controlled study. *Gastrointest Endosc* 53:547, 2001.

61. Freeman ML, Overby C: Selective MRCP and CT-targeted drainage of malignant hilar biliary obstruction with self-expanding metallic stents. *Gastrointest Endosc* 58:41, 2003.

62. Sherman S, Lehman G, Earle D, et al: Multicenter randomized trial of 10-French versus 11.5-French plastic stents for malignant bile duct obstruction. *Gastrointest Endosc* 43:396A, 1996.

63. Tarnasky PR, Miller C, Mauldin P, et al: Comparison of prophylactic versus indicated stent exchange for malignant obstructive jaundice using computer modeling. *Gastrointest Endosc* 43:399A, 1996.

64. Prat F, Chapat O, Ducot B, et al: A randomized trial of endoscopic drainage methods for inoperable malignant strictures of the common bile duct. *Gastrointest Endosc* 47:1, 1998.

65. Mokhashi M, Rawls E, Tarnasky PR, et al: Scheduled vs as required stent exchange for malignant biliary obstruction. A prospective randomized study. *Gastrointest Endosc* 51:142A, 2000.

66. Davids PH, Groen AK, Rauws EA, et al: Randomized trial of self-expanding metal stents versus polyethylene stents for distal malignant biliary obstruction. *Lancet* 340:1488, 1992.

67. Carr-Locke DL, Ball TJ, Connors PJ, et al: Multicenter randomized trial of Wallstent biliary endoprosthesis versus plastic stents. *Gastrointest Endosc* 39:310A, 1993.

68. Knyrim K, Wagner HJ, Pausch J, et al: A prospective, randomized, controlled trial of metal stents for malignant obstruction of the common bile duct. *Endoscopy* 25:207, 1993.

69. Wagner HJ, Knyrim K, Vakil N, et al: Plastic endoprostheses versus metal stents in the palliative treatment of malignant hilar biliary obstruction: A prospective and randomized trial. *Endoscopy* 25:213, 1993.

70. Kaassis M, Boyer J, Dumas R, et al: Plastic or metal stents for malignant stricture of the common bile duct? Results of a randomized prospective study. *Gastrointest Endosc* 57:178, 2003.

71. Speer AG, Cotton PB, Russell RC, et al: Randomized trial of endoscopic versus percutaneous stent insertion in malignant obstructive jaundice. *Lancet* 2:57, 1987.

72. Andersen JR, Sørensen SM, Kruse A, et al: Randomized trial of endoscopic endoprosthesis versus operative bypass in malignant obstructive jaundice. *Gut* 30:1132, 1989.

73. Smith AC, Dowsett JF, Russell RC, et al: Randomized trial of endoscopic stenting versus surgical bypass and malignant low bile duct obstruction. *Lancet* 344:1655, 1994.

74. Shephard HA, Royle G, Ross AP, et al: Endoscopic biliary endoprosthesis in the palliation of malignant obstruction of the distal common bile duct: A randomized trial. *Br J Surg* 75:1166, 1988.

75. Jailwala J, Fogel EL, Sherman S, et al: Triple-tissue sampling at ERCP in malignant biliary obstruction. *Gastrointest Endosc* 51:383, 2000.

76. Sawada Y, Gonda H, Hayashida Y: Combined use of brushing cytology and endoscopic retrograde pancreatography for the early detection of pancreatic cancer. *Acta Cytol* 33:870, 1989.

77. Howell DA, Beveridge RP, Bosco J, et al: Endoscopic needle aspiration biopsy at ERCP in the diagnosis of biliary strictures. *Gastrointest Endosc* 38:531, 1992.

78. Howell DA, Parsons WG, Jones MA, et al: Complete tissue sampling of biliary strictures at ERCP using a new device. *Gastrointest Endosc* 43:498, 1996.

79. DeBellis M, Sherman S, Fogel EL, et al: Tissue sampling at ERCP in suspected malignant biliary strictures (Part 2). *Gastrointest Endosc* 56:720, 2002.

80. Fritcher EG, Kipp BR, Halling KC, et al: A multivariable model using advanced cytologic methods for the evaluation of indeterminate pancreatobiliary strictures. *Gastroenterology* 136:2180, 2009.

81. Funabiki T, Matsubara T, Miyakawa S, et al: Pancreaticobiliary maljunction and carcinogenesis to biliary and pancreatic malignancy. *Langenbecks Arch Surg* 394:159, 2009.

82. Ladas SD, Katsogridakis I, Tassios P, et al: Choledochocele, an overlooked diagnosis: Report of 15 cases and reviews of 56 published reports from 1984 to 1992. *Endoscopy* 27:233, 1995.

83. Elton E, Hanson BL, Biber BP, et al: Dilated common channel syndrome: Endoscopic diagnosis, treatment, and relationship to choledochocele formation. *Gastrointest Endosc* 47:471, 1998.

84. Samavedy R, Sherman S, Lehman GA: Endoscopic therapy in anomalous pancreatobiliary duct junction. *Gastrointest Endosc* 50:623, 1999.

85. Ng WD, Liu K, Wong MK, et al: Endoscopic sphincterotomy in young patients with choledochal dilation and a long common channel: A preliminary report. *Br J Surg* 79:550, 1992.

86. Cremer M, Deviere J, Delhaye M, et al: Stenting in severe chronic pancreatitis: Results of medium-term follow-up in 76 patients. *Endoscopy* 23:171, 1991.

87. Delhaye M, Vandermeeren A, Baize M, et al: Extracorporeal shock-wave lithotripsy of pancreatic calculi. *Gastroenterology* 102:610, 1992.

88. Wilcox CM: Endoscopic therapy for pain in chronic pancreatitis: Is it time for the naysayers to throw in the towel? [Editorial]. *Gastrointest Endosc* 61:582, 2005.

89. Rösch T, Daniel S, Scholz M, et al: Endoscopic treatment of chronic pancreatitis: A multicenter study of 1000 patients with long-term follow-up. *Endoscopy* 34:765, 2002.

90. Dite P, Ruzicka M, Zboril V, et al: A prospective, randomized trial comparing endoscopic and surgical therapy for chronic pancreatitis. *Endoscopy* 35:553, 2003.

91. Eleftherladis N, Dinu F, Delhaye M, et al: Long-term outcome after pancreatic stenting in severe chronic pancreatitis. *Endoscopy* 37:223, 2005.

92. Cremer M, Deviere J, Delhaye M, et al: Non-surgical management of severe chronic pancreatitis. *Scand J Gastroenterol* 25:77, 1990.

93. Sherman S, Lehman GA, Hawes RH, et al: Pancreatic ductal stones: Frequency of successful endoscopic removal and improvement in symptoms. *Gastrointest Endosc* 37:511, 1991.

94. Guda NM, Partington S, Freeman ML: Extracorporeal shockwave lithotripsy in the management of chronic calcific pancreatitis: A meta-analysis. *JOP* 6:6, 2005.

95. Brand B, Kahl M, Sidhu S, et al: Prospective evaluation of morphology, function, and quality of life after extracorporeal shock-wave lithotripsy and endoscopic treatment of chronic calcific pancreatitis. *Am J Gastroenterol* 95:3428, 2000.

96. Cahen DL, Gouma DJ, Rauws EA, et al: Endoscopic versus surgical drainage of the pancreatic duct in chronic pancreatitis. *N Engl J Med* 356:676, 2008.

97. Binmoeller KF, Seifert H, Walter A, et al: Transpapillary and transmural drainage of pancreatic pseudocysts. *Gastrointest Endosc* 42;219, 1995.

98. Catalano MF, Geenen JE, Schmalz MJ, et al: Treatment of pancreatic pseudocysts with ductal communication by transpapillary pancreatic duct endoprosthesis. *Gastrointest Endosc* 42:214, 1995.

99. Cremer M, Deviere J, Engelholm L: Endoscopic management of cysts and pseudocysts in chronic pancreatitis: Long-term follow-up after 7 years of experience. *Gastrointest Endosc* 35:1, 1989.

100. Kozarek RA, Ball TJ, Patterson DJ, et al: Endoscopic transpapillary therapy for disrupted pancreatic duct and peripancreatic fluid collections. *Gastroenterology* 100:1362, 1991.

101. Barthet M, Sahel J, Bodiou-Bertei C, et al: Endoscopic transpapillary drainage of pancreatic pseudocysts. *Gastrointest Endosc* 42:208, 1995.

102. Smits ME, Rauws EAJ, Tytgat GN, et al: The efficacy of endoscopic treatment of pancreatic pseudocysts. *Gastrointest Endosc* 42:202, 1995.

103. Howell DA, Elton E, Parsons WG: Endoscopic management of pseudocysts of the pancreas. *Gastrointest Endosc Clin N Am* 8:143, 1988.

104. Baron TH, Harewood GC, Morgan DE, et al: Outcome differences after endoscopic drainage of pancreatic necrosis, acute pancreatic pseudocysts, and chronic pancreatic pseudocysts. *Gastrointest Endosc* 56:7, 2002.

105. Grimm H, Meyer WH, Nam VC, et al: New modalities for treating chronic pancreatitis. *Endoscopy* 21:70, 1989.

106. Telford JJ, Farrell JJ, Saltzman JR, et al: Pancreatic stent placement for duct disruption. *Gastrointest Endosc* 56:18, 2002.

107. Lans JI, Geenen JE, Johanson JF, et al: Endoscopic therapy in patients with pancreas divisum and acute pancreatitis: A prospective, randomized, controlled trial. *Gastrointest Endosc* 38:430, 1992.

108. Ertan A: Long-term results after endoscopic pancreatic stent placement without pancreatic papillotomy in acute recurrent pancreatitis due to pancreas divisum. *Gastrointest Endosc* 52:9, 2000.

109. Lehman GA, Sherman S, Nisi R, et al: Pancreas divisum: Results of minor papilla sphincterotomy. *Gastrointest Endosc* 39:1, 1993.

110. Heyries L, Barthet M, Delvasto C, et al: Long-term results of endoscopic management of pancreas divisum with recurrent acute pancreatitis. *Gastrointest Endosc* 55:376, 2002.

111. Klein SD, Affronti JP: Pancreas divisum, an evidence-based review: Part II, patient selection and treatment. *Gastrointest Endosc* 60:585, 2004.

Biliary Tract Tumors

Clifford S. Cho | Yuman Fong

BENIGN GALLBLADDER TUMORS

Benign tumors of the gallbladder are relatively common, with up to 5% of patients undergoing abdominal ultrasonography being found to harbor gallbladder polyps.[1] Benign gallbladder tumors can be broadly categorized as epithelial (adenomas), mesenchymal (fibromas, lipomas, hemangiomas), or as pseudotumors (cholesterol polyps, inflammatory polyps, and adenomyomas). Importantly, most gallbladder cancers do not arise from precursor adenomas. Cholesterol polyps are the most common of the benign tumors. Adenomyomas are extensions of Rokitansky-Aschoff sinuses through the muscular layer of the gallbladder wall; they can appear polypoid or infiltrative in morphology, and can be associated with biliary colic–like symptoms.

The likelihood of malignancy in gallbladder polyps increases with increasing polyp size and decreasing polyp number. A review of 182 cases of resected gallbladder polyps identified only 13 cases of malignancy; likelihood of malignancy in this series was associated with patient age more than 50 years and solitary polyps greater than 1 cm in size.[2] In a similar review of 134 cases of gallbladder polyps (from which 6 malignancies were identified), malignancy was noted to be associated with polyp number less than 3.[3]

The management of gallbladder polyps is dictated by the presence of symptoms and their likelihood of harboring occult malignancy. Any patient with symptoms referable to gallbladder polyps should undergo cholecystectomy. In addition, patients with suspicious polyps (size >1 cm, number <3, sessile lesions, or those with sonographic evidence of mucosal invasion) should undergo cholecystectomy. Cholecystectomy for patients with suspicious polyps should be performed via an open approach to minimize the likelihood of tumor spillage. Furthermore, intraoperative frozen-section analysis of the resected gallbladder specimen must be undertaken, as confirmation of malignancy may dictate the performance of an extended oncologic resection. Patients who do not undergo surgical therapy deserve close radiographic followup, with serial sonograms performed at 6-month intervals in order to identify any rapid interval size progression that may indicate the presence of malignancy.

GALLBLADDER CANCER

Cancer of the gallbladder is the most common biliary malignancy, and it is the fifth most common gastrointestinal cancer. In the United States, it has an incidence of approximately 1.2 per 100,000 and is the cause of about 2800 deaths yearly. Because of its aggressive nature

(manifested by its propensity toward nodal metastases, direct hepatic invasion, and seeding of peritoneal surfaces), it is usually diagnosed at an advanced stage, resulting in an overall median survival of less than 6 months. These dismal biological characteristics have historically fostered a cynical nihilism among clinicians caring for patients with this malignancy. However, advances in our understanding of its tumor biology accompanied by progress in diagnostic and surgical extirpative techniques have motivated a fresh, new approach to this once universally fatal disease; indeed, the possibility of cure is a real one for a subset of patients presenting with gallbladder cancer.

EPIDEMIOLOGY

The prevalence of gallbladder cancer appears to be highest in South America, intermediate in Europe, and lower in the United States and United Kingdom. In the United States, Native Americans, patients in urban areas, and those of lower socioeconomic status appear to be affected more commonly. Epidemiologic analysis suggests that processes that promote chronic gallbladder irritation and inflammation are also risk factors for the onset of gallbladder cancer. Indeed, a history of biliary disease, age, female gender, obesity, high carbohydrate diet, ethanol abuse, and tobacco abuse (all of which are associated with calculous biliary disease) have been shown to be associated with a higher risk of developing gallbladder cancer. Moreover, 79% to 98% of patients diagnosed with gallbladder cancer have a personal history of gallstone disease (most commonly large, symptomatic, cholesterol stones). Mirizzi syndrome, characterized by chronic gallbladder irritation from an impacted stone, has been associated with an increased risk of gallbladder cancer. The presence of an abnormal pancreaticobiliary duct junction, thought to promote chronic biliary inflammation, has been associated with both choledochal cyst disease as well as gallbladder cancer.[4] The incidence of gallbladder cancer in the so-called porcelain gallbladder, presumably resulting from chronic inflammation and calcification of the gallbladder wall, was once estimated to be as high as 61%; however, more contemporary analyses suggest that the correct figure is more likely between 7% and 25%.[5,6]

The exact nature of the relationship between chronic inflammation and gallbladder tumorigenesis is unclear. It has been estimated that only 0.3% to 3% of patients with gallstones will develop gallbladder cancer, eliminating any theoretical benefit for prophylactic cholecystectomy (with one possible exception being patients with porcelain gallbladder). Introduction of cholesterol stones into normal gallbladders does not experimentally induce gallbladder cancer in animal models; however, the presence of stones does appear to facilitate the ability of teratogens to induce gallbladder cancer.[7]

ANATOMY

The anatomic relationships of the gallbladder to surrounding structures dictate the surgical strategies that must be employed in its treatment. The gallbladder fossa, against which the fundus and body of the gallbladder lie, is found beneath the junction of hepatic segments IVB and V. As a result, the likelihood of direct hepatic invasion of gallbladder cancer typically mandates resection of these segments. The infundibulum of the gallbladder lies adjacent to the right portal pedicle within the porta hepatis; as a result, tumors arising in the infundibulum commonly invade the right portal pedicle and require a right trisectionectomy for complete surgical extirpation.

The thin gallbladder wall is composed of an inner mucosa, a thin lamina propria, and a single muscularis layer (unlike the two muscle layers that line most hollow viscera). The serosa of the gallbladder is typically opened during a standard cholecystectomy, with the avascular subserosal layer being used as the surgical plane of dissection; the ability of mucosally based tumors to microscopically invade across the serosa explains the high prevalence of positive resection margins after standard cholecystectomy for gallbladder cancer.

The lymphatic drainage of the gallbladder has been well characterized. The pattern of lymphatic flow appears to be directed initially toward the cystic and pericholedochal lymph nodes, then to the posterior pancreaticoduodenal, periportal, and common hepatic artery nodes within the hepatoduodenal ligament, and eventually to the celiac, aortocaval, and superior mesenteric artery nodes. There appears to be no ascending lymphatic drainage into the hilum of the liver. For this reason, meticulous lymphadenectomy within the hepatoduodenal ligament is a critical component of surgical strategy in the management of gallbladder cancer. Unfortunately, the potential for direct drainage from the pericholedochal nodes into the aortocaval nodes explains the difficulty of completely encompassing the extent of lymphatic involvement after surgical resection.

PATHOLOGY

Approximately 60% of gallbladder cancers arise in the fundus, with 30% arising from the body and 10% from the neck. Although it is likely that gallbladder cancer may follow the pathogenetic sequence of mucosal dysplasia to carcinoma in situ to invasive cancer, it is unlikely that most gallbladder cancers arise from precursor adenomata.

Gallbladder cancers have been categorized as infiltrative, nodular, combined nodular-infiltrative, papillary, and combined papillary-infiltrative. Infiltrative tumors, which are the most common variety, initially appear as indurated areas of gallbladder wall thickening that spread into the subserosal plane, which is typically violated during routine cholecystectomy. Nodular tumors invade into adjacent pericholecystic structures early, but unlike infiltrative cancers, induce sharply defined borders that can facilitate curative resection. Papillary tumors tend to grow in a polypoid fashion, often filling into the lumen of the gallbladder with minimal wall invasion; as such, this variety of tumors tends to be associated with more favorable prognoses.

Microscopically, adenocarcinoma is the most common histologic subtype seen with gallbladder malignancies. Other histologic subtypes that have been reported include adenosquamous carcinoma, oat cell carcinoma, sarcoma, carcinoid, lymphoma, and melanoma. Histologic grading for gallbladder cancer, which has been recognized as a significant prognostic variable, is categorized from G1 (well-differentiated) to G4 (undifferentiated); patients most commonly present with G3 (poorly differentiated) tumors.

The propensity of gallbladder cancer to penetrate beyond the single muscle layer of the gallbladder wall results in a high likelihood of tumor penetration into the liver, peritoneal cavity, and lymphovascular spaces at the time of diagnosis. Review of the literature suggests that only 10% of cases are confined to the gallbladder wall at the time of diagnosis; 59% exhibit direct invasion into hepatic parenchyma, 45% demonstrate lymph node metastases, and 20% present with distant extrahepatic metastases.[8] Indeed, a high level of suspicion for occult intraperitoneal metastases should be maintained throughout the diagnostic process for patients with gallbladder cancer. The most common site of extraabdominal spread is the lungs, although pulmonary metastases are rare in the absence of extensive intraperitoneal disease.

DIAGNOSIS

Patients with gallbladder cancer may experience complaints that mimic those of benign biliary colic. Symptoms of persistent pain, weight loss, anorexia, jaundice, and a palpable right upper quadrant mass are typically indicative of advanced disease that is not amenable to surgical resection. A review of the Memorial Sloan-Kettering Cancer Center (MSKCC) experience highlighted the observation that 95% of patients presenting with jaundice were ultimately noted to harbor unresectable disease.[9]

Tumor markers provide limited assistance with diagnosis. In the presence of appropriate symptomatology, carcinoembryonic antigen (CEA) elevations greater than 4 ng/mL have been shown to predict gallbladder cancer with 50% sensitivity and 93% specificity.[10] Similarly, elevations of carbohydrate antigen (CA) 19-9 greater than 20 U/mL are 79.4% sensitive and 79.2% specific.[11]

Radiographic findings on ultrasonography include the presence of a polypoid gallbladder mass (seen in 27% of gallbladder cancer cases) or an invasive gallbladder-based lesion (seen in 50% of cases); other sonographic findings consistent with gallbladder cancer include discontinuous gallbladder mucosa, echogenic mucosa, or submucosal echolucency.[12] Computed tomographic (CT) findings seen in patients with gallbladder cancer include a mass filling the gallbladder lumen in 42% of cases, a polypoid mass in 26%, a mass in the region of the gallbladder fossa without a distinctly recognizable gallbladder in 26%, and diffuse wall thickening in 6% (Figure 108-1).[13] Magnetic resonance imaging (MRI) and magnetic resonance cholangiopancreatography (MRCP) are especially accurate

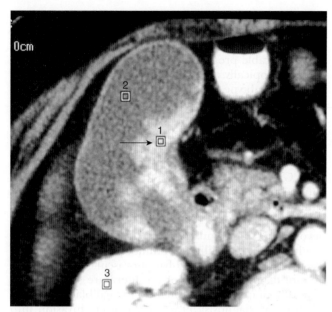

FIGURE 108-1 Appearance of gallbladder cancer on CT: note extensive sessile polypoid lesion within lumen of gallbladder wall.

TABLE 108-1 AJCC System for Gallbladder Cancer

T1a	Tumor invades lamina propria of gallbladder wall
T1b	Tumor invades muscular layer of gallbladder wall
T2	Tumor invades perimuscular connective tissue but not across serosa
T3	Tumor invades across serosa of gallbladder wall and/or invades liver and/or one adjacent structure or organ
T4	Tumor invades main portal vein or hepatic artery or two or more extrahepatic structures or organs
N0	No lymph node involvement
N1	Lymph node involvement within hepatoduodenal ligament
N2	Lymph node involvement beyond hepatoduodenal ligament
M0	No distant metastases
M1	Distant metastases
Stage IA	T1 N0 M0
Stage II	T2 N0 M0
Stage IIIA	T3 N0 M0
Stage IIIB	T1-3 N1 M0
Stage IVA	T4 N0-1 M0
Stage IVB	T1-4 N2 M0
	T1-4 N0-2 M1

means of identifying small hepatic metastases and involvement of the common bile duct.

Despite the high frequency of nodal involvement, definitive preoperative identification of lymph node metastases is challenging. Enlarged benign inflammatory lymph nodes are commonly encountered at the time of laparotomy. Although the CT finding of ring-like or heterogeneous enhancement of a more than 10-mm large lymph node has been found to identify lymph node metastases with 89% accuracy, only 38% of nodal metastases are preoperatively identified by CT.[14] Endoscopic ultrasonography may be useful for assessing peripancreatic and periportal adenopathy. Fluorodeoxyglucose positron emission tomography (PET) may be useful for identifying distant metastases that may contraindicate surgical intervention.

The striking ability of disseminated gallbladder cancer cells to implant within needle tracts limits the utility of percutaneous core biopsy for diagnosis. Percutaneous fine-needle aspiration appears to have a lower incidence of needle tract seeding while providing satisfactory diagnostic accuracy, and it can be employed in cases of surgically unresectable disease where a definitive tissue diagnosis may direct nonoperative therapy.[15] Cytologic analysis of bile samples collected either percutaneously or endoscopically is not often helpful for diagnosing gallbladder cancer, with suboptimal sensitivities of approximately 50%.[15]

STAGING

The most accurate predictor of outcome is tumor stage. With changes and improvements in surgical therapy, the impact of various staging criteria has evolved. For example, previous iterations of the American Joint Committee on Cancer (AJCC) system categorized patients with tumors extending into the liver as having unresectable stage IV disease. With the increased implementation of modern hepatic resection techniques, curative resection is now possible for this subset of patients with gallbladder cancer; the current AJCC system (Table 108-1) now categorizes patients with disease invasive into the liver within stage III. In addition, nodal metastases found outside of the hepatoduodenal ligament (N2) have been shown to carry the same ominous prognostic weight as distant nonnodal metastases (M1)[16]; for this reason, the current AJCC system categorizes any patients with N2 disease within stage IV. In this way, recommended surgical therapy is specifically tailored to the stage of disease present.

SURGERY

The standard template on which all operations for gallbladder cancer should be based is the so-called radical or extended cholecystectomy. This consists of cholecystectomy with en bloc resection of segments IVB and V and lymphadenectomy of the cystic, pericholedochal, periportal, and posterior pancreaticoduodenal lymph nodes residing in the hepatoduodenal ligament and local aortocaval lymph nodes (Figure 108-2). Knowledge of a patient's tumor stage and familiarity with the general biologic proclivities of gallbladder cancer allow the surgeon to specifically tailor surgical therapy to the individual oncologic needs of each patient. For example, lymphadenectomy can often be performed by simply skeletonizing the porta hepatis. However, in cases of prior dissection where cicatricial changes in the porta hepatis might blur any distinction between tumor and postoperative changes, in patients with infundibular tumors extending into the region of the common bile duct, or in very obese patients, resection of the extrahepatic biliary system with Roux-en-Y hepaticojejunostomy

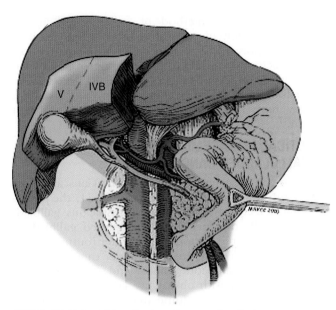

FIGURE 108-2 Portal lymphadenectomy and radical cholecystectomy with en bloc segment IVB/V hepatic resection for gallbladder cancer. (From Bartlett DL, Fong Y: Gallbladder cancer. In Blumgart LH, et al, editors: *Hepatobiliary cancer*. Hamilton, Ontario, 2001, BC Decker, p 216.)

reconstruction may be necessary to accomplish a margin-negative resection and adequate lymphadenectomy.

Analysis of the MSKCC experience demonstrated that only 25% of patients presenting with gallbladder cancer harbored disease ultimately amenable to curative resection. Among those patients who underwent curative resection, a median survival of 26 months and a 5-year actuarial survival of 38% were observed. Factors predictive of poor survival were advanced T stage and N stage.[17]

Staging laparoscopy remains an effective means of identifying patients with unresectable gallbladder cancer. Among 44 patients without preoperative evidence of unresectability who underwent staging laparoscopy at MSKCC, 21 patients were found to have evidence of distant metastatic disease at the time of laparoscopy. Among the 23 patients without laparoscopic evidence of metastatic disease, 15 were ultimately found to harbor unresectable disease due to distant metastases, distant nodal involvement, or locally advanced tumors at the time of laparotomy.[18]

Stage I Disease

The setting in which the surgeon is most apt to encounter stage I gallbladder cancer occurs after routine cholecystectomy for presumed benign stone disease, when pathologic analysis of the resected gallbladder unexpectedly identifies cancer within the muscular layer of the gallbladder wall. As stated earlier, the plane of dissection utilized during a typical cholecystectomy is along the subserosal plane, which should not violate a T1 tumor. The likelihood of N1 disease is vanishingly small for patients with T1 tumors.[19] For this reason, simple cholecystectomy should be curative for patients with pathologically confirmed stage I disease.[20,21] A notable exception to this is the situation in which the cystic duct margin

remains positive, in which case re-resection to negative margins is imperative. On occasion, this may necessitate common bile duct excision with reestablishment of biliary–enteric continuity. A review of 89 patients with stage I gallbladder cancer identified only two patients who recurred after simple cholecystectomy; both had a positive cystic duct margin.[20]

Stage II Disease

The subserosal plane of dissection employed in the standard cholecystectomy is likely to violate T2 tumors; indeed, patients with T2 tumors resected by simple cholecystectomy have a 40% to 50% likelihood of margin positivity.[16,19] Furthermore, approximately one-half of patients with T2 tumors harbor nodal metastases. For these reasons, extended cholecystectomy with portal lymphadenectomy is the procedure of choice for patients with stage II disease. The importance of performing an extended cholecystectomy with negative margins is underscored by the observation that 5-year survival rates are 70% to 90% for patients with stage II disease treated with extended cholecystectomy, as compared with 20% to 40% after simple cholecystectomy alone (with no 5-year survivors among those with positive resection margins).[20,21]

Stage III Disease

Performance of an extended cholecystectomy for patients with stage III disease has been associated with 5-year survival estimates of 33% to 67%.[16,22] Occasionally, tumors localized to the infundibulum of the gallbladder can present unique surgical challenges, as extensive tumor within the region of the adjacent right portal pedicle may necessitate removal of the right hemiliver in addition to resection of segment IVA; this is undertaken in the form of an extended right hepatectomy or right trisectionectomy.

Stage IV Disease

Unfortunately, no long-term survival has been observed among patients with stage IV disease. Involvement of N2 nodes outside of the hepatoduodenal ligament and distant metastases are indicative of a uniquely more aggressive tumor biology than that seen in bulky tumors extending into the hepatic parenchyma or in those with nodal disease confined to the hepatoduodenal ligament.

In practice, the surgeon is often confronted with gallbladder cancer diagnosed incidentally after a routine simple cholecystectomy. As outlined earlier, such patients who are found to harbor T1 tumors do not require repeat resection, provided that all margins of resection (with particular attention paid to the cystic duct margin) are negative. The high likelihood of positive margins and occult nodal metastases among patients with T2 and larger tumors mandates repeat resection in the form of an extended cholecystectomy. The primary challenge confronting the surgeon at this point is the ability to achieve a curative resection. A review of the MSKCC experience with gallbladder cancer patients referred for further surgical therapy after prior laparoscopic cholecystectomy demonstrated that 22 of 42 patients were noted to have unresectable disease at the time of second laparotomy.[23] Laparoscopy trocar site scars are typically excised, although this is done more for staging purposes to identify M1 disease than for any potential therapeutic benefit. In the scenario where the diagnosis of gallbladder cancer is unexpectedly made at the time of laparoscopy, the operating surgeon should either convert to an open exploration for possible extended cholecystectomy, or abort the procedure with subsequent reexploration or referral. A comparison of gallbladder patients presenting for initial definitive operation to those presenting for a second definitive operation identified no adverse survival effect associated with having undergone a prior noncurative exploration.[17]

ADJUVANT THERAPY

Gallbladder cancer is unfortunately highly resistant to chemotherapy, and its proclivity toward diffuse peritoneal spread limits the applicability of radiation therapy. Uncontrolled studies investigating the use of adjuvant chemotherapy and radiation have provided mixed outcomes with no consistent benefit. One phase III trial examining the efficacy of 5-fluorouracil (5-FU)/mitomycin as adjuvant therapy for various pancreaticobiliary malignancies demonstrated a measurable but modest improvement in 5-year overall survival (26% vs. 14%) and 5-year disease-free survival (20% vs. 11%) for patients with gallbladder cancer treated with adjuvant chemotherapy versus those treated with surgical resection alone.[24] Notably, no such survival benefit was observed among patients with pancreatic cancer, cholangiocarcinoma, or ampullary carcinoma in this series.[24] Meta-analysis of studies employing palliative and adjuvant radiation therapy for patients with gallbladder cancer suggests a small benefit in survival for those treated with radiotherapy.[24] One report observed a 5-year survival of 64% among a cohort of 21 gallbladder cancer patients treated with concurrent 5-FU and 54-Gy external beam radiation treatment (EBRT) after resection, suggesting that the use of adjuvant chemoradiation may potentiate the therapeutic benefit of surgical treatment.[25] Unfortunately, there have been no large randomized trials from which recommendations regarding the routine use of adjuvant chemotherapy and/or radiotherapy for gallbladder cancer can be made. In practice, however, patients with positive resection margins or nodal metastases are often offered adjuvant therapy without definitive proof of demonstrable efficacy.

PALLIATION

Because of the very high likelihood of surgical unresectability, comprehensive care for patients with gallbladder cancer must also include an armamentarium of palliative procedures. Unfortunately, the median survival of patients with unresectable gallbladder cancer is typically only 2 to 4 months (with a 1-year survival <5%). Therefore, effective palliation should be accompanied by minimal risk of morbidity. Surgical palliation in the form of a segment III biliary bypass provides a relatively simple means of durable biliary decompression because of its distance from the gallbladder and hepatic hilum.[26] However, percutaneous biliary drainage usually provides

a more reasonable method of palliation when the expected duration of survival is brief. When feasible, resection of port site recurrences after prior laparoscopic cholecystectomy can help to prevent the pain and local cutaneous complications associated with necrotic abdominal wall wounds. Palliative chemotherapy and radiation therapy have not been shown to provide consistent benefit.[27]

PRACTICAL MANAGEMENT OF GALLBLADDER CANCER

There are four scenarios in which clinicians are most often confronted with gallbladder cancer: (1) the preoperatively detected radiographically suspicious gallbladder polyp; (2) the incidentally diagnosed gallbladder cancer encountered postoperatively after routine laparoscopic cholecystectomy; (3) gallbladder cancer presenting as a large gallbladder mass; and (4) gallbladder cancer presenting with obstructive jaundice. In the following comments, we outline interventional strategies for each of these scenarios separately.

Preoperatively Detected Radiographically Suspicious Gallbladder Polyp

These polyps are most often encountered after abdominal ultrasonography that has typically been performed to evaluate symptoms of biliary colic. Ultrasonographic findings that raise the suspicion of malignancy include size greater than 1 cm, polyp number higher than 3, sessile polyps, and polyps with evidence of possible gallbladder mucosal invasion. Prior to operative intervention, diagnostic evaluation should be completed with MRI, which can delineate the biliary anatomy, assess for biliary tumor involvement, and identify small intrahepatic metastases. In the absence of unresectable or metastatic disease, operative intervention should be undertaken in the form of an open cholecystectomy to minimize the likelihood of tumor dissemination resulting from inadvertent bile spillage. Rather than opening the serosa of the gallbladder, the plane of dissection during cholecystectomy is along the cystic plate of the liver, thereby avoiding violation of the gallbladder subserosa. Intraoperative frozen-section analysis is performed to confirm the presence of gallbladder cancer. Theoretically, if frozen-section analysis were to identify a T1 tumor, simple cholecystectomy would suffice (assuming a negative cystic duct margin), given the low likelihood of margin positivity or nodal metastases. In practice, however, definitive demonstration of a T1 tumor is difficult to confirm by frozen-section analysis. Therefore, any pathologic confirmation of malignancy alone is generally sufficient to warrant performance of an extended cholecystectomy, with resection of hepatic segments IVB and V (to encompass the gallbladder fossa) and portal lymphadenectomy (with or without resection of the extrahepatic biliary system).

Gallbladder Cancer Diagnosed Incidentally after Laparoscopic Cholecystectomy

The majority of gallbladder cancers diagnosed incidentally after routine cholecystectomy are early-stage tumors. Depending on particular operative and pathologic variables, repeat resection is often warranted for these patients. The decision-making process begins with careful pathologic analysis of the resected gallbladder. The low likelihood of nodal and distant metastases and the absence of tumor at the subserosal cholecystectomy dissection plane among T1 tumors obviate any need for further surgical therapy after routine cholecystectomy. Two critical exceptions to this rule would be the presence of intraoperative bile spillage and cystic duct margin positivity. The strong propensity of gallbladder cancer to seed the peritoneal cavity considerably raises the possibility of peritoneal dissemination after inadvertent bile spillage. The presence of tumor cells at the cystic duct resection margin warrants repeat resection of the cystic duct and/or common bile duct to pathologically confirmed negative margins.

Repeat operative intervention must therefore be entertained when pathologic analysis identifies T2 or greater disease. Preoperative imaging studies should include MRCP and PET imaging to delineate the relevant biliary anatomy and pathology, and to rule out metastatic disease. If these studies do not identify unresectability, resection of hepatic segments IVB and V and portal lymphadenectomy are undertaken. The presence of peritoneal dissemination will negate any potential benefit of resection; a careful search for occult distant disease is particularly important when the previous laparoscopic cholecystectomy was complicated by bile spillage. Because of the documented ability of disseminated gallbladder cancer to seed laparoscopic incisional sites, trocar scars may be widely excised, particularly in cases where bile spillage may have occurred. As stated, this is primarily a staging maneuver, as identification of tumor infiltration in these areas portends the development of peritoneal metastases.

Gallbladder Cancer Presenting as a Gallbladder Mass

In the situation where the suspicion of gallbladder cancer arises from the radiographic observation of a large mass emanating from the gallbladder, it is imperative to determine resectability. Again, this is best accomplished by MRCP and PET imaging. If resectability is confirmed for these locally advanced lesions, surgical resection is again undertaken. In these cases, effective extirpation will often require a right trisectionectomy with portal lymphadenectomy, extrahepatic biliary resection, and reconstructive Roux-en-Y hepaticojejunostomy, because of the strong likelihood of local hilar involvement by tumor.

Gallbladder Cancer Presenting With Obstructive Jaundice

As stated earlier, the presence of jaundice has been shown to independently predict a very poor likelihood of resectability and long-term survival. In fact, management of this cohort of patients usually centers around palliation. Candidacy for operative intervention can be made on the basis of MRCP and PET imaging. When faced with radiographic evidence of unresectability or other contraindications to surgical treatment, percutaneous external biliary drainage offers a minimally invasive and effective means of palliation. In the limited subset of jaundiced patients demonstrating resectable disease, operative exploration may be undertaken. If operative findings confirm resectability, right trisectionectomy and portal lymphadenectomy with extrahepatic biliary resection and hepaticojejunostomy offer the best chances of complete extirpation.

SURGICAL TECHNIQUE FOR GALLBLADDER CANCER

Surgical therapy is reserved for the subset of patients who demonstrate no evidence of unresectability on preoperative imaging. With the exception of those patients who have undergone cholecystectomy with a pathologically confirmed T1 tumor not extending to the cholecystectomy margins, patients are offered an extended cholecystectomy with portal lymphadenectomy and partial hepatectomy.

The operative strategy begins with deliberate abdominal exploration through a bilateral subcostal or right transverse incision with a vertical extension to the xiphoid process. If no evidence of technically unresectable disease, distant disease, or N2 nodal metastases is identified, the lymphadenectomy is begun by mobilizing the duodenal sweep with an extensive Kocher maneuver. The retroduodenal lymphatic tissue is harvested with care taken to include aortocaval and superior mesenteric nodes. The portal lymphatic tissue may be skeletonized off of the extrahepatic biliary system, but in cases of prior hilar dissection, tumor extension into the bile duct, or extreme obesity, comprehensive portal lymphadenectomy may require excision of the extrahepatic bile ducts. In this scenario, the supraduodenal bile duct is divided and elevated, and its surrounding lymphatic tissue is swept off of the underlying portal vein and hepatic artery as dissection proceeds toward the hepatic hilus.

At the hilus, the hilar plate is lowered by incising Glisson capsule along the base of segment IVB. A determination is made at this point regarding the extent of hepatic resection that will be necessary for complete tumor extirpation. For patients with extensive invasion into the porta hepatis, an extended right hemihepatectomy or right trisectionectomy may be necessary. If the bile duct has been divided, a right hemihepatectomy or trisectionectomy will require division of the left hepatic duct; if the bile duct has been divided and resection of segments IVB and V is sufficient for tumor clearance, the common hepatic duct is typically divided below the confluence of the right and left hepatic ducts.

In the absence of significant tumor extension into the porta hepatis, resection of segments IVB and V is performed. Prior to hepatectomy, care is taken to maintain a low central venous pressure, and the patient is placed into a moderate Trendelenburg position to minimize the risk of air embolism. Inflow control to segment IVB can be obtained by dissection in the region of the umbilical fissure, where the vessels to IVB can be identified and ligated to minimize intraoperative hemorrhage. Control of the segment V vessels is usually achieved after parenchymal transection has commenced; care must be exercised in order to avoid inadvertent injury to the adjacent right anterior sectoral branches or to the segment VIII vessels. Importantly, the middle hepatic vein draining segments IVB and V runs between segments IVA and VIII and enters the portion of liver to be resected; care must be taken to avoid injury to this vessel, which is divided during parenchymal transection. Inflow and outflow control and accurate segmental resection are facilitated by the use of intraoperative ultrasonography, which can identify the anatomy and course of the relevant vessels. In cases where extrahepatic biliary resection has been performed, a retrocolic Roux-en-Y hepaticojejunostomy is constructed to reestablish biliary–enteric continuity. Finally, for patients who have previously undergone laparoscopic cholecystectomy, the surrounding skin and fascia of the laparoscopic port sites may be excised and submitted for pathologic analysis.

BENIGN BILIARY TUMORS

Benign tumors of the biliary tract are exceedingly rare, but can cause symptoms not dissimilar from those resulting from malignant causes. The most common benign biliary tumors are papillomas and adenomas. Less common benign tumors include granular cell myoblastomas, neural tumors, endocrine tumors, and leiomyomas. Because they are found most frequently in the region of the ampulla of Vater or along the common bile duct, benign biliary tumors typically present with jaundice that is slowly progressive or intermittent in nature. Optimal treatment includes local excision with removal of a portion of the duct wall from which they originate, as local recurrences have been reported after subtotal resection.

Bile duct adenomas are benign intrahepatic tumors that are typically found incidentally at the time of laparoscopy or laparotomy. They often appear as well-demarcated white subcapsular lesions ranging from several millimeters to 1 or 2 cm in size. Histologically, they are characterized by numerous well-differentiated bile duct–like structures surrounded by a fibrous stroma. They are generally asymptomatic and have not been proven to be precancerous in nature.

Biliary cystadenomas are unusual benign tumors often characterized by a multiloculated cystic appearance. Most cystadenomas are mucinous in nature; such mucinous cystadenomas may be associated with pancreatic mucinous cystic neoplasms and are histologically also associated with an ovarian-like stroma in females. Far less common are the serous cystadenomas. The occasional presence of dysplasia suggests the possibility that these tumors may harbor a potential for malignant transformation into biliary cystadenocarcinomas.

Several noteworthy benign conditions must be considered in the differential diagnosis of obstructing biliary tract lesions. Primary sclerosing cholangitis is an idiopathic, premalignant disorder characterized by progressive biliary tract fibrosis whose cholangiographic appearance can mimic that of malignant biliary disease. Untreated, it can ultimately progress to cholestatic liver failure and cholangiocarcinoma. Mirizzi syndrome is an unusual benign condition resulting from a chronically impacted stone in the neck of the gallbladder that, over time, induces sufficient pericholecystic inflammation to obstruct the adjacent common hepatic duct or common bile duct. Finally, another unusual benign process that can produce biliary tract obstruction is benign idiopathic focal stenosis, or the so-called malignant masquerade. Because of its propensity to involve the confluence of the hepatic ducts, this benign fibroproliferative disorder is often indistinguishable from cholangiocarcinoma without extensive surgical intervention.[28]

CHOLANGIOCARCINOMA

Cholangiocarcinoma is an uncommon cancer, accounting for only 2% of all reported malignancies. Its incidence in the United States has been estimated at 1 to 2 per 100,000. It may arise anywhere along the entire length of the biliary system; 40% to 60% develop in the hilum (hereafter referred to as hilar cholangiocarcinomas), 20% to 30% in the distal lower biliary tract (distal cholangiocarcinomas), 10% arise intrahepatically (the so-called peripheral or intrahepatic cholangiocarcinomas), and less than 10% develop in a diffuse or multifocal manner. Because of their anatomic differences, these subtypes are associated with distinct patterns of clinical presentation and require distinct strategies for surgical resection. As is the case with gallbladder cancer, the majority of patients with cholangiocarcinoma present with advanced disease that is not amenable to surgical resection; as a result, most patients die within 6 to 12 months of diagnosis from hepatic insufficiency or cholangitis. However, also like gallbladder cancer, improvements in diagnosis and surgical technique have recently given rise to new optimism in their management.

EPIDEMIOLOGY

In the United States, cholangiocarcinoma is more common among Native Americans and Japanese Americans. Most patients are diagnosed after the age of 65, with a peak incidence occurring during the eighth decade of life. Unlike gallbladder cancer, men appear to have cholangiocarcinoma slightly more frequently than women. Known risk factors include primary sclerosing cholangitis, choledochal cyst disease, prior operative transduodenal sphincteroplasty, chronic biliary parasitic infestation, and numerous teratogens, including thorotrast, asbestos, dioxin, and nitrosamines.

PATHOLOGY

Intrahepatic Cholangiocarcinoma

On gross examination, intrahepatic cholangiocarcinomas appear as scirrhous primary hepatic lesions with a nonencapsulated infiltrative pattern of growth that produces poorly defined tumor margins. Their most common histologic type is poorly differentiated adenocarcinoma; as a result, they are not uncommonly misdiagnosed as metastatic adenocarcinomas. Indeed, it is quite likely that many hepatic tumors classified as metastatic adenocarcinoma of unknown primary in the past were truly intrahepatic cholangiocarcinomas. Variants with focal areas of papillary carcinoma, signet ring cells, squamous cells, mucoepidermoid cells, and spindle cells have been described.

Hilar and Extrahepatic Cholangiocarcinoma

Extrahepatic hilar and distal cholangiocarcinomas are categorized into three macroscopic subtypes: sclerosing (the most common subtype, usually hilar in location, characterized by circumferential ductal thickening with periductal fibrosis and inflammation), nodular (firm tumors extending irregularly into the duct lumen, occasionally growing in a nodular-sclerosing pattern), and papillary (soft and friable tumors typically projecting into the duct lumen in a pedunculated fashion, usually distal in location, and associated with higher resectability and more favorable outcomes). Their pattern of growth is insidiously longitudinal, with tumor cells often extending both proximally and distally beneath normal ductal epithelium. This pattern of growth mandates careful microscopic attention to margins at the time of surgical extirpation to ensure complete tumor resection. Another pathologic feature of cholangiocarcinoma is the exuberant desmoplastic reaction that often accompanies these tumors. Histologic analysis of these tumors occasionally identifies only small foci of malignant cells within densely fibrotic stroma. This characteristic can render the analysis of needle biopsy specimens challenging and highly susceptible to sampling error.

The tendency of extrahepatic cholangiocarcinoma to occlude biliary ducts and to invade portal venous branches often results in hepatic atrophy. Gradually progressive segmental or lobar atrophy in the setting of cholangiocarcinoma is indicative of chronic biliary obstruction; comparatively rapid parenchymal atrophy is typically the result of portal obstruction.[29] Distant metastases are not uncommon, perineural and lymphovascular spread are often observed, and up to one-third of patients present with nodal metastases.

PRESENTATION

Symptoms associated with intrahepatic cholangiocarcinomas are nonspecific, including malaise and abdominal pain. Unlike hilar and distal cholangiocarcinomas, a minority of patients develop jaundice. Hilar and distal cholangiocarcinomas can present with nonspecific symptoms of pain, anorexia, and weight loss. Distal cholangiocarcinoma can be clinically indistinguishable from other periampullary neoplasms. Pruritis is a common symptom for patients with extrahepatic cholangiocarcinoma, and it typically precedes clinically apparent jaundice. It is jaundice or the presence of abnormal liver enzymes that usually prompts medical attention. It is helpful to note, however, that although most patients with hilar and distal cholangiocarcinoma ultimately develop jaundice, segmental or incomplete lobar obstruction can produce considerable hepatic atrophy without frank jaundice.

Some of the more nonspecific presenting symptoms of cholangiocarcinoma can closely resemble those associated with benign gallstone disease, and malignant biliary disease can often coexist with benign calculous disease. The level of hyperbilirubinemia can be informative in distinguishing benign from malignant biliary obstruction; benign causes of obstructive jaundice typically produce bilirubin levels ranging from 2 to 4 mg/dL (rarely exceeding 15 mg/dL), whereas biliary obstruction from cholangiocarcinoma usually results in serum bilirubin levels greater than 10 mg/dL (with a mean level of approximately 18 mg/dL).[30] On occasion, intraluminal growth of papillary cholangiocarcinomas (more common among distal tumors) can induce a physiologic ball-valve effect that produces intermittent episodes of obstructive jaundice.

Although a 30% rate of bactibilia has been observed among patients with extrahepatic cholangiocarcinoma, clinically evident cholangitis is unusual as a presenting symptom. The noteworthy variance from this observation comes from patients who undergo biliary instrumentation (either percutaneously or endoscopically), as these patients uniformly develop bactibilia and not uncommonly develop manifestations of cholangitis.

DIAGNOSIS

Cholangiocarcinomas in general are often accompanied by elevations in CA 19-9. Levels of CA 19-9 greater than 100 U/mL have been shown to correspond with the presence of cholangiocarcinoma with a sensitivity of 89% and a specificity of 86%.[31]

Intrahepatic Cholangiocarcinoma

Intrahepatic cholangiocarcinomas often appear as hypovascular masses on standard imaging techniques and can appear similar to other primary and metastatic hepatic malignancies (Figure 108-3). Ultrasonography, CT, and MRI techniques are useful in defining the anatomic relationships between the tumor and adjacent vascular and biliary systems.

Hilar Cholangiocarcinoma

Duplex ultrasonography and MRCP are the principal radiographic techniques used to image hilar cholangiocarcinoma. In experienced hands, duplex ultrasonography can provide data regarding extent of biliary ductal,

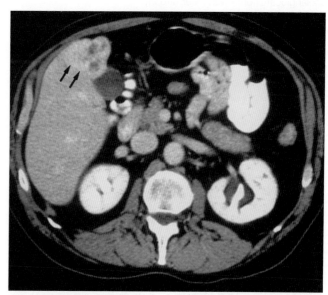

FIGURE 108-3 CT appearance of large intrahepatic cholangiocarcinoma. (From Koea J, Fong Y: Primary hepatic malignancies. In Blumgart LH, et al, editors: *Hepatobiliary cancer.* Hamilton, Ontario, 2001, BC Decker, p 59.)

periductal, and vascular involvement with a sensitivity and specificity matching or exceeding that of CT angiography (Figure 108-4).[32,33] MRCP provides an accurate assessment of biliary ductal anatomy and can evaluate distal or proximal ductal systems that are excluded by the tumor and therefore not imaged by percutaneous or endoscopic cholangiography. MRCP also avoids the biliary instrumentation (and potential infectious complications) associated with invasive cholangiography. The finding of hepatic parenchymal atrophy is indicative of biliary and/or portal venous obstruction from tumor. It is also an indication that partial hepatectomy of the atrophic segment or lobe is likely to be necessary for complete extirpation of disease (Figure 108-5).

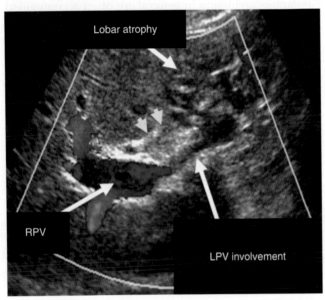

FIGURE 108-4 Ultrasonographic duplex image of hilar cholangiocarcinoma with lobar atrophy.

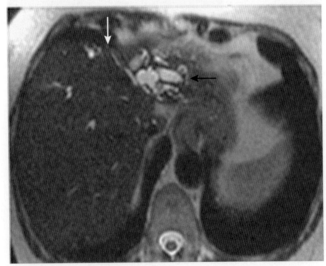

FIGURE 108-5 MRI appearance of hilar cholangiocarcinoma with lobar atrophy. Note crowded, dilated ducts (white arrow) denoting presence of small, hypoperfused left hepatic lobe (black arrow).

Distal Cholangiocarcinoma

Because of its proximity to the duodenum, the radiographic evaluation of distal cholangiocarcinoma more commonly employs endoscopic retrograde cholangiopancreatography (ERCP) and endoscopic ultrasound technology. Although the primary lesions are often too small to be visible on cross-sectional imaging, CT is useful for evaluating the extent of metastatic disease. Endoscopic brushings and biliary cytology are associated with very low diagnostic sensitivity; this, combined with their typical inaccessibility to percutaneous biopsy techniques, often requires that therapeutic intervention be undertaken for extrahepatic cholangiocarcinoma in the absence of a definitive tissue diagnosis.

STAGING

The two major conventional staging systems for cholangiocarcinoma are the Bismuth-Corlette system[34] and the AJCC TNM system (Table 108-2). The Bismuth-Corlette system is an anatomically based, surgically oriented system that is not very predictive of patient outcome. Previous iterations of the AJCC system were pathology-driven constructs that correlated poorly with surgical resectability and patient outcome. The current AJCC system appropriately differentiates hilar and intrahepatic and distal cholangiocarcinoma. Staging criteria for intrahepatic cholangiocarcinoma resemble those used for other primary hepatic tumors, and staging criteria for distal cholangiocarcinoma resemble those used for other periampullary carcinomas. Moreover, as with gallbladder cancer, the new staging systems for cholangiocarcinoma incorporate determinants of surgical resectability and outcome.

In the absence of effective chemotherapy or radiation therapy, surgical resection remains the mainstay of treatment for cholangiocarcinoma. Within this context, the ability to effect a margin-negative R0 complete resection is the best predictor of improved patient survival. A recent trend in which partial hepatectomy has been increasingly utilized in the surgical management of extrahepatic cholangiocarcinoma has largely accounted for increasing rates of R0 resection and improved survival outcomes.[35-38]

The criteria for surgical unresectability for hilar cholangiocarcinoma are listed in Box 108-1.[37] As discussed previously, the presence of hepatic segmental or hemiliver atrophy is indicative of biliary and/or portal venous obstruction, and resection of the atrophic segment or hemiliver is generally required for complete tumor removal. Therefore, the observation of portal venous or biliary obstruction contralateral to an atrophic lobe is suggestive of bilobar tumor involvement that would not be amenable to surgical resection. Importantly, these criteria have been shown to correlate strongly with surgical resectability (Table 108-3).[37] The current iteration of the AJCC staging system for hilar cholangiocarcinoma appropriately incorporates these criteria for resectability.

SURGERY

The goal of surgical therapy for cholangiocarcinoma is complete R0 resection. Complete resection has consistently proven to correlate well with survival.

TABLE 108-2 AJCC Staging System for Cholangiocarcinoma

A. HILAR CHOLANGIOCARCINOMA

T1	Tumor confined to bile duct
T2a	Tumor invades beyond bile duct wall into surrounding adipose tissue
T2b	Tumor invades beyond bile duct wall into adjacent hepatic parenchyma
T3	Tumor invades unilateral portal vein or hepatic artery
T4	Tumor invades bilateral portal veins or hepatic arteries or;
	Tumor invades second-order biliary radicles bilaterally or;
	Tumor invades second-order biliary radicles unilaterally and contralateral portal vein or hepatic artery
N0	No lymph node involvement
N1	Lymph node involvement within hepatoduodenal ligament
N2	Lymph node involvement beyond hepatoduodenal ligament
M0	No distant metastases
M1	Distant metastases
Stage I	T1 N0 M0
Stage II	T2 N0 M0
Stage IIIA	T3 N0 M0
Stage IIIB	T1-3 N1 M0
Stage IVA	T4 N0-1 M0
Stage IVB	T1-4 N2 M0
	T1-4 N0-2 M1

B. INTRAHEPATIC CHOLANGIOCARCINOMA

T1	Solitary tumor without vascular invasion
T2a	Solitary tumor with vascular invasion
T2b	Multiple tumors with or without vascular invasion
T3	Tumor directly invades local extrahepatic structures
T4	Tumor invades periductal tissues
N0	No lymph node involvement
N1	Lymph node involvement
M0	No distant metastases
M1	Distant metastases
Stage I	T1 N0 M0
Stage II	T2 N0 M0
Stage III	T3 N0 M0
Stage IVA	T4 N0 M0
	T1-4 N1 M0
Stage IVB	T1-4 N0-1 M1

C. DISTAL CHOLANGIOCARCINOMA

T1	Tumor confined to bile duct
T2	Tumor invades beyond bile duct
T3	Tumor invades the gallbladder, pancreas, duodenum, or adjacent organs without involvement of the celiac axis or superior mesenteric artery
T4	Tumor invades the celiac axis or superior mesenteric artery
N0	No lymph node involvement
N1	Lymph node involvement
M0	No distant metastases
M1	Distant metastases
Stage I	T1 N0 M0
Stage IB	T2 N0 M0
Stage IIA	T3 N0 M0
Stage IIB	T1-3 N1 M0
Stage III	T4 N0-1 M0
Stage IV	T1-4 N0-1 M1

Intrahepatic Cholangiocarcinoma

Techniques of anatomic hepatic resection for intrahepatic cholangiocarcinoma follow those employed for other hepatic malignancies. A review of the MSKCC experience with 53 patients undergoing operative intervention for intrahepatic cholangiocarcinomas demonstrated a resectability rate of 62%. Patients with disease amenable to surgical resection exhibited a median survival of 37 months and a 3-year actuarial survival of 55%; predictors of poor survival were vascular invasion, positive resection margins, and multiple tumors. Median disease-free survival for this cohort of patients

TABLE 108-3 Correlation of Tumor Extent and Resectability

Biliary Involvement	Ipsilateral Lobar Atrophy	Ipsilateral Portal Vein Involvement	Main Portal Vein Involvement	Resectability (%)
Hilus and/or unilateral bile duct	No	No	No	48
Hilus and/or unilateral bile duct	Yes	No	No	43
Hilus and/or unilateral bile duct	Yes/No	Yes	No	25
Bilateral second-order radicles	Yes/No	Yes/No	Yes	0

From Burke EC, Jarnagin WR, Hochwald SN, et al: Hilar cholangiocarcinoma: Patterns of spread, the importance of hepatic resection for curative operation, and a presurgical clinical staging system. *Ann Surg* 228:385, 1998.

BOX 108-1 Criteria for Unresectability for Cholangiocarcinoma

Medical contraindication to surgical intervention
Advanced cirrhosis/portal hypertension
Bilateral second-order biliary
Main portal vein involvement
Lobar atrophy with contralateral second-order biliary radicle involvement
Lobar atrophy with contralateral portal vein involvement
N2 nodal involvement
Distant metastases

From Burke EC, Jarnagin WR, Hochwald SN, et al: Cholangiocarcinoma: Patterns of spread, the importance of hepatic resection for curative operation, and a presurgical clinical staging system. *Ann Surg* 228:385, 1998.

was 19 months, with a 3-year disease-free survival of 22%; predictors of recurrence were multiple tumors, tumor size, and vascular invasion.[39]

Hilar Cholangiocarcinoma

A prospective evaluation of the ability of staging laparoscopy to identify patients with unresectable disease demonstrated that 14 of 56 patients with hilar cholangiocarcinoma undergoing exploratory laparoscopy at MSKCC were found to have laparoscopic evidence of unresectable disease; of the remaining 42 patients who then underwent laparotomy with curative intent, an additional 19 patients were found to have unresectable tumors for reasons not appreciated laparoscopically.[40]

Because of its propensity for longitudinal ductal spread, partial hepatectomy is often necessary in addition to extrahepatic biliary excision for complete resection of extrahepatic cholangiocarcinoma. As stated previously, review of the relevant literature suggests that the rate of negative-margin resection closely approximates the frequency with which partial hepatectomy is performed. The proximity of the caudate lobe to the hepatic hilus often mandates concomitant caudate lobectomy for hilar tumors; this is particularly evident for left-sided hilar tumors, as the major caudate lobe ducts drain into the left hepatic duct. The MSKCC institutional experience with hilar cholangiocarcinomas showed that only 50% of patients undergoing surgical intervention harbored resectable disease.[41] This number of patients with resectable disease represented only 36% of all patients evaluated at MSKCC with the diagnosis of hilar

cholangiocarcinoma.[41] Patients undergoing resection exhibited an overall median survival of 35 months; predictors of improved survival were well-differentiated tumors, negative resection margin, and the performance of a concomitant hepatic resection. The importance of obtaining negative resection margins is underscored by the observation that patients with histologically positive margins of resection demonstrated survival outcomes indistinguishable from those with locally advanced tumors undergoing operative exploration without attempted resection. It appears that the performance of partial hepatectomy at the time of resection of hilar cholangiocarcinoma is critical for optimizing outcome. Indeed, the 5-year actuarial survival among those patients undergoing partial hepatectomy was 37%, compared with 0% for those treated with bile duct excision alone. Interestingly, even within the cohort of patients who underwent complete R0 resection, the performance of partial hepatectomy conferred a statistically significant survival advantage on multivariate analysis.[41] The correlation between concomitant partial hepatectomy and improved disease-free and disease-specific survival outcomes has been confirmed in other centers as well.[38]

Distal Cholangiocarcinoma

Most distal cholangiocarcinomas will require pancreaticoduodenectomy for complete resection. A review of the MSKCC experience with distal cholangiocarcinomas demonstrated that only 13% of these tumors could be removed with bile duct excision alone.[42] As mentioned previously, distal cholangiocarcinomas are often clinically indistinguishable from other periampullary neoplasms, including pancreatic adenocarcinoma. However, distal cholangiocarcinomas are associated with less frequent lymphovascular invasion, lower margin positivity, higher resectability, and correspondingly better survival compared with pancreatic ductal adenocarcinoma.[42,43] When compared between equivalent stages and resections, there do not appear to be any meaningful survival differences between hilar and distal cholangiocarcinomas.[44]

Orthotopic Liver Transplant

Orthotopic liver transplant for cholangiocarcinoma, often done for patients with underlying primary sclerosing cholangitis, has traditionally been associated with suboptimal survival outcomes. Recently, the Mayo Clinic has demonstrated promising results among a select cohort of patients undergoing neoadjuvant chemoradiation followed by cadaveric or living donor liver transplant. In this clinical protocol, eligibility is reserved for patients with confirmed cholangiocarcinoma who are felt to have technically unresectable disease and no evidence of extrahepatic metastases. Neoadjuvant therapy begins with an initial period of EBRT with intravenous fluorouracil, followed by transcatheter iridium-based brachytherapy, then subsequent maintenance therapy with oral capecitabine. After completion of their neoadjuvant radiotherapy, all patients undergo a staging laparotomy to confirm absence of extrahepatic disease. In their experience, 29% of patients completing neoadjuvant chemoradiation were found to harbor extrahepatic disease, nullifying their continued candidacy for transplant. In a recent update of this experience, among 56 patients initiating therapy under this protocol, 28 ultimately went on to undergo liver transplant. Among this subset of patients, after a mean followup of 43 months, 1- and 5-year actuarial survival has been 88% and 82%, respectively.[45] These novel observations suggest that a highly selective subset of patients with unresectable but nonmetastatic cholangiocarcinoma may experience considerable survival benefit after orthotopic liver transplant.

ADJUVANT THERAPY

As is the case with gallbladder cancer, there have not been sufficiently large or controlled trials rigorously examining the efficacy of adjuvant chemotherapy or radiotherapy for patients undergoing resection of cholangiocarcinoma to dictate general treatment guidelines. A phase III trial examining the effect of 5-FU and mitomycin-C on 139 patients with cholangiocarcinoma demonstrated no survival benefit over surgical resection alone.[41]

PALLIATION

Palliation in the setting of unresectable cholangiocarcinoma is usually directed toward the control of refractory malignant jaundice. Palliation of jaundice is generally indicated for cases of cholangitis, intractable pruritus, or for patients in whom maximization of hepatic function is necessary before initiation of chemotherapy. Several important principles guide the manner in which biliary decompression should be undertaken. First, jaundice is typically not relieved until more than one-third of functional liver mass is effectively decompressed. Because of the propensity of advanced cholangiocarcinoma to obstruct and isolate multiple hepatic segments or lobes, this may necessitate separate drainage of more than one biliary ductal system. Second, decompression of an atrophic segment or hemiliver will not control jaundice. Third, it is possible for jaundice to develop in the absence of biliary obstruction. Portal venous obstruction or thrombosis from cholangiocarcinoma can produce rapid hepatic atrophy and dysfunction; jaundice in such patients will not be relieved by biliary decompression.

Selection of the optimal method of biliary decompression requires a careful balance between the expected duration of treatment benefit and the anticipated length of patient survival, as well as between the potential for treatment-related morbidity and patient quality of life.

Operative bypass options, which include hepaticojejunostomy for hilar cholangiocarcinoma or choledochoenterostomy for distal cholangiocarcinoma, are generally associated with high durability of patency but at the cost of high potential morbidity, mortality, and recovery time. As such, operative biliary bypass is generally reserved for patients in whom unresectability and present or impending biliary obstruction are recognized at the time of attempted surgical resection, or for patients whose expected survival exceeds 6 months. Operative bypass to the segment III ducts is particularly appealing in the setting of unresectable hilar cholangiocarcinoma because of their distance from the hepatic hilus and demonstrates an 80% patency rate at 1 year; bypass to the right anterior or posterior sectional duct can also be performed.[46] For others, percutaneously or endoscopically placed self-expanding metallic biliary stents may be preferable. Percutaneous biliary drainage is generally preferred for patients with hilar cholangiocarcinoma, whose tumors can be difficult to traverse with endoscopically placed stents. Bile duct occlusion from distal cholangiocarcinoma is ideally treated with endobiliary stenting, which can demonstrate 1-year patency rates of up to 89%.[47] Typical duration of patency for permanent metallic stents (8 to 10 months) doubles that of temporary plastic endobiliary stents (4 to 5 months).[48] There is some evidence that intraluminal brachytherapy with iridium-based radiation may prolong patency by delaying ingrowth of tumor into the lumen of the stent. However, the palliative use of intraluminal radiotherapy, even when employed in conjunction with EBRT, has not consistently shown a measurable survival benefit over that seen with biliary decompression alone.[49]

PRACTICAL MANAGEMENT OF CHOLANGIOCARCINOMA

Intrahepatic Cholangiocarcinoma

The presentation of intrahepatic cholangiocarcinoma is not dissimilar to that of other intrahepatic malignancies, and it is often difficult to distinguish cholangiocarcinoma in this setting from other histologic tumor types. The finding of an intrahepatic mass prompts an extensive diagnostic workup that can, in large part, be directed by relevant findings from the patient's history and physical examination. For example, a history of colon cancer or hepatitis might direct the diagnostic evaluation toward hepatic colorectal metastases or hepatocellular carcinoma, respectively. Otherwise, evaluation begins with measurement of tumor markers including CEA, AFP, and CA 19-9, as well as hepatitis B and C viral serologies. Colonoscopic evaluation can be used to identify primary colorectal adenocarcinoma.

Operative planning then begins with staging CT imaging of the chest, abdomen, and pelvis, including triphasic liver imaging. MR imaging can also be used to delineate the extent and anatomic relationships of the intrahepatic pathology. If these imaging studies do not indicate the presence of unresectable disease, surgical extirpation of intrahepatic cholangiocarcinoma uses standard anatomic hepatectomy techniques employed for other liver tumors.

Hilar Cholangiocarcinoma

As stated previously, hilar cholangiocarcinoma most often presents with the clinical finding of jaundice. MRCP and duplex ultrasonography are most effective in the assessment of relevant anatomy and determination of surgical resectability. Patients presenting with acute renal insufficiency or cholangitis, those with unresectable disease, or patients with medical comorbidities that preclude operative intervention, may best be treated with early biliary decompression. Effective relief of jaundice often requires drainage of multiple segments of the biliary tree, which are best identified by ultrasonography and MRCP. Percutaneous drainage generally provides the most effective means of decompression in hilar cholangiocarcinoma; external drains may subsequently be converted to internal stents and drains in a subset of patients. As outlined in Table 108-3, earlier, surgical resectability is determined by the extent of portal venous involvement, biliary radicle involvement, and lobar atrophy. Those patients who are found to harbor resectable disease should undergo operative exploration; complete extirpation will require extrahepatic biliary excision with partial hepatectomy and hepaticojejunostomy.

Distal Cholangiocarcinoma

The typical presentation of distal cholangiocarcinoma is characterized by jaundice, with radiographic evidence of distal biliary obstruction. As stated earlier, the ability to distinguish these tumors from other periampullary neoplasms can be challenging. The initial radiographic assessment should use CT or MR imaging to identify a discrete mass lesion and to determine resectability based on the relationship of the lesion to the adjacent superior mesenteric vein/portal vein confluence and superior mesenteric artery. In the absence of a radiographically demonstrable tumor, ERCP or endoscopic ultrasound (EUS) may be helpful in delineating a lesion in the region of the distal bile duct. Although unusual, patients presenting with liver insufficiency or cholangitis may benefit from early biliary decompression. For patients with resectable disease, this is best performed with temporary endobiliary stenting. Permanent metallic stents provide more durable biliary decompression for patients with technically unresectable disease. Patients with radiographic evidence of resectable distal cholangiocarcinoma are offered surgical exploration with the intention of performing pancreaticoduodenectomy.

SURGICAL TECHNIQUE FOR HILAR CHOLANGIOCARCINOMA

The technique of resection for intrahepatic cholangiocarcinoma follows standard procedures of hepatic resection (Figure 108-6). Similarly, surgical extirpation of distal cholangiocarcinoma is performed by pancreaticoduodenectomy. In this section, we will review the basic technique of surgical management of hilar cholangiocarcinoma.

If preoperative imaging demonstrates no clear evidence of unresectability, operative intervention is undertaken. In selected cases, this may begin with an initial laparoscopic inspection. Alternatively, abdominal exploration through a bilateral subcostal or right transverse incision with a midline extension to the xiphoid process is commenced. Careful visual and manual inspection is performed to identify evidence of distant or N2 nodal metastases that would preclude resection. The ligamentum teres is ligated, divided, and elevated to permit careful inspection of the liver for previously unidentified intrahepatic lesions. The lesser omentum is opened to permit careful inspection of hepatic segment I (the caudate lobe), and a Kocher maneuver is performed to inspect the retroduodenal lymph nodes. Should evidence of unresectable disease be encountered at this point, the surgical strategy turns to one of palliation of biliary obstruction by operative biliary–enteric bypass or nonoperative drainage.

If tumor resectability is confirmed, preparations are begun for possible partial hepatectomy. Low central venous pressure is maintained to minimize blood loss during hepatic parenchymal transection, and the patient is placed in a moderate Trendelenburg position for prevention of air embolism. The supraduodenal bile duct is divided and a cholecystectomy is performed in order to begin mobilization and inspection of the extrahepatic biliary system. The bile duct is dissected free from the underlying portal vein and hepatic artery in an ascending fashion toward the hepatic hilus; direct tumor invasion into the portal vein may preclude resection unless a segmental portal vein resection and reconstruction can be performed with restoration of sufficient portal venous blood flow to the liver. The course of the left hepatic duct is exposed by dividing the bridge of hepatic tissue that typically joins the bases of segments IVB and III, and the hilar plate is lowered by incising Glisson capsule along the base of segment IVB. By exposing the hepatic hilus in this fashion, the need for partial hepatectomy may be determined. If evidence of unilateral second-order biliary radicle involvement or ipsilateral portal vein involvement is detected, partial hepatectomy of the involved lobe is mandated to maximize the likelihood of a complete R0 resection. In the limited number of cases in which second-order biliary radicles are not involved and vascular involvement is absent, segmental extrahepatic bile duct excision may be sufficient.

When segmental bile duct excision can be performed, the right and left bile ducts are divided well above the proximal extent of visible tumor. In certain cases, this may require division of the bile ducts above the level of a sectoral confluence, resulting in more than two duct orifices. Biliary–enteric continuity is then reestablished by construction of a retrocolic Roux-en-Y hepaticojejunostomy. Whenever possible, separated ipsilateral sectoral ducts are first sutured close to one another so that they may be used as a single functional duct when constructing the hepaticojejunostomy. Alternatively, separated sectoral ducts can be sequentially anastomosed into a single enterotomy site. To accomplish this, a row of anterior sutures is first placed along the separated ducts. Retraction of the anterior row of sutures facilitates exposure to the posterior wall of the duct. A posterior row of sutures is then placed along the ducts and the jejunotomy, and serially tied to bring the back wall of the separated ducts into direct apposition against the back wall

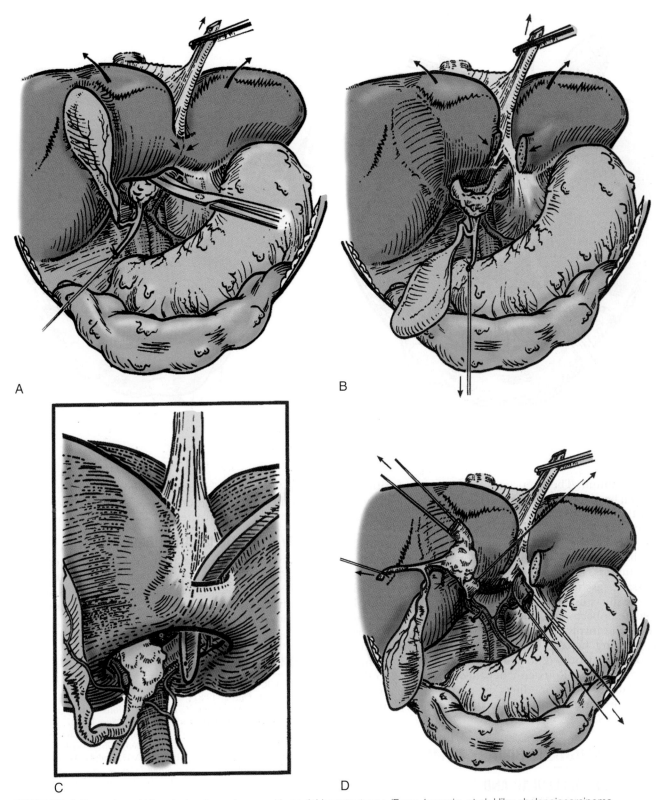

A

B

C

D

FIGURE 108-6 Resection of hilar cholangiocarcinoma with partial hepatectomy. (From Jarnagin, et al: Hilar cholangiocarcinoma. In Blumgart LH, Fong Y, editors: *Surgery of the liver and biliary tract*, UK, 2000, Saunders, p 1033.)

Continued

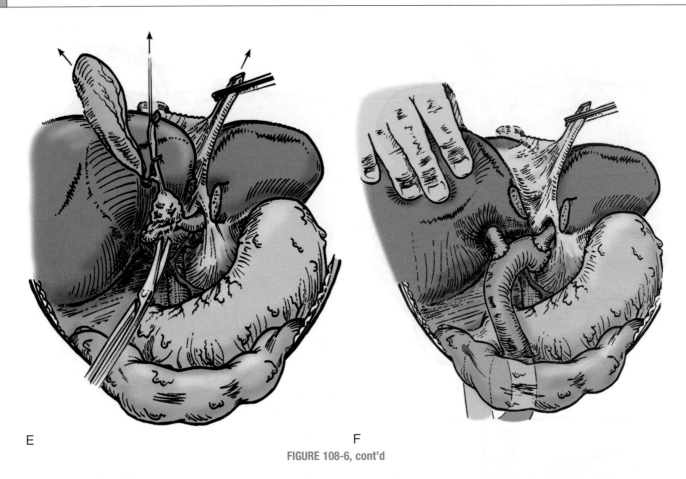

E

F

FIGURE 108-6, cont'd

of the jejunum. The preplaced anterior row of sutures can then be placed along the anterior wall of the jejunum.

In the more common situation in which partial hepatectomy is deemed to be necessary for complete resection, the liver is mobilized by dividing its peritoneal and diaphragmatic attachments. For patients with left-sided tumors, careful inspection of the caudate lobe is necessary, as involvement of the usually left-sided caudate ducts usually requires en bloc segmentectomy I (caudate lobectomy). The hepatic artery and portal vein to the involved lobe or segment are divided, as is the draining hepatic vein. Hepatic parenchymal transection is performed to complete the resection, and construction of a Roux-en-Y hepaticojejunostomy to the contralateral duct or ducts is performed. External drains are routinely placed close to the biliary–enteric anastomoses.

OTHER MALIGNANT BILIARY TUMORS

MIXED HEPATOCELLULAR AND CHOLANGIOCARCINOMA

Limited experience exists with the management of this distinct primary hepatic malignancy. These intrahepatic tumors possess histologic features of both hepatocellular carcinoma and cholangiocarcinoma. Demographics of patients with these mixed tumors appear to be more similar to those with pure intrahepatic cholangiocarcinoma than hepatocellular carcinoma. Furthermore, the

survival outcomes of patients undergoing surgical resection of these mixed tumors appear to more closely parallel those of patients treated for cholangiocarcinoma.[39]

BILIARY CYSTADENOCARCINOMA

Biliary cystadenocarcinomas are rare malignancies that are typically intrahepatic in location. The presence of an associated ovarian-like stroma in female patients appears to signify a favorable prognosis, and these lesions may arise from preexisting biliary cystadenomas.

REFERENCES

1. Boulton RA, Adams DH: Gallbladder polyps: When to wait and when to act. *Lancet* 349:817, 1997.
2. Yang HL, Sun YG, Wang Z: Polypoid lesions of the gallbladder: Diagnosis and indications for surgery. *Br J Surg* 79:227, 1992.
3. Shinkai H, Kimura W, Muto T: Surgical indications for small polypoid lesions of the gallbladder. *Am J Surg* 175:114, 1998.
4. Moerman CJ, Lagerwaard FJ, Bueno DMH, et al: Gallstone size and the risk of gallbladder cancer. *Scand J Gastroenterol* 28:482, 1993.
5. Berk RN, Armbuster TG, Saltzstein SL: Carcinoma in the porcelain gallbladder. *Radiology* 106:29, 1973.
6. Stephen AE, Berger DL: Carcinoma in the porcelain gallbladder: A relationship revisited. *Surgery* 129:699, 2001.
7. Kowalewski K, Todd EF: Carcinoma of the gallbladder induced in hamsters by insertion of cholesterol pellets and feeding dimethylnitrosamine. *Proc Soc Exp Biol Med* 136:482, 1971.
8. Boerma EJ: Towards an oncological resection of gall bladder cancer. *Eur J Surg Oncol* 20:537, 1994.
9. Hawkins WG, DeMatteo RP, Jarnagin WR, et al: Jaundice predicts advanced disease and early mortality in patients with gallbladder cancer. *Ann Surg Oncol* 11:310, 2004.

10. Strom BL, Maislin G, West SL, et al: Serum CEA and CA 19–9: Potential future diagnostic or screening tests for gallbladder cancer? *Int J Cancer* 45:821, 1990.

11. Ritts RE Jr, Nagorney DM, Jacobsen DJ, et al: Comparison of preoperative serum CA19-9 levels with results of diagnostic imaging modalities in patients undergoing laparotomy for suspected pancreatic or gallbladder disease. *Pancreas* 9:707, 1994.

12. Wibbenmeyer LA, Sharafuddin MJ, Wolverson MK, et al: Sonographic diagnosis of unsuspected gallbladder cancer: Imaging findings in comparison with benign gallbladder conditions. *Am J Roentgenol* 165:1169, 1995.

13. Kumar A, Aggarwal S: Carcinoma of the gallbladder: CT findings in 50 cases. *Abdom Imaging* 19:304, 1994.

14. Ohtani T, Shirai Y, Tsukada K, et al: Carcinoma of the gallbladder: CT evaluation of lymphatic spread. *Radiology* 189:875, 1993.

15. Akosa AB, Barker F, Desa L, et al: Cytologic diagnosis in the management of gallbladder carcinoma. *Acta Cytol* 39:494, 1995.

16. Bartlett DL, Fong Y, Fortner JG, et al: Long-term results after resection for gallbladder cancer. Implications for staging and management. *Ann Surg* 224:639, 1996.

17. Fong Y, Jarnagin W, Blumgart LH: Gallbladder cancer: Comparison of patients presenting initially for definitive operation with those presenting after prior noncurative intervention. *Ann Surg* 232:557, 2000.

18. Weber SM, DeMatteo RP, Fong Y, et al: Staging laparoscopy in patients with extrahepatic biliary carcinoma. Analysis of 100 patients. *Ann Surg* 235:392, 2002.

19. Tsukada K, Kurosaki I, Uchida K, et al: Lymph node spread from carcinoma of the gallbladder. *Cancer* 80:661, 1997.

20. Shirai Y, Yoshida K, Tsukada K, et al: Inapparent carcinoma of the gallbladder. An appraisal of a radical second operation after simple cholecystectomy. *Ann Surg* 215:326, 1992.

21. de Aretxabala X, Roa IS, Burgos LA, et al: Curative resection in potentially resectable tumours of the gallbladder. *Eur J Surg* 163:419, 1997.

22. Chijiiwa K, Tanaka M: Carcinoma of the gallbladder: An appraisal of surgical resection. *Surgery* 115:751, 1994.

23. Fong Y, Heffernan N, Blumgart LH: Gallbladder carcinoma discovered during laparoscopic cholecystectomy: Aggressive reresection is beneficial. *Cancer* 83:423, 1998.

24. Takada T, Amano H, Yasuda H, et al: Is postoperative adjuvant chemotherapy useful for gallbladder carcinoma? A phase III multicenter prospective randomized controlled trial in patients with resected pancreaticobiliary carcinoma. *Cancer* 95:1685, 2002.

25. Kresl JJ, Schild SE, Henning GT, et al: Adjuvant external beam radiation therapy with concurrent chemotherapy in the management of gallbladder carcinoma. *Int J Radiat Oncol Biol Phys* 52:167, 2002.

26. Kapoor VK, Pradeep R, Haribhakti SP, et al: Intrahepatic segment III cholangiojejunostomy in advanced carcinoma of the gallbladder. *Br J Surg* 83:1709, 1996.

27. Taal BG, Audisio RA, Bleiberg H, et al: Phase II trial of mitomycin C (MMC) in advanced gallbladder and biliary tree carcinoma. An EORTC gastrointestinal tract cancer cooperative group study. *Ann Oncol* 4:607, 1993.

28. Hadjis NS, Collier NA, Blumgart LH: Malignant masquerade at the hilum of the liver. *Br J Surg* 72:659, 1985.

29. Hadjis NS, Blumgart LH: Role of liver atrophy, hepatic resection and hepatocyte hyperplasia in the development of portal hypertension in biliary disease. *Gut* 28:1022, 1987.

30. Way LW: Biliary tract. In *Appleton and Lange's current surgical diagnosis and treatment*, ed 10. Norwalk, Conn, 1994, Appleton and Lange, p 537.

31. Nichols JC, Gores GJ, LaRusso NF, et al: Diagnostic role of serum CA 19-9 for cholangiocarcinoma in patients with primary sclerosing cholangitis. *Mayo Clin Proc* 68:874, 1993.

32. Hann LE, Greatrex KV, Bach AM, et al: Cholangiocarcinoma at the hepatic hilus: Sonographic findings. *Am J Roentgenol* 168:985, 1997.

33. Bach AM, Hann LE, Brown KT, et al: Portal vein evaluation with US: Comparison to angiography combined with CT arterial portography. *Radiology* 201:149, 1996.

34. Bismuth H, Nakache R, Diamond T: Management strategies in resection for hilar cholangiocarcinoma. *Ann Surg* 215:31, 1992.

35. Hadjis NS, Blenkharn JI, Alexander N, et al: Outcome of radical surgery in hilar cholangiocarcinoma. *Surgery* 107:597, 1990.

36. Klempnauer J, Ridder GJ, von Wasielewski R, et al: Resectional surgery of hilar cholangiocarcinoma: A multivariate analysis of prognostic factors. *J Clin Oncol* 15:947, 1997.

37. Burke EC, Jarnagin WR, Hochwald SN, et al: Hilar cholangiocarcinoma: Patterns of spread, the importance of hepatic resection for curative operation, and a presurgical clinical staging system. *Ann Surg* 228:385, 1998.

38. Ito F, Agni R, Rettammel RJ, et al: Resection of hilar cholangiocarcinoma: Concoomitant liver resection decreases hepatic recurrence. *Ann Surg* 248:273, 2008.

39. Weber SM, Jarnagin WR, Klimstra D, et al: Intrahepatic cholangiocarcinoma: Resectability, recurrence pattern, and outcomes. *J Am Coll Surg* 193:384, 2001.

40. Weber SM, DeMatteo RP, Fong Y, et al: Staging laparoscopy in patients with extrahepatic biliary carcinoma. Analysis of 100 patients. *Ann Surg* 235:392, 2002.

41. Jarnagin WR, Fong Y, DeMatteo RP, et al: Staging, resectability, and outcome in 225 patients with hilar cholangiocarcinoma. *Ann Surg* 234:507, 2001.

42. Fong Y, Blumgart LH, Lin E, et al: Outcome of treatment for distal bile duct cancer. *Br J Surg* 83:1712, 1996.

43. Yeo CJ, Sohn TA, Cameron JL, et al: Periampullary adenocarcinoma: Analysis of 5-year survivors. *Ann Surg* 227:821, 1998.

44. Nagorney DM, Donohue JH, Farnell MB, et al: Outcomes after curative resections of cholangiocarcinoma. *Arch Surg* 128:871, 1993.

45. Heimbach JK, Haddock MG, Alberts SR, et al: Transplantation for hilar cholangiocarcinoma. *Liver Transpl* 10:S65, 2004.

46. Jarnagin WR, Burke E, Powers C, et al: Intrahepatic biliary enteric bypass provides effective palliation in selected patients with malignant obstruction at the hepatic duct confluence. *Am J Surg* 175:453, 1998.

47. Becker CD, Glattli A, Maibach R, et al: Percutaneous palliation of malignant obstructive jaundice with the Wallstent endoprosthesis: Follow-up and reintervention in patients with hilar and non-hilar obstruction. *J Vasc Inter Radiol* 4:597, 1993.

48. Davids PH, Groen AK, Rauws EA, et al: Randomised trial of self-expanding metal stents versus polyethylene stents for distal malignant biliary obstruction. *Lancet* 340:1488, 1992.

49. Kuvshinoff BW, Armstrong JG, Fong Y, et al: Palliation of irresectable hilar cholangiocarcinoma with biliary drainage and radiotherapy. *Br J Surg* 82:1522, 1995.

Prevention and Management of Iatrogenic Bile Duct Injury

Clancy J. Clark | L. William Traverso

Iatrogenic bile duct injury is devastating for both the patient and surgeon. Short- and long-term morbidity is well recognized with associated biloma formation, cholangitis, sepsis, bile duct stricturing, malnutrition (from external loss of bile salts), biliary cirrhosis, or liver atrophy. In some cases, even liver transplantation may be required, and occasionally, there is mortality. Bile duct injury is the most common cause for litigation in laparoscopic gastrointestinal surgery. An increase in iatrogenic bile duct injury from 0.1% to 0.2% up to 0.4% to 0.7% paralleled the rise of laparoscopic cholecystectomy in the 1990s. Despite improvements in surgical technique, optics, and laparoscopic equipment, injury to the biliary tree remains approximately 0.4% worldwide. Successful outcomes and management of biliary injuries require a multidisciplinary team of surgeons, endoscopists, and interventional radiologists with a specific interest and expertise with biliary disease.

Injury to the biliary tree often results in a biliary fistula that must be controlled. Controlling a biliary fistula requires drainage or decompression of the biliary system. The uncontrolled biliary fistula has devastating consequences such as peritonitis, cholangitis, and sepsis. Leakage of sterile bile into the peritoneal cavity is not as important as ongoing loss of bile, secondary infections of a biloma or the biliary system, concomitant hepatic vascular injuries, or hepatic congestion caused by occlusion of the bile duct.

CLASSIFICATION OF BILE DUCT INJURIES

When presented with a bile duct injury, the first task is to define the injury. The ideal injury classification scheme should accurately describe the injury, facilitate an organized approach to managing the injury, and provide insight in the short- and long-term implications of the injury. The original classification scheme described by Bismuth in 1982 outlines five types of biliary stricture following biliary injury and with each type a specific technique of repair.[1] The Bismuth classification scheme was developed before the advent of laparoscopic cholecystectomy and focuses on the extent of healthy bile duct above the injury. To account for newly recognized injuries during the era of laparoscopic cholecystectomy, numerous classification schemes have emerged including: Siewert,[2] McMahon,[3] Strasberg,[4] Amsterdam (Bergman),[5] Neuhaus,[6] Csendes,[7] Stewart-Way,[8] Lau,[9] and Hannover (Bektas).[10]

No standard classification scheme currently exists, but most widely accepted is the Strasberg modification of the Bismuth classification system (Figure 109-1). This scheme expands the Bismuth classification system by including minor leaks from the cystic duct (type A), occlusion of a part of the biliary tree (type B), bile leakage from a duct not in communication with the common bile duct (type C), lateral injuries to the extrahepatic common bile duct (type D), and strictures and/or obstruction of the common bile duct (type E). Importantly, the Strasberg classification scheme did not include a description of vascular injuries. Bektas et al recently published the highly detailed Hannover classification scheme (Figure 109-2) that incorporates vascular injuries.[10] The five categories of the Hannover system are peripheral biliary leaks (type A), incomplete and complete occlusion of the biliary tract (type B), tangential bile duct injuries with or without vascular injury (type C), complete bile duct transection with or without vascular injury (type D), and late biliary tract stenosis (type E).

Although these classification schemes provide detailed anatomic information regarding the injury and facilitate operative planning, no current scheme describes the severity of the injury or the patient's clinical condition at time of presentation. A minor cystic duct leak can have little morbidity with endoscopic management if recognized early, but also can have significant consequences if diagnosis is delayed in an elderly patient with poor performance status. In addition to using the existing classification schemes for operative planning and cross-study comparison, it is equally important to define the patient's clinical status at time of presentation to aid in preparing the patient for subsequent interventions and predicting short- and long-term outcomes.

RISK FACTORS AND CAUSES OF BILE DUCT INJURY

The easiest way to manage a complication is prevention. Recognizing the presence of risk factors for duct injury is essential. In the classic manuscript by Way et al, an analysis of 252 laparoscopic bile duct injuries suggested that misidentification of biliary structures led to inadvertent injury.[8] The classic laparoscopic biliary injury described by Davidoff et al involves misidentification of the cystic duct as the common bile duct, ligation and division of the distal common bile duct, misidentification of the cystic artery as a hepatic artery, injury and ligation of right hepatic artery, and finally ligation and transection of the proximal common hepatic duct.[11] The ligation and transection of the extrahepatic biliary tree in two locations results in complete occlusion of the proximal bile duct and excision of a segment of the

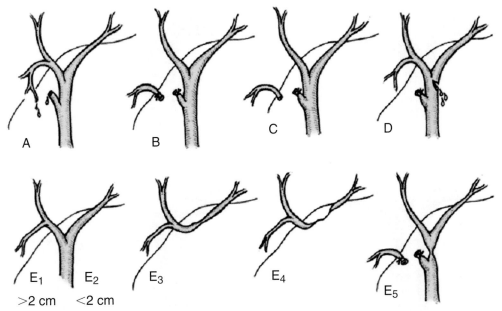

FIGURE 109-1 Strasberg bile duct injury classification scheme. (From Strasberg SM, Hertl M, Soper NJ: An analysis of the problem of biliary injury during laparoscopic cholecystectomy. *J Am Coll Surg* 180:101, 1995.)

extrahepatic bile duct. This unimaginable event is felt to be a result of heuristics, an attempt to make plausible assumptions of the available visual information.[8]

Misperception of the biliary anatomy is one explanation for iatrogenic biliary injury. Population-based studies indicate male gender, advanced age, multiple comorbidities, and inflammation of the gallbladder influence bile duct injury. Aberrant biliary anatomy will also increase the likelihood of injury. The cystic duct inserts into the common bile duct in the conventional fashion in only 83% of patients. Alternatively, the cystic duct may insert into the right hepatic duct, a right subsegmental branch, or the left side of the common bile duct. The cystic duct may be short or run parallel to the common bile duct. Complicated cholecystitis with significant inflammation, scarring, perforation, or Mirizzi syndrome will increase the risk of biliary injury. Aberrant arterial anatomy, such as a replaced right hepatic artery, may result in inadvertent injury and bleeding. Blood within the abdomen will then absorb light, worsening the operative view with the laparoscope.

Specific technical errors resulting in bile duct injury have been well described. Failure to control the retained side of the cystic duct will result in cystic duct stump leak. Such a fistula may result from inadequate clip apposition, clip "scissoring," stump necrosis, or stump "blowout" in the setting of distal bile duct obstruction from persistent or unrecognized common bile duct stone. Thermal injury with excessive or blind application of electrocautery, laser dissection, or ultrasonic scalpel can result in delayed scarring of the common bile duct. Transection of the cystic duct with cautery can lead to arcing to previously placed clips and result in thermal injury. Excessive dissection of the common bile duct may cause local ischemia and stricturing. Injudicious application of clips to control bleeding can lead to obstruction of a part of the biliary tree or the entire extrahepatic bile duct. Excessive lateral traction of the gallbladder can result

in a "tenting" injury where the bile duct is partially or completely occluded by a clip placed at the junction of the cystic duct and common bile duct.

Peripheral hepatic (gallbladder bed) leakage can result from injury to a "subvesical" duct(s). The subvesical duct, frequently misnamed the duct of Luschka, is a small accessory bile duct or group of ducts that course just within the liver parenchyma in the gallbladder fossa and drain into the right hepatic bile ductal system. The subvesical duct is present in about one-third of the population. Too deep of a dissection in the gallbladder fossa can lead to its' inadvertent injury. Identification of the appropriate dissection plane is challenging with acute cholecystitis or the contracted, intrahepatic gallbladder, and deep dissection of the gallbladder bed can lead to injury of a subvesical duct and an unexplained biloma.

Early in the 1990s several reports documented a dramatic rise in iatrogenic bile duct injury with the introduction of laparoscopic cholecystectomy. Surgeon inexperience was attributed to many of these injuries, and it was estimated that 13 cases were required to overcome the laparoscopic cholecystectomy learning curve.[12] Today, laparoscopic cholecystectomy has replaced open cholecystectomy and is an integral part of resident training. It is thus unlikely that inadequate experience and training alone contribute significantly to iatrogenic bile duct injuries.

PREVENTION OF IATROGENIC BILIARY FISTULA

Prevention of bile duct injuries begins during preoperative planning. Recognition of patient factors (older male), local factors (acute cholecystitis), and extrinsic factors (unavailability of intraoperative cholangiography [IOC]) that increase the potential for biliary injury should be identified. As outlined by Strasberg, a

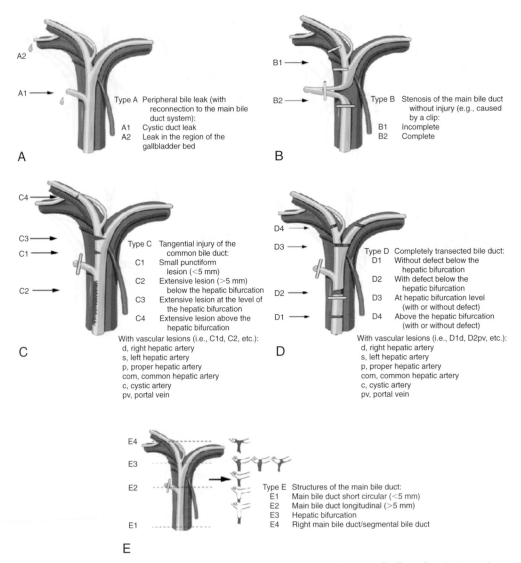

FIGURE 109-2 Hannover bile duct injury classification scheme. **A,** Type A, peripheral bile leak. **B,** Type B, bile duct obstruction. **C,** Type C, tangential bile duct injury. **D,** Type D, transected bile duct. **E,** Type E, late bile duct stenosis. Vascular injury modifiers include right hepatic artery (d), left hepatic artery (s), proper hepatic artery (p), common hepatic artery (com), cystic artery (c), and portal vein (pv). (Bektas H, Schrem H, Winny M, et al: Surgical treatment and outcome of iatrogenic bile duct lesions after cholecystectomy and the impact of different clinical classification systems. *Br J Surg* 94:1119, 2007.)

thoughtful discussion with the patient about the risk of the operation should occur and may incorporate a consent checklist highlighting the rationale for the procedure, description of the procedure, risks of the procedure, and alternative treatments.[13] Although laparoscopic cholecystectomy (as compared to open cholecystectomy) has significant benefits of less pain, shorter hospital stay, and faster return to work, it is not always appropriate. And, to enter the operating room with the attitude that conversion to an open procedure is a failure or a complication is incorrect and unsafe.

Although the elective cholecystectomy rarely needs more than an abdominal ultrasound, we should take advantage of a patient's existing imaging to identify aberrant or anomalous vascular anatomy. Contrast-enhanced, multidetector computed tomography (CT) can provide detailed information regarding hepatic arterial and venous anatomy. Even if preoperative cross-sectional imaging is not available, the surgeon should enter the

operating room knowledgeable of variant vascular and biliary anatomy (the latter which is achieved with frequent observations of normal variants seen during IOC).

Intraoperatively, four strategies are available to minimize the risk of biliary injury: (1) safe surgical technique, (2) routine use of IOC or laparoscopic ultrasonography, (3) intraoperative consultation, and (4) conversion to open procedure.

Multiple intraoperative strategies for safe dissection and identification of the biliary anatomy have been proposed including "visual cholangiography" with dissection of the cystic duct-common bile duct junction; infundibular technique; fundus-first dissection, and the "critical view." Both Hunter and Way have written detailed guidelines to optimize a safe gallbladder dissection.[8,14] The common principles of a safe surgical technique are outlined in Table 109-1.

Current recommendations for safe surgical technique are based on literature of the lower levels of evidence

TABLE 109-1	Safe Surgical Technique in Laparoscopic Cholecystectomy
Optimize visualization	Well-positioned monitor(s)
	Position patient with feet down and slightly rotated to left.
	30-degree scope
Orient and inspect	Define triangle of Calot and the cystic duct–gallbladder junction.
	Evaluate mobility of gallbladder.
	Is the gallbladder inflamed, intrahepatic?
	Decompress gallbladder if tense and difficult to grasp.
	Is the infundibulum redundant or folded?
	Evaluate liver parenchyma, e.g., cirrhosis, steatosis.
	Will hilar or hepatic-duodenal fat impair visualization of biliary anatomy?
Retract	Retract fundus toward diaphragm.
	Retract infundibulum laterally.
Dissect	Divide medial areolar tissue plane between liver and infundibulum.
	Free inferior portion of gallbladder from gallbladder fossa.
	Define cystic duct and artery.
	Minimize electrocautery dissection.
	Avoid dissection and visualization of common bile duct.
	Excessive clip application (>7) may require conversion to open procedure.
Confirm	Establish "critical view."
	(1) Only cystic duct and artery entering gallbladder.
	(2) Visualize inferior gallbladder fossa.
	Perform intraoperative cholangiogram.
Occlude and divide	Occlude cystic duct with two clips.
	Inability to cross cystic duct with clip requires reassessment of anatomy.
	Apply absorbable 0 looped suture around cystic duct if necessary.
	Clip or ligate cystic artery.
	Divide cystic duct with scissors, never with electrocautery.

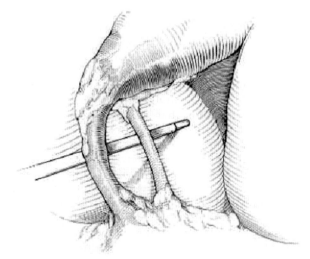

FIGURE 109-3 Critical view. Calot triangle is dissected free of all tissue except for the cystic duct and artery, and the base of the liver bed is exposed. When this view is achieved, the two structures entering the gallbladder can only be the cystic duct and artery. (From Strasberg SM, Hertl M, Soper NJ: An analysis of the problem of biliary injury during laparoscopic cholecystectomy. *J Am Coll Surg* 180:101, 1995.)

(level C recommendations—level 4 case-series studies or extrapolations from level 2 and 3 cohort or case-control studies).[15] Because iatrogenic bile duct injuries are an uncommon event, it is not practical to perform a prospective randomized trial to assess various surgical techniques used to prevent bile duct injury. To have sufficient power, the number of patients required to detect differences in outcomes would be prohibitively high. Large retrospective cohort studies at Kaiser Permanente Los Angeles and Konstantopouleio Hospital Greece have highlighted the benefit of the "critical view" technique.[16,17] Since 2006, the Dutch Society of Surgery has advised that best practices in laparoscopic cholecystectomy include establishing and documenting the "critical view."[18]

We favor recommendations outlined by Hunter[14] and Strasberg's critical view (Figure 109-3). Dissection of the fundus early in the cholecystectomy is discouraged because the fixation of the fundus to the liver facilitates elevation of the liver and exposure. Fundus-first or top-down techniques work well in open procedures because additional retractors can be safety placed on the liver without inadvertent injury to the liver parenchyma. We also discourage excessive dissection in the hilum or hepatoduodenal ligament. We routinely do not expose the common bile duct. Although this can be performed safely in most scenarios, it may result in local ischemia to the tenuous 3 and 9 o'clock anastomosing network of blood vessels leading to delayed stricture of the bile duct.

IOC and intraoperative laparoscopic ultrasound (IUS) are useful in the identification and characterization of biliary anatomy during laparoscopic cholecystectomy. Routine use of IOC in laparoscopic cholecystectomy remains debated and is currently employed based on surgeon preference. In a review by Massarweh and Flum, the arguments for and against IOC are outlined.[19] Although IOC cannot prevent a bile duct injury, it has been strongly associated with lowering the incidence of bile duct injury in large population-based studies. We are strong advocates of routine rather than selective IOC, particularly in a teaching institution. To emphasize the role of routine IOC, a metaanalysis of 40 case series representing 327,523 laparoscopic cholecystectomy operations has demonstrated that routine use of IOC decreased the rate of bile duct injury by 50%.[20] Once again several population-based studies have demonstrated that routine use of IOC is associated with fewer bile duct injuries.[21-23] Flum et al reported that after adjusting for patient-level factors, the relative risk of bile duct injury when IOC was not used was 1.51 (95% confidence interval [CI], 1.44 to 1.58).[22] Interestingly, in this same study, only 21.5% of surgeons used IOC more than 75% of the time.

Arguments against routine IOC for laparoscopic cholecystectomy include cost, longer operative time, unavailable intraoperative fluoroscopy, invasive procedure (requires a ductotomy), potential for injury of the bile duct, and misinterpretation of the cholangiogram. The cost of IOC should not be used to argue against IOC. The $122 cost of IOC is minimal compared with the $87,100 cost per common bile duct injury avoided with routine use of IOC.[22] To avoid delays and lengthening the operative time by IOC, the surgeon should use preoperative planning that includes coordination with radiology and fluoroscopy operators. Availability of intraoperative fluoroscopy should also be considered when planning elective cholecystectomy.

The value of IOC exists only if it is interpreted correctly. Way et al indicate that IOC was misinterpreted in 80% (34 of 43 patients) of bile duct injuries in which IOC was performed.[8] Routine use of IOC increases efficiency in cannulation of the cystic duct and performing an IOC. Cholangiography also teaches us the diversity of biliary anatomy and prepares us for unusual anomalies including the right subsegmental duct, diminutive biliary tree (<4 mm common bile duct), left-sided cystic duct, common wall between cystic duct and common bile duct, and the short cystic duct. The only constant feature of cholangiography is the sigmoid curve formed as the left hepatic duct becomes the common bile duct (Figure 109-4).

IUS in experienced hands may facilitate early identification of hilar anatomy such as the specific relationship of the bile duct to the portal vein and common hepatic artery. Proponents highlight that IUS does not require ductotomy and thus injure the biliary tree. Additionally, IUS does not require extensive dissection and can be performed at any point during the operation. In 2009, Machi et al reported a multiinstitutional prospective study investigating the use of IUS in the prevention of bile duct injury.[24] In 1381 patients, three patients (0.2%) had a bile duct leak from the liver bed and none had common bile duct injury. IUS was not completed in 2% of patients because of inability to identify anatomy,

unclear image of bile duct, equivocal determination of bile duct stones, or technical difficulties with equipment. Although IUS is extremely safe, it has several disadvantages. It does not replace intraoperative cholangiogram, requires special equipment, is operator dependent, and has a slow learning curve. We do not routinely use IUS, but it may become a more realistic option as the quality of transducers and monitors improves.

The final two strategies used to prevent iatrogenic bile duct injury are asking for help and converting to an open procedure. Strasberg defines "stopping rules" when performing cholecystectomy that include failure of progression of the dissection, anatomic disorientation, difficulty in visualization of the field, and inability to perform tasks of dissection with laparoscopic equipment.[13] An additional surgeon or different surgical approach provides a new perspective and decreases the likelihood of misidentifying biliary anatomy. When the dissection is difficult, bleeding pesky, view suboptimal, or anatomy uncertain, consider asking for another set of experienced surgical eyes or convert to an open procedure rather than endangering the bile duct.

PRESENTATION AND RECOGNITION OF BILE DUCT INJURY

Intraoperative recognition of bile duct injury occurs in 20% to 50% of patients. With routine use of IOC, intraoperative injury recognition is as high as 87%. In the Netherlands experience with 151 patients, 22.5% were identified intraoperatively, 41.1% in hospital, and 29.8% after discharge.[25] Unfortunately, the majority of injuries were recognized after the patient had left the operating room.

Bile duct injuries present with biliary fistula or biliary obstruction or a combination of both. Jaundice and abdominal or shoulder pain are the most common

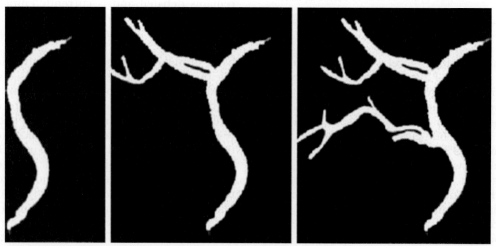

FIGURE 109-4 Sigmoid curve in cholangiography. The sigmoid curve, a constant feature of the biliary tree, is represented in the *left panel*. Then the variables of the biliary tree are added: the right hepatic duct or ducts and the cystic duct. From an actual cholangiogram, the *middle panel* adds the right hepatic duct from an anterosuperior position. Finally, in the *right panel*, a right subsegmental branch connects into the side of cystic duct. The latter anomaly is present in 4% of people. (From Traverso LW: Intraoperative cholangiography lowers the risk of bile duct injury during cholecystectomy. *Surg Endosc* 20:1659, 2006.)

symptoms at presentation followed by anorexia, failure to thrive, fever, nausea, and vomiting. Presentation within 1 week of the operation will more often be accompanied by abdominal pain, cholangitis, biloma or abscess formation, and symptoms consistent with bile leakage. Jaundice is the primary symptom in patients who present more than 1 week from their operation. The majority of patients will have abnormal liver function tests at presentation and this reaches 100% if the duct is strictured.[5] Unlike open cholecystectomy, laparoscopic injuries present earlier (median, 37 days vs. 240 days), will have more persistent biliary fistulas, and higher level injuries.[26]

EVALUATION AND MANAGEMENT OF A BILIARY FISTULA

During the first week after an operation, a patient may call with abdominal pain, nausea, and vomiting. All complaints after laparoscopic cholecystectomy should be taken seriously. The patient should be evaluated with laboratory studies (liver function tests and white blood cell count) and an abdominal ultrasound. Abnormal liver function tests, dilated common bile duct, and fluid collections in the gallbladder fossa, hepatic hilum, or Morison pouch require further evaluation with high-quality CT with intravenous contrast or magnetic resonance imaging (MRI). Magnetic resonance cholangiopancreatography (MRCP) can define the level of injury, condition of proximal and distal bile ducts, vascular involvement, hepatic injury, fluid collections, and aid in operative planning. Hepatobiliary iminodiacetic acid scan may demonstrate a biliary fistula but has limited usefulness and provides little information regarding level and extent of injury.

Once an iatrogenic bile duct injury is recognized, the patient should be cared for by a multidisciplinary team—an interventional radiologist, gastroenterologist, nutritionist, and a hepatobiliary surgeon. Injuries recognized intraoperatively may be repaired immediately. If the technical expertise is not available, a drain should be placed and the patient transferred to a tertiary referral center. If the injury is less than 72 hours, MRCP may be sufficient to define the injury, and early operative repair considered. Otherwise, the anatomy of the biliary injury must be further defined and any fistula controlled. Endoscopic retrograde cholangiopancreatography (ERCP) and percutaneous transhepatic cholangiography (PTC) are essential diagnostic modalities to define the extent and type of bile duct injury. Endoscopic and percutaneous approaches can be diagnostic and therapeutic. Endoscopic stenting is successful in 97% to 99% of patients with peripheral biliary fistula from the gallbladder bed, a subsegmental duct, or the cystic duct (Strasberg-Bismuth type A or C).

At the time of presentation, our practice is to first perform ERCP and define the distal extent of injury. Peripheral leaks, cystic duct leaks, incomplete extrahepatic bile duct transection or obstruction can be stented (preferably endoscopically) to control the fistula and manage the injury. Stents act to decompress the biliary tree and bridge the injury. Complete obstruction of the biliary tree and complete fistulae require PTC to define the proximal biliary tree, level of injury, enable decompression of the liver, and divert the bile flow.

After defining the injury, the biliary fistula must be controlled if immediate operative repair is not planned. Endoscopic stenting and/or transhepatic drainage may be sufficient. If cross-sectional imaging demonstrates a fluid collection or abscess, percutaneous drainage is indicated. This may be performed with CT or ultrasound guidance.

Vascular injuries are commonly associated with iatrogenic biliary injuries. Consequences of a vascular injury are difficult to predict. In a study of 71 injuries during open cholecystectomy, 7% had evidence of hepatic artery injury at autopsy but no evidence of hepatic atrophy.[27] In a case series reported by Gupta et al, biliary anastomotic failure occurred in 3 of 6 cases when the injury included a hepatic artery, compared with no failures in patients with no vascular injury.[28] Vascular injuries can result in ischemia at the anastomosis with early anastomotic leak or late stricture formation. Vascular injuries may also lead to liver failure, necrosis, cholangitis, and intrahepatic abscess formation. Vascular injury may warrant delay in operation as suggested by Wu et al, who wait 2 to 3 months before repair to allow for devascularized bile ducts to declare the new level of integrity.[29]

Aside from defining and controlling an iatrogenic biliary injury, the patient will need to be resuscitated and treated for secondary complications including intraabdominal infections, sepsis, and dehydration. Hepatic insufficiency and coagulopathy may develop acutely or over several weeks if the injury is not recognized or managed appropriately. Electrolyte disturbances are common and should be treated accordingly. The nutritional sequelae of prolonged loss of bile salts with percutaneous drainage of a biliary fistula should be considered. Nutritional assessment should be performed during the initial hospitalization and closely monitored during the preoperative period if surgical intervention is delayed. Adequate nutrition is the foundation for successful healing and avoidance of infection.

OPERATIVE MANAGEMENT

Stewart and Way reported that repair by the primary surgeon was successful in only 17% of patients compared with 94% success by specialty surgeons.[30] Similarly, Carroll et al found that primary surgeons were successful with repair in 27% (6 of 22) of patients compared with 79% (19 of 24) of patients treated at a tertiary referral center with expertise in bile duct repair.[31] If the primary surgeon recognizes a transection injury, the common bile duct should not be intentionally ligated in hopes that it will dilate and facilitate future identification. This maneuver results in dilation in only 10% of patients and more often leads to necrosis of the ligated bile duct and bile leakage. Tangential injuries may be repaired over a T-tube at the initial operation. End-to-end primary ductal repair will usually be unsuccessful because of tension and ischemia at the anastomosis. Cautery injuries will have a larger field of ischemic injury than initially recognized, and primary closure without stenting or T-tube may lead to late stricture formation.

Optimal timing for repair requires careful evaluation and depends highly on the patient's clinical condition, comorbidities, hepatic function, nutritional status, type of injury (biliary fistula vs. obstruction), time from injury, extent of inflammation, and presence of infection or abscess. Patients present at a median of 3 days after laparoscopic cholecystectomy (1 day to 93 weeks).[5] However, referral to a specialized center equipped to manage the biliary injury may be several weeks as in the Johns Hopkins experience (median, 21 days) and at the University of California San Francisco (mean, 20 days).[32,34]

Several studies have examined if the timing of the bile duct repair influences postoperative strictures, complications, and length of stay. Walsh et al indicate that early repair (<7 days from injury) has a higher stricture rate than delayed repair (19% vs. 8%).[34] Sahajpal et al report a high stricture rate in patients repaired between 72 hours and 6 weeks of the injury.[35] However, Stewart and Way indicate success of repair does not depend on timing of repair but rather depends on eradication of intraabdominal infection, complete preoperative cholangiography, use of a single layer end-to-side hepaticojejunostomy with fine absorbable suture, and severity of Stewart-Way injury class.[33] Our practice is to perform immediate repair if less than 72 hours from injury and the patient is clinically stable, can tolerate the operation, and has no sign of infection. Otherwise, we pursue endoscopic management and delay repair for 6 weeks, which allows for decreased inflammation, resolution of infection, and a better understanding of the level and type of injury.

Not all biliary injuries will require biliary-enteric anastomosis. Because 31% to 54% can be successfully managed with closure over a T-tube or endoscopically stented, endoscopic or percutaneous management of the injuries should be considered in some suspected bile duct injuries.[20,36] However, for major bile duct injuries, 93% will require surgical reconstruction with biliary-enteric anastomosis.

Reconstruction and repair methods include biliary bypass with Roux-en-Y hepaticojejunostomy (or rarely hepaticoduodenostomy), closure over T-tube, removal of the obstructing clip, and endoscopic or percutaneous transhepatic dilation and stenting. The level of injury, extent of inflammation, and extent of arterial injury will determine the method of repair. As previously stated for a transected bile duct, primary suture repair or end-to-end primary repair is not advisable.

When inflammation or the level of injury prohibits dissection of the biliary confluence, biliary drainage can be obtained with enteric anastomosis to the left hepatic duct (Hepp-Couinaud technique). The Mayo Clinic reported that the cumulative probability of anastomotic failure was significantly less for the Hepp-Couinaud technique than for other methods of biliary reconstruction.[37] Strasberg et al have described a modified Hepp-Couinaud technique for right-sided hepatic duct injuries.[38] This technique begins with exposure of the left hepatic duct found within the wallerian sheath. With the left hepatic duct identified, it is traced toward the right duct, which enters the liver parenchyma at segment V. The base of segment V is removed to expose the right portal pedicle and the right hepatic duct. Once the right hepatic duct is exposed, a side-to-side or end-to-side right hepaticojejunostomy can be constructed.[38]

Although Roux-en-Y hepaticojejunostomy is most commonly employed for reconstruction, end-to-side hepaticoduodenostomy is equally safe and provides ready access to the biliary anastomosis for endoscopic interventions and is a more physiologic reconstruction. No randomized trials have compared outcomes in hepaticojejunostomy versus hepaticoduodenostomy, but we have found it very useful and applicable to any transection below the bifurcation. (Note that hepaticoduodenostomy is not routinely recommended, as a leak at the anastomosis would not represent a bile-only leak.)

Late anastomotic stricture formation is well recognized and can be managed endoscopically or with a percutaneous transhepatic approach. Alternatively, a Hutson choledojejuno-cutaneous fistula (Hutson loop) can be created at the initial operation to enable postoperative evaluation of a hepaticojejunostomy. With improvements in percutaneous and endoscopic interventions to manage postoperative strictures in balloon dilation, the Hutson loop is no longer necessary.

Transanastomotic stenting at the time of reconstruction is not routinely performed. In our practice, transanastomotic stenting is most useful in small ducts (<4 mm). In a nonrandomized retrospective study by Mercado et al, stented patients had more complications (16% vs. 7%) but fewer reoperations (5% vs. 15%). However, both groups had similar outcomes at 6 months after the operation.[39] If a percutaneous transhepatic cholangiocatheter is in place, we will keep it in place above the anastomosis to allow decompression temporarily in the postoperative period. Perianastomotic drainage with closed suction drain is not routine in our practice, but is used by many following biliary-enteric anastomosis.

Liver transplant, vascular reconstruction, and major hepatic resection may be occasionally required to manage a biliary injury with concomitant arterial injury. Several reports indicate good long-term outcomes with transplantation and major hepatic resection, but the operative morbidity is significant and is likely a reflection of the severity of the injury. Laurent et al report a 61% rate of severe postoperative morbidity in 18 patients who were managed with major liver resection.[40]

POSTOPERATIVE MORBIDITY AND SURGICAL OUTCOMES

Reported overall mortality following bile duct injury ranges from 0 to 4.2%. Operative mortality for bile duct repair is approximately 1.8%. Postoperative complications occur in over 40% of patients. Complications include wound infection (8%), cholangitis (5.7%), stent-related complications (5.7%), and intraabdominal abscess or biloma (2.9%). Predictors of operative failure include history of multiple previous repairs, high-level injury involving the bifurcation, incomplete excision of scarred duct remnant, use of nonabsorbable suture, use

TABLE 109-2 Quality of Life After Bile Duct Injury

Year	Hospital	Treated with Operation	N	Followup	PCS	MCS
2001/2007	Amsterdam[45,49]	30%	82	70 mo	None/lower	Lower
2002	Johns Hopkins[46]	100%	54	59 mo	None	Lower
2004	Vanderbilt[47]	74%	50	62 mo	Lower	Lower
2004	Mayo[48]	100%	45	101 mo	None	None

MCS, Mental component scale; *None*, no difference; *PCS*, physical component scale.

of a two-layer anastomosis, and failure to eradicate infection before repair.

Although single-institution experiences suggest excellent outcomes after biliary reconstruction, stricture remains a particular concern and may present years later. Long-term followup is required to monitor for stricture. Early reintervention may prevent late complications of cholangitis and biliary hepatopathy. In long-term followup, Chapman et al reported that reintervention after hepaticojejunostomy was required in 24% of patients.[41] Metaanalysis by Ludwig et al indicate that 34.8% of patients required reintervention with a followup of 4 years after the bile duct injury.[20] The Mayo Clinic experience with reconstruction using the Hepp-Couinaud technique has resulted in 2- and 5-year stricture-free survival of 95% and 88%, respectively. Likewise, in a series of 142 patients with a median followup of 54.7 months at Johns Hopkins, 129 (90.8%) patients were sucessfully treated by a bile duct repair, 1 required a second reoperation, and 9 were successfully managed with postoperative percutaneous dilation resulting in long-term success in 98% of patients.[42]

Postoperative biliary anastomotic strictures can be managed surgically, percutaneously, and endoscopically. Our preference is to attempt endoscopic balloon dilation and stenting. In selected patients, we can expect an 89% success rate with endoscopic reintervention as demonstrated by Costamagna et al.[43] Endoscopic management will usually require three to four endoscopies with a mean of three stents exchanged over a 12-month period. Percutaneous transhepatic management of anastomotic strictures is an alternative option, with a success rate of 58.8%.[44] Early removal of these percutaneous transhepatic biliary-drainage anastomotic stents (within 4 months) predicted increased likelihood of failure and 90% of failures occurred within 2 years. Despite the success of endoscopic and percutaneous approaches to managing anastomotic strictures, patients should be advised that surgical reintervention may be required in 5% of cases.

QUALITY OF LIFE AFTER BILE DUCT INJURY

The World Health Organization in 1948 defined overall health as being "a state of complete physical, mental, and social well-being and not merely the absence of disease and infirmity." A more comprehensive assessment of overall health after bile duct injury might be to support the doctor-derived information (imaging and blood tests) with patient-derived information, that is, adding the patient's perspective of physical, mental, and social

well-being. The latter assessment has been gathered primarily by the Medical Outcomes Study 36—Item Short Form Health Survey (SF-36). This quality-of-life assessment tool obtains subjective information using 36 items in eight subscales that can be evenly divided into a Physical Component Summary (PCS) and a Mental Component Summary (MCS).

Four studies have assessed quality of life in patients requiring surgical or endoscopic intervention after bile duct injury (Table 109-2).[45-49] These studies used uncomplicated laparoscopic cholecystectomy and healthy age- and sex-matched patients as controls. Comparison between these studies is difficult because of heterogeneity in the treatment strategies, characterization of injuries, and length of followup. Biliary injuries were managed with endoscopy, Roux-en-Y hepaticojejunostomy, or Hepp-Couinaud left hepaticojejunostomy. Many classification schemes were used to define the severity of injury including Bismuth, Strasberg, and Amsterdam classifications schemes. The most significant difference in these studies was the number of "successfully" treated patients with surgery (30% to 100%).

In 2001, the Amsterdam group showed a significantly lower score ($P < 0.05$) in all eight subscales for patients with bile duct injury as compared to either the uncomplicated laparoscopic cholecystectomy or healthy matched controls. In 2007, the Amsterdam group published a correction for their 2001 report by Boerma.[49] Evidently, subscales for the bile duct injury group were calculated on a maximum range of 60 or 80 rather than 100, which made the results seem falsely lower when the bile duct injury group was compared to the control groups. Recalculation showed that two of four physical subscales (PCS) were now no longer significantly different, although all of the four mental subscales (MCS) were still significantly lower but not to the same degree. Findings of the four quality of life studies are summarized in Table 109-2.

The majority of studies indicate that bile duct injury does not result in a sustained physical impact. However, lower MCS scores for bile duct injury patients were seen in the majority of studies, suggesting that the impact of a sudden, unexpected, long-duration, and expensive injury had left its mental mark on these patients.

CONCLUSIONS

Iatrogenic bile duct injury with subsequent biliary fistula or obstruction has significant economic, legal, mental, and physical consequences. Preoperative planning, safe operative technique, routine use of IOC or intraoperative ultrasound, and application of "stopping rules" can decrease the risk of biliary injury. Early recognition and involvement of a multidisciplinary team specialized in biliary disease can result in successful long-term repair of the biliary injury. After identifying the injury with high-quality imaging (CT or MRCP), ERCP, and/or PTC, the appropriate intervention is determined. Endoscopic stenting is a viable treatment option in selected patients. Definitive repair may require biliary-enteric anastomosis. Postoperative complications are increased with hepatic artery injury, and the most common long-term complication is anastomotic stricture. Overall, patients will have good surgical outcomes if treated by a multidisciplinary team of hepatobiliary specialists, but may still have significant negative long-term psychological effects.

REFERENCES

1. Bismuth H, Majno PE: Biliary strictures: Classification based on the principles of surgical treatment. *World J Surg* 25:1241, 2001.
2. Siewert JR, Ungeheuer A, Feussner H: [Bile duct lesions in laparoscopic cholecystectomy]. *Chirurg* 65:748, 1994.
3. McMahon AJ, Fullarton G, Baxter JN, et al: Bile duct injury and bile leakage in laparoscopic cholecystectomy. *Br J Surg* 82:307, 1995.
4. Strasberg SM, Hertl M, Soper NJ: An analysis of the problem of biliary injury during laparoscopic cholecystectomy. *J Am Coll Surg* 180:101, 1995.
5. Bergman JJ, van den Brink GR, Rauws EA, et al: Treatment of bile duct lesions after laparoscopic cholecystectomy. *Gut* 38:141, 1996.
6. Neuhaus P, Schmidt SC, Hintze RE, et al: [Classification and treatment of bile duct injuries after laparoscopic cholecystectomy]. *Chirurg* 71:166, 2000.
7. Csendes A, Navarrete C, Burdiles P, et al: Treatment of common bile duct injuries during laparoscopic cholecystectomy: Endoscopic and surgical management. *World J Surg* 25:1346, 2001.
8. Way LW, Stewart L, Gantert W, et al: Causes and prevention of laparoscopic bile duct injuries: Analysis of 252 cases from a human factors and cognitive psychology perspective. *Ann Surg* 237:460, 2003.
9. Lau WY, Lai ECH, Lau SHY: Management of bile duct injury after laparoscopic cholecystectomy: A review. *Austr N Z J Surg* 80:75, 2010.
10. Bektas H, Schrem H, Winny M, et al: Surgical treatment and outcome of iatrogenic bile duct lesions after cholecystectomy and the impact of different clinical classification systems. *Br J Surg* 94:1119, 2007.
11. Davidoff AM, Pappas TN, Murray EA, et al: Mechanisms of major biliary injury during laparoscopic cholecystectomy. *Ann Surg* 215:196, 1992.
12. A prospective analysis of 1518 laparoscopic cholecystectomies. The Southern Surgeons Club. *N Engl J Med* 324:1073, 1991.
13. Strasberg SM: Biliary injury in laparoscopic surgery: Part 2. Changing the culture of cholecystectomy. *J Am Coll Surg* 201:604, 2005.
14. Hunter JG: Avoidance of bile duct injury during laparoscopic cholecystectomy. *Am J Surg* 162:71, 1991.
15. Philips B, Ball C, Sackett D, et al: Levels of evidence (March 2009). Centre for Evidence Based Medicine, Oxford University, updated 2009, p 1. Available at http://www.cebm.net/index.aspx?o=1025.
16. Avgerinos C, Kelgiorgi D, Touloumis Z, et al: One thousand laparoscopic cholecystectomies in a single surgical unit using the "critical view of safety" technique. *J Gastrointest Surg* 13:498, 2009.
17. Yegiyants S, Collins JC: Operative strategy can reduce the incidence of major bile duct injury in laparoscopic cholecystectomy. *Am Surg* 74:985, 2008.
18. Wauben LS, Goosens RH, van Eijk DJ, et al: Evaluation of protocol uniformity concerning laparoscopic cholecystectomy in the Netherlands. *World J Surg* 32:613, 2008.
19. Massarweh NN, Flum DR: Role of intraoperative cholangiography in avoiding bile duct injury. *J Am Coll Surg* 204:656, 2007.
20. Ludwig K, Bernhardt J, Steffen H, et al: Contribution of intraoperative cholangiography to incidence and outcome of common bile duct injuries during laparoscopic cholecystectomy. *Surg Endosc* 16:1098, 2002.
21. Fletcher DR, Hobbs MS, Tan P, et al: Complications of cholecystectomy: Risks of the laparoscopic approach and protective effects of operative cholangiography: A population-based study. *Ann Surg* 229:449, 1999.
22. Flum DR, Dellinger EP, Cheadle A, et al: Intraoperative cholangiography and risk of common bile duct injury during cholecystectomy. *JAMA* 289:1639, 2003.
23. Flum DR, Koepsell T, Heagerty P, et al: Common bile duct injury during laparoscopic cholecystectomy and the use of intraoperative cholangiography: Adverse outcome or preventable error? *Arch Surg* 136:1287, 2001.
24. Machi J, Johnson JO, Deziel DJ, et al: The routine use of laparoscopic ultrasound decreases bile duct injury: A multicenter study. *Surg Endosc* 23:384, 2009.
25. de Reuver PR, Grossmann I, Busch OR, et al: Referral pattern and timing of repair are risk factors for complications after reconstructive surgery for bile duct injury. *Ann Surg* 245:763, 2007.
26. Chaudhary A, Manisegran M, Chandra A, et al: How do bile duct injuries sustained during laparoscopic cholecystectomy differ from those during open cholecystectomy? *J Laparoendosc Adv Surg Tech Part A* 11:187, 2001.
27. Halasz NA: Cholecystectomy and hepatic artery injuries. *Arch Surg* 126:137, 1991.
28. Gupta N, Solomon H, Fairchild R, et al: Management and outcome of patients with combined bile duct and hepatic artery injuries. *Arch Surg* 133:176, 1998.
29. Wu YV, Linehan DC: Bile duct injuries in the era of laparoscopic cholecystectomies. *Surg Clin North Am* 90:787, 2010.
30. Stewart L, Way LW: Bile duct injuries during laparoscopic cholecystectomy. Factors that influence the results of treatment. *Arch Surg* 130:1123; discussion 1129, 1995.
31. Carroll BJ, Birth M, Phillips EH: Common bile duct injuries during laparoscopic cholecystectomy that result in litigation. *Surg Endosc* 12:310; discussion 314, 1998.
32. Sicklick JK, Camp MS, Lillemoe KD, et al: Surgical management of bile duct injuries sustained during laparoscopic cholecystectomy. *Ann Surg* 241:786, 2005.
33. Stewart L, Way LW: Laparoscopic bile duct injuries: Timing of surgical repair does not influence success rate. A multivariate analysis of factors influencing surgical outcomes. *HPB (Oxford)* 11:516, 2009.
34. Walsh RM, Henderson JM, Vogt DP, et al: Long-term outcome of biliary reconstruction for bile duct injuries from laparoscopic cholecystectomy. *Surgery* 142:450; discussion 456, 2007.
35. Sahajpal AK, Chow SC, Dixon E, et al: Bile duct injuries associated with laparoscopic cholecystectomy: Timing of repair and long-term outcomes. *Arch Surg* 145:757, 2010.
36. Karvonen J, Gullichsen R, Laine S, et al: Bile duct injuries during laparoscopic cholecystectomy: Primary and long-term results from a single institution. *Surg Endosc* 21:1069, 2007.
37. McDonald ML, Farnell MB, Nagorney DM, et al: Benign biliary strictures: Repair and outcome with a contemporary approach. *Surgery* 118:582; discussion 590, 1995.
38. Strasberg SM, Picus DD, Drebin JA: Results of a new strategy for reconstruction of biliary injuries having an isolated right-sided component. *J Gastrointest Surg* 5:266, 2001.
39. Mercado MA, Chan C, Orozco H, et al: To stent or not to stent bilioenteric anastomosis after iatrogenic injury: A dilemma not answered? *Arch Surg* 137:60, 2002.
40. Laurent A, Sauvanet A, Farges O, et al: Major hepatectomy for the treatment of complex bile duct injury. *Ann Surg* 248:77, 2008.
41. Chapman WC, Halevy A, Blumgart LH, et al: Postcholecystectomy bile duct strictures. Management and outcome in 130 patients. *Arch Surg* 130:597; discussion 602, 1995.
42. Lillemoe KD, Melton GB, Cameron JL, et al: Postoperative bile duct strictures: Management and outcome in the 1990s. *Ann Surg* 232:430, 2000.
43. Costamagna G, Pandolfi M, Mutignani M, et al: Long-term results of endoscopic management of postoperative bile duct strictures with increasing numbers of stents. *Gastrointest Endosc* 54:162, 2001.
44. Misra S, Melton GB, Geschwind JF, et al: Percutaneous management of bile duct strictures and injuries associated with laparoscopic cholecystectomy: A decade of experience. *J Am Coll Surg* 198:218, 2004.

45. Boerma D, Rauws EA, Keulemans YC, et al: Impaired quality of life 5 years after bile duct injury during laparoscopic cholecystectomy: A prospective analysis. *Ann Surg* 234:750, 2001.

46. Melton GB, Lillemoe KD, Cameron JL, et al: Major bile duct injuries associated with laparoscopic cholecystectomy: Effect of surgical repair on quality of life. *Ann Surg* 235:888, 2002.

47. Moore DE, Feurer ID, Holzman MD, et al: Long-term detrimental effect of bile duct injury on health-related quality of life. *Arch Surg* 139:476; discussion 481, 2004.

48. Sarmiento JM, Farnell MB, Nagorney DM, et al: Quality-of-life assessment of surgical reconstruction after laparoscopic cholecystectomy-induced bile duct injuries: What happens at 5 years and beyond? *Arch Surg* 139:483; discussion 488, 2004.

49. de Reuver PR, Sprangers MA, Gouma DJ: Quality of life in bile duct injury patients. *Ann Surg* 246:161, 2007.

Biliary Atresia, Biliary Hypoplasia, and Choledochal Cyst

Stephen P. Dunn

Biliary atresia is a disease characterized by progressive obliterative destruction of intrahepatic and extrahepatic biliary structures.[1] It is the most common cause of direct hyperbilirubinemia in infancy and must be quickly and effectively differentiated from the numerous other causes of jaundice.[2] Early surgical intervention and appropriate postoperative medical management are necessary to prolong native liver function.[3] Ultimately, liver transplantation is required in most cases. However, the combination of early surgical intervention and hepatic transplantation has transformed the prognosis in this disease characterized as fatal in the 1960s to one in which the great majority survive with an excellent quality of life.[4,5] *Choledochal cyst* is a congenital dilation of the intrahepatic and/or extrahepatic biliary tree that can cause obstructive jaundice and cholangitis and may result in cholangiocarcinoma. It is commonly recognized now on antenatal ultrasound imaging, and early intervention is effective.[6] *Biliary hypoplasia* is the liver biopsy finding of a paucity of interlobular bile ducts and is most common as a component of Alagille syndrome.[7,8] Many of these patients may have serious cardiac anomalies as well as growth deficiency and decreased renal function. Progressive biliary cirrhosis may occur in the syndromic and nonsyndromic varieties, requiring hepatic transplantation.

DIAGNOSIS

Jaundice is common in newborns and is secondary to immature hepatic enzyme activity resulting in indirect hyperbilirubinemia. Jaundice persisting beyond the age of 2 weeks should be evaluated by fractionated bilirubin determination. Diagnostic evaluation should be initiated promptly if the direct bilirubin fraction is greater than 20% of the total.[9] Infection, especially when caused by gram-negative bacteria, may cause jaundice. Serologic testing for congenital infection, Pi typing for α_1-antitrypsin deficiency, sweat testing or genetic studies for cystic fibrosis, tests to exclude galactosemia, and tests for defects of oxidative enzyme and amino acid metabolism are included in this evaluation.[1,2] Ultrasound examination of the abdomen should be obtained early in the evaluation.[10] In biliary atresia, the gallbladder is normally shrunken, and no common bile duct is visible. A "triangle cord sign" found on ultrasound has a predictive accuracy of 95%.[11] Hepatobiliary scintigraphy with technetium 99m disofenin (hepatic iminodiacetic acid [HIDA]) with 3 to 5 days of preimaging phenobarbital administration demonstrates no intestinal excretion initially or at 24 hours.[12] Percutaneous liver biopsy is helpful. Typical

histology demonstrates intracanalicular cholestasis with proliferation of bile ducts.[9] Findings compatible with neonatal hepatitis, periportal fibrosis, and giant cell formation also may be present.

In the absence of a definitive diagnosis excluding biliary atresia, operative cholangiography must be performed and, if possible, before the age of 60 days. The patient must be prepared for definitive hepatoportoenterostomy at that time.

Choledochal cyst may be discovered on antenatal ultrasound. The cyst is subhepatic and is observed at a mean of 26.9 weeks' gestation.[13] Ultrasound is a useful method of diagnostic imaging in older children presenting with the diagnostic triad of jaundice, abdominal mass, and fever. Confirmation of the ultrasound finding may be done by HIDA testing or computed tomography with intravenous contrast. Hepatic function test results may vary depending on the degree of biliary obstruction, presence of cholangitis, and age at presentation. Pancreatitis may be a common finding at presentation and is postulated to be due to an anomalous common channel at the outflow of the biliary and pancreatic ducts.[14] This finding may be relatively common, although it has not been prominent in the cases diagnosed during the neonatal period. The pancreaticobiliary abnormality probably underlies the etiology of cystic dilation of the biliary tree and injury of the biliary epithelium. Reflux of pancreatic enzymes into the biliary tree may result in injury.[15] Hepatic fibrosis or cirrhosis may be seen in the newborn and is associated with complete obstruction of the biliary tree. Surgical intervention is beneficial in these cases.

Biliary hypoplasia is diagnosed by the findings on liver biopsy and operative cholangiography. A diminished number of interlobular bile ducts and the cholangiography findings of small intrahepatic and extrahepatic biliary structures with the presence of bile in the gallbladder at exploration are typical. The syndromic form of this disease described by Alagille includes several other important findings. These include butterfly-like vertebral arch defects, the ophthalmologic finding of posterior embryotoxon, peculiar facies, and cardiac anomalies, of which the most common is branch pulmonary artery stenosis. Renal tubular abnormalities may also be present on ultrasound. Recent work has identified the abnormal gene *JAGGED1*.[7] Testing for this abnormality is now available.

ETIOLOGY

The cause of biliary atresia remains enigmatic. Although approximately 10% of cases occur in the context of other associated anomalies suggesting a genetic basis, most occur randomly or sporadically, which is consistent with an infectious cause.[1] Animal models of biliary injury have been developed with reovirus and rotavirus as the infectious agent.[16] These agents have not been definitively implicated in biliary atresia in humans. It is suggested that exposure of antigen on biliary epithelium secondary to the consequences of infection leads to an autoimmune-type process. This hypothesis is speculative but is supported by the investigations of the inflammatory process found in biliary atresia. Of particular interest in the sporadic cases is the not-uncommon history that an affected newborn had pigmented stools initially. This history suggests the progressive nature of the biliary injury and is one of the intriguing aspects of this disease. The most common presentation of the syndromic variety of biliary atresia is within the context of heterotaxia now known as *left isomerism*. In these cases, the associated anomalies may include polysplenia; malrotation; situs inversus; interrupted inferior vena cava with azygous continuation; preduodenal portal vein; and cardiac anomalies, including heterotaxia or more severe lesions.[17]

The cause of choledochal cyst is speculative.[18] Malformation of the confluence of the biliary and pancreatic ducts with reflux of the pancreatic enzymes into the biliary tree leading to cystic degeneration is suggested.[19] Cholangiography has demonstrated this anomalous common channel in many patients with choledochal cysts. However, the common channel is not found in all cases and may be found in patients without choledochal cyst.[6] Familial association of choledochal cyst is rare but

does occur.[20] There is also an association of choledochal cyst and biliary atresia. In these cases, cystic dilation of the common bile duct is associated with fibrous obliteration of the proximal hepatic duct. This suggests that a common cause may result in either of these diseases.

The genetic abnormality underlying Alagille syndrome has been discovered during the past decade. Studies of *JAGGED1* expression patterns have shown that the associated abnormalities of Alagille syndrome are not coincidental but related to abnormalities of this gene.[7] The cause of sporadic biliary hypoplasia is not known.

CLASSIFICATION

Ohi et al[21] created an effective classification scheme for the biliary abnormalities found in biliary atresia (Figure 110-1). This scheme allows each case to be designated by the operative findings. Although this classification is important for proper case description, no correlation has been found that associates the various categories with etiology, treatment, or prognosis. The most common findings at operation are atresia at the porta hepatis (type III) with a fibrous common bile duct (subtype b) and a fibrous mass at the hepatic radicles (subgroup v). When biliary atresia was first classified, terms such as *correctable* and *uncorrectable* forms were used. These terms are misleading, as Kasai and Suzuki described their surgical procedure for the "uncorrectable" form of the disease.[22] Most patients have the uncorrectable form of the disease and are still excellent candidates for surgical therapy

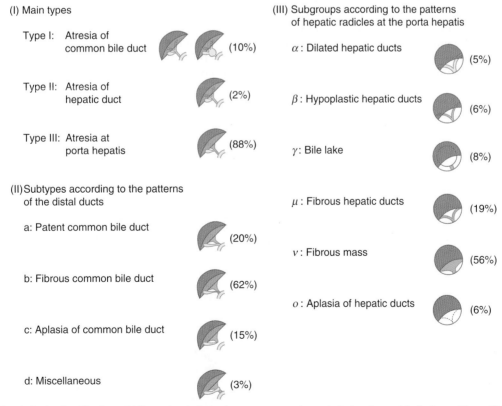

(I) Main types

Type I: Atresia of common bile duct   (10%)

Type II: Atresia of hepatic duct   (2%)

Type III: Atresia at porta hepatis   (88%)

(II) Subtypes according to the patterns of the distal ducts

a: Patent common bile duct   (20%)

b: Fibrous common bile duct   (62%)

c: Aplasia of common bile duct   (15%)

d: Miscellaneous   (3%)

(III) Subgroups according to the patterns of hepatic radicles at the porta hepatis

α : Dilated hepatic ducts   (5%)

β : Hypoplastic hepatic ducts   (6%)

γ : Bile lake   (8%)

μ : Fibrous hepatic ducts   (19%)

ν : Fibrous mass   (56%)

o : Aplasia of hepatic ducts   (6%)

FIGURE 110-1 Morphologic classification of biliary atresia based on macroscopic and cholangiographic findings. (From Ohi R, Nio M: The jaundiced infant: Biliary atresia and other obstructions. In O'Neill JA, Rowe MI, Grosfeld JA, et al, editors: *Pediatric surgery*, ed 5. St. Louis, 1998, Mosby, p 1466.)

with a high expectation of benefit if surgery is performed before 60 days of age. Nevertheless, as many as 10% of all patients never achieve bile drainage because of the damage of the intrahepatic biliary tree, and these cases are correctly identified as uncorrectable. At present, we have no way to identify these cases for whom hepatoportoenterostomy will have no merit. Increased periportal fibrosis is highly correlated with poor response to hepatoportoenterostomy.[23]

Choledochal cyst abnormalities are classified according to location of the cystic dilation of the intrahepatic and extrahepatic structures and gallbladder. The classification scheme of Todani, which is a modification of the Alonzo-Lej classification, has been widely accepted.[24] The most common is type I, which represents 85% of cases (Figure 110-2). The association of type V with hepatic fibrosis and the syndrome of polycystic kidney disease is significant. Also known as *Caroli disease*, this form may be associated with a benign course or may include progressive liver disease with portal hypertension.[25] Careful followup is required in these cases.

OPERATIVE MANAGEMENT

BILIARY ATRESIA

The operation for biliary atresia begins as a diagnostic procedure with a small incision to inspect the gallbladder and biliary tree. In the presence of a small, shrunken, or scarred gallbladder that may contain a small amount of clear fluid, further investigation is not needed. The incision is lengthened to facilitate portal dissection. If the gallbladder is of normal caliber, cholangiography is performed through the dome of the gallbladder. Flow into the duodenum may be encountered, necessitating external pressure to the distal common bile duct to facilitate flow into the proximal ductal structures. If these

structures cannot be seen, dissection of the porta is required. Presence of a fibrous extrahepatic biliary tree and, in some cases, its disruption or absence is consistent with biliary atresia. Portal dissection is facilitated by division of the fibrous remnant of the extrahepatic biliary tree near the duodenum. The fibrous remnant is then lifted off of the portal vein and separated from the hepatic artery branches. Care must be taken not to injure these vessels. The target of the dissection is the fibrous cone of tissue just anterior to the bifurcation of the right and left branches of the portal vein. Removal of the fibrous remnant between the point of entry of the portal vein branches and the hepatic parenchyma is the goal and is the highest safe point for dissection. Gentle traction on the portal vein branches has been advocated to facilitate this dissection. Small vessels from the main portal vein to the biliary plate need to be carefully ligated with fine suture to achieve an adequate dissection (Figure 110-3).

Reconstruction of bile drainage is through a hepaticojejunostomy. A Roux-en-Y limb of jejunum is formed by dividing the proximal jejunum approximately 10 cm from the ligament of Treitz. The distal end is passed through the transverse mesocolon to the area of the porta hepatis. The anastomosis of the proximal jejunum is to the side of the distal jejunum approximately 40 cm from the initial point of jejunal division. The portal reconstruction is performed using an anastomosis of the side of the Roux limb of the jejunum a few centimeters from the blind end to the tissue surrounding the biliary plate. This is usually performed with fine absorbable sutures, especially on the back or inside row with a single layer where the suture knots necessarily are on the inside of the anastomosis. The anastomosis should incorporate the entire biliary plate.

At the completion of the hepaticojejunostomy, the retrocolic tunnel and the mesenteric defects are repaired.

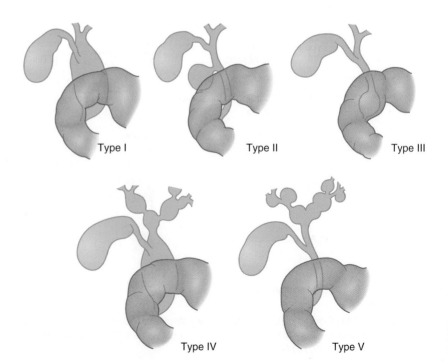

FIGURE 110-2 The five general forms of choledochal cyst that can be found on cholangiography. (From Taylor LA, Ross AJ: Abdominal masses. In Walker AW, Durie PR, Hamilton JR, et al, editors: *Pediatric gastrointestinal disease: Pathophysiology, diagnosis, management.* Philadelphia, 1991, BC Decker, p 134.)

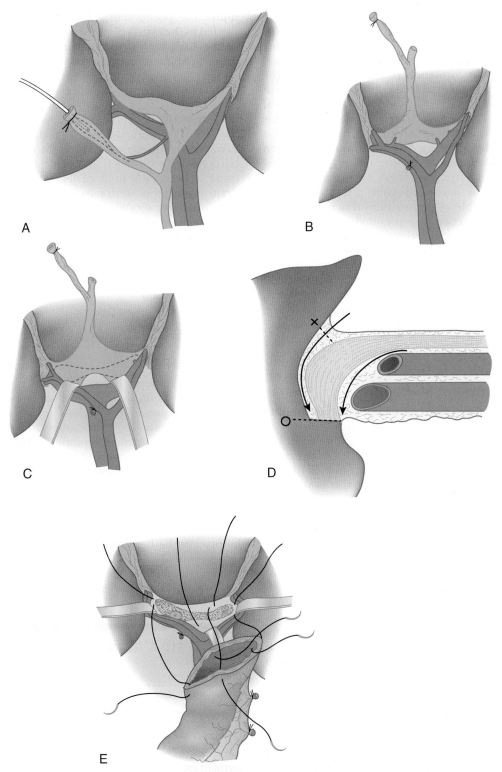

FIGURE 110-3 Sequential depiction of the dissection and reconstruction of the porta hepatis during operation for hepatoportoenterostomy: **A,** Usual finding at exploration with fibrosis of the extrahepatic biliary tree. **B,** Dissection of the fibrous duct off of the portal vein and hepatic artery. **C** and **D,** Level of transection of the fibrous remnant of the bile duct. **E,** Reconstruction of the porta in progress. (From Ohi R, Nio M: The jaundiced infant: Biliary atresia and other obstructions. In O'Neill JA, Rowe MI, Grosfeld JA, et al, editors: *Pediatric surgery*, ed 5. St. Louis, 1998, Mosby, p 1470.)

A single, closed-suction drain is placed posterior to the anastomosis, exiting through the side of the infant. A needle biopsy of the liver is always obtained at the time of operation to document the degree of hepatic fibrosis. Biliary diversion or formation of one-way valves in the Roux limb has not measurably altered the progression of this disease to biliary cirrhosis, although the incidence of cholangitis may be decreased. Heterotaxia findings may complicate the operative procedure. Placement of the initial incision should be guided by ultrasound location of the porta or palpation of the liver under general anesthesia. Malrotation may be found associated with the syndrome and may make retrocolic placement of the Roux limb impossible. Abnormalities of hepatic arterial supply and the presence of a preduodenal portal vein should be anticipated and recognized during portal dissection. Placement of the hepaticojejunostomy is guided by identification of the portal vein bifurcation.

Reports of a laparoscopic approach to hepatoportoenterostomy are found in the literature with initial favorable results.[26] These reports need to be balanced by the technical difficulty of the procedure and the learning curve associated with this approach.[27] Technical accuracy is paramount and large outcome studies of a laparoscopic approach are not available.

CHOLEDOCHAL CYST

The indication for operative intervention is the finding of the choledochal cyst. Antenatal diagnosis has led to the dilemma of the timing of operative intervention. Immediate intervention post delivery is not warranted because it does not appear to improve the benefit of later cyst excision. However, excessive delay also is not warranted because hepatic injury from cholestasis or cholangitis will be the result. Surgery during the first few weeks or months of life can be done safely by experienced surgeons and is probably the best approach. Preoperative intervention with hepatic drainage may be necessary in older patients who have cholangitis. In most cases, treatment with broad-spectrum antibiotics with good biliary penetration is effective. Surgery within a few days after the patient resolves the acute symptoms of cholangitis is usually possible. The incision should provide adequate visualization. A laparoscopic approach is supported by early results.[28] Many children who present with this condition later in life may have quite massive dilation of the choledochal cyst dissecting posteriorly to the duodenum and pancreas. Cholangiography should be performed before dissection specifically to visualize the pancreatic duct location and to identify biliary anatomy. In neonates, the choledochal cyst may not communicate with the hepatic ducts. It should be assumed that these patients have biliary atresia. The choledochal cyst should be excised and the portal dissection completed with drainage by hepatoportoenterostomy. The dissection of the choledochal cyst may be complicated by pericholedochal inflammation, edema, or portal hypertension. The goal of dissection is complete removal of the cyst up to the level of noninflamed biliary ducts, even if they are dilated. The dissection is facilitated by circumferential dissection at a level where the cyst is narrower, with division of the cyst. Care should be taken not to

injure the portal vein, which is usually posterior and medial to the cyst. A dissection plane that leaves a portion of the back wall of the cyst intact while the abnormal mucosal lining is removed has been advocated when necessary. The biliary connection to the common channel of the bile and pancreatic duct should be oversewn when present without narrowing the pancreatic duct. Proximal dissection of the choledochal cyst should proceed to the level of normal-appearing duct epithelium and may require dissection onto right or left hepatic duct branches. Reconstruction is by hepaticojejunostomy using a Roux-en-Y limb of jejunum. A closed suction drain is placed posterior to the anastomosis. Perioperative antibiotics should continue until there are no signs of bile leak or infection. In one report, long-term followup did not reveal cholangiocarcinoma in remnant abnormal ducts after primary choledochal cyst excision. Subsequent choledochojejunal stricture with symptoms of cholangitis and stone formation may occur but is relatively uncommon.[29]

POSTOPERATIVE MANAGEMENT

BILIARY ATRESIA

Bile flow is achieved in most infants who receive surgery before 60 days of life. Bile flow may be slow at first and not reach normal proportions for several months. A medical regimen of corticosteroids, ursodeoxycholic acid, and prophylactic antibiotics to prevent cholangitis appears to enhance and sustain bile flow. Enhanced bile flow is not associated with long-term avoidance of liver transplantation.[30] A recently recommended regimen is included in Table 110-1.[31] Lower doses of corticosteroid may be better tolerated and are as efficacious.[29]

Recurrence of jaundice implies cholangitis. Liver biopsy may be helpful in diagnosis, although presumptive treatment is standard practice. Systemic antibiotics and increased corticosteroids may result in improved bile flow. At one time, repeat operation was advocated for

TABLE 110-1 Medical Regimen to Prevent Cholangitis

Drug or Regimen	Dose	Duration
Methylprednisolone	Taper 10, 8, 6, 5, 4, 3, to 2 mg/kg/day	7 days
Oral prednisone and antibiotics stopped	2 mg/kg/day	8-12 wk after intravenous
ANTIBIOTICS		
Piperacillin/tazobactam	300 mg/kg/day	8-12 wk
Gentamicin	5 mg/kg/day	8-12 wk
Oral trimethoprim/ sulfathiazole and antibiotics stopped	5 mg/kg bid	Indefinite after intravenous
Ursodeoxycholic acid	10 mg/kg bid	Indefinite

From Tsuchida Y, Sato T, Sanjo K, et al: Evaluation of long-term results of Caroli's disease: Twenty-one years' observation of a family with autosomal "dominant" inheritance, and review of the literature. *Hepatogastroenterology* 42:175, 1995.

infants who had drained bile initially and subsequently became jaundiced. This treatment is no longer advocated because it has not had a high rate of success. Infants whose jaundice does not clear or those with recurrent jaundice should be referred for early evaluation for liver transplantation. The average length of survival in those infants whose total bilirubin did not decrease below 5 mg/dL after hepatoportoenterostomy was 18 months.[32] Prevention of malnutrition secondary to fat and fat-soluble vitamin malabsorption avoids unnecessary liver dysfunction, poor growth, bone disease, and coagulopathy.

CHOLEDOCHAL CYST

Excellent bile flow with normal hepatic function is the best deterrent to recurrent cholangitis. Oral antibiotic prophylaxis may be used in the first few weeks or months following operation as well as ursodeoxycholic acid, but these are probably unnecessary as long-term treatment. Annual followup with ultrasound evaluation of the liver and liver function tests may be useful as late recurrence of biliary obstruction, stone formation, and cholangitis may occur. These studies become less interesting after a few years of followup when the patient has developed no signs or symptoms of biliary tract disease.

OUTCOMES

BILIARY ATRESIA

The perioperative mortality rate is approximately 1.5% after hepatoportoenterostomy.[21] Most infants clear their jaundice if operated on before age 60 days. Approximately 35% of children may do well over time with their native liver. However, clearance of jaundice is not curative and may recur. Progression of liver disease to frank cirrhosis may occur over a number of years. Recurrent bouts of cholangitis accelerate the progression of liver disease. Almost one-third of patients have only modest or no improvement in the jaundice after hepatoportoenterostomy. Liver disease progression in these infants is rapid. Liver transplantation is the next line of therapy for the jaundiced child and for those with the sequelae of progressive liver disease.[33]

CHOLEDOCHAL CYST

Generally, outcomes are excellent with a low operative mortality except in the smallest infants.[21] Late recurrence of cholangitis or stone formation may be found, requiring further operative therapy. Cholangiocarcinoma is extremely rare in those treated with cyst excision.[29,34]

LIVER TRANSPLANTATION

Biliary atresia is the most common indication for liver transplantation in children.[5] Most children with biliary atresia require transplantation at some time in their lives because of the progression of liver disease. Transplantation may be required in infancy because of the inability to obtain bile drainage with hepatoportoenterostomy or at the time of initial diagnosis if end-stage liver disease is present. Indications for transplantation are persistent cholangitis, gastrointestinal bleeding from esophageal varices, uncontrolled ascites, and declining synthetic function. Most challenging for the child facing liver transplantation is the inadequacy of the donor organ pool. Segmental transplantation from cadaveric or live donors can meet this need but is neither universally practiced nor possible without the cooperation of adult transplant surgeons. Sadly, the majority of adult donor organs are not split (i.e., separated) into two useable donor grafts suitable for both a child and an adult. Deaths while on the waiting list may be as high as 10% in the youngest age group. Liver transplantation, whether prior to or after hepatoportoenterostomy, is straightforward, although technically challenging. Biliary drainage is by choledochojejunostomy to a Roux-en-Y limb of jejunum. Hepatic artery and portal vein anastomoses are facilitated by operating loupes or microscope. Patient and graft survival rates are excellent. More than 90% of children are alive at 1 year, and of those, most are alive at 10 years.[35]

REFERENCES

1. Kobayashi H, Stringer MD: Biliary atresia. *Semin Neonatol* 8:383, 2003.
2. Suchy FJ: Clinical problems with developmental anomalies of the biliary tract. *Semin Gastrointest Dis* 14:156, 2003.
3. Ohi R: Surgery for biliary atresia. *Liver* 21:175, 2001.
4. Ohi JB, deVille DE, de Goyet J, et al: Sequential treatment of biliary atresia with Kasai portoenterotomy and liver transplantation: A review. *Hepatology* 20:41, 1994.
5. Ryckman FC, Alonso MH, Bucuvalas JC, et al: Biliary atresia: Surgical management and treatment options as they relate to outcome. *Liver Transpl Surg* 4(5 Suppl 1):S24, 1998.
6. Miyano T, Yamataka A: Choledochal cysts. *Curr Opin Pediatr* 9:283, 1977.
7. Hadchouel M: Alagille syndrome. *Indian J Pediatr* 69:815, 2002.
8. Alagille D, Estrada A, Hadchouel M, et al: Syndromatic paucity of interlobal bile ducts (Alagille syndrome or arteriohepatic hypoplasia): Review of 80 cases. *J Pediatr* 110:195, 1987.
9. Balistreri WF: Neonatal cholestasis. *J Pediatr* 106:171, 1985.
10. Gubernick JA, Rosenberg HK, Ilaslan H, et al: US approach to jaundice in infants and children. *Radiographics* 20:173, 2000.
11. Park WH, Choi SO, Lee HJ: Technical innovation for noninvasive and early diagnosis of biliary atresia: The ultrasonographic "triangular cord" sign. *J Hepatobiliary Pancreat Surg* 8:337, 2001.
12. Ohi R, Klingensmith WC III, Lilly JR: Diagnosis of hepatobiliary disease in infants and children with Tc-99m-diethyl-IDA imaging. *Clin Nucl Med* 6:297, 1981.
13. Lugo-Vicente HL: Prenatally diagnosed choledochal cysts: Observation or early surgery? *J Pediatr Surg* 30:1288, 1995.
14. Lipsett PA, Pitt HA: Surgical treatment of choledochal cysts. *J Hepatobiliary Pancreat Surg* 10:352, 2003.
15. Okada A, Hasegawa T, Oguchi Y, et al: Recent advances in pathophysiology and surgical treatment of congenital dilatation of the bile duct. *J Hepatobiliary Pancreat Surg* 9:342, 2002.
16. Sokol RJ, Mack C: Etiopathogenesis of biliary atresia. *Semin Liver Dis* 21:517, 2001.
17. Chandra RS: Biliary atresia and other structural anomalies in congenital polysplenia syndrome. *J Pediatr* 85:649, 1974.
18. Landing BH: Consideration of the pathogenesis of neonatal hepatitis, biliary atresia and choledochal cyst: The concept of infantile obstructive cholangiopathy. *Prog Pediatr Surg* 6:113, 1974.
19. Miyano T, Suruga K, Suda K: Abnormal choledocho-pancreatico-ductal junction related to etiology of infantile obstructive jaundice diseases. *J Pediatr Surg* 14:16, 1980.
20. Iwata F, Uchida A, Miyaki T, et al: Familial occurrence of congenital bile duct cysts. *J Gastroenterol Hepatol* 13:316, 1998.
21. Ohi R, Nio M: The jaundiced infant: Biliary atresia and other obstructions. In O'Neill JA, Rowe MI, Grosfeld JL, et al, editors: *Pediatric surgery*, ed 5. St. Louis, 1998, Mosby, p 1465.

22. Kasai M, Suzuki S: A new operation for "non-correctable" biliary atresia: Hepatic portoenterostomy. *Shujyutsu* 13:733, 1959.

23. Pape L, Olsson K, Peterson C, et al: Prognostic value of computerized quantification of liver fibrosis in children with biliary atresia. *Liver Transpl* 15:876, 2009.

24. Todani T, Watanabe Y, Narusue M, et al: Congenital bile duct cysts: Classification, operative procedures, and review of 37 cases including cancer arising from choledochal cyst. *Am J Surg* 134:263, 1977.

25. Tsuchida Y, Sato T, Sanjo K, et al: Evaluation of long-term results of Caroli's disease: Twenty-one years' observation of a family with autosomal "dominant" inheritance, and review of the literature. *Hepatogastroenterology* 42:175, 1995.

26. Liu SL, Li L, Cheng W, et al: Laparoscopic hepatojejunostomy for biliary atresia. *J Laparoendosc Adv Surg Tech A* (Suppl 1):S31, 2009.

27. Wong KK, Chung PH, Chau KL, et al: Should open Kasai portoenterostomy be performed for biliary atresia in the era of laparoscopy? *Pediatric Surg Int* 24:931, 2008.

28. Nguyen TL, Hieu PD, Dung LA, et al: Laparoscopic repair for choledochal cyst: Lessons learned from 190 cases. *J Pediatr Surg* 45:540, 2010.

29. Ishibashi T, Kasahara K, Yasuda Y, et al: Malignant change in the biliary tract after excision of choledochal cyst. *Br J Surg* 84:1687, 1997.

30. Davenport M, Stringer MD, Tizzard SA, et al: Randomized, double-blind, placebo-controlled trial of corticosteroids after Kasai portoenterostomy for biliary atresia. *Hepatology* 46:1821, 2007.

31. Meyers RL, Book LS, O'Gorman MA, et al: High-dose steroids, ursodeoxycholic acid, and chronic intravenous antibiotics improve bile flow after Kasai procedure in infants with biliary atresia. *J Pediatr Surg* 38:406, 2003.

32. Kasai M, Mochizuki I, Ohkohchi N, et al: Surgical limitation for biliary atresia: Indication for liver transplantation. *J Pediatr Surg* 24:851, 1989.

33. Ohi R: Biliary atresia: A surgical perspective. *Clin Liver Dis* 4:779, 2000.

34. Dabbas N, Davenport M: Congenital choledochal formation: Not just a problem for children. *Ann R Coll Surg Engl* 91:100, 2009.

35. Colombani P, Dunn S, Harmon W, et al: SRTR report on the state of transplantation. Pediatric transplantation. *Am J Transpl* 3(Suppl 4):53, 2003.

Cystic Disorders of the Bile Ducts

Hisami Ando | Tadahiro Takada

In 1959, Alonso-Lej[1] first classified extrahepatic bile duct cysts into the following three types: type I is congenital cystic dilation of the common bile duct (choledochal cyst) where the intrahepatic tree is usually normal; type II is a congenital diverticulum of the common bile duct and is extremely rare; type III is choledochocele, a cystic dilation of the distal segment of the common bile duct protruding into the duodenal lumen. Alonso-Lej's classification, however, did not include intrahepatic bile duct cysts or pancreaticobiliary maljunction, the abnormal union between the pancreatic and common bile duct. Todani et al[2,3] refined the classification of bile duct cysts into five types and included the concept of pancreaticobiliary maljunction. Type IV-A is a choledochal cyst associated with intrahepatic duct dilation. Type V is multiple intrahepatic duct dilations. The frequencies of the types of bile duct cyst are as follows: type I, 73%; type IV-A, 24%; type III, 1.1%; type V, 1.1%; and type II, 0.4% of patients (Figure 111-1).[4]

CHOLEDOCHAL CYST (TYPES I AND IV-A)

GENERAL DESCRIPTION OF CHOLEDOCHAL CYST

The first authentic case of choledochal cyst was reported by Douglas in 1852.[5] Choledochal cysts have generally been considered a rarity, but recently the number of cases reported in the literature has steadily increased. The incidence of choledochal cysts in Western countries is 1 in 100,000 to 190,000 live births,[6] while the incidence is higher in the Japanese population.[7] The preponderance of female patients is well known, with the female-to-male ratio being 3 or 4 to 1.[7,8] Choledochal cysts may be found at any age, but more than two-thirds of cases are diagnosed in children younger than 10 years of age, and some cases are diagnosed prenatally by ultrasonographic examinations as early as the fifteenth week of gestation.[9]

Choledochal cysts are characterized by localized dilation of the common bile duct and are associated with pancreaticobiliary maljunction (Figure 111-2). Pancreaticobiliary maljunction, which was first noted by Kozumi and Kodama[10] in an autopsy case with choledochal cyst in 1916, is a congenital anomaly defined as an abnormal union of the pancreatic and biliary ducts. This initial observation did not attract attention for many years. However, since Babbitt[11] reported the anomaly in 1969, the concept has been accepted widely.[12] Pancreaticobiliary maljunction is thought to develop as a misarrangement of the embryonic connections in the pancreaticobiliary ductal system, with the terminal bile duct joined to the second branch of the ventral pancreas.[13,14] As a consequence, the pancreaticobiliary junction is located outside the duodenal wall, where the normal sphincter does not work (Figure 111-3). This permits reflux of pancreatic juice into the biliary tree and destruction of the bile duct wall. Diagnostic criteria for pancreaticobiliary maljunction by radiography are that (1) the pancreatic duct and choledochus connect with an obviously long common channel or (2) the ducts unite in an apparently anomalous form.[15]

Choledochal cysts have been subdivided into those exhibiting cystic, cylindrical, or fusiform dilation of the common bile duct but there is no difference in symptoms, signs, complications, or surgical care among the types. Many theories have been proposed to explain the origin of bile duct dilation and can be divided into two groups: (1) that due to an obstructive factor localized at the junction of the choledochus with the duodenum as an abnormal angularity or congenital stenosis of the terminal common bile duct and (2) that due to a condition originating in the common bile duct proper. However, the mechanism of bile duct dilation remains uncertain.

The cyst wall is usually 1 to 2 mm thick and composed mainly of a fibromuscular layer. This layer is made up of dense connective tissue that is fibrocollagenous and sometimes contains smooth muscles and elastic elements (Figure 111-4). The epithelium is sometimes lacking, but columnar epithelium is identified by gently manipulating the cyst during surgery. On rare occasion, ectopic pancreatic tissue may be found in the cyst wall.[16]

SYMPTOMS AND SIGNS

Patients with choledochal cysts, including type IV-A, most often present with nonspecific symptoms, and half of the patients appear asymptomatic, particularly adults. In children, the major clinical symptoms are recurrent abdominal pain (82%) that may occur repeatedly for several days, nausea and vomiting (66%), mild jaundice (44%), an abdominal mass (29%), and fever (29%). The simultaneous occurrence of symptoms may be explained by the disturbance in bile and pancreatic secretory flow caused by protein plugs, which resolves spontaneously, in the common channel.[17] The classic triad of abdominal pain, jaundice, and abdominal mass occurs in less than 10% of patients.

DIAGNOSIS

There are no specific laboratory tests to identify a choledochal cyst. Patients with choledochal cysts sometimes temporarily show abnormal values for serum bilirubin levels, serum amylase, and serum hepatic transaminases.

The noninvasiveness and accuracy of ultrasonography support its use as the initial investigative procedure. Ultrasonography typically shows the dilated common bile

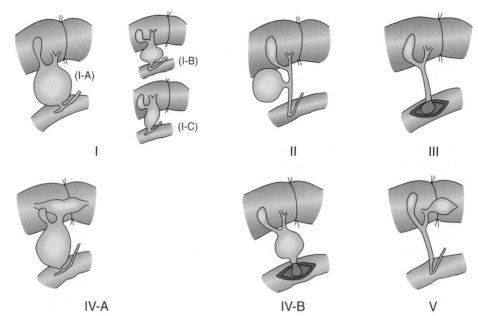

FIGURE 111-1 Classification of cystic disorders of the bile ducts. (From Todani T: Congenital choledochal dilatation: Classification, clinical features, and long-term results. *J Hepatobiliary Pancreat Surg* 4:276, 1997.)

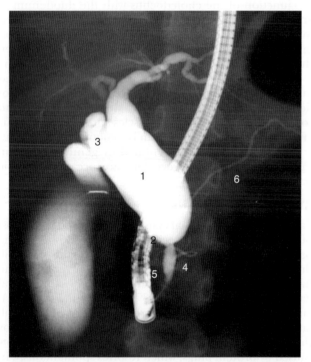

FIGURE 111-2 Endoscopic retrograde cholangiopancreatography provides characteristic images of choledochal cysts: (1) cystic dilation confined to the common bile duct, (2) stenoses at the lower portion of the cyst, (3) dilated cystic duct, (4) abnormal junction of the pancreatic and bile ducts away from the papilla, (5) dilated common channel, and (6) normal dorsal pancreatic duct.

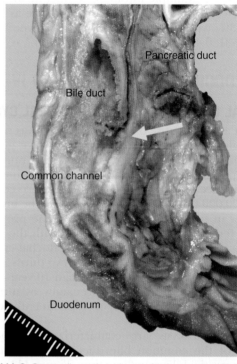

FIGURE 111-3 Gross dissection shows the long common channel and pancreaticobiliary junction *(arrow)* in the extraduodenal region.

duct. Biliary sludge or stones within the cyst also can be identified in some cases. Focal thickening of the cyst wall raises the suspicion of carcinoma.

Endoscopic retrograde cholangiopancreatography (ERCP) gives an excellent visualization of the cyst, duct anatomy, and pancreaticobiliary maljunction (see Figure 111-2). This examination is important in order to avoid intraoperative injury of the pancreatic duct and to recognize protein plugs within the common channel. However, ERCP is invasive and associated with a small risk of complications such as ERCP-induced pancreatitis and must be performed under general anesthesia in children. In adults, ERCP has been used less frequently in recent years.

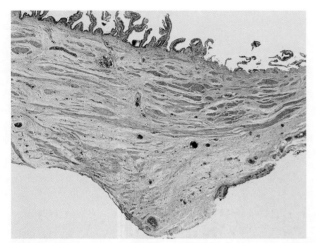

FIGURE 111-4 Hematoxylin-eosin section shows numerous smooth muscle bundles in the lower part of the choledochal cyst wall.

Magnetic resonance cholangiopancreatography (MRCP) provides a noninvasive method to assess the extrahepatic biliary tree and is an attractive alternative to ERCP.[18] However, MRCP can be hindered by the technical difficulty of children holding their breath.[19]

Computed tomography (CT) combined with intravenous cholangiography is useful for the demonstration of a cyst or postoperative evaluation for intrahepatic bile ducts and bilioenteric anastomoses. Helical CT cholangiography is useful for identifying the anastomotic site of hepaticojejunostomy and hepatic ductal stenosis in postoperative followup.[19]

COMPLICATIONS

Stones

Stones are the most frequent complication associated with choledochal cysts. The prevalence of intracystic stones ranges from 11% in children to 41% in adults, with the stone site being cholecystolithiasis in 11%, choledocholithiasis in 21%, and hepatolithiasis in 7% of cases.[20]

Protein Plug

The association of pancreatitis with choledochal cysts is well recognized. A history of clinical pancreatitis is present in nearly 30% of patients.[8] The pattern of pancreatitis can be acute, relapsing, or mild and may be caused by protein plug impaction within the common channel or bile duct, where the plug acts like a ball-valve, producing a transient and abrupt elevation in the intraluminal pressure in both the bile and pancreatic ducts (Figure 111-5).[17]

Spontaneous Perforation of the Bile Duct

Spontaneous perforation of the bile duct is a relatively rare complication of choledochal cysts and has been found in 26 (1.8%) of 1433 patients with choledochal cysts reported in the Japanese literature.[7] Most patients are children, with 60% being younger than 1 year of age. Clinical symptoms and signs are abdominal distention, pain, nausea, vomiting, fever, jaundice, and light-colored stool. Preoperative laboratory investigations show

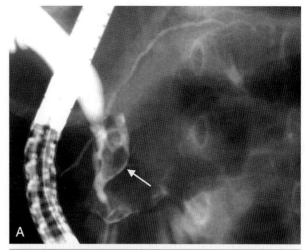
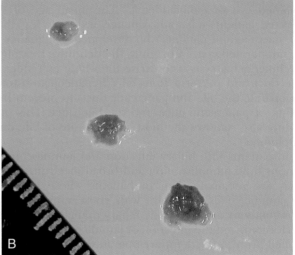

FIGURE 111-5 A, Protein plugs present at the common channel *(arrow).* **B,** The plugs consist mainly of protein, and most are soluble.

elevated white blood count and serum bilirubin levels, serum amylase, and transaminases. Preoperative diagnosis is based on the examination of samples of biliary fluid obtained by paracentesis. An abdominal ultrasound examination, biliary radionuclide scan, or MRCP can be used to make a rapid diagnosis.[21] Perforation of the bile duct occurs as a small, punched-out hole and although found mainly in the anterior aspect, can be found in any part of the cyst. In many cases, cholangiography reveals the presence of protein plugs.[22]

Carcinoma

The association of bile duct carcinoma with choledochal cysts was first reported in 1944.[23] Tumors may develop anywhere within the intrahepatic and extrahepatic bile ducts, but more than one-half occur within the cyst itself. The incidence of hepatobiliary malignancies associated with choledochal cysts ranges from 3.2% to 39.4%.[7,24,25] Malignant degeneration according to age at initial operation has also been reported, and it has been estimated that the risk of cancer in patients who had choledochal cyst diagnosed in the first decade is 0.7%, whereas in those who had choledochal cyst diagnosed at 11 to 20 years of age and at more than 20 years of age it is 6.8% and 14.3%, respectively.[26] The youngest reported patient with primary adenocarcinoma associated with a choledochal cyst was an 3-year-old boy.[27] The pancreaticobiliary maljunction results in free reflux of pancreatic juice into the bile duct and inflammatory changes in the epithelium of the bile duct, and may be a key factor in the pathogenesis of malignant changes in cysts.[28]

SURGICAL MANAGEMENT

General Treatment Before Operation

Historically, internal drainage by cystenterostomy was performed as the standard operation for choledochal cysts. However, internal drainage, particularly cystoduodenostomy, increased the frequency of cholangitis, biliary stones, and the risk of malignant changes in the retained cyst or gallbladder.[29,30] The mean age of the affected patients was approximately a decade less than the mean age of patients who developed malignancy in an unoperated cyst.[29] Currently, the definitive treatment of choledochal cysts is to excise the whole extrahepatic bile duct and perform Roux-en-Y hepaticojejunostomy to separate the bile and pancreatic ducts to prevent free reflux of pancreatic juice into the bile duct. This procedure also removes the most common site of bile duct carcinoma.

In patients with biliary infection and jaundice, intravenous fluid administration and broad-spectrum antibiotics are recommended. In patients whose infection or jaundice fails to resolve with conservative therapy, percutaneous or endoscopic biliary drainage should be performed, and the infection or jaundice should be controlled prior to the definitive operation. In patients with spontaneous perforation of the bile duct, emergency treatment is designed to improve the patient's condition and treat the biliary peritonitis (usually by means of T-tube drainage), followed by delayed surgery once the inflammation has subsided and after the anomalous anatomy has been defined.[22]

Operative Technique

First, the gallbladder is mobilized. Intraoperative choledochoscopy via the cystic duct may be useful to exclude retained ductal stones and to biopsy the abnormal epithelium to exclude malignancy. A cholangiocatheter can be advanced through the cystic duct for bile aspiration and intraoperative cholangiography, which can be used to confirm the orientation of the pancreatic duct and check for protein plugs in the common channel or stenoses of the intrahepatic bile ducts. Dissection of the intrapancreatic cyst proceeds on the outer plane of the epicholedochal plexus, where only loose fibrous tissue exists, so as to leave the plexus with the cyst wall.[31] Further dissection should reveal that the narrow distal segment connecting the cyst and the main pancreatic duct is located not at the bottom of the cyst but almost always to the right and ventral to the cyst (Figure 111-6). Attention must be directed to the main pancreatic duct just ventral to the cyst. The distal narrow segment is ligated carefully with absorbable suture to prevent narrowing of the pancreatic duct. For patients with protein plugs stuck

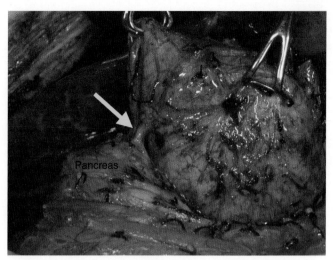

FIGURE 111-6 Operation for choledochal cyst shows the narrow segment *(arrow)* connecting the cyst and the main pancreatic duct, which is located not at the bottom of the cyst but almost always to the right and ventral to the cyst.

in the common channel, irrigation with saline solution through a thin tube placed in the common channel or removal using a blunt spoon through the narrow segment is recommended.[32] As incomplete excision of the cyst causes protein plug formation and may permit malignant change, complete cyst excision is recommended.[33]

Next, the cyst is elevated ventrally off the portal vein and mobilized proximally to the common hepatic duct. The hepatic duct near the bifurcation is transversely incised for assessment of possible stenoses at the orifice of the left and right hepatic ducts. If no stenosis is present at the hepatic ducts, the proximal cyst is transected and the cyst is removed. In patients with Todani type IV-A, stenoses are frequently found at the orifice of the left and right hepatic ducts (Figure 111-7). There are two different types of stenosis: membranous and septal (Figure 111-8).[34] When found, stenoses can be corrected by incising the hepatic ducts laterally to obtain a large anastomosis[35] or by resection.[36] Biliary reconstruction is accomplished by a 45-cm retrocolic Roux-en-Y hepaticojejunostomy.

POSTOPERATIVE COMPLICATIONS

Hepatolithiasis

Early complications can include anastomotic leakage, postoperative bleeding, acute pancreatitis, ileus, gastrointestinal bleeding, and pancreatic fistula. However, few reports on the long-term results of extrahepatic cyst excision are reported.[37] Late complications are cholangitis, intrahepatic lithiasis, and pancreatic stones. Recurrent cholangitis from anastomotic strictures occurs in 10% to 25% of patients.[3,38] The incidence of hepatolithiasis, usually occurring in Todani type IV-A, has been reported in as many as 2.7% to 10.7% of cases after long-term followup.[35,39] Although some cases do have a stricture of the anastomosis, in many other cases, especially type IV-A, calculi occur by residual stenoses near the confluence of the left and right hepatic duct.[36,38]

Carcinoma

Cyst excision has been recognized as the definitive operation for choledochal cyst; however, reports of bile duct cancer after cyst excision are gradually increasing.[7,24,40,41] Watanabe et al[24] reported 23 patients with bile duct cancer developing after cyst excision. Indeed malignant changes may occur before cyst excision or cyst enterostomy and may advance after cyst excision. Long-term followup is important, even after complete cyst excision, as the entire residual biliary tree is believed to be at increased risk for cholangiocarcinoma.

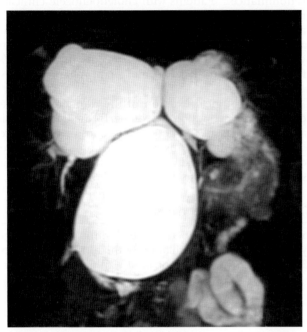

FIGURE 111-7 Magnetic resonance cholangiopancreatography shows the type IV-A choledochal cyst. Characteristics of this type are remarkable dilation of the intrahepatic bile ducts and stenoses at the hepatic hilum.

DIVERTICULUM (TYPE II)

A type II diverticulum arises laterally from the wall of the common bile duct (Figure 111-9). However, because of its rarity, experience with this type is limited.[42] In this type, the weakness factor is limited to one small area of the side of the wall. The treatment of choice is simple cyst excision, a procedure that can be performed open or laparoscopically. Type II diverticulum is not usually associated with pancreaticobiliary maljunction.

CHOLEDOCHOCELE (TYPE III)

Choledochocele is an uncommon abnormality of cystic or diverticular dilation of the terminal intramural portion of the common bile duct, first described by Wheeler in 1940.[43] The term *choledochocele* was introduced by Wheeler, who saw the analogy with congenital ureterocele. The first classification of choledochocele was proposed by Scholz et al in 1976[44] and has been classified by various authors according to this scheme. There are two different types of the internal cyst wall component. One is lined by duodenal mucosa and the other lined by bile duct mucosa. The former type suggests that the choledochocele is a congenital duodenal duplication arising near the main duodenal papilla, which communicates with the common bile duct.[45] The latter type suggests a diverticular enlargement of the terminal portion of the common bile duct.[44] In the latter type, papillary stenosis or congenital or acquired dysfunction of the sphincter of Oddi may cause obstruction of bile flow, resulting in increased pressure within the distal bile duct, which could then evaginate into the duodenum.[46] However, the etiology remains unclear in many cases.

Choledochocele can be diagnosed by duodenoscopic or cholangiographic findings, with a cystic dilation of the distal segment of the common bile duct protruding into the duodenal lumen (Figure 111-10).[47] Some controversy

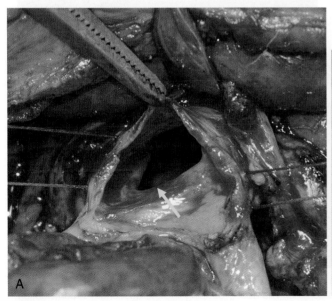

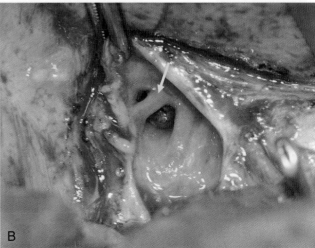

FIGURE 111-8 Two types of stenoses at the right hepatic duct are shown. **A,** The membranous stenosis is characterized by the presence of a thin wall *(arrow).* **B,** The septal stenosis *(arrow)* is characterized by a slender column of tissue.

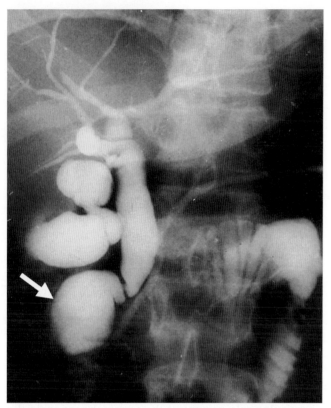

FIGURE 111-9 Endoscopic retrograde cholangiopancreatography shows type II biliary cyst, which is a saccular diverticulum of the common bile duct *(arrow).*

exists concerning the size cutoff for the diagnosis of a choledochocele. Despite the widely recognized view that other biliary cysts are truly congenital, some choledochoceles appear to be acquired. Some authors have stated that an arbitrary 1-cm dividing line may be used to differentiate between a choledochocele and a dilated common channel or normal variants.[48,49] Choledochocele usually shows a normal pancreaticobiliary junction, but is associated with pancreaticobiliary maljunction in rare cases. Patient age may range from 1 to 89 years (median, 40 years), and there appears to be no gender predominance.[45] Patients with choledochocele clinically present with intermittent episodes of upper abdominal pain accompanied by nausea and vomiting, obstructive jaundice, cholangitis, or recurrent acute pancreatitis.[44,45,49] Associated stone disease occurs in about 20% of cases, but the risk of malignant changes is extremely low.[45]

Although surgical excision of the duodenal luminal portion of the cyst wall has been performed, endoscopic papillotomy has been increasingly chosen as the preferred treatment for this type. Asymptomatic choledochoceles, incidentally identified during ERCP examinations, are best left alone and observed.[45]

CAROLI DISEASE (TYPE V)

In 1958, Caroli described a disease entity characterized by (1) segmental cystic dilation of the intrahepatic ducts; (2) increased incidence of biliary lithiasis, cholangitis,

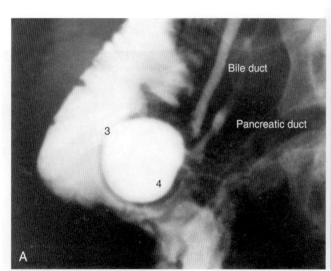

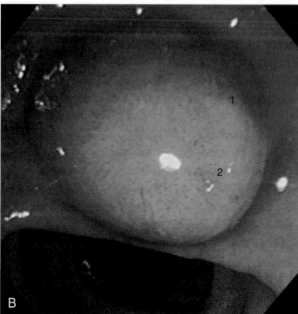

FIGURE 111-10 Endoscopic retrograde cholangiopancreatography **(A)** and endoscopy **(B)** shows characteristic images of a type III choledochal cyst or choledochocele: (1) an intramural segment of the common bile duct protruding into the duodenum in continuation with an enlarged papilla with a spherical shape; (2) soft overlying mucosa with a smooth appearance; (3) ballooning of the papilla during contrast injection; and (4) a rather spherical, cystlike, contrast-filled structure in continuity with the terminal common bile duct.

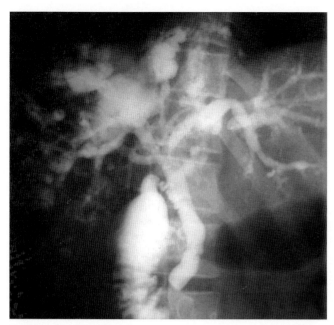

FIGURE 111-11 Endoscopic retrograde cholangiopancreatography shows Caroli disease, with multiple communicating sacculi of the intrahepatic biliary tree. The sacculi are large and are distributed within the right lobe.

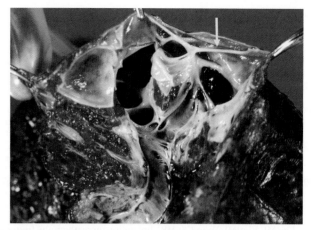

FIGURE 111-12 Gross pathology sections of the liver in Caroli disease show multiple saccular dilations of the intrahepatic bile ducts and black-pigmented calcium bilirubinate stones. Septum-like fibrovascular bundles *(arrow)* are seen on the walls of the cut sacculi.

and abscesses; (3) absence of cirrhosis and portal hypertension; and (4) association of renal tubular ectasia or similar renal cystic disease. Still later, Caroli[50] recognized two entities: a "simple" type and a "periportal fibrosis" type. The so-called simple or pure type, originally described in 1958, is a very rare congenital abnormality, whereas the more common type is associated with congenital hepatic fibrosis, which is present in childhood.[51] However, as a term, *Caroli disease* has been applied broadly to describe patients with segmentally ectatic appearance of the intrahepatic bile ducts, identical to that seen in intrahepatic involvement of the choledochal cyst.

Caroli disease is generally considered autosomal recessive, but there are some cases of autosomal dominant inheritance.[52] The male-to-female ratio is 3 to 2, and the age at diagnosis ranges between 1 and 60 years (median, 25 years).[52] Symptoms include cholangitis (64%), portal hypertension (22%), and abdominal pain in the right upper quadrant (18%).[52,53] The dilated hepatic ducts connect with the common hepatic duct and are liable to become infected and contain stones.

Caroli disease can be diagnosed by the cholangiographic finding of a multiple saccular appearance of intrahepatic bile ducts (Figure 111-11).[54] Ultrasound, magnetic resonance imaging, and CT have been shown to be useful in detecting saccular dilation of the intrahepatic bile ducts. The sacculi may vary greatly in size and distribution within the liver.[51] CT scans of the liver show tiny dots with strong contrast enhancement within the dilated intrahepatic bile ducts or the "central dot sign," which corresponds to intraluminal portal radicles surrounded by the dilated intrahepatic bile ducts (Figure 111-12).[51,55]

The long-term prognosis for patients with Caroli disease is quite poor, with a marked predisposition to septicemia, liver abscess, resultant hepatic failure, portal hypertension, or cholangiocarcinoma.[53] Cholangiocarcinoma has been reported in about 7% of patients.[53,54] The therapeutic management of Caroli disease is difficult, whether using conservative medical management or surgical interventions. Liver transplantation should be considered if the patient's condition deteriorates.[56,57]

REFERENCES

1. Alonso-Lej F, Rever WB, Pessagno DJ: Congenital choledochal cysts, with a report of 2, and an analysis of 94, cases. *Int Abst Surg* 108:1, 1959.
2. Todani T, Wastanabe Y, Narusue M, et al: Congenital bile duct cysts: Classifications, operative procedures, and review of 37 cases including cancer arising from choledochal cyst. *Am J Surg* 134:263, 1977.
3. Todani T: Congenital choledochal dilatation: Classification, clinical features, and long-term results. *J Hepatobiliary Pancreat Surg* 4:276, 1997.
4. Stringer MD: Choledochal cysts. In Howard ED, Stringer MD, Colombani PM, editors: *Surgery of the liver, bile ducts and pancreas in children*, London, 2002, Arnold, p 149.
5. Douglas AH: Case of dilatation of the common bile duct. *Month J Med Sci* 14:97, 1852.
6. Benjamin IS: Biliary cystic disease: The risk of cancer. *J Hepatobiliary Pancreat Surg* 10:335, 2003.
7. Yamaguchi M: Congenital choledochal cyst: Analysis of 1433 patients in the Japanese literature. *Am J Surg* 140:653, 1980.
8. Nagorney DM: Choledochal cysts in adults. In Blumgart LH, Fong Y, editors: *Surgery of the liver and biliary tract*, ed 3, London, 2000, Saunders, p 1229.
9. Lugo-Vicente HL: Prenatally diagnosed choledochal cysts: Observation or early surgery? *J Pediatr Surg* 30:1288, 1995.
10. Kozumi I, Kodama T: A case report and etiology of choledochal cystic dilatation (in Japanesese). *J Tokyo Med Assoc* 30:1413, 1916.
11. Babbitt DP: Congenital choledochal cysts: New etiological concept based on anomalous relationships of common bile duct and pancreatic bulb. *Ann Radiol* 12:231, 1969.
12. Komi N, Takehara H, Kunitomo K, et al: Does the type of anomalous arrangement of pancreaticobiliary ducts influence the surgery and prognosis of choledochal cyst? *J Pediatr Surg* 27:728, 1992.
13. Matsumoto Y, Fujii H, Itakura J, et al: Pancreaticobiliary maljunction: Pathophysiological and clinical aspects and the impact on biliary carcinogenesis. *Arch Surg* 388:122, 2003.
14. Ando H, Kaneko K, Ito F, et al: Embryogenesis of pancreaticobiliary maljunction inferred from development of duodenal atresia. *J Hepatobiliary Pancreat Surg* 6:50, 1999.

15. The Japanese study group on pancreaticobiliary maljunction (JSPBM): Diagnostic criteria of pancreaticobiliary maljunction. *J Hepatobiliary Pancreat Surg* 1:219, 1994.

16. Kattepura S, Nanjegowda NB, Babu MK, et al: Macroscopic pancreatic heterotopia on a congenital biliary dilatation. *Pediatr Surg Int* 26:847, 2010.

17. Kaneko K, Ando H, Ito T, et al: Protein plugs cause symptoms in patients with choledochal cysts. *Am J Gastroenterol* 92:1018, 1997.

18. Kim MJ, Han SJ, Yoon CS, et al: Using MR cholangiopancreatography to reveal anomalous pancreaticobiliary ductal union in infants and children with choledochal cysts. *Am J Roentgenol* 179:209, 2002.

19. Lam WW, Lam TP, Saing H, et al: MR cholangiography and CT cholangiography of pediatric patients with choledochal cysts. *Am J Roentgenol* 173:401, 1999.

20. Aoki H: Pathology of the pancreaticobiliary maljunction. In Aoki H, editor: *Questionnaire survey for bile duct cancer complicated with pancreaticobiliary maljunction*, Toyoake, 1985, The Japanese Study Group on Pancreaticobiliary Maljunction (JSPBM), p 34.

21. Lee MJ, Kim MJ, Yoon CS: MR cholangiopancreatography findings in children with spontaneous bile duct perforation. *Pediatr Radiol* 40:687, 2010.

22. Ando H, Ito T, Watanabe Y, et al: Spontaneous perforation of choledochal cyst. *J Am Coll Surg* 181:125, 1995.

23. Irwin ST, Morison JE: Congenital cyst of the common bile duct containing stones and undergoing cancerous change. *Br J Surg* 32:319, 1944.

24. Watanabe Y, Toki A, Todani T: Bile duct cancer developed after cyst excision for choledochal cyst. *J Hepatobiliary Pancreat Surg* 6:207, 1999.

25. Hasumi A, Matsui H, Sugioka A, et al: Precancerous conditions of biliary tract cancer in patients with pancreaticobiliary maljunction: Reappraisal of nationwide survey in Japan. *J Hepatobiliary Pancreat Surg* 7:551, 2000.

26. Voyles CR, Smadja C, Shands WC, et al: Carcinoma in choledochal cysts. Age-related incidence. *Arch Surg* 118:986, 1983.

27. Lagenbecks S, Kubota M, Yagi M, et al: An 11-year-old male patient demonstrating cholangiocarcinoma associated with congenital biliary dilatation. *J Pediatr Surg* 41:e15, 2006.

28. Kato T, Hebiguchi T, Matsuda K, et al: Action of pancreatic juice on the bile duct: Pathogenesis of congenital choledochal cyst. *J Pediatr Surg* 16:146, 1981.

29. Todani T, Watanabe Y, Toki A, et al: Carcinoma related to choledochal cysts with internal drainage operations. *Surg Gynec Obstet* 164:61, 1987.

30. Tocchi A, Mazzoni G, Liotta G, et al: Late development of bile duct cancer in patients who had biliary-enteric drainage for benign disease: A follow-up study of more than 1,000 patients. *Ann Surg* 234:210, 2001.

31. Ando H, Kaneko K, Ito T, et al: Complete excision of the intrahepatic portion of choledochal cysts. *J Am Coll Surg* 183:317, 1996.

32. Ando H, Kaneko K, Ito F, et al: Surgical removal of protein plugs complicating choledochal cysts: Primary repair after adequate opening of the pancreatic duct. *J Pediatr Surg* 33:1265, 1998.

33. Chiba K, Kamisawa T, Egawa N: Relapsing acute pancreatitis caused by protein plugs in a remnant choledochal cyst. *J Hepatobiliary Pancreat Sci* 17:729, 2010.

34. Ando H, Ito T, Kaneko K, et al: Congenital stenosis of the intrahepatic bile duct associated with choledochal cyst. *J Am Coll Surg* 181:426, 1995.

35. Todani T, Watanabe Y, Toki A, et al: Reoperation for congenital choledochal cyst. *Ann Surg* 207:142, 1988.

36. Ando H, Kaneko K, Ito F, et al: Operative treatment of congenital stenoses of the intrahepatic bile ducts in patients with choledochal cyst. *Am J Surg* 173:491, 1997.

37. Saing H, Han H, Chan KL, et al: Early and late results of excision of choledochal cysts. *J Pediatr Surg* 32:1563, 1997.

38. Uno K, Tsuchida Y, Kawarasaki H, et al: Development of intrahepatic cholelithiasis long after primary excision of choledochal cysts. *J Am Coll Surg* 183:583, 1996.

39. Chijiiwa K, Tanaka M: Late complications after excisional operation in patients with choledochal cyst. *J Am Coll Surg* 179:139, 1994.

40. Ishibashi T, Kasahara K, Yasuda Y, et al: Malignant change in the biliary tract after excision of choledochal cyst. *Br J Surg* 84:1687, 1997.

41. Goto N, Yasuda I, Uematsu, T, et al: Intrahepatic cholangiocarcinoma arising 10 years after the excision of congenital extrahepatic biliary dilatation. *J Gastroenterol* 36:856, 2001.

42. Hewitt PM, Kringe JEJ, Bornman PC, et al: Choledochal cysts in adults. *Br J Surg* 82:382, 1995.

43. Wheeler WIC: An unusual case of obstruction to the common bile-duct (choledochocele?) *Br J Surg* 27:446, 1940.

44. Scholz FJ, Carrera GF, Larsen CR: The choledochocele: Correlation of radiological, clinical and pathological findings. *Radiology* 118:25, 1976.

45. Masetti R, Antinori A, Coppola R, et al: Choledochocele: Changing trends in diagnosis and management. *Surg Today* 26:281, 1996.

46. Schimpl G, Sauer H, Goriupp U, et al: Choledochocele: Importance of histological evaluation. *J Pediatr Surg* 28:1562, 1993.

47. Ladas SD, Katsogridakis I, Tassios P, et al: Choledochocele, an overlooked diagnosis: Report of 15 cases and review of 56 published reports from 1984 to 1992. *Endoscopy* 27:233, 1995.

48. Savader SJ, Benenati JF, Venbrux AC, et al: Choledochal cysts: Classification and cholangiographic appearance. *Am J Roentgenol* 156:237, 1991.

49. Elton E, Hanson BL, Biber BP, et al: Dilated common channel syndrome: Endoscopic diagnosis, treatment, and relationship to choledochocele formation. *Gastrointest Endosc* 47:471, 1998.

50. Caroli J: Diseases of the intrahepatic biliary tree. *Clin Gastroenterol* 2:147, 1973.

51. Miller WJ, Sechtin AG, Campbell WL, et al: Imaging findings in Caroli's disease. *Am J Roentgenol* 165:333, 1995.

52. Tsuchida Y, Sato T, Sanjo K, et al: Evaluation of long-term results of Caroli's disease: 21 years' observation of a family with autosomal "dominant" inheritance, and review of the literature. *Hepatogastroenterology* 42:175, 1995.

53. Dayton MT, Longmire WP, Tompkins RK: Caroli's disease: A premalignant condition? *Am J Surg* 145:41, 1983.

54. Sherlock S, Dooley J: Cysts and congenital biliary abnormalities. In Sherlock S, Dooley J, editors: *Diseases of the liver and biliary system*, ed 10, Oxford, 1997, Blackwell, p 579.

55. Choi BI, Yeon KM, Kim SH, et al: Caroli disease: Central dot sign in CT. *Radiology* 174:161, 1990.

56. Takatsuki M, Umemoto S, Inomata Y, et al: Living-donor liver transplantation for Caroli's disease with intrahepatic adenocarcinoma. *J Hepatobiliary Pancreat Surg* 8:284, 2001.

57. Meier C, Deutscher J, Müller S, et al: Successful liver transplantation in a child with Caroli's disease. *Pediatr Transplant* 12:483, 2008.

Primary Sclerosing Cholangitis

Konstantinos N. Lazaridis | Gregory J. Gores

Primary sclerosing cholangitis (PSC) is a chronic, cholestatic liver disease of unknown cause characterized by diffuse inflammation and fibrosis of the bile ducts and is strongly associated with inflammatory bowel disease.[1] PSC is ultimately progressive, leading to obliteration of the biliary tree and subsequently to biliary cirrhosis.[1] To date, the etiology of PSC remains unknown and effective medical therapy is not currently available. Patients with PSC have shortened life expectancy. Orthotopic liver transplant (OLT) extends the life of patients with advanced-stage PSC. Development of colon cancer, gallbladder cancer, and cholangiocarcinoma are known complications of the disease.

EPIDEMIOLOGY

PSC usually affects more young males than females.[1] The mean age of diagnosis is the late 30s. In the United States, population-based studies have estimated an age-adjusted incidence for PSC to be 1.25 and 0.54 per 100,000 in men and women, respectively.[2] Moreover, the calculated prevalence of PSC was 20.9 and 6.3 per 100,000 in men and women, respectively.[2] About 75% to 80% of northern European origin patients with PSC suffer from inflammatory bowel disease (IBD), with chronic ulcerative colitis (CUC) being more common (approximately 90%) than Crohn disease.

PSC is associated with a lack of smoking. In one study, the incidence of current smoking was 19% in patients with PSC compared with 38% of controls.[3] In another study, 4.9% of PSC patients were reported to smoke compared with 26.1% of controls. The odds of having PSC in current smokers or former and current smokers compared with never-smokers were 0.13 and 0.41, respectively, regardless of the presence or absence of IBD.[4] Studies have also reported that prior appendectomy may delay the onset of PSC but does not affect either the prevalence or severity of the latter.[5]

CLINICAL PRESENTATION

The clinical presentation of PSC is heterogeneous and varies widely depending on the disease stage at the time of diagnosis. Asymptomatic individuals typically come to medical attention because of abnormal liver biochemistry following routine screening. Symptomatic patients present with symptoms/signs of cholestasis and complications of chronic cholestatic liver disease. The symptoms may include fatigue, pruritus, right upper quadrant pain, weight loss, and manifestations related to portal hypertension (i.e., ascites, gastrointestinal bleed from esophageal/gastric varices). Symptoms of bacterial cholangitis are less common, except if the patient has dominant biliary strictures and/or biliary stones. The physical examination of symptomatic patients may reveal jaundice, hepatomegaly, splenomegaly, skin excoriations, ascites, and peripheral edema.

A frequent clinical scenario is a patient with CUC who presents with a cholestatic pattern of liver enzymes. PSC can affect any age group, including children. Children may present with an overlap syndrome of PSC and autoimmune hepatitis (AIH), which can be as high as 35% according to a recent study.[6]

DIAGNOSIS

The diagnosis of PSC is made on the basis of (1) characteristic cholangiographic abnormalities of the biliary tree; (2) clinical and biochemical evidence of ductal cholestasis (i.e., elevated serum alkaline phosphatase of at least 6 months' duration); and (3) exclusion of secondary sclerosing cholangitis (Box 112-1).[1] Currently, the most frequent clinical presentation is an asymptomatic patient with persistently increased levels of alkaline phosphatase noted on routine serum biochemical testing.

Liver biopsy is not always required to make the diagnosis. In a study of 79 patients with a PSC diagnosis established by cholangiography, liver biopsy, performed following diagnosis, did not affect the management in the vast majority of patients.[7] The role of liver biopsy in PSC is to (1) exclude other causes of cholestatic liver disease; (2) diagnose or exclude small-duct PSC; and (3) define the PSC stage, which may have prognostic value. Small-duct PSC is a variant of PSC that accounts for approximately 5% of histologically proven cases.[8] Such patients present with a cholestatic pattern of liver enzymes, but normal cholangiography and liver biopsy reveals evidence of PSC. Small-duct PSC has better long-term prognosis compared with classic PSC. However, a portion of patients with small-duct PSC can progress to classic PSC over time.[8]

In most patients, the history, clinical presentation, serum biochemical profile, and cholangiography distinguish PSC from other causes of chronic cholestatic liver disease. Box 112-2 lists the differential diagnosis of PSC.

BIOCHEMICAL AND SEROLOGIC ABNORMALITIES

In patients with PSC, serum alkaline phosphatase level is elevated three to four times the upper limit of normal. A normal alkaline phosphatase level, however, does not rule out PSC because normal levels have been reported in patients with cholangiographic evidence of disease. PSC patients often have mildly increased aminotransferase levels (less than three times the upper limit of normal).[1]

Serum bilirubin is usually normal. Bilirubin levels will markedly rise as PSC progresses to end-stage liver disease (i.e., biliary cirrhosis). An abrupt, sustained rise of bilirubin may herald the presence of dominant biliary stricture(s), bile duct stone(s), or development of cholangiocarcinoma. Serum copper and ceruloplasmin levels as well as hepatic and urinary copper values are often abnormal. The copper increase is because of prolonged cholestasis. Hepatic copper levels in PSC can be elevated to the same range seen in Wilson disease and primary biliary cirrhosis (PBC).

None of the autoantibodies detected in PSC is pathognomonic. The prevalence of antineutrophil cytoplasmic antibodies, anticardiolipin antibodies, and antinuclear antibodies is 84%, 66%, and 53%, respectively.[9] Autoantibody testing may be helpful to identify those PSC patients with concurrent AIH. However, antibody titers are not important in following PSC activity. Antimitochondrial and anti–smooth muscle antibodies are rare in patients with PSC. Approximately one-fourth of patients have hypergammaglobulinemia with elevated immunoglobulin M (IgM) levels.[10]

IMAGING STUDIES

To diagnose a patient with PSC, cholangiography is required. Among imaging modalities, endoscopic retrograde cholangiopancreatography (ERCP) has been the criterion standard approach to evaluate bile ducts. The classic cholangiographic findings of PSC include multifocal stricturing and beading throughout the biliary tree (Figure 112-1). Strictures are often diffusely distributed with intervening segments of dilated ducts (i.e., ectasia). The cholangiographic findings usually involve both the intra- and extrahepatic bile ducts. Strictures can vary from 1 or 2 mm to several centimeters in length, and 30% to 40% of PSC patients may have mural irregularities, producing a shaggy appearance. These lesions may vary from a "fine brush border" to "frank nodularity." Pseudodiverticula (i.e., tiny diverticulum-like outpouchings) of the extrahepatic bile ducts are nearly pathognomonic for PSC. In approximately 20% of PSC patients, only the intrahepatic and proximal extrahepatic bile ducts are involved, and as many as 15% of PSC patients have involvement of the gallbladder and cystic duct. Moreover, approximately 5% of patients have small-duct PSC (i.e., normal cholangiogram but liver disease detectable on biochemical testing and histology).[8]

Magnetic resonance cholangiography (MRC) is as a noninvasive substitute for ERCP for the diagnosis of PSC.

BOX 112-1 **Causes of Secondary Sclerosing Cholangitis**

Choledocholithiasis (in the absence of PSC)
Biliary trauma/ischemia
Chemicals/drugs (i.e., 5-fluorouracil)
AIDS-associated cholangiopathy
Bile duct neoplasm (in the absence of PSC)
Congenital bile duct abnormalities (i.e., Caroli disease)
Idiopathic adulthood ductopenia
Amyloidosis

BOX 112-2 **Differential Diagnosis of Primary Sclerosing Cholangitis**

Primary biliary cirrhosis
Drug-induced cholestasis
Cholestasis associated with autoimmune hepatitis or alcoholic liver disease
Bile duct carcinoma (i.e., cholangiocarcinoma)
Extrahepatic obstruction
Secondary sclerosing cholangitis
Histiocytosis X
Hyper-IgM syndrome
Autoimmune pancreatitis with involvement of bile ducts

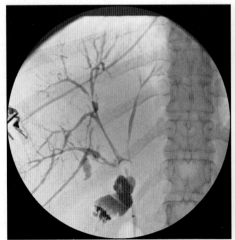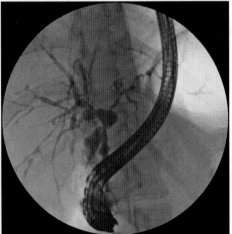

FIGURE 112-1 Endoscopic retrograde cholangiopancreatographic images depicting typical cholangiographic findings of PSC.

In a study of 73 patients with clinically suspected biliary disease, the sensitivity and specificity of MRC for diagnosing PSC were 82% and 98%, respectively.[11] These authors reported that MRC had comparable diagnostic accuracy to ERCP, leading to reduced cost when used as the initial approach to diagnose PSC. In PSC patients, MRC could be used as a noninvasive imaging method for the detection of cholangiocarcinoma. Indeed, MRC has replaced ERCP for the diagnosis of PSC.[1]

Percutaneous transhepatic cholangiography (PTC) is used less frequently to image the bile ducts in patients with suspected PSC. PTC is an alternative approach to access the biliary tree when ERCP is not technically possible. Abdominal ultrasonography is valuable to evaluate the bile ducts for dilation and/or stones, and liver parenchyma for cirrhosis. Computed tomography (CT) can reveal morphologic features of liver cirrhosis. Atrophy of the left lateral segments and hypertrophy of the caudate lobe may differentiate cirrhosis associated with PSC from that seen in other causes of chronic liver disease.[12] CT can also complement cholangiography in evaluating for malignancy, given its ability to detect peripheral, intrahepatic cholangiocarcinoma and metastatic spread within the hepatic parenchyma or the abdomen.[13] It is important to note that perihilar lymphadenopathy is common in PSC, and this finding alone cannot be taken as evidence of malignancy or metastasis.

PATHOLOGY

PSC can affect any portion of the biliary tree. Rarely, PSC may be limited to the small intrahepatic ducts (i.e., small-duct PSC).[8] Liver biopsy specimens from PSC patients show portal tract inflammation and sclerosis. Affected bile ducts are surrounded by a cuff of lightly inflamed sheets of fibrous tissue leading to fibrotic layers and may form the nearly pathognomonic onion-skin appearance. Afflicted biliary ducts will eventually become atrophied and be replaced by rounded cords of scars.

In addition to PSC, other causes of fibroobliterative cholangitis include PBC, mechanical obstruction of large bile ducts, ductopenic rejection following liver transplant, and biliary damage after intraarterial infusion of 5-fluorouracil. Involvement of both the large intrahepatic and extrahepatic ducts usually distinguishes PSC from PBC. Granulomas, once thought to be associated with PBC, may be seen in up to 4% of biopsies from PSC patients.

Canalicular cholestasis is nonspecific to PSC and can occur with any cause of biliary obstruction. As PSC progresses, however, the histopathologic changes of chronic cholestasis spill into the hepatic parenchyma.[14] To this end, the liver histology grading system for PSC is based on the stage of parenchymal changes. For example, in stage 1 (portal stage), there is edema, inflammation, and ductal proliferation. In stage 2 (periportal stage), periportal fibrosis and inflammation are noted. Stage 3 (septal stage) is defined by septal fibrosis or bridging necrosis. Finally, stage 4 (cirrhotic stage) is characterized by biliary cirrhosis (Table 112-1). Unfortunately, histologic changes can be markedly varied from segment to segment of the liver at any given point in time.

TABLE 112-1 Primary Sclerosing Cholangitis Staging

Portal stage (stage I)	Portal edema, inflammation, ductal proliferation; abnormalities do not extend beyond the limiting plate
Periportal stage (stage II)	Periportal fibrosis, inflammation with or without ductular proliferation; piecemeal necrosis may be present
Septal stage (stage III)	Septal fibrosis or bridging necrosis can be identified
Cirrhotic stage (stage IV)	Biliary cirrhosis

ETIOPATHOGENESIS

At present, the exact pathogenesis of PSC is elusive. The consensus working hypothesis postulates that PSC develops in a genetically predisposed individual following exposure(s) to a biliary insult that causes persistent immune-mediated inflammation leading over time to progressive destruction of bile ducts, cholestasis, and cirrhosis.[1] Current proposed etiologies encompass both genetic elements and environmental exposures, thus underscoring the host–environment interaction in the development of PSC. Moreover, it is now widely accepted that biliary epithelia (i.e., the cells that line the bile ducts) are the target cells of PSC.

The strong association of PSC with IBD has drawn much attention to the potential role of the inflamed colon in causing the former. The hypothesis suggests that inflammation of the colon may increase permeability to various intraluminal products (i.e., bacteria, toxins), which ultimately lead to liver disease. Bacteria have been considered, but not conclusively shown, to have a pathogenetic role in PSC development.[15]

Animal models of PSC have demonstrated that bacterial chemotactic peptides can lead to portal inflammation and histologic changes of PSC.[16] Nevertheless, in a pilot study of pentoxifylline, a tumor necrosis factor inhibitor, no beneficial effect on symptoms or liver biochemistry was reported in PSC patients.[17] Moreover, PSC can develop in approximately 25% of patients who have no evidence of IBD despite aggressive endoscopic screening. The lack of association between the seriousness of colonic disease and the likelihood of development and severity of PSC also strengthens the argument that CUC may not directly cause PSC. Finally, failure of proctocolectomy to modify the natural history of PSC disputes against a direct causative role of CUC in PSC.[18] Viral agents and other microorganisms have also been postulated as instigating the development of PSC.

Genetic variation likely contributes to PSC predisposition. To this extent, reports of affected PSC families support the notion of genetic inclination to develop the disease.[19] Moreover, various human leukocyte antigen (HLA) associations have been reported with PSC. A functional variant of stromelysin (i.e., matrix metalloproteinase 3) may also influence PSC susceptibility and disease progression.[20] Moreover, variations in the MICA gene (major histocompatibility complex class I–related MIC gene family) have a role in PSC predisposition. Independent of other HLA haplotypes, the MICA 002 allele appears to significantly reduce the risk of PSC, whereas the MICA 008 allele increases the risk of developing PSC.[21] Recently, the CCR5-Delta 32 mutation, characterized by a 32–base pair deletion in the CCR5 gene of T cells, has been associated with susceptibility to PSC development and severity.[22]

Immune-mediated damage of cholangiocytes seems to be an important step in PSC pathogenesis. Theoretically, certain HLA molecules and haplotypes may contribute to this event by eliciting an immune response against antigenic epitopes present on biliary epithelia. Enhanced expression of major histocompatibility complex (MHC) class II antigens (i.e., HLA DR) on cholangiocytes in early-stage PSC has drawn suspicion toward their role in disease pathogenesis. However, aberrant expression of HLA DR is also apparent in PBC and extrahepatic biliary obstruction, suggesting that this observation is an epiphenomenon rather than an implicit PSC cause.[23,24] Interactions of intracellular adhesion molecule 1 (ICAM-1) present on biliary epithelia with its cognate ligand on T cells (i.e., leukocyte function-associated antigen 1) may be important in PSC development. In fact, genetic polymorphisms of ICAM-1 have been implicated in susceptibility to PSC. For example, homozygote status of the E469E allele for ICAM-1 has been associated with protection against PSC.[25] Enhanced expression of ICAM-1 on proliferating cholangiocytes and increased serum levels of ICAM-1 have been reported in patients with PSC. Recently, a genomewide association study in PSC demonstrated that the HLA region and genes involved in bile homeostasis and other inflammatory conditions represent critical components of the genetic susceptibility to disease.[26]

ASSOCIATED DISEASES

PSC is strongly associated with IBD, most commonly CUC. PSC patients may also present or develop clinical and laboratory features of AIH. In addition, a variety of diseases have been reported to be weakly associated with PSC (Box 112-3).

BOX 112-3 Diseases Associated With Primary Sclerosing Cholangitis

Chronic ulcerative colitis
Crohn disease
Chronic pancreatitis
Sicca syndrome
Hypereosinophilia
Riedel thyroiditis
Celiac disease
Autoimmune hemolytic anemia
Sarcoidosis
Glomerulonephritis
Retroperitoneal fibrosis
Systemic sclerosis

INFLAMMATORY BOWEL DISEASE

IBD is seen in approximately 70% to 80% of patients with PSC.[9] CUC accounts for 85% to 90% of those patients and Crohn disease is responsible for the remaining.[27] Patients with PSC and Crohn disease may have milder hepatic disease than patients with PSC and CUC.[28] Usually, the diagnosis of IBD is established roughly 8 to 10 years before the diagnosis of PSC, although cases of IBD occurring years after the diagnosis of PSC have also been reported.[27] Conventional treatment of IBD does not alter the course of PSC, and severity of the former does not affect the disease seriousness of the latter. Proctocolectomy, the most aggressive treatment for CUC, has had no effect on PSC natural history.[18]

Colitis is usually milder in patients with both CUC and PSC compared with CUC patients alone. However, PSC may play a role in the development of colorectal dysplasia in the setting of CUC. In a Swedish study, patients with both CUC and PSC had an increased risk of colonic dysplasia compared with patients only suffering from CUC.[29] In fact, the absolute cumulative risk of developing colorectal dysplasia/carcinoma in patients with both PSC and CUC was 9%, 31%, and 50% after 10, 20, and 25 years of PSC duration, respectively.[29] On the contrary, patients with CUC alone had 2%, 5%, and 10% absolute cumulative risk to develop colorectal dysplasia/carcinoma following 10, 20, and 25 years' history of CUC, respectively.[29] In a U.S. study, patients with both PSC and CUC were five times more likely to develop colonic dysplasia, compared to patients with CUC alone.[30] In another study, patients with concurrent CUC and PSC had a 16% cumulative risk of colon cancer 10 years after the diagnosis of the liver disease.[31] Nonetheless, it remains unknown whether these observations reflect the fact that patients with PSC have milder pancolonic disease that remained undetected for a longer period of time. Conversely, a retrospective case-control study found similar prevalence of PSC in patients with both CUC and colorectal carcinoma compared with those who had CUC but no neoplasia (carcinoma or dysplasia).[32] Because in patients with both PSC and CUC systematic colon screening and early detection improves survival, annual colonoscopy with surveillance biopsies is recommended.

PSC patients with CUC have increased risk of colorectal dysplasia and neoplasia after OLT.[33] The increased neoplastic potential is of concern in PSC patients following OLT particularly because of the life-long immunosuppression that is required. Thus, in PSC patients who undergo OLT, annual colonoscopy with surveillance biopsies is recommended.

AUTOIMMUNE HEPATITIS

PSC can coexist with AIH.[1] These patients typically fulfill definite criteria for both diseases and have elevated serum alkaline phosphatase and aminotransferases, increased IgG, and antinuclear and/or anti–smooth muscle antibodies. Liver biopsy shows moderate to severe interface hepatitis with or without biliary destruction. Aminotransferase levels are higher than what one would expect for classic PSC. Patients with overlap syndrome may show improvement of AIH with immunosuppressive therapy. Indeed, patients who present with AIH and do not respond entirely to immunosuppressant therapy should be suspected of having concurrent PSC.

NATURAL HISTORY

PSC is an insidious and progressive disease that ultimately leads to end-stage liver disease. Patients with early-stage PSC are virtually asymptomatic. Advanced-stage PSC is described by chronic cholestasis and complications of end-stage liver disease. The median survival from the time of diagnosis is about 12 years if OLT is not available. Asymptomatic PSC patients also have decreased survival compared with matched controls. In a study of 45 PSC patients who were asymptomatic at the time of diagnosis, 34 (76%) patients progressed and 14 (31%) patients developed hepatic failure resulting in death or referral for OLT (mean followup of 6.25 years).[34] The progressive natural history and associated complications of PSC warrant close medical management and intervening treatment.

Small-duct PSC has a more favorable long-term prognosis than classic PSC. Nevertheless, small-duct PSC can progress to classic PSC in a small number of patients.[8] Children with PSC also have progressive disease, with median survival of 12.7 years despite medical therapy.[6]

COMPLICATIONS

Complications of PSC are divided into two categories: PSC-associated and non-PSC associated. Complications of the first group include cholelithiasis, choledocholithiasis, gallbladder polyps and cancer, dominant biliary strictures with or without recurrent bacterial cholangitis, cholangiocarcinoma, and peristomal varices in PSC patients who had undergone proctocolectomy and ileostomy for CUC. Complications of the second group are secondary to chronic cholestasis (i.e., pruritus, steatorrhea, fat-soluble vitamin deficiency, hepatic osteodystrophy) and to the development of end-stage liver disease (i.e., cirrhosis, portal hypertension, ascites).

PSC-ASSOCIATED COMPLICATIONS

CHOLELITHIASIS, CHOLEDOCHOLITHIASIS, AND GALLBLADDER POLYPS

Twenty-five percent to 30% of PSC patients have or will develop calculi in the gallbladder or bile ducts during the course of the disease. In a study of 121 patients with PSC, 32 (26%) patients had gallstones, half of which were pigment stones, and 18 (15%) patients had PSC involving the gallbladder.[35] Gallbladder polyps in patients with PSC require special consideration. In a recent study of 102 PSC patients, 14 (13.7%) patients had an intraluminal gallbladder mass, of which eight (57%) lesions were found to be adenocarcinomas.[36,37] Therefore, in patients with PSC the presence of gallbladder polyps is an indication for cholecystectomy.[1]

Intrahepatic calculi are present in approximately 8% of PSC patients.[38] Biliary calculi can serve as a nidus for the development of bacterial cholangitis in these patients,

although the latter is less common in the absence of dominant biliary strictures or prior bile duct surgery. Following diagnosis of bacterial cholangitis, ERCP is required to remove possible bile duct calculi, and/or to dilate biliary strictures allowing satisfactory bile drainage. Nevertheless, bacterial cholangitis can occur in PSC patients after ERCP. To prevent this complication, we suggest prophylactic coverage with intravenous antibiotics before and oral ciprofloxacin for 10 days after ERCP.

DOMINANT BILIARY STRICTURES

Dominant biliary strictures are present in 20% to 45% of patients with PSC and cause an increased rate of jaundice, pruritus, right upper quadrant pain, and bacterial cholangitis. ERCP is required to assess the bile ducts, rule out the possibility of cholangiocarcinoma, and allow therapeutic dilation with or without biliary stenting to relieve cholestasis. A prospective study of 12 symptomatic PSC patients with major ductal strictures treated with repeated balloon dilation and nasobiliary catheter perfusion showed sustained improvement in 8 patients following an average of three treatment sessions (mean followup, 23 months).[39] A retrospective study of 25 PSC patients with symptomatic dominant strictures reported that endoscopic stenting was technically successful in 21 (84%) patients and was associated with significant improvement of liver function tests. Moreover, 12 (57%) of the 21 PSC patients remained asymptomatic with stable liver biochemistries, whereas 4 (19%) patients had clinical and biochemical relapse over a median followup of 29 months. All 4 patients with relapse did respond positively to additional endoscopic therapy.[40] The same authors reported 16 symptomatic PSC patients treated with short-term biliary stent placement (median duration only 9 days); 13 (81%) patients remained symptom-free and without biochemical evidence of cholestasis after a median followup of 19 months.[41] In spite of these studies, it is uncertain if dominant biliary strictures are directly accountable for cholestasis in PSC patients. The authors of a recent retrospective study of 125 patients with PSC reported that 56 (45%) patients had dominant biliary strictures defined by stenosis of the common bile duct to less than 1.5 mm in diameter and/or stenosis of the right or left hepatic duct to less than 1.0 mm. Of interest, between the 56 patients with and the 69 patients without dominant strictures, alkaline phosphatase and bilirubin levels were not significantly different up to 2 and 12 months after cholangiography.[42]

CHOLANGIOCARCINOMA

The most threatening complication of PSC is the development of cholangiocarcinoma, which occurs in 8% to 15% of PSC patients.[1] In a recent study of 161 PSC patients, approximately 7% developed cholangiocarcinoma during a mean followup of 11.5 years.[43] In patients with PSC, the estimated annual incidence of cholangiocarcinoma is about 1.5%.[44] In one study, the cumulative risk of developing biliary duct malignancy was 11.2% at 10 years after diagnosis of PSC.[31]

Patients with PSC who develop cholangiocarcinoma typically have poor survival. In a retrospective study of 30 patients with PSC, median survival was only 5 months following the diagnosis of cholangiocarcinoma. Additionally, at the time of cholangiocarcinoma diagnosis, 19 of 30 (63%) patients had metastatic disease and 8 of 17 (47%) patients, although believed to have localized malignancy, were found to have abdominal metastases during surgical exploration. Moreover, metastasis or local cholangiocarcinoma extension prevented curative tumor resection in all but one patient who was free of malignancy more than 2 years following resection. For those PSC patients who acquired cholangiocarcinoma, palliative therapies including resection, chemotherapy, and radiotherapy do not improve survival.[44]

Cholangiocarcinoma remains unrecognized in many PSC patients until it is too advanced to cure because of its insidious nature. In fact, many of the signs/symptoms associated with cholangiocarcinoma development are typical of PSC itself, making early detection of the former very challenging.[44] The suspicion for cholangiocarcinoma should be high when a PSC patient reports rapidly progressive jaundice, weight loss, or abdominal discomfort. In a retrospective study, PSC patients who developed cholangiocarcinoma were compared with those who did not. No clinical or biochemical features were found that could herald the onset of biliary cancer in the year before the diagnosis of the malignancy. In PSC patients, risk factors for developing cholangiocarcinoma include age, liver histologic stage, concurrent CUC, smoking, and history of variceal bleeding.[43]

In patients with PSC, dysplasia of the biliary epithelium is likely the main predisposing factor or even a cholangiocarcinoma precursor. In a study from the United Kingdom, biliary dysplasia was detected in 20% of liver biopsies derived from 26 PSC patients with concurrent and subsequent cholangiocarcinoma, but not in a single case of 60 PSC patients without biliary malignancy during a followup period of 2 years.[45] From the same study, recognition of biliary dysplasia by three independent pathologists showed moderate reproducibility, suggesting dysplasia as a feasible indicator of present or future biliary malignancy.[45] Similarly, colonic dysplasia appears to be a risk factor for developing cholangiocarcinoma in PSC; and the risk is significantly increased in patients with both PSC and CUC.[29] Thus, detection of dysplasia in either the bile ducts or colon warrants vigilant surveillance and may deserve consideration for OLT in certain situations.

At this time, early detection of cholangiocarcinoma, and thus hope for cure, is hindered because of the low sensitivity and specificity of standard diagnostic tests. Sclerosing cholangiocarcinoma of the large bile ducts, the type that most commonly develops in PSC patients, presents as biliary stricture and is best detectable by ERCP or PTC.[44] To this end, cholangiographic features suggestive of cholangiocarcinoma have been described, but accurate distinction between benign and malignant biliary stricture is often impossible. In fact, about 10% of malignant-appearing biliary strictures are ultimately benign. Biliary brush cytology and biopsy obtained during ERCP are at best 30% to 40% sensitive for securing the diagnosis of cholangiocarcinoma.[44] One novel test for early detection of cholangiocarcinoma is

fluorescence in situ hybridization (FISH). This test is performed on bile duct cytology specimens. In a study for detection of malignant biliary strictures, FISH had an increased sensitivity (35% to 60%) compared with the sensitivity of conventional cytology (4% to 20%, $P < 0.01$).[46] Therefore, we recommend obtaining biliary brushings from PSC patients during ERCP to carry out FISH, because this test can improve the detection rate of cholangiocarcinoma.

Carbohydrate antigen 19-9 (CA 19-9) is a serum marker for pancreatobiliary malignancies. In patients with PSC, a serum level greater than 129 U/mL has 78.6% sensitivity and 98.5% specificity for diagnosing cholangiocarcinoma in the absence of bacterial cholangitis.[47] However, elevated CA19-9 can be seen in pancreatic malignancies, bacterial cholangitis, and in active smokers. In patients with PSC, we recommend periodic CA 19-9 testing; sustained rise should draw attention for possible development of cholangiocarcinoma. For the future, we need dependable molecular markers to detect cholangiocarcinoma early at a possibly curable stage.

Endoscopic ultrasound (EUS) is better than CT and MRI to evaluate regional lymph nodes for possible cholangiocarcinoma metastasis, and adds the option to biopsy questionable lesions.[44] Positron emission tomography (PET) is another promising tool for detection of cholangiocarcinoma in PSC. In one study, PET was 100% accurate in identifying small cholangiocarcinomas arising in the setting of PSC compared with controls.[48] PET was also proposed as a useful tool for cholangiocarcinoma screening in the pretransplant evaluation of PSC patients.[49] However, more recent data suggest that PET scanning is positive only in approximately 50% of patients with cholangiocarcinoma. Thus, PET scanning should not be considered as "standard of care" in this disease.

NON-PSC–ASSOCIATED COMPLICATIONS

PSC patients may complain of fatigue and pruritus. The etiology of fatigue is unknown and more importantly it can affect patients' quality of life. In patients with PSC the pruritus can be debilitating but its mechanism is not well defined. Endogenous opioids and retention of additional unknown factors usually excreted in the bile may contribute in the development of pruritus.[50] Overall the intensity of pruritus does not parallel the severity of disease. Pruritus may lessen as PSC progresses.

Patients with PSC may also suffer from steatorrhea and ensuing deficiencies of fat-soluble vitamins. In a pretransplant group of PSC patients, deficiencies of vitamins A, D, and E were present in 82%, 57%, and 43% of patients, respectively.[51] In patients with PSC and steatorrhea, consideration should be given to rule out celiac sprue or chronic pancreatitis, because either entity can coexist with PSC and both conditions are treatable causes of fat malabsorption. Metabolic bone disease is also common in PSC. Osteopenic bone disease can be severe in advanced-stage PSC, with 50% of patients having a bone mineral density below the fracture threshold.[52] Although the majority of PSC patients are male, bone biopsies revealed findings consistent with osteoporosis rather than osteomalacia.[52]

Patients with PSC may suffer from complications of portal hypertension, just as patients with other etiologies of liver cirrhosis. In a study of 283 patients with PSC, 102 (36%) patients had esophageal varices, including 57 of 102 (56%) patients deemed to have moderate- to large-size varices.[53] In the same study, platelet count, albumin level, and advanced histologic disease were independent predictors of esophageal varices. Esophageal varices are usually managed with endoscopic banding. If these measures are ineffective, a shunting procedure (i.e., transjugular intrahepatic portosystemic shunt) can be performed, but hopefully as a bridge to OLT. Patients with advanced-stage PSC develop ascites, spontaneous bacterial peritonitis, and encephalopathy. Treatment of these complications is similar to other causes of end-stage liver disease. Liver transplant should be considered as the ultimate therapy for persistent complications.

THERAPY

To date, there is no specific medical therapy for PSC. Medical management should converge on the treatment of specific and nonspecific complications. Clinical trials treating the underlying hepatobiliary disease are currently in progress.

TREATMENT OF PSC-ASSOCIATED COMPLICATIONS

Cholelithiasis, Choledocholithiasis, and Gallbladder Polyps

Symptomatic gallbladder disease in early-stage PSC patients should be treated with cholecystectomy. In an asymptomatic PSC patient, presence of an intraluminal gallbladder mass that cannot be attributed to gallstones requires cholecystectomy. As discussed previously, in a study of PSC patients who underwent cholecystectomy, 13.7% of patients were found to have a gallbladder mass, more than half of which were adenocarcinomas.[36,37] As always, cholecystectomy in patients with liver disease must be embarked on cautiously, both from the surgical aspect and from the anesthetic management aspect.

Following diagnosis of choledocholithiasis, the therapeutic intervention of choice is ERCP. During this procedure, endoscopic sphincterectomy is performed with removal of biliary stones and dilation of possible strictures. Temporary biliary stent placement is recommended, but final decisions should be made based on completeness of stone extraction, as well as the location and nature of biliary strictures.

Dominant Biliary Stricture(s) and Recurrent Bacterial Cholangitis

Dominant biliary stricture(s) should be evaluated by ERCP or PTC to ensure comprehensive imaging of the biliary tree and to permit biliary brushings as well as biopsies of the affected area(s) to exclude cholangiocarcinoma. The main concern is to scrutinize whether the observed biliary stricture(s) represent cholangiocarcinoma or a benign lesion.

The therapeutic management of dominant bile duct stricture(s) includes the combination of biliary dilation and stenting interventions. The preferred approach of intervention (i.e., ERCP vs. PTC) depends on biliary stricture characteristics (i.e., region, length), and experience with the procedures. The majority of bile duct strictures are amenable to endoscopic cholangioplasty followed by biliary stenting. PTC is useful for cholangioplasty of biliary strictures that affect intrahepatic ducts and in cases of prior unsuccessful endoscopic attempts to enter the biliary tree (i.e., patients with history of Roux-en-Y gastrojejunostomy).

PSC patients with frequent episodes of bacterial cholangitis should have cholangiography to evaluate the patency of bile ducts. If strictures are present, they require treatment endoscopically or percutaneously. In patients with PSC, recurrent bacterial cholangitis is not always the result of dominant biliary stricture(s). Edema, inflammatory exudation, and intraluminal debris can result in temporary stenosis of bile ducts leading to obliteration and subsequent recurrent bacterial cholangitis. Patients with relapsing episodes of bacterial cholangitis may be given ciprofloxacin orally as prophylaxis to prevent recurrent events.

THERAPY OF NON-PSC–ASSOCIATED COMPLICATIONS

Pruritus

Patients with advanced-stage PSC frequently complain of intense pruritus. This distressing symptom can improve using various medical therapies (Table 112-2).[54] Cholestyramine is a nonabsorbable resin that decreases the intestinal absorption of bile acids and alleviates pruritus; it is the standard of care. Phenobarbital has rarely been used in conjunction with cholestyramine to treat PSC patients with nocturnal pruritus. Ursodeoxycholic acid (i.e., ursodiol), a hydrophilic bile acid that likely replaces hydrophobic, toxic bile acids from the bile pool, may also improve pruritus in PSC patients. Antihistamines such as hydroxyzine and diphenhydramine have been used as supplements to cholestyramine or ursodeoxycholic acid (UDCA), but are seldom effective because of their sedative properties. Rifampin may also improve pruritus, though its potential side effects (i.e., drug-induced hepatitis) make rifampin a second-line agent following cholestyramine for this upsetting symptom. In patients with PSC, opiate antagonists such as naloxone, nalmefene, and naltrexone have been used to alleviate pruritus but are fraught with psychiatric-type side effects.

TABLE 112-2 Medications for Treatment of Pruritus

Medication	Dosage
Cholestyramine*	4 g three to four times per day, orally
Phenobarbital	120-160 mg per day, orally
Ursodeoxycholic acid	15-20 mg/kg per day, orally
Hydroxyzine	25 mg three to four times per day, orally
Rifampin	150-300 mg twice daily, orally
Naltrexone	50 mg per day, orally

*Should be given 2 hours before or after other medications.

TABLE 112-3 Vitamin Replacement Therapy for Primary Sclerosing Cholangitis

Vitamin A	25,000-50,000 units two to three times per week, orally
Vitamin D	25,000-50,000 units two to three times per week, orally
Vitamin E	100 units twice daily, orally
Vitamin K	5 mg per day, orally

Steatorrhea, Fat-Soluble Vitamin Deficiency, and Hepatic Osteodystrophy

Prolonged cholestasis causes decreased intestinal bile acid concentration. Therefore, patients with advanced-stage PSC may develop fat malabsorption and steatorrhea. PSC patients who develop steatorrhea, however, should first be evaluated for other coexisting causes of steatorrhea, including celiac sprue and pancreatic insufficiency. Steatorrhea, because of intraluminal bile acid deficiency, may improve by dietary changes such as lowering daily fat intake and substituting medium-chain triglycerides for long-chain ones.

Fat-soluble vitamins (i.e., A, D, E, and K) deficiencies are treated by simple oral replacement (Table 112-3). Special consideration must be given in advanced-stage PSC patients who have moderate-to-severe osteopenia. Calcium supplements, replenishment with vitamin D, and use of estrogens all have had therapeutic value. PSC patients deficient in vitamin K have prolonged prothrombin time that usually improves with oral vitamin K supplementation.

Decompensated Cirrhosis and Portal Hypertension

Complications of decompensated cirrhosis and portal hypertension should be managed expectantly as in other end-stage liver diseases. As PSC progresses, the complications of end-stage liver disease become intractable and liver transplantation becomes the only effective cure.

THERAPY OF HEPATOBILIARY DISEASE

Multiple medical therapies have been evaluated for the treatment of PSC including D-penicillamine, cyclosporine, azathioprine, budesonide, silymarin, pentoxifylline, colchicine and UDCA. However, none, thus far, has proven to be effective.

A randomized, controlled study of 105 PSC patients treated with standard dose UDCA (13 to 15 mg/kg body weight/day) did not report any clinical benefit in the treatment group compared with controls (median followup of 2.2 years). However, two independent pilot studies of PSC patients treated with high-dose UDCA have demonstrated promise. A small, double-blind, placebo-controlled study from the United Kingdom reported that 13 PSC patients who received high-dose (20 mg/kg body weight/day) UDCA had significant improvement in liver biochemistries, cholangiographic appearance, and reduction of liver fibrosis compared with 13 PSC patients taking placebo.[55] A U.S. study of 30 PSC patients treated with high-dose UDCA (25 to 30 mg/kg body weight/day) for 12 months

reported improvement of the Mayo PSC risk score at the end of therapy. The observed changes were translated into a significantly better than expected survival at 4 years in the high-dose UDCA group compared with a historic placebo group.[56] To further evaluate these promising results, a multicenter, randomized placebo-controlled trial of long-term, high-dose UDCA (28 to 30 mg/kg/day) was performed, but it did not improve survival and was associated with greater rates of serious adverse events.[57]

Beyond treating the underlying liver disease, UDCA has also been shown to affect the frequency of colonic dysplasia or cancer in patients with PSC and CUC. In a cross-sectional study of 59 patients with both PSC and CUC who were undergoing chronic dysplasia surveillance colonoscopy, UDCA use was correlated with decreased prevalence of colonic dysplasia.[58] In a retrospective analysis of a randomized, placebo-controlled trial of 52 patients with concurrent PSC and CUC, use of UDCA resulted in a reduced relative risk (RR = 0.26; 95% confidence interval = 0.06 to 0.92; $P = 0.049$) for developing colorectal dysplasia or cancer.[59] Additional prospective, randomized placebo-controlled studies are needed to verify the postulated chemopreventive effect of UDCA in patients with PSC and CUC.

SURGICAL THERAPY

In the past three decades, the surgical approach to PSC has evolved tremendously. Earlier, operative cholangiography along with choledochotomy and biopsy were performed to diagnose PSC. The need for these procedures was obviated by the advent of ERCP and percutaneous cholangiography. In the present era of solid organ transplantation, palliative biliary reconstruction has largely been replaced by OLT.

Reconstructive Biliary Surgery

The early surgical approaches to treat PSC advocated prolonged T-tube drainage and use of steroids. Wood and Cuschieri[60] suggested that T-tube drainage and lavage might actually reverse the disease process.

In 1988, Cameron et al reported the Johns Hopkins experience on PSC patients who underwent extended biliary resection in combination with stenting and biliary–enteric anastomosis.[61] This procedure involved excision of the hepatic duct bifurcation and extrahepatic biliary tree, intraoperative dilation of the intrahepatic ducts, insertion of Silastic transhepatic biliary stents, and bilateral hepaticojejunostomies. In that report, two of five (40%) PSC patients with cirrhosis died following the operation; conversely, only one of 26 (3.9%) PSC patients with only liver fibrosis died after the operative procedure. The 1-, 3-, and 5-year actuarial survival rates for PSC patients with cirrhosis and hepatic fibrosis were 20%, 20%, 20% and 92%, 87%, 71%, respectively.[61] The authors recommended that patients with PSC and cirrhosis should be referred for consideration of OLT; however, PSC patients with significant extrahepatic disease and no evidence of cirrhosis should be considered for biliary reconstructive surgery.[61]

In the past decade, biliary reconstructive surgery for PSC has become less common because endoscopic techniques for bile duct dilation and stenting as well as the outcome of OLT have improved. Nevertheless, biliary–enteric anastomosis may still be indicated in noncirrhotic patients with significant but localized extrahepatic disease. However, the reported association of precedent biliary–enteric drainage surgery for benign disease with subsequent development of cholangiocarcinoma has caused skepticism to the proposition for biliary reconstructive surgery in PSC.[62] In addition, there is some hesitation in recommending bile duct reconstructive surgery, after several medical centers reported increased difficulty performing OLT in patients who had previous biliary surgery. In our practice, we refer PSC patients with dominant biliary strictures for endoscopic dilation, given the high degree of success attained by this procedure, its relative ease, and low morbidity/mortality as compared with biliary surgery. We would only recommend biliary reconstructive surgery for those few PSC patients who have extrahepatic strictures not amenable to endoscopic treatment who are not candidates for OLT, and who have no cirrhosis.

Orthotopic Liver Transplantation

OLT remains the most effective treatment for PSC. At our institution, the 1- and 5-year survival rates for PSC patients following OLT are 95% and 86%, respectively. These rates compare favorably with results of OLT for other chronic liver diseases. Risk factors that adversely affected outcomes of patients who underwent OLT for PSC are divided into those that influence the general OLT outcome and the ones specific for PSC.[63] The former include stay in the intensive care unit (ICU) or being on life support prior to OLT, age greater than 65 years old, poor nutritional status, Child's class C, and renal failure requiring dialysis prior to or after OLT. These factors are also predictive of increased operative blood loss, prolonged ICU stay, and major postoperative complications. Risk factors specific for PSC include disease severity, previous biliary or shunt surgery, coexistent cholangiocarcinoma, and presence of IBD. Utilizing the Mayo PSC natural history model as a measure of disease severity, actual survival following transplantation was improved with OLT for all stages of disease.[64] Thus, earlier OLT has been advocated for patients with PSC, as this approach would improve patient outcome and resource utilization.

Controversy exists on the impact of prior biliary surgery on subsequent OLT for PSC. There is little doubt that prior biliary surgery increases the technical difficulty of OLT, but it is unknown if this event affects survival. In a combined series of 216 patients from the University of Pittsburgh and the Mayo Clinic, prior biliary tract and/or portal hypertensive surgery was associated with less favorable survival after OLT, but this event did not reach statistical significance.[64] In a study from the University of California at San Francisco, increased operative time and blood loss, but not mortality, were found in PSC patients with a history of prior colectomy or biliary surgery.[65] These reports suggest that prior biliary tract surgery increases the technical difficulty of OLT for PSC and is associated with a trend toward slightly increased mortality, even when performed at large transplant centers.

Following OLT for PSC, these patients develop unique complications. Increased rates of biliary strictures have been noted; however, not all of these cases represent PSC recurrence, as other factors may also cause biliary stricturing, including ischemia related to chronic rejection or possible chronic low-grade bacterial cholangitis resulting from the Roux-en-Y anastomosis, which is performed much more frequently in PSC patients. However, a study from the University of Pittsburgh found a significantly increased incidence of biliary strictures in allografts of patients transplanted for PSC versus patients who also underwent OLT and choledochojejunostomy for other non-PSC causes of end-stage liver disease.[66] Because cholangiographic, clinical, and biochemical criteria for recurrent disease have not been widely accepted, there is no consensus regarding the incidence of recurrent PSC in liver allografts. Nevertheless, careful analysis of a registry of transplanted PSC patients at our institution concluded that 20% of patients developed recurrent disease based on characteristic cholangiographic and histologic features.[67] Several transplant centers have reported an increased incidence of rejection in patients transplanted for PSC. Acute and chronic ductopenic rejection can be severe and steroid resistant, often leading to graft loss.[65] In a study of 100 consecutive PSC patients undergoing transplants at Baylor University Medical Center, chronic rejection and disease recurrence occurred in 13% and 16% of patients, respectively, following OLT. These events had adversely affected both graft and patient survival, markedly so in those patients with chronic rejection.[68] Five-year graft survival rates were 33% and 65% for patients with chronic rejection and disease recurrence, respectively, compared with 76% for patients free of chronic rejection or recurrence. The authors postulated that chronic rejection and disease recurrence following OLT for PSC are two distinct entities, as evidenced by the difference in outcome, and therefore, these causes should be managed accordingly.[68]

Because many patients with PSC have concurrent CUC, there was concern that life-long immunosuppression after OLT may increase the risk of colorectal carcinoma in such cases. In a study of 108 patients with PSC and concomitant IBD who underwent OLT, Loftus et al reported a fourfold increase in colon carcinoma in the group that did not have a prior colectomy compared with the expected colon cancer rate in a group with comparable (pre-OLT) duration of IBD.[69] This finding, however, was not statistically significant and did not affect patient survival.[69] Goss et al also reported that posttransplant colectomy for dysplasia–carcinoma or symptomatic colitis does not affect PSC patient survival.[70] Given the lack of impact on patient survival, we do not recommend prophylactic proctocolectomy in PSC patients with IBD who undergo OLT. Nonetheless, the high risk of colonic neoplasia in transplanted PSC patients warrants annual surveillance colonoscopy with biopsies, and colectomy in cases where low-grade dysplasia is detected.

Cholangiocarcinoma

In patients with PSC and cholangiocarcinoma, curative therapy for the latter is as disappointing as it is for patients with cholangiocarcinoma alone. In general, cholangiocarcinoma is regarded as a contraindication for OLT, given the reported poor outcome of transplanted patients in the past. However, incidental cholangiocarcinomas (defined as lesions < 1 cm in diameter discovered at the time of pathologic sectioning of explanted liver) have a much better prognosis. In a study of 127 PSC patients who received transplants, 10 (8%) were found to have incidental cholangiocarcinoma, but they enjoyed a 5-year actuarial survival rate of 83%, which is comparable to survival rates of OLT patients without incidental cholangiocarcinoma.[70] Because our ability to detect small cholangiocarcinomas preoperatively will improve, we need to reevaluate the surgical management of these tumors in PSC patients. For example, selected liver transplant centers have shown promising outcome among patients with hilar cholangiocarcinoma (5-year actuarial survival rate of about 80%)[71] using radiation therapy, chemotherapy, and abdominal exploration prior to OLT. For patients with unresectable disease, new chemotherapeutic schemes may be effective.[72,73]

Proctocolectomy

In patients with CUC, development of PSC affects the management of the former. Overall, we recommend proctocolectomy only for indications pertinent to CUC; these being medical failure to control severe symptoms or presence of colon dysplasia. Nevertheless, the decision to perform Brooke ileostomy versus ileal pouch–anal anastomosis (IPAA) is greatly influenced by the presence of PSC. In a retrospective study of 72 patients with PSC and CUC treated with either Brooke ileostomy ($N = 32$) or IPAA ($N = 40$), 8 of 32 (26%) patients who underwent ileostomy developed peristomal varices and subsequent bleeding; however, none of the 40 patients who underwent IPAA developed perianastomotic varices or perineal bleeding.[74] Of interest, the cumulative risk of pouchitis at 10 years after IPAA was 61% for patients with PSC and CUC, as compared with 36% for patients with CUC alone.[75] Therefore, patients with PSC have increased risk of pouchitis if treated for CUC with IPAA. In our practice, in PSC patients who need proctocolectomy, we recommend IPAA and not Brooke ileostomy, because treating pouchitis is simpler than managing bleeding peristomal varices.

CONCLUSION

PSC is a cholestatic liver disease of unknown etiology affecting mainly young men. The disease is characterized by a progressive, fibrous obliteration of ducts resulting in biliary cirrhosis and ultimately liver failure. PSC is strongly associated with CUC. During the course of the illness, patients with PSC develop disease-specific and nonspecific complications. Medical management is challenging and requires a team approach of hepatologists, gastroenterologists, radiologists, and surgeons. At present, we lack an effective medical therapy to treat the primary disease. Nonetheless, OLT is the ultimate cure. Basic and translational research studies are required to better understand the pathogenesis of PSC before we can apply more effective therapies.

SUGGESTED READINGS

Bergasa NV: An approach to the management of the pruritus of cholestasis. *Clin Liver Dis* 8:55, 2004.
A comprehensive review on the therapy of pruritus in cholestatic liver diseases.
Chapman R, Fevery J, Kalloo A, et al: Diagnosis and management of primary sclerosing cholangitis. *Hepatology* 51:660, 2010.
This article is the AASLD Clinical Practice Guidelines for PSC.
Moreno Luna LE, Kipp B, Halling KC, et al: Advanced cytologic techniques for the detection of malignant pancreatobiliary strictures. *Gastroenterology* 131:1064, 2006.
This study describes a novel approach for the detection of malignant biliary strictures in PSC.
Rosen CB, Heimbach JK, Gores GJ: Liver transplantation for cholangiocarcinoma. *Transpl Int* 23:692, 2010.
This article describes the use of liver transplantation for cholangiocarcinoma.

REFERENCES

1. Chapman R, Fevery J, Kalloo A, et al: Diagnosis and management of primary sclerosing cholangitis. *Hepatology* 51:660, 2010.
2. Bambha K, Kim WR, Talwalkar J, et al: Incidence, clinical spectrum, and outcomes of primary sclerosing cholangitis in a United States community. *Gastroenterology* 125:1364, 2003.
3. van Erpecum KJ, Smits SJ, van de Meeberg PC, et al: Risk of primary sclerosing cholangitis is associated with nonsmoking behavior. *Gastroenterology* 110:1503, 1996.
4. Loftus EV Jr, Sandborn WJ, Tremaine WJ, et al: Primary sclerosing cholangitis is associated with nonsmoking: A case-control study. *Gastroenterology* 110:1496, 1996.
5. Florin TH, Pandeya N, Radford-Smith GL: Epidemiology of appendicectomy in primary sclerosing cholangitis and ulcerative colitis: Its influence on the clinical behaviour of these diseases. *Gut* 53:973, 2004.
6. Feldstein AE, Perrault J, El-Youssif M, et al: Primary sclerosing cholangitis in children: A long-term follow-up study. *Hepatology* 38:210, 2003.
7. Burak KW, Angulo P, Lindor KD: Is there a role for liver biopsy in primary sclerosing cholangitis? *Am J Gastroenterol* 98:1155, 2003.
8. Bjornsson E, Olsson R, Bergquist A, et al: The natural history of small-duct primary sclerosing cholangitis. *Gastroenterology* 134:975, 2008.
9. Angulo P, Peter JB, Gershwin ME, et al: Serum autoantibodies in patients with primary sclerosing cholangitis. *J Hepatol* 32:182, 2000.
10. LaRusso NF, Wiesner RH, Ludwig J, et al: Current concepts. Primary sclerosing cholangitis. *N Engl J Med* 310:899, 1984.
11. Talwalkar JA, Angulo P, Johnson CD, et al: Cost-minimization analysis of MRC versus ERCP for the diagnosis of primary sclerosing cholangitis. *Hepatology* 40:39, 2004.
12. Caldwell SH, Hespenheide EE, Harris D, et al: Imaging and clinical characteristics of focal atrophy of segments 2 and 3 in primary sclerosing cholangitis. *J Gastroenterol Hepatol* 16:220, 2001.
13. Campbell WL, Peterson MS, Federle MP, et al: Using CT and cholangiography to diagnose biliary tract carcinoma complicating primary sclerosing cholangitis. *AJR Am J Roentgenol* 177:1095, 2001.
14. Ludwig J, LaRusso NF, Wiesner RH: Primary sclerosing cholangitis. *Contemp Issues Surg Pathol* 8:193, 1986.
15. Palmer KR, Duerden BI, Holdsworth CD: Bacteriological and endotoxin studies in cases of ulcerative colitis submitted to surgery. *Gut* 21:851, 1980.
16. Lichtman SN, Sartor RB, Keku J, et al: Hepatic inflammation in rats with experimental small intestinal bacterial overgrowth. *Gastroenterology* 98:414, 1990.
17. Bharucha AE, Jorgensen R, Lichtman SN, et al: A pilot study of pentoxifylline for the treatment of primary sclerosing cholangitis. *Am J Gastroenterol* 95:2338, 2000.
18. Cangemi JR, Wiesner RH, Beaver SJ, et al: Effect of proctocolectomy for chronic ulcerative colitis on the natural history of primary sclerosing cholangitis. *Gastroenterology* 96:790, 1989.
19. Bergquist A, Lindberg G, Saarinen S, et al: Increased prevalence of primary sclerosing cholangitis among first-degree relatives. *J Hepatol* 42:252, 2005.

20. Satsangi J, Chapman RW, Haldar N, et al: A functional polymorphism of the stromelysin gene (MMP-3) influences susceptibility to primary sclerosing cholangitis. *Gastroenterology* 121:124, 2001.

21. Norris S, Kondeatis E, Collins R, et al: Mapping MHC-encoded susceptibility and resistance in primary sclerosing cholangitis: The role of MICA polymorphism. *Gastroenterology* 120:1475, 2001.

22. Eri R, Jonsson JR, Pandeya N, et al: CCR5-Delta32 mutation is strongly associated with primary sclerosing cholangitis. *Genes Immun* 5:444, 2004.

23. Chapman RW, Kelly PM, Heryet A, et al: Expression of HLA-DR antigens on bile duct epithelium in primary sclerosing cholangitis. *Gut* 29:422, 1988.

24. Broome U, Glaumann H, Hultcrantz R, et al: Distribution of HLA-DR, HLA-DP, HLA-DQ antigens in liver tissue from patients with primary sclerosing cholangitis. *Scand J Gastroenterol* 25:54, 1990.

25. Yang X, Cullen SN, Li JH, et al: Susceptibility to primary sclerosing cholangitis is associated with polymorphisms of intercellular adhesion molecule-1. *J Hepatol* 40:375, 2004.

26. Karlsen TH, Franke A, Melum E, et al: Genome-wide association analysis in primary sclerosing cholangitis. *Gastroenterology* 138:1102, 2010.

27. Loftus EV Jr, Sandborn WJ, Lindor KD: Interactions between chronic liver disease and inflammatory bowel disease. *Inflamm Bowel Dis* 3:288, 1997.

28. Rasmussen HH, Fallingborg JF, Mortensen PB, et al: Hepatobiliary dysfunction and primary sclerosing cholangitis in patients with Crohn's disease. *Scand J Gastroenterol* 32:604, 1997.

29. Broome U, Lofberg R, Veress B, et al: Primary sclerosing cholangitis and ulcerative colitis: Evidence for increased neoplastic potential. *Hepatology* 22:1404, 1995.

30. Brentnall TA, Haggitt RC, Rabinovitch PS, et al: Risk and natural history of colonic neoplasia in patients with primary sclerosing cholangitis and ulcerative colitis. *Gastroenterology* 110:331, 1996.

31. Kornfeld D, Ekbom A, Ihre T: Survival and risk of cholangiocarcinoma in patients with primary sclerosing cholangitis. A population-based study. *Scand J Gastroenterol* 32:1042, 1997.

32. Nuako KW, Ahlquist DA, Sandborn WJ, et al: Primary sclerosing cholangitis and colorectal carcinoma in patients with chronic ulcerative colitis: A case-control study. *Cancer* 82:822, 1998.

33. Bleday R, Lee E, Jessurun J, et al: Increased risk of early colorectal neoplasms after hepatic transplant in patients with inflammatory bowel disease. *Dis Colon Rectum* 36:908, 1993.

34. Porayko MK, Wiesner RH, LaRusso NF, et al: Patients with asymptomatic primary sclerosing cholangitis frequently have progressive disease. *Gastroenterology* 98:1594, 1990.

35. Brandt DJ, MacCarty RL, Charboneau JW, et al: Gallbladder disease in patients with primary sclerosing cholangitis. *AJR Am J Roentgenol* 150:571, 1988.

36. Buckles DC, Lindor KD, Larusso NF, et al: In primary sclerosing cholangitis, gallbladder polyps are frequently malignant. *Am J Gastroenterol* 97:1138, 2002.

37. Karlsen TH, Schrumpf E, Boberg KM: Gallbladder polyps in primary sclerosing cholangitis: Not so benign. *Curr Opin Gastroenterol* 24:395, 2008.

38. Dodd GD 3rd, Niedzwiecki GA, et al: Bile duct calculi in patients with primary sclerosing cholangitis. *Radiology* 203:443, 1997.

39. Wagner S, Gebel M, Meier P, et al: Endoscopic management of biliary tract strictures in primary sclerosing cholangitis. *Endoscopy* 28:546, 1996.

40. van Milligen de Wit AW, van Bracht J, Rauws EA, et al: Endoscopic stent therapy for dominant extrahepatic bile duct strictures in primary sclerosing cholangitis. *Gastrointest Endosc* 44:293, 1996.

41. van Milligen de Wit AW, Rauws EA, van Bracht J, et al: Lack of complications following short-term stent therapy for extrahepatic bile duct strictures in primary sclerosing cholangitis. *Gastrointest Endosc* 46:344, 1997.

42. Bjornsson E, Lindqvist-Ottosson J, Asztely M, et al: Dominant strictures in patients with primary sclerosing cholangitis. *Am J Gastroenterol* 99:502, 2004.

43. Burak K, Angulo P, Pasha TM, et al: Incidence and risk factors for cholangiocarcinoma in primary sclerosing cholangitis. *Am J Gastroenterol* 99:523, 2004.

44. Gores GJ: A spotlight on cholangiocarcinoma. *Gastroenterology* 125:1536, 2003.

45. Fleming KA, Boberg KM, Glaumann H, et al: Biliary dysplasia as a marker of cholangiocarcinoma in primary sclerosing cholangitis. *J Hepatol* 34:360, 2001.

46. Moreno Luna LE, Kipp B, Halling KC, et al: Advanced cytologic techniques for the detection of malignant pancreatobiliary strictures. *Gastroenterology* 131:1064, 2006.

47. Levy C, Lymp J, Angulo P, et al: The value of serum CA 19-9 in predicting cholangiocarcinomas in patients with primary sclerosing cholangitis. *Dig Dis Sci* 50:1734, 2005.

48. Keiding S, Hansen SB, Rasmussen HH, et al: Detection of cholangiocarcinoma in primary sclerosing cholangitis by positron emission tomography. *Hepatology* 28:700, 1998.

49. Prytz H, Keiding S, Bjornsson E, et al: Dynamic FDG-PET is useful for detection of cholangiocarcinoma in patients with PSC listed for liver transplantation. *Hepatology* 44:1572, 2006.

50. Jones EA, Bergasa NV: The pruritus of cholestasis. *Hepatology* 29:1003, 1999.

51. Jorgensen RA, Lindor KD, Sartin JS, et al: Serum lipid and fat-soluble vitamin levels in primary sclerosing cholangitis. *J Clin Gastroenterol* 20:215, 1995.

52. Hay JE, Lindor KD, Wiesner RH, et al: The metabolic bone disease of primary sclerosing cholangitis. *Hepatology* 14:257, 1991.

53. Zein CO, Lindor KD, Angulo P: Prevalence and predictors of esophageal varices in patients with primary sclerosing cholangitis. *Hepatology* 39:204, 2004.

54. Bergasa NV: An approach to the management of the pruritus of cholestasis. *Clin Liver Dis* 8:55, 2004.

55. Mitchell SA, Bansi DS, Hunt N, et al: A preliminary trial of high-dose ursodeoxycholic acid in primary sclerosing cholangitis. *Gastroenterology* 121:900, 2001.

56. Harnois DM, Angulo P, Jorgensen RA, et al: High-dose ursodeoxycholic acid as a therapy for patients with primary sclerosing cholangitis. *Am J Gastroenterol* 96:1558, 2001.

57. Lindor KD, Kowdley KV, Luketic VA, et al: High-dose ursodeoxycholic acid for the treatment of primary sclerosing cholangitis. *Hepatology* 50:808, 2009.

58. Tung BY, Emond MJ, Haggitt RC, et al: Ursodiol use is associated with lower prevalence of colonic neoplasia in patients with ulcerative colitis and primary sclerosing cholangitis. *Ann Intern Med* 134:89, 2001.

59. Pardi DS, Loftus EV Jr, Kremers WK, et al: Ursodeoxycholic acid as a chemopreventive agent in patients with ulcerative colitis and primary sclerosing cholangitis. *Gastroenterology* 124:889, 2003.

60. Wood RA, Cuschieri A: Is sclerosing cholangitis complicating ulcerative colitis a reversible condition? *Lancet* 2:716, 1980.

61. Cameron JL, Pitt HA, Zinner MJ, et al: Resection of hepatic duct bifurcation and transhepatic stenting for sclerosing cholangitis. *Ann Surg* 207:614, 1988.

62. Tocchi A, Mazzoni G, Liotta G, et al: Late development of bile duct cancer in patients who had biliary-enteric drainage for benign disease: A follow-up study of more than 1,000 patients. *Ann Surg* 234:210, 2001.

63. Wiesner RH, Porayko MK, Hay JE, et al: Liver transplantation for primary sclerosing cholangitis: Impact of risk factors on outcome. *Liver Transpl Surg* 2:99, 1996.

64. Abu-Elmagd KM, Malinchoc M, Dickson ER, et al: Efficacy of hepatic transplantation in patients with primary sclerosing cholangitis. *Surg Gynecol Obstet* 177:335, 1993.

65. Narumi S, Roberts JP, Emond JC, et al: Liver transplantation for sclerosing cholangitis. *Hepatology* 22:451, 1995.

66. Sheng R, Zajko AB, Campbell WL, et al: Biliary strictures in hepatic transplants: Prevalence and types in patients with primary sclerosing cholangitis vs those with other liver diseases. *AJR Am J Roentgenol* 161:297, 1993.

67. Graziadei IW, Wiesner RH, Marotta PJ, et al: Long-term results of patients undergoing liver transplantation for primary sclerosing cholangitis. *Hepatology* 30:1121, 1999.

68. Jeyarajah DR, Netto GJ, Lee SP, et al: Recurrent primary sclerosing cholangitis after orthotopic liver transplantation: Is chronic rejection part of the disease process? *Transplantation* 66:1300, 1998.

69. Loftus EV Jr, Aguilar HI, Sandborn WJ, et al: Risk of colorectal neoplasia in patients with primary sclerosing cholangitis and ulcerative colitis following orthotopic liver transplantation. *Hepatology* 27:685, 1998.

70. Goss JA, Shackleton CR, Farmer DG, et al: Orthotopic liver transplantation for primary sclerosing cholangitis. A 12-year single center experience. *Ann Surg* 225:472; discussion 481, 1997.

71. Rosen CB, Heimbach JK, Gores GJ: Liver transplantation for cholangiocarcinoma. *Transpl Int* 23:692, 2010.

72. Williams KJ, Picus J, Trinkhaus K, et al: Gemcitabine with carboplatin for advanced biliary tract cancers: A phase II single institution study. *HPB (Oxford)* 12:418, 2010.

73. Andre T, Reyes-Vidal JM, Fartoux L, et al: Gemcitabine and oxaliplatin in advanced biliary tract carcinoma: A phase II study. *Br J Cancer* 99:862, 2008.

74. Kartheuser AH, Dozois RR, LaRusso NF, et al: Comparison of surgical treatment of ulcerative colitis associated with primary sclerosing cholangitis: Ileal pouch-anal anastomosis versus Brooke ileostomy. *Mayo Clin Proc* 71:748, 1996.

75. Penna C, Dozois R, Tremaine W, et al: Pouchitis after ileal pouch-anal anastomosis for ulcerative colitis occurs with increased frequency in patients with associated primary sclerosing cholangitis. *Gut* 38:234, 1996.

Operative Management of Bile Duct Strictures

Karen Chojnacki | Charles J. Yeo

Bile duct strictures can result from a myriad of conditions, both benign and malignant. These strictures represent a significant clinical problem and if not managed correctly can result in major morbidity, both short and long term, and possible mortality. Complications of untreated or improperly treated strictures include cholangitis, biliary cirrhosis, portal hypertension, and end-stage liver disease. The goal of treatment is to reestablish unobstructed biliary flow into the intestinal tract.

PATHOGENESIS

The most common cause of bile duct stricture is surgery of the gallbladder or biliary tree. In the era of open surgery, the incidence of bile duct injury following cholecystectomy was 0.2% to 0.3%[1,2] Since the introduction of laparoscopic cholecystectomy, the rate of bile duct injury has doubled. Several studies have published an injury rate of 0.4% to 0.6%.[2-4] This rate of injury has remained essentially stable.[5] Less than 30% of bile duct injuries are recognized intraoperatively.[6] Therefore most patients will go on to develop a leak or stricture. The classification of these injuries and strictures has been defined by Strasberg and Bismuth and is shown in Figures 113-1 and 113-2.[2]

Not all bile duct strictures caused by a previous surgery result from laparoscopic cholecystectomy. Endoscopic, percutaneous, and operative procedures on the bile duct may result in stricture. Injury may also occur during gastric and duodenal procedures, liver resection and transplantation, and pancreatic procedures. These injuries typically involve a failure to recognize the extrahepatic biliary tree at the time of antral or duodenal dissection/division. The anatomy in this region may be distorted by inflammation or a neoplastic process. The intrapancreatic bile duct may be injured during surgery of the pancreatic head or ampulla of Vater. Inflammatory or congenital conditions may also cause strictures of the bile duct (Box 113-1). Benign and malignant neoplasms of the biliary tree and surrounding organs are additional causes of biliary stricture (Box 113-2).

CLINICAL PRESENTATION

Patients with postoperative bile duct injuries typically present early after the procedure. In a study of patients with bile duct injury following open cholecystectomy, 69% of patients were diagnosed within the first 6 months and 82% were diagnosed within the first year following surgery.[7] Patients with early postoperative complications have three types of injury: bile leak, obstruction, or a combination of leak and obstruction. Patients with a leak

often complain of vague symptoms such as abdominal fullness, abdominal pain, nausea, vomiting, fever, and/or chills. Their pain is often similar to the biliary colic that brought them to surgery. These patients may have bile leaking from their incisions or operatively placed drains, or the leak may be contained within the abdomen. Any patient who is not improving daily following a cholecystectomy should be suspected of harboring a bile duct injury. Liver function tests can be normal or show only mild elevations of bilirubin. Bilirubin elevation is typically a result of peritoneal absorption. Serum alkaline phosphatase is often elevated as the biliary epithelium is damaged. Levels of alanine aminotransferase and aspartate aminotransferase are usually normal. Patients with obstruction will have evidence of jaundice, scleral icterus, abdominal pain, and/or anorexia. If cholangitis is present, patients will also have fever, chills, and malaise, and these patients will also have abnormalities in their liver function tests. Hyperbilirubinemia is present. Cholangitis will cause leukocytosis. If the obstruction is long-standing with progression to biliary cirrhosis, there will be evidence of decreased hepatic synthetic function (i.e., hypoalbuminemia and prolonged prothrombin time).

Patients undergoing uncomplicated laparoscopic cholecystectomy should recover quickly with minimal discomfort. Most patients have little to no pain in the first postoperative days. There is little requirement for analgesics. Most are back to normal activities within the first week. Any patient with persistent pain, nausea, vomiting, abdominal distention, or declining activity level should be evaluated for a suspected bile duct injury.

RADIOLOGIC WORKUP

Initial radiologic evaluation includes abdominal ultrasound and/or computed tomography (CT). Both can identify intraabdominal fluid collections and dilated intra- or extrahepatic bile ducts. Small fluid collections are found in the gallbladder fossa in 10% to 14% of patients after cholecystectomy, and these typically resolve without intervention.[8,9] Large fluid collections, fluid collections outside of the gallbladder fossa, or ascites are findings worrisome for bile leak. CT and ultrasound cannot distinguish between seroma, lymphocele, hematoma, or biloma. Aspiration, drainage, and/or catheter placement into a fluid collection may be necessary to define the fluid collection. CT and ultrasound can both be used to evaluate for signs of unsuspected malignancy such as mass or adenopathy.

Hepatobiliary iminodiacetic acid (HIDA) scanning can be used to assess for bile leak or biliary obstruction. However, the exact location of a leak or extent of injury cannot be uniformly assessed with HIDA scan. If a drain

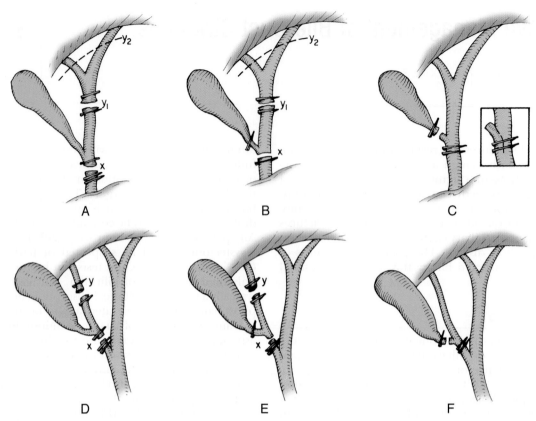

FIGURE 113-1 Various patterns of biliary tract injury. **A,** Classic injury. **B** and **C,** Variants of the classic injury. **D** to **F,** Different injuries resulting from the cystic duct originating from an aberrant right hepatic duct. (From Strasberg SM, Hertl M, Soper NJ: An analysis of the problem of biliary injury during laparoscopic cholecystectomy. *J Am Coll Surg* 180:101, 1995.)

was placed at the time of cholecystectomy, water-soluble contrast can be injected through the catheter (sinography) to define the leak or injury. Alternatively, if a percutaneous drainage catheter has been placed, a sonogram can be obtained via this catheter, to define the leak site and the relevant biliary anatomy.

In most cases, cholangiography will be necessary for accurate evaluation of the biliary tree. Three techniques exist for imaging the bile ducts: percutaneous transhepatic cholangiography (PTC), endoscopic retrograde cholangiography (ERC), and magnetic resonance cholangiopancreatography (MRCP). ERC has the ability to detect the exact location of leak, injury, or obstruction (Figure 113-3, *A*). It is particularly useful in the management of cystic stump leaks and partial injuries to the extrahepatic biliary tree. If a leak or partial injury is detected at ERC, an endoprosthesis can be placed. An endoprosthesis can serve two purposes. As a stent across a leak, the endoprosthesis decreases the pressure gradient between the biliary system and the duodenum by traversing the sphincter of Oddi. This creates a path of least resistance, allowing the bile to flow away from the leak. An endoprosthesis can also bridge and occlude a defect, allowing time to heal and minimize stricture formation.[10] ERC, however, is less valuable in cases of complete common bile duct transection or occlusion. In these cases, the proximal biliary tree cannot be evaluated by ERC (Figure 113-3, *B*). Of note, ERC provides no information about concomitant vascular injuries.

PTC is useful for evaluating the proximal extrahepatic and intrahepatic biliary tree (Figure 113-4). Information gained from this study is essential for planning future reconstruction. First the intrahepatic biliary tree is visualized with a Chiba needle, and then using the Seldinger technique, a wire is passed into the biliary tree. This is followed by the placement of a percutaneous transhepatic catheter. This allows for therapeutic procedures such as drainage, dilation, and control of a bile leak. This is an invasive procedure with a complication rate as high as 6.9%. Complications include bleeding, hemobilia, bile duct injury, and cholangitis. Although challenging, even nondilated intrahepatic ducts can be cannulated safely.[11] At the time of the biliary reconstruction, it is helpful to wedge the catheter at the caudalmost extent of the transected, obstructed extrahepatic biliary tree or advance the catheter for a few centimeters in the subhepatic space in the case of an open proximal biliary tree. This greatly facilitates identification of the injured duct.

MRCP is a noninvasive technique for imaging of the biliary tree. Besides evaluating the bile ducts proximal and distal to an injury, MRCP can also assess for other intraabdominal injuries, fluid collections, vascular injury, and hepatic ischemia or necrosis. These high-quality images have led some to suggest that MRCP is superior to PTC or ERC and should become the initial step in evaluating patients with suspected bile duct strictures.[12,13] Information gained from MRCP can determine which

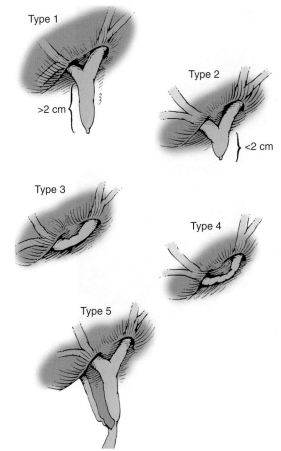

FIGURE 113-2 Classification of bile duct strictures based on the level of the stricture in relation to the confluence of the hepatic ducts. Types 3, 4, and 5 are typically considered complex injuries. (From Bismuth H: Postoperative strictures of the bile ducts. In Blumgart LH, editor: *The biliary tract.* Clinical surgery international series, Vol 5. Edinburgh, 1983, Churchill Livingstone, p 209.)

BOX 113-1 **Causes of Benign Biliary Strictures**

IATROGENIC
Postoperative strictures following biliary procedures
Laparoscopic cholecystectomy
Open cholecystectomy
Common bile duct exploration
Prior stricture repair
Endoscopic retrograde cholangiopancreatography
Endoscopic sphincterotomy
Percutaneous biliary manipulation
Postoperative strictures following other operative procedures
Gastrectomy
   Duodenal ulcer procedures
Hepatic resection
   Hepatic transplantation
   Pancreatic procedures
   Portacaval shunt
   Stricture at biliary-enteric anastomosis

TRAUMATIC
Blunt injury
Penetrating injury

INFLAMMATORY
Chronic pancreatitis
Cholelithiasis and choledocholithiasis
Mirizzi syndrome
Primary sclerosing cholangitis
Duodenal ulcer
Duodenal diverticulum
Crohn disease
Sphincter of Oddi stenosis
Viral infections
Toxic drugs
Radiation fibrosis
Subhepatic abscess
Parasitic infestations

INFLAMMATORY
Choledochal cyst
Caroli disease
Congenital stricture, webs
Biliary atresia

---

patients will have therapeutic benefit from an invasive study (e.g., cystic duct leak requiring biliary endoprosthesis). It can also guide which invasive procedure will most benefit a patient (e.g., PTC for complete common bile duct transection).

The importance of accurate understanding of the biliary anatomy in patients with bile duct stricture cannot be overstated. The success of reconstruction depends on clear delineation of the site of the stricture and the biliary anatomy. In one study, 96% of bile duct reconstructions were unsuccessful when preoperative cholangiography was not obtained. Sixty-nine percent of repairs were unsuccessful if the cholangiographic data were incomplete. When cholangiographic data were complete, 84% of initial repairs were successful.[14]

SURGICAL MANAGEMENT OF BILE DUCT STRICTURES

Once the anatomy of a bile duct stricture has been defined, decisions must be made regarding the timing of repair and the type of repair.

EARLY REPAIR

Patients who present early after surgery, and show no signs of sepsis, intraabdominal collections, or vascular injury, should be considered for early repair within 72 hours. These patients tend to have simpler injuries. The type of injury guides the appropriate intervention. Strasberg type A injuries, cystic duct leaks, can be managed with endoscopic sphincterotomy and stenting, via the placement of a biliary endoprosthesis (typically 8- to 10-French. plastic stent). Leaks from a duct of Luschka can be managed in a similar manner.

Strasberg type D injuries can also be approached in the early postoperative period. These injuries are also amenable to endoscopic sphincterotomy and stenting. Of note, if a partial transection of the common bile duct is recognized at the time of initial surgery, it can be

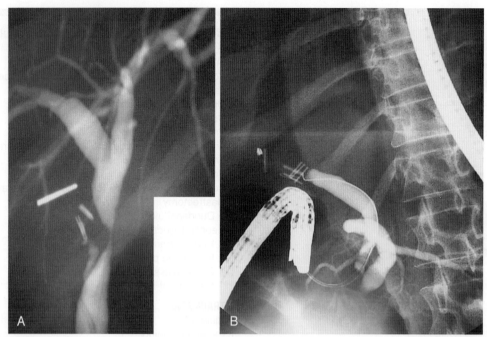

FIGURE 113-3 A, An endoscopic retrograde cholangiopancreatogram from a patient with elevated liver function tests 4 years after open cholecystectomy. Note the extensive narrowing of the bile duct below the bifurcation and the surgical clips close to the strictured area. **B,** A cholangiopancreatogram from a patient with a total transection of the common bile duct during laparoscopic cholecystectomy. Note the multiple clips across the common bile duct and the abrupt termination of the column of contrast medium at the site of the clips.

BOX 113-2 Neoplastic Causes of Biliary Stricture

BENIGN
Bile duct hamartoma
Bile duct adenoma
Benign inflammatory tumors (benign inflammatory
  pseudotumors)

MALIGNANT—INTRINSIC
Cholangiocarcinoma

MALIGNANT—EXTRINSIC
Pancreatic carcinoma
Ampullary carcinoma
Duodenal carcinoma
Gallbladder carcinoma
Lymphoma
Lymphadenopathy from gastric carcinoma, colorectal
  carcinoma

---

repaired primarily over a T-tube. Fine, monofilament, absorbable sutures should be used for the repair. The T-tube should be brought out of the common bile duct at a distant site away from the repair site (Figure 113-5). If the injury is secondary to the use of cautery or results in complete transection of the duct, results of primary repair are poor. One study reported a restricture rate of nearly 100% for end-to-end repairs of the common bile duct.[14] These patients are best managed with a biliary-enteric anastomosis as later described.

DELAYED MANAGEMENT OF BILIARY STRICTURE

If operative repair cannot be completed within 72 hours of injury because of patient condition or inability to complete radiographic workup, delay of repair is often advocated.[15,16] This will allow time for inflammation to subside and infection and sepsis to resolve. Others argue that this approach results in dense adhesions, making definitive repair more difficult.[17] Regardless of timing of repair, intraabdominal sepsis and patient condition must be stabilized before repair of complex injuries.

Patients with a delayed presentation will typically be suffering from an ongoing bile leak or biliary obstruction. Patients with a leak require drainage of intraabdominal collections, volume and electrolyte replacement/correction, correction of anemia, and nutritional assessment. Infection and sepsis will require antibiotic treatment. Patients with obstruction may have signs and symptoms of cholangitis. These patients will require antibiotic therapy and drainage of the biliary tree by percutaneous transhepatic biliary drainage. All patients will require adequate radiologic assessment of the biliary tree. This is most often achieved by percutaneous transhepatic cholangiography. Percutaneous drainage catheters, left in place above the stricture or through the injured, leaking duct, are often useful during reconstruction for identification of the injured/strictured duct.

Successful bile duct enteric reconstruction is dependent on several factors:
1. Adequate preoperative assessment of biliary anatomy
2. Exposure of proximal, healthy bile ducts with adequate blood supply

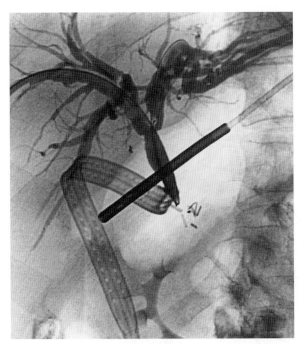

FIGURE 113-4 A percutaneous transhepatic cholangiogram from a patient with a complete transection of the common hepatic duct, which ends close to several surgical clips. A surgical drain is in place, as well as a duodenal feeding tube (which crosses obliquely over the common hepatic duct).

3. The repair must include all injured/strictured ducts to ensure adequate drainage of the entire liver, and control of bile leakage.
4. Use of a healthy segment of intestine that can be brought to the anastomosis without tension (most often a Roux-en-Y jejunal limb)
5. Creation of a tension-free biliary mucosa-to-bowel mucosa anastomosis

Operative intervention is most often done through a midline incision. Careful dissection of the porta hepatis is required. There may be dense adhesions in this area; therefore, the duodenum and hepatic flexure of the colon must be carefully mobilized. Identification of the strictured or injured bile duct can be difficult. Dissection in this area must proceed with caution to avoid injury to the portal vein, proper hepatic artery, or proximal bile duct. Identification of the injured duct can be aided by the presence of a previously placed percutaneous biliary catheter or catheters. If the injured duct(s) is transected, the duct should be dissected circumferentially for a distance of 5 mm. An end-to-side hepaticojejunostomy to the newly created, defunctionalized 50- to 60-cm-long Roux-en-Y jejunal limb is then performed (Figure 113-6). The distal bile duct, if it remains open, is oversewn with absorbable, running suture. Most often, the distal bile duct has been closed with clips at the time of cholecystectomy. If this is the case, the clips are left undisturbed. If the injured duct is strictured or inflamed, the duct proximal to the stricture is cleared anteriorly for 1 to 2 cm. The biliary-enteric anastomosis is accomplished with absorbable monofilament suture in one layer, typically 4-0, 5-0, or 6-0 polydioxanone. If multiple ducts are injured, then more than one anastomosis may be required. Proximal injuries may require the anastomosis to be positioned at the extrahepatic portion of the left hepatic duct after it is lowered by dividing the hepatic plate, the Hepp-Couinaud approach.[18] Continuity of the left and right ducts is required for this approach to work. This technique works well for Bismuth type 2 and 3 strictures. At completion of the anastomosis, a closed suction drain is left in the right upper quadrant to drain any residual collection or small bile leak in the early postoperative period.

If the left and right ducts are not in communication, for example, in Bismuth type 4 and 5 injuries, sufficient exposure of both the right and left ducts or the injured aberrant right duct is required for adequate repair. As the extrahepatic length of the right duct is often quite short, exposure of this duct can be difficult. Dissection along the left duct provides a guide to the coronal plane in which the right ducts will be found. Along this plane, liver tissue can be removed to better expose the right ducts. Exposure can be further improved by dividing the bridge of tissue between liver segments 3 and 4 by fully opening the gallbladder fossa. Partial resection of segments 4b and 5 will open the upper porta hepatic tissue, further exposing the right duct to allow for a standard biliary-enteric anastomosis.

The use of stents across the biliary reconstruction is controversial. Good results have been reported by groups who routinely stent and also by those who do not. Advocates of stenting argue that a transanastomotic stent

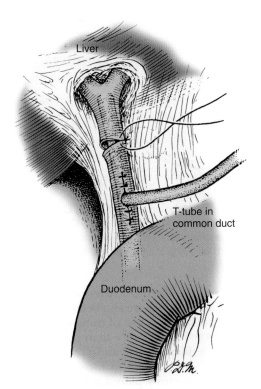

FIGURE 113-5 Primary end-to-end repair of a bile duct injury over a T-tube. In general, this technique is used for partial transections of the bile duct, when there has been no associated loss of ductal length. Note that the T-tube does not exit at the site of injury.

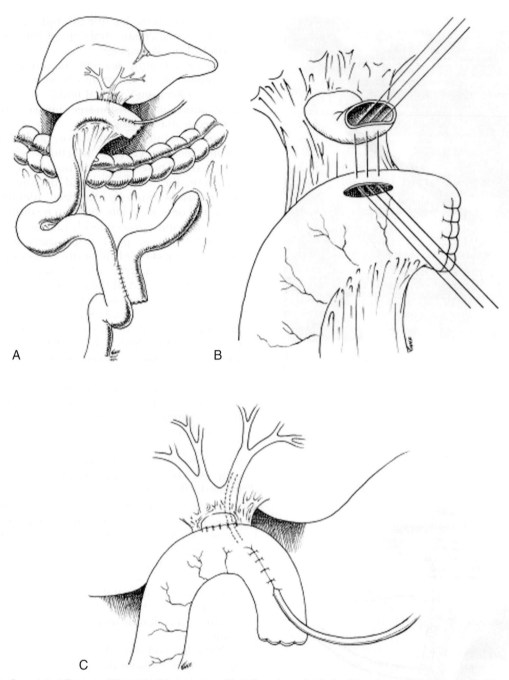

FIGURE 113-6 A, Completed Roux-en-Y hepaticojejunostomy with 5-French pediatric feeding tube as biliary stent. **B,** Closeup view of hepaticojejunostomy using interrupted 5-0 PDS absorbable suture. Note back-wall knots on inside of anastomosis. **C,** Biliary stent secured with Witzel tunnel and used for imaging postoperatively. Omission of stent is acceptable. (From McPartland KJ, Pomposelli JJ: Iatrogenic biliary injuries: Classification, identification, and management. *Surg Clin N Am* 88:1329, 2008, Figure 3, p 1339.)

decompresses the biliary tree and anastomosis, provides a scaffold for scarring of the biliary anastomosis, and maintains patency of the anastomosis.[19] Intraoperatively, transhepatic stents facilitate identification of the bile duct. Postoperatively, stents allow for easy radiologic assessment and intervention at the point of repair. Those arguing against the use of stents note their increased risk of infecting the biliary tree and the increased incidence of hemobilia related to the transhepatic stent. Contaminated bile increases the risk of postoperative infectious complications.[20] Transanastomotic stents may also cause pressure necrosis of the duct. Arterio-biliary and biliary pleural fistula formation have also been reported.[19] Some experts advocate selective use of transanastomotic stents for small ducts (<4 mm), more than one anastomosis, a scarred and/or inflamed duct, and a proximal anastomosis.[21] If the decision is made to use a transanastomotic stent, the percutaneously placed transhepatic stent can be used or a new Silastic stent can be placed. The stent is typically left in place for a minimum of 6 to 8 weeks, occasionally longer. A cholangiogram should be obtained prior to removing the stent. This is best done as an over-the-wire cholangiogram, pulling the transhepatic stent back so that it does not transverse the repair at the time of cholangiography.

In those rare instances where a biliary anastomosis cannot be achieved, hepatectomy/resection of the affected liver segments may be required so as to remove the hepatic parenchyma without continuity to the biliary tree.

POSTOPERATIVE COMPLICATIONS

Complications for bile duct stricture repair range from 20% to 40% in the literature.[22,23] In one large series, the postoperative complication rate was 42.9%, with many complications being minor, including wound infection, cholangitis, anastomotic leak, intraabdominal abscess/biloma, and stent-related complications.[23] Nonsurgical complications typically include cardiopulmonary complications, ileus, and short-term diarrhea. Reported mortality rates ranged from 1.7% to 2.7%.[24,25]

SURGICAL RESULTS

Excellent long-term results of bile duct stricture repair have been reported. Success rates of 80% to 90% for all types of benign strictures have been achieved (Table 113-1). Studies of repair following laparoscopic cholecystectomy have reported similar success rates (Table 113-2). Success is defined by the absence of symptoms, jaundice, and cholangitis. Postoperative stricture formation can occur in the early or late postoperative period.

With long-term followup, recurrent stricture rates of 10% to 14% have been reported.[26,16] Eighty percent of recurrent strictures occur within 5 years of repair. Five percent of strictures occur more than 12 years after repair.[7] The factor most associated with recurrent stricture is the initial injury or stricture level. One-third of injuries proximal to the bile duct bifurcation will develop stricture.[27] A small minority of patients may also develop chronic liver disease following repair of a bile duct stricture. Rates of chronic liver disease have been reported between 6% and 22%.[28,29] Risk factors for the development of chronic liver disease include prolonged interval between injury diagnosis and referral to a tertiary care center, cholangitis, and preexisting liver disease. Patients should be followed closely postoperatively for the development of chronic liver disease and recurrent stricture. Most cases of recurrent stricture can be managed with endoscopic or percutaneous dilation. Rarely, patients with liver failure will require transplantation. In several studies, the long-term quality of life for patients undergoing repair of bile duct injuries approaches the quality of life of the general population.[30]

NONOPERATIVE MANAGEMENT OF BILE DUCT STRICTURES

Endoscopic or percutaneous transhepatic stenting or dilation can be used for simple bile duct injuries or strictures such as cystic stump leaks, duct of Luschka leaks, small partial common bile duct transections, and focal strictures less than 1 cm in length.[31] The success of nonoperative management for more extensive injuries or strictures is less than that of operative repair.

For patients who develop a bile duct stricture following repair, nonoperative therapies may provide relief of the stricture. These patients have developed a stricture after biliary-enteric anastomosis. In one report, 58% of 51 patients with biliary stricture were successfully managed by percutaneous dilation.[32] Another report compared 35 patients managed with surgery to 66 patients treated with endoscopic stenting.[33] The surgical patients were managed with a Roux-en-Y hepaticojejunostomy. Endoscopic therapy involved the placement of an endoprosthesis that was exchanged every 3 months. Excellent results were achieved in 83% of the surgical patients with a recurrent stricture rate of 17% at 40 months. After endoscopic stenting, 72% of patients

TABLE 113-1 Selected Results of Surgical Repair of Bile Duct Strictures

Authors, Year	No. of Patients	Success Rate (%)	Followup (mo)	Reference
Pellegrini et al, 1984	60	78	102	38
Genest et al, 1986	105	82	60	39
Innes et al, 1988	22	95	72	40
Pitt et al, 1989	25	88	57	41
David et al, 1993	35	83	50	33
Chapman et al, 1995	104	76	86	42
McDonald et al, 1995	72	87	<60	43
Tocchi et al, 1996	84	83	108	44
Lillemoe et al, 2000	156	91	58	24

TABLE 113-2 Studies of Repair Following Laparoscopic Cholecystectomy

Authors, Year	No. of Patients	Recognized at Laparoscopic Cholecystectomy (%)	Bismuth Types 3 to 5 (%)	Success Rate (%)	Reference
Walsh et al, 2007[28]	84	43	61	91	28
Bauer et al, 1998[34]	32	31	24	83	34
Lillemoe et al, 1997[35]	52	8	53	92	35
Mirza et al, 1997[36]	27	22	33	81	36
Nealon et al, 1996[37]	23	70	26	100	37

achieved excellent results. Eighteen percent of these patients developed recurrent strictures at a mean of 3 months after stent removal. In cases of stricture following repair, endoscopic stenting should be considered.

SUMMARY

Bile duct injuries and strictures are complex problems requiring a multidisciplinary approach involving surgeons, radiologists, and gastroenterologists. Failure to properly diagnose and/or manage these problems can result in chronic liver disease and/or chronic disabilities. Complete and accurate preoperative imaging is essential to successful outcomes. Appropriate surgical management with careful attention to detail and technique is also imperative. Excellent outcomes can be achieved by following these principles.

REFERENCES

1. Roslyn JJ, Pinns GS, Hughes EF, et al: Open cholecystectomy: A contemporary analysis of 42,474 patients. *Ann Surg* 218:129, 1993.
2. Strasberg SM, Hertl M, Soper NJ: An analysis of the problem of biliary injury during laparoscopic cholecystectomy. *J Am Coll Surg* 180:101, 1995.
3. Fletcher DR, Hobbs MST, Tan P, et al: Complications of cholecystectomy: Risks of the laparoscopic approach and protective effects of cholangiography—a population-based study. *Ann Surg* 229:449, 1999.
4. Deziel DJ, Millikan KW, Economou SG, et al: Complications of laparoscopic cholecystectomy: A national survey of 4,292 hospitals and an analysis of 77,604 cases. *Am J Surg* 165:9, 1993.
5. Wherry DC, Marohn MR, Malansoki MP, et al: An external audit of laparoscopic cholecystectomy in the steady state performed in medical treatment facilities of the Department of Defense. *Ann Surg* 224:145, 1996.
6. Carroll BJ, Birth M, Phillip EH: Common bile duct injuries during laparoscopic cholecystectomy that result in ligation. *Surg Endosc* 12:310, 1998.
7. Pitt HA, Miyamoto T, Parapatis SK, et al: Factors influencing outcome in patients with postoperative biliary strictures. *Am J Surg* 114:14, 1982.
8. McAlister VC: Abdominal fluid collection after laparoscopic cholecystectomy. *Br J Surg* 87:1126, 2000.
9. Moran J, Del Grosso E, Wills J, et al: Laparoscopic cholecystectomy: Imaging of complications and normal postoperative CT appearance. *Abdom Imaging* 19:143, 1994.
10. Weber A, Feussner H, Winkelman F, et al: Long term outcome of endoscopic therapy in patients with bile duct injury after cholecystectomy. *J Gastroenterol Hepatol* 24:762, 2009.
11. Oh HC, Lee SK, Lee TY, et al: Analysis of percutaneous transhepatic cholangioscopy-related complications and the risk factors for those complications. *Endoscopy* 39:731, 2007.
12. Yeh TS, Jan YY, Tseng JH, et al: Value of magnetic resonance cholangiopancreatography in demonstrating major bile duct injuries following laparoscopic cholecystectomy. *Br J Surg* 86:181, 1999.
13. Bujanda L, Calvo MM, Cabriada JL, et al: MRCP in the diagnosis of iatrogenic bile duct injury. *NMR Biomed* 16:475, 2003.
14. Stewart L, Way LW: Bile duct injuries during laparoscopic cholecystectomy. *Arch Surg* 130:1123, 1995.
15. Lillemoe KD: Current management of bile duct injury. *Br J Surg* 95:403, 2008.
16. Sahajpal AK, Chow SC, Dixon E, et al: Bile duct injuries associated with laparoscopic cholecystectomy: Timing of repair and long term outcomes. *Arch Surg* 145:757, 2010.
17. McPartland KJ, Pomposelli JJ: Iatrogenic biliary injuries: Classification, identification, and management. *Surg Clin N Am* 88:1329, 2008.
18. Hepp J, Couinaud C. [Approach to and use of the left hepatic duct in reparation of the common bile duct]. *Presse Med* 64:947, 1956. [in French]
19. Mercado AM, Chan C, Orozco H, et al: To stent or not to stent bilioenteric anastomosis after iatrogenic injury. *Arch Surg* 137:60, 2002.
20. Hochwald SN, Burke EC, Jarnagin WR, et al: Association of preoperative biliary stenting with increased postoperative infectious complications in proximal cholangiocarcinoma. *Arch Surg* 134:261, 1999.
21. Wu YV, Linehan DC: Bile duct injuries in the era of laparoscopic cholecystectomies. *Surg Clin N Am* 90:787, 2010.
22. Robinson TN, Stiegmann GV, Durham JD, et al: Management of major bile duct injury associated with laparoscopic cholecystectomy. *Surg Endosc* 15:1381, 2001.
23. Sicklick JK, Camp MS, Lillemoe KD, et al: Surgical management of bile duct injuries sustained during laparoscopic cholecystectomy: Perioperative results in 200 patients. *Ann Surg* 241:786, 2005.
24. Lillemoe KD, Melto GB, Cameron JL, et al: Postoperative bile duct strictures: Management and outcome in the 1990's. *Ann Surg* 232:430, 2000.
25. Flum DR, Cheadle A, Prela C, et al: Bile duct injury during cholecystectomy and survival in Medicare beneficiaries. *JAMA* 290:2168, 2003.
26. Murr MM, Gigo JF, Nagorney DM, et al: Long-term results of biliary reconstruction after laparoscopic bile duct injuries. *Arch Surg* 134:604, 1999.
27. Mercado MA, Chan C, Orozco H, et al: Prognostic implication of preserved bile duct confluence after iatrogenic injury. *Hepatogastroenterology* 52:40, 2005.
28. Walsh RM, Henderson JM, Voight DP, et al: Long term outcome of biliary reconstruction for bile duct injuries from laparoscopic cholecystectomy. *Surgery* 142:450, 2007.
29. Nordin A, Holme L, Makisalos H, et al: Management and outcome of major bile duct injury after laparoscopic cholecystectomy: From therapeutic endoscopy to liver transplantation. *Liver Transpl* 8:1036, 2002.
30. Melton GB, Lillemoe KD, Cameron JL, et al: Major bile duct injuries associated with laparoscopic cholecystectomy: Effect on quality of life. *Ann Surg* 235:888, 2002.
31. Winslow ER, Fialkowski EA, Linehan DC, et al: Sideways: Results of repair of biliary injuries using a policy of side to side hepaticojejunostomy. *Ann Surg* 94:1119, 2009.
32. Misra S, Melton GB, Beschwind JF, et al: Percutaneous management of bile duct strictures and injuries associated with laparoscopic cholecystectomy: A decade of experience. *J Am Coll Surg* 198:218, 2004.
33. David PHP, Tanka AKF, Rauws EAJ, et al: Benign biliary strictures. Surgery or endoscopy? *Ann Surg* 217:237, 1993.
34. Bauer TW, Morris JB, Lowenstein A, et al: The consequences of a major bile duct injury during laparoscopic cholecystectomy. *J Gastrointest Surg* 2:61, 1998.
35. Lillemoe KD, Martin SA, Cameron JL, et al: Major bile duct injuries during laparoscopic cholecystectomy: Follow-up after combined radiological and surgical management. *Ann Surg* 225:459, discussion 468, 1997.
36. Mirza DF, Narsimhan KL, Ferrazneto BH, et al: Bile duct injury following laparoscopic cholecystectomy: Referral pattern and management. *Br J Surg* 84:786, 1997.
37. Nealon WH, Urrutia F: Long term follow up after bilioenteric anastomosis for benign bile duct stricture. *Ann Surg* 223:639, 1996.
38. Pellegrini CA, Thomas JM, Way IW: Recurrent biliary stricture. Pattern of recurrence and outcome of surgical therapy. *Am J Surg* 147:175, 1984.
39. Genest JF, Nanos E, Grundfest-Broniatowski S, et al: Benign biliary strictures: An analytic review (1970 to 1984). *Surgery* 99:409, 1986.
40. Innes JT, Ferara JJ, Kairey LC: Biliary reconstruction without transanastomotic stent. *Am Surg* 54:27, 1998.
41. Pitt HA, Kaufman Hs, Coleman J, et al: Benign postoperative biliary strictures: Operate or dilate? *Ann Surg* 210:417, 1989.
42. Chapman WC, Halevy A, Blumgart LH, et al: Postcholecystectomy bile duct strictures. Management and outcome in 130 patients. *Arch Surg* 130:597, 1995.
43. McDonald ML, Farnell MB, Nagorney DM, et al: Benign biliary strictures: Repair and outcome with a contemporary approach. *Surgery* 118:582, 1995.
44. Tocchi A, Costa G, Lepre L, et al: The long-term outcome of hepaticojejunostomy in the treatment of benign bile duct stricutres. *Ann Surg* 224:162, 1996.

Anatomy and Physiology of the Liver

Ernesto P. Molmenti | George C. Sotiropoulos | Arnold Radtke |

Jeffrey M. Nicastro | Gene F. Coppa | Eduardo de Santibañes |

Massimo Malagó

Our understanding of functional surgical hepatic anatomy evolved significantly through technical advances in repair of hepatobiliary injury, liver transplantation, hepatic resection, and radiologically guided intervention. This evolution was essential to the development of live-donor and deceased-donor segmental liver transplantation.[1-6] Molmenti described this reconception of hepatic anatomy as derived from an anatomic-physiologic inside-out approach, as opposed to the purely topographic outside-in view of the past (Figure 114-1).[2]

Human anatomy may be classified and is classifiable, but variation is the rule. This chapter reviews basic concepts of hepatic anatomy, with the important caveat that these simple concepts will not always hold true in all circumstances. There are now tools that allow the individual anatomy of the subject to be outlined preoperatively and intraoperatively in cases such as hepatic resection or live liver donation.

MODERN ANATOMIC APPROACH TO LIVER SURGERY

The liver is a single organ that can be functionally regarded as two hemilivers. The parenchyma can be further subdivided into several regions sharing common arterial, portal, and biliary supply and venous drainage. The portal and venous systems define these regions that are named sectors and segments, respectively (Figures 114-2 to 114-5).[2-5] The liver has a rather constant anatomic pattern, the knowledge of which allows for a safe surgical approach. Nevertheless, there are some anatomic irregularities, and in particular instances, exact knowledge of the anatomy specific to the individual patient being examined or operated on is necessary (live donors, left extended or central hepatectomies, caudate lobe masses). In these cases a computed three-dimensional reconstruction of each anatomic detail is possible following an accurate computed tomographic or magnetic resonance imaging contrast scan. Several software packages are currently available that allow for the mapping of the individual anatomy, as well as for the calculation of volumes corresponding to the whole liver, liver sectors, and segments.* The reliability of virtual three-dimensional reconstructions based on standard anatomic landmarks for both surgical planning and graft volume calculations has been demonstrated (Figure 114-6).[7] For standard liver surgery, the operating surgeon should be familiar with the basic anatomic pattern of the liver and the most frequent variations that have been described.

EMBRYOLOGY OF THE LIVER

The liver primordium, also known as *diverticulum hepatis* or *liver bud*, arises from endoderm in weeks 3 through 4 of embryologic development and invades the septum transversum, vitelline (omphalomesenteric) veins, and umbilical veins. Its connection to the embryologic duodenum (foregut) will eventually become the bile duct.[8,9] Embryologically, the liver receives blood from both portal and umbilical veins, themselves connected by the left portal vein.[10,11] Although the primitive portal veins arise from the caudal part of the vitelline veins, the primitive hepatic veins arise from the cranial part of the vitelline veins.[8,12] In humans and many other mammals, the inferior vena cava (IVC), ductus venosus, and umbilical vein are initially surrounded by liver parenchyma and become extrahepatic only in later stages of embryologic development.[11] The arteries develop in conjunction with the bile ducts at a later period than the veins. On the right side, arteries and bile ducts follow the trajectory of the portal venous branches. On the left side, although arterial and biliary branching follows a symmetric pattern similar to

---

*Hepavision, MeVis-Germany, Hitachi-Japan, Hepavis-Slovenia, Université de Starsbourg-France.

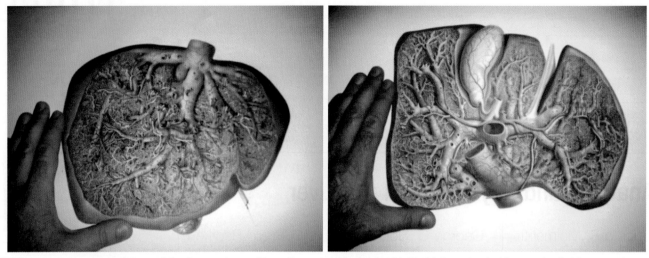

FIGURE 114-1 Classic depictions of the liver anatomy. (From Bourgery JM, Jacob NH: Traité Complet de L'anatomie de L'homme. In Delaunay CA editor: *Tome Cinquième*, Paris, 1839. [Private collection of Ernesto P. Molmenti, MD, PhD, MBA.])

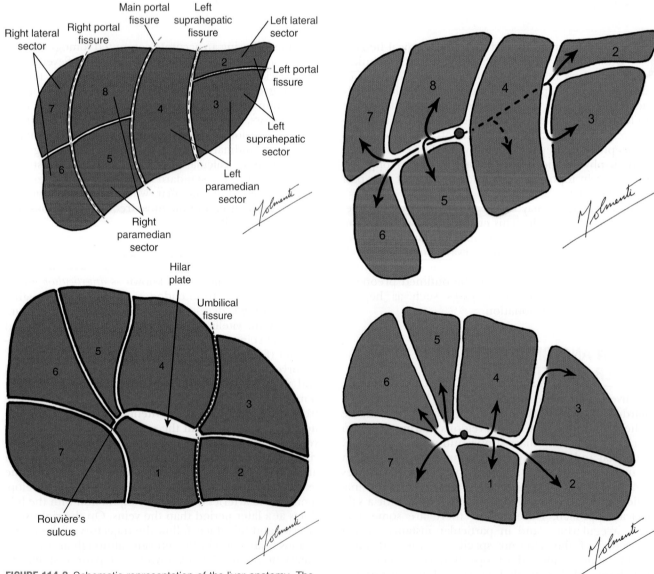

FIGURE 114-2 Schematic representation of the liver anatomy. The hepatic segments have been numbered, and the major structures have been labeled.

FIGURE 114-3 Schematic representation of the arteriobiliary liver anatomy.

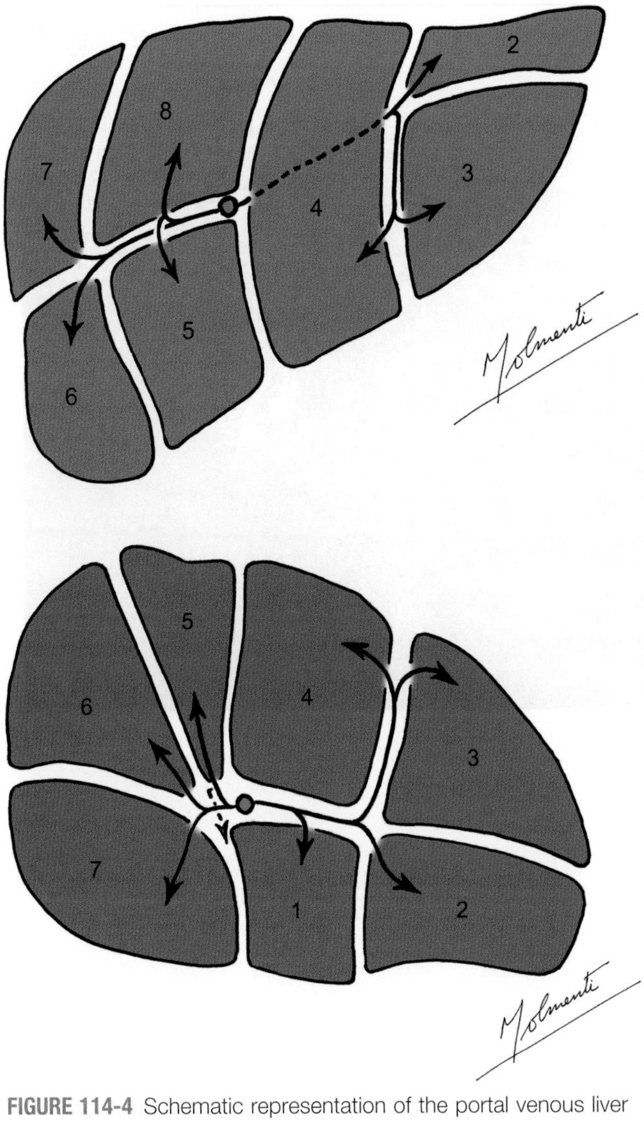

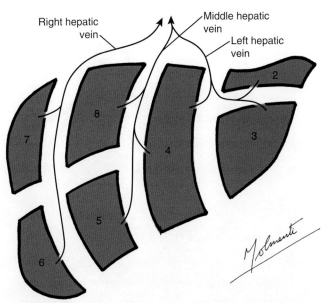

FIGURE 114-5 Schematic representation of the hepatic venous liver anatomy.

FIGURE 114-4 Schematic representation of the portal venous liver anatomy.

that of the right side, the portal vein branches do not.[12] During early stages of development, there are three hepatic arteries: (1) a left hepatic artery arising from the left gastric artery, (2) a middle hepatic artery arising from the celiac trunk, and (3) a right hepatic artery arising from the superior mesenteric artery. Although in most cases the middle artery is the only one that persists, variations in regression and origin of these three early arteries account for the so-called accessory and replaced variants.[11] A complete ductal system is present by the 10th week of intrauterine life.[9,11] The mesoderm of the septum between liver and abdominal wall develops into the *falciform ligament.* The surface of the developing liver in contact with the diaphragm is devoid of peritoneum, and the so-called bare area is a reminder of such association.[8,9] By week 10 of development, the liver is involved in hematopoietic function, an activity that diminishes markedly during gestational months 8 and 9.[8] By week 12 of development, the liver is already producing bile.[8] However, hepatocytes only attain single-cell plate configuration by the age of 5 years.[13] Several events take

place at birth. The *ductus venosus,* which optimized venous return from the placenta to the fetus by connecting the left umbilical and common hepatic vein, closes and becomes the *ligamentum venosus.* Also at birth, the *extrahepatic* umbilical vein closes and becomes the ligamentum teres.[12]

True anomalies of the liver are relatively infrequent. Prolongations of liver tissue from either the right (Riedel lobe) or left lobes usually present as incidental abdominal masses. In other instances, hepatic tissue connected by an isthmus to the liver is found in the chest. Small accessory collections of tissue attached to the liver by a pedicle are also occasionally encountered.[9]

HEPATIC DIVISIONS

Several nomenclatures and topographic divisions have been proposed. According to Couinaud, the right and left hemilivers are supplied by first-order branches. Sectors are supplied by second-order branches. Segments are supplied by third-order branches. Subsegments are supplied by fourth-order or other branches.[11] Segments are numbered in a counterclockwise fashion, from I to VIII.[11] A main portal fissure, a right portal fissure, and a left portal fissure are grossly or conceptually defined, because they may not always be anatomically present.[11,12] Left and right paramedian sectors are adjacent to the main portal fissure. Left and right lateral sectors are located on the outer side of the corresponding paramedian ones (see Figures 114-2 to 114-5).[2-5,11] During our discussion, we follow this nomenclature with some modifications.[11,12]

VASCULOBILIARY SHEATHS

Couinaud referred to the vasculobiliary sheaths that envelop the portal elements as "the most important structure of liver anatomy."[11,14] They seem to have been described initially by Walaeus in 1640, and thus some

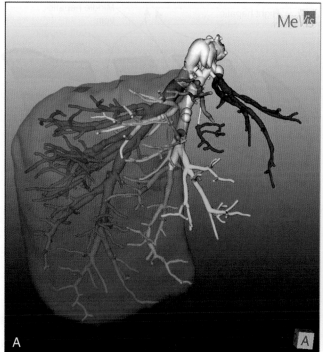

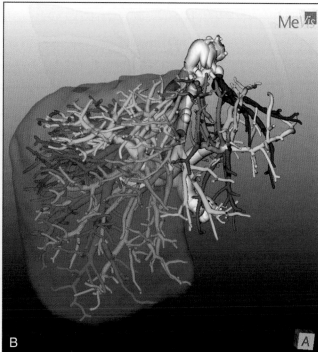

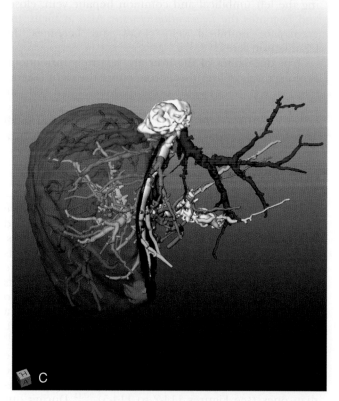

FIGURE 114-6 Virtual three-dimensional reconstruction of the liver anatomy by means of Hepavision, MeVis-Germany software. The right lobe has been reconstructed in a virtual fashion, together with the hepatic veins **(A),** hepatic veins and portal veins **(B),** and hepatic veins and biliary system **(C).**

have used the terms *walaean pedicles* or *walaean sheaths.*[11,15] Glisson published his description of the liver "tunic" in 1642, and Laennec did so in 1803.[11,16,17] The elements of the *portal pedicle* (hepatic artery, portal vein, bile ducts, nerves, and lymphatics) are surrounded throughout their trajectory to the parenchymal plates by connective tissue. Not so the hepatic veins.[11,18] The *hilar plate* is located over the left and right pedicles, and the portal

division, on the hilum of the liver.[11,18] The *umbilical plate* is found in continuity with the hilar plate and the round ligament, covering the left paramedian pedicle in its upper surface.[11] According to Couinaud and others, dissection of the hilar plate allows for the detachment of the hilar contents.[1,2,11,18] Exposure of the umbilical plate is the gateway to the segmental and sectoral pedicles of the left liver. Because dissection at the level of the plates can lead to complications, an approach to the sheaths is recommended.[11] This strategy has been applied by Lazorthes et al in the so-called suprahilar approach for anatomic hepatectomies and segmentectomies.[19] Sheaths originate at the right edge of the hilum, at the umbilical plate, and at the posterior margin of the hilar plate. From these sites they will reach the right liver, the left liver, and the caudate area, respectively.[11,18] In cases of narrow hila or hila of difficult access, consideration should be given to dividing the anterior portion of the main portal fissure. This maneuver does not damage any structures of significance and allows better exposure of the hilar elements.[11]

Couinaud recognized the following three types of approaches to a portal pedicle[11]:

1. Intrafascial—dissection within the sheath, where the elements are identified
2. Extrafascial—dissection around the pedicle sheath
3. Extrafascial and transfissural—dissection of the sheaths at their origin from the hilar and umbilical plates (considered the safest approach, especially for second- and third-order branches)

ARTERIAL AND BILIARY SYSTEMS

According to Couinaud and Houssin, the most frequent arterial and biliary configurations, accounting for almost 90% of cases in their series, are the following[20]:

- A unique artery and bile duct on right and left (24%)
- Two right bile ducts (17%)
- Two left arteries (26%)
- Two right ducts and two left arteries (22%)

Bile ducts are usually located above the portal branches, and arteries below the corresponding veins.[18] The bile ducts derive their blood supply predominantly from arterial branches.[11,13] Preliminary results from our observations in live-donor liver transplantation, however, would point to some differences in the classically accepted (see Figure 114-3) anatomic similarities among arteries and bile ducts.

HEPATIC ARTERIES

Molmenti et al noted that "the occurrence of (arterial) variants that differ from the usual pattern is both surprisingly common and unpredictable."[21] Such findings are especially relevant not only in liver transplantation but in all types of hepatobiliary surgery.[1,2,4,21,22] When addressing arterial polymorphism and nomenclature, it is essential to keep in mind the embryologic reality that the liver has a tripartite arterial supply during developmental life. Although all these structures may not be patent in adulthood, vestigial remnants such as fibrous bands will always be encountered by the hand and sight of gifted surgeons.

The *common hepatic artery* originates from the celiac trunk in more than 80% of cases. In 5% of instances, there is a *replaced common hepatic artery*, most frequently arising from the superior mesenteric artery. In approximately 10% of cases, there is an *absent common hepatic artery*. In such instances, the right and left hepatic arteries originate independently.[21]

The *right hepatic artery* originates from the proper hepatic artery in more than 80% of cases. In approximately 15% to 20% of cases, there is a *replaced right hepatic artery* that arises in most instances from the superior mesenteric artery. In slightly more than 5% of individuals, there is an *accessory right hepatic artery* that may arise from the superior mesenteric artery. The right hepatic artery crosses underneath the common hepatic duct in 65% of cases, anterior to it in approximately 10% of cases, and underneath the common bile duct in approximately 10% of cases.[21,22]

The *left hepatic artery* arises from the hepatic artery proper in more than 80% of instances. In approximately 15% to 20% of cases, there is a *replaced left hepatic artery* that most frequently may arise from the left gastric artery, celiac axis, or replaced common hepatic artery. An *accessory left hepatic artery* may be seen in up to 35% of individuals.[21] Finding such vessels is of help during surgical interventions. Replaced and accessory left hepatic arteries can usually be detected by palpation of the gastrohepatic ligament. Replaced and accessory right hepatic arteries can be identified by palpating the posterior right portion of the hepatoduodenal ligament, with one finger inserted into the foramen of Winslow. The most frequent left-sided arterial distribution is a common trunk formed by the arteries of segments III and IV, which is joined by the artery of segment II. When the latter enters the former near the left-right bifurcation, the left hepatic artery is short. When the entrance occurs at the bifurcation or at the hepatic artery proper, there is a duplication of the left hepatic artery.[20] The hepatic artery is rarely involved by severe atherosclerotic changes, even in elderly individuals.[6]

HEPATIC DUCTS

The *left hepatic duct* drains segments II to IV. It is formed by the junction of ducts from segments II and III into a common trunk that is subsequently joined by the duct from segment IV (see Figure 114-3). Duct IV usually joins at the umbilical fissure, or somewhat to its right. In most cases, the left hepatic duct lies in the most superior location of the left portal pedicle. The most frequent left biliary distribution is a common trunk from segments II and III that is joined by that of segment IV. In cases where duct IV joins late, it may form the upper edge of the left portal pedicle.[11,18,20] In a very small number of cases, the ducts from the left paramedian sector (segments III and IV) may themselves form a trunk, which is joined by the duct of the left lateral sector (segment II) and the caudate lobe (segment I), or the duct from segment IV enters the confluence of the other ducts or the common duct itself. Such variations may lead to the finding of a short left hepatic duct (≈17% of cases) or a double left hepatic duct (≈12% of cases).[11] The left duct has a classic configuration in almost 70% of cases.[18] Biliary drainage may be achieved by performing a bilioenteric anastomosis to the left hepatic duct at the hilum or to ducts III or IV by accessing them at the umbilical fissure (Hepp-Couinaud operation).[23] Variations in anatomic patterns should be kept in mind.[11,18]

The *right hepatic duct* is present in slightly more than 50% of cases (see Figure 114-3). It is harder to reach than its left counterpart, is usually short, and may even be missing in cases of an early second-degree bi-trifurcation (or division). It drains segments V to VIII. The duct draining segments VI and VII has a horizontal trajectory. The duct draining segments V and VIII has a vertical course.[11,18]

The caudate lobe has its own bile drainage.[18]

The *confluence of the hepatic ducts* is observed in front of the portal bifurcation in 57% of cases, in front of the left portal vein in 37% of cases, and in front of the right portal vein in 6% of cases. Isolated segmental or subsegmental bile ducts, usually arising from segments I, IV, and V,[11] can lead to biliary fistulas after interventions in the hilar region. The confluence of the right and left hepatic ducts is described as following a normal configuration in approximately 70% of cases. Other possible configurations and their approximate incidences include trifurcation with left, paramedian and lateral right ducts (10%), right sectoral duct merging into the common bile duct (20%), and right sectoral duct joining the left duct (5%).[18]

PORTAL VEIN AND PORTAL VEIN ANOMALIES

The left portal, left paramedian, left lateral, and right paramedian veins are constant structures within the liver architecture.[11] The absence of the bifurcation of the portal vein can be an extremely dangerous situation. In such cases, the portal vein follows a curvilinear trajectory within the liver, arching from right to left, and giving off collateral branches along the way until it reaches the caudate lobe. Ligation of the presumed right portal vein branch leads to complete interruption of portal blood into the liver.[11,24,25] The classically accepted portal venous branching is illustrated in Figure 114-4.

HILUM, PLATES, FISSURES, AND OTHER STRUCTURES

Couinaud reminded us that "*hilum* meant in Latin a tiny black point seen in beans" and that anatomists in antiquity referred to that region as *porta hepatis*, or gateway of the liver.[11] It contains the bifurcation of the portal elements, with the short right and the long left branches. In approximately 23% of cases, the right portal vein is not present, but rather is replaced by two sectoral branches. In 47% of cases, the right hepatic duct is not present as such.[11]

The location of the *main portal fissure*, described by Rex, may vary (see Figure 114-2). It is identified by the posterior extremity of the cystic plate, and in cases of normal right portal vein anatomy tends to be located to the right of the portal vein, less frequently at the site of the bifurcation of the portal vein, or even less frequently to its left. In cases of right portal vein variants, the fissure is almost always at the level of the bifurcation or at the left portal vein. Its topographic location on the liver is not outlined by superficial markings in humans and can be traced from the gallbladder fossa to the left anterior

surface of the IVC. Furthermore, it has been noted that when the main portal fissure lies on the left, the biliary confluence is located in more than 70% of cases in front of the left portal vein.[11,26,27]

The *hilar plate* (see Figure 114-2) is detached from the liver parenchyma by dissecting in between the left portal pedicle and liver tissue. The left hepatic duct is the structure located in the superior aspect of the portal elements. No major vessels or biliary ducts are encountered in this pathway. Only in the posterior region are there branches to the caudate lobe.[2,11,18,23,28]

The *umbilical fissure and plate* (see Figure 114-2) is the site of origin of segmental and sectoral pedicles to the left liver. Its anatomic landmarks are the falciform ligament and the left longitudinal sulcus. The left paramedian pedicle and the umbilical plate can be identified by following the round ligament in continuity with the left portal vein. No walaean pedicles cross the umbilical fissure.[11] This structure divides the left lobe from the rest of the liver and is a landmark point for the evaluation and performance of left lobectomies and trisectorectomies (trisegmentectomies in the classic diction).[29]

The *sulcus of Rouvière* is an irregular fissure in continuity with the right hilum (see Figure 114-2). It represents the extrahepatic anatomic landmark of the right fissure, usually buried in liver parenchyma. Following this structure leads to the pedicles of segments V and VI and further deeply and posteriorly to the pedicles of segments VII and VIII. The maneuver of isolating these structures is advantageous in the difficult procedures of right sectorectomy (segments VI–VII resection) or left trisectorectomy (trisegmentectomy) (segments I-II-III-IV-V-VIII resection).

The right paramedian portal pedicle is, according to Couinaud, "one of the most constant vessels of the liver."[11]

The *parabiliary venous system* of Couinaud is an accessory venous system with collateral branches to the duodenum, pancreas, and stomach, located within the hilar plate. It is associated with liver parenchyma, especially in the caudate and quadrate lobes, as well as with cystic veins. It may act as a collateral pathway in cases of portal hypertension and may serve as a connection between the right and left livers.[11]

The *cystic vein(s)* usually drain into the right portal vein, but may also drain into the right liver, the left liver, and/or enter the parabiliary venous system.[11,13]

In 20% to 50% of cases, *small ducts* that are not part of a portal pedicle and do not communicate with the gallbladder are encountered in the cystic fossa. These ducts, described by Luschka, represent part of the "vasa aberrantia." They are different from the *cystohepatic ducts*, which are true biliary ducts that traverse from liver tissue to the gallbladder.[11,30]

HEPATIC, SUPRARENAL, AND PHRENIC VEINS

There are three main hepatic veins that drain into the IVC (see Figure 114-5): the right hepatic vein (RHV), the middle hepatic vein (MHV), and the left hepatic vein (LHV). Accessory, inferior, right inferior, right middle, or dorsal hepatic veins also drain directly into the IVC.[31] The MHV and LHV show a relative lack of anatomic diversity, whereas the RHV exhibits multiple variants.[32]

RIGHT HEPATIC VEIN

In most cases, the RHV is single; rarely, it is double. In more than 50% of cases, it has no tributaries within 1 cm of its entrance into the IVC. In such cases, it is possible to ligate it before parenchymal transections. In the other variants, attempts to ligate it may lead to profuse bleeding and potentially air emboli in cases where injuries occur.[18,31]

MIDDLE HEPATIC VEIN

The MHV travels in the liver parenchyma along the main portal fissure (Cantlie line). In approximately 85% of cases, the MHV and the LHV join in a common trunk before their entrance into the IVC. There are five most frequent venous confluence patterns when a length of approximately 1 cm from the IVC is considered (percentiles are approximate numbers)[31]:
- No venous branches (10% of cases)
- Bifurcation (40% of cases)
- Trifurcation (25% of cases)
- Quadrifurcation (5% of cases)
- Independent MHV and LHV (15% of cases)

LEFT HEPATIC VEIN

The LHV has two main tributaries, which usually converge more than 2 cm away from the common trunk's entrance (MHV and LHV) into the IVC.[31] The confluence of the LHV and the MHV represents the posterior part of the sulcus venosus. A posterior vein usually follows the posterior margin of the left lobe.[11] The LHV has a wide variety of branching patterns. However, all principal branches are within the territory limited by the left portal fissure (fissure that separates segments II and III).[11]

INFERIOR HEPATIC VEINS

There are multiple inferior hepatic veins (IHVs) that drain directly into the IVC. According to their location, they can be classified as posterior, posterolateral, posteroinferior, and caudate. Posteroinferior veins were observed in 95% of cases. The veins of the caudate lobe usually range in number from one to four.[31]

RIGHT SUPRARENAL VEIN

There are four frequent suprarenal venous configurations, as follows[31]:
- Single vein flows directly into the IVC, on the right side (75% of cases)
- Single vein merges together with a dorsal hepatic vein before entering the IVC (22% of cases)
- Single vein flows into the confluence of the right renal vein and the IVC (1% of cases)
- Two veins (2% of cases)

PHRENIC VEINS

There are one to five phrenic veins observed. Their confluence into the IVC or hepatic veins was observed with the following frequency patterns (approximate percentages)[31]:

- Supradiaphragmatic IVC, right anterior wall (25% of cases)
- Infradiaphragmatic IVC, right anterior wall (90% of cases)
- Retrohepatic IVC, right posterior wall (50% of cases)
- Supradiaphragmatic IVC, left anterior wall (5% of cases)
- Infradiaphragmatic IVC, left anterior wall (35% of cases)
- Common trunk of MHV and LHV (30% of cases)

ANATOMIC APPROACHES TO HEPATIC RESECTIONS (ACCORDING TO COUINAUD)
(see Figures 114-2 to 114-5)

POSTERIOR LIVER (DORSAL LIVER, SECTOR I)

Couinaud[11] proposed a posterior or dorsal liver that he designated as *sector I*. This area encompasses right and left dorsal segments. The left dorsal segment, also called *segment II*, is the liver parenchyma also known as *caudate lobe, spigelian lobe* (or lobe of Spieghel), or *segment I*. The right dorsal segment, also called *segment Ir*, is the remainder of the liver parenchyma ventral to the IVC, inferior to the right superior and middle hepatic veins, and posterior to the right pedicle.[11] Others view the caudate lobe as "embracing" the IVC and contacting segment VII in approximately half of all cases.[18] Its pathologic involvement may be associated with invasion of the IVC.[4]

Portal vein branches originate from the left portal vein, from the portal bifurcation, from the right portal vein, and from the parabiliary system. There is an artery and bile duct accompanying each vein within the walaean sheaths. Efferent veins drain into the retrohepatic IVC, and hepatic veins.[11]

When attempting to resect part or all of the posterior liver, the sector can be divided into three. The area in front of the IVC, in between the left and middle hepatic veins, can be reached anteriorly by removing segment IV. The area in between the middle and right superior hepatic veins can be reached anteriorly by removing segment VIII (a difficult task). The area below the right superior hepatic vein can be reached anterolaterally by resecting segment VII.[11] Alternatively, a completely posterior approach to the dorsal or paracaval liver can be used after detachment of the liver from the IVC. Caution should be paid to the posterior aspect of the hilum.

LEFT HEMILIVER (SEGMENTS II, III, IV, ±I)

Segment II makes up the left posterior angle, whereas segment III constitutes the left anterior angle of the liver. The left lateral sector encompasses segment II, whereas the left paramedian sector is made up by segments III and IV.[2]

Removal of the left liver along the main portal fissure entails ligation and transection of the left portal pedicle, LHV, and left-sided tributaries of the MHV. The caudate lobe is usually not included when performing a left hepatectomy. The left posterior dissection, dividing the left liver from segment I, is limited by the sulcus of Arantius.

Approximately 40% of the functional liver mass is represented by the left hemiliver.[4,11,18,33] Preoperative imaging studies provide a road map, especially useful when anatomic variations are present. The hilar plate is identified and dissected, ligating and transecting any branches to segment IV. The left portal pedicle is encircled and tied, providing a vascular demarcation of the territory to be resected along the main portal fissure. The left hemiliver is mobilized by transecting its ligaments. As dissection is carried out through the liver parenchyma toward the LHV, collaterals are tied or clipped. A venous branch from segment IV may be encountered posteriorly. The LHV is identified, tied, and transected.[4,11,18]

Potential complications based on liver anatomy include walaean sheaths, variations in hepatic vein topography, portal branches that supply the right liver but arise in the left portal vein or traverse close to it, bile ducts that drain the right liver but end in the left hepatic duct or traverse close to it, and vice versa.[11]

LEFT LOBE (SEGMENTS II AND III)

Access to and knowledge of the *umbilical plate* provides the gateway to left liver surgery. As outlined by Couinaud, the *left portal fissure* separates segments II and III and constitutes the plane where all the main branches of the LHV lie. This fissure should not be confused with the *umbilical (left suprahepatic) fissure*, that runs on the lateral edge of segment IV.[11] Second-order portal branches supply segment II, while third-order ones supply segment III. A large posterior branch of the LHV follows the posterior edge of segment II. Resection of segments II or III individually entails dissection by careful identification of pedicles, preservation of veins, and guidance by means of color demarcation.[4,11] The ligamentum teres (round ligament) joins the terminal part of the left portal vein. In this region, the bile duct lies above while the artery lies anterior and below the left portal vein. The surgical approach always entails the identification of the artery, followed by dissection and division of the most posterior segment III branches of the portal vein, and finally by the identification of the bile duct. In cases where biliary obstruction must be resolved, the bile duct of segment III can be accessed on the left of the ligamentum teres, and a biliary–enteric anastomosis constructed.[2,18,23]

SEGMENT IV

Segment IV can be resected without altering the integrity of the remaining liver mass.[4] Third-order portal branches supply this segment. Resection entails in all cases access to the umbilical fissure, with subsequent ligation and transection of all sheaths arising from the left portal branch and entering segment IV. The liver is divided along the left border of the MHV, allowing for its preservation. However, when necessary it can also be resected.[4,11] If specific cases where pathologic findings demand it, segment IV can be removed in continuity with segments II, III, V, VIII ± I.

RIGHT HEMILIVER (SEGMENTS V, VI, VII, AND VIII)

Segment V constitutes the right border of the gallbladder bed. Segment VI makes the right anterior angle of the liver and is occasionally delimited by the sulcus of Rouvière to the right, while segment VII configures the right posterior angle. Segment VIII is not visible from the inferior surface of the liver.[2] Anatomic variations in portal and hepatic venous configurations are much more frequent in the right than in the left liver.[11] In 1888, Rex described the main portal and the right portal fissures. The *main portal fissure* extends from the anterior-left surface of the IVC to the cystic fossa. The MHV runs within it. In cases where the fissure is at the level of the right portal vein, there is a very low incidence of right portal vein anatomic variants. When the portal vein anatomy shows no variants, the convergence of the right and left hepatic ducts is usually located in front of the bifurcation of the portal vein. In cases of absent right portal vein, the convergence is in front of the left portal vein. The *right portal fissure* has a posterior edge at the RHV but is otherwise devoid of topographic anatomic landmarks. The right superior hepatic vein runs within it.[11,26]

There are several intraoperative ways to outline hepatic territories. Such maneuvers are especially useful in cases of anatomic distortions caused by tumors. Isolating the right (Figure 114-7) or left branches of the portal vein and hepatic artery and clamping them temporarily (*right or left Pringle maneuver*) leads to a color demarcation of the right or left hemilivers, respectively. In the *Malagó maneuver*, the territory of the right hemiliver drained by the MHV is delineated. This maneuver entails the temporary clamping of the right branch of the portal vein, the right branch of the hepatic artery, and subsequently the RHV. Temporary nonperfusion of the area of the liver supplied by the right portal system is achieved and physically demarcated by a darkened color of the liver parenchyma. When the clamp on the right hepatic artery is released, the arterial perfusion will revascularize the right lobe of the liver. However, by maintaining the RHV clamped, its territory will remain demarcated, and only the parenchyma of the right liver drained by the MHV will regain its color. The Malagó maneuver is especially useful in right liver resections in live-donor liver transplantation.

Segmental pedicles on the right, as opposed to what is encountered on the left liver, arise within the liver parenchyma. As such, the gateway to right liver surgery is the right hilar extremity. The right pedicle is short (see Figure 114-7), and sometimes the division of the portal pedicle is so early that it replaces the pedicle itself. The right portal vein is estimated to be missing in slightly more than 20% of cases.[11] Anatomically, the right paramedian portal sheath has an oblique configuration, entering the liver parenchyma from the right area of the hilum. The right paramedian portal vein is a constant structure. The right lateral portal sheath can be found parallel to the inferior surface of the liver.[11,18]

The right hepatic duct is believed to be absent in almost 50% of cases, with variations of trifurcation or right segmental biliary drainage emptying into the left-sided biliary ducts in the majority of the remaining cases.[11,34]

Drainage of the right liver (see Figure 114-5) is by means of the right and middle hepatic veins. The MHV drains segment V on its left side by means of the anterior

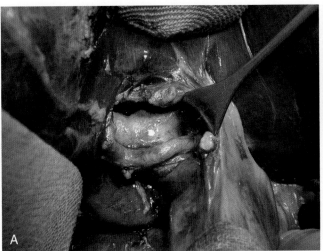
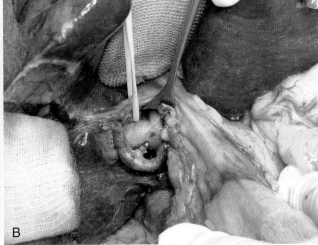

FIGURE 114-7 Surgical dissection of the right portal pedicle. **A,** The right hepatic artery and right portal vein have been dissected. **B,** The right hepatic duct was subsequently isolated and circled with a rubber band.

branches and segment VIII by means of its posterior branches. Couinaud made a distinction between superior, middle, and inferior right hepatic veins and noted their high anatomic variability. Small drainage veins originating in segments VII and VIII can be found to enter the IVC independently.[11] Couinaud related that "the facility and safety of right hepatectomy depends on the length of the right portal pedicle." Broelsch stated that "control of the afferent and efferent vessels is of vital importance." Ease of access to the right pedicle may be encountered by accessing the sulcus of Rouvière, which prolongs the right edge of the hilum, or by addressing its lateral and paramedian pedicles.[4,11,35,36] Small branches that originate from the right portal vein may go toward the precaval parenchyma, segment VII, or the caudate process.[11] Mobilization of the right lobe is of vital importance. Hepatic veins can be approached by rotating the right lobe medially or from the transected parenchyma at the main portal fissure. Approximately 60% of the functional liver mass is represented by the right hemiliver.[4,11]

RIGHT PARAMEDIAN SECTOR (SEGMENTS V AND VIII)

The right paramedian sector is of variable extent. It is limited by the main portal fissure, the right portal fissure, and the dorsal liver. In approximately 75% of cases, interruption of its pedicle has no associated anatomic complications. In the remainder of cases, variants that may lead to surgical challenges include the origin of branches to segments VI or VII, duplication of its usual branches, and absence of the portal vein bifurcation. In most cases in which the main portal fissure is to the right of the portal vein at the level of the hilum, there are no anatomic variants. As suggested by Couinaud, control of the paramedian portal pedicle should be preferably attained through an extrafascial approach at the level of the hilum as it ascends into the liver parenchyma. Variations in branching of the portal distribution manifest as changes in the pattern of color demarcation after occlusion of inflow. When resecting this sector, the RHV (if not atrophic)

should be preserved.[11,18] The right paramedian sector can be resected in continuity with segments IV, VI, and VII.[11]

RIGHT LATERAL SECTOR (SEGMENTS VI AND VII)

The right lateral sector is located lateral to the right portal fissure. On gross inspection, the right margin of the liver is part of the right lateral sector. The plane of the right portal fissure is along the RHV. The RHV, however, may be unusually small in approximately 25% of cases. Couinaud described the fissure as a "very large" fissure, with an oblique orientation, that encompasses "the whole width of the right liver." When performing a resection of the right lateral sector, the portal pedicle can be identified on the right edge of the hilum, usually 2 cm to the right of the main portal fissure. The right lateral pedicle follows a course parallel to the liver surface. Anatomic variations that can be encountered include branches to the right lateral sector originating from the right paramedian sector and duplication of the pedicle of the latter. In more than 80% of cases where the main portal fissure is located to the right of the portal vein, there are no anatomic variations on the right side. The right inferior and middle veins are always part of the right lateral sector. Transection of the hepatic parenchyma is along the line of color demarcation after the pedicle is occluded.[11,18]

Resection of the right lateral sector can be performed together with segments V and VIII.[11]

SEGMENTS V AND VI

When performing an anatomic resection, the pedicles are controlled in an extrafascial way. Segment V is supplied by portal branches arising from the anterior aspect of the right paramedian bundle. Branches to segment VI arise from the anterior aspect of the right lateral pedicle. Occasionally, there is a single pedicle for segment VI. Venous drainage of segment V is into the MHV, while that of segment VI is into the RHV. Resection is guided by the coloration changes associated with vascular occlusion.[11]

SEGMENT VII

The border between segments VII and VIII is the right portal fissure. Segment VII has the peculiarity of being supplied by a single portal pedicle, known as *Rex's ramus arcuatus*. This pedicle originates from the right lateral portal bundle, distal and posterior to the branches for segment VI. Occasionally, such as in cases of right portal trifurcation, it may arise on its own. Venous drainage is usually into the RHV. When resecting this segment, it is recommended to expose the IVC and RHV.[11]

SEGMENT VIII

Segment VIII is supplied by posterior branches of the right paramedian portal bundle. Its venous drainage is mostly through the MHV.[11]

LYMPHATICS

The lymphatic system of the liver is not yet fully understood. Lymphatic channels are encountered in the portal tract and collect lymph that may originate in the spaces of Disse. Lymphatics travel together with other elements of the portal bundle to the hilum of the liver, eventually reaching the aortic lymph nodes and the thoracic duct. Lymphatic vessels also travel with the hepatic veins, along the IVC, and subsequently into the thoracic region. There are also superficial lymphatics within the capsule of the liver.[13,37]

NERVES

The liver receives both sympathetic and parasympathetic innervation. Sympathetic supply is through the celiac plexus. Stimulation leads to increases in glucose and lactate. Parasympathetic innervation is through the vagus nerve. Stimulation leads to glycogen synthesis, decreased glucose release, and gallbladder contraction.[13,37,38]

MICROSCOPIC STRUCTURE

Given the surgical nature of our chapter, we describe here only the basic aspects of the hepatic microscopic structure. The hexagonal lobule, the portal lobule, and the acinus have been described as hepatic functional units by Kiernan, Mall, and Rapaport, respectively.[37] This anatomic-physiologic configuration is associated with topographic variations in hepatocyte metabolic activity, exposure to toxic substances, and oxygen concentrations.[13] It is estimated that the liver has approximately 100 billion hepatocytes that make up 80% of hepatic cells. Hepatocytes are polyhedral in shape and arranged in one-cell-thick plates lining the sinusoids. Hepatocytes have a basolateral (sinusoidal, vascular) domain, a canalicular (apical, biliary) domain, and a lateral domain.[37] The basolateral (vascular, sinusoidal) domain is located toward the sinusoids and space of Disse. The corresponding hepatocytic membrane is lined with microvilli and is a zone of active transport between blood and the hepatocyte. It is responsible in part for maintaining the liver pH around 7.2.[37] The canalicular membrane contains active transport systems and is also responsible in part for maintaining the liver pH around 7.2. This domain contains multiple enzymes with active sites directed toward the exterior of the cell. Bile canaliculi, 1 to 2 μm in diameter, located in between the canalicular domains of hepatocytes, merge into canals of Herring, which in turn drain into bile ductules lined by cholangiocytes. These in turn lead to ducts of larger size and eventually form the common bile duct.[37] The lateral domain separates the former two domains and contains junctional complexes.[37] The perisinusoidal space of Disse is a site where fluids can move freely given the absence of basement membranes in both hepatocytes and sinusoid-lining cells. There are four types of cells in the sinusoids: hepatic sinusoidal endothelial cells, Kupffer cells, lymphocytes, and stellate (Ito) cells. The latter store vitamin A and would contribute to the pathogenesis of cirrhosis.[13,37]

Large and septal bile ducts express blood group antigens.[13] Chronic rejection, toxin reactions, graft-versus-host disease, and other afflictions involve mostly ducts smaller than 0.1 mm.[13]

HEPATIC BLOOD FLOW AND METABOLISM

The liver weighs approximately 1800 g in men and 1400 g in women. It receives approximately 1500 mL of blood per minute, 30% from the hepatic artery and the remaining 70% from the portal vein. There are 25 to 30 mL of blood per 100 g of liver under normal conditions, but that volume may reach up to 60 mL/100 g in cases of congestion. Blood flow also varies as a result of other physiologic conditions, such as ingestion of a meal. Portal blood flow is most sensitive to protein meals. Carbohydrate intake has a moderate effect on increases in portal flow. The influence of lipids is thought to be of minimal importance.[13,37]

The liver is the main site of protein and amino acid metabolism. More than 90% of circulating plasma proteins come from the liver. The liver receives dietary amino acids through the portal circulation. Their availability is limited by hepatocyte membrane transport activity. Hepatocytes are also able to internalize large proteins and other macromolecules by endocytosis. Nonessential amino acids are synthesized in the liver from pathways based on pyruvate, α-ketoglutarate, and oxaloacetate (from the Krebs cycle). Amino acid catabolism occurs mostly in the liver. Those that are not destined to become hepatocytic or plasma proteins are degraded into pyruvate, acetyl coenzyme A (CoA), or members of the tricarboxylic acid cycle intermediaries. The nitrogen from the amino groups is excreted as urea in the urine after being processed by the urea cycle.[37,39]

The liver produces fatty acids from excess sugar. Fatty acids are stored intracellularly mainly as triglycerides. Oxidation of fatty acids in the liver produces ketone bodies.[37] The liver is intimately involved in lipoprotein physiology. It is the site of production of very-low-density lipoprotein (VLDL) and a great part of plasma high-density lipoprotein.[40] Austin Flint was the first to describe hypercholesterolemia in liver disease. Incidentally, he is also credited by some as being the first to report the hepatorenal syndrome.[40,41]

The liver must provide for its own physiologic needs as well as for those of other organs. This is best exemplified when addressing hepatic physiology during fed, postabsorptive, and fasting states.[42] In the *prandial state,* most of the glucose during fed states is converted in the liver to glycogen through three-carbon fragments. The liver can store up to a maximum of 65 g of glycogen for each kilogram of liver tissue. Excess glucose can be directed in a variety of ways. An important such way is the synthesis of fatty acids. Fatty acids are sterified and transported as VLDL to adipocytes.[42] In the *postprandial state,* hepatic glycogen is broken down into glucose mainly at the brain and red blood cells. Adipocytes release fatty acids that act as an energy source for most tissues.[42] In the *fasting state,* glycogen depletion is encountered within 48 hours. Glucose for the brain and red blood cells is produced by means of gluconeogenesis. Gluconeogenesis reaches its peak rate at 24 to 48 hours. In the liver, glycerol, rather than fatty acids, provides the carbon source for gluconeogenesis. During prolonged starvation, glucose use by the brain decreases, and ketone bodies generated by the liver become the major source of energy.[42]

LIVER REGROWTH (REGENERATION)

The liver constitutes the major detoxifying site in the human body and, as such, is prone to significant injury. Loss of liver mass by injury or resection seems to be the inciting event for liver regrowth. The regenerative capacity of the liver seems to find recognition in Greek mythology wherein the titan Prometheus exhibits cyclical hepatic regrowth during his punishment for providing fire to humans.

The liver seems to adapt to the metabolic needs of each individual by reducing or increasing its mass and function. This has been observed in "large for size" liver transplantation in children when a transplanted liver mass greater than needed will shrink by apoptosis. Conversely and most frequently after removal, functional inactivation (ligature or embolization) of large amounts of parenchyma, or after "small for size" transplantation, there is a hyperplastic-trophic response, leading to an increase of liver mass. This finding has been described as consisting of cytokine-dependent and cytokine-independent pathways.[43] This process has become clearly evident in live-donor liver transplantation, where hepatic regrowth is observed in both donor and recipient. Although the liver does not recover its original anatomic morphology with right and left lobes, the volume increases surprisingly quickly up to the point where it is able to accommodate the physiologic needs of the host (Figure 114-8).[3,44] Mean residual volume increased by 88% within 10 days after right hepatectomies in cases of live liver donors.[44] The response, however, varies according to the situation. Hepatocyte injury is associated with a greater inflammatory response than posthepatectomy regeneration. In cirrhosis, although there is regrowth, excessive amounts of collagen are also produced leading to injury rather than a salutary response.[43] It is estimated that hepatocytes have a life span of approximately 1 year, and that in healthy individuals, 1 of every 1000 hepatocytes is replicating at any given time point.[45]

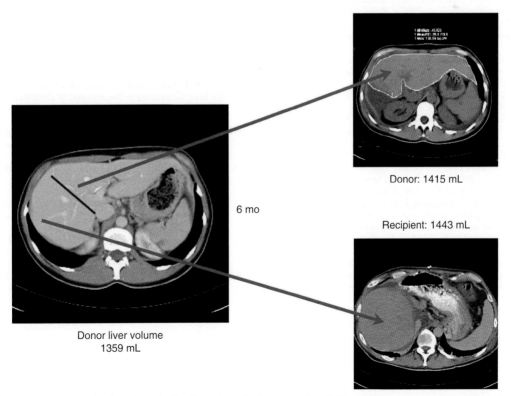

Donor liver volume
1359 mL

6 mo

Donor: 1415 mL

Recipient: 1443 mL

FIGURE 114-8 Computed tomography imaging of a live liver donor before resection *(left)* and the subsequent regrowth of remnant and allograft hemilivers in donor and recipient, respectively *(right).*

BILE FORMATION

Bile consists of an aqueous solution of salts, electrolytes, amino acids, proteins, lipids, vitamins, steroids, toxins, drugs, and heavy metals.[46] It is formed based on an osmotic filtration and the transport of substances that lead to the development of such osmotic gradient. Its function involves absorption and digestion of dietary substances, cholesterol excretion, and the elimination of toxic substances.[46]

REFERENCES

1. Molmenti EP, Klintmalm GB: *Atlas of liver transplantation.* Philadelphia, 2002, Saunders.
2. Lasala AJ, Molmenti LA: *Reoperaciones en vias biliares por lesiones quirurgicas.* Buenos Aires, 1966, Lopez Libreros Editores.
3. Malagó M, Testa G, Frilling A, et al: Right living donor liver transplantation—an option for adult patients: Single-institution experience with 74 patients. *Ann Surg* 238:853; discussion 862, 2003.
4. Broelsch CE: *Atlas of liver surgery.* New York, 1993, Churchill-Livingstone.
5. Lang H, Malagó M, Broelsch CE: Liver transplantation in children and segmental transplantation. In Blumgart LH, Fong Y, editors: *Surgery of the liver and biliary tract,* ed 3. Philadelphia, 2000, Saunders, p 2107.
6. Starzl TE, Putnam CW: *Experience in hepatic transplantation.* Philadelphia, 1969, Saunders.
7. Radtke A, Schroeder T, Molmenti EP, et al: Anatomical and physiological comparison of liver volumes among three frequent types of parenchyma transection in live-donor liver transplantation. *Hepatogastroenterology* 52:333, 2005.
8. Sadler TW: *Langman's medical embryology,* ed 11. Philadelphia, 2010, Lippincott Williams & Wilkins.
9. Skandalakis JE, et al: The liver. In Skandalakis JE, Gray SW, editors: *Embryology for surgeons: The embryological basis of the treatment of congenital anomalies,* ed 2. Baltimore, 1994, Williams & Wilkins, p 283.
10. Sappey C: *Traité d'anatomie descriptive.* Paris, 1889, Lecrosnier er Babe.
11. Couinaud C, editor: *Surgical anatomy of the liver revisited.* Paris, 1989, C. Couinaud.
12. Strasberg SM: Terminology of liver anatomy and liver resection: Coming to grips with hepatic Babel. *J Am Coll Surg* 184:413, 1997.
13. Wanless IR: Physioanatomic considerations. In Schiff ER, et al, editors: *Schiff's diseases of the liver,* ed 10. Philadelphia, 2007, Lippincott Williams & Wilkins.
14. Couinaud C: Les envelopes vasculo-biliaires du foie ou capsule de Glisson: Leur intérêt dans la chirurgie vésiculaire, les resections hépatiques et l'abord du hile du foie. *Lyon Chir* 49:589, 1954.
15. Johannis Walaei epistolae duae de motu chili et sanguinis ad Thomam Bartholeum. In *Thomas Bartholeus Anatomica Lugd.* Bataviae (Leyden), 1640, Franciscus Hackius.
16. Glisson F: *Anatomia hepatis.* London, 1642, O. Pullein.
17. Laennec RTH: Sur les tuniques qui enveloppent certains viscéres, et fournissent des gaines membraneuses à leurs vaisseaux. *J De Méd Chir et Pharm Vendémiaire* an XI:539, et *Germinal* an XI:73, 1803.
18. Blumgart LH, Hann LE: Surgical and radiologic anatomy of the liver and biliary tract. In Blumgart LH, editor: *Surgery of the liver, biliary tract and pancreas,* ed 4. Philadelphia, 2006, Saunders, p 3.
19. Lazorthes F, Chiotasso P, Chevreau P, et al: Hepatectomy with initial suprahilar control of intrahepatic portal pedicles. *Surgery* 113:103, 1993.
20. Couinaud C, Houssin D: *Partition reglee du foie pour transplantation: Contraites anatomiques,* Paris, 1991.
21. Molmenti EP, Pinto PA, Klein J, et al: Normal and variant arterial supply of the liver and gallbladder. *Pediatr Transpl* 7:80, 2003.
22. Molmenti EP, Klein AS, Henry ML: Procurement of liver and pancreas allografts in donors with replaced/accessory right hepatic arteries. *Transplantation* 78:770, 2004.
23. Hepp J, Couinaud C: L'abord et l'utilisation du canal hépatique gauche dans la reparation de la voie biliaire principale. *Presse Méd* 64:947, 1956.
24. Couinaud C: Etude sur la veine porte intrahépatique. *Presse Méd* 61:1434, 1953.
25. Agossou-Veyeme AK: *La segmentation hépatique en tomodensitométrie,* Paris, 1982, Thése, 3e Cycle.
26. Rex H: Beitrage zur Morphologie der Säugerleber. *Morph Jb* 14:517, 1888.
27. Reynaud B, Coucouravas G, Amoros JP, et al: Clampage direct du pedicle glissonien lateral droit. *J Chir* 119:533, 1982.
28. Couinaud C: Recherches sur la chirurgie du confluent biliaire supérieur et des canaux hépatiques. *Presse Méd* 63:669, 1955.
29. http://www.ihpba.org/
30. Luschka H: *Die Anatomie des Menschen. B. II: Die Secretionszelle und der Gallenleitende Apparat.* Tübingen laupp und Siebeckl, 1863.
31. Nakamura S, Tsuzuki T: Surgical anatomy of the hepatic veins and the inferior vena cava. *Surg Gynecol Obstet* 152:43, 1981.
32. Radtke A, Schroeder T, Sotiropoulos GC, et al: Anatomical and physiological classification of hepatic vein dominance applied to liver transplantation. *Eur J Med Res* 10:187, 2005.
33. Couinaud C: A simplified method for controlled left hepatectomy. *Surgery* 105:385, 1985.
34. Tanaka K, et al: *Living-donor liver transplantation: Surgical techniques and innovations,* Barcelona, Spain, 2003, Prous Science.
35. Rouviere H: Sur la configuration et la signification du sillon du processus caudé. *Bull Soc Anat Paris* 60:355, 1924.
36. Couinaud C: Bases anatomiques des hépatectomies droite et gauche: Techniques qui en découlent. *J Chir* 70:933, 1954.
37. Saxena R, et al: Anatomy and physiology of the liver. In Zakim D, Boyer TD, editors: *Hepatology: A textbook of liver disease,* ed 4. Philadelphia, 2003, Saunders, p 3.
38. Bourgery JM, Jacob NH: *Traité complet de l'anatomie de l'homme: Tome cinquième.* Paris, 1839, CA Delaunay (Éditeur).
39. Cooper AJL: Amino acid metabolism and synthesis of urea. In Zakim D, Boyer TD, editors: *Hepatology: A textbook of liver disease,* ed 4. Philadelphia, 2003, Saunders, p 81.
40. Miller JP: Liver disease, alcohol, and lipoprotein metabolism. In Zakim D, Boyer TD, editors: *Hepatology: A textbook of liver disease,* ed 4. Philadelphia, 2003, Saunders, p 127.
41. Flint A: Experimental researches into a new excretory function of the liver: Consisting in the removal of cholesterine from the blood, and its discharge from the body in the form of stercorine. *Am J Med Sci* 44:305, 1862.
42. Zakim D: Metabolism of glucose and fatty acids by the liver. In Zakim D, Boyer TD, editors: *Hepatology: A textbook of liver disease,* ed 4. Philadelphia, 2003, Saunders, p 49.
43. Taub RA: Hepatic regeneration. In Zakim D, Boyer TD, editors: *Hepatology: A textbook of liver disease,* ed 4. Philadelphia, 2003, Saunders, p 31.
44. Nadalin S, Testa G, Malagó M, et al: Volumetric and functional recovery of the liver after right hepatectomy for living donation. *Liver Transpl* 10:1024, 2004.
45. Diehl AME, Rai R: Liver regeneration. In Schiff ER, et al, editors: *Schiff's diseases of the liver,* ed 8. Philadelphia, 1999, Lippincott Williams & Wilkins, p 39.
46. Wolkoff AW, Berk PD: Bilirubin metabolism and jaundice. In Schiff ER, et al, editors: *Schiff's diseases of the liver,* ed 10. Philadelphia, 2007, Lippincott Williams & Wilkins.

Approach to the Patient With Abnormal Hepatic Laboratory Tests

Vivian A. Asamoah | H. Franklin Herlong

The commonly used laboratory tests to detect liver diseases are often referred to as liver function tests (LFTs). However, this terminology is misleading in that many of the tests obtained routinely in the evaluation of liver disease are not true measures of hepatic synthetic function, but are indicators of hepatocellular or biliary tract injury. Furthermore, these tests may be normal in patients with advanced liver disease or abnormal in individuals with a normally functioning liver. It has been estimated that liver biochemical abnormalities occur in approximately 4% of asymptomatic healthy individuals. Consequently, an extensive evaluation of these patients would be unwarranted. Conversely, it is equally important to avoid assuming that minor abnormalities do not indicate serious underlying liver disease. The physician encountering abnormal liver tests must carefully assess the need for further evaluation based on each patient's clinical scenario, including risk factors, data from the physical examination, coexisting diseases, and current medical therapies.

There are few prospective controlled trials that define the optimal approach to the evaluation of patients with abnormal liver tests. In one study of almost 20,000 presumably healthy military recruits, an elevation in alanine aminotransferase (ALT) concentration greater than 2.25 standard deviations above the mean was detected in 99 subjects (0.5%).[1] In only 12 of these individuals was a specific cause identified, such as viral hepatitis, autoimmune hepatitis, or cholelithiasis. In the remainder, no specific diagnosis was made. In a study of 1124 patients referred specifically for evaluation of abnormal liver enzymes, the diagnosis was made noninvasively in 1043 patients. Of the remaining 81 patients whose diagnosis could not be inferred noninvasively, subsequent liver biopsy demonstrated steatosis in 84%.[2] Although it is difficult to extrapolate data from these studies to individual patients, these observations suggest that a specific diagnosis can be made in most asymptomatic patients with abnormal liver enzymes by using laboratory testing alone.

A careful history is essential for the effective evaluation of patients with abnormal liver enzymes. When possible, it is important to determine the onset of abnormalities. Detecting elevated liver enzymes shortly after the initiation of a new medication may establish the diagnosis without further investigation. Exposure to blood or blood products, illicit drug use, tattoos, or intimate contact with high-risk individuals may indicate underlying viral hepatitis. A detailed travel history, family history, and questions concerning occupational exposures and alcohol consumption may help establish a diagnosis.

The physical examination is an important component of the evaluation of patients with abnormal liver enzymes. A thorough skin examination may detect cutaneous stigmata of chronic liver disease, such as spider angiomata, palmar erythema, or dilated abdominal veins. Similarly on abdominal examination, detecting an enlarged spleen implies advanced liver disease with portal hypertension, or a prominent left hepatic lobe may suggest cirrhosis. The physical examination is unreliable in detecting small amounts of ascites, and ultrasonography may be required for documentation. Some diseases have cardinal physical examination findings, such as the bronze skin of hemochromatosis or the Kayser-Fleischer rings of Wilson disease. Thus, clues from the history and physical examination may help determine the sequence in which confirmatory tests should be ordered.

At most centers, the standard "hepatic profile" includes total bilirubin (often fractionated), aspartate aminotransferase (AST), alanine aminotransferase (ALT), alkaline phosphatase, total protein, and albumin levels. Of these tests, only two truly assess hepatic function. The bilirubin concentration measures the liver's ability to take up, conjugate, and excrete bilirubin into the biliary canaliculus. The albumin concentration reflects the liver's synthetic capacity. Instead of focusing on individual laboratory values, it is most helpful to look at patterns of laboratory abnormalities. Using this approach, hepatic diseases have traditionally been classified as "hepatocellular" when the elevation of aminotransferases predominate and "cholestatic" when there is a disproportionate elevation in the alkaline phosphatase concentration. Though useful, this simplistic approach may be limited in circumstances where there are overlapping patterns. In addition, the term *cholestatic* may be inappropriate for "infiltrative" disorders of the liver that may cause a significant elevation in the alkaline phosphatase levels with a normal bilirubin level.

The following sections present guidelines for the initial assessment of patients with varying patterns of hepatic enzyme abnormalities.

ASSESSMENT OF PATIENTS WITH PREDOMINANT ELEVATIONS OF THE AMINOTRANSFERASES

The aminotransferases are a class of enzymes that catalyze the transfer of amino groups to ketoacids to form amino acids. Because of their abundance in hepatocytes, they are sensitive measures of hepatic injury. AST was formerly referred to as *serum glutamate oxaloacetate transaminase* (SGOT), and the term ALT has replaced *serum glutamate pyruvate transaminase* (SGPT). These enzymes are present within hepatocytes but differ in location. ALT is localized in the cytosol, whereas AST is present in both the cytosol and the mitochondria. Consequently, the pattern of enzyme release is determined by the liver cell component affected by the particular disorder. Additionally, the "normal" amounts of both aminotransferases detected in the blood may be affected by gender and body mass, although most reported ranges do not account for these differences.[3]

There are many potential pitfalls in the evaluation of abnormal liver enzymes. Some medications, such as erythromycin estolate or *p*-aminosalicylate, may affect the aminotransferase assays, leading to spurious elevations in the absence of liver disease.[4] In addition, significant quantities of AST are present in nonhepatic tissues including skeletal muscle, heart muscle, kidney, brain, pancreas, lung, leukocytes, and erythrocytes. Although most ALT is found in the liver, small quantities can also be found in other tissues.[5,6] Consequently, elevations in the aminotransferases, particularly AST, may be seen in disorders such as rhabdomyolysis, polymyositis, or hemolysis. Rarely, elevations in the AST and ALT concentrations are encountered in endocrinopathies such as hypothyroidism, hyperthyroidism, and Addison disease.[7] Although the reasons for these abnormalities remain unclear, they seem to resolve once the underlying disease is treated. Similar elevations have also been reported in patients with celiac disease that return to normal on a gluten-free diet.[8,9]

The degree of aminotransferase elevation is a poor indicator of the severity of liver injury. For example, patients with fatal acute alcoholic hepatitis may have minimal aminotransferases elevations, whereas uncomplicated acute viral hepatitis may cause enzyme elevations in the thousands.

Although the degree of aminotransferase elevation is of limited prognostic value, it may be helpful in establishing the etiology of the hepatic injury (Box 115-1). Very high levels (>3000 IU/L) are seen in acute viral hepatitis, toxic or drug-induced liver disease, ischemic liver injury, and, rarely, autoimmune hepatitis and Wilson disease. Transient marked elevations in the AST and ALT concentrations may be seen on occasion with choledocholithiasis. The highest elevations (>10,000 IU/L) are detected in individuals with hepatic ischemia and acetaminophen hepatotoxicity. In both of these settings, the AST will initially predominate but will "cross" with the ALT once the injury ends and recovery ensues. This phenomenon reflects differences in the rates of clearance of the aminotransferases because AST has a shorter half-life than ALT. A rapid decrease in the AST and ALT concentrations in the setting of an increasing bilirubin and/or prothrombin time suggests fulminant hepatitis.

In most patients, mild to moderate elevations of the aminotransferases (<5 times the upper limit of normal) are encountered. Before concluding that the patient has liver disease, the tests should be repeated, preferably within 2 weeks. If the abnormalities persist, then it is highly likely the patient has some form of hepatic injury that should be investigated further.

BOX 115-1 **Approach to the Patient With Abnormal Aminotransferases**

MILD (<500 IU/L)
Nonalcoholic fatty liver disease
Chronic viral hepatitis
Alcoholic hepatitis
Bile duct obstruction
Infiltrating disorder
Nonhepatic sources (e.g., hemolysis, myositis)
Hemochromatosis
Acute fatty liver of pregnancy

MODERATE (500-1000 IU/L)
Autoimmune hepatitis
Wilson disease
Viral hepatitis
Medications

MARKED (>5000 IU/L)
Hepatotoxicity
Ischemia
Acute viral hepatitis

A careful history of use of both prescription and nonprescription medications including herbal preparations and dietary supplements is essential. Correlating hepatic enzyme elevations with the introduction or change in medication dosage may be sufficient to establish a diagnosis, particularly if elimination of the potentially hepatotoxic agent is followed by a decrease in the enzymes within a few weeks. Rechallenge with the medication is usually not recommended, unless there is no substitute for the offending agent and it is medically necessary.

If there is no circumstantial evidence of hepatotoxicity, then the following disorders should be considered: alcoholic liver disease, viral hepatitis, nonalcoholic fatty liver disease (NAFLD), autoimmune hepatitis, hemochromatosis, Wilson disease, and α_1-antitrypsin (A1AT) deficiency.

ALCOHOLIC LIVER DISEASE

Alcohol-related liver disease can range from simple steatosis to alcoholic hepatitis with or without cirrhosis. Consumption of large amounts of alcohol can directly result in liver damage or exacerbate other disorders such as hepatitis C or hemochromatosis. Reliable questionnaires are available to assess the amount of alcohol a patient is consuming and thus estimate its clinical effects.[10] There is no established safe level of alcohol consumption, but there is little evidence to suggest that ingestion of less than 30 g of alcohol per day in the absence of comorbid conditions such as hepatitis C causes significant liver disease. There are gender differences in susceptibility to alcoholic liver disease; women are more susceptible at lower levels of alcohol consumption even when corrected for differences in body mass. The pattern of enzyme elevation may be helpful in establishing the diagnosis of alcoholic liver disease. Alcoholic hepatitis is associated with an increased AST/ALT ratio greater than 2:1. In most cases the AST is less than

300 IU/dL, and the ALT concentration is often normal. The low concentration of ALT results from alcohol's inhibition of the conversion of pyridoxine to pyridoxal phosphate, a cofactor for ALT activity.[11] Superimposed hepatic injury from hepatotoxic agents such as acetaminophen may cause much higher enzyme levels, but the AST/ALT ratio usually remains intact.[12]

Before concluding that a patient with an AST/ALT ratio has alcoholic liver disease, other causes of selective AST elevation should be considered. As previously mentioned, muscle diseases or hemolysis may contribute to the AST elevation. In addition, patients with hepatitis C who have progressed to cirrhosis have higher AST than ALT, but the ratio is usually less than 2.[13]

Additional laboratory observations may help establish the diagnosis of alcoholic liver disease. Patients who consume large quantities of alcohol often have an elevated mean corpuscular volume in the absence of folate or vitamin B_{12} deficiency and will have a disproportionate elevation in the γ-glutamyltransferase (GGT) concentration.

VIRAL HEPATITIS

Chronic viral hepatitis is a common cause of moderate aminotransferase elevations, particularly in asymptomatic individuals. In most patients the ALT predominates, except in those patients with hepatitis C who have progressed to cirrhosis. Approximately 2% of the population has been infected with hepatitis C, making it one of the most common causes of chronic liver disease and the most frequent indication for liver transplantation. It is important to question patients regarding risk factors for transmission, which include blood transfusion before 1992, intravenous or intranasal drug use, tattoo placement, body piercing, or intimate contact with an individual with hepatitis. The diagnosis of chronic hepatitis C is established by detecting hepatitis C virus (HCV) antibody in the blood and confirmed by a positive polymerase chain reaction (PCR) for HCV RNA. A quantitative measure of HCV RNA can assess the level of viremia by reverse transcription PCR or branched DNA assays. HCV genotype is helpful in determining the duration of treatment required and the likelihood of achieving a sustained viral response. Panels of laboratory abnormalities have been devised to predict the degree of inflammation and fibrosis on biopsy and can be used as alternatives to liver biopsy.[14,15] Although these tests appear to accurately predict mild and advanced disease, intermediate grades of injury are difficult to assess without histology.

Hepatitis B virus (HBV) is a common cause of chronic liver disease in the world; however its prevalence in the United States is less than 1%. Risk factors for the acquisition of hepatitis B are similar to those for hepatitis C, although vertical transmission and sexual transmission are more common with hepatitis B. Detecting the hepatitis B surface antigen establishes the diagnosis of hepatitis B. Measuring HBV DNA level, ALT concentration, and the presence or absence of hepatitis B antigen and antibody is helpful in determining which patients should receive antiviral therapy.

NONALCOHOLIC FATTY LIVER DISEASE

Recent studies have suggested that steatosis in the absence of significant alcohol consumption is the most common cause of chronic elevations in the aminotransferases. NAFLD ranges from simple steatosis to nonalcoholic steatohepatitis (NASH) to cirrhosis.

The prevalence of NAFLD in the United States is estimated at 25% and is typically increased in individuals with class III obesity, central adiposity, hypertriglyceridemia, hypertension, glucose intolerance, or type 2 diabetes.[16] The prevalence of NASH, a progressive form of the disease characterized by ballooned hepatocytes on histology, is estimated to be 3% to 5%. Susceptibility to NASH is related to genetic and nongenetic factors. Several studies have shown that NAFLD is responsible for most hepatic enzyme abnormalities once viral hepatitis, autoimmune, metabolic, drug-induced, and alcoholic liver disease have been excluded. At present there is no way to confirm the diagnosis of hepatic steatosis through laboratory tests. There are emerging surrogate markers in the form of expanded laboratory indices, fibrosis markers, and NASH markers of apoptosis such as cytokeratin 18 fragment.[17] Imaging studies may show fatty infiltration, but considerable variations are found among individual interpreters. Weight reduction, glycemic control, lipid-lowering agents, and antihypertensive medications are recommended, although it has been difficult to prove that these therapeutic interventions alter the natural history of NAFLD. A randomized, controlled trial suggests that vitamin E is superior to placebo in reducing hepatic steatosis and lobular inflammation in nondiabetic patients. However no significant improvement in fibrosis scores was noted in these patients.[18] A sustained effect on progression of the disease remains to be proven with other therapies including hypoglycemic agents such as pioglitazone and metformin, ursodeoxycholic acid, or folic acid. The use of probiotic agents, antifibrotic mediators, and certain antihypertensive agents such as angiotensin receptor antagonists (losartan) are currently being studied.

AUTOIMMUNE HEPATITIS

Autoimmune hepatitis is an important disorder to consider in the differential of abnormal hepatic enzymes because immunosuppressive therapy has been shown to dramatically affect the outcome of this disease. With a prevalence of 11% to 23% in patients with chronic liver disease, it occurs most often in young to middle-aged women and is generally associated with other autoimmune disorders. Although most patients are asymptomatic when the disease is initially diagnosed, some patients, particularly older women, may present with symptoms of acute hepatitis such as fatigue, nausea, and low-grade fever. Patients with autoimmune hepatitis usually have a polyclonal increase in immunoglobulins, with the immunoglobulin G (IgG) fraction predominating. Most have a positive antinuclear antibody and smooth muscle (anti-actin) antibody.[19] Prompt diagnosis is essential because significant fibrosis may develop rapidly in untreated patients. A liver biopsy is helpful in establishing the diagnosis and determining the degree of fibrosis. The inflammatory infiltrate often contains numerous plasma cells and can be more extensive than suspected based on the patient's clinical presentation and degree of aminotransferase elevations. Most patients will require long-term immunosuppressive treatment.

HEMOCHROMATOSIS, WILSON DISEASE, AND α₁-ANTITRYPSIN DEFICIENCY

Hereditary hemochromatosis is a common genetic disorder causing elevated hepatic enzymes. It is inherited as an autosomal recessive trait with an increased prevalence among those of Northern European ancestry. Calculating transferrin saturation is the most effective screening test for hemochromatosis. Transferrin saturation greater than 45% should be investigated further.[20] A serum ferritin greater than 400 ng/dL in men and 300 ng/dL in women provides additional evidence of clinically significant iron overload. Most patients with genetic hemochromatosis can be diagnosed through the use of genetic analysis, with the genes *C282Y* and *H63D* being those most commonly associated with genetic hemochromatosis.[21] Detecting homozygosity for the *C282Y* mutation establishes the diagnosis. The *H63D* gene probably represents a polymorphism, because most patients who are homozygous for this gene do not show clinical manifestations of hemochromatosis.

There is no consensus regarding the need for liver biopsy in patients with genetic hemochromatosis. Material obtained from a biopsy can be assessed for iron content with calculation of a hepatic iron index (hepatic iron content divided by the patient's age), with an index greater than 1.9 providing compelling evidence for hemochromatosis even if genetic testing is negative. In addition, the degree of fibrosis can also be assessed. However, many believe that this information is not essential in homozygous patients in order to begin treatment with phlebotomy. A biopsy should be performed when there are comorbid conditions that may require additional or alternative therapeutic interventions such as hepatitis C, obesity, or significant alcohol consumption.

Wilson disease is a rare inherited disorder that may cause abnormal hepatic enzymes. Wilson disease should be considered in patients younger than 45 years of age who have unexplained elevations in the ALT. In some instances, these patients can present with an acute hepatitis with marked elevation of transaminases. Finding a low serum ceruloplasmin warrants additional investigation, including a 24-hour urine collection for quantitation of copper excretion. In patients with a high index of suspicion, an ophthalmic examination should be obtained to look for Kayser-Fleischer rings. If these suggest copper overload, a liver biopsy with quantitation of hepatic copper should be performed. Hepatic copper greater than 250 μg per gram of liver suggests Wilson disease, and the patient should be treated with chelating agents such as penicillamine.[22]

A1AT deficiency is an autosomal recessive disorder caused by defective production of A1AT. This leads to decreases in A1AT activity in the blood and lungs, and deposition of abnormal A1AT protein in the liver cells. Patients with emphysema or a family history of liver disease should have assessment of the A1AT phenotype.

ELEVATED SERUM BILIRUBIN

Bilirubin is a product of the degradation of the heme moiety that is released predominantly from senescent red blood cells. Approximately 30% of serum bilirubin is derived from heme-containing cytochromes or myoglobin. After its initial release into the blood, bilirubin is bound to albumin and thus is not filtered through the glomeruli and does not appear in the urine. It is then taken up by the hepatocytes and conjugated with glucuronic acid to form monoglucuronides and diglucuronides. Conjugated bilirubin is then actively transported across the canalicular membrane into the bile.

Jaundice can develop from alterations in any step in bilirubin metabolism. Because the energy-requiring step in bilirubin metabolism is canalicular transport, most hepatic diseases cause a conjugated (or direct) hyperbilirubinemia, and, conversely, most causes of indirect hyperbilirubinemia are not related to hepatic dysfunction

Unconjugated or indirect hyperbilirubinemia develops from overproduction or ineffective uptake of bilirubin from the blood. The enzymes responsible for bilirubin metabolism are inducible and are capable of handling approximately six times the normal production of bilirubin before it begins to accumulate in the blood. Large hematomas or hemolysis can cause increases in indirect bilirubin, but rarely does the serum bilirubin rise above 5 mg/dL. Evidence supporting hemolysis would include an elevated reticulocyte count, low haptoglobin concentration, and an elevation in lactate dehydrogenase level. As outlined earlier, hemolysis can also cause mild increases in AST.[23] Gilbert syndrome is a common disorder of bilirubin metabolism that affects approximately 5% of the population and is inherited as an autosomal dominant trait. The term *syndrome* is a misnomer because Gilbert's should probably be considered a normal variant in bilirubin metabolism rather than a disease. It results from a polymorphism in the gene encoding the enzyme responsible for bilirubin conjugation.[24] Consequently, mild degrees of unconjugated hyperbilirubinemia (with bilirubin levels typically more than 2 mg/dL but rarely higher than 6 mg/dL) are seen particularly during periods of fasting or systemic illnesses. This becomes important in the patient with Gilbert syndrome who develops acute cholecystitis, because concomitant hyperbilirubinemia is often a result of the preoperative fasting state rather than biliary obstruction from choledocholithiasis. This phenomenon highlights the need to check a fractionated bilirubin in the setting of hyperbilirubinemia. Patients with Gilbert syndrome should be reassured and advised that brief periods of jaundice may occur sporadically.

ELEVATED ALKALINE PHOSPHATASE

Conjugated or direct hyperbilirubinemia can be caused by disorders affecting the hepatocytes or the biliary tract anywhere from the canalicular membrane to the sphincter of Oddi. When conjugated hyperbilirubinemia is seen in the setting of a predominant aminotransferase elevation, injury from a drug, toxin, virus, or metabolic disorder is likely. When bilirubin accumulates because of a disorder of the bile ducts, there is usually a concomitant rise in the alkaline phosphatase concentration. Alkaline phosphatase is an enzyme localized on the sinusoidal membrane of the hepatocyte and the microvilli of the biliary canaliculi. The elevation in serum alkaline phosphatase in hepatobiliary diseases appears to result from an increase in the de novo synthesis in the liver followed by release into the blood in the hepatic sinusoids. Retention of bile salts may be responsible for the induction of alkaline phosphatase synthesis and may also promote its release across the hepatocyte plasma membrane. The normal values for alkaline phosphatase vary based on demographic factors. Individuals older than 60 years of age tend to have higher values than younger adults. In subjects younger than 50 years, the alkaline phosphatase activity is higher in men than in women, whereas in adults older than 60 years, enzyme activity in women is higher than in men.[25]

Alkaline phosphatase is not isolated to the liver and is found in the intestine, bone, and placenta. Assays using heat fractionation or gel fractionation can isolate the individual fractions, thus identifying the specific source, but are seldom used clinically. Instead, measurement of GGT or 5′-nucleotidase are used as surrogate markers for hepatic alkaline phosphatase, as they are not found in extrahepatic tissues. Unfortunately, the usefulness of GGT is limited by its lack of specificity, as many medications and alcohol can elevate the serum GGT concentration in the absence of liver disease.

If an elevation in serum alkaline phosphatase is found to be of hepatic origin, the first step is to exclude obstruction of the biliary tract. The most commonly used modality to detect extrahepatic biliary obstruction is ultrasonography. If the extrahepatic ducts are dilated, magnetic resonance cholangiopancreatography (MRCP) or endoscopic retrograde cholangiopancreatography (ERCP) can define the abnormality more precisely. MRCP is increasingly considered the diagnostic test of choice for choledocholithiasis given its high sensitivity and lower risk profile.[26] In addition to providing important diagnostic information, ERCP may afford the opportunity to relieve the obstruction by performing a sphincterotomy with removal of a biliary calculus or placement of a stent. When an elevation in the alkaline phosphatase concentration is detected in the absence of hyperbilirubinemia, a disorder causing partial obstruction of the biliary tree or affecting the hepatocyte-canalicular membrane, septal or interlobular bile ducts should be considered. Primary sclerosing cholangitis (PSC) should be suspected in individuals with inflammatory bowel disease. The diagnosis of PSC is made when irregularities in the caliber of the extrahepatic biliary ducts are seen on imaging studies. A radiographic appearance similar to PSC, known as *human immunodeficiency virus (HIV) cholangiopathy*, is seen in HIV-infected patients as a complication of opportunistic infections of the biliary tract by *Cryptosporidium* or *Cytomegalovirus*.[27]

If imaging studies show a normal biliary tree in the setting of an elevated alkaline phosphatase, then an intrahepatic disorder is likely present. Infiltration of the liver by granulomata, fat, tumor, or on occasion congestion of the liver from heart failure can cause elevations in hepatic alkaline phosphatase. Appropriate imaging studies can often detect evidence of tumor invasion or steatosis of the liver. Finding tender hepatomegaly with jugular venous distention suggests congestive heart failure. A liver biopsy is required to confirm the presence of hepatic granulomata.

A hepatotoxic reaction to a drug or toxin may cause an elevated alkaline phosphatase with or without jaundice. Such drugs include trimethoprim-sulfamethoxazole, ampicillin, erythromycin, anabolic steroids, chlorpromazine, and estrogens. Patients with sepsis and those receiving hyperalimentation may occasionally develop intrahepatic cholestasis.[28] Modest elevations in alkaline phosphatase and bilirubin have also been seen in patients with a variety of malignancies in the absence of liver involvement, presumably as a result of paraneoplastic syndromes (e.g., Stauffer syndrome).[29]

Primary biliary cirrhosis (PBC) should always be considered in the differential diagnosis of a persistently elevated alkaline phosphatase concentration, particularly in middle-aged women. Presumably an autoimmune disorder, PBC is associated with the detection of antimitochondrial antibodies directed toward the pyruvate dehydrogenase enzyme complex on the inner membrane of the mitochondria of the bile duct epithelium. Finding an antimitochondrial antibody is virtually diagnostic of PBC, and a liver biopsy is usually not necessary to confirm the diagnosis unless there are other disorders that could be causing coexisting hepatic injury such as obesity, alcohol, or certain drugs.[30]

OTHER LABORATORY TESTS USED IN THE ASSESSMENT OF LIVER DISEASES

The prothrombin time measures several of the coagulation factors synthesized in the liver and is helpful in assessing synthetic capacity of the liver. The half-life of factor VII, an important component of the prothrombin time assay, is approximately 6 hours. Consequently, the prothrombin time is particularly useful in the evaluation of patients with acute liver injury such as viral hepatitis or toxic liver injuries. It is also a component of the Child-Pugh score for chronic liver disease and the Model of End-Stage Liver Disease (MELD) score used to assess candidacy for liver transplantation. Prolongation of the prothrombin time can also result from vitamin K deficiency. Traditionally, adequacy of vitamin K stores is assessed by measuring the prothrombin time after parenteral vitamin K administration. Within 24 hours after 1 mg of vitamin K is given subcutaneously, the prothrombin time should decrease by 30%. Consumptive coagulopathies may also cause an abnormal prothrombin time when hepatic synthesis is adequate. Simultaneously measuring a factor VIII level (synthesized by vascular endothelium) may help distinguish hepatic failure from disseminated intravascular coagulation. Factor VIII levels may be inordinately high in cirrhotic patients, while other coagulation factor levels are decreased.[31] A normal or increased factor VIII level in the setting of an abnormal prothrombin time suggests hepatic failure, whereas equal suppression of both implies an underlying coagulopathy.

Albumin is a protein synthesized exclusively by the liver and is another important constituent of the assessment of patients with liver disease. The half-life of albumin is usually 19 to 21 days and therefore is often used to assess hepatic protein synthesis in chronic liver diseases. It is also a component of the Child-Pugh classification. Unfortunately, extrahepatic factors can affect the albumin concentration. The expanded plasma volume that often complicates cirrhosis may falsely lower the albumin concentration, and malnutrition or malabsorption may result in inadequate substrates for protein synthesis despite normal synthetic capacity. Albumin is also an acute-phase reactant that decreases in the setting of systemic inflammation as a result of increased catabolism as well as decreased synthesis.[32]

PERCUTANEOUS LIVER BIOPSY IN THE DIAGNOSIS OF LIVER DISEASE

As previously discussed, performing a liver biopsy can be helpful in establishing the diagnosis and prognosis in a variety of settings where elevated hepatic enzymes are encountered. It is not possible to describe global indications for liver biopsy. Each patient must be assessed for the relative benefit of histologic information compared with the potential risk of performing the procedure. When a biopsy is performed, it is essential to obtain adequate tissue samples for histologic examination, especially when attempting to confirm the presence of cirrhosis. For many diseases, such as steatohepatitis, sampling error is a major problem.

Most liver biopsies are performed safely in outpatient facilities, although complications requiring hospitalization have been reported in up to 4% of patients. Severe complications defined as death, severe hemorrhage, pneumothorax, or bile peritonitis occur in 0.1% to 0.3%, with a mortality rate of 9 : 100,000.

A liver biopsy should not be attempted in an uncooperative patient or when a vascular lesion has been identified. It may be difficult to identify an appropriate site for biopsy in a patient with ascites or a right pleural effusion. A biopsy should not be attempted in patients with a significant coagulopathy, given the high risk of bleeding. There are no published guidelines for a "safe" coagulation profile, although, in general, biopsies are not performed if the prothrombin time exceeds the control value by 3 seconds or the platelet count is less than 60,000/dL.

With increasing frequency, liver biopsies are performed using ultrasound guidance. When a biopsy attempts to sample focal hepatic defects, guidance with computed tomography or ultrasound should be used. Ultrasound guidance is also helpful when ascites is present or when abdominal adiposity renders it difficult to accurately locate the liver on physical examination. At many centers even "routine" liver biopsies are now performed under ultrasonographic guidance, and several studies suggest that this technique can reduce the risk of several potential complications.[33]

SUGGESTED READINGS

American Association for the Study of Liver Diseases (AASLD): Practice guidelines: Liver biopsy. *Hepatology* 49:1017, 2009.

Amini M, Runyon BA: Alcoholic hepatitis 2010: A clinician's guide to diagnosis and therapy. *World J Gastroenterol* 16:4905, 2010.

Czaja AJ, Manns MP: Advances in the diagnosis, pathogenesis, and management of autoimmune hepatitis. *Gastroenterology* 139:58, 2010.

Green RM, Flamm S: AGA technical review on the evaluation of liver chemistry tests. *Gastroenterology* 123:1367, 2002.

Loks AS, McMahon BJ: Chronic hepatitis B: Update 2009. *Hepatology* 50:661, 2009.

Nelson DR, Davis GL: Hepatitis C virus: A critical appraisal of approaches to therapy. *Clin Gastroenterol Hepatol* 7:397, 2009.

Pratt DS, Kaplan MM: Evaluation of abnormal liver-enzyme results in asymptomatic patients. *N Engl J Med* 342:1266, 2000.

REFERENCES

1. Kundrotas LW, Clement DJ: Serum alanine aminotransferase elevation in asymptomatic U.S. Air Force basic trainee blood donors. *Dig Dis Sci* 38:2145, 1993.
2. Daniel S, Ben-Menachem T, Vasudevan G, et al: Prospective evaluation of unexplained chronic liver transaminase abnormalities in asymptomatic and symptomatic patients. *Am J Gastroenterol* 94:3010, 1999.
3. Patt CH, Yoo HY, Dibadj K, et al: Prevalence of transaminase abnormalities in asymptomatic, healthy subjects participating in an executive health-screening program. *Dig Dis Sci* 48:797, 2003.
4. Sabath LD, Gerstein DA, Finland M: Serum glutamic oxaloacetic transaminase: False elevations during administration of erythromycin. *N Engl J Med* 279:1137, 1968.
5. Scola RH, Werneck LC, Prevedello DM, et al: Diagnosis of dermatomyositis and polymyositis: A study of 102 cases. *Arq Neuropsiquiatr* 58:789, 2000.
6. Lin YC, Lee WT, Huang SF, et al: Persistent hypertransaminasemia as the presenting findings of muscular dystrophy in childhood. *Acta Paediatr Taiwan* 40:424, 1999.
7. Burnett JR, Crooke MJ, Delahunt JW, et al: Serum enzymes in hypothyroidism. *N Engl Med J* 107:355, 1994.
8. Novacek G, Miehsler W, Wrba F, et al: Prevalence and clinical importance of hypertransaminasemia in celiac disease. *Eur J Gastroenterol Hepatol* 11:283, 1999.
9. Bardella MT, Fraquelli M, Quatrini M, et al: Prevalence of hypertransaminasemia in adult celiac patients and effect of gluten-free diet. *Hepatology* 22:833, 1995.
10. Taner T, Antony J: Determining positivity of alcohol abuse by Taguchi methods. *Int J Health Care Qual Assur Inc Leadersh Health Serv* 18:83, 2005.
11. Diehl AM, Potter J, Boitnott J, et al: Relationship between pyridoxal 5′-phosphate deficiency and aminotransferase levels in alcoholic hepatitis. *Gastroenterology* 86:632, 1984.
12. Seeff LB, Cuccherini BA, Zimmerman HJ, et al: Acetaminophen hepatotoxicity in alcoholics. *Ann Intern Med* 104:399, 1986.
13. Sheth SG, Flamm SL, Gordon FD, et al: AST/ALT ratio predicts cirrhosis in patients with chronic hepatitis C virus infection. *Am J Gastroenterol* 93:44, 1998.
14. Imbert-Bismut F, Ratziu V, Pieroni L, et al: Biochemical markers of liver fibrosis in patients with hepatitis C virus infection: A prospective study. *Lancet* 357:1069, 2001.

15. Poynard T, McHutchison J, Manns M, et al: Biochemical surrogate markers of liver fibrosis and activity in a randomized trial of peginterferon alfa-2b and ribavirin. *Hepatology* 38:481, 2003.

16. Bacon BR, Farahvash MJ, Janney CG, et al: Nonalcoholic steatohepatitis: An expanded clinical entity. *Gastroenterology* 107:1103, 1994.

17. Feldstein AE, Wieckowska A, Lopez AR, et al: Cytokeratin-18 fragment levels as noninvasive biomarkers for nonalcoholic steatohepatitis: A multicenter validation study. *Hepatology* 50:1072, 2009.

18. Sanyal AJ, Chalasani N, Kowdley KV, et al: Pioglitazone, vitamin E, or placebo for nonalcoholic steatohepatitis. *N Engl J Med* 362:1675, 2010.

19. Meyer zum Büschenfelde KH, Lohse AW, Manns M, et al: Autoimmunity and liver disease. *Hepatology* 12:354, 1990.

20. Powell LW, George DK, McDonnell SM, et al: Diagnosis of hemochromatosis. *Ann Intern Med* 129:925, 1998.

21. Bacon BR: Hemochromatosis: Diagnosis and management. *Gastroenterology* 120:718, 2001.

22. Loudianos G, Gitlin JD: Wilson's disease. *Semin Liver Dis* 20:353, 2000.

23. Shah A: Hemolytic anemia. *Ind J Med Sci* 58:400, 2004.

24. Monaghan G, Ryan M, Seddon R, et al: Genetic variation in bilirubin UPD-glucuronosyltransferase gene promoter and Gilbert's syndrome. *Lancet* 347:578, 1996.

25. Dufour DR, Lott JA, Nolte FS, et al: Diagnosis and monitoring of hepatic injury: I. Performance characteristics of laboratory tests. *Clin Chem* 46:2027, 2000.

26. Guarise A, Baltieri S, Mainardi P, et al: Diagnostic accuracy of MRCP in choledocholithiasis. *Radiol Med* 109:239, 2005.

27. Majahani RV, Uzer MF: Cholangiopathy in HIV-infected patients. *Clin Liver Dis* 3:669, 1999.

28. Mohi-ud-din R, Lewis JH: Drug- and chemical-induced cholestasis. *Clin Liver Dis* 8:95, 2004.

29. Karakolios A, Kasapis C, Kallinikidis T: Cholestatic jaundice as a paraneoplastic manifestation of prostate adenocarcinoma. *Clin Gastroenterol Hepatol* 1:480, 2003.

30. Vierling JM: Primary biliary cirrhosis and autoimmune cholangiopathy. *Clin Liver Dis* 8:177, 2004.

31. Hollestelle MJ, Geertzen HG, Straatsburg IH, et al: Factor VIII expression in liver disease. *Thromb Haemost* 91:267, 2004.

32. Quinlan GJ, Martin GS, Evans TW: Albumin: Biochemical properties and therapeutic potential. *Hepatology* 41:1211, 2005.

33. Pasha T, Gabriel S, Therneau T, et al: Cost-effectiveness of ultrasound-guided liver biopsy. *Hepatology* 27:1220, 1998.

Perioperative Management and Nutrition in Patients With Liver and Biliary Tract Disease

Brendan J. Boland | James R. Ouellette | Steven D. Colquhoun

Even a seemingly innocuous surgical procedure can lead to a catastrophic cascade of complications in the patient with significant underlying liver or biliary disease. The spectrum of portal hypertension, ascites, synthetic dysfunction, coagulopathy, hypersplenism, cholestasis, or biliary obstruction can all be present to varying degrees and should temper enthusiasm for surgical intervention. Liver and biliary tract disease secondarily alter the physiology of other organ systems and create issues that must be considered when planning even the smallest operation, lest an otherwise routine surgical procedure precipitate bleeding, hypotension, and hepatic decompensation. Risks are difficult to quantify, but are related to the degree of underlying dysfunction as well as the magnitude of the anticipated procedure. All phases of perioperative care can be affected. This chapter will focus on the perioperative issues related to patients with various degrees of dysfunction caused by primary liver disease and the consequences of biliary obstruction.

PATHOPHYSIOLOGY OF CIRRHOSIS AND OBSTRUCTIVE JAUNDICE

In classical Greek mythology, the suffering of Prometheus demonstrated the unique regenerative capacity of the liver. Hepatic regeneration in the clinical setting, however, does not always restore the normal anatomic structure of the organ. Liver disease invariably involves some degree of hepatocyte injury and necrosis. Regardless of the etiology, hepatocellular damage leads to fibrosis. Fibrosis occurs in a continuum of severity and when extensive and accompanied by nodule formation is termed *cirrhosis*. Normally, both hepatic arterial and portal blood flow perfuse the sinusoids with a zonal distribution of hepatocytes relative to the nutrient and oxygen-rich blood supply. Single plates of sinusoids are arranged in lobules with a central hepatic vein and portal triads at the periphery. In contrast, regenerating nodules lack this normal architecture, containing only a single source of inflow derived from the hepatic artery, as the portal venule is unable to penetrate the fibrotic collagen rim. As a consequence, single-pass uptake from the gastrointestinal tract is impaired.

In addition to the architectural alteration caused by fibrosis and scarring, there is an overall decrease in secretion of vasodilatory substances, such as nitrous oxide, by the cells lining the sinusoids. This is coupled with activation of hepatic stellate cells in the space of Disse, cells that actively secrete vasoconstrictors. Even normal areas

of hepatocytes suffer from the increased resistance to portal flow. In the splanchnic circulation, the response to this increased resistance to portal flow is a further release of vasodilatory substances, thus increasing overall portal inflow. Portal hypertension is therefore the result of resistance to flow through the liver combined with greater inflow. This increased pressure gradient between the portal and systemic circulation results in the development of collateral pathways for portal venous flow around the liver, and thus the clinical manifestations of portal hypertension.[1]

Pathology at any point between the hepatocyte and the duodenum may give rise to cholestasis.[2] The cholestatic liver appears enlarged, green and rounded, and patients with cholestasis from biliary obstruction are at risk for changes similar to those seen in early cirrhosis. Indeed, in its extreme chronic form, biliary obstruction can lead to secondary biliary cirrhosis. Although the mechanisms are more complex than is appropriate for this discussion, cholestasis causes hepatic dysfunction, and simple relief of obstructive jaundice does not immediately reverse the functional impairment. Cholestasis is also associated with postoperative renal failure, although the precise mechanism remains elusive.[3] Coagulopathy arising from both hepatocellular synthetic dysfunction and malabsorption of vitamin K–dependent coagulation factors develops in patients with jaundice. Cholestasis has profound effects on other organ systems, including the immune response, the central nervous system function, and the gastrointestinal tract.

PREOPERATIVE CONSIDERATIONS

GENERAL ASSESSMENT AND PREOPERATIVE PREPARATION

The successful outcome of any surgical intervention is predicated on the patient's ability to tolerate and recover from the stress of the procedure. Although there are many objective criteria on which to base such an assessment, the subjective impression of an experienced clinician is remarkably accurate. A thorough history should include any personal or family accounts of liver disease. Even a distant or vague history of hepatitis or jaundice should indicate the need for specific laboratory testing. Risk factors for hepatitis, such as past intravenous drug use, tattoos, or blood transfusion, should be documented. Such questioning may elucidate one or more potential risk factors for occult hepatic disease (Table 116-1). Also of particular relevance is a history of recent weight loss, exercise intolerance, shortness of breath, smoking,

TABLE 116-1 Occult Hepatic Disease: Potential Etiologies

Category	Entity	Action/Associations
Infectious	HBV ± delta	History and serology
	HCV	
Metabolic	Fatty liver disease	(See Box 116-1)
	Iron overload	History/specific
	Others	testing
Toxic	Alcohol	History/screen
	Drugs	Amiodarone
	Environmental	Methotrexate
Structural	Cholestasis	Stone or tumor
	Hepatic venous outflow	Budd-Chiari syndrome
		Heart failure
		Pericardial disease
Immune mediated	PSC	IBD/colorectal tumor
	PBC	Cholangiocarcinoma
	Autoimmune	
Others	Granulomatous disease	
	Cryptogenic	

HBV, Hepatitis B virus; HCV, hepatitis C virus; IBD, inflammatory bowel disease; PBC, primary biliary cirrhosis; PSC, primary sclerosing cholangitis.

TABLE 116-3 Laboratory Testing

METABOLIC PANEL	Sodium	Hyponatremia associated with ascites
	BUN/creatinine	Hepatorenal dysfunction
	AST/ALT	Assess ongoing cellular injury
		ETOH: increased ratio
	Alkaline phosphatase	Mass or obstruction
	GGT	Acute ETOH-associated
	Total/direct bilirubin	Assess nature of cholestasis
COAGULATION	INR	Synthetic dysfunction
		Vitamin K deficiency
BLOOD COUNT	Hemoglobin	
	MCV/MCHC	Nature of anemia
	Platelets	Evidence of portal hypertension

ALT, Alanine aminotransferase; AST, aspartate aminotransferase; BUN, blood urea nitrogen; ETOH, ethanol; GGT, γ-glutamyltransferase; INR, international normalized ratio; MCHC, mean corpuscular hemoglobin concentration; MCV, mean corpuscular volume.

TABLE 116-2 Clinical Examination: Evidence of Liver Disease

SKIN	Jaundice
	Spider angiomata
	Dupuytren contracture
HEAD	Scleral icterus
	Temporal wasting
CHEST	Gynecomastia
LUNGS	Right base effusion
ABDOMEN	Caput medusae
	Fluid wave
	Palpable spleen
	Shrunken liver
	Enlarged liver
	Cardiovascular hum
EXTREMITIES	Edema
NEUROLOGIC	Asterixis

BOX 116-1 Fatty Liver Disease Associations

Obesity
Steroid use
Diabetes
Alcohol
Rheumatoid arthritis
Others

gastrointestinal bleeding, easy bruisability, prior surgery, or delayed wound healing. In addition to a good general physical evaluation, a focused examination should seek evidence suggestive of chronic liver disease (Table 116-2 and Box 116-1) such as temporal wasting, scleral icterus, jugular venous distention, supraclavicular adenopathy, diminished breath sounds at the lung bases, gynecomastia, spider angiomata, palmar erythema, splenomegaly, a firm liver edge, peripheral edema, or asterixis.

Basic laboratory tests should include a complete blood count, as well as a comprehensive metabolic panel and coagulation profile. Frequently, in elective circumstances, abnormalities may be able to be corrected before surgery. Even more important may be the clues provided by identified abnormalities with regard to the extent of underlying disease (Table 116-3).

The potential need for intraoperative transfusion should be anticipated during any liver or biliary operation. The use of blood and blood products during liver resection for cancer has been associated with increased rate of recurrence, more postoperative complications, and overall worse survival, but transfusion may be unavoidable in major resections.[4] Efforts should be made to achieve a near-normal hematocrit before operation. Depending on timing, anemia may be treated simply by correcting basic deficiencies such as iron, folic acid, or vitamin B[12]. If time does not permit, it is generally prudent to transfuse packed red blood cells to achieve a hematocrit of at least 30%. If anemia is absent and a delay is acceptable, then autologous blood donation may be an option. Autologous donation has been associated with an improved prognosis in patients with cirrhosis undergoing resection of hepatocellular carcinoma who needed transfusion.[5] Although there is less evidence with autologous transfusion, the use of banked blood has long been controversial from the standpoint of immune function versus recurrence of malignancy.[6,7] Although chronic use in some settings has led to a Food and Drug Administration "black box" warning for increased risk of death, the use of weekly or daily erythropoietin injections in conjunction with repletion of iron stores remains a viable alternative for the correction of preoperative anemia in this setting.[8,9] More recent animal data suggest a protective effect of erythropoietin against ischemic injury to the liver.[10] The use of this drug also remains the preferred strategy for use in patients who subscribe to the Jehovah's Witnesses faith.

Other elements of a complete blood count, such as mean corpuscular volume and mean corpuscular hemoglobin concentration, may yield insights into the nature of an existing anemia or raise suspicion regarding associated diseases or behaviors, such as the megaloblastic anemia associated with chronic alcohol use. Perhaps the most useful is the platelet count. Thrombocytopenia correlates well with diminished hepatocellular function and portal hypertension.[11] Although hypersplenism may be associated with a reduction in any of the formed blood elements, a low platelet count is most common. Indeed, it is not uncommon for patients with occult liver disease and cirrhosis to be referred first to a hematologist for evaluation, including a bone marrow biopsy, before an accurate diagnosis is made. Any degree of thrombocytopenia should be considered a hint to possible underlying portal hypertension. In fact, the platelet count has been colloquially referred to as the "poor man's liver biopsy."

Abnormalities in electrolytes and intravascular volume are common in patients with liver or biliary tract disease. Patients may display a dilutional hyponatremia with peripheral edema and third-space fluid accumulation compounded by hypoalbuminemia. Hypokalemia may result from increased urinary excretion, even with the use of a potassium-sparing diuretic such as spironolactone. Hyponatremia should be corrected with free water restriction, and either supplemental oral or intravenous potassium should be used to correct hypokalemia. Diminished renal function is often associated with liver disease. Serum blood urea nitrogen and creatinine should be measured, and consideration also should be given to assessment of urine electrolytes and 24-hour creatinine clearance. Although it is mostly a diagnosis of exclusion, ominous signs of hepatorenal syndrome should be sought. Hepatorenal syndrome represents a major risk to any contemplated surgical procedure.[12]

Coagulation testing should include a partial thromboplastin time, a prothrombin time, and an international normalized ratio (INR). An additional assessment of fibrinolytic activity requires measuring fibrin degradation products and fibrinogen. Identified abnormalities may better inform preoperative discussion of risks and may prove useful to the anesthesia team.

Finally, thorough assessment of cardiopulmonary function should be performed. An electrocardiogram is indicated in patients with previous heart disease and generally appropriate in those older than age 35 to 40 years, depending on the magnitude of the contemplated procedure. Further cardiac evaluation may be indicated depending on the history, physical examination, or electrocardiogram abnormalities. For older patients undergoing major hepatic surgery, a cardiac stress test is almost always indicated. In high-risk patients, cardiac catheterization may be advisable. Formal pulmonary function testing should be based on history or clinical findings. Room air–blood gas analysis should be performed in those with significant pulmonary risk factors such as smoking, chronic cough, or shortness of breath.

HEPATIC FUNCTIONAL RESERVE

No reliable single test yet exists to assess functional hepatic reserve, and in particular, the adequacy of the postoperative remnant liver.[13] Although often not a major concern when the liver is otherwise healthy or the extent of the planned resection is smaller, assessment of functional reserve becomes critical when a major resection such as trisegmentectomy is required or when underlying liver disease is present in order to avoid a lingering postoperative hepatic failure and death.[14] In the field of liver transplantation, the term *small-for-size* syndrome describes the analogous situation in which an allograft is of inadequate functional capacity.[15] A number of modalities for assessing liver function are available[16] including measurement of the clearance of indocyanine green (ICG), a high first-pass, metabolized drug that is excreted into bile. The rate of ICG clearance correlates with hepatic blood flow and hepatocyte function. Biliary ICG excretion correlates with hepatic adenosine triphosphate (ATP) concentration, and a decrease may reflect a decrease in postresection regenerative capacity. The true clinical usefulness of ICG clearance remains questionable. Over the years a number of other tests have also been employed, including nuclear imaging of the asialoglycoprotein receptor, hippurate ratio determination, the aminopyrine breath test, caffeine-clearance test, galactose-elimination capacity, arterial ketone body ratio, monoethylglycinexylidide, trimethadione, and single-photon emission computed tomography.[17] The current best and most commonly used method is volumetric analysis based on axial imaging. It has been suggested that resection of less than 60% of nontumor-bearing liver is generally acceptable for noncirrhotic livers. When greater than 60% resection is required, preoperative portal vein embolization may be used to increase the size of the anticipated remnant liver.[17] It has been reported that 90% of patients develop hepatic dysfunction if less than 25% of normal liver remains after trisegmentectomy for colorectal hepatic metastases.[18] Volume assessment is most appropriate when there is no underlying parenchymal disease. Any degree of fibrosis, inflammation, or fatty infiltration effectively diminishes the remnant function. In patients with frank cirrhosis, even a small segmental resection may result in hepatic failure.[19] New three-dimensional imaging techniques may offer distinct advantages over prior technologies.

NUTRITIONAL STATUS

Poor nutritional status is associated with a diminished immune response, an increased susceptibility to infection, poor wound healing, increased risk of organ dysfunction, and generally suboptimal outcomes. Despite the significance of nutritional status, none of the many different available methods for its assessment are ideal. The history and physical examination are probably still the most important. Comparison of the patient's current and premorbid state is essential, as an individual who otherwise appears to be of normal weight or build may have started from a baseline of obesity or greater muscular physique. Overt cachexia is common in patients with cirrhosis or malignancy, but more subtle signs of temporal and thenar wasting may be overlooked if not specifically sought.

Objective evaluation of nutritional status includes measurement of serum albumin or other visceral proteins (prealbumin or transferrin), triceps skin fold thickness, total lymphocyte count, and indirect calorimetry. Some of these tests are cumbersome, costly, and not widely available, and none has proven superior to the judgment of an experienced clinician.[20] Characteristics of patients at higher risk include (1) serum albumin less than 3.0 g/dL, (2) weight loss of 10% to 15% over a period of 3 to 4 months, (3) serum transferrin level less than 200 mg/dL, (4) anergy to injected skin antigens, (5) functional impairment for ordinary tasks, and (6) lack of ability to carry out functional tests to normal capacity such as hand dynamometry.[21] In a prospective cross-sectional study, Padillo et al evaluated patients with benign and malignant biliary obstructive diseases and identified protein-calorie malnutrition in 82% of these jaundiced patients. The duration of jaundice correlated with worsening malnutrition, and patients with malignant obstruction were more likely to have moderate or severe malnutrition than those with benign obstruction.[22,23] A number of studies suggest that serum albumin alone may be the best predictor of morbidity for a range of types of major abdominal surgery.[24,25]

PREOPERATIVE NUTRITIONAL INTERVENTION

Enteral and parenteral nutritional supplementation with both enteral and parenteral formulas has been used for decades in an effort to improve surgical outcomes.[21,26] Total parenteral nutrition (TPN) is chosen when the otherwise-preferred enteral route cannot be used. Based on the Veterans Affairs Cooperative Study, a minimum of 2 weeks of TPN is required to obtain nutritional enhancement and improve outcomes in severely malnourished patients.[24] Although mildly malnourished patients also show improvement, it was at the cost of significant increases in non–catheter-related nosocomial infections that negated the benefit. Preoperative TPN has often been found to increase rather than decrease surgical risks.[27] Despite best intentions, patients with cirrhosis or protein and calorie malnutrition resulting from obstructive jaundice are only rarely able to make significant improvement in preoperative nutritional status with a course of enteral supplementation even with detailed instructions. Although decompression of the biliary tree in jaundiced patients can stimulate appetite and caloric intake, the effect is usually insufficient to improve surgical outcome.

Early enteral nutrition in both trauma and burn patients attenuates the inevitable hypercatabolic response.[28] Both animal and human studies have shown that enteral nutrition prevents small bowel disuse atrophy and subsequent bacterial translocation, septic complications, and multisystem organ failure.[29-32] Patients with cirrhosis and biliary obstruction demonstrate reduced capacity to clear translocating bacteria, although the basis for this dysfunction remains to be fully established.[33,34]

PREOPERATIVE MANAGEMENT OF OBSTRUCTIVE JAUNDICE

Patients with obstructive jaundice are inherently at risk for hepatocellular injury and impaired liver function. Preoperative biliary decompression has been advocated to improve hepatic function and decrease the rate of perioperative complications. However, biliary decompression does not always lead to timely, complete normalization of serum bilirubin in the presence of long-standing obstruction and consequent hepatocyte dysfunction. Preoperative biliary decompression has been extensively studied, and the evidence has squarely argued against routine drainage. Preoperative biliary instrumentation has been clearly correlated with an increased rate of postoperative infectious complications, and complications associated with stent placement may delay or otherwise complicate resection.[35] Endoscopic stenting is appropriate in patients otherwise unfit for operation, and in limited circumstances the combination of preoperative decompression and nutritional supplementation may reduce the risk of subsequent resection.[36]

CIRRHOSIS

Cirrhotic patients have multiple interacting medical issues that complicate surgical care (Figure 116-1).

HEMODYNAMICS

Perhaps the most prominent physiologic impact of cirrhosis is hemodynamic. As in sepsis, the hemodynamic changes associated with cirrhosis affect multiple organ systems. Cirrhosis and portal hypertension lead to primary splanchnic arterial vasodilation, resulting in a reduction in systemic vascular resistance and inducing a hyperdynamic state. Vasodilation is caused by production of vasodilatory substances mainly in the splanchnic

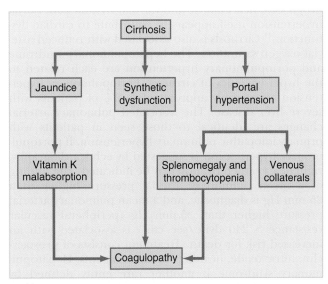

FIGURE 116-1 Schematic showing the interrelationship of multiple physiologic disturbances occurring in patients with portal hypertension and cirrhosis.

circulation including nitric oxide, carbon monoxide, and cannabinoids.[37] In addition to reduced systemic vascular resistance, other changes include increased peripheral blood flow, reduced arteriovenous oxygen saturation difference, decreased effective blood volume with reduced cortical renal blood flow, and activation of the renin-angiotensin axis (leading to sodium and water retention and to ascites formation). Pulmonary artery catheterization may be advisable to guide fluid resuscitation in patients with a distorted difference in right and left heart pressure caused by ascites or other variables. Patients with cirrhosis generally have elevated cardiac output, tachycardia, and low blood pressure. Many of the common physical findings seen in cirrhotic patients, such as palmar erythema and cutaneous spider angiomata, are consequences of these hemodynamic changes.

A variety of approaches may improve overall hemodynamics in cirrhosis. Intravenous administration of colloid can help restore normal intravascular volume, but excess crystalloid administration should be avoided because sodium and free water can exacerbate ascites and peripheral edema. Splanchnic vasoconstrictor therapy, especially in the presence of renal dysfunction, may be of benefit. Improvement of oxygen delivery is also an important goal. Some evidence suggests that N-acetylcysteine can improve oxygen delivery, oxygen extraction, and cardiac output, possibly acting through the nitric oxide–soluble cyclic guanylate monophosphate enzyme system,[38,39] although there are conflicting data on this point.[40] In late stages of cirrhosis, inotropic agents may be required to support sagging blood pressure, but hypotension in the face of adequate filling pressures augurs a poor prognosis.

CARDIOPULMONARY

Cardiac disease is often present in patients with chronic liver disease. Right heart pressures may be elevated because of the hemodynamic disturbances described in the earlier section on Hemodynamics, which can lead to progressive heart failure and valvular dysfunction. Portal hypertension itself appears to contribute to cardiac dysfunction.[41] Cirrhosis is also associated with reduced arterial oxygen saturation. The hepatopulmonary syndrome and portopulmonary hypertension are each related to the hyperdynamics of cirrhosis. Portopulmonary hypertension affects only approximately 2% of patients with severe liver disease. The associated pulmonary arterial changes are identical to those seen in patients with primary idiopathic pulmonary hypertension. If portopulmonary hypertension is suggested by echocardiography, right heart catheterization may be indicated. The finding of a mean pulmonary arterial pressure higher than 25 mm Hg is diagnostic, and a mean pulmonary arterial pressure higher than 35 mm Hg (peripheral vascular resistance > 240 dyne/sec/cm^5) is associated with an increased risk for death. Treatment consists of prostacyclin, nitric oxide, or other vasoactive agents. Hepatopulmonary syndrome is another rare entity defined by the triad of chronic hypoxemia (PaO_2 <60 mm Hg), pulmonary vascular dilation, and severe chronic liver disease. Demonstration of a large pulmonary shunt on ventilation–perfusion scanning or echocardiography is necessary to confirm the diagnosis.

PORTAL HYPERTENSION

The most clinically relevant aspect of cirrhosis is portal hypertension. Complications of portal hypertension are well described and consist mainly of variceal bleeding, usually from the esophagus. These dilated thin-walled vessels develop as a direct result of increased portal pressure and serve to shunt flow around the diseased liver. Approximately 90% of episodes of variceal hemorrhage are successfully treated with endoscopic and/or pharmacologic interventions. Transjugular intrahepatic portosystemic shunt (TIPS) is an interventional radiologic procedure that controls bleeding in more than 90% of patients who fail first-line therapy. Surgical shunts remain appropriate in the nonacute setting, when the most prominent feature of disease is bleeding in an otherwise well-compensated patient. A surgical shunt or TIPS may be contraindicated in the presence of significant hepatic encephalopathy or at serum bilirubin levels greater than 3.0 mg/dL, in which case progressive liver failure may ensue.

Pharmacologic therapy with a splanchnic vasoconstrictor should be started during the initial resuscitation of patients with variceal bleeding. Vasopressin is a potent vasoconstrictor that effectively lowers portal pressure but is associated with multiple side effects, including peripheral and bowel ischemia, that limit its clinical use.[42] Terlipressin is a synthetic analogue of vasopressin that reduces mortality in acute variceal bleeding with significantly fewer side effects, but it is not yet available in the United States. Octreotide, a somatostatin analogue, is widely available and is currently considered the first-line pharmacologic treatment in acute variceal bleeding.[43]

Endotherapy for acutely bleeding varices requires an experienced endoscopist. Multiple approaches have been used, each with a significant risk. Options for endoscopic therapy include banding and sclerotherapy, although both carry the risk of esophageal perforation. If endoscopy is not available, balloon compression with a Sengstaken-Blakemore tube or other device can be used until medical, radiologic, or surgical therapy can be instituted. Ultimately, portal hypertension may require correction by liver transplantation.

ASCITES

The pathogenesis of ascites is complex, but, in essence, it is a consequence of both portal hypertension and hypoalbuminemia, combined with a degree of salt and water retention. Serum albumin is usually less than 3.0 g/dL, and the associated renal excretion of sodium is less than 10 mmol/24 hr. Management includes the use of potassium-sparing diuretics and paracentesis. The goal is an ascites-free peritoneal cavity before undertaking any abdominal operation. Preoperative attempts to control ascites may be complicated by a diuresis-induced renal impairment that can progress to hepatorenal syndrome. Because perioperative fluid management can be challenging, the use of a pulmonary artery catheter is often advisable.

RENAL DYSFUNCTION

Hepatorenal syndrome can be defined as the development of otherwise-unexplained severe renal dysfunction in the setting of end-stage liver disease. It is caused by severe functional renal vasoconstriction, associated with the hemodynamic changes discussed previously, leading to a reduction in glomerular filtration rate without significant renal histologic abnormalities.[44,45] Severe splanchnic vasodilatation in response to portal hypertension causes reduced systemic vascular resistance. Arterial pressure is maintained by increasing cardiac output and activation of endogenous vasoconstrictors including angiotensin, the sympathetic nervous system, and hypersecretion of antidiuretic hormone. The kidney retains sodium and free water in excess of total body needs, exacerbating ascites and anasarca. Intrarenal vasoconstriction and hypoperfusion perpetuate hepatorenal syndrome. Normal renal function is often, but not invariably, restored after liver transplantation. Hepatorenal syndrome often requires hemodialysis. Two subtypes are recognized, based on the pace of functional loss. Type I hepatorenal syndrome, associated with rapidly progressive functional deterioration with a doubling of the initial serum creatinine value in a period of less than 14 days, carries a 90% mortality within 90 days. Type II syndrome progresses less rapidly and generally fares better.

Treatment of hepatorenal syndrome with splanchnic vasoconstrictors to reverse pathologic vasodilatation has met with some success. Terlipressin, a synthetic vasopressin analogue, has been shown to be effective in approximately half of the patients treated for hepatorenal syndrome. There is also evidence that midodrine, an oral α-adrenergic, when combined with octreotide is effective.[46,47]

METABOLIC ABNORMALITIES

Maintenance of fluid and electrolyte balance becomes increasingly difficult for a cirrhotic patient. Multisystem derangements noted earlier contribute to these difficulties. For example, hypoalbuminemia leads to intravascular depletion associated with third spacing of fluids, and cirrhotic patients have increased levels of aldosterone and antidiuretic hormone that favor salt and water retention. The choice of appropriate diuretic should be individualized but, in general, a combination of furosemide and spironolactone is used. Furthermore, thiazide diuretics should be avoided because of a tendency to cause encephalopathy. Renal dysfunction caused by hemodynamic alterations also contributes to fluid and electrolyte imbalance.

HEPATIC ENCEPHALOPATHY

The clinical findings of hepatic encephalopathy can range from subtle personality changes and sleep disturbance to frank coma. Careful questioning of the patient or family member can elicit a suggestive history. Encephalopathy can be acutely exacerbated by infection or a large gastrointestinal protein load, either dietary or from gastrointestinal bleeding. With proper management, even in the most severe circumstance, the mental status changes are potentially reversible. The mechanisms underlying hepatic encephalopathy appear to be related to the accumulation of unmetabolized ammonia because of poor hepatic function and portal-systemic shunting. Other factors may contribute to encephalopathy, including the production of false neurotransmitters, activation of γ-aminobutyric acid receptors, altered cerebral metabolism, and disturbed sodium, potassium, adenylate triphosphatase activity.[48,49]

Lactulose is a nonabsorbable disaccharide that is considered first-line treatment for encephalopathy. It is metabolized by bacteria in the colon to lactic and acetic acid, lowering the intraluminal pH. This makes the colon unfavorable for the growth of bacteria which make ammonia and favors the formation of nonabsorbable NH^{4+}. The result is lower ammonia levels in the blood and colon.[50] It is a powerful laxative, and excessive use can lead to severe volume depletion. Antibiotics such as vancomycin, metronidazole, and neomycin are often used in patients unresponsive or intolerant to disaccharides, although long-term use can be associated with toxicity such as hearing loss (neomycin), peripheral neuropathy (metronidazole), or selection of resistant organisms (vancomycin). Rifaximin is a poorly absorbed oral antibiotic that has proven efficacy in treatment and prevention of encephalopathy, with fewer side effects than other antibiotics.[51]

COAGULOPATHY

Among the potential complications of liver disease, acute hemorrhage is particularly dangerous. Figure 116–1 provides an overview of the factors that contribute to the coagulopathy associated with liver disease. Diminished synthetic capacity for factors II, VII, IX, and X can be recognized by prolongation of the INR or prothrombin time. Whether because of intrinsic parenchymal dysfunction or extrahepatic biliary obstruction, cholestasis further contributes to coagulopathy by inhibiting absorption of vitamin K, on which many clotting factors functionally depend. Thrombocytopenia is also associated with chronic liver disease and is a result of portal hypertension and hypersplenism. The degree of thrombocytopenia appears to roughly correlate with the severity of portal hypertension and cirrhosis. The manifestations of hypersplenism may be improved by TIPS.[52,53]

Treatment of coagulopathy in patients with liver and biliary tract disease is based on the underlying pathology. Parenteral vitamin K replacement corrects coagulopathy related to biliary obstruction, bacterial overgrowth, or malnutrition. Vitamin K is less effective for coagulopathy caused by severe parenchymal liver injury. Transfusion of fresh-frozen plasma (FFP) is the typical treatment for coagulopathy in patients with liver disease and active bleeding. Transfusion of FFP also reverses the moderate to severe coagulopathy of cirrhosis before invasive procedures. It is important to realize that more FFP may be required in patients with chronic liver disease than in those with coagulopathy from unrelated causes.[53] Cryoprecipitate can also be useful for severe coagulopathy with hypofibrinogenemia, especially when avoidance of volume overload is desired. Platelet transfusions, pooled or single donor, are useful in thrombocytopenic patients before performing invasive procedures or in the presence of significant bleeding, especially when the platelet count is below 50,000/mL. The use of recombinant factor VIIa and thrombopoietin therapy for correction of coagulopathy and thrombocytopenia, respectively, in patients with cirrhosis, is currently under investigation. Therapy with prothrombin complex concentrates, 1-deamino-8-D-arginine vasopressin, and antithrombin III concentrates for the management of coagulopathy caused by liver disease is being studied, but such treatment is not standard at this time.[54]

INFECTIOUS DISEASES

Infectious complications are notoriously associated with liver disease. These issues are of particular concern for pretransplant and posttransplant patients because of the need for immunosuppression. The infectious risk is probably multifactorial and related to impaired protein synthesis, malnutrition, and enteric bacterial translocation. Spontaneous bacterial peritonitis is a significant risk in patients with ascites. In cases of suspected spontaneous bacterial peritonitis, broad-spectrum antibiotics should be started without delay. Cholangitis is a major concern in patients with biliary obstruction. Improvement in nutritional status and control of complications may reduce infectious risk.

INTRAOPERATIVE CONSIDERATIONS

ANESTHESIA CONSIDERATIONS

In addition to the altered hemodynamics, coagulopathy, and other systemic effects of liver disease, the hepatic metabolism of many routinely used drugs poses a challenge for intraoperative management. The half-life of drugs cleared by the liver can be significantly prolonged and can thus alter dosage, duration of action, and lipid solubility. Ascites or edema present in cirrhotics can increase the volume of distribution. Conversely, in patients with a history of chronic alcohol use, an increased capacity for enzymatic metabolism may result in larger drug requirements during surgery. Because hepatic impairment also leads to decreased serum albumin concentrations, drugs that are usually protein bound may be present at increased plasma concentrations and give rise to an exaggerated response.

Surgical manipulation of the liver significantly increases the hepatic oxygen extraction ratio in connection with splanchnic vasoconstriction.[55] However, portal blood flow can be preserved despite a 20% to 60% reduction in blood pressure, provided that the cardiac index is maintained during sodium nitroprusside hypotension.[56] Therefore, a well-planned anesthetic that includes the aforementioned considerations and makes use of the now-accepted low central venous pressure technique will allow the greatest success. Low central venous pressure anesthesia is designed to avoid vena cava distention and facilitate hepatic mobilization and dissection of the retrohepatic cava and hepatic veins.[57,58] This is a different outlook from crystalloid fluid loading in the preresection phase. The goal in the loading method is to account for expected blood loss by dilutional bleeding. On the contrary, this technique can lead to more blood loss by distending the cava and making venous repair more difficult. Blood loss greater than 5 L has been associated with excess mortality.[59] Consequently, if central venous pressure is lowered from 15 to 3 mm Hg, caval blood loss from an injury can be theoretically reduced by a factor of 5. This pressure decrease requires fluid restriction until the resection is completed. Therefore, minimal preoperative fluid is given, and small boluses are used to maintain blood pressure. This strategy requires the close availability of a rapid infusion system to provide emergency fluid and blood infusion. Although a low intraoperative urine volume may result, this is not necessarily associated with an increased incidence of postoperative renal failure.[58] The need for effective communication between the surgeon and anesthesiologist cannot be overemphasized.

Inhalational agents such as isoflurane and desflurane have been studied extensively and found to be safe in patients with liver disease. They both undergo negligible hepatic metabolism and result in no free radical formation.[60] Hepatic blood flow and the hepatic artery buffer response are maintained better with isoflurane than with any other volatile anesthetic.[61] In contrast, halothane and other halogenated hydrocarbons must be avoided. Although halothane is a good general anesthetic for most patients, halothane hepatitis may occur from a single exposure,[62] and multiple exposures can result in fulminant hepatic failure. Although the exact cause remains unclear, hypoxic, metabolic, or immunologic mechanisms are likely.[63,64]

The use of local anesthesia should be encouraged, especially for small procedures. Amide-linked local anesthetics undergo hepatic metabolism and should be used with caution. Regional anesthesia is an excellent adjunct, and continuous epidural catheter placement can enhance pain control in the intraoperative and postoperative period. The problem with the widespread use of regional anesthesia in this population is hemostatic impairment, which is a contraindication to spinal or epidural puncture.

OPERATIVE CONSIDERATIONS IN PATIENTS WITH LIVER AND BILIARY DISEASE

Although preparation for surgery is the key to success, some special intraoperative factors must be considered, as well as the basic tenets of abdominal surgery. Adequate exposure is critical, and proper consideration must be given to the type and extent of the incision. Extension of the incision should be performed whenever safety requires. A dependable self-retaining retractor system is essential.

A variety of methods to limit intraoperative blood loss can be used. The most common method used to limit blood loss during liver resection is either intermittent or continuous clamping of the portal triad (Pringle maneuver). Use of this technique is limited by the degree of underlying parenchymal disease. A normal liver may tolerate up to a total cumulative clamping time of 1 hour, but a diseased liver will tolerate much less. The use of total vascular occlusion during major liver resection may be feasible but should be discussed well in advance with the anesthesiologist. Venovenous bypass may be a useful adjunct in selected circumstances, such as in patients with large tumors involving the vena cava.

The use of tubes and drains after liver and biliary surgery is largely idiosyncratic. Consideration of the placement of feeding tubes for postoperative alimentation should be given. Wound closure can be performed by any standard method but special consideration should be given to those patients with ascites or those at risk for its development.

POSTOPERATIVE MANAGEMENT

Advances in anesthesia, surgical technique, and post-operative intensive care have lowered the morbidity and mortality associated with major liver resection to an acceptable level. Jarnagin et al reported on the outcomes of 1803 patients undergoing liver resection at a single institution. In this study the overall operative mortality was 3.1%. The authors found a progressive increase in blood loss as the number of segments resected increased. The perioperative morbidity was 45%, with 19% experiencing multiple complications. Among those experiencing complications, infections occurred in 41%. The most common complications were liver and/or biliary-related (or both), although pulmonary complications were nearly as common.[65]

In general, patients are observed in a surgical intensive care unit postoperatively and ideally are transferred to a specialized liver ward when stable. Hemodynamic monitoring is performed with at minimum a central venous catheter for infusion and measurement of central venous pressure and an arterial line for monitoring blood pressure. The use of pulmonary artery catheters is not routine. Low-volume intravenous fluid hydration is used to maintain adequate blood pressure and urine output. Bolus fluids are given as necessary with a combination of crystalloid, albumin, and blood products. Laboratory values, oxygenation, and urine output are monitored closely to look for early complications.

There are several postoperative issues specifically related to major hepatic resection. Drug metabolism and anesthetic clearance may be altered by resection. Coagulation parameters should be followed closely in the first 48 to 72 hours with close monitoring for postoperative hemorrhage. Vitamin K is given routinely during the hepatic regeneration phase. Phosphorus replacement must be undertaken diligently because life-threatening hypophosphatemia (phosphorus <1.0 mg/dL) has been reported after liver resection.[66] Hypophosphatemia is associated with reversible cardiac dysfunction, hypoventilation, and impaired immunity. Pomposelli and Burns noted almost universal development of hypophosphatemia after elective right hepatic lobectomy for living-donor adult liver transplantation and the degree of hypophosphatemia was associated with an increase in complication rate and worsened surgical outcomes.[67] Hypophosphatemia thus probably occurs to some extent after any major hepatic resection and should be aggressively treated.[66] Liver regeneration involves rapid cell division as early as 24 to 72 hours after resection. This is an ATP-dependent process that probably depletes the remaining stores after resection. For this reason,

potassium phosphate (KPO4) supplementation is undertaken in the immediate postoperative period as an infusion or frequent replacement.

Because perioperative morbidity after major liver operation is so high, vigilance in monitoring for complications is imperative. Operation may trigger or exacerbate any number of problems in patients with chronic liver disease such as jaundice, ascites, encephalopathy, infection, and gastrointestinal bleeding, and these should be recognized and treated promptly.

SUMMARY

Major liver and biliary operations have become safer over recent decades as a result of improved perioperative management. Care of this special group of patients requires a working knowledge of the intricate relationship of many pathophysiologic mechanisms resulting from chronic liver disease and cirrhosis. Experienced teams of surgeons and anesthesiologists have also made great advances in the techniques of hepatic resection and methods to control blood loss. The combination of comprehensive preoperative evaluation, meticulous intraoperative technique, and diligent postoperative care has improved success rates and overall quality of care in complex patients with liver and biliary disease requiring major operation.

REFERENCES

1. Popper H: Pathologic aspects of cirrhosis: A review. *Am J Pathol* 87:228, 1977.
2. Sherlock S, Dooley J: *Diseases of the liver and biliary system*, ed 11, Oxford, 2002, Blackwell.
3. Padillo FJ, Cruz A, Espejo I, et al: Alteration of the renal regulatory hormonal pattern during experimental obstructive jaundice. *Rev Esp Enferm Dig* 101:408, 2009.
4. Cescon M, Vetrone G, Grazi GL, et al: Trends in perioperative outcome after hepatic resection. *Ann Surg* 249:995, 2009.
5. Kato K, Nomoto S, Sugimoto H, et al: Autologous blood storage before hepatectomy for hepatocellular carcinoma. *Hepatogastroenterology* 56:802, 2009.
6. Busch OR, Hop WC, Hoynck van Papendrecht MA, et al: Blood transfusions and prognosis in colorectal cancer. *N Engl J Med* 328:1372, 1993.
7. Marik PE: The hazards of blood transfusion. *Br J Hosp Med* 70:12, 2009.
8. Kosmadakis N, Messaris E, Maris A, et al: Perioperative erythropoietin administration in patients with gastrointestinal tract cancer: Prospective randomized double-blind study. *Ann Surg* 237:417, 2003.
9. Weber RS, Jabbour N, Martin RC 2nd: Anemia and transfusion in patients undergoing surgery for cancer. *Ann Surg Oncol* 15:34, 2008.
10. Luo YH, Li ZD, Liu LX, et al: Pretreatment with erythropoietin reduces hepatic ischemia-reperfusion injury. *Hepatobiliary Pancreat Dis Int* 8:294, 2009.
11. Pluta A, Gutkowski K, Hartleb M: Coagulopathy in liver diseases. *Adv Med Sci* 55:16, 2010.
12. Venkat D, Venkat KK: Hepatorenal syndrome. *South Med J* 103:654, 2010.
13. Garcea G, Ong SL, Maddern GJ: Predicting liver failure following major hepatectomy. *Dig Liver Dis* 41:798, 2009.
14. Garcea G, Maddern GJ: Liver failure after major hepatic resection. *J Hepatobiliary Pancreat Surg* 16:145, 2009.
15. Emond JC, Renz JF, Ferrell LD, et al: Functional analysis of grafts from living donors. Implications for the treatment of older recipients. *Ann Surg* 224:544; discussion 552, 1996.
16. Manizate F, Hiotis SP, Labow D, et al: Liver functional reserve estimation: State of the art and relevance to local treatments. *Oncology* 78:131, 2010.

17. Mullin EJ, Metcalfe MS, Maddern GJ: How much liver resection is too much? *Am J Surg* 190:87, 2005.

18. Shoup M, Gonen M, D'Angelica M, et al: Volumetric analysis predicts hepatic dysfunction in patients undergoing major liver resection. *J Gastrointest Surg* 7:325, 2003.

19. van den Broek MA, Olde Damink SW, Dejong CH, et al: Liver failure after partial hepatic resection: Definition, pathophysiology, risk factors and treatment. *Liver Int* 28:767, 2008.

20. Jeejeebhoy KN, Baker JP, Wolman SL, et al: Critical evaluation of the role of clinical assessment and body composition studies in patients with malnutrition and after total parenteral nutrition. *Am J Clin Nutr* 35:1117, 1982.

21. Sax HC, Souba WW: Enteral and parenteral feedings. Guidelines and recommendations. *Med Clin North Am* 77:863, 1993.

22. Padillo F, Rodríguez M, Hervas A, et al: Nutritional assessment of patients with benign and malignant obstructions of the biliary tract. *Rev Esp Enferm Dig* 91:622, 1999.

23. Padillo FJ, Andicoberry B, Muntane J, et al: Factors predicting nutritional derangements in patients with obstructive jaundice: Multivariate analysis. *World J Surg* 25:413, 2001.

24. Veterans Affairs Total Parenteral Nutrition Cooperative Study Group: Perioperative total parenteral nutrition in surgical patients. *N Engl J Med* 325:525, 1991.

25. Kudsk KA, Tolley EA, DeWitt RC, et al: Preoperative albumin and surgical site identify surgical risk for major postoperative complications. *JPEN J Parenter Enteral Nutr* 27:1, 2003.

26. Moore EE, Jones TN: Benefits of immediate jejunostomy feeding after major abdominal trauma—a prospective, randomized study. *J Trauma* 26:874, 1986.

27. Archer SB, Burnett RJ, Fischer JE, et al: Current uses and abuses of total parenteral nutrition. *Adv Surg* 29:165, 1996.

28. Mochizuki H, Trocki O, Dominioni L, et al: Mechanism of prevention of postburn hypermetabolism and catabolism by early enteral feeding. *Ann Surg* 200:297, 1984.

29. Cerra FB, Cheung NK, Fischer JE, et al: Disease-specific amino acid infusion (F080) in hepatic encephalopathy: A prospective, randomized, double-blind, controlled trial. *JPEN J Parenter Enteral Nutr* 9:288, 1985.

30. Alverdy JC, Saunders J, Chamberlin WH, et al: Diagnostic peritoneal lavage in intra-abdominal sepsis. *Am Surg* 54:456, 1988.

31. Qiu JG, Delany HM, Teh EL, et al: Contrasting effects of identical nutrients given parenterally or enterally after 70% hepatectomy: Bacterial translocation. *Nutrition* 13:431, 1997.

32. Alverdy J, Holbrook C, Rocha F, et al: Gut-derived sepsis occurs when the right pathogen with the right virulence genes meets the right host: Evidence for in vivo virulence expression in *Pseudomonas aeruginosa*. *Ann Surg* 232:480, 2000.

33. Zulfikaroglu B, Zulfikaroglu E, Ozmen MM, et al: The effect of immunonutrition on bacterial translocation, and intestinal villus atrophy in experimental obstructive jaundice. *Clin Nutr* 22:277, 2003.

34. Chuang JH, Shieh CS, Chang NK, et al: Role of parenteral nutrition in preventing malnutrition and decreasing bacterial translocation to liver in obstructive jaundice. *World J Surg* 17:580; discussion 586, 1993.

35. van der Gaag NA, Rauws EA, van Eijck CH, et al: Preoperative biliary drainage for cancer of the head of the pancreas. *N Engl J Med* 362:129, 2010.

36. Wang Q, Gurusamy KS, Lin H, et al: Preoperative biliary drainage for obstructive jaundice. *Cochrane Database Syst Rev* 16, 2008.

37. Gatta A, Bolognesi M, Merkel C: Vasoactive factors and hemodynamic mechanisms in the pathophysiology of portal hypertension in cirrhosis. *Mol Aspects Med* 29:119, 2008.

38. Devlin J, Ellis AE, McPeake J, et al: N-acetylcysteine improves indocyanine green extraction and oxygen transport during hepatic dysfunction. *Crit Care Med* 25:236, 1997.

39. Harrison P, Wendon J, Williams R: Evidence of increased guanylate cyclase activation by acetylcysteine in fulminant hepatic failure. *Hepatology* 23:1067, 1996.

40. Walsh TS, Hopton P, Philips BJ, et al: The effect of N-acetylcysteine on oxygen transport and uptake in patients with fulminant hepatic failure. *Hepatology* 27:1332, 1998.

41. De BK, Majumdar D, Das D, Biswas PK, et al: Cardiac dysfunction in portal hypertension among patients with cirrhosis and noncirrhotic portal fibrosis. *J Hepatol* 39:315, 2003.

42. Gschwantler M, Vavrik J, Gebauer A, et al: Course of platelet counts in cirrhotic patients after implantation of a transjugular intrahepatic portosystemic shunt—a prospective, controlled study. *J Hepatol* 30:254, 1999.

43. Corley DA, Cello JP, Adkisson W, et al: Octreotide for acute esophageal variceal bleeding: A meta-analysis. *Gastroenterology* 120:946, 2001.

44. Gines P, Schrier R: Renal failure in cirrhosis. *N Engl J Med* 361:1279, 2009.

45. Salerno F, Gerbes A, Ginès P, et al: Diagnosis, prevention and treatment of hepatorenal syndrome in cirrhosis. *Gut* 56:1310, 2007.

46. Esrailian E, Pantangco ER, Kyulo NL, et al: Octreotide/midodrine therapy significantly improves renal function and 30-day survival in patients with type 1 hepatorenal syndrome. *Dig Dis Sci* 52:742, 2007.

47. Angeli P, Volpin R, Gerunda G, et al: Reversal of type 1 hepatorenal syndrome with the administration of midodrine and octreotide. *Hepatology* 29:1690, 1999.

48. Riordan SM, Williams R: Treatment of hepatic encephalopathy. *N Engl J Med* 337:473, 1997.

49. Haussinger D: Hepatic encephalopathy. *Acta Gasroenterol Belg* 73:457, 2010.

50. Farrell G, Prendergast D, Murray M: Halothane hepatitis. Detection of a constitutional susceptibility factor. *N Engl J Med* 313:1310, 1985.

51. Bass NM, Mullen KD, Sanyal A, et al: Rifaximin treatment in hepatic encephalopathy. *N Engl J Med* 362:1071, 2010.

52. Karasu Z, Gurakar A, Kerwin B, et al: Effect of transjugular intrahepatic portosystemic shunt on thrombocytopenia associated with cirrhosis. *Dig Dis Sci* 45:1971, 2000.

53. Youssef WI, Salazar F, Dasarathy S, et al: Role of fresh frozen plasma infusion in correction of coagulopathy of chronic liver disease: A dual phase study. *Am J Gastroenterol* 98:1391, 2003.

54. Kaul VV, Munoz SJ: Coagulopathy of liver disease. *Curr Treat Options Gastroenterol* 3:433, 2000.

55. Whittle BJ, Moncada S: Nitric oxide: The elusive mediator of the hyperdynamic circulation of cirrhosis? *Hepatology* 16:1089, 1992.

56. Chauvin M, Bonnet F, Montembault C, et al: Hepatic plasma flow during sodium nitroprusside-induced hypotension in humans. *Anesthesiology* 63:287, 1985.

57. Cunningham JD, Fong Y, Shriver C, et al: One hundred consecutive hepatic resections. Blood loss, transfusion, and operative technique. *Arch Surg* 129:1050, 1994.

58. Melendez JA, Arslan V, Fischer ME, et al: Perioperative outcomes of major hepatic resections under low central venous pressure anesthesia: Blood loss, blood transfusion, and the risk of postoperative renal dysfunction. *J Am Coll Surg* 187:620, 1998.

59. Yanaga K, Kanematsu T, Takenaka K, et al: Hepatic resection for hepatocellular carcinoma in elderly patients. *Am J Surg* 155:238, 1988.

60. Elliott RH, Strunin L: Hepatotoxicity of volatile anaesthetics. *Br J Anaesth* 70:339, 1993.

61. Berendes E, Lippert G, Loick HM, et al: Effects of enflurane and isoflurane on splanchnic oxygenation in humans. *J Clin Anesth* 8:456, 1996.

62. Trey C, Lipworth L, Chalmers TC, et al: Fulminant hepatic failure. Presumable contribution to halothane. *N Engl J Med* 279:798, 1968.

63. Neuberger JM: Halothane and hepatitis. Incidence, predisposing factors and exposure guidelines. *Drug Saf* 5:28, 1990.

64. Hubbard AK, Roth TP, Gandolfi AJ, et al: Halothane hepatitis patients generate an antibody response toward a covalently bound metabolite of halothane. *Anesthesiology* 68:791, 1988.

65. Jarnagin WR, Gonen M, Fong Y, et al: Improvement in perioperative outcome after hepatic resection: Analysis of 1,803 consecutive cases over the past decade. *Ann Surg* 236:397; discussion 406, 2002.

66. Pomposelli JJ, Pomfret EA, Burns DL, et al: Life-threatening hypophosphatemia after right hepatic lobectomy for live donor adult liver transplantation. *Liver Transpl* 7:637, 2001.

67. Pomposelli JJ, Burns DL: Hypophosphatemia and the live liver donor. *Transplantation* 78:305, 2004.

Hepatic Cyst Disease

Michael W. Mulholland | Hero K. Hussain | Danielle M. Fritze

Hepatic cysts are a diverse group of lesions, ranging from developmental to infectious to neoplastic in etiology. The implications of these lesions also vary widely. Advances in abdominal imaging have led to the increasingly common incidental diagnosis of simple hepatic cysts, usually of little clinical consequence. In contrast, malignant hepatic cystadenocarcinomas are life-threatening, and echinococcal cysts remain a major public health problem worldwide. With improving diagnostics and minimally invasive therapies, the management of hepatic cystic disease continues to evolve.

SIMPLE HEPATIC CYSTS

Simple hepatic cysts are presumed to originate from the biliary tree. Current understanding suggests that they develop from microhamartomas or peribiliary glands, which become isolated from the bile ducts. They are lined with a simple cuboidal epithelium and surrounded by a fibrous, hypocellular stroma. Cystic contents are primarily serous; the presence of mucinous or solid contents should prompt consideration of an infectious or neoplastic process.

Hepatic cysts have long been recognized as an incidental finding at laparotomy, during autopsy, or on imaging studies. One early autopsy study noted 28 hepatic cysts in 20,000 examinations, a prevalence of 0.14%.[1] Recent estimates of hepatic cyst prevalence are much higher than previously reported, likely attributable to improvements in the sensitivity of abdominal imaging. A contemporary study of 26,000 patients undergoing upper abdominal ultrasound identified 1235 cysts, corresponding to a prevalence of 4.75%.[2] A similar prospective study using more sophisticated ultrasound equipment revealed cysts in 11.3% of the livers imaged.[3] Cross-sectional imaging with computed tomography (CT) demonstrated cysts in 18% of patients, likely an overestimate of the true prevalence as small hemangiomas may be indistinguishable from simple cysts.[4]

Hepatic cysts become more common with increasing patient age; more than 92% of cysts occur in those older than 40 years of age.[2,3] A higher incidence of cysts in female patients has been repeatedly reported, but has not attained statistical significance in all studies.[3-5]

Although the majority of simple hepatic cysts are asymptomatic and discovered incidentally, up to 15% of patients experience abdominal pain or distention. Symptoms are primarily related to mass effect and are more common in older patients with larger cysts. Progressive cyst enlargement may also lead to early satiety, nausea, and vomiting. Abdominal mass, hepatomegaly, and tenderness are infrequently noted on physical examination.

The laboratory evaluation of patients with simple hepatic cysts typically fails to demonstrate any abnormality. Echinococcal serology should be obtained to exclude infectious etiology. Liver function and coagulation studies are rarely necessary to evaluate for hepatic dysfunction.

Imaging studies are the primary means of characterizing cystic lesions in the liver. Ultrasound, CT, and magnetic resonance imaging (MRI) have varying roles in distinguishing neoplastic from nonneoplastic cysts, identifying echinococcal lesions, and delineating hepatic anatomy.

Hepatic ultrasound is the preferred initial study as it is inexpensive, noninvasive, and highly informative. It reliably distinguishes between cystic and solid hepatic lesions, and can suggest the diagnosis of a cystic neoplasm. Sonographically, simple hepatic cysts appear as anechoic masses with smooth margins and imperceptibly thin walls (Figure 117-1). The differential reflection of ultrasound waves by the cyst wall and cyst fluid leads to back-wall enhancement. Simple cysts have no internal septae; any septation should raise suspicion for a cystic neoplasm. In a recent series, lack of septation was 100% predictive of a simple hepatic cyst.[6] The overall sensitivity and specificity of ultrasound in the diagnosis of hepatic cysts is greater than 90%.[7] Harmonic ultrasound may further characterize lesions that are indeterminate by conventional sonography. In a series of 50 patients, harmonic ultrasound provided additional information in 16% of the patients, leading to a change in management in one third of the patients.[8]

Although ultrasonography is useful in characterizing liver cysts, CT scans provide superior localization and the precise definition of special relationships crucial to surgical planning. Dedicated hepatic CT scans time the administration of contrast to maximize discrimination of the lesion, bile ducts, portal vein, and hepatic vessels. By CT, simple cysts are nonenhancing lesions of water density (0 to 10 Hounsfield units) with smooth, imperceptible walls (Figures 117-2 and 117-3).[9] Wall irregularity, papillary mural projections, internal septations, and intracystic debris are inconsistent with a simple cyst. The limitation of CT lies in its inability to distinguish between cystic and solid lesions less than 1 cm in size because of partial volume averaging with the adjacent liver. In such cases, MRI may be useful.[10]

Similar to CT scan, MRI reveals cyst characteristics as well as significant anatomic detail. Simple hepatic cysts have homogeneous, very low signal intensity relative to surrounding liver parenchyma on T1-weighted images, but very high signal intensity on T2-weighted images. They do not enhance with administration of gadolinium chelates (Figure 117-4).[9,11] Cysts with internal

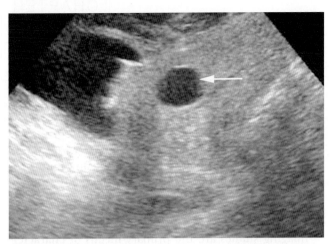

FIGURE 117-1 Simple hepatic cyst. Transverse ultrasound image of the left lobe shows an anechoic cyst *(arrow)* with smooth imperceptible walls and increased through transmission.

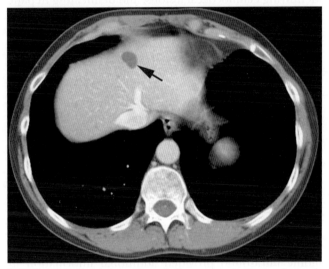

FIGURE 117-2 Simple hepatic cyst. Transverse contrast-enhanced CT image shows a simple cyst *(arrow)* in the left lobe of the liver. The cyst has water attenuation, imperceptible wall, and enhances with contrast.

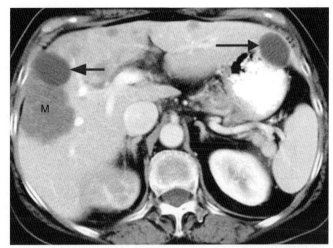

FIGURE 117-3 Two simple hepatic cysts and a liver metastasis. Transverse contrast-enhanced CT image shows two simple hepatic cysts *(arrows)* with water attenuation in the right and left lobes of the liver. The cysts are unenhanced and have imperceptible walls. Compare to the enhanced metastasis *(M)* adjacent to the cyst in the right lobe. Note several other small metastatic lesions in the liver.

hemorrhage will appear hyperintense on both T1- and T2-weighted images, and often demonstrate a fluid–fluid level (Figure 117-5).[11] MRI provides detailed information about internal cystic structure, including septations, papillary nodules, and debris. Additionally, small lesions, which are indeterminate on CT scan, can often be accurately characterized by MRI (Figure 117-6). This modality is particularly useful in distinguishing small hepatic cysts from liver metastases in patients with a history of cancer. A recent study of more than 500 liver lesions evaluated by diffusion-weighted MRI confirmed a statistically significant difference in apparent diffusion coefficient between simple hepatic cysts and other liver lesions including focal nodular hyperplasia, hepatocellular carcinoma, metastases, adenoma, hemangioma, and abscess.[12]

The diagnostic information and anatomic detail provided by ultrasound and cross-sectional imaging have diminished the practical value of more traditional imaging techniques. Angiography, rarely indicated in the evaluation of a simple cyst, demonstrates an avascular mass displacing adjacent vessels. Simple cysts appear as "cold" lesions on nuclear scintigraphy.

The treatment of simple hepatic cysts is predicated on the presence of symptoms. For asymptomatic patients with simple cysts, nonoperative treatment is appropriate. In the long term, 80% to 95% of these patients will remain asymptomatic.

In patients with symptoms attributable to a hepatic cyst, intervention is indicated. Treatment options range from percutaneous ablation to laparoscopic fenestration to formal hepatic resection. The choice of approach is guided by data on recurrence rates and morbidity, as well as patient anatomy and preference.

The least invasive therapies for simple hepatic cysts involve a percutaneous approach. Simple image-guided aspiration is ineffective, with a reported recurrence rate of 100%.[13] The addition of a sclerosant, such as ethanol, following aspiration has resulted in improved recurrence rates. In one prospective study of percutaneous aspiration and ethanol ablation, 80% of patients demonstrated recurrent cysts; however, the majority of these regressed and did not require retreatment.[14] Other small series have reported recurrence in as few as 17% of patients.[15] The majority of cysts treated with percutaneous ablation decrease in size, with a mean volume reduction of 92% to 98% at 30 months followup.[16-18] Placement of closed-suction drains within the cyst cavity following aspiration has not been shown to improve volume reduction or prevent recurrence.[18]

Recently, percutaneous radiofrequency ablation has been proposed as a therapeutic option for patients with symptomatic simple hepatic cysts. In a single case series of 29 patients with 63 cysts, 100% cyst resolution at 1 year was reported for those cysts less than 10 cm in diameter.[19] More rigorous evaluation will be required for

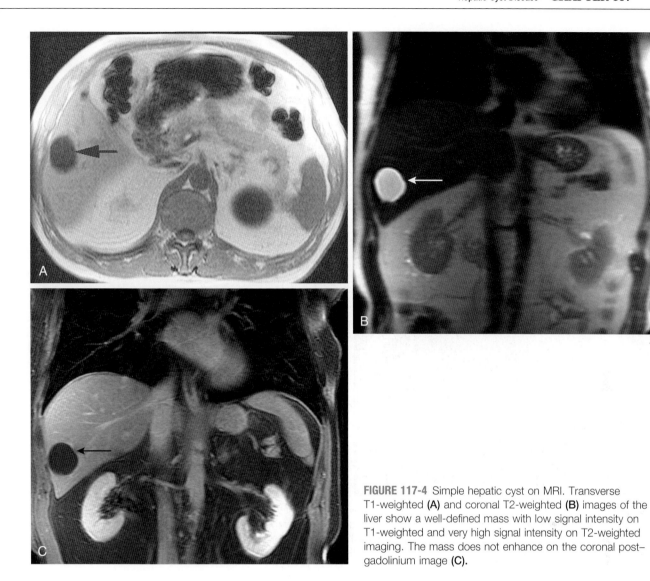

FIGURE 117-4 Simple hepatic cyst on MRI. Transverse T1-weighted **(A)** and coronal T2-weighted **(B)** images of the liver show a well-defined mass with low signal intensity on T1-weighted and very high signal intensity on T2-weighted imaging. The mass does not enhance on the coronal post–gadolinium image **(C).**

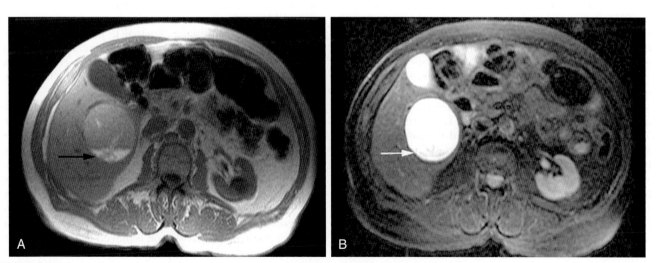

FIGURE 117-5 Hemorrhage within a simple cyst. Transverse T1-weighted **(A)** and T2-weighted **(B)** MRI images show a high attenuation content of the cyst on T1-weighted and T2-weighted imaging with layering high T1, and low T2, signal intensity material *(arrows)* in the dependent portion of the cyst indicating the presence of hemorrhagic products (methemoglobin).

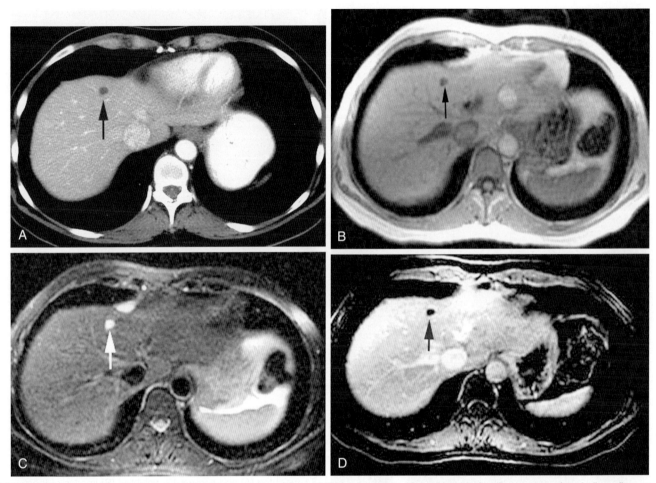

FIGURE 117-6 A small incidentally detected simple cyst on CT and MRI in a patient with no history of malignancy or chronic liver disease. **A,** Transverse contrast-enhanced CT image shows a 1-cm hypodense mass in the medial segment of the left lobe *(arrow).* The mass is too small to be accurately characterized. Transverse T1-weighted **(B)** and T2-weighted MR **(C)** images of the liver show the mass *(arrow)* to be hypointense relative to liver on T1-weighted imaging and markedly hyperintense on T2-weighted imaging. The mass does not enhance on the transverse gadolinium-enhanced image **(D).**

radiofrequency ablation to become a standard treatment option for simple hepatic cysts.

Although the outcomes associated with percutaneous therapies are improving, surgery remains the mainstay of treatment for symptomatic simple hepatic cysts. Procedural options include laparoscopic versus open cyst fenestration or resection.

Regardless of the surgical treatment selected, the operation begins with visual inspection. A superficial cyst may be readily visible as a blue-domed structure protruding from the surface of the liver. Intraoperative Doppler ultrasound can identify and define its relationship to the biliary tree and vasculature. The cyst should then be aspirated with fluid sent for Gram stain, bacterial culture, and cytology. Bilious cyst fluid implies communication with the biliary ductal system. The cyst cavity should be biopsied to definitively exclude neoplasm, with particular focus on any areas of nodularity or projection.

The cyst itself may then be treated with fenestration or resection. Cyst fenestration is achieved by excision of the cyst wall to within 2 cm of the liver parenchyma, allowing the cyst cavity to drain into the peritoneum.

Rarely, bilious cyst aspirate or inspection of the cyst cavity may raise concern for cyst-biliary fistula. The biliary communication should be suture ligated within the cyst cavity if possible, and a Roux-en-Y cystojejunostomy performed to allow enteric drainage. Formal hepatic resections or wedge resections are also an effective means of treating simple hepatic cysts. In this case, cyst-biliary communication does not require additional drainage if the bile ducts are ligated proximally.

Laparoscopic approaches have also been validated in the treatment of simple hepatic cysts. This technique is best suited to lesions in segments II to VI, the anterolateral portion of the liver where visualization and access are easiest. Lesions located centrally or in the posterior aspects of segments VI, VII, or IVa are less accessible, and render laparoscopic therapy more challenging. Typically, the patient is positioned in lithotomy, allowing the surgeon to stand between the legs with assistants at the sides. A 30-degree laparoscope is placed at the umbilicus. Two operating ports surround the umbilicus in a triangulated fashion. A subxiphoid port allows introduction of a fan retractor or suction device. The cyst wall is excised with harmonic scalpel; hemostasis may be obtained with electrocautery. For patients with lesions in segment VII or VIII, positioning and port placement similar to that used for laparoscopic right adrenalectomy may afford improved exposure.[20]

Available data regarding choice of operative procedure for symptomatic simple hepatic cysts are currently limited to case series and prospective observational studies. For patients who undergo cyst fenestration, whether laparoscopic or open, recurrence rates range from 0% to 20%. Mortality is less than 5% for open procedures, and approaches 0% for laparoscopy. Morbidity is correspondingly low at less than 10%.[21-25] One recent case series of laparoscopic fenestration for solitary simple hepatic cysts reported no recurrences with a 7-year mean followup period, and several series have reported success rates exceeding 90%.[24,26] For patients treated with hepatic resection, recurrence is extremely rare, but morbidity and mortality rates exceed those associated with fenestration. A prospective nonrandomized study of 40 patients with simple hepatic cysts demonstrated increased length of stay, operative blood loss, and complication rates in patients treated with resection compared to open fenestration. Laparoscopic fenestration carried the lowest morbidity, with no significant difference in recurrence rates among the different surgical procedures.[27] Excellent recurrence rates coupled with low morbidity, short hospital stay, and decreased postoperative pain make laparoscopic fenestration the procedure of choice for simple hepatic cysts.

POLYCYSTIC LIVER DISEASE

Polycystic liver disease is a benign condition that occurs in close association with polycystic kidney disease (PKD). Patients develop a multitude of cysts that closely resemble their solitary counterparts. In PKD, hepatic cysts become increasingly prevalent with age. They are present in 25% of cases by age 30 years and in 80% by age 60 years. Patients with the greatest renal cyst load and the greatest reduction in renal function exhibit the most extensive hepatic cyst disease.[28]

PKD is most commonly an autosomal dominant condition. Autosomal dominant polycystic kidney disease is caused by defects in two genes, *PKD1* and *PKD2*.[29,30] In murine models, cysts do not form in heterozygous *pkd*[+/−] or *pkd*[+/−] knockout mice. In contrast, severe cystic disease is observed in homozygotes or heterozygotes with a hypermutable normal allele.[31] These observations, coupled with the age-dependence of human hepatic cyst formation, suggest that many human cases may arise as a germline mutation in one *PKD1* or *PKD2* gene coupled with a somatic mutation in the remaining normal allele. In support of this mechanism, most hepatic cysts are clonal in origin. They exhibit somatic mutations in the normal allele with loss of heterozygosity.[32]

In autosomal dominant polycystic disease, hepatic cyst formation is also influenced by the endocrine environment. Polycystic liver disease (PLD) is more common in women, and greater numbers of cysts develop in those having experienced pregnancy or received exogenous hormones. In one study, exposure of patients with polycystic kidney disease to conjugated estrogens

corresponded to a 7% increase in liver cyst size over 1 year relative to untreated controls.[33]

Although remarkably well-tolerated by most, hepatic enlargement does cause symptoms in a minority of patients. Abdominal pain and distention, early satiety, vomiting, respiratory compromise, and lower extremity edema may occur. Although such problems are not life threatening, they may be debilitating and result in a poor quality of life.

Complications attributable to polycystic liver disease are rare, occurring in fewer than 5% of affected individuals. Cyst infection or rupture, portal hypertension with ascites or variceal bleeding, and hepatic venous outflow obstruction secondary to cyst compression occur infrequently. Despite gross distortion of the liver by multiple cysts, liver failure has not been observed.

A classification of liver cysts proposed by Gigot et al is useful in classifying patients and comparing treatments.[34]

- Type 1: Ten or fewer large cysts (>10 cm) with large areas of noninvolved liver parenchyma on CT scan.
- Type 2: Diffuse involvement of liver parenchyma by medium-sized cysts but with large areas of noncystic parenchyma on CT scan.
- Type 3: Massive and diffuse involvement of liver parenchyma with only a few areas of normal substance between cysts (Figure 117-7).

Most patients with polycystic liver disease can be treated nonoperatively. Intervention should be considered only if it can both significantly reduce cyst-associated hepatomegaly and provide long-term relief of symptoms. The form of therapy that will best achieve these goals is uncertain; no prospective trials are available, and the existing surgical literature does not provide consensus.

Cyst aspiration followed by instillation of a sclerosing agent, such as alcohol, has been proposed when a small number of dominant cysts are believed to cause symptoms. This approach is limited by the ability to treat only a small number of cysts per session and by the potential for alcohol extravasation. Experience is limited, and recurrence rates variable, ranging from 30% to 100%.[35,36]

Cyst fenestration or deroofing has been described by multiple surgical investigators.[37] This procedure allows cyst contents to drain into the peritoneal cavity and reduces the overall size of the liver. Both open and laparoscopic approaches have been reported with no clear difference in recurrence rates.[38] Cysts in the right posterior segments and in Couinaud segments VI, VII, and VIII may be more challenging to expose laparoscopically. Deeply situated cysts have been successfully drained through more superficial cysts by penetrating the intervening liver parenchyma. Failure to appreciate intrahepatic veins and portal radicles within the thinned parenchyma may lead to injury and is a major technical complication.

Cyst fenestration is most applicable to patients with type 1 PLD. In properly selected patients with type 1 PLD, a recurrence rate of 11% at 30 months has been reported.[37,38] For patients with type 2 or 3 disease, recurrence rates exceeded 70%. The most common postoperative complication is ascites formation, occurring when

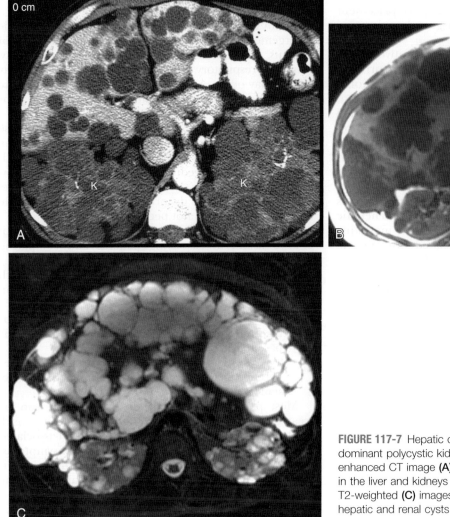

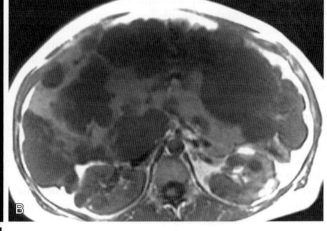

FIGURE 117-7 Hepatic cysts in two patients with autosomal dominant polycystic kidney disease. Transverse contrast-enhanced CT image **(A)** shows numerous nonenhancing cysts in the liver and kidneys *(K)*. Transverse T1-weighted **(B)** and T2-weighted **(C)** images of the liver showing numerous simple hepatic and renal cysts with homogeneous low T1 and high T2 signal intensity.

cyst fluid secretion exceeds the clearance capacity of the peritoneum.

A combination of partial hepatic resection and fenestration has been evaluated in multiple surgical series. Combined resection-fenestration allows treatment of deep-seated cysts that are difficult to access. This approach has the lowest reported recurrence rates, but carries substantial risk. Postoperative ascites, bleeding, and biliary leak are the most frequent complications. A 2009 series of patients treated with hepatic resection for symptomatic or complicated PLD demonstrated morbidity and mortality of 63% and 3%, respectively. After 10 years of followup, 50% of patients had stable or decreased liver volume compared to immediate postoperative imaging, whereas approximately 10% of patients required further surgery for PLD.[39]

Transarterial embolization, a successful therapy for volume reduction in polycystic kidneys, has been recently applied to patients with PLD. In hepatic segments with significant cyst burden, and patent hepatic artery, portal vein occlusion may be performed through interventional radiologic techniques. In a series of 30 symptomatic patients with PLD, 29 had durable symptomatic improvement 1 year after treatment.[40] The safety and efficacy of transcatheter embolization will require further evaluation before it can be considered a standard therapeutic option.

Liver transplantation for PLD was first reported in the 1990s, with more than 120 transplant recipients to date.[38,41] Of these, at least 50 patients received combined liver-kidney transplants. The most appropriate candidates for liver transplantation are those with type 3 disease who have failed other palliative measures and those who are also candidates for renal transplantation. A recent review of published series of patients with PLD reported an 18% mortality rate associated with liver transplantation.[38] Although no survival advantage has been demonstrated for PLD patients undergoing transplant, long-term posttransplant survival does exceed that of patients requiring transplant for other indications.[38,42] Additionally, improved quality of life has been reported in more than 90% of survivors.[38,43] Although lifelong immunosuppression remains a significant risk to accept, particularly for patients who suffer neither malignancy nor hepatic failure, liver transplantation may offer real benefits to a select group of patients with PLD.

CYSTIC NEOPLASMS

Cystic neoplasms include biliary cystadenomas and cystadenocarcinomas and comprise less than 5% of intrahepatic cysts. Although these lesions are believed to arise from the biliary tree, the exact mechanism of their formation is unknown. There is scant evidence to suggest the evolution of simple cysts to cystic neoplasms.[44]

More than 90% of cystadenomas occur in women, and they often express estrogen and progesterone receptors within their stroma.[45] In contrast, cystadenocarcinomas are nearly equally distributed between male and female patients.[46] Both neoplasms are most commonly identified in middle-aged patients.

The majority of patients with a cystic neoplasm present with a history of abdominal pain or mass. The diagnosis is suggested by ultrasonography, CT, or MRI. Internal septations (Figure 117-8), papillary projections from the cyst wall, or mural nodules strongly suggest a cystic neoplasm.[47-49] The cyst contents may have variable signal intensity on MRI T1- and T2-weighted imaging, depending on the presence of hemorrhage, protein content, or solid components (Figure 117-9).[9,11] An enhancing mural nodule and intracystic debris are associated with adenocarcinoma on CT but are not sufficient for diagnosis.[47,50] Invasion of surrounding structures is highly indicative of malignancy, but a rare finding in imaging of cystic neoplasms.

As imaging studies usually do not differentiate between benign and malignant neoplastic cysts, this distinction must be established histologically.[51] Cystadenomas are lined by a simple columnar epithelium resembling bile duct epithelium. In most cases, the stroma underlying the epithelium is distinctive, resembling ovarian stroma or primitive biliary mesenchyme.[52] The subjacent liver parenchyma demonstrates compression atrophy, creating a pseudocapsule separating the cystadenoma and the native tissue.

Cystadenocarcinomas are characterized by a multi-layered malignant epithelium with papillary projections. These tumors are often loculated and may also contain areas of benign epithelium, implying progression from adenoma to adenocarcinoma.[52] Invasion of the basement membrane leads to involvement of the underlying stroma.

Pre- and intraoperative serology, cytology, and cyst fluid analysis have been evaluated in small series as potential means to distinguish between benign and malignant cystic neoplasms. To date, differences in carcinoembryonic antigen and carbohydrate antigen 19-9 levels in serum and cyst fluid have been inconsistently reported and are not reliable.[47,49,53,54] Moreover, percutaneous cyst wall biopsy or aspiration risks biopsy tract or peritoneal dissemination of a possible malignancy.[52,55]

Once the concern for a cystic neoplasm has been raised by imaging findings, operation is indicated.[55] Formal hepatic resection is the only adequate procedure for cystadenocarcinoma; adenomas may be treated with either resection or enucleation. Enucleation requires complete removal of the cyst with a rim of surrounding liver parenchyma. It is recommended over formal resection when anatomically advantageous, particularly for very large or centrally located lesions.[45] Recurrence and complication rates for cystadenomas treated with complete enucleation are approximately equivalent to those reported for formal resection.[56-58] Treatment with incomplete resection or fenestration is uniformly associated with recurrence.[59,60]

Laparoscopy has become an acceptable surgical approach for cystic hepatic neoplasms. Small series report equivalent recurrence rates, shorter hospital stays, and lower complication rates for laparoscopic enucleation or resection as compared to open operation.[53]

ECHINOCOCCAL CYSTS

Hepatic infection with *Echinococcus granulosus* is a major public health problem worldwide and a common cause of cystic liver lesions in endemic areas. Transcontinental travel and immigration make recognition of

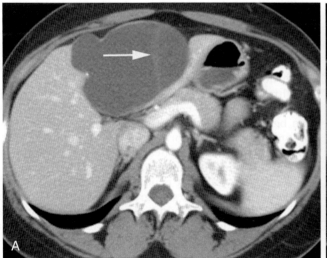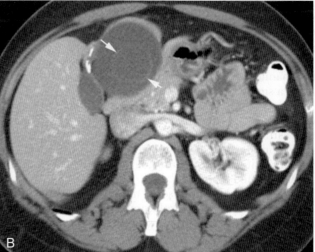

FIGURE 117-8 Biliary cystadenoma. **A** and **B,** Transverse contrast-enhanced CT images show a cystic mass in the left lobe containing thin enhancing septae *(arrows)*. Identification of septae such as these raises suspicion for a cystic neoplasm.

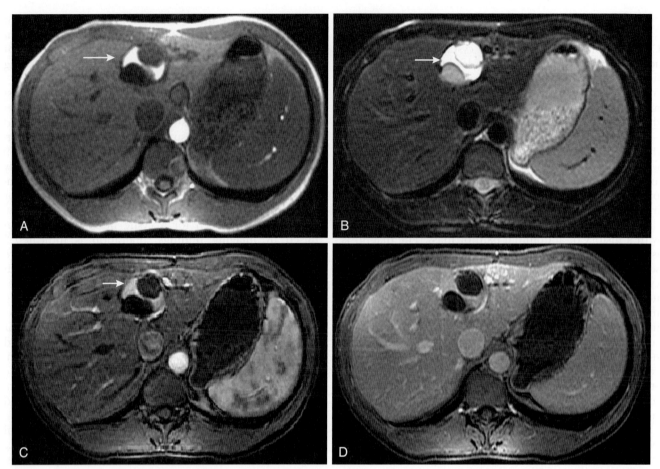

FIGURE 117-9 Hepatobiliary mucinous cystadenoma with ovarian stroma. Transverse T1-weighted **(A)** and T2-weighted **(B)** images of the liver show a complex multilocular mass in the left lobe. The mucinous content of the mass has mixed high and low signal intensity on T1-weighted imaging and high and intermediate signal intensity on T2-weighted imaging. The mass does not enhance on early **(C)** or delayed **(D)** post–gadolinium imaging.

echinococcal liver cysts important in Western countries as well. Human infection occurs following oral intake of cestode eggs. Within the upper gastrointestinal tract, the oncospheres are released, attach to and then penetrate the intestinal wall, and enter the portal venous system. Hematogenous dissemination occurs primarily to the liver, although other organs may also be infected, including lung (20%), brain, and bone (20%). Following tissue lodgment, cestode proliferation occurs in the form of a slowly enlarging cyst. In 80% of affected individuals, the only manifestation of echinococcal disease is a solitary cyst in a single organ.

Cyst expansion is slowly progressive, estimated at 1 to 30 mm yearly.[61] With time, multiple daughter cysts may form within a single larger cyst. The slow cyst growth causes compression atrophy of the adjacent liver. Host reaction incites the formation of a fibrous surrounding capsule, termed a *pericyst*.

Symptoms of hydatid disease may be caused by compression, obstruction, or displacement of adjacent organs or structures. Most commonly, symptoms are neither dramatic nor pathognomic. Malaise, weight loss, and chronic wasting are common. Mass effect from the cyst can cause abdominal pain, early satiety, or obstructive jaundice. Untreated, erosion into surrounding structures or organs

may result in hematogenous dissemination or cyst-biliary fistula. Spontaneous rupture with release of infected material into the peritoneum is rare, but can cause anaphylaxis. Cyst rupture may also be precipitated by minor blunt abdominal trauma.[62]

The diagnosis of echinococcal infection is confirmed by serologic demonstration of an antibody response. Sensitivity and specificity both approximate 90%.[63] Children, in particular, may have a low antibody response. False-positive reactions may occur in individuals infected with other helminthic organisms.

Ultrasonography is an appropriate first-line diagnostic test for patients with echinococcal disease. Hydatid cysts can be distinguished from simple cysts by the presence of internal structures corresponding with daughter cysts and their contained parasites. Although some echinococcal cysts are anechoic, these are often characterized by a thickened cyst wall that is not present in simple cysts.[64] In Western countries, sonography has a specificity of 90%.[65] Although ultrasound allows for the characterization of cysts, it does not provide adequate anatomic information for planning surgical therapy.

CT scanning is superior to ultrasonography in demonstrating the size and depth of cysts, the presence of daughter cysts, and extrahepatic involvement

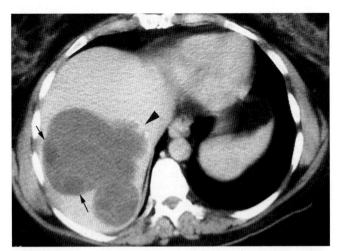

FIGURE 117-10 Hydatid cyst. Transverse nonenhanced CT image shows a cystic mass containing several daughter cysts *(arrows)* and peripheral calcification *(arrowhead)*.

(Figure 117-10).[66] It also allows improved definition of anatomy and relationship to biliary and vascular structures. MRI provides excellent structural detail of hydatid cysts and is superior to CT in demonstrating alteration of the hepatic venous system.[67-69] Magnetic resonance cholangiopancreatography offers the added benefit of possible preoperative diagnosis of cyst-biliary fistula. In one series, sensitivity and specificity were reported as 78% and 100%, respectively for diagnosis of cyst-biliary communication in patients with high pretest probability based on symptoms.[70]

Diagnosis of hydatid disease should prompt therapy to alleviate symptoms, halt progression of infection, and prevent complications. Traditionally, open surgical resection or drainage has been standard therapy. Recently, laparoscopic and percutaneous therapies have been evaluated and gained favor as alternatives to open operation.

Operative goals of hydatid surgery are fourfold: (1) inactivate infectious cyst contents (scolices and the germinative membrane); (2) prevent spillage of cyst contents; (3) evacuate all viable elements; (4) manage the residual cavity. Although these principal goals are widely accepted, debate continues regarding the extent of surgery and optimal management of the cyst cavity.

Radical operations include formal anatomic resection or pericystectomy. The latter involves removal of the infected cyst, pericyst, and a margin of normal surrounding hepatic parenchyma. More conservative procedures seek to sterilize and then evacuate cyst contents, leaving the pericyst intact.

There are conflicting data regarding the most safe and effective operative techniques. Multiple case series report lower recurrence rates following complete resection.[71-73] An association between extent of operation and morbidity has been inconsistently reported.[71,73,74] Metaanalyses suggest that radical and conservative surgical approaches have similar mortality rates (1.2% to 2%).[75] With either approach, morbidity is common (12% to 23%), including wound and intraperitoneal infection, hemorrhage, biliary fistula, and pulmonary complications.[75] The only

randomized controlled trial to date evaluated 32 patients with cystic echinococcus randomized to resection or fenestration. The conservative therapy group had significantly higher rates of recurrence and morbidity, with no difference in operative time, blood loss, or length of hospital stay.[76] Recurrent helminthic infection occurs in 2% to 10% of patients.[75]

Surgery begins by isolating the area immediately adjacent to the cyst with disinfectant-soaked pads to reduce the risk of contamination (see Figure 117-10). In viable cysts, the pressure may reach 75 cm H_2O and aspiration of a small amount of fluid to reduce pressure should be performed before cyst opening.[77] A scolicidal agent is then instilled into the cyst. Ethanol (70% to 95%), hypertonic saline (15% to 20%), and cetrimide solution (5%) have been widely used at acceptably low risk, although no agent is endorsed by the World Health Organization (WHO) for this purpose. In cases of spillage of scolices, WHO does recommend postoperative treatment with albendazole (1 month) or mebendazole (3 months) to reduce the risk of subsequent intraperitoneal recurrence.[61,78]

After total evacuation of infected contents, there are several options for dealing with the residual intrahepatic cavity. The cavity may be left open to the peritoneum, leaving the pericyst intact. The cyst edges may be sutured to prevent bleeding. Omentoplasty fills the cavity with pedicled omentum, and has been associated with fewer postoperative complications than external drainage in two prospective studies.[79,80] Efforts to obliterate the cavity by coapting the walls with sutures risk injury to hepatic veins and bile ducts and should be avoided.

Laparoscopic approaches to hepatic echinococcal cysts employ the same principles as open operations. As with open surgery, both resection and obliterative procedures may be performed with similar options for management of the cyst cavity. Advantages include shorter hospitalization, reduced postoperative pain, and fewer wound complications.[81] Intraoperatively, the laparoscope aids in close inspection of the cyst cavity for communication with the biliary tree.[81] Major disadvantages center on prevention of intraperitoneal spillage and difficulty in aspiration of thick gelatinous cyst contents. Development of innovative laparoscopic devices has decreased the risk of peritoneal contamination.[82] Recurrence rates are low and similar to those reported for open operation.[82,83]

Percutaneous interventions offer an alternative to operative therapy for hydatid cysts. The most extensively evaluated technique is called PAIR, which stands for puncture-aspiration-injection-reaspiration. Cyst contents are aspirated percutaneously under CT or sonographic guidance. A scolicidal agent such as hypertonic saline is injected then reaspirated after a delay of hours to days. This procedure may also be followed by the use of a sclerosing agent such as ethanol. Before percutaneous intervention, cyst-biliary communication should be excluded with cholangiography. Reported cure, recurrence, and complication rates vary widely, and a recent Cochrane review found insufficient evidence to make a recommendation.[84] In certain subgroups of patients, namely those with univesicular and type I cysts, results of PAIR have been particularly favorable.[85-87] Prospective studies directly comparing PAIR with surgical therapy will clarify the optimal treatment for patients with hydatid cysts.

Antihelminthics serve as an important adjunct to surgical or percutaneous therapies.[88-90] Preoperative albendazole is recommended by WHO[78] as it reduces the proportion of viable scolices at operation and cuts postoperative recurrence rates by more than 50%. Albendazole alone is not adequate therapy for cystic echinococcosis because of low cure rates and frequent recurrence. Antihelminthics are contraindicated in pregnancy and carry the risks of elevated liver enzymes and bone marrow suppression.

REFERENCES

1. Eliason EL, Smith DC: Solitary nonparasitic cyst of the liver: Case report. *Clinics* 3:607, 1944.
2. Caremani M, Vincenti A, Benci A, et al: Ecographic epidemiology of non-parasitic hepatic cysts. *J Clin Ultrasound* 21:115, 1993.
3. Larssen TB, Rørvik J, Hoff SR, et al: The occurrence of asymptomatic and symptomatic simple hepatic cysts. A prospective, hospital-based study. *Clin Radiol* 60:1026, 2005.
4. Carrim ZI, Murchison JT: The prevalence of simple renal and hepatic cysts detected by spiral computed tomography. *Clin Radiol* 58:626, 2003.
5. Feldman M: Polycystic disease of the liver. *Am J Gastroenterol* 29:83, 1958.
6. Hansman MF, Ryan JA Jr, Holmes JH 4th, et al: Management and long-term follow-up of hepatic cysts. *Am J Surg* 181:404, 2001.
7. Spiegel RM, King DL, Green WM: Ultrasonography of primary cysts of the liver. *AJR Am J Roentgenol* 131:235, 1978.
8. Sodhi KS, Sidhu R, Gulati M, et al: Role of tissue harmonic imaging in focal hepatic lesions: Comparison with conventional sonography. *J Gastroenterol Hepatol* 20:1488, 2005.
9. Horton KM, Bluemke DA, Hruban RH, et al: CT and MR imaging of benign hepatic and biliary tumors. *Radiographics* 19:431, 1999.
10. Mueller GC, Hussain HK, Carlos RC, et al: Effectiveness of MR imaging in characterizing small hepatic lesions: Routine versus expert interpretation. *AJR Am J Roentgenol* 180:673, 2003.
11. Mortele KJ, Ros PR: Cystic focal liver lesions in the adult: Differential CT and MR imaging features. *Radiographics* 21:895, 2001.
12. Miller FH, Hammond N, Siddiqi AJ, et al: Utility of diffusion-weighted MRI in distinguishing benign and malignant hepatic lesions. *J Magn Reson Imaging* 32:138, 2010.
13. Saini S, Mueller PR, Ferrucci JT Jr, et al: Percutaneous aspiration of hepatic cysts does not provide definitive therapy. *AJR Am J Roentgenol* 141:559, 1983.
14. Hahn ST, Han SY, Yun EH, et al: Recurrence after percutaneous ethanol ablation of simple hepatic, renal, and splenic cysts: Is it true recurrence requiring an additional treatment? *Acta Radiol* 49:982, 2008.
15. Simonetti G, Profili S, Sergiacomi GL, et al: Percutaneous treatment of hepatic cysts by aspiration and sclerotherapy. *Cardiovasc Intervent Radiol* 16:81, 1993.
16. Larssen TB, Rosendahl K, Horn A, et al: Single-session alcohol sclerotherapy in symptomatic benign hepatic cysts performed with a time of exposure to alcohol of 10 min: Initial results. *Eur Radiol* 13:2627, 2003.
17. Yang CF, Liang HL, Pan HB, et al: Single-session prolonged alcohol-retention sclerotherapy for large hepatic cysts. *AJR Am J Roentgenol* 187:940, 2006.
18. Zerem E, Imamović G, Omerović S: Percutaneous treatment of symptomatic non-parasitic benign liver cysts: Single-session alcohol sclerotherapy versus prolonged catheter drainage with negative pressure. *Eur Radiol* 18:400, 2008.
19. Du XL, Ma QJ, Wu T, et al: Treatment of hepatic cysts by B-ultrasound-guided radiofrequency ablation. *Hepatobiliary Pancreat Dis Int* 6:330, 2007.
20. Weber T, Sendt W, Scheele J: Laparoscopic unroofing of nonparasitic liver cysts within segments VII and VIII: Technical considerations. *J Laparoendosc Adv Surg Tech A* 14:37, 2004.
21. Cowles RA, Mulholland MW: Solitary hepatic cysts. *J Am Coll Surg* 191:311, 2000.
22. Koea JB: Cystic lesions of the liver: 6 years of surgical management in New Zealand. *N Z Med J* 121:61, 2008.
23. Mazza OM, Fernandez DL, Pekolj J, et al: Management of nonparasitic hepatic cysts. *J Am Coll Surg* 209:733, 2009.
24. Palanivelu C, Jani K, Malladi V: Laparoscopic management of benign nonparasitic hepatic cysts: A prospective nonrandomized study. *South Med J* 99:1063, 2006.
25. Szabó LS, Takács I, Arkosy P, et al: Laparoscopic treatment of non-parasitic hepatic cysts. *Surg Endosc* 20:595, 2006.
26. Katkhouda N, Mavor E: Laparoscopic management of benign liver disease. *Surg Clin North Am* 80:1203, 2000.
27. Tan YM, Chung A, Mack P, et al: Role of fenestration and resection for symptomatic solitary liver cysts. *Aust N Z J Surg* 75:577, 2005.
28. Tan YM, Ooi LL, Mack PO: Current status in the surgical management of adult polycystic liver disease. *Ann Acad Med Singapore* 31:217, 2002.
29. The polycystic kidney disease 1 gene encodes a 14 kb transcript and lies within a duplicated region on chromosome 16. European Polycystic Kidney Disease Consortium. *Cell* 77:881, 1994.
30. Mochizuki T, Wu G, Hayashi T, et al: PKD2, a gene for polycystic kidney disease that encodes an integral membrane protein. *Science* 272:1339, 1996.
31. Wu G, D'Agati V, Cai Y, et al: Somatic inactivation of Pkd2 results in polycystic kidney disease. *Cell* 93:177, 1998.
32. Watnick TJ, Torres VE, Gandolph MA, et al: Somatic mutation in individual liver cysts supports a two-hit model of cystogenesis in autosomal dominant polycystic kidney disease. *Mol Cell* 2:247, 1998.
33. Sherstha R, McKinley C, Russ P, et al: Postmenopausal estrogen therapy selectively stimulates hepatic enlargement in women with autosomal dominant polycystic kidney disease. *Hepatology* 26:1282, 1997.
34. Gigot JF, Jadoul P, Que F, et al: Adult polycystic liver disease: Is fenestration the most adequate operation for long-term management? *Ann Surg* 225:286, 1997.
35. Tikkakoski T, Mäkelä JT, Leinonen S, et al: Treatment of symptomatic congenital hepatic cysts with single-session percutaneous drainage and ethanol sclerosis: Technique and outcome. *J Vasc Interv Radiol* 7:235, 1996.
36. Bistritz L, Tamboli C, Bigam D, et al: Polycystic liver disease: Experience at a teaching hospital. *Am J Gastroenterol* 100:2212, 2005.
37. Katkhouda N, Hurwitz M, Gugenheim J, et al: Laparoscopic management of benign solid and cystic lesions of the liver. *Ann Surg* 229:460, 1999.
38. Russell RT, Pinson CW: Surgical management of polycystic liver disease. *World J Gastroenterol* 13:5052, 2007.
39. Schnelldorfer T, Torres VE, Zakaria S, et al: Polycystic liver disease: A critical appraisal of hepatic resection, cyst fenestration, and liver transplantation. *Ann Surg* 250:112, 2009.
40. Takei R, Ubara Y, Hoshino J, et al: Percutaneous transcatheter hepatic artery embolization for liver cysts in autosomal dominant polycystic kidney disease. *Am J Kidney Dis* 49:744, 2007.
41. Lang H, von Woellwarth J, Oldhafer KJ, et al: Liver transplantation in patients with polycystic liver disease. *Transplant Proc* 29:2832, 1997.
42. Krohn PS, Hillingsø JG, Kirkegaard P: Liver transplantation in polycystic liver disease: A relevant treatment modality for adults? *Scand J Gastroenterol* 43:89, 2008.
43. Kirchner GI, Rifai K, Cantz T, et al: Outcome and quality of life in patients with polycystic liver disease after liver or combined liver-kidney transplantation. *Liver Transpl* 12:1268, 2006.
44. Akiyoshi T, Yamaguchi K, Chijiiwa K, et al: Cystadenocarcinoma of the liver without mesenchymal stroma: Possible progression from a benign cystic lesion suspected by follow-up imagings. *J Gastroenterol* 38:588, 2003.
45. Daniels JA, Coad JE, Payne WD, et al: Biliary cystadenomas: Hormone receptor expression and clinical management. *Dig Dis Sci* 51:623, 2006.
46. Ishak KG, Willis GW, Cummins SD, et al: Biliary cystadenoma and cystadenocarcinoma: Report of 14 cases and review of the literature. *Cancer* 39:322, 1977.
47. Seo JK, Kim SH, Lee SH, et al: Appropriate diagnosis of biliary cystic tumors: Comparison with atypical hepatic simple cysts. *Eur J Gastroenterol Hepatol* 22:989, 2010.

48. Korobkin M, Stephens DH, Lee JK, et al: Biliary cystadenoma and cystadenocarcinoma: CT and sonographic findings. *AJR Am J Roentgenol* 153:507, 1989.

49. Choi HK, Lee JK, Lee KH, et al: Differential diagnosis for intrahepatic biliary cystadenoma and hepatic simple cyst: Significance of cystic fluid analysis and radiologic findings. *J Clin Gastroenterol* 44:289, 2010.

50. Pojchamarnwiputh S, Na Chiangmai W, Chotirosniramit A, et al: Computed tomography of biliary cystadenoma and biliary cystadenocarcinoma. *Singapore Med J* 49:392, 2008.

51. Devaney K, Goodman ZD, Ishak KG: Hepatobiliary cystadenoma and cystadenocarcinoma. A light microscopic and immunohistochemical study of 70 patients. *Am J Surg Pathol* 18:1078, 1994.

52. Manouras A, Markogiannakis H, Lagoudianakis E, et al: Biliary cystadenoma with mesenchymal stroma: Report of a case and review of the literature. *World J Gastroenterol* 12:6062, 2006.

53. Koffron A, Rao S, Ferrario M, et al: Intrahepatic biliary cystadenoma: Role of cyst fluid analysis and surgical management in the laparoscopic era. *Surgery* 136:926, 2004.

54. Yu Q, Chen T, Wan YL, et al: Intrahepatic biliary cystadenocarcinoma: Clinical analysis of 4 cases. *Hepatobiliary Pancreat Dis Int* 8:71, 2009.

55. Hai S, Hirohashi K, Uenishi T, et al: Surgical management of cystic hepatic neoplasms. *J Gastroenterol* 38:759, 2003.

56. Lau WY, Chow CH, Leung ML: Total excision of mucinous biliary cystadenoma. *Aust N Z J Surg* 60:226, 1990.

57. Pinson CW, Munson JL, Rossi RL, et al: Enucleation of intrahepatic biliary cystadenomas. *Surg Gynecol Obstet* 168:534, 1989.

58. Thomas KT, Welch D, Trueblood A, et al: Effective treatment of biliary cystadenoma. *Ann Surg* 241:769; discussion 773, 2005.

59. Lewis WD, Jenkins RL, Rossi RL, et al: Surgical treatment of biliary cystadenoma. A report of 15 cases. *Arch Surg* 123:563, 1988.

60. Teoh AY, Ng SS, Lee KF, et al: Biliary cystadenoma and other complicated cystic lesions of the liver: Diagnostic and therapeutic challenges. *World J Surg* 30:1560, 2006.

61. Guidelines for treatment of cystic and alveolar echinococcosis in humans. WHO Informal Working Group on Echinococcosis. *Bull World Health Organ* 74:231, 1996.

62. Kurt N, Oncel M, Gulmez S, et al: Spontaneous and traumatic intra-peritoneal perforations of hepatic hydatid cysts: A case series. *J Gastrointest Surg* 7:635, 2003.

63. Sbihi Y, Rmiqui A, Rodriguez-Cabezas MN, et al: Comparative sensitivity of six serological tests and diagnostic value of ELISA using purified antigen in hydatidosis. *J Clin Lab Anal* 15:14, 2001.

64. Caremani M, Lapini L, Caremani D, et al: Sonographic diagnosis of hydatidosis: The sign of the cyst wall. *Eur J Ultrasound* 16:217, 2003.

65. Sayek I, Onat D: Diagnosis and treatment of uncomplicated hydatid cyst of the liver. *World J Surg* 25:21, 2001.

66. Polat P, Kantarci M, Alper F, et al: Hydatid disease from head to toe. *Radiographics* 23:475, 2003.

67. Proietti S, Abdelmoumene A, Genevay M, et al: Echinococcal cyst. *Radiographics* 24:861, 2004.

68. Mortele KJ, Peters HE: Multimodality imaging of common and uncommon cystic focal liver lesions. *Semin Ultrasound CT MR* 30:368, 2009.

69. Czermak BV, Akhan O, Hiemetzberger R, et al: Echinococcosis of the liver. *Abdom Imaging* 33:133, 2008.

70. Hosch W, Stojkovic M, Jänisch T, et al: MR imaging for diagnosing cysto-biliary fistulas in cystic echinococcosis. *Eur J Radiol* 66:262, 2008.

71. Akbulut S, Senol A, Sezgin A, et al: Radical vs conservative surgery for hydatid liver cysts: Experience from single center. *World J Gastroenterol* 16:953, 2010.

72. Aydin U, Yazici P, Onen Z, et al: The optimal treatment of hydatid cyst of the liver: Radical surgery with a significant reduced risk of recurrence. *Turk J Gastroenterol* 19:33, 2008.

73. Safioleas MC, Misiakos EP, Kouvaraki M, et al: Hydatid disease of the liver: A continuing surgical problem. *Arch Surg* 141:1101, 2006.

74. Daradkeh S, El-Muhtaseb H, Farah G, et al: Predictors of morbidity and mortality in the surgical management of hydatid cyst of the liver. *Langenbecks Arch Surg* 392:35, 2007.

75. Buttenschoen K, Carli Buttenschoen D: Echinococcus granulosus infection: The challenge of surgical treatment. *Langenbecks Arch Surg* 388:218, 2003.

76. Yüksel O, Akyürek N, Sahin T, et al: Efficacy of radical surgery in preventing early local recurrence and cavity-related complications in hydatic liver disease. *J Gastrointest Surg* 12:483, 2008.

77. Tsimoyiannis EC, Siakas P, Glantzounis G, et al: Intracystic pressure and viability in hydatid disease of the liver. *Int Surg* 85:234, 2000.

78. World Health Organization, World Organization for Animal Health: WHO/OIE Manual on echinococcosis in humans and animals: A public health problem of global concern. http://whqlibdoc.who.int/publications/2001/929044522X.pdf, 2001.

79. Dziri C, Paquet JC, Hay JM, et al: Omentoplasty in the prevention of deep abdominal complications after surgery for hydatid disease of the liver: A multicenter, prospective, randomized trial. French Associations for Surgical Research. *J Am Coll Surg* 188:281, 1999.

80. Ozacmak ID, Ekiz F, Ozmen V, et al: Management of residual cavity after partial cystectomy for hepatic hydatidosis: Comparison of omentoplasty with external drainage. *Eur J Surg* 166:696, 2000.

81. Yagci G, Ustunsoz B, Kaymakcioglu N, et al: Results of surgical, laparoscopic, and percutaneous treatment for hydatid disease of the liver: 10 years experience with 355 patients. *World J Surg* 29:1670, 2005.

82. Palanivelu C, Jani K, Malladi V, et al: Laparoscopic management of hepatic hydatid disease. *JSLS* 10:56, 2006.

83. Chen W, Xusheng L: Laparoscopic surgical techniques in patients with hepatic hydatid cyst. *Am J Surg* 194:243, 2007.

84. Nasseri Moghaddam S, Abrishami A, Malekzadeh R: Percutaneous needle aspiration, injection, and reaspiration with or without benzimidazole coverage for uncomplicated hepatic hydatid cysts. *Cochrane Database Syst Rev* (2):CD003623, 2006.

85. Giorgio A, Di Sarno A, de Stefano G, et al: Sonography and clinical outcome of viable hydatid liver cysts treated with double percutaneous aspiration and ethanol injection as first-line therapy: Efficacy and long-term follow-up. *AJR Am J Roentgenol* 193:W186, 2009.

86. Kabaalioğlu A, Ceken K, Alimoglu E, et al: Percutaneous imaging-guided treatment of hydatid liver cysts: Do long-term results make it a first choice? *Eur J Radiol* 59:65, 2006.

87. Zerem E, Jusufovic R: Percutaneous treatment of univesicular versus multivesicular hepatic hydatid cysts. *Surg Endosc* 20:1543, 2006.

88. Kapan S, Turhan AN, Kalayci MU, et al: Albendazole is not effective for primary treatment of hepatic hydatid cysts. *J Gastrointest Surg* 12:867, 2008.

89. Bildik N, Cevik A, Altintaş M, et al: Efficacy of preoperative albendazole use according to months in hydatid cyst of the liver. *J Clin Gastroenterol* 41:312, 2007.

90. Arif SH, Shams-Ul-Bari, Wani NA, et al: Albendazole as an adjuvant to the standard surgical management of hydatid cyst liver. *Int J Surg* 6:448, 2008.

Liver Abscess

Sylvester M. Black | Sangeetha Prabhakaran | Selwyn M. Vickers

Liver abscess is an uncommon entity that over the past 100 years has seen fairly dramatic changes in demographics, etiology, diagnosis, and treatment. While the mortality from liver abscess has decreased significantly since the early 20th century, the incidence appears to be increasing.[1] Traditionally, it has been useful to think of hepatic abscesses in two broad categories: those of bacterial origin, otherwise known as pyogenic liver abscess (PLA) or those of parasitic origin primarily caused by *Entamoeba histolytica* leading to amebic liver abscess (ALA). Obviously, with the increase in the number of patients with various forms of immunosuppression, including but not limited to neutropenia from anticancer treatments and transplant immunosuppression, the reports of other unusual types of liver abscess such as mycobacterial abscess and fungal abscess, though rare, also appear to be increasing. Improvements in mortality and morbidity appear to be centered on improvements in early diagnosis, with refinements in diagnostic imaging in the form of ultrasound and CT scan as well as the evolution of minimally invasive percutaneous aspiration and drainage techniques. Very likely and no less important are general improvements in antibiotic usage and the development of critical care medicine in further reducing the mortality from these diseases.

The seminal paper by Ochsner in 1938 was the first attempt to rigorously classify, categorize, and offer treatment strategies in the form of surgical drainage for PLA.[2] In his series, Ochsner noted that ALA was about three times more common than PLA. However, currently PLAs account for a majority of hepatic abscesses observed in most series in the Western literature, in contrast to ALA, which accounts for the largest number of liver abscesses observed worldwide. Currently in Western literature, amebic abscess is not as common and presumably this is because of significant improvements in hygiene and sanitation leading to decreases in invasive amebiasis. Medical therapy in the form of metronidazole has been so effective in the treatment of ALA that surgical intervention has become rare.

PYOGENIC LIVER ABSCESSES

PLA has long been recognized as a morbid disease, which was associated with significant mortality. Lack of understanding of PLA as a disease contributed to these poor outcomes. Ochsner in 1938 demonstrated that surgical drainage combined with antibiotic therapy could considerably improve survival in patients with PLA. Ochsner reported that patients undergoing surgical drainage in addition to antibiotic therapy had a 62% survival rate compared to nearly a 100% mortality in those that did not receive this treatment.[2] The standard of care until

the 1950s was surgical drainage combined with antibiotic therapy. The mortality rate from PLA continued to remain high although significantly improved when compared with the results at the turn of the century. Improvement in patient survival with PLA remained elusive and the likely contributing factors included the relatively late presentation of patients combined with the inaccuracy of localization, which was primarily by manual palpation and detection of induration and/or fluctuance during surgery. Thus, further advancement in the treatment of PLA would depend on refinement in diagnostic imaging, localization, and minimally invasive techniques. In 1953 McFadzean reported 14 patients who received percutaneous drainage for PLA in which all patients survived.[3] Percutaneous drainage of PLA, however, would not be widely advocated and was seldom discussed in the literature until the 1980s when several reports of percutaneous drainage combined with antibiotics showed improved survival in patients with PLA.[4,5]

Early detection and localization advanced the treatment of PLA considerably and ran concurrently with advancements in computed tomography (CT) and ultrasonography. These refined imaging techniques allowed for more precise localization and thus facilitated accurate drainage of PLA such that source control was usually achieved. Furthermore, percutaneous aspiration or drain placement could be done with minimal morbidity when compared with open operation, which was important when considering the general condition of many of these patients. Thus percutaneous treatment of PLA, whether single or multiple abscesses are present, has become the standard of care. Open operation is reserved primarily for cases of failure of nonoperative treatment, presence of fungal growth on culture, or communication of the abscess cavity with an obstructed biliary tree that cannot be managed nonoperatively.[6,7] The mortality associated with open operation under these circumstances is very high.

INCIDENCE AND DEMOGRAPHICS

PLA is associated with significant morbidity, mortality, and medical costs. The incidence varies from 1.1 to 3.6 per 100,000 population in the Western literature to 17.6 per 100,000 population in the Eastern literature and it appears that incidence of PLA is increasing.[1] The recently reported incidence of PLA in the United States is 3.6 per 100,000 with an increase in PLA-based hospitalizations between 1994 and 2005 from 2.7 to 4.1 per 100,000 population.[1] The mortality from PLA has decreased significantly from Ochsner's series in 1938 where the mortality from PLA was reported to be about 72% (Table 118-1). Currently, mortality from PLA in most North American

TABLE 118-1 Selected Series of Pyogenic Hepatic Abscesses

Author, Year	Location	No. of Cases	Time Period	Age (yr)	Male-to-Female Ratio	Incidence	Mortality Rate (%)
Oschner et al, 1938[2]	New Orleans	47	1928-1937	30-39 (mean)	2.35:1.0	47/540,776 admissions	72.3
Pitt and Zuidema, 1975[8]	Baltimore	80	1952-1972	60	1.0:1.0	13/100,000	65
Branum et al, 1990[5]	Durham	73	1970-1986	53 (median)	1.1:1.0	*1970-1978:* 11.5/100,000 *1979-1986:* 22/100,000	19
Seeto and Rockey, 1996[9]	San Francisco	142	1979-1994	51 (median)	1.3:1.0	22/100,000 admissions	11
Huang et al, 1996[10]	Baltimore	153	1973-1993	55.5 (mean)	1.3:1.0	20/100,000 admissions	31
Alvarez et al, 2001[11]	Spain	133	1985-1997	58.1-64.9 (mean)	1.6:1.0	Not reported	14
Mohsen et al, 2002[12]	United Kingdom	65	1988-1999	64 (median)	1.3:1.0	18.5/100,000	12.3
Wong et al, 2002[13]	Hong Kong	80	1991-2001	63.4 (mean)	1.67:1.0	Not reported	6

and European series ranges from 5.6% to 10%, whereas mortality worldwide ranges from 3% to 30%. Importantly, although incidence of PLA appears to be increasing, mortality has remained stable and the demographics of the patient with PLA have changed significantly.[1] At the turn of the century, the patient with PLA was typically a 20- to 30-year-old male with pylephlebitis secondary to appendicitis, diverticulitis, or another intraabdominal infectious process. With improved management of the underlying cause of the intraabdominal infection in the form of early diagnosis and with improvements in antibiotic therapy, the demographics of PLA have shifted considerably. Now the typical patient with PLA is predominately male in his 60s with either an actively treated advanced hepatobiliary malignancy or benign biliary tract pathology as the underlying cause of PLA.[1,2,6,7]

ETIOLOGY AND PATHOGENESIS

Although there are multiple etiologies of PLA, patients with ascending infection of the biliary tree associated with obstruction are currently the most commonly identified cause of PLA.[6,7,9] Differences in geographic location can account for differences observed in the etiology of the obstruction leading to the ascending infection and subsequent PLA. In many Asian countries, hepatolithiasis with associated biliary strictures accounts for most of the cases of PLA,[14,15] whereas in Western countries obstruction secondary to underlying malignancy such as an obstructing cholangiocarcinoma (Figure 118-1) with associated ascending cholangitis is a very common scenario leading to PLA.[6,7,10] Furthermore, the widespread use of bile duct stents and biliary tract manipulation in these situations has also greatly increased the risk of cholangitis and thus PLA.

Other causes of PLA include hematogenous spread from sources other than the gastrointestinal tract such as bacterial endocarditis, intravenous drug use, and other

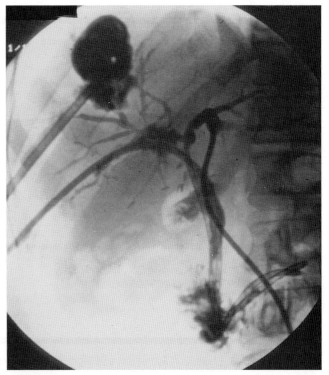

FIGURE 118-1 Cholangiogram demonstrating a perihilar cholangiocarcinoma as well as an abscess near the dome of the right lobe of the liver.

infectious processes that can produce bacteremia. Radiofrequency ablation and transarterial chemoembolization (TACE) of liver tumors can also lead to liver necrosis, which may then become secondarily infected, leading to PLA. Traumatic liver injury that results in necrosis may predispose a patient to development of PLA. Prior biliary reconstructive procedures may lead to biliary stricture and subsequent biliary tract infection, predisposing the patient to the development of PLA.

When no identifiable cause of PLA is found, the abscess is described as cryptogenic. Cryptogenic PLA is currently reported to represent approximately 25% of all liver abscesses in some series (Table 118-2).

CLINICAL PRESENTATION

The clinical presentation of PLA can be quite variable, so that the early presentation of symptoms is nonspecific or vague. Prodromal symptoms such as weight loss, fever, fatigue, malaise, anorexia, and myalgia may occur many weeks before more specific symptoms, which may localize the process such as right upper quadrant pain, hepatomegaly, or jaundice. Classically the presentation is described as a triad of right upper quadrant pain, fever or chills, and generalized malaise; however, this triad is not universally seen. Fever is the most common presenting sign, which is present in 67% to 99% of patients. Right upper quadrant pain is also present in approximately 35% to 74% of patients (Table 118-3). Other signs or symptoms are quite variable across different series. PLA most often occurs in the setting of other intraabdominal pathology, such as hepatobiliary malignancy or ascending biliary tract infection with obstruction, in which the underlying disease process influences the severity and duration of the symptoms.

DIAGNOSIS

Laboratory investigations in most cases of PLA are non-specific. Many patients will present with an elevated white blood cell count ranging from 64% to 88%. Hypoalbuminemia is also present in most patients ranging from 50% to 94% and likely reflects the chronicity of the underlying disease process (Table 118-4). Transaminases and alkaline phosphatase are also frequently elevated in the setting of PLA. Bilirubin may or may not be elevated in PLA. An elevation of bilirubin in the context of jaundice would suggest underlying biliary obstruction as an etiologic factor in the disease process. Although liver-specific laboratory results can serve to help localize the disease process, other laboratory findings such as leukocytosis, anemia, and hypoalbuminemia reflect the systemic nature of the disease. Therefore, it becomes difficult based on laboratory results alone to make the diagnosis or predict outcome in patients with PLA.

TABLE 118-2 Etiology of Pyogenic Hepatic Abscess

Author, Year	No. of Cases	Cryptogenic, %	Hepatobiliary (%)	Portal (%)	Hepatic Artery (%)	Other (%)
Oschner et al, 1938[2]	47	60	6	19	N/A	15
Pitt and Zuidema, 1975[8]	80	20	51	15	1	<10[†]
Branum et al, 1990[5]	73	27	31.4	18.2	10	14[‡]
Huang et al, 1996[10]	153	16	60	<10	10	<10[†]
Seeto and Rockey*, 1996[9]	142	40	37	11	N/A	12*
Alvarez et al, 2001[11]	133	26	25[§]	13	2	33[¶]
Mohsen et al, 2002[12]	65	24 (18 uninvestigated)	28	48	N/A	N/A
Wong et al, 2002[13]	80	N/A	61	N/A	1.25	N/A

N/A, Not available.
*Includes direct extension, abdominal trauma, and chronic granulomatous disease.
[†]Trauma.
[‡]Trauma, other solid tumors, direct extension, Crohn disease.
[§]Includes seven patients with recent hepatic surgery.
[¶]Trauma, direct extension.

TABLE 118-3 Presenting Symptoms and Signs in Pyogenic Hepatic Abscess

Author, Year	No. of Cases	Fever (%)	Abdominal Pain (%)	Nausea/Vomiting (%)	Weight Loss (%)	Diarrhea (%)	Jaundice (%)	Hepatomegaly (%)
Pitt and Zuidema, 1975[8]	80	92	74	N/A	51	23	54	48
Branum et al, 1990[5]	73	75	55	27	29	8	23	38
Huang et al, 1996[10]	153	89	55	N/A	43	10	50	35
Seeto and Rockey, 1996[9]	142	79	55	30/37	28	20	22	28
Alvarez et al, 2001[11]	133	92	69	29	42	N/A	21	24
Mohsen et al, 2002[12]	65	67	67	41	35	23	14	30
Wong et al, 2002[13]	80	99	35	N/A	10	N/A	14	18

N/A, Not available.

TABLE 118-4 Laboratory Findings in Pyogenic Hepatic Abscesses

Author, Year	Leukocytosis (%)	Elevated Alkaline Phosphatase Level (%)	Hypoalbuminemia (%)	Hyperbilirubinemia (%)	ALT (%)	AST (%)	Anemia (%)
Pitt and Zuidema, 1975[8]	69	90	62	68	82	90	N/A
Branum et al, 1990[5]	68	78	N/A	36	N/A	57	67
Huang et al, 1996[10]	77	70	71	49	67	64	N/A
Seeto and Rockey, 1996[9]	64	80	>67	N/A*	69[†]	57[†]	75
Alvarez et al, 2001[11]	65	56	50	23	N/A	41	56
Mohsen et al, 2002[12]	88	64	N/A	36	67	49	*Male:* 74 *Female:* 47
Wong et al, 2002[13]	84	73	94	48	50-63	N/A	76

ALT, Alanine aminotransferase; *AST*, aspartate aminotransferase; *N/A*, not available.
*Exact numbers not provided, but was present in most patients with biliary tract disease and hepatic abscess.
[†]Specific to patients with biliary tract and hepatic abscess.

Plain chest or abdominal radiographs are nonspecific and usually not diagnostic for PLA. Chest radiographic examination in 50% of the cases may show an elevated right hemidiaphragm, subdiaphragmatic air–fluid levels if gas-forming organisms are present, pleural effusions, and atelectasis.[9] Abdominal radiography is usually not helpful unless there is an abscess with gas-forming organisms present, in which air–fluid levels may be visible. Ultrasonography is usually the initial study of choice for imaging of the liver and biliary tree. The low cost, lack of exposure to ionizing radiation, and the high sensitivity for diagnosis of PLA make ultrasonography an excellent choice for initial evaluation of the liver. Ultrasonography has a reported sensitivity of 83% to 95% for the diagnosis of PLA.[10,11] Ultrasonography can also characterize the liver abscess, with the appearance of the abscess varying by the stage of maturation. Early in the formation of a PLA, the abscess is hyperechoic and not distinct. However, as the abscess matures with the formation of pus, a distinct wall forms and the abscess becomes hypoechoic.[16] Another advantage of ultrasonography is the ability to characterize underlying biliary pathology such as dilated bile ducts, hepatolithiasis, and choledocholithiasis, which would subsequently affect the treatment of PLA.

CT scanning is highly sensitive in its ability to distinguish PLA from other intrahepatic lesions. The reported sensitivity for detection of PLA is between 93% and 100%.[9,16] In addition to high sensitivity for detection of PLA, CT scanning is also efficient at detecting small PLAs with a diameter of less than 2 cm, the so-called microabscess. CT scanning can detect abscesses within the liver parenchyma as small as 0.5 cm. Based on size, PLAs are classified as either microabscesses (<2 cm) or macroabscesses (>2 cm). Microabscesses will appear as small, multiple, hypodense lesions with distribution throughout the liver parenchyma. During CT scan and especially during the portal venous phase with intravenous contrast, PLAs will often exhibit peripheral rim enhancement, whereby the PLA will appear as a hypodense cystic lesion demonstrating segmental wall enhancement with surrounding low-density edema (Figure 118-2). There is often a

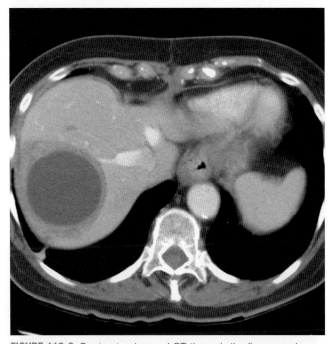

FIGURE 118-2 Contrast-enhanced CT through the liver reveals a unilocular low-density mass near the dome representing a pyogenic abscess. Note the peripheral enhancing rim, which is relatively narrow.

transition zone between the low-density center of the abscess and the peripheral rim. This transition zone is typically narrow, which is a feature that can help differentiate PLA from necrotic metastasis.[16,17]

Classically microabscesses have been described as having two distinct appearances on CT scan. First, microabscesses may appear as multiple, widely scattered, miliary-type lesions or they may appear as adjacent "daughter" abscesses clustering around central larger abscesses. The clustering phenomenon may represent coalescence of multiple smaller abscesses and has been postulated to represent an early stage in the evolution of the PLA cavity.[17] Many of these multifocal clustered abscesses tend to form intercommunicating cavities, essentially forming larger multiseptate abscesses (Figure 118-3).

Magnetic resonance (MR) imaging does not appear to offer any significant advantage in the detection of PLA when compared with ultrasonography and CT. The high sensitivity of CT scanning and ultrasonography limits the utility of MR imaging in the diagnosis of PLA. However,

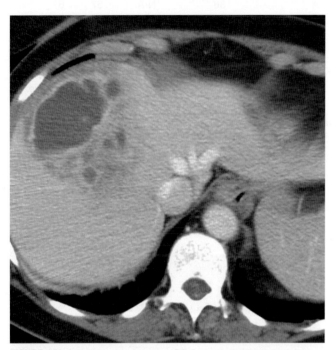

FIGURE 118-3 Contrast-enhanced CT through the liver reveals the "cluster" appearance of a pyogenic hepatic abscess with several smaller peripheral abscesses that have coalesced.

if there is diagnostic uncertainty, MR imaging may be able to better characterize intrahepatic lesions and delineate differences between PLA and cystic or necrotic lesions. PLA tends to be hypointense on T1-weighted MR images and hyperintense on T2-weighted MR images (Figure 118-4). Another area where MR imaging may be beneficial is magnetic resonance cholangiopancreatography (MRCP). If biliary obstruction is suggested clinically, MRCP may help identify the level of obstruction, making planning of the appropriate intervention more precise. However, the high cost, length of the study, and lack of availability in many medical centers serve to limit the usefulness of MR imaging in the routine management of PLA.

MICROBIOLOGY

Culture techniques and microbiology culture technology have evolved considerably since the early part of the 20th century. Bacteria may be cultured from the abscess cavity itself using percutaneous techniques or from the blood. Bacteria are more likely to be isolated from the abscess cavity than from blood culture.[9] Reports in the literature describe varying rates of monomicrobial versus polymicrobial isolates in PLA, with 33% to 55% of hepatic abscess cultures being polymicrobial, compared with a lower rate of polymicrobial blood culture isolates.[9,12,18,19] There have been many series of PLA in the literature, which have identified multiple species of bacterial flora presumed to be etiologic agents responsible for hepatic abscesses (Box 118-1). *Escherichia coli*, *Streptococcus*, *Enterococcus*, and *Klebsiella* are often cultured in patients with PLA, with *E. coli* and *Streptococcus* being the most frequently isolated bacterial flora in most series in the Western literature.[18] There also appears to be some

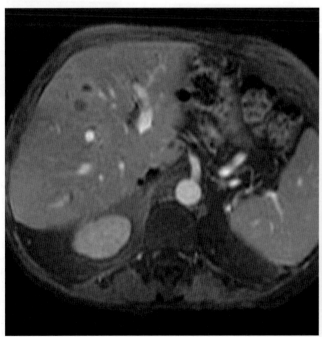
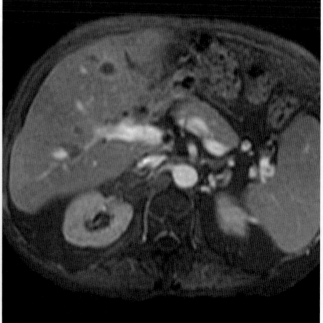

FIGURE 118-4 Gadolinium-enhanced T1-weighted MR imaging through the liver reveals multiple low-signal lesions with a thin peripheral ring of enhancement in this patient with multiple pyogenic microabscesses.

BOX 118-1 Microbiology of Pyogenic Liver Abscess

GRAM-POSITIVE ORGANISMS
Streptococcus
Staphylococcus
Pneumococcus
Enterococcus
  Mycobacterium

GRAM-NEGATIVE ORGANISMS
Escherichia
Klebsiella
Pseudomonas

Proteus
Haemophilus
Serratia

ANAEROBIC ORGANISMS
Bacteroides
Fusobacterium
Pasteurella

POLYMICROBIAL

YEAST

---

geographic correlation with culture isolates in patients with PLA, as *Klebsiella pneumoniae* is especially prevalent in Asia when compared to Western populations.[14,20]

However, there are many confounding factors that make it difficult to generalize regarding the etiology of PLA. Most patients receive antibiotic therapy prior to obtaining liver abscess or blood culture, which may make it difficult to isolate the offending pathogen. Furthermore, there is a wide variation in culture techniques and quality among the different series investigating PLA. A population-based study of PLA in the United States revealed that rural hospitals were less likely to obtain positive culture results (42%) when compared with urban teaching (45%) and nonteaching hospitals (49%).[1] In this study, rural hospitals were also less likely to utilize radiologic-guided aspiration and culture. In fact, most previous studies were performed in tertiary medical centers with a relatively high level of experience in the treatment of PLA. These medical centers had access to advanced diagnostic tools such as CT scan and ultrasonography with interventional radiology support. These findings serve to highlight the relative heterogeneity in culture results and the difficulty in generalizing the findings from one series to the next.

Evolution and refinement of culture technique have led to the increasing identification of anaerobic and microaerophilic organisms in PLA. This is well illustrated by changes that have occurred in anaerobic culture techniques where Sabbaj et al in 1972 demonstrated that when using strict anaerobic culture techniques, 45% of cultures obtained from hepatic abscesses were in fact anaerobic, a finding that was much higher than prior studies.[21] Huang et al demonstrated a significant increase in anaerobic isolates over a period of 42 years from 1952 to 1993 at Johns Hopkins.[10] Similarly, Chemaly et al identified *Streptococcus milleri*, a microaerophilic or anaerobic collection of streptococcal bacteria, and anaerobic gram-negative bacilli as the most common bacterial isolates from culture.[22] In recent studies, *Bacteroides* species are the most commonly isolated anaerobes in PLA.[23] The improvement in culture technique, especially anaerobic techniques, suggests that abscesses, which were previously thought to be "sterile" or cryptogenic, may in fact be caused by anaerobic organisms that were not previously identified secondary to inadequate technique.

PLA due to hematogenous spread not associated with a gastrointestinal source is often monomicrobial, the result of infection with *Staphylococcus aureus* or *Streptococcus* species and tends to form solitary abscesses. In contrast, infections that are from enteric or biliary sources tend to be polymicrobial and associated with aerobic gram-negative bacteria and anaerobes.[9,12,18] The clinician should be mindful that, as with many infections, bacteria associated with PLA have developed increased resistance to many antimicrobial agents. This antimicrobial resistance is likely the result of increasing use of indwelling biliary stents and biliary tract manipulation with recurrent episodes of cholangitis treated with antibiotics. PLA may contain multiple species of bacteria, and antibiotic choices should initially have broad coverage to reflect this fact until definitive culture results can be obtained. Abscess cavity culture is not usually immediately available. However, Gram stain of liver abscess aspirates in addition to blood culture provides useful information for the initiation of therapy for PLA. Gram stain of liver abscess aspirates is reported to have sensitivity of 90% with a specificity of 100% for gram-positive cocci. The reported sensitivity and specificity for gram-negative bacilli is 52% and 94%, respectively.[22] Blood culture and Gram stain of the abscess cavity contents are useful tests that can guide appropriate antimicrobial therapy until liver abscess culture results are made available.

TREATMENT

In the early part of the 20th century, PLA was associated with a nearly 100% mortality rate. Ochsner et al demonstrated that with surgical drainage, a significant reduction in mortality could be achieved.[2] With the introduction of antibiotics and advancements in diagnostic imaging modalities such as ultrasonography and CT scan, earlier and more accurate diagnosis of PLA was possible. Percutaneous aspiration and drainage, made possible by these same advancements in diagnostic imaging, further reduced morbidity and mortality. Open surgical drainage is now considered second-line therapy, utilized after failure of percutaneous drainage, and remains associated with a high mortality.[6,7] Therefore, the principles of treatment of PLA are to drain the abscess cavity, identify the pathogen, start appropriate antibiotic therapy, and treat any underlying disease process associated with the abscess.

ANTIBIOTIC THERAPY

Once the diagnosis of PLA is suspected, blood cultures should be immediately obtained. Diagnostic imaging in the form of ultrasonography and/or CT scanning is helpful in localizing the process and in identifying any associated intraabdominal pathology. If a hepatic abscess is identified by diagnostic imaging, *E. histolytica* serology should be obtained to assist in differentiating between the two major types of hepatic abscess, as amebic abscesses usually do not require drainage. Percutaneous aspiration or drainage with Gram stain of abscess cavity contents is helpful in guiding initial antibiotic management. As noted earlier, Gram stain has a high sensitivity and specificity for gram-positive organisms and a moderate sensitivity and high specificity for gram-negative organisms.

Therapy should not be delayed while waiting for blood or abscess culture results, but rather initiation of broad-based empiric antibiotic coverage should be the goal. An understanding of the underlying cause of the abscess is helpful in guiding initial antimicrobial therapy. Biliary disorders commonly yield gram-negative bacteria, whereas abscesses as a result of pylephlebitis often yield gram-negative and anaerobic bacteria. Antimicrobials such as the extended-spectrum penicillins (piperacillin-tazobactam, ticarcillin-clavulanate, ampicillin-sulbactam), carbapenems (imipenem, meropenem, ertapenem), or second-generation cephalosporins with or without metronidazole depending on antimicrobial anaerobic coverage are good initial antibiotic choices for the treatment of PLA. Modifications of the antibiotic regimen can be made later once the speciation and sensitivities are obtained from the blood cultures or abscess cavity aspirate cultures. Antimicrobial therapy is usually initiated parenterally for a duration of 2 to 3 weeks, with conversion to oral antibiotics to complete a 4- to 6-week course.[24] It is important to individualize the antimicrobial therapeutic regimen to the patient, with consideration given to factors such as the number of abscesses, underlying pathology, toxicity of the antibiotic regimen, and clinical response. In situations where there are multiple PLAs that are very small and widespread in distribution, and therefore impossible to percutaneously drain, antimicrobial therapy may be the only treatment option available. In this instance, duration of therapy is likely to be longer and the mortality rate has been reported to be as high as 29%.[14]

DRAINAGE PROCEDURES

Percutaneous aspiration and/or catheter-based drainage along with antibiotic therapy is the mainstay of treatment for PLA. Morbidity from percutaneous aspiration and catheter-based drainage is very low and the effectiveness in treating PLA is well established.[3,5-7,25] The vast majority of PLA can be treated with percutaneous procedures, either by aspiration or percutaneous catheter-based drain placement. Both treatment strategies are efficacious, so consideration of when to use aspiration over drain placement depends on a multitude of factors such as abscess size, location, number, and viscosity of abscess cavity contents. Previously, multiple abscesses were an indication to utilize surgical drainage; however, placement of multiple percutaneous drains or multiple aspirations has been shown to be quite effective.[25] It is important to consider underlying disorders, especially biliary obstruction, which has been associated with a high rate of failure for percutaneous drainage.[7] Underlying biliary obstruction requires treatment either by endoscopic, percutaneous, or surgical means in addition to abscess drainage for resolution of the PLA.

PERCUTANEOUS ASPIRATION AND PERCUTANEOUS CATHETER DRAINAGE

The first description in the literature of percutaneous aspiration for PLA was in 1953. McFadzean et al published a series that reported percutaneous intervention in 14 patients with PLA who were treated with closed-needle aspiration and intracavitary antibiotics. There was

no mortality in this series, with all patients recovering.[3] Percutaneous intervention has become the first-line treatment of PLA with diminished need for open surgical drainage. There has been some debate concerning whether catheter-based drain placement is superior to aspiration. Arguments for the advantages of needle aspiration include procedure simplicity, patient comfort, and price.[25] Yu et al demonstrated that intermittent needle aspiration of PLA was equivalent to percutaneous catheter-based drainage. This study included 64 patients over a period of 5 years treated with intravenous antibiotics and randomized to either percutaneous catheter drain placement or percutaneous needle aspiration. The percutaneous needle aspiration group trended toward a higher treatment success rate, a shorter duration of hospital stay, and a lower mortality rate, although these findings did not reach statistical significance. O'Farrell et al reported that in 61 patients, 82% were successfully treated with percutaneous intervention for PLA, with 15% managed medically and 1 patient requiring operative intervention. In this series, there were no mortalities and the average hospital stay was 23 days.[6]

Particularly difficult subsets of patients are those with hepatobiliary malignancies, which have traditionally been associated with high failure rates for percutaneous drainage and high mortality rates in general. However, when the often-associated underlying biliary communication or obstruction is treated, percutaneous drainage becomes an effective and safe therapeutic option. Mezhir et al reported that in 51 patients with a history of actively treated pancreatic cancer, cholangiocarcinoma, or colon or gallbladder cancer, 66% of the time percutaneous drainage was successful. In the 26% of the patients who died with their drainage catheters in place, more than 60% had cancer progression and had no clinical evidence of sepsis. In this series, 9% of the patients required operative intervention and 3% died postoperatively of sepsis.[7] Predictors of failure with percutaneous drainage included abscess culture isolates containing yeast and communication of the abscess cavity with the biliary tree.[7] Although percutaneous methods are safe and effective, attention must be paid to patients worsening clinically or failing to improve, in which case surgical drainage and/or hepatic resection may be the most effective option.

SURGICAL DRAINAGE AND HEPATIC RESECTION

The role of surgical therapy for the treatment of PLA has changed dramatically since the early part of the 20th century. In Ochsner's original series,[2] surgery was the primary treatment modality; currently, however, open operation is primarily indicated for failure of medical management, failure of percutaneous drainage, and complications secondary to percutaneous treatments such as bleeding or spillage of pus into the peritoneal cavity. Primary surgical treatment may be required to treat abdominal pathology responsible for the PLA such as diverticulitis, appendicitis, and PLA rupture into the peritoneal cavity with subsequent peritonitis or an obstructed biliary tree, which cannot be treated by endoscopic or interventional means.

Traditionally, the open surgical approach to hepatic abscess is through a midline laparotomy or an extended subcostal incision. Exploration of the abdomen with control of any associated intraabdominal pathology is then performed. Localization of all hepatic abscesses with palpation of the liver and intraoperative ultrasound is performed next. At this point, it is often useful to perform needle aspiration to confirm location of the abscess and obtain material for culture and Gram stain. The area of the liver containing the abscess is then isolated from the rest of the abdomen with laparotomy sponges. The abscess cavity is then entered with electrocautery in an area that will allow it to drain in a dependent fashion. A suction catheter is then inserted into the abscess cavity to evacuate the pus and gently break up any loculations. Biopsies of the abscess wall should be obtained at this time to rule out a neoplasm as the etiology for the PLA. Drainage catheters are then placed into the abscess cavity in as dependent a position as possible to ensure adequate drainage. These catheters are brought through the abdominal wall with separate incisions. These drains can be used for drainage, irrigation, or radiologic contrast studies to ensure collapse of the abscess cavity. Omentum may also be placed in the abscess cavity as an adjunct to drain placement.

There are circumstances where single or multiple PLA is associated with severe hepatic destruction and in these instances partial hepatectomy may be the best therapeutic option. Chou et al[14] have advocated hepatic resection in these circumstances and have reported a low mortality rate in patients undergoing partial hepatectomy.[9] Likely outcomes in these particular cases are largely dependent on the underlying cause of the PLA and the general condition of the patient. Patients with underlying malignancies who require hepatectomy for liver destruction secondary to PLA generally have poor outcomes.

OUTCOMES

Mortality rates vary from series to series and typically range in North American and European series from 5.6% to 10% and worldwide from 3% to 30%. The difference likely reflects the different patient populations of the series reported and differences in the underlying disease processes responsible for the PLA. When considering the change in demographics from a younger to an older patient and the change in etiology to a patient with actively treated malignancy or biliary tract disease, it is not surprising that a recent population-based study noted increased incidence of PLA without a decrease in mortality from 1994 to 2005.[1] In this study, as could be expected, mortality was increased in elderly patients, and those with multiple medical comorbidities including cirrhosis, renal failure, sepsis, and malignancy. Interestingly, patients who were culture positive for bacteria had a negative association with mortality, suggesting the importance of early culture and speciation in guiding antimicrobial therapy. Patients who underwent percutaneous aspiration or drainage for PLA had half the mortality of patients who did not undergo drainage. Surgical drainage, however, was not associated negatively or positively with mortality.

In summary, PLA is a relatively rare condition that can have a somewhat vague initial clinical presentation and be associated with a myriad of underlying pathologies. If one suspects PLA, it is critical to rapidly obtain cultures, start appropriate antimicrobial therapy, drain the abscess, and treat any underlying disorders as PLA can have a high mortality if not promptly recognized.

AMEBIC LIVER ABSCESS

Amebiasis is a parasitic infection caused by *E. histolytica*, the third leading parasitic cause of death worldwide affecting approximately 50 million people, resulting in approximately 100,000 deaths per year. In some countries, the antibody prevalence rate exceeds 50%; in the United States, the seroprevalence is estimated at only 4%. The majority of those who are infected (90%) remain relatively asymptomatic. The liver is the most common site of extraintestinal amebiasis. The incidence of hepatic abscess in amebiasis is 3% to 9%. The long-held concept that 10% of the world's population are infected with *E. histolytica* is now thought to be incorrect. Another species, *Entamoeba dispar*, is morphologically indistinguishable from *E. histolytica* and more common in humans in many parts of the world. Similarly *Entamoeba moshkovskii*, which was long considered to be a free-living ameba, is also morphologically identical to *E. histolytica* and *E. dispar* and is highly prevalent in some *E. histolytica*–endemic countries. However, the only species to cause invasive amebiasis and clinical disease in humans is *E. histolytica*. Most older epidemiologic data on *E. histolytica* are unusable as the techniques employed do not differentiate between these three *Entamoeba* species. Molecular tools are now available not only to diagnose these species accurately but also to study intraspecies genetic diversity.[26]

DEMOGRAPHICS

The highest prevalence of amebiasis is found in developing countries, particularly in Mexico, India, Central and South America, and tropical areas of Asia and Africa. The incidence is increased in areas with high poverty and is a reflection of poor sanitation and hygiene. Risk factors for infection include travel or residence in endemic areas. In industrialized countries, risk groups include male homosexuals, travelers and recent immigrants, and institutionalized populations. There is a 7 to 12 times higher incidence in males than females despite an equal sex distribution of noninvasive colonic amebic disease among adults. Possible reasons include heavy alcohol consumption in men, hormonal effects in premenopausal women, and a possible protective effect of iron-deficiency anemia in menstruating women. Individuals in their fourth and fifth decades of life are most commonly affected. The prevalence of infection is higher than 5% to 10% in endemic areas. In a 4-year observational study of 289 preschool children in an urban slum in Bangladesh, *E. histolytica* infection was detected at least once in 80%, and repeat infection in 53%, after 4 years of observation.[27] According to the World Health Organization (WHO) in 1996, in Mexico, intestinal amebiasis ranked third as a cause for outpatient visits in 1.3 million cases (rate of 1.5 cases per 100 population) next only to respiratory infections and intestinal infectious diarrhea.

The impact of the acquired immunodeficiency syndrome (AIDS) pandemic on the prevalence of invasive amebiasis remains controversial. Although the incidence of invasive amebiasis in human immunodeficiency virus (HIV) is rare, reports suggest that ALA is an emerging parasitic infection in individuals with HIV infection in disease-endemic areas.[28] Despite immunosuppression, amebic liver abscesses and colitis responded favorably to medical treatment.[29]

ETIOLOGY AND PATHOGENESIS

Infection by *E. histolytica* occurs by ingestion of mature quadrinucleate cysts in fecally contaminated food, water,

or hands (Figure 118-5). The cysts are resistant to the acidic pH of the stomach. Excystation occurs in the alkaline pH of the small intestine and trophozoites are released, which migrate to the large intestine. The trophozoites multiply by binary fission and produce cysts (Figure 118-6). Both stages are passed in the feces and the cysts can survive days to weeks in the external environment. However, trophozoites passed in the stool are rapidly destroyed once outside the body, and if ingested would not survive exposure to the gastric environment. In many cases, the trophozoites remain confined to the intestinal lumen of individuals who are asymptomatic carriers, passing cysts in their stool. Depending on the genetic and immunoenzymatic profile, and the parasite's

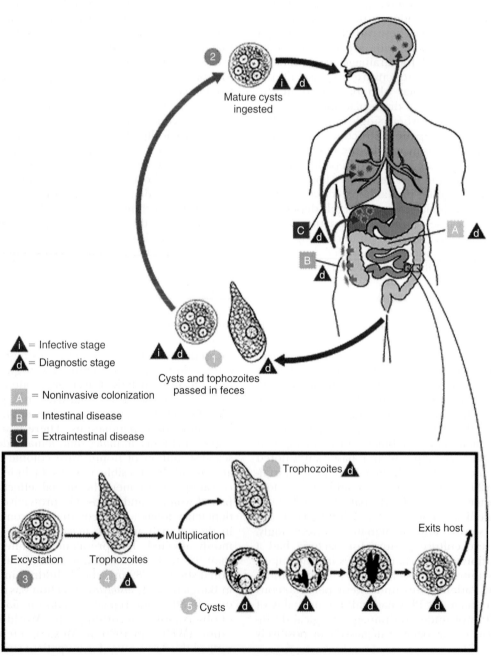

FIGURE 118-5 Lifecycle of *Entamoeba histolytica*. (From US Centers for Disease Control and Prevention. http://www.dpd.cdc.gov/dpdx/HTML/Amebiasis.htm.)

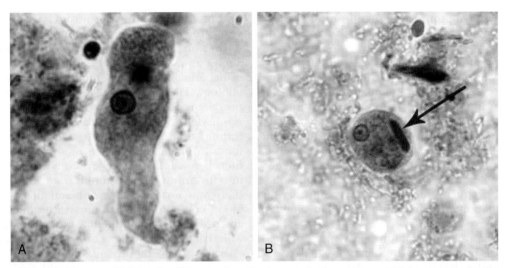

FIGURE 118-6 **A,** *Entamoeba histolytica/Entamoeba dispar* trophozoites have a single nucleus, which has a centrally placed karyosome and uniformly distributed peripheral chromatin. **B,** Mature *E. histolytica/E. dispar* cysts have four nuclei that characteristically have centrally located karyosomes and fine, uniformly distributed peripheral chromatin. Cysts usually measure 12 to 15 μm. (From US Centers for Disease Control and Prevention. http://www.dpd.cdc.gov/dpdx/HTML/ImageLibrary/Amebiasis_il.htm.)

ability to produce proteolytic enzymes and resist complement-mediated lysis, the trophozoite becomes virulent and starts its invasion of the intestinal mucosa. Spread is usually through the portal venous radicles to the liver. The hepatic lesion is usually solitary and most frequently is located in the right lobe. In some cases, it may occupy more than 80% of the whole liver surface. This may be explained by the larger volume of the right lobe, which receives most of the venous drainage from the right colon, a segment of the bowel frequently affected by intestinal amebiasis. Lesions of the left lobe are less common, and occasionally multiple abscesses may occur in advanced cases.

Amebic-induced lysis of neutrophils at the edge of the lesion releases cytotoxic mediators leading to hepatocyte death, extending the damage to distant hepatic cells and thereby increasing the number of small lesions that coalesce to develop a larger ALA. The content of its central cavity is a thick, viscous exudate. This is generally homogeneous, and varies in color, ranging from creamy white to dirty brown and pink, which is often described as "anchovy paste" (Figure 118-7). This material is almost always sterile, except when a secondary infection has occurred, allowing differential diagnosis from a pyogenic abscess. The amebae can be found at the edge of the lesion but are rarely detected in the pus or within the abscess cavity itself.

IMMUNOPATHOLOGY

During the establishment of infection, *E. histolytica* confronts a series of innate host defenses, such as the intestinal epithelial barrier, leukocytes, and the complement system.[30] While the host cells elaborate diverse mechanisms of defense, amebae have also developed complex strategies to evade host defenses and facilitate their own survival.[31]

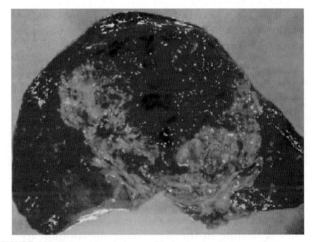

FIGURE 118-7 Amebic abscess. Photograph of a gross liver specimen shows an amebic abscess filled with a chocolate-colored, pasty material (anchovy paste). (From Mortele KJ, Segatto E, Ros PR: The infected liver: Radiologic-pathologic correlation. *Radiographics* 24:937, 2004.)

The early stage of the ALA lesion is characterized by a dominant infiltration of polymorphonuclear leukocytes surrounding the trophozoites. In later stages of ALA formation, usually occurring after 3 days, lymphocytes, macrophages, and epithelioid cells are recruited to the developing lesion, which leads to the formation of granuloma. This process contributes to the confinement of invading trophozoites.

CLINICAL PRESENTATION

Most patients with amebiasis are asymptomatic and clear their infection without any sign of disease. Clinical amebiasis usually has a subacute presentation, which occurs over 1 to 3 weeks. Symptoms can range from mild diarrhea to severe dysentery with abdominal pain. High-grade fever and right upper quadrant abdominal pain are the main presenting symptoms in ALA, and a history of gastroenteritis is often noted. Pleuritic and right scapular pain are present if the diaphragmatic surface of the liver is involved with or is close to the abscess. It is important to distinguish ALA from PLA because their treatment and prognosis differ. In a retrospective review of 577 adults with liver abscesses, 82% of whom had amebic abscesses, patients with amebic abscess were more likely to be young males with a tender, solitary, right-lobe abscess.[32] This is frequently accompanied by a history of diarrhea and abdominal pain/tenderness, and amebic serology titers above 1:256 IU.

Jaundice is relatively uncommon and if present is a marker of abscess erosion into the biliary tract. Varying incidence of jaundice has been reported in patients with ALA. The most commonly accepted pathogenetic mechanism is obstruction of the biliary system by the abscess. Multiple, large abscesses, especially on the inferior surface of the liver, have also been directly related to elevation of serum bilirubin levels. The prolonged duration and poor response to drug therapy allow the abscess to enlarge; compress biliary radicles, producing jaundice; and finally penetrate the tough fibrous vasculobiliary sheath that surrounds the portal triad structures, with resultant biliary communication.

LABORATORY FINDINGS

Light microscopic examination of fecal specimens is often the first step in diagnosis.[33] In the stages of dysentery/amebic colitis, trophozoites are readily detected in submucosal tissue or fecal samples by permanent stains. Submission of three stool specimens on different days over a period of 10 days is recommended. Because *E. histolytica* invades the colonic mucosa, feces are almost universally positive for occult blood. The presence of Charcot-Leyden crystals and blood is the most common finding in the acute stage. In addition to the red blood cells, macrophages and polymorphonuclear cells can also be seen on microscopy in cases of amebic dysentery. Microscopy alone cannot differentiate *E. histolytica* from *E. dispar* and *E. moshkovskii*, and additional tests are required for definitive speciation. Identification methods include biopsy, serology, antigen detection, and molecular assays.

Diagnosis of liver abscess is confirmed by a positive serologic test, as amebic serology is highly sensitive (>94%) and highly specific (>95%). A false-negative serologic test can be obtained early during infection (within the first 7 to 10 days), but a repeat test is usually positive. Many different assays have been developed for the detection of antibodies, including indirect hemagglutination assay (IHA), latex agglutination, immunoelectrophoresis, counterimmunoelectrophoresis (CIE), the amebic gel diffusion test, immunodiffusion, complement fixation, indirect immunofluorescence assay (IFA), and enzyme-linked immunosorbent assay (ELISA). Of these, ELISA is the most popular assay throughout the world and has been used to study the epidemiology of asymptomatic disease. Serum IgG antibodies persist for years after *E. histolytica* infection.

In nonendemic areas, a positive amebic serology almost always reflects acute infection, and in the setting of hepatic abscess is essentially diagnostic of an amebic etiology. However, in regions where amebiasis is very prevalent, positive serology does not carry the same diagnostic yield. Serologic IHA titers usually become negative within 1 year of acute infection, but may remain elevated for 5 to 6 years after cure in some patients. Serologic titers below 1:256 IU were predictive of pyogenic abscess in both univariate and multivariate analyses.[32] Although there was no difference between the peripheral white blood cell counts in patients with amebic or pyogenic abscesses, hypoalbuminemia was more severe in those with bacterial abscess. Lodhi et al found serum liver enzymes to be of no value in distinguishing between amebic and pyogenic abscess, although bacterial abscesses may be more frequently associated with greater elevations of serum alanine transferase and alkaline phosphatase.[32]

Polymerase chain reaction (PCR)–based approaches are the method of choice for clinical and epidemiologic studies in the developed countries and are endorsed by the WHO.[33] *E. histolytica* can be identified in a variety of clinical specimens, including feces, tissues, and liver abscess aspirate. They offer the highest sensitivity and specificity and can also differentiate between the various *Entamoeba* species.

IMAGING

Chest radiographic examination is abnormal in 50% of the cases, showing elevated right hemidiaphragm, subdiaphragmatic air-fluid levels, pleural effusions, and consolidating infiltrates. Ultrasonography reveals hypoechoic and well-defined lesions with rounded edges and has a diagnostic accuracy of 90%.[34] CT is more sensitive in detecting hepatic abscesses and contiguous organ extension and is the imaging study of choice (Figure 118-8). CT and MRI also allow for better detection of smaller lesions. All three techniques may facilitate guided needle biopsy and drainage if indicated. An abscess can usually be distinguished from solid lesions and biliary tract disease, but the differentiation between bacterial and amebic abscesses is less clear. Gallium scans (a rarely used test in the current era) may have a role in this differential diagnosis because amebic abscesses are usually "cold" on scan because of the lack of white blood cells in the abscess, whereas bacterial abscesses are typically "hot."

The average time to radiologic resolution is 3 to 9 months and can take as long as years in some patients. Studies have shown that more than 90% of the visible lesions disappear radiologically, but a small percentage of patients are left with a clinically irrelevant residual lesion.[35]

SITES OF AMEBIC ABSCESSES

The liver is the most common site of extraintestinal amebiasis. *E. histolytica* also has been reported to cause brain abscesses from hematogenous spread. Cerebral

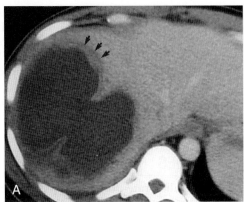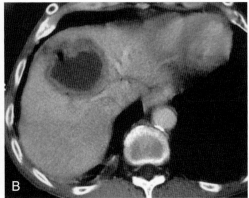

FIGURE 118-8 Amebic abscess. **A,** Contrast-enhanced CT scan demonstrates a large, lobulated, well-defined cystic mass in the right hepatic lobe. Note the enhanced, thickened wall of the lesion *(arrows).* **B,** Contrast-enhanced CT scan obtained in a different patient shows a rounded, well-defined low-attenuation lesion in the right hepatic lobe with a small focus of air and mild hyperemia of the adjacent liver parenchyma. (From Mortele KJ, Segatto E, Ros PR: The infected liver: Radiologic-pathologic correlation. *Radiographics* 24:937, 2004.)

amebiasis has an abrupt onset and rapid progression to death in 12 to 72 hours. Presentation is with altered consciousness and focal neurologic signs. CT scanning reveals irregular lesions without a surrounding capsule or enhancement. A tissue biopsy sample reveals the trophozoites. Amebomas are localized masses of infected granulation tissue in the intestine whose appearance can mimic colon cancers, and these masses can extend to involve the perianal skin. There is even a report of a rectovaginal fistula developing from an ameboma. A case of duodenal ameboma involving the second and third portions of the duodenum, causing gastrointestinal bleeding, has been reported. Rare presentation of amebiasis as acute appendicitis has also been reported.

AMEBIC LIVER ABSCESS IN CHILDREN

Pyogenic abscesses constitute the majority of hepatic abscesses in children. Studies suggest that amebic abscesses are rare in children. The treatment of amebic liver abscess in children is by amebicides. Metronidazole is currently the amebicide of choice. All uncomplicated ALAs can be managed medically and do not require aspiration. Rupture of an ALA is relatively rare in children. Surgical drainage is necessary when the abscess has ruptured. Porras-Ramirez et al conducted a study that determined criteria for percutaneous aspiration, which included the following: no clinical improvement, the abscess is 6 cm or more in diameter, and the patient is septic, or there is imminent risk of rupture.[36] Sharma et al suggest surgical drainage for (1) children who have failed percutaneous drainage, (2) those who require management for an underlying abdominal problem, (3) selected patients with multiple macroscopic abscesses, (4) those on steroids, and (5) patients with ascites.[37]

TREATMENT

The mainstay of treatment for uncomplicated amebic hepatic abscesses are amebicidal drugs (Table 118-5). The discovery of systemic amebicides, mainly in the

TABLE 118-5 Treatment of Amebic Liver Abscess

Drug treatment	Uncomplicated amebic hepatic abscess
	Both amebic colitis and liver abscess— nitroimidazole derivatives (e.g., metronidazole)
	Amebic colitis—luminal agents such as paromomycin, diloxanide furoate, iodoquinol
Percutaneous drainage	Deterioration in clinical condition despite adequate treatment
	Bacterial superinfection
	Abscess with high risk of rupture
Surgery	Ruptured abscess
	Impending rupture
	Inadequate catheter drainage

nitroimidazole group, with high tissue diffusion, and enhanced capability to cross the wall and reach the interior of the abscess at a very high concentration (four times the minimum inhibitory concentration [MIC] for *E. histolytica*), have been responsible for a dramatic change in the treatment of invasive amebiasis, reducing complications and therefore mortality. The drugs of choice for amebic colitis and amebic liver abscess include nitroimidazole derivatives (metronidazole, tinidazole, and ornidazole), of which only metronidazole is available in the United States. It is given in doses of 750 mg three times a day by mouth or intravenously for 5 to 10 days. It is activated in anaerobic organisms by reduction, and when activated damages DNA. The main side effects include metallic aftertaste, nausea, vomiting, and diarrhea. Dehydroemetine is an additional drug that inhibits protein synthesis and is mainly used in fulminant colitis or patients with ruptured ALA when administered in combination with metronidazole, but controlled trials are lacking. The drugs for amebic colitis include luminal agents such as paromomycin, which is the drug of choice; diloxanide furoate; and iodoquinol. The conventional indications for percutaneous drainage include deterioration in clinical condition on adequate treatment, bacterial superinfection, and an abscess having a high risk of rupture, whereas surgery is reserved for patients with ruptured abscess, impending rupture, or inadequate drainage through a catheter.

In a retrospective analysis of 966 patients, 68% of whom had ALAs, the predictive factors for aspiration of liver abscess included age 55 years or older, size 5 cm or more, involvement of both lobes of the liver, and duration of symptoms of at least 7 days. Hospital stay in the aspiration group was longer than that in the nonaspiration group, and no statistically significant difference in mortality was observed between the two groups.[38]

A metaanalysis of seven low-quality randomized trials was performed.[39] Pooled analysis of three homogeneous trials showed that needle aspiration did not significantly increase the proportion of patients with fever resolution. The benefits in the number of days to resolution of pain, number of days to resolution of abdominal tenderness, and duration of hospitalization were observed in the needle aspiration group only. However, the value of therapeutic aspiration in addition to metronidazole to hasten clinical or radiologic resolution of uncomplicated ALAs cannot be supported or refuted by the current evidence. A prospective study of 200 patients with confirmed ALA comparing ultrasound-guided needle aspiration and medications to drug treatment alone showed initial response (after 15 days) being better in the aspirated group, but resolution of abscess after 6 months was similar. This rapid clinical response was particularly noted in those with larger (>6 cm) abscesses and there were no complications.[40]

One of the reasons for nonresolution of amebic abscesses seems to be the presence of communication with the biliary tree. In a study of 13 patients who underwent catheter drainage of ALA with persistent drainage after the procedure probably due to abscess–biliary communication, therapeutic endoscopic retrograde cholangiopancreatography was done with sphincterotomy followed by placement of either a pigtail biliary stent or a nasobiliary drain. The procedure resulted in decrease in drainage in 48 hours, and in 11 of 13 patients, the drainage catheter was removed by 1 week and after 10 days in the remaining 2 patients. Clinical improvement and significant decrease was noted in the volume of the abscess cavity, and no recurrence of abscess was noted after 9 to 25 months of followup.[41]

Patients with abscesses communicating with the biliary tree presented more frequently with jaundice (67% vs. 0%), with a longer duration of illness (median, 20 vs. 12 days), had larger lesions, and required catheter drainage for longer periods (median, 17 vs. 6.5 days).[42]

COMPLICATIONS

The failure of medical therapy for amebic liver abscess may be heralded by abscess perforation, a complication associated with high mortality. Rupture into the thorax or abdomen are the most common. Factors used to predict rupture include diameter 5 to 10 cm, progressive increase in size, and left lobe location. Rupture into the peritoneal cavity occurs in 18% to 70% of cases. Amebic pericarditis accounts for 4% of all extraintestinal amebiasis, with a mortality rate of approximately 30%. Other rare complications of ALA include hepatic vein and inferior vena cava thrombosis. Bacterial superinfection, anemia, acute respiratory distress syndrome (ARDS), and sepsis also can develop in severe cases.

OUTCOMES

The mortality rate for all patients with amebic liver abscess is about 5% and does not appear to be affected by the addition of aspiration to metronidazole therapy or chronicity of symptoms. For ruptured abscess, the mortality rate is reported to be from 6% to as high as 50%. Factors independently associated with poor outcome are elevated serum bilirubin (>3.5 mg/dL), encephalopathy, hypoalbuminemia (<2.0 g/dL), multiple abscess cavities, abscess volume greater than 500 mL, anemia, and diabetes.[43] Followup imaging should be used to monitor response to therapy; continue treatment until CT scan shows complete or near-complete resolution of cavity. Using PCR-based method of genotyping, Ali et al found that parasite genome might play a role in determining the outcome of infection with *E. histolytica*.[44]

In summary, amebiasis is a disease of high prevalence and morbidity in developing countries. In industrialized nations, risk groups include male homosexuals, travelers and recent immigrants, and institutionalized populations. ALA is the commonest manifestation of extraintestinal amebiasis. Presentation of ALA varies from PLA in that patients with ALA are more likely to be young males with tender, solitary right-lobe abscess. Presence of jaundice is more common in PLA and if present in ALA is indicative of biliary tract obstruction or abscess erosion into the biliary tract. Patients are also more likely to have a history of fever, right upper quadrant abdominal pain, and diarrhea. Tender hepatomegaly is twice as common in ALA compared with PLA, and amebic serology titers above 1:256 IU are diagnostic (Tables 118-6 and 118-7). Amebic serology is highly sensitive and specific as a diagnostic tool. Ultrasonographic and CT scans have good diagnostic accuracy and also facilitate needle biopsy and drainage if needed. PCR-based studies can also differentiate between various *Entamoeba* species. Most patients with uncomplicated ALA can be treated with medical management alone. This is in contrast to PLA, which is usually treated with percutaneous drainage. Drainage procedures should be reserved for those patients who do not respond to medical therapy, whose abscess appears to have a high likelihood of rupture, or those whose diagnosis is in question. Surgical procedures are used for patients who fail these management approaches or experience complications of the abscess, such as peritoneal rupture or empyema. Prevention efforts would include improvement of sanitation and hygiene, use of safe sexual practices, etc. Vaccination strategies especially with recombinant antigens are being studied as well.

TABLE 118-6 Selected Signs and Symptoms in Series Comparing Pyogenic and Amebic Hepatic Abscesses*

	CONTER ET AL, 1986[45] (UNIVERSITY OF CALIFORNIA, LOS ANGELES): DATA PERIOD 1968-1983		BARNES ET AL, 1987[46] (UNIVERSITY OF SOUTHERN CALIFORNIA, LOS ANGELES): DATA PERIOD 1979-1985		LODHI ET AL, 2004[32] (KARACHI, PAKISTAN): DATA PERIOD 1988-1998	
	Pyogenic Abscess	*Amebic Abscess*	*Pyogenic Abscess*	*Amebic Abscess*	*Pyogenic Abscess*	*Amebic Abscess*
STUDY DESCRIPTORS						
No. of cases	42	40	48	96	106	471
Age (yr, mean)	46.5	37.6	44	28	51	40
Male-to-female ratio	2.5:1.0	3.4:1.0	1.4:1.0	18.2:1.0	2.9:1.0	6.1:1.0
SYMPTOMS						
Fever (%)	88	93	77	87	48	67
Abdominal pain (%)	64	93	66	90 ($P < 0.001$)	N/A	N/A
Diarrhea (%)	12	60 ($P < 0.005$)	32	35	22	30
Symptom duration (%)	N/A	N/A	63 <14 d 37 >14 d	86 <14 d 14 >14 d	N/A	N/A
Nausea/vomiting (%)	31	50	62/43	85/32	N/A	N/A
SIGNS						
Abdominal tenderness (%)	50	75	42	67	77	87
Jaundice (%)	36	5	22	10	43	32
Shock/sepsis (%)	26	0	N/A	N/A	N/A	N/A
Hepatomegaly (%)	26	53	18	25	67	74

N/A, Not available.
*Listed *P* value indicates significant difference between pyogenic and amebic abscesses in that specific study.

TABLE 118-7 Selected Laboratory Parameters in Series Comparing Pyogenic and Amebic Hepatic Abscesses*

Laboratory Parameter	CONTER ET AL, 1986[45] (UNIVERSITY OF CALIFORNIA, LOS ANGELES): DATA PERIOD 1968-1983		BARNES ET AL, 1987[46] (UNIVERSITY OF SOUTHERN CALIFORNIA, LOS ANGELES): DATA PERIOD 1979-1985		LODHI ET AL, 2004[32] (KARACHI, PAKISTAN): DATA PERIOD 1988-1998	
	Pyogenic Abscess	*Amebic Abscess*	*Pyogenic Abscess*	*Amebic Abscess*	*Pyogenic Abscess*	*Amebic Abscess*
Amebic serology (% positive)	0	95	4	94	33	72
Mean alkaline phosphate or % with elevation	319 IU	198 IU	50% > 220 U/L	35% > 220 U/L	236 IU	211 IU
Mean total bilirubin or % elevated	4.1 mg/dL	0.9 mg/dL	15%	2% ($P < 0.005$)	2.4 mg/dL	1.9 mg/dL
Albumin level or % with hypoalbuminemia	2.7 g/dL	2.9 g/dL	50%	16%	2.1 g/dL	2.4 g/dL
WBC × 10³/mm³ or % elevation > 10³/mm³	13.4	13.5	91%	92%	18.9	19.1

WBC, White blood cell.
*Listed *P* value indicates difference between pyogenic and amebic hepatic abscesses.

REFERENCES

1. Meddings L, Myers RP, Hubbard J, et al: A population-based study of pyogenic liver abscesses in the United States: Incidence, mortality, and temporal trends. *Am J Gastroenterol* 105:117, 2010.
2. Ochsner A, DeBakey M, Murray S: Pyogenic abscess of the liver. *Am J Surg* 40:292, 1988.
3. McFadzean AJ, Chang KP, Wong CC: Solitary pyogenic abscess of the liver treated by closed aspiration and antibiotics; a report of 14 consecutive cases with recovery. *Br J Surg* 41:141, 1953.
4. Bertel CK, van Heerden JA, Sheedy PF 2nd: Treatment of pyogenic hepatic abscesses. Surgical vs percutaneous drainage. *Arch Surg* 121:554, 1986.
5. Branum GD, Tyson GS, Branum MA, et al: Hepatic abscess. Changes in etiology, diagnosis, and management. *Ann Surg* 212:655, 1990.
6. O'Farrell N, Collins CG, McEntee GP: Pyogenic liver abscesses: Diminished role for operative treatment. *Surgeon* 8:192, 2010.
7. Mezhir JJ, Fong Y, Jacks LM, et al: Current management of pyogenic liver abscess: Surgery is now second-line treatment. *J Am Coll Surg* 210:975, 2010.
8. Pitt HA, Zuidema GD: Factors influencing mortality in the treatment of pyogenic hepatic abscess. *Surg Gynecol Obstet* 140:228, 1975.
9. Seeto RK, Rockey DC: Pyogenic liver abscess. Changes in etiology, management, and outcome. *Medicine (Baltimore)* 75:99, 1996.
10. Huang CJ, Pitt HA, Lipsett PA, et al: Pyogenic hepatic abscess. Changing trends over 42 years. *Ann Surg* 223:600; discussion 607, 1996.
11. Alvarez JA, Gonzalez JJ, Baldonedo RF, et al: Single and multiple pyogenic liver abscesses: Etiology, clinical course, and outcome. *Dig Surg* 18:283, 2001.
12. Mohsen AH, Green ST, Read RC, et al: Liver abscess in adults: Ten years experience in a UK centre. *QJM* 95:797, 2002.
13. Wong WM, Wong BC, Hui CK, et al: Pyogenic liver abscess: Retrospective analysis of 80 cases over a 10-year period. *J Gastroenterol Hepatol* 17:1001, 2002.
14. Chou FF, Sheen-Chen SM, Chen YS, et al: Single and multiple pyogenic liver abscesses: Clinical course, etiology, and results of treatment. *World J Surg* 21:384; discussion 388, 1997.
15. Chu KM, Fan ST, Lai EC, et al: Pyogenic liver abscess. An audit of experience over the past decade. *Arch Surg* 131:148, 1996.
16. Saini S: Imaging of the hepatobiliary tract. *N Engl J Med* 336:1889, 1997.
17. Benedetti NJ, Desser TS, Jeffrey RB: Imaging of hepatic infections. *Ultrasound Q* 24:267, 2008.
18. Alvarez Perez JA, Gonzalez JJ, Baldonedo RF, et al: Clinical course, treatment, and multivariate analysis of risk factors for pyogenic liver abscess. *Am J Surg* 181:177, 2001.
19. Rahimian J, Wilson T, Oram V, et al: Pyogenic liver abscess: Recent trends in etiology and mortality. *Clin Infect Dis* 39:1654, 2004.
20. Wang JH, Liu YC, Lee SS, et al: Primary liver abscess due to *Klebsiella pneumoniae* in Taiwan. *Clin Infect Dis* 26:1434, 1998.
21. Sabbaj J, Sutter VL, Finegold SM: Anaerobic pyogenic liver abscess. *Ann Intern Med* 77:627, 1972.
22. Chemaly RF, Hall GS, Keys TF, et al: Microbiology of liver abscesses and the predictive value of abscess Gram stain and associated blood cultures. *Diagn Microbiol Infect Dis* 46:245, 2003.
23. Johannsen EC, Sifri CD, Madoff LC: Pyogenic liver abscesses. *Infect Dis Clin North Am* 14:547, 2000.
24. Ng FH, Wong WM, Wong BC, et al: Sequential intravenous/oral antibiotic vs. continuous intravenous antibiotic in the treatment of pyogenic liver abscess. *Aliment Pharmacol Ther* 16:1083, 2002.
25. Yu SC, Ho SS, Lau WY, et al: Treatment of pyogenic liver abscess: Prospective randomized comparison of catheter drainage and needle aspiration. *Hepatology* 39:932, 2004.
26. Ali IK, Clark CG, Petri WA Jr: Molecular epidemiology of amebiasis. *Infect Genet Evol* 8:698, 2008.
27. Haque R, Mondal D, Duggal P, et al: *Entamoeba histolytica* infection in children and protection from subsequent amebiasis. *Infect Immun* 74:904, 2006.
28. Hung CC, Chen PJ, Hsieh SM, et al: Invasive amoebiasis: An emerging parasitic disease in patients infected with HIV in an area endemic for amoebic infection. *AIDS* 13:2421, 1999.
29. Hung CC, Ji DD, Sun HY, et al: Increased risk for *Entamoeba histolytica* infection and invasive amebiasis in HIV seropositive men who have sex with men in Taiwan. *PLoS Negl Trop Dis* 2:e175, 2008.
30. Guo X, Houpt E, Petri WA Jr: Crosstalk at the initial encounter: Interplay between host defense and ameba survival strategies. *Curr Opin Immunol* 19:376, 2007.
31. Santi-Rocca J, Rigothier MC, Guillen N: Host-microbe interactions and defense mechanisms in the development of amoebic liver abscesses. *Clin Microbiol Rev* 22:65, 2009.
32. Lodhi S, Sarwari AR, Muzammil M, et al: Features distinguishing amoebic from pyogenic liver abscess: A review of 577 adult cases. *Trop Med Int Health* 9:718, 2004.
33. Fotedar R, Stark D, Beebe N, et al: Laboratory diagnostic techniques for *Entamoeba* species. *Clin Microbiol Rev* 20:511, 2007.
34. Reid-Lombardo KM, Khan S, Sclabas G: Hepatic cysts and liver abscess. *Surg Clin North Am* 90:679, 2010.
35. Blessmann J, Khoa ND, Van An L, et al: Ultrasound patterns and frequency of focal liver lesions after successful treatment of amoebic liver abscess. *Trop Med Int Health* 11:504, 2006.
36. Porras-Ramirez G, Hernandez-Herrera MH, Porras-Hernandez JD: Amebic hepatic abscess in children. *J Pediatr Surg* 30:662, 1995.
37. Sharma MP, Kumar A: Liver abscess in children. *Indian J Pediatr* 73:813, 2006.
38. Khan R, Hamid S, Abid S, et al: Predictive factors for early aspiration in liver abscess. *World J Gastroenterol* 14:2089, 2008.
39. Chavez-Tapia NC, Hernandez-Calleros J, Tellez-Avila FI, et al: Image-guided percutaneous procedure plus metronidazole versus metronidazole alone for uncomplicated amoebic liver abscess. *Cochrane Database Syst Rev* 1:CD004886, 2009.
40. Ramani A, Ramani R, Kumar MS, et al: Ultrasound-guided needle aspiration of amoebic liver abscess. *Postgrad Med J* 69:381, 1993.
41. Sandeep SM, Banait VS, Thakur SK, et al: Endoscopic biliary drainage in patients with amebic liver abscess and biliary communication. *Indian J Gastroenterol* 25:125, 2006.
42. Agarwal DK, Baijal SS, Roy S, et al: Percutaneous catheter drainage of amebic liver abscesses with and without intrahepatic biliary communication: A comparative study. *Eur J Radiol* 20:61, 1995.
43. Hughes MA, Petri WA Jr: Amebic liver abscess. *Infect Dis Clin North Am* 14:565, 2000.
44. Ali IK, Mondal U, Roy S, et al: Evidence for a link between parasite genotype and outcome of infection with *Entamoeba histolytica*. *J Clin Microbiol* 45:285, 2007.
45. Conter RL, Pitt HA, Tompkins RK, et al: Differentiation of pyogenic from amebic hepatic abscesses. *Surg Gynecol Obstet* 162:114, 1986.
46. Barnes PF, De Cock KM, Reynolds TN, et al: A comparison of amebic and pyogenic abscess of the liver. *Medicine (Baltimore)* 66:472, 1987.

Management of Hepatobiliary Trauma

Jason Smith | J. David Richardson

Injuries to the liver are quite common and have been reported to occur in 35% to 45% of patients with severe abdominal trauma. Throughout the past century, the treatment of hepatic injuries has often been a divisive and contentious issue in the management of the trauma patient.[1] Changes from nonoperative management for blunt trauma in the early part of the 20th century to aggressive operative treatment after World War II with a more recent return to the frequent use of nonoperative strategies have led to significant confusion over the appropriate method of treating hepatobiliary trauma. With improved modalities for abdominal imaging and acceptance of nonoperative management for blunt injuries in the modern era, the primary focus for the surgeon has shifted to the selection of appropriate patients for this type of treatment with operative options reserved for failure of observational strategies. The treatment of penetrating hepatic injuries has generally remained standard with reliance on an operative approach.

HISTORICAL PERSPECTIVE

FROM ANTIQUITY TO WORLD WAR II

To understand the controversies and contemporary management of hepatobiliary trauma, an examination of the historical management of these injuries is informative. Although most of the major advances in the treatment of patients with liver injuries have taken place in the past century, there is significant historical literature describing hepatobiliary injuries. Some of the first descriptions of liver injuries and their treatment can be traced back to both Greek and Arabic medical literature near the turn of the first millennium. However, the first successful treatment of a liver injury is attributed to Hildanus in the early 17th century. Hildanus described a young man who had been stabbed in the abdomen with resultant severe hemorrhage. A large piece of liver that eviscerated through the wound was removed and cauterized, and the patient subsequently recovered. Otis[2] painstakingly reviewed Civil War injuries in which he documented 37 individuals who recovered after gunshot wounds (GSWs) of the liver. Twenty-three of these cases were complicated by injury of other viscera in the abdomen. Bruns treated a GSW of the liver by resection of the lacerated portion in 1870. In 1902, Beck summed up various treatment methodologies for liver injuries, including the use of cautery to treat hemorrhage and ligature of some vessels that continued bleeding after cauterization. In 1904, Tilton[3] reported on 189 injuries of the liver, emphasizing that wounds to the liver are very frequently associated with concomitant injuries to other visceral organs. One of his most important observations noted, "there are

many mild cases of laceration of the liver to go onto recovery without complications and with very few symptoms. The number of these cases is, I think, larger than is generally supposed." Tilton's review of the literature at that time showed that injury of the liver was associated with a 78.1% mortality if the wound was caused by blunt forces, 39% if caused by GSWs, and 37.5% if caused by stab wounds. In addition, he reviewed all of the New York hospitals with large accident services over a 10-year period and found there were 25 liver injuries: 12 were caused by blunt injuries, 9 by GSWs, and 4 by stab wounds, with an overall mortality of 44%. Twenty of the 25 patients were operated on, with a mortality of 40%. In his paper, he discussed current therapy of the day and acknowledged that some surgeons recommended nonoperative management. Tilton stated, "This seems a wrong principle to work on. Many cases might recover without interference but others will prove fatal from oversight, an intestinal perforation or foreign body or from insufficient drainage of the wound in the liver." He also made the point that the surgeon "has no choice" but to operate on those patients with aggressive symptoms of internal hemorrhage. His recommended method of stopping hemorrhage was to use sutures or gauze packing. He stated "the thermal cautery is of very little value in arresting hemorrhage from the liver." His opinion on the treatment of these injuries would shape the management of hepatobiliary injuries for the next 75 years.

Despite these early advances, hepatobiliary trauma during the first half of the 20th century was marked by high morbidity and mortality, with reported mortality for patients with liver injuries during World War I being greater than 66%. Packing of liver wounds was frequently practiced and often resulted in perihepatic sepsis. However, during World War II, major advances in resuscitation, anesthetic techniques, early operation, hemorrhage control, establishment of liver drainage, and use of antibiotics reduced the mortality rate. In their book *Trauma to the Liver*, which referenced their World War II experience, Madding and Kennedy[4] stated that "before the war, house surgeons advocated expectant or conservative treatment, or no treatment at all for the majority of wounds of the liver.... Peritonitis, hepatitis, fistulas and numerous other complications often followed this form of treatment." In an 18-month period during the later part of World War II, they cared for 829 wounds of the liver in 3154 patients with abdominal and thoracoabdominal wounds. Overall mortality was reduced to 27%, a significant improvement because of the use of drainage and "aggressive resectional debridement" as needed. They further stated that "use of packing either with gauze or absorbable hemostatic agents should be avoided, except for temporary purposes." The work of these authors brought the notion of uniform drainage as a standard of care to the forefront and in the years following World War II; celiotomy to establish drainage alone was the rule. The lessons that were advocated for the next four decades could be summarized as follows: (1) most patients with liver wounds require operation, (2) all wounds should be drained, (3) hepatic tissue should be judiciously debrided, and (4) liver packing should not be performed.

POST–WORLD WAR II: THE ERA OF AGGRESSIVE SURGICAL MANAGEMENT

Following World War II, the mortality from hepatic injuries decreased greatly.[5,6] Much of that decrease was due to a decline in death from infection. Although many authors attributed this to uniform hepatic drainage, it was likely due to several factors, including earlier transport, better resuscitation, advances in antibiotic therapy, and improved supportive care. A 36-year view of liver injury mortality from the Ben Taub Hospital in Houston, Texas, noted that the mortality declined from 20.6% in 1939 to 9.2% by the early 1970s.[7] However, as highway speeds increased and civilian GSWs became more prevalent, deaths from infection were supplanted to a large extent by deaths from hemorrhage. From the 1960s to the early 1990s, a series of aggressive operative maneuvers were employed to treat liver injuries.[8-11] These included major hepatic resections including hepatic lobectomy, hepatic artery ligation for hemorrhage control, atriocaval shunting, tractomy to expose deep bleeding, and a variety of other aggressive operative strategies. Although all of these still have a place in the treatment of major hepatic injuries, their use is now much less common than 20 years ago. These techniques are now generally used only for the difficult case rather than as a routine practice.

By the 1960s, there was a great concern about missed abdominal injuries, and the diagnosis of solid organ disruption by physical examination alone was widely recognized as inadequate. The development of diagnostic peritoneal lavage (DPL) solved this dilemma by providing a rapid means of determining the presence of blood within the abdomen. This technique was an extremely valuable diagnostic tool in the pre-CT era and it had an extremely high sensitivity for intraperitoneal blood. However, it was fraught with a low specificity for patients actually requiring therapeutic maneuvers at operation and a high incidence of nontherapeutic celiotomies.

At the other end of the spectrum, the aforementioned aggressive operative strategies often failed to prevent deaths from hemorrhage. Even if operative treatment was prompt and efficient, the vascularity of the liver was such that ongoing bleeding not amenable to control by standard maneuvers often occurred. Deaths from ongoing bleeding often followed the cascade of major hemorrhage, rapid development of coagulopathy due to loss of clotting factors and hypothermia.

By the 1990s it was recognized that there were two distinct problems in the management of hepatic injuries; many patients were receiving operations that were not therapeutic and some patients had bleeding that could not be controlled by standard surgical maneuvers alone.[12] The former problems will be further addressed in the section on nonoperative management, whereas the latter will be discussed under damage control strategies.

INITIAL EVALUATION

The assessment and resuscitation of trauma patients undergoing evaluation for hepatobiliary injury are initially no different than for any other injured patient. General principles of the Advanced Trauma Life Support Program as promulgated by the American College of Surgeons should be followed and the response to resuscitation monitored. Special attention is paid to the patient's abdominal examination, vital signs, and response to resuscitation. The specific goals of the initial resuscitation in all patients entail (1) determining, in an efficient manner, the presence of potentially life-threatening injuries; (2) assessing the hemodynamic stability of the patient; and (3) initiating a therapeutic plan that is based on the initial response to resuscitation and findings on the initial surgeon-performed ultrasound, DPL, or abdominal computed tomography (CT) scan. The response to resuscitation serves as an early decision point in the initial treatment of patients with hepatobiliary injuries.

EVALUATION

The evaluation of the patient will be dependent to a considerable degree on the mechanism of injury. Patients with GSWs that enter the peritoneal cavity will require a celiotomy in virtually all circumstances. There are a few highly selected reports of a small number of patients with hepatic GSW that are followed without operation, but this treatment in no way constitutes the standard of care (see later discussion). In addition to concerns about the liver injury itself, the risk of associated intraperitoneal injury is so high that celiotomy should generally be practiced. Hemodynamically stable patients with stab wounds can often be followed if their physical examination is unremarkable, with operative treatment reserved for those with a change in their clinical status.

Patients who sustain blunt trauma and have hemodynamic instability or signs of peritonitis on examination are candidates for urgent operative intervention. However, with the exception of shock, blunt hepatic trauma rarely causes findings on physical examination that mandate the need for surgical exploration. Bruising over the right thoracoabdominal area may suggest blunt force application in the area of the liver, and right lower rib fractures should arouse suspicion for hepatic trauma, but most patients who require an operation for a blunt hepatic injury have relatively few specific abdominal findings. Therefore, additional diagnostic tests are useful for the initial triage and management of those at risk for liver injury. In most trauma centers, the diagnostic modality of choice is an ultrasound evaluation preferably performed by a surgeon (although many emergency physicians may have such training and skills as well). The focused abdominal sonogram for trauma (FAST) is an effective technique for rapid imaging in hemodynamically stable or unstable patients with possible hepatic injuries. A sagittal view of the right upper quadrant is performed by placing the transducer on the anterior axillary line between the tenth and eleventh ribs. The presence of an anechoic stripe in the hepatorenal fossa or in the right subdiaphragmatic area is strongly suggestive of blood accumulation in the right upper quadrant. While this fluid may represent hemorrhage from other organs in the abdomen, the patient with blunt trauma to the right upper quadrant or flank is likely to have an injury to the liver. The hemodynamically stable patient with a "positive" ultrasound then undergoes a spiral CT of the abdomen to document the presence and magnitude of injuries to the liver and other intraabdominal viscera, whereas the hemodynamically unstable patient with a "positive" ultrasound is moved directly to the operating room without further imaging. A search for extraabdominal injuries contributing to shock should be undertaken in patients with persistent hemodynamic instability with a negative FAST. If extraabdominal sources of shock are not present or if hemoperitoneum remains a concern in an unstable patient with a negative FAST, a diagnostic peritoneal aspirate could be performed or the patient may require an exploratory celiotomy.

In emergency departments where major trauma is encountered less frequently, the use of ultrasound occurs infrequently in the United States because of lack of equipment and an experienced operator. In these circumstances, CT scanning is generally employed as the primary diagnostic modality in stable patients. A spiral CT of the abdomen and pelvis in the hemodynamically stable patient performed after the intravenous injection of contrast remains the most sensitive and specific imaging modality for the evaluation of hepatobiliary trauma. The value of administering oral contrast before initiation of the scan is debated continuously in the United States but is generally not necessary for the evaluation of traumatic injuries. Spiral CT findings of interest to the surgeon include the presence and magnitude of the hepatic parenchymal injury, the presence and magnitude of intraperitoneal blood, and the presence and magnitude of associated intraperitoneal and retroperitoneal visceral, mesenteric, and vascular injuries. Hepatic injuries typically noted on a spiral CT study include a parenchymal laceration, intrahepatic hematoma, or subcapsular hematoma with or without active extravasation of intravenous contrast (Figure 119-1).

Although studies in the early 1990s questioned the reliability of CT scanning as a means to accurately stage injuries, experience gained in the past two decades has demonstrated that CT scans are highly accurate in detecting the liver injury itself and aiding the decisions on the need for further intervention—either operation or angiographic embolization. A study from Maryland[13] compared CT and angiography for the ability to detect arterial vascular injury; they noted 65% sensitivity and 85% specificity for CT scanning with arteriography as the criterion standard. Numerous subsequent studies have confirmed the reliability of CT scanning as an accurate tool for the diagnosis and assessment of blunt hepatic injuries. There are three issues that occasionally arise that the surgeon must consider in using this tool: (1) the occasional lack of correlation between the CT scan and the clinical or operative findings; (2) the controversy surrounding intraparenchymal extravasation; and (3)

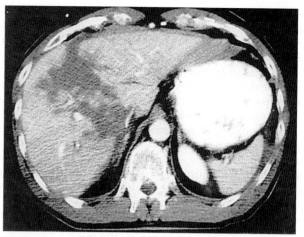

FIGURE 119-1 Computed tomography scan discloses a large intraparenchymal disruption with contrast pooling within the area of injury.

the reliability of scanning in the detection of associated hollow viscus injuries.

Although CT scanning is highly reliable for the diagnosis of hepatic injuries, it may be less accurate in grading injuries.[14] Whether there are patterns of injury on CT scans that are particularly ominous remains controversial, but it is clear that on many occasions the CT scan does *not* provide accurate guidance as to the need for operation. Occasionally, patients with trivial-appearing parenchymal injuries on CT scan are hemodynamically unstable and require a celiotomy. Likewise, most experienced trauma surgeons have observed patients with major injuries obvious on CT scan who are hemodynamically stable often with little hemoperitoneum. Thus, the need for operation should be determined by clinical factors, most notably hemodynamic stability, rather than CT findings.

A second area of note regarding CT scanning involves the findings of suspected intraparenchymal hemorrhage or pseudoaneurysms within the liver.[13] If an area of suspected hemorrhage as identified by a contrast blush is noted in a hemodynamically unstable patient, then an intervention is clearly needed. This may involve angiographic embolization, although most surgeons loathe transporting an unstable patient to an angiography suite. Patients who can be stabilized may have selective embolization if that capability is available or if no operation likely will be required. On occasion, a patient has CT evidence of extravasation but is very stable and has little evidence of blood loss. Whether that patient requires angiography and embolization is problematic although most algorithms follow such a course.

The third area of concern regarding CT scanning of suspected liver injuries involves its reliability in detecting visceral injuries. Associated intestinal injuries occur in about 2% to 6% of most series of liver injuries, and their diagnosis may be problematic. Our extensive experience suggests that hollow viscus injuries occur in about 1% of patients with blunt liver injuries. The blood from a hepatic injury may obscure the fluid from a perforated intestinal segment and clinical findings of intestinal injury may be masked by sedation, need for mechanical ventilation, or associated injuries causing distracting pain. It is imperative that intestinal injuries be considered in appropriate clinical circumstances, regardless of negative CT findings.

DPL was once the mainstay of the diagnosis of intraperitoneal bleeding but its use has been greatly curtailed in the past two decades. Although some units continue to use it selectively, others do so rarely, and currently it is rarely considered indicated in the evaluation of hepatic injuries. Laparoscopy has been useful in selected circumstances for the diagnosis and possible treatment of some intraabdominal injuries but its role in the primary management of liver injury is minimal if any. Our unit frequently uses laparoscopy as an adjunct to manage bile ascites postinjury (see later discussion).

CLASSIFICATIONS OF LIVER INJURIES

The American Association for the Surgery of Trauma (AAST) developed the Hepatic Organ Injury Scale in 1989 and revised this system in 1994.[15] At the time of its development, the scoring system was based on operative findings (Table 119-1). Grade I injuries were generally minor and they increased in severity to a grade VI injury, which denoted complete avulsion of the liver. In an ideal system, as severity increases, the need for more aggressive interventions increases, as does mortality. Although the classification system for liver injuries has many useful features, it has some inherent problems. First, the system was developed for operative findings and there is less evidence of its applicability to CT scan evaluation of injuries. Second, although there is a general worsening of outcomes with more severe injuries, that is, grade IV and V injuries are more likely to require operation, the majority of even these more severe injuries still do not require operative treatment. On occasion, less severe grades may injure a peripheral vascular structure with consequent major bleeding requiring operation. Thus, the system has general utility for the management of liver injuries and a greater value in reporting the results of

treatment, but it is not specific enough to be useful in a protocol for the treatment of these problems. Several authors have noted this lack of correlation and have suggested other systems, but to date a better grading mechanism has not been adopted.

Anatomic classifications of the liver have been developed by Couinaud and Bismuth based on segmental anatomy of vessels and bile ducts. These classifications are widely used in planning elective operative treatments and describing outcomes for a number of hepatic operative procedures. Occasionally, a surgical oncologist with an interest in the liver will editorialize on the failure of those interested in hepatic trauma to use these anatomic classifications in either the treatment or reporting of liver injury. Generally, injuries to the liver do not correspond to anatomic segments and most trauma surgeons have not found these classifications useful in their treatment of hepatic injuries.

PRINCIPLES OF OPERATIVE TREATMENT

Operations for trauma should utilize a midline incision (whether done for blunt or penetrating injury) to permit rapid exploration of the entire abdomen.[16] Transverse incisions, which we commonly use in our elective hepatic procedures, do not permit a thorough abdominal evaluation and are not the standard incision for trauma patients. The use of an upper abdominal retraction system will greatly facilitate exposure of the liver. If further exposure is required, the incision may be extended cephalad either partially or completely through the sternum. If a full cephalad sternotomy is required to control life-threatening bleeding it is certainly justified, but opening the sternum for a bicavitary procedure does increase evaporative heat loss and potentially worsens coagulopathy. Therefore, it should not be done unless it is expected to offer a major advantage in exposure. The conduct of the operation will be determined to a considerable degree by the extent of hemoperitoneum encountered and the site of the presumed source of bleeding. If a large volume of free blood is encountered, packs should be placed in the four quadrants of the abdomen in an attempt to determine the primary site of bleeding. If liver bleeding can be controlled with packs, these can be left in place while other potential injuries are evaluated and/or addressed. A seriously injured spleen should be removed promptly and any concomitant gastrointestinal injuries rapidly evaluated and managed.

Minor bleeding from hepatic trauma may occur in association with other intraabdominal injuries and is often due to low-grade (I and II) liver injuries. These minor injuries can usually be managed by compression and temporary packing alone or with electrocautery, argon beam coagulation, or topical hemostatic agents as adjuncts to speed hemorrhage control. Packing with temporary abdominal closure will rarely be required for these low-grade injuries. However, for more severe hepatic injuries (grade III to V) a stepwise approach to the patient with massive bleeding is required for successful outcome. One such algorithm was recently described by the Western Trauma Association and is outlined in Figure 119-2. The primary method of hemorrhage

TABLE 119-1 AAST Liver Injury Scale	
Grade	**Description**
I. Hematoma	Subcapsular, nonexpanding <10 cm surface area
Laceration	Capsule tear, nonbleeding <1 cm depth
II. Hematoma	Subcapsular, nonexpanding 10% to 50% surface area Intraparenchymal nonexpanding <10 cm diameter
III. Hematoma	Subcapsular, >50% surface area or expanding, ruptured
Laceration	<3 cm depth (parenchyma)
IV. Hematoma	Ruptured intraparenchymal hematoma with active bleeding
Laceration	Parenchymal disruption 25% to 75% of lobe
V. Laceration	<75% parenchymal disruption
Vascular	Juxtahepatic venous injury
VI. Vascular	Hepatic avulsion

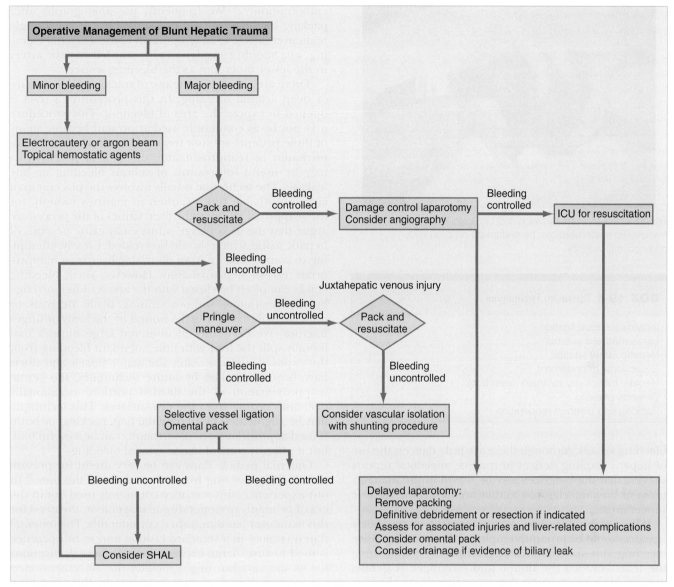

FIGURE 119-2 The Western Trauma Association proposed this algorithm for management of blunt liver injuries requiring operation. *SHAL,* Selective hepatic artery ligation. (From Kozar RA, Moore FA, Moore EE, et al: Western Trauma Association critical decision in trauma: Non-operative management of blunt hepatic trauma. *J Trauma* 67:1144, 2009.)

control is manual compression followed by perihepatic packing. The surgeon compresses the injured parenchyma between two hands and places laparotomy pads around the liver to both compress the injury and to assist in hemostasis (Figure 119-3). Operative treatment can often be successfully rendered on a nonbleeding liver with appropriate compression. If massive bleeding not amenable to temporary control is encountered, it must be addressed immediately. Bimanual compression usually permits arrest of most parenchymal bleeding and will permit resuscitative efforts by the anesthesiologist. The operative strategy will then be determined by the extent of the hepatic injury and the amount of bleeding encountered. If significant bleeding occurs, activation of a massive transfusion protocol should be strongly considered, as early activation has been shown to reduce mortality, as has the transfusion of a balanced ratio of blood

products (1:1:1, red blood cells/plasma/platelets ratio). Additionally, prevention and correction of hypothermia and acidosis should be instituted to minimize blood loss from coagulopathy.

There is no single method or technique that will ensure successful control of hepatic bleeding.[16] Therefore, the surgeon may need to consider a variety of options depending on the geometry and depth of the wound and the nature of vessels injured (Box 119-1). Bleeding parenchymal injuries are best managed by vessel ligation if feasible. In our experience, the use of surgical clips is less than satisfactory because of ease of dislodgement with hepatic manipulation. Bleeding from within the depths of the parenchyma may require removal of liver tissue to expose the bleeding vessels. The use of the finger fracture technique will remove devitalized liver tissue and permit exposure to perform suture ligation of

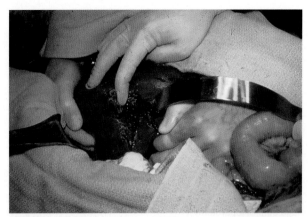

FIGURE 119-3 With mobilization and bimanual compression, hemostatic maneuvers can be performed on even deep parenchymal wounds.

BOX 19-1 Operative Techniques

Individual vessel ligation
Large mattress sutures
Hepatic artery ligation
Resectional debridement
Hepatic lobectomy (or major resection)
Omental packing
Packing and planned reoperation

bleeding vessels. Although there are little data on the use of hepatic stapling devices in trauma, anecdotal reports suggest that these devices may be useful in the management of liver injuries, just as they are in elective hepatic procedures.

When major bleeding occurs, control of the porta hepatis should be promptly employed. In cases of massive bleeding, this may be initially performed by compressing the triad between the thumb and forefinger. A gentle, noncrushing fine vascular clamp can then be applied for more secure control. Although some texts mention dissection of the portal triad with vessel loop placement around individual structures, it would be difficult to envision an emergency situation where a Pringle maneuver was required that would permit such a tedious dissection. It appears the Pringle maneuver can be safely employed for an hour at least. In our experience, if the bleeding cannot be controlled surgically or by packing within that interval, it is doubtful further clamping of the triad with surgical maneuvers will salvage the patient.

If there is arterial bleeding from deep within the parenchyma not amenable to suture control, there are several options. If the arterial bleeding is arrested with portal triad compression, selective hepatic artery ligation (SHAL) can be performed. Though employed frequently at our institution three decades ago,[8,9] it is now used approximately one to two times annually but remains an important consideration for the occasional patient with arterial bleeding that is controlled with unilateral vascular occlusion. Some units manage uncontrolled arterial hemorrhage by packing the patient and taking him or her to the angiography suite for selective

embolization.[17,18] We frequently use angiography after packing in a damage control situation.[19] If the Pringle maneuver fails to even temporarily control arterial bleeding, one should consider an aberrant left hepatic artery in the lesser omentum as the bleeding source.

There are reports on the use of tractomy for exposure of deep arterial bleeding. In this procedure, a tract is opened to expose the area of bleeding. This procedure may not be as commonly used at present because many of these patients are now treated by embolization. Hepatorrhaphy or reapproximation of the liver parenchyma may be useful for control of venous bleeding or bile leakage. The technique usually involves the placement of large absorbable sutures, often in mattress fashion, for the reapproximation of the liver. Critics of the procedure argue that the use of large sutures may cause necrosis of hepatic tissue, which should be avoided. Clearly, attempting to control oozing from nonviable liver is an inappropriate use of hepatorrhaphy. However, small bleeding cracks can often be closed with the arrest of hemorrhage by this technique without causing tissue necrosis or unnecessarily extending the wound by tractomy or finger fracture. We have also encountered large injuries that literally split the liver with little attendant bleeding from the exposed surfaces. After the major vessels and ducts have been controlled by suture techniques, the gentle reapproximation of the divided portions occasionally decreases oozing from the raw surfaces. This technique may be augmented by an omental flap, packing, or both. If used appropriately, hepatorrhaphy can be a useful tool, but it will not control major arterial bleeding.

Omental pedicle flaps can be very useful for prevention of diffuse oozing from raw surfaces of the liver.[20] In our experience, this was once commonly used but in the era of primarily nonoperative management, the need for this maneuver has diminished considerably. The omental flap is created in a standard fashion and in our practice is used to cover large exposed liver surfaces. Indications for its use vary but might include the aforementioned crevasses in hepatic tissues, coverage of the remaining surface following resection or debridement of hepatic tissue, and for any larger area where there is no liver capsule. In the unusual instance where a subcapsular hematoma has ruptured or been surgically entered, diffuse bleeding from the exposed liver surface liver usually ensues. The use of an omental flap in this circumstance may be extremely useful.

Formal anatomic resection of the liver is not commonly indicated for trauma as it would be for oncologic issues. Several decades ago, there was a rush of enthusiasm for hepatic lobectomy for trauma. This was followed by several reports with extremely high mortality and its general disuse. However, there are several instances where a major hepatic resection is indicated: devitalizing injuries along anatomic planes, completion lobectomy when the injury has transected the liver along lobar anatomy, and for exposure of major venous bleeding associated with a major hepatic parenchymal injury. The use of hepatic artery embolization has occasionally resulted in lobar hepatic necrosis that requires a formal lobectomy for resolution. Unlike a planned lobar resection for hepatic tumors, major resections for injury must often be performed under an emergent, less-than-optimal situation in a patient who is at grave risk for exsanguination. In this circumstance, operative speed is imperative. The use of techniques employed by elective hepatic surgeons such as vascular and hepatic staplers is a useful adjunct in such cases.

MAJOR VENOUS BLEEDING

Although major arterial hemorrhage must be controlled by surgical or radiologic means and is not amenable to cessation by packing, major venous bleeding is a great impediment to patient survival as well.[10,21-23] Major venous bleeding may result from injury to one of the main hepatic veins, from a major injury associated with the vena cava, or from a retrohepatic vena cava wound itself. Isolated vena cava lacerations without involvement of a hepatic vein branch are unusual in blunt trauma but may occur with a GSW. Major hepatic venous injuries confined to the liver parenchyma can generally be successfully managed by suture ligation. If the injury is not readily apparent and blood is welling up from a deep crevasse, it may be necessary to expose the venous injury more clearly with finger fracture or tractomy. Suture ligation can generally be used to control hemorrhage. Once major bleeding has been lessened, packing may be used to control the remaining bleeding.

Avulsion of the hepatic veins from the vena cava is potentially a lethal injury. On occasion, this problem can be solved by packing the area of injury and allowing the low-pressure venous system to tamponade. We have had several successes with packing for serious hepatic venous injuries.[23,24] However, the packing may not succeed in hemorrhage control and if the packs are placed too aggressively, the venous return from the lower body may be totally interrupted, with resultant unsustainably low cardiac output. Using inflow occlusion, the bleeding may be decreased enough to allow suture control but inflow occlusion of the portal triad does not prevent back-bleeding from the vena cava. Our group[25] has reported on the direct application of fine vascular clamps to reapproximate the anterior wall of the vena cava and the major hepatic veins with good success. The clamps can be allowed to remain in place with the abdomen packed in a damage control strategy. We have noted markedly decreased bleeding when the packs are removed; in a couple of cases, removal of the clamps produced no bleeding and the patients survived. There have also been a few reports of successful management by the use of fenestrated endovascular stent grafts. This method usually involves a contained injury, in which extravasation was demonstrated on a CT scan.

Historically, the method of choice for management of juxtahepatic major venous injuries has involved the use of an atriocaval shunt.[10,21] The concept involves the placement of a tube of some type (usually a thoracostomy or endotracheal tube) through the right atrium into the inferior vena cava. Snares are used around the cavae above and below the liver in an attempt to divert flow through the tube and away from the area of injury, permitting a bloodless field and, theoretically, a more controlled repair. This operation requires an incredible amount of skill and good fortune to be successful. It

requires opening a second body cavity (the thorax), which worsens hypothermia and bleeding, and many wounds are difficult to repair even if the shunt is functioning. The best reported results emanated from San Francisco in the 1980s in which 45% of 27 patients survived. A review of the world's literature disclosed 412 cases with 88% mortality.[1] Suffice it to say, juxtahepatic venous injuries remain an unsolved problem in hepatic trauma, no single technique is successful, and no algorithm for management can be constructed with a reasonable likelihood of patient survival.

PERIHEPATIC PACKING AND DAMAGE CONTROL STRATEGIES

Prior to World War II, perihepatic packing was often used to control bleeding around the liver but in the next several decades perihepatic packing was denigrated as a method of managing liver hemorrhage. However, it became obvious that many patients were dying from bleeding that could not be surgically controlled often because of the associated triad of shock, hypothermia, and coagulopathy. In the early 1980s, several reports[24,26,27] presenting a reappraisal of perihepatic packing occurred, which demonstrated a major survival advantage in patients who would have likely died with conventional surgical treatment. The term *damage control*, in which packing was an integral part of that strategy, became a recognized and accepted concept.[28]

The tenets of liver packing begin with the choice of an appropriate patient; arterial hemorrhage will likely require control by suture or embolization. Good judgment is required to not forego appropriate attempts at technical control of bleeding without delaying for an inappropriate time, which might prevent patient survival.[29] Other technical features we have found useful are outlined in Box 119-2. Secondary effects of abdominal compartment syndrome can generally be ameliorated by avoiding fascial closure, often accompanied by some method of temporary closure usually involving a dressing or vacuum pack technique.[30] Some advocate return to the operating suite for pack removal when the patient is rewarmed and coagulopathy corrected. These goals may be accomplished within 6 hours. However, we prefer to leave packs for 24 hours to allow for coagulation of

---

BOX 19-2 Tenets of Hepatic Packing

Choose appropriate patient
   Control arterial bleeding surgically/arteriographically
   Ideal for lesser venous bleeding, coagulopathy
Use before excess bleeding and coagulopathy develops
   (patients often have acidosis and abnormal coagulation
   profile in the emergency department—unlikely to control
   bleeding surgically)
Pack to compress liver in superior to inferior plane;
   anteroposterior packing tends to compress the vena cava
Count sponges (if feasible; facilitates later removal)
Some use nonadherent material over liver
Temporary abdominal closure must avoid tension and
   secondary abdominal compartment syndrome

exposed vessels that may rebleed with early pack removal. Issues regarding abdominal compartment syndrome and management of the open abdomen may complicate the decision for perihepatic packing, but are outside the scope of this discussion.[31]

NONOPERATIVE MANAGEMENT

By the late 1980s it was clear that although some problems remained with management of hemorrhage from the liver, many patients were undergoing celiotomy for injuries that did not require operative treatment. Diagnostic peritoneal lavage was extremely sensitive and its widespread use led to many nontherapeutic operations for liver injury. As imaging with CT scans became prevalent, it allowed a diagnosis to be made without DPL and also permitted evaluation of other intraabdominal injuries. Pediatric surgeons initiated nonoperative management (NOM) for splenic injuries to avoid the complications of splenectomy and, buoyed by the success of that strategy, began to extend the concept to the management of hepatic injuries. Experienced surgeons then began to cautiously adopt similar protocols in older patients with liver injuries.

Several series of selected patients were reported with near uniform success, and the concept was rapidly extended and guidelines for its use liberalized.[32-35] A literature review of collected contemporary series disclosed that about 80% to 90% of hepatic injuries can be safely managed without operation.[36] Although the guidelines for NOM may vary slightly, the principles are fairly well standardized. Initially, most centers required a hemodynamically stable patient who did not require a blood transfusion; many centers desired the patient to be alert and able to cooperate with physical examination. These criteria generally are not required in most contemporary protocols. The key factor in determining whether NOM can be safely used is hemodynamic stability.[37] Most trauma centers will permit up to four units of blood transfusion to be given before celiotomy is required. There should be no evidence of visceral injuries on CT scan. Although a baseline CT scan is almost always performed, operation is usually mandated by the clinical findings of hemodynamic instability and/or ongoing transfusion requirements, and not by the injury grade on CT scan. While patients with a higher-grade injury (as judged by CT) have an increased rate of operation, many patients with high-grade injuries on CT scan do not need operation. Conversely, an occasional patient with a relatively innocuous injury may have bleeding requiring an emergent celiotomy. In our experience, most patients who fail NOM tend to do so quickly and delayed bleeding is rather uncommon.[38]

Patients who are selected for NOM should be in an intensive care unit environment with careful monitoring of vital signs and hemoglobin level for the first several days postinjury. There are several controversial areas regarding followup care that remain unresolved. It is unclear whether patients require a follow-up CT scan. Many studies show no change in management, with additional scans if patients are clinically improving. Likewise, there is a wide range of opinion and little data on the permitted level of activity following treatment. Most centers limit activity for 4 to 6 weeks and perhaps longer for contact sports, but these recommendations (though likely reasonable) are not data driven.

The failure rate after 36 hours for NOM is in the 2% to 3% range. A few patients have ongoing bleeding and some require operations for associated injuries including those to the spleen and delayed recognition of a visceral injury. Abdominal compartment syndrome may also require operative decompression.[39]

The avoidance of operation for injured patients who require blood transfusions would certainly have been heretical 20 years ago, but there is inferential evidence that NOM may not only avoid an operation but actually lower mortality in blunt trauma patients. One substantiation for this hypothesis is that deaths from liver-related injuries improved somewhat with the advent of NOM (Figure 119-4). Second, there is anecdotal evidence that suggests venous injuries, which are low pressure in nature, may actually heal if operation is avoided. From 1975 to 1990, we treated 54 juxtahepatic venous injuries operatively for a rate of 2.7 per year with an 18% survival rate. In the past 15 years, we have treated 28 (1.3 per year) such patients despite an actual increase in hepatic injuries seen at our trauma center.[23] The survival rate has improved to 61%. Although experience and technical improvement of operative treatment has undoubtedly occurred, avoidance of operation may have allowed juxtahepatic venous injuries to heal spontaneously.

REQUIREMENTS OF ADJUNCTIVE INVASIVE TREATMENT

The use of NOM does not imply that other types of invasive treatments may not be required to treat the patients. Therefore, the mindset for NOM should not be to avoid needed therapeutic interventions but to allow the patient to recover as rapidly as possible, which may require adjunctive procedures. Angiography has been previously discussed and may be very useful for patients with an arterial blush on CT or evidence of arterial extravasation on angiography. Delayed bleeding from hemobilia may require angiographic treatment as well. Patients with prolonged bile leaks may be improved by endoscopic retrograde cholangiography with possible sphincterotomy and biliary stent placement.[19,40]

Patients with perihepatic fluid collections may benefit from percutaneous drainage. However, the radiologic placement of small-caliber drains around the liver will not remove the liters of blood and bile distributed in all four abdominal quadrants and the pelvis. When large accumulations of blood and bile are present, they may cause bile peritonitis, a systemic inflammatory response syndrome (SIRS), or an abdominal compartment syndrome. To prevent and/or treat these problems, we perform laparoscopy for evacuation of a major accumulation of blood and bile.[41] When the patient is stable after 3 or 4 days, a followup CT scan is performed and if a large amount of fluid is present we perform laparoscopy. We generally use a gasless system to prevent the theoretical problem of gas embolism. Laparoscopy permits the evacuation of virtually all of the fluid from the abdominal quadrants and the pelvis itself. We do not attempt to remove organized clot from around the liver and

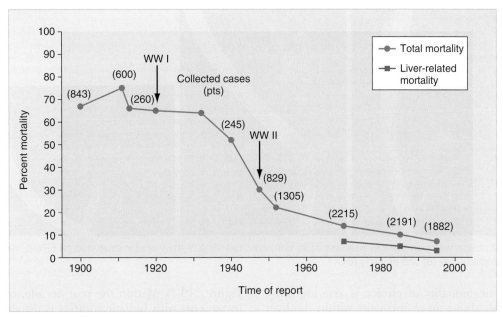

FIGURE 119-4 A review of several thousand cases of liver injury from the early 20th century to the present demonstrates a progressively downward trend. Mortality related to liver injury itself is in the 2% to 4% range at present.

generally place a perihepatic drain to monitor subsequent bile output.

Our experience[42] with a large number of such procedures demonstrates an improvement in respiratory parameters, decreased temperature and pulse rate, and the amelioration of SIRS associated with the presence of a large amount of blood and bile. We have not experienced any complications with this approach, and patients are often dramatically improved immediately after the operation.

NONOPERATIVE MANAGEMENT FOR PENETRATING INJURIES

There have been a few reports on the use of NOM for penetrating hepatic injuries. Stab wounds to the right upper quadrant can be safely managed in an evaluable patient who is stable and does not exhibit findings of peritonitis. A few small series on NOM for GSWs have also been reported. In 1998, Demetriades et al[43] reported on 16 patients with GSW managed nonoperatively from a much larger group of patients who required operation. Five (31%) required delayed operation for peritonitis (four patients) and abdominal compartment syndrome (one patient). In 2009, Navsaria et al[44] treated 63 patients with GSW by NOM. Associated injuries to the kidney (22%), diaphragm (69%), and lung (80%) were very common but only five required delayed celiotomy. Ten patients had complications. Both of these reports stressed the safety of this approach. However, given the fairly high rate of failure and associated injury, such an approach has not become widely accepted.

SPECIAL PROBLEMS

SUBCAPSULAR HEMATOMAS

Subcapsular hematomas occur in about 2% to 3% of major blunt liver injuries. The natural history of subcapsular hematomas is not clearly defined, but unlike a similar injury to the spleen, which has a real risk of delayed rupture, subsequent bleeding seems to be much less in common hepatic hematomas. In the previous era of uniform operation for suspected liver injury, it was advised to leave these lesions intact if they were encountered. Two papers[45,46] from pediatric surgeons urged nonoperative management several decades ago. If subcapsular hematomas are encountered, indications for further operative intervention include continued expansion of the hematoma and management of its rupture. Arteriography and embolization may be useful for expanding lesions. If a suspected subcapsular hematoma is detected on CT scan, no therapy is recommended unless it is associated with an arterial blush, suggesting the possibility of continued bleeding. In such instances, angiographic embolization is recommended. If the capsule is ruptured, then operation may be required to control the diffuse bleeding from the exposed surface of the liver. Temporary packing will usually control such bleeding and an omental flap may be useful to prevent rebleeding.

HEMOBILIA

Hemobilia is defined as bleeding from the liver which is expressed from the biliary tree. Since the classic review by Sandblom[47] in 1972 in which he described the phenomenon and reviewed its etiology and clinical presentation, several hundred cases have been described in the literature. Typically, the bleeding begins several days to a few weeks postinjury and may be manifested by several clinical presentations. Occasionally, patients may present with brisk upper gastrointestinal bleeding, although melena is somewhat more common. Jaundice or subclinical evaluation of bilirubin is frequently present. Hemobilia should be suspected in those who sustained recent liver injury with gastrointestinal bleeding and/or jaundice.

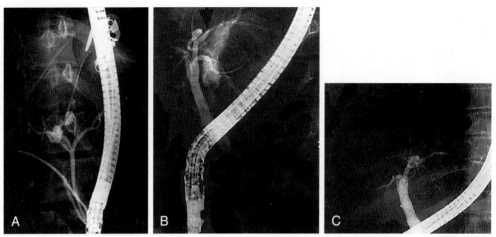

FIGURE 119-5 **A,** A patient with high bilirubin after liver injury demonstrated filling of the vascular structures on ERCP. Venous filling obliterated by sphincterotomy (**B**) and stenting (**C**).

The diagnostic modality of choice is arteriography, which commonly shows an abnormality within the liver parenchyma. Selective embolization of the vascular abnormality is nearly always effective in treating this problem, and operation is rarely required. Operative treatment is indicated for failure of angiographic treatment, for debridement of associated necrotic liver, or for intrahepatic sepsis.

BILEHEMIA

In contradistinction to hemobilia where bleeding occurs through the biliary system, bilehemia is an abnormal communication between an intrahepatic bile duct and a vein. The bile flows into the venous system (Figure 119-5, *A* and *B*) and may result in profound jaundice. There are few reports of bilehemia in the literature, but most require a two-pronged approach aimed at obliterating the offending vessel through angiographic techniques and decompression of the biliary system through endoscopic retrograde cholangiography and stenting.

AVULSION OF THE LIVER

Grade VI injuries consist of total avulsion of the liver. Although most of these injuries are rapidly fatal, an occasional patient survives his or her operative treatment. There are several reports of successful venovenous bypass with the patient in an anhepatic state followed by emergency liver transplantation. These cases require a mindset of preparedness and ingenuity to salvage an otherwise fatal situation.

MORTALITY FROM HEPATIC INJURIES

The mortality from liver injuries has declined considerably in the past several decades. In World War II, the fatality rate was 66%; by the Vietnam War, it had declined to 15% to 20%. As large civilian experiences with liver injuries were reported after midcentury, the mortality was often reported as 8% to 15%. The concept of "liver-related mortality" was introduced in an attempt to define those deaths likely due to the liver injury itself versus those related to associated trauma such as head injury. A comprehensive review of major series published since 1900 shows the downward trend in mortality[1] (see

Figure 119-4). Within the past decade, overall mortality in patients with hepatic injuries is usually in the 5% to 8% range, whereas the liver-related mortality is about 3% to 4%.

SUMMARY

As mentioned throughout the text, there are a myriad of presentations of liver injuries that require a variety of therapeutic maneuvers. A simplified strategy is outlined in Figure 119-6.

GALLBLADDER INJURY

Injuries to the gallbladder may result from either blunt or penetrating trauma. Regardless of mechanism, isolated gallbladder injuries are relatively uncommon. The treatment of choice should be cholecystectomy, and the outcome will be determined by the presence and extent of associated injuries. Attempts to repair even minor gallbladder injuries should generally be avoided because of the propensity for bile leakage and the risk of gallstone formation engendered by the inflammation around the suture used for repair.

Acalculous cholecystitis may also follow treatment modalities that interrupt the gallbladder's blood supply. Both selective hepatic artery ligation and angiographic embolization of the hepatic artery commonly lead to acalculous cholecystitis and may result in gallbladder necrosis. Although this problem is more commonly encountered with interruption of the right hepatic artery flow, our unit has encountered the problem with left hepatic artery embolization as well. If a selective right hepatic artery ligation is performed, we recommend concomitant cholecystectomy to prevent this problem.

INJURIES OF THE EXTRAHEPATIC BILE DUCTS

Injuries of the extrahepatic bile ducts may follow both blunt and penetrating injuries and, as in the case of gallbladder injuries, rarely occur in isolation.[48] Several textbooks suggest these injuries may be managed by techniques commonly employed to manage iatrogenic complications such as bile duct injury occurring during a cholecystectomy. In our experience of more than 35

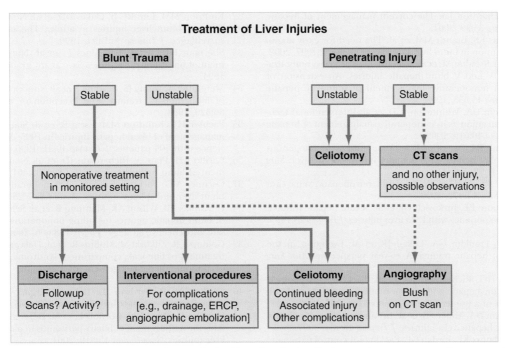

Treatment of Liver Injuries

FIGURE 119-6 Most gunshot wounds are managed operatively although select patients may have a nonoperative approach if stable *(broken arrow)*. The key decision point in blunt trauma is hemodynamic stability or not.

years of managing such injuries (which are fortunately not common), the parallels between iatrogenic injuries and either blunt or penetrating trauma have little in common. When the extrahepatic ductal system is injured by penetrating injuries, other structures are invariably injured, and given the close approximation of the bile ducts to major vessels, massive hemorrhage often accompanies such injuries. Embarking on a choledochojejunostomy to definitively repair a ductal injury may not be prudent with a patient recently in hemorrhagic shock or cold and coagulopathic.

When the extrahepatic ductal injury is due to blunt trauma, a tremendous force is required to produce extrahepatic ductal injury. This usually results in associated injuries to the liver, pancreas, duodenum, or other structure and/or a devastating ductal injury. Clean transections of the ductal system are rarely, if ever, encountered and the duct is often totally devascularized or completely avulsed from the liver bed or duodenum.

Given both the complexities of these injuries, the diversity of anatomic disruptions, the myriad of associated injuries, and, fortunately, their rarity, it is not practical to propose an algorithm for the management of extrahepatic ductal injuries. The axiom "if you have seen one ductal injury, you have seen one ductal injury" might well apply. If the patient were stable, had no other major injuries to address and had a structural configuration amenable to early repair with choledochojejunostomy, or hepaticojejunostomy, such would be a logical approach. Since these conditions rarely are encountered, other strategies are often necessary. If it is feasible to place a T-tube or some type of tube in the remaining biliary structures for drainage, that is a step we recommend. Unfortunately, given the aforementioned difficulties each case may present, the surgeon must often be creative in attempting to manage these most challenging

problems. After the patient has been stabilized, the ductal system can be evaluated by ERCP, via a T-tube if that was placed intraoperatively or by a transhepatic route. Delayed reconstruction can then be planned as needed.

REFERENCES

1. Richardson JD: Changes in the management of injuries to the liver and spleen. *J Am Coll Surg* 200:648, 2005.
2. Otis GA: *Medical and surgical history of the rebellion*, Vol. 2, pt. 2, 1877, p 129.
3. Tilton BJ: Considerations regarding wounds of the liver. *Ann Surg* 61:20, 1905.
4. Madding GF, Kennedy PA: *Trauma to the liver. Major problem in clinical surgery*. Philadelphia, 1965, Saunders.
5. Peitzman AB, Richardson JD: Surgical treatment of injuries to the solid abdominal organs: A 50-year perspective from the *Journal of Trauma*. *J Trauma* 69:1011, 2010.
6. Trunkey DD, Shires GT, McClellan RN: Management of liver trauma in 811 consecutive patients. *Am J Surg* 197:727, 1974.
7. Defore WW, Mattox KL, Jordan GL, et al: Management of 1590 consecutive cases of liver trauma. *Arch Surg* 111:493, 1976.
8. Mays ET, Conti S, Fallahzadkh H, et al: Hepatic artery ligation. *Surgery* 86:536, 1979.
9. Flint LM, Polk HC Jr: Selective hepatic artery ligation: Limitations and failures. *J Trauma* 19:319, 1978.
10. Shrock T, Blaisdell FW, Mathewson C Jr, et al: Management of blunt trauma to the liver and hepatic veins. *Arch Surg* 96:698, 1968.
11. Carillo EH, Wohltmann C, Richardson JD, et al: Evolution in the management of complex liver injuries. *Curr Probl Surg* 38:1, 2001.
12. Beal SL: Fatal hepatic hemorrhage is an unresolved problem in the management of complex liver injuries. *J Trauma* 30:163, 1990.
13. Poletti PA, Mirvis SE, Shanmuganathan K, et al: CT criteria for management of blunt liver trauma: Correlation with angiographic and surgical findings. *Radiology* 216:418, 2000.
14. Croce MA, Fabian TC, Kudsk KA, et al: AAST injury scale: Correlation of CT-graded liver injuries and operative findings. *J Trauma* 31:806, 1991.
15. Moore EE, Cogbill TH, Jurkovich GJ, et al: Organ injury scaling: Spleen and liver (1994 Revision). *J Trauma* 38:433, 1995.

16. Carillo EH, Richardson JD: The current management of hepatic trauma. *Adv Surg* 35:39, 2001.
17. Wahl WL, Ahrns KS, Brandt MM, et al: The need for early angiographic intervention in blunt liver injuries. *J Trauma* 52:1097, 2002.
18. Ciraulo DL, Luk S, Palter M, et al: Selective hepatic artery embolization of grade IV and V blunt hepatic injuries: An extension of resuscitation in nonoperative management of traumatic hepatic injuries. *J Trauma* 45:353, 1998.
19. Carillo EH, Spain DA, Wohltmann CD, et al: Interventional techniques are useful adjuncts in nonoperative management of hepatic injuries. *J Trauma* 46:619, 1999.
20. Stone HH, Lamb JM: Use of pedicled omentum as an autogenous pack for control of hemorrhage in major injuries of the liver. *Surg Gynecol Obstet* 141:92, 1975.
21. Ciresi KF, Lim RC Jr: Hepatic vein and retrohepatic vena cava injury. *World J Surg* 14:472, 1990.
22. Cogbill TH, Moore EE, Jurkovich GJ, et al: Severe hepatic trauma: A multi-center experience with 1335 liver injuries. *J Trauma* 28:1433, 1988.
23. Richardson JD, Franklin GA, Lukan JK, et al: Evolution in the management of hepatic trauma: A 25-year perspective. *Ann Surg* 232:324, 2000.
24. Cue JI, Cryer HG, Richardson JD, et al: Packing and planned re-exploration for hepatic and retroperitoneal hemorrhage: Critical refinements of a use technique. *J Trauma* 30:1007, 1990.
25. Carillo EH, Spain DA, Miller FB, et al: Intrahepatic vascular clamping in complex hepatic vein injuries. *J Trauma* 43:131, 1997.
26. Feliciano DV, Mattox KL, Jordan GL: Packing for control of hepatic hemorrhage: A reappraisal. *J Trauma* 21:285, 1981.
27. Carmona RH, Peck DZ, Lim RC Jr: The role of packing and planned reoperation in severe hepatic trauma. *J Trauma* 24:779, 1984.
28. Rotondo MF, Schwab CW, McGonigal MD, et al: "Damage control": An approach for improved survival in exsanguinating penetrating abdominal injury. *J Trauma* 35:375, 1993.
29. Garrison JR, Richardson JD, Hilakos AS, et al: Predicting the need to pack early for severe intra-abdominal hemorrhage. *J Trauma* 40:923, 1996.
30. Barker DE, Kaufman HJ, Smith LA, et al: Vacuum pack technique of temporary abdominal closure: A 7-year experience with 112 patients. *J Trauma* 48:201, 2000.
31. Campbell A, Chang M, Fabian T, et al: Open Abdomen Advisory Panel: Management of the open abdomen: From initial operation to definitive closure. *Am Surg* 75(11 Suppl):S1, 2009.
32. Knudson MM, Lim RC Jr, Oakes DD, et al: Nonoperative management of blunt liver injuries in adults: The need for continued surveillance. *J Trauma* 30:1494, 1990.
33. Sherman HF, Savage BA, Jones L, et al: Nonoperative management of blunt hepatic injuries: Save at any grade? *J Trauma* 37:616, 1994.
34. Meredith JW, Young JS, Bowling J, et al: Nonoperative management of blunt hepatic trauma: The exception or the rule? *J Trauma* 36:529, 1994.
35. Pachter HL, Knudson MM, Esrig B, et al: Status of nonoperative management of blunt hepatic injuries in 1995: A multi-center experience with 404 patients. *J Trauma* 40:31, 1996.
36. Carillo EH, Platz A, Richardson JD, et al: Nonoperative management of blunt hepatic trauma. *Br J Surg* 85:461, 1997.
37. Oschner MG: Factors of failure of nonoperative management of blunt liver and splenic injuries. *World J Surg* 25:1393, 2001.
38. Christmas AB, Wilson AK, Manning B, et al: Selective management of blunt hepatic injuries including nonoperative management is a safe and effective strategy. *Surgery* 138:606, 2006.
39. Goldman R, Zilkoski M, Mullins R, et al: Delayed celiotomy for the treatment of bile leak, compartment syndrome, and other hazards of nonoperative management of blunt liver injury. *Am J Surg* 185:492, 2003.
40. Carillo EH, Richardson JD: Delayed surgery and interventional procedures in complex liver injuries. *J Trauma* 46:978, 1999.
41. Carillo EH, Reed DN, Gordon L, et al: Delayed laparoscopy facilitates the management of biliary peritonitis in patients with complex liver injuries. *Surg Endosc* 15:319, 2001.
42. Franklin G, Richardson JD, Brown AL, et al: Prevention of bile peritonitis by laparoscopic evacuation and lavage of nonoperative treatment of liver injuries. *Am Surg* 73:611, 2007.
43. Demetriades D, Gomez H, Chahwan S, et al: Gunshot wounds to the liver: The role of selective nonoperative management. *J Am Coll Surg* 188:427, 1998.
44. Navsaria P, Nicol AJ, Krige JG, et al: Selective nonoperative management of liver gunshot injuries. *Ann Surg* 249:653, 2009.
45. Richie JP, Fonkalsrud EW: Subcapsular hematoma of the liver—nonoperative management. *Arch Surg* 104:781, 1972.
46. Cheatham JE Jr, Smith EI, Tunnell WP: Nonoperative management of subcapsular hematoma of the liver. *Am J Surg* 140:852, 1980.
47. Sandblom P: *Hemobilia (biliary tract hemorrhage).* Springfield, Ill, 1972, Charles C Thomas.
48. Felicino DV, Ritondo CG, Burch JM, et al: Management of traumatic injuries of the biliary ducts. *Am J Surg* 150:705, 1985.

Diagnostic Operations of the Liver and Techniques of Hepatic Resection

Richard D. Schulick | Aram N. Demirjian

LIVER BIOPSY

PERCUTANEOUS AND TRANSJUGULAR LIVER BIOPSY

It is often necessary to obtain liver tissue for either gross or microscopic examination to aid in diagnosis and treatment planning. Liver biopsy was originally described by Ehrlich in 1883 to determine glycogen stores in patients with diabetes.[1] There are multiple approaches for performing liver biopsy, including percutaneous, transjugular, laparoscopic, and open techniques. If the liver abnormality is relatively diffuse, then a percutaneous biopsy without image guidance can be contemplated. Image-guided percutaneous biopsies are required for focal lesions. When performed by experienced physicians, percutaneous hollow-needle liver biopsy is safe and reliable and can provide a cylindrical core of tissue, generally with good preservation of hepatic architecture and minimal artifact.

When a percutaneous biopsy is contraindicated, for example in the presence of significant ascites or with coagulopathy, a transjugular biopsy can be performed. A transjugular biopsy allows also the measurement of intrahepatic portal pressures. However, transjugular biopsies are often smaller and more fragmented than core biopsies, making pathologic assessment more difficult. Additionally, transjugular biopsy techniques cannot be used for small focal lesions because of the inability to accurately place the needle.

If multiple percutaneous attempts have failed to obtain adequate material, if there is suspicion that a liver lesion is highly vascularized and prone to bleeding, if there is a need to obtain tissue from multiple sites, or if it is otherwise preferable to biopsy the liver under direct vision, then either laparoscopic or open liver biopsy may be used.

LAPAROSCOPY AND BIOPSY

Laparoscopic examination of the liver is performed using standard laparoscopic equipment along with laparoscopic ultrasound probes. Laparoscopic examination consists of visual inspection, "palpation" using the instrumentation, and tissue biopsy. In general, fine-needle aspiration should be avoided during laparoscopy because of the superior results of core biopsies and the ability to directly address bleeding problems resultant from the more aggressive core biopsies. Superficial lesions can be directly biopsied under visualization using cupped biopsy forceps, and deeper lesions can be biopsied percutaneously under laparoscopic ultrasound guidance.

There has developed a great deal of interest in the role of laparoscopy in hepatobiliary malignancies to identify disease that is unresectable, thus avoiding unnecessary laparotomy. Hepatobiliary malignancies are associated with particularly high rates of unresectability, and although preoperative imaging is improving, it is relatively insensitive for small liver lesions, peritoneal disease, and sometimes even vascular invasion.

Patients with extrahepatic cholangiocarcinomas or gallbladder cancer often present with unresectable disease. Even with state-of-the-art preoperative imaging, they are often found to have occult metastatic disease at the time of exploration. In a series from Memorial Sloan-Kettering Cancer Center (MSKCC), the yield of laparoscopy for occult unresectable disease in gallbladder cancer was approximately 50%.[2] Even in patients whose gallbladder cancer had been incidentally identified after recent laparoscopic cholecystectomy, the yield of relaparoscoping the patient was about 20%. In the same study, the yield of staging laparoscopy for hilar cholangiocarcinomas was about 25%. For gallbladder and hilar cholangiocarcinomas, the yield of staging laparoscopy and ultrasonography is relatively high and the value of surgical palliation is relatively low and therefore staging laparoscopy should be considered.

Because hepatocellular carcinoma rarely presents with peritoneal dissemination, the potential value of laparoscopy and ultrasonography should be its ability to identify additional liver lesions and the assessment of cirrhosis. Again, in the study from MSKCC the use of laparoscopy and ultrasound was able to avoid unnecessary laparotomy in 29% of patients who had cirrhosis or stage IVA disease.[2] However, if the patients had neither of these factors, then in only 5% of the patients did laparoscopy and ultrasonography avoid unnecessary laparotomy. In another series from Hong Kong, laparoscopy and ultrasonography was performed in 91 patients taken to the operating room for planned curative resection of liver tumors.[3] Laparoscopy and ultrasonography correctly identified 15 of 24 patients whose tumors subsequently proved unresectable. Of the 15 patients identified to have contraindications to resection, 11 had bilateral metastases, 6 had severe cirrhosis or inadequate liver remnant, 2 had main portal vein tumor thrombus, 1 had inferior vena cava (IVC) thrombus, and 1 had peritoneal metastases (some had multiple findings). Of the 9 patients with unresectable disease not detected by laparoscopy and ultrasonography, 3 had main portal vein tumor thrombus, 3 had involvement of adjacent organs, 2 had bilateral metastases, 1 had inadequate liver remnant, and 1 had IVC thrombus. Lai et al from Hong Kong reported another series of 122 patients with resectable hepatocellular carcinoma by imaging criteria. They were able to perform staging laparoscopy with laparoscopic ultrasound in 119 of these patients, and thereby identified 44 of them to be unresectable. By contrast, of the remaining patients who went on to laparotomy, only 2 further cases proved to be unresectable. This led the authors to conclude that a significant percentage of patients were incorrectly deemed resectable by noninvasive techniques and could be saved laparotomy. They also found laparoscopy to be an extremely useful tool in the armamentarium of further treatment planning.[4] Staging laparoscopy and ultrasonography is more likely to benefit patients with hepatocellular carcinoma who have cirrhosis and central lesions.

In one of the largest studies in 103 patients on the use of staging laparoscopy and ultrasonography for resection of colorectal metastases to the liver, only 14% of patients overall had unresectable disease identified, and only 10% were spared laparotomy.[5] An additional 8% of patients had unresectable disease missed by laparoscopy. The authors concluded that staging laparoscopy and ultrasound should be used selectively in patients at highest risk of having unresectable disease.

OPEN LIVER BIOPSY AND EXAMINATION

An open liver biopsy can be performed through a limited right subcostal incision. The incision should be placed over the inferior edge of the liver but should be at least 3 cm below the costal margin to allow for adequate fascial closure. The liver can be examined both visually and by palpation, but care should be taken to not disturb any portosystemic collateral vessels. If these friable vessels are disrupted, or if the hepatic capsule is ruptured during examination, a major abdominal operation may be required to gain control. Visual inspection for gross evidence of cirrhosis, nodularity, abnormal color or texture, or neoplasm may be revealing. A laparoscopic ultrasound probe can be used through a small incision, or if the incision is large enough, the regular probe may be used. A wedge biopsy can be obtained using a no. 15 scalpel and removing a specimen measuring about 1 cm at its base. A core-needle biopsy can be obtained through the same site, directed deeper into the liver parenchyma but away from the porta hepatis. If significant bleeding is expected, hemostatic 2-0 chromic catgut or Vicryl mattress sutures can be placed in an interlock "V" shape outside the biopsy site prior to biopsy. Once the biopsies are taken, the base of the biopsy site is treated with the argon beam coagulator for hemostasis. The fascia should be closed with running permanent suture if ascites is anticipated. Similarly, the skin should be closed with a running long-lasting suture if ascites is anticipated.

INCISIONS FOR LIVER OPERATIONS

SUBCOSTAL APPROACH

Most hepatectomies can be accomplished via a right subcostal incision made 3 to 4 cm below the right costal margin with an upper midline extension in a supine patient. The right rectus abdominis muscle is completely divided, as are the medial portions of the external oblique, internal oblique, and transversus abdominis muscles. Depending on the exposure required, the incision can be made up to and beyond the midaxillary line between the costal margin and the iliac bone. This incision exposes the anterior and inferior surfaces of the right and left liver and provides good access to the porta hepatis. For exposure to the dome of the liver, a midline extension over and above the xiphoid is performed and the xiphoid removed. For even more exposure, the incision can be extended under the left subcostal area (Figures 120-1 and 120-2). With this full incision, the surgeon has excellent exposure to the entire upper abdomen, including the liver as well as the retrohepatic and suprahepatic IVC. Because of the appearance when closed, this incision is often referred to as the *Mercedes incision*.

In extreme circumstances, a median sternotomy or right thoracotomy through the costal margin can even further increase access and exposure.

MIDLINE APPROACH

The midline incision is sometimes used in thin patients, when a pelvic procedure such as low anterior resection is being performed at the same time, or if the hepatic resection will be limited to the left half of the liver. The patient is positioned supine. It does not generally afford good access to the retrohepatic vena cava, the right hepatic vein, or the right posterior sector of the liver until the liver is completely mobilized off the diaphragm and retroperitoneum. It is commonly used in exploration for trauma where hepatic injury may be found. If greater exposure is required, a median sternotomy or right thoracotomy through the costal margin can be performed.

RIGHT THORACOABDOMINAL APPROACH

The thoracoabdominal incision is sometimes used in patients with large bulky lesions involving the right dome or right posterior sector of the liver. It gives the best access to the suprahepatic and retrohepatic vena cava as well as the right hepatic vein. Additionally, it is sometimes used in instances of significant right diaphragmatic involvement. The patient is positioned on a bean bag with the chest in a lateral position but the hips at 45 degrees. The incision is made from the umbilicus to the right costal margin, and depending on the location of the lesion, the seventh, eighth, or even ninth rib interspace is opened. If keeping the right lung unventilated will help, then a double-lumen endotracheal tube should be used. The diaphragm should be incised circumferentially to avoid the neurovascular bundle supplying it. Care should be taken to leave 3 to 4 cm of diaphragm on the rib cage to allow for later closure.

PORT PLACEMENT FOR THE LAPAROSCOPIC APPROACH

Given the greater difficulty of mobilization and retraction, especially in the case of a purely laparoscopic approach, trocar placement is of great importance. Placement of the camera port can vary, though in a recent

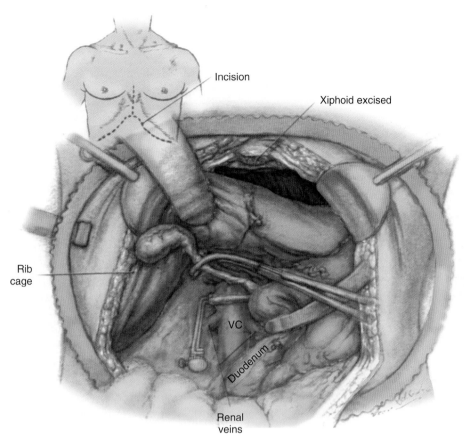

FIGURE 120-1 Bilateral subcostal incision with a short midline extension. This is a versatile incision appropriate for most major hepatic resections and portosystemic shunts. *VC,* Vena cava.

review paper, Gumbs et al recommend placing this trocar a hand-breadth caudad to the costal margin, partway between the midclavicular line and the midline.[6] A second large trocar is placed near the liver to facilitate ultrasonography, then two to three working ports on either side of the camera, and a right lateral port for the option of placing a self-retaining liver retractor (Figure 120-3).[6]

MORPHOLOGIC AND FUNCTIONAL ANATOMY

It is important that the surgeon performing a hepatectomy intimately understands the anatomy of the liver. The reader is strongly encouraged to review Chapter 114 detailing the anatomy of the liver. However, a brief review and overview are presented here to clarify this topic. The description and definition of the anatomic divisions of the liver have been revised and written about numerous times in the past 100 years.[7-10] At present, there is still confusion between the various hepatic anatomic nomenclatures in the literature. Based only on morphologic criteria and surface anatomy, the liver can be divided into right and left halves by forming a plane through the gallbladder fossa (Cantlie line) and the IVC (Figure 120-4). This plane approximates the true division between the right and left halves using the more strict definition of a plane through the middle hepatic vein and IVC, but the middle hepatic vein is not obvious by direct inspection of the surface. Further subdivisions of the right half

of the liver into a right anterior section and a right posterior section are not possible based only on surface anatomy. The left half of the liver can be further subdivided into a left medial section and left lateral section based on the umbilical fissure and falciform ligament. The caudate of the liver is identified as lying posterior to the gastrohepatic ligament and emanating from a process of liver situated posterior to the main portal pedicle and anterior to the IVC.

The most widely accepted nomenclature of liver anatomy is based on Couinaud's description of the eight discrete anatomic segments of the liver (Figure 120-5).[11] The eight segments of a liver can be determined using surface anatomy, the location of the three main hepatic veins, the location of the portal pedicle bifurcation, and the location of the umbilical fissure and falciform ligament. The right and left halves of the liver are delineated by a plane through the middle hepatic vein and IVC. Segments II, III, and IV lie to the left of this plane and form the left half of the liver. Segments V, VI, VII, and VIII lie to the right of this plane and form the right half of the liver. Segment I, or the caudate, is morphologically distinct from the two halves of the liver and emanates from a process of liver lying posterior to the portal pedicle and anterior to the IVC. Whereas the right and left halves of the liver derive blood supply from the corresponding right and left portal veins and hepatic arteries, respectively, segment I derives blood supply from both. Additionally, the right half of the liver has venous

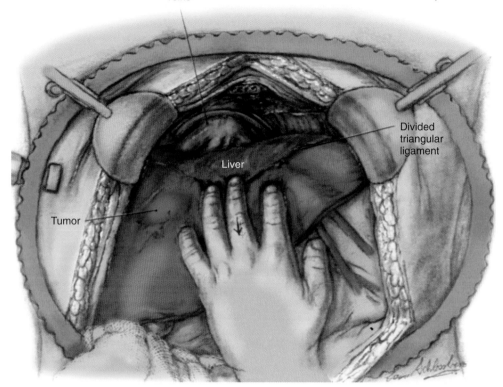

Suprahepatic inferior vena cava and right, middle, and left hepatic veins

Divided triangular ligament

Liver

Tumor

FIGURE 120-2 "Mercedes sign" incision. Excision of the xiphoid process and downward traction on the liver provide excellent exposure of the hepatic veins and suprahepatic inferior vena cava.

drainage mostly through the right and middle hepatic veins, and the left half of the liver has drainage mostly through the left and middle hepatic veins. Segment I, however, drains directly via small branches into the IVC.

The right half of the liver can be further subdivided using a plane through the right hepatic vein and the IVC. The liver anterior to this plane forms the right anterior sector of the liver, and liver posterior to this plane forms the right posterior sector. The right anterior sector of the liver comprises segment V (caudal to the portal bifurcation) and segment VIII (cephalad to the portal bifurcation). The right posterior sector of the liver comprises segment VI (caudal to the portal bifurcation) and segment VII (cephalad to the portal bifurcation).

The left half of the liver can be further subdivided using a plane through the umbilical fissure and falciform ligament. Liver medial to this plane forms the left medial section of the liver or segment IV, and liver lateral to this plane forms the left lateral section of the liver. The left lateral section of the liver is further subdivided into segment II (closer to segment I) and segment III (closer to segment IV), which are supplied by separate portal pedicles from the umbilical fissure.

PREOPERATIVE EVALUATION OF HEPATIC RESERVE

When a surgical resection is planned, the future remnant liver should be sufficient and healthy enough to

regenerate and sustain the patient long term. Up to 70% to 75% of the hepatic volume may be resected with good recovery in patients with relatively normal hepatic parenchyma (without active hepatitis, cirrhosis, or metabolic defects), as long as the remnant liver has adequate portal venous and hepatic arterial inflow, adequate hepatic venous outflow, and adequate biliary drainage. Different groups have used various strategies to try to predict hepatic reserve, including the following:

- Child-Pugh score that assesses synthetic ability (albumin, prothrombin time, and ascites), bile excretory function (total bilirubin), and metabolic function (changes in mental status from ammonia retention) (Table 120-1).[12]
- Volumetric measurements of the liver and predicted liver remnant after resection based on three-dimensional reconstructions from computed tomographic scan and magnetic resonance imaging.[13]
- Clearance of galactose or organic anionic dyes, such as indocyanine green.[14,15]
- Tests of microsomal function, such as caffeine clearance,[16] lidocaine clearance,[17] or aminopyrine breath tests.[18,19]

None of these tests or strategies has demonstrated better ability to predict outcome than another. Many hepatobiliary centers in the United States rely simply on the Child-Pugh score and the prediction of adequate liver remnant volume after resection. In select circumstances, it may be of benefit to perform portal vein embolization to the right or left half of the liver in the hopes

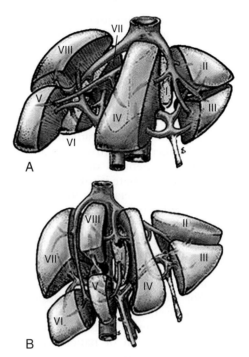

A

B

FIGURE 120-5 Couinaud's eight anatomic segments of the liver: anterior (**A**) and posterior (**B**) views. (From Blumgart LH, Fong Y: *Surgery of the liver and biliary tract: Selected operative procedures*, CD-ROM, ed 3. London, 2000, Harcourt.)

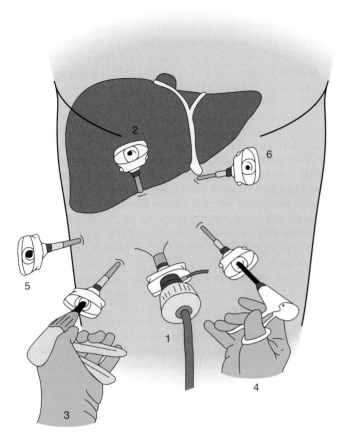

FIGURE 120-3 Optimal port placement for laparoscopic hepatectomy. (From Gumbs AA, Gayet B, Gagner M: Laparoscopic liver resection: When to use the laparoscopic stapler device. *HPB (Oxford)* 10:296, 2008.)

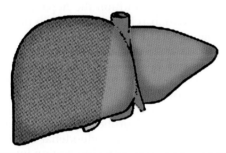

FIGURE 120-4 The liver can be divided into right and left halves by forming a plane through the gallbladder fossa (Cantlie line) and inferior vena cava. (From Blumgart LH, Fong Y: *Surgery of the liver and biliary tract: Selected operative procedures*. CD-ROM, ed 3, London, 2000, Harcourt.)

TABLE 120-1 Child-Pugh Classification*

| | SCORE | | |
Parameter	1	2	3
Bilirubin (mg/dL)	<2	2-3	>3
Albumin (g/dL)	>3.5	2.8-3.5	<2.8
Ascites	Absent	Moderate	Severe
Encephalopathy	Absent	Moderate	Severe
PROTHROMBIN TIME			
Seconds prolonged	<4	4-6	>6
INR	<1.7	1.7-2.3	>2.3

INR, International normalized ratio.
*The Child-Pugh classification: Grade A = 5-6 points; Grade B = 7-9 points; Grade C = 10-15 points.

ONCOLOGIC CONSIDERATIONS IN HEPATIC RESECTION

of obtaining compensatory hypertrophy of the other side prior to resection.[20,21] This is especially useful when the predicted liver remnant after resection is small or if the patient has an underlying hepatic dysfunction that may not allow the remnant to fully regenerate and sustain the patient long term. The disadvantage of portal vein embolization includes the need to wait 4 to 6 weeks prior to resection to allow the compensatory hypertrophy to occur. Additionally, the surgeon must commit to taking out one or the other side without the benefit of intraoperative evaluation.

The decision of whether and when to operate is as important as the technical details of successfully performing a hepatectomy. In making these decisions, it is important to consider the diagnosis. For example, a solitary liver lesion presenting in an elderly patient with a rising carcinoembryonic antigen level and a recent history of a resected colon cancer should be approached and treated differently from a young woman with a solitary lesion with radiologic characteristics of a focal nodular hyperplasia. It is also important to consider the biology of the tumor within the patient. An extreme example of this are two patients, the first of whom re-presents with a solitary hepatic colorectal cancer metastasis 4 years after resection of the primary, and the second who presents with 12 synchronous lesions in the liver at the time of diagnosis of the primary. The former patient is much more likely to benefit from surgical resection than the latter.

It is also important to consider if the goal of resection is curative or palliative. Patients with neuroendocrine tumor metastatic to the liver may be debulked of disease, but the disease is rarely totally eradicated. If the tumor is functional and difficult to control medically, then there may be significant benefit to debulking. Even if the tumor is not functional, there is some evidence that surgical debulking of liver metastases in carefully selected patients may benefit long-term survival.[22,23] It is important to exclude other distant extrahepatic disease with a reasonable number of preoperative tests. For example, prior to performing hepatic resection for colorectal cancer metastases, it is often helpful to obtain a positron emission tomographic scan to exclude extrahepatic metastases.[24] For patients with neuroendocrine tumors metastatic to the liver, it is often helpful to obtain an octreotide scan to survey for extent of disease.[25] These tests allow better selection of patients most likely to benefit from hepatic resection.

The comorbid status of the patient is also important. Extended hepatic resections with or without biliary reconstruction can exert a toll on even very fit patients. It is important to identify patients who may have difficulties with hepatic regeneration such as those with a history of hepatitis, cirrhosis, or metabolic disorders. Patients with suspected cardiopulmonary disease should undergo appropriate preoperative evaluation and treatment prior to hepatic resection. Finally, other effective treatments and the optimal sequence of treatments should be considered. For example, in the treatment of hepatocellular carcinoma the possibilities include liver transplantation, liver resection, liver ablation (radiofrequency, cryotherapy, or ethanol), embolization, and systemic chemotherapies. A patient with poor hepatic reserve due to chronic liver disease and a single small hepatocellular carcinoma may be best treated with liver transplantation, whereas a patient with normal liver parenchyma and a resectable lesion may be best treated with liver resection. Additionally, some patients may best be treated with ablative techniques, especially if they have extremely small lesions that are easily approached percutaneously. Some patients are treated with a combination of these modalities. For example, some patients will first be treated with ethanol ablation and embolization prior to liver transplantation or resection for hepatocellular carcinoma.

INTRAOPERATIVE ASSESSMENT

Incisions for hepatic resections usually involve a right subcostal incision. Significant exposure can be obtained with a trifurcated incision as previously discussed. However, in most cases, all that is needed is an extended right subcostal incision with a vertical extension to the base of the xiphoid. The xiphoid may be resected for better exposure. For bulky lesions on the left or if the left half of the liver extends significantly to the left upper quadrant, a left subcostal component can be added. In

rare circumstances, especially for lesions high on the dome, an intercostal extension or even median sternotomy may improve exposure. This is especially true for lesions involving the hepatic vein and IVC confluences.

Several versions of self-retaining costal margin retractors or ringed retractors are available that provide good access to the subdiaphragmatic surface. For complete intraoperative ultrasonography and for major resections, mobilization of the liver is required. The round ligament is divided and the falciform ligament divided close to the liver parenchyma. The right and left triangular ligaments are then divided to expose the bare areas of the liver. During exposure of the bare areas of the liver, care should be taken to not enter the right or left chest through the ligamentous portions of the diaphragm, as this will cause excessive bellowing of the diaphragm and poor exposure until a chest tube is placed on that side. Additionally, the right and left phrenic veins are very superficial on the hemidiaphragms and are prone to injury. The right colon can be mobilized out of the field by dividing the Gerota fascia over the right kidney and pulling the hepatic flexure inferiorly. To completely assess the caudate lobe, the overlying lesser omentum should be divided. Care should be taken to not inadvertently divide a replaced or accessory left hepatic artery running in this plane. After mobilization, a thorough bimanual examination should be performed and intraoperative ultrasonography used.

Hepatic ultrasonography can be quite useful in identifying lesions within the hepatic parenchyma, and at most centers intraoperative ultrasonography is used routinely to assess the anatomy of the pedicles (portal vein, hepatic artery, bile duct), the hepatic veins, and the hepatic parenchyma. It is both useful to further identify and characterize lesions within the hepatic parenchyma and to delineate their relationships within the eight anatomic segments of the liver. Additionally, it is often helpful to delineate proximity of lesions to major vascular structures and to survey for abnormal anatomy in planning a resection. With radiofrequency ablation more commonly employed, ultrasound has become indispensable in directing its use.

Using the ultrasound probe, the main portal pedicle is identified within the hepatoduodenal ligament. It is followed cephalad to the portal bifurcation into the main right and left pedicles. The portal pedicles are invested with the Glisson capsule and have a very echogenic covering to them in contrast to hepatic vein branches. The main right portal pedicle is followed toward the right, where it gives off an anterior and posterior branch (Figure 120-6). The right anterior branch gives off separate pedicles to segment V (caudal) and to segment VIII (cephalad). The right posterior branch gives off separate pedicles to segment VI (caudal) and to segment VII (cephalad). The main left pedicle is usually much longer and courses intact to the base of the umbilical fissure before branching into various segmental pedicles. At the base of the umbilical fissure, the main left pedicle courses anteriorly toward the round ligament and gives off a pedicle to segment IV medially and pedicles to segments II and III laterally. Next, if the bare areas around the junction of the hepatic veins and IVC have been well

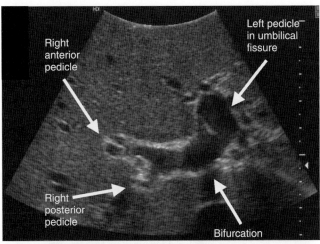

FIGURE 120-6 Intraoperative ultrasound image of bifurcation of the main portal pedicle into the right and left branches.

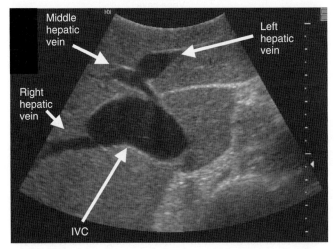

FIGURE 120-7 Intraoperative ultrasound image of the three main hepatic veins. The left and middle hepatic veins often join together before emptying into the inferior vena cava (IVC).

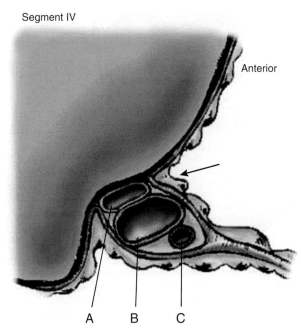

FIGURE 120-8 The hilar plate of the liver can be "lowered" by dividing the Glisson capsule at the lowest edge of segment IV. This maneuver gains access to the most cephalad portion of the bifurcation of the porta hepatis. **A,** Left hepatic duct. **B,** Portal vein. **C,** Hepatic artery. (Adapted from Blumgart LH, Fong Y: *Surgery of the liver and biliary tract: Selected operative procedures*, CD-ROM, ed 3. London, 2000, Harcourt.)

mobilized, the hepatic veins can easily be visualized using intraoperative ultrasonography (Figure 120-7). As described previously, usually a larger right hepatic vein can be delineated and smaller left and middle hepatic veins joining into a common trunk before emptying into the IVC are seen. Commonly, an umbilical hepatic vein branch can be identified coursing between the middle and left hepatic veins and running under the falciform ligament. Not uncommonly, significant accessory right hepatic veins can be seen emptying from the posterior surface of the right liver directly into the IVC as it courses posterior to the liver. The identification of these accessory right hepatic veins is quite important for both vascular control and preservation of outflow from the liver. Finally, the hepatic parenchyma is systematically scanned to identify lesions within the liver. It is sometimes useful to adjust the ultrasound settings on a known lesion defined preoperatively to maximize the echogenicity in the hopes of identifying other occult lesions not identified preoperatively.

GENERAL MANEUVERS FOR HEPATECTOMY

The porta hepatis can be dissected to identify the main bifurcations of the hepatic artery, bile duct, and portal vein and to allow individual ligation of these. Ligation of the hepatic artery and portal vein to one side causes the liver parenchyma to demarcate between the right and left liver. Greater exposure of the cephalad aspect of the hepatic hilum and exposure of a high or intraparenchymal bifurcation of portal triad structures may be aided by lowering the hilar plate (Figure 120-8) and dividing the Glisson capsule at the most inferior border of segment IV.

Control of the inflow hepatic artery and portal vein branches to a specific anatomic section of the liver may also be obtained by pedicle ligations in which small hepatotomies are made around the main right pedicle, main left pedicle, right anterior pedicle, or right posterior pedicle after identification with ultrasound (Figure 120-9).[26] The pedicle of interest can be dissected out bluntly with a right angle or by finger fracture. The pedicle should be test clamped atraumatically to confirm that it does indeed supply the area of liver of interest. If the proper pedicle is clamped, the appropriate portion of the liver (i.e., right half, left half, right anterior section, or right posterior section) should demarcate. Once confirmed, it can be divided. Alternatively, the specific inflow pedicles can be divided as they are encountered during parenchymal transection. With this technique, hemorrhage can be minimized by intermittent portal inflow

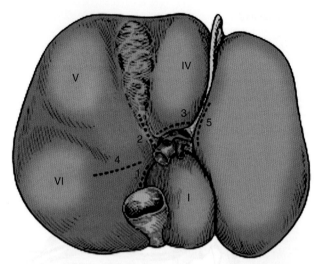

FIGURE 120-9 Sites for intraparenchymal portal pedicle ligation. Incisions at 1 and 2 allow isolation of the main right pedicle. Incisions at 1 and 4 allow isolation of the right posterior pedicle. Incisions at 2 and 4 allow isolation of the right anterior pedicle. Incisions at 3 and 5 allow isolation of the left pedicle. (From Fong Y, Blumgart LH: Useful stapling techniques in liver surgery. *J Am Coll Surg* 185:93, 1997.)

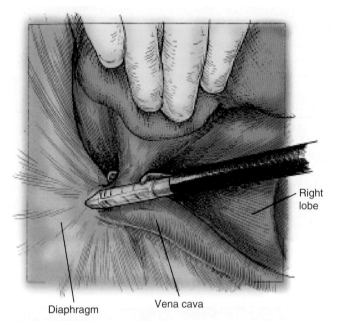

FIGURE 120-10 The right hepatic vein can be divided with the aid of an endoscopic stapling device with a vascular load. (From Fong Y, Blumgart LH: Useful stapling techniques in liver surgery. *J Am Coll Surg* 185:93, 1997.)

occlusion accomplished by atraumatically clamping the main portal triad within the hepatoduodenal ligament (Pringle maneuver).

Outflow control of the hepatic veins can be obtained at differing time points depending on the situation. If there is a sufficient length of extraparenchymal hepatic vein, often it is easier to divide the hepatic vein early and prior to parenchymal transection (but after inflow control). If the extraparenchymal portion of the hepatic vein is short (or absent), it may be easier and safer to divide the hepatic vein or veins within the hepatic parenchyma after most of the parenchymal transection has been performed. The use of endoscopic vascular stapling devices has made the ligation of hepatic veins whether extraparenchymally or intraparenchymally much quicker and safer (Figure 120-10).[26] Another technique used to minimize blood loss is a low central venous pressure technique where the central venous pressure of the patient is kept low (<5 mm Hg) until after parenchymal transection.[27] Once the parenchymal transection is complete and the bleeding is controlled, the patient is made euvolemic. This minimizes the bleeding coming from the hepatic vein branches.

MAJOR HEPATECTOMIES

To develop a uniform nomenclature understood by all, the American Hepato-Pancreato-Biliary Association (AHPBA) and the International Hepato-Pancreato-Biliary Association (IHPBA) have adopted the Brisbane 2000 terminology of hepatic anatomy and resections.[28] Right hepatectomy or right hemihepatectomy involves the resection of segments V through VIII; left hepatectomy or hemihepatectomy involves the resection of segments II through IV. Either of these resections may or may not include resection of segment I, which should be

stipulated. Extended right hepatectomy involves the resection of segments IV through VIII; extended left hepatectomy involves the resection of segments II through V plus VIII. Again, either of these extended resections may or may not include resection of segment I, which should be stipulated.

Right anterior sectionectomy includes segments V and VIII. Right posterior sectionectomy includes segments VI and VII. Left medial sectionectomy removes segment IV. Left lateral sectionectomy includes segments II and III. A segmentectomy involves the resection of a single segment, and a bisegmentectomy involves the resection of two contiguous segments.

The steps involved in major hepatectomies include optimal exposure, vascular inflow control, vascular outflow control, and parenchymal transection. Vascular inflow control may be obtained by directly ligating the main right or left branches of the hepatic artery and portal vein in the hilum and/or by intermittent 10- to 20-minute intervals of a Pringle maneuver with 3 minutes in between to reestablish blood flow. I prefer to encircle the hepatoduodenal ligament twice with a ¼-inch Penrose drain that is tightened and clamped for a Pringle maneuver. Alternatively, pedicle ligations can be performed as described previously, or the pedicles can be controlled as they are encountered during parenchymal transection. I prefer to obtain vascular inflow by ligating the appropriate vessels in the hilum or by pedicle ligations and to supplement this with intermittent Pringle maneuvers as necessary during parenchymal transection for hemihepatectomies. Vascular outflow to the right or left liver can be obtained by exposing and ligating the hepatic veins as previously described or by ligating the vessels intraparenchymally during transection of the liver tissue.

TRANSECTING THE HEPATIC PARENCHYMA

There are many possibilities with regard to the technique of transecting the liver. Regardless of the method to be employed, certain principles must be adhered to. These include safety, speed, minimization of blood loss, and avoidance of significant liver injury. Traditionally, a finger-fracture or crush-clamp technique has been used. These continue to be popular and extensively practiced; however, developing technologies have made significant additions to the armamentarium. Devices based on ultrasound, high-pressure liquid, tissue-sealing, and radiofrequency are all in common use, in addition to surgical staplers. With such a wide array of choices, the natural question of whether one method is superior to the others quickly arises. In fact, many studies have been undertaken to compare techniques, and born from these, a large metaanalysis. In the seven trials assessed in this metaanalysis, the primary endpoints focus on operative mortality (which is difficult to assess as it is relatively uncommon, and therefore challenging to adequately power the study), morbidity, intraoperative blood loss, parenchymal transection time/speed, and overall cost.[29] Most of the studies compared the crush-clamp technique to newer technologies such as the Cavitronic Ultrasonic Surgical Aspirator (CUSA),[30] radiofrequency (RF)-based dissectors/sealers,[31,32] and hydrojet.[33] A general conclusion seems to endorse the crush-clamp technique as the fastest, least bloody, and cheapest option. In all previously done studies, the crush-clamp technique is used in conjunction with a Pringle maneuver, whereas many of the newer technologies are employed without portal triad occlusion. The precise reason for this is unclear as the Pringle maneuver has been historically shown to be safe, and in comparisons of biochemical liver abnormalities, there is no significant difference with regard to the risk of permanent liver injury. A couple of key points deserve mention. Studies demonstrated a higher rate of intraabdominal abscess formation with the use of an RF-assisted device. This was theorized to occur as a result of excess nonviable tissue created by the large "burn area" associated with this technique. Also, CUSA and RF-assisted devices have fairly high cost as a consequence of their use, and more complex equipment that requires additional training of both the operator and the operating room staff.

One particular technique of hepatic parenchymal transection not covered by the aforementioned metaanalysis is the use of surgical stapling devices. This is an especially important consideration in the discussion of laparoscopic liver resection. A recent study of 62 patients who underwent partial hepatectomies using endoGIA stapling devices showed this to be a safe, effective, and efficient method of liver transection.[34] Technology continues to evolve in this arena as more efficient and less costly devices are sought. One feature of all of the aforementioned techniques is that they require more than one instrument, at times multiple, to achieve parenchymal division as well as hemostasis. A new device utilizing RF technology, which can simultaneously cut and coagulate liver tissue, has been tested with promising results in the areas of transection speed and limiting blood loss.[35]

With these techniques, individual blood vessels and bile ducts are cauterized, clipped, or sutured in rapid succession as they are encountered. Constant reevaluation of the direction of transection is important both to not injure vital structures to the remnant liver and to maintain a negative margin. After parenchymal transection and removal of the specimen, the raw surface of the liver is carefully inspected for bleeding and bile leakage, which can then be controlled by suture ligation and argon beam coagulation. New formulations of fibrin glues are constantly being developed to aid in hemostasis and prevention of biliary leak. Whether they are indeed a cost-effective way of controlling bleeding and maintaining hemostasis has yet to be determined.[36-38] A recent prospective study involving 300 patients undergoing hepatectomy randomized them to the use of fibrin glue or no sealant (150 in each arm). More than 50% of those in each group underwent a major hepatectomy, though the percentage of minor hepatectomies was still high. With this in mind, the authors found no difference in the two groups when considering the endpoints of bleeding, bile leak, postoperative drain output, or overall morbidity.[39] The authors prefer to place closed-suction drains near resected liver surfaces to monitor and drain unrecognized postoperative bile leaks, but some centers do not routinely place drains, and their routine use is controversial.[40,41]

RIGHT HEPATECTOMY WITH HILAR DISSECTION

A right hepatectomy can usually be accomplished through a right subcostal incision with upper midline extension and involves resection of segments V, VI, VII, and VIII. If greater exposure toward the left is required, a trifurcated incision can be used. The hepatic flexure of the colon is mobilized caudad. The round ligament and falciform ligament are divided. The right bare area of the liver is exposed by dividing the right triangular ligament. The right inferior liver edge is mobilized out of the retroperitoneum. This dissection reveals the upper pole of the right kidney, right adrenal gland, and suprahepatic IVC. The liver is then rotated to the left, and the subhepatic IVC is dissected by controlling the small venous branches draining directly from the liver. There is often an IVC ligament that extends from the right liver and around the right side of the IVC just caudad to the right hepatic vein. This can often be controlled with an endoscopic stapler with a vascular load after it is dissected out. At this point, the right hepatic vein can be identified and dissected out, whereupon a vessel loop can be placed around it. If dissection of the right hepatic vein is not safe at this time, it can be controlled later after parenchymal transection.

A cholecystectomy is then performed. The hepatic artery bifurcation is localized. The right hepatic artery is ligated. The common hepatic duct is then dissected and mobilized anteriorly and to the left to expose the portal vein (Figure 120-11). Dissection is then carried out into the hilum of the liver to expose the bifurcation of the portal vein. The right portal vein is circumferentially dissected (Figure 120-12). Care should be taken to make sure that the left portal vein takeoff is clear of the dissection and that small branches draining the caudate are

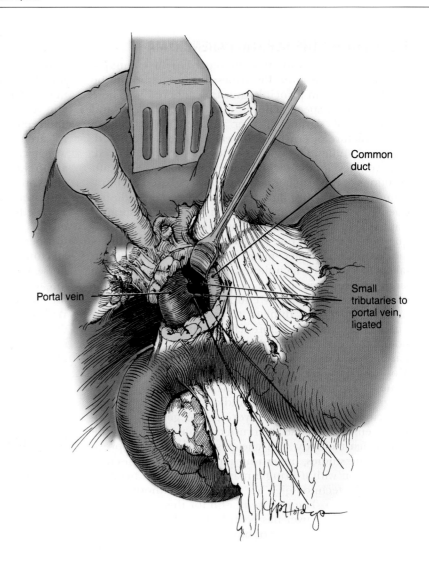

FIGURE 120-11 Right hepatectomy. Initial exposure of the portal vein before hilar ligation of its right branch is shown. The area to be dissected, closer to the hilus of the liver than shown, has no branches. (From Nora PE: *Operative surgery: Principles and techniques.* Philadelphia, 1980, Lea and Febiger, p 647.)

sufficiently controlled and divided. The right portal vein can be divided with ties with a reinforcing suture ligature on the stump or with an endoscopic stapler with a vascular load. Hilar dissection is then completed by identifying and isolating the right hepatic duct, which is next ligated and divided.

The liver is then rotated to the left and the previously isolated right hepatic vein is divided between vascular clamps or an endoscopic stapler with a vascular load. If vascular clamps are used, the caval stump is closed with a running 4-0 Prolene suture and the specimen side simply suture-ligated. Several minutes after the right hepatic artery and portal vein are ligated, the right liver should become devascularized and turn dusky. The Glisson capsule is then scored with the electrocautery device starting at the level of the divided right hepatic vein to the gallbladder fossa on the anterior surface. If preservation of the middle hepatic vein is intended, then the line of transection should be moved slightly lateral. If the intention is to take the middle hepatic vein, then the line of transection should be moved medially. Intraoperative ultrasound can be used to carefully map this out. On the posterior surface of the liver, the liver is scored along the right lateral border of the IVC toward

the portal bifurcation. Parenchymal transection is then performed by any of the previously described techniques. Intermittent portal inflow clamping, as described previously, can be used to help decrease blood loss if this is a problem during parenchymal transection. During parenchymal transection vascular and biliary structures are controlled by the appropriate combination of clips, sutures, suture ligatures, and stapling devices. Once the parenchyma is transected, the specimen can be removed.

LEFT HEPATECTOMY WITH HILAR DISSECTION

A left hepatectomy can also be accomplished through a right subcostal incision with an upper midline extension and involves resection of segments II, III, and IV. For large bulky tumors on the left or if the left liver extends significantly laterally, a left subcostal component may be needed to trifurcate the incision. Alternatively, a midline incision can be used, but this may limit exposure to the right liver should unexpected findings be encountered during exploration. The round ligament and falciform ligament are divided. The left bare area is next exposed by dissecting the left triangular ligament. Usually the left hepatic vein and middle hepatic vein join together within the parenchyma of the liver before emptying into the

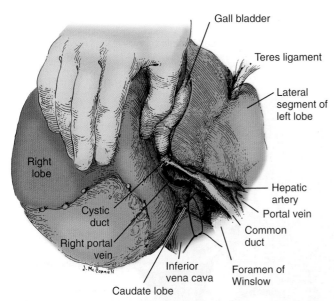

FIGURE 120-12 Right hepatectomy: Exposure of the right branch of the portal vein from the posterior approach. The liver has been retracted anteriorly and to the left. The looped ligature is around a branch to the caudate lobe. (From Starzl TE, Bell RH, Baert RW: Hepatic trisegmentectomy and other liver resections. *Surg Gynecol Obstet* 141:429, 1975.)

IVC, which precludes extrahepatic dissection of this vessel without taking the middle hepatic vein. If it is separate and dissectible, a vessel loop is encircled around it. A cholecystectomy is performed. The lesser omentum is divided to fully expose the margins of the hepatoduodenal ligament. Care should be taken to note a replaced or accessory left hepatic artery running in this location. The proper hepatic artery is identified and dissected above the bifurcation of the right and left branches. The left hepatic artery is then divided.

The common hepatic duct is next exposed, and the left hepatic duct is divided above the bifurcation. The left portal vein can then be identified at the base of segment IV and traced to the hilus of the liver. It is circumferentially dissected and can be ligated or controlled with an endoscopic stapler with a vascular load. The left liver should become devascularized and turn dusky. If the left hepatic vein was previously successfully dissected then it can be divided with either ligatures or an endoscopic stapler with a vascular load. The anterior surface of the liver is then scored with the electrocautery device from the left hepatic vein (or stump) to the top of the gallbladder fossa. The posterior surface of the liver is then scored with the electrocautery device from the top of the gallbladder fossa to the portal bifurcation. If preservation of the middle hepatic vein is intended, then the line of transection should be moved slightly to the left; if the intention is to take the middle hepatic vein, then the line of transection should be moved to the right. Intraoperative ultrasound can be used to carefully map this out. Parenchymal transection is then performed by any of the previously described techniques. Intermittent portal inflow clamping as described previously can be used to help decrease blood loss if this is a problem

during parenchymal transection. During parenchymal transection, vascular and biliary structures are controlled by the appropriate combination of clips, sutures, suture ligatures, and stapling devices. Once the parenchyma is transected, the specimen can be removed (Figure 120-13). If the caudate must also be removed to provide adequate tumor clearance, it can be mobilized off the IVC by sequentially dividing the short veins that directly drain into the IVC.

LEFT LATERAL SECTIONECTOMY

Left lateral sectionectomy can usually be performed through an upper midline incision and involves resection of segments II and III of the liver. If unexpected findings in the right liver are discovered during exploration, however, a midline incision may be limiting. Alternatively, a bilateral subcostal incision can be used. The round ligament and falciform ligament are divided. The bridge of liver parenchyma between segments III and IV over the round ligament is divided either with electrocautery or with an endoscopic stapler with a vascular load. The left bare area is next exposed by dissecting the left triangular ligament.

For resection of tumor, the surface of the liver is then scored 1 cm to the left of the falciform ligament and to the left of the umbilical fissure (provided that the margin is adequate). This preserves the blood supply and biliary drainage to segment IV of the remnant liver. For donor hepatectomy, the anterior surface of the liver is scored 1 cm to the right of the falciform ligament and to the right of the umbilical fissure. This preserves the blood supply and biliary drainage to segments II and III of the donor liver. Parenchymal transection is then performed by any of the previously described techniques. Intermittent portal inflow clamping is usually not required for left lateral sectionectomy. As the main portal pedicles to the segments are encountered within the parenchyma, they are controlled with clamps, divided, and ligated or stapled with an endoscopic stapler with a vascular load. The left hepatic vein can then be finally controlled within the hepatic parenchyma either with ligatures or a stapler.

EXTENDED RIGHT AND LEFT HEPATECTOMIES

Extended right and left hepatectomies are perhaps the most difficult and complicated types of liver resections and are covered in classic manuscripts.[42,43] The initial maneuvers for the extended right hepatectomy are similar to right hepatectomy. The cystic artery and duct are ligated and divided, but the gallbladder can be left attached to the specimen because segments IV, V, VI, VII, and VIII are to be resected in continuity. The portal structures are dissected and divided as before. The right hepatic vein is controlled and divided, if possible, as before. Because the line of parenchymal transection is just to the right of the umbilical fissure and falciform ligament, the feedback structures to segment IV must be controlled. The bridge of liver parenchyma between segments III and IV is divided. The liver parenchyma is scored with the electrocautery device along the plane of transection. Parenchymal transection is then performed by any of the previously described techniques. As the

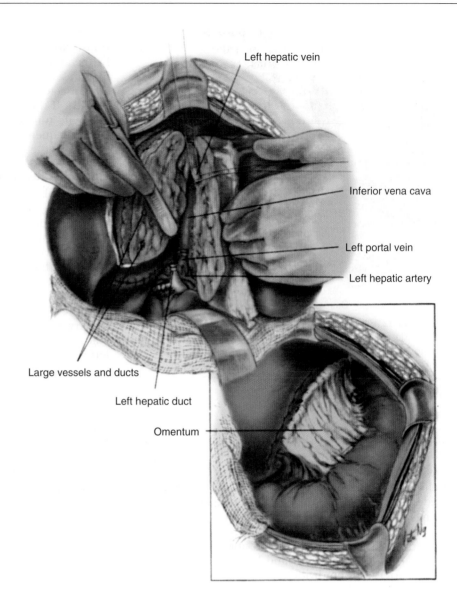

Left hepatic vein

Inferior vena cava

Left portal vein

Left hepatic artery

Large vessels and ducts

Left hepatic duct

Omentum

FIGURE 120-13 Left hepatectomy. The hilar structures have been dissected and ligated, and the parenchymal transection is complete. In this case, the left hepatic vein has been left for last. This also depicts a resection that includes the caudate lobe. (From Schwartz SI: *Surgical diseases of the liver*. New York, 1964, McGraw-Hill, p 254.)

main portal pedicles to segment IV are encountered within the parenchyma, they are controlled with clamps, divided, and ligated or stapled with an endoscopic stapler with a vascular load. This dissection is carried to the base of the umbilical fissure (Figure 120-14). Parenchymal transection is continued posteriorly ligating the middle hepatic vein and/or its branches. Great care is taken to preserve the left hepatic vein (Figure 120-15). Intermittent portal inflow clamping as described previously can be used to help decrease blood loss if this is a problem during parenchymal transection. The caudate is either preserved or resected with the specimen. Because of the risk of torsion of the liver remnant, it should be attached back to the falciform ligament.

The initial maneuvers for an extended left hepatectomy are similar to left hepatectomy. The cystic artery and duct are ligated and divided, but the gallbladder can be left attached to the specimen as segments II, III, IV, V, and VIII are to be resected in continuity. The right triangular ligament, in addition to the left, is also divided. The portal structures are dissected and divided as before.

The left hepatic vein (with the middle hepatic veins) is controlled and divided, if possible, as before. The difficulty with extended left hepatectomy is performing the parenchymal transection to preserve the right posterior pedicle and the right hepatic vein while taking the right anterior sector of the liver (segments V and VIII). Intraoperative ultrasound is useful in locating and protecting these structures. Intermittent portal inflow clamping as described previously is usually required because of the magnitude of parenchymal transection and difficulty in early control of the right anterior pedicle. Parenchymal transection is then performed by any of the previously described techniques (Figures 120-16 and 120-17).

SEGMENTAL RESECTIONS

To maximize functional reserve, (multi)segmental or subsegmental (or nonanatomic) hepatectomies can be performed. For example, left lateral sectionectomy (segments II and III), central hepatectomy to remove the right anterior section (segments V and VIII) and left medial section (segment IV), right posterior sectionectomy (segments VI and VII), or caudate resection (segment I) are examples in which one, two, or three contiguous segments are removed to eradicate tumors within those regions of the liver. These resections are often done with intermittent Pringle maneuver until the specific pedicles supplying these areas are controlled.

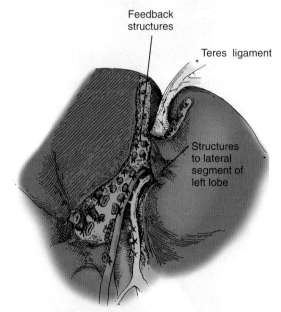

FIGURE 120-14 Right extended hepatectomy. Control of the feedback vessels to segment IV. Blunt dissection in liver substance just to the right of the umbilical fissure exposes these vessels. Each vascular and biliary structure is ligated individually to complete devascularization of segment IV. (From Starzl TE, Bell RH, Baert RW: Hepatic trisegmentectomy and other liver resections. *Surg Gynecol Obstet* 141:429, 1975.)

WEDGE RESECTIONS

When a simple wedge resection of the liver is appropriate, the area to be resected is isolated between two interlocking mattress sutures of heavy absorbable material (Figure 120-18). The two mattress sutures are placed in the form of a "V" intersecting at the apex. After the wedge resection is performed, the mattress sutures can be tied to each other to approximate the two opposing raw liver surfaces.

LAPAROSCOPIC LIVER RESECTION

As is the case with all operations, significant attention has been given to developing and furthering minimally invasive approaches to liver resection in recent years. This has ranged from minor procedures such as wedge resections, to more extensive segmentectomies, sectionectomies, and even hemihepatectomies. The first laparoscopic liver resection was reported in 1992,[44] a volume that has now grown in excess of 3000 reported cases (as of 2010).[44] With regard to hepatic resection, the term *laparoscopic* actually encompasses a number of techniques: pure laparoscopy, hand-assisted laparoscopy, and hybrid techniques where both laparoscopic and open approaches are utilized during the procedure.[44] The same anatomic and oncologic principles apply as with open approaches. It should be noted, however, that laparoscopy may introduce limitations in the areas of ultrasonographic evaluation, information gathered through tactile sensation, and maneuvers of mobilization and retraction. Similar to any other operation, proper patient selection is of paramount importance to a safe and successful procedure. To that end, the recommendations of one author included specific guidelines when considering laparoscopy as the method of resection: solitary masses, 5 cm or

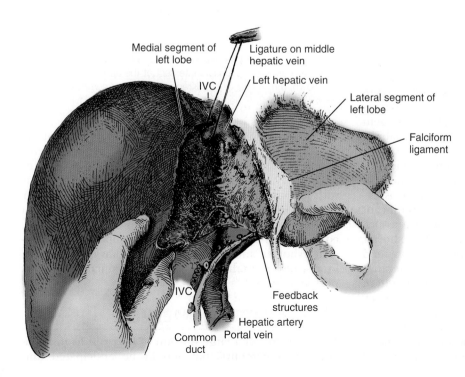

FIGURE 120-15 Right extended hepatectomy. Parenchymal transection is nearly complete. The main trunk of the middle hepatic vein is exposed, with a ligature around it. At this juncture, the caudate still may be left in situ. *Ivc,* Inferior vena cava. (From Starzl TE, Bell RH, Baert RW: Hepatic trisegmentectomy and other liver resections. *Surg Gynecol Obstet* 141:429, 1975.)

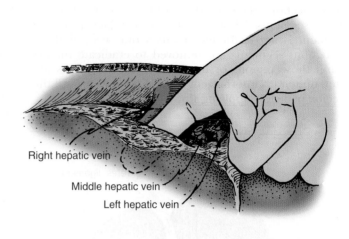

FIGURE 120-16 Left extended hepatectomy: superior-to-inferior dissection between the right anterior sector and right posterior sector. The dissecting finger is kept anterior to the right hepatic vein. The left and middle hepatic veins have been ligated or sutured. (From Starzl TE, Iwatsuki S, Shaw BW, Jr, et al: Left hepatic trisegmentectomy. *Surg Gynecol Obstet* 155:25, 1982.)

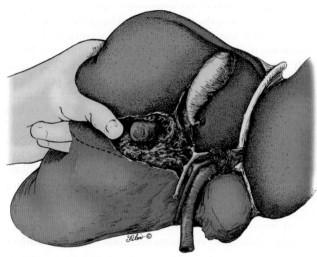

FIGURE 120-17 Left extended hepatectomy. Further development of the plane between the anterior and posterior sectors of the right liver. (From Starzl TE, Iwatsuki S, Shaw BW, Jr, et al: Left hepatic trisegmentectomy. *Surg Gynecol Obstet* 155:25, 1982.)

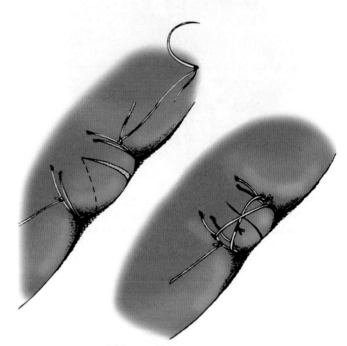

FIGURE 120-18 Wedge biopsy of the free margin of the liver. The two mattress sutures of heavy absorbable material actually should be placed as a V and should intersect at the apex, not run parallel as shown. (From Grewe HE, Kremer K: *Atlas of surgical operations*, vol 2. Philadelphia, 1980, Saunders, p 321.)

smaller in diameter, considered to be anatomically peripheral (segments II to VI).[44] Multiple studies have compared the group of techniques referred to using the umbrella term *laparoscopic* to the traditional open approach. As has been previously written, these papers must be evaluated while carefully considering patient selection, especially given the tremendous variability among those in need of liver resection. Key factors include not only the size, location, and number of lesions but just as importantly the quality of the background liver and the overall health of the patient. Larger retrospective series and metaanalyses reveal some significant findings. As a whole, laparoscopic hepatectomy is associated with lower estimated blood loss, possibly shorter operative times, markedly shorter hospital stays, and no significant differences in operative or postoperative morbidity.[45-47] As Jensen and Vickers astutely highlight in an invited critique of one of the aforementioned metaanalyses, the overall evaluation does not assign proper weight to certain vital considerations: namely the size and location of a given lesion and the degree of background liver disease in cirrhotic patients.[48] There are smaller studies that have aimed to eliminate some of the confounding variables by attempting to match patients based on tumor size, number, location, and severity of cirrhosis. While this inherently will still select patients with less complex disease, authors have reached similar conclusions. Operative time appears to correlate with surgeon/operative team experience, blood loss is less, complication rates are equivalent, hospital stay is significantly shorter, and in one paper, there was no difference in all-cause mortality as late as (approximately) 3 years postoperatively.[49,50]

POSTOPERATIVE MANAGEMENT

The resection of a large portion of liver results in metabolic derangements that should be anticipated and treated. Jaundice is not uncommon and is secondary to loss of hepatic parenchyma and to effects from blood transfusion if used. Hyperbilirubinemia usually peaks 3 to 4 days postoperatively and then begins to resolve as the liver remnant recovers and regenerates. Serum transaminase elevations are expected but generally plateau at less than 1000 units/L and are not usually ominous in the absence of severe prolongation in international normalized ratio (INR), decreased fibrinogen, hepatic encephalopathy, acidosis, and elevated serum ammonia levels. Hypophosphatemia and hypokalemia are common after liver resection, and these electrolytes should be monitored closely and repleted. Hypoglycemia is sometimes observed after massive liver resection, as is hypoalbuminemia.

Coagulopathies are often noted after hepatic resection, because of a combination of blood loss, dilution of clotting factors, blood product transfusion, and inadequate liver function. Vitamin K is administered commonly to patients after liver resection, although a patient with a prolonged prothrombin time often does not respond to this therapy if the primary cause is liver failure. Patients with coagulopathy and ongoing bleeding may require support with blood, plasma, cryoprecipitate, and platelets as appropriate.

Most surgeons use parenteral antibiotics prior to incision and for one or two doses intraoperatively. Antibiotics are typically not given after the case concludes. In general, diets can be advanced relatively quickly once patients can tolerate liquids. Patients may need to be salt restricted if fluid retention is significant. Some patients benefit from diuresis after the acute postoperative period.

POSTOPERATIVE COMPLICATIONS

Postoperative complication rates vary greatly depending on what population of patients is being studied. For example, mortality and morbidity following donor hepatectomy are appropriately very low, whereas those following liver resection in patients with cirrhosis are high. The degree of hepatic resection as well as whether the biliary tree requires reconstruction or not also will affect morbidity and mortality.

Mortality rates following liver resection in many modern series are now less than 5%. Not uncommon complications following liver resection are bile leak, intraabdominal abscess, bleeding, pneumonia, and cardiac complications.

SUMMARY

It is important for surgeons performing liver resections to be familiar with normal anatomy as well as the specific anatomic variations for each patient. Patient selection is paramount, so that those most likely to benefit can be appropriately taken to the operating room. The indications for performing a liver resection are myriad and cover many primary and secondary conditions of the liver. An operative plan should be formulated based on preoperative imaging and intraoperative findings after visualization, examination, and intraoperative ultrasound where appropriate. A strategy of resection including

inflow vascular control, outflow vascular control, and parenchymal transection should be formulated that will remove the lesion(s) with appropriate margins but that will leave the patient with an adequate liver remnant that has good vascular inflow, vascular outflow, and biliary drainage. Although laparoscopic and hybrid techniques have advanced and enjoy increasing popularity, they must be considered within the context of the disease and the patient, and are just additional tools in the surgeon's arsenal.

REFERENCES

1. von Frerichs FT: *Uber den Diabetes.* Berlin, 1884, Hirschwald.
2. Weitz J, D'Angelica M, Jarnagin W, et al: Selective use of diagnostic laparoscopy prior to planned hepatectomy for patients with hepatocellular carcinoma. *Surgery* 135:273, 2004.
3. Lo CM, Lai EC, Liu CL, et al: Laparoscopy and laparoscopic ultrasonography avoid exploratory laparotomy in patients with hepatocellular carcinoma. *Ann Surg* 227:527, 1998.
4. Lai EC, Tang CN, Ha JP, et al: The evolving influence of laparoscopy and laparoscopic ultrasonography on patients with hepatocellular carcinoma. *Am J Surg* 196:736, 2008.
5. Jarnagin WR, Conlon K, Bodniewicz J, et al: A clinical scoring system predicts the yield of diagnostic laparoscopy in patients with potentially resectable hepatic colorectal metastases. *Cancer* 91:1121, 2001.
6. Gumbs AA, Gayet B, Gagner M: Laparoscopic liver resection: When to use the laparoscopic stapler device. *HPB (Oxford)* 10:296, 2008.
7. McIndoe AH, Counseller VX: A report on the bilaterality of the liver. *Arch Surg* 15:589, 1927.
8. Healey JE Jr, Schroy PC: Anatomy of the biliary ducts within the human liver: Analysis of the prevailing pattern of branchings and the major variations of the biliary ducts. *AMA Arch Surg* 66:599, 1953.
9. Goldsmith NA, Woodburne RT: The surgical anatomy pertaining to liver resection. *Surg Gynecol Obstet* 105:310, 1957.
10. Bismuth H, Houssin D, Castaing D: Major and minor segmentectomies "reglees" in liver surgery. *World J Surg* 6:10, 1982.
11. Couinaud C: *Le foi: Etudes anatomogiques et chirurgicales.* Paris, 1957, Masson.
12. Pugh RN, Murray-Lyon IM, Dawson JL, et al: Transection of the oesophagus for bleeding oesophageal varices. *Br J Surg* 60:646, 1973.
13. Shoup M, Gonen M, D'Angelica M, et al: Volumetric analysis predicts hepatic dysfunction in patients undergoing major liver resection. *J Gastrointest Surg* 7:325, 2003.
14. Schneider PD: Preoperative assessment of liver function. *Surg Clin North Am* 84:355, 2004.
15. Hsieh CB, Chen CJ, Chen TW, et al: Accuracy of indocyanine green pulse spectrophotometry clearance test for liver function prediction in transplanted patients. *World J Gastroenterol* 10:2394, 2004.
16. Shrestha R, McKinley C, Showalter R, et al: Quantitative liver function tests define the functional severity of liver disease in early-stage cirrhosis. *Liver Transpl Surg* 3:166, 1997.
17. Lee WC, Chen MF: Assessment of hepatic reserve for indication of hepatic resection: How I do it. *J Hepatobiliary Pancreat Surg* 12:23, 2005.
18. Lau H, Man K, Fan ST, et al: Evaluation of preoperative hepatic function in patients with hepatocellular carcinoma undergoing hepatectomy. *Br J Surg* 84:1255, 1997.
19. Lau W, Leung K, Leung TW, et al: A logical approach to hepatocellular carcinoma presenting with jaundice. *Ann Surg* 225:281, 1997.
20. Covey AM, Tuorto S, Brody LA, et al: Safety and efficacy of preoperative portal vein embolization with polyvinyl alcohol in 58 patients with liver metastases. *AJR Am J Roentgenol* 185:1620, 2005.
21. Khatri VP, Petrelli NJ, Belghiti J: Extending the frontiers of surgical therapy for hepatic colorectal metastases: Is there a limit? *J Clin Oncol* 23:8490, 2005.
22. Sutcliffe R, Maguire D, Ramage J, et al: Management of neuroendocrine liver metastases. *Am J Surg* 187:39, 2004.

23. Sarmiento JM, Heywood G, Rubin J, et al: Surgical treatment of neuroendocrine metastases to the liver: A plea for resection to increase survival. *J Am Coll Surg* 197:29, 2003.

24. Fernandez FG, Drebin JA, Linehan DC, et al: Five-year survival after resection of hepatic metastases from colorectal cancer in patients screened by positron emission tomography with F-18 fluorodeoxyglucose (FDG-PET). *Ann Surg* 240:438; discussion 47, 2004.

25. Kwekkeboom DJ, Krenning EP: Somatostatin receptor imaging. *Semin Nucl Med* 32:84, 2002.

26. Fong Y, Blumgart LH: Useful stapling techniques in liver surgery. *J Am Coll Surg* 185:93, 1997.

27. Melendez JA, Arslan V, Fischer ME, et al: Perioperative outcomes of major hepatic resections under low central venous pressure anesthesia: Blood loss, blood transfusion, and the risk of postoperative renal dysfunction. *J Am Coll Surg* 187:620, 1998.

28. The Terminology Committee of the IHPBA: The Brisbane 2000 terminology of hepatic anatomy and resections. *HPB* 2:333, 2000.

29. Pamecha V, Gurusamy KS, Sharma D, et al: Techniques for liver parenchymal transection: A meta-analysis of randomized controlled trials. *HPB (Oxford)* 11:275, 2009.

30. Takayama T, Makuuchi M, Kubota K, et al: Randomized comparison of ultrasonic vs clamp transection of the liver. *Arch Surg* 136:922, 2001.

31. Arita J, Hasegawa K, Kokudo N, et al: Randomized clinical trial of the effect of a saline-linked radiofrequency coagulator on blood loss during hepatic resection. *Br J Surg* 92:954, 2005.

32. Lupo L, Gallerani A, Panzera P, et al: Randomized clinical trial of radiofrequency-assisted versus clamp-crushing liver resection. *Br J Surg* 94:287, 2007.

33. Lesurtel M, Selzner M, Petrowsky H, et al: How should transection of the liver be performed?: A prospective randomized study in 100 consecutive patients: Comparing four different transection strategies. *Ann Surg* 242:814; discussion 22, 2005.

34. Delis SG, Bakoyiannis A, Karakaxas D, et al: Hepatic parenchyma resection using stapling devices: Peri-operative and long-term outcome. *HPB (Oxford)* 11:38, 2009.

35. Burdio F, Grande L, Berjano E, et al: A new single-instrument technique for parenchyma division and hemostasis in liver resection: A clinical feasibility study. *Am J Surg* 200:e75, 2010.

36. Schwartz M, Madariaga J, Hirose R, et al: Comparison of a new fibrin sealant with standard topical hemostatic agents. *Arch Surg* 139:1148, 2004.

37. Chapman WC, Clavien PA, Fung J, et al: Effective control of hepatic bleeding with a novel collagen-based composite combined with autologous plasma: Results of a randomized controlled trial. *Arch Surg* 135:1200; discussion 1205, 2000.

38. Noun R, Elias D, Balladur P, et al: Fibrin glue effectiveness and tolerance after elective liver resection: A randomized trial. *Hepatogastroenterology* 43:221, 1996.

39. Figueras J, Llado L, Miro M, et al: Application of fibrin glue sealant after hepatectomy does not seem justified: Results of a randomized study in 300 patients. *Ann Surg* 245:536, 2007.

40. Fuster J, Llovet JM, Garcia-Valdecasas JC, et al: Abdominal drainage after liver resection for hepatocellular carcinoma in cirrhotic patients: A randomized controlled study. *Hepatogastroenterology* 51:536, 2004.

41. Fong Y, Brennan MF, Brown K, et al: Drainage is unnecessary after elective liver resection. *Am J Surg* 171:158, 1996.

42. Starzl TE, Koep LJ, Weil R 3rd, et al: Right trisegmentectomy for hepatic neoplasms. *Surg Gynecol Obstet* 150:208, 1980.

43. Starzl TE, Iwatsuki S, Shaw BW Jr, et al: Left hepatic trisegmentectomy. *Surg Gynecol Obstet* 155:21, 1982.

44. Nguyen KT, Geller DA: Laparoscopic liver resection—current update. *Surg Clin North Am* 90:749, 2010.

45. Buell JF, Thomas MT, Rudich S, et al: Experience with more than 500 minimally invasive hepatic procedures. *Ann Surg* 248:475, 2008.

46. Simillis C, Constantinides VA, Tekkis PP, et al: Laparoscopic versus open hepatic resections for benign and malignant neoplasms—a meta-analysis. *Surgery* 141:203, 2007.

47. Croome KP, Yamashita MH: Laparoscopic vs open hepatic resection for benign and malignant tumors: An updated meta-analysis. *Arch Surg* 145:1109, 2010.

48. Jensen EH, Vickers SM: The maximally invasive hepatobiliary surgeon: A dying breed?: Comment on "Laparoscopic vs open hepatectomy for benign and malignant tumors." *Arch Surg* 145:1118, 2010.

49. Tsinberg M, Tellioglu G, Simpfendorfer CH, et al: Comparison of laparoscopic versus open liver tumor resection: A case-controlled study. *Surg Endosc* 23:847, 2009.

50. Aldrighetti L, Guzzetti E, Pulitano C, et al: Case-matched analysis of totally laparoscopic versus open liver resection for HCC: Short and middle term results. *J Surg Oncol* 102:82, 2010.

Minimally Invasive Techniques of Hepatic Resection

Ido Nachmany | David Geller

The field of hepatobiliary surgery has evolved dramatically in the past few decades, with improved understanding of the anatomic segments of the liver, advancements in modern imaging techniques, and improved anesthesia support as well as postoperative management. At the same time, minimally invasive surgery has become an integral part of each surgical subspecialty. However, the application of minimally invasive techniques to liver surgery has been slow to develop, and is still far from being a standard option for most practicing hepatobiliary surgeons. This reluctance stems in part from the complexity of liver surgery, the concern for significant bleeding or gas embolism, and the lack of formal training in minimally invasive surgery for the more "senior" hepatobiliary surgeons.

However, dramatic progress in minimally invasive hepatic surgery has been made in recent years, with nearly 3000 cases reported in the English-language literature.[1] Large reviews and series now report on the safety and feasibility of laparoscopic liver surgery for both benign lesions and malignant tumors,[2-17] including anatomic right hepatectomies,[18-22] left hepatectomies,[1,23,24] and even extended hepatectomies.[25,26] In a world review of 2804 cases of laparoscopic liver resection, 50% of the resections were done for malignancy, with the majority being performed for hepatocellular carcinoma (HCC) or colorectal cancer (CRC) metastases.[1] Although no randomized clinical trial comparing laparoscopic to open hepatic resection for cancer has been performed, the feasibility of conducting such a trial was recently discussed at the First International Conference on Laparoscopic Liver Resection Surgery in Louisville, Kentucky, in November 2008.[2]

The panel acknowledged that although there may be a role for a prospective randomized trial, the difficulties in defining the relevant study questions, and the size and length of time to perform the trial may make this impracticable. There was consensus that understanding the role and safety of laparoscopic liver surgery would be advanced through a cooperative patient registry.

INDICATIONS FOR LAPAROSCOPIC LIVER SURGERY

An important principle of minimally invasive surgery is that the availability of this technique does not alter the indication. Therefore, a laparoscopic liver resection should be considered only for lesions that would otherwise be treated with open hepatic surgery. Indications and contraindications for laparoscopic liver surgery are shown in Table 121-1. For benign liver lesions, symptomatic hemangioma or FNH, and adenomas larger than

4 cm should be resected. Ideally suited lesions are masses located in the right anterior segments (V and VI) or left lateral segments (II and III). However, experienced groups have shown that even laparoscopic major hepatectomies can be accomplished.[18-21] The main differences between benign and malignant lesions are related to achieving adequate margins and avoidance of tumor rupture. For malignant liver tumors, lesions abutting major vasculature or tumors that are too large to be manipulated laparoscopically should be resected by an open approach. Hilar cholangiocarcinomas are often challenging even by an open approach, and in general should not be done with a minimally invasive technique. The presence of dense adhesions that prevent safe dissection, unexpected difficulty in manipulating the liver, or failure to make progress are indications for conversion to an open technique. Such a decision is never considered a failure, but rather a good judgment call, employed in order to prevent a complication. Another indication for laparoscopic liver resection is live donor hepatectomy for liver transplant. This has been described for live donor left lateral sectionectomy,[27] and adult-to-adult live donor right hepatectomy.[28,29] Caution is noted in that these operations should only be done by transplant teams with extensive open live donor liver transplant expertise as well as minimally invasive liver resection experience.

TECHNICAL APPROACHES TO LAPAROSCOPIC LIVER RESECTION

There are two main approaches for performing minimally invasive liver resection—pure laparoscopic and hand assisted. A third option is using the laparoscopic technique for mobilization of the liver before opening the abdomen and completing the resection through a relatively small laparotomy incision (so-called hybrid technique).[30] Some authors use a hand port for all cases, others use it selectively, and some never use it at all. The benefits of the hand-assisted technique are the relative ease of manipulation of the liver, palpation for improved tactile sensation, and the ability for faster control of bleeding in the case of a major vascular injury. Because most specimens mandate a utility incision for intact specimen extraction, the main difference between hand-assisted and pure laparoscopy is the position of the incision. There are no comparative studies to support benefit or inferiority of hand-assisted versus purely laparoscopic technique and the choice is strictly surgeon preference. In a large review of more than 2800 laparoscopic liver resections,[1] the majority of minimally invasive liver resections were pure laparoscopic (75%), hand-assisted

TABLE 121-1 Indications and Contraindications for Laparoscopic Liver Resection

Indications	Contraindications
Benign liver lesions	Any contraindications to open
Symptomatic hemangioma	liver resection
Symptomatic focal nodular	Patients who cannot tolerate
hyperplasia (FNH)	pneumoperitoneum
Adenoma	Dense adhesions that cannot
Symptomatic giant hepatic	be lysed laparoscopically
cyst	Lesion too close to
Malignant liver lesions	vasculature
Hepatocellular carcinoma	Lesion too large to be safely
(HCC)	manipulated laparoscopically
Colorectal cancer liver	Resection that requires
metastasis (CRC)	extensive portal
Other malignant lesions	lymphadenectomy
Live donor hepatectomy for	
liver transplant	
Indeterminate lesions—	
cannot rule out cancer	

Reprinted with permission from Nguyen KT, Gamblin TC, Geller DA: World review of laparoscopic liver resection—2804 patients. *Ann Surg* 250:831, 2009.

TABLE 121-2 Types of Laparoscopic Liver Resection in the Published Literature

Total No. of Reported Cases	2804
INDICATIONS FOR LAPAROSCOPIC LIVER RESECTION	
Malignant lesions	1395 (49.8%)
Benign lesions	1253 (44.7%)
Live donor hepatectomies for liver transplant	49 (1.7%)
Indeterminant	107 (3.8%)
MINIMALLY INVASIVE APPROACHES TO LIVER RESECTION	
Totally laparoscopic	2105 (75.1%)
Hand-assisted laparoscopic	463 (16.5%)
Laparoscopy-assisted open (hybrid)	60 (2.1%)
Gasless laparoscopic	52 (1.8%)
Thoracoscopic	5 (0.2%)
Robotics-assisted	3 (0.1%)
Converted to open	116 (4.1%)
TYPES OF RESECTIONS PERFORMED LAPAROSCOPICALLY	
Wedge resection/Segmentectomy	1258 (44.9%)
Left lateral sectionectomy	570 (20.3%)
Right hepatectomy	253 (9.0%)
Bisegmentectomy	209 (7.4%)
Left hepatectomy	191 (6.8%)
Deroofing/enucleation	142 (5.1%)
Extended right hepatectomy	19 (0.7%)
Caudate lobectomy	18 (0.6%)
Central hepatectomy	8 (0.3%)
Extended left hepatectomy	3 (0.1%)
Other	16 (0.6%)
Not documented	117 (4.2%)

Reprinted with permission from Nguyen KT, Gamblin TC, Geller DA: World review of laparoscopic liver resection—2804 patients. *Ann Surg* 250:831, 2009.

approach was the next most common (17%), and the "hybrid" technique was used rarely (2%) (Table 121-2).

In the operating room, the patient is placed in the supine position with both arms extended. Some authors favor the French lithotomy position. The preparation is similar to that of major liver resection, including line placement, bladder catheterization, and nasogastric tube insertion. We use a foot board and strapping that allow for steep rotation of the table. In the case of a planned major hepatectomy, we use a hand port and place it at the beginning of the procedure, as a supraumbilical midline incision (Figure 121-1). In the case of a small patient (e.g., less than 5'8" in height), the incision can be infraumbilical. The pneumoperitoneum is established via a trocar inserted through the hand port. The hand port incision may be used for a rapid conversion, by extending it to a longer midline.

LAPAROSCOPIC RIGHT HEPATECTOMY

After inserting the hand port and establishing the pneumoperitoneum to a pressure limit of 14 mm Hg, four additional trocars are placed, as depicted (see Figure 121-1). The falciform ligament is divided with endoshears and the round ligament divided using a stapler or with LigaSure or harmonic scalpel. The falciform ligament is left long on the liver side to facilitate retraction. Intraoperative ultrasound is performed to identify the lesion and mark the parenchymal transection line. After taking down the right coronary and triangular ligaments, the right lobe is gradually rotated off the retroperitoneum and lifted from the inferior vena cava (IVC). Short hepatic veins are clipped with 5-mm hemolocks. Small veins can be divided with the LigaSure. At that stage, the right hepatic vein is exposed and can be divided with a vascular stapler. If the exposure of the right hepatic vein is not optimal, it can be divided inside the liver at the end of the procedure after the parenchymal transection.

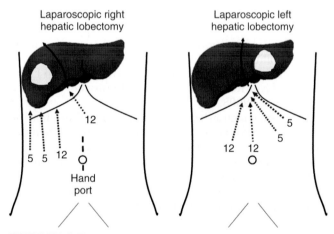

FIGURE 121-1 Trocar placement for laparoscopic right and left hepatic lobectomy.

The next step is the hilar dissection. It is started with the cholecystectomy and exposure of the right hepatic artery, right portal vein, and bile duct. The right hepatic artery is doubly secured with locking clips. The right portal vein is dissected and encircled. It can be transected with the vascular stapler; however, if the angle precludes safe stapling, it can be left to the end of the procedure and controlled with a small bulldog clamp inserted through the hand port to allow for an ipsilateral Pringle maneuver. Next, the parenchymal transection is started with the harmonic scalpel or LigaSure. The deeper parenchyma with crossing middle hepatic vein branches is divided with vascular stapler. Some surgeons utilize a bipolar pinching forceps and/or Cavitron ultrasonic surgical aspirator (CUSA) or hydrojet to help divide the parenchyma. During the parenchymal transection, as in an open hepatic resection, the central venous pressure is kept low in order to minimize blood loss. Also, the pneumoperitoneum tends to decrease oozing from the cut edge of the liver. If not already done, the right portal vein and right hepatic veins are divided as the parenchymal transection is deepened, along with the right hepatic duct inside the liver. If a hand port is utilized, the hand can provide a laparoscopic "hanging maneuver" to facilitate exposure and transection. Any oozing from the cut edge is controlled with cautery or TissueLink sealing device. Any visible bile leaks are oversewn with 4-0 absorbable suture. The specimen is extracted through the hand port, and the abdomen is reinspected for bleeding. A closed suction drain is left next to the cut surface of the liver and brought out through one of the 5-mm trocar sites.

LAPAROSCOPIC LEFT HEPATECTOMY

The technique of laparoscopic left hepatectomy is similar to that of the right lobe. The position of the trocars is depicted (see Figure 121-1). Often laparoscopic left lateral sectionectomy and left lobectomy can be done with a pure laparoscopic approach, with the hand port being reserved for a large tumor or difficult case. Care must be given to avoiding injury to the left phrenic and left hepatic veins when taking down the left triangular ligament. Next, the gastrohepatic ligament is divided (watching for a replaced left hepatic artery), and the left hilum is dissected at the base of the falciform ligament after opening the liver bridge from segment III to IVb. The left hepatic artery is doubly clipped and divided, followed by dissection of the left portal vein. The left portal vein can be controlled/divided in a manner similar to the description of the right portal vein. The left hepatic duct is transected laterally at the base of the umbilical fissure to avoid injury to a not infrequent right posterior (or right anterior) duct coming off the proximal end of the left hepatic duct. A hepatotomy is made in segment IVb and stapler insinuated to divide the left hepatic duct. Parenchymal transection is done using LigaSure or harmonic scalpel, followed by vascular staplers to divide the left hepatic vein after the parenchyma is divided.

CLINICAL BENEFITS OF LAPAROSCOPIC LIVER SURGERY

More than 150 publications have shown the safety and efficacy of laparoscopic liver resection. In the world review of laparoscopic liver resection in 2804 patients, overall mortality was 0.3% (9/2804 patients) and morbidity was 10.5%.[1] Two recent studies reviewed the clinical benefits of laparoscopic liver resection (LLR) versus open liver resection (OLR). The first study is a critical appraisal of 31 publications that directly compared LLR with OLR in 2473 patients.[31] In case-cohort studies of well-matched patients, LLR was associated with less blood loss, less packed red blood cell transfusion, quicker resumption of oral diet, less pain medication requirement, and shorter length of stay, as compared to OLR. Further, seven publications in this analysis reported a lower morbidity (complication rate) in LLR versus OLR, while the remaining studies found no difference in complication rates.[31] Other potential advantages include better cosmetic result and potentially a lesser physiologic stress response.

In those patients undergoing laparoscopic hepatic resection for cancer, there was no difference in 3- or 5-year overall survival when compared with well-matched open hepatic resection cases.

The second recent review is a metaanalysis of 26 articles comparing LLR to OLR from 1998 to 2009.[32] In this study, the LLR group had a lower operative blood loss, shorter hospital stay, less intravenous narcotic use, fewer days until oral intake, and lower relative risk of postoperative complications compared to the OLR group. Further, the hazards ratio for recurrence of malignant tumors was not significantly different between the two groups (HR = 0.79, $P = 0.37$).[32] In another recent study, Martin et al reported on 90 laparoscopic versus 360 open formal hepatic lobectomies.[33] Patients in the two arms were matched in a 1:4 ratio for age, American Society of Anesthesiology (ASA) class, tumor size, histology, and tumor location. Benign tumors were more common in the laparoscopic group. Estimated intraoperative blood loss, Pringle time, total and pulmonary complication rates, and hospital length of stay were significantly lower for the laparoscopic group.

ONCOLOGIC OUTCOMES FOR LAPAROSCOPIC LIVER RESECTION

To date, no randomized clinical trial comparing laparoscopic to open liver resection for cancer has been performed. Given the large number of cases already performed, as well as multiple case-cohort matched studies reported, it may be challenging to accrue patients to a randomized clinical trial, especially given the large number of patients required, and difficulties in managing patient preference of suitable LLR candidates. Suffice it to say, from the vast body of literature available, there is no current evidence for trocar or peritoneal tumor seeding, compromise of tumor margins or R0 resection rates, or worse oncologic outcomes using 5-year overall or disease-free survival when comparing LLR to OLR for CRC metastases or HCC (Table 121-3). A brief summary of a few noteworthy studies is provided.

COLORECTAL CANCER METASTASES

In a multicenter international series, Nguyen et al described 109 patients who underwent minimally invasive liver resection for CRC metastasis, in four American and two French centers.[9] Major liver resections (three or more segments) were performed in 45% of patients. Median operating room time was 234 minutes (range, 60 to 555 minutes) and blood loss was 200 mL (range, 20

TABLE 121-3 Overall Survival After Laparoscopic Liver Resection Versus Open Liver Resection for Cancer in Comparative Studies

Reference	Year	Country	Journal	Tumor	OVERALL SURVIVAL			
					LLR	OLR	F/U (yr)	P
Belli et al[34]	2009	Italy	Br J Surgery	HCC	67	61	3	NS
Ito et al[35]	2009	USA	J GI Surgery	CRC	72	56	3	NS
Lai et al[36]	2009	Hong Kong	Arch Surgery	HCC	60	60	3	NS
Lee et al[37]	2007	Hong Kong	Hong Kong Med J	CRC	81	79	3	NS
Laurent et al[15]	2003	France	Arch Surgery	HCC	89	70	3	NS
Castaing et al[38]	2009	France	Ann Surgery	CRC	64	56	5	NS
Endo et al[39]	2009	Japan	Surg Lap Endo Tech	HCC	57	48	5	NS
Sarpel et al[40]	2009	USA	Ann Surg Oncology	HCC	95	75	5	NS
Tranchart et al[41]	2010	France	Surg Endosc	HCC	46	37	5	NS
Cai et al[42]	2008	China	Surg Endosc	mix*	50	51	5	NS
Kaneko et al[16]	2005	Japan	Am J Surgery	HCC	61	62	5	NS
Shimada et al[43]	2001	Japan	Surg Endosc	HCC	50	38	5	NS

Reprinted with permission from Nguyen KT, Marsh JW, Tsung A, et al: Comparative benefits of laparoscopic versus open hepatic resection: A critical appraisal. *Arch Surg* 146:346, 2011.
CRC, Colorectal carcinoma; *F/U,* followup; *HCC,* hepatocellular carcinoma; *LLR,* laparoscopic liver resection; *OLR,* open liver resection; *NS,* not significant; *n/a,* not available.
*Survival analysis of patents with malignant liver tumors (24 HCC, 2 CRC, 1 breast cancer metastasis, and 4 intrahepatic cholangiocarcinoma).

to 2500 mL), with 10% receiving a blood transfusion. There were four conversions to open surgery (3.7%), all due to bleeding. Median length of postoperative hospital stay for the entire series was 4 days (range, 1 to 22 days). The median interval from primary colon surgery to liver metastasectomy was 12 months (range, 0 to 60 months). The median tumor size was 3.0 cm, and negative margins were achieved in 94.4% of patients, with a median margin of 10 mm. At 1, 3, and 5 years, overall survival rates were 88%, 69%, and 50%, respectively, whereas disease-free survival rates were 65%, 43%, and 43%, respectively.

Other recent studies by Sasaki et al[10] and Kazaryan et al[44] report similar 5-year overall survival rates of 64% and 51%, respectively, after laparoscopic liver resection performed for CRC metastases. The report by Kazaryan et al reflects a 12-year Norwegian single-center experience in 122 patients. The R0 resection rate was 93.4%, and the median tumor resection margin was 6 mm. These 5-year overall survival rates after laparoscopic liver resection of CRC metastases are comparable to 5-year overall survival rates in the range of 37% to 50% reported in modern open hepatic resection series from large liver cancer centers.

In a prospective, head-to-head study, Castaing et al described the results of two French groups, one performing laparoscopic and the other open hepatectomy, for metastatic CRC.[38] They matched 60 laparoscopic to 60 open cases, based on 9 preoperative prognostic criteria predictive of survival: sex, age, primary tumor localization, number, size, and distribution of metastases, presence of extrahepatic disease, initial resectability, and prehepatectomy chemotherapy administration. The mean operative time, 60-day mortality (1.7% in both groups), general and hepatic complication rates, and median postoperative length of stay (10 days for the laparoscopic vs. 11 days for the open group), and mean resection margin were similar between the groups. The transfusion rate was significantly lower in the

laparoscopic group (15% vs. 36%; $P < 0.007$). At a median followup of 30 months, the 5-year overall survival for the laparoscopic group was 64%, versus 56% for the open group ($P = 0.32$). The recurrence-free survival at 5 years was 30% for the laparoscopic and 20% for the open group ($P = 0.13$).

HEPATOCELLULAR CARCINOMA

Five different studies report 5-year overall survival after laparoscopic liver resection performed for HCC in the range of 50% to 75%, and 5-year disease-free survival ranging from 31% to 38%.[1] Kaneko et al reported the results of 30 LLR versus 28 OLR for HCC.[16] The strength of this study is that all patients were offered a laparoscopic approach, but some elected open hepatectomy at the time of informed consent, thereby minimizing surgeon selection bias. The patients were well matched in age, gender, degree of cirrhosis, tumor size, ICG clearance, and extent of surgery between the two groups. The laparoscopic group had a shorter time to ambulation, oral intake, and length of hospital stay. There were no significant differences in 5-year overall (61% vs. 62%) or disease-free (31% vs. 29%) survival between the LLR and OLR groups.

Tranchart et al reported a case-control matched comparison of 42 patients who underwent LLR versus 42 patients undergoing OLR for HCC.[41] The LLR group had significantly less intraoperative blood loss (364 vs. 724 mL, $P < 0.0001$) and postoperative ascites (7.1% vs. 26.1%, $P = 0.03$), and shorter length of hospital stay (6.7 vs. 9.6 days, $P < 0.0001$). There were no differences in transfusion rates, or resection margins. With a median followup of 30 months, there were no differences in overall survival. Sarpel et al reported a case-cohort study of 20 LLR versus 56 OLR for HCC.[40] The two groups were well matched with no significant difference in age, gender, degree of cirrhosis, or tumor size between the groups. There were no significant differences in rates of blood transfusion, operative time, or positive margins between the groups. The LLR group had a shorter length of stay, and there were no differences in overall or disease-free survival between the groups.

In a large series of 163 LLR for HCC, Dagher et al reported the results from three European centers from 1998 to 2008.[45] Seventy-four percent of patients were cirrhotic, and the liver resection was anatomic in 107 (65.6%) patients and was a major resection (three or more segments) in 16 (9.8%). A totally laparoscopic approach was used in 155 (95.1%) patients. Median OR time was 180 minutes. Median blood loss was 250 mL, and 16 (9.8%) patients received a blood transfusion. Conversion to open surgery was required in 15 (9.2%) patients. Median tumor size was 3.6 cm and median surgical margin was 12 mm. Liver-specific and general complications occurred in 19 (11.6%) and 17 (10.4%) patients, respectively. Postoperative hospital length of stay was 7 days. The 5-year overall survival was 64.9%, and 5-year recurrence-free survival was 32.2%, respectively. Similar to LLR for CRC metastases, the 5-year overall survival for HCC reported in LLR are comparable to the best data available for OLR for HCC.

Moreover, a recent study from an experienced hepatobiliary center showed that prior LLR (vs. OLR) for HCC facilitated subsequent salvage liver transplantation with decreased morbidity.[46] Of 24 patients who underwent salvage liver transplant after prior LLR (12 patients) or OLR (12 patients), patients that had previous LLR had shorter explant hepatectomy and total operative time, less blood loss, and reduced need for blood transfusions, as compared to the OLR patients.

ECONOMIC ASPECTS OF LAPAROSCOPIC LIVER SURGERY

One of the concerns regarding laparoscopic surgery is related to the cost of the procedure, particularly with the added costs of the laparoscopic instruments in the operating room, many of which are single-use, disposables. Koffron et al showed that the operating room costs for minimally invasive liver resections were higher than open liver resections; however, the nonoperating room costs were higher in the open cases, with the primary determinant being greater length of hospital stay, leading to higher costs.[8] Vanounou et al compared 44 laparoscopic left lateral sectionectomies (LLS) to 29 open hepatic LLS at the University of Pittsburgh Medical Center.[47] A deviation-based cost modeling (DBCM) approach was utilized to compare the economic impact of LLR to OLR approaches. The LLR cases had a shorter length of stay (3 vs. 5 days, $P < 0.001$) and a weighted average median cost savings of $2939 as compared to the OLR group. Likewise, in a comparative analysis from Dundee, United Kingdom, 25 patients undergoing LLR were compared to 25 well-matched OLR patients between 2005 and 2007.[48] The two groups were homogeneous by age, sex, coexistent morbidity, magnitude of resection, prevalence of liver cirrhosis, and indications. Hospital costs were obtained from the Scottish Health Service Costs Book (ISD Scotland). Overall hospital cost was significantly lower in the laparoscopic group by an average of 2571 pounds sterling ($P < 0.04$).

SUMMARY

Laparoscopic liver surgery is an evolving discipline in the field of hepatobiliary surgery. Multiple studies have shown that laparoscopic liver resection is safe and effective in the hands of experienced surgeons in selected patients. Clinical benefits to the patients include reduced blood loss, postoperative pain, narcotic use, and earlier discharge, with no overall financial disadvantage. From the oncologic standpoint, laparoscopic liver resections have been shown to yield equivalent cancer outcomes for HCC and CRC metastases with similar rates of negative margins, as well as 5-year overall and disease-free survival.

REFERENCES

1. Nguyen KT, Gamblin TC, Geller DA: World review of laparoscopic liver resection—2804 patients. *Ann Surg* 250:831, 2009.
2. Buell JF, Cherqui D, Geller DA, et al: The International Position on Laparoscopic Liver Surgery: The Louisville Statement, 2008. *Ann Surg* 250:825, 2009.
3. Viganò L, Tayar C, Laurent A, et al: Laparoscopic liver resection: A systematic review. *J Hepatobiliary Pancreat Surg* 16:410, 2009.
4. Pulitanò C, Aldrighetti L: The current role of laparoscopic liver resection for the treatment of liver tumors. *Nat Clin Pract Gastroenterol Hepatol* 5:648, 2008.
5. Koffron AJ, Geller DA, Gamblin TC, et al: Laparoscopic liver surgery: Shifting the management of liver tumors. *Hepatology* 44:1694, 2006.
6. Cherqui D, Laurent A, Tayar C, et al: Laparoscopic liver resection for peripheral hepatocellular carcinoma in patients with chronic liver disease: Midterm results and perspectives. *Ann Surg* 243:499, 2006.
7. Buell JF, Thomas MT, Rudich S, et al: Experience with more than 500 minimally invasive hepatic procedures. *Ann Surg* 248:475, 2008.
8. Koffron AJ, Auffenberg G, Kung R, et al: Evaluation of 300 minimally invasive liver resections at a single institution: Less is more. *Ann Surg* 246:385, 2007.
9. Nguyen KT, Laurent A, Dagher I, et al: Minimally invasive liver resection for metastatic colorectal cancer: A multi-institutional, international report of safety, feasibility, and early outcomes. *Ann Surg* 250:842, 2009.
10. Sasaki A, Nitta H, Otsuka K, Takahara T, et al: Ten-year experience of totally laparoscopic liver resection in a single institution. *Br J Surg* 96:274, 2009.
11. Kazaryan AM, Pavlik Marangos I, Rosseland AR, et al: Laparoscopic liver resection for malignant and benign lesions: Ten-year Norwegian single-center experience. *Arch Surg* 145:34, 2010.
12. Descottes B, Glineur D, Lachachi F, et al: Laparoscopic liver resection of benign liver tumors. *Surg Endosc* 17:23, 2003.
13. Gamblin TC, Holloway SE, Heckman JT, et al: Laparoscopic resection of benign hepatic cysts: A new standard. *J Am Coll Surg* 207:731, 2008.
14. Gigot JF, Glineur D, Santiago Azagra J, et al: Laparoscopic liver resection for malignant liver tumors: Preliminary results of a multicenter European study. *Ann Surg* 236:90, 2002.
15. Laurent A, Cherqui D, Lesurtel M, et al: Laparoscopic liver resection for subcapsular hepatocellular carcinoma complicating chronic liver disease. *Arch Surg* 138:763, 2003.
16. Kaneko H, Takagi S, Otsuka Y, et al: Laparoscopic liver resection of hepatocellular carcinoma. *Am J Surg* 189:190, 2005.
17. Nguyen KT, Gamblin TC, Geller DA: Laparoscopic liver resection for cancer. *Future Oncol* 4:661, 2008.
18. Dagher I, O'Rourke N, Geller DA, et al: Laparoscopic major hepatectomy: An evolution in standard of care. *Ann Surg* 250:856, 2009.

19. O'Rourke N, Fielding G: Laparoscopic right hepatectomy: Surgical technique. *J Gastrointest Surg* 8:213, 2004.

20. Topal B, Aerts R, Penninckx F: Laparoscopic intrahepatic Glissonian approach for right hepatectomy is safe, simple, and reproducible. *Surg Endosc* 21:2111, 2007.

21. Gayet B, Cavaliere D, Vibert E, et al: Totally laparoscopic right hepatectomy. *Am J Surg* 194:685, 2007.

22. Dagher I, DiGiuro G, Dubrez J, et al: Laparoscopic versus open right hepatectomy: A comparative study. *Am J Surg* 198:173, 2009.

23. Samama G, Chiche L, Brefort JL, et al: Laparoscopic anatomical hepatic resection. Report of four left lobectomies for solid tumors. *Surg Endosc* 12:76, 1998.

24. Vibert E, Perniceni T, Levard H, et al: Laparoscopic liver resection. *Br J Surg* 93:67, 2006.

25. Gumbs AA, Bar-Zakai B, Gayet B: Totally laparoscopic extended left hepatectomy. *J Gastrointest Surg* 12:1152, 2008.

26. Gumbs AA, Gayet B: Totally laparoscopic extended right hepatectomy. *Surg Endosc* 22:2076, 2008.

27. Soubrane O, Cherqui D, Scatton O, et al: Laparoscopic left lateral sectionectomy in living donors: Safety and reproducibility of the technique in a single center. *Ann Surg* 244:815, 2006.

28. Kurosaki I, Yamamoto S, Kitami C, et al: Video-assisted living donor hemihepatectomy through a 12-cm incision for adult-to-adult liver transplantation. *Surgery* 139:695, 2006.

29. Koffron AJ, Kung R, Baker T, et al: Laparoscopic-assisted right lobe donor hepatectomy. *Am J Transplant* 6:2522, 2006.

30. Koffron AJ, Kung RD, Auffenberg GB, et al: Laparoscopic liver surgery for everyone: The hybrid method. *Surgery* 142:463, 2007.

31. Nguyen KT, Marsh JW, Tsung A, et al: Comparative benefits of laparoscopic versus open hepatic resection: A critical appraisal. *Arch Surg* 146:348, 2011.

32. Kris PC, Michael HY: Laparoscopic vs open hepatic resection for benign and malignant tumors: An updated meta-analysis. *Arch Surg* 145:1109, 2010.

33. Martin RC, Scoggins CR, McMasters KM: Laparoscopic hepatic lobectomy: Advantages of a minimally invasive approach. *J Am Coll Surg* 210:627, 2010.

34. Belli G, Limongelli P, Fantini C, et al: Laparoscopic and open treatment of hepatocellular carcinoma in patients with cirrhosis. *Br J Surg* 96:1041, 2009.

35. Ito K, Ito H, Are C, et al: Laparoscopic versus open liver resection: A matched-pair case control study. *J Gastrointest Surg* 3:2276, 2009.

36. Lai EC, Tang CN, Ha JP, Li MK: Laparoscopic liver resection for hepatocellular carcinoma: Ten-year experience in a single center. *Arch Surg* 144:143, 2009.

37. Lee KF, Cheung YS, Chong CN, et al: Laparoscopic versus open hepatectomy for liver tumours: A case control study. *Hong Kong Med J* 13:442, 2007.

38. Castaing D, Vibert E, Ricca L, et al: Oncologic results of laparoscopic versus open hepatectomy for colorectal liver metastases in two specialized centers. *Ann Surg* 250:849, 2009.

39. Endo Y, Ohta M, Sasaki A, et al: A comparative study of the long-term outcomes after laparoscopy-assisted and open left lateral hepatectomy for hepatocellular carcinoma. *Surg Laparosc Endosc Percutan Tech* 19:171, 2009.

40. Sarpel U, Hefti MM, Wisnievsky JP, et al: Outcome for patients treated with laparoscopic versus open resection of hepatocellular carcinoma: Case-matched analysis. *Ann Surg Oncol* 16:1572, 2009.

41. Tranchart H, Di Giuro G, Lainas P, et al: Laparoscopic resection for hepatocellular carcinoma: A matched-pair comparative study. *Surg Endosc* 24:1170, 2010.

42. Cai XJ, Yang J, Yu H, et al: Clinical study of laparoscopic versus open hepatectomy for malignant liver tumors. *Surg Endosc* 22:2350, 2008.

43. Shimada M, Hashizume M, Maehara S, et al: Laparoscopic hepatectomy for hepatocellular carcinoma. *Surg Endosc* 15:541, 2001.

44. Kazaryan AM, Marangos IP, Røsok BI, et al: Laparoscopic resection of colorectal liver metastases: Surgical and long-term oncologic outcome. *Ann Surg* 252:1005, 2010.

45. Dagher I, Belli G, Fantini C, et al: Laparoscopic hepatectomy for hepatocellular carcinoma: A European experience. *J Am Coll Surg* 211:16, 2010.

46. Laurent A, Tayar C, Andreoletti M, et al: Laparoscopic liver resection facilitates salvage liver transplantation for hepatocellular carcinoma. *J Hepatobiliary Pancreat Surg* 16:310, 2009.

47. Vanounou T, Steel JL, Nguyen KT, et al: Comparing the clinical and economic impact of laparoscopic versus open liver resection. *Ann Surg Oncol* 17:998, 2010.

48. Polignano FM, Quyn AJ, de Figueiredo RS, et al: Laparoscopic versus open liver segmentectomy: Prospective, case-matched, intention-to-treat analysis of clinical outcomes and cost effectiveness. *Surg Endosc* 22:2564, 2008.

Ablative Therapies for Hepatic Neoplasms

David M. Mahvi | Seth B. Krantz

The liver is a frequent site of both primary and metastatic neoplastic disease. The gastrointestinal (GI) tract drains through the mesenteric portal system, and thus ultimately to the liver. Presumably because of this shower of shed tumor cells, the liver is the primary site for hematologic spread of all GI cancers. Colorectal cancer (CRC) is the most common GI malignancy in the United States, with more than 140,000 new cases each year.[1] Approximately 30% of patients have either synchronous or metachronous liver metastases.[2] With improved surgical techniques and chemotherapy, the 5-year survival rates for patients with stage IV disease continue to improve and have been reported to be as high as 40%.[3] Gastric and pancreatic cancer also frequently metastasize to the liver; however, given patients' uniformly poor survival rates, liver-directed therapy has had no impact on survival in noncolorectal cancer metastatic disease.

Primary hepatocellular carcinoma (HCC) is less common in the United States but more common in the developing world. Resection, ablation, and transplantation do appear to improve survival in selected patients. As HCC is almost uniformly a result of cirrhosis, it is geographically associated with regions endemic for hepatitis B such as Southeast Asia and Sub-Saharan Africa.[4] Hepatitis C incidence has increased in the United States and other Western countries and is now the primary cause of both cirrhosis and HCC in the West.[4,5]

For both metastatic disease and HCC, resection remains the first-line therapy. However, unlike other GI malignancies, where radical resection is possible, the amount of liver that can be safely removed is limited. Thus, a significant portion of patients have disease not amenable to surgical resection. Resection is not attempted either because of underlying cirrhosis or multiple bilobar metastases. For these patients, ablation procedures are an important adjunct to systemic therapy.

Ablative technologies for hepatic malignancies have been commercially available for only the past two decades. Initial enthusiasm for cryoablation has been supplanted by multiple different platforms for radiofrequency ablation (RFA). Newer techniques that may ultimately replace RFA include microwave ablation (MWA), high-intensity focused ultrasound (HIFU), and irreversible electroporation (IRE). RFA, MWA, and cryotherapy can be performed during open surgery, laparoscopically, or percutaneously. HIFU can be done with a surgical approach though one of its primary advantages is the ability to perform it completely extracorporeally. All of these therapies can also be used in combination with surgical resection.

In this chapter, we will provide an overview of the strengths and weaknesses of current technology. The focus will be on local recurrence within the first year after ablation. Survival is driven by many different variables and, though critical, is less likely to determine the most effective modality. We will place in context the various malignancies that are amenable to ablative therapies. Finally, we will speculate on where future technology may be headed.

RADIOFREQUENCY ABLATION

Radiofrequency ablation (RFA) is the most widely used method of liver-directed therapy for those patients who are not candidates for surgical resection. It can be performed during open exploration, during laparoscopic exploration, or percutaneously under image guidance. Metal probes are placed in the liver parenchyma. An alternating electrical current (5000 to 9000 MHz) is then used for treatment. This alternating current generates heat sufficient for tissue destruction by coagulative necrosis (Figure 122-1). The heat generated by the probe decreases as the inverse square of distance from the probe, limiting the efficacy of RFA for larger tumors. RFA is also ineffective for tumors located near major vascular structures. Major vascular structures act as heat sinks, which lead to relative cooling of the liver, thus preventing adequate heat production and tissue destruction. The heat sink of smaller vessels may contribute to the somewhat patchy nature of tissue destruction seen with RFA. Pathologic review of ablated liver tumors that were subsequently resected have shown that within areas of tissue destruction there are nests of still viable cells residing near small blood vessels. These islands of residual tumor may be one source of recurrence after RFA.

Like all ablation techniques, RFA is used almost exclusively in patients who are not surgically resectable and thus there is very little comparison data on RFA in patients with tumors amenable to resection. Local recurrence is probably a better surrogate for tumor destruction than survival given this disparity in patient populations.

No prospective randomized trials comparing RFA and any other modality have been performed in patients with colorectal cancer. A 2009 systematic review evaluated the results of RFA in colorectal adenocarcinoma liver metastases.[6] There were numerous single-modality studies, nonrandomized comparison trials between resection and RFA, and nonrandomized trials comparing RFA and liver-directed therapies other than resection. The extreme heterogeneity of the studies made any comparison difficult, specifically with respect to selection criteria. The criteria for unresectability varied greatly between studies. The extent of hepatic disease, the presence of previous hepatic surgery, and prohibitive surgical risk

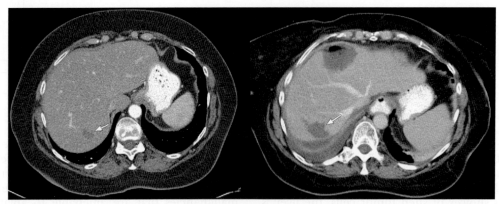

FIGURE 122-1 CT scan of a liver tumor before *(left arrow)* and 1 month after *(right arrow)* radiofrequency ablation. (Courtesy Dr. David J. Bentrem, Department of Surgery, Northwestern University Feinberg School of Medicine.)

TABLE 122-1 Local Recurrence for Radiofrequency Ablation According to Size and Approach

Size	Percutaneous (%)	Laparoscopy/Laparotomy (%)
<3 cm	16.0	3.6
3-5 cm	25.9	21.7
>5 cm	60.0	50.0

Adapted from Mulier S, Ni Y, Jamart J, et al: Local recurrence after hepatic radiofrequency coagulation: Multivariate meta-analysis and review of contributing factors. *Ann Surg* 242:158, 2005, Table 2.

were typical selection criteria, but tumors that seemed unresectable in some series were resectable in others.

Overall, in comparative studies, RFA was inferior to resection in both local recurrence (0% to 9.5% vs. 12% to 37%) and median overall survival (31 to 36 months vs. 41 to 80 months).[6] In all of these comparative studies, however, patients who underwent RFA were not randomized, and thus their poor results may reflect their underlying biology rather than an effect of treatment modality. When compared to other patients with unresectable disease, RFA fares better. In several studies that compared RFA and chemotherapy, RFA alone or RFA with chemotherapy was better than chemotherapy alone, with 5-year overall survival ranging from 22% to 30% for RFA alone versus 9% to 15% for chemotherapy alone.[6] RFA, when used as part of a first-line treatment strategy, as opposed to second-line after failed chemotherapy, showed overall survival improvements of up to 30 months.

The most significant factor associated with recurrence is tumor size. A 2005 metaanalysis evaluated multiple variables in multiple series (Table 122-1).[7] In univariate analysis, size, tumor location, histology, and approach (percutaneous vs. surgical) were all significant variables. However, in multivariate analysis, only small tumor size (<3 cm) and surgical approach (open or laparoscopic) were associated with decreased recurrence.[7] The advantage from a surgical approach likely stems from superior overlapping of burn zones aided by intraoperative ultrasound, the ability to restrict hepatic blood flow (via either a full Pringle maneuver or occlusion of the hepatic artery), thereby reducing heat sink, and the surgical oncologic dictum of achieving 1-cm margins. Each of

these factors was also significant in univariate analysis and were more likely to occur during a surgical as opposed to percutaneous approach.

The significance of this increased local recurrence on systemic disease progression and survival in patients treated with systemic chemotherapy after ablation or resection is more difficult to discern. A nonrandomized study comparing RFA to resection as a first-line therapy for patients with early (within 1 year of colon resection) liver metastases showed significantly higher treatment site recurrence for RFA compared with resection (32% vs. 4%) (Figure 122-2).[8] RFA-treated patients also had an increased rate of new metastases and shorter time to progression. Despite these differences, the rates of systemic recurrence were not significantly different, and the 3-year overall survival was 60% in both groups.[8]

The treatment of hepatocellular carcinoma with RFA has been compared to resection in a few small series. A randomized trial comparing RFA with resection for HCC less than 5 cm showed no difference in overall survival or recurrence between the two groups. Four-year overall survival was 67.9% for ablation and 64% for resection, and recurrence was 53.6% and 48.4% for RFA and resection, respectively.[9] Similar results were seen in a smaller prospective study[10] and in a recent nonrandomized study in 218 patients who underwent RFA for HCC less than 2 cm and who were technically "resectable."[11] For lesions larger than 5 cm, the recurrence rate is much higher and treatment failure is much more common. Of note, the review by Mulier et al found similar recurrence rates for HCC as for CRC metastases, both close to 14%. In that review, size rather than pathology was the dominant factor, as both small HCC and CRC lesions had very low recurrence rates.[7]

MICROWAVE ABLATION

The other primary ablative therapy based on heating of tissue and coagulative necrosis is MWA. MWA uses high-frequency (900- to 2500-MHz) microwaves to agitate water molecules, creating friction and generating heat. The probe acts as a microwave antenna to "broadcast" the energy throughout the targeted region. Compared with RFA, MWA has several theoretical advantages. The

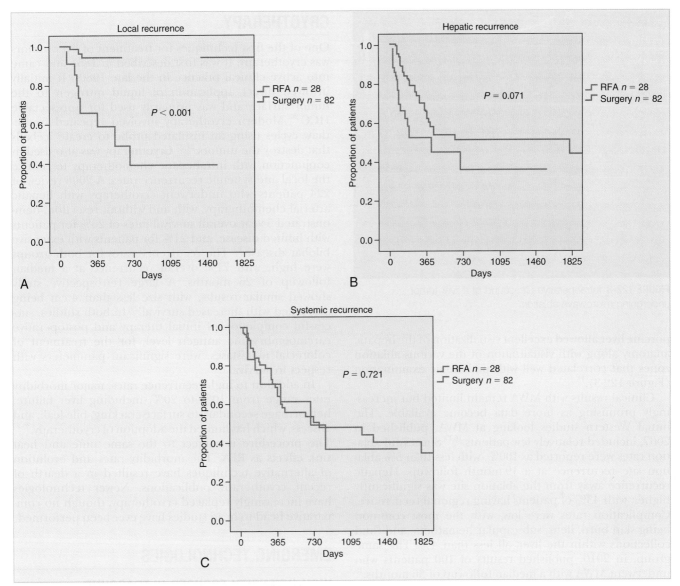

FIGURE 122-2 Local **(A)**, hepatic **(B)**, and systemic **(C)** recurrences in patients treated with radiofrequency ablation versus hepatic resection for early occurring colorectal liver metastases. (From Otto G, Düber C, Hoppe-Lotichius M, et al: Radiofrequency ablation as first-line treatment in patients with early colorectal liver metastases amenable to surgery. *Ann Surg* 251:796, 2010, Figure 1.)

first is the ablation area. Radiofrequency, which works by creating an electric current through the tissue, heats via friction from electrons moving within the current. The tissue is actively heating within 1 to 2 mm of the probe, with the surrounding tissue heated through passive conduction. Thus, the ablation zone is relatively limited and results in the need for multiple overlapping zones. In contrast, MWA affects all tissue within the antennae range actively and can thus generate heat more quickly over an area of 10 to 20 mm. This provides a more homogenous zone of tumor destruction.

Active heating of the tissue rather than passive conduction makes MWA less affected by the "heat sink" phenomena that adversely affects RFA. Because radiofrequency relies on conduction of heat through the tissue, high-blood-flow areas rapidly carry away the transmitted heat, frequently leading to incomplete ablation in the vicinity of vessels as small as 3 mm. In several porcine models of

MWA, the heat sink effect was significantly less than that typically seen with RFA.[12-14] In the majority of cases, there was no appreciable heat sink. As with RFA, the heat sink effect was related to the size of the vessel producing the effect; however, even with hepatic veins larger than 6 mm, nearly 40% of specimens showed no heat sink effect, whereas an additional third of the specimens had only mild heat sink.[12] In a study directly comparing the two modalities in a porcine model, they showed similar ablation zones; however, RFA showed nearly 25% more susceptibility to the heat sink effect.[14] A separate study comparing RFA and MWA in a porcine model showed larger ablation zones, higher temperatures 5 mm from the probe, and a more rapid rise in temperature, all markers suggesting more complete and efficient tissue destruction.[15] MWA also has less tissue charring than RFA and causes significantly less distortion on ultrasound. Use of a 12-MHz ultrasound transducer during MWA on

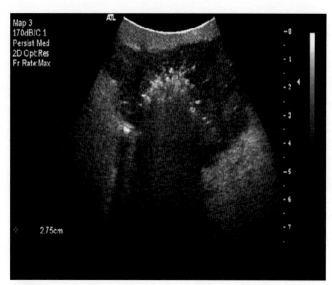

FIGURE 122-3 Intraoperative ultrasound of a liver tumor undergoing microwave ablation.

porcine liver allowed excellent visualization of the hepatic anatomy along with visualization of the various ablation zones that correlated well with pathologic examination (Figure 122-3).[13]

Clinical results with MWA remain limited but increasingly promising as more data become available. The initial Western studies looking at MWA, published in 2007, included relatively few patients.[16,17] Successful ablation rates were reported as 100%, with less than 3% ablation site recurrence at a 19-month followup. Hepatic recurrence away from the ablation site was significantly higher, with 43% of patients having regional recurrence. Complication rates were low, with the most common being skin burn, ileus, subscapular hematoma, and fluid collections within the liver, all less than 4%. The same group, in 2010, published results of 100 patients who underwent MWA with a median followup of 36 months.[18] Ablation site recurrence remained low at only 2%, whereas overall hepatic recurrence, at 37%, was also similar to the earlier studies.[18] With respect to complication rates, the data are somewhat difficult to interpret as the majority of patients had combined ablation and resection, with nearly 70% of patients having a laparotomy. The overall complication rate was 35%; however, complications specific to ablation, such as hepatic abscess, were only 2%. Data from a large Chinese study of 1100 patients who underwent exclusively percutaneous MWA also showed a major complication rate of only 2%.[19]

Outcomes for both colorectal metastases and hepatocellular carcinoma are similar. Definitive conclusions are difficult secondary to the size of the subgroups in early studies. In a recent series, 50 patients underwent treatment for CRC metastases, whereas 17 had primary HCC. Initial ablation rates, site-specific recurrence, and overall survival, respectively, were similar for CRC and HCC: 98% versus 100%, 6% versus 6%, 38 versus 41 months.[18] Patients with CRC had a higher complication rate; however, 60% in this study had concomitant hepatectomy, whereas 30% had resection of extrahepatic disease.

CRYOTHERAPY

One of the first techniques for treatment of liver tumors was cryotherapy. It was first described in 1851 and came into active clinical practice in the late 1980s. It initially involved direct application of liquid nitrogen to the tumor surface and was primarily used for unresectable HCC.[20] Modern cryotherapy involved repeated freeze-thaw cycles using an insulated probe to create iceballs that destroy the tumors.[21,22] Cryotherapy was also used in conjunction with intrahepatic chemotherapy to reduce the local and systemic recurrence rates. A 2006 review of 224 patients who underwent cryotherapy with hepatic arterial chemotherapy, with and without resection, demonstrated 5-year overall survival rates of 26% for patients with limited disease, and 21% for patients with extensive bilobar disease.[23] The recurrence rates for both groups were high, with 71% overall recurrence at a median followup of 26 months. A large retrospective study showed similar results, with size less than 4 cm being associated with increased survival.[24] In both studies, successful completion of initial therapy and postoperative carcinoembryonic antigen level, for the treatment of colorectal metastases, were significant parameters with respect to survival.

In addition to high recurrence rates, major morbidity rates range from 10% to 20%, including liver failure, hemorrhage secondary to surface cracking, bile leak, and abscess, which has limited the adoption of cryotherapy.[20-25] The procedure is subject to the same time and heat sink effects as RFA. The morbidity rates and evolution of alternative techniques have resulted in a dearth of recent cryotherapy publications. Newer technologies have increasingly replaced cryotherapy, though no comparative head-to-head studies have ever been performed.

EMERGING TECHNOLOGIES

HIGH-INTENSITY FOCUSED ULTRASOUND

The ultimate aim of nonresective liver tumor therapy is the avoidance of tumor puncture by a probe. High-intensity focused ultrasound (HIFU) was developed as a noninvasive method of tumor ablation. HIFU utilizes high-intensity ultrasound waves from multiple transducers to focus the ultrasound beam to highly selective areas of hepatic parenchyma. Tumor destruction is via coagulative necrosis due to heat. The technique was initially described in the early 1990s, though most of the early studies involved experimental animal models.[26] With improved visualization and better ultrasound probes leading to higher temperatures and shorter ablation times, recent studies have begun to look at the efficacy of treating a variety of neoplasms in humans.

Early clinical results of HIFU are promising. A study of 55 patients with unresectable HCC who underwent HIFU demonstrated a good local tumor response with improved long-term survival.[27] The majority of tumors were greater than 5 cm. Over 18 months of followup, tumor size was reduced by an average of 92%, 75%, and 68% in patients with stage II, IIIa, and IIIc disease, respectively. Overall 1-year survival was 86%, and

18-month survival was 35%.[27] The primary limitation was ablation time, which took up to 8 hours and had an average time of 5.5 hours. Several adjuvant techniques, such as utilizing a contrast-type material to improve ablation, or reducing hepatic blood flow, with preoperative transarterial chemoembolization (which was utilized in this study), along with improved transducers, may eventually reduce ablation time and therefore improve both its clinical efficacy and its attractiveness as a viable technology.

Experimental results of the newest devices show promising results, with excellent tissue destruction, rapid ablation times, scalability to larger lesions, and minimal heat sink effect. One group, utilizing an open approach in a porcine model, was able to generate ablation zones with a volume of 7 cm^3 with a single 40-second burn, generating temperatures greater than 80° C. Given the excellent visibility because of minimal tissue charring, greater than 90% of the time, precise overlapping burns were feasible, generating ablation zones up to 6 cm in maximum diameter.[28] Utilization of ultrasound contrast agents, which involve the intravenous injection of microbubbles, has been shown to increase the volume of tumor ablated. In a rabbit model of liver tumors, one group was able to double the ablation volume with use of such a contrast agent.[29] Another benefit of ultrasound is the ability to vary the depth of ablation. By adjusting the multiple transducers that make up these devises, tumors from the liver surface to up to 9 cm in depth can be successfully targeted without requiring penetration of the liver parenchyma by ablation probes.[28] This technique can thus be used in a completely extracorporeal approach with either ultrasound or MR guidance.[27,30-32] HIFU remains a new technology, with limited clinical studies; however, given its high ablation rates, the potential for completely extracorporeal use, and low complication rate, it will likely play an increasing role in the treatment of hepatic neoplasms.

IRREVERSIBLE ELECTROPORATION

Irreversible electroporation (IRE) is the newest and least-studied technology that has been tested clinically. IRE is based on the concept of disrupting the proper functioning of the cell membrane using electrical pulses targeted to specific anatomic locations, such as liver tumors. By applying repeated electrical pulses, the lipid bilayer can be made irreversibly permeable, leading to necrotic cell death. In several animal models, this technology has shown promising results with respect to ablation zone, sparing of adjacent structures, and time necessary to achieve ablation.[20-25] A clinical trial evaluating the clinical efficacy of this technology began recruiting patients in 2010. This represents an exciting emerging technology for the treatment of hepatic neoplasms.

SUMMARY

The standard of care for hepatic neoplasms remains resection. For HCC, this includes segmental and lobar resection in addition to transplant for properly selected patients. Although there are data to suggest that RFA may also be appropriate as primary therapy for HCC less than 2 cm in diameter, for those patients able to tolerate it, surgical resection should still be considered primary therapy.

The patient with unresectable cancer has by definition no options for resection. The definition of unresectable disease varies widely, but primarily includes patients with bilobar disease, patients unfit for surgery, and those patients who would have insufficient residual liver. In these patients, a measurable survival advantage can be gained from ablative therapies.

All ablative therapies have advantages and disadvantages. RFA remains the most common and best studied, but is limited by high recurrence rates, considerable heat sink effect, and poor visualization from charring. MWA, HIFU, and IRE have the potential for lower recurrence and are less affected by heat sink, though only MWA is in wide clinical practice. For all modalities and across tumor types, recurrence is related to lesion size and number. In general, RFA and MWA are appropriate for lesions smaller than 3 cm. Larger lesions are frequently treated, but high recurrence rates should be anticipated. Improved imaging and faster ablation times with new technologies will allow the easier creation of more optimal overlapping ablation zones, perhaps allowing the ablation of larger lesions with low recurrence and improved survival.

Ablative techniques are probably most applicable in colorectal cancer in combination with resection. Ablative techniques are effective at treating small lesions distant from a larger lesion that may be amenable to resection. This is particularly true in patients with limited bilobar disease, who may have a single large lesion in one lobe combined with two or three small lesions amenable to ablative destruction in the other lobe.

The treatment of hepatic neoplasms remains a rapidly evolving field without clear consensus guidelines or standard practices to treat these complex problems. As such, treatment decisions will continue to require the collaboration of experienced multidisciplinary teams. Ablative therapies remain a useful adjunct in the treatment of these diseases, either as alternative therapy for patients with advanced disease, in combination with resection to improve its efficacy, and as technologies continue to improve, perhaps as primary therapy. Resection, however, at least for now, remains the gold standard for the treatment of primary and metastatic colorectal cancer.

REFERENCES

1. Jemal A, Siegel R, Xu J, et al: Cancer statistics, 2010. *CA Cancer J Clin* 60:277, 2010.
2. Manfredi S, Lepage C, Hatem C, et al: Epidemiology and management of liver metastases from colorectal cancer. *Ann Surg* 244:254, 2006.
3. van der Pool AEM, Lalmahomed ZS, de Wilt JHW, et al: Trends in treatment for synchronous colorectal liver metastases: Differences in outcome before and after 2000. *J Surg Oncol* 102:413, 2010.
4. Nordenstedt H, White DL, El-Serag HB: The changing pattern of epidemiology in hepatocellular carcinoma. *Dig Liver Dis* 42:S206, 2010.
5. (CDC) CfDCaP: Hepatocellular carcinoma: United States, 2001-2006. *MMWR Morb Mortal Wkly Rep* 59:517, 2010.
6. Stang A, Fischbach R, Teichmann W, et al: A systematic review on the clinical benefit and role of radiofrequency ablation as treatment of colorectal liver metastases. *Eur J Cancer* 45:1748, 2009.

7. Mulier S, Ni Y, Jamart J, et al: Local recurrence after hepatic radio-frequency coagulation: Multivariate meta-analysis and review of contributing factors. *Ann Surg* 242:158, 2005.

8. Otto G, Düber C, Hoppe-Lotichius M, et al: Radiofrequency ablation as first-line treatment in patients with early colorectal liver metastases amenable to surgery. *Ann Surg* 251:796, 2010.

9. Chen M-S, Li J-Q, Zheng Y, et al: A prospective randomized trial comparing percutaneous local ablative therapy and partial hepatectomy for small hepatocellular carcinoma. *Ann Surg* 243:321, 2006.

10. Shibata T, Iimuro Y, Yamamoto Y, et al: Small hepatocellular carcinoma: Comparison of radio-frequency ablation and percutaneous microwave coagulation therapy. *Radiology* 223:331, 2002.

11. Livraghi T, Meloni F, Di Stasi M, et al: Sustained complete response and complications rates after radiofrequency ablation of very early hepatocellular carcinoma in cirrhosis: Is resection still the treatment of choice? *Hepatology* 47:82, 2008.

12. Yu NC, Raman SS, Kim YJ, et al: Microwave liver ablation: Influence of hepatic vein size on heat-sink effect in a porcine model. *J Vasc Interv Radiol* 19:1087, 2008.

13. Garrean S, Hering J, Saied A, et al: Ultrasound monitoring of a novel microwave ablation (MWA) device in porcine liver: Lessons learned and phenomena observed on ablative effects near major intrahepatic vessels. *J Gastrointest Surg* 13:334, 2009.

14. Wright AS, Sampson LA, Warner TF, et al: Radiofrequency versus microwave ablation in a hepatic porcine model. *Radiology* 236:132, 2005.

15. Yu J, Liang P, Yu X, et al: A comparison of microwave ablation and bipolar radiofrequency ablation both with an internally cooled probe: Results in ex vivo and in vivo porcine livers. *Eur J Radiol* 79:124, 2011.

16. Martin RCG, Scoggins CR, McMasters KM: Microwave hepatic ablation: Initial experience of safety and efficacy. *J Surg Oncol* 96:481, 2007.

17. Iannitti DA, Martin RCG, Simon CJ, et al: Hepatic tumor ablation with clustered microwave antennae: The US Phase II trial. *HPB (Oxford)* 9:120, 2007.

18. Martin RCG, Scoggins CR, McMasters KM: Safety and efficacy of microwave ablation of hepatic tumors: A prospective review of a 5-year experience. *Ann Surg Oncol* 17:171, 2010.

19. Liang P, Wang Y, Yu X, et al: Malignant liver tumors: Treatment with percutaneous microwave ablation: Complications among cohort of 1136 patients. *Radiology* 251:933, 2009.

20. Zhou XD, Tang ZY, Yu YQ, et al: Clinical evaluation of cryosurgery in the treatment of primary liver cancer. Report of 60 cases. *Cancer* 61:1889, 1988.

21. Kohli V, Clavien PA: Cryoablation of liver tumours. *Br J Surg* 85:1171, 1998.

22. Morris DL, Horton MD, Dilley AV, et al: Treatment of hepatic metastases by cryotherapy and regional cytotoxic perfusion. *Gut* 34:1156, 1993.

23. Yan TD, Padang R, Morris DL: Longterm results and prognostic indicators after cryotherapy and hepatic arterial chemotherapy with or without resection for colorectal liver metastases in 224 patients: Longterm survival can be achieved in patients with multiple bilateral liver metastases. *J Am Coll Surg* 202:100, 2006.

24. Niu R, Yan TD, Zhu JC, et al: Recurrence and survival outcomes after hepatic resection with or without cryotherapy for liver metastases from colorectal carcinoma. *Ann Surg Oncol* 14:2078, 2007.

25. Sheen AJ, Poston GJ, Sherlock DJ: Cryotherapeutic ablation of liver tumours. *Br J Surg* 89:1396, 2002.

26. Yang R, Reilly CR, Rescorla FJ, et al: High-intensity focused ultrasound in the treatment of experimental liver cancer. *Arch Surg* 126:1002, discussion 1009, 1991.

27. Wu F, Wang Z-B, Chen W-Z, et al: Extracorporeal high intensity focused ultrasound ablation in the treatment of patients with large hepatocellular carcinoma. *Ann Surg Oncol* 11:1061, 2004.

28. Parmentier H, Hubert P, Melodelima D, et al: High-intensity focused ultrasound ablation for the treatment of colorectal liver metastases during an open procedure: Study on the pig. *Ann Surg* 249:129, 2009.

29. Luo W, Zhou X, Yu M, et al: Ablation of high-intensity focused ultrasound assisted with SonoVue on Rabbit VX2 liver tumors: Sequential findings with histopathology, immunohistochemistry, and enzyme histochemistry. *Ann Surg Oncol* 16:2359, 2009.

30. Bradley WG: MR-guided focused ultrasound: A potentially disruptive technology. *J Am Coll Radiol* 6:510, 2009.

31. Zhang L, Zhu H, Jin C, et al: High-intensity focused ultrasound (HIFU): Effective and safe therapy for hepatocellular carcinoma adjacent to major hepatic veins. *Eur Radiol* 19:437, 2009.

32. Illing RO, Kennedy JE, Wu F, et al: The safety and feasibility of extracorporeal high-intensity focused ultrasound (HIFU) for the treatment of liver and kidney tumours in a Western population. *Br J Cancer* 93:890, 2005.

Hepatic Transplantation

Steven D. Colquhoun | Nicholas N. Nissen | Andrew S. Klein

Liver transplantation has now been the accepted standard of care for the treatment of end-stage liver disease and related conditions for more than 25 years. Although it was in 1963 that Thomas Starzl and his team performed the first successful human liver transplant, it was not until 1967 that the first 1-year survival was celebrated.[1] Indeed, acceptable and reliable outcomes came significantly later. Starzl and others went on to refine and overcome most of the technical aspects of the procedure, but truly satisfactory results became possible only after 1979. It was in that year that advances in immunosuppression and the efforts of Sir Roy Calne, another pioneer surgeon, made the availability of cyclosporine possible. Ultimately the National Institutes of Health (NIH) convened a consensus development conference in 1984 to evaluate this new clinical option and concluded "that liver transplantation is a therapeutic modality for end-stage liver disease that deserves broader application."[2] With this endorsement, a "broader application" unquestionably occurred as evidenced by the rather swift growth in the United States from a single liver transplant center, to eventually more than 120 programs nationwide. Most importantly, liver transplantation was firmly established as the standard of care for selected patients with end-stage cirrhosis. Patients who would have succumbed to their disease a few years earlier now completely recovered, and once again enjoyed normal and productive lives.

In the years intervening to the present, surgical techniques have continued to evolve along with a better understanding of disease processes, immunosuppression, prophylaxis against infection, and the general sophistication of patient management before, during, and after transplantation. With these advances, outcomes have also continuously improved, with current national statistics for 1-year patient survival approaching 90%, and 3-year survival being nearly 80%. Although in the earlier days of liver transplantation, the goal was simply that of survival, in the current era the focus has shifted to quality of life and other long-term issues facing transplant recipients.

Ironically, improved results, expanded indications, and wider availability of expertise have all led to undoubtedly the single greatest ongoing challenge facing the field of liver transplantation: the persistent shortage of suitable organs for transplantation. At its worst, in the span of 5 years between 1996 and 2001, the number of patients awaiting liver transplantation increased at a seemingly exponential rate from just more than 7000 to an all-time high of more than 18,000 (Figure 123-1). In the absence of a commensurate increase in the availability of suitable donor organs, there was a predictable corresponding increase in deaths among potential recipients waiting for organs.

These frustrating facts have led to a number of strategies for increasing the number of available organs, including improved nationwide donor awareness campaigns, dividing deceased donor organs to provide allografts to two recipients, the acceptance of increasingly "marginal" or "extended criteria" deceased donors, the use of "non-heartbeating" donors, and finally, the general acceptance of adult-to-adult living donor liver transplantation.

In this chapter, many of the clinically relevant details of liver transplantation will be discussed, including the current challenges and opportunities faced by those in the field.

EPIDEMIOLOGY

Chronic end-stage cirrhotic liver disease is the most frequent indication for orthotopic liver transplantation. In the United States, the overall incidence of cirrhosis of any etiology is in the range of 70 to 100,000, with rates higher for men than women (95 vs. 50 to 100,000). Currently in the United States there are estimated to be nearly 6 million individuals with cirrhosis and the most recent National Vital Statistics Reports lists a rate of 9.7 deaths per 100,000.[3] Viral hepatitis, cholestatic liver diseases, and alcoholic and fatty liver diseases are some of the more common causes of end-stage liver failure (Table 123-1).

ETIOLOGIES OF END-STAGE LIVER DISEASE

HEPATITIS C

Estimates vary, but worldwide there are likely more than 200 million individuals infected with the hepatitis C virus (HCV). According to the Centers for Disease Control and Prevention (CDC), the prevalence of hepatitis C in the United States is estimated to be much more than 3 million. In fact, cirrhosis from HCV remains the most common indication for liver transplantation in the United States, accounting for roughly 40% of the activity at most centers.[4] HCV is a parenterally transmitted RNA virus with no DNA intermediates. The HCV genome was elucidated in 1989 and screening of blood products began shortly thereafter. Acute HCV infections are usually subclinical with no icteric phase. The disease becomes chronic in the majority of those infected, with cirrhosis developing between one and two decades later. The interval to cirrhosis is greatly accelerated by heavy alcohol consumption.[5] In the United States, 1% to 2% of the population is infected with HCV: from blood transfusions prior to 1990, intravenous drug use, or other parenteral routes, such as tattoos. Despite blood product screening and efforts at greater public awareness, and

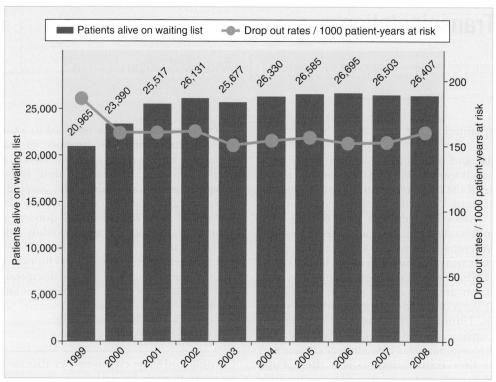

FIGURE 123-1 Patients alive on the waiting list at any time during the year and annual dropout (removal for death or being too sick) rates from the liver waiting list per 1000 patient-years. (From SRTR Analysis, Data as of May 2009.)

TABLE 123-1 Chronic End-Stage Liver Disease: Etiologies

Category	Disease	Frequency
Hepatitis	(Hepatitis A)	Never chronic
	Hepatitis B	10% to 15%
	Hepatitis C	40%
Noncholestatic	Laennec cirrhosis	
	Cryptogenic cirrhosis	
	Autoimmune hepatitis	
Cholestatic	Primary sclerosing cholangitis	
	Primary biliary cirrhosis	
Metabolic	Hemochromatosis	
	Wilson disease	
	α_1-Antitrypsin deficiency	
Malignancies	Hepatocellular carcinoma	Adults
	Hepatoblastoma	Children
	Cholangiocarcinoma	Investigational
	Carcinoid/neuroendocrine	Rare
	Hemangioendothelioma	Rare
	Hemangiosarcoma	
Atresia: children	Biliary atresia	50%
Others	Budd-Chiari	Rare
	Cystic fibrosis	
	Congenital hepatic fibrosis	
	Benign tumors	

because of the prolonged course of the disease, HCV is predicted to be an increasing problem for at least another decade. Effective treatment options are available and soon will include new HCV protease inhibitors. These drugs can block viral replication and, in conjunction with other treatments, may finally displace HCV from its prominent role in the realm of liver transplantation.

HEPATITIS B

Hepatitis B is a DNA virus endemic in many countries, especially those of the Pacific Rim. Although effective vaccines have been available for more than 20 years, it continues to be a major worldwide health problem, due especially to vertical transmission. HBV-related liver disease currently accounts for up to 15% of transplant activity at most centers. In the earlier days of liver transplantation, postoperative reinfection was a major issue leading to dismal results and the general acceptance of HBV as a relative contraindication to transplant. A dramatic success story followed first the development of improved prophylactic strategies utilizing HBV immune globulin, and the subsequent availability of effective antiviral agents. Hepatic allograft reinfection with HBV is no longer a significant clinical problem.[6]

CHOLESTATIC DISEASES

Collectively, primary biliary cirrhosis (PBC) and primary sclerosing cholangitis (PSC) are referred to as the cholestatic liver diseases. Although both are idiopathic, each has a genetic/autoimmune element, and overlap syndromes with autoimmune hepatitis can occur. Together they account for upwards of 25% of transplant activity at most centers.[4]

Ninety percent of patients with PBC are female, presenting at an average age of 50 years and not uncommonly with familial clustering. Pruritus is the most common presenting symptom, while the diagnostic hallmark is the presence of antimitochondrial antibodies, which are present in virtually 100% of those with the disease.[7]

Men are twice as likely as women to be afflicted with PSC, usually presenting between 25 and 45 years of age. Many cases are discovered incidentally on routine blood tests with the finding of an elevated serum alkaline phosphatase. Patients with symptoms are equally likely to present with either pruritus or jaundice. In the proper clinical context, diagnosis is confirmed with endoscopic retrograde cholangiography showing irregular stricturing and beading of the intrahepatic biliary tree. As discussed in some detail later, there is a strong association between PSC and inflammatory bowel disease. A major concern among patients with PSC is the 15% to 30% overall associated risk for the development of cholangiocarcinoma (CCA).[8] Unfortunately, there is as yet no reliable method for predicting or detecting this malignancy in its early stages. Ironically, demonstrable disease was, until relatively recently, considered a contraindication for transplantation because of generally dismal outcomes. However, those transplanted and found to have incidental CCA actually fare quite well.[9] As of November 2009, organ allocation policies now facilitate transplantation in highly selected patients with early-stage CCA in the context of aggressive adjuvant therapy.

ALCOHOLIC LIVER DISEASE

Alcoholic liver disease ranks as one of the most common causes of death in the Untied States and the second most common indication for liver transplantation in adults.[10] Interestingly, only between 10% and 15% of alcoholics develop cirrhosis. Nevertheless, it has been determined that upwards of 80 g of alcohol per day for more than 5 years will put most individuals at risk. As already noted, alcohol acts synergistically with HCV or HBV infection. Alcohol-related liver injury can manifest across a spectrum, from acute alcoholic hepatitis to chronic fatty changes and on to cirrhosis and hepatocellular carcinoma. Most transplant centers maintain strict abstinence guidelines for determining candidacy when alcohol is the cause of liver failure. Most often, a 6-month a period of sobriety is required to allow demonstration of insight and compliance. Another very practical reason for period of abstinence is to avoid transplanting those who will recover from the acute effects of alcohol and no longer meet transplant criteria.

UNRESECTABLE HEPATOCELLULAR CARCINOMA

Hepatocellular carcinoma (HCC) is one of the most common malignancies worldwide, ranking eighth among all cancers while accounting for approximately 90% of those that are primary to the liver. The incidence of HCC in endemic regions of Asia and Africa can be as high as 150 cases per 100,000. Although rates found in the United States and Western Europe are much lower (1 to 5 cases per 100,000) the incidence is rising. In the United States, the incidence of HCC is currently estimated to be from 8500 to 11,500 new cases per year.[11-15]

Even though environmental toxins pose a major risk in some parts of the world, the incidence of HCC is primarily related to the prevalence of cirrhosis from chronic viral hepatitis B and C, with a relative risk several-hundred-fold greater than those unaffected. Cirrhosis per se is a premalignant condition, regardless of etiology. Although cirrhosis remains the common denominator, the DNA intermediates in the replicative cycle of the hepatitis B virus may be directly carcinogenic, even in the absence of cirrhosis. The irony of HCC is that such tumors are typically multifocal and almost exclusive to those with underlying cirrhosis that precludes resection. The intuitive appeal of orthotopic liver transplant (OLT) is the elimination of tumor as well as the underlying liver disease, which creates a fertile environment for developing neoplasms.

UNUSUAL TUMORS

The early transplant experience in patients with secondary hepatic malignancy was dismal, and consequently metastatic tumors are generally still considered an absolute contraindication. However, few exceptions do exist. Although largely anecdotal, acceptable outcomes have been described in patients with metastatic midgut carcinoid tumors, whereas patients transplanted for other unresectable neuroendocrine tumors have generally not fared as well. Hepatic epithelioid hemangioendothelioma have also been successfully treated using OLT but outcomes have been unpredictable. Outcomes for primary hepatic angiosarcoma as well as biliary cystadenocarcinoma have been disappointing. Hepatic epithelioid hemangioendothelioma has also been successfully treated using OLT but outcomes are unpredictable.[16] When considering OLT in this setting of secondary tumors, the tradeoff is between the survival advantages offered by traditional therapies for otherwise slowly progressive tumors versus the potential for rapid progression of occult residual disease under the influence of posttransplant immunosuppression. A small number of symptomatic and otherwise unresectable benign tumors, or those with the potential for malignant degeneration, such as adenomas, have also been treated with transplantation.[17]

OTHER ETIOLOGIES

A number of other chronic disorders, which can also lead to liver failure and the need for transplantation, do exist, but are beyond the scope of this discussion. Metabolic abnormalities of iron and copper underlie the disorders of hemochromatosis and Wilson disease, respectively. Other entities include autoimmune hepatitis, α_1-antitrypsin deficiency, nonalcoholic fatty liver disease, and the Budd-Chiari syndrome. In addition, there are a host of other disorders that occur in the pediatric population, the most common of which is biliary atresia.

TABLE 123-2 Acute Liver Failure: Etiologies

Toxic	Infectious	Metabolic	Cardiovascular
Drugs or chemicals	Viral hepatitis	Wilson disease	Acute Budd-Chiari syndrome
Acetaminophen	Yellow fever	Acute fatty liver of pregnancy	Portal vein thrombosis
Halothane	Q fever	Reye syndrome	"Shock" liver
Isoniazid	Other viruses	Other inborn errors	Heat stroke
Valproate			
Amanita phalloides			

ACUTE LIVER FAILURE

Although the vast majority of patients undergoing liver transplantation suffer from chronic diseases, an estimated 2000 individuals in the United States each year present with conditions leading to acute or "fulminant" liver failure (ALF) (Table 123-2). The most common etiologies include toxic drug exposures such as acetaminophen or idiosyncratic reactions to other drugs. Mushroom poisoning (e.g., *Amanita phalloides*) and industrial or environmental toxins have also led to ALF. Other causes include acute hepatitis A, acute or reactivated hepatitis B, and Wilson disease (a hereditary disease of copper metabolism). Other conditions, such as an acute Budd-Chiari syndrome, fatty liver of pregnancy, autoimmune conditions, and even shock can give rise to ALF. In up to 20% of cases, no apparent etiology can be identified. As discussed later, patients presenting with ALF must undergo urgent evaluation and listing for transplantation, as death can occur within hours.[18]

EVALUATION PROCESS

There is unlikely to be another area in the field of medicine in which the word *team* more aptly applies. Organ transplantation in general, and liver transplantation in particular, is so complex as to only be possible through the coordinated efforts of many individuals with special expertise, working in concert. The patient's first encounter through the evaluation process is illustrative. The three goals of evaluation are to (1) confirm the presence of end-stage liver disease and the indications for transplant, (2) exclude contraindications, and (3) initiate patient and family education regarding the transplantation process. To that end, each patient is seen by a core group of individuals composed of a transplant hepatologist, a transplant surgeon, a psychiatrist, a social worker, a certified transplant nursing coordinator, and a nutritionist. Additional consultations are obtained as indicated in cardiology, pulmonology, nephrology, neurology, anesthesiology, dentistry, and infectious disease. Each of the consultants has acknowledged experience in working with liver failure patients, and understands the special concerns and challenges presented by liver disease and transplantation. In the evaluation of healthy volunteer candidates for living-donor liver donation, a team composed of a physician, social worker, and nurse coordinator, all independent from the team of individuals caring for the recipient, act as dispassionate advocates for the potential donor. Increasingly, transplant programs are engaging in regular interactions with hospital ethicists to ensure the appropriateness of details related to living donation and other aspects of transplantation.[19]

TRANSPLANT CANDIDACY

There are three interrelated aspects of determining transplant candidacy, including criteria defining indications and contraindications, but also the appropriate prioritization of candidates in the context of the limited resource of available organs. There has been an ongoing effort and continuous evolution of policies to better prioritize potential recipients and to maintain the spirit of "sickest first" in organ allocation. Specifically there has been a determined progression toward more objective and evidence-based criteria.

INDICATIONS FOR TRANSPLANTATION

CHRONIC DISEASE

The basic clinical indications for liver transplant candidacy among patients with chronic disease have remained relatively constant over the past two and a half decades. They include (1) progressive hyperbilirubinemia, (2) portal hypertension as evidenced by signs of gastrointestinal bleeding (usually from esophageal or gastric varices), hypersplenism with thrombocytopenia, (3) disabling symptoms of portosystemic or hepatic encephalopathy, and finally (4) synthetic dysfunction as assessed by ProTime or international normalized ratio (INR). More subjective criteria include general wasting or a "failure-to-thrive" condition, which certainly can afflict patients with the constellation of problems associated with end-stage liver disease, as well as poor quality of life (secondary to fatigue, weakness, intractable pruritis, etc.).

ACUTE DISEASE

Patients presenting with ALF have a much more dramatic clinical presentation. In such circumstances, there is a prominent defining role for encephalopathy, which in contrast to the chronic setting, can progress to cerebral edema with herniation. In the acute setting more than chronic, clinical jaundice parallels the degree of hepatocyte injury. Fundamentally, any previously healthy individual presenting with a rapid decline in liver function associated with coagulopathy and an altered mental status meets the criteria defining ALF.[18] There are two standard definitions for fulminant liver failure and both

TABLE 123-3 Acute Liver Failure: Definitions

Jaundice to Encephalopathy	Days
Hyperacute	≤ 7
Subacute	8 to 28
Subacute	29 to 60

TABLE 123-4 Preoperative Assessment

Labs	Tests	Consultations
CMP	CXR	Surgery
CBC	ECG	Hepatology
INR/ProTime	PFT w/ ABG	Psychiatry
Hepatitis serologies	Axial imaging	Nursing
	Doppler ultrasonography	Social Work
Iron	PPD/*Candida*/Mumps/	Nutrition
AMA, ANA	Tetanus	Cardiology PRN
CMV	Mammogram >45 years	Pulmonology
EBV	Echocardiogram >45	PRN
	years	Nephrology PRN
TSH/T$_3$/T$_4$	CT chest if tumor	Infectious
HIV	Bone scan if tumor >	disease PRN
	stage II	
CEA/AFP		
U/A		
Type & screen		
VDRL		

ABG, Arterial blood gas; *AMA,* antimitochondrial antibody; *ANA,* antinuclear antibody; *CBC,* complete blood count; *CEA/AFP,* carcinoembryonic antigen/α-fetoprotein; *CMP,* comprehensive metabolic panel; *CMV,* cytomegalovirus; *CXR,* chest x-ray; *ECG,* electrocardiograph; *EBV,* Epstein-Barr virus; *INR,* international normalized ratio; *PFT,* pulmonary function testing; *PPD,* purified protein derivative; *PRN,* as needed; *TSH,* thyroid-stimulating hormone; *VDRL,* Venereal Disease Research Laboratory.

require the absence of any preexisting chronic liver disease. The first includes a clinical presentation with encephalopathy 8 weeks or less from the onset of symptoms and the second is based on the development of encephalopathy 2 weeks or less from the onset of clinical jaundice (Table 123-3). Interestingly, a longer interval between the development of jaundice and encephalopathy is associated with a poorer clinical prognosis.

CONTRAINDICATIONS

The contraindications to liver transplantation can be relative or absolute, but both lists continue to diminish. Extremes of age, for example, were once limitations that have since broadened dramatically. Human immunodeficiency virus disease was once considered an absolute contraindication, but this too has been reconsidered.[20,21] More so than the other organs, candidacy for liver transplantation weighs equally the medical and the psychosocial considerations. Transplant centers must be compassionate but deliberate and consistent in light of the ongoing shortage of organs, government oversight, and the court of public opinion with a history of misunderstanding regarding issues of substance abuse and mischaracterized celebrity transplants.

In general, the contraindications to OLT are those comorbid conditions that would preclude an operative procedure of its magnitude. The hemodynamic changes that can occur during a liver transplantation may be extreme, stressing any or all of the major organ systems (Table 123-4).

Severe cardiac and pulmonary conditions are the most frequently identified medical contraindications. Although advanced age per se is uncommonly cited as a contraindication, it is rare for most programs to consider candidates aged much beyond the midseventies. Many centers do adhere to programmatically agreed-on age thresholds. More important than age is the overall condition of a potential recipient. This assessment can be difficult, in that liver failure has dramatic systemic effects that may lead to severe deconditioning. At first glance, the inexperienced clinician might consider many typical transplant candidates to be "too sick." Careful consideration often finds that organ dysfunction is attributable to the liver disease and will reverse with a normally functioning allograft.

The shortage of organs and the methodology of the organ allocation algorithm, which provides priority to the "sickest first," makes it increasingly common that patients undergoing OLT are extremely ill, often hospitalized, or in an intensive care unit setting. For such patients with decompensated chronic disease, or those with fulminant liver failure, other more specific, acute

criteria are applicable (Tables 123-5 and 123-6). Patients must display adequate hemodynamics and be maintained on no more than a single pressor agent. Those on a ventilator should have oxygen requirements not greater than an FiO$_2$ of 50%. As noted earlier, patients with acute liver failure can develop cerebral edema. In such circumstances, if cerebral perfusion pressures have been inadequate, then an acceptable outcome is unlikely, and the use of an organ is unwarranted. Infectious issues can also present acute contraindications, such as an active pneumonia or other systemic processes. Occasionally, severe psychiatric or extreme social conditions may also present as relative contraindications. In the common circumstance of acetaminophen overdose, for example, multiple prior suicide attempts despite adequate psychiatric therapy would likely contraindicate proceeding to transplant. Similarly, patients with a history of liver failure related to substance abuse but without an adequate period of abstinence, or the patient with no evidence of social support, may also be denied candidacy.

One final, but extremely important, potential contraindication to transplantation is any prior history of extrahepatic malignancy in the candidate. Early in the experience of organ transplantation, it was appreciated that immunosuppression can have profound effects on the growth of a malignancy, including subclinical residual tumor. Many common cancers may recur, even years after definitive treatment. Despite modern imaging technology, in many cases only the passage of time can be the determinant of cure. The histologic cell type, the stage and grade of a tumor, as well as the interval between treatment and transplantation, are the factors considered in the selection process. Based on the propensity to

TABLE 123-5 Contraindications: Acute

Organ System	Observation	Contraindication
Cardiac	CAD risks	Recent MI
	Unstable hemodynamics	Inadequate CO
		≥Single pressor required
Pulmonary	Pneumonia	Active/progressive
	ARDS	PEEP ≥10 mm Hg
	Ventilator dependency	FiO₂ ≥50%
Neurologic	Altered mental status	Recent/acute CVA
	Acute encephalopathy/ cerebral edema	Herniation or CPP ≤50
	Seizures	Uncontrolled activity
Infectious disease	Chronic condition	Untreated TB or similar
	Acute infection	Untreated or progressive
Renal	Azotemia	Inadequate renal replacement therapy
	Hyperkalemia	
	Acidosis	
	Hypervolemia	
Psychiatric*	Substance abuse	Inadequate abstinence period
	Suicide attempt(s)	
	Schizophrenia or bipolar (refractory)	Repeated despite therapy
		Jeopardy to followup care
Social*	Inadequate support	Jeopardy to followup care

ARDS, Acute respiratory distress syndrome; *CAD*, coronary artery disease; *CO*, cardiac output; *CPP*, cerebral perfusion pressure; *CVA*, cerebrovascular accident; *FiO₂*, fraction of inspired oxygen; *MI*, myocardial infarction; *PEEP*, positive end-expiratory pressure; *TB*, tuberculosis.
*Relative.

TABLE 123-6 Contraindications: Severe Chronic

Organ System	Contraindication*
Cardiac	CAD
	Valvular disease
	Cardiomyopathy
Pulmonary	COPD
	Pulmonary HTN
	Hepatopulmonary
	Pulmonary fibrosis
Infectious diseases	HIV
	Untreated TB
	Syphilis
	Other
Psychiatric	Jeopardy to followup care
Social	Inadequate transportation
	Inadequate communication
	Homeless
	Inadequate support general

CAD, Coronary artery disease; *COPD*, chronic obstructive pulmonary disease; *HTN*, hypertension; *TB*, tuberculosis.
*Relative/evolving.

TABLE 123-7 Preexisting Malignancy: Risk of Post-OLT Recurrence

Low (0% to 10%)	Intermediate (11% to 22%)	High (≥23%)
Renal cell	Lymphoma	Breast
Uterine	Wilms	Bladder
Testicular	Prostate	Renal cell (large)
Uterine cervix	Colon	Sarcoma
Papillary thyroid	Melanoma	Myeloma

OLT, Orthotopic liver transplant.

recur after transplantation, various tumor cell types have been categorized as low (0% to 10%), intermediate (11% to 25%), or high (>25%) risk (Table 123-7). Most programs avoid transplants in patients with a history of histologically aggressive tumors.

A key consideration in evaluating patients with a prior history of extrahepatic malignancy is determining the likelihood of recurrence absent a liver transplant. Predicted recurrence rates of less than 5% over the next 2 years are generally required. For the majority of the more commonly occurring malignancies, a 2- to 5-year waiting period is usually imposed.[11] Of those who do recur after transplantation, the majority are evident within 2 years of transplantation.

LIVER ALLOCATION

In the earliest days of organ transplantation, there were no systems in place to facilitate the placement of available donor organs to appropriate recipients. In the mid-1960s, center-to-center phone calls for matching donated kidneys with potential recipients evolved into essentially two confederations of transplant centers: one in the eastern part of the United States, and one in the west. By the early 1970s, the use of a computerized database to track patient information was implemented in the east and, with further refinements in 1977 it was named the "United Network of Organ Sharing" (UNOS). As of 1984, UNOS had evolved into a nationwide transplant candidate registry and was incorporated as a private, nonprofit organization. Finally, in 1986, UNOS was awarded a federal contract by the Department of Health and Human Services to establish the Organ Procurement and Transplant Network (OPTN).[12]

In an ongoing effort to balance utility with equity and optimize outcomes, the algorithms for allocating livers have been under constant revision. To minimize ischemia times, organs have always been first utilized locally, followed by regional and then national placement. Unlike the past, patients with acute conditions are currently prioritized above those with chronic disease, and now also take precedence regionally over local primacy.[22] Originally, time on the waiting list was weighed heavily in determining priority. This has since been essentially eliminated and replaced by a greater emphasis on the philosophy of "sickest first." Initially, the Child-Turcotte-Pugh (CTP) (Table 123-8) system was used to prioritize patients but was found to be excessively subjective while also inadequately partitioning patients into only four

TABLE 123-8 Child-Turcotte-Pugh Scoring

Points	1 Points	2 Points	3 Points
Encephalopathy	None	Stage 1 or 2	Stage 3 or 4
Bilirubin (noncholestatic disease)	<2	2 to 3	>3
Bilirubin (cholestatic disease)	<4	4 to 10	>10
Albumin	>3.5	3.5 to 2.8	<2.8
Ascites	None	Moderate	Severe
INR/(ProTime)	<1.7 (4 sec)	1.7 (4 sec) to 2.3 (6 sec)	>2.3 (6 sec)

TABLE 123-9 Model for End-Stage Liver Disease (MELD): Formula*

MELD Score =	$0.957 \times \log$ (creatinine mg/dL)
+	$0.378 \times \log$ (bilirubin mg/dL)
+	$1.120 \times \log$ (INR)
+	0.643

*Multiply score × 10 and round to nearest whole number. Lab test <1.0 is set to 1.0.

TABLE 123-10 Pediatric End-Stage Liver Disease (PELD): Formula*

PELD score =	$0.480 \times \log$ (bilirubin mg/dL)
+	$1.857 \times \log$ (INR)
+	$0.687 \times \log$ (albumin g/dL)
+	0.436 if patient < 1 year of age
+	0.667 if growth failure (≤2 standard deviations)

*Multiply score × 10 and round to nearest whole number. Lab test <1.0 is set to 1.0.

TABLE 123-11 UNOS Hepatocellular TNM/Staging

T1	Single nodule <1.9 cm	Stage I
T2	Single nodule 2.0–5.0 cm or up to three nodules all <3.0 cm	Stage II
T3	Single nodule >5.0 cm or up to three nodules, one >3.0 cm	Stage III
T4a	Four or more nodules	Stage IVA
T4b	Any of the above with portal vein involvement on imaging	Stage IVA2
	Any N1 or M1	Stage IVB

Despite the significant improvements offered by the MELD system, allocation remains imperfect.[17] It has been estimated that up to 10% of patients have conditions that are underappraised. The best example of such a deficiency is the circumstance of hepatocellular carcinoma (HCC). Because cirrhosis of any etiology may predispose to the development of HCC, many patients present with or develop such tumors (Table 123-11).

Even in those who are well compensated, only about 15% are amenable to liver resection because of issues of tumor size and location in the context of underlying cirrhosis and portal hypertension. Because allocation schemes have been designed to assess the degree of liver failure, patients with HCC were thus disadvantaged. Importantly, patients with early-stage HCC were shown to have excellent long-term survival and a low incidence of tumor recurrence after liver transplantation. With the introduction of the MELD, its limited ability to adequately prioritize HCC patients was acknowledged and additional MELD points were granted for patients with stage 1 to 2 HCC. HCC patients with more advanced clinical staging have a poorer prognosis following OLT and thus fail the utility criteria on which allocation policy is based. Such patients are not afforded additional MELD points. Currently, automatic increases in MELD points are given to early-stage HCC candidates on the waiting list every 3 months, based on a defined statistical likelihood of receiving an organ over the ensuing 3 months. This is in effect until transplantation occurs or the tumor stage has progressed beyond acceptable limits. With adjustments, this system has worked well for tumor patients.

More recently, some additional conditions have been considered for incremental MELD point assignment similar to HCC. In general, these are also conditions in which the MELD system inadequately captures the magnitude of the patient's need (Table 123-12). There are still other diseases and conditions that have been discussed as appropriate for granting additional MELD points. However, the list is long and the concern is that the MELD system could be rendered unwieldy and unreasonably complex if too many exceptions are applied (Table 123-13). Benefits of the current MELD system are that it is objective, simple, easily understood, and readily verifiable. Discussions regarding such changes are ongoing, but a complete resolution of these issues seems unlikely in the near future. Currently, additional MELD points may be granted to specific patients with special considerations through an appeals process to a "jury of

categories and failing to account for a vast spectrum of disease severity.

Under government pressure to decrease the disparity of waiting times between regions, the Model for End-stage Liver Disease (MELD) was introduced in February of 2002. Despite its development for another purpose, the MELD system was shown to be predictive of death on the waiting list, had the advantage of utilizing only objective criteria (Table 123-9), and allowed improved patient discrimination by severity of disease.[23] The more discrete data offered by MELD has also facilitated statistical analyses providing additional insights such as the risk–benefit threshold of illness versus transplantation. The Pediatric End-stage Liver Disease (PELD) provides a similar objective system for children. The current liver allocation scheme is outlined in Tables 123-9 and 123-10. In summary, patients can be placed on the UNOS transplant waiting list with a minimum MELD score of 6, organs are offered first to patients above the "minimum transplant" MELD score of 15, and the maximum score rests at 40. With exceptions, organs are offered within blood groups only.

TABLE 123-12 Current Exceptions to MELD

Diagnosis	Rationale
HCC (stage T2)	Disease disproportionate to liver failure, primary malignancy removed with OLT (Milan criteria)
HCC (not stage T2)	Disease disproportionate to liver failure, primary malignancy downstaged to Milan criteria
Hepatopulmonary syndrome	Disease disproportionate to liver failure, reversible posttransplant ($PaO_2 <$ 60 mm Hg at rest)
Portopulmonary hypertension	Disease disproportionate to liver failure, reversible posttransplant (mPAP > 35 mm Hg)
Familial amyloidosis	Disease disproportionate to liver failure, metabolic disorder restored with OLT
Primary oxaluria	Associated renal disease recurs without liver transplant, metabolic disorder restored with OLT
Cholangiocarcinoma	Confined to proximal ducts, Small size, meets approved institutional protocol
Hepatic artery thrombosis (<10 days post-OLT)	Early arterial thrombosis, MELD 40 to expedite re-OLT without competing with status 1 candidates

HCC, Hepatocellular carcinoma; *OLT,* orthotopic liver transplant; PaO_2, partial pressure of oxygen in arterial blood; *MELD,* Model for End-stage Liver Disease; *mPAP,* mean pulmonary artery pressure.

TABLE 123-13 Potential Future MELD Exceptions

Diagnosis	Problem
Ascites	Failed/contraindicated TIPS Frequent large volume paracentesis
Hyponatremia	Alternative to ascites
Encephalopathy	Repeated hospitalizations Refractory to therapy
Budd-Chiari	Chronic TIPS/Shunt failed/not feasible
Cystic fibrosis	Cirrhosis alone With lung transplant
Polycystic disease	Malnutrition With/without renal disease
Pruritus (intractable)	Cholestatic diseases
Primary sclerosing cholangitis	Recurrent cholangitis Repeated hospitalizations/sepsis
Small-for-size syndrome	Inadequate volume: – Living donor – Split deceased donor
Unusual tumors	Carcinoid /NET Sarcoma Epithelioid hemangioendothelioma Other
Refractory GI hemorrhage	Failed conservative measures Failed/contraindicated TIPS
Hereditary hemorrhagic telangiectasia	High output failure Portal hypertension Biliary stricture
Familial amyloidotic polyneuropathy	With/without combined cardiac transplant

MELD, Model for End-stage Liver Disease; *TIPS,* transjugular intrahepatic portosystemic shunt.

peers" provided by the UNOS Regional Review Board (RRB). Presently, no unusual primary or metastatic tumors are given special consideration for additional or automatic MELD points, except within the RRB process. The search for the perfect allocation system continues.[19]

ASSOCIATED CONDITIONS AND SPECIAL CONSIDERATIONS

Patients with end-stage liver disease often have significant associated conditions affecting other organ systems. Those that are more common, surprising, or sinister are briefly mentioned here by organ system. An understanding of these conditions can be critical to the management of a patient's severe cirrhosis and the maintenance of transplant candidacy.

HEMODYNAMICS

Perhaps the most pervasive physiologic changes associated with cirrhosis are those affecting hemodynamics which, in turn, can affect each of the organ systems.[24] Cirrhosis leads to a generalized vasodilation and hyperdynamic state. In addition to a reduced systemic vascular resistance, a host of attendant changes can occur, including increased peripheral blood flow, reduced arteriovenous oxygen difference, reduced effective blood volume with reduced cortical renal blood flow, and activation of the renin-angiotensin axis with sodium and water retention contributing to ascites formation. Patients with cirrhosis are generally observed to have an elevated cardiac output, tachycardia, and a low blood pressure. As

cirrhosis progresses, patients with a history of hypertension no longer require antihypertensive medications. Many of the common physical findings seen in cirrhotic patients, such as palmar erythema and cutaneous spider angiomata, are also explained by these vascular changes.

HEART

Iron overload states, such as that seen with genetic hemochromatosis, can lead to cardiac iron deposition. Although overt abnormalities may be discovered with echocardiography, those afflicted are at risk for conduction abnormalities, severe dysrhythmias, and right heart failure, especially during the significant stress of surgery. Magnetic resonance imaging can detect cardiac iron overload, and cardiac catheterization is usually required to determine transplant candidacy. In some circumstances, patients have been considered for simultaneous dual-organ (heart-liver) transplantation. As a group, those with either primary or secondary iron overload fare worse with transplantation than those without iron overload.[25]

LUNG

Up to one-third of patients with cirrhosis may be found to have reduced arterial oxygen saturation. A number of conditions common to cirrhosis may affect pulmonary function (Box 123-1). Two of the most serious conditions

BOX 123-1 Pulmonary Issues in Cirrhosis

Hepatopulmonary syndrome
Pulmonary hypertension
Pleural effusions
Raised hemidiaphragm
Basal atelectasis
Ventilation-perfusion mismatch

TABLE 123-14 Stages of Encephalopathy

Stage	Clinical Findings
I	Irritability, altered sleep cycles
II	Disorientation, asterixis
III	Confusion, somnolence
IV	Coma

are portopulmonary hypertension and the hepatopulmonary syndrome. Both are likely related to the hyperdynamics of cirrhosis.[26]

Although the etiology of portopulmonary hypertension is unclear and the incidence is low, 2% of patients with severe liver disease are at risk for developing pulmonary arterial changes indistinguishable from those seen in primary idiopathic pulmonary hypertension. If suspected based on echocardiography, right heart catheterization must be performed. A mean pulmonary arterial pressure (MPAP) greater than 25 mm Hg defines the disease, whereas an MPAP >35 mm Hg (peripheral vascular resistance [PVR] $\geq$240 dynes·s^{-1}·cm^{-5}) is considered the threshold for an increased risk of death. Treatment with prostacyclins, nitric oxide, or similarly active agents can be used in an attempt to lower pressures and facilitate a safe OLT.

Hepatopulmonary syndrome is another uncommon entity defined by the triad of (1) chronic hypoxemia (PaO$_2$ < 60 mm Hg), (2) pulmonary vascular dilation as seen on examinations such as angiography or bubble echo, both in the context of (3) severe underlying chronic liver disease. This is a progressive condition that can be reversed following transplantation. Some patients with advanced disease are clearly in jeopardy for death at surgery, but for those with acceptable risks, current UNOS regulations do provide additional MELD priority points to facilitate transplantation within a 3-month period.[4]

GASTROINTESTINAL

Portal hypertensive bleeding is a well-known complication of cirrhosis and about 90% of such episodes can be successfully treated with endoscopic and/or pharmacologic interventions. When indicated, an experienced interventional radiologist can place transjugular intrahepatic portal systemic shunts (TIPSS).[27] Surgical shunts remain appropriate in the nonacute setting when the most prominent feature of disease is bleeding in an otherwise well-compensated patient. TIPSS may be contraindicated by significant hepatic encephalopathy or bilirubin levels elevated much higher than 3.0 mg/dL, in which case progressive liver failure may ensue without shunt reversal.

Inflammatory bowel disease is strongly associated with PSC.[8] Among patients with PSC, there is a 75% prevalence of ulcerative colitis (UC), whereas the converse is true in only 5%. PSC may also be associated with colonic Crohn disease. In those with PSC and UC, the risk for colonic malignancy may be greater than for those with UC alone and is an indication for vigilant screening colonoscopy, both before and after transplantation.

BONE

Hepatic osteodystrophy can be a complication of end-stage liver disease, especially among those with cholestatic diagnoses. Steroid treatments before or after transplantation can also exacerbate this problem. Consequences include bone pain, fractures, and vertebral collapse.[24] Aggressive calcium replacement and hormonal therapy are usually indicated.

KIDNEY

In the absence of other identifiable pathology, the development of severe renal dysfunction in the presence of end-stage liver failure defines the hepatorenal syndrome.[28] Although the etiology remains uncertain, it is likely related to the hemodynamic changes noted earlier. Because this is largely a functional problem, renal failure can be expected to resolve after liver transplantation. However, in patients with long-standing hepatorenal dysfunction, normalization may be unpredictable. The hepatorenal syndrome has been subdivided into type I and type II based on the pace of functional loss. Patients with type I hepatorenal syndrome experience a rapidly progressive deterioration, with a doubling of the initial serum creatinine in a period of less than 14 days. Such patients have 90% mortality within 90 days. Those with type II syndrome have a less rapid progression and fare better as a group. In either case, patients often require hemodialysis. When renal dysfunction is severe and of a long-standing nature, consideration must be given to combined liver and kidney transplantation. Because one of the parameters for the MELD calculation is serum creatinine, such patients are favored and nationwide there are an increasing number of patients undergoing dialysis at the time of transplantation as well as a growing population of liver transplant recipients receiving simultaneous renal transplants.

BRAIN

Hepatic encephalopathy is a neuropsychiatric condition associated with severe liver disease.[29] It can have manifestations that affect the spectrum of neurologic function from changes in personality and intellect to altered levels of consciousness (Table 123-14). Although it can complicate either chronic liver disease or acute liver failure, there are distinct clinical differences between the two conditions. In chronic disease, symptoms of encephalopathy may wax and wane with dietary indiscretion, poor compliance to medications, gastrointestinal bleeding, or infection. In the worst scenario, stage IV coma may require endotracheal intubation for airway protection. However, with proper management, even in the most severe circumstance, the mental status changes are temporary and reversible. On the other hand, encephalopathy associated with *acute* liver failure may also lead to coma, but unlike its counterpart, it is also associated with cerebral edema and acute brainstem herniation. The optimal management of acute hepatic encephalopathy may require intracranial pressure monitoring, which is not indicated in the chronic setting.

INFECTIOUS DISEASES

Cholangitis can be a significant pretransplant issue, especially in those patients with biliary strictures, such as those seen with PSC or other more rare congenital or acquired conditions. Such patients may require repeated endoscopic balloon dilations or stenting of prominent strictures. Occasionally, the chronic administration of rotating antibiotics may be necessary. Repeated hospitalizations, episodes of biliary sepsis with positive blood cultures, and associated hypotension may be factors considered for requesting additional MELD points. Although extrahepatic infection is a contraindication to liver transplantation, it may be impossible to clear cholangitis in a patient with biliary strictures and chronic liver disease until the liver is removed. In the absence of florid sepsis, such patients may still remain candidates for liver transplantation.

SKIN

Intractable pruritus is occasionally seen in patients with cholestatic liver disease. Curiously, the symptoms do not correlate well with the level of cholestasis, and the exact etiology remains unclear. A variety of treatment options can be used, but none with predictable results. These include ursodeoxycholate, cholestyramine, rifampin, opioid receptor antagonists such as naloxone, or serotonin receptor agonists such as ondansetron.[24] Some patients may be driven to the point of considering suicide, and despite the fact that liver transplantation provides definitive relief, additional MELD points are rarely considered appropriate. Patients with chronic HCV cirrhosis may develop small vessel vasculitis and cryoglobulinemia, manifest by palpable cutaneous purpura. In addition to those mentioned here and earlier, a number of other skin changes can be associated with specific liver diseases.

ADULT-TO-ADULT LIVING DONOR TRANSPLANTATION

The first living donor liver transplants were performed from adults to children in the late 1980s, but the evolution to adult-to-adult living donor liver transplants in the United States has been much more recent. Only after the shortage of organs reached a critical threshold was consideration given to performing such a procedure, which poses substantial perioperative and perhaps long-term risks to the healthy donor. Many ethical issues continue to be raised including the age, relationship to recipient, and the social circumstances of potential donors.[30] The advantages of this procedure are primarily twofold. First, transplantation can be timed to intervene before a recipient becomes severely decompensated, thereby

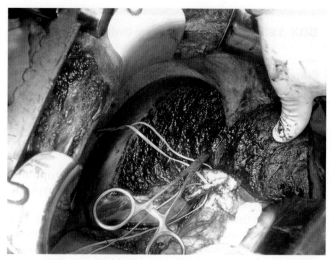

FIGURE 123-2 The magnitude of the living donor procedure is evident in this intraoperative photograph. The *blue tape* surrounds the vascular pedicle while a vascular clamp has been temporarily placed on a segment VIII hepatic vein.

minimizing the risks of certain complications, avoiding repeated hospitalizations, and even minimizing costs. Second, the quality of the allograft should be optimal with minimal cold-ischemia and without the physiologic insults often suffered by deceased donors. On the other hand, the relatively smaller volume and the increased technical anastomotic challenges presented by partial grafts create a new set of potential recipient problems. Add to that the most paramount concern of donor health, and the advantages of living versus deceased donors become less distinct. Indeed, data from the Scientific Registry of Transplant Recipients (SRTR) has shown inferior outcomes for right lobe allografts compared to those from deceased-donor whole organs.[31] The magnitude of this surgery and its potential impact on the donor is evident when viewing an intraoperative photograph (Figure 123-2).

One of the greatest concerns regarding adult-to-adult living donor transplantation is the adequacy of the liver volume provided by a partial allograft. A pattern of graft failure is now recognized and referred to as the *small-for-size (SFS) syndrome*.[32,33] This can occur when the actual or functional volume of an allograft is inadequate for the recipient. As a general rule, the liver is approximately 2% to 3% of body weight in healthy individuals, but there is considerable individual variability. An SFS graft is now generally accepted to have a graft-to-recipient weight ratio of less than 0.8%, or less than 30% to 50% of the standard estimated liver volume required by the recipient. Factors such as fatty change, the donor's age, duration of ischemia and the adequacy of venous drainage, can all contribute to a functionally diminished graft volume. Severe cholestasis, ongoing coagulopathy, and ascites are all prominent features of the SFS syndrome. Although recovery is possible, outcomes are unpredictable and survival without retransplantation may be uncertain. Sepsis and multiorgan failure can follow, and retransplantation must often be performed within a narrow window of time. Because recipients of living donors have otherwise not drawn from the "pool" of deceased-donor organs, generally RRBs grant additional points when necessary to ensure timely retransplantation in such circumstances.

The Adult-to-Adult Living Donor Liver Transplant Cohort (A2ALL) is a multicenter prospective study, funded by the NIH, undertaken to assess risks and outcomes for this procedure.[34] The most recent results indicate a 1-year graft survival of 81% in which 13.2% of grafts failed within 90 days. Biliary complications were most common, with 30% early and 11% late. Graft failure was notably greater among transplant programs with less experience.

In the United States, the initial enthusiasm for adult-to-adult living donor transplantation has waned, as indicated by the number of such transplants performed each year and the number of centers actively involved. At this juncture, only a handful of higher volume programs exist, yet recent donor deaths have been reported in the media. The role for this procedure in the armamentarium for liver transplant surgeons is still in evolution.

LIVER TRANSPLANT PROCEDURE

TOTAL NATIVE HEPATECTOMY

Because of the location of the liver in the right upper quadrant, a number of different incisions have been employed to gain adequate access for the transplant procedure. One of the more commonly used is the bilateral subcostal incision with an upward midline extension to the xiphoid process, euphemistically referred to as the "Mercedes-Benz" incision. Although this incision offers excellent exposure, it carries a significant risk of incisional hernia. A hockey stick incision in the right subcostal and midline area can also provide excellent exposure in many patients and has a lower risk of hernia. Often the xiphoid process is removed, both to increase exposure and to prevent lacerating the graft during manipulation. All ligamentous attachments to the liver are divided with cautery. The hepatoduodenal ligament is opened and the hepatic artery and bile duct are divided close to the liver to leave maximal length with the recipient. The gastrohepatic ligament is divided and the suprahepatic and infrahepatic IVC are isolated. If a standard orthotopic approach is utilized, the infrahepatic and suprahepatic IVC will be clamped and the intrahepatic portion of the IVC will be resected with the native liver. If a "piggyback" approach is used, the liver is separated from the intrahepatic IVC by dividing all penetrating hepatic veins up to the level of the main hepatic vein orifices and the native IVC is then left in situ.

The decision as to whether to proceed with a piggyback approach must obviously be made during the explant phase, and a number of factors should be considered. In cases in which tumor is close to the hepatic vein and IVC, a standard approach (removal of the intrahepatic IVC) is favored to allow a better resection margin. Obesity or other factors making the infrahepatic IVC anastomosis difficult to complete may make the piggyback option attractive. Living donor liver transplant must use a piggyback technique, because the donor graft has no caval component. If the piggyback technique can be performed without complete caval occlusion, there may also be hemodynamic benefits because of improved preload during the anhepatic phase, but this benefit is obviated in patients undergoing venovenous bypass. In the majority of cases, the decision on which option to use is largely one of surgeon familiarity and personal preference.

VENOVENOUS BYPASS

Venovenous bypass is a technique that reroutes blood from the clamped splanchnic and lower extremity venous circulation to the right heart, using a nonheparinized centrifugal pump circuit. The decision to utilize venovenous bypass should be made prior to dividing the portal vein during the total hepatectomy. The use of such bypass is a matter of preference and patient selection. Once considered a major technical advance in liver transplantation, some transplant programs routinely utilize venovenous bypass, whereas in others it is virtually never used.[35] A third approach is selective use in those cases in which the recipient demonstrates hemodynamic compromise during a test clamp of the portal vein and infrahepatic vena cava. Another factor considered in using bypass is the size of the allograft versus the recipient's abdominal space. On occasion, bypass may be required to minimize edematous enlargement of the intestines, which might otherwise leave inadequate room for a relatively large allograft, or when there is unmanageable portal hypertensive bleeding.

If a decision for venovenous bypass is made, an inflow cannula is placed in the saphenous or femoral vein and an outflow cannula is inserted into the jugular, subclavian, or axillary vein to bypass the occluded IVC and to maintain cardiac filling during clamping. Bypass cannulae may be placed either using a cutdown technique or percutaneous techniques. In the former, the cannulation sites are usually saphenous vein and axillary veins, whereas the latter utilize the femoral and jugular or cephalic veins. Flow rates of 1 to 1.5 L/min can be achieved without difficulties using a simple centrifugal pump. Portal vein inflow is easily added to the inflow circuit using an additional cannula if portal vein decompression is needed. In cases in which cannulation of the portal vein is difficult or dangerous, such as during retransplantation, portal decompression can be accomplished by cannulation of the inferior mesenteric vein. A heat exchanger is often safely added to the circuit to reduce ambient heat loss in the extracorporeal tubing.[36]

BACK-TABLE PREPARATION OF THE DONOR ORGAN

Prior to implantation, the donor organ is prepared in a saline ice slush "back table" basin to minimize rewarming. All extraneous peritoneal and diaphragmatic tissue is excised and phrenic and adrenal veins on the vena cava are ligated. The portal vein and hepatic artery are skeletonized and side branches are ligated to facilitate efficient vascular anastomoses during implantation. When using the piggyback technique, the inferior vena cava is ligated because it will not be used during implantation.

A small cannula is typically placed in the portal vein to allow perfusion of the organ with cold saline during implantation, which flushes out retained preservative solution before organ reperfusion. Aberrant arterial anatomy is managed by reconstructing the vessels to provide a single inflow to all hepatic arteries.[37] It is paramount that all vessels be preserved to prevent segmental biliary ischemic changes or graft dysfunction.[38] Most aberrant left hepatic arteries do not need reconstruction because the left gastric artery from which they arise is preserved with the donor celiac trunk. The standard approach to reconstructing an accessory right hepatic artery is to either attach the aberrant right vessel to the splenic or gastroduodenal artery off the celiac trunk or to put the aortic sides of the celiac and superior mesenteric artery stumps together to create a single inflow through the more distal superior mesenteric artery trunk. Because the superior mesenteric artery trunk is also used during pancreas transplantation, the finding of an aberrant right hepatic vessel during organ recovery may have implications for whether the pancreas can be successfully transplanted. Recovery teams and transplant teams should be in contact during the donor surgery to resolve these issues, but priority and final approval is always given to the liver procurement.

VASCULAR RECONSTRUCTION

Implantation of the donor organ must be accomplished quickly and efficiently to minimize ischemic time. Cold ischemic time is considered the time from cessation of endogenous organ perfusion in the donor (which typically occurs at the time of aortic cross-clamp) to the time that the donor organ is removed from cold storage for implantation in the recipient. The maximal allowable cold ischemic time for any given liver varies with the quality of the graft. In general, low-risk organs can tolerate cold ischemic times of up to 12 hours, whereas higher risk organs should be implanted within 8 hours or less. Warm ischemic time is considered the time from which the organ is removed from cold storage until the time the organ is reperfused in the recipient.

Vascular reattachment of the donor organ follows a logical sequence with emphasis on both quality and speed. The first anastomosis is created between the suprahepatic cuff of the IVC of the allograft and the recipient IVC (or the hepatic vein confluence if the piggyback technique is used). The second anastomosis is an end-to-end anastomosis between the infrahepatic IVC of the donor and recipient (this is eliminated in piggyback technique). These anastomoses are usually performed with running nonabsorbable suture. During completion of the IVC anastomosis the donor organ is flushed with cold saline through the portal vein cannula to remove preservative solution. The third step is an end-to-end anastomosis between donor and recipient portal veins. This is also performed with a running suture with care taken to avoid excessive redundancy that could predispose to kinking and thrombosis. A growth factor roughly half the circumference of the portal vein is usually included in the anastomosis to allow maximal dilation and to prevent a purse-string compromise of the vessel caliber. The organ is typically reperfused with portal flow

after completion of the portal vein anastomosis, followed by immediate arterial reconstruction and subsequent arterial reperfusion. However, if the hepatic arterial anastomosis can be completed quickly, some prefer to proceed to this anastomosis before portal reperfusion, which allows the graft to have complete simultaneous portal and arterial reperfusion. The arterial anastomosis can be performed in a number of different ways but should always adhere to vascular surgery principles of maximizing vessel caliber, minimizing intimal injury, and avoiding vessel kinking. A common approach which can be performed quickly is to create a running end-to-end anastomosis between the celiac trunk of the donor organ and a branch patch of the common hepatic artery/gastroduodenal artery junction of the recipient.

REPERFUSION SYNDROME

With the reintroduction of blood flow to the allograft, significant hypotension and/or cardiac dysrhythmia can occur, which is collectively termed "reperfusion syndrome."[39] Such changes can occur across a spectrum from very mild and transient bradycardia and peaked T-waves, to cardiac failure and asystole. Sudden exposure of the heart to cold, hyperkalemic fluid and the milieu of cytokines released from the transplanted organ are the likely causes. An ominous sign is that of an escalating pulmonary artery pressure associated with a falling systolic blood pressure. This scenario is more common in recipients with preexisting pulmonary hypertension, diastolic dysfunction, or any other condition leading to fixed cardiac output or limited cardiac reserve.

CONTROL OF BLEEDING

Once the organ has been fully reperfused, attention is turned to obtaining hemostasis in a systematic and safe fashion. The vascular anastomoses are inspected individually, along with the retroperitoneal area along the diaphragmatic attachments and the bare area. Overaggressive attempts to inspect the retroperitoneum or suprahepatic IVC with a liver rotation maneuver can lead to kinking of the IVC and sudden drop in blood pressure, and this should always be done with attention of the anesthesia team. Even more problematic is the fragile liver that is firm, fatty, or develops subcapsular blebs, as in these cases aggressive rotation can lead to liver fracture and catastrophic bleeding. This degree of bleeding is rarely amenable to surgical control and is best handled with packing. In rare cases, this degree of bleeding and liver injury may require urgent retransplantation.

BILIARY RECONSTRUCTION

The final phase of the transplant procedure is creation of the biliary anastomosis. The donor gallbladder is removed and the donor and recipient bile ducts are trimmed to appropriate lengths and to the point of demonstrating healthy bleeding from periductal vessels. Most often, an end-to-end anastomosis between donor and recipient ducts is fashioned with interrupted absorbable suture. In the past, T-tubes were used commonly but were associated with a number of biliary complications.[40] Most programs now avoid the use of T-tubes except in unusual circumstances, such as concern over distal drainage because of stones or pancreatitis. In the circumstance of an unhealthy or unusable recipient duct, Roux-en-Y hepaticojejunostomy reconstruction is performed.

INTRAOPERATIVE PROBLEM SOLVING

Portal Vein Thrombosis

Preoperative assessment of recipient portal vein patency is vital to planning the transplant procedure. Patients with preexisting portal vein thrombosis (PVT) can be expected to have higher blood product requirements and more postoperative complications. When preoperative PVT is present, several management options exist. Most acute and chronic thrombi can be removed with eversion atherectomy with restoration of portal venous inflow. If the lumen is obliterated or the occlusion extends substantially into the superior mesenteric vein, this technique may not be sufficient, and consideration should be given to use of an interposition venous graft. Iliac veins from the deceased donor should always be obtained at the time of organ procurement for just this purpose. The inability to identify a vessel with adequate portal flow to reperfuse the allograft is a rare but potentially catastrophic occurrence. In such circumstances, flow from the inferior vena cava can be diverted to the allograft with a cava-portal anastomosis. In these cases the retrohepatic IVC is constricted or even ligated to increase portal perfusion pressure. Although this technique may allow the patient to survive surgery, they are left with persistent portal hypertension as well as vena caval obstruction and its sequelae.[41]

Hepatic Artery Insufficiency

During preparation of the recipient hepatic artery, the dissection is usually carried back to at least the common hepatic artery in order to allow for an anastomosis of adequate size. If the inflow at this level is inadequate, then it may be necessary to create alternative hepatic arterial inflow. Donor iliac artery can be used to fashion a conduit from other sources, most commonly the infrarenal aorta. Other options include taking a graft off the recipient splenic artery or the supraceliac aorta. The latter option carries a risk of paralysis due to compromised spinal artery flow. In some cases, hepatic artery flow may be compromised by the recipient arcuate ligament, which is most often identified by noting a significant variation in arterial flow with each ventilator breath. A dramatic improvement can be effected with release of the celiac axis from this ligament at its origin at the aorta.

Split Grafts

The increasing shortage of deceased donor organs has led to a number of methods to expand the donor organ pool. One such option is that of dividing a healthy donor liver into two portions for use in two recipients. Most often the liver is split into a left lateral segment (Couinaud segments 2 and 3) for use in a child while the remaining right-trisegmentectomy (Couinaud segments 1, 4 to 8) is utilized for an appropriate-sized adult. On rare occasions, an organ may be of adequate size and quality to split into true right and left lobar grafts if appropriate size-matched recipients are identified.

Because a split graft carries the additional risk of a bile leak from the cut edge, a T-tube or internal stent may be useful to maximally decompress the biliary tree.

Perhaps the most important factor when considering split liver transplantation is patient selection. Technical aspects to consider include the possible need for a piggyback technique (depending on which half of the split is being used), the shortened and smaller vessels that may accompany a split graft, and the increased risk of SFS syndrome and bile leak following split liver transplantation. These factors may lead to increased morbidity and mortality in the severely ill recipient, and split grafts should be used sparingly in this group.[42] Patients with high risk of vascular complications, such as those with preexisiting portal vein or hepatic artery thrombosis (HAT), may also be at higher risk with split grafts.

Graft Function and Primary Nonfunction

The assessment of graft function employs clinical signs, laboratory analysis, and a certain amount of intuition. In the ideal scenario, the graft shows a healthy perfusion pattern and starts producing bile within 30 minutes of reperfusion. The organ should be soft, and hemostasis and hypothermia should improve rapidly. Over the next 12 to 24 hours acidosis should resolve, and hemodynamics, mental status, and urine output should improve. INR should correct within 24 to 48 hours and the peak AST elevation should be under 3000 IU/L.

When a transplanted organ shows signs of dysfunction in the first several hours or days after transplant, several factors must be considered. Vascular and other technical complications are discussed later. In the absence of any technical complications, severe graft dysfunction within the first 7 days is termed "primary nonfunction" (PNF).[43] This poorly defined circumstance is a diagnosis of exclusion and can occur across a spectrum from mild to catastrophic. Although most grafts do show at least partial function, the signs and symptoms of a truly nonfunctional graft are easy to recognize. These grafts appear hyperemic, "blebbed," and firm, and may fracture with manipulation. Recipient acidosis, persistent vasodilation, renal failure, coagulopathy, and even cerebral edema may occur. Aspartate aminotransferase (AST) levels are usually greater than 5000 IU/mL. By definition, the end result of PNF is either retransplantation or recipient death. In extreme circumstances, if no suitable replacement organ is available and a patient is unstable, removal of the nonfunctional graft and creation of a temporary portocaval shunt may allow the patient to stabilize. Other manipulations, such as plasmapheresis or utilization of experimental artificial hepatic support devices have been attempted with varying degrees of success.[44] Because of this risk of rapid deterioration and death from PNF, UNOS guidelines allow for these patients to be listed for retransplantation at the highest priority level (status 1).

Much more common than the patient with PNF is the patient with delayed graft function, which manifests as failure of INR to correct, persistently climbing bilirubin, and moderate elevations of AST (3000 to 5000 IU/L). Graft dysfunction of this sort is often accompanied by ileus and renal insufficiency, and if a T-tube is present, by poor bile output. Some of these grafts may recover, provided other major complications such as infection do not destabilize the patient. In other cases, graft dysfunction leads to a cascade of events leading to multiorgan dysfunction and a "failure to thrive," which may ultimately lead to sepsis and death. It is up to the transplant team to weigh the risks of watchful waiting versus that of retransplantation. Although early retransplantation can be technically straightforward, it is not to be taken lightly as it removes another donor organ from the pool and subjects the recipient to a renewed period of intense immunosuppression.

EARLY COMPLICATIONS

Hepatic Artery Thrombosis

Thrombosis of the hepatic artery occurs in 2% to 10% of liver transplants and usually results in early or delayed graft loss.[45] Because the hepatic artery is the sole blood supply to the biliary tree, HAT causes biliary ischemia, which has several manifestations depending on the interval since transplant. HAT within the first 1 to 2 weeks after transplant, before anastomotic healing is secure, often leads to breakdown of the biliary anastomosis and bile leak. Occasionally, in a liver heavily reliant on hepatic arterial flow, thrombosis of the hepatic artery will result in a picture of graft failure similar to PNF. HAT occurring more than 30 days after transplant typically presents as mild elevation in liver tests or as biliary stricture with cholangitis or hepatic abscess.

The diagnosis of HAT should be considered in the presence of unexplained changes in liver function tests or if biliary complications are identified. Doppler ultrasound is performed at the first suspicion of HAT at most transplant centers, but is very operator dependent. Definitive diagnosis is often obtained by surgical exploration, angiography, or cross-sectional imaging. If the interval between diagnosis and discovery of HAT is less than 24 hours, there may be value to surgical thrombectomy and attempted hepatic revascularization. Biliary damage occurs quickly, however, and most patients with established HAT are best served with timely retransplantation.[46,47]

The mechanism by which HAT occurs is not always clear. Small donor arteries and the need for revision of the arterial anastomosis are risk factors for HAT, supporting the contention that technical factors play a significant role. Other risk factors suggested by some studies, which are less intuitive, include an HCV-positive recipient, cytomegalovirus infection, and female donor organ into a male recipient.[45,48] HAT may also be higher in those with conditions causing postoperative abdominal inflammation such as bacterial peritonitis or pancreatitis.

In the past, UNOS guidelines allowed patients with HAT diagnosed within 7 days of transplant to be listed at the highest priority (status 1). In recent years, it has become increasingly appreciated that HAT is rarely associated with PNF-like organ dysfunction.[49] For this reason, current UNOS guidelines allow for HAT that occurs within 7 days of transplant to receive a MELD score of 40, but not to receive status 1 designation unless PNF criteria are met.

Portal Vein Thrombosis

Fortunately, PVT is exceptionally uncommon after liver transplantation, occurring in only about 1% of cases.[50] Because the portal vein provides the majority of oxygen delivery to the parenchyma, severe parenchymal injury, graft loss, and patient death are common in the face of PVT. Occasionally, thrombectomy may be possible if detected early. The main risk factor for PVT is the need for thrombectomy at the time of the initial transplant.

Biliary Complications

Complications related to the biliary tree occur in up to 15% of deceased-donor liver transplant patients, and with a reported incidence often greater than 30% among recipients of living donor transplants.[51,52] Biliary strictures are the most common complication, which usually occur at the site of the biliary anastomosis. Strictures at this level can often be managed with endoscopic or percutaneous interventional radiology techniques, but occasionally surgical revision with hepaticojejunostomy is required. Intrahepatic strictures and those that are remote from the anastomosis generally reflect a more diffusely diseased biliary tree. Hepatic artery thrombosis and recurrent PSC should be excluded. Other factors such as the use of extended criteria grafts, long ischemic times during transplantation, cytomegalovirus infection, and primary choledocholithiasis should also be considered. Many grafts with intrahepatic strictures can be temporized with aggressive and repeated percutaneous or endoscopic interventions, but some will require repeat transplantation because of recurrent cholangitis or secondary biliary cirrhosis.

Bile leaks typically occur within the first 1 to 2 weeks after transplant and usually reflect either technical error or HAT. If the bile leak is of a large volume or is associated with peritonitis, surgical repair should be attempted promptly. A skilled endoscopist or radiologist can often manage smaller volume leaks by stenting the anastomosis and decompressing the biliary tree.[53]

LATE COMPLICATIONS

Late complications of liver transplantation can be divided into those due to rejection, those due to immunosuppressant medications, and those due to recurrent liver disease.[54]

Rejection

The number of medications available for preventing and treating rejection, as well as knowledge regarding mechanism of action and optimal drug combinations, is growing rapidly.[55] Acute cellular rejection occurs with a reported incidence of 10% to 20% in the first 6 months after liver transplant. Typically an episode of rejection is asymptomatic and the diagnosis is suspected based on abnormal liver tests. The diagnosis is confirmed by liver biopsy. Treatment options include simply increasing the maintenance immunosuppression in mild cases, and initiating a steroid pulse in cases that are more severe. Although acute rejection itself does not appear to impact long-term graft function, diseases such as hepatitis C have greater risk of recurrence in those requiring treatment of acute rejection. The augmented immunosuppression used to treat rejection is thought to play a role in viral replication and the more aggressive return of viral hepatitis.

Chronic rejection is a poorly understood entity often referred to as "vanishing bile duct syndrome." This condition is characterized by a cholestatic pattern typically occurring several years after transplantation and is diagnosed by paucity of bile ducts on liver biopsy. There is no effective therapy and some of these patients may ultimately require retransplantation.

Complications of Immunosuppressive Medications

Infection. Not surprisingly, the use of medications designed to disrupt immune competence puts individuals at increased risk for infection. The nature of that risk depends on a number of parameters including the interval since transplantation, the intensity of immunosuppression, preexisting exposures to certain infectious agents, the age of the recipient, and the nature and extent of other comorbid conditions (Table 123-15). As with other surgical procedures, the risk for bacterial infections is greatest in the first few weeks after transplant. Fungal infections peak during the first 1 to 2 months posttransplant and are largely related to the patient's nutritional state, the extent of antibiotic use in the perioperative period, and the need for massive transfusions or reoperations at the time of transplant.[56]

High-risk donor/recipient cytomegalovirus (CMV) exposure history can also predispose to CMV infection or reactivation.[57] Three to 4 months after transplantation, *Pneumocystis*, CMV, Epstein-Barr virus (EBV), and varicella-zoster virus (VZV) all become a concern. Because of their impaired cell-mediated immunity, transplant patients remain at higher than normal risk for viral and fungal infections for life. Prophylactic antibiotics are given after transplant, although the exact agent and duration varies between programs. An example of the success of prophylaxis is in the treatment of cytomegalovirus. This agent was once a common cause of morbidity and death of liver transplant but now is seen with an incidence of less than 5%.

Malignancy. Although the exact mechanisms are still incompletely understood, immunosuppression clearly increases the risk of some types of malignancy.

Transplant immunosuppression places recipients at a three- to fourfold increased incidence of cancer compared with age-matched controls. The largest increases are in skin cancers in sun-exposed areas. Although the incidence of other primary neoplasms, such as those of the breast and colon, are not increased in solid organ recipients, they tend to demonstrate a more aggressive behavior in the transplant patient when they do occur. All transplant patients should undergo vigilant screening for breast, prostate, colorectal, gynecologic, and skin cancer.

Cardiovascular Side Effects

Cardiovascular disease has become one of the leading causes of long-term morbidity in liver transplant survivors.[58] Several factors likely contribute to this morbidity, including the increasing frequency of older and obese transplant recipients and medication-related dyslipidemias and diabetes mellitus.

DISEASE RECURRENCE

Recurrence of underlying liver disease is a common cause of long-term morbidity and mortality in liver transplant recipients. Because of its prevalence as an indication for transplantation, its propensity to reinfect the new allograft, and our relatively ineffectual ability to treat in the posttransplant setting, recurrence of hepatitis C is a significant problem facing liver transplant physicians.[59] In patients with active replication of hepatitis C, graft reinfection is virtually guaranteed, although for most patients no treatment is needed for several years. An unfortunate unpredictable subgroup will manifest early aggressive recurrence, often leading to graft failure within the first year. The mainstay of treatment at the present is interferon-based viral suppression. Specific guidelines for optimal treatment of recurrent HCV after transplant remain elusive. Clearly more effective HCV treatment strategies such as protease inhibitors will represent a major advance in the field of liver transplantation.

Although the recurrence of HCV after transplant is the most widely recognized, virtually every condition for

TABLE 123-15 Immunosuppression Profiles

Agent	Use	Toxicity	Typical Duration
Corticosteroids	Primary immunosuppressant	Diabetes, hypertension, wound healing	6 mo
Cyclosporin A	Primary immunosuppressant	Nephrotoxicity, neurotoxicity, hyperkalemia	Lifelong
Tacrolimus	Primary immunosuppressant	Nephrotoxicity, neurotoxicity, hyperkalemia	Lifelong
Mycophenolate	Used as adjunct to primary agent	Diarrhea, leukopenia	As needed
OKT3	Induction	Cytokine storm, pulmonary edema	5 d
IL-2 receptor antibodies	Induction		2 wk

which transplant is undertaken can recur after transplant. Hepatitis B activation, once common after transplant, is now rare because of improved antiviral regimens. PBC, PSC, and autoimmune hepatitis can also recur and may even require retransplantation.

ORGAN SHORTAGE AND THE FUTURE OF LIVER TRANSPLANTATION

As stated earlier, the greatest crisis facing the field of liver transplantation remains the donor organ shortage. Although adult-to-adult living donor liver transplantation has made some impact, the number of such transplants performed yearly has plateaued in the United States in recent years. In light of this, the best option for most recipients, especially those who are severely ill, is to receive a whole-organ allograft from a brain dead donor.

There are ongoing efforts to increase the deceased donor organ pool by several distinct pathways. The first approach is to increase the number of potential donors by improving intensive care unit and resuscitation protocols of patients with lethal brain injury, so that organ quality is maintained until organ recovery can be coordinated. The second approach is to decrease the number of donors that are lost because of lack of family consent by using a variety of public educational and public health measures. The third approach is to increase the utilization of organs that are not ideal and that might otherwise not be recovered. These marginal, or "extended criteria" donors, include older or less hemodynamically stable donors, non-heart-beating donors, or those with comorbid conditions such as severe hepatic steatosis (Box 123-2). Use of these organs, however, carries an increased risk of death and graft loss, and these results are available to the public and to third-party payers through the current UNOS Internet portal. Although this system of reporting has many benefits, it also disincentivizes the use of marginal grafts, because these grafts by definition carry an increased risk of graft failure, retransplantation, and death.

SUMMARY

To witness the transplant process from recipient evaluation through organ procurement, the transplant procedure, recovery, and return to health is to be humbled by the miracles of life and our collective ability to overcome devastating disease. Nothing in modern medicine is more dramatic.

BOX 123-2 Deceased Donor Extended Criteria

Steatosis
Hepatitis B core antibody positive
Hepatitis C positive
Age >65
Non-heart-beating donor

REFERENCES

1. Starzl TE, Groth CG, Brettschneider L, et al: Orthotopic homotransplantation of the human liver. *Ann Surg* 168:392, 1968.
2. Kolata G: Liver transplants endorsed. An NIH consensus panel recommends more transplants but does not say who will pay. *Science* 221:139, 1983.
3. Xu J, Kenneth D, Kochanek MA, et al: Deaths: Final data for 2007. *National Vital Statistics* 58, 2010.
4. United Network of Organ Sharing, 2010. http://www.unos.org.
5. Day CP: Heavy drinking greatly increases the risk of cirrhosis in patients with HCV hepatitis. *Gut* 49:750, 2001.
6. Colquhoun SD, Belle SH, Samuel D, et al: Transplantation in the hepatitis B patient and current therapies to prevent recurrence. *Semin Liver Dis* 20:7, 2000.
7. Neuberger J, Bradwell AR: Anti-mitochondrial antibodies in primary biliary cirrhosis. *J Hepatol* 37:712, 2002.
8. Wiesner RH: Liver transplantation for primary sclerosing cholangitis: Timing, outcome, impact of inflammatory bowel disease and recurrence of disease. *Best Pract Res Clin Gastroenterol* 15:667, 2001.
9. Rea DJ, Heimbach JK, Rosen CB, et al: Liver transplantation with neoadjuvant chemoradiation is more effective than resection for hilar cholangiocarcinoma. *Ann Surg* 242:458, 2005.
10. Vong S, Bell BP: Chronic liver disease mortality in the United States, 1990-1998. *Hepatology* 39:476, 2004.
11. Penn I: Evaluation of transplant candidates with pre-existing malignancies. *Ann Transplant* 2:14, 1997.
12. Williams MC, Creger JH, Belton AM, et al: The organ center of the United Network for Organ Sharing and twenty years of organ sharing in the United States. *Transplantation* 77:641, 2004.
13. El-Serag HB, Mason AC: Rising incidence of hepatocellular carcinoma in the United States. *N Engl J Med* 340:745, 1999.
14. El-Serag HB: Hepatocellular carcinoma: Recent trends in the United States. *Gastroenterology* 127:S27, 2004.
15. Thomas M, Jaffe D, Choti D: Hepatocelluar carcinoma: Consensus recommendations of the National Cancer Institute Clinical Trials Planning Meeting. *J Clin Oncol* 28:3994, 2010.
16. Grossman E, Millis JM: Liver transplantation for non-hepatocellular carcinoma malignancy: Indications, limitations, and analysis of the current literature. *Liver Transpl* 16:930, 2010.
17. Olthoff KM, Brown RS Jr, Delmonico FL, et al: Summary report of a national conference: Evolving concepts in liver allocation in the MELD and PELD era. December 8, 2003, Washington, DC, USA. *Liver Transpl* 10:A6, 2004.
18. *Practice Guidlines.* 2010. http://www.aasld.org/practiceguideline/documents/acuteliverfailure.
19. Freeman RB: MELD: The holy grail of organ allocation? *J Hepatol* 42:16, 2005.
20. Coffin CS, Stock PG, Dove LM, et al: Virologic and clinical outcomes of hepatitis B virus infection in HIV-HBV coinfected transplant recipients. *Am J Transplant* 10:1268, 2010.
21. Schreibman I, Gaynor JJ, Jayaweera D, et al: Outcomes after orthotopic liver transplantation in 15 HIV-infected patients. *Transplantation* 84:697, 2007.
22. United Network of Organ Sharing. www.UNOS.org, 2005.
23. Wiesner RH, McDiarmid SV, Kamath PS, et al: MELD and PELD: Application of survival models to liver allocation. *Liver Transpl* 7:567, 2001.
24. Sherlock SAD, Dooley J: *Diseases of the liver and biliary system,* ed 11. Oxford, 2002, Blackwell Science.
25. Kowdley KV, Brandhagen DJ, Gish RG, et al; National Hemochromatosis Transplant Registry: Survival after liver transplantation in patients with hepatic iron overload: The national hemochromatosis transplant registry. *Gastroenterology* 129:494, 2005.
26. Mandell MS: Hepatopulmonary syndrome and portopulmonary hypertension in the model for end-stage liver disease (MELD) era. *Liver Transpl* 10:S54, 2004.
27. Bass NM, Yao FY: The role of the interventional radiologist. Transjugular procedures. *Gastrointest Endosc Clin N Am* 11:131, 2001.
28. Cardenas A: Hepatorenal syndrome: A dreaded complication of end-stage liver disease. *Am J Gastroenterol* 100:460, 2005.
29. Colquhoun SD, Lipkin C, Connelly CA: The pathophysiology, diagnosis, and management of acute hepatic encephalopathy. *Adv Intern Med* 46:155, 2001.

30. Truog RD: The ethics of organ donation by living donors. *N Engl J Med* 353:444, 2005.

31. Brown RS, Jr, Russo MW, Lai M, et al: A survey of liver transplantation from living adult donors in the United States. *N Engl J Med* 348:818, 2003.

32. Emond JC, Renz JF, Ferrell LD, et al: Functional analysis of grafts from living donors. Implications for the treatment of older recipients. *Ann Surg* 224:544; discussion 552, 1996.

33. Kiuchi T, Tanaka K, Ito T, et al: Small-for-size graft in living donor liver transplantation: How far should we go? *Liver Transpl* 9:S29, 2003.

34. Olthoff KM, Merion RM, Ghobrial RM, et al; A2ALL Study Group: Outcomes of 385 adult-to-adult living donor liver transplant recipients: A report from the A2ALL Consortium. *Ann Surg* 242:314; discussion 323, 2005.

35. Griffith BP, Shaw BW, Jr, Hardesty RL, et al: Veno-venous bypass without systemic anticoagulation for transplantation of the human liver. *Surg Gynecol Obstet* 160:270, 1985.

36. Neelakanta G, Colquhoun S, Csete M, et al: Efficacy and safety of heat exchanger added to venovenous bypass circuit during orthotopic liver transplantation. *Liver Transpl Surg* 4:506, 1998.

37. Melada E, Maggi U, Rossi G, et al: Back-table arterial reconstructions in liver transplantation: Single-center experience. *Transplant Proc* 37:2587, 2005.

38. Margarit C, Hidalgo E, Lázaro JL, et al: Biliary complications secondary to late hepatic artery thrombosis in adult liver transplant patients. *Transpl Int* 11:S251, 1998.

39. Aggarwal S, Kang Y, Freeman JA, et al: Postreperfusion syndrome: Hypotension after reperfusion of the transplanted liver. *J Crit Care* 8:154, 1993.

40. Shimoda M, Saab S, Morrisey M, et al: A cost-effectiveness analysis of biliary anastomosis with or without T-tube after orthotopic liver transplantation. *Am J Transplant* 1:157, 2001.

41. Tzakis AG, Kirkegaard P, Pinna AD, et al: Liver transplantation with cavoportal hemitransposition in the presence of diffuse portal vein thrombosis. *Transplantation* 65:619, 1998.

42. Renz JF, Emond JC, Yersiz H, et al: Split-liver transplantation in the United States: Outcomes of a national survey. *Ann Surg* 239:172, 2004.

43. Nissen NN, Colquhoun S: Graft failure: Cause, etiology, recognition and treatment, In Busuttil RW, Klintmalm GB, editors, *Transplantation of the liver*. Philadelphia, 2005, Saunders.

44. Mandal AK, King KE, Humphreys SL, et al: Plasmapheresis: An effective therapy for primary allograft nonfunction after liver transplantation. *Transplantation* 70:216, 2000.

45. Vivarelli M, Cucchetti A, La Barba G, et al: Ischemic arterial complications after liver transplantation in the adult: Multivariate analysis of risk factors. *Arch Surg* 139:1069, 2004.

46. Drazan K, Shaked A, Olthoff KM, et al: Etiology and management of symptomatic adult hepatic artery thrombosis after orthotopic liver transplantation (OLT). *Am Surg* 62:237, 1996.

47. Stange B, Glanemann M, Nuessler NC, et al: Hepatic artery thrombosis after adult liver transplantation. *Liver Transpl* 9:612, 2003.

48. Madalosso C, Souza NF Jr, Ilstrup DM, et al: Cytomegalovirus and its association with hepatic artery thrombosis after liver transplantation. *Transplantation* 66:294, 1998.

49. Wiesner RH: MELD/PELD and the allocation of deceased donor livers for status 1 recipients with acute fulminant hepatic failure, primary nonfunction, hepatic artery thrombosis, and acute Wilson's disease. *Liver Transpl* 10:S17, 2004.

50. Varotti G, Grazi GL, Vetrone G, et al: Causes of early acute graft failure after liver transplantation: Analysis of a 17-year single-centre experience. *Clin Transplant* 19:492, 2005.

51. Guichelaar MM, Benson JT, Malinchoc M, et al: Risk factors for and clinical course of non-anastomotic biliary strictures after liver transplantation. *Am J Transplant* 3:885, 2003.

52. Fondevila C, Ghobrial RM, Fuster J, et al: Biliary complications after adult living donor liver transplantation. *Transplant Proc* 35:1902, 2003.

53. Thethy S, Thomson BN, Pleass H, et al: Management of biliary tract complications after orthotopic liver transplantation. *Clin Transplant* 18:647, 2004.

54. Jain A, Reyes J, Kashyap R, et al: Long-term survival after liver transplantation in 4,000 consecutive patients at a single center. *Ann Surg* 232:490, 2000.

55. Fung J, Kelly D, Kadry Z, et al: Immunosuppression in liver transplantation: Beyond calcineurin inhibitors. *Liver Transpl* 11:267, 2005.

56. Winston DJ, Pakrasi A, Busuttil RW: Prophylactic fluconazole in liver transplant recipients. A randomized, double-blind, placebo-controlled trial. *Ann Intern Med* 131:729, 1999.

57. Winston DJ, Busuttil RW: Randomized controlled trial of sequential intravenous and oral ganciclovir versus prolonged intravenous ganciclovir for long-term prophylaxis of cytomegalovirus disease in high-risk cytomegalovirus-seronegative liver transplant recipients with cytomegalovirus-seropositive donors. *Transplantation* 77:305, 2004.

58. Rabkin JM, de la Melena V, Orloff SL, et al: Late mortality after orthotopic liver transplantation. *Am J Surg* 181:475, 2001.

59. NIH Consensus Statement on Management of Hepatitis C: 2002. *NIH Consens State Sci Statements* 19:1, 2002.

Fulminant Hepatic Failure and Liver Support Systems

James Fisher | Joseph Lillegard | Scott Nyberg

FULMINANT HEPATIC FAILURE

The failing liver represents a syndrome with profound morbidity and mortality. The morbidity of liver failure is secondary to the tremendous decline in metabolic and synthetic functions inherent to the liver. With the decline in metabolic activity, accumulation of toxic substances occurs. The most notable of these toxins is ammonia. Cerebral edema (the most feared complication) is strongly associated with elevated levels of ammonia.[1] In addition to ammonia accumulation, drugs metabolized by the liver require strict regulation, if they are used at all. One of the leading synthetic functions of the liver is the production of coagulation factors. As the time in failure progresses, the patient will become more coagulopathic. Also, the liver is home to an abundant source of resident macrophages, Kupffer cells,[2,3] which are believed to produce cytokines leading to systemic inflammation in the setting of the failing liver.[4-6] The systemic inflammatory response syndrome (SIRS) occurs in approximately 60% of patients with a failing liver.[7] The SIRS can lead to failure of other organ systems (kidneys, lungs, etc.), further complicating the course and treatment of patients with failing livers.

The failing liver can be separated into two groups: acute liver failure (ALF) and acute decompensation of a cirrhotic liver (Figure 124-1). Patients suffering from an acutely failing liver have the possibility of recovering spontaneously. However, for the patients who are not likely to recover spontaneously, the only proven treatment is liver transplantation. Before liver transplantation, the mortality rate of patients with acutely failing livers was higher than 80%.[8] Today, this mortality rate has decreased to about 30% as a result of liver transplantation and the high level of intensive care now available.[8] Nonetheless, there are still issues with liver transplantation. For example, these patients are fated to lifetime immunosuppression. More importantly, there is shortage of livers for patients on the transplant waiting list. Thus, adding patients in ALF or acute decompensation to this already overextended list only worsens the problem. According to work done by the U.S. ALF Study Group, patients with ALF currently wait a median of 1 day for transplant after listing. However, ALF patients on the transplant list who waited 3 days or longer had a much greater risk of death.[8]

The solution to this shortage is unclear but likely requires multiple advances, including improved knowledge of the etiology, high-quality medical care, and some form of artificial liver support until the supply of donor liver organs can be increased. Over the course of this chapter, the most common etiologies of ALF will be reviewed, current medical protocols will be listed, artificial liver support systems will be described, and potential future directions will be explored.

ETIOLOGY OF ACUTE LIVER FAILURE

The incidence of ALF in the United States has been estimated to be 2000 to 3000 per year.[9] However, defining good estimates of the causes of ALF in the United States was difficult because of small sample sizes. In an effort to better define and treat ALF in the United States, the Food and Drug Administration and the National Institutes of Health allotted funding for the development of the U.S. ALF Study Group. As a consequence, a robust sampling of ALF patients (1147 patients) between 1998 and 2007 in the United States occurred.[8] This sampling has allowed for a high-quality estimation of the various etiologies of ALF common to the United States.

Drug Induced

Acetaminophen overdose leads to a buildup of its reactive intermediate N-para-aminoquinonimine (NAPQI). The sulfhydryl groups of glutathione bind to NAPQI and form nontoxic by-products. Once glutathione is depleted from hepatocytes, a centrilobular pattern of hepatocyte necrosis ensues.[10,11] According to the results from the U.S. ALF Study Group, 46% of the cases of ALF sampled were secondary to acetaminophen overdose. Nearly two-thirds of these patients recovered spontaneously, about one-tenth were transplanted, and about one-quarter died without transplantation. Besides advances in intensive care, the use of N-acetylcysteine has proven efficacious in preventing liver injury and has shown promise in improving brain dysfunction (encephalopathy) in animal models. Another 11% of the cases of ALF from the U.S. ALF Study Group were caused by other drug toxicities. The outcome from these other drugs is less favorable than acetaminophen overdose. Only about three-tenths of these patients spontaneously recovered (less than half of those who had acetaminophen-induced ALF), and approximately 40% of these patients required transplantation[8] (about four times the number compared to acetaminophen-induced ALF).

Viral

The two main causes of viral hepatitis leading to ALF are hepatitis A (HAV) and hepatitis B (HBV). Combined, these two viral etiologies account for 10% (HAV 3%, HBV 7%) of the ALF cases seen in the United States. Patients with HAV-induced ALF have a better prognosis, both with spontaneous recovery (58% vs. 24%) and

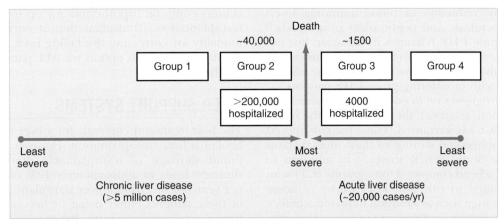

FIGURE 124-1 Continuum of severity of liver disease, U.S. data. Liver disease is separated into acute and chronic forms with prevalences of approximately 20,000 and 5 million cases per year, respectively. The cases requiring hospitalization are shown here on a spectrum of severity. Groups 1 and 4 represent those cases that do not lead to hospitalization. However, group 2 (acute decompensation) and group 3 (acute liver failure) are recognized as those cases that lead to hospitalization. Unfortunately, about 35% of the acute liver failure group and 20% of the acutely decompensated group die as a result of their failing liver.

overall survival (87% vs. 61%) as compared to those with HBV-induced ALF.[8] Because of the lower spontaneous recovery and the need for more transplantation, patients with HBV-induced ALF may be considered for antiviral therapy.[12]

Indeterminate and Other Causes

The remaining one-third of patients in the U.S. ALF Study Group developed ALF secondary to indeterminate causes (14%), autoimmune causes (5%), ischemic events (4%), Wilson disease (2%), or various other causes (7%).[8] Etiology-specific treatments can help with spontaneous recovery in some of these groups although transplantation may still be required. Even if the cause of a patient's ALF may be indeterminate, there is some evidence that administration of *N*-acetylcysteine can help with recovery or bridge the time to transplant as many of these indeterminate cases may have a combination of causes that include acetaminophen.[13]

Surgical Causes of Acute Liver Failure

Acute liver failure can occur following massive hepatic resection in otherwise healthy patients or with smaller resections in patients with marginal hepatic function. In a large retrospective study from Memorial Sloan-Kettering Cancer Center, the rate of acute liver failure following hepatic resection was 1% (19 of 1803 patients). This study included consecutive resections ranging from non-anatomic wedge resections to extended hepatectomies (up to six segments). The incidence of failure was not listed for the number of segments resected; however, 583 patients had five or six segments resected.[14] To answer the question of how much liver is safe to resect, a study from M.D. Anderson Cancer Center looked at outcomes from 301 consecutive extended right hepatectomies. Three groups were identified and compared according to the ratio of future liver remnant (FLR) to standardized liver volume (SLV) prior to resection: FLR/SLV ≤ 20%; 20% < FLR/SLV ≤ 30%; and FLR/SLV > 30%. Of the 301

patients receiving extended right hepatectomy, 44 patients were determined to have liver insufficiency following resection. The FLR/SLV ≤ 20% group had a significantly higher percentage of patients (34%) with liver insufficiency compared to the 20% < FLR/SLV ≤ 30% group (10%, P < 0.001) and the FLR/SLV > 30% group (15%, P = 0.01).[15] For patients who develop liver failure after resection, supportive therapies may provide time by facilitating remnant hypertrophy and recovery, or bridge the patient to liver transplantation.

MEDICAL THERAPY

Medical therapy for the failing liver has seen improvement over the past decades. Much credit is given to improvement in the quality of intensive care delivered to ALF patients. Effective medical management requires early recognition of a failing liver. Once recognized, coordination is a necessity between primary care and referral centers, and medical and surgical disciplines at the referral center. Quality intensive care aims to counteract hemodynamic instability and prevent extrahepatic manifestation of liver failure, including cerebral edema, and potentially allow for recovery or sufficient time for transplant.

The current definition of ALF is acute liver injury associated with an international normalized ratio (INR) of 1.5 or greater in a patient with altered mental status for less than 26 weeks and no history of liver disease.[16] Once a patient has been defined as having ALF, management ensues based on the level of encephalopathy and the specific etiology (if identified). The most complete set of guidelines for acutely failing liver management are listed in a position paper[16] on the American Association for the Study of Liver Diseases website (www.aasld.org).

Management common to all grades of hepatic encephalopathy (HE) includes baseline and routine laboratory work (CBC, electrolytes, arterial blood gas, lactate, liver function tests, LDH, ammonia, albumin, and a coagulation panel), routine glucose measurements, correction of coagulopathy, reduction of blood ammonia levels using enteral lactulose, and peptic ulcer prophylaxis.[16] Patients with grade I HE (changes in behavior, but not level of consciousness) can appropriately be managed in a setting other than the intensive care unit if the staffing has experience with monitoring grade I HE patients.[16]

If a patient progresses on to grade II HE (disoriented, delayed mentation, asterixis), then transfer to the intensive care unit (ICU) is warranted. These patients should have routinely scheduled scoring of their mental status (Glascow Coma Scale, FOUR score).[17] In addition to clinical scoring, a head computed tomography (CT) scan should be obtained to rule out other causes of acute mental status change such as subdural hematoma before placement of an intracranial pressure monitor. However, CT scanning is not routinely used to evaluate cerebral edema because it is a late finding in ALF and transport of patients in advanced ALF to radiology for scanning can be problematic. Nutrition (enteral or parenteral) should be initiated at this juncture to maintain intake of calories, prevent hypoglycemia, stabilize ammonia production, and assist in healing the injured liver.[18] Also, prophylactic antibiotics (antibacterial, antifungal, and antiviral) may be considered because of high infection rates and future possibility of further immunosuppression should transplantation occur.[19] During grades I and II HE, sedation should be avoided to allow for accurate scoring of the patient's mental status; however, short-acting agents such as propofol may be effective and safe when needed for procedures.[20] If renal dysfunction occurs, then continuous venovenous hemodialysis is preferred over intermittent hemodialysis, as intermittent hemodialysis can cause hemodynamic changes with worsening cerebral perfusion pressure (CPP).[21]

With progression of cerebral edema to grade III (in and out of consciousness, confusion), protection of the patient's airway via endotracheal intubation becomes necessary. Grade III HE marks the point at which aggressive measures to both monitor and lower intracranial pressure (ICP) are initiated.[22,23] In preparation for ICP monitor placement, the patient's coagulation profile should be corrected to an INR of 1.5 or less to avoid intracranial hemorrhage during ICP catheter placement. INR may be allowed to rise after ICP catheter placement to assess liver synthetic function, but an INR above 3.0 should be avoided with the catheter in place. A rising INR is a poor prognostic sign, while stabilization or decline in INR is a useful measure of liver recovery from acute injury. With the ICP monitor in place, the goal-directed therapy is now maintaining a CCP greater than 60 mm Hg. The patient should have the head of the bed elevated to 30 to 45 degrees, minimal stimulation from lighting and noise, and sedation with propofol. Hyperventilation ($PaCO_2$ between 25 and 30 mm Hg) can help reduce ICP but only for a limited period.[24] Given the hemodynamic changes that occur with ALF, vasopressors are initiated to help increase the mean arterial pressure (MAP) to maintain adequate CPP. If these measures are inadequate to reduce ICP or maintain CPP higher than 60 mm Hg, then hypothermia may be started to halt the progression of cerebral edema.[25] However, there is no set standard for the duration of hypothermia. Some centers continue hypothermia for up to 24 hours after transplantation. Transplantation is currently the best modality for correcting the failing liver; however, transplantation is not an option for ALF patients with brain death.

LIVER SUPPORT SYSTEMS

The best treatment currently for a liver that will inevitably fail is liver transplantation. However, there is a profound shortage of transplantable donor livers. This shortage leads to approximately 40% of listed patients per year not receiving a liver transplant, with a majority of these patients either dying or becoming too sick to transplant (www.unos.org). Patients in ALF are given status 1 priority on the recipient list. One potential solution for decreasing the number of ALF patients requiring liver transplantation is a liver support system that would allow time for recovery and avoid transplantation. The ideal liver support system would detoxify blood to physiologic levels, accomplish all hepatic synthetic functions, attenuate systemic inflammation, and allow for the regenerative capacity of the liver.

The most important identified toxin requiring clearance by the liver is ammonia. Ammonia accumulation correlates with the most feared complication of the acutely failing liver, cerebral edema. For ammonia to be effectively detoxified and eliminated by the body, a functioning urea cycle must be present (Figure 124-2). During the development of a potentially successful liver support system, investigators should document urea cycle function not only by measuring levels of urea production and ammonia removal but also by showing effective levels of urea cycle gene expression by hepatocytes in the liver support device.

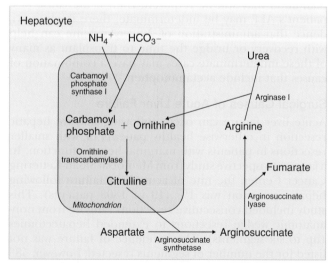

FIGURE 124-2 The urea cycle occurs within hepatocytes. Ammonia (in the form of ammonium, NH_4^+) enters into the hepatocyte and then is transported into the mitochondria. The first two steps of the urea cycle occur within the mitochondria. The remaining three steps occur in the cytosol of the hepatocyte. Once urea and ornithine are produced from arginine, the urea diffuses out of the hepatocyte and ornithine is transported back into the mitochondria to continue the cycle.

Two important synthetic functions of the liver are the production of albumin and coagulation proteins. Albumin production serves as a useful marker of liver-specific protein production in support systems utilizing hepatocytes. Coagulation pathway restoration is an important part of the ideal liver support system. An effective coagulation pathway profile by a bioartificial liver not only prevents bleeding complications but also reduces the use of transfused blood products, avoids complications of their usage, and saves resources for other patient populations (e.g., trauma patients requiring fresh-frozen plasma).

Important design features of any liver support system include free passage of toxins requiring breakdown, free passage of newly synthesized proteins (bioartificial support system), exclusion of the patient's antibodies/complement components to prevent cytotoxic effects (bioartificial support system), and prevention of cells in the support system entering the patient's circulation (bioartificial support system) (Figure 124-3). To control the passage or exclusion of various molecules, the permeability of the filter separating the patient's blood from the detoxifying agent compartment (dialyzer or cells), and the flow rate of the patient's blood passing by the detoxifying agent compartment are adjusted for optimal performance. In the setting of a bioartificial liver support system, this concept of controlling the flow rate can be demonstrated in two models (the diffusion model and the convection model). The diffusion model considers the transfer of waste molecules and product molecules across a semipermeable membrane according to concentration gradients of these molecules. In this model, the semipermeable membrane separates the patient's blood from the hepatocyte compartment. On the other hand, the convection model considers the transfer of waste molecules and product molecules according to pressure gradients and fluid flow. The convection model incorporates pumps that force flow across the semipermeable membrane and allow for a theoretical advantage of increased passage of larger toxins and liver-synthesized proteins into and out of the hepatocyte compartment.

Work done by Nedredal et al demonstrated that optimal toxin removal in a bioartificial liver support

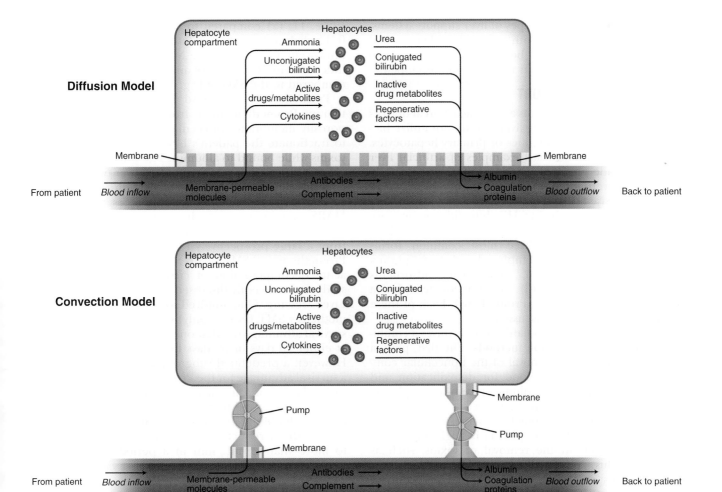

FIGURE 124-3 Two conceptual models are displayed for bioartificial liver (BAL) support devices. The *top model* is based on diffusion—molecules filter from high concentration to low concentration. The *bottom model* relies on pumps (convection) to allow for increased filtration of larger molecules. Both models contain a semipermeable membrane that allows for passage of nonimmunologic molecules. Toxins from the patient are metabolized and proteins are synthesized within the hepatocyte compartment and returned back to the patient.

system (the spheroid reservoir bioartificial liver) occurred with a 400-kDa (kilodalton) membrane incorporating mass transport by both diffusion and high-flow-rate convection. Under these conditions, ammonia, direct and indirect bilirubin, tumor necrosis factor (TNF), and albumin were shown to cross the membrane at high rates. Equally important, IgG and IgM were shown to cross at negligible levels, thus significantly reducing the risks of cytotoxic effects.[26]

In addition to detoxifying and maintaining synthetic function, the support system should help attenuate the SIRS associated with the acutely failing liver, as well as promote liver regeneration within the patient. Various cytokines have been shown to play pivotal roles in both the SIRS of the acutely failing liver and liver regeneration.[4-6] To successfully treat the SIRS of ALF, the liver support device should lower high circulating levels of proinflammatory cytokines such as interleukin (IL)-1β and TNF-α, while maintaining levels of both proinflammatory and regenerative cytokines, such as IL-6, which favor liver regeneration. Failure to attenuate the SIRS will accentuate the extrahepatic manifestations of liver failure and inflammation and worsen the inability to recover adequate functioning liver mass to maintain homeostasis.

There are currently two types of liver support systems, artificial and bioartificial. Both systems have been tested in various trials, which will be discussed. However, the ideal liver support system has not yet been developed.

ARTIFICIAL LIVER SUPPORT

Artificial liver support systems are extracorporeal devices intended to assist the failing liver that do not utilize biologic material, such as cell lines or primary hepatocytes, to remove toxins. Historical examples of artificial liver support include charcoal hemoperfusion and hemodialysis. Both were used in an effort to remove small toxins that cause HE and improve survival. Early devices were successful in reducing HE, but did not improve survival in controlled studies in the era before liver transplantation.[27-29] The three most common forms of artificial liver support employed today are plasma exchange/hemodiafiltration, molecular adsorbents recirculating system (MARS), and fractionated plasma separation and absorption (Prometheus). Each of these forms of therapy will be discussed.

Plasma exchange/hemodiafiltration involves a combination of two detoxification methods. The first, plasma exchange, involves the removal of the noncellular components of the patient's blood for detoxification and replacement with an equal volume of fresh-frozen plasma containing liver-specific synthetic factors. The second, hemodiafiltration (a combination of hemodialysis and hemofiltration), washes the plasma in high volumes of dialysate and aids in the removal of toxins, such as ammonia. This combined method of artificial liver support is most commonly employed in Japan secondary to the low number of cadaveric organ donations performed in that country. In a recent study by Inoue et al, 12 patients (7 with indeterminate etiology and 5 with acute HBV infection) received artificial liver support using plasma exchange/hemodiafiltration. The overall survival was 42% (5/12), with 7 patients dying from lack

of donor livers. All patients had reduction of HE and regained consciousness during treatments.[30]

MARS utilizes albumin dialysis within a three-circuit system. The extracorporeal blood circuit is separated from the albumin dialysate circuit by a restrictive 70-kDa-pore-size membrane that allows for selective removal of water-soluble and albumin-bound molecules from the patient's blood. The third circuit then allows for removal of water-soluble toxins from the second albumin circuit.[31] Toxins are also removed from the second albumin circuit by a charcoal filter and resin-binding column placed in the second circuit. The majority of the studies testing MARS have been conducted in the setting of acute decompensation of the cirrhotic patient. Multiple randomized studies have demonstrated significant recovery from HE with MARS plus standard medical therapy (SMT) compared to SMT alone.[32-34] For example, the pivotal U.S. trial by Hassanein et al showed that HE improvement occurred more quickly in the MARS treatment group than SMT alone; the median time to improve two grades in HE occurred 36 hours sooner in the MARS treatment group (72 vs. 108 hours).[32] In another study, Heemann et al showed a statistically significant improvement in survival at 30 days for the MARS plus SMT group (92%, 11/12) compared to the SMT-only group (55%, 6/11).[33] Interestingly, Sen et al demonstrated that the improvement in HE in the MARS plus SMT group was independent of changes of ammonia and cytokine levels compared to the SMT-only group.[34]

Prometheus is a second form of albumin dialysis therapy. Prometheus differs from MARS by using a larger-porosity membrane (molecular weight cutoff, 200 kDa) to fractionate the patient's blood and allow removal of toxins while bound to albumin. The fractionated plasma (containing albumin) is then passed over two adsorption columns allowing for direct detoxification of the albumin. In contrast, the patient's albumin does not cross the MARS membrane, so toxins must enter the albumin circuit of MARS as free, unbound molecules.[35] Results from a large prospectively randomized trial comparing Prometheus and SMT versus SMT alone in the setting of acute decompensation of cirrhotic patients (HELIOS study) were recently discussed at the 2010 International Liver Meeting. One-hundred forty-five patients (77 Prometheus + SMT, 68 SMT only) were enrolled. Overall, no survival advantage was demonstrated between the groups at either 28 days or 90 days following initial treatment. However, a predefined subgroup analysis demonstrated a survival advantage for the Prometheus group in patients with a Model of End-Stage Liver Disease (MELD) score greater than 30 and patients with hepatorenal syndrome type I (doubling of serum creatinine to more than 2.5 mg/dL or reduction of creatinine clearance by 50% to more than 20 mL/min in a period of less than 2 weeks).[36]

BIOARTIFICIAL LIVER SUPPORT

The most important difference between an artificial liver support system and a bioartificial liver support system is the use of cells in the latter. The ideal bioartificial liver support system would utilize human hepatocytes; however, a high-quality source of large numbers of human hepatocytes is currently not available. Most human hepatocytes currently come from unused cadaveric donors (discarded because of poor quality) or from nondiseased partial-hepatectomy specimens, which are relatively uncommon. Good-quality donor livers are not available because they are in great demand for use in liver transplantation. Novel solutions to expand the availability of human hepatocytes will be discussed later in this chapter. Currently, the two cell sources with the most use in human clinical trials of bioartificial liver therapy are the human hepatoblastoma cell line HepG2/C3A and primary hepatocytes from healthy pig livers.

The use of HepG2/C3A cells comprises the foundation of the extracorporeal liver assist device (ELAD). This device allows for hemoperfusion from the patient through columns containing immortalized C3A cells. By use of ultrafiltration, toxins can be detoxified and synthesized proteins can return to the patient. The device contains two acellular membranes to prevent the spread of hepatoblastoma cells back to the patient. Work by Kelly et al from 1991 to 1993 using the Hepatix ELAD demonstrated the potential safety for patients suffering from ALF. However, this device was composed of a single cartridge containing 100 g of HepG2/C3A cells.[37] Ellis et al then conducted a small randomized controlled trial using two 100-g Hepatix HepG2/C3A cartridges in a single circuit. A total of 24 patients were enrolled in the study with 12 treated with ELAD plus SMT and 12 with SMT only. Groups were stratified based on who met criteria for transplantation and who did not. Overall, the survival was not different between the two groups (ELAD plus SMT 67%, 8/12 vs. SMT only 58%, 7/12). There was also no difference between the groups when they were further separated based on meeting or not meeting transplantation criteria.[38] More recently, the use of the HepG2/C3A cell line in the ELAD device has been improved. The latest generation of ELAD utilizes four HepG2/C3A columns. A promising trial of ELAD was recently conducted in China on cirrhotic patients with acute decompensation. Interim results from this study were presented at the 2007 AASLD meeting in Boston. Of the 60 patients reported in this study, 6 were excluded because of breaks in protocol. From the remaining 54 patients, 35 were randomized to the ELAD plus SMT and 19 to the SMT alone. The primary endpoint of overall survival free of transplant was statistically higher for the treatment group (86%, 30/35) versus the control group (47%, 9/19).[39] These results are awaiting confirmation by current randomized trials in the United States, the United Kingdom, and Saudi Arabia.

The largest trial to date using a bioartificial liver (BAL) support device was the HepatAssist device trial.[40] This BAL device used 70 g of cryopreserved porcine hepatocytes. The trial was conducted at 20 institutions (11 in the United States and 9 in Europe) in which 171 patients were prospectively randomized (85 to BAL plus SMT and 86 to SMT alone). The primary endpoint for this study was the overall 30-day survival. There was no statistically significant difference between the two groups in overall 30-day survival (BAL plus SMT 71%, 60/85 vs. SMT alone 62%, 53/86). On further analysis, 147 of the 171 patients enrolled suffered from fulminant or subfulminant hepatic failure. The overall survival between these patients favored the BAL plus SMT group (73%, 53/73) over the SMT alone group (59%, 44/74); however, this 14% improvement in survival did not reach statistical significance.[40] A further post hoc analysis of 83 patients with known causes of ALF did show significance in survival of BAL therapy over SMT ($P < 0.009$). The HepatAssist device first performed plasmapheresis before pumping the patient's fractionated plasma into an activated charcoal column for initial detoxification. The charcoal effluent was then oxygenated and passed through the hepatocyte bioreactor before returning back to the patient's circulation.

Despite the promising results from these two methods of BAL therapy for both ALF patients and acutely decompensated cirrhotic patients, concerns exist for both therapies. The biggest concern for the ELAD is the theoretical risk of HepG2/C3A tumor cell migration into the patient's circulation. Another concern of ELAD therapy is the inability of HepG2/C3A cells to perform all functions specific to primary hepatocytes. Nyberg et al demonstrated that primary rat hepatocytes had statistically higher ureagenesis and drug metabolism compared to HepG2/C3A in the setting of a gel entrapment BAL device.[41] As for the therapeutic use of porcine hepatocytes, the greatest concern is the possibility of zoonotic infections, such as porcine endogenous retrovirus (PERV) transmission to the patient. During the large trial with the HepatAssist device, there was no detection of PERV transmission to a patient.[40] The other concern with isolated primary hepatocytes is that they have been shown to lose function and undergo apoptosis under ex vivo conditions.[42-44] However, culturing hepatocytes as spheroids (three-dimensional clusters) has been shown to maintain function and prevent apoptosis longer than in monolayer systems.[45,46] Although hepatocyte spheroids have been shown to maintain function longer than isolated hepatocytes, no randomized controlled trials have been performed yet to test BAL support devices utilizing this culturing technique.

FUTURE EFFORTS

The ideal therapy for a patient suffering from an acutely failing liver should perform liver-specific detoxification and synthetic functions, attenuate the SIRS often associated with the failing liver, and allow for regeneration of the injured liver. Thus, the ideal therapy should either increase the likelihood of spontaneous recovery or effectively serve as a bridge to transplant with the ultimate goal of improved survival. The device that best fulfills these criteria is likely a cell-based support device, such as BAL. Cellular transplantation of 10^7 to 10^{10} allogeneic hepatocytes has also been tested as therapy for human liver failure with modest results.[47] Our discussion of future efforts will focus on those related to improving extracorporeal BAL devices, but these efforts may also have application in the field of hepatocyte transplantation. Efforts to improve BAL therapy continue to modify the microenvironment and architecture of the cells within the device to optimize long-term functionality. The optimal architecture of the hepatocytes will need to prevent cell death and dedifferentiation secondary to the lack of normal cell-to-cell and cell-to-matrix adhesion.

More importantly, the functionality of the cells in the BAL device should resemble that of human hepatocytes as closely as possible. For example, investigators working with the metabolic defect seen in human hereditary tyrosinemia type 1 have recently shown successful engraftment and rapid expansion of human hepatocytes in the livers of knockout mice with this defect. These mice are deficient of the enzyme fumarylacetoacetate hydrolase (Fah), which provides a selective advantage to normal transplanted human hepatocytes over FAH-deficient mouse hepatocytes in a tyrosine-rich environment.[48] Ideally, a large animal (i.e., pig) version of this model could potentially allow for large-scale production of high-quality and readily available human hepatocytes for use in BAL support systems. Besides using repopulation models, advancements have been made in the field of induced pluripotent stem cells (iPSCs), making an individualized approach possible to the treatment of liver disease.[49] iPSCs involve reprogramming normal somatic cells to multipotent stem cells that can then be differentiated back to cells that closely resemble human hepatocytes in function (hepatocyte-like cells).[50] These new hepatocytes-like cells have the same genetic makeup as the donor, making cellular therapies such as hepatocyte transplantation possible without the need for immunosuppression. These patients could either undergo cell transplantation using their own hepatocytes or their own hepatocyte-like cells following genetic correction of the inherent deficiency in these cells. Hepatocyte-like cells may also serve as an autologous cell source for a BAL support system.

REFERENCES

1. Clemmesen J, Larsen F, Kondrug J, et al: Cerebral herniation in patients with acute liver failure is correlated with arterial ammonia concentration. *Hepatology* 29:648, 1999.
2. Correll PH, Morrison AC, Lutz MA: Receptor tyrosine kinases and the regulation of macrophage activation. *J Leukoc Biol* 75:731, 2004.
3. Mackay IR: Hepatoimmunology: A perspective. *Immunol Cell Biol* 80:36, 2002.
4. Schmidt L, Larson F: Prognostic implications of hyperlactemia, multiple organ failure, and systemic inflammatory response syndrome in patients with acetaminophen-induced liver failure. *Crit Care Med* 34:337, 2006.
5. Boermeester MA, Houdijk AP, Meyer S, et al: Liver failure induces a systemic inflammatory response. Prevention by recombinant N-terminal bactericidal/permeability-increasing protein. *Am J Pathol* 147:1428, 1995.
6. Sekiyama KD, Yoshiba M, Thomson AW: Circulating proinflammatory cytokines (IL-1 beta, TNF-alpha, and IL-6) and IL-1 receptor antagonist (IL-1Ra) in fulminant hepatic failure and acute hepatitis. *Clin Exp Immunol* 98:71, 1994.
7. Rolando N, Wade J, Davalos M, et al: The systemic inflammatory response syndrome in acute liver failure. *Hepatology* 32:734, 2000.
8. Lee WM, Squires RH, Jr, Nyberg SL, et al: Acute liver failure: Summary of a workshop. *Hepatology* 47:1401, 2008.
9. Ostapowicz G, Fontana RJ, Schiodt FV, et al: Results of a prospective study of acute liver failure at 17 tertiary care centers in the United States. *Ann Intern Med* 137:947, 2002.
10. Mitchell JR, Thorgeirsson SS, Potter WZ, et al: Acetaminophen-induced hepatic injury: Protective role of glutathione in man and rationale for therapy. *Clin Pharmacol Ther* 16:676, 1974.
11. Pumford NR, Hinson JA, Benson RW, et al: Immunoblot analysis of protein containing 3-(cystein-S-yl)acetaminophen adducts in serum and subcellular liver fractions from acetaminophen-treated mice. *Toxicol Appl Pharmacol* 104:521, 1990.
12. Jochum C, Gieseler RK, Gawlista I, et al: Hepatitis B-associated acute liver failure: Immediate treatment with entecavir inhibits hepatitis B virus replication and potentially its sequelae. *Digestion* 80:235, 2009.
13. Lee WM, Hynan LS, Rossaro L, et al: Intravenous N-acetylcysteine improves transplant-free survival in early stage non-acetaminophen acute liver failure. *Gastroenterology* 137:856, 64, 2002.
14. Jarnagin WR, Gonen M, Fong Y, et al: Improvement in perioperative outcome after hepatic resection: Analysis of 1,803 consecutive cases over the past decade. *Ann Surg* 236:397, discussion 406, 2002.
15. Kishi Y, Abdalla EK, Chun YS, et al: Three hundred and one consecutive extended right hepatectomies: Evaluation of outcome based on systematic liver volumetry. *Ann Surg* 250:540, 2009.
16. Polson J, Lee WM: AASLD position paper: The management of acute liver failure. *Hepatology* 41:1179, 2005.
17. Wijdicks EF, Bamlet WR, Maramattom BV, et al: Validation of a new coma scale: The FOUR score. *Ann Neurol* 58:585, 2005.
18. Merli M, Riggio O: Dietary and nutritional indications in hepatic encephalopathy. *Metab Brain Dis* 24:211, 2009.
19. Vaquero J, Polson J, Chung C, et al: Infection and the progression of hepatic encephalopathy in acute liver failure. *Gastroenterology* 125:755, 2003.
20. Wijdicks E, Nyberg S: Propofol to control intracranial pressure in fulminant hepatic failure. *Transpl Proc* 73:1965, 2002.
21. Davenport A, Will EJ, Davidson AM: Improved cardiovascular stability during continuous modes of renal replacement therapy in critically ill patients with acute hepatic and renal failure. *Crit Care Med* 21:328, 1993.
22. Lidofsky SD, Bass NM, Prager MC, et al: Intracranial pressure monitoring and liver transplantation for fulminant hepatic failure. *Hepatology* 16:1, 1992.
23. Daas M, Plevak DJ, Wijdicks EFM, et al: Acute liver failure: Results of a 5-year clinical protocol. *Liver Transpl Surg* 1:210, 1995.
24. Laffey JG, Kavanagh BP: Hypocapnia. *N Engl J Med* 347:43, 2002.
25. Jalan R, Olde Damink SW, Deutz NE, et al: Moderate hypothermia in patients with acute liver failure and uncontrolled intracranial hypertension. *Gastroenterology* 127:1338, 2004.
26. Nedredal GI, Amiot BP, Nyberg P, et al: Optimization of mass transfer for toxin removal and immunoprotection of hepatocytes in a bioartificial liver. *Biotechnol Bioeng* 104:995, 2009.
27. Kiley JE, Pender JC, Welch HF, et al: Ammonia intoxication treated by hemodialysis. *N Engl J Med* 259:1156, 1958.
28. Merrill JP, Smith S 3rd, Callahan EJ 3rd, et al: The use of an artificial kidney. II. Clinical experience. *J Clin Invest* 29:425, 1950.
29. O'Grady J, Gimson A, O'Brien C, et al: Controlled trials of charcoal hemoperfusion and prognostic factors in fulminant hepatic failure. *Gastroenterology* 94:1186, 1988.
30. Inoue K, Kourin A, Watanabe T, et al: Artificial liver support system using large buffer volumes removes significant glutamine and is an ideal bridge to liver transplantation. *Transpl Proc* 41:259, 2009.
31. Stange J, Mitzner S, Risler T, et al: Molecular adsorbent recycling system (MARS): Clinical results of a new membrane-based blood purification system for bioartificial liver support. *Artificial Organs* 23:319, 1999.
32. Hassanein T, Tofteng F, Brown RJ, et al: Randomized controlled study of extracorporeal albumin dialysis for hepatic encephalopathy in advanced cirrhosis. *Hepatology* 46:1853, 2007.
33. Heemann U, Treichel U, Loock J, et al: Albumin dialysis in cirrhosis with superimposed acute liver injury: A prospective, controlled study. *Hepatology* 36:949, 2002.
34. Sen S, Davies NA, Mookerjee RP, et al: Pathophysiological effects of albumin dialysis in acute-on-chronic liver failure: A randomized controlled study. *Liver Transpl* 10:1109, 2004.
35. Rifai K, Ernst T, Kretschmer U, et al: Prometheus: A new extracorporeal system for the treatment of liver failure. *J Hepatol* 39:984, 2003.
36. Rifai K, Kribben A, Gerken G, et al: Extracorporeal liver support by fractionated plasma separation and adsorption (Prometheus) in patients with acute-on-chronic liver failure (HELIOS Study): A prospective randomized controlled multicenter study. *J Hepatol* 52:S3, 2010.
37. Kelly JH, Sussman NL. The Hepatix extracorporeal liver assist device in the treatment of fulminant hepatic failure. *ASAIO J* 40:83, 1994.

38. Ellis A, Highes R, Wendon J, et al: Pilot-controlled trial of the extracorporeal liver assist device in acute liver failure. *Hepatology* 24:1446, 1996.

39. Duan Z, Zhang J, Xin S, et al: Interim results of randomized controlled trial of ELAD™ in acute on chronic liver disease. *Hepatology* 46:1.2007.

40. Demetriou AA, Brown RS, Jr, Busuttil RW, et al: Prospective, randomized, multicenter, controlled trial of a bioartificial liver in treating acute liver failure. *Ann Surg* 239:660, discussion 667, 2004.

41. Nyberg SL, Remmel RP, Mann HJ, et al: Primary hepatocytes outperform Hep G2 cells as the source of biotransformation functions in a bioartificial liver. *Ann Surg* 220:59, 1994.

42. Frisch SM, Francis H: Disruption of epithelial cell-matrix interactions induces apoptosis. *J Cell Biol* 124:619, 1994.

43. Grossmann J: Molecular mechanisms of "detachment-induced apoptosis: Anoikis." *Apoptosis* 7:247, 2002.

44. Zvibel I, Smets F, Soriano H: Anoikis: Roadblock to cell transplantation? *Cell Transplant* 11:621, 2002.

45. Ambrosino G, Basso S, Varotto S, et al: Isolated hepatocytes versus hepatocyte spheroids: In vitro culture of rat hepatocytes. *Cell Transplant* 14:397, 2005.

46. Sakai Y, Yamagami S, Nakazawa K: Comparative analysis of gene expression in rat liver tissue and monolayer- and spheroid-cultured hepatocytes. *Cells Tissues Organs* 191:281, 2010.

47. Fox IJ, Roy-Chowdhury J: Hepatocyte transplantation. *J Hepatol* 40:878, 2004.

48. Azuma H, Paulk N, Ranade A, et al: Robust expansion of human hepatocytes in Fah-/-/Rag2-/-/Il2rg-/- mice. *Nature Biotechnology* 25:903, 2007.

49. Yu J, Hu K, Smuga-Otto K, et al: Human induced pluripotent stem cells free of vector and transgene sequences. *Science* 324:797, 2009.

50. Si-Tayeb K, Noto F, Nagaoka M, et al: Highly efficient generation of human hepatocyte-like cells from induced pluripotent stem cells. *Hepatology* 51:297, 2010.

Vascular Diseases of the Liver

David M. Levi | Andreas G. Tzakis

The topic *vascular diseases of the liver* encompasses an array of disparate clinicopathologic entities with the common thread that they specifically affect the hepatic vasculature. They can be arbitrarily classified into those that involve the hepatic arterial blood supply, those that involve the portal vein, and those that involve the hepatic veins. The topics *portal hypertension* and *portal vein thrombosis* are addressed separately in Chapter 131.

HEPATIC ARTERY DISORDERS

ANEURYSMS OF THE HEPATIC ARTERY

Hepatic artery aneurysms are rare, comprising about 20% of all visceral aneurysms. True aneurysms may be a manifestation of systemic diseases including atherosclerosis or vasculitides such as polyarteritis nodosa[1] and systemic lupus erythematosus.[2] Pseudoaneurysms of the hepatic artery can result from hepatic trauma[3] or may be iatrogenic, occurring as a procedure-related injury to the artery.[4] Mycotic pseudoaneurysms, resulting from bacterial endocarditis[5] or following liver transplantation,[6] have also been reported.

Most commonly, hepatic artery aneurysms are solitary, involve the extrahepatic portion of the artery, and are 3 to 4 cm in diameter at the time of presentation.[7,8] The clinical presentation varies considerably. Some are discovered incidentally by noninvasive imaging studies (Figure 125-1). Patients with mycotic pseudoaneurysms may present with pain, fever, or other signs of infection. Hemobilia following laparoscopic cholecystectomy,[9] liver biopsy, or interventional radiologic procedures can result from rupture of a pseudoaneurysm into the biliary tree. Intraperitoneal or gastrointestinal hemorrhage-related rupture is associated with a high mortality rate.[10]

The diagnosis may be suspected based on the presentation but is confirmed by Doppler ultrasonography, intravenous contrast-enhanced computed tomography (CT), or magnetic resonance (MR) imaging. Angiography can be diagnostic, and with the aid of interventional radiologic techniques, can be therapeutic as well.[3,4]

The treatment of hepatic artery aneurysms is dictated by their cause, size, location, and patient condition. Although the natural history of these aneurysms is unclear, it seems that size correlates with the risk of rupture. Additionally, the ubiquitous use of high-quality imaging techniques has led to an increased detection of small, asymptomatic aneurysms. The concern of eventual complications, especially hemorrhage, warrants the consideration of treating all of these lesions, even those that are asymptomatic or are discovered incidentally.[7] The underlying condition needs to be addressed, and

adequate resuscitation is required for patients presenting with intraperitoneal or gastrointestinal hemorrhage.

Aneurysms of the extrahepatic portion of the artery are classically managed surgically. Those affecting the common hepatic artery may be ligated proximally and distally if adequate collateral circulation to the liver is afforded by the gastroduodenal artery via the pancreaticoduodenal arcade. Those originating distal to the gastroduodenal artery, affecting the proper hepatic artery, can be treated by ligation and aneurysmectomy and revascularization of the liver. A pseudoaneurysm of the hepatic artery anastomosis following liver transplantation is a serious complication. The usual treatment is revascularization of the liver with resection of the pseudoaneurysm. In an emergency, ligation of the artery proximally and distally may be the only option. Urgent retransplantation may be necessary.[11] Of note, as interventional radiological techniques have developed, cases of extrahepatic aneurysms treated by percutaneous transarterial catheter embolization or endovascular stent placement have been reported.[4,12]

Intrahepatic aneurysms can be managed by percutaneous transarterial catheter embolization (Figure 125-2). This approach is especially useful if the lesions are multiple, as seen in cases of polyarteritis nodosa.[1] The risk of significant hepatic ischemia is minimized if there is adequate portal venous blood flow and the affected artery branch or branches are distal within the liver. Solitary, posttraumatic intrahepatic pseudoaneurysms, confined to a hepatic segment or lobe, may be treated by hepatic resection if an interventional radiologic approach is not possible.[13]

HEPATIC ARTERY INJURY

Traumatic injury of the hepatic artery is uncommon. Penetrating injuries to the portal triad outnumber blunt injuries, and associated injuries are the rule.[14] The diagnosis is usually made at the time of laparotomy or postmortem. Portal triad injuries carry a high mortality rate because of exsanguinating hemorrhage or refractory shock. Successful treatment requires control of bleeding, aggressive resuscitation, and temporization of other injuries. Often concomitant biliary tract and/or portal vein injury must be addressed.[14] Treatment options for the injured artery include ligation or primary repair. Better survival has been reported with hepatic artery ligation as compared to repair.[15] The late sequelae of portal triad injuries including hepatic ischemia, biliary strictures, portal hypertension, and liver failure may mandate liver transplantation.[16]

Iatrogenic injury of the hepatic artery is an uncommon but potentially devastating complication of laparoscopic cholecystectomy. At least one-fifth of

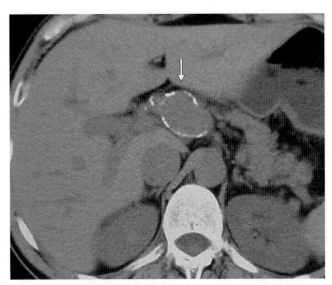

FIGURE 125-1 CT demonstration of a large, solitary, calcified hepatic artery aneurysm *(arrow)*.

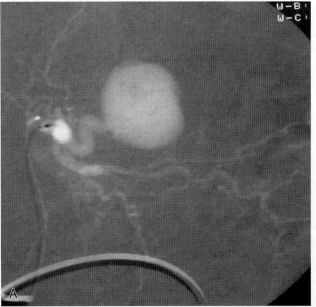

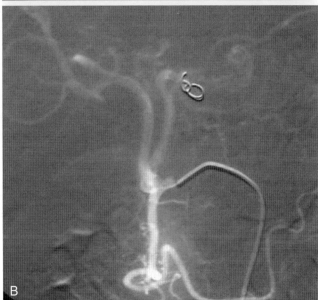

FIGURE 125-2 A and **B,** Transarterial catheter embolization of a traumatic pseudoaneurysm of the left hepatic artery.

cholecystectomy-related bile duct injuries have an associated hepatic artery injury. The addition of an injury to the artery portends a higher complication rate after biliary reconstruction and a greater risk of mortality.[17] The injury is often not recognized at the time of surgery, even if the biliary injury is identified and corrected immediately. In the patient presenting with bile duct strictures after cholecystectomy, the presence of a concomitant arterial injury should be suspected based on the severity of the bile duct injury and the discovery of a report of difficulty gaining hemostasis during the cholecystectomy. Angiography can demonstrate the interrupted vessel, but this study is not necessary if it will not alter patient management.

The treatment of these injuries is usually directed toward repairing the bile duct, either primarily or by Roux-en-Y hepaticojejunostomy. Arterial reconstruction, except when noted immediately, is seldom indicated or performed. Rarely, an injury to the right hepatic artery results in acute necrosis of the right hepatic lobe or right-sided intrahepatic strictures and cholangitis, both amenable to hepatic resection.[18]

HEPATIC ARTERY THROMBOSIS

Hepatic artery thrombosis is the most dreaded vascular complication following liver transplantation. With an incidence of 2% to 8% of cases, it has a high associated morbidity and mortality. Pediatric recipients and cases requiring arterial conduits are at increased risk for the development of this complication.[19] Advanced donor age increases the risk of liver graft loss from hepatic artery thrombosis.[20] When it occurs early, within the first month following transplantation, it usually results in acute graft necrosis necessitating urgent retransplantation (Figure 125-3). Protocol surveillance of the hepatic artery using Doppler ultrasound may detect early or impending thrombosis allowing for immediate revascularization and potential graft salvage.[21]

Late hepatic artery thrombosis is less well understood than early thrombosis and has a wider spectrum of presentation. Some patients are asymptomatic and the diagnosis is discovered incidentally. For others, the sequelae are biliary tract complications including stricture formation, bile leak, cholangitis, hemobilia, and hepatic biloma/abscess. Cholangitis can be managed by percutaneous or endoscopic catheter decompression of the biliary tree. Infected bilomas are treated by percutaneous drainage and antibiotics. Attempts at biliary reconstruction or hepatic artery revascularization are rarely successful. Although some asymptomatic patients spontaneously develop arterial collaterals, most survivors with late hepatic artery thrombosis will ultimately require retransplantation.[22]

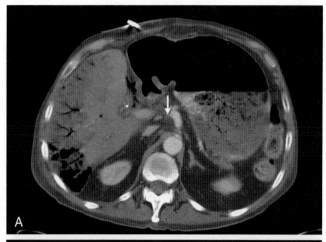

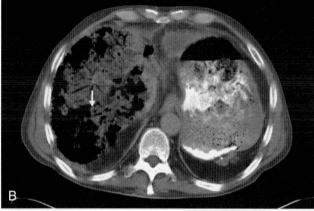

FIGURE 125-3 CT scan images of hepatic artery thrombosis after liver transplantation. **A,** The *arrow* marks the thrombus in the hepatic artery. **B,** The *arrow* denotes the gangrenous liver allograft.

HEPATIC ARTERIOPORTAL AND ARTERIOVENOUS SHUNTS

Aberrant communication between the hepatic artery and either portal or hepatic venous branches is seen in a variety of diseases and is of variable clinical significance. These shunts can result from iatrogenic, penetrating, or blunt liver trauma,[23] benign and malignant hepatic neoplasms, or may develop congenitally,[24] such as in patients with portal hypertension or hereditary hemorrhagic telangiectasia (Rendu-Osler-Weber disease). Iatrogenic causes include core liver biopsy, hepatic resection, and radiofrequency tumor ablation. Hepatocellular carcinoma can produce a vascular fistula by eroding into a vein branch,[25] and tumors such as cavernous hemangioma, focal nodular hyperplasia, and infantile hepatic hemangioendothelioma can develop abnormal shunts. Hereditary hemorrhagic telangiectasia is an autosomal dominant disorder characterized by microscopic and macroscopic arteriovenous malformations with rare but well-described liver involvement (Figure 125-4).[26]

The pathophysiologic and clinical impact of these shunts depends on their type and hemodynamic magnitude. A large shunt from the high-pressure hepatic artery to the low-pressure portal vein can lead to the development of portal hypertension and its consequences,

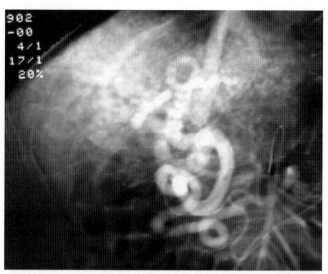

FIGURE 125-4 This angiogram of a patient with hereditary hemorrhagic telangiectasia with liver involvement depicts an enlarged, tortuous hepatic artery with shunting to the hepatic veins.

particularly variceal hemorrhage.[27] Additionally, the increase in portal venous blood flow can cause fibrous tissue proliferation and nodular regeneration within the liver. A large shunt from the hepatic artery to the hepatic venous system can have two main effects. First, this arteriovenous shunt siphons oxygenated blood away from the hepatic parenchyma and biliary tree. Hepatic necrosis and/or ischemic biliary injury can result. Second, the shunt can provoke a hyperdynamic response eventually leading to high-output cardiac failure. This is typically seen in infantile hepatic hemangioendothelioma.[28]

The treatment of arterioportal and arteriovenous shunts is dependent on the size, location, and cause of the shunt. Small, focal, hemodynamically insignificant shunts may be found incidentally on radiologic imaging studies and may not require specific treatment. Shunts that are confined to one lobe or segment of the liver, such as those related to a hepatic tumor, may be amenable to resection. Those shunts resulting from trauma or iatrogenic injury affecting the extrahepatic artery and portal vein may be treated by surgical interruption of the fistula and primary repair of the vessels. As interventional radiologic techniques have improved, more shunts have been treated by percutaneous transarterial catheter embolization.[23,29] Finally, those patients presenting with multifocal or diffuse intrahepatic arteriovenous shunts, as seen in infantile hemangioendothelioma and hereditary hemorrhagic telangiectasia, may be candidates for liver transplantation.[30]

PORTAL VEIN DISORDERS

PORTAL VEIN ANEURYSM

Aneurysmal dilation of the portal vein is an exceedingly rare entity. Venous aneurysms are possibly congenital in nature or may develop as a result of trauma to the portal vein. They can develop in the absence of portal

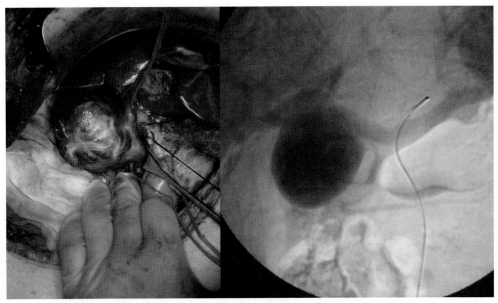

FIGURE 125-5 Images of a symptomatic, saccular aneurysm of the portal vein.

hypertension. Most present with epigastric abdominal pain or cause symptoms by compressing adjacent structures, typically the common bile duct, duodenum, or inferior vena cava.[31] Many are discovered incidentally (Figure 125-5). Rupture is rare but has been reported, and even spontaneous resolution has been documented. Although their etiology and natural history are not clear, it is reasonable to suspect that the incidence of compressive symptoms and risk of complications correlate with the size of the aneurysm. There is no consensus regarding the treatment of these lesions but asymptomatic, small (<3 cm) aneurysms of the portal vein can be observed.[32] Larger-diameter aneurysms that compress adjacent structures should be addressed surgically. Resection and repair with or without an interposition graft has described on numerous occasions and even liver transplant has been reported.[31]

HEPATIC VEIN DISORDERS

BUDD-CHIARI SYNDROME

Budd-Chiari syndrome can result from an array of disorders and has a variable clinical presentation. The common denominator in the pathogenesis of this syndrome is hepatic venous outflow obstruction characterized by the classic clinical triad of abdominal pain, hepatomegaly, and ascites.

The list of disorders that can cause the syndrome includes various inherited and acquired hypercoagulable states, tumor invasion of the hepatic outflow tract typically by liver,[33] adrenal, or renal malignancies,[34] iatrogenic outflow obstruction following liver surgery or transplantation, vascular webs, and trauma. Myeloproliferative disorders, especially polycythemia vera, are the most common underlying cause.[35]

Hepatic vein occlusion results in increased sinusoidal pressure and decreased sinusoidal blood flow. Hepatic congestion can cause liver enlargement and abdominal pain. Diminished sinusoidal blood flow is thought to be important in the pathogenic progression of fibrosis and regenerative nodule formation leading to cirrhosis. Portal hypertension contributes to ascites formation and the development of varices. Concomitant portal vein thrombosis is present in approximately 20% of cases.[36] Because the venous outflow for the caudate lobe is separate from the major hepatic veins, compensatory hypertrophy of this hepatic segment is common. The enlarged caudate lobe can extrinsically compress the adjacent inferior vena cava (IVC), producing a pressure gradient across it.

The clinical presentation of patients with Budd-Chiari syndrome varies depending on the extent and acuity of the obstruction to the hepatic venous outflow. Sudden-onset, complete hepatic vein thrombosis may on occasion present as fulminant liver failure. If the onset is gradual and/or the degree of obstruction is incomplete, there is the opportunity for the development of venous collaterals. The degree to which these collaterals decompress the portal venous system impacts the clinical manifestations of the syndrome and determines the preferred treatment. Some patients develop liver enlargement and intractable ascites with relatively preserved hepatic function, whereas others develop cirrhosis with hepatic decompensation.[37]

The diagnosis of Budd-Chiari syndrome should be considered in any patient with hepatomegaly and ascites. Laboratory investigation of liver function may reveal abnormalities, but these tests are nonspecific. Doppler ultrasonography is excellent for visualizing the hepatic vasculature revealing the level and extent of the obstruction of the hepatic outflow.[38] It is also useful for evaluating the retrohepatic vena cava and the portal vein. CT and MR imaging may reveal obliterated hepatic veins, heterogeneously perfused hepatic parenchyma and areas of necrosis, hepatomegaly, caudate lobe hypertrophy,

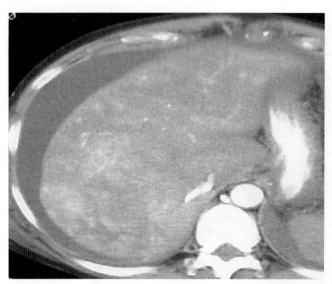

FIGURE 125-6 CT image of a patient with Budd-Chiari syndrome characterized by heterogeneously appearing hepatic parenchyma, caudate lobe enlargement, ascites, and no visualization of the hepatic veins.

narrowing of the retrohepatic vena cava, and ascites (Figure 125-6). When the underlying cause is tumor invasion of the hepatic veins, these imaging studies are important for determining the local extent of the disease. Hepatic venography is often not needed for establishing a diagnosis but may be useful for direct measurement of a pressure gradient across a narrowed IVC or stenotic hepatic outflow tract. Interventional radiologic techniques including transluminal angioplasty, vein stenting, and transjugular intrahepatic portosystemic shunt (TIPS) placement may be employed therapeutically at the time of hepatic venography.[39]

The treatment of Budd-Chiari syndrome must be individualized to the patient and is enhanced by a multidisciplinary team approach.[40] The principles of treatment include addressing the underlying cause, decreasing hepatic sinusoidal pressure and congestion, and preserving liver function. Once the diagnosis is established, a liver biopsy may be needed to determine the extent of hepatic fibrosis and cirrhosis. Because the hepatic parenchyma may not be uniformly affected, bilobar biopsies have been advocated to avoid sampling error.[36] Liver biopsy is unnecessary in cases where it is clear that the liver cannot be salvaged, such as those with fulminant liver failure or decompensated cirrhosis.

A variety of medical therapies, interventional radiologic techniques, and surgical procedures are available for the patient with Budd-Chiari syndrome. The best therapy or combination of therapies depends on the patient's individual anatomic and physiologic condition as much as the expertise and bias of the team caring for the patient. Medical therapies include thrombolysis, anticoagulation, and pharmacologic treatment of ascites and portal hypertension. Interventional radiologic techniques that have been developed include percutaneous transluminal angioplasty with or without stent placement and TIPS. Surgical procedures include a variety of portosystemic shunts and liver transplantation.

Thrombolysis alone has been attempted for acute hepatic vein thrombosis anecdotally but with limited success.[41] Its best place in therapy may be as a prelude to a more definitive procedure such as a TIPS or a surgical shunt. Vein angioplasty with or without stent placement also has been tried in selected cases. It is indicated for short-segment stenoses of a hepatic vein or veins, hepatic venous outflow tract stenosis following liver transplantation,[42] or IVC webs. Angioplasty with stenting of the retrohepatic IVC has been performed in conjunction with surgical portosystemic shunting when a pressure gradient exists across this segment of the IVC from caudate lobe compression.[43]

Physiologically, a TIPS is a central portosystemic shunt. It is indicated in the patient with Budd-Chiari syndrome and chronic, well-compensated liver disease to relieve portal hypertension and treat intractable ascites. Some patients that have presented with acute liver failure have been treated with TIPS with excellent long-term survival.[44] For patients with fulminant liver failure or decompensated cirrhosis, the procedure has a high incidence of complications.[45] Disadvantages of the TIPS procedure are that its placement may be technically difficult, especially if the ostia of the hepatic veins are occluded, and it often needs revision over time. The introduction of covered stents may yield better results.[46]

Although interventional radiology techniques have evolved and improved, surgical intervention remains the standard for the definitive treatment of Budd-Chiari syndrome. However, there is no consensus as to the best procedure for the disease. The decision between TIPS or a surgical shunt and which shunt depends largely on the experience of the treatment team. For those patients with chronic, symptomatic Budd-Chiari syndrome, a variety of surgical shunts are available to decompress the portal venous system and preserve liver function. Survival following these procedures is determined primarily by the rate of progression of the liver disease and the long-term patency of the shunt.

If the IVC is widely patent, either a mesocaval shunt, a central splenorenal shunt, or a side-to-side portocaval shunt are the available options. Mesocaval and splenorenal shunts are employed most commonly. Mesocaval shunts require an interposition graft of synthetic material or autologous vein between the superior mesenteric vein and the infrahepatic IVC. If the graft thromboses, the superior mesenteric vein will probably not be available should liver transplant eventually become warranted. A direct, side-to-side splenorenal shunt preserves the hepatic hilum and does not require a vein graft. Although side-to-side portocaval shunts have a reported high-patency rate,[47] hypertrophy of the caudate lobe can make direct shunting impossible. Also, dissection of the hepatic hilum can make subsequent liver transplantation difficult. Finally, portal vein thrombosis is an obvious contraindication for the procedure.

The long-term patency of these surgical shunts depends on the presence of a pressure gradient between a high-pressure portal venous system and a low-pressure infrahepatic IVC. If the retrohepatic vena cava is stenotic or thrombosed, this pressure gradient may be insufficient. In this situation, the retrohepatic vena cava may be stented prior to the surgical shunt.[43] Another procedure developed to address this situation is a mesoatrial shunt or one of its variations.[48]

Most would agree that liver transplantation is the procedure of choice for the patient with fulminant liver failure or decompensated cirrhosis related to the Budd-Chiari syndrome.[36] The shortage of available organs for transplant and the need for immunosuppression after transplant are the main reasons for reserving this option for those patients with liver failure. Depending on the underlying cause, liver replacement may correct the hypercoagulable state providing a phenotypic cure. For the remaining patients, long-term anticoagulation is essential after transplantation to avoid recurrence of the syndrome. Regardless of the treatment—TIPS, surgical shunt, or liver transplantation—the eventual outcome depends largely on the ability to control the underlying disorder.

ACKNOWLEDGMENT

The authors are grateful to Victor Javier Casillas, MD, for providing us with the radiologic images for this chapter.

REFERENCES

1. Stambo GW, Guiney MJ, Cannella XF, et al: Coil embolization of multiple hepatic artery aneurysms in a patient with undiagnosed polyarteritis nodosa. *J Vasc Surg* 39:1122, 2004.
2. Pollono EN, Madoff DC, Spence SC, et al: Multiple hepatic artery aneurysms in a patient with systemic lupus erythematosus. *Lupus* 19:93, 2010.
3. Yi IK, Miao FL, Wong J, et al: Prophylactic embolization of hepatic artery pseudoaneurysm after blunt abdominal trauma in a child. *J Pediatr Surg* 45:837, 2010.
4. Hylton JR, Pevec WC: Successful treatment of an iatrogenic right hepatic artery pseudoaneurysm and stenosis with a stent graft. *J Vasc Surg* 51:1510, 2010.
5. Jordan M, Razvi S, Worthington M: Mycotic hepatic artery aneurysm complicating *Staphylococcus aureus* endocarditis: Successful diagnosis and treatment. *Clin Infect Dis* 39:756, 2004.
6. Alamo JM, Gomez MA, Tamayo MJ, et al: Mycotic pseudoaneurysms after liver transplantation. *Transplant Proc* 37:1512, 2005.
7. Puilli R, Dorigo W, Troisi N, et al: Surgical treatment of visceral artery aneurysms: A 25-year experience. *J Vasc Surg* 48:334, 2008.
8. Abbas MA, Fowl RJ, Stone WM, et al: Hepatic artery aneurysm: Factors that predict complications. *J Vasc Surg* 38:41, 2003.
9. Yao CA, Arnell TD. Hepatic artery pseudoaneurysm following laparoscopic cholecystectomy. *Am J Surg* 199:e10, 2010.
10. Sebastian JJ, Pena E, Blas JM, et al: Fatal upper gastrointestinal bleeding due to hepatic artery pseudoaneurysm diagnosed by endoscopy. *Dig Dis Sci* 53:1152, 2008.
11. Lee CC, Jeng LB, Poon KS, et al: Fatal duodenal hemorrhage complicated after living donor liver transplantation: Case report. *Transplant Proc* 40:2840, 2008.
12. Tulsyan N, Kashyap VS, Greenberg RK, et al: The endovascular management of visceral artery aneurysms and pseudoaneurysms. *J Vasc Surg* 45:276, 2007.
13. Croce MA, Fabian TC, Spiers JP, et al: Traumatic hepatic artery pseudoaneurysm with hemobilia. *Am J Surg* 168:235, 1994.
14. Pearl J, Chao A, Kennedy S, et al: Traumatic injuries to the portal vein: Case study. *J Trauma* 56:779, 2004.
15. Croce MA, Fabian TC, Spiers JP, et al: Traumatic hepatic artery pseudoaneurysm with hemobilia. *Am J Surg* 168:235, 1994.
16. Delis SG, Bakoyiannis A, Selvaggi G, et al: Liver transplantation for severe hepatic trauma: Experience from a single center. *World J Gastroenterol* 15:1641, 2009.
17. Schmidt SC, Settmacher U, Langrehr JM, et al: Management and outcome of patients with combined bile duct and hepatic arterial injuries after laparoscopic cholecystectomy. *Surgery* 135:613, 2004.
18. Li J, Frilling A, Nadalin S, et al: Management of concomitant hepatic artery injury in patients with iatrogenic major bile duct injury after laparoscopic cholecystectomy. *Br J Surg* 95:460, 2008.
19. Bekker J, Ploem S, de Jong KP: Early hepatic artery thrombosis after liver transplantation: A systematic review of the incidence, outcome and risk factors. *Am J Transplant* 9:746, 2009.
20. Stewart ZA, Locke JE, Segev DL, et al: Increased risk of graft loss from hepatic artery thrombosis after liver transplantation with older donors. *Liver Transpl* 15:1688, 2009.
21. Nishida S, Kato T, Levi D, et al: Effect of protocol Doppler ultrasonography and urgent revascularization on early hepatic artery thrombosis after pediatric liver transplantation. *Arch Surg* 137:1279, 2002.
22. Gunsar F, Rolando N, Pastacaldi S, et al: Late hepatic artery thrombosis after liver transplantation. *Liver Transpl* 9:605, 2003.
23. O'Hanlon DM, McDonnell CO, Walsh T, et al: Traumatic arteriovenous fistula of the liver. *J Am Coll Surg* 193:575, 2001.
24. Sutcliffe R, Mieli-Vergani G, Dhawan A, et al: A novel treatment of congenital hepatoportal arteriovenous fistula. *J Pediatr Surg* 43:571, 2008.
25. Ishii H, Sonoyama T, Nakashima S, et al: Surgical treatment of hepatocellular carcinoma with severe intratumoral arterioportal shunt. *World J Gastroenterol* 16:3211, 2010.
26. Khalid SK, Garcia-Tsao G: Hepatic vascular malformations in hereditary hemorrhagic telangiectasia. *Semin Liver Dis* 28:247, 2008.
27. Kobayashi S, Asano T, Kenmochi T, et al: Arterio-portal shunt in liver rescued by hepatectomy after arterial embolization. *Hepatogastroenterology* 48:1730, 2001.
28. Moon SB, Kwon HJ, Park KW, et al: Clinical experience with infantile hepatic hemangioendothelioma. *World J Surg* 33:597, 2009.
29. Warmann S, Bertram H, Kardorff R, et al: Interventional treatment of infantile hepatic hemangioendothelioma. *J Pediatr Surg* 38:1177, 2003.
30. Dupuis-Girod S, Chesnais AL, Ginon I, et al: Long-term outcome of patients with hereditary hemorrhagic telangiectasia and severe hepatic involvement and orthotopic liver transplantation: A single-center study. *Liver Transpl* 16:340, 2010.
31. Cho SW, Marsh JW, Fontes PA, et al: Extrahepatic portal vein aneurysm: Report of six patients and review of the literature. *J Gastrointest Surg* 12:145, 2008.
32. Moreno JA, Fleming MD, Farnell MB, et al: Extrahepatic portal vein aneurysm. *J Vasc Surg* 2010 Aug 4. [Epub ahead of print].
33. Kao WY, Hung HH, Lu HC, et al: Hepatocellular carcinoma with presentation of Budd-Chiari syndrome. *J Chin Med Assoc* 73:93, 2010.
34. Cerwinka WH, Ciancio G, Salerno TA, et al: Renal cell cancer with invasive atrial tumor thrombus excised off-pump. *Urology* 66:1319, 2005.
35. Buzas C, Sparchez Z, Cucuianu A, et al: Budd-Chiari syndrome secondary to polycythemia vera. A case report. *J Gastrointestin Liver Dis* 18:363, 2009.
36. Klein AS, Molmenti EP: Surgical treatment of Budd-Chiari syndrome. *Liver Transpl* 9:891, 2003.
37. Menon KV, Shah V, Kamath PS: The Budd-Chiari syndrome. *N Engl J Med* 350:578, 2004.
38. Boozari B, Bahr MJ, Kubicka S, et al: Ultrasonography in patients with Budd-Chiari syndrome: Diagnostic signs and prognostic implications. *J Hepatol* 49:572, 2008.
39. Cura M, Haskal Z, Lopera J: Diagnostic and interventional radiology for Budd-Chiari syndrome. *Radiographics* 29:669, 2009.
40. Plessier A, Valla DC: Budd-Chiari syndrome. *Semin Liver Dis* 28:259, 2008.
41. Sharma S, Texeira A, Texeira P, et al: Pharmacological thrombolysis in Budd-Chiari syndrome: A single-centre experience with review of the literature. *J Hepatol* 40:172, 2004.
42. Liu XL, Li FQ, Li X, et al: Treatment of hepatic venous outflow stenosis after living donor liver transplantation by insertion of an expandable metallic stent. *Hepatobiliary Pancreat Dis Int* 8:424, 2009.
43. Oldhafer KJ, Frerker M, Prokop M, et al: Two-step procedure in Budd-Chiari syndrome with severe intrahepatic vena cava stenosis: Vena cava stenting and portocaval shunt. *Am J Gastroenterol* 93:1165, 1998.
44. Rossle M, Olschewski M, Siegerstetter V, et al: The Budd-Chiari syndrome: Outcome after treatment with transjugular intrahepatic portosystemic shunt. *Surgery* 135:394, 2004.

45. Mancuso A, Fung K, Mela M, et al: TIPS for acute and chronic Budd-Chiari syndrome: A single-centre experience. *J Hepatol* 38:751, 2003.

46. Murad SD, Luong TK, Pattynama PM, et al: Long-term outcome of a covered vs. uncovered transjugular intrahepatic portosystemic shunt in Budd-Chiari syndrome. *Liver Int* 28:249, 2008.

47. Orloff MJ, Daily PO, Orloff SL. A 27-year experience with surgical treatment of Budd-Chiari syndrome. *Ann Surg* 232:340, 2000.

48. Xu PQ, Ma XX, Ye XX, et al: Surgical treatment of 1360 cases of Budd-Chiari syndrome: 20-year experience. *Hepatobiliary Pancreat Dis Int* 3:391, 2004.

Drug-Induced Liver Disease

Rudra Rai | Anurag Maheshwari

Drug-induced hepatotoxicity is a frequent cause of liver injury.[1-4] It is the most frequent reason for withdrawal from the market of an approved drug and accounts for one-third to one-half of the cases of acute liver failure in the United States.[5] It can mimic both acute and chronic forms of liver disease and often represents an important diagnostic and therapeutic challenge for the treating physician. Although more than 1000 drugs are thought to have the potential to cause hepatotoxicity, only a handful have caused acute liver failure with resultant death or liver transplantation.[2,4]

EPIDEMIOLOGY

Drug-induced hepatotoxicity for most agents is relatively rare with the incidence ranging from 1 to 10 per 100,000 persons exposed.[1-5] It is higher for some agents such as isoniazid (INH) that can cause some form of liver injury in up to 2% of the exposed population. In general drugs that cause liver injury can be divided into two categories: (1) those that cause dose-dependent toxicity such as acetaminophen or tetracycline and (2) the vast majority of others that cause idiosyncratic reactions. For the former group, factors such as dose, blood level, and duration of intake play an important role in determining toxicity. For the latter group host factors such as age, gender, concomitant diseases, and other drug exposure are important factors.[6-8]

Age. Hepatic drug reactions are more common in the elderly and much less frequent among children. The exceptions include valproic acid, where hepatotoxicity is frequently seen among children younger than 3 years of age. Salicylic acid–induced Reye syndrome is also exclusively seen in children.

Gender. Women seem to be particularly predisposed to drug-induced hepatotoxicity, and a recent study noted that women comprised 76% of all transplant recipients for acute liver failure caused by drugs.[9]

Past Drug History. Cross-reactivity to related agents in cases of drug-induced liver injury are uncommon but have been reported, particularly with erythromycin-related compounds.

Concomitant Drugs. Recipients of polypharmacy are more likely to experience liver toxicity because of various mechanisms including enhanced cytochrome P450[7] metabolism that results in accumulation of the toxic metabolite, or delayed biliary excretion. Chronic alcohol ingestion can increase the severity of liver injury from certain agents such as acetaminophen and INH.[10-13]

Concomitant Illnesses. In general, preexisting liver disease[14] including cirrhosis is not a predisposition to adverse hepatic reactions with some exceptions. Human immunodeficiency virus (HIV) infection increases the risk of sulfonamide toxicity,[15-17] and renal transplantation is a risk factor for azathioprine-induced vascular injury.

PATHOPHYSIOLOGY

The liver is the site of first-pass metabolism and is highly exposed to drugs that are absorbed from the gastrointestinal tract. Drugs tend to be lipophilic compounds that are not readily excreted in bile or urine, so one of the functions of drug metabolism in the liver is its conversion to a hydrophilic substrate.[5,9,18-26] Drug metabolism in the liver is divided into three series of pathways: Phase 1 metabolism alters the parent molecule, phase 2 produces a conjugate of the drug or its metabolite, and phase 3 metabolism comprises energy-dependent pathways for excretion of the conjugate from the hepatocyte.

Phase 1. Phase 1 pathways include oxidation, reduction, and hydrolytic reactions. Most reactions are catalyzed by microsomal drug oxidases that act by way of the cytochrome P450 system. Reduced nicotinamide adenine dinucleotide phosphate in the cytosol acts as cofactor. A typical example is the production of N-acetyl-p-benzoquinone imine from acetaminophen mediated by the CYP2E1 pathway. Enzyme inducers include barbiturates, alcohol, anticonvulsants, rifampin, inhaled anesthetics, and oral hypoglycemic agents. Enzyme induction has implications for metabolism of other drugs and mechanisms for drug-induced liver injury.

Phase 2. These reactions involve the conjugation of the parent drug or its metabolite with a small endogenous molecule. The conjugates are highly water soluble and readily excreted in bile or urine. Conjugation is dependent on cofactors such as glucuronic acid and can be impaired by their depletion.

Phase 3. This involves the active excretion of drug and drug metabolites into bile or sinusoids and involves energy-dependent pathways mediated by the adenosine triphosphate binding cassette transport proteins. This system is located at the biliary pole of the hepatocyte and can be saturated, with implications for drug accumulation and cholestatic drug-induced liver injury.

MECHANISMS OF LIVER INJURY

Various mechanisms of drug-induced injury, as follows, have been identified that involve the hepatocyte,[5] and the manner in which the intracellular organelles are affected defines the pattern of disease:

1. Disruption of calcium homeostasis can result in actin disruption and loss of ionic gradient, which results in cell swelling and rupture.
2. Covalent binding of drug to the cytochrome P450 system involving high-energy reactions can lead to

the formation of nonfunctioning adducts. Such covalent binding may inactivate key enzymes in the cell; the protein-drug adducts may serve as immune targets inducing the formation of antibodies, or they can evoke a direct cytolytic T-cell response.

3. Oxidative stress in the liver can produce reactive oxygen species that disrupt mitochondrial DNA and microsomal electron transport systems. This results in the disruption of fatty acid metabolism and energy production with ensuing anaerobic metabolism and can result in lactic acidosis as well as microvesicular steatosis.

4. Drugs that affect transport proteins at the canalicular membrane can interrupt bile flow. Interruption of transport pumps such as multidrug resistance–associated protein 3 prevents the excretion of bilirubin, resulting in intracellular cholestasis causing secondary injury to the hepatocytes.

5. Other cells within the liver may be targets of injury or serve as modulators of injury. Activation of Kupffer cells may release reactive oxygen species and cytokines that amplify the injury to hepatocytes. Injury to hepatic sinusoidal endothelium can result in drug-induced vascular injury and the development of venoocclusive disease. Activation of hepatic stellate cells by methotrexate or vitamin A can result in increased matrix deposition with resultant fibrosis and cirrhosis.

Drugs can be divided into dose-dependent hepatotoxins or dose-independent (idiosyncratic) hepatotoxins. Dose-dependent hepatotoxins require activation to a toxic metabolite and interference with the function of intracellular organelles such as the mitochondria or canalicular biliary secretion. Liver injury caused by these drugs occurs after a short latent period, is characterized by zonal necrosis, and can be reproduced in other species. In contrast, idiosyncratic reactions cause a wide variety of histologic changes, exhibit a variable latent period to onset of injury, and cannot be reliably reproduced. Idiosyncratic hepatotoxicity is thought to occur by two major mechanisms: metabolic idiosyncrasy or immunoallergy. Metabolic idiosyncrasy is the susceptibility of rare individuals to a drug, which in conventional doses is usually safe. This susceptibility may be the result of genetic or acquired differences in drug metabolism or excretion. Immunoallergy indicates immune-mediated injury in response to the formation of adducts or hapten molecules, which may result from the interaction between the drug metabolite and the cell proteins or cytochrome P450 enzyme.

DIAGNOSIS AND TREATMENT OF DRUG-INDUCED LIVER DISEASE

Almost any drug has the potential for hepatotoxicity and should be suspected when considering the diagnosis.[5,27-42] Clinicians must have a high index of suspicion, and the history should include the dose, route, duration, and concomitant administration of all drugs (Table 126-1). Particular interest should be paid to the use of alternative and complementary medications because that history is

not easily forthcoming. The onset of injury is usually within 5 to 90 days of exposure to the drug. A positive dechallenge is defined as a drop in serum transaminase levels by 50% within days or weeks of cessation of the offending drug. Although a deliberate rechallenge is logistically and ethically impossible, an inadvertent rechallenge may give valuable evidence of a drug's hepatotoxicity. Other causes of liver disease such as viral hepatitis, autoimmune liver disease, or biliary obstruction must be excluded, and in difficult cases a liver biopsy may be useful. Although not universally recommended in all cases of drug-induced liver injury, certain findings such as steatosis, granulomas, zonal hepatic necrosis, bile duct lesions, and mixed hepatocellular necrosis with cholestasis may point toward a drug reaction. The treatment of drug-induced liver disease obviously includes cessation of the offending drug, and continuation of therapy after development of hepatotoxicity is a predictor of poor outcome. There is no role for glucocorticoids, although few reports have indicated benefit in cases of chronic hepatitis with autoimmune features. Ursodeoxycholic acid and cholestyramine may be useful for the treatment of pruritus in cases of cholestasis, along with supportive care for liver failure. Resolution of liver damage can take weeks to months after cessation of offending drug, although immediate improvement is the norm.

CONDITIONS ASSOCIATED WITH DRUG-INDUCED LIVER DAMAGE

HEPATOCELLULAR ZONE 3 NECROSIS

Liver injury observed in zone 3 is caused by dose-dependent hepatotoxins such as acetaminophen, carbon tetrachloride, *Amanita* mushrooms, and salicylates. Injury is rarely caused by the drug itself, and a toxic metabolite is usually responsible. The cytochrome P450 enzymes produce electrophilic drug metabolites. These metabolites then bind covalently to liver molecules that are essential to the life of a hepatocyte and necrosis occurs. In addition, exhaustion of intracellular substances (e.g., glutathione) capable of conjugating the toxic metabolite contributes to further damage. Histologically, damage is greatest in zone 3 where the cytochrome P450 enzymes are present in highest concentration and sinusoidal oxygen tension is the lowest. Hepatic necrosis is dose dependent, and marked elevations in serum transaminases are seen. Enzyme induction enhances drug toxicity as evidenced by chronic alcohol ingestion that induces the CYP2E1 enzyme, which is important in generating toxic metabolites of acetaminophen. As a result, as little as 4 g can cause serious liver toxicity in chronic alcoholics. Rats pretreated with phenobarbital show increased zone 3 necrosis following carbon tetrachloride ingestion, and cimetidine can modify the hepatotoxicity of acetaminophen by inhibition of the cytochrome P450 system.

Carbon Tetrachloride. Ingestion of this toxic solvent may be accidental or suicidal. It is used in dry-cleaning liquids and fire extinguishers. Liver injury is induced by a toxic metabolite, and its production depends on the cytochrome P450 oxygenase enzyme. This enzyme can be

TABLE 126-1 Classification of Drug-Induced Liver Injury Based on Histologic Damage

Histologic Damage	Histologic Features	Commonly Associated Drugs
Zone 3 necrosis	Hepatocellular necrosis in zone 3 (region of lowest sinusoidal O₂ tension)	*Amanita* mushroom, CCl₄, acetaminophen
Zone 1 necrosis	Periportal hepatocellular necrosis	Yellow phosphorus
Mitochondrial cytopathies	Steatosis, occasional cholestasis with focal hepatocellular cell death	Valproate, HAART, tetracyclines
Steatohepatitis	NASH, fibrosis, and cirrhosis	Amiodarone, tamoxifen, methotrexate, perhexiline
Acute hepatitis	Acute hepatocellular necrosis, occasional plasma cells, submassive to massive necrosis	Nitrofurantoin, phenytoin, methyldopa, disulfiram, sulfonamides, isoniazid, ketoconazole, troglitazone
Chronic hepatitis	Spotty hepatocellular necrosis, occasional plasma cells, bridging fibrosis	Nitrofurantoin, methyldopa, diclofenac, minocycline, isoniazid, dantrolene
Canalicular cholestasis	Cholestasis without associated hepatitis	Synthetic estrogens, androgens, cyclosporine
Hepatocanalicular cholestasis	Cholestasis with associated hepatitis and inflammation	Chlorpromazine, clavulanic acid, dextropropoxyphene, erythromycin
Venoocclusive disease	Zone 3 inflammation and fibrosis with intimal edema and sclerosis	Cyclophosphamide, busulfan, carmustine, etoposide, azathioprine, total-body irradiation, Jamaican bush tea, comfrey
Nodular regenerative hyperplasia	Endotheliitis of hepatic arterioles and portal venules	Chemotherapeutic agents, especially alkylating agents
Noncirrhotic portal hypertension	Portal venular sclerosis with periportal fibrosis	Arsenic, vitamin A, methotrexate, vinyl chloride
Peliosis hepatis	Blood-filled cavities without endothelial lining	Androgens, azathioprine, tamoxifen, estrogens, vitamin A
Hepatic adenoma	Single or multiple adenomas	Estrogens, anabolic steroids, danazol
Hepatocellular carcinoma	Overlap with adenoma	Long-term estrogen use (>8 yr)
Angiosarcoma	Malignant transformation of endothelium	Androgenic metabolic steroids, vinyl chloride, arsenic salts, thorium and copper salts

HAART, Highly active antiretroviral therapy; *NASH,* nonalcoholic steatohepatitis.

induced by prior alcohol and barbiturate intake and may potentiate toxicity. Clinical features include vomiting, abdominal pain, and diarrhea followed by jaundice. In severe cases, acute renal failure overshadows the liver toxicity and death is usual. If the patient survives, there seems to be no evidence for chronic liver damage in humans. Acute poisoning is treated by a high-carbohydrate diet in addition to supportive therapy for hepatic and renal failure. Prompt administration of acetylcysteine may help minimize hepatic damage.

Amanita **Mushrooms.** Ingestion of a single *Amanita* mushroom can cause acute liver failure, and the syndrome is common in Western Europe where mushroom hunting is more popular than in the United States. Clinical features include nausea, cramping, abdominal pain, and watery diarrhea. This can last for 3 to 5 days and is usually followed by massive hepatorenal and nervous system necrosis. Spontaneous recovery can occur, although patients usually require liver transplantation. Silymarin has been used as an antidote for the mushroom toxin phalloidin.

Acetaminophen. Liver toxicity is caused by the toxic metabolite, *N*-acetyl-*p*-benzoquinone imine. This metabolite is generated by the CYP2E1 enzyme and is inactivated by glutathione. Cell damage follows the depletion of glutathione, and enzyme induction by alcohol or drugs such as INH or anticonvulsants increases toxicity. As a result, as little as 4 to 8 g/day may produce liver damage in an alcoholic patient, whereas a minimum of 8 to 10 g is necessary to produce hepatic necrosis in adults. Clinical features include nausea and emesis soon after ingestion followed by an apparent period of recovery for 48 hours. Thereafter the patient deteriorates and develops jaundice, and significant elevations of serum transaminases are seen. Renal failure follows in as many as one-third of cases, and hypoglycemia is a prominent feature late in the disease. The Kings College criteria for fulminant hepatic failure identifies those patients with a poor prognosis who usually require transplantation, although spontaneous recovery is the norm without late sequelae. Specific treatment of acetaminophen overdose includes the use of *N*-acetylcysteine, which should be given as early as possible after ingestion.[43,44] Guidelines for its use are based on a nomogram plotting serum acetaminophen levels against time from ingestion. Although maximum benefit is achieved when *N*-acetylcysteine is given within 16 hours of ingestion, its use is recommended for all patients with evidence of significant liver injury irrespective of time from ingestion. The mechanism of action is the replenishment of glutathione reserves in the hepatocyte.[45] Fulminant hepatic failure requires liver transplantation, although its necessity is diminishing with time.[2,5,46]

HEPATOCELLULAR ZONE 1 NECROSIS

Yellow Phosphorus. Approximately 50 to 60 g may be a lethal dose, and ingestion is usually suicidal or accidental. Necrosis is predominantly in zone 1 (periportal areas), and patients develop jaundice 2 to 4 days after ingestion. There is no specific antidote, and fulminant hepatic failure often develops with mortality rates as high as 50%. No late sequelae have been described.

MITOCHONDRIAL CYTOPATHIES

Some drugs predominantly inhibit mitochondrial function causing lactic acidosis and hypoglycemia. β-Oxidation of fatty acids in the mitochondria is associated with microvesicular steatosis.

Valproic Acid. Younger patients are more susceptible to valproic acid–associated liver damage, which can be severe and sometimes fatal. More than two-thirds of reported cases have been younger than 10 years of age. Males are particularly affected, and clinical presentation occurs between 2 and 12 months of onset of therapy. Sodium valproate or its metabolites interfere with mitochondrial function and the susceptibility may be genetic. Some reports have suggested that patients with severe reactions to valproate may have inborn deficiencies of urea cycle enzymes. Liver biopsy usually demonstrates microvesicular steatosis with hepatocellular necrosis in zone 3, and electron microscopy shows mitochondrial destruction.

Tetracyclines. Large intravenous doses have been associated with hepatic failure, particularly in pregnant women. It has also been associated with acute fatty liver of pregnancy and therefore should be avoided during pregnancy.

Highly Active Antiretroviral Therapy. The frequency of hepatic injury with combination therapy is estimated to be 10% or more. Whether concomitant hepatitis C infection increases the risk of drug-induced toxicity is unclear. All nucleoside and nucleotide analogues can inhibit mitochondrial DNA polymerase causing cell death. Although zidovudine and didanosine are the most commonly reported hepatotoxins, all drugs in this category can cause liver injury with the exception of lamivudine. Several cases of fulminant liver failure associated with didanosine have been reported, and the clinical course is characterized by severe metabolic acidosis with multiorgan failure leading to death. Drug combinations seem more likely to result in hepatotoxicity compared to monotherapy. Among the protease inhibitors, indinavir and ritonavir have been most commonly reported to cause liver injury. The pattern of injury is usually mixed with prominent steatosis, associated with cholestasis and focal hepatic injury. Recovery from protease inhibitor–associated liver injury is slower when compared to other antiretroviral drugs.

STEATOHEPATITIS, FIBROSIS, AND CIRRHOSIS

Nonalcoholic steatohepatitis (NASH) can produce focal liver injury, Mallory hyaline, and inflammation with fibrosis.

Amiodarone. Amiodarone can cause a variety of adverse effects with abnormal liver tests seen in 15% to 50% of treated patients. There are rare cases of acute liver failure, although the typical lesion is steatohepatitis. Cirrhosis may develop in rare cases, and progression of disease may occur after drug discontinuation because of prolonged storage of the drug in the liver. Liver disease is usually detected a year after beginning therapy, and symptoms may range from asymptomatic elevations of liver function tests (LFTs) to jaundice with features of cirrhosis. Serial LFT monitoring is recommended in all patients treated with this drug.

Tamoxifen. The development of steatosis in women administered tamoxifen correlates with other risk factors for NASH such as obesity and insulin resistance. Tamoxifen may play a synergistic role with other risk factors to produce NASH. Although steatosis is the most commonly reported form of liver injury, it has been associated with cholestasis, acute hepatitis, peliosis hepatis, and fulminant hepatic failure. Although most cases of abnormal LFTs improve after cessation of tamoxifen, underlying NASH or metastatic breast cancer may be the cause in other cases. Monitoring for patients on tamoxifen should include periodic LFT determinations with yearly imaging tests.

Methotrexate. Methotrexate causes dose-dependent liver injury resulting in fibrosis and cirrhosis. Risk factors for methotrexate-induced fibrosis include total dose, alcohol intake, and preexisting liver disease. Cirrhosis can be complicated by the development of hepatocellular cancer. Serum transaminases correlate poorly with the degree of fibrosis but should be monitored routinely because elevations may indicate the need for a liver biopsy. It is now recommended that liver biopsy be performed after 4 g of cumulative dose or 2 years of therapy, and strict avoidance of alcohol should be emphasized. There have been reports of liver transplantation for severe methotrexate-associated liver injury.

Other Drugs. Other drugs associated with the development of steatosis include perhexiline, synthetic estrogens in large doses, calcium channel blockers, and methyldopa. Perhexiline has now been withdrawn from the market, and the association with other drugs may be anecdotal and related to other risk factors for NASH such as diabetes, obesity, and hyperlipidemia.

ACUTE HEPATITIS

The reaction is characterized by acute cell death and associated inflammation.[47-52] Severe forms of acute hepatitis can cause fulminant hepatic failure. Acute hepatitis is the most commonly reported drug reaction. The reaction is usually immunoallergic, although some drugs cause reactions by metabolic idiosyncrasy and lack typical features of the immunoallergic reaction. The immunoallergic reaction occurs more commonly in women and usually presents with prodromal symptoms after a latent period of 2 to 10 weeks. Eosinophilia is a common feature, and extrahepatic manifestations such as rash and lymphadenopathy are also seen. Autoantibodies may be detected in the serum and improvement after discontinuation of the drug is prompt. In contrast, the idiosyncratic reaction lacks the classic prodromal symptoms and extrahepatic manifestations and eosinophilia is rarely observed. Other drugs (e.g., alcohol, rifampin) may exacerbate the reaction, and improvement after drug discontinuation is variable.

IMMUNOALLERGY

Nitrofurantoin. This drug can cause liver toxicity ranging from acute hepatitis to chronic hepatitis, cholestasis, granulomatous hepatitis, and cirrhosis. The frequency of liver damage increases with age and is more common in women. Chronicity usually depends on the duration of drug ingestion. Early symptoms are frequently nonspecific (e.g., fever, weight loss, and anorexia) and are followed by more specific symptoms of liver disease such as jaundice, pruritus, and high-colored urine. Patients with chronic hepatitis may show signs such as spider angiomata, splenomegaly, and ascites. Autoantibodies are frequently noted, as is an increase in serum globulins. Eosinophilia may also be present in one-third of cases. Recovery is rapid after drug discontinuation, and systemic steroids have not proven useful even in cases of chronic hepatitis associated with autoimmune features.

Methyldopa. The clinical features of hepatotoxicity are similar to those noted with nitrofurantoin. Hepatic damage can range from acute hepatitis, cholestasis, chronic hepatitis, and cirrhosis.

Phenytoin. Drug toxicity occurs in equal frequency among children and adults. The systemic features of immunoallergy such as fever, rash, eosinophilia, and lymphadenopathy are common. A familial enzyme defect in the metabolism of phenytoin has been identified, suggesting that not all reactions are immunoallergic. The mortality rate is high among patients with jaundice. The most common reaction associated with phenytoin is related to microsomal induction with elevated γ-glutamyl transpeptidase and alkaline phosphatase levels in a large proportion of cases.

Sulfonamides. Hepatotoxicity usually occurs as part of the broader serum sickness (Stevens-Johnson syndrome) reaction caused by the sulfa moiety. Reactions may be severe and have caused death due to hepatic failure. Patients infected with HIV have a higher predilection for sulfa toxicity. Hepatotoxicity caused by sulfamethoxazole plus trimethoprim (Bactrim) is frequently due to trimethoprim, which causes a cholestatic picture.

Minocycline. Tetracycline can rarely cause acute hepatitis, and minocycline has been associated with the development of drug-induced autoimmune hepatitis.

Disulfiram. A drug used to treat alcoholism itself is associated with acute hepatitis that can be fatal and has required liver transplantation.

Etretinate. This is a synthetic retinoid used for dermatologic conditions that has been associated with abnormal LFTs in up to one-fourth of cases. A few cases of severe acute hepatitis have been reported mostly in older women. LFTs may improve with dose reduction implying dose-dependent toxicity, but the compound has a long half-life, necessitating periodic monitoring of alanine aminotransferase (ALT) levels.

Zafirlukast. This leukotriene antagonist used in the treatment of asthma has been associated with rare cases of acute liver failure and patients treated with it should have periodic monitoring of ALT levels.

METABOLIC IDIOSYNCRASY

Isoniazid. Ten percent to 36% of persons taking INH develop asymptomatic elevations of LFTs in the first 8 weeks that resolve spontaneously. Acute hepatitis is seen in up to 2% of individuals, with the highest risk for women older than 50 years of age and those on combination drug regimens using rifampin and pyrazinamide.

Chronic excessive alcohol intake and acetaminophen use also increase the risk of toxicity, as may concomitant illnesses such as malnutrition and chronic hepatitis B and C. Clinical symptoms include nonspecific anorexia and weight loss preceding jaundice 8 to 12 weeks after starting therapy. Although the hepatitis resolves rapidly on stopping the drug, prognosis is poorer for those with high bilirubin levels. The severity of reaction is higher in cases of continued ingestion after development of symptoms and has required transplantation on occasion. Rechallenge has not been proved to cause recurrent hepatitis especially with slow reintroduction of the drug. Biweekly or monthly monitoring of LFTs during therapy has been advocated to monitor for hepatotoxicity. Rifampin and pyrazinamide have both been associated with hepatotoxicity, although most often in combination with INH.

Antifungals. Ketoconazole is associated with increased LFTs in up to 17% of patients treated for onychomycosis. Symptomatic hepatitis is rare and seen more frequently in older women. LFTs improve rapidly after drug discontinuation, although rare cases requiring transplantation have been reported. Terbinafine has been reported to cause prolonged cholestasis occurring 4 to 6 weeks after starting therapy. Periodic monitoring of LFTs during therapy is recommended. Fluconazole and itraconazole have also rarely been associated with hepatotoxicity, although the frequency is much lower than that seen with ketoconazole.

Troglitazone. This drug seemed free of hepatotoxicity in early clinical trials, but postmarketing data found significant cases of fatal hepatotoxicity. The mechanism of injury seems to be metabolic idiosyncrasy, although immunologic injury may play a role in some cases, and cross-reaction with rosiglitazone has been observed. There is no clear relationship of toxicity to dose or timing. Nor has screening by ALT monitoring always proven useful in preventing the development of acute hepatitis. Mortality is higher in older patients and several cases requiring liver transplantation have been reported. The drug was withdrawn from the U.S. market in March 2000.

CHRONIC HEPATITIS

Although the true definition of chronicity is persistence of inflammation more than 6 months after its onset, in cases of drug-induced hepatitis, clinical and biochemical evidence of liver injury associated with histologic changes of fibrosis confirms the diagnosis of drug-induced chronic hepatitis.[47-52] There are two distinct clinical pictures associated with this form of drug toxicity. The first scenario resembles acute hepatitis that either persists longer or is delayed in recognition without signs or symptoms of chronic liver disease. The second syndrome resembles autoimmune hepatitis in serologic and histologic features. The management of both syndromes consists of drug withdrawal and supportive care, although glucocorticoids have shown to benefit those with autoimmune features. The drugs most commonly associated with chronic hepatitis include nitrofurantoin, methyldopa, diclofenac, minocycline, INH, dantrolene, and etretinate. Indeed, a large number of patients thought to have chronic drug-induced hepatitis in the past were found to have chronic hepatitis C, and the evidence for causality is not always convincing.

CHOLESTASIS

Drugs can cause cholestasis with or without concomitant hepatitis. Clinical and biochemical features resemble many hepatobiliary conditions, and imaging is often necessary to exclude biliary obstruction. A liver biopsy is often helpful in the diagnostic algorithm and histologic features of acute hepatitis with cholestasis are highly suggestive of a drug reaction. Clinical features include pruritus, jaundice, and dark-colored urine. Glucocorticoids have no role in management, and resolution of jaundice may take a few weeks after discontinuation of the drug. Cholestyramine and ursodeoxycholic acid are first-line therapies for pruritus, although phenobarbital, antihistamines, rifampin, phototherapy, plasmapheresis, and naloxone all have been attempted with variable success.

Canalicular Cholestasis

Cholestasis without associated hepatitis is caused by the retention of bile within the biliary canaliculi. This represents a primary disturbance in biliary flow and susceptibility may be related to genetic variations in biliary transporters. Various androgens and estrogens are the typical causative agent. The cause is usually, although not always, a C-17 alkylated testosterone, and the reaction is dose dependent and reversible. Cyclosporine also inhibits adenosine triphosphate–dependent bile salt transport. Hyperbilirubinemia is common with features of cholestasis. The reaction is frequently mild and reverses rapidly with dose reduction.

Hepatocanalicular Cholestasis

The histologic picture of cholestasis predominates but is associated with hepatocellular features including cell death and inflammation. There is considerable overlap with drug-induced hepatitis, and the immunodestructive injury focuses on the bile ducts. The acute reaction may resolve in 3 months, but cases of protracted cholestasis have been reported, some requiring liver transplantation caused by progressive ductopenia.

Chlorpromazine. Up to 2% of patients taking the drug may develop cholestatic hepatitis. There is no relationship to dose, and the onset is usually within 4 weeks of starting therapy. Female predominance suggests an autoimmune cause. Patients present with pruritus preceding jaundice in a syndrome that resembles acute viral hepatitis. Recovery is usual with discontinuation; however, a few cases of prolonged cholestasis with ductopenia requiring transplantation have been reported.

Amoxicillin/Clavulanic Acid. Clavulanic acid is the hepatotoxic agent because liver injury caused by amoxicillin is rare. Cholestasis is noted predominantly in older men on long-term therapy and may evolve into prolonged cholestasis with vanishing bile duct syndrome. Recovery after drug discontinuation is usual.

Dextropropoxyphene. This is an opioid analgesic that can cause cholestatic hepatitis associated with injury to the bile ducts. The onset of symptoms is within 2 weeks of the first dose and consists of abdominal pain as the presenting sign. This can be followed by recurrent jaundice and rigors mimicking structural biliary disease. Biliary imaging is usually normal and LFTs improve within a couple of months after stopping the drug.

Erythromycin. Hepatotoxicity seems more common with the estolate salt of the drug and is associated with fever, jaundice, and pruritus. Eosinophilia may be observed suggesting autoimmune disease. The predominant histologic feature is cholestasis with acidophil bodies, and recurrent jaundice may be noted with distant administration of other erythromycin derivatives.

VASCULAR TOXICITY

Venoocclusive Disease

The terminal hepatic venules and the small zone 3 hepatic veins are sensitive to endothelial damage by alkylating agents that cause intimal edema and subsequent collagen deposition. This can result in hepatic venous outflow tract obstruction, and patients present with painful hepatomegaly, jaundice, and ascites. Venoocclusive disease is particularly associated with the use of anticancer drugs such as cyclophosphamide, busulfan, carmustine, etoposide, and azathioprine, and total-body irradiation. Recipients of allogeneic bone marrow transplantation are frequently afflicted, and the onset is usually 2 to 10 weeks after therapy. Occasional cases may recover; however, prognosis is generally poor with death caused by liver failure a few weeks later. The condition was first described in association with Jamaican bush teas (that contain pyrrolizidine alkaloids) and later with comfrey as well.

Nodular Regenerative Hyperplasia

The condition is characterized by the development of regenerating nodules in the absence of fibrosis. The underlying lesion seems to be endothelial damage to the terminal hepatic arterioles and portal venules with the resulting ischemia inducing regenerative changes. The drugs implicated are similar to those implicated in the development of venoocclusive disease, and the two conditions frequently overlap. The clinical features are those of portal hypertension with esophageal varices. The overall prognosis is better than with venoocclusive disease, and complete reversal can occur with cessation of the offending drug.

Noncirrhotic Portal Hypertension

Noncirrhotic portal hypertension caused by drugs is usually the result of obstruction to portal blood flow. This is usually caused by sclerosis of the portal vein branches and is associated with a variable degree of periportal fibrosis. Agents associated with this condition include arsenic, vitamin A, methotrexate, and vinyl chloride. Clinical features of portal hypertension including splenomegaly, esophageal varices, and thrombocytopenia predominate. Angiosarcoma may be an occasional complication and has been reported with the use of arsenic and vinyl chloride.

Peliosis Hepatis

Peliosis hepatis refers to blood-filled cavities without endothelial lining. The lesions vary from a few millimeters to several centimeters. The disruption of normal sinusoidal architecture is the underlying disease. Peliosis hepatis has been associated with androgens, azathioprine, tamoxifen, estrogens, and possibly vitamin A. The condition has also complicated danazol therapy and is rarely suspected before surgery or liver biopsy. Rare cases of shock and abdominal pain because of rupture have been reported. Helical computed tomography or magnetic resonance imaging that can identify the lesion should be used to investigate unexplained hepatomegaly in a patient taking an implicated drug.

HEPATIC TUMORS

Hepatic Adenoma

High-dose estrogens in oral contraceptive pills, as well as anabolic steroids, have been implicated in the genesis of hepatic adenomas. Danazol, a synthetic steroid used for the treatment of hereditary angioedema, has been associated with the development of hepatic adenomas. Although regression of smaller lesions after withdrawal of steroids has been noted, resection may be necessary for larger or symptomatic lesions. Transition to hepatocellular cancer has been documented, and recurrence rate is high with pregnancy or continued steroid use.

Focal Nodular Hyperplasia

Although commonly observed in women in their reproductive years, the association between focal nodular hyperplasia and exogenous sex hormones is unproven. Estrogen has been shown to have a trophic effect on established lesions, and larger lesions should undergo resection especially if associated with symptoms.

Hepatocellular Carcinoma

The risk of hepatocellular carcinoma in patients on long-term (>8 years) estrogen use is higher, but estrogen-related hepatocellular carcinoma is rare as compared to other causative etiologies such as viral hepatitis. There have been cases reported of concomitant adenoma and carcinoma in the same liver, and recurrence rate of estrogen-induced tumors is high.

Angiosarcoma

Angiosarcoma is a rare liver tumor associated with androgenic metabolic steroids, vinyl chloride, arsenic salts, and thorium and copper salts. Cases are diagnosed 2 to 3 decades after exposure to toxic agents, and periodic hepatic imaging is indicated among patients with chronic liver disease and high levels of exposure.

ALTERNATIVE REMEDIES, RECREATIONAL DRUGS, AND ENVIRONMENTAL AGENTS

Numerous other medicinal and nonmedicinal compounds including vitamins, herbal remedies, environmental agents, and recreational drugs can cause various forms of hepatotoxicity. The increasing popularity of alternative medicines has led to many reports of associated toxicity. In most cases, the hepatotoxin is not readily apparent, and many preparations contain more than one ingredient that may be the culprit. The spectrum of toxicity ranges from acute hepatitis, chronic hepatitis with cirrhosis, cholestasis, and vascular injury. Chinese herbal

teas and other mixed preparations can cause a host of toxic reactions, and patient self-reporting may be unreliable to establish temporal relationships. Recreational drugs such as ecstasy and cocaine have been associated with hepatotoxicity severe enough to require liver transplantation. Hypervitaminosis A is now more commonly recognized as secondary to self-medication of large doses of vitamin A over prolonged periods. The pathologic spectrum of liver disease caused by vitamin A toxicity can range from abnormal LFTs, stellate cell hyperplasia, noncirrhotic portal hypertension, cirrhosis, and rare cases of peliosis hepatis. The prognosis is poorer in cases with established cirrhosis and portal hypertension, and patients with chronic liver diseases should be cautioned against vitamin A supplementation.

Update on Drug-Induced Acute Liver Failure

The Acute Liver Failure Study Group recently published an article looking at prospectively collected cases of all forms of acute liver failure since 1998 in a U.S. multicenter study.[53] They described subjects with idiosyncratic drug-induced liver injury–associated acute liver failure who were enrolled during a 10.5-year period. Data were collected prospectively, using detailed case report forms, from 1198 subjects enrolled at 23 sites in the United States, all of whom had transplant services. A total of 133 (11.1%) Acute Liver Failure Study Group subjects were deemed by expert opinion to have drug-induced liver injury; 81.1% were considered highly likely, 15.0% probable, and 3.8% possible. Subjects were mostly women (70.7%), and there was overrepresentation of minorities for unclear reasons. More than 60 individual agents were implicated; the most common were antimicrobials (46%) and to a lesser extent antiepileptics, antimetabolites, statins, and herbal products (Table 126-2). Presentations are subacute, and although spontaneous survival is infrequent, for many patients liver transplantation is often feasible and highly successful. Survival is determined by the degree of liver dysfunction.

CONCLUSION

Clinical trials are often inadequate in identifying a drug's potential for liver injury, and this may be evident only after the drug has been approved for public use.[5,54,55] The Food and Drug Administration has provided guidance for the pharmaceutical industry about drug-induced liver injury. Indeed, it acknowledges that during premarketing clinical evaluation, only the most overt hepatotoxins can be expected to show cases of severe liver injury in the 1000 to 3000 subjects typically studied and described in a new drug application. Although several drugs cause asymptomatic transient elevations of LFTs, the safety of such a reaction is questionable. LFTs should be monitored 3 to 4 weeks after commencing therapy with any drug that has the potential to cause liver toxicity. Continued administration of the offending drug after development of liver toxicity is the most common cause of poor outcome necessitating early recognition of the syndrome. The increasing use of complementary medications has raised awareness of their potential for liver toxicity among the medical community, although the lay public

TABLE 126-2 Causes of Drug-Induced Liver Injury–Associated Acute Liver Failure

A. ANTIMICROBIAL AGENTS	Cases (n)
Antituberculosis Drugs	25
Isoniazid alone	15
Isoniazid combined with 2 of 3: rifampin, pyrazinamide, and ethambutol	6
Rifampin and pyrazinamide with or without ethambutol	3
Dapsone	1
Sulfur-Containing Drugs	12
Trimethoprim/sulfamethoxazole alone	6
Trimethoprim/sulfamethoxazole in combination with azithromycin, statin, and/or antiretroviral drugs	3
Sulfasalazine	3
Other Antibiotics	19
Nitrofurantoin alone	11
Nitrofurantoin with a statin	1
Amoxicillin (2), doxycycline (2), ciprofloxacin (1), clarithromycin (1), cefepime (1)	7
Antifungal Agents	6
Terbinafine	3
Itraconazole	1
Ketoconazole alone	1
Ketoconazole with ezetimibe	1
Antiretroviral Drugs	4
Stavudine with didanosine	2
Lamivudine with stavudine and nelfinavir	1
Abacavir	1

B. CAMs AND ILLICIT SUBSTANCES, NEUROPSYCHOTROPIC DRUGS, AND ANESTHETICS	Cases (n)
CAMs and Illicit Substances	14
Unspecified herbal preparations	3
Usnic acid	2
Thermoslim (contains saw palmetto)	1
Herbal mixture (contains blue-green algae)	1
Ma-Huang	1
Horny goat weed	1
Black cohosh	1
Hydroxycut	1
Uva-ursi	1
Cocaine	1
Ecstasy	1

	Cases (n)
Antiepileptic Drugs	13
Phenytoin	8
Divalproic acid	2
Carbamazepine	3
Psychotropic Agents	4
Quetiapine	1
Nefazodone	1
Fluoxetine	1
Venlafaxine	1
Anesthetics	2
Halothane	1
Isoflurane	1

C. ANTIMETABOLITES AND ENZYME INHIBITORS, NSAIDS, BIOLOGICAL AGENTS, STATINS, AND OTHER DRUGS	Cases (n)
Antimetabolites and Enzyme Inhibitors	11
Disulfiram	4
Propylthiouracil	5
Allopurinol	1
Melphalan	1
NSAIDs	7
Bromfenac	4
Diclofenac	2
Etodolac	1
Biological Agents and Leukotriene Inhibitors	4
Gemtuzumab	1
Zafirlukast	1
Interferon β	1
Bacille-Calmette-Guérin (BCG)	1
*Statins And Ezetimibe**	6
Cerivastatin	2
Simvastatin (±ezetimibe)	2
Atorvastatin	2
Other Drugs	8
Troglitazone	4
Oxyiminoalkanoic acid derivative	1
Methyldopa	2
Hydralazine	1

*Reprinted with permission from Reuben A, Koch DG, Lee WM, et al: Drug-induced acute liver failure: Results of a U.S. multicenter, prospective study. *Hepatology* 52:2065-2076, 2010.
CAM, Complementary and alternative medicine; *NSAID*, nonsteroidal antiinflammatory drug.

must also be cautioned about the dangers of unregulated nonproprietary preparations. Practitioners are encouraged to report suspected drug reactions because underreporting is common, and improved reporting may help early recognition of drug toxicity.

REFERENCES

1. Lazarou J, Pomeranz BH, Corey PN: Incidence of adverse drug reactions in hospitalized patients. *JAMA* 279:1200, 1998.
2. Ostapowicz G, Fontana RJ, Schiødt FV, et al: Results of a prospective study of acute liver failure at 17 tertiary care centers in the United States. *Ann Intern Med* 137:947, 2002.
3. Bissell DM, Gores GJ, Laskin DL, et al: Drug-induced liver injury: Mechanisms and test systems. *Hepatology* 33:1009, 2001.
4. Center for Drug Evaluation and Research: Drug-induced liver toxicity. www.fda.gov/cder/livertox/default.htm.
5. Lee WM: Drug-induced hepatotoxicity. *N Engl J Med* 349:474, 2003.
6. Weinshilboum R: Inheritance and drug response. *N Engl J Med* 348:529, 2003.
7. Guengerich FP: Common and uncommon cytochrome P450 reactions related to metabolism and chemical toxicity. *Chem Res Toxicol* 14:611, 2001.

8. Hunt CM, Westerkam WR, Stave GM: Effect of age and gender on the activity of human hepatic CYP3A. *Biochem Pharmacol* 44:275, 1992.

9. Russo MW, Galanko JA, Shrestha R, et al: Liver transplantation for acute liver failure from drug-induced liver injury in the United States. *Liver Transpl* 10:1018, 2004.

10. Ikemoto S, Imaoka S, Hayahara N, et al: Expression of hepatic microsomal cytochrome P450s as altered by uremia. *Biochem Pharmacol* 43:2407, 1992.

11. Moss AJ: The QT interval and torsades de pointes. *Drug Saf* 21:5, 1999.

12. Thummel KE, Slattery JT, Ro H, et al: Ethanol and production of the hepatotoxic metabolite of acetaminophen in healthy adults. *Clin Pharmacol Ther* 67:591, 2000.

13. Welch KD, Wen B, Goodlett DR, et al: Proteomic identification of potential susceptibility factors in drug-induced liver disease. *Chem Res Toxicol* 18:924, 2005.

14. Powell EE, Jonsson JR, Clouston AD: Steatosis: Co-factor in other liver diseases. *Hepatology* 42:5, 2005.

15. Dieterich DT, Robinson PA, Love J, et al: Drug-induced liver injury associated with the use of nonnucleoside reverse-transcriptase inhibitors. *Clin Infect Dis* 38:S80, 2004.

16. Pol S, Lebray P, Vallet-Pichard A: HIV infection and hepatic enzyme abnormalities: Intricacies of the pathogenic mechanisms. *Clin Infect Dis* 38:S65, 2004.

17. Ena J, Amador C, Benito C, et al: Risk and determinants of developing severe liver toxicity during therapy with nevirapine-and efavirenz-containing regimens in HIV-infected patients. *Int J STD AIDS* 14:776, 2003.

18. Korenblat KM, Berk PD: Hyperbilirubinemia in the setting of antiviral therapy. *Clin Gastroenterol Hepatol* 3:303, 2005.

19. Lazerow SK, Abdi MS, Lewis JH: Drug-induced liver disease 2004. *Curr Opin Gastroenterol* 21:283, 2005.

20. Fernández-Villar A, Sopeña B, Fernández-Villar J, et al: The influence of risk factors on the severity of anti-tuberculosis drug-induced hepatotoxicity. *Int J Tuberc Lung Dis* 8:1499, 2004.

21. Anfossi G, Massucco P, Bonomo K, et al: Prescription of statins to dyslipidemic patients affected by liver diseases: A subtle balance between risks and benefits. *Nutr Metab Cardiovasc Dis* 14:215, 2004.

22. Sniderman AD: Is there value in liver function test and creatine phosphokinase monitoring with statin use? *Am J Cardiol* 94:30F, 2004.

23. Lee WM: Acetaminophen and the U.S. Acute Liver Failure Study Group: Lowering the risks of hepatic failure. *Hepatology* 40:6, 2004.

24. Arora A, Shukla Y: Induction of preneoplastic altered hepatic foci following dietary sulphur supplementation. *Hum Exp Toxicol* 23:229, 2004.

25. de Abajo FJ, Montero D, Madurga M, et al: Acute and clinically relevant drug-induced liver injury: A population-based case-control study. *Br J Clin Pharmacol* 58:71, 2004.

26. Shakya R, Rao BS, Shrestha B: Incidence of hepatotoxicity due to antitubercular medicines and assessment of risk factors. *Ann Pharmacother* 38:1074, 2004.

27. Pollak PT, Shafer SL: Use of population modeling to define rational monitoring of amiodarone hepatic effects. *Clin Pharmacol Ther* 75:342, 2004.

28. Nygaard U, Toft N, Schmiegelow K: Methylated metabolites of 6-mercaptopurine are associated with hepatotoxicity. *Clin Pharmacol Ther* 75:274, 2004.

29. Linnebur SA, Parnes BL: Pulmonary and hepatic toxicity due to nitrofurantoin and fluconazole treatment. *Ann Pharmacother* 38:612, 2004.

30. Robinson K, Lambiase L, Li J, et al: Fatal cholestatic liver failure associated with gemcitabine therapy. *Dig Dis Sci* 48:1804, 2003.

31. Velayudham LS, Farrell GC: Drug-induced cholestasis. *Expert Opin Drug Saf* 2:287, 2003.

32. Kontorinis N, Dieterich D: Hepatotoxicity of antiretroviral therapy. *AIDS Rev* 5:36, 2003.

33. Spigset O, Hägg S, Bate A: Hepatic injury and pancreatitis during treatment with serotonin reuptake inhibitors: Data from the World Health Organization (WHO) database of adverse drug reactions. *Int Clin Psychopharmacol* 18:157, 2003.

34. Shukla Y, Arora A: Enhancing effects of mustard oil on preneoplastic hepatic foci development in Wistar rats. *Hum Exp Toxicol* 22:51, 2003.

35. Chan KA, Truman A, Gurwitz JH, et al: A cohort study of the incidence of serious acute liver injury in diabetic patients treated with hypoglycemic agents. *Arch Intern Med* 163:728, 2003.

36. Pollak PT, You YD: Monitoring of hepatic function during amiodarone therapy. *Am J Cardiol* 91:613, 2003.

37. Angles A, Bagheri H, Montastruc JL, et al: Le Reseau Francais des Centres Regionaux de Pharmacovigilance. [Adverse drug reactions (ADRs) to antimalarial drugs. Analysis of spontaneous report from the French pharmacovigilance database (1996-2000).] *Presse Med* 32:106, 2003.

38. Graham DJ, Drinkard CR, Shatin D: Incidence of idiopathic acute liver failure and hospitalized liver injury in patients treated with troglitazone. *Am J Gastroenterol* 98:175, 2003.

39. Bull RJ, Orner GA, Cheng RS, et al: Contribution of dichloroacetate and trichloroacetate to liver tumor induction in mice by trichloroethylene. *Toxicol Appl Pharmacol* 182:55, 2002.

40. Clark DW, Layton D, Wilton LV, et al: Profiles of hepatic and dysrhythmic cardiovascular events following use of fluoroquinolone antibacterials: Experience from large cohorts from the Drug Safety Research Unit Prescription-Event Monitoring database. *Drug Saf* 24:1143, 2001.

41. Ward E, Boffetta P, Andersen A, et al: Update of the follow-up of mortality and cancer incidence among European workers employed in the vinyl chloride industry. *Epidemiology* 12:710, 2001.

42. Roy B, Chowdhury A, Kundu S, et al: Increased risk of antituberculosis drug-induced hepatotoxicity in individuals with glutathione S-transferase M1 "null" mutation. *J Gastroenterol Hepatol* 16:1033, 2001.

43. James LP, Wells E, Beard RH, et al: Predictors of outcome after acetaminophen poisoning in children and adolescents. *J Pediatr* 140:522, 2002.

44. Mitchell I, Bihari D, Chang R, et al: Earlier identification of patients at risk from acetaminophen-induced acute liver failure. *Crit Care Med* 26:279, 1998.

45. Kerr F, Dawson A, Whyte IM, et al: The Australasian Clinical Toxicology Investigators Collaboration randomized trial of different loading infusion rates of N-acetylcysteine. *Ann Emerg Med* 45:402, 2005.

46. Lee WS, McKiernan P, Kelly DA: Etiology, outcome and prognostic indicators of childhood fulminant hepatic failure in the United Kingdom. *J Pediatr Gastroenterol Nutr* 40:575, 2005.

47. Cullen JM: Mechanistic classification of liver injury. *Toxicol Pathol* 33:6, 2005.

48. Watkins PB: Idiosyncratic liver injury: Challenges and approaches. *Toxicol Pathol* 33:1, 2005.

49. Chalasani N: Statins and hepatotoxicity: Focus on patients with fatty liver. *Hepatology* 41:690, 2005.

50. Klein C, Wüstefeld T, Assmus U, et al: The IL-6-gp130-STAT3 pathway in hepatocytes triggers liver protection in T cell–mediated liver injury. *J Clin Invest* 115:860, 2005.

51. Saito T, Kwon AH, Qiu Z, et al: Protective effect of fibronectin for endotoxin-induced liver injury after partial hepatectomy in rats. *J Surg Res* 124:79, 2005.

52. Roth RA, Ganey PE: Successes and frustrations in developing animal models of idiosyncratic drug reactions. *Chem Biol Interact* 152:165, 2005.

53. Reuben A, Koch DG, Lee WM, et al: Drug-induced acute liver failure: Results of a U.S. multicenter, prospective study. *Hepatology* 52:2065, 2010.

54. Ruiz Montero A, Durán Quintana JA, Jiménez Sáenz M, et al: A strategy to improve the detection of drug-induced hepatotoxicity. *Rev Esp Enferm Dig* 97:155, 2005.

55. Lee WM, Senior JR: Recognizing drug-induced liver injury: Current problems, possible solutions. *Toxicol Pathol* 33:155, 2005.

Benign Hepatic Neoplasms

Georg Lurje | Philipp Dutkowski | Pierre-Alain Clavien

Widespread use and progress in modern imaging modalities (especially ultrasound) have led to a more frequent discovery of incidental hepatic lesions. Despite refinements in contrast-enhanced computed tomography (ce-CT) and magnetic resonance imaging (MRI), the differential diagnosis of patients presenting with focal liver lesions is broad and remains a challenge in the management of these patients. As such, a correct evaluation of the lesion is critical, as further management depends on the exact diagnosis and differentiation from a malignant process. In this regard, life-long followup of a young patient might be more distressing and costly than definitive resection and may therefore represent a good indication for laparoscopy if the location is suitable (i.e., the lesion is in the lateral and anterior segments). Therefore, an interdisciplinary approach (past medical history, clinical symptoms, imaging studies) remains the gold standard in the management of patients with focal liver lesions. This was also illustrated in a Japanese study involving patients with hepatic lesions in whom initial evaluation could not exclude a malignant process. All patients underwent extensive laboratory and imaging workup studies and were referred for surgical resection. Interestingly, preoperative diagnoses proved to be correct in 156 of 160 patients (98%).[1] Nevertheless, an aggressive surgical approach is warranted when there is any suspicion of malignancy. Clinically, the most important benign liver lesions are hemangioma, focal nodular hyperplasia (FNH), and hepatic adenoma, but a variety of other rare lesions have also been described.

HEMANGIOMA

Hepatic hemangiomas (also referred to as cavernous hemangiomas) are the most common benign neoplasms of the liver. Estimates of the prevalence range from 0.4% to 10% of the population, although one autopsy series explicitly searching for hepatic lesions suggested a prevalence as high as 20%.[2] Hepatic hemangiomas are usually small (<5 cm) and incidentally discovered during abdominal imaging studies for unrelated causes. Lesions larger than 5 cm have been arbitrarily termed giant hemangiomas. Patients presenting for evaluation of hepatic hemangioma are predominantly female (2:1 to 4:1) and 60% to 80% of cases are diagnosed in patients who are in their fourth and fifth decade of life. Hemangiomas are often solitary and located in the right hemiliver, even though multiple lesions may be present in up to 40% of patients.[3] If more than one lesion is present, these are typically located in the same hepatic lobe.[3,4]

Macroscopically, hemangiomas may vary in size from a few millimeters to many centimeters. They are dark purple, soft, and compressible lesions that are well demarcated and frequently surrounded by a thin capsule. Histologically they consist of cavernous vascular spaces lined by endothelium and separated by connective tissue, totally lacking biliary or portal structures. By immunohistochemistry, the endothelium displays vascular as opposed to sinusoidal differentiation.[5] Large tumors can have central thromboses, necrotic areas, or dystrophic calcifications.

ETIOLOGY

The cause of hepatic hemangioma is unknown, but they are considered to be vascular malformations or hamartomas of congenital origin. Enlargement occurs by ectasia rather than hypertrophy or hyperplasia. As there is a predilection for females, and enlargement of existing hemangioma has been reported during pregnancy, there might be a relationship with female hormonal factors such as endogenous or exogenous estrogen and progesterone exposure. In fact, Glinkova et al reported that enlargement occurred over time in 23% of patients receiving estrogen hormone therapy as compared to only 10% of the control group. On the other hand, estrogen receptors have not been detected in all tumors and tumor growth has also been demonstrated in the absence of estrogen therapy and postmenopausal women.[6,7] As such, the risk associated with the use of oral contraceptives or pregnancy is poorly understood and there is still insufficient evidence to conclusively link estrogens to the development or progression of hepatic hemangiomas. Kasabach-Merritt syndrome was originally described as purpura associated with thrombocytopenia and "capillary hemangioma." Newer analyses have identified these tumors as tufted angioma or kaposiform hemangioendothelioma rather than typical hemangioma.[8]

DIAGNOSIS

Hemangiomas are typically asymptomatic hepatic lesions that are incidentally discovered at laparotomy, autopsy, or during routine imaging studies for unrelated reasons. If symptoms are present, right upper quadrant pain and discomfort are most frequent. However, nonspecific abdominal symptoms and hepatic hemangioma are both common conditions; therefore, the likelihood of a coincidence is high. Often these symptoms have been found unrelated to the hemangioma itself,[9] and young women are more likely to complain of symptoms. Very large hemangiomas can cause symptoms due to their size, such as early satiety by gastric compression, biliary stasis, or vascular obstruction.[10] Rapid onset of symptoms is a sign of bleeding or thrombosis. Rupture is an extremely rare complication, even in very large hemangiomas or during pregnancy.[11] Liver function tests and tumor markers (carcinoembryonic antigen, α-fetoprotein) are usually normal.[12]

Hemangiomas can often be unequivocally identified by imaging studies because of their typical radiographic features. Ultrasonography displays a well-defined hyperechoic lesion, although larger lesions are often more complicated because of calcifications, thromboses, or hemorrhage. In a fatty liver, the lesion might actually appear hypoechoic compared with the surrounding parenchyma. Typical findings by contrast-enhanced ultrasonography are rapid peripheral globular-nodular enhancement, followed by centripetal filling of the lesion.[13] As blood flow within hemangiomas can be detected in only 10% to 50% of cases, Doppler sonography does not add any predictive value.[14] Noncontrast computed tomographic (CT) scanning shows a well-demarcated hypodense mass. In ce-CT a peripheral nodular enhancement is evident, followed by centripetal filling over minutes (Figure 127-1). Late images show the lesion as isodense or hyperdense to surrounding tissue. Small hemangiomas (<3 cm) can lack the characteristic filling pattern, and it can be difficult to discriminate them from hypervascular malignant tumors.[15] The best imaging modality for the detection and characterization of hemangioma is MR.[16] Typical findings are hypointensity on T1-weighted sequences and hyperintensity on T2-weighted sequences. Contrast enhancement with gadolinium leads to centripetal filling similar to CT. Scintigraphy with technetium 99m pertechnetate–labeled erythrocytes documents gradual accumulation of red blood cells inside the hepatic lesion.[17] Although the specificity is extremely high and can be further improved by using single-photon emission CT (SPECT), the technique is cumbersome and rarely used today. Hepatic angiography is rarely used for diagnosis; yet it can be helpful in selected cases where definitive diagnosis cannot be established by noninvasive imaging modalities. Classic angiographic features include the characteristic "cotton wool" appearance that circumscribes a large feeding vessel with displacement and diffuse pooling of intravenous contrast material. Percutaneous biopsy has a low diagnostic yield[18] and carries the risk of severe bleeding complications. Therefore, biopsies are contraindicated when there is a suspicion of hemangioma (Table 127-1).

TREATMENT

Complications of hepatic hemangiomas are extremely rare,[19] and malignant transformation has never been reported. Therefore, most patients, particularly those with lesions less than 1.5 cm, can be followed safely without any therapeutic intervention (Figure 127-2).[20] One series observed 97% of 249 patients with liver hemangioma for up to 14 years without adverse events or morphologic changes of the lesions.[4] As such, patients without risk factors for hepatic malignancy and typical features of hemangioma on ultrasound do not need to undergo further imaging studies and can be followed clinically safely. It is prudent to follow up patients with clear hemangioma once or twice in 6-month intervals and then refrain from further imaging. Women should neither discontinue oral contraception nor refrain from pregnancy.

Surgical intervention is necessary in only a small subset of patients.[9] The most common indications for surgical resection include symptomatic lesions of unclear etiology, new-onset tumor growth, and extrinsic compression of adjacent structures. Large superficial hemangiomas in physically active individuals are often considered for surgery because of the perceived danger of rupture, although there is no evidence to support this approach.

Surgical interventions include formal resection or enucleation. Enucleation is possible because of a pseudocapsule of compressed hepatic parenchyma between the hemangioma and the surrounding tissue.[21] In theory, this technique spares hepatic parenchyma and does not

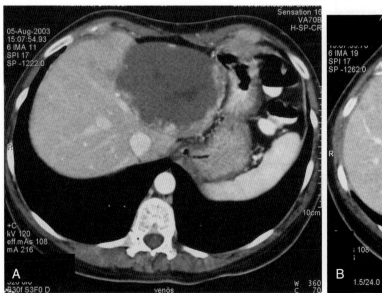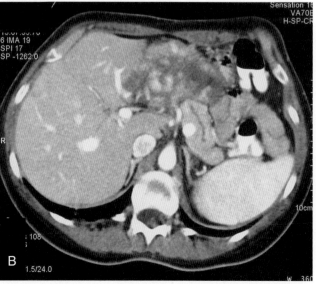

FIGURE 127-1 Contrast-enhanced CT of large hemangioma in the left hemiliver displaying hypoattenuation on early scans **(A)** and centripetal filling on delayed images **(B)**.

TABLE 127-1 Differential Diagnosis of Benign Hepatic Neoplasms

	Cavernous Hemangioma	Focal Nodular Hyperplasia	Hepatocellular Adenoma
Incidence	0.4%-20%	3%	1%
Solitary	80%-90%	80%-90%	80%-90%
Pathogenesis	Unknown (vascular malformations, congenital)	Unknown (vascular malformations, congenital)	Steroid hormones (estrogen, progesterone, androgen)
Imaging	US, ce-CT, MRI, ^{99m}Tc, RBC-SPECT	US, ce-CT, MRI, ^{99m}Tc	US, ce-CT, MRI, ^{99m}Tc
α-Fetoprotein	Normal	Normal	Normal
Macroscopic features	Dark purple, soft, compressible lesions that are well demarcated and frequently surrounded by a thin capsule (blood-filled "cyst")	Light brown, well-circumscribed lobulated tumor without capsule (central scar)	Well-circumscribed masses with a pseudocapsule of compressed hepatic parenchyma. Areas of inhomogeneous, yellow-brown lipid-rich tissue, as well as hemorrhage, necrosis, and calcifications
Microscopic features	Cavernous vascular spaces lined by endothelium and separated by connective tissue, totally lacking biliary or portal structures	Normal hepatocytes arranged in thickened plates, containing Kupffer cells and hepatocyte-derived biliary ductules at the interface between fibrous bands and nodules, totally lacking actual bile ducts	Composed of large lipid and glycogen-containing hepatocytes arranged in plates, separated by dilated sinusoids that are fed by arterial perfusion
Treatment	Surgical resection only if symptomatic or >10 cm	Discontinue estrogens, periodic imaging	Discontinue estrogens, resect if possible (malignant potential)

ce-CT, Contrast-enhanced computed tomography; *MRI*, magnetic resonance imaging; ^{99m}Tc, 99m-technetium-labeled sulfur colloid scan; *RBC-SPECT*, red blood cell study using single photon emission computed tomography; *US*, ultrasonography.

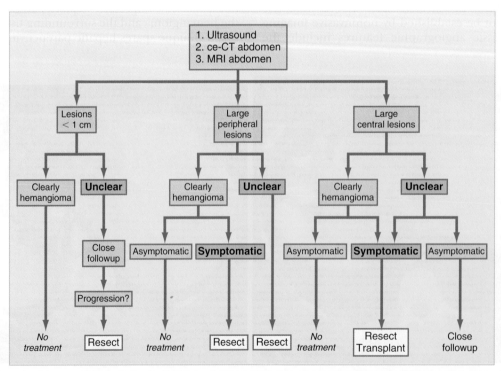

FIGURE 127-2 Flow chart for noncirrhotic patients: Focal non-hepatocellular carcinoma liver lesion (hemangioma, focal nodular hyperplasia, adenoma).

transect any biliary structures.[22] Overall the advantages of enucleation are minor, and we prefer standard liver resection for hemangioma. Occasionally, giant hemangiomas can be technically challenging to resect, and special surgical techniques such as total vascular exclusion must be employed. Recurrence after enucleation or resection requiring reoperation is extremely rare.[23] With both techniques, small residual hemangioma at the resection margin is not uncommon, particularly in extended resections for very large lesions.

Arterial embolization[24] and radiation therapy[25] of hepatic hemangiomas are rarely used therapeutic modalities. In patients who do not qualify for surgical resection because of medical or technical reasons, arterial embolization or radiation therapy may be appropriate therapeutic alternatives. Liver transplantation is an exceptional treatment modality described for symptomatic but unresectable hemangioma.[26]

FOCAL NODULAR HYPERPLASIA

FNH, the second most common benign hepatic tumor, is more prevalent in women (about 8:1) and presents in the third to fifth decades of life.[27] Lesions are usually less than 5 cm in diameter and solitary in 80% of cases. Only 3% are larger than 10 cm, although FNH of up to 19 cm have been reported.[27] Macroscopically, FNH appears as a light brown, well-circumscribed lobulated tumor. In contrast to hemangiomas, FNH lacks a capsule and has a central scar around a prominent arterial vessel with fibrous septa radiating outward. Histology reveals morphologically normal hepatocytes arranged in thickened plates. FNH contains Kupffer cells and hepatocyte-derived biliary ductules at the interface between fibrous bands and nodules but lacks actual bile ducts. Atypical or nonclassic forms of FNH exist, constituting as much as 20% in series of resected cases; these include telangiectatic FNH, a mixed hyperplastic and adenomatous form, and FNH with cytologic atypia.[27]

ETIOLOGY

The pathogenesis of FNH is controversial. Originally FNH was considered a neoplasm, a hamartoma, or a hyperplastic regenerative response to ischemia. Today it is generally accepted that FNH develops as a hyperplastic (regenerative) response to malformed vascular structures. An association of FNH with other vascular malformations and hereditary diseases strengthens this theory, as existence with hepatic hemangioma[28] and hereditary hemorrhagic telangiectasia (Osler-Weber-Rendu disease)[29] are frequently reported phenomena. A possible association with female hormonal factors has been suggested because of its predominant occurrence in women of childbearing age. In contrast, an Italian case-control study illustrated that the use of oral contraceptive pills (OCPs) did not appear to influence the size, number, or natural history of the disease in 216 women with FNH.[30]

DIAGNOSIS

The most important aspect in the management of patients with FNH is to discriminate it from other focal hepatic lesions, especially from hepatic adenoma and fibrolamellar carcinoma, both of which require surgical resection. FNH is asymptomatic in most cases and the majority are identified incidentally.[20] In contrast to hepatic adenomas, complications such as rupture, bleeding, and malignant transformation do not occur. Clinical findings and laboratory test results are usually normal. Although ultrasonography is often the initial diagnostic evaluation, the diagnosis of FNH cannot be confidently made for lack of specific signs. In fact, in 20% of all cases, the pathognomonic central scar is missing and FNH may appear as hyperechoic, isoechoic, or hypoechoic on conventional ultrasound.[31] Contrast-enhanced ultrasound seems to be more useful, because of unique portal and arterial perfusion patterns within FNH.[32] Noncontrast CT displays an isodense or hypodense lobulated tumor. Via CT, FNH becomes hyperattenuating in the arterial phase, sparing the central scar.[33] The scar may show some enhancement on portal or later phases, when the remainder of the lesion has already returned to baseline attenuation. By MRI, FNH is typically isointense or hypointense on T1-weighted images and isointense or hyperintense on T2-weighted images, with the central scar being hyperintense on the T2 images.[34] The pattern after MR contrast application is equal to CT imaging: rapid hyperintensity sparing the central scar, which shows increased signal intensity in later acquisitions (Figure 127-3). The presence of Kupffer cells in FNH leads to an uptake of superparamagnetic iron oxide (SPIO) contrast agents, distinguishing it from adenoma on MRI. The same effect can be used by scintigraphy with 99m-technetium–sulfur colloid. Angiography demonstrates a "spoked wheel" appearance but is usually not indicated for diagnosis. We do not advocate biopsy because of its low diagnostic yield.

TREATMENT

FNH has a benign and stable natural history and therefore should be treated conservatively. After establishing the diagnosis, followup imaging should be performed

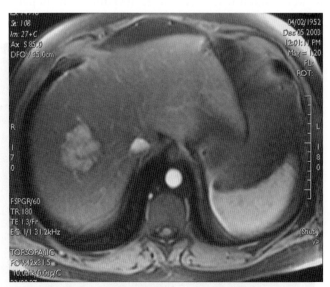

FIGURE 127-3 Dynamic contrast-enhanced MRI of focal nodular hyperplasia presenting as a hypervascular lesion with a central scar.

after 6 to 12 months. If the lesion remains stable and asymptomatic, no further imaging is required. If symptoms can be confidently linked to FNH, or if the benignity of the lesion is in doubt, resection is indicated. This can be performed laparoscopically or by traditional open partial hepatectomy.

HEPATIC ADENOMA

Hepatic adenomas, or hepatocellular adenomas, are rare benign hepatic neoplasms that typically affect young women of childbearing age. They are frequently located in the right hemiliver and are solitary in up to 80%. Since the introduction of oral contraceptive pills (OCPs) in the early 1960s, it has become increasingly apparent that long-term use of OCPs is associated with a 30-fold increase in hepatic adenoma incidence as illustrated by numerous epidemiologic outcome studies.[35] With the advent of newer low-dose estrogen and/or progesterone formulations, the incidence of hepatic adenomas is declining again. Adenomatosis refers to the presence of more than 10 hepatic adenomas and represents a distinct disease entity because there is no relationship with hormone exposure.[36]

Macroscopically, adenomas are well-circumscribed masses with a pseudocapsule of compressed hepatic parenchyma. The cut surface is inhomogeneous, displaying areas of yellow-brown lipid-rich tissue, as well as hemorrhage, necrosis, and calcifications. Histologically, adenomas are composed of large lipid- and glycogen-containing hepatocytes arranged in plates, separated by dilated sinusoids that are fed by arterial perfusion. In contrast to FNH, adenoma contains few or no Kupffer cells and contains no bile ductules.

ETIOLOGY

Although the underlying molecular mechanisms are not well understood, the association of steroid hormones and OCP use with the development of hepatic adenomas is well established.[37] As such, two-thirds of hepatic adenomas express estrogen and progesterone receptors,[38] and enlargement or even rupture has been reported during pregnancy. An increased risk of hepatic adenoma has also been noted with the use of androgen preparations, such as in aplastic anemia, hypogonadism, hypopituitarism, and other endocrine disorders.[39] Furthermore, the illicit use of androgens by bodybuilders has also been reported to promote hepatic adenoma formation.[40] Other predisposing conditions are type I and III glycogen storage disease, where adenomas predominantly affect male patients.[41]

DIAGNOSIS

Similar to hepatic hemangiomas and FNH, about half of all hepatic adenomas are discovered incidentally during imaging studies for unrelated medical conditions.[20] The larger the tumor, the more likely it will be symptomatic as evidenced by right upper quadrant or epigastric pain. As with other benign hepatic neoplasms, adenomas are usually asymptomatic and acute onset of pain is usually related to rupture or bleeding, which can lead to dramatic manifestations of acute abdomen and shock. Adenomatosis is more often symptomatic and has a higher tendency for bleeding complications.[36]

The initial evaluation is often done by ultrasound, yet this modality does not permit a final diagnosis. Adenomas appear hyperechoic, with hypoechoic and cystic areas with occasional intratumoral calcifications. In contrast to FNH, CT scanning shows a heterogeneous, mostly hypodense, mass interspersed with hyperdense regions of hemorrhage and hypodense areas of necrosis.[42] Contrast administration leads to a rapid enhancement in the arterial phase, which is often pronounced at the margin because of peripheral vascularization and then proceeds centrally. MRI shows a similarly heterogeneous lesion, which is predominantly hyperintense in both T1- and T2-weighted sequences but can also be hypointense (Figure 127-4, *A*). Dynamic contrast-enhanced MR sequences display rapid arterial enhancement. As adenomas contain none or few Kupffer cells, special imaging

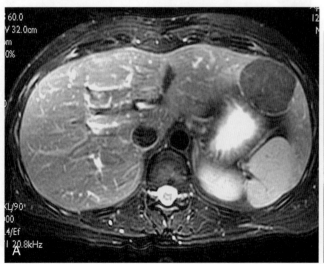
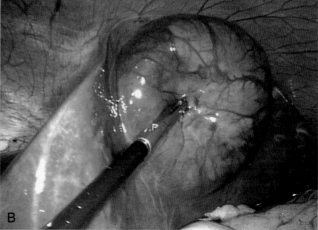

FIGURE 127-4 A, Hepatic adenoma in the left lateral segment presenting as a T2-weighted hypointense encapsulated lesion. **B,** Laparoscopic view of the adenoma depicted in **A.**

techniques such as MRI with superparamagnetic iron oxide contrast or 99m-technetium–sulfur colloid scanning can be used to distinguish them from FNH.[43] MRI with gadobenate dimeglumine can also differentiate between adenoma and FNH because its uptake and excretion are reduced in adenoma, rendering the lesion hypointense on delayed scans. Laboratory analyses including tumor markers are usually normal. Biopsy has a low diagnostic yield,[20] especially if diagnostic uncertainty exists after several imaging modalities, and it carries a risk of bleeding.

TREATMENT

Because hepatic adenomas display a different natural history of disease than FNH, they pose a significant risk of rupture and bleeding. Furthermore, there is a certain risk of malignant transformation into hepatocellular carcinoma.[44] As such, we advocate surgical resection of all hepatic adenomas, as well as of all cases of diagnostic uncertainty. Others have proposed a less aggressive approach for asymptomatic adenoma by discontinuing contraceptive therapy and following patients with serial imaging and α-fetoprotein determinations.[45] Radiofrequency ablation is a possibility, but followup data are lacking to support routine clinical use.[46] However, the standard of care is surgical resection, which can be achieved by open or laparoscopic resections (Figure 127-4, B). Adenomatosis associated with glycogen storage disease can be an indication for liver transplantation, especially because of the high risk of malignant transformation.[47]

OTHER BENIGN TUMORS

A variety of rare benign tumors have been described to occur in the liver. In contrast to hepatocellular tumors, the benign variant of a biliary tumor is exceedingly rare. Bile duct adenoma is usually asymptomatic, but obstructive jaundice can be the presenting symptom depending on location and size.[48] As the diagnosis is rarely accurate preoperatively, and bile duct adenoma is considered a premalignant lesion, management should consist of surgical resection with clear margins. Biliary hamartomas (von Meyenburg complexes) are more common benign malformations of the biliary tract. The only relevance of these small lesions (<1 cm) consisting of cystic spaces and fibrous stroma is to distinguish them from metastases (Figure 127-5). The diagnosis can be made by high-frequency ultrasound or by MRI.[49]

Angiomyolipomas are tumors derived from perivascular epithelioid cells, which are associated with tuberous sclerosis and mostly occur in the kidney. Hepatic angiomyolipomas are rarely diagnosed correctly by imaging procedures. They are a premalignant lesion and should be resected.[50]

Peliosis hepatis refers to a vascular disorder that can appear as a tumor.[51] It is associated with the use of steroid hormones, malignancy, transplantation, and chronic inflammation. Histology reveals multiple blood-filled cysts of different sizes. The natural history is not known, but rupture has been reported, and this lesion should probably be resected.

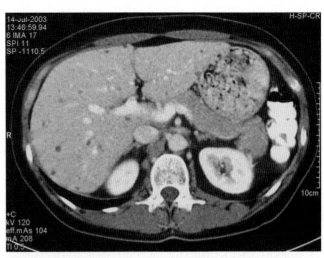

FIGURE 127-5 Contrast-enhanced CT scan of multiple biliary hamartomas (von Meyenburg complexes) evident as multiple cystic lesions.

Other benign primary tumors that have been described in the liver include solitary fibrous tumors, schwannoma, lipoma, leiomyoma, teratoma, and lymphangioma.

REFERENCES

1. Torzilli G, Minagawa M, Takayama T, et al: Accurate preoperative evaluation of liver mass lesions without fine-needle biopsy. *Hepatology* 30:889, 1999.
2. Karhunen PJ: Benign hepatic tumours and tumour like conditions in men. *J Clin Pathol* 39:183, 1986.
3. Tait N, Richardson AJ, Muguti G, et al: Hepatic cavernous haemangioma: A 10 year review. *Aust N Z J Surg* 62:521, 1992.
4. Herman P, Costa ML, Machado MA, et al: Management of hepatic hemangiomas: A 14-year experience. *J Gastrointest Surg* 9:853, 2005.
5. Duff B, Weigel JA, Bourne P, et al: Endothelium in hepatic cavernous hemangiomas does not express the hyaluronan receptor for endocytosis. *Hum Pathol* 33:265, 2002.
6. Glinkova V, Shevah O, Boaz M, et al: Hepatic haemangiomas: Possible association with female sex hormones. *Gut* 53:1352, 2004.
7. Gemer O, Moscovici O, Ben-Horin CL, et al: Oral contraceptives and liver hemangioma: A case-control study. *Acta Obstet Gynecol Scand* 83:1199, 2004.
8. Enjolras O, Wassef M, Mazoyer E, et al: Infants with Kasabach-Merritt syndrome do not have "true" hemangiomas. *J Pediatr* 130:631, 1997.
9. Farges O, Daradkeh S, Bismuth H: Cavernous hemangiomas of the liver: Are there any indications for resection? *World J Surg* 19:19, 1995.
10. Kim DY, Pantelic MV, Yoshida A, et al: Cavernous hemangioma presenting as Budd-Chiari syndrome. *J Am Coll Surg* 200:470, 2005.
11. Cobey FC, Salem RR: A review of liver masses in pregnancy and a proposed algorithm for their diagnosis and management. *Am J Surg* 187:181, 2004.
12. Terkivatan T, de Wilt JH, de Man RA, et al: Indications and long-term outcome of treatment for benign hepatic tumors: A critical appraisal. *Arch Surg* 136:1033, 2001.
13. von Herbay A, Vogt C, Willers R, et al: Real-time imaging with the sonographic contrast agent SonoVue: Differentiation between benign and malignant hepatic lesions. *J Ultrasound Med* 23:1557, 2004.
14. Perkins AB, Imam K, Smith WJ, et al: Color and power Doppler sonography of liver hemangiomas: A dream unfulfilled? *J Clin Ultrasound* 28:159, 2000.
15. Kim T, Federle MP, Baron RL, et al: Discrimination of small hepatic hemangiomas from hypervascular malignant tumors smaller than 3 cm with three-phase helical CT. *Radiology* 219:699, 2001.
16. Semelka RC, Martin DR, Balci C, et al: Focal liver lesions: Comparison of dual-phase CT and multisequence multiplanar MR imaging

including dynamic gadolinium enhancement. *J Magn Reson Imaging* 13:397, 2001.

17. Farlow DC, Chapman PR, Gruenewald SM, et al: Investigation of focal hepatic lesions: Is tomographic red blood cell imaging useful? *World J Surg* 14:463, 1990.

18. Yoon SS, Charny CK, Fong Y, et al: Diagnosis, management, and outcomes of 115 patients with hepatic hemangioma. *J Am Coll Surg* 197:392, 2003.

19. Yamamoto T, Kawarada Y, Yano T, et al: Spontaneous rupture of hemangioma of the liver: Treatment with transcatheter hepatic arterial embolization. *Am J Gastroenterol* 86:1645, 1991.

20. Charny CK, Jarnagin WR, Schwartz LH, et al: Management of 155 patients with benign liver tumours. *Br J Surg* 88:808, 2001.

21. Baer HU, Dennison AR, Mouton W, et al: Enucleation of giant hemangiomas of the liver. Technical and pathologic aspects of a neglected procedure. *Ann Surg* 216:673, 1992.

22. Kuo PC, Lewis WD, Jenkins RL: Treatment of giant hemangiomas of the liver by enucleation. *J Am Coll Surg* 178:49, 1994.

23. Ozden I, Emre A, Alper A, et al: Long-term results of surgery for liver hemangiomas. *Arch Surg* 135:978, 2000.

24. Deutsch GS, Yeh KA, Bates WB 3rd, et al: Embolization for management of hepatic hemangiomas. *Am Surg* 67:159, 2001.

25. Gaspar L, Mascarenhas F, da Costa MS, et al: Radiation therapy in the unresectable cavernous hemangioma of the liver. *Radiother Oncol* 29:45, 1993.

26. Tepetes K, Selby R, Webb M, et al: Orthotopic liver transplantation for benign hepatic neoplasms. *Arch Surg* 130:153, 1995.

27. Nguyen BN, Flejou JF, Terris B, et al: Focal nodular hyperplasia of the liver: A comprehensive pathologic study of 305 lesions and recognition of new histologic forms. *Am J Surg Pathol* 23:1441, 1999.

28. Mathieu D, Zafrani ES, Anglade MC, et al: Association of focal nodular hyperplasia and hepatic hemangioma. *Gastroenterology* 97:154, 1989.

29. Buscarini E, Danesino C, Plauchu H, et al: High prevalence of hepatic focal nodular hyperplasia in subjects with hereditary hemorrhagic telangiectasia. *Ultrasound Med Biol* 30:1089, 2004.

30. Scalori A, Tavani A, Gallus S, et al: Oral contraceptives and the risk of focal nodular hyperplasia of the liver: A case-control study. *Am J Obstet Gynecol* 186:195, 2002.

31. Shamsi K, De Schepper A, Degryse H, et al: Focal nodular hyperplasia of the liver: Radiologic findings. *Abdom Imaging* 18:32, 1993.

32. Dietrich CF, Schuessler G, Trojan J, et al: Differentiation of focal nodular hyperplasia and hepatocellular adenoma by contrast-enhanced ultrasound. *Br J Radiol* 78:704, 2005.

33. Hussain SM, Terkivatan T, Zondervan PE, et al: Focal nodular hyperplasia: Findings at state-of-the-art MR imaging, US, CT, and pathologic analysis. *Radiographics* 24:3; discussion 8, 2004.

34. Mortele KJ, Praet M, Van Vlierberghe H, et al: CT and MR imaging findings in focal nodular hyperplasia of the liver: Radiologic-pathologic correlation. *AJR Am J Roentgenol* 175:687, 2000.

35. Rooks JB, Ory HW, Ishak KG, et al: Epidemiology of hepatocellular adenoma. The role of oral contraceptive use. *JAMA* 242:644, 1979.

36. Ribeiro A, Burgart LJ, Nagorney DM, et al: Management of liver adenomatosis: Results with a conservative surgical approach. *Liver Transpl Surg* 4:388, 1998.

37. Zucman-Rossi J: Genetic alterations in hepatocellular adenomas: Recent findings and new challenges. *J Hepatol* 40:1036, 2004.

38. Torbenson M, Lee JH, Choti M, et al: Hepatic adenomas: Analysis of sex steroid receptor status and the Wnt signaling pathway. *Mod Pathol* 15:189, 2002.

39. Velazquez I, Alter BP: Androgens and liver tumors: Fanconi's anemia and non-Fanconi's conditions. *Am J Hematol* 77:257, 2004.

40. Socas L, Zumbado M, Perez-Luzardo O, et al: Hepatocellular adenomas associated with anabolic androgenic steroid abuse in bodybuilders: A report of two cases and a review of the literature. *Br J Sports Med* 39:e27, 2005.

41. Labrune P, Trioche P, Duvaltier I, et al: Hepatocellular adenomas in glycogen storage disease type I and III: A series of 43 patients and review of the literature. *J Pediatr Gastroenterol Nutr* 24:276, 1997.

42. Grazioli L, Federle MP, Brancatelli G, et al: Hepatic adenomas: Imaging and pathologic findings. *Radiographics* 21:877; discussion 892, 2001.

43. Laumonier H, Bioulac-Sage P, Laurent C, et al: Hepatocellular adenomas: Magnetic resonance imaging features as a function of molecular pathological classification. *Hepatology* 48:808, 2008.

44. Ito M, Sasaki M, Wen CY, et al: Liver cell adenoma with malignant transformation: A case report. *World J Gastroenterol* 9:2379, 2003.

45. Ault GT, Wren SM, Ralls PW, et al: Selective management of hepatic adenomas. *Am Surg* 62:825, 1996.

46. Atwell TD, Brandhagen DJ, Charboneau JW, et al: Successful treatment of hepatocellular adenoma with percutaneous radiofrequency ablation. *AJR Am J Roentgenol* 184:828, 2005.

47. Lerut JP, Ciccarelli O, Sempoux C, et al: Glycogenosis storage type I diseases and evolutive adenomatosis: An indication for liver transplantation. *Transpl Int* 16:879, 2003.

48. Allaire GS, Rabin L, Ishak KG, et al: Bile duct adenoma. A study of 152 cases. *Am J Surg Pathol* 12:708, 1988.

49. Troltzsch M, Borte G, Kahn T, et al: Non-invasive diagnosis of von Meyenburg complexes. *J Hepatol* 39:129, 2003.

50. Flemming P, Lehmann U, Becker T, et al: Common and epithelioid variants of hepatic angiomyolipoma exhibit clonal growth and share a distinctive immunophenotype. *Hepatology* 32:213, 2000.

51. Savastano S, San Bortolo O, Velo E, et al: Pseudotumoral appearance of peliosis hepatis. *AJR Am J Roentgenol* 185:558, 2005.

Hepatocellular Carcinoma

Elika Kashef | John Paul Roberts

EPIDEMIOLOGY AND ETIOLOGY

Hepatocellular carcinoma (HCC) is the sixth most common malignancy in the world and third commonest cause of death from cancer.[1] More common among men, the incidence of HCC in the United States has increased since 1975 to 2000 from 1.4 to more than 5 per 100,000, respectively (Figure 128-1).[2]

Of the 600,000 deaths per annum worldwide, 50% occur in China. Hepatitis B and C viruses are both strongly associated with the development of HCC. This association increases significantly with coinfection of both these viruses. Hepatitis B has a higher prevalence in Asia and Africa, whereas hepatitis C is more prevalent in Japan, Europe, and America, where up to 60% of HCC patients are infected with hepatitis C.[3]

The average age at the time of diagnosis of HCC in the United States is 65 years, with a 75% male predominance.[4] In the United States, hepatitis C and B and alcohol consumption are the commonest causes of HCC. The rise of HCC in the United States and other Western countries has been fueled by the increase in the prevalence of hepatitis C. The greatest incidence of hepatitis C infection was during the late 1970s and early 1980s, with a dramatic drop in incidence in the late 1980s (Figure 128-2). Because of the time necessary for cancer to develop in infected patients and the increased risk in older patients, the number of patients with HCC has risen rapidly (Figure 128-3).[5]

STEATOHEPATITIS

In addition to the increasing number of patients with HCC associated with hepatitis C, there is an increasing number of patients with HCC whose only risk factor is steatohepatitis associated with obesity. With the explosion of obesity in the United States, it is expected that a large population of obese patients will develop steatohepatitis and progress to cirrhosis, which puts them at risk for hepatocellular carcinoma. A recent paper looking at a health claims database found that 59% of the 4400 patients with HCC had associated nonalcoholic steatohepatitis, as compared to only 22% of patients having the liver cancer associated with hepatitis C.[6] Although these results probably are affected by the selection bias of cases in the claims database, the results are worrisome for a marked increase in HCC over time related to obesity.

OTHER RISK FACTORS

In sub-Saharan Africa, Southeast Asia, and China, aflatoxin, a contaminant in maize and nuts, produced by the fungi *Aspergillus*, is a potent carcinogen for liver cancer. The carcinogenic potential is greatly enhanced in the presence of chronic HBV infection, where the combination creates a thirtyfold increased risk of HCC

(Table 128-1). The estimate of the percentage of HCC related to aflatoxin ranges between 5% and 28%.[7]

The incidence of hepatocellular carcinoma related to risk factors other than viral hepatitis, aflatoxin, and steatohepatitis is relatively small. It is probably true that any patient with cirrhosis from any etiology is at risk for hepatocellular carcinoma. In children, the viral etiologies are the most common causes of HCC.

PATHOLOGY

Hepatitis B, a DNA virus, integrates itself into hepatocyte DNA and is thought to increase the rate of oncogene transcription. Hepatitis C, an RNA virus, does not incorporate into DNA of the hepatocytes. Its relationship with HCC is thought to be through chronic inflammation leading to cirrhosis. After cirrhosis develops, hepatitis C virus continues to replicate, which sustains inflammation and a rapid cell turnover, resulting in mutation and dysplastic changes that lead to neoplastic growth.[8] The pathogenesis in steatohepatitis is poorly understood, although the associated chronic inflammation is thought to contribute in large part to development of HCC.

The three aspects that one must take into consideration in the pathophysiology of HCC are cirrhosis, arterial angiogenesis, and portal vein invasion.

CIRRHOSIS

More than 90% of patients who develop HCC have evidence of fibrosis in the liver. In patients with hepatitis C, almost all the patients have cirrhosis, and the risk of developing hepatocellular carcinoma once cirrhosis is established is about 3% to 5% per year.

The cirrhotic liver consists of regenerative nodules surrounded by fibrosis. It appears that because of chronic inflammation, progression from regenerative nodules to dysplasia and finally to HCC occurs. Dysplastic nodules generally range from 1 to 2 cm and contain areas of dysplasia or carcinoma in situ.[9] Because the risk of liver cancer is generalized to the entire organ, the carcinogenic potential is termed a "field effect." This "field effect" is responsible for the high rate of recurrence after resection of HCC because of the remaining unresected liver being at risk. The recurrences after resection are most commonly second primary lesions rather than recurrence of the resected lesion.[10]

ARTERIAL ANGIOGENESIS

Unlike the cirrhotic liver and dysplastic nodules that are predominantly supplied by the portal vein, HCC gets its blood supply from the hepatic artery. This propensity for HCC to undergo neoangiogenesis and derive much of its blood supply from hepatic arterial perfusion is one of the features that allow recognition and diagnosis on

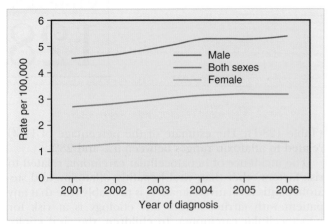

FIGURE 128-1 Hepatocellular carcinoma incidence rate by gender—United States, 2001–2006. (From CDC's National Program of Cancer Registries and the National Cancer Institute's Surveillance, Epidemiology, and End Results surveillance system; data from 45 cancer registries covering 90.4% of the U.S. population. Centers for Disease Control and Prevention: Hepatocellular carcinoma—United States, 2001-2006. *Morb Mortal Wkly Rep* 59:517, 2010. www.cdc.gov/mmwr/preview/mmwrhtml/mm5917a3.htm.)

TABLE 128-1 Major Risk Factors for Hepatocellular Carcinoma

Infection	Hepatitis B
	Hepatitis C
Toxin/drug	Alcoholic cirrhosis
	Alfatoxins
	Anabolic steroids
Genetic	Hemochromatosis
	α_1-Antitrypsin deficiency
Immunologic	Autoimmune chronic active hepatitis
	Primary biliary cirrhosis
Other	Obesity
	Nonalcoholic steatohepatitis
	Cirrhosis (other causes and idiopathic)

imaging. Thus on computed tomography (CT), the HCC lesion appears hyperdense during the arterial phase, whereas the liver is higher in attenuation during the portovenous phase. Because the portal venous phase is later than the arterial phase, the HCC lesions tend to show washout or loss of contrast during the portal venous phase. On angiographic imaging, the vessels have an unusual and irregular pattern in both size and branch pattern, which is different than normal hepatic arterial supply. This abnormal arterial perfusion allows for treatment of HCC via embolization of the feeding artery(ies). These radiographic findings are due to the dysregulation of the angiogenesis pathway and lack of a basement membrane that occurs with malignant tumors.[11]

PORTAL VEIN INVASION

Another characteristic of HCC involving the blood supply of the liver is its propensity to invade the portal vein.[12] Tumors measuring more than 2 cm have an increased

risk of portal vein invasion, which can be assessed on imaging.[13]

Predictably, the outcome of patients with evidence of microscopic and macroscopic portal venous invasion is worse, as their risk of recurrence both in the liver and systemically following resection or transplantation is significantly higher. Macroscopic portal vein invasion is thought to be a contraindication to transplantation and in many cases to resection. It is likely that portal venous invasion is either a mechanism for a diffusion of the tumor elsewhere in the liver and the body and/or that the phenotypes of the cells that can invade the portal vein are cells that can disseminate and implant in other organs such as the lung or bone.

It is well recognized that the recurrence of HCC after transplantation is related to the size and number of lesions in the liver. This finding is probably a reflection of the increased probability of having vascular invasion and/or dedifferentiation of cells in the tumor when the tumor is larger or is multifocal.

CLINICAL PRESENTATION

Because of the known risk factors for HCC, there is usually a history of viral hepatitis, alcohol or drug abuse, obesity and/or diabetes, or past history of HCC. Many patients have a history of complications of cirrhosis.

Hepatocellular carcinoma can present in varying ways: as an incidental finding during ultrasound for right upper quadrant pain, abdominal mass, weight loss, anorexia, onset of ascites, or while screening for patients at risk for HCC, with or without evidence of cirrhosis.

A patient with known cirrhosis who develops any of the symptoms previously mentioned should be suspected of having developed HCC. The finding of small asymptomatic liver lesions during the radiologic evaluation for liver transplantation is another common presentation, particularly in patients with hepatitis C.

Physical examination can reveal jaundice, ascites, cachexia, splenomegaly, hepatomegaly, or it may be normal. Owing to the strong association between cirrhosis and HCC, examination can reveal more subtle stigmata of liver disease, such as spider angiomata or palmar erythema.

LABORATORY FINDINGS

Blood tests can reveal abnormal liver function tests and enzymes. Viral serology including hepatitis B surface antigen and hepatitis C antibody tests are also necessary. Patients with cirrhosis may also demonstrate thrombocytopenia, which is a marker of portal hypertension.

α-Fetoprotein (AFP) may be elevated in HCC; however, this is not highly sensitive or specific. The American Association for the Study of Liver Disease (AASLD) recommended that serum AFP not be used as a screening tool, although it still plays a diagnostic role. AFP is best used as a confirmatory test in cases of cirrhosis and a liver mass, bearing in mind that in lesions less than 2 cm the levels may be normal.[14] A level greater than 400 ng/mL is diagnostic when there is a liver mass greater than 2 cm present.

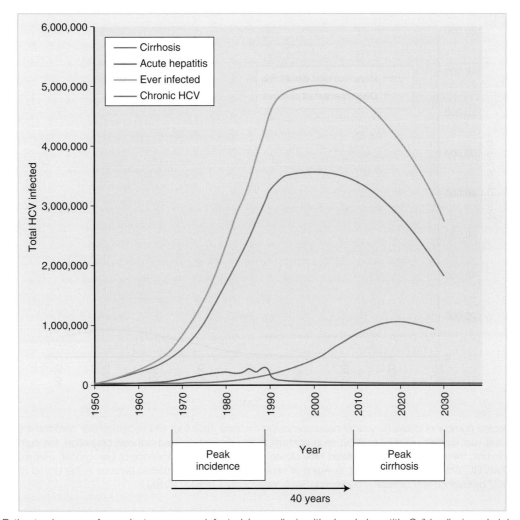

FIGURE 128-2 Estimates by year of prevalent cases ever infected *(green line)*, with chronic hepatitis C *(blue line)*, and cirrhosis *(red line)*. Acute infections *(purple line)* peaked between 1970 and 1990. The peak of chronic hepatitis prevalence was 2001, whereas the highest prevalence of cirrhosis is projected to be between 2010 and 2030, about 40 years after the peak of acute infections. (Reprinted with permission from Davis GL, Alter MJ, El-Seraq H, et al: Aging of hepatitis C virus (HCV)-infected persons in the United States: A multiple cohort model of HCV prevalence and disease progression. *Gastroenterology* 138:513, 2010.)

The Des-carboxyprothrombin (DCP) is a test that is thought to be specific in differentiating benign from malignant lesions, and is elevated in about 40% of patients with HCC lesions less than 2 cm. There is no correlation between DCP and AFP levels.[15]

IMAGING

The purpose of imaging in the cirrhotic patient is three-fold: diagnosis, staging, and excluding complications of cirrhosis.

LESIONS LESS THAN 2 CM

With a background of cirrhosis and the associated findings of regenerating nodules, diagnosis and identifying HCC can be difficult, particularly if the lesion is less than 2 cm in diameter. In a cirrhotic liver, a lesion measuring less than 1 cm on imaging carries less than 50% risk of being malignant transformation. Thus, ultrasound surveillance every 3 months is recommended in these patients until lesions grow above 1 cm. If the appearance

remains stable at 24 months, then the imaging interval can increase to every 6 months to 1 year.[16]

For lesions between 1 and 2 cm, if on two modalities the image findings such as arterialization and washout are characteristic for HCC, then HCC is assumed. If one modality or both modalities are atypical for HCC, then tissue biopsy is recommended.[16,17]

The controversy with biopsying small lesions is that the differentiation between dysplasia and highly differentiated HCC overlaps or that the lesion could be missed, providing a false sense of security. In cases of negative biopsy findings, regular enhanced imaging is recommended for followup instead of ultrasound.

LESIONS GREATER THAN 2 CM

Due to advances in imaging, the combination of clinical features and image findings provides a positive predictive value of 95%, and is thus reliable.[16] Current diagnostic consensus is that with an elevated AFP (>200 ng/mL) with typical imaging features (see later) in a lesion greater than 2 cm, the probability of HCC is so high that

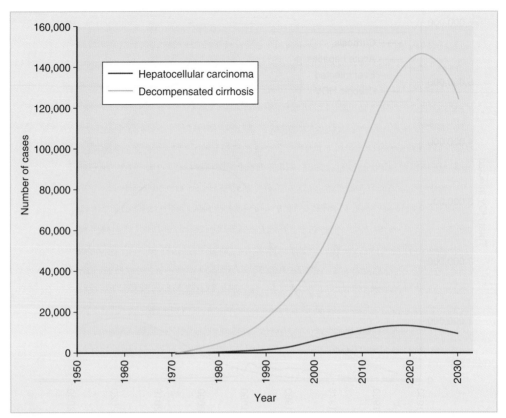

FIGURE 128-3 Projected number of cases by year of decompensated cirrhosis *(blue line)* and hepatocellular carcinoma *(purple line)*. The model assumes a first-year mortality of 80% to 85%, so in contrast to the decompensated cirrhosis projection, the number of cases of hepatocellular carcinoma, the prevalence demonstrated here closely resembles annual incidence of liver cancer. (Reprinted with permission from Davis GL, Alter MJ, El-Seraq H, et al: Aging of hepatitis C virus (HCV)-infected persons in the United States: A multiple cohort model of HCV prevalence and disease progression. *Gastroenterology* 138:513, 2010.)

biopsy is not required and management can be commenced following staging. However, atypical image findings do require tissue biopsy.

ULTRASOUND

The primary use for ultrasonography is in screening populations for HCC. The value of doing so is primarily related to the low cost, availability, and no use of radiation. As a radiologic screening tool, it has a sensitivity of 65% to 85% and a specificity greater than 90%.[18] A prospective randomized controlled trial suggested that surveillance of high-risk individuals with ultrasound and AFP every 6 months reduces HCC-related mortality by close to 40%. However, the screening compliance was only approximately 60%.[19]

For screening populations in which the incidence of HCC may be quite high and the picture complicated by the nodular pattern of the cirrhotic liver, such as patients awaiting liver transplantation, ultrasound may be less useful.[20]

The finding of a lesion less than 1 cm on ultrasound should result in frequent followup monitoring of the lesion. The finding of a lesion 1 to 2 cm or greater than 2 cm should be confirmed with another imaging modality.[21] Ultrasound cannot differentiate between benign and malignant lesions but can differentiate between solid and cystic nodules, and it can be used to guide needle biopsies. The use of contrast agents containing microbubbles may increase the value of ultrasound in distinguishing between liver masses, as these agents will allow demonstration of arterialization of the lesions.

The role of ultrasound in the management of HCC for directing the use of ablative techniques is discussed later.

COMPUTED TOMOGRAPHY

Because of recent advances in helical CT, including faster scanning time with lower radiation dose, this modality can accurately diagnose HCC, as well as stage the extent of the hepatic disease. The cost and radiation exposure issues limit the use of CT scan in most screening protocols. The use of CT scan in screening may be of benefit in the cirrhotic patient, but MRI has the same efficacy without the radiation risk. Unenhanced CT of the liver can demonstrate fatty infiltration and nodular appearance. Calcification within lesions (or posttreatment presence of Lipiodol) can be better demonstrated using precontrast images. The current imaging guidelines for liver and pancreatic disease include precontrast axial images of the upper abdomen. After completion of the unenhanced CT, contrast is then injected intravenously; then scanning at the early or true arterial phase is performed. This usually occurs at 12 to 30 seconds after injection depending on the CT and the patient's hemodynamic status. Because of the arterial angiogenesis of the tumor and its main supply of blood from the hepatic artery, the arterial phase can demonstrate enhancement, whereas the liver shows maximal enhancement during the portovenous phase because 70% of the liver's blood supply comes from the portal vein.[22]

The current sensitivity of identifying HCC on multidetector CT is about 86%, which drops to about 60% with lesions less than 2 cm in size.[23] However, recently more invasive combination techniques such as intraarterial CT angiograms and CT arterial portography have shown a sensitivity and specificity of up to 93% and 97%, respectively, as demonstrated by posthepatic explantation/resection.[24]

Intravenous ionized poppyseed oil (Lipiodol) is no longer used for planning and staging. Lipiodol, however, is still injected when transarterial embolization therapy is delivered, and is used as a marker of treatment on followup CT as the lesions can be identified on the noncontrast phase of the CT scan. The Lipiodol is normally cleared by lymphatic vessels and Kupffer cells that the tumor lacks and can be retained by the tumor for months or weeks after arterial injection. Heterogeneous uptake of Lipiodol on followup CT with residual tumor enhancement is suggestive of presence of viable tumor. Followup CT is also used to assess for complications of embolization therapy such as hepatic or gallbladder necrosis.[25]

MAGNETIC RESONANCE IMAGING

MRI is becoming the predominant imaging modality in characterizing and differentiating malignant liver tumors. MRI can be used to assess fat and iron content as well as acquiring angiographic images and enhancement patterns postcontrast. Classically HCC has high signal intensity on T2-weighted sequences with strong early arterial enhancement and delayed washout; however, studies have shown that smaller HCCs can vary in their appearance on MRI.[26] The capsule surrounding HCC may be of low signal intensity. The lesion may show a "mosaic" appearance because of combined areas of growth and necrosis. Early malignant growth within dysplastic nodules can be identified simply as an area within a nodule that has a different intensity and arterial enhancement in comparison to the remainder of the nodule. This is known as a "nodule within a nodule" appearance.

MRI needs less contrast volume than CT, and injection time is shorter. There is also no ionizing radiation in MRI. Contrast agents used include gadolinium chelates, superparamagnetic iron oxide, and hepatocyte-directed agents (mangafodipir trisodium). Gadolinium should be avoided in patients with renal dysfunction.

STAGING

Staging of hepatocellular carcinoma is important because acquiring information about the degree of spread/metastases can help plan management and predict prognosis and outcome. The staging system can act as a prognostic tool and can be used to ascertain which patient should get which treatment modality. It can also be used for research purposes and response to therapy in clinical trials.

The commonest classifications used are the following:

- *Barcelona Clinic Liver Cancer Staging System (BCLC)* provides information on prognosis and aids with planning patient's treatment. It takes into account a variety of factors including clinically relevant portal hypertension. Stage A (early tumor) is suitable for all treatment modalities; stages B (intermediate) and C (advanced) are more suitable for palliative care and use of new agents; and stage D (end-stage) should be treated symptomatically only (Figure 128-4).[21]
- *Tumor, node, metastasis (TNM)*, which only assesses the tumor and not the function of the remaining liver. TNM is difficult to use in the preoperative patient because it relies on histologic assessment of the liver. Currently in the United States, this staging system has been modified for use to prioritize patients with HCC based on radiologic imaging. This modified staging system is used to allow for prioritization of patients with HCC for transplantation.
- *Okuda classification* assesses both the tumor and the liver. It takes into account the tumor size and liver function tests, such as albumin and bilirubin levels. It does *not* take into account vascular invasion or whether or not the tumor is single or multiple. This is a commonly used staging system (stages I, II and III).
- *Cancer of the Liver Italian Program (CLIP)* includes the Child-Pugh stage, tumor extension, AFP levels, and portal vein thrombosis. The CLIP staging has been viewed as an easy and acceptable method of staging hepatocellular carcinoma, which takes into account all the factors needed to allow assessment and management in a patient with the tumor. It is, however, poor at staging patients undergoing surgery or transplantation.

The use of staging systems is exemplified by the use of the modified TNM classification in prioritizing patients with HCC for transplantation in the United States. In this classification, patients are stratified by the size and number of the tumor. Patients with a single lesion between 2 and 5 cm in size are given priority for transplantation. If more than one lesion is present, there must be fewer than three lesions with no individual lesion greater than 3 cm in size in order for the patient to be given priority for transplantation. Patients with single lesions greater than 5 cm, with more than three lesions, with multiple lesions where one lesion is greater than 3 cm, or with radiologic evidence of vascular invasion are not given priority for transplantation.

MANAGEMENT

As with most cancers, treatment decisions in patients with HCC need to be based on the overall health status of the patient, the extent of the disease, and the data regarding the results of any particular treatment. In addition to these considerations, it should be remembered that HCC frequently arises in a cirrhotic liver. Decompensation or the risk of decompensation because of the chosen therapy of the cirrhosis can limit potential therapies. Further, because of the field effect created by the associated liver disease, patients with hepatocellular carcinoma are at high risk to develop a second primary lesion. The risk of

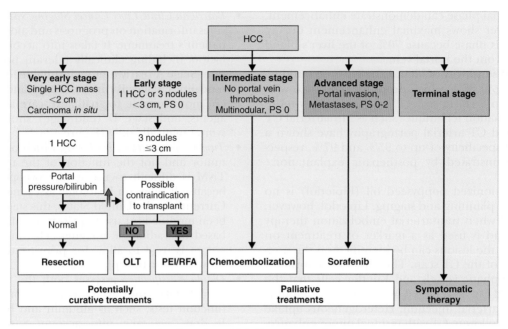

FIGURE 128-4 Management guideline using modified Barcelona Clinic Liver Cancer Staging System. (Reprinted with permission from El-Seraq HB, Marrero JA, Rudolph L, Reddy KR: Diagnosis and treatment of hepatocellular carcinoma. *Gastroenterology* 134:1752, 2008.)

developing a second primary after resection for HCC is about 35% at 1 year, 40% to 50% over 3 years, and as high as 70% at 5 years.[28,29]

Much of the future of therapy for this disease will be aimed at reducing the risk of second primary lesions. These therapies may either identify patients at risk for development of a second primary lesion or prevent the ongoing production of new cancers by limiting viral damage, inflammation, or progression of dysplasia to cancer. Unfortunately, 80% of patients will present at a stage too advanced for surgical resection or transplantation. These patients may be candidates for other types of locoregional therapy or systemic chemotherapy.

SYSTEMIC CHEMOTHERAPY

In patients with intermediate or advanced HCC, surgical intervention is often contraindicated, and thus chemotherapy has a potential role. However, HCC invariably arises from a diseased liver, which reduces potential tolerance to chemotherapy. This, in combination with the known chemoresistant character of HCC, has previously limited the role of chemotherapy in the management of HCC. Recently, Food and Drug Administration approval has been received for the use of sorafenib. This drug, which has been proven effective for treatment of advanced renal cell carcinoma, has been shown to reduce radiologic disease progression in patients with advanced HCC when compared to a placebo group (5.5 vs. 2.8 months respectively).[30] Better survival rates were also demonstrated in the study in comparison with the placebo group, with an increase in the median survival (10.7 vs. 7.9 months). At this time, the effectiveness of using sorafenib in patients with less advanced disease, especially in the adjuvant or neoadjuvant setting, is unknown. Current trials are examining the use of this

agent as an adjuvant to resection and/or ablation to prevent recurrence or development of second primary lesions after therapy. The estimated cost of the drug is about $5000 per month.

ABLATIVE THERAPIES

Ablation is the use of either energy (radiofrequency or microwave) or toxic substance, such as alcohol, to destroy the lesions. One of the attractive aspects of this class of therapies is that they can be used to destroy a cancer in a cirrhotic liver with a relatively low risk of decompensation of the remaining liver as compared to resection. These therapies are particularly attractive if they can be done percutaneously, though the positioning of the lesion sometimes requires either a laparoscopic or open approach. These techniques have undergone rapid improvement in the past 10 years. It has been suggested that for small lesions, radiofrequency ablation may be equivalent to resection in terms of patient outcome.[31]

Radiofrequency Ablation

Radiofrequency ablation (RFA) consists of a high-frequency alternating current that causes agitation and frictional heat up to 120° C, resulting in denaturing of proteins and the tumor cells' bilayer lipid, resulting in tissue destruction and coagulative necrosis. Once temperatures reach 60° C, complete circumferential tissue damage between 0.5 and 3 cm begins, with a further 8-mm rim of partial destruction.[27]

The stainless-steel insulated needle is inserted into the tumor site, and the prongs are then deployed to provide heating over a larger area. Repeated applications of the heating can be used to treat larger tumors.[32] There are reports that the diameter coagulated by radiofrequency is greater in bigger tumors, because of a conductive "oven effect." When the needles are withdrawn, diathermy is used to prevent tumor seeding.

Indications and Advantages of RFA. Indications for RFA include reducing tumor bulk in patients with unresectable disease in preparation for surgery or transplantation, or in patients who cannot tolerate surgery because of other comorbidities and/or coagulopathies. Recently, a study demonstrated similar outcome in patients receiving RFA vs. resection in HCC lesions less than 5 cm.[33] If the outcome of this study can be verified, percutaneous ablation may become preferred to resection for management of these patients.

Limitations and Disadvantages of RFA. Percutaneous RFA may be limited in lesions that are close to the right hemidiaphragm, near the portal triad or extrahepatic structures, such as the duodenum or colon. The use of a laparoscopic or open surgical approach offers the advantage of being able to inspect the surface of the liver and the ability to move extrahepatic structures such as the colon away from the planned ablation site, as well as simultaneous insertion of multiple electrodes into satellite lesions.

Complete ablation is difficult for tumors near large vessels because of the perfusion of the tissue, which results in protective cooling of the tumor. The use of occlusion of the portal triad (Pringle maneuver) may decrease the effect of the flowing blood removing heat and allowing adequate heating of tumors.

One further limitation of RFA is incomplete tumor destruction. This may occur because of large disease volume and the poor visibility that occurs during the procedure secondary to the gas produced as tissue is ablated. Consequently, patients who undergo RFA must be monitored every 3 months with CT scans or MR images to detect any recurrence.

Percutaneous Ethanol Injection

Ethanol causes cell damage by coagulative necrosis, cell dehydration, and denaturation. It is relatively inexpensive and has few side effects. Percutaneous injection takes place under ultrasound guidance using 95% alcohol. The tumor is injected and the needle is left in situ for 1 to 2 minutes and then withdrawn with negative pressure. Because this procedure can be difficult for lesions near the dome of the liver, CT- or MRI-guided injection is preferred. Percutaneous ethanol injection (PEI) causes complete necrosis in tumors of less than 3 cm, and 50% necrosis in 3- to 5-cm tumors.

Side effects of the procedure include pain, transient hyperthermia, intoxication, portal venous system thrombosis, right pleural effusion, and hemobilia. PEI should not be carried out in patients with bleeding tendencies or advanced cirrhosis.

Radiofrequency ablation has largely replaced PEI. In tumors of less than 2 cm, the outcome is similar for both treatments; however, RFA has better survival rates and lower local recurrence in tumors larger than 4 cm.[34] After PEI, CT scans are obtained for followup. Because necrotic tissue does not enhance on CT, any enhancement is a sign of residual viable tissue. AFP levels, if previously elevated, are checked 2 to 3 weeks after PEI to monitor the effect of therapy.

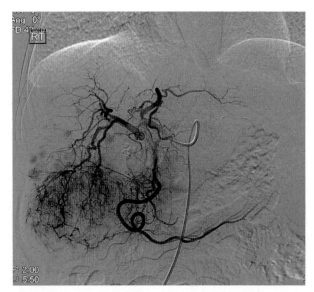

FIGURE 128-5 Digital subtraction angiography demonstrating right hepatic lobe hepatocellular carcinoma with characteristic angiogenesis.

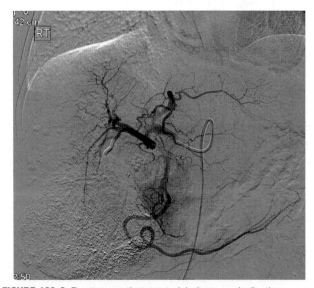

FIGURE 128-6 Posttranscatheter arterial chemoembolization showing complete occlusion of the feeding vessels and hepatocellular carcinoma no longer visualized. The "grainy" appearance shown at the site of the known tumor is residual Lipiodol.

Transcatheter Arterial Chemoembolization

Transcatheter arterial embolization/chemoembolization (TAE/TACE) has become the first line of treatment for managing unresectable or advanced HCC (Figures 128-5 and 128-6). It takes almost all the blood to the tumor. The technique involves occlusion of the hepatic artery supplying the tumor with or without local delivery of chemotherapeutic agent. The expectation is that the occlusion may increase the tumor's susceptibility to the chemotherapeutic agent. Selective arterial catheterization is performed under digital subtraction angiography followed by infusion of chemotherapy (e.g., doxorubicin or cisplatin) suspended in Lipiodol (oily contrast agent) followed by occlusion of the artery using polyvinyl alcohol (PVA) or gelatin sponge.[35] Lipiodol has the tendency to remain in the tumor, and its pattern of distribution is assessed on followup CT scanning. Tissue enhancement within areas of Lipiodol uptake is a sign of recurrence, as the tissue in between areas of uptake either reduce in size or do not enhance on followup.

This procedure is used in patients who are not suitable candidates for anesthesia and/or transplantation. However, patients with portal vein thrombosis are not usually suitable for this technique because there is increased risk of hepatic ischemia. Use of highly selective arterial catheterization may decrease the risk of liver failure after TACE. A study by Llovet and Bruix have shown promising survival rates in use of TACE in unresectable HCC at 1, 2, and 3 years at 96%, 77%, and 47%, respectively.[36] The role of TACE as a bridge to transplantation remains controversial.[37] Because tumor progression can result in patient ineligibility for liver transplantation, patients awaiting a transplant can undergo this procedure in an attempt to prevent tumor progression and vascular invasion. When the waiting time to transplant is relatively short, there may not be a great advantage to providing TACE because the theoretical advantage of TACE is to prevent progression of the disease beyond the stage for which transplantation is effective therapy. In geographic areas where the waiting time to transplantation is quite long, TACE or radiofrequency ablation may prevent progression of small tumors to large tumors, which can prevent transplantation.

Transcatheter Arterial Chemoembolization/ Radiofrequency Ablation Combination Therapy

Studies suggest that combining the tissue necrosis achieved with RFA with the tissue hypoxia secondary to vessel occlusion during TACE results in better survival.[38,39] A recent paper reported the midterm results of a randomized trial of TACE/RFA compared to RFA alone. Although there was not a statistically significant improvement in survival, 3-year survival rates of the patients in the RFA and TACE-RFA groups were 80% and 93%, respectively ($P = 0.369$). The rates of local tumor progression at the end of the third year in the RFA and TACE-RFA groups were 39% and 6%, respectively ($P = 0.012$) (Figures 128-7 and 128-8).[40]

Other Treatments

Microwave Therapy. In radiofrequency ablation therapy, the electrodes act as an active source of energy, whereas in microwave thermotherapy, which causes kinetic energy among molecules that converts into heat energy, the probe inserted into the tumor site acts as a transmitter of energy from an external source. Microwave therapy can be delivered percutaneously, laparoscopically, or via open surgery. Microwave therapy is thought to penetrate tissue better than radiofrequency therapy, resulting in larger areas of ablation, which, unlike RFA, is not limited by areas of tissue desiccation.

Complications include pain, fever, hematoma formation, and bleeding.

Several studies have reported the efficacy of microwave ablation. A recent study reported 1-year and 5-year survival rates of 93% and 51%, respectively.[41]

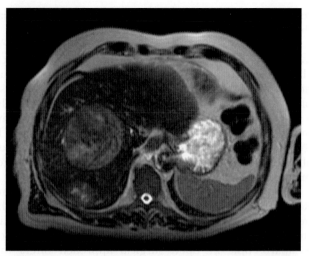

FIGURE 128-7 MRI—two hepatocellular carcinoma lesions within the right hepatic lobe.

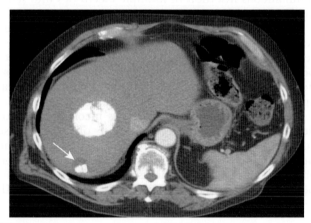

FIGURE 128-8 Contrast enhanced CT followup imaging posttranscatheter arterial chemoembolization. The larger lesions demonstrate Lipiodol within the lesion. Although the smaller lesion, posteriorly, demonstrates a smaller, nonenhanced area *(white arrow)*, the appearances are in keeping with response to treatment. Both lesions show tumor size reduction.

Laser Ablation. This technique requires use of light fibers transferring energy into tissue, causing tissue dehydration and necrosis. A further probe causes focal cooling to avoid local overheating. No randomized controlled trials have been performed on long-term outcome and efficacy with laser ablation.

Resection. If the HCC tumor is limited to one lobe and there is no extrahepatic invasion, the remaining liver is functional enough to support life, and the tumor is surgically accessible, then surgical resection should be considered.

EVALUATING HEPATIC FUNCTION AND RESERVE

Usually the advanced nature of HCC at the time of presentation means that most patients are not suitable for surgical resection, because of concurrent cirrhosis and hepatic impairment. Postoperatively, patients are at risk of hepatic failure. Therefore, the determining factor of whether a patient is a candidate for resection is adequate hepatic function, which must be assessed pre-operatively. Careful preoperative planning and correct patient selection result in perioperative mortality as low as 1% and 5-year survival of 40% to 70% depending on disease stage.

Several tests have been used to assess hepatic function before resection to determine the appropriate extent of hepatic resection. Indocyanine green (ICG) clearance is used in patients with normal synthetic function (bilirubin, albumin, and prothrombin time). If hepatic ICG retention is greater than 20% at 15 minutes after injection, no more than one-sixth of the liver should be resected. If ICG retention is greater than 30%, then limited resection or RFA is appropriate.[42] Although the ICG test has its advocates, it is not widely used in the United States.

When assessing cirrhotic patients for resection, a rule of thumb is that patients with Child-Pugh score A can have up to 50% of their liver resected. This value decreases to 25% for Child-Pugh B and is contraindicated in Child-Pugh C.[43] Using this general guideline, it is not certain that more complex testing has a greater predictive value than this rule of thumb.

The presence of portal hypertension as measured by the hepatic vein wedge pressure and an abnormal bilirubin appear to be a combined risk factor for postoperative decompensation and may predict patient suitability for resection. The presence of portal hypertension prevents adequate regeneration of the liver.

More recently, portal vein embolization has been used to assess and minimize the risk of liver failure after resection.[44] This technique consists of accessing the portal vein percutaneously and embolizing the branch of the portal vein that supplies the lobe to be resected. In theory, portal vein embolization allows the portal blood to be diverted from the lobe to be resected and allows compensatory hypertrophy of the lobe that is to remain after resection. Significant growth of the lobe contralateral to the embolized portal branch appears to signify that the liver is capable of regeneration. Failure of growth suggests that the liver that would be left behind after resection may not be capable of regeneration. The technique may allow for improved postoperative survival in patients with fibrosis or cirrhosis who undergo resection. Portal vein embolization is not efficacious in patients who clearly have portal hypertension.

Intraoperative ultrasonography has been used to ascertain vessel orientation, which, when combined with preoperative knowledge of the tumor and its blood supply, makes accurate resection of the tumor and its associated segments possible. Once the tumor and its associated vessels are identified, the surface markings are made on the liver using diathermy. The information gained by this technique may allow for segmental or subsegmental resections that are oncologically correct but spare as much residual liver as possible.

OPERATIVE TECHNIQUES

There are many ways of performing liver surgery. The appropriate technique depends on the location of the tumor, the degree of cirrhosis, and the experience of the surgeon. The principles are the prevention of blood loss and the preservation of as much functional liver as possible. It does appear that margins greater than 5 to 10 mm are adequate.

Several techniques are used to minimize blood loss. These include inflow occlusion, total vascular isolation, and the use of clamps to compress the parenchyma. The intermittent inflow occlusion technique (Pringle maneuver) is used to minimize blood loss during hepatectomies. Fifteen minutes of occlusion followed by 5 minutes of reperfusion is usually used. Another technique is total vascular isolation of the liver in which occlusion of the infrahepatic and suprahepatic vena cava is combined with occlusion of portal triad inflow. This technique can be helpful when the resection requires dividing parenchyma that is close to a major hepatic vein that cannot be sacrificed.

The expectation is that as instrumentation improves and surgeons get more experience with laparoscopic resection of the liver, it will become much more common. Currently both right and left lobes of the liver can be resected laparoscopically. Laparoscopic resection is less invasive and results in shorter postoperative hospital stays as a result of earlier patient mobilization and restoration of normal bowel function.

Outcome of Resection

HCC recurrence after resection/partial hepatectomy is common with reported figures between 50% and 80% of patients recurring within 5 years, with the majority recurring within 2 years. Recurrence may be in the form of residual lesion or, because of the field effect, a second primary lesion. Of these two possibilities, the more common is a second primary lesion. Thus it is crucial to scrutinize all imaging preoperatively. Given the relative lack of sensitivity of the CT scan for small lesions, it is not surprising that small lesions, that later grow to recognizable size, are missed in the preoperative staging. Some additional lesions may be found by the use of intraoperative ultrasound, but the specificity of the technique is limited in a nodular liver.

Transplantation

Hepatic transplantation is an effective way to remove both the carcinoma and the remaining cirrhotic liver with its propensity for tumorigenesis. Overall survival and recurrence-free survival after transplantation are better than resection for selected tumor stages. Criteria stated by Mazzaferro et al,[45] also known as the *Milan criteria* (Figure 128-9), propose transplantation for patients who have a single tumor smaller than 5 cm or fewer than three tumors, each of which are smaller than 3 cm. Using these criteria resulted in an overall 4-year survival rate of 74%, similar to that for patients who received a liver transplant but did not have HCC. The 4-year survival rate for patients outside of the Milan criteria is only about 40%. Because of these poorer results, patients with larger tumors are excluded from deceased donor transplantation in the United States.

There has been criticism that the Milan criteria may be too strict, eliminating patients from transplantation

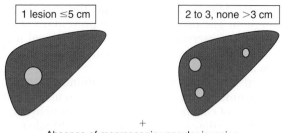

FIGURE 128-9 Milan Criteria. (From Mazzaferro V, Regalia E, Doci R, et al: Liver transplantation for the treatment of small hepatocellular carcinomas in patients with cirrhosis. *N Engl J Med* 334:693, 1996.)

who would have equivalent survival. Alternative criteria, known as the *University of California San Francisco (UCSF) criteria*, were proposed by Yao et al.[46] These criteria offered transplantation to patients with a single tumor less than 6.5 cm or fewer than three tumors, the total diameter of all being less than 8 cm and the largest tumor less than 4.5 cm. The 1- and 5-year survival rates for these patients posttransplant were 90% and 75%, respectively.

In February 2002, the United Network for Organ Sharing (UNOS) modified their criteria, giving priority to patients with HCC. This has increased the number of liver transplants among patients with HCC. It is estimated that 20% of the liver transplants done in the United States are for patients with HCC. Patients meeting the Milan criteria gain a priority for transplantation if one of the tumors is greater than 2 cm in diameter. Patients with single lesions less than 2 cm do not receive priority.

While patients are on the waiting list for a liver transplant, tumor progression or even death may occur. As noted earlier, a major obstacle for patients for whom a transplant is suitable is the lengthy waiting time during which tumor growth may result in the tumor progressing beyond the Milan criteria and having to drop off the waiting list. Ideally, waiting times should be less than 6 months, but because of the donor shortage, waiting times can exceed 12 months in some areas of the country. The median waiting time for transplantation in the United States is currently about 3 months. Dropout rates for patients with HCC have been reported to be as high as 70% depending on the length of time the patient waits for transplantation.[47]

Living donor liver transplantation (LDLT) has provided a new source of organs for transplantation. Originally, LDLT was performed in children, with an organ donated from a parent or other relative; however, adult-to-adult LDLT is now performed throughout the world. Some studies suggest similar outcomes in cadaveric and LDLT, whereas other studies have shown an increased risk following LDLT.[48] Because the waiting time before transplantation can be quite short, there is a concern that LDLT may produce more risk of recurrence. More studies are needed on the natural history of HCC and its recurrence rate in such cases.[49]

The advantages of LDLT for patients with HCC include little or no time on the waiting list, thus avoiding the risk of tumor progression while waiting. Decision analyses have shown that LDLT for patients with HCC improves life expectancy and is more cost-effective than waiting on the transplant list for more than 7 months.[50]

LDLT raises a number of ethical issues that need to be dealt with on an individual basis. These include (1) ascertaining that a donor's decision to donate part of their organ is voluntary; (2) ensuring a clear understanding by the donor that the procedure, unlike most operations, is not being done for their own medical problem; (3) noting that donation is associated with complications both intraoperatively and postoperatively; and (d) that there is uncertainty about the long-term survival of donors and the effect on their quality of life.

Resection Versus Transplantation

In many parts of the world, the lack of resources available for transplantation makes this question moot. In countries that have available resources, controversy continues about whether a patient with HCC should undergo resection or liver transplantation. Although patients with HCC usually have portal hypertension and hepatic decompensation, making most patients suitable only for transplantation, a small group of patients with small tumors with hepatic reserve are potentially suitable for either resection or transplantation. To date, however, no randomized controlled studies have been published comparing resection and transplantation in such groups of patients. It appears that for tumors that fit the Milan or UCSF criteria, the outcome after transplantation is better than the outcome 5 years after resection. A recent literature review by Morris-Stiff et al[49] demonstrated that disease-free survival rates postresection at 1, 3, and 5 years were 64%, 38%, and 27%, respectively. The disease-free survival rates following liver transplantation at the same time intervals were 79%, 62.5%, and 54.5%.

However, a major issue is that the patients on the transplant waiting list have a risk of tumor progression during the waiting time. Patients who have a liver cancer are at risk for developing a second lesion. As the Milan criteria limit the size and number of primaries where transplantation is indicated, this progression may result in a patient being unsuitable for transplantation. In addition, patients with cirrhosis generally have progression of their disease and are at risk for developing liver failure. One factor that merits consideration in the decision about resection versus liver transplantation is the waiting time to obtain a liver transplant; an immediate resection has a better outcome than waiting a year for a liver transplant, because the immediate resection prevents progression of the disease (Figure 128-10).[51]

In about half of the United States, the waiting time to transplantation is less than 3 months. In this situation, liver transplantation has a better survival at a lower cost per life-year than resection.[52]

Controversy exists about the strategy of initially resecting patients who would be transplant candidates and having transplantation as a means of salvage if the tumor recurs.

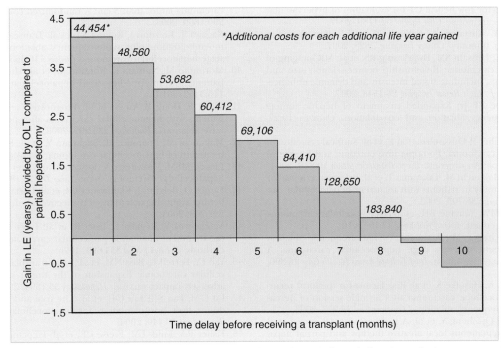

FIGURE 128-10 Tabular demonstration of life expectancy in patients who undergo orthotopic liver transplant versus resection. (From Sarasin FP, Giostra E, Mentha G, et al: Partial hepatectomy or orthotopic liver transplantation for the treatment of resectable hepatocellular carcinoma? A cost-effectiveness perspective. *Hepatology* 28:436, 1998.)

This strategy attempts to take advantage of the fact that about 30% of patients who undergo resection or ablation will be alive and disease free 5 years after resection. Currently, there is no way to prospectively select the patients who will survive. This presupposes that transplantation after resection (secondary transplantation) does not have a significantly different survival rate than transplantation without resection (primary transplantation) and that patients with recurrence are frequently transplant candidates.

REFERENCES

1. Ferenci P, Fried M, Labrecque D, et al: Hepatocellular carcinoma (HCC): A global perspective. *J Clin Gastroenterol* 44:239, 2010.
2. Centers for Disease Control and Prevention: Hepatocellular carcinoma—United States, 2001-2006. *Morb Mortal Wkly Rep* 59:517, 2010. Available from: http://www.cdc.gov/mmwr/preview/mmwrhtml/mm5917a3.htm.
3. Marrero CR, Marrero JA: Viral Hepatitis and Hepatocellular Carcinoma. *Arch Med Res* 38:612, 2007.
4. El-Serag HB: Hepatocellular carcinoma: Recent trends in the United States. *Gastroenterology* 127:S27, 2004.
5. Davis GL, Alter MJ, El-Serag H, et al: Aging of hepatitis C virus (HCV)-infected persons in the United States: A multiple cohort model of HCV prevalence and disease progression. *Gastroenterology* 138:513, 2010.
6. Sanyal A, Poklepovic A, Moyneur E, et al: Population-based risk factors and resource utilization for HCC: US perspective. *Curr Med Res Opin* 26:2183, 2010.
7. Liu YWF: Global burden of aflatoxin-induced hepatocellular carcinoma: A risk assessment. *Environ Health Perspect* 118:818, 2010.
8. Di Bisceglie AM: Natural history of hepatitis C: Its impact on clinical management. *Hepatology* 31:1014, 2000.
9. Röcken C, Carl-McGrath S: Pathology and pathogenesis of hepatocellular carcinoma. *Dig Dis* 19:269, 2001.
10. Koike Y, Shiratori Y, Sato S, et al: Risk factors for recurring hepatocellular carcinoma differ according to infected hepatitis virus—An analysis of 236 consecutive patients with a single lesion. *Hepatology* 32:1216, 2000.
11. Semela D, Dufour J-F: Angiogenesis and hepatocellular carcinoma. *J Hepatol* 41:864, 2004.
12. Esnaola NF, Lauwers GY, Mirza NQ, et al: Predictors of microvascular invasion in patients with hepatocellular carcinoma who are candidates for orthotopic liver transplantation. *J Gastrointest Surg* 6:224, 2002.
13. Sakata J, Shirai Y, Wakai T, et al: Preoperative predictors of vascular invasion in hepatocellular carcinoma. *Eur J Surg Oncol (EJSO)* 34:900, 2008.
14. Talwalkar JA, Gores GJ: Diagnosis and staging of hepatocellular carcinoma. *Gastroenterology* 127:S126, 2004.
15. Saitoh S, Ikeda K, Koida I, et al: Small hepatocellular carcinoma: Evaluation of portal blood flow with CT during arterial portography performed with balloon occlusion of the hepatic artery. *Radiology* 193:67, 1994.
16. Bruix J, Sherman M: Management of hepatocellular carcinoma. *Hepatology* 42:1208, 2005.
17. Llovet JM, Burroughs A, Bruix J: Hepatocellular carcinoma. *Lancet* 362:1907, 2003.
18. Bolondi LSS, Siringo S, Gaiani S, et al: Surveillance programme of cirrhotic patients for early diagnosis and treatment of hepatocellular carcinoma: A cost effectiveness analysis. *Gut* 48:251, 2001.
19. Zhang B-H, Yang B-H, Tang Z-Y: Randomized controlled trial of screening for hepatocellular carcinoma. *J Cancer Res Clin Oncol* 130:417, 2004.
20. Van Thiel DH, Yong S, Li SD, et al: The development of de novo hepatocellular carcinoma in patients on a liver transplant list: Frequency, size, and assessment of current screening methods. *Liver Transplant* 10:631, 2004.
21. El-Serag HB, Marrero JA, Rudolph L, et al: Diagnosis and treatment of hepatocellular carcinoma. *Gastroenterology* 134:1752, 2008.
22. Perez-Johnston R, Lenhart DK, Sahani DV: CT Angiography of the hepatic and pancreatic circulation. *Radiol Clin North Am* 48:311, 2010.
23. Murakami T, Kim T, Takamura M, et al: Hypervascular hepatocellular carcinoma: Detection with double arterial phase multidetector row helical CT. *Radiology* 218:763, 2001.
24. Tsurusaki M, Sugimoto K, Fujii M, et al: Combination of CT during arterial portography and double-phase CT hepatic arteriography

with multi-detector row helical CT for evaluation of hypervascular hepatocellular carcinoma. *Clin Radiol* 62:1189, 2007.

25. Schima WB-SA, Kurtaran A, Schindl M, et al: Post-treatment imaging of liver tumours. *Cancer Imaging* 7:S28, 2007.

26. van den Bos IC, Hussain SM, Dwarkasing RS, et al: MR imaging of hepatocellular carcinoma: Relationship between lesion size and imaging findings, including signal intensity and dynamic enhancement patterns. *J Magn Reson Imaging* 26:1548, 2007.

27. Weber SM, Lee FT Jr: Expanded treatment of hepatic tumors with radiofrequency ablation and cryoablation. *Oncology* 19:27, 2005.

28. Jaeck D, Bachellier P, Oussoultzoglou E, et al: Surgical resection of hepatocellular carcinoma. Post-operative outcome and long-term results in Europe: An overview. *Liver Transplantation* 10:S58, 2004.

29. Minagawa M, Makuuchi M, Takayama T, et al: Selection criteria for repeat hepatectomy in patients with recurrent hepatocellular carcinoma. *Ann Surg* 238:703, 2003.

30. Cha CH, Saif MW, Yamane BH, et al: Hepatocellular carcinoma: Current management. *Curr Probl Surg* 47:10, 2010.

31. Zie XDN, McGregor M: Percutaneous radiofrequency ablation for the treatment of early stage hepatocellular carcinoma: A health technology assessment. *Int J Technol Assess Health Care* 26:390, 2010.

32. Hori T, Nagata K, Hasuike S, et al: Risk factors for the local recurrence of hepatocellular carcinoma after a single session of percutaneous radiofrequency ablation. *J Gastroenterol* 38:977, 2003.

33. Chen M-S, Li J-Q, Zheng Y, et al: A prospective randomized trial comparing percutaneous local ablative therapy and partial hepatectomy for small hepatocellular carcinoma. *Ann Surg* 243:321, 2006.

34. Lin S-M, Lin C-J, Lin C-C, et al: Radiofrequency ablation improves prognosis compared with ethanol injection for hepatocellular carcinoma ≤4 cm. *Gastroenterology* 127:1714, 2004.

35. Vogl TJ, Naguib NN, Nour-Eldin N-E, et al: Review on transarterial chemoembolization in hepatocellular carcinoma: Palliative, combined, neoadjuvant, bridging, and symptomatic indications. *Eur J Radiol* 72:505, 2009.

36. Llovet JM, Bruix J: Systematic review of randomized trials for unresectable hepatocellular carcinoma: Chemoembolization improves survival. *Hepatology* 37:429, 2003.

37. Ravaioli M, Grazi GL, Ercolani G, et al: Partial necrosis on hepatocellular carcinoma nodules facilitates tumor recurrence after liver transplantation. *Transplantation* 78:1780, 2004.

38. Cheng B-Q, Jia C-Q, Liu C-T, et al: Chemoembolization combined with radiofrequency ablation for patients with hepatocellular carcinoma larger than 3 cm: A randomized controlled trial. *JAMA* 299:1669, 2008.

39. Kagawa T, Koizumi J, Kojima S-I, et al: Transcatheter arterial chemoembolization plus radiofrequency ablation therapy for early stage hepatocellular carcinoma. *Cancer* 116:3638, 2010.

40. Morimoto M, Numata K, Kondou M, et al: Midterm outcomes in patients with intermediate-sized hepatocellular carcinoma. *Cancer* 116:5452, 2010.

41. Liang P, Dong B, Yu X, et al: Prognostic factors for survival in patients with hepatocellular carcinoma after percutaneous microwave ablation1. *Radiology* 235:299, 2005.

42. Makuuchi M, Imamura H, Sugawara Y, et al: Progress in surgical treatment of hepatocellular carcinoma. *Oncology* 62:74, 2002.

43. Llovet JMSM, Mazzaferro V: Resection and liver transplantation for hepatocellular carcinoma. *Semin Liver Dis* 25:181, 2005.

44. Farges O, Belghiti J, Kianmanesh R, et al: Portal vein embolization before right hepatectomy: Prospective clinical trial. *Ann Surg* 237:208, 2003.

45. Mazzaferro V, Regalia E, Doci R, et al: Liver transplantation for the treatment of small hepatocellular carcinomas in patients with cirrhosis. *N Engl J Med* 334:693, 1996.

46. Yao FY, Ferrell L, Bass NM, et al: Liver transplantation for hepatocellular carcinoma: Expansion of the tumor size limits does not adversely impact survival. *Hepatology* 33:1394, 2001.

47. Lo C-M, Fan S-T, Liu C-L, et al: The role and limitation of living donor liver transplantation for hepatocellular carcinoma. *Liver Transplant* 10:440, 2004.

48. Fisher RA, Kulik LM, Freise CE, et al: Hepatocellular Carcinoma Recurrence and Death Following Living and Deceased Donor Liver Transplantation. *Am J Transplant* 7:1601, 2007.

49. Morris-Stiff G, Gomez D, de Liguori Carino N, et al: Surgical management of hepatocellular carcinoma: Is the jury still out? *Surg Oncol* 18:298, 2009.

50. Sarasin FP, Majno PE, Llovet JM, et al: Living donor liver transplantation for early hepatocellular carcinoma: A life-expectancy and cost-effectiveness perspective. *Hepatology* 33:1073, 2001.

51. Sarasin FP, Giostra E, Mentha G, et al: Partial hepatectomy or orthotopic liver transplantation for the treatment of resectable hepatocellular carcinoma? A cost-effectiveness perspective. *Hepatology* 28:436, 1998.

52. Majno PE, Sarasin FP, Mentha G, et al: Primary liver resection and salvage transplantation or primary liver transplantation in patients with single, small hepatocellular carcinoma and preserved liver function: An outcome-oriented decision analysis. *Hepatology* 31:899, 2000.

Management of Malignant Hepatic Neoplasms Other Than Hepatocellular Carcinoma

Michael A. Choti

Any variety of primary malignancies can arise from the liver because of cellular heterogeneity present in this complex organ. In addition to hepatocytes, the liver is made up of cholangiocytes, neuroendocrine cells, hepatic progenitors, myofibroblastic mesenchymal cells, and vascular endothelial cells. Hepatocellular carcinoma (HCC) comprises an estimated 80% to 90% of primary liver cancers,[1] whereas all other primary malignancies of the liver, including cholangiocarcinoma, account for the remaining 10% to 20%.[2] Table 129-1 outlines the primary hepatic neoplasms based on the presumed cell of origin. This chapter will focus on nonhepatocellular primary malignancies of the liver. Though less common than HCC, these tumor types can be aggressive and are being seen with increasing frequency. The clinician should have a better understanding in the recognition and management of these malignancies (Box 129-1).

INTRAHEPATIC CHOLANGIOCARCINOMA

Intrahepatic cholangiocarcinoma (ICC) is the second most common primary liver malignancy, accounting for up to 15% of all primary liver cancers.[3] Although the incidence of extrahepatic cholangiocarcinoma (hilar and distal bile duct cancer) is decreasing in the United States and worldwide, ICC has more than doubled in incidence over recent decades (from 0.32 per 100,000 in 1975 to 0.85 per 100,000 in 1999).[3] Reasons for the rise in incidence are likely multifactorial but may in part be related to improved radiographic and pathologic determination of many patients in the past who were classified as having metastases to the liver, frequently called "adenocarcinoma of unknown origin." Yet, recent epidemiologic evidence suggests the true incidence of ICC to be increasing as well.[4]

The evaluation and staging of ICC is based on serologic, radiologic, and histologic findings. Previous studies have demonstrated that elevated serum concentration of CA 19-9, a tumor-associated antigen, has good sensitivity and specificity for cholangiocarcinoma in patients and is a useful adjunct to the workup of cholangiocarcinoma. Patel et al have shown in 36 patients with sporadic cholangiocarcinoma that serum CA19-9 values greater than 100 U/mL are associated with sensitivity of 53% and specificity of 75% to 90% for the diagnosis of malignancy, compared to those with benign liver disease or benign biliary strictures.[5]

Radiologic evaluation is also critical in the evaluation of an ICC.[6,7] As with other intrahepatic malignancies,

computed tomography (CT) or magnetic resonance imaging (MRI) can identify a mass lesion within the liver (Figure 129-1, A). In most cases, ICC has imaging characteristics similar to hepatic metastases, including peripheral venous enhancement and central necrosis. Less commonly, ICC can appear with arterial enhancement or intravascular thrombus, mimicking radiologic findings of HCC.[7,8] More recently, fluoro-deoxyglucose positron emission tomography (FDG-PET) is emerging as a potentially useful adjunctive imaging modality in patients being considered for surgical therapy for ICC.[9-11] These reports suggest the nodular ICC morphology to be more avid in FDG uptake than the infiltrating form and, in general, PET is most valuable for detecting regional lymph node involvement and unsuspected distant metastases. Unlike for the evaluation and management of hilar cholangiocarcinoma, percutaneous or endoscopic cholangiography is seldom required for the management of ICC.

When a biopsy of a suspicious liver tumor reveals adenocarcinoma, perhaps the most common diagnostic dilemma is differentiating ICC from hepatic metastasis of known or unknown site. In such cases, careful history of a previous malignancy, identification of other risk factors, and scrutiny of tumor markers can be helpful. Moreover, multifocal lesions within the liver increase the likelihood that these are metastases. Staging of the chest and abdomen using CT scanning are useful to help rule out other potential primary tumors as well as metastatic disease. Upper and lower endoscopy should be considered to rule out an intestinal origin and, in women, mammography and gynecologic screening should be considered.

Intraoperatively, ICC can appear much like other hepatic malignancies, often with normal-appearing surrounding liver (Figure 129-1, B). Careful intraoperative assessment is important to rule out extrahepatic disease and other tumors within the liver. As with most liver surgery, intraoperative ultrasonography plays an important role in assessment and planning of liver surgery for ICC. When possible, surgical resection is the treatment of choice for ICC. The goal of resection is the complete extirpation of all gross disease with negative margins while maintaining adequate portal and arterial inflow, hepatic venous outflow, intact biliary drainage, and sufficient uninvolved remnant liver volume. Inclusion of a resection of the extrahepatic biliary tree with reconstruction may be required in some circumstances when the disease extends into the porta hepatis. In one study from Memorial Sloan-Kettering Cancer Center, among the 82

TABLE 129-1 Cellular Phenotype and Primary Hepatic Neoplasms

Cellular Phenotype	Primary Hepatic Tumor
Epithelial	
Hepatocellular	Hepatocellular carcinoma
Hepatic progenitor	Hepatoblastoma
Cholangiocellular	Intrahepatic cholangiocarcinoma
	Hepatic cystadenocarcinoma
Mixed	Mixed cholangiohepatocellular carcinoma
Other	Primary squamous cell carcinoma
Mesenchymal	
Muscular	Leiomyosarcoma
	Rhabdomyosarcoma
Fibroblastic	Fibrosarcoma
Adipose	Liposarcoma
Neural	Schwannoma
Vascular	Angiosarcoma
	Epithelioid hemangioendothelioma

BOX 129-1 Management Options and Therapies for Primary Hepatic Neoplasms

SURGICAL RESECTION
Major hepatectomy
Minor hepatectomy (anatomic or wedge)
Laparoscopic liver resection
Total hepatectomy with orthotopic liver transplantation

ABLATION (OPERATIVE, LAPAROSCOPIC, OR PERCUTANEOUS)
Radiofrequency ablation
Microwave ablation
Laser hyperthermia
Cryotherapy
Irreversible electroporation

NONOPERATIVE
Chemotherapy
  Systemic therapy
  Transarterial chemoembolization (TACE)
  Hepatic artery infusion (HAI)
Radiotherapy
  Yttrium-90 intraarterial radioembolization
  Stereotactic external-beam radiotherapy
Chemical therapy
  Percutaneous ethanol injection

patients who underwent resection for ICC, 78% required major hepatectomy and 21% required a concomitant biliary resection.[12]

Complete resection is associated with improved long-term survival in patients with ICC, with reported 5-year overall survival rates of 18% to 34%.[13-17] Outcomes seem to be improving more recently. Endo et al reported improved disease-free survival when comparing patients resected between 2000 and 2006 compared to those resected between 1990 and 1999 (14% vs. 21%, $P = 0.043$).[12] Similarly, Nathan et al reported in a review of ICC outcomes in the United States using the Surveillance Epidemiology and End Results (SEER) database, a trend toward better outcome following resection, in spite of overall poorer outcome in patients with ICC.[15]

Intrahepatic cholangiocarcinoma is commonly associated with regional lymph node involvement.[18] Moreover, nodal involvement is an important predictor of poor long-term outcome following resection.[15,19] Based on these data, some have questioned the value of surgical resection in patients with ICC and lymph node involvement. Uenishi et al found, however, that although patients with negative nodes had the best survival, patients with positive lymph node involvement and solitary tumors enjoyed long-term survival in some cases, with a 5-year survival rate of 26%.[20] Though controversial, these and other reports have promoted the position by some that surgical resection should be offered to patients even with preoperative evidence of nodal involvement, provided all disease can be completely removed. In addition, many now recommend routine hilar and periportal lymphadenectomy in all patients undergoing surgical resection for ICC.

Similar to the management of other primary liver tumors and hepatic metastases, a variety of locoregional approaches can be considered in patients with unresectable disease. Thermal ablation has been reported in small series of patients with ICC.[21,22] However, this approach is only useful in small tumors (<5 cm) and unlike HCC or hepatic metastases, ICC rarely presents with low-volume disease amenable to interstitial ablation. In addition, although ablation has been shown to play a role in other liver malignancies, there are no studies with sufficient sample size to know the long-term benefit of tumor ablation in ICC. In contrast, regional intraarterial approaches are being reported with increasing frequency. In particular, transarterial chemoembolization for ICC is promising, with response rates ranging from 40% to 70% and median survival times of 12 to 29 months.[23-26] This modality should generally be used for unresectable patients with liver-only or liver-dominant disease. The role of other intraarterial approaches, including hepatic arterial infusion and yttrium-90 radioembolization, are equally promising but less well studied.

Systemic therapies have also improved in the management of advanced ICC. Specifically, several recent studies have demonstrated benefit of the combination of gemcitabine plus cisplatin over gemcitabine alone for patients with advanced or metastatic biliary tract cancer.[27,28] Studies are underway examining the role of novel targeted agents combined with cytotoxic chemotherapy in patients with advanced disease, as well as examining the role of adjuvant or neoadjuvant systemic therapies in patients undergoing surgical therapy.

MIXED CHOLANGIOHEPATOCELLULAR CARCINOMA

Over recent years, an increased understanding of stem cell theories has shed light on how cancer develops in the liver.[29,30] Given that bipotential liver progenitors exist in the adult liver that can differentiate toward hepatocytic or biliary lineages, it is conceivable that these cells

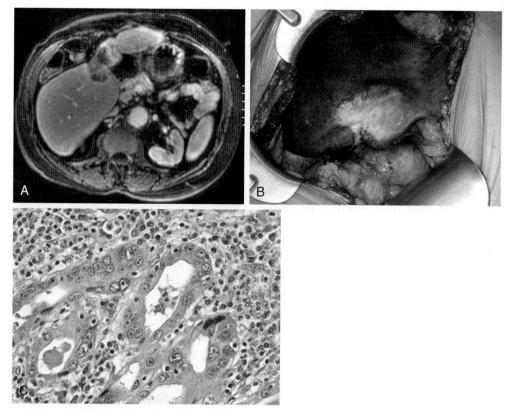

FIGURE 129-1 A, Magnetic resonance imaging demonstrating a 6-cm intrahepatic cholangiocarcinoma involving the left hemiliver. **B,** Intraoperative photograph demonstrating the same tumor before planned resection. **C,** Photomicrograph of an intrahepatic cholangiocarcinoma. Small glandular structures with nuclei that are oval and vesicular can be seen. There is also demonstrable mucin production within the ducts. (Courtesy M.S. Torbenson, Department of Pathology, Johns Hopkins Hospital.)

may give rise to tumors of heterogeneous cellularity or mixed cholangiohepatocellular carcinoma. On the basis of the concomitant cytokeratin profile consistent with a bile ductular lineage, albumin expression consistent with a hepatocytic lineage, as well as carcinoembryonic antigen (CEA) and α-fetoprotein (AFP) levels, mixed cholangiohepatocellular carcinomas exist and can be distinguished from ICC and HCC. Like HCC, these rare tumors are commonly associated with chronic viral hepatitis as well as cirrhosis suggesting that chronic injury and expansion of hepatic progenitors may be earlier events in tumor progression. However, this is not always the case.[31] Cross-sectional imaging of mixed tumors typically appears much like HCC, with arterial enhancement and heterogeneous necrosis (Figure 129-2). Histologically, although two cellular patterns are recognized, this tumor has features of both HCC and ICC within one discrete mass. They can be classified into two types: "collision tumors," which demonstrate more discrete areas of domination by hepatocytic or biliary cells, and "transition tumors," which have a more uniform heterogeneity.[32,33]

Given the similarity of mixed cholangiohepatocellular carcinomas with HCC, in general, the recommended management is comparable. Liver resection should be considered as the treatment of choice when possible based on staging and health of the surrounding uninvolved liver. Similarly, liver transplantation can be considered based on similar criteria to that of HCC (e.g., Milan criteria). Predicting outcomes (e.g., disease progression,

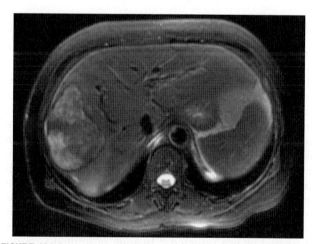

FIGURE 129-2 Abdominal MRI revealing a large right liver mass. Pathologic analysis following resection demonstrated findings consistent with a mixed cholangiohepatocellular carcinoma.

metastasis, and prognosis) based on histopathology is difficult given the infrequency of these tumors.

HEPATIC CYSTADENOCARCINOMA

In addition to the ICC and mixed cholangiohepatocellular carcinoma, the hepatic or biliary cystadenocarcinoma is a tumor with an epithelioid phenotype. The hepatic cystadenocarcinoma is uncommon, with fewer than 200 cases reported in the literature.[34-36] Cystadenocarcinomas are felt to arise from intrahepatic bile ducts and possibly from a benign cystadenoma, although the relationship between cystadenoma and cystadenocarcinoma is not clear. Unlike the benign condition that mostly occurs in women, the incidence of cystadenocarcinoma occurs equally among males and females.[34,37] Yet, given the potential association, most experts recommend complete resection of hepatic cystadenoma because of the potential risk for malignant transformation.

Hepatic cystadenocarcinoma can present with localized symptoms or with advanced disease. With increasing frequency, this tumor is presenting as an incidental finding on radiologic imaging such as CT, MRI, and ultrasonography. Cystadenocarcinoma tends to be larger in size than their benign counterpart but this feature is not reliable. The radiologic appearance of a hepatic cystic mass with features of a thick or irregular wall, peripheral enhancement, associated mass, or papillary tumor projections into the cyst cavity should lead one to suspect cystadenocarcinoma. Histologically, these tumors are characterized by cellular pleomorphism, anaplasia, and evidence of invasiveness. The cyst fluid can be helpful to distinguish benign from malignant cystic tumors[36,38] but with suboptimal accuracy and risk of peritoneal seeding. Consequently, cyst aspiration is not recommended in most cases.

The only potentially curative treatment for cystadenocarcinomas is complete removal, usually by a major liver resection with clear margins.[34,36] Survival rates for this disease have been reported in the range of 25% to 100% at 5 years.

SQUAMOUS CELL CARCINOMA OF THE LIVER

Primary squamous cell carcinoma of the liver is extremely rare, with fewer than 30 cases reported in the literature.[39-41] Most patients with this histologic finding within the liver suffer from metastatic deposits from another primary site, and the diagnosis should be made only without evidence of a primary epidermoid malignancy elsewhere, including skin, oropharynx, or anus. Primary SCC of the liver has been reported to be associated with hepatic teratoma, hepatic cyst, or hepatolithiasis.[41-43] Histologically, these tumors are described with keratinized-type cellular features, often with benign-appearing metaplastic squamous epithelium. Overall, survival is poor in these patients with median survival of 6 months when left untreated or not resected.[44] In spite of limited supporting evidence, liver resection is generally recommended when possible, with several reports of long-term survival in selected patients following hepatectomy.[21,26]

PRIMARY HEPATIC SARCOMA: LEIOMYOSARCOMA, RHABDOMYOSARCOMA, FIBROSARCOMA, LIPOSARCOMA

Sarcomas represent only about 2% of primary liver malignancies. Care must be taken not to confuse such primary hepatic malignancy with sarcoma liver metastases, which can arise from gastrointestinal, retroperitoneal, or gynecologic primary sites. Yet, primary hepatic sarcomas do occur, more commonly in children, and can arise from any type of connective tissue, including smooth muscle, liver mesenchymal cells, and fatty tissue. Sarcomas are more often hypervascular in appearance on contrast imaging. However, the pattern of vascularization and a lack of venous invasion can often differentiate primary hepatic sarcomas from HCC, especially in noncirrhotic patients.[45] Histologic or cytologic evaluation with immunohistochemical staining for vimentin, a mesenchymal marker, without staining for epithelial markers can help to confirm the diagnosis.

Again, resection or ablation appears to be the optimal treatment option when possible, with small series reporting some long-term survivors. Careful evaluation of the extent of disease, both within and outside of the liver, is important when evaluating such a patient. Though reasonable to consider, the role of transarterial chemoembolization (TACE) or systemic chemotherapy is unproven.

VASCULAR HEPATIC MALIGNANCIES

Vascular malignancies are exceedingly uncommon primary tumors of the liver. Among these, *angiosarcoma* (Figure 129-3) is the most common, accounting for 1.8% of primary hepatic malignancies. Although the cause is unknown in most patients, some relate a recognized association with exposure to carcinogens such as thorium dioxide (Thorotrast), arsenicals, and vinyl chloride.[46,47] When present, the period from exposure to disease is on the order of several decades. The presenting symptoms are similar to those of most other hepatic malignancies, but spontaneous hemorrhage from the tumor may occur. There are two classic presentations of angiosarcoma: multiple nodules, or as a solitary tumor. Though historically confused with hepatic hemangioma on contrast imaging, more recent reports suggest that these tumors are rarely confused. In particular, MR imaging of angiosarcoma demonstrates heterogeneous signal intensities and septally progressing enhancement.[45] When multifocal and unresectable, operative biopsy via an open or laparoscopic approach is recommended for tissue diagnosis because of the high risk of bleeding during percutaneous interventions.

Most patients with angiosarcoma are not candidates for surgical therapy and overall survival rates for these patients are poor, with a median survival of 6 months and a 2-year survival rate of only 3%.[48,49] Yet, in selected patients with apparently localized and resectable disease, surgical therapy should be considered. In others, consideration for regional or systemic approaches can be offered.

Hepatic epithelioid hemangioendothelioma (HEH) is another rare vascular hepatic neoplasm accounting for less than 1% of primary hepatic malignancies. These tumors most commonly occur in women in the fifth decade of life without underlying chronic liver disease. Risk factors for HEH are unknown, although some have reported an association with vinyl chloride and oral contraceptives.[50] The clinical presentation is variable, and up to 25% can present incidentally. In approximately one-half of cases, cutaneous hemangiomas are also present.

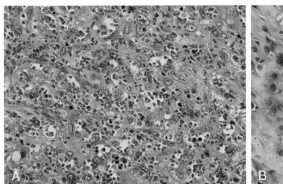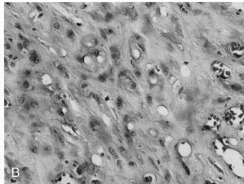

FIGURE 129-3 Comparison of vascular tumors of the liver. **A,** Photomicrograph of an angiosarcoma. Note the small, highly aggressive–appearing cells with disruption of the hepatic parenchymal architecture. **B,** Photomicrograph of an epithelioid hemangioendothelioma. Note the tumor cells' abundant cytoplasm. Although the tumor cells are often surrounded by sclerotic stroma with diffuse hepatic involvement, the liver architecture is preserved. (Courtesy M.S. Torbenson, Department of Pathology, Johns Hopkins Hospital.)

Radiologic evaluation can be helpful in identifying HEH and distinguishing it from angiosarcoma. CT scan can show irregular hypodense lesions that may have hypervascular enhancement in the periphery following injection of intravenous contrast.[45] Tumor calcification can occasionally be seen. The extent of the tumor can often be difficult to evaluate radiologically because they tend to be multifocal and widespread within the liver at the time of diagnosis.

Although imaging studies can distinguish these vascular tumors from other liver neoplasias, diagnosis is confirmed by histologic examination. When not resectable, operative biopsy via an open or laparoscopic approach is recommended for tissue diagnosis, because of the high risk of bleeding during percutaneous procedures. HEH stain strongly positive for coagulation factor VIII expression. The cells are typically epithelioid with abundant cytoplasm, but a dendritic cell type has also been recognized.

The diffuse nature of these tumors often precludes surgical resection and, therefore, survival rates following liver resection are poor. Unlike angiosarcoma, some patients with HEH may benefit from liver transplantation or partial hepatectomy.[51] Grotz et al found that liver transplantation and resection achieved comparable results in the treatment of HEH. When apparently confined to the liver, surgical therapy should be considered.

SUMMARY

Although the worldwide incidence of HCC is rising, clinicians treating patients with liver disease should be aware of the variety of other types of primary hepatic malignancies. Most common among these, intrahepatic cholangiocarcinoma appears to be increasing in incidence. As with HCC and liver metastatic disease, the evaluation and staging should be done based on the potential treatment options available to the patient. When surgical resection is being considered, careful imaging of both the liver and extrahepatic site is important in order to determine resectability. While many of these diseases are rare and therapeutic decisions cannot be based on large prospective studies, hepatic resection should generally be considered when possible for most of these diseases. The

role of liver transplantation, tumor ablation, regional intraarterial approaches, and systemic chemotherapy is poorly established. As with other diseases, it is prudent when managing these patients to do so with a multidisciplinary team involving hepatic surgeons, medical and radiation oncologists, diagnostic and interventional radiologists, and hepatologists.

REFERENCES

1. Nordenstedt H, White DL, El-Serag HB: The changing pattern of epidemiology in hepatocellular carcinoma. *Dig Liver Dis* 42:S206, 2010.
2. Charbel H, Al-Kawas FH: Cholangiocarcinoma: Epidemiology, risk factors, pathogenesis, and diagnosis. *Curr Gastroenterol Rep* 13:182, 2011.
3. Shaib YH, El-Serag HB, Davila JA, et al: Risk factors of intrahepatic cholangiocarcinoma in the United States: A case-control study. *Gastroenterology* 128:620, 2005.
4. Welzel TM, Graubard BI, El-Serag HB, et al: Risk factors for intrahepatic and extrahepatic cholangiocarcinoma in the United States: A population-based case-control study. *Clin Gastroenterol Hepatol* 5:1221, 2007.
5. Patel AH, Harnois DM, Klee GG, et al: The utility of CA 19-9 in the diagnoses of cholangiocarcinoma in patients without primary sclerosing cholangitis. *Am J Gastroenterol* 95:204, 2000.
6. Ariff B, Lloyd CR, Khan S, et al: Imaging of liver cancer. *World J Gastroenterol* 15:1289, 2009.
7. Lee JW, Han JK, Kim TK, et al: CT features of intraductal intrahepatic cholangiocarcinoma. *AJR Am J Roentgenol* 175:721, 2000.
8. Kim SA, Lee JM, Lee KB, et al: Intrahepatic mass-forming cholangiocarcinomas: Enhancement patterns at multiphasic CT, with special emphasis on arterial enhancement pattern—correlation with clinicopathologic findings. *Radiology* 260:148, 2011.
9. Seo S, Hatano E, Higashi T, et al: Fluorine-18 fluorodeoxyglucose positron emission tomography predicts lymph node metastasis, P-glycoprotein expression, and recurrence after resection in mass-forming intrahepatic cholangiocarcinoma. *Surgery* 143:769, 2008.
10. Lee SW, Kim HJ, Park JH, et al: Clinical usefulness of ^{18}F-FDG PET-CT for patients with gallbladder cancer and cholangiocarcinoma. *J Gastroenterol* 45:560, 2010.
11. Anderson CD, Rice MH, Pinson CW, et al: Fluorodeoxyglucose PET imaging in the evaluation of gallbladder carcinoma and cholangiocarcinoma. *J Gastrointest Surg* 8:90, 2004.
12. Endo I, Gonen M, Yopp AC, et al: Intrahepatic cholangiocarcinoma: Rising frequency, improved survival, and determinants of outcome after resection. *Ann Surg* 248:84, 2008.
13. Weimann A, Varnholt H, Schlitt HJ, et al: Retrospective analysis of prognostic factors after liver resection and transplantation for cholangiocellular carcinoma. *Br J Surg* 87:1182, 2000.

14. Inoue K, Makuuchi M, Takayama T, et al: Long-term survival and prognostic factors in the surgical treatment of mass-forming type cholangiocarcinoma. *Surgery* 127:498, 2000.

15. Nathan H, Aloia TA, Vauthey JN, et al: A proposed staging system for intrahepatic cholangiocarcinoma. *Ann Surg Oncol* 16:14, 2009.

16. Shimada K, Sano T, Nara S, et al: Therapeutic value of lymph node dissection during hepatectomy in patients with intrahepatic cholangiocellular carcinoma with negative lymph node involvement. *Surgery* 145:411, 2009.

17. Lang H, Sotiropoulos GC, Sgourakis G, et al: Operations for intrahepatic cholangiocarcinoma: Single-institution experience of 158 patients. *J Am Coll Surg* 208:218, 2009.

18. Poultsides GA, Zhu AX, Choti MA, et al: Intrahepatic cholangiocarcinoma. *Surg Clin North Am* 90:817, 2010.

19. Guglielmi A, Ruzzenente A, Campagnaro T, et al: Intrahepatic cholangiocarcinoma: Prognostic factors after surgical resection. *World J Surg* 33:1247, 2009.

20. Uenishi T, Kubo S, Yamazaki O, et al: Indications for surgical treatment of intrahepatic cholangiocarcinoma with lymph node metastases. *J Hepatobiliary Pancreat Surg* 15:417, 2008.

21. Yokoyama T, Egami K, Miyamoto M, et al: Percutaneous and laparoscopic approaches of radiofrequency ablation treatment for liver cancer. *J Hepatobiliary Pancreat Surg* 10:425, 2003.

22. Kim JH, Won HJ, Shin YM, et al: Radiofrequency ablation for the treatment of primary intrahepatic cholangiocarcinoma. *AJR Am J Roentgenol* 196:W205, 2011.

23. Cantore M, Mambrini A, Fiorentini G, et al: Phase II study of hepatic intraarterial epirubicin and cisplatin, with systemic 5-fluorouracil in patients with unresectable biliary tract tumors. *Cancer* 103:1402, 2005.

24. Burger I, Hong K, Schulick R, et al: Transcatheter arterial chemoembolization in unresectable cholangiocarcinoma: Initial experience in a single institution. *J Vasc Interv Radiol* 16:353, 2005.

25. Gusani NJ, Balaa FK, Steel JL, et al: Treatment of unresectable cholangiocarcinoma with gemcitabine-based transcatheter arterial chemoembolization (TACE): A single-institution experience. *J Gastrointest Surg* 12:129, 2008.

26. Kim JH, Yoon HK, Ko GY, et al: Nonresectable combined hepatocellular carcinoma and cholangiocarcinoma: Analysis of the response and prognostic factors after transcatheter arterial chemoembolization. *Radiology* 255:270, 2010.

27. Valle J, Wasan H, Palmer DH, et al: Cisplatin plus gemcitabine versus gemcitabine for biliary tract cancer. *N Engl J Med* 362:1273, 2010.

28. Okusaka T, Nakachi K, Fukutomi A, et al: Gemcitabine alone or in combination with cisplatin in patients with biliary tract cancer: A comparative multicentre study in Japan. *Br J Cancer* 103:469, 2010.

29. Sell S: Alpha-fetoprotein, stem cells and cancer: How study of the production of alpha-fetoprotein during chemical hepatocarcinogenesis led to reaffirmation of the stem cell theory of cancer. *Tumour Biol* 29:161, 2008.

30. Alison MR: Liver stem cells: Implications for hepatocarcinogenesis. *Stem Cell Rev* 1:253, 2005.

31. Tickoo SK, Zee SY, Obiekwe S, et al: Combined hepatocellular-cholangiocarcinoma: A histopathologic, immunohistochemical, and in situ hybridization study. *Am J Surg Pathol* 26:989, 2002.

32. Goodman ZD, Ishak KG, Langloss JM, et al: Combined hepatocellular-cholangiocarcinoma. A histologic and immunohistochemical study. *Cancer* 55:124, 1985.

33. Kwon Y, Lee SK, Kim JS, et al: Synchronous hepatocellular carcinoma and cholangiocarcinoma arising in two different dysplastic nodules. *Mod Pathol* 15:1096, 2002.

34. Vogt DP, Henderson JM, Chmielewski E: Cystadenoma and cystadenocarcinoma of the liver: A single center experience. *J Am Coll Surg* 200:727, 2005.

35. Lauffer JM, Baer HU, Maurer CA, et al: Biliary cystadenocarcinoma of the liver: The need for complete resection. *Eur J Cancer* 34:1845, 1998.

36. Lee JH, Lee KG, Park HK, et al: Biliary cystadenoma and cystadenocarcinoma of the liver: 10 cases of a single center experience. *Hepatogastroenterology* 56:844, 2009.

37. Ishak KG, Willis GW, Cummins SD, et al: Biliary cystadenoma and cystadenocarcinoma: Report of 14 cases and review of the literature. *Cancer* 39:322, 1977.

38. Seo JK, Kim SH, Lee SH, et al: Appropriate diagnosis of biliary cystic tumors: Comparison with atypical hepatic simple cysts. *Eur J Gastroenterol Hepatol* 22:989, 2010.

39. Naik S, Waris W, Carmosino L, et al: Primary squamous cell carcinoma of the liver. *J Gastrointest Liver Dis* 18:487, 2009.

40. Clements D, Newman P, Etherington R, et al: Squamous carcinoma in the liver. *Gut* 31:1333, 1990.

41. Yagi H, Ueda M, Kawachi S, et al: Squamous cell carcinoma of the liver originating from non-parasitic cysts after a 15 year follow-up. *Eur J Gastroenterol Hepatol* 16:1051, 2004.

42. Lombardo FP, Hertford DE, Tan LK, et al: Epidermoid cyst of the liver complicated by microscopic squamous cell carcinoma: CT, ultrasound, and pathology. *J Comput Assist Tomogr* 19:131, 1995.

43. Caratozzolo E, Massani M, Recordare A, et al: Squamous cell liver cancer arising from an epidermoid cyst. *J Hepatobiliary Pancreat Surg* 8:490, 2001.

44. Weimann A, Klempnauer J, Gebel M, et al: Squamous cell carcinoma of the liver originating from a solitary non-parasitic cyst case report and review of the literature. *HPB Surg* 10:45, 1996.

45. Yu RS, Chen Y, Jiang B, et al: Primary hepatic sarcomas: CT findings. *Eur Radiol* 18:2196, 2008.

46. Lipshutz GS, Brennan TV, Warren RS: Thorotrast-induced liver neoplasia: A collective review. *J Am Coll Surg* 195:713, 2002.

47. Sherman M: Vinyl chloride and the liver. *J Hepatol* 51:1074, 2009.

48. Falk H, Herbert J, Crowley S, et al: Epidemiology of hepatic angiosarcoma in the United States: 1964-1974. *Environ Health Perspect* 41:107, 1981.

49. O'Grady JG: Treatment options for other hepatic malignancies. *Liver Transpl* 6:S23, 2000.

50. Mehrabi A, Kashfi A, Fonouni H, et al: Primary malignant hepatic epithelioid hemangioendothelioma: A comprehensive review of the literature with emphasis on the surgical therapy. *Cancer* 107:2108, 2006.

51. Grotz TE, Nagorney D, Donohue J, et al: Hepatic epithelioid haemangioendothelioma: Is transplantation the only treatment option? *HPB (Oxford)* 12:546, 2010.

Management of Secondary Hepatic Neoplasms

Juan Camilo Barreto Andrade | Mitchell C. Posner | Kevin K. Roggin

Secondary hepatic neoplasms refer to a heterogeneous collection of tumors that all metastasize to the liver. By definition, these cancers develop from other organs, but share a common metastatic pathway. Tumors that hematogenously disseminate to the liver include carcinomas (e.g., colorectal, pancreatic, gastric, breast, lung), neuroendocrine cancers, and certain types of retroperitoneal sarcomas and gastrointestinal stromal tumors. Systemic chemotherapy may be associated with improved survival compared to untreated patients, but rarely results in cure. The enhanced efficacy of systemic chemotherapeutic regimens has increased tumor response rates and improved the progression-free and overall survival of patients with these malignancies. The ability to effectively control systemic disease with chemotherapy and reduce either the size of large or number of diffuse hepatic metastases has expanded the pool of patients eligible to receive curative surgical therapy. Recent advances in the perioperative management of patients undergoing liver surgery undoubtedly contribute to these improved outcomes. Most importantly, our enhanced collective understanding of the molecular and biologic behavior of these tumors facilitates the appropriate use, combination, and sequencing of cancer-directed treatments. Although much of our knowledge has been drawn from retrospective analyses, several recent prospective, randomized trials have provided an evidence-based rationale for therapy.

As the primary drainage basin of the portal circulatory system, the liver is the most common site of gastrointestinal tract metastases. Colorectal cancer (CRC) is the third-leading worldwide cause of cancer-specific mortality and the most frequent tumor type classified as secondary hepatic neoplasm. Up to half of patients with CRC develop hepatic metastases during the course of their disease. Combination treatment with systemic chemotherapy and complete hepatic metastasectomy has been associated with long-term (5-year) survival rates that may approach 40% to 50%.[1] A smaller percentage of patients are completely cured of their disease.[2] In neuroendocrine carcinomas with spread to the hepatic parenchyma, complete surgical resection of isolated metastases has been associated with improved survival. Although hepatectomy and locoregional ablative therapies have been used for noncolorectal, nonneuroendocrine metastases (NCNN), the biology of these tumors is variable, and surgical resection should be reserved for patients with an excellent performance status, adequate control of the primary lesion, and in select clinical scenarios where the disease-free interval can be measured in years.

Generally accepted criteria for hepatic metastasectomy include (1) acceptable patient performance status to tolerate the necessary hepatic resection; (2) the liver as the only or predominant site of metastatic disease; (3) the primary tumor (and all other sites of disease) must be completely resectable and not progressing on the most effective systemic chemotherapy regimen; (4) favorable tumor biology, such that rapid progression or widespread micrometastatic disease is unlikely; (5) resection of metastasis will provide either the possibility of a long-term disease-free state or cure. Factors that influence the extent of hepatic resection are the number, size, and location of hepatic lesions, baseline hepatic function, and size of the anticipated postresection liver remnant. Traditionally, the presence of bilobar hepatic metastases and extrahepatic disease (in distant nodal basins or lungs) had been considered absolute contraindications to complete hepatic metastasectomy. The combination of effective neoadjuvant chemotherapy, increasingly effective local ablative therapies, and aggressive surgical resection have broadened the indications for surgical resection. The ability to achieve an R0 (negative gross and microscopic margins) appears to be a significant factor that is associated with improved disease-free survival rates. Although hepatic recurrence rates have been shown to be higher when the microscopic margins are positive for residual disease, several retrospective reports suggest that this may not influence long-term survival.[3] Positive margins likely reflect poor tumor biology and increased risk of hepatic recurrence. Anatomic resections, along the vascular inflow and outflow structures and biliary ducts, are indicated for metastatic disease where subanatomic or "wedge" resections would lead to a higher probability of positive margins, major blood loss, or a bile leak. The unique capability of the liver parenchyma to regenerate after hepatectomy allows the surgeon to resect up to 80% of the original volume if the baseline hepatic function is normal. The oncologic principles regarding CRC, neuroendocrine, and other hepatic metastasis will be discussed here, as a separate chapter will address the surgical and technical details of liver resection more thoroughly.

COLORECTAL CANCER METASTASES

The liver is the most common site of distant metastatic disease in CRC patients. Approximately half of patients with CRC will develop metastases during their course of disease, and up to 25% will have liver metastases at the time of presentation.[4] The historical results of resection, before the development of current-day chemotherapeutic regimens, typically yielded 5-year survival rates between 20% and 40%.[5] Selected patients undergoing modern chemotherapeutic regimens in combination with complete metastasectomy can achieve durable 5-year survival rates exceeding 50%.[1,6] Approximately 10% to 15% of these patients are cured of their disease.[2] These improved survival trends are likely related to improved patient selection with favorable tumor biology, dramatic improvement in the systemic chemotherapeutic regimens, and the concomitant development of new targeted therapeutics.

The historical selection criteria used to identify stage IV patients who might benefit from metastasectomy have focused on disease burden: number and size of metastatic lesions, bilateral hepatic disease, lymph-node positive primary tumors, and high carcinoembryonic antigen (CEA) levels. The Fong Clinical Risk Score consolidates these factors into prognostic elements that can be used to select patients for hepatic metastasectomy. Patients who have 0 to 2 of these risk factors have 5-year survival rates of 40% to 60%, whereas patients with a score of 3 or higher have less than a 25% chance of surviving beyond the same time interval.[7] Because the data to construct these scoring systems were generated before the advent of modern combination chemotherapy, the clinical usefulness of this model has been debated. Recent retrospective data suggest that tumor response to induction or "neoadjuvant" therapy as a marker of favorable biology may have more value than the aforementioned variables.[8] Improved perioperative therapy, concentrating on minimizing blood loss, maintaining an appropriate and functional remnant liver volume, and maximizing hepatic regeneration and recovery through state-of-the-art surgical intensive care techniques, likely has contributed to the improved results in recent retrospective case series. Patients with normal hepatic and renal function can tolerate up to an 85% hepatectomy without significant perioperative mortality. The selective use of portal vein embolization to induce in vivo hepatic regeneration of the anticipated remnant liver is an evolving technique that is both predictive of the response to hepatectomy and can help select patients who could tolerate complete metastasectomy. Portal vein embolization can be combined with neoadjuvant chemotherapy without compromising liver growth.[9] Furthermore, our improved understanding of hepatic anatomy, physiology, and the factors responsible for regeneration has expanded the indications for operation and allowed more patients with stage IV disease to be considered for combination therapy. The ability to achieve a complete resection (i.e., R0 resection) with both gross and microscopically negative margins has been associated with improved recurrence-free survival. It no longer appears necessary to perform anatomic or segmental resections on all patients with hepatic metastases to achieve disease control.[3]

ROLE OF SYSTEMIC CHEMOTHERAPY IN RESECTABLE METASTATIC DISEASE

The most effective single agent as first-line therapy for metastatic CRC has historically been the fluoropyrimidine analogue, 5-fluorouracil (5-FU). For over two decades, the synergistic combination of 5-FU and leucovorin or folinic acid (which inhibits thymidylate synthase) was the standard of care both as an adjuvant treatment for node-positive, resected colon cancers and as treatment for metastatic disease. The addition of

oxaliplatin, a platinum-based alkylating agent, to the 5-FU–leucovorin backbone (FOLFOX), has increased the response rates and progression-free survival with lower rates of nephrotoxicity and myelosuppression. In some studies, FOLFOX has shown benefit in overall survival in the metastatic setting.[10] Irinotecan is a topoisomerase inhibitor that when combined with 5-FU and leucovorin (FOLFIRI) is superior to 5-FU alone and comparable to FOLFOX.[11] Capecitabine, an oral fluoropyrimidine antimetabolite with similar efficacy to 5-FU, is an equivalent, orally administered, substitute for 5-FU in most regimens.[12] Several novel biologic agents have recently been added to these combination regimens in an attempt to improve survival in patients with metastatic disease. Bevacizumab, a recombinant monoclonal antibody that blocks the activity of vascular endothelial growth factor A, has proved of benefit in extending survival in patients with metastatic disease[13] and is frequently added to the FOLFOX and FOLFIRI regimens. Cetuximab and panitumumab are monoclonal antibodies that block the epidermal growth factor receptor (EGFR) pathway. These anti-EGFR agents have efficacy against primary tumors that lack activating mutations in the *KRAS* gene.[14]

The surgeon treating patients with metastatic CRC must be familiar with safety profiles and potential deleterious effects of these regimens. The extended use of these agents (usually >6 to 12 weeks) may be associated with higher rates of postoperative complications and liver insufficiency. Irinotecan has been associated with both drug-induced steatosis and steatohepatitis, which may lead to increased morbidity and mortality.[15] Oxaliplatin may produce sinusoidal dilatation, which can also increase the risk of postoperative complications.[16] The rare, but potentially lethal side effects of bevacizumab include hypertension, increased risk of arterial thromboembolism, gastrointestinal bleeding, and perforation.[17] Its antiangiogenic effects and long circulating half-life (approximately 6 to 8 weeks) have been associated with delayed wound healing. Most physicians interrupt bevacizumab therapy at least 4 to 6 weeks before surgical metastasectomy.[18] Anti-EGFR agents, in particular cetuximab, have not been associated with the same risk profile or increase in postoperative morbidity or mortality.[19]

Patients with unresectable CRC liver metastases who are treated with modern systemic chemotherapy alone have a median survival of 22 months,[20] compared to the dismal natural history of the disease in untreated patients (median survival of 6 to 12 months). Several randomized, controlled, multicenter trials have established the efficacy of the current standards of care for the treatment of metastatic disease.[10,11,13]

The rate of complete pathologic response to chemotherapy has been estimated to be less than 5%.[21] In addition, there is a poor correlation between complete radiologic and pathologic responses; residual disease (documented by pathologic examination of the resected liver) is present in more than 80% of lesions that disappear on state-of-the-art cross-sectional and metabolic imaging studies.[22] Surgical metastasectomy alone can yield disease-free survival rates in the range of 20% and 5-year survival rates of 25% to 40%.[5] Unfortunately, recurrence after resection is common. In approximately 50% of these cases, the recurrence occurs within the liver, and it is the only site of disease.[5] Long-term disease-free survival is unlikely without a combination of complete metastasectomy and modern chemotherapy. The proper sequencing of surgery and chemotherapy remains unclear. The European Organization for Research and Treatment of Cancer (EORTC) trial 40983, a randomized, controlled phase III trial of perioperative FOLFOX versus surgery alone in patients with resectable hepatic CRC metastases, showed a significant improvement in progression-free survival from 28% to 36%, with an objective tumor response rate in all treated patients of 43%. The possible beneficial impact on overall survival is still being monitored. Postoperative complications were more frequent in the chemotherapy group, although they were reversible and there was no increase in mortality.[23] The National Surgical Adjuvant Breast and Bowel Project C-11 trial has been designed to determine the optimal timing of systemic treatment. It will compare postoperative treatment with FOLFOX or FOLFIRI and bevacizumab with pre- and postoperative treatment with the same regimen. The impact of biologic agents on survival after resection of hepatic metastases is still being analyzed in prospective trials. A summary of the outcomes of current combined-modality treatment is shown in Table 130-1. Many of these studies included patients who initially had unresectable disease and became resectable after chemotherapy.

There are potential advantages and disadvantages to the neoadjuvant approach. The theoretical advantages include eliminating micrometastatic disease, in vivo cytoreduction to reduce the amount of hepatic parenchyma required for complete resection, the ability to individualize the chemotherapeutic efficacy, and most importantly, to select patients who may benefit from metastasectomy. The potential disadvantages are biologic or chemotherapy-induced toxicity, inducing a complete radiologic response making the lesion(s) difficult to identify intraoperatively, and missing a window of opportunity to cure patients with resectable lesions that may progress on therapy and become unresectable.

SYNCHRONOUS VERSUS METACHRONOUS DISEASE

Fifteen to 25% of CRC patients have synchronous liver metastases at the time of diagnosis.[4] In most cases, metastatic disease is recognized within the first year (or >6 months) after diagnosis. The biologic importance of synchronous metastatic disease remains controversial. One hypothesis is that there may be no significant difference between synchronous and metastatic disease (i.e., lead-time bias). Several recent studies suggest that the presence of synchronous disease may be associated with a more adverse prognosis secondary to more aggressive tumor behavior (i.e., higher incidence of bilobar liver and extrahepatic metastases).[31] The optimal treatment of synchronous metastases is not clear. Most patients are treated with a limited period (>3 months) of systemic chemotherapy and are restaged. Surgical resection may be appropriate in the absence of disease progression and if both the primary and all sites of metastatic disease can be resected with acceptable morbidity and mortality.

The concept of staged resection has evolved in response to retrospective data that suggest higher rates of morbidity and mortality with combined resections. There are now single-institution, retrospective data to

TABLE 130-1 Survival Outcomes in Patients With Metastatic Colorectal Cancer Treated With Modern Combined Chemotherapy and Resection

Study	No. of Patients	Initially Resectable	Regimen	Disease-Free Survival	Overall Survival
EORTC 40983[23] phase III RCT	152 151	Yes	Surgery Surgery + FOLFOX	28.1% $P = 0.041$ 36.2% (3 yr)	NA
Ychou et al[24] phase III RCT	153 153	Yes	5-FU + leucovorin FOLFIRI	46% $P = 0.44$ 51% (2 yr)	71.6% $P = 0.69$ 72.7% (3 yr)
Adam et al[25]	701	No	FOLFOX	NA	34% (5 yr)
Wein et al[26] phase II trial	20	Yes	FOLFOX	52% (2 yr)	80% (2-yr DSS)
Taieb et al[27] phase II trial	47	Yes	FOLFOX followed by FOLFIRI	47% (2 yr)	89% (2 yr)
Barone et al[28]	40	No	FOLFIRI	NA	63.5% (2 yr)
Masi et al[29]	196	No	FOLFOX/FOLFIRI?	29% (5 yr)	42% (5 yr)
First-BEAT trial[30]	107	No	Bev + 5-FU based	NA	89% (2 yr)
N016966 study[30]	34 44	No	Placebo + XELOX/FOLFOX Bev + XELOX/FOLFOX	NA	82.3% 90.9% (2 yr)

BEAT, Bevacizumab Expanded Access Trial; *Bev*, bevacizumab; *DSS*, disease-specific survival; *EORTC*, European Organization for Research and Treatment of Cancer; *FOLFIRI*, 5-fluorouracil, leucovorin, and irinotecan; *FOLFOX*, 5-fluorouracil, leucovorin, and oxaliplatin; *5-FU*, 5-fluorouracil; *NA*, not available or not reported; *RCT*, randomized, controlled trial; *XELOX*, capecitabine and oxaliplatin.

suggest that simultaneous resections are not only feasible, but may be advantageous in selected cases and in high-volume centers. More recent reports have shown that morbidity and mortality are not increased in simultaneous hepatic and colorectal resections, even when major liver resections are performed. These are retrospective reports, and simultaneous resections were more frequently performed in patients with fewer or smaller metastases, with more proximal tumors, and better prognostic factors.[32] In the absence of evidence-based data, most treatment decisions are individualized based on tumor biology, patient factors (e.g., performance status, liver health), and the location and distribution of metastatic disease.

LIVER RESECTION IN THE PRESENCE OF EXTRAHEPATIC DISEASE

Traditionally, patients with CRC liver metastases and extrahepatic disease (EHD) have not been considered as candidates for metastasectomy. The improved efficacy of chemotherapy has allowed some to reconsider the role of surgical resection in these individuals. The most prudent approach involves a limited period of neoadjuvant chemotherapy to allow patients with favorable tumor biology to be selected for aggressive surgical intervention.

Five-year survival rates of up to 20% to 30% have been reported in patients with EHD.[33] The largest series of patients undergoing liver resection and extrahepatic metastasectomy to date reported a 5-year predicted survival of 27%, which is consistent with the previous reports and encouraging. The vast majority (>95%) of patients eventually developed recurrence, emphasizing that liver resection in the presence of EHD is likely not curative.[34]

The value of removing metastatic disease in "distant" regional lymphatic basins (e.g., periaortic or hepatic pedicle) remains controversial. It is likely that this clinical situation reflects adverse tumor biology associated with poor long-term survival. Recent reports of hepatic resection and aggressive portal lymphadenectomy in combination with chemotherapy have been associated with 5-year survival rate approaching 20% when lymph node metastases are limited to the portal basin, with no long-term survivors found among patients with celiac or retroperitoneal metastases.[35]

The evolution of hyperthermic intraperitoneal chemotherapy in combination with cytoreductive surgery offers another possible aggressive treatment for selected patients with peritoneal disease. The value of this treatment in metastatic CRC is unknown, especially in the setting of concomitant solid organ metastases.[36]

TREATMENT OF UNRESECTABLE DISEASE: SYSTEMIC THERAPY AND ABLATION TECHNIQUES

Unfortunately, most patients with metastatic CRC are not candidates for surgical resection. Some patients with "unresectable" disease treated with modern chemotherapy have been converted to a resectable state resulting in a durable disease-free interval with the combination of neoadjuvant chemotherapy and aggressive surgical metastasectomy. In a large series of 1439 patients with metastatic CRC and disease limited to the liver, a regimen of FOLFOX or FOLFIRI induced a favorable response in 138 patients allowing subsequent resection. Although 80% of patients developed eventual recurrence, survival at 5 years was 33%.[37] Defining the criteria for "unresectable" disease in this era remains a challenging proposition. Nonsurgical treatment options for patients who are truly unresectable or have progressed after treatment with either first- or second-line combination systemic therapy include regional chemotherapy (i.e., hepatic arterial infusion [HAI]), percutaneous ablative therapies (i.e. radiofrequency [RFA] or microwave ablation), and experimental therapies. Novel investigational modalities include the use of radiation therapies (including intensity modulated radiation therapy, proton- and gamma-beam irradiation, chemoembolization, and hepatic-arterial injection of radioactive materials (e.g., yttrium 90 glass microspheres). The technical aspects of ablative techniques are described in a separate chapter. Table 130-2 summarizes the results of nonsurgical regional therapies. Direct comparison between resection and ablation techniques is difficult, because the latter is usually offered to patients who are not optimal surgical candidates. Aside from the selection bias and retrospective nature of the data, most published studies suggest a higher risk of recurrence after ablative techniques, with variable rates across studies.[43] A small, randomized, phase II comparative trial compared the combination of RFA and chemotherapy with systemic therapy alone. Progression-free survival was improved in the group that included RFA (10 months compared to 17 months), and overall survival was still under evaluation.[44]

HAI has generated interest among some investigators because liver metastases derive most of their blood supply from the hepatic artery. Several randomized trials demonstrated a superior response rate from chemotherapeutic HAI compared to systemic chemotherapy. In the Cancer and Leukemia Group B 9481 trial, systemic chemotherapy using 5-FU and leucovorin was compared to HAI using floxuridine, leucovorin, and dexamethasone in 135 patients. HAI prolonged survival from 20 to 24 months, increased the response rate from 24% to 47%, and was associated with improved physical functioning.[45] Other multiinstitutional clinical trials have attempted to establish the role of adjuvant or neoadjuvant HAI chemotherapy (in combination with 5-FU chemotherapy) and hepatic resection versus resection alone. Phase III trials have shown an improvement in disease-free, but not overall survival, when compared to resection alone.[46] In the era of current-day chemotherapy, which yields enhanced response rates and improved survival, the role of HAI in the management of CRC hepatic metastases remains unclear and has not been embraced by most medical oncologists.

SURVEILLANCE AFTER LIVER RESECTION FOR CRC

The recommended guidelines for surveillance of stage IV CRC patients are based on the results of several clinical trials comparing low- and high-intensity followup programs.[47] A history and physical examination should be performed every 3 to 6 months for the first 2 years, and then every 6 months up to 5 years; serum CEA

TABLE 130-2 Nonsurgical Regional Therapies for Metastatic Colorectal Cancer to the Liver

Treatment Modality	Limitations	Outcomes	Complications
RFA[38]	Higher recurrence compared to resection Lesion proximity to blood vessels Lesion size >5 cm	Up to 84% local recurrence rate Survival benefit not established	Morbidity 5%-30%: abscess, hemorrhage, bile leak
Cryoablation[39]	Similar to RFA, but possible higher rate of complications	Local recurrence rate: 10%-60%	Morbidity 15%-30%: hemorrhage, bile leak, cryoshock syndrome, myoglobinuria
HAI[40]	Laparotomy needed to implant infusion device Limited centers with experience	Response rate >50% No proven survival benefit	Hepatobiliary toxicity Pump complications Gastritis/duodenitis
Radioembolization (yttrium 90 microspheres)[41]	Emerging experience	Response rate: 44% Progression-free survival: 16–18 mo Combined with systemic chemotherapy or HAI	Morbidity: 24% Abdominal pain and fever Gastritis/duodenitis Radiation hepatitis
Conformal/stereotactic radiotherapy[42]	Low liver tolerance to radiation Lesion proximity to adjacent organs	Median survival: 17 mo Local control rates >60%	Radiation hepatitis: 5% Skin erythema Chest wall pain

HAI, Hepatic artery infusion; *RFA*, radiofrequency ablation.

measurements should occur at each of these visits. This only applies to patients with an abnormally elevated baseline CEA level at diagnosis. These evidence-based recommendations also apply to patients who underwent resection of their primary tumor. Because 2% to 5% of patients with CRC will develop metachronous primary lesions, an interval colonoscopy to detect new colorectal cancers and to evaluate for local (anastomotic) recurrence appears reasonable. In the setting of resected metastatic disease, other experts have recommended more intensive imaging surveillance with computed tomography (CT) scan of the chest, abdomen, and pelvis in each of these visits.[48] However, this approach is not supported by data and subjects patients to the harmful and cumulative effects of CT-induced radiation exposure. Magnetic resonance imaging can be used as an effective substitute for CT surveillance without the deleterious effects of radiation exposure. In patients with elevated or rising CEA levels, the use of positron emission tomography scans combined with the anatomic detail of noncontrast-enhanced CT may be helpful to detect the site of recurrent disease.

NEUROENDOCRINE METASTASES

Neuroendocrine tumors (NET) are malignant gastroenteropancreatic neoplasms of the amine precursor uptake and decarboxylation cells. These heterogeneous collections of tumors include carcinoid tumors, pancreatic endocrine tumors, and all other NET (e.g., pheochromocytoma, neuroblastoma, medullary thyroid carcinoma). These tumor subtypes are further classified by their location, cell of origin, functionality, and by their specific production of hormones. Carcinoid tumors are usually slow-growing neuroendocrine tumors that arise from the enterochromaffin cells along the GI tract. They typically

secrete a range of hormones, but primarily elaborate serotonin (5-HT). The majority (approximately 70%) of pancreatic endocrine tumors or islet cell tumors of the pancreas secrete specific hormones that may have characteristic physiologic and biologic consequences. Approximately one-third of pancreatic endocrine tumors are completely nonfunctional.

Malignant NET frequently metastasize to the liver. Their biologic behavior often is strikingly different from adenocarcinomas of the colon, rectum, small bowel, and pancreas. The role of metastasectomy or debulking is determined by the distribution of disease, presence of symptoms, and the anticipated impact of resection on long-term disease control or palliation.

Ninety percent of NET have receptors to somatostatin or its analogue, octreotide. Approximately 60% to 80% of patients have either an objective tumor response or symptomatic improvement with the subcutaneous administration of somatostatin analogues.[49] Several large retrospective reports suggest a progression-free and possible overall survival benefit with the administration of radiolabeled octreotide compared to patients treated with best medical care.[50] The duration of response can range from weeks to years, but the vast majority of patients eventually become refractory to its effect.[51] In the absence of symptomatic control with somatostatin analogues, a palliative resection may be considered to remove or debulk intrahepatic metastatic disease. Nonoperative ablative techniques (e.g., RFA, ethanol injection), chemoembolization, and systemic chemotherapy have been used in patients who have failed somatostatin therapy and are not candidates for surgical resection.[52] In asymptomatic patients, curative resection should be considered in patients with an excellent performance status and in clinical situations where both the primary and all sites of metastatic disease can be safely extirpated. The goal of surgery (curative versus palliative) should be established before operative intervention. Unfortunately, most of the data that influences management is nonevidence-based, and therefore most treatment decisions are individualized and generated within the context of multidisciplinary tumor boards.

Medical management of NET typically results in 5-year survival rates that range from 20% to 30%.[53] When resection is performed with curative intent, durable long-term survival is associated with the complete removal of all disease and reported to be as high as 70% at 5 years.[54] Liver transplantation has been attempted in selected patients with hepatic metastases from NET. The reported actuarial 5-year survival for patients with carcinoid tumors is significantly higher (69%) than for patients with other types of NET (36%). These outcomes may not be reproducible and are tempered by the high reported postoperative mortality rate (19% overall; 7% for carcinoid, 31% other NET) and limited supply of donor organs.[55]

The most common NET that metastasize to the liver are carcinoids and gastrinomas, which are discussed in more detail subsequently.

CARCINOID TUMORS

Carcinoid tumors give rise to two thirds of NET liver metastases. After the regional lymph nodes, the liver is the most common site of metastasis, although this only occurs in 5% of patients. These enterochromaffin cell tumors most commonly arise from the small bowel and tend to have an indolent nature. There is a correlation between their metastatic potential and their size and location. Rectal carcinoids have the highest risk of metastasis, and appendiceal have the lowest. The clinical course of patients with metastatic liver disease is variable. Patients may remain completely asymptomatic for extended time periods before their disease burden produces hepatic failure, metabolic disturbances, or cachexia. Ninety-percent of symptomatic patients have metastatic disease. A minority (<10%) of patients with metastatic disease to the liver develop the classic "carcinoid syndrome" manifest by flushing, diarrhea, bronchospasm, and/or right-sided heart failure. An elevated serum chromogranin A level has been associated with a worse prognosis.[56]

As with all NET, treatment options are dictated by the extent of disease, presence of symptoms, and surgical risk for the patient. Prolonged survival can be obtained with complete resection of the primary and metastatic disease.[57] To prevent a life-threatening carcinoid crisis exacerbated by anesthesia, surgery or invasive procedures, intravenous octreotide should be readily available for administration during any of these interventions. In addition, it is recommended that all patients with carcinoid tumors in whom the use of somatostatin analogues is anticipated, have their gallbladder removed at the time of surgery, because somatostatin analogues increase the risk of developing gallstones.

GASTRINOMAS

Gastrinomas (Zollinger-Ellison syndrome) are foregut NET that produce excess gastrin, which is a potent stimulator of hydrochloric acid secretion from the parietal cells of the stomach. Peptic ulceration is common, and the disease has both sporadic and inherited forms. Sixty to eighty percent of gastrinomas are malignant, but less than 10% metastasize to the liver. Hepatic metastases are the most important predictor of survival and primary cause of death in the majority of patients.[58] As is the case in other NET, complete resection can result in long-term survival in more than 70% of patients.[59] Unfortunately, less than 15% of patients are candidates for curative resection. In the past, complications of gastrin secretion resulted in significant morbidity and mortality, and palliative surgery was indicated in cases refractory to acid suppression therapy. The use of proton pump inhibitors can control symptomatic disease in many patients by near-complete suppression of gastric acid production.

OTHER NEUROENDOCRINE TUMORS

The remainder of NET that cause liver metastases are far more uncommon. Insulinomas are the most common islet cell tumor, although only 10% are malignant. Even with widely disseminated disease, aggressive surgical debulking may improve hypoglycemic episodes. Fifty percent of vasoactive intestinal peptide tumors (NET producing VIPomas), and the majority of glucagonomas, somatostatinomas, and pancreatic-polypeptide (PPomas) are malignant. Specific data regarding their surgical management in the setting of metastatic liver disease is limited, but the same principles used in patients with all NET can be extrapolated to these clinical situations.

RESULTS OF LOCAL ABLATIVE THERAPY FOR NEUROENDOCRINE TUMORS

In patients who are not candidates for curative resection or cytoreduction, ablative modalities offer a possibility of palliation of symptoms. Laparoscopic RFA has been reported as successful in amelioration of symptoms in more than 90% of patients, with minimal risk of morbidity and mortality.[60] Hepatic artery embolization has been described as well in patients who have failed RFA, because the blood supply to neuroendocrine metastases arises from the hepatic artery. It has been used in combination with cytotoxic chemotherapy or alone to improve pain or hormonal symptoms.[61] A small phase II study showed a decrease in size of lesions in 33% of patients and symptomatic relief in most, with a median duration of the response of 14 months.[62] Complications with RFA are common and include infection, bleeding, ileus, abdominal pain, fever, elevated liver enzymes, and cholecystitis. Treatment-related mortality ranges from 2% to 5%.[62]

NONCOLORECTAL, NONNEUROENDOCRINE METASTASES

NCNN metastases represent a heterogeneous collection of all other nonprimary hepatic metastases. This group includes metastatic extremity and retroperitoneal sarcomas, renal cell carcinomas, breast cancers, gastrointestinal stromal tumors, melanoma, non-CRC gastrointestinal tumors, and non–small cell lung carcinoma. Although the biologic spectrum of NCNN metastatic disease is variable, centers of experience have attempted to collectively group these tumors en masse to provide retrospective data that may influence medical and surgical therapy.

The role of hepatic resection for NCNN metastases is more controversial, and it is generally not considered to be the standard of care. Although reports of actuarial 3-year cancer-specific survival rates over 50% have been reported, these numbers likely cannot be extrapolated to all patients with NCNN.[63] Favorable prognostic factors included a long disease-free interval, the ability to perform a complete metastasectomy, and a primary tumor originating from the reproductive tract.[63] In summary, current data suggest that in highly selected patients, resection can be associated with favorable outcomes.

CONCLUSIONS

The progress in the management of patients with metastatic liver disease has been significant and continues to evolve. Resection is the current standard of care for patients with limited metastatic disease from colorectal cancer, and combined treatment has resulted in improved survival rates. There is a role for resection in selected patients with neuroendocrine tumors and in rare patients with NCNN and favorable risk factors. Despite these advances, most patients with liver metastases have incurable disease, and further development of novel therapies is awaited.

ACKNOWLEDGMENT

The authors would like to thank Roberta Carden for proofreading and editing this manuscript.

REFERENCES

1. Adam R, Vibert E, Pitombo M: Induction chemotherapy and surgery of colorectal liver metastases. *Bull Cancer* 93:S45, 2006.
2. Tomlinson JS, Jarnagin WR, DeMatteo RP, et al: Actual 10-year survival after resection of colorectal liver metastases defines cure. *J Clin Oncol* 25:4575, 2007.
3. Pawlik TM, Scoggins CR, Zorzi D, et al: Effect of surgical margin status on survival and site of recurrence after hepatic resection for colorectal metastases. *Ann Surg* 241:715, 2005.
4. Reddy SK, Barbas AS, Clary BM: Synchronous colorectal liver metastases: Is it time to reconsider traditional paradigms of management? *Ann Surg Oncol* 16:2395, 2009.
5. Fong Y, Cohen AM, Fortner JG, et al: Liver resection for colorectal metastases. *J Clin Oncol* 15:938, 1997.
6. Choti MA, Sitzmann JV, Tiburi MF, et al: Trends in long-term survival following liver resection for hepatic colorectal metastases. *Ann Surg* 235:759, 2002.
7. Fong Y, Fortner J, Sun RL, et al: Clinical score for predicting recurrence after hepatic resection for metastatic colorectal cancer. Analysis of 1001 consecutive cases. *Ann Surg* 230:309, discussion 318, 1999.
8. Allen PJ, Kemeny N, Jarnagin W, et al: Importance of response to neoadjuvant chemotherapy in patients undergoing resection of synchronous colorectal liver metastases. *J Gastrointest Surg* 7:109, 2003.
9. Covey AM, Brown KT, Jarnagin WR, et al: Combined portal vein embolization and neoadjuvant chemotherapy as a treatment strategy for resectable hepatic colorectal metastases. *Ann Surg* 247:451, 2008.
10. Goldberg RM, Sargent DJ, Morton RF, et al: A randomized controlled trial of fluorouracil plus leucovorin, irinotecan, and oxaliplatin combinations in patients with previously untreated metastatic colorectal cancer. *J Clin Oncol* 22:23, 2004.
11. Douillard JY, Cunningham D, Roth AD, et al: Irinotecan combined with fluorouracil compared with fluorouracil alone as first-line treatment for metastatic colorectal cancer: A multicentre randomized trial. *Lancet* 355:1041, 2000.
12. Twelves C, Wong A, Nowacki MP, et al: Capecitabine as adjuvant treatment for stage III colon cancer. *N Engl J Med* 352:2696, 2005.
13. Hurwitz H, Fehrenbacher L, Novotny W, et al: Bevacizumab plus irinotecan, fluorouracil, and leucovorin for metastatic colorectal cancer. *N Engl J Med* 350:2335, 2004.
14. Van Cutsem E, Köhne CH, Hitre E, et al: Cetuximab and chemotherapy as initial treatment for metastatic colorectal cancer. *N Engl J Med* 360:1408, 2009.
15. Vauthey JN, Pawlik TM, Ribero D, et al: Chemotherapy regimen predicts steatohepatitis and an increase in 90-day mortality after surgery for hepatic colorectal metastases. *J Clin Oncol* 24:2065, 2006.
16. Aloia T, Sebagh M, Plasse M, et al: Liver histology and surgical outcomes after preoperative chemotherapy with fluorouracil plus oxaliplatin in colorectal cancer liver metastases. *J Clin Oncol* 24:4983, 2006.
17. Scappaticci FA, Skillings JR, Holden SN, et al: Arterial thromboembolic events in patients with metastatic carcinoma treated with chemotherapy and bevacizumab. *J Natl Cancer Inst* 99:1232, 2007.
18. Kesmodel SB, Ellis LM, Lin E, et al: Preoperative bevacizumab does not significantly increase postoperative complication rates in patients undergoing hepatic surgery for colorectal cancer liver metastases. *J Clin Oncol* 26:5254, 2008.
19. Adam R, Aloia T, Lévi F, et al: Hepatic resection after rescue cetuximab treatment for colorectal liver metastases previously refractory to conventional systemic therapy. *J Clin Oncol* 25:4593, 2007.
20. Meyerhardt JA, Mayer RJ: Systemic therapy for colorectal cancer. *N Engl J Med* 352:476, 2005.
21. Adam R, Wicherts DA, de Haas RJ, et al: Complete pathologic response after preoperative chemotherapy for colorectal liver metastases: Myth or reality? *J Clin Oncol* 26:1635, 2008.
22. Benoist S, Brouquet A, Penna C, et al: Complete response of colorectal liver metastases after chemotherapy: Does it mean cure? *J Clin Oncol* 24:3939, 2006.
23. Nordlinger B, Sorbye H, Glimelius B, et al: Perioperative chemotherapy with FOLFOX4 and surgery versus surgery alone for resectable liver metastases from colorectal cancer (EORTC Intergroup trial 40983): A randomised controlled trial. *Lancet* 371:1007, 2008.
24. Ychou M, Hohenberger W, Thezenas S, et al: A randomized phase III study comparing adjuvant 5-fluorouracil/folinic acid with FOLFIRI in patients following complete resection of liver metastases from colorectal cancer. *Ann Oncol* 20:1964, 2009.
25. Adam R, Avisar E, Ariche A, et al: Five-year survival following hepatic resection after neoadjuvant therapy for nonresectable colorectal liver metastases. *Ann Surg Oncol* 8:347, 2001.
26. Wein A, Riedel C, Brückl W, et al: Neoadjuvant treatment with weekly high-dose 5-fluorouracil as 24-hour infusion, folinic acid and oxaliplatin in patients with primary resectable liver metastases of colorectal cancer. *Oncology* 64:131, 2003.
27. Taïeb J, Artru P, Paye F, et al: Intensive systemic chemotherapy combined with surgery for metastatic colorectal cancer: Results of a phase II study. *J Clin Oncol* 23:502, 2005.
28. Barone C, Nuzzo G, Cassano A, et al: Final analysis of colorectal cancer patients treated with irinotecan and 5-fluorouracil plus folinic acid neoadjuvant chemotherapy for unresectable liver metastases. *Br J Cancer* 97:1035, 2007.
29. Masi G, Loupakis F, Pollina L, et al: Long-term outcome of initially unresectable metastatic colorectal cancer patients treated with 5-fluorouracil/leucovorin, oxaliplatin, and irinotecan (FOLFOX-IRI) followed by radical surgery of metastases. *Ann Surg* 249:420, 2009.
30. Okines A, Puerto OD, Cunningham D, et al: Surgery with curative-intent in patients treated with first-line chemotherapy plus bevacizumab for metastatic colorectal cancer. First BEAT and the randomised phase-III N016966 trial. *Br J Cancer* 101:1033, 2009.
31. Tsai MS, Su YH, Ho MC, et al: Clinicopathological features and prognosis in resectable synchronous and metachronous colorectal liver metastases. *Ann Surg Oncol* 14:786, 2007.
32. Martin R, Paty P, Fong YG, et al: Simultaneous liver and colorectal resections are safe for synchronous colorectal liver metastasis. *J Am Coll Surg* 197:233, 2003.
33. Elias D, Ouellet JF, Bellon N, et al: Extrahepatic disease does not contraindicate hepatectomy for colorectal liver metastases. *Br J Surg* 90:567, 2003.

34. Carpizo DR, Are C, Jarnagin W, et al: Liver resection for metastatic colorectal cancer in patients with concurrent extrahepatic disease: Results in 127 patients treated at a single center. *Ann Surg Oncol* 16:2138, 2009.

35. Adam R, de Haas RJ, Wicherts DA, et al: Is hepatic resection justified after chemotherapy in patients with colorectal liver metastases and lymph node involvement? *J Clin Oncol* 26:3672, 2008.

36. Yan TD, Black D, Savady R, et al: Systematic review on the efficacy of cytoreductive surgery combined with perioperative intraperitoneal chemotherapy for peritoneal carcinomatosis from colorectal carcinoma. *J Clin Oncol* 24:4011, 2006.

37. Adam R, Delvart V, Pascal G, et al: Rescue surgery for unresectable colorectal liver metastases downstaged by chemotherapy. A model to predict long-term survival. *Ann Surg* 240:644, 2004.

38. Abdalla EK, Vauthey JN, Ellis LM, et al: Recurrence and outcomes following hepatic resection, radiofrequency ablation, and combined resection/ablation for colorectal liver metastases. *Ann Surg* 239:818, 2004.

39. Pearson AS, Izzo F, Fleming RY, et al: Intraoperative radiofrequency ablation or cryoablation for hepatic malignancies. *Am J Surg* 178:592, 1999.

40. Lorenz M, Muller HH: Randomized, multicenter trial of fluorouracil plus leucovorin administered either via hepatic artery or intravenous infusion versus fluorodeoxyuridine administered via hepatic artery infusion in patients with nonresectable liver metastases from colorectal carcinoma. *J Clin Oncol* 18:243, 2000.

41. Gulec SA, Fong Y: Yttrium 90 microsphere selective internal radiation treatment of hepatic colorectal metastases. *Arch Surg* 142:675, 2007.

42. Swaminath A, Dawson LA: Emerging role of radiotherapy in the management of liver metastases. *Cancer J* 16:150, 2010.

43. Abdalla EK, Adam R, Bilchik AJ, et al: Improving respectability of hepatic colorectal metastases: Expert consensus statement. *Ann Surg Oncol* 13:1271, 2006.

44. Ruers T, Punt CJ, et al: Final results of the EORTC intergroup randomized study 40004 (CLOCC) evaluating the benefit of radiofrequency ablation combined with chemotherapy for unresectable colorectal liver metastases. *J Clin Oncol* 28:15s, 2010.

45. Kemeny NE, Niedzwiecki D, Hollis DR, et al: Hepatic arterial infusion versus systemic therapy for hepatic metastases from colorectal cancer: A randomized trial of efficacy, quality of life, and molecular markers (CALGB 9481). *J Clin Oncol* 24:1395, 2006.

46. Lorenz M, Müller HH, Schramm H, et al: Randomized trial of surgery versus surgery followed by adjuvant hepatic arterial infusion with 5-fluorouracil and folinic acid for liver metastases of colorectal cancer: German Cooperative on Liver Metastases (Arbeitsgruppe Lebermetastasen). *Ann Surg* 228:756, 1998.

47. Desch CE, Benson AB 3rd, Somerfield MR, et al: Colorectal cancer surveillance: 2005 update of an American Society of Clinical Oncology practice guideline. *J Clin Oncol* 23:8512, 2005.

48 Engstrom PF, Arnoletti JP, Benson AB 3rd, et al: NCCN colon cancer clinical practice guidelines in oncology, 2010, www.nccn.org.

49. Sarmiento JM, Heywood G, Rubin J, et al: Surgical treatment of neuroendocrine metastases to the liver: A plea for resection to increase survival. *J Am Coll Surg* 197:29, 2003.

50. Kwekkeboom DJ, de Herder WW, Kam BL, et al: Treatment with the radiolabeled somatostatin analog [177Lu-DOTA0,Tyr3] octreotate: Toxicity, efficacy, and survival. *J Clin Oncol* 26:2124, 2008.

51. Wynick D, Anderson JV, Williams SJ, et al: Resistance of metastatic pancreatic endocrine tumours after long-term treatment with the somatostatin analogue octreotide (SMS 201–995). *Clin Endocrinol (Oxf)* 30:385, 1989.

52. Eriksson BK, Larsson EG, Skogseid BM, et al: Liver embolizations of patients with malignant neuroendocrine gastrointestinal tumors. *Cancer* 83:2293, 1998.

53. Chamberlain RS, Canes D, Brown KT, et al: Hepatic neuroendocrine metastases: Does intervention alter outcomes? *J Am Coll Surg* 190:432, 2000.

54. Mayo SC, de Jong MC, Pulitano C, et al: Surgical management of hepatic neuroendocrine tumor metastasis: Results from an international multi-institutional analysis. *Ann Surg Oncol* 17:3129, 2010.

55. Le Treut YP, Delpero JR, Dousset B, et al: Results of liver transplantation in the treatment of metastatic neuroendocrine tumors. A 31-case French multicentric report. *Ann Surg* 225:355, 1997.

56. Janson ET, Holmberg L, Stridsberg M, et al: Carcinoid tumors: Analysis of prognostic factors and survival in 301 patients from a referral center. *Ann Oncol* 8:685, 1997.

57. Chen H, Hardacre JM, Uzar A, et al: Isolated liver metastases from neuroendocrine tumors: Does resection prolong survival? *J Am Coll Surg* 187:88, 1998.

58. Yu F, Venzon DJ, Serrano J, et al: Prospective study of the clinical course, prognostic factors and survival in patients with longstanding Zollinger-Ellison syndrome. *J Clin Oncol* 17:615, 1999.

59. Norton JA, Warren RS, Kelly MG, et al: Aggressive surgery for metastatic liver neuroendocrine tumors. *Surgery* 134:1057, 2003.

60. Berber E, Flesher N, Siperstein AE: Laparoscopic radiofrequency ablation of neuroendocrine liver metastases. *World J Surg* 26:985, 2002.

61. Yao KA, Talamonti MS, Nemcek A, et al: Indications and results of liver resection and hepatic chemoembolization for metastatic gastrointestinal neuroendocrine tumors. *Surgery* 130:677, 2001.

62. Ruszniewski P, Rougier P, Roche A, et al: Hepatic arterial chemoembolization in patients with liver metastases of endocrine tumors. A prospective phase II study in 24 patients. *Cancer* 71:2624, 1993.

63. Weitz J, Blumgart LH, Fong Y, et al: Partial hepatectomy for metastases from noncolorectal, nonneuroendocrine carcinoma. *Ann Surg* 241:269, 2005.

Multidisciplinary Approach to the Management of Portal Hypertension

J. Michael Henderson

The management of portal hypertension has changed dramatically in the past two decades with improved understanding of the pathophysiology, better and more logical approaches to patient evaluation, and many new and improved treatment modalities. By definition, portal hypertension is present when the portal pressure rises above 8 mm Hg, but the wide spectrum of etiologies leading to this broad clinical syndrome mandates the need for a multidisciplinary approach to identification, evaluation, and management of these patients. The clinical manifestations of portal hypertension are variceal bleeding, ascites, liver failure and hepatic encephalopathy, hepatoma, and the hepatopulmonary syndromes (HPSs). These cover every field of medicine, with the main players in the multidisciplinary team being the following:

- Hepatologists
- Gastroenterologists/Endoscopists
- Radiologists
- Surgeons
- Pathologists
- Anesthesia/Critical care staff
- Nurse clinicians/Support team

The role of the surgeon has changed dramatically over the past two decades in this multidisciplinary team, with the main role now being in liver transplantation as compared to a role in operative decompressive shunts for such patients 20 to 30 years ago. The goal of this chapter is to present current status of knowledge for the pathophysiology of portal hypertension, present a logical approach to the evaluation of such patients, and give an assessment of current treatment modalities and when they should be used.

HISTORY

The early history of portal hypertension has been well documented by Reuben and Groszmann.[1] The liver was recognized as a highly vascular organ in ancient times with writings from the ancient Egyptians, the Greeks, and the Romans. However, most misunderstood the liver, its vasculature, and its physiologic role. Francis Glisson and William Harvey gave structural proof and functional demonstration of the anatomy and blood flow through the liver. It was not until microscopic examination became possible that the liver lobule with its hexagonal appearance, portal venous and hepatic arterial inflow from the periphery, and hepatic venous drainage from the center could be fully understood.

Ascites was the first clinical complication of portal hypertension to be recognized long before its pathogenesis was understood. Ascites is mentioned in the ancient texts of Egypt and the Central American Mayans and acquired its name from the ancient Greeks. Gastro-esophageal varices were not recognized until the mid-19th century, and even then they were believed to be a rare entity. Much confusion reigned over the next 100 years as to the pathophysiology of portal hypertension. It was recognized that there was elevated pressure in the portal venous system, but it was not recognized that this occurred secondary to cirrhosis. For a long time, the so-called forward theory of portal hypertension popularized by Banti was accepted.[2] Banti believed that patients with splenomegaly, anemia, and leukopenia suffered from a splenopathy that in turn injured the liver and caused cirrhosis; this led to the term *hepatosplenopathy*. It was in the 1920s that McIndoe[3] postulated a "backward flow" theory for portal hypertension based on the primary pathology being in the liver—cirrhosis obstructing portal flow—and a buildup of portal pressure behind this obstruction.

The treatment of these conditions had focused on splenectomy, omentopexy, or other "preobstructive" operations while the forward flow theory held. Recognition that a blockage to portal flow within the liver—usually due to cirrhosis—led to portal hypertension initiated an era of decompressive operations to manage the overall syndrome. Portacaval shunt was initially performed in dogs by Nicolai Eck in St. Petersburg in 1890, but it was another Russian, Pavlov, who documented the risks of such portal diversion leading to progressive liver failure, inanition, and hepatic encephalopathy. However, a new era of surgery for portal hypertension started in the 1930s when it was believed that careful technique could circumvent these issues and provide a viable treatment modality with portacaval shunt. The pioneering work of Whipple[2] and his colleagues at Columbia in New York significantly advanced the field. However, they soon recognized that such shunts, though controlling bleeding and ascites, led to acceleration of liver failure with no survival advantage to their patients. This initiated the era of randomized controlled trials in portal hypertension.

Portal hypertension has evolved over the past 50 years because of the multiple randomized controlled trials performed for all treatment modalities introduced. This was one of the earliest fields of medicine to receive such scrutiny, and as a result the progress in managing patients has been based on level 1 evidence since the 1950s. Initial trials compared surgical shunts to medical therapy in patients who had not bled and showed that mortality was increased with such intervention. Subsequent studies comparing medical therapy and surgical shunts in patients following their initial variceal bleed showed no improvement in overall survival, but a change in the mode of death from variceal bleeding to liver failure. These observations stimulated the investigators of that time to look for new treatment modalities.

Selective shunts were pioneered by Warren et al[3] and Inokuchi,[4] who showed that variceal decompression could be achieved while maintaining portal perfusion to the cirrhotic liver. Partial shunts were carefully studied and championed by Sarfeh et al,[5] who documented that they could achieve adequate decompression of varices and maintain some portal flow. Preservation of portal flow with both selective and partial shunts resulted in lower encephalopathy and liver failure. Endoscopic therapy was initially introduced by surgeons using rigid esophagoscopes but rapidly moved to flexible endoscopy in the 1980s as this technology was introduced. Sclerotherapy of varices became the realm of the gastroenterologist, but it was a surgeon (Steigmann et al[6]) who introduced variceal banding as a further significant advance in endoscopic therapy for bleeding varices.

Even as these multiple therapeutic interventions were evolving, the pathophysiology of portal hypertension was becoming better understood.[7] The recognition that the perpetuation and even increase in portal pressure is mediated through splanchnic hyperemia and a hyperdynamic systemic circulation (see Pathophysiology, later) not only resurrected a component of Banti's forward-flow hypothesis but also led to the introduction of pharmacologic means of reducing portal hypertension. Lebrec et al[8] introduced noncardioselective β-blockers to ameliorate these changes and reduce portal pressure. This has become one of the mainstays of managing such patients.

Technology has also contributed to radiologic decompressive shunts for portal hypertension following the lead of cardiac and peripheral vascular stents. Transjugular intrahepatic portosystemic shunts (TIPSs) were pioneered by Rosche, and became widely used in the 1990s. "Minimally invasive" shunting has come of age and is clearly part of the treatment armamentarium for these patients.

Finally, the history of portal hypertension must recognize the role of liver transplantation introduced by Starzl and Calne in the 1970s and coming of age in the mid-1980s and 1990s. Their perseverance and pioneering work to resolve many of the technical issues of liver transplantation bore fruit. But it was really the immunologic advances and the introduction of powerful new immunosuppressants that gave life to liver transplantation. The clinical reality is that many patients with significant liver disease have only their complications of portal hypertension and their survival improved by liver transplantation. For the surgeon, this brings the management of such patients full circle where the surgeon's role is now largely in the field of liver transplantation as part of the multidisciplinary team taking care of such patients.

ANATOMY

The portal vein has complex embryologic development from the vitelline and umbilical veins.[9] The vitelline veins

intercommunicate in the septum transversum, which is the site of development of liver sinusoids. The left vitelline vein forms most of the extrahepatic portal venous system, whereas the left umbilical vein plays a critical role in utero as the ductus venosus, which communicates directly from the rudimentary portovenous system to the hepatic veins, bypassing the hepatic sinusoids.

The portal vein is formed behind the neck of the pancreas by the joining of the superior mesenteric and splenic veins. It is normally 10 to 20 mm in diameter, but in portal hypertension may enlarge up to 20 mm. It courses along the free edge of the gastrohepatic ligament to the liver hilus, where it divides into right and left branches (Figure 131-1). Its feeding tributaries have some variability, with the inferior mesenteric vein entering the splenic vein in approximately two-thirds of persons and superior mesenteric vein in one-third. Similarly, the left gastric or coronary vein enters the portal vein in approximately two-thirds and the splenic vein in one-third. The latter may vary considerably in size in portal hypertension and is often one of the major veins feeding into gastroesophageal varices. The umbilical vein is remarkably constant in its communication with the left branch of the portal vein, and in portal hypertension when recanalized this may be quite large. The major changes of clinical significance are around the gastroesophageal junction in portal hypertension. Radiologic studies using corrosion casting and morphometry have clarified the venous pathologic changes at this location

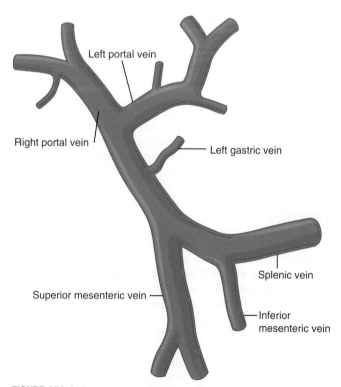

FIGURE 131-1 Portal venous anatomy. The portal vein is formed by the union of the superior mesenteric and splenic veins behind the neck of the pancreas. The inferior mesenteric vein enters the splenic vein in two-thirds of patients, and the left gastric vein enters the portal vein in two-thirds of patients.

in portal hypertension. These are schematically represented in Figure 131-2, where the following four zones are recognized:

1. The gastric zone extends 2 to 3 cm below the gastroesophageal junction. These veins run longitudinally in the submucosa and lamina propria to the short gastric and left gastric veins.
2. The palisade zone extends 2 to 3 cm superiorly from the gastric zone in the lower esophagus. These

parallel palisades run longitudinally and correspond to the esophageal mucosal folds. There are multiple communications between these veins in the lamina propria, but there are no perforating veins in the palisade zone linking the intrinsic and extrinsic venous plexuses.

3. The perforating zone extends approximately 2 cm higher up the esophagus just superior to the palisade zone. In this zone, the vessels perforate through the esophageal wall linking the internal and external veins.
4. The truncal zone extends 8 to 10 cm up the esophagus and is characterized by four or five longitudinal veins in the lamina propria. In this zone, there are irregular perforating veins from the submucosa to the external esophageal venous plexuses.

Hepatic arterial anatomy is highly variable, with anomalies being of clinical importance to transplant surgeons, particularly during donor hepatectomy. The normal arterial anatomy is a common hepatic artery arising from the celiac axis that gives rise to a right and left artery just above the gastroduodenal artery. In approximately 20% of persons there is an anomalous right accessory or replaced hepatic artery arising from the superior mesenteric artery. Similarly, there is an approximately 20% incidence for an accessory or replaced left hepatic artery arising from the left gastric artery. These two anomalies may coexist (Figure 131-3).

The segmental anatomy of the liver is of importance to the surgeon in liver resection and in living donor liver transplant. The liver has eight segments, each with its own hepatic arterial and portal venous inflow and hepatic venous drainage (Figure 131-4).[10] This allows for division in these planes with functional segments for liver remnant or for donor grafts. At a physiologic level, each of these segments has smaller microscopic functional units of the liver lobules. At this level, the portal vein and hepatic artery enter the periphery of hexagonal-shaped liver lobules, with blood traversing the sinusoids and draining through central hepatic veins.

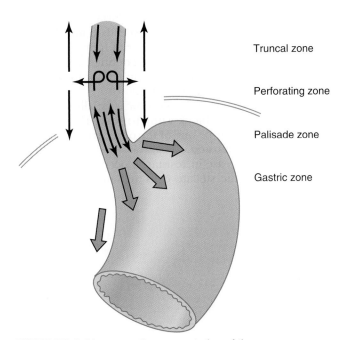

Truncal zone

Perforating zone

Palisade zone

Gastric zone

FIGURE 131-2 Diagrammatic representation of the venous zones at the gastroesophageal junction. The perforating zone is the site of highest variceal bleeding risk. Details of the zones are given in the text. (Modified from Vianna A, Hayes PC, Moscoso G, et al: Normal venous circulation of the gastroesophageal junction. A route to understanding varices. *Gastroenterology* 93:876, 1987.)

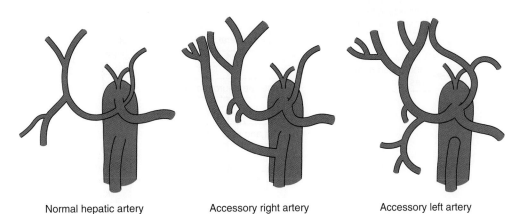

Normal hepatic artery   Accessory right artery   Accessory left artery

FIGURE 131-3 Hepatic arterial anatomy is highly variable. The most common anomalies are accessory—or replaced—right and left hepatic arteries arising from the superior mesenteric and left gastric arteries, respectively. These occur in approximately 20% of the population each; they may coexist. (Redrawn from Henderson JM: Atlas of liver surgery. In Bell RH, Rikkers LF, Mulholland MW, editors: *Digestive tract surgery: A text and atlas*. Philadelphia, 1995, Lippincott-Raven.)

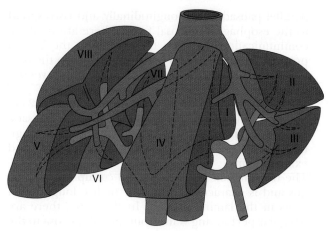

FIGURE 131-4 Liver segmental anatomy is based on portal inflow and hepatic venous outflow. Each of the eight segments is its own functional anatomic unit. (Redrawn from Henderson JM: *Atlas of liver surgery*. In Bell RH, Rikkers LF, Mulholland MW, editors: *Digestive tract surgery: A text and atlas*. Philadelphia, 1995, Lippincott-Raven.)

PATHOPHYSIOLOGY

Normal portal venous pressure is 5 to 8 mm Hg, with the normal portal flow in the 1 to 1.5 L/min range. The portal vein is a passive conduit from the gut that carries blood back to the liver. Total liver blood flow is regulated by intrinsic and extrinsic mechanisms with alteration of portal venous flow having a direct reciprocal increase or decrease in hepatic arterial flow. The changes in portal hypertension occur on this physiologic background. The steps in the development of the pathophysiology of portal hypertension have been carefully elucidated in the past two decades in animal models. Portal hypertension is present when portal pressure exceeds 8 mm Hg, but variceal bleeding rarely occurs until portal pressure exceeds 12 mm Hg. There is a well-defined sequence of events, as follows, that occurs in the pathophysiology of portal hypertension (Figure 131-5):

- Obstruction to portal venous flow is usually secondary to an intrahepatic block with cirrhosis. However, the inciting event may be one of the other etiologic causes of portal hypertension.
- Functional increase in resistance occurs secondary to activated hepatic stellate cells and myofibroblasts in

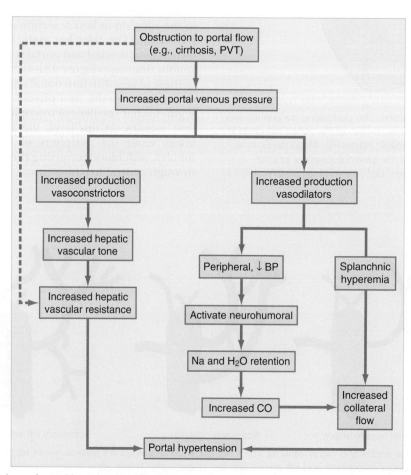

FIGURE 131-5 Pathophysiology of portal hypertension. Complex vascular and neurohumoral responses that affect splanchnic, renal, and peripheral vascular control are shown. *BP,* Blood pressure; *CO,* cardiac output; *PVT,* portal vein thrombosis.

the fibrous septa of the sinusoid. These represent a potentially reversible component to intrahepatic resistance.

- There is an imbalanced production of vasoconstrictors such as endothelin, norepinephrine, and angiotensin, with an insufficient release of hepatic vasodilators such as nitric oxide and prostaglandins.
- Splanchnic vasodilation occurs with increased splanchnic flow aggravating and contributing to the portal hypertensive syndrome. This is multifactorial, with neurogenic, humoral, and local mediators.
- Portosystemic collaterals develop not only at the gastroesophageal junction but in the abdominal wall and retroperitoneum.
- There is an increase in plasma volume secondary to the vascular changes.
- A systemic hyperdynamic circulation develops with increased cardiac output, low total systemic vascular resistance, and further aggravation of the splanchnic hyperemia and overall hyperdynamic state.

This sequence of pathophysiologic changes in the hepatic, splanchnic, and finally systemic circulation offers an opportunity for pharmacologic manipulation and management of portal hypertension.

CLINICAL PRESENTATIONS IN PORTAL HYPERTENSION

Variceal bleeding is one of the most lethal complications of portal hypertension. An improved understanding of the natural history of varices has helped put logic into their management.[11,12] The following points apply:

- Thirty percent of patients with cirrhosis develop varices.
- Thirty percent of patients with varices bleed from varices.
- Patients with large varices are more at risk for bleeding than patients with small varices.
- Patients with variceal bleeding and well-preserved liver function have a broader range of treatment options and better outcomes than patients with variceal bleeding and poor liver function.

All patients with documented or suspected cirrhosis should have an upper endoscopy to document whether or not they have varices. Documentation of varices may lead to treatment at the following time points:

- Prophylactic therapy, prior to the initial bleed
- Management of an acute variceal bleeding episode
- Therapy to prevent a recurrent variceal bleed

The details of evaluation and management for patients are dealt with in the following discussion.

Ascites develops in patients with cirrhosis at a more advanced stage than may be the case for variceal bleeding.[13] Ascites is a sign of "decompensation" of the underlying liver disease. From a clinical perspective, it is the responsiveness of ascites to simple treatment with salt restriction and diuretics versus refractory ascites that is important in patient management. The diagnosis and management of ascites are discussed in later sections.

Liver failure and encephalopathy are common complications of portal hypertension, are caused by progressive liver disease, and are the most definitive markers of end-stage disease. From a clinical perspective, recurring encephalopathy or signs of liver failure are an indication for evaluation for liver transplant. If the patient is not a candidate for liver transplant, their treatment options are limited once this clinical presentation occurs.

Hepatocellular carcinoma (HCC) is an increasingly frequent complication of cirrhosis seen in patients with portal hypertension.[14] The epidemic of HCC is largely due to the increased incidence of hepatitis C, but this complication of chronic liver disease can occur with cirrhosis of any etiology. From a clinical perspective, hepatoma should be looked for in all patients with a documented cirrhosis by serial scanning with ultrasound and evaluation of α-fetoprotein. If HCC is the initial presentation of the patient, it is important for the clinician to document if the rest of the liver is normal or indeed has an established cirrhosis. The management options for hepatoma are dictated by the rest of the liver as much as by the tumor itself.

The *portopulmonary syndromes* have more recently been recognized as an important component of the clinical presentation of patients with portal hypertension.[15] There are two broad groups of patients: (1) those with HPS that is marked by hypoxemia secondary to intrapulmonary shunting in patients with chronic liver disease, in the absence of pulmonary hypertension, and (2) patients with pulmonary hypertension and chronic underlying liver disease who have a more sinister syndrome with a poor prognosis.

ETIOLOGY OF PORTAL HYPERTENSION

The etiologies of portal hypertension are summarized in Box 131-1. Broadly, the etiologies fall into the categories of (1) prehepatic block raising portal pressure, (2) intrahepatic obstruction to portal flow, and (3) posthepatic venous outflow block.

Prehepatic portal hypertension comprises 5% to 10% of portal hypertension patients in the United States and Europe.[16] In other parts of the world such as India, this may be the etiology in a higher percentage of portal hypertension patients. The importance of identifying patients with this etiology is that the liver is usually

---

BOX 131-1 Etiology of Portal Hypertension

PREHEPATIC
Portal or splenic vein thrombosis
Extrinsic portal vein compression
Arteriovenous fistula

INTRAHEPATIC
Cirrhosis: multiple etiologies
Schistosomiasis
Congenital hepatic fibrosis
Rare causes

POSTHEPATIC
Budd-Chiari syndrome
Constrictive pericarditis

normal, which is a major factor in overall prognosis. The most common prehepatic block is portal and/or splenic vein thrombosis. Portal vein thrombosis may be associated with umbilical vein catheterization or other causes of sepsis and dehydration in infancy. In the adult patient, the hypercoagulable syndromes should be sought in patients with a newly diagnosed portal or splenic vein thrombosis, with a full hematologic workup. Other etiologies include pancreatitis and pancreatic tumors, with the later portending a poor prognosis related to the cancer. Occasionally, extrinsic pressure on the portal vein from lymph nodes or other tumors can lead to portal hypertension, but this is unusual. Finally, hepatic artery–to–portal venous fistulas, usually secondary to a liver biopsy, can occur and if large can lead to portal hypertension. Fistulas are diagnosed with radiologic imaging and can usually be managed with endoluminal angiographic techniques for their occlusion.

One important variant of portal hypertension is left-sided (sinistral) portal hypertension with isolated splenic vein thrombosis, a normal portal vein, and no intrahepatic block. The most common causes of this are pancreatitis and carcinoma of the body and tail of the pancreas. This is increasingly recognized on computed tomographic (CT) scan, with large collaterals coming from the splenic hilus up to the fundus of the stomach. From a portal hypertension perspective, this is readily handled with splenectomy, but clearly an understanding of the underlying pathology is most important in prognosis.

The intrahepatic causes of portal hypertension account for 90% of the cases in the United States and Europe. Most patients with an intrahepatic block have cirrhosis, which has multiple etiologies. These include alcohol, hepatitis B, hepatitis C, the cholestatic liver diseases (primary sclerosing cholangitis and primary biliary cirrhosis), hemochromatosis, and the other metabolic causes of cirrhosis. In the course of patient evaluation, full definition of the underlying disease is important for management. It is the natural history, activity, and rate of progression of the underlying liver disease that ultimately sets the prognosis.

Schistosomiasis is still an important cause of portal hypertension on a world-wide basis. Still seen in the Middle and Far East and in South America, the pathologic block in schistosomiasis is fibrosis of the terminal portal venules. Although pathologically an intrahepatic block, it is presinusoidal, and lobular architecture is maintained with well-preserved liver function. However, many patients with schistosomiasis may also have hepatitis as a concomitant disease with implications of liver function impairment.

Congenital hepatic fibrosis is a relatively rare cause of an intrahepatic block in the United States and Europe, but it is important to recognize because it is usually associated with preserved liver function. However, more recently there have been reports of progression of congenital hepatic fibrosis to end-stage liver disease requiring liver transplantation. A similar entity is seen in India as noncirrhotic portal fibrosis, which is a cause for portal hypertension in that country.[17] The implication of preserved liver function is that there is a broader range of options for treatment, particularly for variceal bleeding.

The posthepatic causes of portal hypertension fall into the broad category of Budd-Chiari syndrome[18] and the occasional patient with a constrictive pericarditis. The common feature is hepatic venous outflow block. Classic Budd-Chiari syndrome involves thrombosis of the main hepatic veins, but other etiologies such as inferior vena caval (IVC) webs may cause this syndrome. The outflow block leads to an increase in sinusoidal pressure, centrilobular hepatocyte damage, and ultimately fibrosis, scarring, and cirrhosis. These are exceedingly rare syndromes, accounting for 1% to 2% of the cases of portal hypertension.

EVALUATION

Evaluation of patients with portal hypertension requires a multidisciplinary approach focused on the clinical presentations. All patients with cirrhosis should have some component of this evaluation, with the depth of evaluation determined by the specific presentation as outlined earlier. The essential components of such evaluation are summarized in Box 131-2.

Endoscopy plays a key role in the evaluation because varices and bleeding are the most serious complications of portal hypertension. Any patient with cirrhosis should have an endoscopy to assess for varices. The presence of varices may be the first indication that a patient does have portal hypertension. Even if the patient has not bled, this evaluation will identify some patients with moderate to large varices who should receive prophylactic therapy. Endoscopy should assess the size of the varices, their extent, and risk factors.[19] Risk factors are red-color signs that indicate thin-walled varices that are at increased risk of bleeding. In addition, the gastric mucosa should be assessed for portal gastropathy, which also has risk factor grading with red-color signs that indicate an increased risk of bleeding. Grading systems to classify bleeding risk for gastroesophageal varices, portal

---

BOX 131-2 Evaluation of Patients With Portal Hypertension

ENDOSCOPY
Size of varices
Extent of varices
Risk factor, red-color signs
Portal gastropathy

IMAGING
Doppler ultrasound
CT scan
HVPG and imaging
Angiography

LIVER FUNCTION
Clinical: ascites, encephalopathy, jaundice, muscle wasting
Laboratory data
Child score
MELD score

HVPG, Hepatic venous pressure gradient; *MELD,* model for end-stage liver disease.

hypertension gastropathy, and gastric varices help standardize patient populations.[20]

Radiologic evaluation of the portal venous system is the next important step. Initially done with Doppler ultrasound,[21] this method visualizes the portal vein and its main tributaries as well as assessing flow patterns in the portal venous system. This is also the best method for assessing the hepatic veins both for patency and their wave-flow patterns. Ultrasound is the most useful screening modality for liver morphology, defining the cirrhotic liver, but focal lesions suggestive of HCC can also be assessed.

Further imaging of the liver and its vasculature may be done with either CT scan or magnetic resonance (MR) imaging. The choice is largely made by institutional preference and experience. Both provide good methods of imaging the normal and cirrhotic liver. Morphologic assessment for liver tumors, particularly with the increasing incidence of hepatoma, is increasingly accurate with these imaging modalities. Both also provide a further means to evaluate the portal venous system, with the ability to look at flow patterns with faster scanners and more sophisticated postimage processing. These have largely replaced the need for visceral angiography in this population.

Arteriography and hepatic venous studies still play some role in evaluation of these patients.[22] Hepatic venous pressures are measured with a balloon occlusion catheter in the hepatic vein, measuring the occluded and free hepatic vein pressures. The difference between these gives the hepatic venous pressure gradient (HVPG), which is an indirect measure of portal venous pressure akin to pulmonary artery pressure in the lungs. Increasing emphasis is being placed on the value of this measurement in the era of more sophisticated pharmacologic therapies. If the HVPG can be reduced to 10 mm Hg or less, variceal bleeding will not occur. Occasionally visceral arteriography followed through to the venous phase is required for full clarification of portal hypertension. When there remains doubt after CT or MR imaging as to patency and flow patterns in the superior mesenteric, splenic, or portal veins, angiography may clarify this. It also gives dynamic imaging of the flow patterns in the major tributaries and collaterals associated with portal hypertension. This may be of importance to the surgeon considering intervention.

Liver function assessment is the final phase of evaluation. The components of this are clinical, laboratory data, and calculation of prognostic indices. The important parts in clinical assessment of liver function are the detection of ascites, evaluation for encephalopathy, detection of clinical jaundice, and assessment of muscle wasting. All of these clinical signs are indications of advanced liver disease.

Laboratory data that are important are those that directly assess liver status: bilirubin, albumin, prothrombin time, aspartate aminotransferase, alanine transaminase, and alkaline phosphatase. In addition, hematologic parameters (i.e., hemoglobin, platelet count, and white blood cell count) may be affected by portal hypertension. A platelet count lower than 100,000 is indicative of significant portal hypertension. A prothrombin time

TABLE 131-1 Child-Pugh Grading of Severity of Liver Disease*

CLINICAL AND LABORATORY MEASUREMENT	PATIENT SCORE FOR INCREASING ABNORMALITY		
	1	2	3
Encephalopathy (grade)	None	1 or 2	3 or 4
Ascites	None	Mild	Moderate
Bilirubin (mg/dL)	1-2	2.1-3	≥3.1
Albumin (g/dL)	≥3.5	2.8-3.5	≤2.7
Prothrombin time (increase, seconds)	1-4	4.1-6	≥6.1

*Grade A, 5-6 points; Grade B, 7-9 points; Grade C, 10-15 points.

BOX 131-3 Model for End-Stage Liver Disease Score for Liver Disease Severity

Score = 0.957 × log$_e$ creatinine (mg/dL) + 0.378 × log$_e$ bilirubin (mg/dL) + 1.120 log$_e$ INR

---

international normalized ratio (INR) of 1.5 indicates poor liver function. All patients should have checks made of specific liver disease markers, including hepatitis panels, antinuclear antibody, antimitochondrial antibody, and metabolic disease markers for iron, copper, and α_1-antitrypsin. Finally, hepatoma risk can be assessed with α-fetoprotein.

The prognostic indices that are used in patients with portal hypertension are the Child-Pugh score (Table 131-1),[23] and the model for end-stage liver disease (MELD) score (Box 131-3).[24] The Child-Pugh score, developed to assess prognosis of patients undergoing portal decompressive surgery, has stood the test of time for more than 50 years as a useful index of disease severity. More recently, the MELD score has come into being as a more objective way of assessing mortality risk for patients with more advanced disease. Its genesis was the need for a better method for grading disease severity for liver transplantation.

MANAGEMENT OF VARICEAL BLEEDING

PROPHYLAXIS OF VARICEAL BLEEDING[25]

Figure 131-6 shows an algorithm for the investigation and management of patients with cirrhosis and varices that have not bled. The initial step, as indicated earlier, is endoscopic evaluation of all patients with cirrhosis. If patients have no varices, they should have a followup endoscopy at 2 years. If they have small (5-mm) varices, they should receive no prophylactic therapy and have a followup endoscopy in 1 year. If they have moderate to large varices (>5 mm) and/or red-color risk factors, they should receive prophylactic therapy. Standard prophylactic therapy to reduce the risk of an initial bleed is with a noncardioselective β-blocker—propranolol or nadolol. In patients who are intolerant to β-blockers or who have large, high-risk varices, a course of endoscopic banding

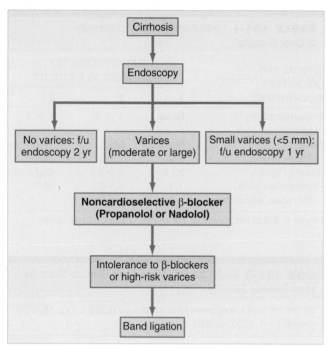

FIGURE 131-6 Algorithm for prophylaxis of the first variceal bleed. Diagnosis of varices is step 1; grading of size determines the need for therapy. Moderate or large varices should be treated. *f/u*, Followup.

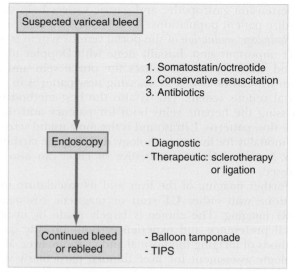

FIGURE 131-7 Algorithm for managing acute variceal bleeding. This falls into (1) general measures, (2) endoscopic therapy, and (3) salvage of refractory/recurrent bleeding. *TIPS*, Transjugular intrahepatic portosystemic shunt.

may be appropriate. Both of these approaches reduce the risk of initial bleed from 30% to approximately 15% to 18%.

ACUTE VARICEAL BLEEDING

Figure 131-7 shows a management algorithm for acute variceal bleeding.[26] This falls into the following three broad steps:

1. General measures for managing the patient when it is still not certain if they are bleeding from varices
2. An endoscopic assessment and treatment
3. Those patients who need further treatment if they are not controlled with endoscopic and pharmacologic therapy or rebleed through endoscopic treatment

The general measures for a suspected variceal bleed are initial pharmacologic therapy with either somatostatin or its analogue octreotide as a continuous infusion at 50 µg/hr. These drugs have virtually replaced vasopressin/nitroglycerin, although triglycyl lysine vasopressin (Terlipressin) is available and used in Europe. Patient resuscitation should be on the conservative side with underresuscitation rather than overresuscitation. It is better to have a patient with a slightly reduced intravascular volume rather than overexpanded volume, which increases the risk of a recurrent variceal bleed. In practical terms, this means that a systolic blood pressure of 100 to 110 mm Hg is preferable to 120 to 130 mm Hg. Ideally, patients should be placed in an intensive care unit (ICU) for ongoing monitoring. A Foley catheter should be placed so that urine output can be monitored. Finally, it has been increasingly recognized that sepsis plays an important role in prognosis at this time and all patients with cirrhosis and an acute variceal bleed should

receive antibiotics—a systemic cephalosporin should be given for 3 to 5 days.

Endoscopy at the time of an acute variceal bleed is initially diagnostic but, if appropriate, becomes therapeutic. Diagnostic endoscopy focuses on the presence of varices, their risk factors, and identification of an actively bleeding or a recently bleeding site. The latter are identified by a platelet plug on a varix. In addition, other sites of upper gastrointestinal bleeding such as peptic ulcer disease should be excluded. Frequently an active site is not identified, and a recently bleeding site may not be seen. In the absence of any other bleeding source, it is thus assumed that bleeding was from varices and treatment initiated. The therapeutic component of endoscopy is usually endoscopic banding of the varices. This should be aggressively undertaken with serial spiral banding of all varices around the gastroesophageal junction (Figure 131-8). If banding is not available, direct endoscopic sclerotherapy can be completed at this time to control acute bleeding.

For the 5% to 10% of patients in whom the acute variceal bleed is not controlled, or the 10% to 15% of patients in whom there is early rebleeding after the management discussed earlier, balloon tamponade may play a role to stabilize patients before moving to decompression. Balloon tamponade requires a knowledgeable team and careful protocols for its use. Patients requiring balloon tamponade should have endotracheal intubation for control of their airway. The tube can either be passed through the nose or the mouth. The position of the gastric balloon in the stomach should be confirmed with a radiograph after inflating it with 25 to 30 mL of air. Once the position is confirmed, the gastric balloon is inflated to approximately 200 mL and brought up snugly in the gastric fundus. Occasionally, the esophageal balloon may need to be inflated to 40 mm Hg

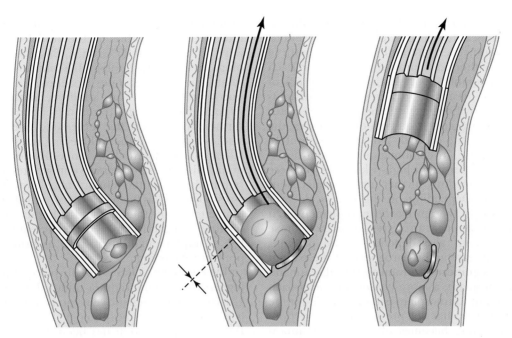

FIGURE 131-8 Diagnostic representation of variceal banding. The varix is sucked into the "cup" at the end of the endoscope and a tight band is fired around the base of the varix. The bands slough off in 5 to 10 days. (From Sanyal AJ, Shah VH, editors: *Portal hypertension.* Totowa, NJ, 2005, Humana Press, p 227.)

(monitored through a pressure cuff) but usually this is not required. Placement of a tamponade balloon mandates a further step within 12 to 24 hours to control bleeding, which is usually done with an urgent TIPS. Once the patient is stabilized, an urgent TIPS should be done. This must be viewed as similar to taking the patient to the operating room—intubation, sedation, and careful monitoring should be performed. TIPS is therefore indicated in a very small number of patients in the acute setting who do not respond to pharmacologic and endoscopic therapy.

A recent randomized trial of early TIPS in Child B and C patients with acute variceal bleeding—not just patients who failed endoscopic therapy—showed significantly lower rebleeding and better survival in patients randomized to early TIPS compared to endoscopic therapy with TIPS salvage.[27]

PREVENTION OF RECURRENT VARICEAL BLEEDING

Figure 131-9 presents an algorithm for management to prevent recurrent variceal bleeding. Following stabilization of an acute bleeding episode, patients should undergo evaluation, as outlined earlier.[26]

PRIMARY THERAPY

The initial management to prevent recurrent bleeding should be a combination of pharmacologic and endoscopic therapy. The aggressive banding session at the time of the acute bleed should be followed in 7 to 10 days with further variceal ligation and repeat sessions until the varices are obliterated. Usually two or three sessions suffice. Banding has been shown to be better than sclerotherapy,[28] with better bleeding control and fewer

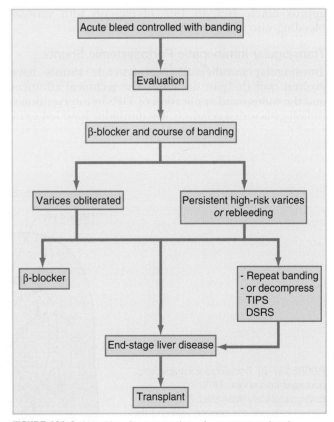

FIGURE 131-9 Algorithm for prevention of recurrent variceal bleeding. Primary therapy for all patients is with β-blockers and banding. Secondary therapy may be variceal decompression for recurrent bleeding or transplant for advanced disease and recurrent bleeding. *DSRS,* Distal splenorenal shunt; *TIPS,* transjugular intrahepatic portosystemic shunt.

complications. Concurrently, the patient should be started on a noncardioselective β-blocker to reduce portal hypertension. There are multiple trials of both of these modalities either on their own, compared to each other, or used in combination.[26] Both reduce the risk of further bleeding at 1 year from 70% in untreated patients to 30%. The combination may reduce the risk to closer to 20%. If the banding course obliterates the varices, the patient should continue on their β-blocker indefinitely. If the banding course, in combination with pharmacologic therapy, leaves persistent high-risk varices, or there is an episode of rebleeding, further treatment decisions need to be made. Depending on the time scale over which the endoscopic therapy has been implemented, it may be reasonable to repeat an aggressive further course of banding. Decisions also depend on the patient's underlying liver disease and its prognosis. If the patient has moderate or significantly advanced liver disease and is headed for transplant, a more conservative approach bridging the patient to transplant is indicated. If, on the other hand, the patient has well-preserved liver function, stopping the bleeding becomes of paramount importance so that the liver disease is not accelerated. Such patients may be candidates for decompression.

DECOMPRESSION OF VARICES

The current recommendations for variceal decompression are to use either TIPS or a surgical shunt. It is only approximately 10% to 15% of patients with variceal bleeding who will need this level of treatment.

Transjugular Intrahepatic Portosystemic Shunts

Transjugular intrahepatic portosystemic shunts have evolved over the past decade.[29] The technical advances and the widespread application of TIPS by interventional radiologists with a relatively low morbidity have led to its general acceptance. This is being supported by data as indicated later. Although the initial rebleeding rates were in the 20% to 25% range, this appears to be dropping. First, the technology has improved and covered stents have a lower rate of stenosis than the original uncovered stents.[30] In addition, data indicate that ongoing monitoring with reintervention for stenosis will further bring down the rebleeding rates. More recent studies have shown that rebleeding rates with TIPS have fallen to the 11% to 15% range. However, the costs of doing this in terms of reintervention rates and the dollars required for reintervention have not yet been fully assessed. TIPS has been shown to control bleeding better than endoscopic therapy, but the higher rate of encephalopathy, and the lack of a difference in survival has not led to implementation of TIPS as primary therapy to prevent rebleeding.[31]

The Procedure. TIPS is usually placed via a right transjugular route to the right or middle hepatic vein (Figure 131-10), but any hepatic vein can be used and the choice is dictated by liver morphology. Direct access from the IVC to the portal vein has been used in some cases of Budd-Chiari syndrome. Next, the hepatic parenchyma is traversed with a needle to puncture the portal vein; ultrasound guidance can be used, but experienced interventional radiologists can usually access the portal vein readily. It is important to enter the right or left portal vein within the liver cephalad to the bifurcation that sits outside the liver—puncture and dilation of the tract at the bifurcation can result in a major intraabdominal bleed. A catheter is placed over a guidewire into the portal vein, pressure is measured, and a portogram contrast study performed. The transparenchymal tract is dilated and the stent(s) placed to keep the tract open. The stent is dilated to reduce the portal-to-right atrial gradient to equal 10 mm Hg. Stent placement is

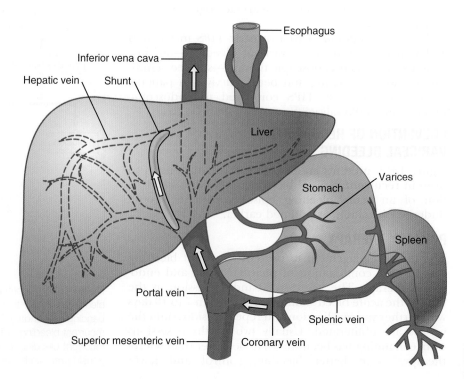

FIGURE 131-10 Transjugular intrahepatic portosystemic shunt (TIPS) is diagrammatically illustrated. The stent is placed between the hepatic vein and the portal vein, dilated to 10 to 12 mm, and the portal-to-right atrial pressure gradient is reduced to less than 10 mm Hg. (From Henderson JM: Portal hypertension. In Corson JD, Williamson R, editors: *Surgery*. London, 2001, Mosby.)

important: not too low into the portal vein and not too high into the suprahepatic IVC, both of which can create technical problems if subsequent transplant is needed. However, the tract must be adequately stented because the most common site for subsequent stenosis is the hepatic vein end of the stent. Covered stents require more fastidious placement to be sure the covered components do not protrude into the portal vein or IVC. Covered stents have a short uncovered segment at the end. A completion study should document patency and appropriate pressure gradient reduction (to ≤10 mm Hg).

Followup requires careful monitoring. Doppler ultrasound is adequate for screening and documenting total thrombosis. Covered stents do not transmit the Doppler signal for several days, so initial evaluation should be 3 to 4 days after the procedure. Ultrasound does not always document stenosis, which requires stent recatheterization and pressure measurement and possibly imaging. Gradients greater than 12 mm Hg or stenosis greater than 50% require dilation. Additional stents may be required if the stenosis is refractory to dilation or occurs at either end of the initial stents(s). The necessary frequency of recatheterization is undefined: current indications are when Doppler ultrasound studies change—increased or decreased velocities. The study with the lowest rebleeding rate after TIPS (11%) included protocol recatheterization at yearly intervals—this may set a standard.[32]

Surgical Shunts

Surgical shunts fall into three broad categories: total,[33] partial,[5] and selective shunts.[3,4] There are few indications for total surgical shunts at the current time. Partial shunts have been used successfully by some groups, with rebleeding rates in the 5% to 10% range, and because some portal perfusion is preserved, encephalopathy rates are lower with partial shunts than total shunts.[34] Selective shunts are most commonly done with the distal splenorenal shunt (DSRS), which selectively decompresses gastroesophageal varices while maintaining portal hypertension in the splanchnic-to-portal axis, thereby maintaining portal flow. DSRS controlled bleeding better than sclerotherapy in controlled trials, with equivalent encephalopathy.[35] Several uncontrolled series of DSRS in the 1990s to early 2000s showed rebleeding rates of 5% to 6%, encephalopathy rates around 15%, and 1- and 3-year survival rates of 85% and 75%, respectively, in good-risk Child Class A and B patients.[36-38] Selective shunts remain the most widely used surgical shunts at the present time.

Distal Splenorenal Shunt

The Procedure. DSRS is performed through a long left subcostal incision carried across the midline to the right rectus muscle (Figure 131-11). Exposure of the splenic and left renal veins is key. Access to the pancreas is obtained through the lesser sac, taking down the gastroepiploic vessels from the pylorus to the short gastric veins—this also serves as part of the portal/azygos disconnection. In addition, the splenic flexure of the colon should be taken down from the spleen—this both

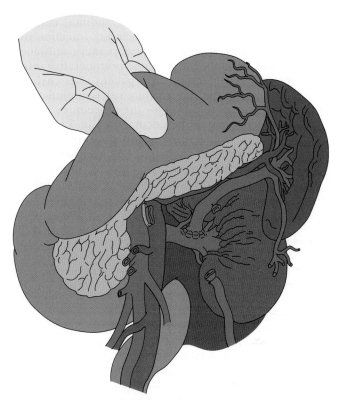

FIGURE 131-11 Distal splenorenal shunt selectively decompresses gastroesophageal varices through the spleen and splenic vein to the left renal vein. Portal hypertension and portal perfusion of the liver are maintained in the superior mesenteric and portal veins.

improves access to the posterior surface of the pancreas and interrupts potential collaterals to the shunt. The pancreas is fully mobilized along its inferior margin from the superior mesenteric vein to the splenic hilus—it is turned cephalad to expose its posterior surface and the splenic vein. Dissection of the splenic vein from the pancreas is done from the superior mesenteric vein over sufficient distance to mobilize enough vein to come down to the left renal vein without kinking. The posteroinferior surface is cleared first, then the small draining tributaries from the pancreas are isolated and ligated. The left renal vein is then identified in the retroperitoneum—a move made easier by preoperative venographic imaging. The left renal vein is mobilized with the left adrenal vein ligated and the gonadal vein left intact. This mobilization must be sufficient to allow the vein to come up into a side-biting clamp. The splenic vein is then divided at the splenic–superior mesenteric–portal junction and brought down for end-to-side anastomosis to the renal vein. We recommend interrupted sutures to the anterior row of the anastomosis to avoid purse-stringing. The shunt is opened, and the spleen can be seen to decompress. The operation is completed with further portal/azygos dissection mainly by interrupting the left gastric vein both at the portal vein and above the pancreas.

Management. Perioperative and postoperative details in care are important for patients with cirrhosis having major operative procedures. The major risks are ascites, infection, and liver failure. Ascites risk is minimized by careful fluid management: minimize sodium, run the patient "dry," and use diuretics judiciously. Infection risk is minimized with appropriate perioperative antibiotic coverage and vigilance for potential postoperative infection, always a consideration in a patient with cirrhosis who is "not doing well." Liver failure risk is minimized by appropriate patient selection for the procedure.

Shunt patency should be documented in 5 to 7 days by direct shunt catheterization and pressure measurements before hospital discharge. Full variceal decompression takes 4 to 8 weeks, so knowing shunt status before discharge is important. If the shunt is working well at this time, late stenosis/thrombosis is unusual.

Followup. Patients are discharged on a low-sodium, low-fat diet—the latter because of the risk of chylous ascites in the first 6 to 8 weeks. Medications are spironolactone (Aldactone), 100 mg/day, and an H_2 blocker for gastric acid suppression. Blood work—liver function tests and electrolytes—should be monitored carefully for the first 2 to 3 months. Long-term followup is dictated by the underlying liver disease.

A National Institutes of Health–funded prospective, randomized, controlled trial has just been completed comparing TIPS and DSRS.[32] This study in Child Class A and B patients who were refractory to endoscopic and pharmacologic therapy ran over 7 years, with a median followup of 42 months. The rebleeding rates were not significantly different (5.6% in the DSRS group and 11.5% in the TIPS group). Encephalopathy rates were not significantly different, with 50% of patients in each group having at least one clinical encephalopathy event by 5 years. The survival rates were not significantly different, with 85% survival at 1 year and 65% survival at 5 years. What was significantly different was the reintervention rate, which was 82% in the TIPS group and 11% in the DSRS group ($P < 0.001$). It was the careful surveillance, protocol recatheterizations of TIPS at annual intervals, and completeness of followup that contributed to the low rebleeding rate in the TIPS group. This trial was conducted with uncovered stents. A European multicenter trial compared covered and uncovered TIPS—the reintervention rate with covered stents dropped to 15% at 1 year.[30] The issue remains, however, of how to identify those patients who do have a stenosis that does require reintervention.

A trial compared TIPS to the 8-mm H-graft interposition portacaval shunt in an "all-comers" population.[34] This trial entered patients who had failed primary therapy; 50% were Child C and 63% had alcoholic cirrhosis. At late followup, the rebleeding rate was significantly lower ($P < 0.01$) in the surgical shunt group (3%) compared to the TIPS group (17%), and fewer patients in the surgical shunt group came to transplant ($P < 0.01$). Mortality was not significantly different but in both groups was significantly better at 2-year followup than the predicted mortality by MELD score at study entry.

Devascularization Procedures

Devascularization procedures have been more extensively used in Japan and Egypt than in the United States and Europe. The goal of this group of operations is to reduce variceal inflow and to have the following components:

- Splenectomy
- Esophageal devascularization—at least 7 cm
- Gastric devascularization—all the greater curvature and the upper two-thirds of the lesser curvature

The advantage of these procedures is that they maintain portal hypertension and perfusion of the cirrhotic liver, provided there is no portal vein thrombosis, which occurs in up to 20%. Maintaining portal flow has been associated with lower encephalopathy rates.

The results have been better in Japan[39] than in the United States and Europe, but good results have also been achieved in Mexico.[40] Although not widely used in good-risk cirrhotic patients who have "shuntable" veins, an indication for this operation at the present time is in patients with extensive portal venous system thrombosis and recurrent variceal bleeding—many of these patients have a normal liver.

Transplant

Finally, in preventing variceal rebleeding, it is clear that transplant has played a major role over the past two decades.[41] Although variceal bleeding per se is not an indication for transplant, progression of liver disease, often with variceal bleeding as a component, is an indication for transplant. Transplant is the best shunt for variceal bleeding in patients with advanced liver disease and provides excellent control of bleeding. However, not all patients with variceal bleeding are candidates for transplant, and there are not enough livers available to provide transplantation for every patient with portal hypertension and variceal bleeding. Appropriate listing criteria have been developed by the United Network for Organ Sharing (UNOS), and allocation of organs to the sickest patients has improved the overall outcome and utility of organs available for transplantation. This is a field that continues to evolve and is an area in which surgeons still play a role in the management of patients with variceal bleeding.

Summary for Variceal Bleeding

At the present time, the management of variceal bleeding falls into the following three time points:
1. Prophylaxis with pharmacologic β-blockers
2. Acute bleed treated with pharmacologic and endoscopic therapy
3. Prevention of rebleeding with initial pharmacologic and endoscopic therapy, with decompression reserved for the 10% to 15% of patients who rebleed

Finally, liver transplantation is the treatment of choice for patients with variceal bleeding and advanced liver disease.

ASCITES

Ascites is the most common complication of cirrhosis, with approximately two-thirds of patients with compensated cirrhosis developing ascites within 10 years. Once a patient with cirrhosis develops ascites, particularly as it becomes increasingly difficult to manage, there is an approximately 50% mortality over the next 3 years without liver transplantation.[13]

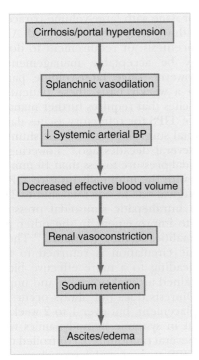

```
┌─────────────────────────────────┐
│  Cirrhosis/portal hypertension  │
└─────────────────────────────────┘
               ↓
      ┌────────────────────┐
      │ Splanchnic vasodilation │
      └────────────────────┘
               ↓
      ┌────────────────────┐
      │  ↓ Systemic arterial BP  │
      └────────────────────┘
               ↓
   ┌──────────────────────────────┐
   │ Decreased effective blood volume │
   └──────────────────────────────┘
               ↓
      ┌────────────────────┐
      │  Renal vasoconstriction  │
      └────────────────────┘
               ↓
      ┌────────────────────┐
      │   Sodium retention   │
      └────────────────────┘
               ↓
      ┌────────────────────┐
      │    Ascites/edema     │
      └────────────────────┘
```

FIGURE 131-12 Pathogenesis of ascites. Sequential changes in local and systemic vascular beds play a major role. *BP*, Blood pressure.

PATHOPHYSIOLOGY

Ascites develops in patients with cirrhosis because of overall hemodynamic changes, vasoconstrictor and sodium-retaining systems being triggered in the kidneys, and the accompanying renal dysfunction. The pathophysiologic sequence in the development of ascites is summarized in Figure 131-12. As indicated earlier in this chapter, one of the early vascular responses to portal hypertension is marked arterial vasodilation of the splanchnic circulation. This in turn leads to a hyperdynamic systemic circulation, decreased systemic vascular resistance, and lowered blood pressure. This in turn activates the vasoconstrictor and antinatriuretic systems that affect the kidneys, with sodium and water retention and renal vasoconstriction. The inability of the kidneys to excrete sodium is thus the first event, with water retention subsequently leading to dilutional hyponatremia. This gives the deceptive laboratory picture of low serum sodium yet high total body sodium.

The secondary component of pathophysiology in the development of ascites is the hepatic sinusoidal change. Cirrhosis results in high intrasinusoidal pressure and further damage to the already discontinuous endothelium of the sinusoid. This high pressure leads to excess fluid filtration through the sinusoid, and much of the ascitic fluid forms from the liver surface.

DIAGNOSIS

Traditionally, ascites is a clinical diagnosis.[42] However, in patients with cirrhosis, ascites is increasingly recognized at evaluation imaging ultrasound and CT scan. Ascites volume as low as 100 mL can be detected on ultrasound. However, it is clinical ascites that is important to the patient, and the first sign of this is often an unexpected and unanticipated weight gain. There may be associated peripheral edema.

A diagnostic paracentesis should be performed on all patients with cirrhosis when they first present with ascites. This is done to characterize the ascites and to exclude the diagnosis of spontaneous bacterial peritonitis (SBP), the most lethal complication of cirrhotic ascites. The fluid (30 to 50 mL) should be sent for the following diagnostic tests:

- Appearance of the fluid
- Ascites albumin concentration (a concurrent serum albumin should be measured)
- Total protein content
- White blood cell count and differential
- Culture

Ascites total protein level of less than 2.5 g/dL with a serum/ascites albumin gradient greater than 1.1 is highly indicative of ascites being of cirrhotic origin. In malignant ascites, the total protein content is usually higher than 2.5 g/dL and the serum/ascites albumin gradient is less than 1.1. The white blood cell count is important in differentiating SBP, with a count of $500/mm^3$ being diagnostic and the 250 to $500/mm^3$ range being highly suspicious. Samples for culture should be placed in blood culture bottles with both aerobic and anaerobic media. The minimum amount of ascitic fluid in these bottles should be 10 mL.

MANAGEMENT

The management of ascites[42,43] falls into the following phases:

1. Treat the underlying liver disease
2. Take simple steps to manage ascites
3. Take major steps to manage intractable ascites

A summary of these is given in Figure 131-13.

Patients with mild to moderate ascites require dietary sodium restriction and appropriate diuretic management. Ascites is a disease of sodium retention; therefore, limiting sodium intake is important. This requires patient education on how to achieve a 2 g/day sodium diet and where they can obtain appropriate products. Water restriction is not usually required unless patients become significantly hyponatremic (serum sodium <120 mmol/L). Initial diuretic management is with an aldosterone antagonist because hyperaldosteronism is a major factor in their sodium retention. Starting with spironolactone 100 mg/day, this may be titrated up to a maximum of 400 mg/day. It takes approximately 48 to 72 hours for the effect of spironolactone to occur, unlike the rapid response within hours with loop diuretics. An indication as to whether sodium reabsorption is being blocked in the tubules can be obtained from a spot sodium-to-potassium ratio in the urine. If there is more sodium than potassium being excreted, the spironolactone is probably at an adequate dosage. Some patients develop significant gynecomastia with spironolactone, and in such patients amiloride is an alternative, starting at 5 mg/day and titrating up to 25 mg/day.

A loop diuretic such as furosemide may be added to the spironolactone. Furosemide has a quick onset of action (within the first hour of administration) and is

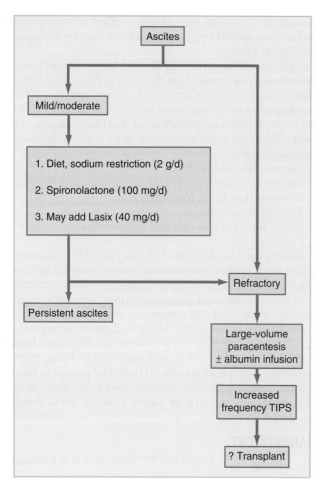

FIGURE 131-13 Treatment of ascites. Most patients are managed with diet and diuretics. Refractory ascites portends a poor prognosis and the need for more aggressive therapy. *TIPS,* Transjugular intrahepatic portosystemic shunt.

given only if the spironolactone is ineffective. Started at 40 mg/day, it may be increased up to 160 mg/day. Although spironolactone retains potassium, furosemide will promote potassium loss. Hence, the use of these in combination is often optimal for patients. Much has been written about the optimal combination of diet and diuretics in managing ascites—this is an art form rather than an exact science.

Refractory ascites is defined as ascites that cannot be mobilized with adequate medical therapy.[44] This term really only applies to approximately 10% of patients who are unresponsive to the regimen discussed earlier. This group of patients are candidates for large-volume paracentesis, TIPS, or transplantation.

Large-volume paracentesis entails removal of 4 to 6 L of ascites at a single sitting. This may or may not be associated with albumin reinfusion. The argument for concomitant albumin infusion is that it will minimize the circulatory dysfunction associated with loss of a large volume at the time of paracentesis, but it is expensive. Although most patients have some circulatory dysfunction if they do not receive albumin, this is not considered sufficiently severe in most patients to warrant its use. This remains an ongoing controversy in this field.

The major issue with large-volume paracentesis is the frequency with which it needs to be used. A single large-volume paracentesis, or requirement to do this once a month, may be acceptable management for many patients. However, once large-volume paracentesis is required on a weekly basis, these patients have truly refractory ascites that requires further management.

The use of TIPS for refractory ascites dates from the success of total surgical portosystemic shunts in managing ascites several decades ago.[45] Lowering of intrahepatic sinusoidal pressure to less than 10 mm Hg can now be achieved with the minimally invasive TIPS compared with open surgical side-to-side total shunts. TIPS not only reduces the intrahepatic sinusoidal pressure but also contributes to improvement in the other pathophysiologic abnormalities leading to ascites.[46] The splanchnic hyperdynamic circulation is returned to the systemic circulation leading to a more effective blood volume, better-maintained arterial pressure, and improved renal perfusion. Diuresis does not always occur immediately after TIPS placement, but over 1 to 2 weeks the overall improvement in systemic hemodynamics will initiate a natriuresis. Several randomized, controlled trials[44,45] have compared TIPS to repeated large-volume paracentesis and have shown an advantage with TIPS with control of ascites, although there was not a survival advantage in all trials. It is clear that TIPS is not the panacea for all ascites, a major concern being that it will accelerate liver failure and encephalopathy with the portal diversion that occurs with TIPS. Data are conflicting on this, and at the present time TIPS remains widely used for ascites. Long-term followup remains important, and recurrence of ascites is usually the first sign of a TIPS stenosis that requires dilation in such patients. Some caution in selecting patients is indicated, and as general guidelines TIPS has been reserved for patients younger than 65 years of age with normal cardiac and renal function, bilirubin less than 6.0, and an INR less than 2.0 and the absence of any evidence of systemic infection or SBP.

Liver transplantation is the only definitive treatment for patients with cirrhosis who develop moderate or refractory ascites. As indicated at the beginning of this section, ascites is an ominous sign for a patient with cirrhosis. Unless easily managed, ascites is a trigger for transplant evaluation. Liver transplant not only replaces the diseased liver but also totally relieves the portal hypertension and reverses the majority of the hemodynamic consequences. The goal is to perform liver transplant on these patients before they have severely impaired renal function, which will limit the options for managing immunosuppression in such patients posttransplantation. Liver transplant is the one therapy that has been clearly shown to have survival benefit in patients with cirrhosis and ascites.

PULMONARY SYNDROMES IN LIVER DISEASE

Lung dysfunction has been recognized in some patients with liver disease for more than a century, but it is only in the past two decades that two distinct pulmonary

TABLE 131-2 Pulmonary Syndromes in Liver Disease

Variables	Hepatopulmonary Syndrome	Portopulmonary Hypertension
Prevalence	8%-20% of cirrhosis	3%-12% of cirrhosis
Pulmonary vascular changes	Vasodilation	Vasoconstriction
Contributing factors	Liver dysfunction, portal hypertension	Portal hypertension
Place of transplant	Curative	Contraindicated

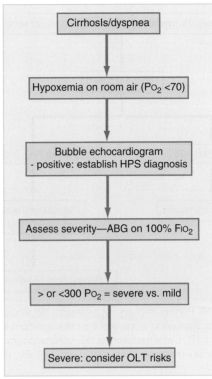

FIGURE 131-14 Diagnosis and management of hepatopulmonary syndrome (HPS). The sequential steps in diagnosis, with their management implications are illustrated. *ABG,* Arterial blood gas; *FIO₂,* fraction of inspired oxygen; *OLT,* orthotopic liver transplant; *PO₂,* partial pressure of oxygen.

vascular disorders have been better understood.[15] HPS occurs when there is a pulmonary vascular vasodilation and hypoxemia, whereas portopulmonary hypertension (PPH) occurs when there is pulmonary vasoconstriction and increased pulmonary artery pressure. The major features of these two syndromes are summarized in Table 131-2.

PATHOPHYSIOLOGY

Both HPS and PPH occur in the setting of cirrhosis and portal hypertension.[47] The comparative contributions of liver dysfunction and portal hypertension vary with these syndromes. HPS can occur without severe portal hypertension and has also been recognized in some patients with prehepatic and postsinusoidal blocks. PPH can occur when the degree of liver dysfunction is relatively minor in the presence of established portal hypertension.

The mechanisms for development of both disorders remain unclear. Chronic liver disease and its associated systemic hemodynamic changes probably induce changes in the pulmonary vasculature mediated by shear stress, cytokine release, and local endothelin 1 release. Local overproduction of nitric oxide in the pulmonary vasculature appears to contribute to the vasodilation of HPS. Although no clear evidence exists as to the role of cytokines and inflammatory responses in the pulmonary vasculature in PPH, these have been postulated as contributory.

CLINICAL PRESENTATION

Shortness of breath is the most common presentation for either HPS or PPH.[48] Increased dyspnea on standing, cyanosis, and finger clubbing are often present with HPS and should lead to evaluation for this syndrome in patients with cirrhosis. Although patients with PPH may present with dyspnea, they are more likely to be asymptomatic, are not usually cyanotic, and do not develop finger clubbing but may have chest pain and syncopal episodes.

It is important to differentiate these pulmonary syndromes from other causes of dyspnea in patients with cirrhosis. Intrinsic cardiopulmonary diseases such as chronic obstructive pulmonary disease or congestive heart failure are more common than either of these syndromes. Appropriate evaluation of cardiac and other pulmonary causes needs to be made.

HEPATOPULMONARY SYNDROME

Figure 131-14 outlines the diagnostic and management steps for this syndrome. Patients with cirrhosis and shortness of breath in whom pulmonary and cardiac disease causes of dyspnea have been excluded should be considered as potentially having HPS. If a patient is hypoxemic on room air (PO₂ <70 mm Hg), the next study should be a bubble-contrast echocardiogram. If this is positive as judged by delayed visualization (occurring after the third heartbeat) of intravenously administered microbubbles in the left cardiac chamber, the patient has HPS. Evaluation of the severity of the syndrome can be assessed by measuring arterial oxygenation on 100% oxygen inspiration. If the patients have a PO₂ higher than 300 mm Hg, they have mild disease, whereas below this level they have severe disease.[48] Patients with HPS require oxygen therapy. Many other pharmacologic therapies have been tried with little effect. The only effective treatment for HPS is liver transplant, which results in resolution of the syndrome over several months. Patients with PO₂ less than 50 mm Hg going into liver transplant have poorer survival rates than those with PO₂ higher than 50 mm Hg. Currently this syndrome gives patients priority scores on the MELD system for liver transplantation to ensure timely transplant within 3 to 6 months in the United States.[49]

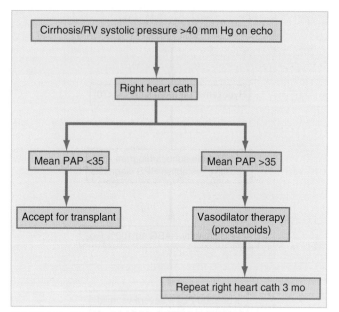

FIGURE 131-15 Portopulmonary hypertension: diagnosis and management. Evaluation steps and their management implications are defined. *cath*, Catheterization; *echo*, echocardiogram; *PAP*, pulmonary artery pressure (measured in mm Hg); *RV*, right ventricular.

PORTOPULMONARY HYPERTENSION

The diagnosis of PPH (Figure 131-15) requires documentation of elevated pulmonary arterial pressures. Echocardiography is used for screening for elevated right heart pressure, but when the estimate is equal to or greater than 40 mm Hg, direct pulmonary artery pressure measurements should be made with right heart catheterization. At right heart catheterization, a mean pulmonary artery pressure greater than 25 mm Hg with a capillary wedge pressure less than 15 mm Hg confirms a diagnosis of pulmonary arterial hypertension. Mild degrees of pulmonary artery hypertension up to 35 mm Hg do not preclude liver transplantation in otherwise acceptable candidates, but pressures greater than 35 mm Hg require aggressive evaluation and treatment. At the present time, pulmonary artery pressures greater than 50 mm Hg are considered an absolute contraindication to liver transplantation because of the high perioperative mortality. For patients with pulmonary artery pressure greater than 35 mm Hg, prostanoid therapy should be considered, with reassessment of patients after 3 months.[50] Response to this treatment may make such patients candidates for liver transplantation.

THE MULTIDISCIPLINARY TEAM

The content of this chapter has involved many specialists to take care of the complications of portal hypertension, including the following:

Hepatologists are in the front line for diagnosing and directing the management for many of the clinical presentations.

Endoscopists play an important role diagnostically and in primary therapy for managing variceal bleeding. Endoscopic banding requires significant expertise.

Radiologists, both imaging and interventional, play roles in diagnosis, directed biopsy, and procedural (TIPS) management of these patients.

Surgeons play a major role in liver transplant but should also have a place in shunting good-risk patients with refractory variceal bleeding.

Pathologists with an interest in liver pathology are important in the accurate diagnosis and staging of disease severity.

Critical care physicians and anesthesiologists are vital team members when patients with portal hypertension have "acute events" and in their perioperative management. The different pathophysiologies of portal hypertension can be challenging in the ICU and operating room.

Nephrologists, cardiologists, and pulmonologists all play a role in the management of some of these patients, and in major centers it is important to have members of all these specialties "on the team" who understand the pathophysiologic changes of portal hypertension.

Finally, who coordinates? In a complex multidisciplinary team such as described, it is frequently the nurse clinicians or "coordinators" who help bring these specialists together. Undoubtedly, it is the coordinators that patients turn to for help in navigating their way through management in this complex field.

REFERENCES

1. Reuben A, Groszmann RJ: Portal hypertension: A history. In Sanyal AJ, Shah VH, editors: *Portal hypertension: Pathobiology, evaluation, and treatment.* Totowa, NJ, 2005, Humana Press, p 3.
2. Whipple AO: The problem of portal hypertension in relation to the hepatosplenopathies. *Ann Surg* 122:449, 1945.
3. Warren WD, Zeppa R, Fomon JJ: Selective trans-splenic decompression of gastroesophageal varices by distal splenorenal shunt. *Ann Surg* 166:437, 1967.
4. Inokuchi K: A selective portacaval shunt. *Lancet* 2:51, 1968.
5. Sarfeh IJ, Rypins EB, Mason GR: A systematic appraisal of portocaval H-graft diameters: Clinical and hemodynamic perspectives. *Ann Surg* 204:356, 1986.
6. Steigmann GV, Goff JS, Sunn JH, et al: Endoscopic variceal ligation: An alternative to sclerotherapy. *Gastrointest Endosc* 35:431, 1989.
7. Garcia-Pagan JC, Groszmann RJ, Bosch J: Portal hypertension. In Weinstein WM, Hawkey CJ, Bosch J, editors: *Clinical gastroenterology and hepatology, Part 2, Section 4: Diseases of the gut and liver.* Philadelphia, 2005, Elsevier, p 707.
8. Lebrec D, Nouel O, Corbic M, et al: Propranolol: A medical treatment for portal hypertension? *Lancet* 2:180, 1980.
9. Henderson JM: Anatomy of the portal venous system in portal hypertension. In Bircher J, Benhannan JP, McIntyre N, et al, editors: *Oxford textbook of clinical hepatology,* ed 2. London, 1999, Oxford University Press, p 645.
10. Couinaud C: *Le foie: Anatomique et chirugicasles.* Paris, 1957, Masson.
11. Zoli M, Merkel C, Magalotti D, et al: Natural history of cirrhotic patients with small esophageal varices: A prospective study. *Am J Gastroenterol* 95:503, 2000.
12. DeFranchis R: Evaluation and follow-up of patients with cirrhosis and esophageal varices. *J Hepatol* 38:361, 2003.
13. Fernandez-Esparrach G, Sanchez-Fueyo A, Gines P, et al: A prognostic model for predicting survival in cirrhosis with ascites. *J Hepatol* 34:46, 2001.
14. Bruix J, Sherman M, Llovet JM, et al: Clinical management of hepatocellular carcinoma: Conclusions of the Barcelona EASL Conference. *J Hepatol* 35:421, 2001.
15. Krowka MJ: Hepatopulmonary syndromes. *Gut* 40:1, 2000.
16. Valla DC, Condat B: Portal vein thrombosis in adults: Pathophysiology, pathogenesis and management. *J Hepatol* 32:865, 2000.

17. Sarin SK, Kapoor D: Non-cirrhotic portal fibrosis: Current concepts and management. *J Gastroenterol Hepatol* 17:526, 2002.
18. Zeitoun G, Escolano S, Hadengue A, et al: Outcome of Budd-Chiari syndrome: A multivariate analysis of factors related to survival including surgical portosystemic shunting. *Hepatology* 30:84, 1999.
19. The North Italian Endoscopic Club for the Study and Treatment of Esophageal Varices: Prediction of the first variceal hemorrhage in patients with cirrhosis of the liver and esophageal varices. *N Engl J Med* 319:983, 1988.
20. Stewart C, Sanyal A: Grading portal gastropathy: A validation of a gastropathy scoring system. *Am J Gastroenterol* 98:1758, 2003.
21. Bolondi L, Gatta A, Groszmann RJ, et al: Imaging techniques and hemodynamic measurements in portal hypertension. Baveno II consensus statement. In De Francis R, editor: *Baveno II Consensus Workshop*, Oxford, 1996, Blackwell Science, p 67.
22. Groszmann RJ, Wangcharatrawee S: The hepatic venous pressure gradient: Anything worth doing should be done right. *Hepatology* 39:280, 2004.
23. Pugh RN, Murray-Lyon IM, Dawson JL, et al: Transection of the oesophagus for bleeding oesophageal varices. *Br J Surg* 60:646, 1973.
24. Kamath PS, Wiesner RH, Malinchoc M, et al: A model to predict survival in patients with end-stage liver disease. *Hepatology* 33:464, 2001.
25. Chalasani N, Boyer TD: Primary prophylaxis against variceal bleeding: beta-blockers, endoscopic ligation, or both? *Am J Gastroenterol* 100:805, 2005.
26. D'Amico G, Criscuoli V, Fili D, et al: Meta-analysis of trials for variceal bleeding. *Hepatology* 36:1023, 2002.
27. Garcia-Pagan JC, Caca K, Bureau C, et al: Early TIPS (Transjugular Intrahepatic Portosystemic Shunt) Cooperative Study Group. Early use of TIPS in patients with cirrhosis and variceal bleeding. *N Engl J Med* 362:2370, 2010.
28. Laine L, Cook D: Endoscopic ligation compared with sclerotherapy for treatment of esophageal variceal bleeding. *Ann Intern Med* 123:280, 1995.
29. Boyer TD, Haskal ZJ: The role of transjugular intrahepatic portosystemic shunt in the management of portal hypertension: update 2009. *Hepatology* 51:306, 2010.
30. Bureau C, Garcia-Pagan JC, Otal P, et al: Improved clinical outcome using polytetrafluoroethylene-coated stents for TIPS: Results of a randomized study. *Gastroenterology* 126:469, 2004.
31. Burroughs AK, Vangoli M: Transjugular intrahepatic portosystemic shunt versus endoscopic therapy: Randomized trials for secondary prophylaxis of variceal bleeding—an updated meta-analysis. *Scand J Gastroenterol* 37:249, 2002.
32. Henderson JM, Boyer TD, Kutner MH, et al: DSRS versus TIPS for refractory variceal bleeding: A randomized trial. *Gastroenterology* 130:1643, 2006.
33. Orloff MJ, Orloff MS, Orloff SL, et al: Three decades of experience with emergency portacaval shunt for acutely bleeding esophageal varices in 400 unselected patients with cirrhosis of the liver. *J Am Coll Surg* 180:257, 1995.
34. Rosemurgy AS, Bloomston M, Clark WC, et al: H-graft portacaval shunts versus TIPS: Ten-year follow-up of a randomized trial with comparison to predicted survivals. *Ann Surg* 241:238, 2005.
35. Spina GP, Henderson JM, Rikkers LF, et al: Distal spleno-renal shunts versus endoscopic sclerotherapy in the prevention of variceal rebleeding: A meta-analysis of four randomized clinical trials. *J Hepatol* 16:338, 1992.
36. Jenkins RL, Gedaly R, Pomposelli JJ, et al: Distal spleno-renal shunt: Role, indications, and utility in the era of liver transplantation. *Arch Surg* 134:416, 1999.
37. Orozco H, Mercado MA, Garcia JG, et al: Selective shunts for portal hypertension: Current role of a 21-year experience. *Liver Transplant Surg* 3:475, 1997.
38. Rikkers LF, Jin G, Langnas AN, et al: Shunt surgery during the era of liver transplantation. *Ann Surg* 226:51, 1997.
39. Idezuki Y, Kokudo N, Sanjo K, et al: Sugiura procedure for management of variceal bleeding in Japan. *World J Surg* 18:216, 1994.
40. Orozco H, Mercado MA, Takahashi T, et al: Elective treatment of bleeding varices with the Sugiura operation over 10 years. *Am J Surg* 13:585, 1992.
41. Abu-Elmagd K, Iwatsuki S: Portal hypertension: role of liver transplantation. In Cameron J, editor: *Current surgical therapy*, ed 7. St. Louis, 2001, Mosby, p 406.
42. Hou W, Sanyal AJ: Ascites: Diagnosis and management. *Med Clin North Am* 93:801, 2009.
43. Moore KP, Wong F, Gines P, et al: The management of ascites in cirrhosis: Report on the consensus conference of the International Ascites Club. *Hepatology* 38:258, 2003.
44. Arroyo V, Gines P, Gerbes AL, et al: Definition and diagnostic criteria of refractory ascites and hepatorenal syndrome in cirrhosis. *Hepatology* 23:164, 1996.
45. Sanyal AJ, Genning C, Reddy KR, et al: The North American Study for the Treatment of Refractory Ascites. *Gastroenterology* 124:634, 2003.
46. Rossle M, Oclis A, Gulberg V, et al: A comparison of paracentesis and transjugular intrahepatic portosystemic shunting in patients with ascites. *N Engl J Med* 342:1701, 2000.
47. Swanson KL, Krawka MJ: Pulmonary complications associated with portal hypertension. In Sanyal AJ, Shah VH, editors: *Portal hypertension*. Totowa, NJ, 2005, Humana Press, p 455.
48. Singh C, Sager JS: Pulmonary complications of cirrhosis. *Med Clin North Am* 93:871, 2009.
49. Taille C, Cadranel J, Bellocq A, et al: Liver transplantation for hepatopulmonary syndrome: A ten-year experience in Paris, France. *Transplantation* 75:1482, 2003.
50. Krowka MJ, Frantz RP, McGoon MD, et al: Improvement in pulmonary hemodynamics during intravenous epoprostenol (prostacyclin): Study of 15 patients with moderate to severe portopulmonary hypertension. *Hepatology* 30:641, 1999.

Anatomy and Physiology of the Spleen

Ernesto P. Molmenti | Donald O. Christensen | Jeffrey M. Nicastro |

Gene F. Coppa | Hugo V. Villar

The spleen has been associated throughout history with melancholy, laughter, discomfort, and impaired athletic abilities.[1] In 350 BC Aristotle associated the "hot character" of the spleen with digestion.[2] Hippocrates described the anatomy of the spleen in 421 BC. Approximately 600 years later, Galen called it an "organ of mystery" and believed that it extracted "melancholy" from blood and liver, purified it, and released it through the splenogastric vessels into the stomach. During the 17th and 18th centuries, Malpighi, Glisson, Harvey, and Morton further described the structure of the spleen. The spleen was associated with the lymphatic system by Hewson in 1777; and in 1846 Virchow demonstrated that the Malpighian follicles were involved in the formation of white cells. Ponchif, in 1885, recognized that the spleen was involved in the removal of red blood cells. Quittenbaum is credited with the first removal of a spleen in 1826, although the rationale for performing it remains unclear.[3] Pean, in 1865, performed a successful splenectomy in a patient with a splenic cyst,[1] and Spencer Wells in 1887 successfully removed the spleen from a young woman with hereditary spherocytosis, achieving lifelong remission of the disease. By 1921, as stated by Lord Moynihan, splenectomy was considered to be of value for hematologic diseases such as "leukaemia, pernicious anaemia, Hodgkin's disease, splenic anaemia (Banti's disease), haemolytic jaundice, Gaucher's diseases, and polycythaemia."[3]

The two main functions of the spleen are phagocytosis and the development of both humoral and cellular immunity.[4] However, the spleen is also associated with multiple nonimmunologic functions. Such functions include being the differentiation site for platelets, reticulocytes, and monocytes; the reservoir for granulocytes and erythrocytes; and the removal site for aged and deformed red blood cells.[4]

The spleen is the largest reticuloendothelial organ.[2] It consists of vascular and lymphoid tissue derived from the primitive mesoderm, and it is surrounded by a thin capsule. Although present in other mammals, smooth muscle cells are not a feature of the human splenic capsule.[1,2] The spleen lies underneath the ninth, tenth, and eleventh ribs on the left, measures 7 to 11 cm in length, and weighs an average of 150 g, although normal weights range from 70 to 300 g. Splenomegaly is usually considered for weights greater than 500 g and/or lengths greater than 15 cm. Its weight decreases with advancing age.[1,2,5] It becomes palpable underneath the left costal margin in instances where its size is at least double the normal.[1,2] The spleen receives at least 5% of the cardiac output[6] and contains 20 to 40 mL of blood.[7] Approximately 20% of the population has one or more accessory spleens, usually located within the splenic hilar region. The incidence of accessory spleens may be as high as 30% in individuals with hematologic pathology.[2] The spleen is covered by a fibrous capsule. Trabeculae arising from the inner aspect of the capsule divide the spleen into communicating compartments.[4] Surrounding the arteries within the splenic parenchyma is a central area known as the *white pulp*. The larger surrounding area is known as the *red pulp*. In between red and white pulp is the marginal zone, which contains lymphatics and macrophages.[1] Externally, the spleen is enveloped almost entirely by peritoneum, which is adherent to the splenic capsule and forms several ligaments to surrounding structures.[5] These ligaments develop collateral vessels in cases of portal hypertension.[2] Transection of these ligaments is necessary when mobilizing the spleen. The tail of the pancreas lies within 1 cm of the splenic hilum in more than 70% of cases and is in direct contact with the spleen in 30% of cases.[1,2]

EMBRYOLOGY

The splenic primordium appears during the fifth week of development as a mesodermal proliferation between the two leaves of the dorsal mesogastrium. As the stomach rotates around an anteroposterior axis, with its caudal portion moving upward and to the right and its cephalic portion moving downward and to the left, a portion of the dorsal mesogastrium eventually fuses with the peritoneum of the posterior abdominal wall. The spleen remains intraperitoneal and is connected to the kidney by the lienorenal (splenorenal) ligament and to the stomach by the gastrolienal (gastrosplenic) ligament (Figure 132-1).[8] The splenic primordium is eventually infiltrated by lymphoid cells. Hematopoiesis is prominent in the spleen from the third to the fifth months of embryonic life. By the fourth month, the red pulp structure begins to appear.[9]

BLOOD SUPPLY, LYMPHATIC DRAINAGE, AND INNERVATION

The spleen receives its arterial supply from the splenic artery, the largest of the three branches of the celiac trunk. The accessory supply is from the left gastroepiploic artery.[1,5] The splenic artery lies posterior to the superior border of the body of the pancreas, forming multiple coils, and eventually divides into two or three main branches that penetrate through the hilum of the spleen (Figure 132-2). These branches in turn divide into segmental arteries that enter along the splenic trabeculae

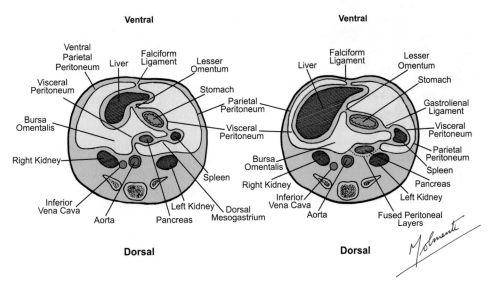

FIGURE 132-1 Transverse schematic sections through the region of the stomach, liver, and spleen during embryologic development. It is possible to visualize the lesser peritoneal sac, the rotation of the stomach, and the positioning of the spleen and tail of the pancreas between the two leaves of the dorsal mesogastrium. The pancreas eventually assumes a secondary retroperitoneal position.

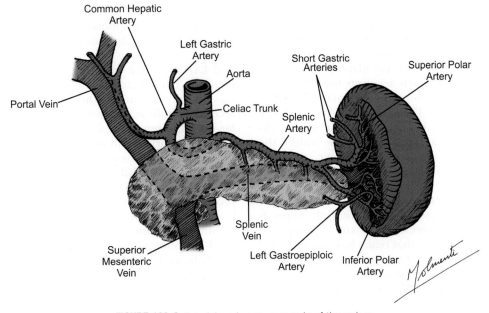

FIGURE 132-2 Arterial and venous supply of the spleen.

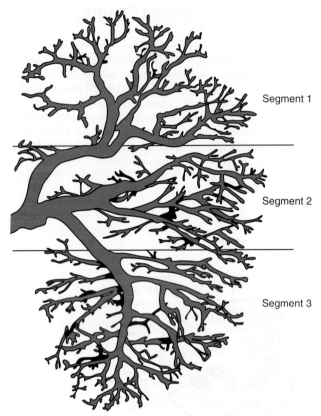

Segment 1

Segment 2

Segment 3

FIGURE 132-3 Segmental splenic arterial supply showing a division into three distinct segments. (From Morgenstern L: Splenic repair and partial splenectomy. In Nyhus LM, Baker RJ, editors: *Mastery of surgery*, ed 2, vol 2. Boston, 1992, Little, Brown, p 1103.)

(Figure 132-3). There is little collateral circulation at this level, and occlusion of one of these arteries usually is associated with infarction of the corresponding region of the spleen. Segmental arteries give rise to trabecular arteries, which in turn, and by means of perpendicular branches, give origin to central arteries.[1,5] Veins leave the spleen through fibrous bands, or trabeculae, attached to the capsule, and coalesce to form the splenic vein. This vein joins the superior mesenteric vein behind the neck of the pancreas to give origin to the portal vein (see Figure 132-2). Two types of circulation have been described. The *fast flow*, which accounts for about 10% of blood flow and has a predominance of plasma, returns blood rapidly to the veins. The *slow flow*, with a predominance of erythrocytes, makes up 90% of the splenic circulation and leads to a filtration process within the fenestrated red pulp network.[1] Lymphatic drainage follows the vasculature. Drainage is into the splenic hilar and celiac nodes.[1,5]

The splenic nervous plexus is formed by branches of the celiac plexus, left celiac ganglion, and right vagus. It runs together with the splenic artery and is composed mainly of sympathetic fibers that reach blood vessels and nonstriated muscle of the capsule and trabeculae. Sympathetic activity seems to be associated with an increase in the "fast" circulation of the spleen. Referred pain from the spleen is frequently localized in the central epigastrium.[5]

FUNCTIONS OF THE SPLEEN

The spleen has an acidotic, hypoxic, and hypoglycemic environment and performs several erythrocyte-associated functions. Culling, or the destruction of erythrocytes, is one of them. Another is pitting, or the removal, of erythrocytic inclusions. Platelets and leukocytes are not usually removed in the spleen. The spleen has a major role in the recognition of antigens, in the production of antibodies, and in the removal from the bloodstream of particles coated with antibodies. Under nonpathologic conditions, hematopoiesis is not encountered in the adult spleen.[7]

NORMAL BASIC HISTOLOGY AND IMMUNOPHENOTYPE OF THE SPLEEN

The human spleen is composed of red and white pulp (Figure 132-4). The red pulp makes up approximately 75% of the spleen and is predominantly composed of splenic cords, capillaries, and venous sinuses, which express endothelial markers (e.g., clotting factor VIII), within loose reticular tissue. This richly vascular, specialized portion of the spleen enables it to function as a filter of blood. The white pulp, including the lymphoid follicles (mostly B lymphocytes) and the periarterial lymphoid sheath (PALS) (mostly T lymphocytes), along with the lymphoid, nonfiltering red pulp (both B and T lymphocytes), are responsible for the spleen's immunologic function. Although comprising only a minority of the overall mass, this lymphoid compartment plays an important role in the early immunologic response against blood-borne antigens and is the compartment primarily responsible for splenic involvement with lymphoproliferative disorders.[10-14]

The primary follicle and secondary follicle mantle zone comprise "naive" (nonimmunologically challenged) B lymphocytes that have small, round nuclei with condensed chromatin, inconspicuous nucleoli, and scant cytoplasm. These lymphocytes characteristically have the following immunophenotype (Table 132-1): surface immunoglobulin (sIg) positive, both sIgD and sIgM; CD5 positive; positive for pan–B-cell antigens (CD19, CD20, and CD79a); CD23 positive; BCL2 positive; and BCL6 negative. These mantle zone cells undergo blast transformation and migrate to the germinal center, forming a secondary follicle. Centroblasts are large cells with vesicular nuclei, often multiple, prominent, peripheral nucleoli, with a narrow rim of basophilic cytoplasm. Changes in the immunophenotype of these cells include the switching on of BCL6 expression and the switching off of BCL2 expression. Centroblasts express CD10 and pan B-cell antigens and express low levels of sIg. Centroblasts mature into centrocytes (cleaved follicular center cells) within the germinal center. Centrocytes are medium-sized lymphocytes with irregular nuclei, inconspicuous nucleoli, and scant cytoplasm. As part of the germinal center reaction, the immune globulin variable region (*IGVR*) gene and the *BCL6* gene undergo somatic mutations. The resulting centrocytes reexpress sIg, which has altered antigen affinity. Decreased affinity results in

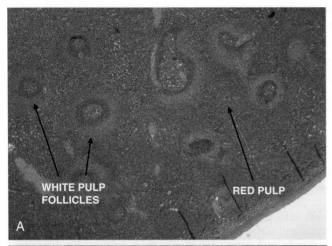

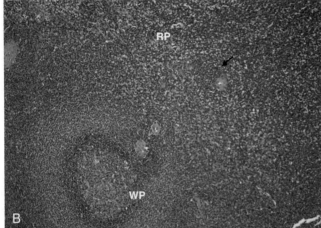

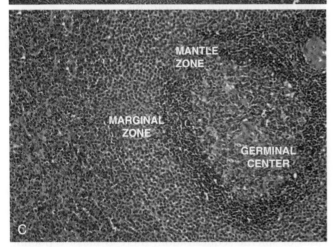

FIGURE 132-4 Normal human spleen on hematoxylin-eosin staining. **A,** Low-power photomicrograph showing relationship and relative proportions of red and white pulp. **B,** Medium-power photomicrograph (*arrow* indicates periarterial lymphoid sheath). *RP,* Red pulp; *WP,* white pulp (secondary follicle). **C,** High-power photomicrograph showing detailed secondary follicle architecture.

apoptosis, whereas increased affinity results in "rescue" of the cell by antigen-mediated binding to the follicular dendritic cell processes. The rescued centrocytes reexpress *BCL2.* Centrocytes switch off *BCL6* expression and mature into memory B cells, which then migrate to the

marginal zone. Memory B cells (marginal zone B cells) have round to slightly irregular nuclei and a moderate amount of cytoplasm. These cells characteristically express sIgM (but not sIgD), lack CD5 and CD10, and express the pan–B-cell antigens. The lymphoid follicles contain a small number of scattered CD3-positive T lymphocytes, which are predominantly CD4-positive T-helper cells.[10-12,14]

Peripheral to the marginal zone and abutting the red pulp is the perifollicular zone, made up of reticular tissue, capillaries, red blood cells, and leukocytes. Within this perifollicular zone, as well as within the red pulp surrounded by its own perifollicular zone, are PALSs. PALSs are composed of antigen-presenting cells and small polymorphic CD3-positive T lymphocytes (of both subsets—CD4 and CD8—with T-helper cells predominating). The lymphoid, nonfiltering red pulp contains a mixture of mature B and T lymphocytes, with a T-cell predominance. As in the PALS and peripheral blood, the CD4-positive T-helper cells outnumber the CD8-positive T cells.[10-12,14]

Understanding the normal lymphoid morphology and immunophenotypic distribution (see Table 132-1) within the spleen is important when discriminating between normal and pathologic states (Figure 132-5). For example, the spleen is a frequent site of involvement with mature B-cell neoplasms—clonal proliferations of B cells, which, to some extent, reflect the stages of physiologic B-cell maturation. Classification of these neoplasms is based, in part, on this relationship between normal physiology and its neoplastic counterparts. Characterizing the departure from the physiologic state (by means of histologic, immunohistochemical, flow cytometric, cytogenetic, polymerase chain reaction, and/or fluorescence in situ hybridization analysis) can confirm the process as pathologic, demonstrate genotypic and phenotypic alterations, and identify the cell from which the tumor originated. This information has significant implications regarding the expected course of the disease, available treatments, and overall prognosis. Similarly, as the spleen receives a significant percentage of the total cardiac output, it is not an uncommon site for hematogenously spread metastatic carcinoma. Such neoplasms differ not only in cytologic morphology from both normal and lymphomatous spleen but have reliably distinctive immunohistochemical staining patterns. Specifically, a splenic nodule from a patient with occult primary neoplasm, which stains positive for cytokeratin and negative for leukocyte common antigen (CD45) should be considered nonnative splenic tissue—confirming metastatic disease. A more extensive immunohistochemical workup could then be performed in an effort to determine the site of origin.[10-12,14]

SPLENIC CIRCULATION

There is an ongoing and still unresolved debate regarding whether the spleen has an open or a closed circulation (Figure 132-6). The closed circulation concept entails continuity of the endothelium from arteries to sinuses. The open circulation theory proposes that blood empties into the marginal zone and red pulp cords,

TABLE 132-1 Significant Cluster Designations (CD Markers) and Other Antigens: Description of Function and Clarification of Cell Type Typically Expressing the Antigen

Cluster Designation	Function	Physiologic Staining
CD3	Antigen recognition	Thymocytes, peripheral T cells, NK cells
CD4	T-cell activation	Thymocytes, mature T cells (~65%, T-helper subset), macrophages, Langerhans cells, dendritic cells, granulocytes
CD5	Signal transducer	B cells of mantle zone of spleen and lymph nodes, almost all T cells
CD8	Increases avidity of cell-to-cell interactions	Mature T cells (~35% of peripheral T cells, most cytotoxic T cells), NK cells, cortical thymocytes (70%-80%)
CD10	Inactivates bioactive peptides	Pre-B cells, cortical thymocytes; follicular center cells; granulocytes; lymphohematopoietic precursors; neutrophils
CD19	Regulates B-cell development, activation, differentiation	Pre-B cells, B cells, first B-cell antigen after HLA-DR, follicular dendritic cells
CD20	Early activation of B cells	Most B cells (after CD19 and CD10 expression, before CD21/22 expression and surface immunoglobulin expression), retained on mature B cells until plasma cell development, follicular dendritic cells
CD23	Regulates IgE synthesis; B-cell growth factor	Activated mature B cells expressing IgM or IgD, monocytes/macrophages, T-cell subsets, platelets, eosinophils, Langerhans cells, follicular dendritic cells
CD45	T- and B-cell antigen receptor–mediated activation	All hematopoietic cells; stronger in lymphocytes (10% of surface area)
CD79a	Encodes Ig proteins	Early in B-cell differentiation (often positive when mature B-cell markers are negative), plasma cells
BCL2	Induces apoptosis	Mantle zone B cells, germinal center centrocytes
BCL6	Regulates transcription	Germinal center centroblasts and centrocytes

HLA-DR, Human leukocyte antigen D-related; *IgD*, immunoglobulin D; *IgM*, immunoglobulin M; *NK*, natural killer.

travels through the cavernous spaces, and finally reenters the vasculature through interendothelial slits.[4]

PERIPHERAL BLOOD SMEAR AND SPLENIC FUNCTION

The peripheral blood smear is a very useful way to evaluate splenic function. The presence of Howell-Jolly bodies, or nuclear remnants removed by the spleen, indicates hyposplenism (or asplenia). The exception is in infants, who commonly have them. Pappenheimer bodies, or siderotic particles removed by the spleen, are also seen in cases of hyposplenism, especially in those associated with hemolysis. The presence of acanthocytes and target cells represents lack of membrane polishing by the spleen. The number of pitted cells is inversely proportional to splenic function. Pits represent vesicles containing hemoglobin, ferritin, and mitochondrial remnants. Under normal circumstances, there are less than 2% pitted cells. The number of platelets and granulocytes is typically increased in asplenia.[7]

IMAGING TECHNIQUES

A liver-spleen scan uses intravenous ^{99m}Tc–sulfur colloid that is taken up by macrophages at these two sites. Ultrasonography is a noninvasive, rapid, and cost-effective way that can assess splenic anatomy without imparting any radiation. Duplex ultrasonography allows for the assessment of vascular flow. Computed tomographic (CT) scanning demonstrates anatomy, volume, lesions, and

some aspects of splenic function. Magnetic resonance imaging has no associated radiation, and is useful in some infections such as candidiasis.[7]

PATHOLOGIC FINDINGS

Congenital asplenia may occur in an isolated fashion or in conjunction with severe congenital cardiac disease. Administration of polysaccharide vaccine and early prescription of antibiotics is recommended in these individuals to prevent an overwhelming sepsis.[7] Polysplenia is also associated with congenital defects, both of vascular and nonvascular nature. It has not been shown to be associated with an increased risk of infection.[7] In sickle cell disease, the hypoxic, hypoglycemic, and acidotic environment of the spleen is associated with erythrocyte sickling. This in turn leads to blockage of the splenic microcirculation and subsequent splenic infarcts. In cases of splenic sequestration, there is massive pooling of blood secondary to occlusion of the venous drainage. In such potentially life-threatening cases, splenectomy is recommended.[7]

Hypersplenism is a term used to define the nonimmune destruction of formed blood elements by an enlarged spleen, with or without the presence of portal hypertension. Splenectomy corrects the low cell counts in such cases.[7] Splenic hypertrophy leads to pooling of blood and the premature destruction of cells by splenic macrophages.[7] *Hyposplenism* associated with decreased phagocytic function and increased risk of infections is seen in rheumatoid arthritis, systemic lupus erythematosus, systemic vasculitis, sarcoidosis, celiac disease, ulcerative

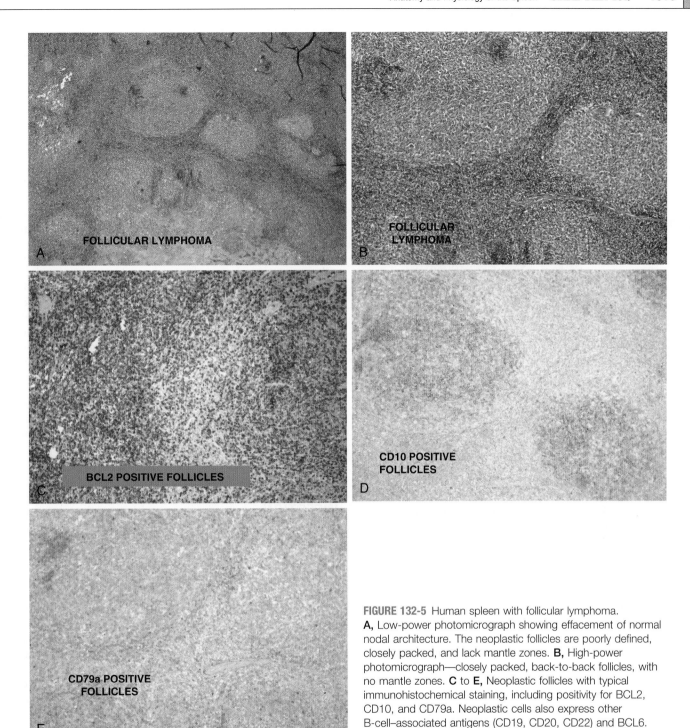

FIGURE 132-5 Human spleen with follicular lymphoma. **A,** Low-power photomicrograph showing effacement of normal nodal architecture. The neoplastic follicles are poorly defined, closely packed, and lack mantle zones. **B,** High-power photomicrograph—closely packed, back-to-back follicles, with no mantle zones. **C** to **E,** Neoplastic follicles with typical immunohistochemical staining, including positivity for BCL2, CD10, and CD79a. Neoplastic cells also express other B-cell–associated antigens (CD19, CD20, CD22) and BCL6. The tumor cells are usually CD5 and CD43 negative.

colitis, amyloidosis, mastocytosis, combined immunodeficiency, and chronic graft-versus-host disease.[7] Radiation therapy affects splenic function. Although phagocytic cells are not usually affected by irradiation, lymphoid cells are. Corticosteroid therapy impairs the function of splenic macrophages. Intravenous IgG is also known to impair splenic function.[7] Splenomegaly of anatomic origin is rare and may be caused by cysts, pseudocysts, hamartomas, hemangiomas, and peliosis. In most cases, however, splenomegaly represents the manifestation of an underlying pathology that should be diagnosed.[7]

SPLENECTOMY

The indications for splenectomy are usually clinical. The decision to proceed with this intervention should be based on specific clinical indices and parameters. Pathologic entities that benefit from splenectomy include some instances of trauma, idiopathic thrombocytopenic purpura, hemolytic anemias caused by intrinsic erythrocyte membrane or enzyme disorders (pyruvate kinase deficiency and hereditary spherocytosis), and chronic conditions such as those seen in storage diseases (Gaucher

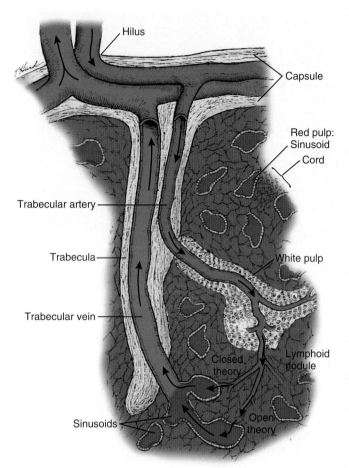

FIGURE 132-6 Structure of the sinusal spleen. (From the Microcirculatory Society Eugene M. Landis Award Lecture—Microcirculature of the spleen: New concepts, new challenges. *Microvasc Res* 34:270, 1987.)

disease).[7] Left-sided (sinistral) portal hypertension constitutes another indication for splenectomy.

Laparoscopic splenectomy is considered the technique of choice in cases of intractable benign hematologic disorders. Although its efficacy, morbidity, and mortality rates are comparable to those of open splenectomy, parameters such as return of intestinal function and length of hospital stay are significantly shorter.[15-17] Its popularity is especially associated with diseases such as idiopathic thrombocytopenic purpura, hereditary spherocytosis, autoimmune hemolytic anemia, and thrombotic thrombocytopenic purpura. One series reported significant resolution of thrombocytopenia in more than 80% of patients with idiopathic thrombocytopenic purpura, improvement in hematocrit levels in 70% of patients with chronic hemolytic anemia, and a positive response in more than 90% of patients with hereditary spherocytosis.[18] Elective laparoscopic splenectomy was found to have a greater incidence of postoperative thrombosis of the portal venous system than the elective open technique. In such instances, diagnosis was established by contrast-enhanced CT scanning and successful treatment achieved with anticoagulation therapy.[17] Laparoscopic splenectomy has also been found to be safe and

effective in cases of splenomegaly.[19] It should be mentioned, however, that body mass index, underlying hematologic pathologies, and splenic size have been found in some series to be predictors of surgical complications in laparoscopic splenectomy.[20,21]

Leukocytosis is usually observed after splenectomy and may last up to a few months. It is characterized by a preponderance of granulocytes. Thrombocytosis is also encountered in most patients, but is rarely associated with thrombotic events.[6] Extramedullary hematopoiesis, found in diseases such as malignant osteoporosis in children and myelofibrosis in adults, constitutes a relative contraindication to splenectomy. In such cases, it should be determined that the patient is not dependent on splenic hematopoiesis.[7]

Complications associated with splenectomy include splenic rupture, hemorrhage, postsplenectomy septicemia, subphrenic abscesses, necrosis of the fundus of the stomach, injury to the tail of the pancreas, and atherosclerotic heart disease. The presence of remnant accessory spleens in instances of splenectomy for hematologic disorders may be associated with relapse of the underlying disease.[6] Splenosis, or the regeneration of miniscule splenic remnants in the peritoneal cavity, may be encountered in cases of traumatic rupture where splenic tissue disseminates throughout the peritoneal cavity. Its protective effect against sepsis in humans is still unclear.[7] Intraoperative diagnosis is by means of frozen section.

OVERWHELMING POSTSPLENECTOMY INFECTION

Overwhelming postsplenectomy infection (OPSI) is a life-threatening potential complication seen in asplenic individuals that gained significant acceptance in 1953 after an observation by King and Shumacker.[22] OPSI is encountered with greatest frequency within 2 years after splenectomy, in the very young, in patients with other medical complications, and in those with malignancies.[22] The risk of postsplenectomy sepsis increases according to the specific indications for splenectomy; trauma, hematologic disorders, portal hypertension, Hodgkin disease, sickle cell disease, and thalassemia are associated with increasing cumulative indices of sepsis, ranging from 1.5% to 25%, respectively.[7] OPSI occurs mostly in association with encapsulated organisms that require opsonization for effective phagocytosis. The most frequent such pathogens are *Neisseria meningitides, Haemophilus influenzae* type b, and *Streptococcus pneumoniae.* There are effective vaccines against all of them, and it is recommended that they be administered 3 weeks before splenectomy to allow for a more effective immune response.[7] Focal infections such as meningitis are more frequent in children younger than 5 years of age.[22] OPSI usually follows a rapid course, evolving into sepsis and disseminated intravascular coagulation; 80% of deaths occur within the first 48 hours. Asplenic patients who develop fever should be immediately evaluated and promptly treated with broad-spectrum intravenous antibiotics.[22]

MASSIVE SPLENOMEGALY

Massively enlarged spleens constitute a special surgical challenge because of their size and risk of bleeding or fracture at the time of splenectomy. A generous midline incision rather than a transverse one is preferable, to allow for the pivoting of the inferior pole of the spleen and the subsequent ligation and division of the enlarged and usually lengthened short gastric vessels. Opening the gastrocolic omentum allows access to the splenic artery that is subsequently ligated in continuity. The artery is approached with greater ease halfway along the superior pancreatic border. Although this maneuver will not routinely diminish the size of the spleen, it will make it softer and easier to handle and will diminish blood loss in cases of splenic fractures or tears associated with mobilization. The upper two or three short gastric vessels are hard to reach because the massive spleen blocks the view and may be safely divided after the spleen is exteriorized and the splenic hilum divided. Division of the attachments to the colon may also facilitate safer mobilization. Division of the phrenosplenic ligament allows safe exteriorization of massively enlarged spleens and ligation under full view of the splenic artery and vein. Often the spleen is wrapping the tail of the pancreas, and "carving" the vessels into the spleen will avoid damage to the tail of the pancreas. Because of the significant weight of the spleen while still attached to the hilum, caution should be exercised to prevent the splenic vessels from tearing by unexpected traction or tilting of the spleen. Seroserosal invagination of the greater curvature of the stomach where the short gastric vessels were tied is a good way to prevent a tie from coming off and causing postoperative hemorrhage, as well as to minimize the chances of gastric necrosis and fistulas from ties placed too close to the stomach. In cases where platelet counts are below 10,000 to 50,000/µL and during splenectomy platelet replacement is desired, platelet transfusions are usually given after ligation of the splenic artery, to prevent the immediate sequestration of the transfused platelets in the spleen.

REFERENCES

1. Fraker DL: Spleen. In Mulholland MW, et al, editors: *Greenfield's surgery: Scientific principles and practice*, ed 4. Philadelphia, 2006, Lippincott Williams & Wilkins, p 1222.
2. Park AE, Godinez CD Jr: Spleen. In Brunicardi FC, et al, editors: *Schwartz's principles of surgery*, ed 9. New York, 2009, McGraw-Hill, p 1501.
3. Lewis SM: The spleen: Mysteries solved and unresolved. *Clin Haematol* 12:363, 1983.
4. Paraskevas F: Lymphocytes and lymphatic organs. In Greer JP, et al, editors: *Wintrobe's clinical hematology*, ed 12. Philadelphia, 2009, Lippincott Williams & Wilkins, p 300.
5. Standring S, editor: *Gray's anatomy: The anatomical basis of clinical practice*, ed 40. Philadelphia, 2008, Elsevier Churchill Livingstone, p 1225.
6. Molmenti EP, et al: Anatomy and physiology of the spleen. In Yeo CJ, et al, editors: *Shackelford's surgery of the alimentary tract*, ed 6. Philadelphia, 2006, Saunders Elsevier, p 1771.
7. Shurin SB: The spleen and its disorders. In Hoffman R, et al, editors: *Hematology: Basic principles and practice*, ed 5. Philadelphia, 2008, Elsevier, p 2419.
8. Sadler TW: *Langman's medical embryology*, ed 11. Philadelphia, 2009, Lippincott Williams & Wilkins, p 209.
9. Carlson BM: *Human embryology and developmental biology*, ed 3. St. Louis, 2004, Mosby.
10. Han J, et al: Spleen. In Mills SE, editor: *Histology for pathologists*, ed 3. Philadelphia, 2007, Lippincott Williams and Wilkins, p 783.
11. Tablin F, et al: The microanatomy of the mammalian spleen. In Bowdler AJ, editor: *The complete spleen*, ed 2. Totowa, NJ, 2002, Humana, p 11.
12. Dailey MO: The immune functions of the spleen. In Bowdler AJ, editor: *The complete spleen*, ed 2. Totowa, NJ, 2002, Humana, p 51.
13. Jaffe ES: Introduction and overview of the classification of the lymphoid neoplasms. In Swerdlow SH, et al, editors: *WHO classification of tumours of haematopoietic and lymphoid tissues*, ed 4. Lyon, 2008, IARC.
14. PathologyOutlines.com: "CD Markers, CD1 to CD49," "CD Markers, CD50 to CD99," and "Stains and molecular markers." Accessed September 7, 2010. Available at http://pathologyoutlines.com/.
15. Rhodes M, et al: Laparoscopic splenectomy and lymph node biopsy for hematologic disorders. *Ann Surg* 222:43, 1995.
16. Flowers JL, et al: Laparoscopic splenectomy in patients with hematologic diseases. *Ann Surg* 224:19, 1996.
17. Ikeda M, et al: High incidence of thrombosis of the portal venous system after laparoscopic splenectomy: A prospective study with contrast-enhanced CT scan. *Ann Surg* 241:208, 2005.
18. Katkhouda N, et al: Laparoscopic splenectomy: Outcome and efficacy in 103 consecutive patients. *Ann Surg* 228:568, 1998.
19. Targarona EM, et al: Splenomegaly should not be considered a contraindication for laparoscopic splenectomy. *Ann Surg* 228:35, 1998.
20. Casaccia M, et al; IRLSS Centers: Putative predictive parameters for the outcome of laparoscopic splenectomy: A multicenter analysis performed on the Italian Registry of Laparoscopic Surgery of the Spleen. *Ann Surg* 251:287, 2010.
21. Patel AG, et al: Massive splenomegaly is associated with significant morbidity after laparoscopic splenectomy. *Ann Surg* 238:235, 2003.
22. Porembka MR, et al: Disorders of the spleen. In Greer JP, et al, editors: *Wintrobe's clinical hematology*, ed 12. Philadelphia, 2009, Lippincott Williams & Wilkins, p 1637.

Minimally Invasive Surgical and Image-Guided Interventional Approaches to the Spleen

Michael R. Marohn | Kimberly E. Steele | Leo P. Lawler

Modern surgical treatment of disorders of the spleen requires familiarity with traditional "open" surgical approaches, minimally invasive surgical approaches, and image-guided interventional approaches that can be tailored to manage specific splenic problems. Minimally invasive surgical and image-guided interventional approaches to the spleen form the focus of this chapter's two sections.

Minimally invasive surgery approaches to the spleen accompanied the rapid expansion of laparoscopic surgery in the early 1990s. Laparoscopic splenectomy rapidly became the procedure of choice for elective splenectomy for spleens of normal size. Because the spleen is a fragile solid organ, with a rich blood supply, situated close to the colon, stomach, pancreas, and kidney, it poses special challenges for minimally invasive surgery. Improvements in laparoscopic techniques and instrumentation have enabled more challenging cases to become amenable to a minimally invasive surgical approach.

Minimally invasive vascular/percutaneous interventional techniques for disorders of the spleen evolved from the 1970s and 1980s and continue to play an important role in managing splenic problems. The contemporary surgeon and image-guided interventionalist share complementary tools for the modern management of splenic disorders.

MINIMALLY INVASIVE SURGERY FOR THE SPLEEN

Laparoscopic splenectomy, first described in 1991 by Delaitre and Maignien, rapidly gained acceptance as the first-line approach for patients requiring elective splenectomy for normal-sized spleens. Conversion to open splenectomy is reported in less than 5% of cases—hemorrhage being the usual cause for conversion. Improvements in laparoscopic techniques and instrumentation enable more challenging cases, including patients with larger spleens, or spleens in complex reoperative settings, to be accessible to a laparoscopic approach. Benefits from a minimally invasive approach are those of minimally invasive surgery established for other procedures and include reduced blood loss, better pain control, decreased perioperative morbidity, and shorter hospital length of stay.[1-3]

INDICATIONS

Trauma

The most common indication for splenectomy is splenic trauma, and the vast majority of these are performed via open laparotomy. However, over the past 30 years, efforts to preserve functional splenic tissue wherever feasible have been increasingly emphasized. Reports of laparoscopic techniques in the management of the injured spleen are uncommon, and this approach appears to have limited if any indications in current practice. Most trauma surgeons view minimally invasive surgery contraindicated in major abdominal trauma.[4] Minor splenic injuries from blunt trauma can be treated nonoperatively. A small series of laparoscopic splenectomy in the setting of blunt trauma, without conversion or major morbidity, has been reported, and it has been suggested that laparoscopic splenectomy may be reasonable in hemodynamically stable patients who have radiographic evidence of severe organ damage and/or large hemoperitoneum.[5] Delayed laparoscopic splenectomy for blunt trauma may be safe especially if combined with adjunctive preoperative embolization, which appears to reduce the risk of continued or delayed hemorrhage. Delayed splenectomy is required in some of these patients because of continued bleeding or infarction with abscess formation, and successful delayed laparoscopic splenectomy in this setting has been reported.[6] Penetrating splenic injury usually mandates open laparotomy, but occasional reports of successful laparoscopic repair of penetrating splenic injury in hemodynamically stable patients have appeared.[7] Laparoscopy has been used to confirm the diagnosis of splenic injury and to determine the extent of splenic injury. Laparoscopic techniques can be used to selectively apply electrocautery, fibrin, Gelfoam, suture repair, or other maneuvers to avoid splenectomy.[8-10]

No prospective randomized trials have compared selective laparoscopic approaches to splenic trauma to nonoperative management. Further experience is needed to define selection criteria for laparoscopy in trauma patients with splenic injury, just as criteria were developed for nonoperative management.[11]

Hematologic Disorders

Indications for elective laparoscopic splenectomy are similar to "open" splenectomy, and the most common is hematologic disorders. For a normal-sized spleen, laparoscopic splenectomy has now achieved standard of care status. Among hematologic disorders, the most common indication is idiopathic thrombocytopenic purpura (ITP).[12,13,14] Kovaleva et al reviewed their 20-year experience with more than 1000 ITP patients. First-line therapy for ITP remains medical therapy, usually steroids. Second-line treatment after failure of medical therapy is splenectomy, which achieves 80% remission, with long-term (60

BOX 133-1   Indications for Laparoscopic Splenectomy

PLATELET DISORDERS
Idiopathic thrombocytopenic purpura (ITP)
Human immunodeficiency virus–related ITP
Thrombotic thrombocytopenic purpura
Evans syndrome

ANEMIAS/RED BLOOD CELL DISORDERS
Autoimmune hemolytic anemia
Hereditary spherocytosis
Hereditary elliptocytosis
Hereditary pyropoikilocytosis
White blood cell disorders/malignancy
Hodgkin lymphoma
Non-Hodgkin lymphoma
Chronic myeloid leukemia
Chronic lymphocytic leukemia
Hairy cell leukemia
Myelofibrosis
Primary splenic tumors

MISCELLANEOUS
Splenic abscess
Splenic cysts
Splenic trauma
Sarcoidosis
Hypersplenism—Gaucher disease, Felty syndrome, SLE,
   splenic vein thrombosis

SLE, Systemic lupus erythematosus.

months or longer) remission in 32%. Resistance occurs in about 6% of patients.[15]

Other indications for laparoscopic splenectomy include disorders of red blood cells, white blood cells, platelets, and malignancy.[12] Box 133-1 summarizes indications for laparoscopic splenectomy. Evolving techniques, technology, instrumentation, and experience continue to expand the scope of splenic surgeries amenable to a minimally invasive approach.

Contraindications

Contraindications include acute coagulopathic states or inability to tolerate general anesthesia. Acute hemorrhage limits safe laparoscopic splenectomy, which is a major factor limiting the application of laparoscopic splenectomy in the trauma setting. Portal hypertension, though not an absolute contraindication to laparoscopic splenectomy, should be approached cautiously. Cai's group reported 24 successful cases of splenectomy for hypersplenism in cirrhotic patients.[16]

PATIENT SELECTION

Spleen size remains the most important determinant in patient selection for open versus laparoscopic splenectomy, as well as predicting success of a minimally invasive surgical approach. At a threshold of 500 g for defining a "large" spleen, there are no differences in conversion rates, lengths of stay, or complications.[17] However, at a threshold of 1000 g, conversion rates for large spleens may approach 60%.[18] Some surgeons use 2 kg as an

exclusion criteria for laparoscopic splenectomy, citing similar outcome variables of higher conversion rates, greater blood loss, longer hospitalization, and increased morbidity with larger spleens.[19] Splenic weight, however, is difficult to assess preoperatively. Further, the role of experience is undoubtedly important, and emerging technologies continually improve minimally invasive capabilities.

Although spleen weight retrospectively can powerfully correlate with minimally invasive splenectomy success or failure, spleen size based on computed tomography (CT) or ultrasound imaging measurements provides a more practical preoperative selection criterion. As a guideline, spleen size on ultrasound or CT scan should be less than 20 to 25 cm in the craniocaudal axis.[18-20] Larger spleens have been removed laparoscopically, but are technically challenging, requiring experience in managing larger spleens and may require special pre- and intraoperative strategies. Spleens measuring greater than 30 cm leave little room for favorable port placement and limit working space. Laparoscopic success in this setting may be improved by preoperative splenic artery embolization, and a hand-assisted technique. Experience remains a key predictor of successful laparoscopic splenectomy. Grahn reported a 10-year retrospective review of laparoscopic splenectomy for 85 patients of whom 25 (29%) had massive or supermassive spleens, with an increasing number of these (40% to 50%) approached laparoscopically during the later years of the study. Despite the increase in giant spleens in the minimally invasive group, conversion rates declined from 33% halfway through the 10-year period to 0% for the final 2 years of the study, with no reoperations for bleeding and no deaths.[13]

Specimen removal for massive spleens can require either an incision comparable to the open technique, which may obviate benefits of the minimally invasive approach, or may require use of a morcellation device.

PREOPERATIVE CONSIDERATIONS

Imaging

Preoperative ultrasound or CT imaging is critical for operative planning. Imaging can not only help assess spleen size but can delineate useful anatomic relationships that impact the conduct of surgery. The normal spleen measures about 11 cm in length. Moderate splenomegaly, from 11 to 20 cm, should be noted in preoperative planning. Massive splenomegaly, greater than 20 cm length, may alter preoperative and intraoperative strategy. Preoperative imaging may also identify accessory spleens, reported in from 10% to 20% of patients.

Although not indicated for a normal-sized spleen, preoperative splenic artery embolization can be a useful adjunct in cases of massive splenomegaly. Timing is important, because patients can develop significant pain from infarcted splenic tissue; angioembolization coordinated within 24 hours of surgery is helpful. Preoperative angioembolization of the splenic artery for laparoscopic splenectomy appears to be safe and facilitates a low conversion rate.[14]

General Considerations: Antibiotic Prophylaxis, Deep Venous Thrombosis Prophylaxis, Bowel Preparation

A broad-spectrum antibiotic should be administered approximately 30 minutes before skin incision. Patients undergoing splenectomy for a hematologic disorder should undergo the same preparation that they would for open splenectomy, which may include administration of steroids, immune globulin, fresh-frozen plasma, cryoprecipitate, or platelets. Blood products should be available intraoperatively, especially platelets for intraoperative transfusion in patients with severe thrombocytopenia. Prophylactic platelet transfusions are typically given only for patients with platelet counts below 50,000, and the platelets are administered only after the splenic artery has been ligated.[12]

All patients require deep venous thrombosis (DVT) prophylaxis, including pneumatic sequential compression devices placed before induction of anesthesia, pre- and postoperative heparin prophylaxis following established national guidelines, and early postoperative ambulation. Controversy remains over how long postoperatively to continue thromboembolism prophylaxis. For high-risk patients, DVT prophylaxis should be considered up to and beyond 14 days after surgery.

Mechanical bowel preparation before splenectomy is not mandatory. A limited prep the night before surgery may clear the left colon of stool bulk, with the objectives of both improving ease of intraoperative splenic flexure colon mobilization and of avoiding postoperative constipation given that nearly all patients will be on postoperative constipating narcotic pain management.

Immunization Against Overwhelming Postsplenectomy Infection

Patients who undergo splenectomy are at increased risk for overwhelming postsplenectomy infection (OPSI), reported by most experts at 3% to 5% lifetime risk. The annual incidence of OPSI is reported at between 0.23% and 0.42%. Risk is highest in three groups: (1) patients at the extremes of age, (2) immunocompromised patients, and (3) patients with hematologic disorders. Previously healthy trauma patients who require splenectomy are the lowest risk groups for OPSI. When OPSI occurs, it is a true emergency, can be lethal, and requires immediate parenteral antibiotics and intensive care support. Intravenous immunoglobulin may play a beneficial role. OPSI carries a mortality rate of 38% to 69%. In general, OPSI results from decreased antigen clearance in postsplenectomy patients, loss of opsonization, and decreased antigen response. *Streptococcus pneumoniae* is the most common infective agent, recovered in 50% to 90% of isolates from OPSI patients, followed by *Haemophilus influenzae* type B, *Streptococcus* group B, *Staphylococcus aureus*, and *Escherichia coli* and coliforms. Increased susceptibility to parasites and malaria is noted in endemic areas. Hypothesized increased risk of *Neisseria meningitidis* has not been documented but remains a theoretical risk.[21,22]

Optimally, immunization against encapsulated organisms is given 14 days prior to surgery. Recommended immunizations include polyvalent pneumococcal, meningococcal, and *Haemophilus* vaccinations.[22] Pneumovax provides protection against 73% of OPSI-causing organisms. Data on revaccination remain unclear, but current consensus favors a Pneumovax booster every 5 to 10 years, which may be protective against all OPSI bacteria. Hib/Meningococcal/Influenza vaccine benefit is unproven but is recommended. For patients who do not receive recommended OPSI immunizations prior to surgery (such as trauma patients), immunization is performed just before hospital discharge and is preferred over relying on patient compliance with outpatient immunizations in case these patients are lost to follow-up.

OPERATIVE APPROACH

There is wide variation in the technique of laparoscopic splenectomy with respect to approach, patient positioning, port site placement, number of ports, and instrumentation for controlling splenic vessels.

Minimally invasive surgery requires a high-technology environment. The surgeon should review with the operative team the required equipment and instruments as part of the "time out" before the procedure starts, systematically going through a checklist to ensure that all needed, or potentially needed, equipment and instruments are available, including video towers with high definition camera, insufflator, high-intensity light source, video-capture device, preferred energy sources (Harmonic Scalpel, LigaSure, etc.), angled telescope (we favor a 45-degree angled telescope to optimize visualization in three dimensions; we also favor availability of a 5-mm, 45-degree angled telescope option for use through 5-mm ports if needed), suction irrigator, access device, additional laparoscopic ports (if needed), special laparoscopic instruments (including, e.g., preferred dissectors, right-angle dissector), laparoscopic retractor, specimen retrieval bags, endoscopic staplers, endoclips, morcellator (if needed), and other devices (such as hand-assist devices) potentially anticipated for the procedure.

Anatomic Considerations

Laparoscopic splenectomy is not a forgiving procedure. Methodical maintenance of hemostasis, both during division and control of splenic vasculature, and as the spleen is mobilized, is key to successful minimal access splenectomy. The splenic parenchyma is fragile, has a rich blood supply, and is particularly vulnerable to capsular tear and procedure-limiting bleeding, because bleeding can lead to loss of visualization and hemodynamic instability. Understanding variable splenic anatomy is essential to safe intraoperative management.

Michels' 1942 review of 100 spleens suggested that no two spleens have the same anatomy.[23] Michels divided splenic blood supply into two types: distributed and magistral, with the distributed type present in 70% of patients. Splenic size does not correlate with the number or distribution of splenic arteries, although the number of splenic notches and tubercles does. Splenic hilar anatomy can include numerous branches with various division levels. In addition, six or more short gastric arteries may be found in the gastrosplenic ligament arising from the fundus of the stomach. The lienorenal ligament contains hilar vessels and the tail of the pancreas. In nearly three-quarters of patients, the tail of the pancreas lies within 1 cm of the spleen, and direct contact between the pancreas and spleen is found in about one-third of patients.[23]

Technique of Laparoscopic Splenectomy

There are nine steps to laparoscopic splenectomy:
1. Positioning and safe access to establish pneumoperitoneum
2. Diagnostic laparoscopy, including a search for accessory spleens
3. Mobilization of the spleen with dissection of splenic ligaments
4. Division of the splenic vessels, including splenic hilum and short gastric vessels
5. Division of remaining attachments completely detaching the spleen and spleen placement within a specimen bag
6. Extraction of the spleen within the specimen bag from the peritoneal cavity
7. Inspection of the operative field for hemostasis, pancreatic injury, etc.
8. Removal of trocars, pneumoperitoneum desufflation, and port site closure

Step 1: Positioning and Safe Access for Pneumoperitoneum

Anterior Approach. The anterior approach was the first laparoscopic splenectomy technique to be described. However, after 15 years of experience with laparoscopic splenectomy worldwide, the more frequent approach is lateral. The anterior approach may be better suited for dealing with a giant spleen, particularly with prior splenic artery embolization. It may be preferable for clearance of accessory spleens when these are suspected. The anterior approach may also be preferable if other procedures such as diagnostic laparoscopy or cholecystectomy are planned, as may be indicated for disorders with a high association with gallstones, such as spherocytosis.

We favor use of a combined Veress "closed" technique approach to obtain pneumoperitoneum, followed by use of a "direct optical visualization" device, taking advantage of the safety afforded by the already established pneumoperitoneum from the Veress needle. We avoid prior scars, hoping to avoid adherent bowel and minimize risk of bowel injury, making the assumption that bowel will be adherent wherever there is a previous scar or incision. With the anterior approach, initial insufflation is at the umbilicus using a Veress needle, with the subsequent direct-visualization optical device placed in the left abdomen, approximately one-third of the distance between the umbilicus and xiphoid process in the midclavicular line. The laparoscopic insufflator is preset for abdominal pressure at 12 mm Hg or less to minimize the untoward effects of intraabdominal hypertension.

Four or five total laparoscopic ports are placed—all under direct visualization. Laparoscopic port size is the surgeon's choice. We place at least one 10- to 12-mm port to have immediate access for use of either an endoscopic stapler or large endoclips device. Configuration of the port placement for the anterior approach is typically in a "V," with the initial port for the camera at the base of the "V," positioned approximately one-third of the distance between the umbilicus and the left costal margin in a line directly toward the splenic hilum. One line of the "V" extends from the initial port to the xiphoid process; the other line of the "V" extends from the initial port to the most lateral left subcostal region. After the initial port placement for the camera, all ports are placed under direct visualization. Two dissection ports are placed, one near the midline approximately half the distance between the umbilicus and the xiphoid process, and one along the lateral "V" line in the left midabdomen at about the midclavicular line. We use a 10- to 12-mm port at this location, because it is the likely port for introduction of an endoscopic stapler or endoclips device. An additional port for retraction is placed further lateral along the lateral "V" line in the anterior axillary line. If a fifth port is necessary for retraction, it is placed in the subxiphoid position. The patient is then placed in reverse Trendelenburg position and tilted slightly to the right. The surgeon stands between the legs if the patient is in low lithotomy, and adjacent to the patient's right hip if the patient is supine, with the surgeon's video monitor placed at the head of the bed to the patient's left. Surgical assistants and the scrub nurse are positioned at the patient's sides.[24,25]

Lateral Approach. The lateral approach is useful for normal and moderately enlarged spleens. The lateral laparoscopic approach to splenectomy has the advantages that it is technically easier, allows access to the splenic vasculature through the relatively avascular retroperitoneum, and decreases inadvertent trauma to the spleen as it allows gravity to achieve retraction more than instruments. Dissection planes open more easily, enhancing identification of key ligaments and dissection planes, and the tail of the pancreas is more accessible and less susceptible to injury. Operative times may be shorter, and the lateral approach increases dissection strategy options.

Positioning for the lateral approach to laparoscopic splenectomy is similar to that used for posterolateral thoracotomy and/or laparoscopic left adrenalectomy. Patients are initially positioned supine on a beanbag. Once anesthesia-monitoring devices are placed and general endotracheal anesthesia is established and the airway is secured, the operative team repositions the patient in lateral decubitus position with the right side down. Care is taken to ensure adequate padding, including placing an axillary roll. The beanbag is desufflated, and additional tape with padding is placed to secure the patient. Security and safety of patient positioning is tested by moving the electric operating table to different planned positions before scrubbing to ensure adequacy of positioning and taping. The kidney rest is raised, and the operating table is flexed. The positioning goal is to maximize the working space between the left costal margin and the left anterior superior iliac spine.

As with the anterior approach, we use a combination of Veress closed and direct-visualization optical device techniques. In the lateral decubitus position, however, the umbilicus is avoided, as we favor an access position approximately one-third the distance from the umbilicus to the splenic hilum in a line between the umbilicus and spleen. After securing access to the peritoneal cavity, typically three additional ports are placed along the costal margin. Depending on spleen size and body habitus, it may be necessary to site the trocars inferiorly or medially to accommodate the spleen size. We typically place a 10- to 12-mm port capable of accommodating an endostapler or large endoclips device in the left subcostal anterior axillary line. A 5-mm port is placed in the left subcostal region in the midaxillary line. A fourth port, usually 5 mm, is placed in the far left lateral subcostal position. Occasionally an additional port is required for retraction toward the midline near the xiphoid process.

Step 2: Diagnostic Laparoscopy, Including a Search for Accessory Spleens. Diagnostic laparoscopy is performed to survey the abdominal cavity, confirm location of the spleen, assess anatomic relationships of adjacent organs (colon, stomach, pancreas, etc.), search for accessory spleens, and plan operative strategy.

Up to 20% of people harbor an accessory spleen. The majority of patients with accessory spleens have only one. However, as many as 20% of patients with accessory spleens have two, and up to 17% have three or more. Accessory spleens range in size from 0.2 cm to 10 cm but typically are small, less than 1.5 cm, and appear as miniature spleens in gross appearance. Approximately two-thirds of accessory spleens are located at or near the splenic hilum. Twenty percent are within the substance of the tail of the pancreas. The remainder of accessory spleens are found in the omentum, along the splenic artery, in the mesentery, or along the left gonadal vessels.[26,27] When accessory spleens are suspected and the underlying hematologic disorder would be compromised by incomplete splenectomy, preoperative imaging with technetium scan may be helpful, even supplemented by intraoperative localization with a laparoscopic gamma probe after preoperative technetium administration within 2 hours of surgery.

Step 3: Mobilization of the Spleen With Dissection of Splenic Ligaments. Although some surgeons describe a step-by-step approach to the laparoscopic dissection, variable splenic anatomy often forces a "strategy of opportunity." Laparoscopic dissection begins by partially mobilizing the splenic flexure of the left colon, dividing the splenocolic ligament, the distal phrenocolic ligament, and the sustentaculum lienis. This dissection can be accomplished with endoscopic scissors, harmonic scalpel, or various endosurgical electrocautery devices. This dissection creates access to the gastrosplenic ligament, which is then easily separated from the splenorenal ligament. The lower pole of the spleen is carefully elevated. Dissection continues medially and cephalad, opening the space like a book, with the spleen gradually rolling laterally as access to the splenic hilum increases. Gentle handling of traction on the spleen is required to avoid capsular tear and ensuant bleeding. As the spleen is gently elevated and rolled laterally, pertinent dissection targets come into view. Gravity is an invaluable adjunct to exposure, taking advantage of patient positioning on an electric bed. Some authors describe a "splenic tent," with the gastrosplenic ligament making up the left side, the lienorenal ligament the right side, and the stomach the floor of the tent. A cautious, stepwise approach is taken to divide the phrenocolic ligament, enabling the spleen to be rolled laterally away from the tail of the pancreas, enabling visualization of the splenic hilum.

Step 4: Division of the Splenic Vessels, Including Splenic Hilum and Short Gastric Vessels. No two spleens are alike. Spleen size, shape, and vasculature vary. Vascular anatomy can be "distributed" or "magistral." The vascular pattern can usually be recognized by inspecting the inner surface of the spleen during initial laparoscopy. If the vessels appear to cover more than three-quarters of the surface, a distributed pattern is present. If the vessels appear to enter the spleen more uniformly and cover only one-third of the splenic surface, a magistral pattern is present. In the more commonly encountered distributed variant, there is a short splenic vascular trunk and many long branches entering along the medial surface of the spleen. Division of the distributed array of splenic vessels can be performed using sequential applications of an energy source device and endoclips. We typically use the harmonic scalpel, but caution is advised that it must be used to completely traverse each vessel, and only a single vessel at a time.

The less common magistral pattern is characterized by a long main splenic artery that divides into short branches close to the hilum.[24,26,28] The optimal approach for this pattern is to isolate the hilum as much as possible, preparing a window for access with an endoscopic linear stapler with a vascular load applied across the splenic hilum, ideally identifying and isolating the splenic artery and the splenic vein for separate vascular control to avoid the theoretical concern of an arteriovenous fistula, but also the more concerning risk of bleeding, as the mismatch in tissue thickness of the splenic artery and splenic vein has the potential for inadequate closure of the vein, resulting in post–staple fire splenic vein bleeding. Before firing the endoscopic linear stapler, careful inspection must ensure that the tail of the pancreas has been dissected free and is not included within the stapler to avoid possible pancreatic injury or fistula.

Short gastric vessels are divided sequentially, individually, to the most cephalad portion of the spleen, noting that the length of short gastric vessels often becomes shorter as this dissection proceeds, with progressively less distance between the stomach and the spleen. Care must be exercised with the placement of energy devices adjacent to the stomach while dividing short gastric vessels to avoid later gastric necrosis and resultant gastric fistula.

Step 5: Division of Remaining Attachments and Spleen Placement Within a Specimen Bag. Final mobilization of the spleen is completed by dividing the proximal phrenocolic ligament along its entire length to the diaphragm and left crus. Careful inspection ensures complete mobilization and freedom of the now-completely detached spleen for safe placement in the specimen bag. Some surgeons prefer leaving the superiormost portion of the phrenosplenic ligament intact until placement of the spleen within the specimen bag. This tactic leaves the spleen tethered to the diaphragm, which can facilitate placement of the spleen within the endoscopic specimen bag.

A large endoscopic specimen bag is introduced through the larger left midabdominal port. Several vendors have designed large endoscopic specimen bags that are especially strong for removal of the spleen. Some surgeons have used sterilized medium or large heavy-duty plastic freezer bags as an acceptable alternative.[25] The spleen is placed in the endoscopic specimen bag and extracted under direct laparoscopic visualization.

Step 6: Extraction of the Spleen Within the Specimen Bag from the Peritoneal Cavity. Preoperative discussion with the patient care team, including the hematologist and pathologist, should be held to determine if morcellation of the spleen specimen is appropriate. When laparoscopic splenectomy is performed for malignancy, morcellation of the specimen may make histologic evaluation of the specimen difficult. The endoscopic specimen bag is grasped and extracted through an appropriate port site. When the anterior approach is used, the extraction site is the umbilicus. When the lateral approach is used, extraction of the specimen bag is often through one of the lateral left subcostal ports. Typically, the specimen bag is continuously observed as it is elevated to the abdominal wall, enabling the surgeon to morcellate the spleen within the bag, allowing extraction of the fragmented specimen within the specimen bag through a small incision. Care is taken not to rupture the bag, as peritoneal spillage of the fragmented spleen can lead to later splenosis (disseminated splenic implantation), a particularly troubling problem after splenectomy for hematologic disorders. To enable delivery of the spleen and specimen bag, it is rarely necessary to enlarge the extraction port incision more than a few centimeters. For larger spleens, extraction may be preferred through a Pfannenstiel incision, or through a hand port incision, if a hand-assisted laparoscopic surgery (HALS) device has been used.

Step 7: Inspection of the Operative Field. After the spleen has been successfully delivered, or possibly prior to final laparoscopic specimen bag extraction and loss of pneumoperitoneum, the operative field is carefully inspected for hemostasis, previously undetected accessory spleens, or for other unexpected mischief. No surgical drains are placed, reflecting the established experience from open surgery. The exception to this guideline is if inspection suggests an evident pancreatic tail injury, in which case a closed suction drain along the pancreatic tail in the splenic bed is recommended, exteriorized through one of the lateral laparoscopic port sites.

Step 8: Removal of Trocars, Pneumoperitoneum Desufflation, and Port Site Closure. Once the operative team is satisfied with inspection of the operative field, all ports are removed under direct visualization. The pneumoperitoneum is desufflated. Fascia at all port sites greater than 5 mm diameter is closed. Port sites are irrigated, injected with local anesthetic, skin edges are closed with subcuticular closure, and Steri-Strips or tissue sealant is placed, followed by placement of simple dressings.

Tips Regarding Evolving Instrumentation and Energy Sources. Twenty-five years of laparoscopy has resulted in significant evolution in instrumentation and energy source options for the minimally invasive surgeon. Surgeon experience and preference guide selection of instruments for dissection and division of splenic vessels. Twenty years ago, vascular control options were limited to isolation of individual vessels and division between endoloops or endoclips. Larger vessels, however, are often challenging for standard endoclip control, even with larger metallic endoclips. Self-locking endoclips are available and provide a larger vessel size control capability. Energy devices such as the harmonic scalpel and LigaSure electrocautery devices have evolved; both can be used to divide and seal vessels up to 7 mm in diameter. Each device has strengths and weaknesses. The 10-mm-diameter LigaSure device has a low degree of adjacent collateral tissue damage, but at 10 mm with no curve, it is cumbersome to use through a splenic hilar dissection. The 5-mm-diameter LigaSure device is easier to use but results in higher adjacent collateral tissue damage because of its smaller surface area to absorb the impedance of the device. The 5-mm-diameter harmonic scalpel device has a gentle curve to facilitate dissection but should be used with caution to avoid past-pointing with the device tip to avoid contact with adjacent tissues, and to ensure that the device is completely across target vessels, because unlike LigaSure technology, the harmonic scalpel must be completely across a vessel to seal the vessel. Both harmonic scalpel and LigaSure technologies are effective and have shortened operative times compared with historical tools.

Minimally Invasive Surgery Approaches to Massive Spleens

Hand-Assisted Laparoscopic Splenectomy. Laparoscopic splenectomy is the standard of care for normal to moderately enlarged spleens. However, to successfully manage massive spleens, minimal-access splenectomy employing hybrid technologies such as HALS is increasingly reported to be an effective adjunct for spleens significantly larger than 25 cm in length.

HALS utilizes a combination of laparoscopic and open splenectomy techniques. HALS employs a device to enable intraabdominal placement of a hand and forearm through a small incision through a HALS device, while maintaining pneumoperitoneum, to facilitate performing laparoscopic surgery. HALS advocates argue that use of a hand-assisted device enables tactile (haptic) feedback and helps the surgeon better judge the extent of disease, identify underlying structures, and palpate anatomic landmarks. HALS improves manipulation of instruments intraabdominally, assists in restoring depth perception and three-dimensional (3D) orientation, and can serve as a bridge to enhance laparoscopic skills. For large spleens, it helps the surgeon manipulate the spleen more safely than laparoscopic instrumentation alone. Vendors have developed a variety of commercially available hand port devices with a wide range in cost. Length of the required hand port incision correlates mainly with the breadth of the surgeon's palm, usually the required HALS incision length being determined by the size of the surgeon's glove (6.5 to 8.0 cm), subtracting 2 cm if the marking was prior to the pneumoperitoneum. The surgeon's hand and forearm size are key, and can be limiting for surgeons with large hands, with respect to both how far the surgeon's hand can reach from the hand port, and in terms of how much working and visual space the surgeon's hand occupies—both factors can be limiting.

Optimal placement of the hand port is important. There is a need for "stand-off" distance between the hand port and the target organ or operative field, so that the surgeon's hand has working room within the abdomen and does not interfere with laparoscopic instruments and visualization. Options for hand port placement for left upper quadrant surgery include the midline just above the umbilicus, the lower midline or left lower quadrant using a muscle splitting incision, or even a Pfannenstiel incision for surgeons with small hands. Patient positioning for HALS splenectomy can be approached either from the anterior or lateral approach. The most common location for the hand port is in the midline, between the xiphoid and the umbilicus. For massive spleens, the incision has also been described in a Pfannenstiel position.[20,28,29]

Pneumoperitoneum is established after the hand port is placed. Additional laparoscopic port placement must be planned carefully to enable visualization and working access while maintaining hand port access.

Once the hand port and additional laparoscopic ports have been placed and pneumoperitoneum established, the principles for splenectomy remain the same. The biggest technical challenge is avoiding hemorrhage. Small series have reported successful HALS splenectomy for severe splenomegaly, with spleen mean length of 27.9 cm (range, 23 to 32 cm), with acceptable operative times, morbidity, and outcomes.[29] Pietrabissa et al reported a more recent 10-year retrospective registry review of 85 laparoscopic splenectomies comparing 43 patients who underwent HALS splenectomy and 43 patients who underwent conventional laparoscopic splenectomy, with larger spleens weighing more than 700 g in the HALS group. Rates of conversion to open surgery and operative mortality were similar. Of interest, portal venous thrombosis remained common, but similar in both groups. With the HALS option, even patients with massive splenomegaly can be offered a minimally invasive surgical option.[30,31]

Emerging Minimally Invasive Options

Single-Port Laparoscopic Splenectomy. Single-port access (SPA) developed as an alternative to traditional multiport laparoscopy, with the goal of exploiting proven benefits of minimally invasive surgery through a single umbilical incision. Controversy continues surrounding SPA procedures regarding cost of SPA devices and long-term outcomes at the SPA site regarding hernia/wound problems. Challenging technical issues relate to the decreased triangulation forced by the more coaxial alignment of visualization and instrumentation during SPA surgery. Evolution of flexible and/or curved instruments as well as adoption of crossing instrument techniques can help address these challenges.

Curcillo's group, one of the pioneering SPA teams, reported single-port splenectomy for staging with a normal-sized spleen using standard instrumentation and trocars to maintain cost and familiarity of the procedure, with a good early outcome and 18-month follow-up with no hernia.[32] Targarona's group reported a subsequent series of eight single-incision laparoscopic surgeries (SILS), with SILS technique for splenectomy successful in six of eight patients. SILS may provide safe operative

visualization, hilar transection using endostapling devices, and spleen removal, decreasing abdominal wall trauma to a single site.[33] Successful single-port laparoscopic partial splenectomy has also been reported.[34]

Robot-Assisted Laparoscopic Splenectomy. Robotic surgery restores a three-dimensional view and permits greater instrument degrees of freedom, with the potential for improved precision. Limitations of haptics, limited multi-quadrant mobility, cost, and unproven benefit for other general surgery procedures, particularly given the high levels of established success for most advanced complex laparoscopic procedures, has limited the rapid expansion of robotics usage. Robot-assisted laparoscopic splenectomy has been reported, though the role and/or need for robotic splenectomy remains to be established in the spectrum of minimally invasive surgery approaches to the spleen.[35] An early retrospective review compared six robot-assisted laparoscopic splenectomies against six laparoscopic splenectomies—all for ITP, with patients matched for age, American Society of Anesthesiologists score, body mass index (BMI), and preoperative platelet levels. There were no conversions. No complications were reported. Medium postoperative stay was 1 day longer in the robotic group. Mean average costs were almost one-third higher in the robotic group. Operative times were approximately 20% longer in the robotic group. In this analysis, robot-assisted laparoscopic splenectomy resulted in prolonged operative time, length of stay, and procedural costs, and though feasible, no relevant benefit was demonstrated.[36] A contemporary updated comparative study of laparoscopic versus robotic splenectomy by Gelmini's group retrospectively reviewed two well-matched groups of 45 patients, finding no significant differences in intraoperative blood loss, conversion to laparotomy, return to diet, morbidity, and length of stay, with no differences at 6-month assessment.[37]

Natural Orifice Transluminal Endoscopic Surgery (NOTES) Splenectomy. NOTES represents another potential step in the evolution of minimally invasive surgery, with the promise of "no scar." NOTES remains early in clinical experience and application. Since Reddy and Rau's first video of a NOTES appendectomy in 2004, NOTES evolution has been slow to translate into clinical practice. Transvaginal extraction of laparoscopically removed spleens was described in the early 1990s but has not been widely adopted.[38-40] Feasibility and patient benefit of NOTES approaches await further study and further instrument development.

MINIMALLY INVASIVE SPLENECTOMY POSTOPERATIVE CARE

Postoperative care following a laparoscopic splenectomy is straightforward provided that the procedure is uneventful. Orogastric tubes and urinary catheters are removed immediately. Routine postoperative chest radiograph is not required. Pneumothorax following laparoscopic splenectomy is rare. DVT prophylaxis is continued postoperatively with both pneumatic sequential compression devices, and heparin, or enoxaparin, unless contraindicated. A diet is resumed as tolerated. Typical length of stay following laparoscopic splenectomy is currently 1 day, although most series report average length of stay of 2 to 3 days.

All patients undergoing splenectomy should be counseled regarding their increased lifetime risk of OPSI. Patients should be advised to seek medical care immediately if they develop a febrile illness. Asplenic patients in general have poor knowledge about their condition and risks. Information on the Internet for asplenic patients is a resource they are likely to access, and although many websites have incomplete information, almost all discuss the long-term risk of serious infection and need for vaccination.[41]

The use of long-term prophylactic antibiotics after splenectomy remains controversial. Long-term antibiotic therapy risks selection of resistant microbial strains. Pediatric hematologists often recommend treatment for 2 years postsplenectomy with a penicillin-based regimen. Studies have demonstrated benefit from OPSI antibiotic prophylaxis in children with sickle cell disease, but there have been no studies in adults. We discharge patients with a supply of oral antibiotics, with instructions to initiate therapy at the onset of symptoms of infection as they simultaneously seek urgent medical attention.

SURGICAL COMPLICATIONS

Laparoscopic splenectomy is unforgiving. Intraoperative complications, particularly hemorrhage, can be challenging to manage. Recognition that splenic vascular anatomy is variable and complex, and that the spleen is a fragile solid organ with a delicate capsule underscore preemptive efforts to avoid bleeding. Dissection should be methodical—identifying, isolating, and individually controlling vessels sequentially. The lateral approach decreases traction requirements on the spleen, decreasing traction-related splenic capsular tears. Constant intraoperative monitoring for hemostasis is important. Energy sources have limitations, as do clip and linear stapler devices. Improper cautery application can cause injury to adjacent organs. Improper harmonic scalpel application can result in hemorrhage from a partially sectioned vessel. Improper clip application can result in injury to an adjacent vessel. Blind linear stapler application can result in damage to the tail of the pancreas. The tip of the linear stapler should always be clearly seen before it is fired. Hemorrhage can occur from partial division of a major splenic vessel after release of the stapler. Instruments should be introduced to the operative field under direct visualization, avoiding inadvertent injury to the delicate splenic parenchyma.

Postoperative complications for laparoscopic splenectomy are similar to those for the open procedure, although most recent series report lower morbidity and mortality compared to open splenectomy. Early complications include bleeding, pneumonia, left pleural effusions, atelectasis, and, rarely, injury to other organs (colon, small bowel, stomach, liver, and pancreas). Late complications include subphrenic abscesses, splenic vein and/or portal vein thrombosis, failure of the procedure to control the primary disease, recurrent disease due to accessory spleens, and OPSI. A recent multicenter analysis of laparoscopic splenectomy reported data from 1993 to 2007 including 25 centers and 676 cases. Conversion to open splenectomy was reported in 6%, complications in 17%, and perioperative death in 0.4%. Multivariate analysis found that BMI and presence of hematologic malignancy were independent predictors for intraoperative complications and surgical conversion. Spleen longitudinal size and surgical conversion were independent predictors of postoperative complications.[42]

Approximately 6% to 10% of open splenectomy patients develop splenic or portal vein thrombosis.[28] The incidence of portal vein thrombosis after laparoscopic splenectomy has been reported to be higher at 14%.[43,44] However, a prospective comparison of open and laparoscopic splenectomy using helical CT imaging pre- and postoperatively identified portal venous thrombosis in 19% of the open group, and 55% of the laparoscopic group.[45] Most instances of splenoportal venous thrombosis are asymptomatic. When present, symptoms are vague and include fatigue, nausea, vomiting, and nonspecific abdominal pain. The overall risk of *symptomatic* postsplenectomy splenic or portal vein thrombosis is about 3%. Risk factors include splenomegaly and hereditary hemolytic anemias, whereas risk may be lower in autoimmune thrombocytopenia and trauma. Treatment of splenic/portal vein thrombosis with heparin and warfarin leads to complete or partial resolution of thrombosis in 80%, with persistent occlusion, portal hypertension, or cavernoma in 20%. The long-term outcome of treatment failure is unknown. Well-designed prospective studies on prophylaxis of visceral venous thrombosis following splenectomy are lacking.[46,47]

Patients with persistent postoperative fever, increased white blood cell count, and abdominal pain should undergo computed tomography of the abdomen. Subphrenic abscesses are treated with drainage and intravenous antibiotics. Missed accessory spleens appear no more frequent with laparoscopic than open splenectomy.

IMAGE-GUIDED INTERVENTIONAL THERAPY FOR THE SPLEEN

The spleen possesses a single, accessible feeding artery with a relatively simple branching pattern, making the splenic artery well suited to routine, safe catheter access. Its brisk blood flow and rich vascular parenchyma provides high-quality arteriograms, parenchymal opacification, and portal venous imaging using digital subtraction angiography (DSA). Minimally invasive vascular interventional techniques for the spleen were rapidly popularized in the 1970s and 1980s and play an increasing role in algorithms of contemporary surgical practice, particularly with the shift toward preservation of functioning splenic tissue through nonoperative management. This section reviews techniques and provides updates on clinical applications of image-guided splenic interventions, which include splenic trauma, splenic artery pseudoaneurysm, hypersplenism, drainage of splenic collections, and splenic biopsy, with focus on the complementary role of image-guided interventions for the spleen as adjuncts to expanding minimally invasive surgery applications—particularly in splenic trauma and in managing giant spleens.

TRANSARTERIAL SPLENIC EMBOLIZATION

Anatomy

Although surgical splenectomy can be performed efficiently and safely, it is now clear that removal of this reticuloendothelial organ is accompanied by significant risks of OPSI. Catheter-directed therapies provide an adjunct to surgery intervention to achieve therapeutic goals while preserving adequate functioning splenic tissue for host immunity. In some cases, image-guided splenic intervention, such as splenic embolization, can obviate the need for surgery, as described in the previous section as an adjunct in nonoperative blunt splenic trauma management.[48] In other cases, splenic embolization can facilitate laparoscopic splenectomy, as described previously for the subset of patients failing nonoperative splenic trauma management[49]; embolization can also be used for patients with giant spleens being prepared for laparoscopic or HALS splenectomy.[50] The splenic artery is usually a large single vessel arising anterolaterally from the celiac axis trunk. Splenic artery anatomic variants are uncommon but include a separate origin from the aorta.[51] The artery corkscrews clockwise or anticlockwise while undulating across the posterosuperior aspect of the pancreas body. It gives off sequentially the dorsal pancreatic and pancreatica magna arteries before dividing into extrasplenic polar branches in the region of the pancreatic tail (Figure 133-1). One should note that the pancreas also receives a blood supply from the pancreaticoduodenal and transverse pancreatic arcades, and the spleen has a rich vascular network from the short gastric and gastroepiploic arteries. This anatomy may be depicted on current 3D multidetector-row CT angiography (CTA) and MR angiography (MRA) with a diagnostic quality comparable to invasive splenic angiography (Figure 133-2).

Technique

Most splenic interventions can be performed with conscious sedation, though pediatric patients may require general anesthesia. An initial aortogram is performed with a 5-French (5F) flush catheter through a 5F sheath in the femoral artery. This assesses globally for sites of bleeding and depicts the normal and variant anatomy for selective angiography. The celiac axis and splenic artery are selected using a combination of 5F Simmons 1 or Cobra glide catheter and an 0.035 glide wire. With proximal placement of the catheter, a selective splenic angiogram is performed with arterial, parenchymal, and portal venous phase timing of the contrast bolus. Smaller, more distal hilar and branch vessels may be selected with the 5F catheter combined with a 3F microcatheter over a 0.014 to 0.018 microwire. Standard DSA suffices, though newer 3D fluoroscopy units may benefit cases with difficult anatomy (Figure 133-3).

Embolization is performed from distal to proximal within the artery. Embolic materials available include Gelfoam, particles, and coils. Smaller, more distal arteries and parenchyma may be temporarily embolized with gelatin sponge pledgets or slurry or autologous blood clot. Permanent distal parenchymal vascular occlusion is achieved with 300- to 900-μm particulate polyvinyl alcohol, silicone, or acrylic embolic spheres. The embolic agents may be soaked in antibiotic to decrease the risk of abscess formation. The splenic artery may be permanently embolized with metallic coils from the second-order branches into the main splenic artery. Coils are deployed distal to the dorsal pancreatic and pancreatica magna arteries in an effort to avoid splenic infarction by preserving collateral supply to functioning splenic pulp.[52] Coils must be sized to the target vessel to avoid inadvertent distal embolization to nontarget vessels or proximal migration into the celiac axis or aorta. Depending on the indication a combination approach of coil and embolic agents may be employed. One must remain cognizant that proximally placed coils may limit future interventions if required.

SPLENIC BLEEDING AND TRANSARTERIAL SPLENIC EMBOLIZATION

Most cases of splenic bleeding result from blunt or penetrating trauma of the normal-sized spleen. The spleen represents the most commonly injured organ presenting for transarterial embolization, first described by Sclafani et al in 1995.[53] The algorithm for managing the patient with splenic injury is an evolving practice, reflected by decreased splenectomies in adults and children and expansion of the number of patients managed nonoperatively by observation and transarterial splenic embolization (TASE). Nonoperative management has become the treatment of choice for hemodynamically stable patients with blunt splenic trauma. Outcomes are predominantly based on large-volume studies from level 1 trauma centers in the United States, but emerging data suggest good outcomes even from smaller centers.[48] Assignment of patients to operative or nonoperative groups and to interventional and noninterventional groups is best achieved through reconciliation of the clinical picture, imaging findings, and injury scale (American Association for the Surgery of Trauma [AAST] Organ Injury Scale [OIS])[54] in consultation between surgeon and interventionalist.[53] CT has largely eliminated the application of admission diagnostic angiography as a routine measure for all splenic injuries. Grading of the injury is now largely based on CT which has some interobserver variation, is limited in depicting active bleeding on a single study, and cannot reliably distinguish arterial and venous extravasation. CT imaging findings cannot be viewed in isolation for the management algorithm. Temporal change that is clinically occult may indicate intervention, but less remarkable features should not deny intervention when discordant with the clinical picture.

Clinical features of patient age, grade of splenic injury,[54,55] size of retroperitoneal bleed,[56] and the need for resuscitation as well as associated injuries[57,58] are no longer absolute indications for surgery nor do they absolutely preclude an interventional approach.[53,56] Broadly speaking, most would agree that the hypotensive, unstable patient refractory to resuscitation mandates surgical exploration (usually grade III to V injury).[54] The majority of injuries present as hemodynamically stable patients

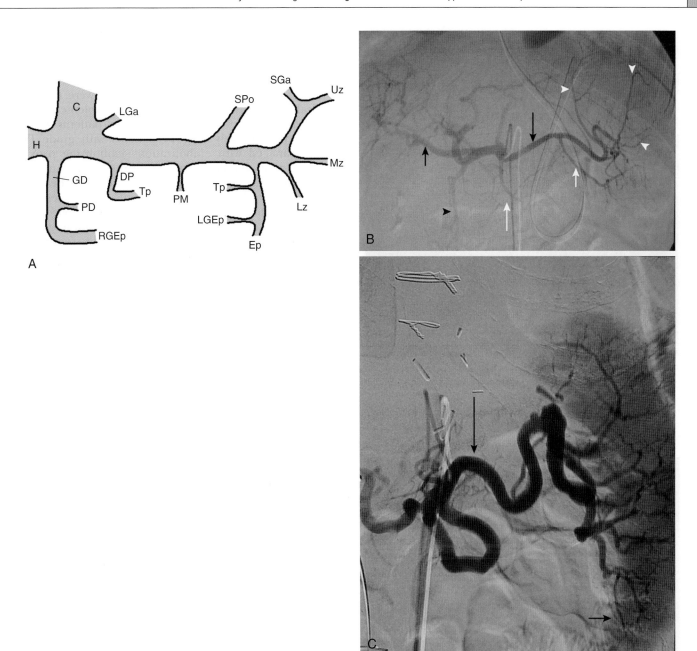

FIGURE 133-1 A, Schematic illustration of the splenic artery and its branches seen at splenic arteriography. *C,* Celiac artery; *Ep,* epiploic artery; *GD,* gastroduodenal artery; *H,* hepatic artery; *LGa,* left gastric artery; *LGEp,* left gastro-epiploic artery; *Lz,* inferior pole of splenic artery; *Mz,* midzone splenic artery; *PD,* pancreaticoduodenal artery; *PM,* pancreatica magna; *RGEp,* right gastroepiploic artery; *SGa,* short gastric arteries; *SPo,* superior polar artery; *Tp,* transverse pancreatic artery; *Uz,* upper pole splenic artery. **B,** Forty-one-year-old woman with gastrointestinal bleeding. Normal anteroposterior celiac arteriogram demonstrating splenic artery *(long black arrow),* dorsal pancreatic artery *(long white arrow),* pancreatica magna *(short white arrow),* splenic artery hilar branches *(white arrowheads),* hepatic artery *(short black arrowhead),* and gastroduodenal artery *(arrowhead).* **C,** Fifty-year-old man with pancreatic carcinoma. Normal anteroposterior celiac arteriogram demonstrates the splenic artery *(long arrow)* and parenchymal phase enhancement of the spleen *(short arrow).*

with a grade I or II injury and no signs of continued bleeding and may be managed conservatively with observation.[59,60] The role of endovascular therapy lies between these broadly defined groups and is still actively debated. Management today largely depends on local expertise and trauma team organization, which evaluates each case on its individual merits. Most splenic injuries treated by embolization are grade 2.8 to 3.[54,56,59] TASE has little role

in the shattered or devascularized spleen. In centers with rapid access to interventional services as part of trauma triage, there is some evidence to support TASE in patients who respond transiently to minimal resuscitation[61] and in endovascular treatment of higher-grade injuries. Up to 10% of hemodynamically stable patients may have imaging signs of continued bleeding from grade III injuries and are potential candidates for TASE. The

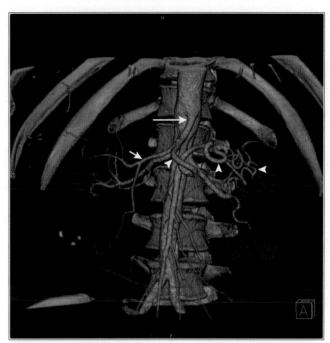

FIGURE 133-2 Thirty-year-old woman being evaluated for renal organ donation. Three-dimensional volume-rendered anteroposterior projection multidetector-row computed tomography of the splenic artery *(arrowheads)*. Celiac axis *(long arrow)* and hepatic artery *(short arrow)*.

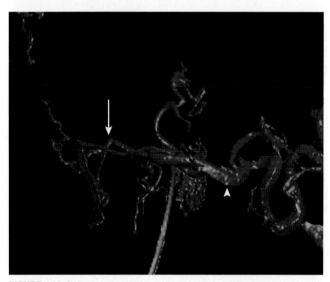

FIGURE 133-3 Forty-year-old woman receiving hepatic chemoembolization. Three-dimensional fluoroscopic digital subtraction angiography that offers infinite planes and projections for interpretation and can unravel complex anatomy. Hepatic artery *(arrow)* and splenic artery *(arrowhead)*.

impact of splenic embolization in the algorithm for nonoperative management of splenic trauma is not well established. A retrospective study over 7 years at a level 1 trauma center reviewing 499 patients who suffered blunt splenic trauma found 407 (81.6%) with successful nonoperative management and 92 (18.4%) failed nonoperative management criteria and underwent splenectomy within 1 hour of admission. Splenic embolization

was protective against splenectomy for lower-grade injures.[51] Early experience with splenic embolization for higher-grade splenic trauma is favorable, but requires a vigilant team and algorithm. One group reported 46 patients with splenic trauma of whom 17 were treated surgically, 15 conservatively, and 14 with splenic artery embolization. Hemodynamically stable patients were treated conservatively with 14 patients with grade IV injury managed with embolization—embolizing proximally the main splenic artery with diffuse organ damage, and embolizing distally selective splenic branches for localized injury. In 13 of the 14 patients (92.9%), embolization was successful and there were no periprocedural complications, with the remaining patient undergoing splenectomy within 24 hours because of recurrent bleeding.[52]

Endovascular therapy for splenic trauma begins with review of the contrast-enhanced CT or magnetic resonance imaimg (MRI). The aortogram may demonstrate generalized vasoconstriction and renal retention of contrast in the patient in shock. Splenic angiography findings include abrupt termination of vessels, vasospasm, pseudoaneurysm, and arteriovenous fistula formation. Intrasplenic vessels may be displaced and the extrasplenic artery may be "accordioned" from the hematoma. The parenchymal phase may demonstrate contrast extravasation, avascular segments, abnormal accumulation of contrast within the pulp, and loss of the smooth splenic contour. In the setting of large subcapsular hematoma, the spleen will be displaced anteromedially and the left kidney may be displaced inferiorly. Bleeding may initially be treated with a temporary distal particulate agent to slow the cut surface bleed but the definitive therapy is permanent coil embolization of the splenic artery. If there are only two to three identifiable bleeding sites, they may be selectively coiled distally. However, if there are multiple sites, a more proximal embolization will be required. Embolization slows arterial inflow and permits distal clot to form,[62] and Haan et al noted no difference in outcomes between proximal and distal embolization.[57] After therapy, one may see complete stasis or markedly slowed flow. Absence of extravasation at angiography is a reliable sign of successful therapy,[53] and such patients will not likely need later laparotomy.

The success of TASE and its contribution to nonoperative management is largely from retrospective data. Patients failing nonoperative management (3% to 17%) and requiring splenectomy are decreasing.[56,57] Overall the success of TASE for controlling splenic bleeding and splenic salvage is more than 80% in adults and children.[53,58,63,64] Haan et al reviewed 648 patients with blunt splenic injury of whom 132 had embolization with salvage rates of 90%.[57] The presence of an arteriovenous fistula may predict operative failure,[57] but this will depend on how aggressively the fistula is treated. Those who fail an initial TASE may yet be considered for a second therapy if they remain stable and can account for 2% to 5% of patients treated (Figure 133-4).[57] One would expect the failure rates to increase as the technique is increasingly applied to higher injury grades.

Complications of TASE include a failure to treat where delayed recurrent bleeding occurs either due to

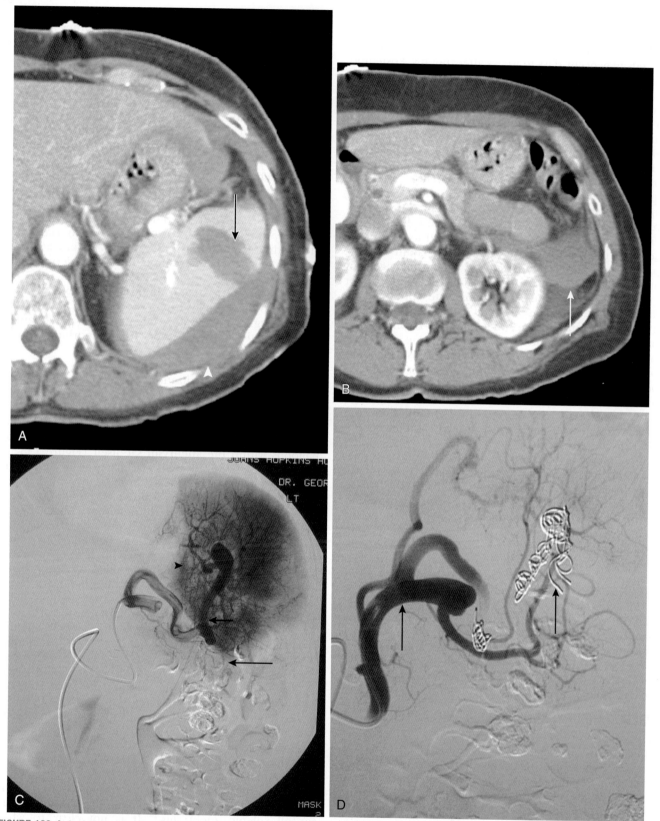

FIGURE 133-4 **A,** Axial contrast-enhanced computed tomography (CT) scan in a 32-year-old female who fell from a horse and had active splenic bleeding. Grade IV laceration *(black arrow)* and subcapsular hematoma *(white arrowhead)* of the spleen. **B,** Axial contrast-enhanced CT. Moderate retroperitoneal hematoma in the left anterior pararenal space *(arrow).* **C,** Anteroposterior digital subtraction angiography (DSA) of splenic arteriogram demonstrates splenic artery *(short arrow)* supplying remaining upper-pole splenic pulp *(arrowhead)* though there is a sharp cutoff from the avascular lower-pole segment because of the expanding hematoma *(long arrow).* **D,** Treatment with transarterial splenic embolization. Hemostasis was achieved with coil embolization of the splenic artery. Splenic artery DSA demonstrates decreased splenic perfusion and coils in the distal lobar branch of the splenic artery *(black arrows).*

continued bleeding through the embolization, lysis of the clot at the injured site, pseudoaneurysm rupture, or relaxation of acutely vasospastic vessels.[65,66] Delayed bleeds may occur days to weeks after therapy. Postembolization syndrome comprises abdominal pain and fever and may be associated with CT findings of necrotic, air-containing parenchyma and left-side pleural effusion. This is usually self-limited unless superimposed with infection. Bacterial peritonitis, septicemia, splenic abscesses, and rupture are recognized complications. Hematomata may evolve into calcified splenic hematomata or cysts. Postembolization infarction rates are quoted to be up to 20% but depend on the site of injury and the extent of embolization required.[65-67] Controversy remains regarding proximal versus distal splenic artery embolization. A recent metaanalysis tried to specifically address this issue. Studies evaluating adult trauma patients sustaining blunt splenic injury managed by angioembolization were systematically evaluated for grade of splenic injury, indication, site (proximal vs. distal), and outcomes. Fifteen of 147 studies were included, all retrospective, for a cohort of 479 embolized patients. Overall embolization failure rate was 10% (range, 0.0% to 33.3%). Rebleeding was the most common reason for failure but did not differ statistically between distal and proximal angioembolization techniques. Minor complications occurred statistically more often after distal than after proximal embolization, primarily explained by higher rate of segmental infarctions after distal embolization.[68]

Nonoperative management of splenic trauma assumes that splenic preservation preserves splenic function. To test this assumption, immune function of the spleen posttrauma was assessed in 43 patients with splenic injury (grades I to IV) comparing patients undergoing nonoperative management, splenectomy, splenectomy with autotransplantation, or splenic embolization—analyzing for lymphocyte subpopulations and antibody responses to *Streptococcus pneumoniae* and *Haemophilus influenzae* vaccinations. Splenectomy patients exhibited significant decrease in CD4[+] T lymphocytes and in IgM and IgD/B cells compared with splenic preservation patients, reinforcing the importance of conservative options in splenic trauma. Better measurement markers, however, are needed to predict splenic function and vaccination response after nonoperative splenic trauma management.[69]

PSEUDOANEURYSM OF THE SPLENIC ARTERY

The splenic artery is the most common visceral artery affected by aneurysms and pseudoaneurysms and is second only to aortoiliac aneurysm formation. They share some etiologies with aneurysms elsewhere but are specifically associated with pancreatitis, hypersplenism, and pregnancy. Traumatic pseudoaneurysms presumably occur from deceleration of the spleen on its vascular pedicle during blunt abdominal trauma.[70] It has been suggested that the increased nonoperative management of splenic injuries may lead to a greater prevalence of traumatic pseudoaneurysms that would otherwise have been resected[71] but there is also an increased detection of incidental splenic aneurysms because of the

widespread application of cross-sectional imaging. There is an increased prevalence in women and they are more prone to rupture in pregnancy. Splenic aneurysms are typically saccular and situated in the distal third of the splenic artery. Rarely, intrasplenic aneurysms have been reported.[72] They contain a variable amount of mural thrombus, are frequently calcified, but they don't affect splenic perfusion. CT angiography is highly accurate for detection and characterization of splenic aneurysms though 3D reconstructions are required to differentiate the false positive of normal vessel tortuosity and atherosclerotic change. There is some debate on which pseudoaneurysms should be treated. Most agree that aneurysms larger than 2 to 2.5 cm and enlarging or symptomatic aneurysms should be treated, as up to 60% of those who bleed will be unstable and the mortality rate of bleeding is quoted as high as 15%.[71] Many advocate therapy for smaller aneurysms in those considering childbearing also. Some argue that lesions less than 2.5 cm and small pediatric splenic aneurysms may be managed conservatively with close followup imaging and surveillance though some authors suggest that all pseudoaneurysms be actively treated given the low morbidity of the procedure.[71,73]

The majority of splenic aneurysms may be treated by TASE, with embolization of the aneurysmal sac directly or its feeding artery. For broad-necked, saccular, or fusiform aneurysms, coils are deployed from distal to proximal within the splenic artery. In saccular lesions with a narrow neck, one may deploy detachable coils or balloons within the aneurysm sac itself (Figure 133-5). More recently, covered stents placed across the aneurysm neck have been suggested as a form of therapy that will exclude the aneurysm and preserve blood flow and future access.[74] This procedure, however, may be of higher risk in very tortuous and diseased arteries and requires careful patient selection. Percutaneous injection of thrombin has been reported but is an uncommon approach and perhaps less controlled as one cannot compress the neck as is done in peripheral arteries.[75] Localized treatment of pseudoaneurysm and its neck preserves splenic function through more proximal branches. A recent retrospective review of 38 splenic artery aneurysm patients (all >2 cm in diameter) included 9 treated with transcatheter embolization, 8 treated by open repair, and 21 observed. Success rates were 100% in both the transcatheter embolizaton and open surgical repair groups, with shorter length of stay (8 vs. 16 days) in the angioembolization group, with no recurrence in either group at 45 and 57 months, respectively, with authors recommending transcatheter embolization as first-line strategy for all splenic artery aneurysms requiring treatment.[76,77]

The results of endovascular management have matured and it is now a recommended consideration for all splenic aneurysms.[76] It is not clear to what extent splenic artery integrity is undermined by its proximity to the pancreas in pancreatitis, but it has been suggested that pseudoaneurysms related to pancreatitis may be better treated surgically. If surgery is anticipated, balloon occlusion catheters may control bleeding intraoperatively.[71]

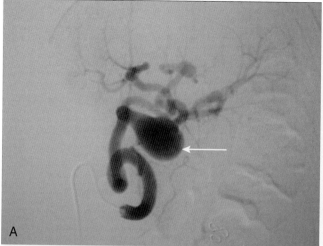

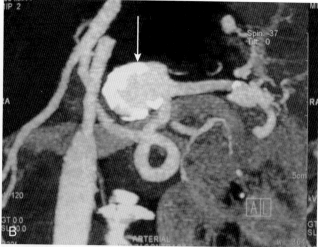

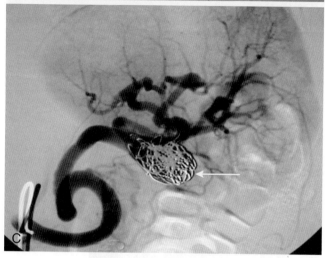

FIGURE 133-5 Pseudoaneurysm of the distal splenic artery. **A,** Anteroposterior digital subtraction angiography (DSA) demonstrates a large saccular pseudoaneurysm *(arrow)*. **B,** Anteroposterior maximum-intensity multidetector-row CT arteriogram demonstrates the saccular pseudoaneurysm *(arrow)*. **C,** Anteroposterior DSA demonstrates successful coil embolization with detachable coils *(arrow)*. (Courtesy Dr. A. Arapally, Johns Hopkins Hospital.)

Splenic artery and vein aneurysm with splenic arteriovenous fistula is rare, but amenable to image-guided intervention. Surgical ligation and percutaneous embolization have been reported to be equally effective. In addition, percutaneous placement of an occlusion device has been reported as yet another emerging alternative.[78]

HYPERSPLENISM AND PARTIAL SPLENIC EMBOLIZATION

Splenic embolization was introduced in the early 1970s and is considered for hypersplenism and pancytopenia with or without massive splenomegaly (e.g., thalassemia, myelofibrosis).[79] In addition to improving hematologic parameters and decreasing splenic size, it may improve liver function and decrease gastric or splenic variceal bleeding though this will depend on the baseline disease and hepatic reserve.[67,80,81] Though initially complete embolization was performed, the combination of antibiotic prophylaxis and partial splenic embolization (PSE)[82] led to an effective, safer alternative to surgical splenectomy.

Treatment is usually with small (300 to 900 μm) permanent particulate embolic agents (e.g., polyvinyl alcohol, silicone, or acrylic embolic spheres) that seek to deprive peripheral, intraparenchymal segmental regions of the spleen of their blood flow. Coils are not used because it is harder to gauge and stage the percentage of parenchyma treated and they limit access for future treatments that are frequently required. The risk of pancreatitis is reduced by placement of the catheter as distal as possible to avoid particulate agent going to nontarget sites and one may select individual hilar branches to better distribute the embolic agent throughout the spleen. The percentage embolization is judged from parenchymal phase angiography after particulate injection. It has been suggested that embolization of less than 50% predisposes to relapse[67,83] but with embolization of more than 70% of the splenic pulp, greater long-term efficacy may be achieved.[80] Most achieve this 70% in staged therapies to limit postembolization syndrome and complications. The response in organ size is best appreciated from CT or MRI and will be noticed within 2 to 4 months of therapy. The hematologic response may be seen within weeks[84] but a prolonged long-term response has also been demonstrated (Figure 133-6).[85] Though Nio et al noted relapse of thrombocytopenia after a single PSE treatment, they noted long-term efficacy in

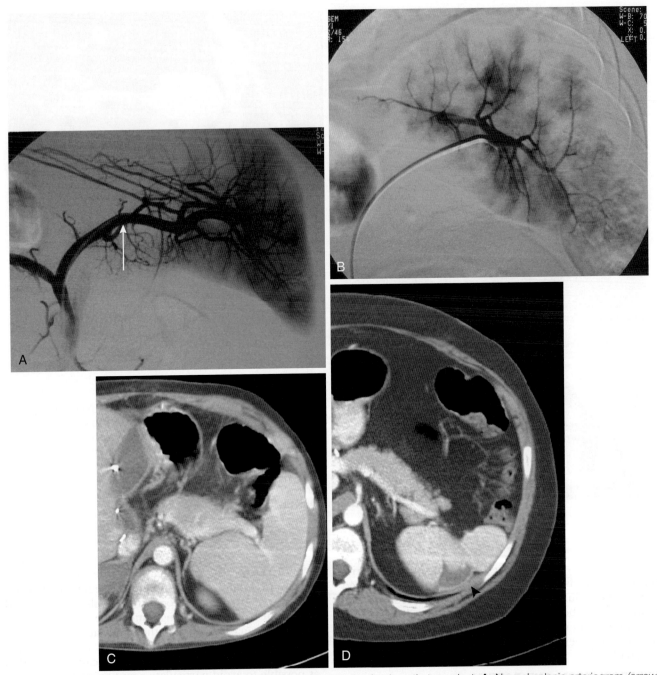

FIGURE 133-6 Fourteen-year-old with hypersplenism and thrombocytopenia after hepatic transplant. **A,** Normal splenic arteriogram *(arrow)* with parenchymal phase enhancement. **B,** Splenic arteriogram digital subtraction angiography after 70% embolization demonstrating mottled enhancement pattern. **C,** Contrast-enhanced CT before embolization. Note the size of the spleen. **D,** Contrast-enhanced CT 3 months after embolization. Note the decreased size of the spleen and small peripheral infarct *(arrowhead).* (**A** courtesy Dr. A. Arapally, Johns Hopkins Hospital.)

70% of patients. Success rates are higher for decreased variceal bleeding and improved liver function. Relapse may be related to the rate of splenic regeneration. Reported complications of the procedure include splenoportal venous thrombosis, splenic necrosis, abscess, and septicemia, which are potentially lethal in this patient population.[67,84]

A similar technique is used for presplenectomy splenic embolization. In general, the surgical approach to

splenectomy permits good control of bleeding and limited blood loss (Figure 133-7). However, it may be more challenging in the patient with massive splenomegaly (lymphoma or leukemia) where access to the hilum is more difficult. Coil embolization proximally may limit blood flow into the hilar vessels. Although the coils may affect placement of surgical clamps and ligatures, they can be removed easily if placed close to the time of operation. Intraparenchymal particulate

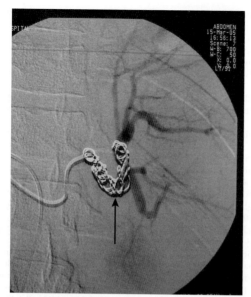

FIGURE 133-7 Sixty-two-year-old man who presented for preoperative embolization before splenectomy for lymphoma and splenomegaly. Note coils in the splenic artery *(arrow)* and decreased blood flow distally.

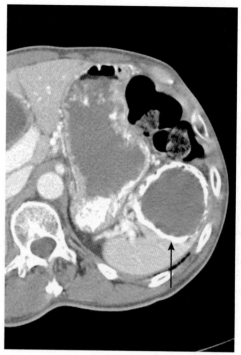

FIGURE 133-8 Axial contrast-enhanced CT demonstrating a calcified splenic hematoma *(arrow)*.

Gelfoam slurry embolization may limit bleeding of an intrasplenic mass (hemangiosarcoma or fibrosarcoma). Typically embolization is performed close to the time of operation.

As referenced in the first section of this chapter on minimally invasive surgery special considerations for laparoscopic splenectomy in the giant spleen, preoperative splenic artery embolization can aide laparoscopic or hand-assisted laparoscopic splenectomy.[50]

SPLENIC ABSCESS AND PSEUDOCYST

The commonest splenic collections are old hematoma, pseudocysts and cysts (Figure 133-8), and splenic abscesses (Figure 133-9). Cysts commonly seen on cross-sectional imaging require therapy only when they are large enough to cause early satiety or left shoulder pain. Noninfected splenic cysts may be treated by percutaneous puncture and aspiration with sclerosis. The volume of aspirate is replaced with 100% dehydrated ethanol or doxycycline and the patient is placed in alternate postures for an hour before the fluid is aspirated.[86,87] Repeat therapy may be required. Splenic abscess may be iatrogenic and may be complicated by mycotic pseudoaneurysm. They are usually accessed by ultrasound guidance, with a single-wall 18-gauge needle, followed by a 10F drain placed over a 0.035 guidewire. When drainage tapers off, repeat imaging indicates when the cavity has collapsed to allow drain removal.[88,89] Sterile collections that repeatedly reaccumulate may be sclerosed with tetracycline.[89]

IMAGE-GUIDED BIOPSY OF THE SPLEEN

Controversy surrounds the use of percutaneous image-guided biopsy of the spleen. Traditional opinion has been that the risk of bleeding is too high. Metaanalysis has shown high diagnostic accuracy, with pooled major

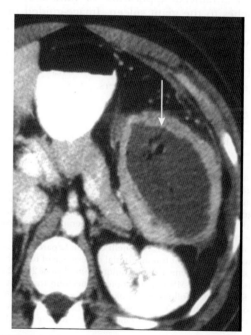

FIGURE 133-9 Axial contrast-enhanced CT demonstrating an air-containing splenic abscess *(arrow)*.

complication rate (hemorrhage most frequently, followed by pain) of only about 1% for needles 18 gauge or smaller, similar to that reported for image-guided biopsy of the liver or kidney. Percutaneous image-guided splenic biopsy is thus a reasonable option and favored over splenectomy "biopsy," unless the biopsy result would not change the decision for splenectomy.[90]

SUMMARY

Laparoscopic splenectomy is the criterion standard for most elective splenectomies for normal and slightly enlarged spleens. Conditions once considered relative or absolute contraindications to laparoscopic splenectomy have been reduced by surgical innovation, technology, and experience. There remain limited applications for laparoscopic splenectomy in the acute, unstable trauma patient, but with increased adoption of nonoperative management pathways and adjunctive therapy such as embolization, delayed laparoscopic splenectomy for failed nonoperative management in selected patients may become a preferred option. For elective splenectomy, the minimally invasive approach is applied to increasingly complex splenic disorders, reoperative settings, and massive splenomegaly, often with the application of hand-assist devices. Single-port, robotic, and NOTES splenectomy require further study of safety and cost-effectiveness.

Diagnostic splenic angiography is shifting from interventional diagnostic techniques to noninvasive 3D CT and MRI, which produce studies of similar quality. Therapeutic image-guided percutaneous interventions for the spleen continue to expand. There has been growth in splenic artery therapeutic embolization in trauma, helping to achieve organ preservation. Angioembolization has enhanced application of minimally invasive approaches to the giant spleen. Image-guided management of splenic artery aneurysm is emerging as a first-line strategy, as is selected application of image-guided splenic biopsy. Collaboration between the surgeon and image-guided interventionalist is essential in contemporary management of splenic disorders.

REFERENCES

1. Delaitre B, Maignien B: Splenectomy by the laparoscopic approach. Report of a case. *Presse Med* 20:2263, 1991.
2. Park A, Marcaccio M, Sternbach M, et al: Laparoscopic vs open splenectomy. *Arch Surg* 134:1263, 1999.
3. Targarona EM, Espert JJ, Cerdan G, et al: Effect of spleen size on splenectomy outcome. A comparison of open and laparoscopic surgery. *Surg Endosc Ultrasound Intervent Tech* 13:559, 1999.
4. Smith RS, Fry WR, Morabito DJ, et al: Therapeutic laparoscopy in trauma. *Am J Surg* 170:632, 1995.
5. Carobbi A, Romagnani F, Antonelli G, et al: Laparoscopic splenectomy for severe blunt trauma: Initial experience of ten consecutive cases with a fast hemostatic technique. *Surg Endosc* 24:1325, 2010.
6. Ransom KJ, Kavic MS: Laparoscopic splenectomy for blunt trauma: A safe operation following embolization. *Surg Endosc* 23:352, 2009.
7. Davoodi P, Budde C, Minshall CT: Laparoscopic repair of penetrating splenic injury. *J Laparoendosc Adv Surg Tech A* 19:795, 2009.
8. Isaev AF, Alimov AN, Safronov EP, et al: Evaluation of status severity in patients with isolated and combined injury of abdomen associated with spleen disruption. *Khirurgiia (Mosk)* 9:31, 2005.
9. Shen HB, Lu XM, Zheng QC, et al: Clinical application of laparoscopic spleen-preserving operation in traumatic spleen rupture. *Chin J Traumatol* 8:293, 2005.
10. Mostofa G, Matthews BD, Sing RF, et al: Elective laparoscopic splenectomy for grade III splenic injury in an athlete. *Surg Laparosc Endosc Percutan Tech* 12:283, 2002.
11. Longo WE, Baker CC, McMillen MA, et al: Nonoperative management of adult blunt splenic trauma: Criteria for successful outcome. *Ann Surg* 210:626, 1989.
12. Cameron JL: Current surgical therapy. In Park AE, editor: *Laparoscopic splenectomy*. Philadelphia, 2004, Elsevier Mosby, p 1254.
13. Grahn SW, Alvarez J 3rd, Kirkwood K: Trends in laparoscopic splenectomy for massive splenomegaly. *Arch Surg* 141:755, 2006.
14. Reso A, Brar MS, Church N, et al: Outcome of laparoscopic splenectomy with preoperative splenic artery embolization for massive splenomegaly. *Surg Endosc* 24:2008, 2010.
15. Uranues S, Alimoglu O: Laparoscopic surgery of the spleen. *Surg Clin North Am* 85:75, 2005.
16. Friedman R, Hiatt J, Korman J, et al: Laparoscopic or open splenectomy for hematologic disease: Which approach is superior? *J Am Coll Surg* 185:52, 1997.
17. Heniford BT, Park A, Walsh RM, et al: Laparoscopic splenectomy with normal-sized spleens versus splenomegaly: Does size matter? *Am Surg* 67:854, 2001.
18. Mahon D, Rhodes M: Laparoscopic splenectomy: Size matters. *Ann R Coll Surg Engl* 85:248, 2003.
19. Terrosu G, Baccarani U, Bresadola V, et al: The impact of splenic weight on laparoscopic splenectomy for splenomegaly. *Surg Endosc* 16:103, 2002.
20. Kercher KW, Matthews BD, Walsh RM, et al: Laparoscopic splenectomy for massive splenomegaly. *Am J Surg* 183:192, 2002.
21. Davidson RN, Wall RA: Prevention and management of infections in patients without a spleen. *Clin Microbiol Infect* 7:657, 2001.
22. Recommendations of the Advisory Committee on Immunization Practices (ACIP): Use of vaccines and immune globulins in persons with altered immunocompetence. *Morb Mortal Wkly Rep* 42:4, 1993.
23. Michels NA: The variational anatomy of the spleen and splenic artery. *Am J Anat* 70:21, 1942.
24. Scott-Conner CE: The SAGES manual—fundamentals of laparoscopy and GI endoscopy. In Rege RV, editor: *Laparoscopic splenectomy*. New York, 1999, Springer-Verlag, p 327.
25. Soper NJ: Mastery of endoscopic and laparoscopic surgery. In Poulin EC, editor: *Laparoscopic splenectomy*, ed 2, Philadelphia, 2005, Lippincott Williams & Wilkins, p 374.
26. Skandalakis JE: *Surgical anatomy and technique. Accessory spleens.* New York, 2000, Springer-Verlag, p 621.
27. Barawi M, Bekal P, et al: Accessory spleen: A potential cause of misdiagnosis at EUS. *Gastrointest Endosc* 52:769, 2000.
28. Souba WW, et al: ACS surgery principles and practice. In Poulin EC, Schlachta CM, Mamazza J, editors: *Laparoscopic splenectomy*. New York, 2005, Web MD Professional Publishing, p 578.
29. Borrazzo EC, Daly JM, Morrisey KP, et al: Hand-assisted laparoscopic splenectomy for giant spleens. *Surg Endosc* 17:918, 2003.
30. Pietrabissa A, Moreeli L, Peri A, et al: Laparoscopic treatment for splenomegaly: A case for hand assisted laparoscopic surgery. *Arch Surg* 146:818, 2011.
31. Swanson TW, Meneghetti AT, Sampath S, et al: Hand-assisted laparoscopic splenectomy versus open splenectomy for massive splenomegaly: 20-year experience at a Canadian centre. *Can J Surg* 54:189, 2011.
32. Rottman SJ, Podolsky ER, Kim E, et al: Single port access (SPA) splenectomy. *JSLS* 14:48, 2010.
33. Targarona EM, Pallares JL, Balague C, et al: Single incision approach for splenic diseases: A preliminary report on a series of 8 cases. *Surg Endosc* 24:2236, 2010.
34. Hong TH, Lee SK, You YK, et al: Single-port laparoscopic partial splenectomy: A case report. *Surg Laparosc Endosc Percutan Tech* 20:e164, 2010.
35. Chapman W, Albrecht R, Kim V, et al: Computer-assisted laparoscopic splenectomy with the da Vinci surgical robot. *J Laparoendosc Adv Surg Tech A* 12:155, 2002.
36. Bodner J, Kafka-Ritsch R, Lucciarini P, et al: A critical comparison of robotic versus conventional laparoscopic splenectomies. *World J Surg* 29:982, 2005.
37. Gelmini R, Franzoni C, Spaziani A, et al: Laparoscopic splenectomy: Conventional versus robotic approach—a comparative study. *J Laparoendosc Adv Surg Tech A* 21:393, 2011.
38. Zornig C, Emmermann A, Von Waldenfels HA, et al: Colpotomy for specimen removal in laparoscopic surgery. *Chirurg* 65:883, 1994.
39. Vereczkei A, Illenyi L, Arany A, et al: Transvaginal extraction of the laparoscopically removed spleen. *Surg Endosc* 17:157, 2003.
40. Targarona EM, Gomez C, Rovira R, et al: NOTES-assisted transvaginal splenectomy: The next step in the minimally invasive approach to the spleen. *Surg Innov* 16:218, 2009.
41. Downing MA, Omar AH, Sabri E, et al: Information on the internet for asplenic patients: A systematic review. *Can J Surg* 54:5510, 2011.

42. Casaccia M, Torelli P, Pasa A, et al: Putative predictive parameters for the outcome of laparoscopic splenectomy: A multicenter analysis performed on the Italian Registry of Laparoscopic Surgery of the Spleen. *Ann Surg* 252:287, 2010.

43. Ikeda M, Sekimoto M, Takiguchi S, et al: High incidence of thrombosis of the portal venous system after laparoscopic splenectomy. A prospective study with contrast-enhanced CT scan. *Ann Surg* 241:208, 2005.

44. Harris W, Marcaccio M: Incidence of portal vein thrombosis after laparoscopic splenectomy. *Can J Surg* 48:352, 2005.

45. Ikeda M, Sekimoto M, Takiguchi S, et al: High incidence of thrombosis of the portal venous system after laparoscopic splenectomy: A prospective study with contrast-enhanced CT scan. *Ann Surg* 241:208, 2005.

46. Krauth MT, Lechner K, Neugebauer EA, et al: The postoperative splenic/portal vein thrombosis after splenectomy and its prevention—an unresolved issue. *Haematologica* 93:1227, 2008.

47. Wang H, Kopac D, Brisebois R, et al: Randomized controlled trial to investigate the impact of anticoagulation on the incidence of splenic or portal vein thrombosis after laparoscopic splenectomy. *Can J Surg* 54:227, 2011.

48. van der Vlies CH, Hoekstra J, Ponsen KJ, et al: Impact of splenic artery embolization on the success rate of nonoperative management for blunt splenic injury. *Cardiovasc Intervent Radiol* 35:76, 2012.

49. Ransom KJ, Kavic MS: Laparoscopic splenectomy for blunt trauma: A safe operation following embolization. *Surg Endosc* 23:352, 2009.

50. Reso A, Brar MS, Church N, et al: Outcome of laparoscopic splenectomy with preoperative splenic artery embolization for massive splenectomy. *Surg Endosc* 24:2008, 2010.

51. Jeremitsky E, Kao A, Carlton C, et al: Does splenic embolization and grade of splenic injury impact nonoperative management in patients sustaining blunt splenic trauma? *Am Surg* 77:215, 2011.

52. Franco F, Monaco D, Volpi A, et al: The role of arterial embolization in blunt splenic injury. *Radiol Med* 116:454, 2011.

53. Sclafani SJ, Shaftan GW, Scalea TM, et al: Nonoperative salvage of computed tomography-diagnosed splenic injuries: Utilization of angiography for triage and embolization for hemostasis. *J Trauma* 39:818; discussion 826, 1995.

54. Moore EE, Cogbill TH, Jurkovich GJ, et al: Organ injury scaling: Spleen and liver (1994 revision). *J Trauma* 38:323, 1995.

55. Haan JM, Biffl W, Knudson MM, et al: Splenic embolization revisited: A multicenter review. *J Trauma* 56:542, 2004.

56. Wahl WL, Ahrns KS, Chen S, et al: Blunt splenic injury: Operation versus angiographic embolization. *Surgery* 136:891, 2004.

57. Haan JM, Bochicchio GV, Kramer N, et al: Nonoperative management of blunt splenic injury: A 5-year experience. *J Trauma* 58:492, 2005.

58. Sekikawa Z, Takebayashi S, Kurihara H, et al: Factors affecting clinical outcome of patients who undergo transcatheter arterial embolisation in splenic injury. *Br J Radiol* 77:308, 2004.

59. Brasel KJ, DeLisle CM, Olson CJ, et al: Splenic injury: Trends in evaluation and management. *J Trauma* 44:283, 1998.

60. Gaunt WT, McCarthy MC, Lambert CS, et al: Traditional criteria for observation of splenic trauma should be challenged. *Am Surg* 65:689; discussion 691, 1999.

61. Peitzman AB, Heil B, Rivera L, et al: Blunt splenic injury in adults: Multi-institutional study of the Eastern Association for the Surgery of Trauma. *J Trauma* 49:177; discussion 187, 2000.

62. Lawler LP, Fishman EK: Celiomesenteric anomaly demonstration by multidetector CT and volume rendering. *J Comput Assist Tomogr* 25:802, 2001.

63. Hagiwara A, Murata A, Matsuda T, et al: The usefulness of transcatheter arterial embolization for patients with blunt polytrauma showing transient response to fluid resuscitation. *J Trauma* 57:271; discussion 276, 2004.

64. Liu PP, Lee WC, Cheng YF, et al: Use of splenic artery embolization as an adjunct to nonsurgical management of blunt splenic injury. *J Trauma* 56:768; discussion 773, 2004.

65. Frumiento C, Sartorelli K, Vane D: Complications of splenic injuries: Expansion of the nonoperative theorem. *J Pediatr Surg* 35:788, 2000.

66. Cocanour CS, Moore FA, Ware DN, et al: Delayed complications of nonoperative management of blunt adult splenic trauma. *Arch Surg* 133:619; discussion 624, 1998.

67. Sakai T, Shiraki K, Inoue H, et al: Complications of partial splenic embolization in cirrhotic patients. *Dig Dis Sci* 47:388, 2002.

68. Schnuriger B, Inaba K, Konstantinidis A, et al: Outcomes of proximal versus distal splenic artery embolization after trauma: A systematic review and meta-analysis. *J Trauma* 70:252, 2011.

69. Oller-Sales B, Troya-Diaz J, Martinez-Arconada MJ, et al: Post-traumatic splenic function depending on severity of injury and management. *Trans Res* 158:118, 2011.

70. Goffette PP, Laterre PF: Traumatic injuries: Imaging and intervention in post-traumatic complications (delayed intervention). *Eur Radiol* 12:994, 2002.

71. Tessier DJ, Stone WM, Fowl RJ, et al: Clinical features and management of splenic artery pseudoaneurysm: Case series and cumulative review of literature. *J Vasc Surg* 38:969, 2003.

72. Gorg C, Colle J, Wied M, et al: Spontaneous nontraumatic intrasplenic pseudoaneurysm: Causes, sonographic diagnosis, and prognosis. *J Clin Ultrasound* 31:129, 2003.

73. Yardeni D, Polley TZ Jr, Coran AG: Splenic artery embolization for post-traumatic splenic artery pseudoaneurysm in children. *J Trauma* 57:404, 2004.

74. Arepally A, Dagli M, Hofmann LV, et al: Treatment of splenic artery aneurysm with use of a stent-graft. *J Vasc Interv Radiol* 13:631, 2002.

75. Huang IH, Zuckerman DA, Matthews JB: Occlusion of a giant splenic artery pseudoaneurysm with percutaneous thrombin-collagen injection. *J Vasc Surg* 40:574, 2004.

76. Davis KA, Fabian TC, Croce MA, et al: Improved success in nonoperative management of blunt splenic injuries: Embolization of splenic artery pseudoaneurysms. *J Trauma* 44:1008; discussion 1013, 1998.

77. Kagaya H, Miyata T, Hoshina K, et al: Long-term results of endovascular treatment for splenic artery aneurysms. *Int Angiol* 30:359, 2011.

78. Moghaddam MB, Kalra M, Bjarnason H, et al: Review: Splenic arteriovenous fistula: Successful treatment with an Amplatz occlusion device. *Ann Vasc Surg* 25:556.e17, 2011.

79. Mozes MF, Spigos DG, Pollak R, et al: Partial splenic embolization, an alternative to splenectomy—results of a prospective, randomized study. *Surgery* 96:694, 1984.

80. Nio M, Hayashi Y, Sano N, et al: Long-term efficacy of partial splenic embolization in children. *J Pediatr Surg* 38:1760, 2003.

81. Sakata K, Hirai K, Tanikawa K: A long-term investigation of transcatheter splenic arterial embolization for hypersplenism. *Hepatogastroenterology* 43:309, 1996.

82. Kumpe DA, Rumack CM, Pretorius DH, et al: Partial splenic embolization in children with hypersplenism. *Radiology* 155:357, 1985.

83. Sangro B, Bilbao I, Herrero I, et al: Partial splenic embolization for the treatment of hypersplenism in cirrhosis. *Hepatology* 18:309, 1993.

84. N'Kontchou G, Seror O, Bourcier V, et al: Partial splenic embolization in patients with cirrhosis: Efficacy, tolerance and long-term outcome in 32 patients. *Eur J Gastroenterol Hepatol* 17:179, 2005.

85. Palsson B, Hallen M, Forsberg AM, et al: Partial splenic embolization: Long-term outcome. *Langenbecks Arch Surg* 387:421, 2003.

86. Akhan O, Baykan Z, Oguzkurt L, et al: Percutaneous treatment of a congenital splenic cyst with alcohol: A new therapeutic approach. *Eur Radiol* 7:1067, 1997.

87. Moir C, Guttman F, Jequier S, et al: Splenic cysts: Aspiration, sclerosis, or resection. *J Pediatr Surg* 24:646, 1989.

88. Chou YH, Tiu CM, Chiou HJ, et al: Ultrasound-guided interventional procedures in splenic abscesses. *Eur J Radiol* 28:167, 1998.

89. Green BT: Splenic abscess: Report of six cases and review of the literature. *Am Surg* 67:80, 2001.

90. McInnes MD, Kielar AZ, Macdonald DB.: Percutaneous image-guided biopsy of the spleen: Systematic review and meta-analysis of the complication rate and diagnostic accuracy. *Radiology* 260:699, 2011.

Management of Splenic Trauma in Adults

Amy P. Rushing | Anne Lidor

The spleen, an important component of the reticuloendothelial system in normal adults, is a highly vascular solid organ that arises as a mass of differentiated mesenchymal tissue during early embryonic development. The normal adult spleen weighs between 75 and 100 g and receives an average blood flow of 300 mL/min. It functions as the primary filter of the reticuloendothelial system by sequestering and removing antigens, bacteria, and senescent or damaged cellular elements from the circulation. In addition, the spleen has an important role in humoral immunity as it produces immunoglobulin M and opsonins for the complement activation system.[1]

Although the spleen resides under the confines of the left lower rib cage, it is frequently subject to both blunt and penetrating trauma. Isolated splenic injury after blunt trauma is common in children, whereas the adult trauma population will often sustain associated injuries to the thorax, kidneys, extremities, and head.[2] The mechanism of injury in blunt trauma stems from abrupt deceleration resulting in vascular torsion of the splenic hilum, shearing of the short gastric vessels within the gastrosplenic ligament, or capsular tearing at sites of ligamentous fixation. Clinical features that suggest splenic trauma include left upper quadrant or flank ecchymosis and abrasions as well as left shoulder pain caused by irritation of the left hemidiaphragm by subphrenic blood (Kehr sign). In instances of penetrating trauma, a wound track traversing the left upper quadrant raises the suspicion for splenic injury. Regardless of mechanism, all trauma patients should receive the primary survey followed by the appropriate secondary evaluation and ancillary studies.

Currently, the accepted standard of care for most splenic trauma is expectant management with close observation. Operative intervention is reserved for the hemodynamically labile patient who shows signs of active hemorrhage and who does not respond appropriately to fluid resuscitation. While these clinical scenarios seem straightforward, it is often the condition of the patient who falls in between the two ends of the spectrum that can be the most challenging to manage. In the setting of advanced imaging techniques and interventional radiology, the trauma surgeon has more diagnostic information as well as more treatment options for the patient with splenic trauma.

DIAGNOSIS

Patients who present with evidence of ongoing intraabdominal hemorrhage should undergo immediate operative exploration. For those who present with normal hemodynamics, a thorough diagnostic evaluation should be performed. Following the primary survey, a focused abdominal examination should be performed looking for signs of significant intraabdominal injuries: abdominal wall ecchymosis, abrasions, flank pain, and distention should raise suspicion for an injury and prompt further diagnostic workup. Additionally, the patient who presents with left-sided rib fractures should also be evaluated for a concomitant splenic laceration.

A laboratory panel should be sent to obtain an index hemoglobin and hematocrit, platelet count, and coagulation profile. While in the emergency department, the focused abdominal sonography for trauma (FAST) exam offers a rapid and noninvasive approach to detecting intraperitoneal blood. The sensitivity of FAST has been reported between 42% and 93%, whereas its specificity ranges in various reports between 90% and 98%.[3] The primary limitations of FAST are the heavy operator dependence of the ultrasonographic exam as well as the technical limitations caused by the patient's body habitus or intestinal gas. In spite of these obstacles, the FAST exam is helpful in the preliminary evaluation of the patient, especially when the patient cannot undergo further imaging because of hemodynamic instability.

Unlike ultrasonography, computed tomography (CT) has dramatically changed the way we characterize splenic injuries. The CT scan is the diagnostic modality of choice for the hemodynamically stable patient in whom a splenic injury is suspected. The sensitivity and specificity of CT imaging approaches 100% and 98%, respectively.[4] Current-generation multislice scanners provide a detailed survey of the splenic architecture and allow the clinician to differentiate simple subcapsular hematomas from more severe parenchymal and vascular injuries. CT imaging has become such an integral part of the management of splenic trauma that certain radiographic features are starting to guide treatment algorithms. This will be described later in the chapter.

Several grading systems have been employed for classifying splenic injuries and these have important implications in both the operative and nonoperative management decisions. The Organ Injury Scaling Committee of the American Association for the Surgery of Trauma (OISC-AAST) devised an anatomic grading system that defines the severity of splenic injuries. The system incorporates both CT scan findings and intraoperative assessment of the spleen and consists of five grades (Table 134-1). This grading scale provides universal definitions that all clinicians can understand and it becomes particularly useful when a patient requires transfer to a tertiary trauma center from an acute care hospital as the severity of injury is readily appreciated. Although the trauma community recognizes that the primary predictor of operative intervention is hemodynamic instability, the organ

TABLE 134-1 Splenic Injury Scale: 1994 Revision[1]

Grade and Type of Injury	Injury Description
I Hematoma	Subcapsular, <10% surface area
Laceration	Capsular tear, <1 cm parenchymal depth
II Hematoma	Subcapsular, 10%-50% surface area; intraparenchymal, <5 cm diameter
Laceration	1-3 cm parenchymal depth, does not involve trabecular vessel
III Hematoma	Subcapsular, >50% surface area or expanding; ruptured subcapsular or parenchymal hematoma; intraparenchymal hematoma ≥5 cm or expanding
Laceration	>3 cm parenchymal depth or involving trabecular vessels
IV Laceration	Laceration involving hilar vessels producing >25% devascularization of spleen
V Laceration	Completely shattered spleen
Vascular	Hilar vascular injury, spleen devascularized

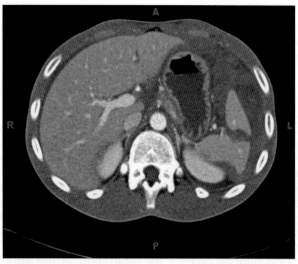

FIGURE 134-1 CT scan of the abdomen featuring grade V splenic laceration with hilar injury and large hemoperitoneum.

injury severity scale can also serve as a predictor of further therapeutic intervention. Haan et al reported a splenic salvage rate of 94% over a 5-year period; however, they found that the salvage rate decreased with increased splenic injury grade.[5]

NONOPERATIVE MANAGEMENT

The increased availability of high-resolution CT scan and advances in arterial angiography and embolization techniques have contributed to the success of nonoperative management of splenic injuries. The hemodynamically stable patient with blunt splenic trauma can be adequately managed with bed rest, serial abdominal exams, and hemoglobin and hematocrit monitoring. This approach, in combination with occasional angiography, confers a splenic salvage rate of up to 90%.[6] In the setting of expectant management, indications for angiography have been delineated by several studies and include the following CT scan features: contrast extravasation, the presence of a pseudoaneurysm, significant hemoperitoneum, high-grade injury (Figure 134-1), and evidence of a vascular injury.[7] The goal of angiography is to localize bleeding and embolize the source with coils or a gelatin foam product. Embolization can occur either at the main splenic artery just distal to the dorsal pancreatic portion of the vessel—known as proximal embolization—or selectively at the distal branch of the injured vessel. The goal behind the former technique is to decrease the perfusion pressure to the spleen to encourage hemostasis. The disadvantage to this technique is global splenic ischemia, and many have questioned the spleen's immunocompetence following proximal embolization. Malhotra et al recently examined the effects of angioembolization on splenic function by looking at serum levels of a particular T-cell line. This preliminary study

compared T-cell proportions between patients who had undergone splenic embolization with asplenic patients and healthy controls. The data suggest that the patients who underwent embolization maintained splenic immunocompetency as they had T cells that are only present among individuals with normal splenic function.[8] A Norwegian study comparing blood samples from patients who had undergone angioembolization with healthy controls demonstrated that the study samples had similar levels of pneumococcal immunoglobulins and no Howell-Jolly bodies suggesting normal splenic function.[9] While these preliminary studies remain encouraging, there is no definitive evidence that splenic immunocompetency is fully maintained following angioembolization.

There is no question that advancements in interventional techniques have contributed to the successful nonoperative management of splenic injuries. This has certainly changed the strategy, but it has not completely replaced operative intervention. The challenge now remains predicting those patients who will ultimately require splenectomy. Many groups have studied potential predictors of nonoperative failure. Earlier studies found that a higher injury grade, increased transfusion requirement, and hypotension on initial presentation consistently predicted failure of nonoperative management. More recent literature reflects the use of advanced imaging techniques for predicting which patients will ultimately require splenectomy. Haan looked at the overall outcomes of patients admitted with blunt splenic trauma and reported several radiographic findings that were prevalent among patients requiring splenectomy after angioembolization: contrast extravasation, pseudoaneurysm, significant hemoperitoneum, and arteriovenous fistula. Among these characteristics, an arteriovenous fistula had the highest rate of nonoperative failure at 40%.[10] Aside from radiographic findings, some groups have also examined the mechanism of injury and its association with nonoperative failure. Plurad et al conducted a retrospective review over a 15-year period and found that patients who were victims of blunt assault were more likely to fail nonoperative management: 36%

of these patients required splenectomy versus 11.5% of patients from all other mechanisms combined. These findings suggest that regardless of overall injury severity, individuals who sustain a direct transfer of injury to the left torso are more likely to require splenectomy.[11]

OPERATIVE MANAGEMENT

When a patient presents with hemodynamic lability in spite of timely resuscitation, operative intervention remains the most prudent course of treatment. In this situation, standard principles of trauma care are followed: the patient should have reliable intravenous access, appropriate volume resuscitation, preparation of type and crossmatched packed red blood cells, nasogastric decompression, and preoperative intravenous antibiotic administration. It is standard practice to utilize a vertical midline incision for laparotomy as this affords the quickest access to the peritoneal cavity. If this incision proves to be insufficient, it can be extended cephalad and to the left of the xiphoid process. Additionally, the left triangular ligament of the liver may be incised to allow reflection of the liver away from the area of interest. While it may seem practical, an oblique left upper quadrant incision for a presumed isolated splenic injury is more time-consuming and offers little access to the remainder of the peritoneal cavity should a concomitant injury present itself.

After entering the peritoneal cavity, a standard initial survey should be performed. All four quadrants should be packed and systematically inspected for bleeding or enteric contamination. If other injuries are recognized and require more urgent attention, one can achieve adequate hemostasis of the spleen with proper packing. Multiple laparotomy tapes should be placed around the splenic parenchyma in such a manner that a tamponade effect is maintained between the diaphragm, lateral abdominal wall, and retroperitoneum. When it is time to address the injury, mobilization is achieved by placing laparotomy tapes posterior to the spleen and lifting it directly into the operative field. Following its inspection, the spleen's ligamentous attachments to the diaphragm, kidney, and colon should be sharply incised. These connections are avascular and can be divided with impunity in most circumstances. The spleen can then be rotated to the midline and further elevated, thus enabling complete access to its anterior and posterior surfaces as well as to the hilum. Once accomplished, the operator can easily achieve virtually complete hemostasis of any splenic injury by direct manual compression of the splenic parenchyma or by control of the splenic artery and vein at the hilum. At this point, a decision is made regarding splenectomy or splenorrhaphy.

Once the spleen has been fully mobilized, one may proceed with splenectomy by first individually ligating and dividing the short gastric vessels. These vessels should be addressed far from the greater curvature of the stomach so that the risk of gastric wall necrosis is minimized. As the short gastric vessels are divided and the splenic hilum is skeletonized, one must pay attention to the tail of the pancreas. Careless technique can result in disruption of the pancreatic capsule and the development of a pancreatic fistula with subsequent morbidity. Following the division of the short gastric vessels, the splenic artery is then doubly ligated and divided within the splenic hilum. The splenic vein is dealt with in the same manner and the splenectomy is completed. After removal of the spleen, the splenic bed should be thoroughly irrigated and inspected for hemostasis. These steps are essential to minimize the chances of postoperative splenic bed hematoma, which in turn predisposes to the risk of a subphrenic abscess. Although there are no conclusive data regarding the use of closed-suction drains in the surgical bed, we do not routinely drain the splenic fossa following splenectomy. Meticulous hemostasis tends to be the best method in avoiding splenic bed complications.

The term *splenorrhaphy* refers to a variety of "spleen-sparing" techniques aimed at controlling hemorrhage so that the patient may retain the immunologic benefits of the spleen. The intraoperative decision to attempt splenorrhaphy should be made only after the spleen has been fully mobilized and inspected.[12,13] As a general rule, splenorrhaphy is most appropriately considered in cases of less severe injury (e.g., grades I and II, and occasionally grade III). Splenorrhaphy should not be attempted to repair extensive or complex injuries of the spleen, nor is it well advised to undertake splenorrhaphy in the face of multiple concomitant injuries or associated hypotension. With the spleen fully mobilized and controlled in the surgeon's hand, splenorrhaphy may consist of mere manual compression of the parenchyma to achieve hemostasis of simple lacerations. In addition, there are a variety of topical hemostatic agents that may be applied directly to the bleeding parenchymal surface. Other options include suture repair of the spleen using a monofilament suture in a mattress technique, where one can also incorporate a piece of omentum or gelatin sponge product into the repair. Alternatively, wrapping the entire spleen in absorbable mesh has been described as a means of effective tamponade and has not been associated with a significant increase in infectious complications.[13] Examining splenic salvage rates over a 9-year period, Feliciano et al found that the majority of splenorrhaphy cases were accomplished with simple techniques and less than 10% required a mesh wrap. In this series, the incidence of rebleeding was 1.3%.[14]

POSTOPERATIVE CONSIDERATIONS

Overwhelming postsplenectomy sepsis (OPSS), first described by Diamond in 1969, is an infrequent but potentially catastrophic complication of splenectomy resulting from an increased susceptibility to infection by encapsulated microorganisms.[15] Although the precise incidence of OPSS is not well defined, one retrospective review of 5902 postsplenectomy patients studied between 1952 and 1987 documented an incidence of OPSS of 4.4% in children less than 16 years of age and 0.9% in adults.[16] Schwartz et al estimated the risk of developing fulminant sepsis following splenectomy to be just 1 case per 500 person-years of observation; however, the cumulative incidence of infections requiring hospitalization was 33% over a 10-year period.[17] Early reports of OPSS indicated mortality rates of 50% to 70% in spite of the use of intravenous antibiotics and intensive therapeutic intervention. With advances in antibiotic therapy and intensive care, the mortality rate of OPSS can be expected to be approximately 10%, with more than half of all fatalities occurring within 48 hours of presentation.[1,18] Given these findings, it is a widely accepted practice to immunize patients with pneumococcal vaccine shortly after undergoing emergency splenectomy prior to discharge from the hospital.[19] The efficacy and clinical importance of meningococcal and *Haemophilus influenzae* type b vaccination in splenectomized individuals is unknown, but should be considered in patients who are deemed more likely to encounter these organisms.[19] We typically administer all three of the vaccines to patients undergoing emergency splenectomy. Although these patients should take all necessary precautions to avoid serious infections, prophylactic antibiotics are not thought to be necessary following splenectomy in adults.[20]

REFERENCES

1. Lynch AM, Kapila R: Overwhelming postsplenectomy infection. *Infect Dis Clin North Am* 10:693, 1996.
2. Miller PR, Croce MA, Bee TK, et al: Associated injuries in blunt solid organ trauma: Implications for missed injury in nonoperative management. *J Trauma* 53:238, 2002.
3. Rozycki GS, Ballard RB, Feliciano DV, et al: Surgeon-performed ultrasound for the assessment of truncal injuries: Lessons learned from 1540 patients. *Ann Surg* 228:557, 1998.
4. Wing VW, Federle MP, Morris JA Jr, et al: The clinical impact of CT for blunt abdominal trauma. *AJR Am J Roentgenol* 145:1191, 1985.
5. Haan JM, Bochicchio GV, Kramer N, et al: Nonoperative management of blunt splenic injury: A 5-year experience. *J Trauma* 58:492, 2005.
6. Renzulli P, Gross T, Schnurger B, et al: Management of blunt injuries to the spleen. *Br J Surg* 97:1696, 2010.
7. Haan JM, Biffl W, Knudson MM, et al: Splenic embolization revisited: A multicenter review. *J Trauma* 56:542, 2004.
8. Malhotra AK, Carter RF, Lebman DA, et al: Preservation of splenic immunocompetence after splenic artery angioembolization for blunt splenic injury. *J Trauma* 69:1126, 2010.
9. Skattum J, Titze TL, Dormagen JB, et al: Preserved splenic function after angioembolisation of high grade injury. *Injury* 2010 July 29 [Epub ahead of print].
10. Haan JM, Bochicchio GV, Kramer N, et al: Nonoperative management of blunt splenic injury: A 5-year experience. *J Trauma* 58:492, 2005.
11. Plurad DS, Green DJ, Inaba K, et al: Blunt assault is associated with failure of nonoperative management of the spleen independent of organ injury grade and despite lower overall injury severity. *J Trauma* 66:630, 2009.
12. Berry MF, Rosato EF, Williams NN: Dexon mesh splenorrhaphy for intraoperative splenic injuries. *Am Surg* 69:176, 2003.
13. Pachter HL, Hofstetter SR, Spencer FC: Evolving concepts in splenic surgery: Splenorrhaphy versus splenectomy and postsplenectomy drainage—experience in 105 patients. *Ann Surg* 194:262, 1981.
14. Feliciano DV, Spjut-Patrinely V, Burch JM, et al: Splenorrhaphy—the alternative. *Ann Surg* 211:569, 1990.
15. Diamond LK: Splenectomy in childhood and the hazard of overwhelming infection. *Pediatrics* 43:886, 1969.
16. Holdsworth RJ, Irving AD, Cuschieri A: Postsplenectomy sepsis and its mortality rate: Actual versus perceived risks. *Br J Surg* 78:1031, 1991.
17. Schwartz PE, Sterioff S, Mucha P, et al: Postsplenectomy sepsis and mortality in adults. *JAMA* 248:2279, 1982.
18. Brigden ML, Pattullo AL: Prevention and management of overwhelming postsplenectomy infection—an update. *Crit Care Med* 27:836, 1999.
19. Shatz DV: Vaccination practices among North American trauma surgeons in splenectomy for trauma. *J Trauma* 53:950, 2002.
20. Guidelines for the prevention and treatment of infection in patients with an absent or dysfunctional spleen. Working Party of the British Committee for Standards in Haematology Clinical Haematology Task Force. *BMJ* 312:430, 1996.

Management of Splenic Trauma in Children

Mindy B. Statter | Donald C. Liu

To quote the book of Jewish mysticism Zohar (3:234), "the spleen produces laughter in children." Perhaps it is not a coincidence that according to the Midrash (Ecclesiastes Rabbah 7:19), the spleen is among the "ten organs that minister to the soul" because of its relationship to laughter.[1] Yet far beyond its abstract significance, the spleen is clinically not an expendable organ. The immunologic importance of the spleen became evident in cases of overwhelming postsplenectomy sepsis, leading to the trend to preserve the spleen, particularly in children. In 1952, King and Shumacher reported two deaths among five infants who developed severe sepsis following splenectomy for hereditary spherocytosis.[2] Evaluations of "quality-adjusted life expectancy" for management strategies after blunt splenic trauma, including the options of observation, splenorrhaphy, and splenectomy, have shown a decreased life expectancy for patients undergoing splenectomy.[3] In light of these studies and the observation that bleeding from splenic injuries ceases by the time of laparotomy, the treatment of children with blunt splenic injuries evolved from routine splenectomy to splenic preservation. Upadayaya and Simpson pioneered selective nonoperative management of splenic injuries in children sustaining blunt trauma.[4] Since that time, nonoperative management is now the standard of care, with success rates of nonoperative management of blunt splenic injuries exceeding 90% in children. This chapter will review the relevance of splenic anatomy to the management of traumatic injury, the evaluation of the child with blunt splenic injury, operative and nonoperative management of splenic injury in the child, and the ongoing controversies regarding the necessity of followup imaging, and timing of return to play. Despite the development of consensus guidelines for children with blunt splenic injuries, there remains significant practice variation in the care of the pediatric trauma patient with splenic injury.

SPLEEN ANATOMY AND ITS RELEVANCE TO MANAGEMENT OF TRAUMATIC INJURY

The unique segmental arterial inflow and venous drainage of the spleen permits repair and resection of the injured spleen. Corrosion casts of human splenic arterial trees demonstrated a superior and an inferior splenic segment in 84% of specimens and a superior, middle, and inferior segment in 16% of specimens (Figure 135-1). These arterial segments are separated by avascular planes. The avascular plane of separation passes obliquely relative to the longitudinal axis of the spleen and often does not traverse the full thickness of the spleen from the parietal to visceral surfaces. The same segmental pattern has been observed in the venous drainage. Doubly injected (arteries and veins) specimens confirmed that neither the arterial supply nor the venous supply to segments crossed to adjacent parenchyma. Intrasplenic vessels are lobar, segmented, and generally without intersegmental communication according to Dixon et al. These authors divided the spleen into three-dimensional cones with hilar, intermediate, and peripheral zones with each zone requiring a specific technique for hemostasis. Bleeding from the peripheral zone may be managed with topical agents, and ligation is recommended for the trabecular and segmental vessels in the intermediate and hilar zones (Figure 135-2).[5,6]

The splenic capsule in children is relatively thicker than that of the adult and contains abundant myoepithelial cells that favor hemostatic control of hemorrhage.[7] The lack of atherosclerosis confers greater vascular compliance, with greater contraction leading to more effective hemostasis. Lower rib fractures are commonly associated with splenic injuries in adults; the broken terminus of the rib penetrates the splenic capsule. In contrast, the ribs of children have greater elasticity and after deformation due to a traumatic force will recoil rather than fracture, reducing the risk of penetrating the spleen.[8]

EVALUATION OF SPLENIC TRAUMA IN THE CHILD

Evaluation of the pediatric trauma patient proceeds systematically as outlined by Advanced Trauma Life Support, prioritizing the assessment and management of the airway, breathing, and circulation.[9] The sequential assessment and maintenance of airway patency, adequacy of gas exchange, and perfusion are the priorities of resuscitation, preventing and/or correcting hypoxemia due to inadequate oxygen delivery. Many children with abdominal injuries have either equivocal or absent physical findings; the overall accuracy of initial physical examination varies from 16% to 45%. Root, in 1965, developed diagnostic peritoneal lavage (DPL) in adults to supplement the physical examination; DPL served as a means to reliably detect or exclude peritoneal injury. A DPL positive for blood indicates the presence of hemoperitoneum without identifying the source of the blood. Although it has a greater than 95% reported accuracy, DPL has a number of limitations, including invasiveness, nonspecificity, and the frequent overestimation of trivial injuries that did not require laparotomy. These limitations are magnified in children. Because many solid organ injuries

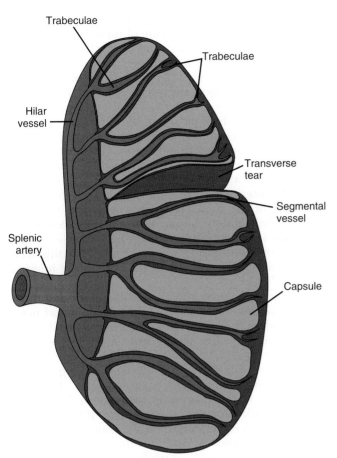

FIGURE 135-1 Diagram of segmental splenic vasculature.

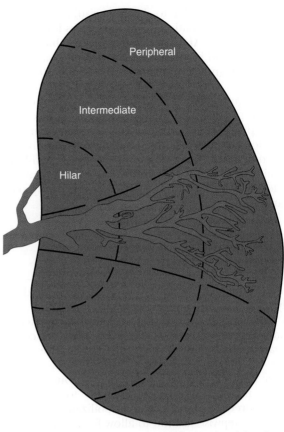

FIGURE 135-2 Diagram of hilar, intermediate, and peripheral zones.

may be successfully managed nonoperatively in children, the presence of blood in the abdomen is not an indication for operation in the hemodynamically stable child. DPL provides no information regarding the retroperitoneum. It is apparent that reliance on physical examination alone is an inadequate evaluation of the child with potential abdominal injury. Diagnostic adjuncts in the assessment of abdominal trauma include focused assessment sonography in trauma (FAST) and computed tomography (CT). CT scanning has been the standard of care for the evaluation of the peritoneal cavity and retroperitoneum. To obtain maximal information regarding organ perfusion, presence of free intraperitoneal fluid, and the characteristics of the bowel, intravenous contrast is recommended. There is a direct correlation between the severity of the isolated injury and the likelihood and volume of associated free fluid.[10] FAST is limited in that it does not identify the injured organ or the quality of the intraperitoneal fluid (blood, succus, urine). In a systematic review and metaanalysis of the test performance of ultrasonography in the identification of intraabdominal injuries in children sustaining blunt trauma, abdominal ultrasound has a modest sensitivity in the detection of hemoperitoneum (66%). A negative ultrasound examination has questionable utility as the sole diagnostic test to rule out intraabdominal injuries in the pediatric trauma patient.[11] In algorithms for the management of blunt abdominal injuries in pediatric trauma

patients, if the patient is hemodynamically unstable, the child undergoes immediate surgical exploration. If the patient responds to resuscitation, the patient then undergoes definitive diagnostic imaging with CT.

Although CT is an essential imaging modality in children, there is an obligatory exposure to ionizing radiation during this examination. Ionizing radiation has been demonstrated to increase the risk of cancer in individuals exposed to high doses of radiation. The 2005 Biologic Effects of Ionizing Radiation (BEIR) IV Report of the National Academy of Sciences summarizes risk estimates for cancer from exposure to low-level ionizing radiation. The BEIR IV concludes that "current scientific evidence is consistent with the hypothesis that, at the low doses of interest in this report, there is a linear dose relationship between exposure to ionizing radiation and the development of solid cancers in humans.[12] For a given dose, there are several reasons for the difference in cancer risk from radiation exposure in children compared to adults. Tissues and organs that are growing and developing are more sensitive to radiation effects than mature tissue. The oncologic effect of radiation may have a longer latent period, for example, decades, and this latent period varies with the type of malignancy. An infant or child has a longer life expectancy during which to manifest the potential oncologic effects of radiation compared to the adult. The radiation exposure from a fixed set of CT parameters results in relatively higher dose for a child's smaller cross-sectional area compared to the adult. In order to decrease radiation exposure, radiologists use radiation doses that are as low as reasonably achievable (ALARA), which means that no more radiation should be used than is required to achieve the necessary diagnostic information and to perform these studies only when they are necessary. The potential benefit from an indicated CT scan is clinically recognized and is far greater than the potential cancer risk.[13]

The presence of intraperitoneal blood on CT or FAST does not necessarily mandate exploration. Bleeding from solid organ injury is generally self-limited. Overall, less than 10% of children with solid organ injury and less than 15% of those with hemoperitoneum require laparotomy.

OPERATIVE MANAGEMENT INCLUDING LAPAROSCOPY

Operative management is indicated in the hemodynamically unstable child and in those children with a packed red blood cell transfusion requirement exceeding 40 mL/kg, and in those children with concomitant intraabdominal injury. The goal of operative management is splenic preservation. Laparotomy for blunt splenic injury is generally performed through an upper midline incision allowing accessibility to other potentially injured organs. Splenic mobilization should be done in a stepwise fashion to allow for adequate inspection of the spleen while minimizing the chance of increased injury. With splenic trauma, hematoma has generally dissected the ligamentous attachments and rapid delivery of the spleen into the wound is facilitated. The first step in mobilizing the spleen is to divide the lateral attachments, the splenophrenic and splenorenal ligaments. The spleen and tail of the pancreas are then delivered as a unit from lateral to medial. The short gastric vessels are then divided; because of the dual blood supply of the spleen, it is possible to divide the short gastric vessels without compromising splenic viability. The final step in splenic mobilization is the division of the splenocolic ligament. The spleen is then inspected in its entirety and a decision is then made regarding splenic preservation (splenorrhaphy) versus splenectomy. The factors in this decision include the degree of splenic injury, the overall condition of the patient, and the presence of associated injuries. Small lacerations can be managed by compression and topical application of hemostatic agents such as oxidized regenerated cellulose, absorbable gelatin sponge (plain or saturated with thrombin), or microfibrillar collagen. Tissue adhesives such as fibrin glue are another adjunct for topical hemostasis. Hemorrhage from exposed areas of splenic parenchyma can be controlled using electrocautery. Arcing the current onto the spleen is generally more effective because the cautery tip when directly applied becomes adherent and pulls away tissue, deepening the injury as the cautery tip is withdrawn. The argon beam coagulator is effective in controlling hemorrhage from larger oozing raw surface. Severe disruptions of the splenic parenchyma with intact capsule can be managed with absorbable sutures that traverse the capsule and incorporate the

parenchyma; use of pledgets to buttress the repair is recommended in adults because of their thinner splenic capsule. Omentum can be sutured over the raw surface of the spleen or packed into a defect. Partial splenectomy is possible because of the segmental nature of the splenic blood supply. Wrapping the spleen with absorbable mesh is another technique. The most common complication after splenorrhaphy is persistent bleeding or rebleeding. Splenectomy is generally performed with a technique of mobilization and dissection down to an ultimate pedicle of splenic artery and vein. After splenectomy, hemostasis is checked in a specific fashion assessing three major areas: the inferior surface of the diaphragm, the greater curvature of the stomach and the region of the short gastric vessels, and the hilum. Autotransplantation is controversial; reports of overwhelming postsplenectomy sepsis after autotransplantation suggest that this technique is not universally successful in restoring immune function.[14,15]

Emergency laparoscopy is a safe diagnostic and therapeutic modality in the management of blunt and penetrating abdominal injuries in the hemodynamically stable child. A retrospective review from a level 1 pediatric trauma center database over a 5-year interval reported 113 children with abdominal injuries requiring exploration; 32 (28%) underwent laparoscopy. In this study, laparoscopy had a diagnostic accuracy of 100%, and avoided nontherapeutic laparotomy in 40%, and laparotomy in 57% of patients. Over the course of the study, a greater proportion of patients who required operative intervention (20 to 29 annually) underwent laparoscopy.[16] Therapeutic laparoscopic splenic salvage with delivery and application of fibrin glue[17] and collagen fleece-bound sealants in the management of blunt splenic injury has been reported.[18]

NONOPERATIVE MANAGEMENT

Wesson et al described one of the first algorithms for nonoperative management of blunt splenic injuries in children with the decision to operate based on physical examination, for example, increased abdominal girth, hemodynamic instability, or decreasing hematocrit. They found that the need for operative intervention was apparent within 16 hours; those patients demonstrating ongoing bleeding with a transfusion requirement of 40 mL/kg of blood within 24 hours of injury also required operative intervention.[19-21] Nonoperative management, by a surgical team, has become the standard of care for solid organ injury in the hemodynamically stable child, with success rates greater than 90%. Disparities in practice patterns were noted among physicians caring for children with solid organ injury.[22,23] In 1998, the American Pediatric Surgery Association (APSA) Trauma Committee defined evidence-based guidelines for resource utilization in hemodynamically stable children with isolated liver or spleen injury based on multiinstitutional data analysis. Clinical guidelines were stratified according to CT grade of injury[24] (Table 135-1). These guidelines were prospectively applied from 1998 to 2000 at 16 centers in 312 children with isolated liver and spleen injuries treated nonoperatively, resulting in validation of

TABLE 135-1	Spleen Injury Scale (1994 Revision)	
Grade	Injury Type	Description of Injury
I	Hematoma	Subcapsular, <10% surface area
	Laceration	Capsular tear, <1 cm parenchymal depth
II	Hematoma	Subcapsular, 10%-50% surface area intraparenchymal, <5 cm in diameter
	Laceration	Capsular tear, 1-3 cm parenchymal depth that does not involve a trabecular vessel
III	Hematoma	Subcapsular, >50% surface area or expanding; ruptured subcapsular or parenchymal hematoma; intraparenchymal hematoma ≥5 cm or expanding
	Laceration	>3 cm parenchymal depth or involving trabecular vessels
IV	Laceration	Laceration involving segmental or hilar vessels producing major devascularization (>25% of spleen)
V	Laceration	Completely shattered spleen
	Vascular	Hilar vascular injury with devascularized spleen

From Moore EE, Cogbill TH, Jurkovich GJ, et al: Organ injury scaling: Spleen and liver (1994 revision). *J Trauma* 38:323, 1995.

guideline safety, conformity in patient management, and improved resource utilization.[25] Implementation of the guidelines also resulted in significant reductions in intensive care unit stay, length of hospital stay, postdischarge imaging, and length of activity restrictions without adverse consequences. These studies support the concept that the physiologic response to resuscitation is more important than the radiologic findings.

Subsequent to the development of the guidelines, there has been discussion that nonoperative management of solid organ injury in children be based on physiologic rather than radiologic parameters. The contraindication to nonoperative management is hemodynamic instability unresponsive to fluid and blood resuscitation or the presence of associated injuries requiring laparotomy. Grade of injury and volume of hemoperitoneum correlate with injury severity but do not necessarily correlate with the need for immediate operative intervention or failure of nonoperative management. Mehall et al prospectively applied a standardized management algorithm for hemodynamically stable children with isolated blunt liver or spleen injury and showed that the hemodynamically stable child did not require intensive care unit monitoring or prolonged hospitalization. They concluded that the management of pediatric solid organ injury should be based on hemodynamic stability rather than CT grade of organ injury.[26] This center retrospectively reviewed the utilization of this protocol over a 5-year interval and concluded that the nonoperative management of children with isolated splenic injuries, based on the physiologic response to resuscitation and hemodynamic status of the patient, is not only safe but results in decreased hospital length of

stay compared with the current guidelines.[27] An abbreviated protocol for the management of blunt splenic injuries recommends that the number of days of bed rest equal the grade of injury plus 1 for grade 1 and 2 injuries and two additional days for higher grades, with the exception of grade 5 injuries. It was projected that implementation of the abbreviated protocol would have affected 65.8% of their patients and would have saved a mean of 2.0 ± 1.5 hospital days per patient.[28] The Hospital for Sick Children in Toronto, where nonoperative management was first proposed in 1948, summarized their five-decade institutional experience. Four eras were reviewed—1956-1965, 1972-1977, 1981-1986, and 1992-2006—for demographics, injury patterns, management, and complications. Their review included 486 patients with blunt splenic injury; an increase in the number of blunt splenic injuries observed per year is likely related to the centralization of pediatric trauma care to their hospital in the 1980s and 1990s. The proportion of patients being managed nonoperatively increased to 99% in the most recent era. The mortality rate and the use of blood products have steadily decreased through the series. The observed decrease in hospital stay was attributed not only to surgeon comfort but additionally to resource restraints with a mean length of stay of 5 days.[29]

Hemodynamic instability in the child being managed nonoperatively for a blunt splenic injury has been an indication for blood transfusion and operative intervention. The need for blood products with the attendant risk of posttransfusion hepatitis and its sequelae is the compelling reason to choose splenectomy over nonoperative therapy. One of the criticisms of nonoperative management was the potential for increased utilization of blood transfusions with the inherent risks of transmission of infection (hepatitis and human immunodeficiency virus). Patients managed nonoperatively require less transfusion of blood products compared to those managed surgically; those children being managed nonoperatively who required transfusion often had multiple injuries. This aspect of management may reflect that over time pediatric surgeons have become more comfortable managing solid organ injury, particularly blunt splenic injuries. Routine blood transfusion in order to maintain an arbitrary optimum hematocrit level has also declined.[26,30,31]

Nonoperative management has also been successful in the multiply injured child with splenic injury, and other injuries remote from the abdomen. Even multiply injured patients with unreliable abdominal examinations and altered mental status may be candidates for nonoperative management. Multiply injured patients who failed nonoperative management demonstrated sufficient evidence of ongoing intraabdominal blood loss with a decreasing hematocrit despite blood transfusion or unexplained hypotension.[32] Studies have not substantiated concerns regarding missing intraabdominal injuries.[33] There is no indication for operative intervention, exploratory laparotomy, to avoid missing potential associated injuries. There are no absolute contraindications to nonoperative management of blunt solid organ injury in the hemodynamically stable child with a concomitant closed head injury.[34] In theory, head injury may complicate the management of children with blunt solid organ injury because the altered level of consciousness results in an unreliable abdominal examination. With head trauma and the release of tissue thromboplastin from damaged neuronal tissue, there is the theoretical concern of possible coagulopathy and increased transfusion requirement. However, hemorrhagic hypotension worsens neurologic outcome. Using the guidelines for the medical management of acute traumatic brain injury in infants, children, and adolescents and the definition of hypotension (systolic blood pressure <5th percentile), a retrospective study showed that hypotension occurring during the early period (<6 hours after traumatic brain injury) may be more detrimental than hypotension occurring later in the course, representing a critical period on the resuscitation of the patient with traumatic brain injury and associated injuries.[35]

Another area of controversy in the nonoperative management of children with splenic injury is the length and type of activity restriction after hospital discharge and the indication and need for followup imaging. Pranikoff et al reported CT-demonstrated complete healing 6 weeks after injury in 10 of 13 (77%) grade I and grade II injuries, but in only 1 of 12 (8%) grade III, IV, or V injuries managed nonoperatively. The 6-week followup CT showed disappearance of the majority of splenic fractures and reperfusion of previously nonperfused regions of the spleen. They recommended 3 months of restricted activity for all patients without followup CT scan evaluation. In those patients with grade I and II injuries, followup CT scan demonstrating injury resolution at 6 weeks would allow resumption of full activities.[36] Lynch et al prospectively evaluated the role of serial ultrasounds in assessing healing in CT-demonstrated splenic injuries managed nonoperatively. Baseline ultrasonographies were obtained on the day prior to discharge, and then at 4- to 6-week intervals until complete homogeneity of the splenic tissue was observed without residual defect or fluid. Mean time to ultrasound healing of grade I, II, III, and IV injuries was 3.1, 8.2, 12.1, and 20.7 weeks, respectively. They concluded that the time to radiographic healing was proportional to the severity of the CT-graded splenic injury.[37] Radiographic evidence of healing does not necessarily correlate with histopathologic healing.

There are no definite data to suggest a correlation between the initial grade of splenic injury and the incidence of long-term complications. Nonoperative management of pediatric blunt splenic injury is associated with minimal complications. In a series of 228 patients with blunt splenic injury, and a mean followup of 5 years, there was a 0.44% incidence of long-term complications. In this cohort of patients, 18% of grade II, 27% of grade III, and 13% of grade IV injured patients returned to full activity earlier than the APSA guidelines recommended, suggesting that prolonged periods of restricted activity (e.g., 6 months or greater) is not necessary.[38] The incidence of delayed complications (e.g., splenic artery pseudoaneurysms, splenic abscesses, and delayed bleeding) ranges from 0% to 7.5%.[39] Splenic artery pseudoaneurysms appear as actively bleeding intraparenchymal hematomas seen as a contrast blush on CT scan and can

be detected by Doppler ultrasound. In adults, a significant proportion of these pseudoaneurysms are thought to expand and rupture. The incidence of splenic artery pseudoaneurysm appears to be lower in children with greater likelihood of spontaneous resolution attributed to self-tamponade and thrombosis. The severity of the splenic injury does not have predictive value for the development of splenic artery pseudoaneurysms in children.[40] Interventional radiology may represent an adjunct to the nonoperative management algorithm of blunt splenic trauma in children. Splenic artery embolization in the management of splenic artery pseudoaneurysm is an alternative to observation, in light of the potential risk of rupture, versus splenectomy.[41] Delayed splenic bleeding was defined by McIndoe in 1931[42] as hemorrhage from a ruptured spleen occurring more than 48 hours after trauma but remains a controversial entity, it being difficult to differentiate between true delayed ruptures and delayed presentation of acute injuries. In a retrospective 14-year review of a single center's series of 303 consecutive blunt splenic injuries in children managed nonoperatively, the incidence of delayed splenic bleeding was 0.33% (1/303). The authors' review of the literature found 14 cases of delayed splenic bleeding since 1980 and the advent of nonoperative management, and suggested that although this may reflect bias in publication, the relatively few cases of delayed splenic bleeding may be an actual decrease in incidence of this complication due to possible improved splenic healing with the current protocols including bed rest and activity restriction.[43] A literature review from 1970 to 1999 extracted a study population of 1083 children managed nonoperatively for blunt splenic injuries; 920 (85%) underwent routine followup imaging (ultrasound, CT, or scintigraphy) and in the remaining 15% imaging was either not performed or selectively performed. The maximum risk of delayed splenic rupture was 0.3%. It was concluded that the findings did not support the use of routine followup imaging of children with blunt splenic trauma.[44]

Multiple studies have aimed at determining if the radiologic contrast blush on initial CT evaluation is associated with negative outcomes in children with blunt splenic injury, specifically, failure of nonoperative management and/or the need for operative intervention. This sign is seen during an intravenous contrast-enhanced CT scan and is indicative of active bleeding. The identification of a radiologic sign may provide an opportunity to identify a subset of children with blunt splenic injury who require intervention; however, overemphasis on the predictive value of the contrast blush could potentially result in unnecessary surgical intervention with splenectomy.[45] Cox et al[41] in their review of five cases of blunt solid organ injury considered the contrast blush an anatomic lesion that predisposes the patient to subsequent deterioration but not an absolute indication for laparotomy. They concluded that earlier operative intervention was indicated in those patients with a contrast blush that demonstrates any significant change in hemodynamic stability. Nwomeh et al[46] reported the detection of a contrast blush in 12.5% of their study population (27/216) and that 46% of this group underwent operative splenic intervention. They note that the presence of a contrast blush was not a factor in the surgical decision making. They concluded that the child with blunt splenic injury who has a contrast blush on CT is more likely to require surgical intervention than the patient without a contrast blush; however, this finding without associated hemodynamic instability was insufficient to determine the need for operative intervention. Lutz et al[47] noted the presence of blush sign in 7% (6/86) of children with blunt splenic injury. This finding was associated with higher grades of injury but did not mandate embolization or surgery, and the nonoperative management of blunt splenic injury was successful in 98% of cases. These findings concurred with those of Cloutier reported in the same year.[48]

Davies et al[29] reported a contrast blush in 6.5% of their 123 patients with blunt splenic injury. Contrast extravasation was associated with higher grades of injury, lower initial hemoglobin levels, without the need for increased transfusion rate. Their institutional rate of successful nonoperative management of pediatric blunt splenic injury was 97%. In a limited retrospective study of blunt abdominal solid organ injuries from a pediatric trauma center, angiographic embolization was shown to be an effective and safe adjunct in the nonoperative management of blunt splenic injury in hemodynamically stable children with evidence of ongoing hemorrhage as evidenced by decreasing hemoglobin/hematocrit levels.[49] Van der Vlies et al[50] in their systematic review of the literature published between 1985 and 2009 assessed the failure rate of nonoperative management without angio-embolization in children with blunt liver and/or splenic injury when a contrast blush is present on CT and secondarily to determine the failure of nonoperative management after angioembolization. The combined data of the studies reporting nonoperative management with or without angioembolization showed a failure rate of 21%. They note that if only the two studies reporting nonoperative management supplemented by angioembolization were analyzed, the failure rate was 6.5%, suggesting that angioembolization leads to fewer failures. Because of the low level of evidence found, the authors suggest that the definitive answer about optimal management strategy should come from a randomized trial in which nonoperative management without, and nonoperative management with, angioembolization should be compared in hemodynamically stable children with solid organ injuries.

The management of the traumatized diseased spleen and the management of spontaneous rupture of the diseased spleen remain controversial. Advocates of nonoperative management in the hemodynamically stable patient suggest that the patient with a pathologically enlarged spleen, either due to infectious mononucleosis, HIV/AIDS, leukemia, or sickle cell anemia, and spontaneous rupture may be particularly susceptible to post-splenectomy infection and may benefit from splenic preservation. Successful nonoperative management has been reported in patients with pathologic splenomegaly secondary to infectious mononucleosis and leukemia with spontaneous rupture, and in similar patients sustaining blunt splenic injury.[51] Patients with hemophilia and blunt splenic injury do not always require splenectomy;

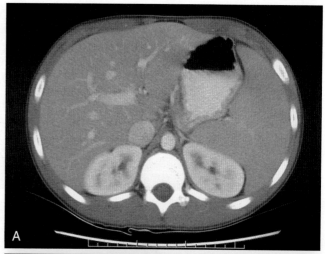
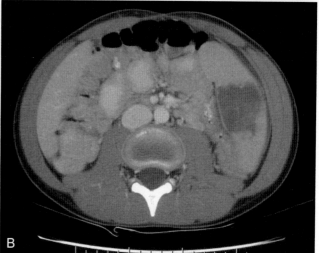

FIGURE 135-3 Abdominal CT scan demonstrating pathologic splenomegaly due to infectious mononucleosis **(A)**, and the traumatic laceration in the same diseased spleen **(B)**.

operative splenic salvage with perioperative correction of the coagulopathy has been reported[52] (Figure 135-3).

The primary indication for operative management in children who continue to have hemodynamic instability is a transfusion requirement that exceeds half of the child's blood volume, or 40 mL/kg, during the first 24 hours after injury. In most children who require operation for solid organ injury, the necessity for operative exploration presents itself generally within 24 hours. Nonoperative management of confirmed abdominal visceral injuries is a surgical decision made by surgeons, as is the decision to operate. The decision to operate continues to be based on abnormal physiologic parameters and the volume of blood lost (Figure 135-4).

OUTCOMES

Nonoperative management of blunt splenic injury has become the standard of care in the hemodynamically stable child with success rates greater than 90%. Only a small percentage of children will require laparotomy, and studies have attempted to characterize the cohort of

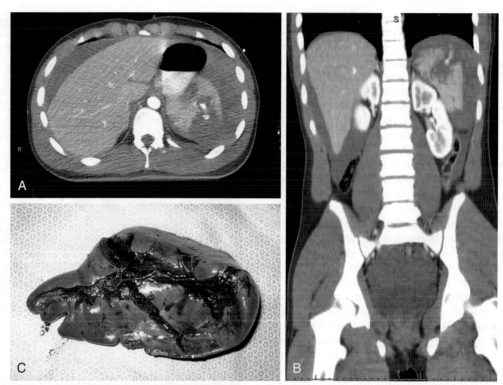

FIGURE 135-4 Abdominal CT scan demonstrating laceration with extravasation of contrast: cross section **(A)**, coronal **(B)**. This patient had an associated closed head injury with two episodes of hypotension and because of his hemodynamic instability underwent splenectomy; operative photo **(C)**.

children who require operative intervention. A retrospective review of the Pennsylvania Trauma Outcome Study database identified 754 children who sustained blunt splenic injury. These patients were stratified into three groups according to the mode of management: splenectomy, splenorrhaphy, or nonoperative. Overall, 15.1% of children underwent splenectomy, 7.4% underwent splenorrhaphy, and 77.5% were managed nonoperatively. The authors' data showed that children undergoing splenectomy were older (15 to 16 years of age), and sustained more severe injury overall in motor vehicle or pedal cycle crashes and sports-related activities. In contrast, children injured by falls, assault, or abuse had significantly lower rates of splenectomy. The independent determinants of splenectomy included Glasgow Coma Scale scores 3 to 8, high spleen injury grade, nonspleen abdominal injury, and age 15 to 16 years. The authors also noted that treatment at a pediatric trauma center was associated with a lower risk of splenectomy.[53]

Holmes et al[54] identified 1880 pediatric patients with solid organ injury from the trauma registries of seven designated level I pediatric trauma centers over a 6-year interval. Nonoperative management was successful in 1729 patients and failed in 89 patients for a nonoperative failure rate of 5%. The failure rate for isolated splenic injury was 4%. Children who failed nonoperative management had greater overall injury severity (higher mean Injury Severity Score [ISS]) and higher organ injury grade. The authors found that the majority of children (60%) who fail nonoperative management do so early in their hospital course, with an overall peak failure rate at 4 hours postadmission.

Retrospective cohorts from seven designated level I pediatric trauma centers identified 2944 children younger than age 19 years over a 10-year interval who sustained blunt abdominal trauma. There were a total of 2981 organ injuries due to multiplicity of organ injuries in a given patient; 1392 were splenic injuries (46.7%). Two groups were characterized: immediate operation and failed nonoperative management, the latter defined as laparotomy more than 3 hours after arrival. The characteristics of those patients requiring laparotomy were compared to controls managed nonoperatively. The overall rate of operation was low, with 140 of the 2944 patients requiring laparotomy (4.8%); 50% of the patients in this group had splenic injuries. The mean age did not differ in the control versus operative groups (8.9 vs. 9.1 years). The patients requiring operation had greater injury severity indicated by higher ISS (28.7 vs. 14.6) and a significantly lower median Glasgow Coma Scale score—12 for patients requiring operation versus 14 in controls. Of the 140 patients requiring operative intervention, 81 (59%) required immediate operation, and of this group 54.3% had splenic injuries, and 59 patients failed nonoperative management with 44.1% splenic injuries. The most common indication for operation in both groups was hemodynamic instability or bleeding. Their analysis showed no adverse outcomes in terms of mortality, blood transfusion requirements, or hospital and intensive care unit length of stay if nonoperative management was initially attempted but then failed.[55]

The operative treatment varies widely depending on the expertise of the treating physician and institution. Mooney et al used the Kids' Inpatient Database 2000 to examine the existence and variation of management of pediatric splenic injuries and the factors associated with splenectomy. There were 2191 children identified with splenic injuries who were discharged from one of 734 of the 2784 KID 2000 hospitals in 25 states covering 68% of the nation's population for the year 2000. Three types of pediatric hospitals were recognized: freestanding pediatric, pediatric unit within an adult hospital, and adult hospital. The distribution of hospitals was 25 freestanding (3%), 68 pediatric unit (9%), and 641 adult (88%). The patient distribution, however, was different, with 339 (15%) admitted to freestanding pediatric hospitals, 525 (24%) to pediatric units within an adult hospital, and 1327 (61%) to adult hospitals. Overall, the rate of splenectomy was 12% (253/2191). The crude splenectomy rate varied significantly among the pediatric hospital types: 3% (11/339) at freestanding children's hospitals, 9% (45/525) at pediatric units within an adult hospital, and 15% (197/1327) at adult hospitals. Teaching hospitals and hospitals with higher patient volume were associated with lower risk for splenectomy. The odds of splenectomy at an adult facility were 2.8 times that of a freestanding children's hospital, whereas that at a pediatric unit within an adult hospital was 2.6 times that of a freestanding children's hospital.[56] Stylianos et al used a four-state database (California, Florida, New Jersey, and New York) to determine variations in the treatment of children with blunt spleen injury from 2000 to 2002. There were 3232 pediatric patients identified, including 1933 patients with isolated spleen injury. Although nearly two-thirds (65.8%) of the patients were treated at trauma centers, only 15% of these patients were treated at designated children's hospitals. Trauma centers had a significantly lower rate of operation for both multiply injured patients and those with isolated injury compared to nontrauma centers. The operative rates at both trauma centers and nontrauma centers exceeded the published APSA benchmarks for all children with spleen injury (5% to 11%) and those with isolated spleen injury (0% to 3%). The authors suggested that better strategies are needed for the dissemination and implementation of benchmarks and guidelines to optimize care of children and to salvage spleens.[57]

ETHICAL DILEMMA: REQUEST FOR SPLENECTOMY BY ATHLETES

A case report describes a collegiate football player who sustained a grade III splenic laceration while playing football.[58] The high-grade splenic injury mandated avoidance of vigorous activity for a period of time that was not acceptable to the patient, who was unwilling to sacrifice his opportunity to become a professional athlete. He underwent laparoscopic splenectomy on postinjury day 8, was discharged 20 hours after surgery, played in a collegiate football game 12 days after surgery, was drafted into the National Football League 9 months later and signed a lucrative contract. Laparoscopic splenectomy allows quicker return to sports participation but carries the risk of postsplenectomy sepsis. Nonoperative management is considered the standard of care for hemodynamically stable patients. However, there remains no clear consensus regarding return to vigorous activity. Radiographic and physiologic splenic healing does not necessarily correlate.[59] There is an ethical dilemma regarding the hemodynamically stable patient's request for a minimally invasive surgical procedure, laparoscopic splenectomy, to expedite recovery and rapid return to normal activities.

REFERENCES

1. McClusky DA, Skandalakis LJ, Colburn GL, et al: Tribute to a triad: History of splenic anatomy, Physiology, and surgery. Part 1. *World J Surg* 23:211, 1999.
2. King H, Shumacher HB: Splenic studies. I. Susceptibility to infection after splenectomy performed in infancy. *Ann Surg* 136:239, 1952.
3. Velanovich V, Tapper D: Decision analysis in children with blunt splenic trauma: The effects of observation, splenorrhaphy, or splenectomy on quality-adjusted life expectancy. *J Pediatr Surg* 28:179, 1993.
4. Upadyaya P, Simpson JS: Splenic trauma in children. *Surg Gynecol Obstet* 126:781, 1968.
5. Dixon JA, Miller F, McCloskey D, et al: Anatomy and techniques in segmental splenectomy. *Surg Gynecol Obstet* 150:516, 1980.
6. Skandalakis JE, Gray SW: *Embryology for surgeons.* Baltimore, MD, 1994, Williams & Wilkins, p 334.
7. Rodrigues CJ, Sacchetti JC, Rodrigues AJ: Age-related changes in the elastic fiber network of the human splenic capsule. *Lymphology* 32:64, 1999.
8. Mazel MS: Traumatic rupture of spleen, with special reference to its characteristics in young children. *J Pediatr* 26:82, 1945.
9. American College of Surgeons: *Advanced Trauma Life Support,* ed 8. Chicago, 2008, American College of Surgeons.
10. Nance ML, Mahboubi S, Wickstrom M, et al: Pattern of abdominal free fluid following isolated blunt spleen and liver injury in the pediatric patient. *J Trauma* 52:85, 2002.
11. Holmes JF, Gladman A, Chang CH: Performance of abdominal ultrasonography in pediatric blunt trauma patients: a meta-analysis. *J Pediatr Surg* 42:1588, 2007.
12. Rice HE, Frush DP, Farmer D, et al, APSA Education Committee: Review of radiation risks from computed tomography: essentials for the pediatric surgeon. *J Pediatr Surg* 42:603, 2007.
13. Brody AS, Frush DP, Huda W, et al, AAP Section on Radiology: Radiation risk to children from computed tomography. *Pediatrics* 120:677, 2007.
14. Jacoby RC, Wisner DH: Injury to the spleen. In Feliciano DV, Mattox KL, Moore EE, editors: *Trauma,* ed 6. New York, 2008, McGraw Hill.
15. Mucha P: Splenic repair and partial splenectomy (preservation of splenic function). In Baker RJ, Fischer JE, editors: *Mastery of surgery.* Philadelphia, 2001, Lippincott Williams & Wilkins.
16. Feliz A, Shultz B, McKenna C, et al: Diagnostic and therapeutic laparoscopy in pediatric abdominal trauma. *J Pediatr Surg* 41:72, 2006.
17. Schmal H, Geiger G: Laparoscopic splenic salvage in delayed rupture by application of fibrin glue in a 10 year old boy. *J Trauma* 58:628, 2005.
18. Carbon RT, Baar S, Waldschmidt J, et al: Innovative minimally invasive pediatric surgery is of therapeutic value for splenic injury. *J Pediatr Surg* 37:1146, 2002.
19. Ein SH, Shandling B, Simpson JS, et al: Non-operative management of traumatized spleen in children: How and why. *J Pediatr Surg* 13:117, 1978.
20. Wesson DE, Filler RM, Ein SH, et al: Ruptured spleen—when to operate? *J Pediatr Surg* 16:324, 1981.
21. Pearl RH, Wesson DE, Spence LJ, et al: Splenic injury: A 5-year update with improved results and changing criteria for conservative management. *J Pediatr Surg* 24:121, 1989.

22. Fallat ME, Casale AJ: Practice patterns of pediatric surgeons caring for stable patients with traumatic solid organ injury. *J Trauma* 43:820, 1997.

23. Stylianos S: APSA Trauma Committee. Evidence-based guidelines for resource utilization in children with isolated spleen or liver injury. *J Pediatr Surg* 35:164, 2000.

24. Moore EE, Cogbill TH, Jurkovich GJ, et al: Organ injury scaling: Spleen and liver (1994 revision). *J Trauma* 38:323, 1995.

25. Stylianos S: Compliance with evidence-based guidelines in children with isolated spleen or liver injury: A prospective study. *J Pediatr Surg* 37:453, 2002.

26. Mehall JR, Ennis JS, Saltzman DA, et al: Prospective results of a standardized algorithm based on hemodynamic status for managing pediatric solid organ injury. *J Am Coll Surg* 193:347, 2001.

27. McVay MR, Kokoska ER, Jackson RJ, et al: Throwing out the "grade" book: management of isolated spleen and liver injury based on hemodynamic status. *J Pediatr Surg* 43:1072, 2008.

28. St Peter SD, Keckler SJ, Spilde TL, et al: Justification for an abbreviated protocol in the management of blunt spleen and liver injury in children. *J Pediatr Surg* 43:191, 2008.

29. Davies DA, Pearl RH, Ein SH, et al: Management of blunt splenic injury in children: Evolution of the nonoperative approach. *J Pediatr Surg* 44:1005, 2009.

30. Schwartz MZ, Kangah R: Splenic injury in children after blunt trauma: Blood transfusion requirements and length of hospitalization for laparotomy versus observation. *J Pediatr Surg* 29:596, 1994.

31. Partrick DA, Bensard DD, Moore EE, et al: Nonoperative management of solid organ injuries in children results in decreased blood transfusion. *J Pediatr Surg* 34:1695, 1999.

32. Coburn MC, Pfeifer J, DeLuca FG: Nonoperative management of splenic and hepatic trauma in the multiply injured pediatric and adolescent patient. *Arch Surg* 130:332, 1995.

33. Morse MA, Garcia VF: Selective nonoperative management of pediatric blunt splenic trauma: Risk for missed associated injuries. *J Pediatr Surg* 29:23, 1994.

34. Keller MS, Sartorelli KH, Vane DW: Associated head injury should not prevent nonoperative management of spleen or liver injury in children. *J Trauma* 41:471, 1996.

35. Samant UB 4th, Mack CD, Koepsell T, et al: Time of hypotension and discharge outcome in children with traumatic brain injury. *J Neurotrauma* 25:495, 2008.

36. Pranikoff T, Hirschl RB, Schlesinger AE, et al: Resolution of splenic injury after nonoperative management. *J Pediatr Surg* 29:1366, 1994.

37. Lynch JM, Meza MP, Newman B, et al: Computed tomography grade of splenic injury is predictive of the time required for radiographic healing. *J Pediatr Surg* 32:1093, 1997.

38. Kristoffersen KW, Mooney DP: Long-term outcome of nonoperative pediatric splenic injury management. *J Pediatr Surg* 42:1038, 2007.

39. Frumiento C, Sartorelli K, Vane D: Complications of splenic injuries: Expansion of the nonoperative theorem. *J Pediatr Surg* 35:788, 2000.

40. Yardeni D, Polley TZ Jr, Coran AG: Splenic artery embolization for post-traumatic splenic artery pseudoaneurysm. *J Trauma* 57:404, 2004.

41. Cox CC, Geiger JD, Liu DC, et al: Pediatric blunt abdominal trauma: Role of computed tomography vascular blush. *J Pediatr Surg* 32:1196, 1997.

42. McIndoe AH: Delayed haemorrhage following traumatic rupture of the spleen. *Br J Surg* 20:249, 1931.

43. Davies DA, Fecteau A, Himidan S, et al: What is the incidence of delayed splenic bleeding in children after blunt trauma? An institutional experience and review of the literature. *J Trauma* 67:573, 2009.

44. Huebner S, Reed MH: Analysis of the value of imaging as part of the follow-up of splenic injury in children. *Pediatr Radiol* 31:852, 2001.

45. Davies DA, Ein SH, Pearl R, et al: What is the significance of contrast "blush" in pediatric blunt splenic trauma. *J Pediatr Surg* 45:916, 2010.

46. Nwomeh BC, Nadler EP, Meza MP, et al: Contrast extravasation predicts the need for operative intervention in children with blunt splenic trauma. *J Trauma* 56:537, 2004.

47. Lutz N, Mahboubi S, Nance ML, et al: The significance of contrast blush on computed tomography in children with splenic injuries. *J Pediatr Surg* 39:491, 2004.

48. Cloutier DR, Baird TB, Gormley P, et al: Pediatric splenic injuries with a contrast blush: Successful nonoperative management without angiography and embolization. *J Pediatr Surg* 39:969, 2004.

49. Kiankhooy A, Sartorelli KH, Vane DM, et al: Angiographic embolization is safe and effective therapy in blunt abdominal solid organ injury in children. *J Trauma* 68:526, 2010.

50. Van der Vlies CH, Saltzherr TP, Wilde JCH, et al: The failure rate of nonoperative management in children with splenic or liver injury with contrast blush on computed tomography: A systematic review. *J Pediatr Surg* 45:1044, 2010.

51. Statter MB, Liu DC: Nonoperative management of blunt splenic injury in infectious mononucleosis. *Am Surg* 71:376, 2005.

52. Koren JP, Klein RL, Kavic MS, et al: Management of splenic trauma in the pediatric hemophiliac patient: Case series and review of the literature. *J Pediatr Surg* 37:568, 2002.

53. Potoka DA, Schall LC, Ford HR: Risk factors for splenectomy in children with blunt splenic trauma. *J Pediatr Surg* 37:294, 2002.

54. Holmes JH, Wiebe DJ, Tataria M, et al: The failure of nonoperative management in pediatric solid organ injury: A multi-institutional experience. *J Trauma* 59:1309, 2005.

55. Tataria M, Nance ML, Holmes JH, et al: Pediatric blunt abdominal injury: Age is irrelevant and delayed operation is not detrimental. *J Trauma* 63:608, 2007.

56. Mooney DP, Rothstein DH, Forbes MA: Variation in the management of pediatric splenic injuries in the United States. *J Trauma* 61:330, 2006.

57. Stylianos S, Egorova N, Guice KS, et al: Variation in treatment of pediatric spleen injury at trauma centers versus nontrauma centers: A call for dissemination of American Pediatric Surgical Association benchmarks and guidelines. *J Am Coll Surg* 202:247, 2006.

58. Mostafa G, Matthews B, Sing RF, et al: Elective laparoscopic splenectomy for grade III splenic injury in an athlete. *Surg Laparosc Endosc* 12:283, 2002.

59. Terrell TR, Lundquist B: Management of splenic rupture and return-to-play decisions in a college football player. *Clin J Sport Med* 12:400, 2002.

Cysts and Tumors of the Spleen

Michael S. Thomas | Douglas P. Slakey

Cysts and tumors of the spleen are uncommonly encountered in clinical practice and continue to present challenges in both surgical workup and treatment. Perhaps the continuing evolution of surgical traditions associated with splenic maladies can be partly explained by the relative rarity of these conditions. Literature references provide benchmarks to the myriad of supposed functions and attributes of the spleen as our experience and understanding of the organ continue to advance. For an excellent timeline of the medical and scientific inquiry as to the function of the spleen, the reader is directed to the two-part review by McClusky et al entitled *Tribute to a Triad: History of Splenic Anatomy, Physiology, and Surgery*.[1] Historically it has been questioned whether the spleen is required at all for survival. It was only within the latter half of the 20th century that the spleen came to be regarded as vital. For the majority of recorded history the spleen, although often described as having diverse functions, was regarded as wholly unnecessary. This is reflected in early surgical approaches to splenic maladies. Although the veracity of the recording has been questioned,[2] Adrian Zacarelli is thought to have performed the first splenectomy in 1549 on a 24-year-old woman who had developed splenomegaly. Later, Buliemi Ballonii (Ballonius) asked in a report of another splenectomy performed by an unknown barber-surgeon in 1578, "*Este igitur spelnatar necessarisu* [Is the spleen so necessary for life]?" Ultimately, Edwin Beer would argue in 1928 that any splenic operation must be extirpative to be considered satisfactory.[3]

Traumatic injury to the spleen provided the majority of earliest opportunities to evaluate splenectomy as a successful treatment of splenic conditions. A testament to the rarity of splenic interventions is the observation that only 10 surgeons had followed in Zacarelli's footsteps during the next two and a half centuries. Almost invariably these reports concluded with success stories of patients returning to healthy lives. However, in 1826 Karl Quittenbaum performed an elective splenectomy on a 22-year-old female with splenomegaly, presumably from portal hypertension, that serves as the first recorded failure resulting in postoperative death. He was admonished for both his patient selection, given the patient had ascites and anasarca, as well as technique, in that a portion of the pancreas was found in the resected spleen.[2] It was the author of those admonitions, Sir Thomas Spencer Wells, who would go on to note through his own failures that the spleen may have some necessary but as of yet unknown hematologic role, and that an elective total splenectomy may only be appropriate for the treatment of life-threatening leukemia. He based these speculations on the observation that enlarged spleens were often found in conjunction with an abundance of leukocytes and that by removing the spleen the surgeon may cut off the production of these cells. His caution to those who would perform these procedures was in contrast to the long-held view of the nonnecessity of the organ. His hypothesis, although incorrect, was important to the beginning of applying methodology in evaluation of surgical treatments for conditions involving the spleen. A subsequent review of 49 splenectomies performed for the treatment of leukemia suggested an almost 90% mortality rate, and splenectomy as a treatment of choice for this condition would be later replaced by irradiation.[4]

During the 20th century clinicians continued to question the prevailing view that the spleen was unimportant. By 1952 King had observed increased rates of infection in children who had undergone splenectomy.[5] Recognition of the spleen's immunologic role and the description of overwhelming postsplenectomy infection (OPSI) encouraged surgeons to consider alternatives to extirpative surgery. Morgenstern and Shapiro are credited with the first successful open partial splenectomy for an epidermoid cyst in 1980.[6] Continuing advances in minimally invasive surgery allowed Seshadri et al to complete the first successful laparoscopic partial splenectomy in 2000.[7] Advances in surgical technology have increased the number of management options for pathologic lesions of the spleen.[8,9] Paralleled technologic improvements in radiologic imaging, along with an increase in abdominal imaging have led to more frequent diagnosis of splenic abnormalities, especially cystic and solid lesions.

APPROACH TO THE SPLENIC MASS

As with any medical condition, a history and physical provide the basic foundation for the evaluation of the patient with a splenic lesion. Before one determines the most appropriate treatment, the nature or type of mass must be ascertained. Splenic masses are very rare when compared to masses involving other solid organs such as the ovary, liver or kidney, so the physician may benefit from a simplified approach that assists in the correct diagnosis and timely treatment. Patients may present to the surgeon's office with classic complaints of left upper quadrant pain or otherwise vague abdominal discomfort; however, they frequently are asymptomatic with a mass incidentally discovered in imaging obtained for other purposes. Noninvasive radiographic imaging is necessary in assisting the initial classification of the lesion as cystic or solid as well as providing size measurements. Ultrasound (US) can demonstrate the internal echoes indicative of an abscess or hematoma versus the round homogeneous, anechoic enhancing signal that is the hallmark of a cystic structure. Computed tomography

(CT) scanning with intravenous contrast or magnetic resonance imaging (MRI) can better delineate the trabeculated or septated nature of the cyst wall and wall calcification and has a superior specificity in defining whether a mass is cystic or solid. Cysts observed on CT typically demonstrate attenuation near water without rim enhancement. CT scanning may be especially useful when US views are limited by obesity, or signal distortion from overlying bowel gas or the lower ribs.[10]

Both cysts and solid tumors are further divided each into two broad categories. Cysts are classified as either a primary (true) cyst containing an epithelial lining or more commonly, as a secondary cyst (pseudocyst), which lacks an epithelial lining. True cysts are either parasitic or nonparasitic, whereas pseudocysts most commonly arise as the result of blunt abdominal trauma. Tumors of the spleen are divided into either lymphoid or nonlymphoid. Lymphoid tumors are mainly of the Hodgkin or non-Hodgkin variety, while nonlymphoid tumors most commonly are of vascular origin and may be either benign or malignant. This broad schema may serve as a starting point to understand the etiology of the mass and thereby provide the most appropriate course of treatment without undue risk of immunologic complication to the patient (Table 136-1).

Options for treatment include medical management with continued observation and/or surgical intervention. The varied types of intervention available include splenectomy, either complete or partial, percutaneous drainage, fenestration or marsupialization. Management decisions will be based in part on the presentation of the patient, but also by the etiology of the lesion.

CYSTIC MASSES

Splenic cysts are most common in the second and third decade of life, although they have been noted in all age groups including infants. An asymptomatic abdominal mass is the presenting feature in 30% to 45% of cases. Abdominal symptoms such as pain or physical examination findings are present in children when cysts are larger than 8 cm and possibly larger in adults. Signs may arise from the compression on adjacent structures by an enlarging mass. For example, poorly controlled hypertension may arise because of compression of the left renal artery or vague urinary complaints caused

by compression and/or pressure on the left kidney or ureteropelvic junction. The pain may either be localized or referred, classically to the left shoulder. A review of systems may yield complaints of gastrointestinal distress that are neither associated with meals nor helped by antacids. Respiratory complaints may include shortness of breath, pleuritic chest pain, or even a history of left lower lobe pneumonia. Sudden onset of abdominal pain and peritoneal signs caused by rupture may occur in previously asymptomatic patients as the risk of rupture is 25% in cysts larger than 5 cm.[11]

Fowler is credited with the first classification system for splenic cysts after reviewing more than 400 cases. There have been attempts to simplify his system most recently by Hansen and Moller who collectively reviewed 800 reported cases.[9] It is important to note that the prevalence of primary versus secondary cysts differs in the United States versus other parts of the world, especially in areas endemic for *Echinococcus* such as south central Europe, South America, and Australia. Worldwide (but not in the United States) the vast majority of primary or "true" splenic cysts are parasitic, two thirds or more being caused by echinococci, with *Echinococcus granulosus* being the most common species. The echinococcal splenic cyst is composed of an inner germinal layer and an outer laminated layer surrounded by a fibrous capsule, characteristically multilocular in appearance, and filled with fluid under pressure. It may contain daughter cysts and infective scolices. Echinococcal cysts may be asymptomatic or may cause pressure symptoms when they reach a large enough size, become secondarily infected, or rupture. Diagnosis is suggested by a history of travel to an endemic area and may be confirmed by indirect hemagglutination or enzyme-linked immunosorbent assay tests, which are positive in approximately 90% of patients with echinococcal cysts. Although hepatic hydatid cysts of echinococcal disease may be treated with percutaneous drainage and systemic treatment with albendazole,[12] the treatment of choice for splenic hydatid cysts is splenectomy. However, there have been reports of limited success in small (<5 cm) single cysts with chemical sterilization with cetrimide, 3% sodium chloride, or ethanol and cyst evacuation in order to achieve splenic salvage.[13] Whichever method is chosen, care must be taken to avoid intraperitoneal spillage and the resultant potential for anaphylaxis and hypotension. Low morbidity rates have been reported in patients needing to undergo simultaneous surgical treatment of splenic and hepatic hydatid cysts.[14]

The remaining causes of nonparasitic primary cysts include congenital and neoplastic cysts. Congenital causes account for approximately 10% of all splenic cysts and 25% of nonparasitic cysts. Primary nonparasitic congenital cysts are present predominantly in children and young adults. The developmental model proposed for development of these cysts suggests they arise as a result of invaginations of the mesothelium-lined splenic capsule and are primary in nature.[15] Neoplastic nonparasitic cysts are much less common and historically have included epidermoid, dermoid, and endodermoid cysts, the latter being the most common Endodermoid lesions are not

Solid Masses	Cystic Masses
LYMPHOID	**PRIMARY OR "TRUE"**
Hodgkin	*Parasitic*
Non-Hodgkin	*Nonparasitic*
NONLYMPHOID	Congenital
Benign	Neoplastic
Malignant	
	PSEUDOCYSTS
	Posttraumatic
	Other

TABLE 136-1 Classification of Splenic Masses

true cysts and include lymphangiomas and hemangiomas and will be discussed later as solid masses. Dermoid cysts are exceedingly rare and are characterized by structures derived from all three germ layers similar to a cystic teratoma. These lesions may be observed if they are small (<5 cm) and followed with ultrasound. Larger lesions should be surgically removed.

Three-quarters of nonparasitic splenic cysts are termed secondary cysts (pseudocysts) and thought to be attributed to trauma,[16] although 30% of these patients may not recall the specific event,[17] suggesting that causes other than trauma (such as splenic infarcts or infection) may play a larger role than originally thought. Secondary cysts typically occur in young and middle-aged adults. Women are more affected than men for unknown reasons, although hormonal effects and changes during pregnancy are presumed to play a role. Secondary cysts are thought to be formed by encapsulation of a splenic hematoma and subsequent absorption of the blood and persistence of a false cyst wall.[18] Clinically it is difficult to differentiate primary from secondary cysts given the similarity of complaints, the overlap of the age groups, and the frequent omission of trauma from the patient's history. However, the treatment guidelines are also similar for primary and secondary cysts, in that masses smaller than 5 cm may be observed and followed with serial US, whereas a surgical approach should be chosen for larger masses.

Tumor markers carcinoembryonic antigen (CEA) and carbohydrate antigen 19-9 (CA 19-9) may be elevated in primary cysts, and studies have shown immunoreactivity of the cyst's inner lining to anti-CA 19-9.[19,20] Because increased CEA or CA 19-9 levels may be from either benign or malignant processes, preoperative and postoperative levels documenting change are at times useful.

SOLID TUMORS

Tumors of the spleen are uncommon lesions and are categorized as either lymphoid or nonlymphoid. Lymphoid tumors of the spleen are mainly Hodgkin disease or non-Hodgkin lymphoma. As primary lesions of the spleen, these tumors are rare; however, the spleen is often the site of secondary involvement. Regardless of whether primary or secondary, lymphoid lesions are first observed in the white pulp. The process may be diffuse, as seen with nodular lymphoma, or localized with large irregular tumors, as seen with large cell lymphomas. Surgical treatment invariably involves complete splenectomy, either as part of a staging operation in the case of Hodgkin disease or as an attempt at palliation for symptomatic splenomegaly or hypersplenism. It is notable that the usefulness of a staging laparotomy and/or a splenectomy for Hodgkin disease remains controversial and is outside the scope of this chapter.

Nonlymphoid tumors may be either primary or secondary (metastatic). It is important to distinguish benign from malignant lesions. The most common nonlymphoid primary tumors are vascular tumors consisting of benign and malignant hemangiomas, lymphangiomas, and hemangioendotheliomas. Other tumors include hamartomas, fibrosarcomas, inflammatory pseudotumors, and lipomas, although these are all rarely reported lesions. Secondary or metastatic tumors are most commonly from melanoma and breast and lung tumors. Although the spleen is one of the most vascular organs in the body, metastatic disease is uncommon.

Hemangiomas are the most common benign tumor of the spleen. Typically, these tumors are asymptomatic, found incidentally at autopsy, or in spleens removed for other reasons. They may be single, multiple, or involving the entire organ. As noted, symptoms may be present when the lesion increases in size sufficient to compress adjacent structures or grows large enough to rupture spontaneously. A hematologic clue to the existence of splenic hemangioma may present as unexplained consumptive coagulopathy caused by platelet trapping. Radiographic findings can be seen as "laking" on angiography or contrast CT similar to hepatic hemangiomas. Lymphangiomas are less common and are thought to be congenital malformations of the lymphatic system. These malformations may fill with eosinophilic proteinaceous material contributing to increased weight of the spleen. These lesions usually become symptomatic because of a mass effect. They may be differentiated from the hemangiomas by the absence of the "lakes" associated with the latter. Treatment considerations for both benign conditions are based on symptomatology, with observation for small asymptomatic lesions and complete splenectomy for larger symptomatic hemangiomas and lymphangiomas.

Primary hemangiosarcoma, although rare, is the most common primary malignancy of the spleen. Historically, these lesions have been referred to as angiosarcoma; however, hemangiosarcoma is now the preferred nomenclature to distinguish them from lymphangiosarcoma. Hemangiosarcomas grow rapidly and metastasize to regional lymph nodes, liver, bone marrow, and lungs. In addition to the clinical presentation associated with splenomegaly, these patients may develop cachexia because of the aggressive nature of the malignancy. Ascites and pleural effusion are less common findings. Spontaneous rupture may be the initial presenting feature. Imaging may be similar to hemangiomas on angiography, but care must be taken to attempt differentiation as the prognosis of hemangiosarcoma remains poor in almost all cases. Treatment, if appropriate, remains splenectomy.

The reported incidence of metastatic disease varies from 0.3% to 7.3% depending on the location of the primary tumor. Speculation as to reasons for such a relatively low rate of metastatic lesions are based on both anatomic features such as the acute angle the splenic artery presents to tumor emboli as well as a lack of afferent lymphatics, and functional peculiarities such as the rhythmic contractions of the spleen and high antitumoral activity of the splenic lymphoid tissue. The finding of metastatic disease in the spleen mandates a thorough evaluation of the rest of the body, as it is extremely rare to find the spleen as the initial site of metastasis. Like other splenic lesions, symptoms are often attributable to mass effects and the progression of disease before clinical presentation may be variable. Spontaneous rupture is a feared, although exceedingly rare and devastating complication.[21] Splenectomy is the treatment of choice to assist in relieving symptoms of compression.

SURGICAL PLANNING

Since 1952, with the demonstration of the increased mortality of splenectomized patients (mainly children) because of OPSI, there has been an interest in splenic salvage.[5] The incidence of OPSI is reported to 0.2% to 4.3%, with a lifetime risk of 5%.[22] Although the overall incidence may be low, the risk of developing an overwhelming infection is 200 times greater as compared to the background population.[23] The organisms responsible are most often *Streptococcus pneumoniae, Neisseria meningitidis, Haemophilus influenzae,* and *Escherichia coli.*[24] Vaccines directed toward the first three bacteria species are available in case a complete splenectomy is unavoidable.[25] Partial splenectomy has been reported only for solitary cysts of the spleen. Complete splenectomy for splenic cysts would be indicated in cases of polycystic disease.

In the case of solid tumors, sound surgical principles should be followed meaning good exposure, removal of the entire tumor without rupture, adequate margins, and perfect homeostasis must be achieved for a successful tumor operation. In staging operations such as for Hodgkin disease, the risk of a negative staging error with partial splenectomy has been reported, and it is advised against. For primary splenic tumors, these principles are best achieved with a total splenectomy. If the spleen has tumors that are clearly part of disseminated metastatic disease, splenic biopsy is sufficient, as there is no survival benefit to splenectomy to justify the risk.

COMPLETE SPLENECTOMY

Splenectomy may be performed by the traditional open or laparoscopic (including hand-assisted) approaches. The experience of the surgical team and history of previous abdominal surgeries are factors influencing the choice. For open splenectomy, a left subcostal incision or midline incision can be used to expose the spleen, although Morgenstern et al believe the subcostal incision to be the best approach; the midline incision may offer better exposure in patients with marked splenomegaly.[26] The midline view allows for better isolation of the lower pole if it extends down into the pelvis. The first step is the transection of the ligamentous attachments, including the splenophrenic ligament at the superior pole, the splenocolic and splenorenal ligaments at the inferior pole, and lateral retroperitoneal attachments. Either blunt dissection or sharp dissection in the case of thickened ligaments accomplishes these tasks. Early ligation of the splenic artery or arteries in the hilum allows for possible reduction of spleen size, decrease in venous outflow, and easier delivery of the spleen into the wound. Ligation of the readily accessible veins including the short gastric veins, vessels to the anterior hilum, and lower pole should be accomplished before mobilization is attempted. An endovascular stapler with a 30 mm or 60 mm vascular load may offer an advantage over individual isolation of short gastric and hilar vessels, especially in cases of splenomegaly or portal hypertension. Rarely, it might be necessary to remove a portion of the parietal peritoneum or diaphragm if the spleen is not easily separable from these areas. Once the spleen has been sufficiently mobilized to the midline and the posterior hilar surface exposed, it is advisable to control the large posterior splenic veins. Attempts at control of the fragile veins from the anterior approach may result in venous disruption and massive bleeding, and an increased risk of injuring the tail of the pancreas. On removal of the spleen, attempts at sampling the hilar lymph nodes should be made. These are usually located near the major hilar vessels and may be useful in grading of splenic tumors.[26,27]

Complete splenectomy using the laparoscopic approach for tumors has also been reported.[28,29] The principles for open tumor surgery apply for laparoscopy. In the past, opponents of the laparoscopic splenectomy criticized the necessity of splenic morcellation for the removal of the spleen from the peritoneal cavity. However, with a small 3-cm extension of one of the trocar sites, most spleens can be removed intact. Carroll et al proved that the staging surgery for Hodgkin disease could be performed entirely laparoscopically.[28] It is essential that the spleen be removed intact to avoid peritoneal dissemination of potentially malignant cells. Proponents of the laparoscopic approach believe that the spleen can be more cleanly dissected and because of better visualization, vessels more safely ligated earlier in the course of the operation to prevent hematologic spread with dissection. Flowers et al warned, however, that a learning curve of 20 laparoscopic splenectomies was usual before surgeons felt comfortable with the technique.[29] The authors of this chapter have successfully used the hand-assisted laparoscope technique to remove spleens as large as 25 cm. The patient is placed in a semidecubitus position with the left side elevated approximately 45 degrees. The hand port incision is made in the midline just above the umbilicus.

Given the relative rarity of these splenic lesions and the technical difficulty associated with traditional laparoscopic techniques, the hand-assisted laparoscopic splenectomy may be a more practical alternative. This offers both the benefits of close inspection with the laparoscope and palpation of the organ and tumor as in open surgery. The hand offers easy exposure, more complete exploration of regional lymph nodes, stomach, and pancreas by palpation, and immediate hemostasis with manual compression. Intact removal is easily accomplished through the hand port, and the patient receives many of the same benefits attributed to the laparoscopic approach.

PARTIAL SPLENECTOMY

As noted in Surgical Planning, earlier, partial splenectomy is typically suitable only in treating splenic cysts. The surgeon must bear in mind that at least 25% of the spleen is required to maintain immunity against pneumococcus, the most common organism associated with OPSI. Immunization against *S. pneumoniae* is recommended in all patients 10 days to 2 weeks before undergoing a splenic operation, with a booster in 5 to 10 years. *H. inflenzae* type b and meningococcal vaccinations are also available and recommended.[22] Partial splenectomy with a thoracoabdominal (TA) stapler or harmonic scalpel makes organ conservation possible[30,31] and has proved superior to alternatives such as autotransplantation.[32] Depending on the location, the technique may be either open or laparoscopic; however, care to control the vessels supporting the cyst must be taken regardless of the chosen technique. Additionally, it is often difficult to control bleeding in a partial splenectomy. It is recommended to have an argon beam coagulator available in conjunction with commercially available hemostatic agents to effectively stop all bleeding. Excessive bleeding caused by a partial splenectomy that requires blood transfusions may negate any theoretic advantages. Surgical judgment is critical in determining when to abandon partial splenectomy in favor of total.

OTHER TECHNIQUES

When the location of the cyst is superficial, definitive treatment may be accomplished with less invasive techniques. However, care must be taken in both patient selection, as well as selection of appropriate technique, so as not to increase the risk of recurrence. Percutaneous laparoscopic aspiration or drainage with indwelling catheters has been suggested especially as a bridging technique in the management of pseudocysts that will eventually undergo operative resection.[33,34] Fenestration involves resection of the extrasplenic cyst wall to create a permanent opening into the peritoneum, accomplished either by open or laparoscopic surgical techniques. Care must be taken to remove a large enough piece of the cyst wall to prevent recurrence, and the omentum may be attached to cover the parenchyma defect. A better alternative involves partial splenic decapsulation, also known as marsupialization. This approach involves the trocar decompression of the cyst with removal of the outer splenic capsule. A running locking suture in the splenic wall is used to ensure hemostasis and external drainage may also be performed. Surgeons must prepare in advance in using these and other puncture techniques for the occasion of anaphylaxis because of a missed parasitic cyst with subsequent spillage of fluid into the peritoneal cavity. This risk and the observation that a subsequent dense inflammatory reaction can make future operations for recurrence more difficult makes simple puncture techniques contraindicated.

CONCLUSION

When faced with a splenic lesion, care must be taken to ensure that the mass is correctly identified as either cystic or solid. Fortunately, this task is easily accomplished by current imaging modalities. With the knowledge of the nature of the lesion as cystic or solid, the surgical management is greatly simplified as total splenectomy is indicated for symptomatic or potentially malignant solid tumors. For cystic structures, exposure to regions endemic for culpable parasites or a history of blunt trauma may assist in determining the appropriate treatment, which may not involve complete removal of this

historically underappreciated organ. Additionally, observation alone may suffice in the case of smaller splenic cysts, sparing the patient unneeded procedures. If an operation should be indicated, laparoscopic and open techniques are equally effective and safe as long as the surgeon has the requisite experience.

REFERENCES

1. McClusky DA 3rd, Skandalakis LJ, Colborn GL, et al: Tribute to a triad: History of splenic anatomy, physiology, and surgery. *World J Surg* 23:311, 1999.
2. Wells TS: On excision of enlarged spleen, with a case in which the operation was performed. *Med Times Gaz* 1:2, 1866.
3. Beer E: Development and progress of surgery of the spleen. *Ann Surg* 88:335, 1928.
4. Johnston GB: Splenectomy. *Ann Surg* 88:409, 1908.
5. King H, Shumacker HB Jr: Splenic studies I. Susceptibility to infection after splenectomy performed in infancy. *Am J Surg* 136:239, 1952.
6. Morgenstern L, Shapiro SJ: Partial splenectomy for non-parasitic splenic cysts. *Am J Surg* 139:278, 1980.
7. Seshadri PA, Poulin EC, Mamazza J, et al: Technique for laparoscopic partial splenectomy. *Surg Laparosc Endosc Percutan Tech* 10:106, 2000.
8. Uchida H, Ohta M, Shibata K, et al: Laparoscopic splenectomy in patients with inflammatory pseudotumor of the spleen: Report of 2 cases and review of the literature. *Surg Laparosc Endosc Percutan Tech* 16:3, 2006.
9. Hansen MB, Moller AC: Splenic cysts. *Surg Laparosc Endosc Percutan Tech* 14:316, 2004.
10. Robertson F, Leander P, Ekberg O: Radiology of the spleen. *Eur Radiol* 11:80, 2001.
11. Qureshi MA, Hafner CD, Dorchak Jr: Nonparasitic cysts of the spleen: Report of 14 cases. *Arch Surg* 89:570, 1964.
12. Khuroo MS, Wani NA, Javid G, et al: Percutaneous drainage compared with surgery for hepatic hydatid cysts. *N Engl J Med* 337:881, 1997.
13. Khoury G, Abiad F, Geagea T, et al: Laparoscopic treatment of hydatid cysts of the liver and spleen. *Surg Endosc* 14:243, 2000.
14. Meimarakis G, Grigolia G, Loehe F, et al: Surgical management of splenic echinococcal disease. *Eur J Med Res* 14:165, 2009.
15. Ough YD: Mesothelial cysts of the spleen with squamous metaplasia. *Am J Clin Pathol* 76:666, 1981.
16. Andrews MW: Ultrasound of the spleen. *World J Surg* 24:183, 2000.
17. Boesby S: Spontaneous rupture of benign non-parasitic cyst of the spleen. *Ugeskr Laeger* 134:2596, 1977.
18. Dawes LG, Malangoni MA: Cystic masses of the spleen. *Am Surg* 52:333, 1986.
19. Madia C, Lumachi F, Veroux M, et al: Giant splenic epithelial cyst with elevated tumor markers CEA and CA 19-9: An incidental association? *Anticancer Res* 23:773, 2003.
20. Trompetas V, Panagopoulos E, Priovolou-Papaevangelou M, et al: Giant benign true cyst of the spleen with high serum levels of CA 19-9. *Eur J Gastroenterol Hepatol* 14:85, 2002.
21. Lam KY: Metastatic tumors of the spleen: A twenty-five clinicopathologic study. *Arch Pathol Lab Med* 124:526, 2000.
22. Davidson RN, Wall RA: Prevention and management of infections in patients without a spleen. *Clin Microbiol Infect* 7:657, 2001.
23. Grinblat J, Gilboa Y: Overwhelming pneumococcal sepsis 25 years after splenectomy. *Am J Med Sci* 270:523, 1974.
24. Eadie PA: Conservative treatment of splenic cysts. *Ir Med J* 79:11, 1986.
25. Smith ST, Scott DJ, Burdick JS, et al: Laparoscopic marsupialization and hemisplenectomy for splenic cysts. *J Laparoendosc Adv Surg Tech A* 11:243, 2001.
26. Morgenstern L, Rosenberg J, Geller SA: Tumors of the spleen. *World J Surg* 9:468, 1985.
27. Schwartz SI, Cooper RA Jr: Surgery in the diagnosis and treatment of Hodgkin disease. *Adv Surg* 6:175, 1972.
28. Carroll BJ, Phillips EH, Semel CJ, et al: Laparoscopic splenectomy. *Surg Endosc* 6:183, 1992.

29. Flowers JL, Lefor AT, Steers J, et al: Laparoscopic splenectomy in patients with hematologic diseases. *Ann Surg* 224:19, 1996.

30. Uranŭs S, Kronberger L, Kraft-Kine J: Partial splenic resection with a TA-stapler. *Am J Surg* 168:49, 1994.

31. Sardi A, Ojeda HF, King D Jr: Laparoscopic resection of a benign true cyst of the spleen with the harmonic scalpel producing high levels of CA 19-9 and carcinoembryonic antigen. *Am Surg* 64:1159, 1994.

32. Balzan SM, Riedner CE, Santos LM, et al: Posttraumatic splenic cysts and partial splenectomy: Report of a case. *Surg Today* 31:262, 2001.

33. Pachter HL, Hofstetter SR, Elkowitz A, et al: Traumatic cysts of the spleen-the role of cystectomy and splenic preservation: Experience with seven consecutive patients. *J Trauma* 35:430, 1993.

34. Moir C, Guttman F, Jequier S, et al: Splenic cysts: Aspiration, sclerosis, or resection. *J Pediatr Surg* 24:646, 1989.

Management of Splenic Abscess

Jeffrey L. Ponsky | Adheesh Sabnis

Splenic abscesses are rare, with small case series comprising a majority of the subject's literature. Splenic abscesses were lethal prior to the era of antibiotics and were usually diagnosed at autopsy[1] with incidences of 0.14% to 0.7%.[2,3] In recent times, the incidence of splenic abscess has increased because of the growing number of immunocompromised patients.[4] However, with the development of new imaging techniques and improved antibiotics comes an advance in the management and resolution of splenic abscesses.

PRESENTING SYMPTOMS AND SIGNS

The clinical triad of fever, left upper quadrant pain, and leukocytosis is seen only in one-third to two-thirds of patients with splenic abscess.[5,6] At the time of diagnosis, patients may present with a variety of signs and symptoms or none at all. Reported symptoms and signs include nausea, vomiting, weight loss, decreased left-sided breath sounds, splenomegaly, and a new systolic murmur.[4,7-9] Immunocompromised patients usually present further along in the disease process with generalized symptoms and signs such as fever, abdominal pain, and weight loss.[4]

DIAGNOSIS

The diagnosis of splenic abscess can be supported by microbiology and laboratory data. Leukocytosis (white blood cell count >12,000/mm^3) is reported in 60% of cases.[5] Idiopathic thrombocytosis in septic patients may suggest a splenic abscess.[10] Cultures of abscess fluid identify the offending organism 80% of the time.[5] However, blood cultures isolate the infecting organism in less than half of all cases.[5,7] Moreover, in 66% of cases, different organisms are identified from the abscess and blood cultures.[5,7] These factors need to be considered when choosing a patient's antibiotic regimen. Imaging studies can be invaluable when diagnosing splenic abscess. Plain chest radiographs cannot give a definitive diagnosis, however, because there are nonspecific findings in 33% to 80% of cases.[2,3,7,11,12] These findings include left pleural effusion, left pleural thickening, left basilar pulmonary infiltrate, and an elevated left hemidiaphragm.[4,7,11,13] Nonspecific findings are also seen in about 25% to 69% of abdominal radiographs.[2,3,7,11,12] These studies may demonstrate a soft tissue mass, extraluminal gas shadow, or a nongastric air–fluid level in the left upper quadrant.[11,13] There is one reported case of a gas-forming splenic abscess causing pneumoperitoneum and generalized peritonitis in an immunocompromised patient, in which the plain abdominal film showed free air and extraluminal air bubbles in the left upper quadrant.[14] Ultrasound (Figure 137-1) has a sensitivity of 75% to 90%

for detecting splenic abscess.[3,11,15] Sonographic findings include an anechoic (13%) or hypoechoic (87%) mass, with an irregular wall, with or without internal echogenic foci that may represent septations, debris, or layering.[5,16-18] Computed tomography (CT) is more accurate than ultrasound, with a sensitivity of up to 96%[3] and specificity of 90% to 95%.[3,5] In addition, CT has a greater specificity over ultrasound in detecting gas, a diagnostic finding for splenic abscess.[5] CT also offers the advantage of being able to localize abscesses as small as several millimeters and enables the examiner to determine whether the abscesses are unilocular (Figures 137-2 and 137-3) or multilocular (Figure 137-4). Another advantage to CT is being able to identify the anatomic location of the abscess in relation to the spleen and other organs, thus aiding in determining the appropriate management option. Findings on CT scan include low-density parenchymal areas with peripheral enhancement after intravenous contrast administration.[11,13] These scans can help differentiate splenic abscess from other diseases such as splenic cysts and infarctions and can be used serially to follow abscess response to therapy.[4] Furthermore, CT- or ultrasound-guided intervention can be used for both diagnosis and therapy.

In situations where the diagnosis remains unclear after the imaging and laboratory studies, fine-needle aspiration is recommended.[5]

ABSCESS CHARACTERISTICS

The pathogenesis of splenic abscess includes hematogenous spread of a remote infection, hemoglobinopathy resulting in embolization/infarction, chemotherapy and other immunodeficiency states, trauma, and contiguous infection from adjacent organs.[2,19-21] Traditionally, the pathogenesis is related to the spread of microorganisms from an infectious source via a hematogenous route. This route of infection has been reported in 49% to 68% of cases.[11,19,21] Metastatic hematogenous infections from endocarditis account for greater than 66% of splenic abscesses.[8] However, in recent times, 18% to 28% of splenic abscess cases are found in immunocompromised patients.[11,21] In this patient population, splenic abscesses are usually multilocular. Secondary to the increased population of immunocompromised patients, opportunistic pathogens such as fungi and gram-positive aerobes are more often identified than in the past.[21] Splenic abscess due to a contiguous septic process from adjacent organs such as the stomach, colon, pancreas, or kidney is seen less frequently, with an incidence of only 6% to 15% of reported cases.[3,11,21] Hemoglobinopathies such as sickle cell, thalassemia, and leukemia are known to predispose patients to splenic abscess.[11] These disorders are recently

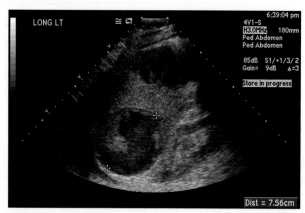

FIGURE 137-1 Ultrasound of the upper abdomen showing a 7.6-cm unilocular abscess of the spleen.

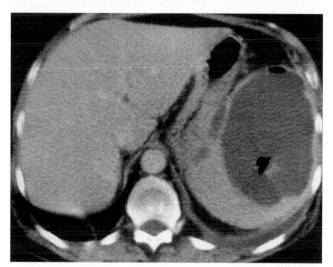

FIGURE 137-2 CT of the upper abdomen following intravenous contrast medium administration. There is a large fluid-filled cavity with enhancing borders and containing gas, consistent with an abscess of the spleen. (Courtesy GE Healthcare BioSciences—Medical Diagnostics, www.medcyclopaedia.com.)

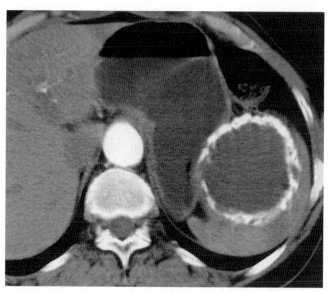

FIGURE 137-3 CT of the upper abdomen following intravenous contrast medium administration. There is a chronic abscess cavity with irregular and thick calcifications of the wall. (Courtesy GE Healthcare BioSciences—Medical Diagnostics, www.medcyclopaedia.com.)

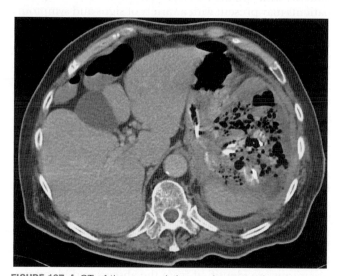

FIGURE 137-4 CT of the upper abdomen demonstrating a multilocular splenic abscess after splenic flexure lymphoma resection. There is a Penrose drain centrally.

reported in 6% or less of cases.[3,11,19,21] Unilocular splenic abscess has a more favorable prognosis and is usually present with subacute bacterial endocarditis, drug abuse, trauma, or other septic episodes.[5]

There are a large variety of both aerobic and anaerobic bacteria responsible for splenic abscess. The most common bacteria are *Staphylococcus aureus, Streptococcus, Salmonella, Escherichia coli,* and anaerobes.[2,3,22] Polymicrobial abscesses have been found in 11% to 36% of cases,[22] with anaerobic bacteria being present most often.[3,22] With the increased number of immunodeficient patients, there has been an increase in fungal abscesses in up to 25% of cases.[3,11,21] *Candida* accounts for more than 70% of fungal abscesses with other isolates including *Aspergillus, Cryptococcus neoformans, Aureobasidium pullulans,* and *Blastomyces dermatitidis.*[3,11] Fungal abscesses tend to be multilocular in 90% of patients,[11,23] whereas bacterial abscesses are multilocular in 26% of patients.[3,11,19] Splenic abscess involvement with *Mycobacterium* species was once rare but recently has been reported in 4% to 7.8% of cases, mostly in immunocompromised patients.[3,11]

MANAGEMENT

If left untreated, splenic abscesses are universally fatal. Combined medical therapy and drainage is used to treat many splenic abscesses. Drainage can be accomplished by either splenectomy or percutaneously using radiographic guidance. Medical management (antibiotics) alone is generally ineffective and is associated with a mortality rate as high as 80%.[4] However, splenic abscess caused by *Mycobacterium* species, *Pneumocystis jiroveci,* or fungal infection may be treated successfully with antibiotics or antifungals alone.[21]

The traditional treatment for splenic abscess is splenectomy (Figures 137-5 and 137-6), but this is associated

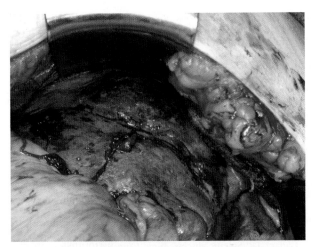

FIGURE 137-5 This patient has a splenic abscess due to pneumococcal bacteremia. Note that the massively enlarged spleen is readily visible, with minimal retraction in the left upper quadrant. (From eMedicine from WebMD—Medscape, emedicine.medscape.com/article/194655-media.)

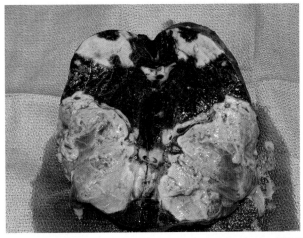

FIGURE 137-6 Resected spleen (same patient as in Figure 137-5) with abscesses caused by pneumococcal bacteremia. Note the discrete abscesses adjacent to normal parenchyma. (From eMedicine from WebMD—Medscape, emedicine.medscape.com/article/194655-media.)

with morbidity and mortality rates of 11% to 28% and 6% to 14%, respectively, secondary to underlying disease and intraabdominal rupture during operation.[3,5,7,21] Mortality is even greater in critically ill and immunocompromised patients.[4,5,21] Furthermore, splenectomy may be difficult in some patients because of extensive parasplenic inflammation and adhesions. In these situations, early ligation of the splenic artery through an opening in the gastrosplenic ligament may be desirable prior to splenic mobilization and splenectomy. After splenectomy, the left subphrenic space should be drained. At the time of exploration, if dense adhesions prevent a safe splenectomy, the abscess can be aspirated or drained, and interval splenectomy performed at a later date. Infrequently, it may be necessary to remove the tenth and eleventh ribs to gain access to a high-lying abscess, taking caution not to enter the pleural cavity.

Laparoscopic drainage of splenic abscess may be indicated when percutaneous drainage is not an option because of location or access or when prior percutaneous drainage attempts have failed. In such cases, laparoscopic drainage of splenic abscess can offer a minimally invasive alternative to open surgery. Additionally, with laparoscopic drainage, abscesses can be aspirated, larger drains placed, and if warranted, a total splenectomy completed. When using laparoscopic therapy for splenic abscess, the abscess may be aspirated at the onset of the procedure to facilitate splenectomy. Laparoscopic splenectomy[24] or drainage may also be successfully and safely implemented for cases of splenic abscess, with outcomes comparing favorably to open series.

An alternative to splenectomy is CT- or ultrasound-guided percutaneous drainage. This carries a lower morbidity and mortality rate of 5% and 1%, respectively.[3,5,21] Reported complications associated with this modality include pneumothorax and hemothorax.[21] The advantage of the low mortality rate must be weighed against the disadvantage of the 30% recurrence rate from percutaneous drainage.[3] Multiple drain placements have been required in some patients for complete resolution of an abscess. Moreover, percutaneous drainage with serial attempts may be implemented as initial therapy for many cases of unilocular abscesses. Response to therapy is monitored with CT or ultrasound, and failure of response can be followed by splenectomy. Techniques of percutaneous drainage may offer advantages over splenectomy in that the therapy is tolerated even in severely debilitated, elderly, or critically ill patients.[4] Additionally, preservation of the spleen is vital in children and immunocompromised patients.[4] Adequate percutaneous drainage of a splenic abscess can be usually achieved by using 12- to 14-French catheters.[4,20]

Abscesses appropriate for percutaneous drainage are usually unilocular, solitary, and possess a well-defined wall with homogeneous-appearing contents. Proper localization of the abscess is also essential for CT- or ultrasound-guided percutaneous drainage. For abscesses that are multiple, septated, or anatomically inaccessible, percutaneous drainage is relatively contraindicated.[4] Percutaneous drainage is not recommended in patients with coagulopathies, ascites, or associated diseases requiring surgical management.[4,6] Percutaneous drainage carries a risk of iatrogenic injury to the spleen and surrounding organs such as the colon, stomach, left kidney, and diaphragm. Additional iatrogenic complications may include hemorrhage, pleural empyema, pneumothorax, and enteric fistula.[25,26]

Selection of antibiotics in patients with splenic abscess should be guided by the sensitivity of isolates or by the most likely pathogens in culture-negative isolates.[11] The most common length of antibiotic therapy is 10 to 14 days.[11]

OUTCOMES AND FOLLOWUP

A complete peer-reviewed clinical algorithm for splenic abscess does not yet exist. This is secondary to the relatively low incidence of splenic abscess and subsequent lack of randomized or prospective studies evaluating diagnostic and treatment modalities. The current literature suggests a universal theme that early diagnosis, targeted management, and employment of minimally invasive techniques may decrease the morbidity and mortality of splenic abscess.

REFERENCES

1. Lawhorne TW Jr, Zuidema GD: Splenic abscess. *Surgery* 79:686, 1976.
2. Chun CH, Raff MJ, Contreras L, et al: Splenic abscess. *Medicine (Baltimore)* 59:50, 1980.
3. Nelken N, Ignatius J, Skinner M, et al: Changing clinical spectrum of splenic abscess. A multicenter study and review of the literature. *Am J Surg* 154:27, 1987.
4. Farres H, Felsher J, Banbury M, et al: Management of splenic abscess in a critically ill patient. *Surg Laparosc Endosc Percutan Tech* 14:49, 2004.
5. Ng KK, Lee TY, Wan YL, et al: Splenic abscess: Diagnosis and management. *Hepatogastroenterology* 49:567, 2002.
6. Sarr MG, Zuidema GD: Splenic abscess: Presentation, diagnosis, and treatment. *Surgery* 92:480, 1982.
7. Faught WE, Gilbertson JJ, Nelson EW: Splenic abscess: Presentation, treatment options, and results. *Am J Surg* 158:612, 1989.
8. Robinson SL, Saxe JM, Lucas CE, et al: Splenic abscess associated with endocarditis. *Surgery* 112:781; discussion 786, 1992.
9. Saadeh AM, Abu-Farsakh NA, Omari HZ: Infective endocarditis and occult splenic abscess caused by Brucella melitensis infection: A case report and review of the literature. *Acta Cardiol* 51:279, 1996.
10. Ho HS, Wisner DH: Splenic abscess in the intensive care unit. *Arch Surg* 128:842; discussion 846, 1993.
11. Green BT: Splenic abscess: Report of six cases and review of the literature. *Am Surg* 67:80, 2001.
12. Johnson JD, Raff MJ, Barnwell PA, et al: Splenic abscess complicating infectious endocarditis. *Arch Intern Med* 143:906, 1983.
13. Johnson JD, Raff MJ, Chun CH, et al: Surgical management of splenic abscess in endocarditis. *Arch Intern Med* 145:370, 1985.
14. Ishigami K, Decker GT, Bolton-Smith JA, et al: Ruptured splenic abscess: A cause of pneumoperitoneum in a patient with AIDS. *Emerg Radiol* 10:163, 2003.
15. Tikkakoski T, Siniluoto T, Paivansalo M, et al: Splenic abscess. Imaging and intervention. *Acta Radiol* 33:561, 1992.
16. Goerg C, Schwerk WB, Goerg K: Sonography of focal lesions of the spleen. *AJR Am J Roentgenol* 156:949, 1991.
17. Hertzanu Y, Mendelsohn DB, Goudie E, et al: Splenic abscess: A review with the value of ultrasound. *Clin Radiol* 34:661, 1983.
18. Ralls PW, Quinn MF, Colletti P, et al: Sonography of pyogenic splenic abscess. *AJR Am J Roentgenol* 138:523, 1982.
19. Alonso Cohen MA, Galera MJ, Ruiz M, et al: Splenic abscess. *World J Surg* 14:513; discussion 516, 1990.
20. Gadacz TR: Splenic abscess. *World J Surg* 9:410, 1985.
21. Phillips GS, Radosevich MD, Lipsett PA: Splenic abscess: Another look at an old disease. *Arch Surg* 132:1331; discussion 1335, 1997.
22. Chang KW, Chiu CH, Jaing TH, et al: Splenic abscess caused by group A beta-haemolytic streptococcus. *Acta Paediatr* 92:510, 2003.
23. Helton WS, Carrico CJ, Zaveruha PA, et al: Diagnosis and treatment of splenic fungal abscesses in the immune-suppressed patient. *Arch Surg* 121:580, 1986.
24. Rosen M, Brody F, Walsh RM, et al: Outcome of laparoscopic splenectomy based on hematologic indication. *Surg Endosc* 16:272, 2002.
25. Choudhury SR, Rajiv C, Pitamber S, et al: Management of splenic abscess in children by percutaneous drainage. *J Pediatr Surg* 41:e53, 2006.
26. Schaberle W, Eisele R: [Percutaneous ultrasound controlled drainage of large splenic abscesses]. *Chirurg* 68:744, 1997.

Splenectomy for Conditions Other Than Trauma

Yi-Qian Nancy You | John H. Donohue | David M. Nagorney

Splenectomy for nontraumatic disorders demands careful risk-benefit analysis and surgical planning. Crucial factors considered include the nature of the underlying disease, the severity of symptoms, alternative therapeutic options, the operative risk, and the success rate of splenectomy. During the past decade, the underlying diseases have become better understood; more and effective medical therapies have become available; laparoscopic techniques have decreased operative risks; and prophylaxis has minimized the risk of postsplenectomy infections. These advances have challenged some of the traditional concepts regarding splenectomy. This chapter aims to summarize the current indications and contemporary outcomes of splenectomy for nontraumatic conditions encountered by surgeons in consultation. These conditions mainly include hematologic disorders but also splenic mass lesions, splenic vascular disease, iatrogenic injuries, and other rare diseases.

SPLENECTOMY FOR HEMATOLOGIC DISORDERS

The spleen performs important hematologic and immunologic functions. It maintains the circulating blood components by filtering and removing damaged or senescent cells. As the largest aggregate of lymphoid tissue in the reticuloendothelial system, the spleen functions in both antibody production and phagocytosis. Accordingly, cytopenia and splenomegaly are two common manifestations of hematologic disorders involving the spleen. Cytopenia is associated with hypersplenism, the excessive destruction of one or more blood components. Splenomegaly, defined as splenic weight of more than 175 g (normal, 90 to 150 g), can become massive (>1000 to 15,000 g). Mechanical symptoms of splenomegaly include pain and early satiety. When the spleen is the sole site of the disease or a major contributor to the underlying pathophysiology, splenectomy is performed with curative intent. In most conditions, it is performed for effective palliation of symptoms and complications.

DISORDERS CAUSING THROMBOCYTOPENIA

Thrombocytopenia is defined as platelet count less than 150×10^9/L. Patients with platelet counts of 50×10^9/L or greater are usually asymptomatic and are discovered incidentally. Excessive oozing after surgery or bruising after minor trauma usually does not occur until the platelet count is below 30 to 50×10^9/L. Spontaneous internal bleeding may occur with platelet counts of 10 to 20×10^9/L. Response of thrombocytopenia to therapy has been variably defined in previous studies. Complete response (CR) is most commonly defined as achieving platelet counts of 150×10^9/L for at least 30 days after splenectomy without additional therapy. Partial response (PR) results when platelet counts of at least 50×10^9/L are achieved, whereas no response (NR) is defined when counts remain below 50×10^9/L for 30 days. Relapse occurs when thrombocytopenia recurs after achieving a normal platelet count.[1]

Idiopathic Thrombocytopenic Purpura

Idiopathic thrombocytopenic purpura (ITP) is the most common hematologic disease for which splenectomy is indicated. Affected patients may be asymptomatic or may present with petechiae, ecchymosis, epistaxis, gastrointestinal bleeding, or menorrhagia. Subarachnoid or intracranial hemorrhage suggests severe thrombocytopenia. ITP is mediated by autoantibodies, typically against multiple platelet membrane glycoproteins such as IIb/IIIa, Ib/Ix, Ia/IIa, IV, and V. Splenic macrophages clear platelets coated with IgG autoantibodies in an accelerated fashion.[2] When compensatory platelet production is impaired or outstripped, thrombocytopenia ensues. The test for antiplatelet antibodies has a sensitivity of only 49% to 66% and a specificity of 78% to 92%.[2,3] A positive test does not definitively diagnose ITP, whereas a negative result cannot exclude it. ITP remains a clinical diagnosis of exclusion. A search for a secondary cause for thrombocytopenia should be prompted by a history of drug or toxin exposure, recent viral infections, splenomegaly on physical examination, an abnormal peripheral smear, or a hypoplastic bone marrow. Although a peripheral blood smear has been required as a diagnostic test, bone marrow aspiration is considered for patients older than age 60 years with atypical presentations and in whom other disorders are suspected and splenectomy is contemplated.[4]

The time of disease onset in childhood or adulthood determines the clinical presentation, natural history, and treatment approaches. Childhood ITP most commonly affects children between 2 and 5 years of age without a gender bias. In approximately 90% of the patients, the disease manifests as acute thrombocytopenia, associated with a sudden onset of petechiae occurring 4 to 8 weeks after the prodrome of viral illness, allergies, or immunizations.[5] Antibodies formed during the preceding illnesses cross-react against platelets. The natural history of childhood ITP is favorable; a vast majority (83%) spontaneously recover within 8 weeks without therapy, with approximately 10% to 15% persisting as chronic ITP.[6] Therefore, aggressive therapy is avoided. Typical management includes observation and avoidance of platelet-inhibiting medications and of activities predisposing to trauma. The decision to initiate any form of therapy is typically driven by a concern for the risk of intracranial hemorrhage, the development of refractory clinical symptoms, and activity restrictions that compromise a child's quality of life. First-line therapy is medical and includes intravenous immunoglobulin (IVIG), corticosteroids, anti-IgD, and platelet transfusion. Splenectomy is delayed for as long as possible.[5] However, when it is performed, response rates of 63% to 86% may be expected. The response is sustained in the long term in 45% to 60% of the patients.[7,8] Benefit from splenectomy may be predicted by preoperative response to IVIG, with positive predictive values of 74% to 91% and negative predictive values of 75% to 100%.[9,10] In the pediatric population, laparoscopic splenectomy does not compromise the response rates, can be safely performed, and allows faster recovery without increasing costs.[11]

Adult ITP has an insidious onset and affects women between 18 and 40 years of age most commonly. The natural history contrasts with that of childhood ITP, in that spontaneous remission occurs in only 2% to 9% of all patients.[12] The majority develop chronic ITP. Although the disease course is usually benign, those with severe or refractory thrombocytopenia face four times the risk of mortality than the general population.[13] The decision to initiate therapy depends on the bleeding risk, estimated from patient's age, lifestyle, platelet count, and concomitant diseases.[4] Standard first-line options include corticosteroids, intravenous immune globulin (IVIG), and anti-IgD. Each therapy suffers from limitations: (1) corticosteroids may induce remission in 66% of the patients initially, but less than 20% maintain remission in the long term; (2) IVIG is costly and is reserved for when steroids are ineffective or contraindicated (e.g., pregnancy); and (3) anti-IgD is only effective in Rh-D–positive nonsplenectomized patients.[4,13] Splenectomy is the most likely curative therapy for ITP. Currently, it is indicated when disease is refractory to 6 weeks of corticosteroid therapy, when maintenance of platelets is dependent on 10 mg or more of prednisone daily, or when options for alternative therapy are limited.[4]

Outcomes of splenectomy for ITP have been summarized in a systematic review by Kojouri et al reporting on 130 articles.[1] The overall rate of platelet response to splenectomy is 67% (range, 37% to 100%), with a sustained response rate of 64% after 7 years (range, 5 to 12.75 years) of followup. The average relapse rate after splenectomy is 15% (range, 0% to 51%), most occurring within the first postoperative year. One single-center experience of 140 adults revealed an overall complete platelet response rate of 78% initially and 74% after 1 year.[4] Corticosteroids, danazol, and/or IVIG salvaged 81% of those who relapsed.[14] Factors predictive of successful outcome after splenectomy have also been investigated.[1,12] Younger age (<30 years) at splenectomy and previous response to glucocorticoids most consistently correlated with good response. Additionally, when platelets are mainly sequestered in the spleen rather than the liver and other lymphoid organs, as identified by indium-labeled platelet scans,[4] a superior response rate has been observed.

Laparoscopic splenectomy has become the criterion standard for ITP patients. Operative mortality has

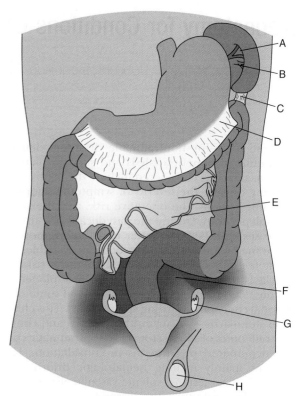

FIGURE 138-1 Common locations for accessory spleens: hilus of the spleen *(A)*; along the splenic vessels *(B)*; splenocolic ligament *(C)*; omentum *(D)*; mesentery *(E)*; presacral region *(F)*; adrenal region *(G)*; and gonads *(H)*. The weight of the dot corresponds to the frequency an accessory spleen may be found at that location. (From Martin JK: Staging laparotomy. In Donohue J, van Heerden J, Monson J, editors: *Atlas of surgical oncology.* Cambridge, Mass, 1995, Blackwell Science, p 150.)

decreased from 1% for open splenectomy to 0.2% for laparoscopic splenectomy. Similarly, operative morbidity has decreased from 12.9% to 9.6%.[1] Postoperative recovery is superior, with less pain and earlier hospital discharge. These benefits are realized without increased cost and without compromising hematologic response rates.[15] In debilitated patients who are unsuitable for an operation, splenic irradiation or partial splenic embolization may be considered, but the experience with this treatment is limited.

Accessory splenic tissue may be present in 16% to 29% of patients with ITP.[1] The most common locations for accessory splenic tissue include the splenic hilum, the gastrosplenic ligament, gastrocolic ligament, greater omentum, mesentery, and presacral space (Figure 138-1).[16] A thorough search should be conducted intraoperatively whether the operative approach is open or laparoscopic, because a missed accessory spleen may be the cause for relapse of ITP. The presence of residual functioning splenic tissue after splenectomy is indicated by the absence of Howell-Jolly bodies on a peripheral smear.

ITP occurs in every 1 to 2 per 1000 pregnancies, with or without a preexisting diagnosis. Differential diagnosis should exclude hereditary thrombocytopenia, gestational thrombocytopenia, and syndrome of hemolysis with elevated liver enzymes and low platelets. In pregnant ITP patients, bleeding risks for both the mother and the fetus must be considered, because maternal IgG antibodies cross the placenta and can cause fetal thrombocytopenia. Treatment consists of careful monitoring of maternal platelet counts that typically reach a nadir in the third trimester. Intervention is generally not needed in patients with platelet counts greater than $20 \times 10^9/L$ until before delivery. A maternal count greater than $50 \times 10^9/L$ is considered safe for any mode of delivery and is the goal of therapy. Treatment options of low teratogenic risk include corticosteroids or IVIG, but their side effects may be exacerbated in pregnancy and should be carefully monitored. Splenectomy is usually avoided, but if necessary, splenectomy should be performed during the second trimester. With maternal platelet count greater than $50 \times 10^9/L$, the incidence of fetal thrombocytopenia is 10% to 15% and that of fetal hemorrhage is less than 1%.[4,17]

Emergent intervention for ITP is indicated for patients with neurologic symptoms suggestive of intracranial bleeding, with evidence of internal or widespread mucocutaneous bleeding, and for those requiring an emergency operation for other reasons. First-line therapy consists of IVIG (1 g/kg/day for 2 days), intravenous methylprednisolone (1 g/day for 3 days), and platelet transfusions. Emergency splenectomy for refractory patients is rarely needed.[4]

Thrombotic Thrombocytopenia Purpura

Unlike ITP, thrombotic thrombocytopenia purpura (TTP) can be a highly lethal disorder. TTP is characterized by the pentad of thrombocytopenia, hemolytic anemia, fever, renal dysfunction, and less commonly, neurologic impairment. Characteristic findings include peripheral schistocytes (fragmented erythrocytes) and evidence of microvascular thrombosis. The pathophysiology of TTP involves an undefined trigger of vascular endothelial injury, leading to the release of unusually large forms of the von Willebrand factor. Abnormal platelet agglutination and marked intrasplenic phagocytosis follow. Currently, the first-line therapy consists of total plasma exchange in conjunction with corticosteroids and antiplatelet drugs such as aspirin or dipyridamole. Total plasma exchange has revolutionized the care of TTP by increasing the previously dismal survival rate to approximately 70% to 85%.[18,19] Relapse rates remain as high as 36% over 10 years.[20] Splenectomy has also been advocated for patients who are refractory to or suffer a relapse after plasma exchange. In several small series of patients, splenectomy induced remission of TTP in 50% of refractory patients[21] and reduced the risk of relapse by 70% to 95%.[21,22] However, the operative morbidity in this patient population may be substantial at 17% to 39%. Only recent reports have suggested that laparoscopic splenectomy has lowered these operative risks.[22,23]

Systemic Lupus Erythematosus

Systemic lupus erythematosus (SLE) is a chronic autoimmune disease of unknown cause. Antiplatelet antibodies are demonstrable in 78% of SLE patients. These pathogenic autoantibodies and immune complexes affect virtually every body system. Destruction of antibody-coated platelets leads to severe thrombocytopenia in 8% to 20% of these patients.[24] First-line therapy involves agents aimed at reducing the pathogenic immune response: corticosteroids, danazol, IVIG, and immunosuppressive (e.g., CellCept) and antineoplastic (e.g., cyclophosphamide, vincristine) drugs. Response rates to medical therapy have been variable and transient. Splenectomy is considered for patients who are refractory to dependent, or intolerant of medical therapy. Despite previous concerns, the operative risks of splenectomy are acceptable. The largest recent single-center experience of 25 patients undergoing splenectomy reported a 30-day mortality of 0% and morbidity of 24%, with hemorrhage and infection the most common complications.[24] The hematologic response was comparable to splenectomy for ITP, with an initial response rate of 88% and a relapse-free long-term response rate of 64%. Previously reported initial response rates ranged from 21% to 93% and prior sustained response rates were only 10% to 32%.[24] Although 36% of the patients relapsed after initial response (consistent with previously reported rates of 6% to 79%), additional medical therapy successfully salvaged 55% of these patients.[24] Because splenomegaly is typically not present, laparoscopic splenectomy is the procedure of choice in this patient population.

Human Immunodeficiency Virus

Chronic thrombocytopenia affects approximately 10% of patients infected with the human immunodeficiency virus (HIV) and 33% of those with acquired immunodeficiency syndrome (AIDS). Bleeding complications are infrequent and rarely severe even in the 1% to 5% of the patients with severe thrombocytopenia.[25] Most patients have platelet counts higher than $50 \times 10^9/L$; some may even spontaneously correct their thrombocytopenia. The pathogenesis of HIV-thrombocytopenia involves (1) immune-mediated platelet destruction, similar to that in ITP, and (2) impaired platelet production due to infected megakaryocytes in the bone marrow.[26] Accordingly, first-line therapy consists of (1) corticosteroids, IVIG and anti-D, similar to ITP, and (2) antiviral agents such as azidothymidine (AZT) or combination highly active antiretroviral therapy to treat the primary disease.[25,27] The immunosuppressive effects of corticosteroids make them unsuitable for long-term administration. Splenectomy is indicated in patients unresponsive, refractory, or intolerant of medical therapy. Operative mortality is minimal,[28] though the complication rate approaches 24%.[29] Favorable response is achieved in 83% of HIV patients[28,30] and slightly fewer AIDS patients.[29] Splenectomy has not been shown to adversely impact the progression to AIDS, overall survival, and AIDS-free survival.[29] Despite encouraging results, the timing and patient selection for splenectomy during the course of HIV infection remain controversial.

Wiskott-Aldrich Syndrome

Wiskott-Aldrich syndrome (WAS) is an X-linked immunodeficiency disorder characterized by thrombocytopenia, eczema, vasculitis, progressive immunodeficiency, and increased risk for malignancy. Its pathogenesis

TABLE 138-1 Classification of Hereditary Spherocytosis

Variable	Trait/Carrier	Mild	Moderate	Severe
Hemoglobin, g/dL	Normal	11-15	8-12	6-8
Reticulocyte, %	<3	3-6	>6	>10
Bilirubin, μmol/L	<17	17-34	>34	>51
Spectrin per RBC, % normal	100	80-100	50-80	40-60
Splenectomy	Not indicated	Usually not indicated	Consider before puberty	Usually necessary, delay until age 6 yr if possible

RBC, Red blood cell.

involves defective cytoplasmic scaffolding proteins.[31] Although phenotypic expression varies, thrombocytopenia is the most common manifestation of WAS. For patients with severe symptoms and available human leukocyte antigen (HLA)-matched donors, bone marrow transplant is performed with curative intent. For symptomatic patients without appropriate donors, splenectomy is indicated in combination with prophylactic antibiotics and immunization. Median survival of up to 25 years has been reported,[32,33] representing substantial improvement over the previously dismal median survival of less than 5 years. IVIG may be used alone or in combination with splenectomy.

DISORDERS CAUSING ANEMIA

Hereditary Anemia

Hereditary anemias can be categorized by (1) defects of the erythrocyte membrane (e.g., hereditary spherocytosis, hereditary elliptocytosis); (2) defects of an erythrocyte enzyme (e.g., pyruvate kinase deficiency, glucose-6-phsophase dehydrogenase deficiency); and (3) defects of hemoglobin synthesis (e.g., thalassemias, sickle cell anemia). All of these mutations result in abnormal erythrocyte morphology and stability and lead to increased hemolysis and phagocytosis by the spleen. The benefit and use of splenectomy vary depending on the diagnosis.

Red Blood Cell Membrane Defects. Hereditary spherocytosis (HS) is the most common inherited hemolytic disorder in North America and Europe. It is transmitted mainly as an autosomal dominant trait. The pathogenesis of HS involves deficiencies in membrane structural proteins. The affected family of spectrin proteins, including β spectrin, ankyrin, band 3, and protein 4-2, normally forms the supportive cytoskeleton of the red blood cell (RBC). Dysfunction of these proteins results in abnormal RBC morphology, increased cell membrane fragility, and shortened life span. Clinical findings are variable and include anemia, jaundice, and splenomegaly. Pigmented gallstones form in up to 41% of patients screened with ultrasonography, and their prevalence is higher in patients who coinherit Gilbert disease.[34] HS is distinguished from other anemias by the findings of elevated reticulocyte counts, hyperbilirubinemia, negative direct antiglobulin test (DAT), spherocytes on peripheral smear, and increased erythrocyte osmotic fragility.[35,36]

The indication for splenectomy is not based on the diagnosis of HS, per se, but on its symptoms and complications (Table 138-1).[37] For patients with mild HS and no gallstones, splenectomy has no benefit.[38] For patients with moderate or severe disease, splenectomy is indicated but usually delayed until after the sixth year of life but before puberty to minimize the risk of postsplenectomy sepsis.[36] Children with accelerating anemia, frequent hemolytic crises, transfusion dependency, or intractable leg ulcers may require earlier intervention.[35] For patients with symptomatic cholelithiasis, laparoscopic splenectomy and cholecystectomy are indicated and can be performed safely together.[39] When gallstones are asymptomatic or found incidentally, the best approach has not been established. Options include observation, cholecystotomy with stone removal, or cholecystectomy.[40]

The optimal approach for splenectomy remains controversial. Laparoscopic splenectomy offers a faster postoperative recovery in the pediatric population. It should be the approach of choice when splenomegaly is not present to increase the operative risks.[12,41] Partial (80% to 90%) open[42] or laparoscopic[43] splenectomy has been advocated for very young patients with severe disease, but preservation of splenic function must be balanced against the risks of disease recurrence. Recently, near-total splenectomy (98%) has been proposed as a means to optimize this balance.[44]

Hereditary elliptocytosis is a variant of HS also involving defective spectrin proteins. These patients typically have mild anemia requiring no intervention. Splenectomy does not correct the abnormal RBC morphology but is effective for the rare patient with severe transfusion-dependent anemia. HS must also be differentiated from other rare disorders of RBC membrane permeability, such as hereditary stomatocytosis or cryohydrocytosis. Splenectomy is ineffective and unwarranted and carries a high risk of postsplenectomy venous thrombosis in these patients.[35]

Red Blood Cell Enzymatic Defects. Glucose-6-phosphate dehydrogenase deficiency is the most common RBC enzymatic defect. It manifests as a mild anemia and rarely splenomegaly. Experience with splenectomy in this disease is limited. Pyruvate kinase deficiency results in reduced energy generation in RBCs. The homozygous form of this disease results in a severe anemia with splenomegaly. Splenectomy is effective in reducing transfusion requirements.[45]

Hemoglobinopathies. Sickle cell disease includes sickle cell anemia (SS), hemoglobin C disease (SC), and the sickle β thalassemia. The inherited point mutation on the sickle gene leads to an abnormal β-chain forming a hemoglobin with decreased solubility in its deoxygenated form. Pathogenesis of sickle disease results from abnormal polymerization of hemoglobin S with low cellular oxygen content. Exponential propagation of this process stiffens and distorts erythrocytes. Further compounding factors include abnormal endothelial adhesion, formation of heterocellular aggregates, dysregulation of nitric oxide–mediated vasodilation, and local inflammation. All of these factors lead to slowed RBC transit and their entrapment in the vasculature and in the spleen.[46] Microvascular occlusion results, and sickle patients suffer from end-organ damage of the eyes, kidneys, subcutaneous tissue, and bone. Splenic sequestration occurs when the RBC is trapped in the enlarged spleen, which then undergoes autoinfarction; it is observed in 7% to 30% of SS patients between 2 and 5 years of life. Acute manifestation, known as *acute splenic sequestration crisis* (ASSC), is potentially fatal. Patients present with profound acute anemia (decrease in hemoglobin by >2 g/dL), reticulocytosis, and thrombocytopenia. Acute therapy requires resuscitation by RBC transfusions. However, recurrence carries a 20% mortality rate and can occur in 50% of those who survive ASSC.[46] As a means to prevent future ASSC, elective splenectomy has been indicated in children older than 2 or 3 years of age after the first episode of ASSC. The operative mortality is 7%, and 5-year mortality is 3.4%.[47,48] The risk of postsplenectomy sepsis is approximately 2% in this patient population but increases substantially if splenectomy is performed before 4 years of age.[49-51] Although splenectomy has not been proven to increase survival, its benefits include reducing transfusion dependency, relief from pain from splenomegaly, and treatment of splenic abscesses resulting from splenic infarctions.[47,52]

Patients with thalassemia major (or homozygous β thalassemia) synthesize structurally abnormal hemoglobin that deforms erythrocytes. They typically depend on multiple transfusions to maintain a hemoglobin level above 10 g/dL. When complications of hypersplenism develop, as measured by transfusion requirement of greater than 250 mL/kg/year and iron overload, splenectomy is indicated.[53] Splenectomy reduces the requirements for both transfusions and deferoxamine (an iron chelator) in 32% of patients.[54] More than 80% of children with thalassemia regain normal weight and growth rates after splenectomy.[55] The risk for overwhelming postsplenectomy sepsis (OPSS) is high in this patient population, approximately 10% in the long term.[56] Therefore, splenectomy is usually delayed until after 6 to 8 years of age. Partial splenectomy has been advocated in younger children,[57] and laparoscopic splenectomy is definitely feasible in these patients.[58]

Acquired Hemolytic Anemia

Hemolytic anemia may result from numerous etiologies. Autoimmune hemolytic anemia (AIHA) is an IgG-mediated (so-called warm agglutinin) hemolytic anemia with a positive Coombs antiglobulin test. Erythrocyte destruction is mediated by splenic macrophages. AIHA may be idiopathic or a manifestation of a systemic disease, such as viral infection, SLE, rheumatoid arthritis,

ulcerative colitis, or chronic lymphocytic leukemia (CLL). Splenectomy is indicated when disease is refractory to corticosteroids. It succeeds in up to 64% of patients and reduces the steroid requirement in an additional 21%.[45] The success rate is higher when AIHA is associated with systemic disease.[59] In contrast, so-called cold agglutinin hemolytic anemia is mediated by IgM. Erythrocytes are sequestered and destroyed in the liver, and splenectomy therefore plays no role in this condition.

MISCELLANEOUS HEMATOLOGIC DISORDERS

Evans Syndrome

Patients with Evans syndrome present with a combination of autoimmune thrombocytopenia (ITP) and autoimmune hemolytic anemia (AIHA). Medical therapy typically involves multiple agents, with corticosteroids and IVIG being used most commonly.[60,61] Experience with splenectomy for this rare disease is limited.[62] Although long-term remission has been reported,[63] one study observed the median duration of response following splenectomy to be only 1 month.[61]

Felty Syndrome

Felty syndrome, defined as a combination of rheumatoid arthritis, splenomegaly, and neutropenia, affects a small subset of patients, particularly those with destructive rheumatoid arthritis, severe extraarticular symptoms, and an HLA-DR4 haplotype.[64] Neutropenic sepsis is the main cause of patient demise. First-line therapy consists of hematopoietic growth factors and often leads to rapid, favorable responses.[65] Splenectomy is indicated when the neutropenia fails to improve adequately or rapidly enough. Neutropenia is corrected by splenectomy in 80% of patients, and active preoperative infections resolve in nearly half of patients.[65]

Autoimmune Neutropenia

Patients affected by autoimmune neutropenia, a rare disorder, usually have neutrophil counts of 500 to 1000/μL but manifest granulocyte-specific antibodies. It commonly presents in infancy as recurrent infections. When present in adults, it may be associated with underlying diseases such as viral infection, collagen vascular diseases, ITP, or AIHA. Autoimmune neutropenia is typically characterized by spontaneous disappearance of autoantibodies and does not require specific intervention. However, for acute infections or operative procedures, granulocyte colony-stimulating factors effectively improve the neutrophil counts. Fifty percent to 60% of the patients also respond to corticosteroids and IVIG.[62] Therefore, the role for splenectomy is limited only to the rare patient who is refractory to medical interventions.

LYMPHOPROLIFERATIVE DISORDERS

Lymphoma

Lymphomas are categorized into two distinct types: Hodgkin disease (HD) and non-Hodgkin lymphoma (NHL). The surgeon's role in HD is to provide disease staging, a rare indication for splenectomy today, since

TABLE 138-2 Hodgkin Disease: Ann Arbor Classification With Cotswold Modification

Classification Stage	Description of Involvement	MODIFYING FEATURES		
		Classification Letter	Description	
I	1 lymph node/tissue (e.g., spleen, thymus, Waldeyer ring)	A	No symptoms	
II	≥2 lymph nodes/tissue, on same side of the diaphragm	B	Fever, night sweats, weight loss >10% in 6 mo	
III	Lymph node/tissue, on opposite side of the diaphragm	X	Bulky disease	
1	Splenic, celiac, portal nodes			
2	Paraaortic, iliac, mesenteric nodes			
IV	Extranodal sites	E	Involves single, contiguous, or proximal extranodal site	

most HD patients now receive chemotherapy. Splenectomy provides palliative and therapeutic benefits in several subtypes of NHL.

Hodgkin Disease: The diagnosis of HD is made when a tissue biopsy demonstrates Reed-Sternberg cells surrounded by reactive lymphocytes. Molecular alterations in the BCL2 or the NFκB pathways enable the malignant Reed-Steinberg cells to evade apoptosis and account for the pathogenesis of HD.[66] The clinical manifestations and course of HD are largely dependent on its histopathology. Classic HD includes the following histologic subtypes:

1. The most common nodular-sclerosing form affects the mediastinum predominantly and carries a favorable prognosis.
2. The mixed-cellularity subtype is the second most common and has a high frequency of abdominal involvement.
3. The diffuse lymphocyte-predominant subtype is distinguished from the nodular lymphocyte-predominant form in its involvement of multiple anatomic regions.
4. The least common, lymphocyte-deplete subtype, is usually a subdiaphragmatic disease characterized by pancytopenia, abnormal liver function, minimal peripheral adenopathy, and poor prognosis.

Apart from classic HD, the nodular lymphocyte-predominant form of HD affects a minority (5%) of patients with limited cervical or inguinal disease and carries a favorable prognosis. Regardless of the histologic type, 30% to 60% of all patients with HD experience systemic symptoms consisting of fever, night sweats, and weight loss.

The therapy of HD depends on its clinical and pathologic stage, according to the Ann Arbor staging system with Cotswold modification (Table 138-2). Patients with advanced disease (stage III or IV) receive combination chemotherapy and radiation. The current criterion standard therapeutic regimen is ABVD (doxorubicin, bleomycin, vinblastine, and dacarbazine), with more intense drug regimens used for refractory disease. Patients with localized disease (stage I or II) may receive only radiation therapy to the involved fields. Short-cycle chemotherapy (ABVD) is added for high-risk disease.

Clinical staging of HD can be ascertained by physical examination; laboratory tests; bone marrow biopsy; chest radiograph; computed tomographic (CT) or magnetic resonance (MR) imaging scan of the chest, abdomen, and pelvis; lymphangiogram; and positron emission tomography. Pathologic confirmation of the disease extent is undertaken only when the information gained would change therapy. Surgical staging is indicated when patients are potential candidates for radiation as their sole therapy based on their clinical stage.[67] The goal of laparotomy is to rule out occult subdiaphragmatic disease that would upstage the disease and require systemic chemotherapy. It has been reported to detect occult splenic or upper abdominal disease in 20% to 35% of the patients with clinical stage I or II disease. Currently, however, surgical staging plays only a limited role in HD because the use of radiation-only treatment regimens has decreased and accurate imaging and percutaneous biopsies are well developed. Current indication for surgical staging is limited to patients in whom tissue sampling is inadequate.

The components of staging laparotomy are summarized in Figure 138-2.[16,17,67] Exploration is performed through an upper midline incision and includes palpation of the liver, spleen, bowel, mesentery, and major nodal groups. Splenectomy is performed with nodal clearance from the splenic hilum. The tied ends of the splenic vessels are marked with metal clips to guide postoperative radiation therapy. Both wedge and core-needle biopsies are obtained from each lobe of the liver, plus a wedge biopsy of any abnormality. Finally, all abnormal nodes identified by preoperative lymphangiogram are removed. Systemic nodal biopsies then follow with celiac axis, hepatic artery, hepatoduodenal, bilateral paraaortic, and iliac nodes being sampled. All areas are marked with metal clips for future localization. Oophoropexy behind the uterus in the midline has been recommended for women of childbearing age to exclude the ovaries from the radiation field. Operative complications (~10%) include small bowel obstruction, venous thrombosis, and subphrenic abscess.[17] Staging laparoscopy is now preferred over laparotomy. Adequate tissue biopsies, similar to those of traditional laparotomy, are readily

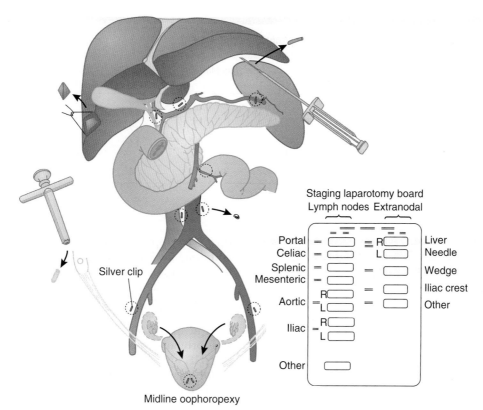

Staging laparotomy board				
Lymph nodes		Extranodal		
Portal	= ☐	≅ R☐	Liver	
Celiac	= ☐	L☐	Needle	
Splenic	= ☐	= ☐	Wedge	
Mesenteric	= ☐			
Aortic	R☐ = ☐	= ☐	Iliac crest	
	=L☐	= ☐	Other	
Iliac	R☐ =L☐			
Other	☐			

Silver clip

Midline oophoropexy

FIGURE 138-2 Components of a staging laparotomy for Hodgkin lymphoma. These include splenectomy, bilobar liver biopsies (needle and wedge), and nodal sampling (including celiac, porta hepatitis, mesenteric, paraaortic, and iliac nodes). Oophoropexy to the midline is performed in women to exclude ovaries from the radiation field. Bone marrow biopsy may be performed as a part of the procedure. (From Martin JK: Staging laparotomy. In Donohue J, van Heerden J, Monson J, editors: *Atlas of surgical oncology.* Cambridge, Mass, 1995, Blackwell Science, p 150.)

obtained.[68] Laparoscopic ultrasonography may supplant digital palpation in doubtful areas. In experienced hands, staging laparoscopy can achieve an accuracy rate of 96% to 100% for primary or relapsed HD, without false-negative results[69,70] and lower complication rates. The reported rates of conversion to laparotomy range from 0% to 20%, mainly because of hemorrhage during splenectomy.[69]

Non-Hodgkin Lymphoma. NHL is a diverse group of more than 20 malignancies originating from B lymphocytes (~80%), T lymphocytes (~15% to 20%), or natural killer cells (<5%). A specific NHL diagnosis requires histologic examination of lymphoid tissue plus flow cytometry and molecular marker studies. Patients with NHL frequently present with nonspecific symptoms of fever, night sweats, malaise, and weight loss. Peripheral lymphadenopathy is variably present and lymphatic spread is often noncontiguous. The spleen is involved in 30% to 40% of NHL patients.[70] Although NHL shares the same Ann Arbor staging system as HD, clinical staging is less crucial in NHL treatment because most patients present with advanced disease. There is no role for staging laparotomy in NHL because therapy is seldom redirected by staging information.[67]

There are three indications for splenectomy in NHL patients: (1) to correct hypersplenism and the resultant cytopenia(s), thereby allowing aggressive chemotherapy and/or independence from transfusions; (2) to relieve symptoms of splenomegaly from lymphocytic infiltration; and (3) tumor debulking when the spleen is the main site of disease involvement, either as primary treatment or for residual disease. Operative mortality ranges between 0% and 3.5%, and reported operative morbidity is higher at 11% to 37% in studies published since 1990 (Table 138-3).[71-75] The most common severe complications are venous thrombosis and subphrenic abscess. A laparoscopic splenectomy is associated with reduced morbidity but requires technical expertise, particularly when splenomegaly is present.[75] Blood counts normalize in 72% to 89% of patients with NHL within the first postoperative month. A durable response is observed in a substantial proportion of patients (see Table 138-3). Finally, these potential benefits and risks of splenectomy must be balanced against the prognosis of the primary disease. The proposed World Health Organization classification system (Box 138-1)[76] categorizes subtypes of NHL by clinical behavior: indolent subtypes have mean expected survivals measured in years, but aggressive subtypes generally have survivals measured only in months.

The spleen is the primary site of disease in several subtypes of NHL. Mantle cell lymphoma (MCL), an uncommon type, constitutes only 5% to 8% of NHL. Patients with MCL may have minimal adenopathy but prominent extranodal disease.[77] Up to 60% develop

TABLE 138-3 Experience With Splenectomy in NHL, Published Since 1990

Authors, Year	No. of Patients	Operative Technique	Operative Mortality (%)	Morbidity (%)	Initial Response (1 mo) (%)	Durable Response Followup (%)
Delpero et al, 1990[71]	62	Open	1.6	29	89	63 (26 mo)
Lehne et al, 1994[73]	35	Open	2.9	37	72	14
Brodsky et al, 1996[72]	12	Open	0	17	80 (3 mo)	N/A
Walsh and Heniford, 1999[75]	9	Laparoscopic	0	11	N/A	N/A
Xiros et al, 2000[74]	29	Open	3.5	14	88	N/A

NHL, Non-Hodgkin lymphoma; *N/A*, not available.

BOX 138-1 Proposed World Health Organization Classification of Lymphoid Neoplasms

INDOLENT LYMPHOMAS

B-Cell Neoplasms

Small lymphocytic lymphoma/B-cell chronic lymphocytic leukemia

Lymphoplasmacytic lymphoma (± Waldenström macroglobulinemia)

Plasma cell myeloma/plasmacytoma

Hairy cell leukemia

Follicular lymphoma (grades I and II)

Marginal zone B-cell lymphoma

Mantle cell lymphoma

T-Cell Neoplasms

T-cell large granular lymphocyte leukemia

Mycosis fungoides

T-cell prolymphocytic leukemia

Natural Killer Cell Neoplasms

Natural killer cell large granular lymphocyte leukemia

AGGRESSIVE LYMPHOMAS

B-Cell Neoplasms

Follicular lymphoma (grade III)

Diffuse large B-cell lymphoma

T-Cell Neoplasms

Peripheral T-cell lymphoma

Anaplastic large cell lymphoma, T/null cell

HIGHLY AGGRESSIVE LYMPHOMAS

B-Cell Neoplasms

Burkitt lymphoma

Precursor B lymphoblastic leukemia/lymphoma

T-Cell Neoplasms

Adult T-cell lymphoma/leukemia

Precursor T-lymphoblastic leukemia/lymphoma

massive splenomegaly.[78] For patients with splenic-predominant MCL, splenectomy should be considered to palliate either hypersplenism or splenomegaly or both. Splenectomy may further benefit patients by stabilizing their disease, delaying the start of chemotherapy, and prolonging survival. A retrospective study of 26 patients[77] found that splenectomy is safe (no operative mortality and morbidity of 24%). Hypersplenism was corrected in 69% of patients with anemia, 90% with thrombocytopenia, and 50% of patients with both. In addition, 90% did not require chemotherapy until at least a year after splenectomy. The median survival is 5.5 years (typically 3 to 4 years), and splenectomy was the sole therapy in 15% of the patients.

The therapeutic role of splenectomy is more prominent in splenic marginal zone B-cell lymphoma (MZL). This primary lymphoma of the spleen comprises only 1% of NHL and is characterized by massive splenomegaly, lymphocytes with villous projections, anemia, thrombocytopenia, and mild monoclonal gammopathy.[79] Reversal of cytopenia occurs in 82% to 95% of patients following splenectomy,[79-83] with a median survival of 8.5 years[80,82] and 3-year survival of 82%[79] in patients with spleen-only MZL. These results suggest that clinically localized MZL patients behave like those with localized stage I NHL. Longer overall survival correlated with prompt correction of cytopenia during the immediate postoperative period.[80] Splenectomy is a treatment of choice in patients with localized MZL.

Leukemias. Leukemia is characterized by a malignant clonal proliferation of hematopoietic stem cells. For patients with acute lymphocytic or acute myelogenous leukemia, there is consensus that splenectomy plays no role except for splenic rupture with hemorrhage.[17] For patients with chronic forms of leukemia, splenectomy may be indicated to palliate symptoms of splenomegaly or cytopenias. The survival benefit of splenectomy in patients with leukemia remains controversial.

CLL is the most common chronic leukemia. CLL is characterized by the accumulation of morphologically normal but functionally incompetent B lymphocytes. Patients follow either an indolent course requiring no therapy or an accelerated course with severe symptoms that require intervention.[84] CLL patients present with painless lymphadenopathy alone or with additional features including splenomegaly, cytopenia, and constitutional symptoms, as defined by the Rai classification (Table 138-4). Patients with stage 0 disease require no therapy, but selected patients with stage I or II disease and all patients with stage III or IV disease should receive chemotherapy, typically fludarabine.[71] Although cytopenia in CLL may result from bone marrow failure, hypersplenism, autoimmune destruction, chemotherapy, or any combination,[85] splenectomy is an efficacious method of reversing cytopenia (Table 138-5). A durable response of cytopenia in CLL is observed in at least 80% of patients, with higher response rates when splenectomy is performed for thrombocytopenia rather than for anemia.[78,85-89] However, no predicative factor of a hematologic response to splenectomy has been consistently identified.[90] The overall survival is longer in patients with a hematologic response than those who fail to respond,[86,89,90] but the survival benefit of splenectomy in patients with advanced CLL remains controversial. No significant difference in survival was observed in a case-matched study,[89] though in subgroup analysis of patients with severe anemia (hemoglobin <10 g/dL) or thrombocytopenia (platelet count <50 × 10⁹/L), splenectomy did significantly prolong median survival (19 vs. 10 months and 17 vs. 4 months, respectively). These results suggest that splenectomy should be considered for all CLL patients with cytopenia, particularly those with severe anemia or thrombocytopenia.

Chronic myelogenous leukemia (CML) consists of a chronic benign phase followed by an acute blast transformation phase. Patients usually present during the chronic phase with systemic symptoms, splenomegaly, leukocytosis, and cytopenias. Chromosomal translocation t(9;22) (i.e., Philadelphia chromosome) is present in 90% of the CML patients; and treatment efficacy is monitored by decreased expression of the abnormal chromosome.[67] Therapeutic options in CML include chemotherapy (e.g., hydroxyurea or busulfan), interferon-α, and bone marrow transplant.[17] Splenectomy is used only for palliation of refractory cytopenia or painful splenomegaly. Splenectomy does not seem to increase survival or delay the onset of the acute blastic transformation. Acute blastic crisis, marked by prolonged fever of unknown origin, leukocytosis, thrombocytopenia, and greater than 30% blasts in peripheral circulation, carries a grim prognosis, with median survival measured in months. Splenectomy is contraindicated during the acute phase. However, when necessary for emergency indications, a low 30-day mortality rate of 3.5% can be achieved.[91] Additionally, splenectomy does not have an adverse impact on the incidence of infections, graft versus host disease, or overall survival if a bone marrow transplant is performed after splenectomy.[92]

Hairy cell leukemia (HCL) comprises 2% to 5% of leukemias and is a chronic B-lymphocyte disorder characterized by peripheral cytopenia and massive splenomegaly. The malignant cells have hairlike projections and accumulate mainly in the red pulp of the spleen but can be identified elsewhere by their positive tartrate-resistant acid phosphatase staining.[90] Cytopenia in HCL may result from hypersplenism, bone marrow failure, or other reasons. Before 1990, splenectomy was the only known effective therapy for HCL. Cytopenia improved after splenectomy in 60% to 100%,[90] with a potential survival benefit. In the early 1990s, interferon-α was shown to be superior to splenectomy for cytopenia in a randomized trial.[93] Currently, medical therapies of interferon-α and purine analogues are efficacious. The indications for splenectomy in HCL are, therefore, limited to those patients with an uncertain diagnosis, splenic rupture, severe

---

TABLE 138-4 Rai Classification of Chronic Lymphocytic Leukemia

Stage	Description
0	Lymphocytosis (WBC >150,000/mL, >40% lymphocytes in bone marrow)
I	Lymphocytosis and lymphadenopathy
II	Lymphocytosis and splenomegaly/hepatomegaly
III	Lymphocytosis and anemia (hemoglobin <11 g/dL)
IV	Lymphocytosis, lymphadenopathy, anemia, and thrombocytopenia (platelet <100,000/mL)

WBC, White blood cell count.

TABLE 138-5 Experiences With Splenectomy for Chronic Lymphocytic Leukemia, Published Since 1990

Authors, Year	No. of Patients	Operative Mortality (%)	Operative Morbidity (%)	Response for Cytopenia (Response %)	Long-Term Cytopenia (Response %)	Median Survival (mo)
Thiruvengadam et al, 1990[84]	30	N/A	N/A	N/A	71-87	36 (18-62)
Neal et al, 1992[85]	50	4	26	64-77 (3 mo)	84-86	36 (41, responders; 14, nonresponders)
Majumdar et al, 1992[86]	14	0	28.5	84.6 (2-3 mo)	N/A	44
Pegourie-Bandelier et al, 1995[87]	29	0	34	N/A	85-100	N/A
Seymour et al, 1997[88]	55*	9	25	38-81	N/A	27 (vs. 23, *P* = 0.96)
Cusack et al, 1997[89]	77*	7.8	54	61-69	N/A	34 (vs. 24, *P* = 0.27)
Ruchlemer et al, 2002[78]	47	6.4	35	47 (3 mo)	N/A	56.4

N/A, Not available.
*Case matched with patients treated with fludarabine.

splenomegaly with symptomatic cytopenia, or disease refractory to chemotherapy. Resection of residual splenic disease after interferon therapy may prolong progression-free survival.[94] The contemporary experience with splenectomy for HCL is limited.

MYELOPROLIFERATIVE DISORDERS

Chronic myeloproliferative disorders are marked by abnormal clonal proliferation of hematopoietic stem cells. Myelofibrosis with myeloid metaplasia (MMM) occurs when bone marrow develops a fibrotic reaction to the stem cell disease and can be divided into agnogenic (AMM), postthrombocythemic (PTMM), and postpolycythemic (PPMM) types. PTMM and PPMM are preceded by essential thrombocythemia and polycythemic rubra vera, respectively, and splenectomy generally does not benefit these patients.[17,95,96] AMM is characterized by peripheral cytopenia and progressive extramedullary hematopoiesis in the spleen and the liver. Associated features include painful splenomegaly, increased portal blood flow, portal hypertension from venous thrombosis (~7%),[97] and cytopenia from splenic sequestration. The prognosis of AMM is poor, with median survival ranging from 3 to 5 years. Nonoperative therapy options are limited. Bone marrow transplant is frequently not an option for elderly AMM patients. Transfusions, androgens, corticosteroids, and interferon-α are largely palliative, and splenic irradiation is only transiently effective. Therefore, splenectomy should be considered in symptomatic patients. Symptomatic splenomegaly, constitutional symptoms, and portal hypertension improve in 100%, 67%, and 50% of the respective patients at 1 year postsplenectomy. Among those patients with transfusion-dependent anemia, 30% remain independent of transfusions for 6 months. No benefit for splenectomy is seen with thrombocytopenic patients.[98] Despite potential benefits, splenectomy in this patient population is a high-risk procedure.[99] Before 1940, operative mortality was prohibitively high at 40%. Currently, it ranges from 8% to 11%, with postoperative morbidity ranging from 31% to 40%.[94,98-100] Hemorrhage, infection, and thrombosis are the most common nonfatal complications. Several complications characteristic of this patient population have also been described.[98] Progressive hepatomegaly develops in 12% to 29% of the patients after splenectomy; as extramedullary hematopoiesis increases in the liver, 7% develop fatal hepatic failure. Severe thrombocytosis affects 18% to 50% of AMM patients after splenectomy, particularly if the preoperative platelet count is greater than 50×10^9/L. Postsplenectomy leukemic transformation occurs in 11% to 20% of patients and manifests as an accumulation of blasts in the bone marrow and peripheral blood.[95] Whether postsplenectomy blast transformation affects overall patient survival remains controversial[95,96,98,101,102] and should not deter the surgeon from performing an otherwise appropriate splenectomy. The median overall postsplenectomy survival is 2.3 years.[98] The main causes of death include infection, thrombosis, bleeding, and acute leukemia. Current indications for splenectomy in patients with AMM remain palliative and include severe constitutional symptoms, mechanical symptoms of splenomegaly, portal hypertension complicated by ascites and variceal hemorrhage, and transfusion-dependent anemia.[95]

SPLENECTOMY FOR TUMORS, CYSTS, AND ABSCESSES

TUMORS

Splenic masses are usually discovered incidentally. They present for surgical intervention with an unknown diagnosis, when the spleen ruptures, or when symptoms develop from their large size or associated hypersplenism.

The most common cause of a malignant splenic mass is metastasis from a primary carcinoma. Splenic metastases are present in 7% of patients dying from cancers of the breast, lung, ovary, stomach, and prostate.[17] Melanoma and other skin cancers also spread to the spleen. When the spleen is the only site of metastasis, splenectomy may prolong patient survival.

Primary, nonlymphatic, malignant tumors of the spleen include angiosarcoma, hemangioendothelioma, and malignant fibrous histiocytoma. Angiosarcoma is the most common of these rare tumors. Patients present at a median age of 60 years, with abdominal pain, splenomegaly, and microangiopathic hemolytic anemia. The tumors appear as well-circumscribed nodules with central necrosis or hemorrhage. The prognosis for splenic angiosarcoma patients is dismal. Eighty-nine percent of patients die of metastatic disease, with a median survival of 5 months.[103] Splenectomy is indicated for palliation and for splenic rupture, which may occur in 25% of patients. The rarity of the disease has hindered identification of risk factors, but exposure to thorium dioxide (Thorotrast), vinyl chloride, and anabolic steroids has been implicated in isolated reports.[103]

Benign tumors of the spleen are uncommon and include hamartoma, inflammatory pseudotumor, and vascular lesions (hemangioma, lymphangioma, peliosis). Hemangiomas are the most common benign splenic lesions and arise from the red pulp of the spleen. They can become very large, with prominent cystic components. Nonexpanding and asymptomatic hemangiomas less than 4 cm are safely observed.[104] Splenectomy may be considered to prevent or treat complications such as hypersplenism and splenomegaly. Peliosis of the spleen occurs alone or in association with peliosis of the liver. It occurs more frequently in men and is the result of the exogenous androgens and oral contraceptives, and accompanies chronic debilitation from tuberculosis, diabetes, or a neoplasm.[17] Complications of peliosis include thrombosis and fatal hemorrhage from splenic rupture. Splenectomy is indicated when peliosis is incidentally discovered. Splenic hamartomas as large as 2 kg have been reported and require surgical intervention for diagnosis. Inflammatory pseudotumors are a poorly understood entity. Patients present with fever, night sweats, and weight loss. These tumors must be distinguished from malignant lymphoma by immunohistologic studies, making splenectomy necessary for diagnosis in many patients. Additional rare benign splenic lesions include littoral cell angioma, hemangioendothelioma, and angiomyolipoma.

CYSTS

Parasitic Cysts

Echinococcus cysts are common in endemic disease areas but rare in the United States. Humans serve as intermediate hosts after ingestion of food contaminated with feces laden with tapeworm eggs. Hydatid cysts most commonly develop in the liver and the lungs; their daughter cysts contain multiplying larvae called *scolices*. Cysts of *Echinococcus granulosus* are unilocular, but those of *Echinococcus multilocularis* and *Echinococcus volegi* are multilocular.[12] Intervention is indicated when the disease is refractory to the antiparasitic drug albendazole or when cysts become large enough to risk rupture. Cystectomy or splenectomy should be performed with care to avoid cyst rupture or leakage. Anaphylaxis and disseminated scolices infection are serious operative complications. Administration of albendazole and instillation of hypertonic saline or ethanol before cyst manipulation have been advocated to decrease these risks.[12]

Nonparasitic Cysts

Nonparasitic splenic cysts were previously classified as true cysts (~20%) or pseudocysts (~80%) based on the presence or absence of an epithelial lining. True cysts may be epidermoid or, less commonly, dermoid in origin, resulting from splenic inclusion of embryonic tissue. They may also be associated with benign splenic hemangiomas or lymphangiomas. Pseudocysts are typically associated with antecedent splenic trauma or splenic infarction.[17] Splenic infarction occurs with hematologic disorders (most commonly sickle cell disease) in younger patients or with arterial emboli (the most common cause being atrial fibrillation) in patients older than age 40 years.[105] Recently, however, the reliability of identifying the cyst lining has been questioned. A newly proposed system classifies splenic cysts based on cause into congenital, neoplastic, true traumatic, and degenerative cysts.[106]

Intervention is not necessary for asymptomatic, small (<5 cm) splenic cysts that have imaging characteristics of a benign cyst, namely, a smooth, regular cyst wall, with no solid component within the cyst interior or wall, either with or without calcification.[106] Total splenectomy is typically considered for patients with low operative risk who develop pain or early satiety because of their splenic cysts. Recently developed minimally invasive treatment options include cyst aspiration with sclerosis using alcohol or tetracycline, cyst marsupialization, and local cyst resection with or without a portion of the cyst wall contiguous with splenic parenchyma. There is significant risk of cyst recurrence with these techniques. Laparoscopic or partial splenectomy is now the preferred treatment because of their low complication and cyst recurrence rates.[107]

ABSCESSES

Although splenic abscess remains a rare entity, it is uniformly fatal if unrecognized or untreated. With an increasing incidence of immunosuppressive diseases and medications, splenic abscesses have become more common.[108] A high index of suspicion is required for timely diagnosis and favorable outcome. Patients able to mount an immune response present with the triad of fever, leukocytosis, and left upper quadrant pain. Chest or abdominal radiographs often show a left-sided pleural effusion, elevated hemidiaphragm, left upper quadrant mass, and extraluminal air. A CT scan has a very high sensitivity and is the imaging modality of choice. A splenic abscess typically has a thick, irregular rim with a hypodense center, but multiple or miliary abscesses may be difficult to identify.

Splenic abscesses are classified by their cause.[12,108] The most common cause is primary hematogenous seeding from a distant septic source (common sources include bacterial endocarditis associated with valvular disease, intravenous drug use, bacteremia, and postoperative or primary intraabdominal infection). The most common organisms causing a splenic abscess are *Streptococcus* and *Staphylococcus* species, but *Salmonella* species, gram-negative *Escherichia coli*, and *Enterococcus* species, plus fungal infections also lead to splenic abscesses.[109] Although most splenic abscesses are solitary, multiple abscesses more frequently develop from hematogenous spread. Secondary infection of a splenic infarction is another cause of splenic abscess. Patients with an architecturally or functionally abnormal spleen are most susceptible to this type of infection. Common associated conditions include sickle cell anemia, lymphoproliferative and myeloproliferative diseases, trauma, and systemic arterial embolization. Patients with sickle cell anemia characteristically develop splenic abscesses with *Salmonella* species. The direct extension of a local septic focus may also result in a splenic abscess. These infections originate from a gastric, colonic, pancreatic, or perinephric source. Posttraumatic splenic abscesses occur after conservative management of splenic trauma or an iatrogenic intraoperative injury. Immunocompromised host accounts for up to 35% of patients with splenic abscesses. Associated conditions include malignancy, organ transplantation, chronic steroid use, and HIV/AIDS.

The treatment of choice for splenic abscess consists of broad-spectrum antibiotics, splenectomy, and drainage of the left upper quadrant. In critically ill patients unable to tolerate a surgical procedure, image-guided drainage should be attempted. When the abscess is discrete, unilocular, and filled with thin fluid, the success rate of nonoperative therapy is as high as 51%.[108] Occasionally, dense inflammatory adhesions preclude splenectomy, leaving splenotomy or surgical drainage as the only surgical options. In this setting, a delayed splenectomy is necessary because intravenous antibiotics are almost never sufficient treatment for a splenic abscess. Mortality from splenic abscess still ranges from 0% to 24%. Poor outcomes occur with immunocompromised patients, delayed diagnosis, and postponed operative intervention.[108]

SPLENECTOMY FOR VASCULAR DISORDERS

SPLENIC ARTERY ANEURYSM

Splenic artery aneurysm (SAA) constitutes 60% of all visceral arterial aneurysms and is the third most common abdominal aneurysm after aortic and iliac artery aneurysms. The typical patient with SAA is a multiparous woman (in a series of 87 women, the average number of pregnancies per patient was 4.5).[110] Other associated conditions include portal hypertension, congenital vascular or connective tissue diseases, and trauma. SAA presents (1) after rupture with hemodynamic instability; (2) as a symptomatic mass; or (3) as an incidental finding. Rupture occurs most commonly in the third trimester of pregnancy and may be forewarned by a sentinel hemorrhage in 20% to 30% of patients.[111] In pregnant patients, the mortality rate after rupture is 70% for the mother and approaches 100% for the fetus.[112] In nonpregnant patients, the mortality rate for SAA rupture is 25%.[17] As soon as rupture is suspected, prompt resuscitation, emergent splenectomy, and resection of the aneurysm are indicated. All symptomatic aneurysms require surgical intervention. For incidental and asymptomatic aneurysms, surgical treatment is indicated if the SAA is larger than 2.5 cm in diameter and if the patient is pregnant or of childbearing potential.[17,113] Operative treatment differs by location of the SAA. Proximal SAAs are excised after proximal and distal ligation. Mid-SAAs are excluded by proximal and distal ligation of the splenic artery and all collateral vessels. The spleen blood flow is preserved by the short gastric arteries. Distal or hilar SAAs are the most common and are treated with aneurysmectomy and splenectomy.[110,112,114] For patients unable to tolerate an operation, transcatheter embolization is utilized. This results in splenic infarction and has the risks of distant embolization, arterial disruption, and arterial recanalization with potential future rupture.[111,113] Successful laparoscopic ligation and splenectomy have been reported.[115,116] The optimal approach to elective treatment of SAA depends on patient variables and physician expertise.

SPLENIC VENOUS THROMBOSIS

Splenic venous thrombosis (SVT) complicates acute pancreatitis and pancreatic neoplasms in 7% to 20% of patients. Nonpancreatic diseases, including primary retroperitoneal fibrosis, peptic ulcer disease, and a hypercoagulable state, may also be associated with SVT.[117] SVT results in a localized form of portal hypertension termed *sinistral portal hypertension*.[118] Collateral flow through the short gastric vessels leads to engorgement of submucosal veins of the gastric fundus (gastric varices). Esophageal varices may arise if the left gastric vein is also occluded by the thrombus. The diagnosis of SVT should be suspected in patients with upper gastrointestinal hemorrhage following pancreatitis, in patients with splenomegaly but no hepatic or hematologic disease, and when isolated gastric varices are noted on upper endoscopy. Ultrasonography, CT scan, and visceral angiography all can confirm the diagnosis. In patients presenting with hemorrhage, urgent splenectomy is indicated. The operative bleeding risk is substantial because of the perigastric varices and inflammation. To reduce this risk, some surgeons advocate preoperative splenic artery embolization.[118] In unstable patients or those not fit for an operation, endoscopic variceal sclerotherapy or banding may be performed but this is usually ineffective.[119]

In asymptomatic patients with SVT, the indication for splenectomy is controversial. Prophylactic splenectomy used to be uniformly recommended, because up to 51% of asymptomatic patients with SVT were thought to develop acute variceal bleeding.[120] Recent studies have found a more benign natural history of SVT with a 4% to 18% prevalence of clinical hemorrhage.[118,120] Expectant management, initially advocated by Loftus et al,[121] has generally been adopted. Prophylactic splenectomy should be considered for noncompliant patients, those undergoing an abdominal operation for another cause, and patients who have endoscopic features such as "red wale markings" indicating a higher risk of hemorrhage.[118,119]

PORTAL HYPERTENSION

Patients with portal hypertension often develop thrombocytopenia from platelet sequestration in the splenic sinusoids.[17] Splenectomy should be considered with a devascularization or shunting procedure when the bleeding risk from thrombocytopenia is excessive, when medical therapy cannot be administered, or when the varices are resistant to nonoperative management.[122] Portal hypertension is not an absolute contraindication to laparoscopic splenectomy, but higher conversion (9.6%) and morbidity (11%) rates have been reported.[122]

"WANDERING SPLEEN" AND SPLENIC TORSION

A "wandering spleen" occurs when the spleen is attached only by a long, loose vascular pedicle. The spleen may be ectopic on imaging studies. Wandering spleens in children arise from congenital atresia of the dorsal mesogastrium. In women between 20 and 40 years of age, wandering spleens result from an acquired tissue laxity associated with pregnancy.[123] This condition may result in acute torsion around the vascular pedicle, which manifests as acute abdominal pain, fever, vomiting, acute pancreatitis, and gastric compression. Without detorsion, splenic infarction and gangrene ensue. Chronic torsion typically causes venous congestion and splenomegaly. In children without splenic infarction, the therapeutic procedure of choice is splenopexy, suturing the spleen to the diaphragm, abdominal wall, or omentum.[124] Laparoscopic splenopexy has been reported.[125] Although splenopexy allows for splenic preservation, the long-term results are unknown. For adults, splenectomy is preferred.

SPLENECTOMY FOR IATROGENIC INJURY

An iatrogenic splenic injury is an unintentional injury caused by the operator during either an interventional radiologic or surgical procedure. The surgical operations most commonly associated with iatrogenic splenic injury include distal esophageal and stomach procedures, colon surgery, left nephrectomy, and upper abdominal vascular procedures.[17] Risk factors for iatrogenic injury include a prior left upper quadrant operation, malignant or inflammatory diseases, and obese body habitus.[126] The spleen tethered by its peritoneal ligaments plus dense adhesions is prone to injury by inappropriate traction, retractor placement, or instrumentation.

When an iatrogenic splenic injury occurs, exposure to the left upper quadrant should be optimized, blood and clots are gently removed, and severe bleeding is temporized by pressure on the splenic artery at the superior edge of the pancreas. Limited splenic capsular tears may be treated successfully by packing, by electrocautery, argon beam coagulation, or hemostatic agents such as fibrin adhesive, thrombin-soaked Gelfoam, and microfibrillar collagen. Deeper lacerations may be salvaged with argon beam coagulation, mattress sutures in the spleen with or without pledgets, wrapping the spleen in an absorbent mesh, or segmental splenectomy. If the initial attempt at repair is unsuccessful, splenectomy should be performed.[127] In patients with severe (>grade 4) splenic injury, hemodynamic instability, or in those requiring postoperative anticoagulation, splenectomy is indicated. Splenectomy for iatrogenic injury prolongs hospital stay and increases morbidity from 0% to 32% and from 16% to 84% in various series.[126] Whether incidental splenectomy compromises immune function and decreases survival in cancer patients is uncertain. The incidence of sepsis is low after unplanned splenectomy in adults: 1 per 545 adult-years.[126] Measures to prevent iatrogenic injury include placement of the incisions and ports to maximize exposure, gentle retraction, careful medial or downward traction on the peritoneal attachments, and manipulation of stomach and colon only after dividing splenic ligaments and perisplenic adhesions.[126]

SPLENECTOMY FOR MISCELLANEOUS DISORDERS

Gaucher disease is an inherited metabolic disorder manifesting with anemia, thrombocytopenia, hepatosplenomegaly, and bone dysplasia. The genetic deficiency in lysosomal glucocerebrosidase leads to accumulation of glucosyl ceramide-laden macrophages in the reticuloendothelial cells of the liver, bone, and spleen. Enzyme replacement therapy (alglucerase or imiglucerase) effectively ameliorates symptoms of Gaucher disease.[128] Splenectomy is reserved for patients with compressive symptoms from massive splenomegaly or refractory cytopenia. The largest series to date reports operative mortality of 2.1% and morbidity of 27%.[129] In children with Gaucher disease, partial splenectomy or another spleen-preserving technique is advocated.

Splenomegaly complicates 6% of patients with sarcoidosis and is associated with anemia, neutropenia, or pancytopenia. Most patients have mild and asymptomatic splenomegaly and do not require treatment. Splenectomy is considered for massive or painful splenomegaly, refractory hypersplenism, to exclude lymphoma or other malignancy, and prophylaxis against splenic rupture. Outcome of splenectomy for sarcoidosis is favorable in isolated case reports.[130]

Amyloidosis is a systemic infiltrative disease. Splenic rupture may occur as amyloid deposits distend the capsule and increase vascular fragility.[131] Emergent splenectomy may be necessary for splenic rupture.

OPERATIVE CONSIDERATIONS FOR SPLENECTOMY

PREOPERATIVE PREPARATION

The indication for splenectomy, the underlying disease, and the patient's comorbidities, hematologic status, and previous therapy must be clearly reviewed.

Vaccinations are indicated whenever splenectomy or impaired splenic function is anticipated. They should be administered at least 2 weeks before splenectomy because the vaccine immunogenicity may be reduced if given after the splenectomy.[132] Pneumococcal vaccine is indicated for all patients; meningococcal and *Haemophilus influenzae* vaccinations are added for younger patients and those not previously immunized. The normal host defense against these encapsulated species involves antipolysaccharide antibodies and opsonization. Splenectomy renders both processes deficient and the patient more susceptible to infection without vaccination. If the splenectomy is emergent and preoperative vaccination is precluded, postoperative immunization is necessary.

Patients' hematologic reserve and the operative risks must be considered. The need for blood component transfusion is anticipated. Laboratory tests (e.g., cross-match) are performed and appropriate blood components reserved. One unit of platelets usually elevates the platelet count by 5×10^9/L, whereas 1 unit of erythrocytes elevates hemoglobin by 1 g/dL. In selected high-risk patients with severe thrombocytopenia (platelet count $<20 \times 10^9$/L), transfusion of 6 units of platelets may be considered before anesthetic induction to reduce the risk of laryngeal hematoma during endotracheal intubation. Preoperative platelet transfusion should be avoided in patients with ITP because transfused platelets will not survive splenic circulation until the splenic vessels are ligated.[17] In patients with portal hypertension and massive splenomegaly, preoperative splenic artery embolization can be performed to reduce the bleeding risk. However, its potential benefit must be balanced against the risk for pancreatitis, splenic abscess from infarction, hematoma formation, and pain.

Immediately before splenectomy, several medications are administered in the operating room. Patients on chronic steroid therapy should receive a bolus of exogenous steroid for operative stress. Prophylactic antibiotics are indicated in immunocompromised patients or when the gastrointestinal tract may be opened. In patients prone to thrombosis (e.g., myeloproliferative disorders), administration of unfractionated heparin (5000 IU subcutaneously three times daily), low-molecular-weight heparin, or antiplatelet agent (e.g., aspirin) may be beneficial.[133]

OPERATIVE CONSIDERATIONS

Splenectomy can be performed via the open, hand-assisted, or totally laparoscopic approach. The surgeon's experience and size of spleen generally determine the surgical method used. The larger the spleen, the more likely an open operation will be needed to safely remove it.

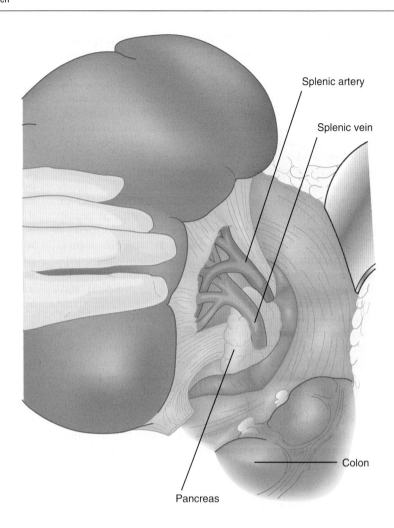

FIGURE 138-3 Mobilization of the spleen from its peritoneal ligamentous attachments. (From Scott-Conner CEH: *Chassin's operative strategy in general surgery: An expositive atlas*. Stamford, Conn, 2002, Springer, p 736.)

OPEN SPLENECTOMY

The most commonly used surgical incisions for open splenectomy are the left subcostal and the midline incisions. The latter is preferred for patients with narrow costal arches or with marked splenomegaly. A left thoracoabdominal incision with a midline vertical extension has been described but is rarely needed.[133] Most surgeons prefer gastric decompression via an orogastric or nasogastric tube.

The initial steps of splenectomy generally involve mobilizing the spleen. The stomach and the spleen are retracted medially to expose the splenophrenic and splenorenal ligaments. Unless venous varices are present, the ligaments are avascular and can be divided by blunt or sharp dissection. After the spleen is freed from its posterior attachments to the diaphragm and Gerota fascia, the splenocolic ligament is divided, releasing the splenic flexure and the omentum from the inferior splenic pole. The spleen can then be lifted into the abdominal incision (Figure 138-3). This maneuver should not be performed with excessive force, to avoid a capsular tear or avulsion of the splenic vessels. The splenogastric ligament is divided with identification, clamping, division, and ligation of the short gastric vessels. Suture ligation of these vessels on the gastric wall has been advocated by some surgeons to prevent postoperative loosening of the ligatures if the stomach becomes distended. The spleen is now attached only by the hilar vessels.

An alternative approach to splenectomy involves control of the splenic vessels at the hilum as the initial step. The gastrocolic omentum is opened lateral to the gastroepiploic arcade (Figure 138-4, *A*). The splenic artery is palpated along the superior border of the pancreas. Dissection of the vessels should be performed close to the splenic hilum to avoid injury to the tail of the pancreas (Figure 138-4, *B* to *D*). The splenic artery and vein may be divided together; however, separate division is preferable to prevent the formation of an arteriovenous fistula. The splenic artery should be controlled by double ligation, with one suture ligature. The splenic vein is divided after double ligation; a continuous vascular suture or a vascular stapler is used when the vein is markedly enlarged. This approach of initial vascular control may be particularly suitable in the presence of massive splenomegaly, marked hilar lymphadenopathy, or dense perisplenic adhesions. It has also been advocated for ITP, where early ligation of the vessels allows earlier administration of platelet transfusion. Similarly, it may be preferred for splenic malignancies, because it can prevent inadvertent tearing of the vessels during splenic mobilization and spillage of malignant cells.

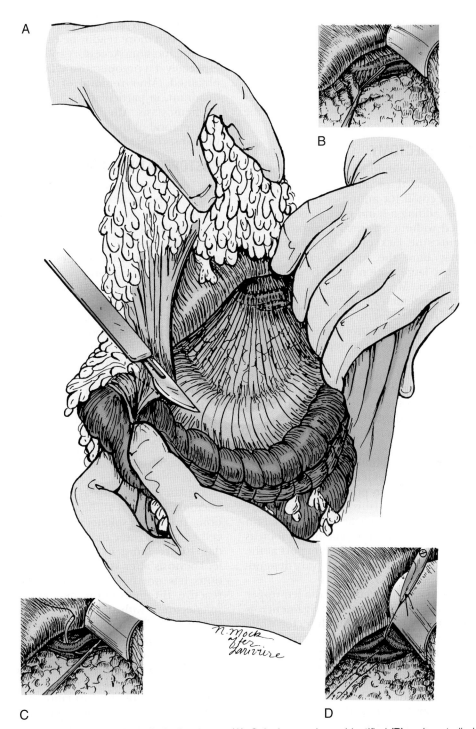

FIGURE 138-4 Approach to the splenic hilum through the lesser sac (**A**). Splenic vessels are identified (**B**) and controlled (**C** and **D**) along the superior border of the pancreas. (From Schwartz S: The spleen. In Zinner MJ, Schwartz SI, Ellis H, editors: *Maingot's abdominal operations*. Stamford, Conn, 1997, Appleton & Lange, p 2058.)

When a partial splenectomy is considered, branches of the vasculature are identified before they enter the spleen and ligated separately. Once the plane of vascular demarcation is recognized and marked, transection of the splenic parenchyma should be performed with total hilar occlusion to reduce hemorrhage on the transection surface. Placement of pledgets on through-and-through sutures with inflow occlusion reduces hemorrhage during partial splenectomy.

After removal of the spleen for hematologic diseases, the abdomen should be explored for accessory splenic tissue at the common locations (see Figure 138-1).

Prior to closure, hemostasis in the left upper quadrant should be ascertained by inspection of the inferior surface of the diaphragm, the left cephalad retroperitoneum, the greater curvature of the stomach, and the splenic hilum. The left upper quadrant may be packed to promote hemostasis. The greater curvature of the stomach should be imbricated with interrupted Lembert sutures if any serosal damage has occurred to prevent a gastric fistula. Closed-suction drainage of the left upper quadrant is not indicated unless injury to the tail of the pancreas is suspected or documented.

LAPAROSCOPIC SPLENECTOMY

Laparoscopic splenectomy should be considered for any spleen that is normal-sized or mildly to moderately enlarged. No distinct cutoff for an upper limit of size is used, because (1) by adding a hand port, larger spleens can still be removed without a formal laparotomy and (2) in small patients, the lack of space to maneuver laparoscopically may limit the options, whereas the same-size spleen in a large patient may be amenable to laparoscopic excision. Most spleens occupying the entire left half of the abdomen or crossing the midline with the patient supine are best treated by open splenectomy. Occasionally postoperative adhesions from open operations or infection will preclude laparoscopic splenectomy.

Laparoscopic splenectomy can be performed with the patient supine, in semi–right lateral decubitus or full right lateral decubitus position. The lateral or hanging spleen approach is performed with larger spleens because it is easier to manipulate the spleen anteriorly than with the patient supine.

Three ports are used, one 12-mm working port in the upper midline, which can be extended for hand port placement as indicated, a 10-mm port in the left upper quadrant for the laparoscope (this position will vary based on spleen size, ranging from near the costal margin to even in the right lower quadrant near the umbilicus with a very large spleen) and a second 12-mm port at the left anterior axillary line (the site will again vary depending on spleen size) (Figure 138-5, A).

After port placement and inspection of the left upper quadrant, the caudal pole (splenocolic ligament) is incised with electrocautery or ultrasonic dissector while lifting the spleen (see Figure 138-5, A). Continuing posterior to the spleen, the splenorenal and splenophrenic ligaments are divided by the dissector in the surgeon's right hand, retracting the spleen anterior with a blunt instrument in the left hand. The tissues are generally flimsy and rapidly separated once the peritoneum is divided. Care must be taken to avoid injury to the hilar vessels at this time (Figure 138-5, C). After switching instruments, the spleen is retracted posteriorly with the right hand and the splenogastric ligament divided from caudad to cephalad with an ultrasonic dissector. (Vessels make monopolar cautery a less suitable option with this tissue dissection.) The short gastric vessels are likewise serially divided up to the cephalad pole of the spleen (see Figure 138-5, C). The splenic hilum is then inspected, evaluating for the location of the tail of the pancreas. Once the hilar vessels are adequately skeletonized, they can be readily transected with vascular loads of a linear endoscopic stapler (Figure 138-5, D).

The detached spleen is placed in a specimen bag and morcellated. If a hand port has been placed, larger spleens can more readily be removed through the upper midline incision. Accessory spleens should be looked for, especially if a preoperative CT or MRI scan has not been obtained. After removal of the spleen, the left upper quadrant, in particular the hilar staple line, is inspected for hemostasis. After release of the pneumoperitoneum and removal of the cannulae, all the incisions are closed with absorbable fascial and subcutaneous sutures.

POSTOPERATIVE COURSE AND COMPLICATIONS

The highest rate of postoperative complications is anticipated in patients with massive splenomegaly (splenic weight >1500 mg) or myeloproliferative diseases, where a morbidity of up to 52% has been reported.[134,135]

All patients are closely monitored during the early postoperative period for hemorrhage. Immediate postoperative bleeding most commonly arises from an unligated short gastric vessel high on the greater curvature or from small veins around the tail of the pancreas. When indicated by a fall in hemoglobin and signs of hypovolemia, exploration should be promptly performed. Another common complication, pulmonary atelectasis, can be prevented with adequate pain control and incentive spirometry. A subphrenic abscess occurs rarely but may develop with poor hemostasis and clot formation in the splenic bed or when the gastrointestinal tract is opened. Percutaneous drainage plus parenteral antibiotics is usually adequate therapy. A gastric or pancreatic fistula occurs in less than 1% of splenectomy patients and is associated with iatrogenic injury to these organs.

Leukocytosis occurs as a physiologic response to splenectomy. It may be difficult to distinguish from an infection. Traumatic splenectomy patients with white blood cell counts greater than 20×10^9/L after postoperative day 10 are more likely to harbor an infection,[136] but leukocytosis after splenectomy for nontraumatic indications has not been thoroughly investigated. Similarly, reactive thrombocytosis may occur immediately postsplenectomy, with the platelets peaking at 2 to 3 weeks postoperatively. In the absence of hemostatic or vascular complications, therapy is not routinely indicated for secondary thrombocytosis.

Venous thrombosis involving the mesenteric and portal veins is a serious complication after splenectomy. The incidence of clot formation may be as high as 50% if all patients are screened, but only 8% become symptomatic. Predisposing factors include a myeloproliferative disease or hemolytic anemia, postoperative thrombocytosis, a previously undiagnosed systemic hypercoagulable state, and a long splenic vein stump.[137] Laparoscopic splenectomy may be associated with a higher incidence of portal and splenic vein thrombosis than the open technique (55% vs. 12% in one retrospective series).[138] Patients usually present within 10 days of splenectomy with vague symptoms, including generalized abdominal pain and distention, fever, nausea, and anorexia. The diagnosis is best obtained by contrast-enhanced abdominal CT, MRI, or ultrasonography. Systemic anticoagulation is initiated promptly and maintained for 6 months.

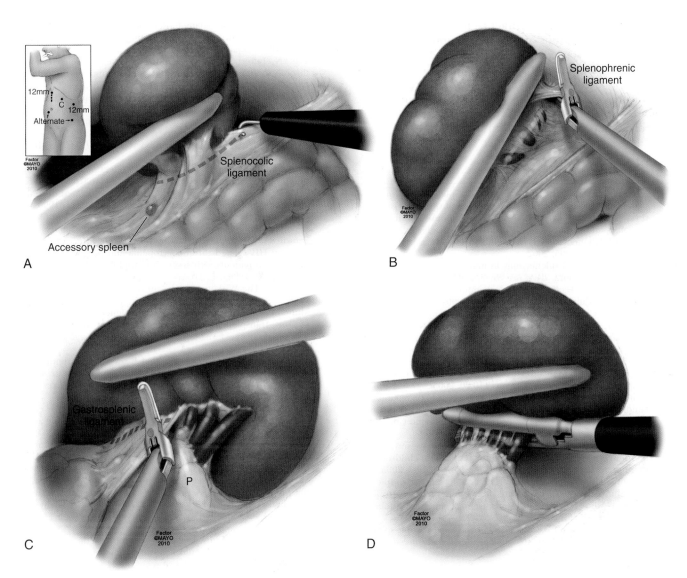

FIGURE 138-5 Laparoscopic splenectomy: **A,** The patient is placed in right lateral decubitus position. Three ports, two 12-mm and a 10-mm camera (C) port are placed *(inset)*. With splenomegaly, the ports may need to be placed more inferiorly (alternate). The dissection of the spleen is started by retracting the spleen medially and dividing the inferior and posterior peritoneum reflections. An accessory spleen is present near the inferior pole of the spleen. **B,** The dissection is continued posterior to the superior pole of the spleen, dividing the peritoneal reflection up to the diaphragm. **C,** The spleen is now retracted posteriorly with a blunt instrument and the anterior peritoneal reflection divided, being careful to avoid injuring the splenic hilar vessels. **D,** Once the hilar vessels are isolated, they can be readily divided with one or more applications of a linear stapler. The spleen is then placed in a specimen bag and morcellated. (Illustrated by David Factor of the Mayo Section of Medical Illustrations.)

Recannulation occurs in 90% of those on appropriate anticoagulation.[139]

All asplenic patients are at risk for overwhelming postsplenectomy sepsis (OPSS). The incidence of OPSS ranges between 1% and 2.4% and is fatal in 45% to 75% of patients. The elevated risk of mortality is lifelong.[44] Any febrile asplenic patient must be promptly evaluated and initiated on a broad-spectrum antibiotic regimen such as a third-generation cephalosporin.[132] Measures to prevent OPSS include vaccination and prophylactic antibiotics.[140] Preoperative vaccination is preferred. When the vaccines are administered postoperatively, they are conventionally given on the day of dismissal to avoid confusing febrile reactions to the vaccine with a

postoperative complication. In the absence of established guidelines, repeat vaccination should be considered every 5 years. Prophylactic antibiotics have been advocated for children and include two commonly used strategies. First, a daily prophylactic antibiotic is given to asplenic children (<5 years old) for the first 2 years after splenectomy. The traditional regimen has been a single daily dose of penicillin, amoxicillin, or erythromycin. Recently, antibiotics with broader spectrum, including amoxicillin/clavulanic acid, cefuroxime, and trimethoprim/sulfamethoxazole, have been used. Prophylactic antibiotics can reduce the infection rate by 47% and mortality rate by 88%.[141] Concerns of increasing pneumococcal resistance and poor patient compliance have recently brought this practice into question. Alternatively, asplenic adults are given a supply of "standby" antibiotics to be started if symptoms of infection develop. It should be emphasized that these patients seek immediate medical attention. All patients and caretakers should be educated regarding OPSS, as well as documenting the patients' asplenic state and vaccination status, plus issuing a medical alert bracelet to help recognition of OPSS.

REFERENCES

1. Kojouri K, Vesely SK, Terrell DR, et al: Splenectomy for adult patients with idiopathic thrombocytopenic purpura: A systematic review to assess long-term platelet count responses, prediction of response, and surgical complications. *Blood* 104:2623, 2004.
2. Cines DB, Blanchette VS: Immune thrombocytopenic purpura. *N Engl J Med* 346:995, 2002.
3. Bell WR Jr: Role of splenectomy in immune (idiopathic) thrombocytopenic purpura. *Blood Rev* 16:39, 2002.
4. Stasi R, Provan D: Management of immune thrombocytopenic purpura in adults. *Mayo Clin Proc* 79:504, 2004.
5. Nugent DJ: Childhood immune thrombocytopenic purpura. *Blood Rev* 16:27, 2002.
6. McFarland J: Pathophysiology of platelet destruction in immune (idiopathic) thrombocytopenic purpura. *Blood Rev* 16:1, 2002.
7. El-Alfy MS, El-Tawil MM, Shahein N: Five- to sixteen-year follow-up following splenectomy in chronic immune thrombocytopenic purpura in children. *Acta Haematol* 110:20, 2003.
8. Kuhne T, Blanchettte GR, Buchanan U, et al: Splenectomy in children with idiopathic thrombocytopenic purpura: A prospective study of 134 children from the Intercontinental Childhood ITP Study Group. *Pediatr Blood Cancer* 49:829. 2007.
9. Holt D, Brown J, Terrill K, et al: Response to intravenous immunoglobulin predicts splenectomy response in children with immune thrombocytopenic purpura. *Pediatrics* 111:87, 2003.
10. Hemmila MR, Foley DS, Castle VP, et al: The response to splenectomy in pediatric patients with idiopathic thrombocytopenic purpura who fail high-dose intravenous immune globulin. *J Pediatr Surg* 35:967; discussion 971, 2000.
11. Hicks BA, Thompson WR, Rogers ZR, et al: Laparoscopic splenectomy in childhood hematologic disorders. *J Laparoendosc Surg* 6:S31, 1996.
12. Gargiulo N III, Zenilman ME: Spleen. In Cameron J, editor: *Current surgical therapy.* St Louis, 2001, CV Mosby, p 587.
13. Provan D, Newland A: Fifty years of idiopathic thrombocytopenic purpura (ITP): Management of refractory ITP in adults. *Br J Haematol* 118:933, 2002.
14. Kumar S, Diehn FE, Gertz MA, et al: Splenectomy for immune thrombocytopenic purpura: Long-term results and treatment of postsplenectomy relapses. *Ann Hematol* 81:312, 2002.
15. Cordera F, Long KH, Nagorney DM, et al: Open versus laparoscopic splenectomy for idiopathic thrombocytopenic purpura: Clinical and economic analysis. *Surgery* 134:45, 2003.
16. Donohue JH, van Heerden JA, Monson JR: *Atlas of surgical oncology.* Cambridge, MA, 1995, Blackwell Science.
17. Coon WW: Surgical aspects of splenic disease and lymphoma. *Curr Probl Surg* 35:543, 1998.
18. Rock GA: Management of thrombotic thrombocytopenic purpura. *Br J Haematol* 109:496, 2000.
19. Rock GA, Shumak KH, Buskard NA, et al: Comparison of plasma exchange with plasma infusion in the treatment of thrombotic thrombocytopenic purpura. Canadian Apheresis Study Group. *N Engl J Med* 325:393, 1991.
20. Rock GA, Shumak KH, Nair RC: Late relapses in patients successfully treated for thrombotic thrombocytopenic purpura. Canadian Apheresis Study Group. *Ann Intern Med* 122:569, 1995.
21. Aqui NA, Stein SH, Konkle BA, et al: Role of splenectomy in patients with refractory or relapsed thrombotic thrombocytopenic purpura. *J Clin Apheresis* 18:51, 2003.
22. Schwartz J, Eldor A, Szold A: Laparoscopic splenectomy in patients with refractory or relapsing thrombotic thrombocytopenic purpura. *Arch Surg* 136:1236; discussion 1239, 2001.
23. Essien FA, Ojeda HF, Salameh JR, et al: Laparoscopic splenectomy for chronic recurrent thrombotic thrombocytopenic purpura. *Surg Laparosc Endosc Percutan Tech* 13:218, 2003.
24. You YN, Tefferi A, Nagorney DM: Outcome of splenectomy for thrombocytopenia associated with systemic lupus erythematosus. *Ann Surg* 240:286, 2004.
25. The Swiss Group for Clinical Studies on the Acquired Immunodeficiency Syndrome (AIDS): Zidovudine for the treatment of thrombocytopenia associated with human immunodeficiency virus (HIV): A prospective study. *Ann Intern Med* 109:718, 1988.
26. Scaradavou A: HIV-related thrombocytopenia. *Blood Rev* 16:73, 2002.
27. Hymes KB, Greene JB, Karpatkin S: The effect of azidothymidine on HIV-related thrombocytopenia. *N Engl J Med* 318:516. 1988.
28. Tyler DS, Shaunak S, Bartlett JA, et al: HIV-1-associated thrombocytopenia: The role of splenectomy. *Ann Surg* 211:211, 1990.
29. Aboolian A, Ricci M, Shapiro K, et al: Surgical treatment of HIV-related immune thrombocytopenia. *Int Surg* 84:81, 1999.
30. Brown SA, Majumdar G, Harrington C, et al: Effect of splenectomy on HIV-related thrombocytopenia and progression of HIV infection in patients with severe haemophilia. *Blood Coagul Fibrinolysis* 5:393, 1994.
31. Ochs HD: The Wiskott-Aldrich syndrome. *Semin Hematol* 35:332, 1998.
32. Mullen CA, Anderson KD, Blaese RM: Splenectomy and/or bone marrow transplantation in the management of the Wiskott-Aldrich syndrome: Long-term follow-up of 62 cases. *Blood* 82:2961, 1993.
33. Dupuis-Girod S, Medioni J, Haddad E, et al: Autoimmunity in Wiskott-Aldrich syndrome: Risk factors, clinical features, and outcome in a single-center cohort of 55 patients. *Pediatrics* 111: e622, 2003.
34. Tamary H, Aviner S, Freud E, et al: High incidence of early cholelithiasis detected by ultrasonography in children and young adults with hereditary spherocytosis. *J Pediatr Hematol Oncol* 25:952, 2003.
35. Bolton-Maggs PH, Stevens RF, Dodd NJ, et al: Guidelines for the diagnosis and management of hereditary spherocytosis. *Br J Haematol* 126:455, 2004.
36. Shah S, Vega R: Hereditary spherocytosis. *Pediatr Rev* 25:168, 2004.
37. Eber SW, Armbrust R, Schroter W: Variable clinical severity of hereditary spherocytosis: Relation to erythrocytic spectrin concentration, osmotic fragility, and autohemolysis. *J Pediatr* 117:409. 1990.
38. Marchetti M, Quaglini S, Barosi G: Prophylactic splenectomy and cholecystectomy in mild hereditary spherocytosis: Analyzing the decision in different clinical scenarios. *J Intern Med* 244:217, 1998.
39. Caprotti R, Franciosi C, Romano F, et al: Combined laparoscopic splenectomy and cholecystectomy for the treatment of hereditary spherocytosis: Is it safe and effective? *Surg Laparosc Endosc Percutan Tech* 9:203, 1999.
40. Sandler A, Winkel G, Kimura K, et al: The role of prophylactic cholecystectomy during splenectomy in children with hereditary spherocytosis. *J Pediatr Surg* 34:1077, 1999.
41. Rescorla FJ, West KW, Engum SA, et al: Laparoscopic splenic procedures in children: experience in 231 children. *Ann Surg* 246:683, 2007.
42. de Lagausie P, Bonnard A, Benkerrou M, et al: Pediatric laparoscopic splenectomy: Benefits of the anterior approach. *Surg Endosc* 18:80, 2004.
43. Vasilescu C, Stanciulea O, Tudor S, et al: Laparoscopic subtotal splenectomy in hereditary spherocytosis: To preserve the upper or the lower pole of the spleen? *Surg Endosc* 20:748, 2006.
44. Stoehr GA, Stauffer UG, Eber SW: Near-total splenectomy: A new technique for the management of hereditary spherocytosis. *Ann Surg* 241:40, 2005.
45. Coon WW: Splenectomy in the treatment of hemolytic anemia. *Arch Surg* 120:625, 1985.
46. Stuart MJ, Nagel RL: Sickle-cell disease. *Lancet* 364:1343, 2004.
47. al-Salem AH, Qaisaruddin S, Nasserallah Z, et al: Splenectomy in patients with sickle-cell disease. *Am J Surg* 172:254, 1996.
48. Sorrells DL, Morrissey TB, Brown MF: Septic complications after splenectomy for sickle cell sequestration crisis. *Pediatr Surg Int* 13:100, 1998.
49. Wright JG, Hambleton IR, Thomas PW, et al: Postsplenectomy course in homozygous sickle cell disease. *J Pediatr* 134:304, 1999.

50. Emond AM, Morais P, Venugopal S, et al: Role of splenectomy in homozygous sickle cell disease in childhood. *Lancet* 1:88, 1984.

51. Lesher AP, Kalpatthi R, Glenn JB, et al: Outcome of splenectomy in children younger than 4 years with sickle cell disease. *J Pediatr Surg* 44:1134, 2009.

52. Kar BC: Splenectomy in sickle cell disease. *J Assoc Phys India* 47:890, 1999.

53. Graziano JH, Piomelli S, Hilgartner M, et al: Chelation therapy in beta-thalassemia major: III. The role of splenectomy in achieving iron balance. *J Pediatr* 99:695, 1981.

54. Yang XY, Qu Q, Yang TY, et al: Treatment of the thalassemia syndrome with splenectomy. *Hemoglobin* 12:601, 1988.

55. Hathirat P, Isarangkura P, Numhom S, et al: Results of the splenectomy in children with thalassemia. *J Med Assoc Thai* 72:133, 1989.

56. Pinna AD, Argiolu F, Marongiu L, et al: Indications and results for splenectomy for beta thalassemia in two hundred twenty-one pediatric patients. *Surg Gynecol Obstet* 167:109, 1988.

57. al-Salem AH, al-Dabbous I, Bhamidibati P: The role of partial splenectomy in children with thalassemia. *Eur J Pediatr Surg* 8:334, 1998.

58. Laopodis V, Kritikos E, Rizzoti L, et al: Laparoscopic splenectomy in beta-thalassemia major patients: Advantages and disadvantages. *Surg Endosc* 12:944, 1998.

59. Akpek G, McAneny D, Weintraub L: Comparative response to splenectomy in Coombs-positive autoimmune hemolytic anemia with or without associated disease. *Am J Hematol* 61:98, 1999.

60. Wang WC: Evans syndrome: Pathophysiology, clinical course, and treatment. *Am J Pediatr Hematol Oncol* 10:330, 1988.

61. Mathew P, Chen G, Wang W: Evans syndrome: Results of a national survey. *J Pediatr Hematol Oncol* 19:433, 1997.

62. Bux J, Behrens G, Jaeger G, Welte K: Diagnosis and clinical course of autoimmune neutropenia in infancy: Analysis of 240 cases. *Blood* 91:181, 1998.

63. Duperier T, Felsher J, Brody F: Laparoscopic splenectomy for Evans syndrome. *Surg Laparosc Endosc Percutan Tech* 13:45, 2003.

64. Campion G, Maddison PJ, Goulding N, et al: The Felty syndrome: A case-matched study of clinical manifestations and outcome, serologic features, and immunogenetic associations. *Medicine (Baltimore)* 69:69, 1990.

65. Rashba EJ, Rowe JM, Packman CH: Treatment of the neutropenia of Felty syndrome. *Blood Rev* 10:177, 1996.

66. Swerdlow AJ, Douglas AJ, Vaughan Hudson G, et al: Risk of second primary cancer after Hodgkin's disease in patients in the British National Lymphoma Investigation: Relationships to host factors, histology and stage of Hodgkin's disease, and splenectomy. *Br J Cancer* 68:1006, 1993.

67. Frederick W: Hematologic malignancies and splenic tumors. In Feig BW, Fuhrman GM, editors: *The M.D. Anderson surgical oncology handbook.* Philadelphia, 2003, Lippincott Williams & Wilkins, p 393.

68. Strickler JG, Donohue JH, Porter LE, et al: Laparoscopic biopsy for suspected abdominal lymphoma. *Mod Pathol* 11:831, 1998.

69. Silecchia G, Raparelli L, Perrotta N, et al: Accuracy of laparoscopy in the diagnosis and staging of lymphoproliferative diseases. *World J Surg* 27:653, 2003.

70. Walsh RM, Brody F, Brown N: Laparoscopic splenectomy for lymphoproliferative disease. *Surg Endosc* 18:272, 2004.

71. Delpero JR, Houvenaeghel G, Gastaut JA, et al: Splenectomy for hypersplenism in chronic lymphocytic leukemia and malignant non-Hodgkin's lymphoma. *Br J Surg* 77:443, 1990.

72. Brodsky J, Abcar A, Styler M: Splenectomy for non-Hodgkin's lymphoma. *Am J Clin Oncol* 19:558, 1996.

73. Lehne G, Hannisdal E, Langholm R, et al: A 10-year experience with splenectomy in patients with malignant non-Hodgkin's lymphoma at the Norwegian Radium Hospital. *Cancer* 74:933, 1994.

74. Xiros N, Economopoulos T, Christodoulidis C, et al: Splenectomy in patients with malignant non-Hodgkin's lymphoma. *Eur J Haematol* 64:145, 2000.

75. Walsh RM, Heniford BT: Laparoscopic splenectomy for non-Hodgkin's lymphoma. *J Surg Oncol* 70:116, 1999.

76. Zelenetz A: Non-Hodgkin's Lymphoma. National Comprehensive Cancer Network Practice Guidelines in Oncology 2005. Version 1. www.nccn.org

77. Yoong Y, Kurtin PJ, Allmer C, et al: Efficacy of splenectomy for patients with mantle cell non-Hodgkin's lymphoma. *Leuk Lymphoma* 42:1235, 2001.

78. Ruchlemer R, Wotherspoon AC, Thompson JN, et al: Splenectomy in mantle cell lymphoma with leukaemia: A comparison with chronic lymphocytic leukaemia. *Br J Haematol* 118:952, 2002.

79. Mulligan SP, Matutes E, Dearden C, et al: Splenic lymphoma with villous lymphocytes: Natural history and response to therapy in 50 cases. *Br J Haematol* 78:206, 1991.

80. Morel P, Dupriez B, Gosselin B, et al: Role of early splenectomy in malignant lymphomas with prominent splenic involvement (primary lymphomas of the spleen): A study of 59 cases. *Cancer* 71:207, 1993.

81. Thieblemont C, Felman P, Berger F, et al: Treatment of splenic marginal zone B-cell lymphoma: An analysis of 81 patients. *Clin Lymphoma* 3:41, 2002.

82. Chacon JI, Mollejo M, Munoz E, et al: Splenic marginal zone lymphoma: Clinical characteristics and prognostic factors in a series of 60 patients. *Blood* 100:1648, 2002.

83. Hamblin T: Is chronic lymphocytic leukemia one disease? *Haematologica* 87:1235, 2002.

84. Thiruvengadam R, Piedmonte M, Barcos M, et al: Splenectomy in advanced chronic lymphocytic leukemia. *Leukemia* 4:758, 1990.

85. Neal TF Jr, Tefferi A, Witzig TE, et al: Splenectomy in advanced chronic lymphocytic leukemia: A single-institution experience with 50 patients. *Am J Med* 93:435, 1992.

86. Majumdar G, Singh AK: Role of splenectomy in chronic lymphocytic leukaemia with massive splenomegaly and cytopenia. *Leuk Lymphoma* 7:131, 1992.

87. Pegourie-Bandelier B, Sotto JJ, Hollard D, et al: Therapy program for patients with advanced stages of chronic lymphocytic leukemia: Chlorambucil, splenectomy, and total lymph node irradiation. *Cancer* 75:2853, 1995.

88. Seymour JF, Cusack JD, Lerner SA, et al: Case/control study of the role of splenectomy in chronic lymphocytic leukemia. *J Clin Oncol* 15:52, 1997.

89. Cusack JC Jr, Seymour JF, Lerner S, et al: Role of splenectomy in chronic lymphocytic leukemia. *J Am Coll Surg* 185:237, 1997.

90. Van Norman AS, Nagorney DM, Martin JK, et al: Splenectomy for hairy cell leukemia: A clinical review of 63 patients. *Cancer* 57:644, 1986.

91. Bouvet M, Babiera GV, Termuhlen PM, et al: Splenectomy in the accelerated or blastic phase of chronic myelogenous leukemia: A single-institution, 25-year experience. *Surgery* 122:20, 1997.

92. Kalhs P, Schwarzinger I, Anderson G, et al: A retrospective analysis of the long-term effect of splenectomy on late infections, graft-versus-host disease, relapse, and survival after allogeneic marrow transplantation for chronic myelogenous leukemia. *Blood* 86:2028, 1995.

93. Zakarija A, Peterson LC, Tallman MS: Splenectomy and treatments of historical interest. *Best Pract Res Clin Haematol* 16:57, 2003.

94. Barosi G, Ambrosetti A, Buratti A, et al: Splenectomy for patients with myelofibrosis with myeloid metaplasia: Pretreatment variables and outcome prediction. *Leukemia* 7:200, 1993.

95. Mesa RA, Elliott MA, Tefferi A: Splenectomy in chronic myeloid leukemia and myelofibrosis with myeloid metaplasia. *Blood Rev* 14:121, 2000.

96. Mesa RA, Tefferi A: Palliative splenectomy in myelofibrosis with myeloid metaplasia. *Leuk Lymphoma* 42:901, 2001.

97. Tefferi A, Barrett SM, Silverstein MN, et al: Outcome of portal-systemic shunt surgery for portal hypertension associated with intrahepatic obstruction in patients with agnogenic myeloid metaplasia. *Am J Hematol* 46:325, 1994.

98. Tefferi A, Mesa RA, Nagorney DM, et al: Splenectomy in myelofibrosis with myeloid metaplasia: A single-institution experience with 223 patients. *Blood* 95:2226, 2000.

99. Lafaye F, Rain JD, Clot P, et al: Risks and benefits of splenectomy in myelofibrosis: An analysis of 39 cases. *Nouv Rev Fr Hematol* 36:359, 1994.

100. Akpek G, McAneny D, Weintraub L: Risks and benefits of splenectomy in myelofibrosis with myeloid metaplasia: A retrospective analysis of 26 cases. *J Surg Oncol* 77:42, 2001.

101. Barosi G, Ambrosetti A, Centra A, et al: Splenectomy and risk of blast transformation in myelofibrosis with myeloid metaplasia. Italian Cooperative Study Group on Myeloid with Myeloid Metaplasia. *Blood* 91:3630, 1998.

102. Mesa RA, Nagorney DS, Schwager S, et al: Palliative goals, patient selection, and perioperative platelet management: Outcomes and

lessons from 3 decades of splenectomy for myelofibrosis with myeloid metaplasia at the Mayo Clinic. *Cancer* 107:361, 2006.

103. Neuhauser TS, Derringer GA, Thompson LD, et al: Splenic angiosarcoma: A clinicopathologic and immunophenotypic study of 28 cases. *Mod Pathol* 13:978, 2000.

104. Willcox TM, Speer RW, Schlinkert RT, et al: Hemangioma of the spleen: Presentation, diagnosis, and management. *J Gastrointest Surg* 4:611, 2000.

105. Jaroch MT, Broughan TA, Hermann RE: The natural history of splenic infarction. *Surgery* 100:743, 1986.

106. Morgenstern L: Nonparasitic splenic cysts: Pathogenesis, classification, and treatment. *J Am Coll Surg* 194:306, 2002.

107. Pachter HL, Hofstetter SR, Elkowitz A, et al: Traumatic cysts of the spleen—the role of cystectomy and splenic preservation: Experience with seven consecutive patients. *J Trauma* 35:430, 1993.

108. Ooi LL, Leong SS: Splenic abscesses from 1987 to 1995. *Am J Surg* 174:87, 1997.

109. Phillips G, Radosevich MD, Lipsett PA: Splenic abscess: Another look at an old disease. *Arch Surg* 132:1331, 1997.

110. Trastek VF, Pairolero PC, Bernatz PE: Splenic artery aneurysms. *World J Surg* 9:378, 1985.

111. Dave S, Reis ED, Hossain A, et al: Splenic artery aneurysm in the 1990s. *Ann Vasc Surg* 14:223, 2000.

112. Selo-Ojeme D, Welch CC: Review: Spontaneous rupture of splenic artery aneurysm in pregnancy. *Eur J Obstet Gynecol Reprod Biol* 109:124, 2003.

113. Hallett JW Jr: Splenic artery aneurysms. *Semin Vasc Surg* 8:321, 1995.

114. Abbas MA, Stone WM, Fowl RJ, et al: Splenic artery aneurysms: Two decades' experience at Mayo Clinic. *Ann Vasc Surg* 16:442, 2002.

115. Obuchi T, Sasaki A, Nakajim J, et al: Laparoscopic surgery for splenic artery aneurysm. *Surg Laparosc Endosc Percutan Tech* 19:338, 2009.

116. Pietrabissa A, Ferrari M, Berchiolli R, et al: Laparoscopic treatment of splenic artery aneurysms. *J Vasc Surg* 50:275, 2009.

117. Han DC, Feliciano DV: The clinical complexity of splenic vein thrombosis. *Am Surg* 64:558; discussion 561, 1998.

118. Sakorafas GH, Sarr MG, Farley DR, et al: The significance of sinistral portal hypertension complicating chronic pancreatitis. *Am J Surg* 179:129, 2000.

119. Weber SM, Rikkers LF: Splenic vein thrombosis and gastrointestinal bleeding in chronic pancreatitis. *World J Surg* 27:1271, 2003.

120. Heider TR, Azeem S, Galanko JA, et al: The natural history of pancreatitis-induced splenic vein thrombosis. *Ann Surg* 239:876; discussion 880, 2004.

121. Loftus JP, Nagorney DM, Ilstrup D, et al: Sinistral portal hypertension: Splenectomy or expectant management. *Ann Surg* 217:35, 1993.

122. Hashizume M, Tomikawa M, Akahoshi T, et al: Laparoscopic splenectomy for portal hypertension. *Hepatogastroenterology* 49:847, 2002.

123. Desai DC, Hebra A, Davidoff AM, et al: Wandering spleen: A challenging diagnosis. *South Med J* 90:439, 1997.

124. Cohen MS, Soper NJ, Underwood RA, et al: Laparoscopic splenopexy for wandering (pelvic) spleen. *Surg Laparosc Endosc* 8:286, 1998.

125. Peitgen K, Majetschak M, Walz MK: Laparoscopic splenopexy by peritoneal and omental pouch construction for intermittent splenic torsion ("wandering spleen"). *Surg Endosc* 15:413, 2001.

126. Cassar K, Munro A: Iatrogenic splenic injury. *J R Coll Surg Edinb* 47:731, 2002.

127. Holubar SD, Wang JK, Wolff BG, et al: Splenic salvage after intraoperative splenic injury during colectomy. *Arch Surg* 144:1040, 2009.

128. Weinreb NJ, Charrow J, Andersson HC, et al: Effectiveness of enzyme replacement therapy in 1028 patients with type 1 Gaucher disease after 2 to 5 years of treatment: A report from the Gaucher registry. *Am J Med* 113:112, 2002.

129. Fleshner PR, Aufses AH Jr, Grabowski GA, et al: A 27-year experience with splenectomy for Gaucher's disease. *Am J Surg* 161:69, 1991.

130. Sharma OP, Vucinic V, James DG: Splenectomy in sarcoidosis: Indications, complications, and long-term follow-up. *Sarcoidosis Vasc Diffuse Lung Dis* 19:66, 2002.

131. Khan AZ, Escofet X, Roberts KM, et al: Spontaneous splenic rupture: A rare complication of amyloidosis. *Swiss Surg* 9:92, 2003.

132. Brigden ML: Detection, education and management of the asplenic or hyposplenic patient. *Am Fam Physician* 63:499, 2001.

133. Schwartz S: Splenectomy and splenorrhaphy. In Baker RJ, Fischer JE, editors: *Mastery of surgery*, Vol II. Philadelphia, 2001, Lippincott Williams & Wilkins, p 1691.

134. Arnoletti JP, Karam J, Brodsky J: Early postoperative complications of splenectomy for hematologic disease. *Am J Clin Oncol* 22:114, 1999.

135. Horowitz J, Smith JL, Weber TK, et al: Postoperative complications after splenectomy for hematologic malignancies. *Ann Surg* 223:290, 1996.

136. Rutherford EJ, Morris JA Jr, van Aalst J, et al: The white blood cell response to splenectomy and bacteraemia. *Injury* 25:289, 1994.

137. Franciosi C, Romano F, Caprotti R, et al: Splenoportal thrombosis as a complication after laparoscopic splenectomy. *J Laparoendosc Adv Surg Tech A* 12:273, 2002.

138. Ikeda M, Sekimoto M, Takiguchi S, et al: High incidence of thrombosis of the portal venous system after laparoscopic splenectomy: A prospective study with contrast-enhanced CT scan. *Ann Surg* 241:208, 2005.

139. Winslow ER, Brunt LM, Drebin JA, et al: Portal vein thrombosis after splenectomy. *Am J Surg* 184:631; discussion 635, 2002.

140. Working Party of the British Committee for Standards in Haematology Clinical Haematology Task Force: Guidelines for the prevention and treatment of infection in patients with an absent or dysfunctional spleen. *BMJ* 312:430, 1996.

141. Gaston MH, Verter JI, Woods G, et al: Prophylaxis with oral penicillin in children with sickle cell anemia: A randomized trial. *N Engl J Med* 314:1593, 1986.

PART ONE

Anatomy, Physiology, and Diagnosis of Colorectal and Anal Disease

Anatomy and Embryology of the Colon

Trevor M. Yeung | Luca Stocchi | Neil J. Mortensen

ANATOMY OF THE COLON

The colon extends from the end of the ileum to the junction of the sigmoid colon with the rectum and includes the ileocecal valve and appendix. It may be considered from its proximal end to be made up of cecum, which leads into the ascending, transverse, descending, and sigmoid colon. Together with the rectum and anus, they make up the large intestine (Figures 139-1 and 139-2) which differs considerably from the small intestine. Whereas these landmarks have been widely accepted, their definition is more controversial. At the proximal end, the term ileocecal valve is considered a misnomer by several authors,[1] who postulate that the valve mechanism is located entirely in the terminal ileum. On the other hand, the delimitation between the colon and the rectum is not uniformly accepted. Some surgeons consider the sacral promontory or the changes in the characteristics of the longitudinal muscular layer at the end of the sigmoid to be landmarks. Others simply measure the rectum as the last 10, 12, or 15 cm of the large bowel from the anal verge and consider as colon the entire remaining large bowel.

The location of the colon in the peritoneal cavity varies greatly based on individual shape and extent of mesenteric attachments. In most cases, the hepatic flexure lies lower than the splenic flexure, as can be seen on barium enema. In general, the ascending and descending colons are retroperitoneally located, whereas the transverse and sigmoid colons have mesenteries.

The colonic length is approximately 150 cm, but it ranges between 120 and 200 cm depending on gender as well as individual variations. The greatest caliber of the colon is in the range of 7.5 cm at the cecum, from where it gradually diminishes to 2.5 cm at the rectosigmoid. In a study that compared colonic length as measured on barium enema, despite a significantly smaller stature, women had a longer colon than men, with a median of 155 versus 145 cm. In addition, women have a longer transverse colon, which also carries an increased likelihood of location within the pelvis.[2] These anatomic data might explain why colonoscopies are generally more difficult to perform in women than in men. Similarly, there is evidence that Western patients have an increased incidence of sigmoid colonic adhesions compared with Asian counterparts, which again would confirm the increased technical difficulty in performing colonoscopy that is observed in Western patients.[3] It has been reported that the transverse colon lies below the umbilicus in as many as 10% of women, a detail that might carry importance for laparoscopic surgery.[4] A recent study based on CT colonography demonstrated that the transverse colon was the major determinant in length differences, and was significantly longer in older adults, women, and thinner adults.[5]

Three distinctive basic macroscopic features in the colon help differentiate it from the small bowel: the presence of taeniae coli, the presence of haustra coli, and appendices epiploicae (or fatty appendices) (Figure 139-3). The taeniae coli are condensations of the longitudinal muscular layer of the large bowel into three bundles that are macroscopically visible and equidistant from each other, although a thinner longitudinal layer remains to completely encircle the lumen. The taeniae extend from the tip of the cecum to the rectosigmoid junction and are approximately 6 mm wide. The taeniae are traditionally named after their location in the transverse colon. The taenia mesocolica is connected to the mesocolon; the taenia omentalis is attached to the greater omentum; and the taenia libera has no attachments and is more clearly identifiable on the surface of the bowel wall. The taeniae are shorter than the length of the bowel wall, causing the circular muscle coat to be puckered, contributing to the configuration of the haustra as convex folds of colonic wall, which confer to the colon its saccular appearance. Most of the colon, other than the appendix and cecum, is peppered with peritoneum-covered adipose pieces known as appendices epiploicae. They are most numerous along the taeniae and are relatively flat in the right-sided colon, but they are elongated, pedunculated, and most prominent in the sigmoid, and become absent in the rectum.

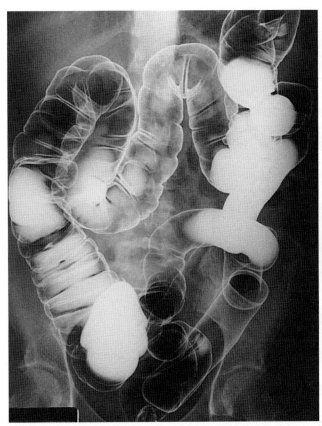

FIGURE 139-1 Double-contrast barium enema demonstrating the tortuous route that is commonly followed by the colon.

SURFACE ANATOMY

The surface projection of the cecum (Figure 139-4) is bounded by the right lateral plane, the transtubercular plane, and the inguinal ligament. From here, the ascending colon moves up to the right of the lateral plane until a point midway between the subcostal and transpyloric planes at the hepatic flexure. Here, the ascending colon meets the transverse colon, which drops toward the umbilicus before passing upward and to the left to a point (splenic flexure) above and lateral to where the left lateral and transpyloric planes meet. The transverse colon may show both intraindividual and interindividual differences in position, varying by as much as 17 cm in the same person between standing upright and lying flat.[6] The descending colon then passes down just lateral to the left lateral plane to the inguinal ligament, where it becomes the sigmoid colon. Surface projections of the sigmoid colon vary considerably because of its length, movement on its mesocolon, its distention, and the condition of other pelvic viscera (rectum, bladder, and uterus in females).

CECUM

The cecum is the commencement of the large intestine and is the portion located below a transverse line passing just above the ileocecal valve. The ileum, the vermiform appendix, and the ascending colon all are continuous with the cecum. Its average axial diameter is approximately 6 cm, with a breadth of about 7.5 cm. It is related posteriorly to the iliacus and psoas major muscles and to the lateral cutaneous nerve of the thigh, which lies on the iliacus. Anteriorly, the cecum is in contact with the anterior abdominal wall, but may have greater omentum or coils of small intestine overlying it.

The cecum is mobile and has a complete covering of peritoneum, although this may be absent at the superior part of the posterior surface, which is then connected to iliac fascia by areolar tissue. Although the mesocecum is usually short, the mobility of the cecum may cause it to twist on its mesenteric axis to form a cecal volvulus or to herniate through the right inguinal canal. The area of tenderness in acute appendicitis may be unusually located if the cecum has a long mesocecum.

Externally, the junction between the ileum and the cecum is associated with a number of peritoneal folds and recesses. The superior ileocecal fold extends anteriorly as a mesenteric appendage where the anterior cecal artery runs. The fold covers the corresponding superior ileocecal recess. Inferiorly, the inferior ileocecal fold connects the antimesenteric aspect of the terminal ileum with the mesenteriolum of the appendix. Because this fold does not contain any vessel, it is also referred to as the bloodless fold of Treves. A small inferior ileocecal recess lies inferior and posterior to the corresponding fold.[7]

The lowest haustrum corresponds to what can be endoscopically viewed as the cecal fundus, where the appendiceal orifice is generally visible and is a useful indicator of a complete colonoscopic exploration. A mucosal fold referred to as Gerlach's valve inconsistently covers the appendiceal orifice. An additional landmark visible endoscopically is the ileocecal valve, with the ileal orifice delimited by two distinct lips: the ileocolic, or superior, lip and the ileocecal, or inferior, lip.

ILEOCECAL VALVE

The ileum opens into the large intestine through the ileocecal valve medially and posteriorly where the cecum joins the ascending colon. This "valve" forms a sphincter as a result of the continuation of the circular and longitudinal muscle layers of the terminal ileum. The valve not only prevents reflux from the cecum into the ileum but probably also acts as a terminal ileum sphincter that prevents small intestinal contents from passing too quickly into the cecum. An absolutely competent ileocecal valve together with a colonic obstruction results in a closed-loop obstruction, and in the absence of surgical intervention this will result in perforation of the colon. Barium enema studies have shown that the ileocecal valve is frequently incompetent in persons without any disease.

Although the term ileocecal valve is still largely used, some authors have objected to its accuracy in consideration that the valve mechanism might actually lie in the terminal ileum. On the other hand, Faussone Pellegrini et al performed functional anatomy studies on 100 patients (including an endoscopic examination in vivo and both macroscopic and microscopic examinations of the ileocecocolonic region from surgical specimens) and concluded that the cecocolonic junction contained both sphincter morphology and function.[8] The existence of a

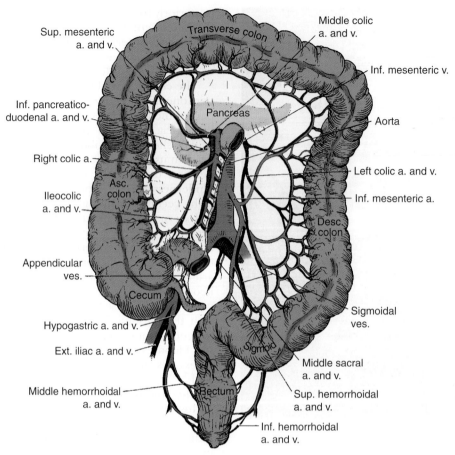

FIGURE 139-2 The colon, showing its anatomic divisions and its blood supply (the veins are shown in black lines). (Modified from Jones T, Shepard WC: *A manual of surgical anatomy.* Philadelphia, 1945, Saunders.)

physiologic sphincter zone at the cecocolonic junction has been suggested based on manometric studies performed during right hemicolectomy.[9]

VERMIFORM APPENDIX

The vermiform appendix is a blind-ending tube in continuation with the cecum through the appendiceal orifice, opening below and behind the ileocecal valve. It is surrounded by a continuous longitudinal muscular layer, which results from the union of the three taeniae. It varies from 2 to 20 cm in length (it is longer in the child), with an average length of about 9 cm. While the lumen is relatively wide in infants, it gradually narrows throughout life. The appendix generally arises from the posteromedial wall of the cecum about 2 cm below the end of the ileum, although it can be connected to the cecal fundus or even located in close proximity to the ileocecal valve. Its serous coat is complete except for the attachment of its mesentery. Although the position of the appendix base is constant, the appendix itself may occupy one of the following positions (Figure 139-5):

1. Anterior to the terminal ileum and in relation to the anterior abdominal wall (preileal)
2. Posterior to the terminal ileum (postileal)
3. Descending over the pelvic brim (pelvic/descending)
4. Below the cecum (subcecal)

5. Posterior to the cecum and lower part of the ascending colon (retrocecal and retrocolic)

Despite much anatomic and surgical literature, there remains debate as to the incidence of each appendix position. In a large study of 10,000 subjects in 1933,[10] the appendix was retrocecal or retrocolic in 65%. McBurney point, the junction of the lateral and middle thirds of the line that joins the right anterior superior iliac spine to the umbilicus, is used as a surface marking for the base of the appendix. The three taeniae coli converge at the tip of the cecum to form the continuous longitudinal muscle layer of the appendix. The base of the appendix can be located by tracing the anterior taenia coli to the tip of the cecum. The ileocecal fold of peritoneum (also known as the "bloodless fold of Treves"), which connects the terminal 2.5 cm of ileum to the cecum, can also be used to locate the base of the appendix. A short, triangular mesoappendix extends along the length of the appendix and connects it to the lower portion of the mesentery of the ileum. The mesoappendix contains the main artery to the appendix, which is a branch of the lower division of the ileocolic artery. It is postulated that this anatomic condition predisposes to inflammatory damage because of the inability to meet the demand for an increased blood supply. Conversely, branches derived from the anterior and posterior cecal arteries provide additional blood supply to the base

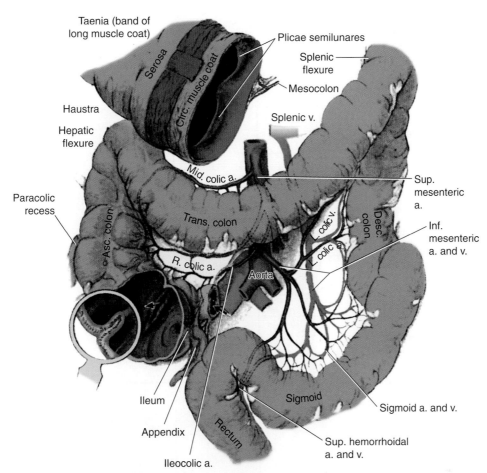

FIGURE 139-3 The large intestine. The position of the colon as shown is based on radiographic study in living humans. The anterior wall of the cecum is removed to show the ileocolic valve, characteristic folds, and opening of the appendix. Note that the blood supply is from two sources: (1) the superior (sup) mesenteric artery through the middle, right, and ileocolic branches and (2) the inferior (inf) mesenteric artery through the left colic, sigmoid, and superior hemorrhoidal branches. An enlarged segment of transverse colon is shown above with details of the wall and plicae. A magnified portion of cecum wall is seen at the *lower left*. (From Bockus HL: *Gastroenterology*, vol 2, ed 3. Philadelphia, 1976, Saunders.)

of the appendix. The venous circulation drains into the ileocolic and the right colic veins, whereas the lymphatics drain into the ileocecal nodes and then along the SMA nodes into the celiac nodes.

ASCENDING COLON

The ascending colon lies on the right side of the abdominal cavity, in front of the quadratus lumborum and transversus abdominis muscle. It extends from the cecum to the hepatic flexure and averages 12 to 20 cm in length. The ascending colon is narrower than the cecum at its origin, ascending to the inferior surface of the right lobe of the liver. It then turns down, forward, and to the left, forming the hepatic flexure.

The ascending colon is related posteriorly to the iliacus, iliolumbar ligament, quadratus lumborum, the origin of the transversus abdominis, the perirenal fat, and Gerota fascia anterior to the inferolateral part of the right kidney, the lateral cutaneous nerve of the thigh, the fourth lumbar artery, and the ilioinguinal and iliohypogastric nerves. It also relates posteriorly to the right

ureter and gonadal vessels, which lie on the surface of the psoas muscle (Figure 139-6). Anteriorly, it is related to the small intestine, the right edge of the greater omentum, and the anterior abdominal wall. The ascending colon is covered on all sides except its posterior surface and is bound by areolar tissue to the posterior abdominal wall (Figure 139-7). It is not uncommon for it to be completely covered with peritoneum and to contain a narrow mesocolon. Treves[11] found an ascending mesocolon in 12% of cadavers, a descending mesocolon in 22%, and both mesocolons in 14%. Rarely, a tenuous adhesion from the right abdominal wall to the anterior taeniae of the ascending colon has been observed, which is referred to as Jackson membrane.

At the lower margin of the liver and lateral or adherent to the gallbladder, the ascending colon turns to the left at the hepatic flexure (Figure 139-8). The hepatic flexure lies immediately above the second portion of the duodenum, to which it is sometimes attached by a peritoneal fold referred to as the duodenocolic ligament. In addition, a hepatocolic ligament can be occasionally

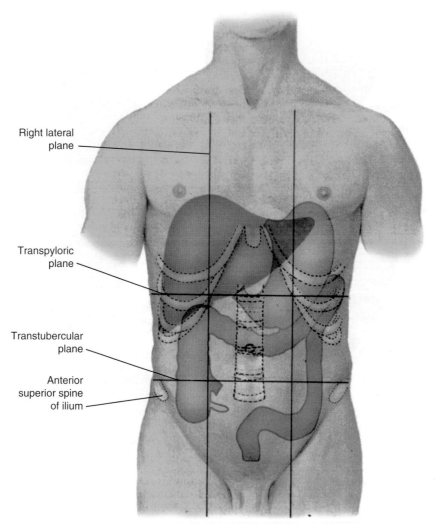

FIGURE 139-4 Surface projection of the stomach, liver, and colon. The outlines of the lumbar vertebral bodies, lower ribs, xiphoid process, and parts of the iliac crests are indicated. (From Williams PL, Warwick R: *Gray's anatomy*, ed 36. London, 1980, Saunders.)

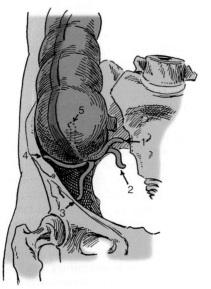

FIGURE 139-5 Various positions (1-5) occupied by the appendix.

found, in continuity with the lesser omentum. The posterior aspect of the hepatic flexure is in direct contact with the inferolateral part of the right kidney, whereas above and anterolaterally, it is related to the right lobe of the liver. The descending portions of the duodenum and fundus of the gallbladder lie anteromedially. The hepatic flexure has a vertical mobility of 2.5 to 7.5 cm with respiration.[12]

TRANSVERSE COLON

The transverse colon begins at the hepatic flexure and passes across the abdomen into the left upper quadrant, where it curves acutely onto itself (more so than at the hepatic flexure), down and backward, to form the splenic flexure. It is about 50 cm long, and in its course across the abdomen, it forms an arch with its concavity facing backward and up.

The transverse colon is almost completely covered with peritoneum between the head of the pancreas and the splenic flexure and is attached to the posterior

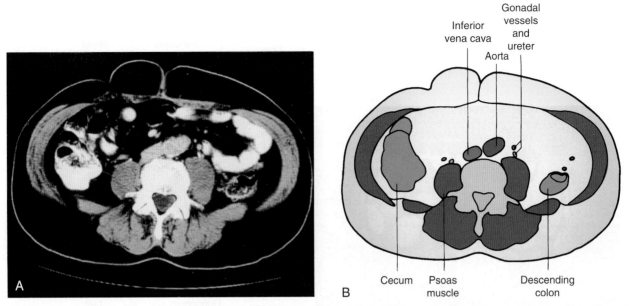

FIGURE 139-6 A and **B,** The right colon is related posteriorly to the right ureter, gonadal vessels, duodenum, and kidney. (From Fozard JBJ, Pemberton JH: Applied surgical anatomy: Intraabdominal contents. In Fielding LP, Goldberg SM, editors: *Rob and Smith's operative surgery of the colon, rectum, and anus*, ed 5. Philadelphia, 1994, Chapman & Hall.)

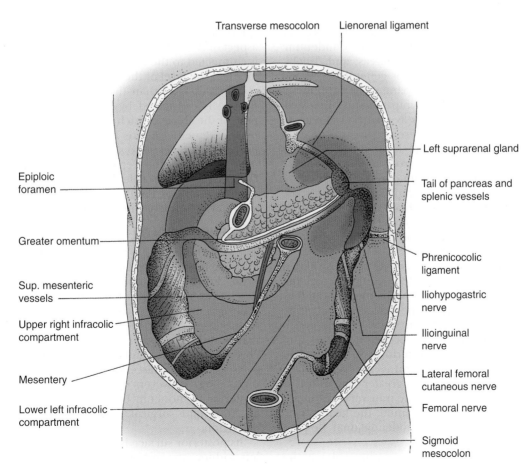

FIGURE 139-7 Posterior abdominal wall. The colon is removed, demonstrating the attachments of the parietal peritoneum.

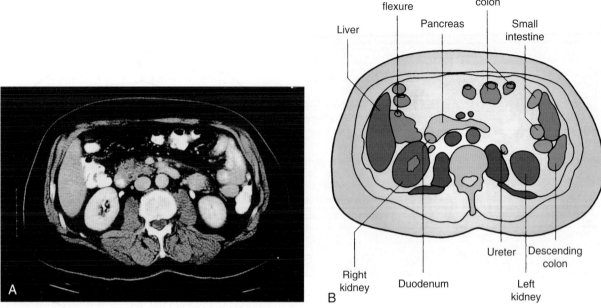

FIGURE 139-8 A and **B,** If the peritoneum is divided along the line of Toldt and the right colon is mobilized medially, the root of the small intestinal mesentery is exposed. The right ureter and gonadal vessels run on the surface of the psoas muscle. The hepatic flexure may be free or adherent to the gallbladder. The hepatic flexure mesentery crosses over the second and third portions of the duodenum. (From Fozard JBJ, Pemberton JH: Applied surgical anatomy: Intra-abdominal contents. In Fielding LP, Goldberg SM, editors: *Rob and Smith's operative surgery of the colon, rectum, and anus*, ed 5. Philadelphia, 1994, Chapman & Hall.)

abdominal wall by a long mesentery, which renders it extremely flexible. The root of the transverse mesocolon lies anteriorly to the lower pole of the right kidney and extends over the second portion of the duodenum; the head, body, and tail of the pancreas; and, finally, on the hilum of the left kidney. It is generally accepted as the anatomic landmark that separates the supramesocolic from the inframesocolic compartments. This division of the abdominal cavity acts as a natural barrier to reciprocal infections between these two areas. The duodenojejunal junction, where the ligament of Treitz is located, lies just inferior to the root of the transverse mesocolon. The greater omentum covers the transverse colon along almost its entire length and contains the gastrocolic ligament, which runs from the greater curvature of the stomach to the transverse colon. This structure is usually dissected in cases of transverse colectomy or to obtain access to the lesser sac.

The right extremity of the transverse colon is related posteriorly to the front of the descending part of the duodenum and head of the pancreas, being separated by areolar tissue. On its superior aspect, it is related to the liver and gallbladder, the greater curvature of the stomach (to which it is attached by the gastrocolic omentum), and the lateral end of the spleen. Inferiorly, it is related to the small intestine. It is covered on its anterior surface with the posterior layers of the greater omentum to which it is attached. Posterior to the transverse colon are the descending part of the duodenum, the head of the pancreas, the mesentery, the duodenojejunal flexure, and the small intestine.

The transverse colon joins the descending colon at the splenic flexure. This may be so acute that the distal transverse colon lies anterior to the descending colon. Superior to the splenic flexure is the lower part of the spleen and the tail of the pancreas, whereas the anterior aspect of the left kidney lies medially. The splenic flexure is connected to the diaphragm by the phrenicocolic ligament, at the level of the tenth and eleventh ribs, and lies at a higher level than the hepatic flexure. The splenic flexure is connected by flimsy adhesions to the lower pole of the spleen, which contributes to render it a fixed bowel segment (Figure 139-9). Such an anatomic location is often difficult to access, which poses the spleen at increased risk of inadvertent tears during splenic flexure takedown. A retrosplenic colon variation has been described in 3 of 1000 patients examined by thoracoabdominal computed tomography (CT) scan.[13]

DESCENDING COLON

The descending colon is approximately 25 cm long and extends from the splenic flexure down to the pelvic brim. From the lateral border of the left kidney, it descends vertically and slightly toward the midline in the groove between the psoas and the quadratus lumborum to the iliac crest. It then turns medially in front of the iliacus and psoas major to end in the sigmoid colon. It is covered by peritoneum over its anterior surface and sides, and, like the ascending colon, it may have a narrow mesocolon. However, in most cases, it is fixed on the posterior peritoneum through the Toldt fascia. This is an important surgical plane to allow for a bloodless dissection.

Its posterior surface is related to the lower pole of the left kidney, the origin of the transversus abdominis, the quadratus lumborum, the iliacus and psoas major,

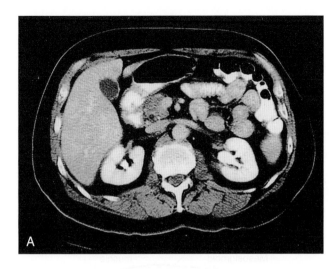

the subcostal vessels and nerve, the iliohypogastric and ilioinguinal nerves, the fourth lumbar artery, the lateral femoral cutaneous, the femoral and genitofemoral nerves, the gonadal vessels, and the external iliac artery. On its anterior aspect, it is related to the coils of the small intestine, and in its lower portion, it is related to the anterior abdominal wall. The descending colon is both narrower and more deeply placed than the ascending colon, and tends to be in a more posterolateral position in young women.[14]

SIGMOID COLON

The sigmoid colon begins at the pelvic brim and forms a loop of about 40 cm that lies within the pelvis. The diameter of the sigmoid colon decreases along its course, and its length, position, and fixation are extremely variable. The definition of the border between the sigmoid colon and rectum is variable. Some surgeons consider it to be at the level of the third sacral vertebra, while others use the sacral promontory as the landmark. The sigmoid loop is made up of the following parts:

1. Descending in contact with the left pelvic wall
2. Crossing the pelvic cavity between rectum and bladder (or uterus in the female), where it may reach the right pelvic wall
3. Arching backward to reach the median plane

The sigmoid colon is completely surrounded by peritoneum, which forms the sigmoid mesocolon (Figure 139-10). The sigmoid mesocolon usually has an inverted V-shaped attachment (although it can be U-shaped or straight),[15] extending from the left iliac fossa to the pelvic brim and then across the left sacroiliac joint at the second or third sacral space, with the apex of the "V" at the bifurcation of the common iliac vessels that overlies the sacroiliac joint. The left ureter lies between the peritoneum and common iliac artery at this point and is an important landmark for the identification of this structure.

The mesocolon is greatest in length at its center and decreases in length toward the end of the loop, so that the sigmoid colon is relatively fixed at its junctions with the descending colon and rectum. It is commonly accepted that a long mesocolon with a short base

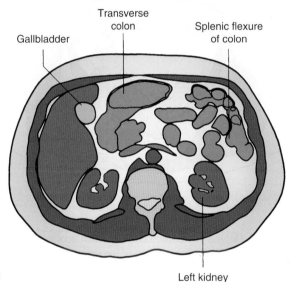

FIGURE 139-9 A and **B,** The splenic flexure is related to the left kidney, adrenal gland, and tail of the pancreas. (From Fozard JBJ, Pemberton JH: Applied surgical anatomy: Intra-abdominal contents. In Fielding LP, Goldberg SM, editors: *Rob and Smith's operative surgery of the colon, rectum, and anus*, ed 5. Philadelphia, 1994, Chapman & Hall.)

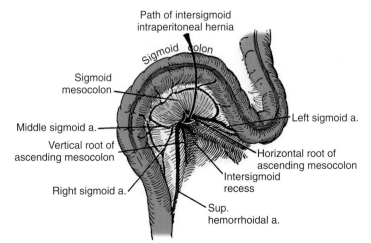

FIGURE 139-10 Sigmoid colon, its mesentery and arterial supply, and the intersigmoid recess. The sigmoid colon and mesocolon are raised forward and upward to show the vertical and horizontal attachments of its two roots. The *arrow* indicates the apex of the intersigmoid recess into which a loop of small bowel may insinuate and travel up behind a partially unfused descending mesocolon to form an intraperitoneal hernia. The superior hemorrhoidal artery, which is the main arterial supply to the rectum, lies between the leaves of the vertical root of the sigmoid mesocolon.

predisposes to the onset of sigmoid volvulus, whereas a long convoluted sigmoid has been implicated in the origin of constipation. The lateral limb of the mesocolon passes forward along the pelvic brim midway to the inguinal ligament. The medial limb slopes down into the hollow of the sacrum, where it reaches the median plane at the level of the third sacral vertebra.

As a consequence of the mobility of the loops, the sigmoid colon has variable anatomic relations. On its posterior aspect are the left internal iliac vessels, the ureter, the piriformis, and the sacral plexus. Laterally, it is related to the left external iliac vessels, the obturator nerve, the ovary or ductus deferens, and the lateral pelvic wall. The bladder (and uterus in the female) lies inferior. Above and medially, the sigmoid colon is related to the coils of the small intestine.

The rectosigmoid junction has the following six distinguishing features:
1. The diameter of the large intestine narrows.
2. There is an absence of complete peritoneal investment.
3. There is no true mesentery.
4. The three taeniae coli converge to form a continuous longitudinal muscle coat on the rectum.
5. There are no appendices epiploicae.
6. Endoscopically, an acute angle is encountered at the narrowing of the rectosigmoid and the rectal mucosa, which is smooth and flat, whereas the mucosa of the sigmoid forms prominent rugal folds.

In a study on the anatomic dimensions of the sigmoid colon of 70 North Indian subjects, the sigmoid colon of females tended to be wider rather than long, whereas the opposite was true for male subjects.[16] The lateral wall of the sigmoid often presents with adhesion to the lateral wall of the iliac fossa (Figure 139-11), which must be freed to allow mobilization of the left colon. Once lateral adhesions are taken down and the lateral peritoneal reflection is incised, the fascia of Toldt can generally be appreciated. The mesosigmoid contains a recess, referred to as the intersigmoid fossa, which can be used as a landmark for identification of the ureter. In fact, the ureter can usually be identified deep to the intersigmoid fossa, where it courses along the surface of the psoas muscle and grossly parallel to the gonadal vessels, as it descends and crosses medially into the pelvis above the common iliac artery bifurcation. However, the intersigmoid fossa can also be the location of internal hernias, when a small bowel loop remains entrapped into this blind pouch. The presence of distinct colosigmoid and sigmoidorectal sphincters is generally not recognized, although Shafik et al have identified distinct, thickened smooth muscle bundles in these areas.[17,18]

ENDOSCOPIC VIEW OF THE COLON

The cecum is identified on colonoscopy by the following three distinct features:
1. Ileocecal valve—This is typically located on the last fold prior to entry into the cecum, and appears as "pouting lips," which lie transversely. These in part are responsible for the valvular continence in that reflux back to the small bowel is prevented. It is viewed "side on" from the colonoscope. It may have a lobular

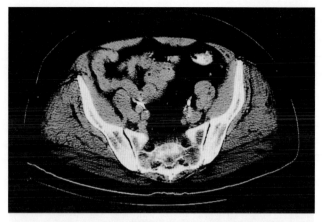

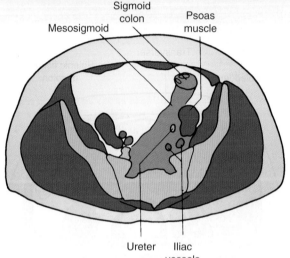

FIGURE 139-11 Near the pelvic brim, the colon acquires a mesentery. This marks the junction of the descending with the sigmoid colon, which in turn becomes the rectum at the sacral promontory. The sigmoid colon is variable in length and position. A long mesosigmoid colon with a short base predisposes to volvulus. Commonly, the sigmoid colon loops down into the pelvis to lie anterior to the rectum. (From Fozard JBJ, Pemberton JH: Applied surgical anatomy: Intra-abdominal contents. In Fielding LP, Goldberg SM, editors: *Rob and Smith's operative surgery of the colon, rectum, and anus*, ed 5. Philadelphia, 1994, Chapman & Hall.)

appearance that resembles a lipoma, and the mucosa appears more velvety, typical of small bowel. It moves rhythmically, and this movement can often be accentuated by inflating and deflating the cecum with the colonoscope. Finally, bile-stained ileal effluent may be seen discharging intermittently.
2. "Mercedes-Benz" sign—The convergence of the three taeniae at the cecum results in a three-pointed star, which has been associated with the German marque. The three taeniae are located anteriorly, posteromedially, and posterolaterally.
3. Appendiceal orifice—At the site of convergence of the taeniae should be the orifice of the appendix with a curvilinear indent. The "bow and arrow" sign uses this curve to point toward the direction of the ileocecal valve, and the colonoscope can be passed in this direction to intubate the terminal ileum.

Two of these three signs are usually sufficient for a diagnosis of the cecum endoscopically, because occasionally one of the signs may be obscured by a less-than-perfect bowel preparation.

On withdrawal up the ascending colon, the hepatic flexure may be recognized by the bluish indentation of the liver. In addition, once past the flexure, the easiest way to advance the colonoscope is usually to shorten the endoscope while applying suction. This causes a "paradoxical advance," allowing the ascending colon to concertina over the colonoscope.

The transverse colon has a highly characteristic endoscopic triangular shape. This is the result of the attachment of the peritoneum at three points to the colon (e.g., gastrocolic omentum, greater omentum, and transverse mesocolon). Occasionally, the length of the transverse colon may cause difficulty in advancement of the colonoscope through because of the resulting "looping." External pressure on the colonoscope in the epigastrium often fixes the transverse colon, facilitating intubation. However, the best way to avoid this situation completely is to insufflate the colon minimally, thus avoiding lengthening it. Suction applied here often allows advancement of the colonoscope without pushing. This, in addition to avoiding looping, also makes the procedure less uncomfortable.

Further distally, the splenic flexure may be difficult to negotiate and is marked by a turn at the end of the descending colon as well as the bluish tinge of the spleen. The sigmoid–descending colon junction is probably the most difficult curve to negotiate endoscopically. It marks the end of the free sigmoid and ends in a tunnel-like appearance of the descending colon. Finally, the sigmoid is easily identified, because of the multiple turns and bends that occur as soon as the rectosigmoid junction is negotiated. Moreover, the haustra of the sigmoid colon are quite thickened (muscular).

ARTERIAL SUPPLY

The colon receives its arterial supply from two main branches of the aorta (Figures 139-12 to 139-14). The superior mesenteric artery (SMA) is the artery of the midgut, and it supplies the colon (and the small intestine from the level of the entrance of the bile duct into the duodenum) to a level just short of the splenic flexure. The inferior mesenteric artery (IMA) is the artery of the hindgut, and it supplies the large distal intestine as far as the mucous membrane of the upper third of the anal canal.

The SMA arises at the level of the L1 vertebra, approximately 1 cm below the celiac trunk. It descends behind the splenic vein and neck of the pancreas and accompanies the superior mesenteric vein (which lies on its right side) into the upper end of the small intestine mesentery, with the left renal vein, uncinate process of the pancreas, and third part of the duodenum lying behind them. They continue to a point approximately 60 cm from the cecum, passing to the right along the root of the mesentery. The following branches are responsible for supplying the colon:

1. The ileocolic artery branches early from the superior mesenteric trunk in the base of the mesentery. Having

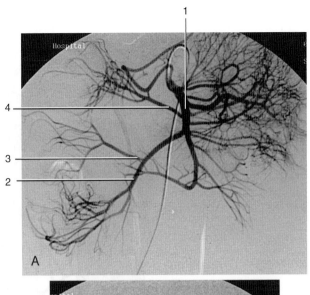

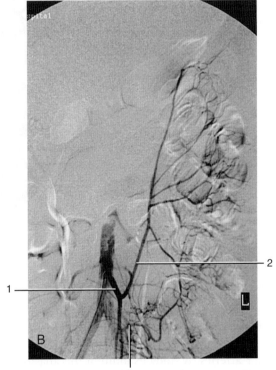

FIGURE 139-12 A, Superior mesenteric angiogram: superior mesenteric artery (1), ileocolic artery (2), right colic artery (3), and middle colic artery (4). **B,** Inferior mesenteric angiogram: inferior mesenteric artery (1), left colic artery (2), and sigmoid artery (3).

reached the ileocecal junction, it gives off ileal and colic branches (Figure 139-15). The colic branch follows the left side of the ascending colon behind the peritoneal floor to anastomose with the right colic artery. The artery then divides into anterior and posterior cecal arteries to supply the cecum. The larger posterior cecal artery supplies the medial, lateral, and posterior walls of the cecum and gives off the appendicular artery, which passes toward the tip of the appendix in the mesoappendix. The appendicular artery is an end artery and does not anastomose with

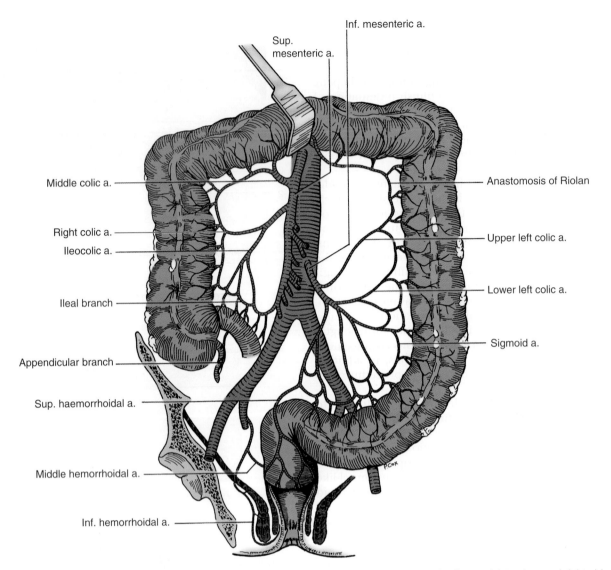

FIGURE 139-13 The arterial supply to the colon and rectum. The normal distribution of supply to the ileum, right colon, and right side of transverse colon from the middle colic artery and ileocolic arteries is shown. The distribution of the arterial supply from the inferior mesenteric artery to the left side of the transverse colon, the descending colon, the sigmoid, and the upper rectum is also demonstrated. (From Keighley MRB, Williams NS: *Surgery of the anus, rectum, and colon.* Philadelphia, 1995, Saunders.)

other arteries. A study examining the anastomosis at the ileocecal valve showed that the anterior cecal artery was present in 100% of specimens, and the posterior cecal artery was present in 89%.[19] There was a rich anastomosis between the vessels at the ileocecal valve, and the authors concluded that preservation of the anterior cecal artery would ensure a vascularized ileocecal valve following a right hemicolectomy.

2. The right colic artery (RCA) has its origin at the right side of the root of the SMA in the mesentery. It runs behind the peritoneal floor to the ascending colon lying anterior to the right psoas muscle, gonadal vessels, ureter, genitofemoral nerve, and quadratus lumborum. At the left side of the colon, it divides into a descending branch, which anastomoses with the colic branch of the ileocolic artery, and an ascending branch, which runs anterior to the lower pole of the right kidney to the hepatic flexure, where it anastomoses with a branch of the middle colic artery.

3. The middle colic artery (MCA) is the most proximal branch of the SMA, and it arises from the artery at the lower border of the neck of the pancreas, passing into the transverse mesocolon. It travels to the right of the midline in the transverse mesocolon and divides into right and left branches at the transverse colon that run along its length. The right branch anastomoses with the ascending branch of the RCA, whereas the left branch anastomoses with a branch of the left colic artery (branch of IMA) just proximal to the splenic flexure. A large avascular window is left in the transverse mesocolon to the left of the MCA and is often used for surgical access to the lesser sac and posterior wall of the stomach. Unrecognized injury to the MCA will usually result in gangrene of a significant portion of the transverse colon.

The IMA arises opposite the L3 vertebra from the front of the aorta at the lower border of the third part of the duodenum. It is smaller than the SMA and

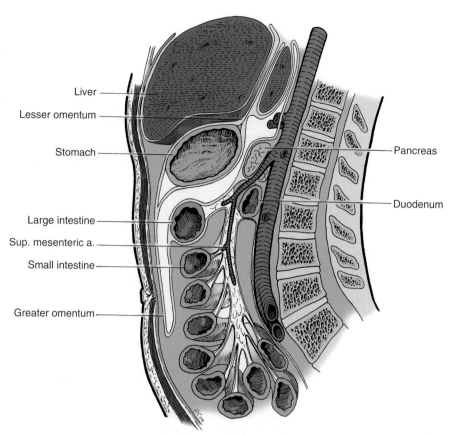

FIGURE 139-14 Sagittal section of the abdomen to demonstrate the blood supply to the transverse colon and small bowel, the greater omentum, the greater sac, and the lesser sac. (From Keighley MRB, Williams NS: *Surgery of the anus, rectum, and colon*. Philadelphia, 1995, Saunders.)

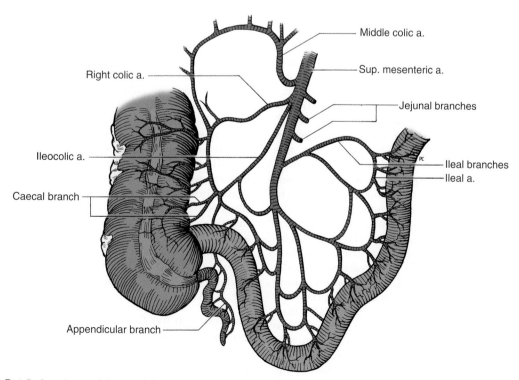

FIGURE 139-15 Detailed anatomy of the arterial supply to the terminal ileum and right colon is shown. In particular, the normal divisions of the ileocolic artery and arcade with the middle colic artery are demonstrated. (From Keighley MRB, Williams NS: *Surgery of the anus, rectum, and colon*. Philadelphia, 1995, Saunders.)

runs beneath the peritoneal floor of the left infracolic compartment to the pelvic brim. Here, it crosses the bifurcation of the left common iliac vessels and converges on the left ureter. In its descent, it lies anterior to the aorta, left psoas muscle, left sympathetic trunk, left common iliac artery, and hypogastric nerve. On crossing the pelvic brim, the IMA becomes the superior rectal artery (supplying the rectum) and continues along the pelvic wall in the root of the sigmoid mesocolon. Branches of the IMA pass to the left in front of the ureter in the floor of the left infracolic compartment. The following branches supply the left side of the colon:

1. The first branch is the left colic artery (LCA), which, lying beneath the peritoneal floor, passes up and laterally to the splenic flexure. It branches after a short course into the ascending branch, which continues laterally and up, and a descending branch. The ascending branch lies anterior to the left psoas muscle, gonadal vessels, ureter, genitofemoral nerve, and quadratus lumborum and is crossed by the inferior mesenteric vein. It then divides into the upper branch, which crosses the lower pole of the left kidney on its way to the splenic flexure, and the lower branch, which passes across to the descending colon. Both branches further divide into branches that anastomose with the left branch of the MCA. The descending branch passes laterally and down (anterior to the same structures as the ascending branch), and at the pelvic brim, it divides into two or three branches that pass laterally behind the peritoneal floor of the left iliac fossa and form anastomoses with each other to supply the lower portion of the descending colon.

2. The sigmoid arteries are three or four branches that arise from a common origin at the IMA below the LCA. They pass forward in the sigmoid mesocolon and supply the sigmoid colon.

The marginal artery of Drummond is the name given to a single arterial trunk made up of anastomoses around the concave border of the large intestine from the ileocecal junction to the rectosigmoid junction. The marginal artery is therefore made up of branches of both the superior and inferior mesenteric arteries. Moynihan[20] remarked that the importance of the marginal artery "cannot be overemphasized." Vessels arise from this artery that run perpendicular to and sink into the walls of the colon to supply the large intestine. Short vessels supply the mesocolic two-thirds of the large bowel circumference, whereas the long vessels penetrate the serosa, encircling the bowel to supply the antimesenteric third of the large bowel circumference (Figure 139-16). The vasa recta arise from the marginal artery and show variability in their spacing and in their collaterals. At the splenic flexure and the proximal and mid–descending colon, the vasa recta are spaced 2 cm apart and have few collaterals. In contrast, at the right, transverse, distal descending and sigmoid colon, the vasa recta are less than 1 cm apart and have more extensive collaterals. Unrecognized disruption of these small artery collaterals could result in anastomotic leakage.[21] Branches of the vasa recta merge in the colon wall, pierce the muscular layer, and spread out as the submucous plexus, extending throughout the whole intestine. The mucosa is supplied

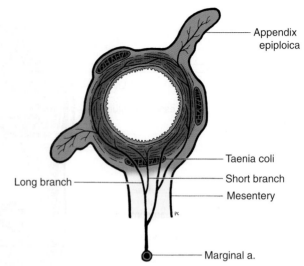

FIGURE 139-16 The terminal arterial supply to the colon and its relation to the taeniae coli and appendices epiploicae are demonstrated. (From Keighley MRB, Williams NS: *Surgery of the anus, rectum, and colon.* Philadelphia, 1995, Saunders.)

by the mucous plexus, and the vascular bed of the intestinal glands is arranged in a regular hexagonal pattern.[22]

The weakest link in the marginal artery is the anastomosis between the middle and left colic arteries in the region of the splenic flexure, where the vascular arcades connecting these two arteries are often absent, in a critical colonic segment that has been described as Griffith point. Hall et al measured tissue oxygen tension and showed that after "high tie" of the IMA (flush with the aorta), the marginal artery remains able to adequately supply the transverse and descending colon but not the sigmoid colon.[23] Furthermore, Dworkin and Allen-Mersh demonstrated with the use of laser Doppler flowmetry that there is a 50% reduction in blood perfusion of the sigmoid colon after ligation of the IMA.[24]

It has been speculated that an inconsistent marginal artery might also enhance a more tenuous vascular supply at the junction of the lowest sigmoid branch and the superior rectal artery, referred to as Sudeck point. Van Tonder et al examined Sudeck point in 64 cadavers and identified the absence of macroscopic anastomosis in 4.7%, with a mean diameter of 1.9 mm.[25] They deduced that although the anastomosis was present in most cases, the vessel was very small and may not be sufficient to meet the demands of a caudal stump. The meandering artery or arc of Riolan is an additional collateral branch that can occasionally be observed intraoperatively. This branch connects the proximal MCA to the LCA and runs in the transverse mesocolon parallel to the left branch of the MCA.

Variations in the Arterial Supply Based on Anatomic Studies

Angiographic and autopsy studies have often challenged the vascular anatomy as traditionally accepted. Yada et al reported on 344 patients with colon cancer who were preoperatively studied with angiography. Four possible branching patterns of the RCA were detected. In 41% of cases, the RCA arose from the SMA; in 19%, it originated from the MCA; and in 14%, it arose from the ileocolic artery. It is of note that the RCA was absent in 26% of cases.[26] In two different smaller series, although the ileocolic artery was ubiquitously found, an RCA emanating from the SMA was encountered in only 11% and 30% of cases, respectively.[27,28]

Based on a superior mesenteric angiogram conducted in 273 patients, the MCA forked into the right and left branches in 160 cases (59%). Of these, 3 patients had a completely replaced MCA originating from the IMA. The remaining 113 patients had an independent origin for the left branch of the MCA, mainly from the SMA (90%) and less commonly from the IMA, dorsal pancreatic artery, or splenic artery.[26] Rare cases of an MCA originating from the celiac trunk[29] or a common trunk from which celiac, SMA, and IMA originate[30] have been reported. For every possible anatomic configuration, it is important to ensure that before resection of the right colon, the proximal vascular ligation is properly carried out at the level of the ileocolic artery. An excessively proximal ligation would actually occur at the level of the SMA and imperil the blood supply of all or part of the small bowel.

Similar anatomic variations have been observed in the IMA, which has important implications for laparoscopic colorectal surgery. In 1971, Zebrowski et al examined 115 patients and identified four different arrangements of IMA[31] (Figure 139-17). In type I, the IMA divides into the LCA and the common rectal sigmoid trunk (RST). In type II, the IMA divides into the colosigmoid trunk and the superior rectal artery. In type III, sigmoid arteries arise from both divisions of the IMA, that is, the colosigmoid and rectosigmoid trunks. In type IV, the IMA divides simultaneously into three branches: LCA, superior rectal, and sigmoid trunk.

VENOUS DRAINAGE

Venous blood returns from the colon in veins with names that correspond to those of the artery, having drained an area similar to that supplied with arterial blood (Figure 139-18).

Veins from the right side of the colon flow into the superior mesenteric vein (SMV), which drains the midgut. This large vein lies to the right side of the artery, crossing ventral to the third part of the duodenum and ascending between the uncinate process and the neck of the pancreas to join with the splenic vein and to form the portal vein. The portal vein continues up behind the first part of the duodenum to its position in the hepatoduodenal ligament.

Veins from the left side of the colon flow into the inferior mesenteric vein (IMV), which drains the hindgut. The inferior mesenteric vein is the continuation of the superior rectal vein, which lies to the left of its artery. The inferior mesenteric vein runs vertically up beneath the peritoneal floor of the left infracolic compartment and is well to the left side of the artery. It lies anterior to the left psoas muscle, gonadal vessels, ureter, and genitofemoral nerve. The vein continues to the left side of the duodenojejunal flexure and passes behind the lower border of the body of the pancreas (anterior to the left

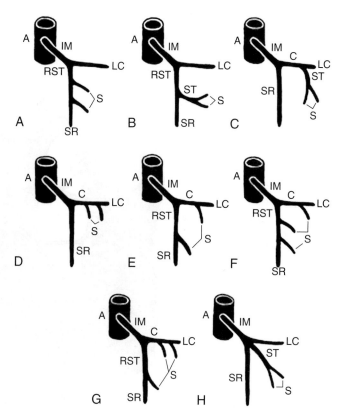

FIGURE 139-17 Anatomic variations of the IMA. In type I, the IMA divides into LC and RST (**A** and **B**). In type II, the IMA divides into SR and the colosigmoid trunk (**C** and **D**). In type III, the sigmoid arteries arise from both divisions of IMA, that is, the colosigmoid trunk and RST (**E, F,** and **G**). In type IV, the IMA divides simultaneously into three branches: SR, LC, and sigmoid trunk (**H**). *A,* Aorta; *C,* colosigmoid trunk; *IM,* inferior mesenteric; *LC,* left colic; *RST,* rectosigmoid trunk; *S,* sigmoid; *SR,* superior rectal; *ST,* sigmoid trunk. (From Anatomy Atlases, www.anatomyatlases.org/AnatomicVariants/Cardiovascular/Text/Arteries/InferiorMesenteric.shtml.)

renal vein) and joins the splenic vein. The inferior mesenteric vein may alternatively open directly into the superior mesenteric vein, having taken a course farther to the right and passing behind the pancreas, below and parallel with the splenic vein.

In a study examining the venous anatomy of the right colon on 58 cadavers, there was a single ileocolic vein in all cases. The right colic vein was absent in 57% of cadavers and single in the remainder. When present, the right colic vein joined the SMV in 56% of cases and the gastrocolic trunk in the remaining 44%. The middle colic vein was double in 50% of cases, but it could also be single or triple. It generally drained in the SMV (85%) but could also drain into the gastrocolic trunk and more rarely into the splenic vein or IMV.[32]

LYMPHATIC DRAINAGE

Lymph vessels of the gastrointestinal tract run along arteries, in the reverse direction, to their draining lymph nodes. Colonic lymphatics are traditionally divided into four drainage levels (Figure 139-19). The lymphatic plexuses located on the bowel wall drain first into the epicolic

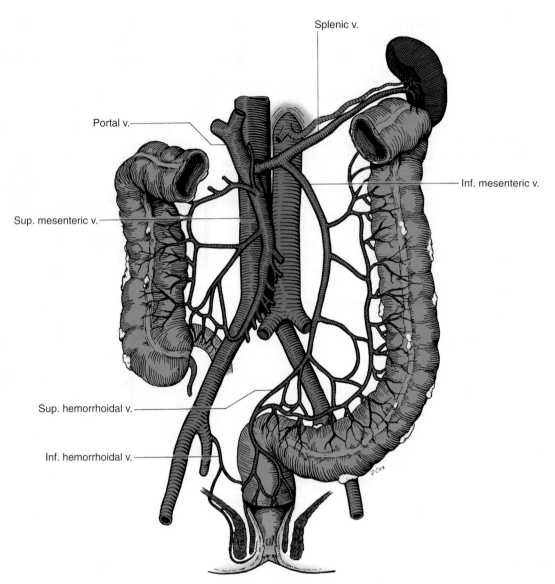

FIGURE 139-18 The venous drainage of the large bowel and rectum is illustrated; in particular, the drainage of the left colon via the inferior mesenteric vein to the splenic vein is shown. (From Keighley MRB, Williams NS: *Surgery of the anus, rectum, and colon*. Philadelphia, 1995, Saunders.)

nodes, located in the epiploic appendages and subserosally. The epiploic nodes then drain into the paracolic nodes, which are located behind the peritoneum on the upper border of the transverse and on the mesenteric side of the remaining colon. The intermediate nodes are the third lymphatic station and are encountered along the course of the main colonic vessels, namely, the ICA, RCA, MCA, LCA, and sigmoid branches. The intermediate nodes ultimately drain into the lymph nodes that accompany the two main colonic tributaries, that is, the SMA and IMA. From these two main trunks, the lymphatic drainage continues to the paraaortic lymph nodes, the cisterna chyli, and then into the thoracic duct.

The lymphatic vessels of the left colon drain into lymph nodes at the inferior mesenteric trunk, which drain into the superior mesenteric trunk, which drains the right colon (and most of the small intestine).

In particular, the appendix drains into lymph nodes in the mesoappendix and from there into paracolic nodes that lie along the ileocolic artery. The cecum and ascending colon drain into epicolic nodes that lie along the left side of the bowel, into the paracolic nodes along the ileocolic and right colic arteries behind the peritoneal floor, and then into the superior mesenteric group of preaortic lymph nodes. The transverse colon drains via epicolic nodes into the paracolic nodes along the middle colic artery in the transverse mesocolon and then into the superior mesenteric nodes.

The lymphatic vessels of the left side of the colon from the splenic flexure to the start of the rectum drain into epicolic nodes along the right side of the bowel. From here, they drain into paracolic nodes that lie along branches of the IMA behind the peritoneal floor (although the paracolic nodes draining the sigmoid

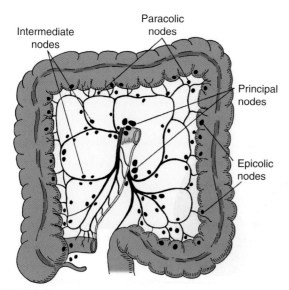

FIGURE 139-19 Diagram showing the epicolic, paracolic, intermediate, and principal lymph node groups that accompany the vessels of the colon. (From Grinnell RS: Lymphatic metastases of carcinoma of the colon and rectum. *Ann Surg* 131:494, 1950.)

colon lie in the root of the sigmoid mesocolon) and then into the inferior mesenteric nodes.

INNERVATION

The colon is innervated by both the sympathetic (from the eleventh and twelfth thoracic and first and second lumbar nerves) and parasympathetic (from the vagus and second, third, and fourth sacral nerves) divisions of the autonomic nervous system, and the nerves follow the arterial distribution (Figure 139-20). The sympathetic nerves are thought to have an inhibitory effect on colonic peristalsis and secretions, whereas the parasympathetic nerves increase colonic peristalsis and secretions, as well as inhibiting sphincteric musculature.

The sympathetic preganglionic nerves proceed to the respective paravertebral chains of ganglia and then organize themselves into bundles, which give origin to the splanchnic nerves. The splanchnic nerves form distinct network-like structures referred to as prevertebral ganglia, such as the celiac, the superior, and the inferior mesenteric ones, which follow the course of the respective arteries. In these structures, synapses occur, and the emerging postganglionic fibers travel as mesenteric nerves into the mesocolon to reach the bowel wall. The proximal half of the colon is supplied by the celiac plexus through the superior mesenteric plexus, whereas the distal colon receives its sympathetic fibers from the lumbar part of the sympathetic trunk, via the superior hypogastric plexus, which sends nerves along branches of the IMA. The superior hypogastric plexus is often referred to as the presacral nerve, but it is a misnomer as it is prelumbar, not presacral, and it is a plexus, not a nerve.

The parasympathetic innervation of the proximal colon is derived from the celiac branch of the right vagus nerve, which reaches the celiac plexus. Fibers that exit this plexus move to the preaortic and superior mesenteric plexuses and then follow the course of the SMA and its branches and ultimately reach the bowel wall. The distal colon and rectum receive their parasympathetic innervation through the nervi erigentes, also referred to as pelvic splanchnic nerves, which originate from S2 to S4. Fibers that exit from the nervi erigentes then move cranially into the superior hypogastric plexus (nerves to the rectum and anus pass to the inferior hypogastric plexus) and supply the distal transverse, descending, and sigmoid colon, traveling in close proximity to the IMA. Preganglionic fibers enter the bowel wall and synapse in the myenteric and submucosal plexuses. The splenic flexure and descending colon also receive branches of the pelvic splanchnic nerves, which have traveled up behind the peritoneal floor and independent of the IMA.[33]

Colonic pain may be referred to a site distant to the organic insult. Nash described a study of intestinal pain reference in which a balloon was inflated at various points of the gastrointestinal tract. Pain from the cecum is referred to McBurney point with spread to the epigastrium, whereas pain from the hepatic flexure is referred to the right upper quadrant. Pain from the ascending, transverse, and descending colons is referred to the lower abdomen in the midline and to the left. Rectosigmoid pain is referred to the suprapubic and coccygeal areas.[34]

EMBRYOLOGY OF THE COLON

The colon develops from the primitive midgut, which opens ventrally into the yolk sac. Starting at the fifth gestational week, the midgut rapidly grows and reorganizes to delineate the permanent gastrointestinal tract structures, including the colon. This progression is traditionally divided into three separate stages (Figure 139-21). In the first stage, the elongated midgut loop enters the extraembryonic coelom into the umbilical cord, a process referred to as physiologic umbilical herniation. The SMA also exits the abdominal cavity along with this bowel loop and within its corresponding mesentery. The SMA thus separates the midgut in a proximal and anterior portion, referred to as prearterial, which carries the omphalomesenteric duct at its apex, and a posterior and distal portion. The herniated intestine then rotates counterclockwise by 180 degrees around the SMA axis. In particular, the prearterial segment moves posteriorly and to the left of the SMA and delineates what will become the third and fourth portions of the duodenum.

In the second stage, the primitive intestine returns into the abdominal cavity and undergoes an additional 90 degrees of rotation, thus completing a total of 270 degrees. At this point, the duodenum has rotated counterclockwise around and below the SMA, and the small bowel is located mostly on the right side of the midline. At variance with that, the primitive colon rotates over the SMA, starting from the left. In particular, the cecum is the last segment to reenter the abdominal cavity, where it is initially located right below the liver and then migrates toward its permanent position in the right iliac

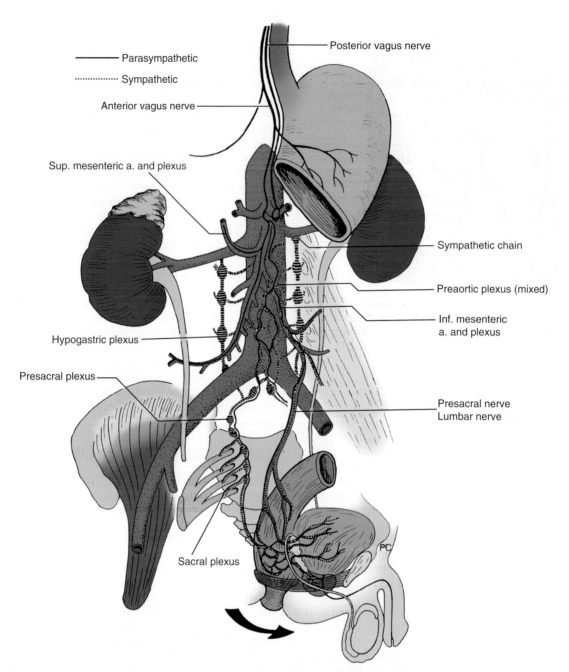

Parasympathetic

Sympathetic

Anterior vagus nerve

Posterior vagus nerve

Sup. mesenteric a. and plexus

Sympathetic chain

Preaortic plexus (mixed)

Inf. mesenteric a. and plexus

Hypogastric plexus

Presacral plexus

Presacral nerve
Lumbar nerve

Sacral plexus

PC

FIGURE 139-20 The autonomic supply to the colon and rectum is diagrammatically illustrated in an oblique plane. The contribution of the vagus nerve and the nervi erigentes to the parasympathetic supply to the pelvis is demonstrated. The sympathetic chain is shown together with the perivascular plexus to provide the autonomic innervation to the large bowel and rectum. (From Keighley MRB, Williams NS: *Surgery of the anus, rectum, and colon*. Philadelphia, 1995, Saunders.)

fossa. Meanwhile, the small bowel elongates while its mesentery shortens, before becoming fixed to the posterior peritoneum.

A number of anomalies of rotation can occur at this stage, including nonrotation, incomplete rotation, reversed rotation, and the range of intermediate conditions collectively considered under the definition of malrotation (Figure 139-22).[35] In general, individuals with anomalies of rotation are at an increased risk for

mesenteric volvulus and extrinsic duodenal compression from abnormal peritoneal attachments, also referred to as Ladd bands. In the nonrotation, the midgut is unable to complete the physiologic 270 degrees of rotation and lies at 0 or 90 degrees with the colon in the left abdomen, the cecum near the midline, and the small bowel to the right. This anomaly can be encountered in approximately 0.2% of radiologic studies and predisposes to midgut volvulus and extrinsic compression of

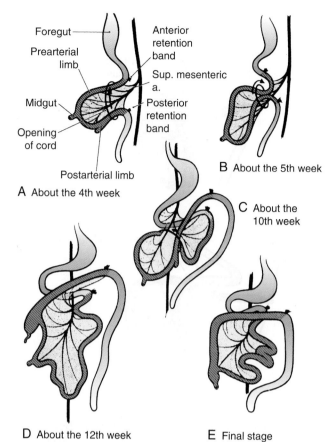

FIGURE 139-21 Normal rotation. **A,** Human embryo at the 4th or 5th week. Note that the midgut supplied by the superior mesenteric artery has "herniated" into the cord. The foregut and hindgut derivatives do not enter this "hernia"; the retention bands are points of fixation. **B,** The prearterial segment of the midgut loop has returned into the abdomen first, as the gut has rotated counterclockwise. The duodenum thus comes to lie behind the superior mesenteric artery. Note the splenic flexure is fixed on the left. **C,** Embryo at the 10th week. The postarterial segment has also reduced and comes to lie in front of the superior mesenteric artery. The cecum is in the upper abdomen and must migrate to the right lower quadrant as counterclockwise rotation continues to 270 degrees. **D,** Embryo at the 12th week. Rotation has been completed; the viscera have attained their normal relationships. **E,** Gradually, fusion of parts of the primitive mesentery occurs fixing the duodenum and ascending and descending portions of the colon to the posterior abdominal wall. (From Haller JD, Morgenstern L: Anomalous rotation and fixation of the left colon: Embryogenesis and surgical management. *Am J Surg* 108:331, 1964.)

the duodenum. In incomplete rotation, the rotation progresses to approximately 180 degrees. Therefore, the prearterial segment does not reach the posterior location, and the cecum does not rotate anteriorly to the SMA but typically remains in the left upper abdomen. The colon becomes fixed to the posterior wall by abnormal peritoneal bands, which can cause duodenal obstruction. The reversed rotation is the result of a clockwise

rotation around the SMA, with the prearterial segment ending up anteriorly to the posterior segment, which can become entrapped in a mesocolic hernia. The transverse colon lies posteriorly to the duodenum and the SMA, in a tunnel beneath the mesentery, which predisposes to the onset of intestinal obstruction (Figure 139-23).

The third and final developmental stage occurs at approximately the twelfth week of gestation and consists of cecal descent and colon fixation to the posterior peritoneum. In particular, the cecum reaches the right iliac fossa, whereas the ligament of Treitz becomes an identifiable anatomic structure located to the left of the aorta, and the small bowel mesentery retracts in its permanent oblique and broad-based position. When the migration of the colon is complete, the posterior mesentery of the ascending and descending colon fuses with the posterior abdominal wall and forms the fascia of Toldt, also referred to as the white line of Toldt, which is an essential landmark for a bloodless dissection (Figure 139-24).

Anomalies of the third phase include undescended, mobile, or hyperdescended cecum; persistent colon mesentery; and ileocecal mesentery. In these anomalies, the laxity of the posterior attachments increases the risk of volvulus.

ANOMALIES OF FIXATION

When the posterior fixation of the colon is incomplete, abnormal spaces result that may favor the onset of internal hernias. The most common types of internal hernias are referred to as mesocolic or paraduodenal hernias, which can occur either on the right or to the left (Figure 139-25).[36-39] A right mesocolic hernia results from a failure of the prearterial limb to rotate around the SMA so that the intestinal loops become entrapped into the right colon mesentery. Surgical repair is accomplished by mobilization of the right colon and rotation to the left, which is essential to free the small bowel.

The more frequent left mesocolic hernia results from migration and protrusion of the small intestine through the space between the SMV and the descending colon mesentery. In such a case, the surgical repair consists of mobilization of the IMV and reduction of the hernia through the sac, which is then closed to prevent the creation of an empty space.

Rarely, anomalies of rotation and fixation coexist, and these can occur in the left colon. The primary disorder is fixation of the left colon on the right side, followed by a physiologic counterclockwise rotation of the transverse colon, which concludes its trajectory behind the SMA and the duodenum.

ATRESIA OF THE COLON

Atresia of the colon is a rare disorder that resembles the analogous condition of the small bowel and constitutes 5% to 12% of all the intestinal atresias. Three different types have been described. In type I, there is simple mucosal diaphragm, whereas in type II, two blind ends are connected by a fibrous cord derived from the mesentery. In type III, the two blind ends are associated with

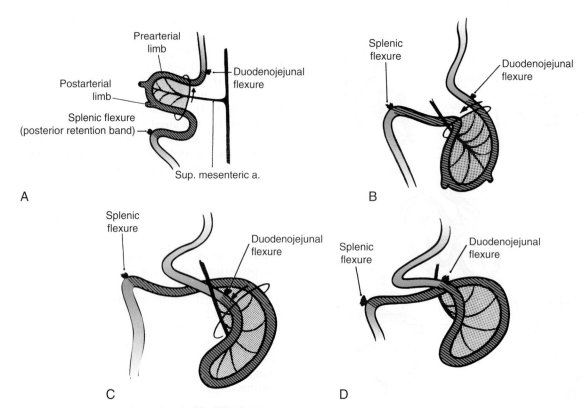

FIGURE 139-22 Mechanism for producing anomalies of rotation and fixation of the entire left colon. **A,** The splenic flexure fixes on the right side rather than on the left. This is the first and basic anomaly. **B,** Rotation begins in the normal counterclockwise direction. Because the splenic flexure is already fixed on the right, the adjacent segment of bowel, the transverse colon, reduces first and comes to lie behind the superior mesenteric artery. Thus, the first anomaly of fixation has produced the second anomaly of rotation. **C,** The next loop to reduce is the duodenum, as is normal. By projecting from this diagram, one can see that the reduction of the cecum last, as also is normal, will throw the proximal transverse colon in front of all of the other structures. **D,** If duodenal reduction is delayed or its rotation is incomplete, it may reenter the abdomen later and come to lie anterior to the superior mesenteric artery. (From Haller JD, Morgenstern L: Anomalous rotation and fixation of the left colon: Embryogenesis and surgical management. *Am J Surg* 108:331, 1964.)

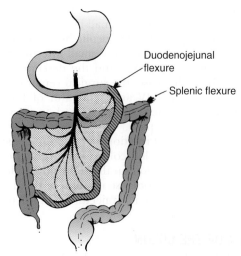

FIGURE 139-23 Reversed rotation. Note that (1) the locations of all parts of the large and small bowel are normal and (2) the only anomaly is the reversed relationship of the transverse colon and duodenum with the superior mesenteric artery; the colon is posterior and the duodenum is anterior. (From Haller JD, Morgenstern L: Anomalous rotation and fixation of the left colon: Embryogenesis and surgical management. *Am J Surg* 108:331, 1964.)

a corresponding mesenteric gap. The most accepted pathogenetic theory postulates that this disorder originates from an intrauterine derangement in the development of the vascular supply to the involved segment of bowel. A more recent theory supported by experimental evidence correlates colonic atresia to the absence of embryonic expression of fibroblast growth factor or its corresponding receptor.[40] The three types occur with approximately similar frequency without any gender predilection.

In approximately 20% of cases, a number of associated congenital abnormalities have been described, including Hirschsprung disease, duodenal atresia, bladder exstrophy, and ophthalmic defects. Symptoms are not distinctively different from other types of intestinal obstruction and include bilious vomiting, abdominal distention without bowel movements, and absent or minimal passage of meconium. Barium enema is diagnostic and should be promptly followed by surgery to avoid the risk of necrosis and perforation. A delayed diagnosis predisposes to profound dehydration and electrolyte imbalance. Colonic atresia may be associated with multiple atresias involving the gastrointestinal tract from stomach to rectum and may be hereditary.[41]

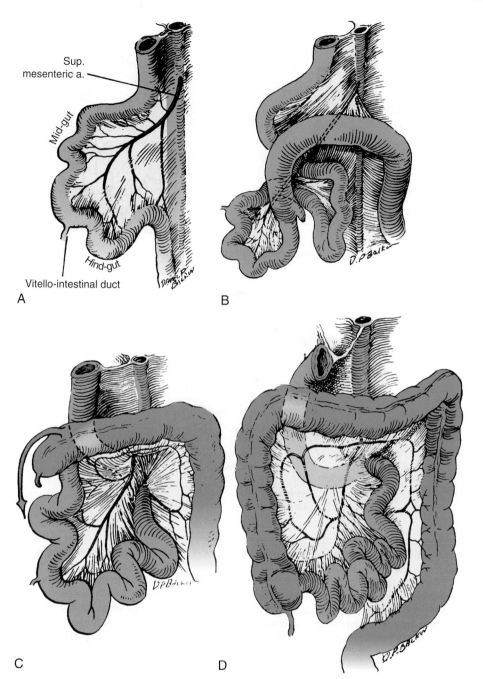

FIGURE 139-24 Normal intestinal rotation. **A,** Loop formed by midgut. **B,** Rotation of midgut and extracoelomic position. **C,** Orderly return of intestinal loops into peritoneal cavity below the transverse mesocolon and further rotation of 180 degrees in counterclockwise direction. **D,** Descent of cecum and fixation of ascending colon to posterior parietal peritoneum. *Sup mes a,* Superior mesenteric artery. (From Zimmerman LM, Laufman H: Intra-abdominal hernias due to developmental and rotational anomalies. *Ann Surg* 138:82, 1953.)

DUPLICATION OF THE COLON

A number of different disorders are included in this category; they are basically divided into mesenteric cysts, colonic diverticula, and true colon duplications.

Mesenteric cysts are generally located in the mesocolon. They are rare and account for only 1 in 100,000 acute adult hospital admissions. They can communicate or not with the intestinal lumen and can have an independent blood supply. They are lined with intestinal epithelium and present as palpable masses or with symptoms of intestinal obstruction.[42] Although most of the cysts are benign, they may contain foci of malignancy or gastrointestinal stromal tumor.[43]

A different variant of colonic duplication is the presence of colonic diverticula. Congenital disorders are often difficult to differentiate from acquired diverticula,

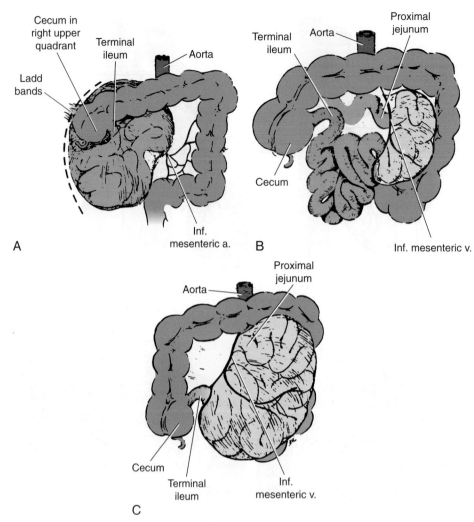

FIGURE 139-25 Mesocolic hernias. **A,** Right mesocolic hernia. Prearterial segment of the midgut has failed to rotate. Postarterial segment does not rotate and traps most of the small bowel behind the right mesocolon. The *dashed line* indicates the surgical incision used to reduce the hernia. **B,** Left mesocolic hernia. Initial rotation of the small intestine is normal. During migration to the left superior portion of the abdomen, the bowel invaginates into an avascular portion of the left mesocolon posterior to the inferior mesenteric vein. **C,** Left mesocolic hernia. Small intestine, except for portions of the distal ileum, is trapped beneath the left mesocolon. Note that the inferior mesenteric vein delineates the right margin of the sac and is an integral part of the neck of the sac. (**A** from Willwerth BM, Zollinger RM, Izant RJ: Congenital mesocolic (paraduodenal) hernias: Embryologic basis of repair. *Am J Surg* 128:358, 1974. **B** and **C** adapted from Callander CL, Rusk R, Nemir A: Mechanism, symptoms, and treatment of hernia into the descending mesocolon. *Surg Gynecol Obstet* 60:1052, 1935.)

a quite common condition in elderly individuals living in Western countries. Acquired diverticula are common and generally located in the sigmoid colon and tend to increase in frequency with age. In contrast, right colon diverticula are much rarer and are equally frequent in elderly and younger patients. Therefore, it has been speculated that right colon diverticula are most likely congenital. In general, congenital diverticula can be located on the mesenteric or antimesenteric border of the colon and can undergo mucosal metaplasia, most frequently gastric or pancreatic. Accumulation of fecal material can increase the dimensions of the diverticulum, which becomes manifest as an abdominal mass. Alternatively, the diverticulum can present with bleeding

from gastric ectopic mucosa, obstruction related to colonic intussusception, or may even perforate.[44]

A truly bilateral colon duplication is a rare disorder often accompanied by duplication of other structures, most frequently the spine, bladder, and vagina (Figure 139-26). In its complete form, two distinct gastrointestinal tubules are encountered from the terminal ileum to the rectum. The two proceed distally while sharing a common wall and terminate in two separate anal openings.[45] However, in most cases, the duplication is incomplete and involves only a segment of the large bowel, which can terminate in one anus or an anus and a fistula.[46] Other anomalies may coexist, such as horseshoe or absent kidney and clubfoot.

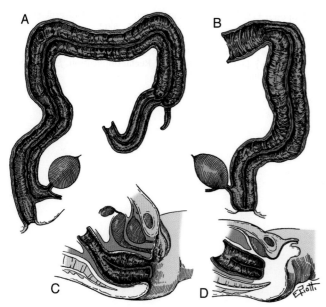

FIGURE 139-26 Examples of tubular duplications of the intestine. **A,** Duplication from ileum to rectum. One canal ends at a normal anus, and the other ends in a fistula to the urethra. **B,** Duplication of the descending colon with double anus and a fistula to the urethra. **C,** Short duplication of the rectum, with two anal openings. **D,** Duplication of the rectum, with both canals ending blindly (more frequently, the cranial end of the duplication is blind). (From Skandalakis JE, Gray SW, editors: *Embryology for surgeons*, ed 2. Baltimore, 1994, Williams & Wilkins, p 249.)

REFERENCES

1. Terminology FCoA: *Terminologia anatomica: International anatomical terminology.* New York, 1998, Thieme.
2. Saunders BP, Fukumoto M, Halligan S, et al: Why is colonoscopy more difficult in women? *Gastrointest Endosc* 43:124, 1996.
3. Saunders BP, Masaki T, Sawada T, et al: A preoperative comparison of Western and Oriental colonic anatomy and mesentery attachments. *Int J Colorectal Dis* 10:216, 1995.
4. Chee SS, Godfrey CD, Hurteau JA, et al: Location of the transverse colon in relationship to the umbilicus: Implications for laparoscopic techniques. *J Am Assoc Gynecol Laparosc* 5:385, 1998.
5. Khashab MA, Pickhardt PJ, Kim DH, et al: Colorectal anatomy in adults at computed tomography colonography: Normal distribution and the effect of age, sex, and body mass index. *Endoscopy* 41:674, 2009.
6. Moody RO: The position of the abdominal viscera in healthy, young British and American Adults. *J Anat* 61:223, 1927.
7. Schumpelick V, Dreuw B, Ophoff K, et al: Appendix and cecum. Embryology, anatomy, and surgical applications. *Surg Clin North Am* 80:295, 2000.
8. Faussone Pellegrini MS, Manneschi LI, Manneschi L: The caecocolonic junction in humans has a sphincteric anatomy and function. *Gut* 37:493, 1995.
9. Shafik A, Mostafa RM, Shafik AA, et al: Study of the functional activity of the cecocolonic junction with identification of a "physiologic sphincter", "cecocolonic inhibitory reflex" and "colocecal excitatory reflex". *Surg Radiol Anat* 25:16, 2003.
10. Wakeley CP: The position of the vermiform appendix as ascertained by an analysis of 10,000 cases. *J Anat* 67:277, 1933.
11. Treves F: Lectures on the anatomy of the intestinal canal and peritoneum in man. *BMJ* 1:580, 1885.
12. Kantor JL, Schechter S: Colon studies: VIII. Variations in fixation of the cecocolon: Their clinical significance. *AJR Am J Roentgenol* 31:751, 1934.
13. Oyar O, Yesildag A, Malas MA, et al: Splenodiaphragmatic interposition of the descending colon. *Surg Radiol Anat* 25:434, 2003.
14. Faure JP, Richer JP, Chansigaud JP, et al: A prospective radiological anatomical study of the variations of the position of the colon in the left pararenal space. *Surg Radiol Anat* 23:335, 2001.
15. Madiba TE, Haffajee MR: Anatomical variations in the level of origin of the sigmoid colon from the descending colon and the attachment of the sigmoid mesocolon. *Clin Anat* 23:179, 2010.
16. Bhatnagar BN, Sharma CL, Gupta SN, et al: Study on the anatomical dimensions of the human sigmoid colon. *Clin Anat* 17:236, 2004.
17. Shafik AA, Asaad S, Loka MM, et al: Colosigmoid junction: Morphohistologic, morphometric, and endoscopic study with identification of colosigmoid canal with sphincter. *Clin Anat* 22:243, 2009.
18. Shafik A, Asaad S, Doss S: Identification of a sphincter at the sigmoidorectal canal in humans: Histomorphologic and morphometric studies. *Clin Anat* 16:138, 2003.
19. Fernando ED, Deen KI: Consideration of the blood supply of the ileocecal segment in valve preserving right hemicolectomy. *Clin Anat* 22:712, 2009.
20. Moynihan B: Remarks on the surgery of the large intestine. *Lancet* 2:1, 1913.
21. Allison AS, Bloor C, Faux W, et al: The angiographic anatomy of the small arteries and their collaterals in colorectal resections: Some insights into anastomotic perfusion. *Ann Surg* 251:1092, 2010.
22. Kachlik D, Baca V, Stingl J: The spatial arrangement of the human large intestinal wall blood circulation. *J Anat* 216:335, 2010.
23. Hall NR, Finan PJ, Stephenson BM, et al: High tie of the inferior mesenteric artery in distal colorectal resections—a safe vascular procedure. *Int J Colorectal Dis* 10:29, 1995.
24. Dworkin MJ, Allen-Mersh TG: Effect of inferior mesenteric artery ligation on blood flow in the marginal artery-dependent sigmoid colon. *J Am Coll Surg* 183:357, 1996.
25. van Tonder JJ, Boon JM, Becker JH, et al: Anatomical considerations on Sudeck's critical point and its relevance to colorectal surgery. *Clin Anat* 20:424, 2007.
26. Yada H, Sawai K, Taniguchi H, et al: Analysis of vascular anatomy and lymph node metastases warrants radical segmental bowel resection for colon cancer. *World J Surg* 21:109, 1997.
27. Garcia-Ruiz A, Milsom JW, Ludwig KA, et al: Right colonic arterial anatomy. Implications for laparoscopic surgery. *Dis Colon Rectum* 39:906, 1996.
28. Shatari T, Fujita M, Nozawa K, et al: Vascular anatomy for right colon lymphadenectomy. *Surg Radiol Anat* 25:86, 2003.
29. Yildirim M, Celik HH, Yildiz Z, et al: The middle colic artery originating from the coeliac trunk. *Folia Morphol (Warsz)* 63:363, 2004.
30. Nonent M, Larroche P, Forlodou P, et al: Celiac-bimesenteric trunk: Anatomic and radiologic description—case report. *Radiology* 220:489, 2001.
31. Zebrowski W, Augustyniak E, Zajac S: [Variations of origin and branching of the inferior mesenteric artery and its anastomoses]. *Folia Morphol (Warsz)* 30:575, 1971.
32. Yamaguchi S, Kuroyanagi H, Milsom JW, et al: Venous anatomy of the right colon: Precise structure of the major veins and gastrocolic trunk in 58 cadavers. *Dis Colon Rectum* 45:1337, 2002.
33. Mitchell GAG: *Anatomy of the autonomic nervous system.* Edinburgh, 1953, Churchill-Livingstone.
34. Nash J: *Surgical physiology.* Springfield, IL, Charles C Thomas. 1942.
35. Kapfer SA, Rappold JF: Intestinal malrotation—not just the pediatric surgeon's problem. *J Am Coll Surg* 199:628, 2004.
36. Hendrickson RJ, Koniaris LG, Schoeniger LO, et al: Small bowel obstruction due to a paracolonic retroperitoneal hernia. *Am Surg* 68:756, 2002.
37. Papaziogas B, Souparis A, Makris J, et al: Surgical images: Soft tissue, right paraduodenal hernia. *Can J Surg* 47:195, 2004.
38. Rollins MD, Glasgow RE: Left paraduodenal hernia. *J Am Coll Surg* 198:492, 2004.
39. Osadchy A, Weisenberg N, Wiener Y, et al: Small bowel obstruction related to left-side paraduodenal hernia: CT findings. *Abdom Imaging* 30:53, 2005.
40. Fairbanks TJ, Kanard RC, Del Moral PM, et al: Colonic atresia without mesenteric vascular occlusion. The role of the fibroblast growth factor 10 signaling pathway. *J Pediatr Surg* 40:390, 2005.

41. Conrad C, Freitas A, Clifton MS, et al: Hereditary multiple intestinal atresias: 2 new cases and review of the literature. *J Pediatr Surg* 45:E21, 2010.
42. Grimison P, Goldstein D, Yeo B: An unusual abdominal mass. *Gut* 54:478, 2005.
43. Tan JJ, Tan KK, Chew SP: Mesenteric cysts: An institution experience over 14 years and review of literature. *World J Surg* 33:1961, 2009.
44. Jeppesen GA, Willerth M: Perforated congenital diverticulum of the sigmoid colon. *J Pediatr Surg* 37:E35, 2002.
45. Sarpel U, Le MN, Morotti RA, et al: Complete colorectal duplication. *J Am Coll Surg* 200:304, 2005.
46. Knudtson J, Jackson R, Grewal H: Rectal duplication. *J Pediatr Surg* 38:1119, 2003.

Anatomy and Physiology of the Rectum and Anus Including Applied Anatomy

David Beddy | Luca Stocchi | John H. Pemberton

Excellent results from surgical management of rectal cancer with precise anatomic dissection have sparked renewed interest in the anatomy and physiology of the anorectum. There is little doubt that an "anatomic" rectal dissection is the key factor that minimizes the chance of local recurrence. It is quite necessary, at this juncture, to consider again the rectum, its anatomy, and its relations within the pelvis. Moreover, a better understanding of the complex mechanisms that subserve continence and defecation is important; increasing numbers of patients are seeking surgical intervention to ameliorate functional problems.

ANATOMY

RECTUM

The definition of what truly constitutes the rectum varies. Most surgeons agree that the rectum extends from the sacral promontory to the anorectal ring (Figure 140-1).[1] The *anorectal ring* is defined as the site at which the muscles that form the levator ani (pubococcygeus, ileococcygeus, and puborectalis) merge with the cranial portion of the anal sphincter mechanism. The point at which the taeniae coli coalesce to form a diffuse longitudinal layer and the epiploic appendages disappear has been considered as the upper margin of the rectum, but it is more convenient to consider a measurement for the purpose of data comparison.

The length of the rectum is a matter of controversy. According to some, it can extend well above 15 cm from the anal verge.[2] However, the National Cancer Institute guidelines recommended considering the upper limit of the rectum as 12 cm from the anal verge. Measurements should be carried out with rigid proctoscopy to minimize technical variability encountered when flexible instruments are used for measurement.[3] Evidence suggests that a carcinoma located more than 10 cm from the anal verge is biologically more similar to a carcinoma in the sigmoid colon than to a rectal carcinoma. Therefore, it has been suggested that the rectum be considered only the most distal 10 cm.[4]

Traditionally, the rectum has been described as covered by peritoneum in its top third (Figure 140-2) only anteriorly and laterally and only anteriorly in its middle third, with the distal third completely devoid of peritoneum. The peritoneal reflection is located 7 to 9 cm from the anal verge in men and 5 to 7.5 cm from the anal verge in women.[5,6]

The rectum has been defined by anatomists as starting opposite the body of S3, or 14 to 16 cm from the anal verge. These definitions have no relevance to the surgeon, who would be better off using the sacral promontory as the point of reference. The upper rectum has peritoneum on the anterior and lateral sides, the midrectum has peritoneum only on its anterior wall, and the lower rectum is extraperitoneal, being below the peritoneal reflection. The latter is an important surgical landmark, because the difference between a high and low anterior resection is defined as having the anastomosis above or below the peritoneal reflection, respectively. A new term, *an ultralow anterior resection*, has been coined to define an anastomosis at the level of the puborectalis muscle, or pelvic floor. This can then be distinguished from a hand-sewn or stapled coloanal anastomosis, which is performed at the level of the dentate line. The various definitions are important, because reports that detail surgical technique and results can then be compared logically.

The rectum is surrounded for most of its length by the mesorectum. This is a fibrofatty tissue entity that contains the vessels, nerves, and lymph nodes of the rectum. Although it generally lies posterior to the rectum, it extends laterally to include three-fourths of the rectal circumference, from 2 to 10 o'clock.[7] The mesorectum disappears in the most distal few centimeters of rectum at the level of the pelvic floor.[8]

Three curvatures have been described in the rectum, with two of them having their convexity (Figure 140-3) on the right and one having the convexity on the left, corresponding to three intraluminal mucosal folds known as the valves of Houston. The second valve is located at the peritoneal reflection.[5] The valves are not identifiable after rectal mobilization.

The wall of the rectum is composed of four layers: mucosa, submucosa, and circular and longitudinal muscles. An additional serosal layer is present at the peritoneal reflection.[9]

Endoscopic View

The ampulla of the rectum is immediately obvious on insertion and insufflation of the scope. The mucosa is smooth, which differentiates it from the sigmoid colon, which has transverse crescentic folds because of the presence of the haustra. The cavernous capacity of the rectum allows retroflexion of the colonoscope and examination of the lower rectum and anal canal, which often are missed on insertion.

Fascial Relationships and Attachments

The parietal pelvic fascia, or endopelvic fascia, covers the surface of the sacrum, coccyx, and muscles of the pelvic side walls (piriformis, coccygeal). It is thickened over the sacrum and coccyx, where it forms a protective cover over troublesome presacral veins that may bleed

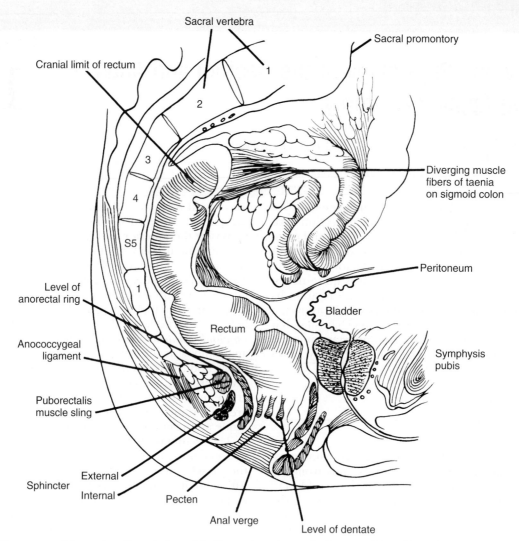

Sacral vertebra

Sacral promontory

Cranial limit of rectum

1

2

Diverging muscle
fibers of taenia
on sigmoid colon

3

4

S5

1

Peritoneum

Bladder

Level of
anorectal ring

Rectum

Symphysis
pubis

Anococcygeal
ligament

Puborectalis
muscle sling

External

Sphincter

Internal

Pecten

Anal verge

Level of dentate

FIGURE 140-1 The course of the rectum through the pelvis. The rectum descends downward from S3 to the most proximal level of the coccyx and then downward and forward to end at the level of the anorectal ring. The fibers of the taeniae coli diverge at the level of S2–3, providing an external visual landmark indicating the beginning of the proper rectum.

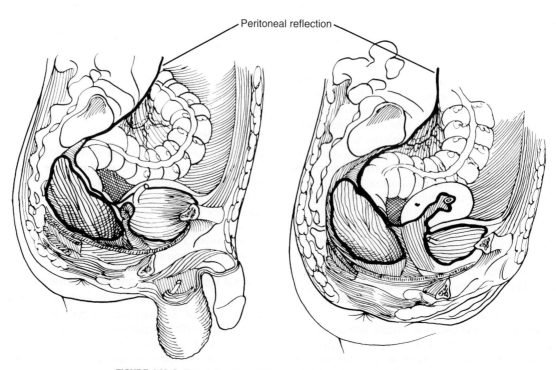

Peritoneal reflection

FIGURE 140-2 The reflections of the peritoneum in men and women.

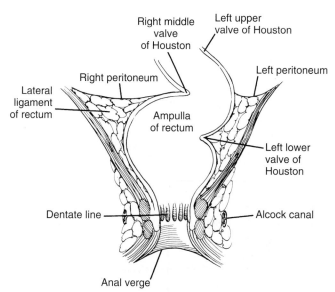

FIGURE 140-3 The curves of the rectum. The upper and lower curves are convex to the right, whereas the middle curve is convex to the left. The three valves of Houston are also seen. Note the peritoneum is reflected from the rectum at the level of the middle valve.

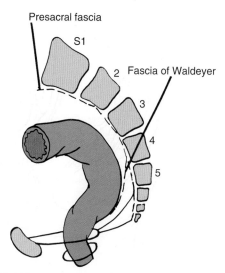

FIGURE 140-4 The presacral and Waldeyer fascia. Waldeyer fascia reflects from the presacral fascia above the anorectal ring.

during inaccurate rectal mobilization. The rectum itself is surrounded by the *fascia propria*, or visceral rectal fascia, which is a thin layer enveloping the mesorectum as well as its anterior wall. In the lower rectum, the visceral fascia merges with Waldeyer fascia, forming a single fascial plane behind the rectum (Figure 140-4).[10] This rectosacral fascia is an anteroinferiorly directed thick fascial reflection from the presacral fascia at the S4 level to the fascia propria of the rectum just above the anorectal ring. The rectosacral fascia described by Crapp and Cuthbertson in 1974, classically known as Waldeyer fascia, is an important landmark during posterior rectal mobilization.[11] It has been postulated that an inaccurate blunt dissection can result in violation of the mesorectum with potential cancer spread because the hand moving down is redirected anteriorly into the mesorectum by this strong fascial structure. In addition, inadvertent tearing of Waldeyer fascia from the sacrum can produce prodigious bleeding from the presacral veins. More distal to this, the visceral fascia becomes bilayered with an anterior and posterior leaf.[12] Another discrete fascial structure, the prostatoperitoneal fascia, lies just behind the prostate, in front of the rectum, and was described in men by Denonvilliers (Figure 140-5). This probably arises from fusion of the embryonic peritoneum of the rectovesical cul-de-sac. Although less evident, the rectovaginal septum is the counterpart of Denonvilliers fascia in women. Denonvilliers fascia has been described by some as composed by two leaves separated by a cleavage plane.[13] The anterior leaf adheres to the prostate and the seminal vesicles in men. Posteriorly to Denonvilliers fascia lies a thin layer of areolar tissue that is the anterior mesorectum, whereas deeper is the fascia propria that covers the rectum.[14]

Gross Relations of the Rectum

Knowledge of the gross relations, including the fascial planes surrounding the rectum, forms the foundation of good rectal surgery. Rectal dissection begins with complete mobilization of the sigmoid colon as described, which brings the sigmoid colon to the midline.

With the sigmoid colon mobilized, the sigmoid mesentery is stretched, and the inferior mesenteric artery, which continues into the mesorectum as the superior rectal artery, is identified. The fascial plane just below the vessels is identified, and a window is created. It is important to dissect just below the vessels, because additional fascial planes contain the hypogastric nerves, which run from the plexus around the inferior mesenteric artery. The window in the sigmoid mesentery can now be developed caudally with sharp dissection to enter the retrorectal space. This space is directed initially down, following the curve of the sacrum with cautery. A long narrow pelvic retractor (St. Marks) is indeed useful in that when inserted into the presacral space and pulled anteriorly, dissection of the areolar presacral plane is enhanced.

At the level of S4, the rectum curves forward. Here, it is attached to the sacrum by Waldeyer fascia or the rectosacral fascia (Figure 140-6). This must be divided sharply so the dissection can be completed down to the puborectalis or pelvic floor. The mesorectum is enveloped by a fascia propria. The oncologic plane of dissection should be just outside the fascia propria, preserving an intact mesorectum, visualized as a shiny bilobed structure. Local recurrence is significantly lower in rectal cancer when the mesorectum is dissected intact compared with intramesorectal or close rectal dissection.[15] The nervi erigentes lie posterior to this plane. More caudal is the presacral venous plexus. Care must be taken while dividing Waldeyer fascia to not tear this plexus because troublesome bleeding may ensue. Overwhelming, life-threatening sacral bleeding is nearly always stopped with the use of sterile thumbtacks.

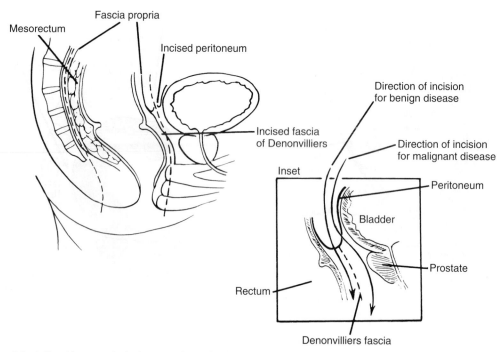

FIGURE 140-5 Fascial relationships anteriorly. In men, the peritoneum reflects from the bladder onto the rectum. Denonvilliers fascia runs *parallel* to the rectum, separating the rectum from anterior structures. *Anterior* mobilization is accomplished by incising posteriorly through Denonvilliers fascia; the "correct" plane can be readily developed by blunt dissection.

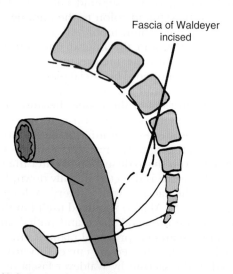

FIGURE 140-6 Cutting the fascia frees the rectum *posteriorly*, facilitating complete mobilization.

The fascia propria on the lateral walls of the rectum is not as distinct as in the retrorectal space. The location of this plane is enhanced by first developing the posterior retrorectal plane and then continuing it forward. Traction of the rectum to the contralateral side helps to further define this plane. This dissection can be brought around the front at the level of the peritoneal reflection. Anteriorly, the rectovesical, or Denonvilliers, fascia must be entered. This condensation of areolar tissue separates the anterior rectum from the base of the bladder, seminal vesicles, prostate, ureters, and ductus deferens. Laterally,

this condensation may appear as discrete lateral ligaments of the rectum. The lateral ligaments may contain accessory branches of the middle rectal artery. Deep to the lateral ligaments are the pelvic plexus of autonomic nerves controlling bladder and sexual function. In women, the rectovaginal septum corresponds to the rectovesical and Denonvilliers fascia and, like the latter, offers a plane to avoid the anterior plexus of veins (vaginal or prostatic).

Complete mobilization of the rectum straightens the bowel and "lengthens" it by about 5 cm (Figure 140-7). This is crucial in a low anterior resection of the rectum.

Anatomic Rectal Mobilization

Complication-free mobilization of the rectum can be achieved rapidly and safely through "anatomic" dissection of the perirectal structures (Figure 140-8).

Elevation of the Sigmoid. After the sigmoid colon is freed from any developmental lateral abdominal wall attachments, the white line of Toldt is incised, and the gonadal vessels and underlying left ureter are swept laterally (Figure 140-9, *A* and *B*). With firm elevation of the sigmoid loop, the inferior mesenteric artery is then placed on stretch, making identification of the superior hemorrhoidal artery easier. With the forceps, the tissue that is clinging to the superior hemorrhoidal artery (superior rectal artery) is swept directly posteriorly, opening a window in the sigmoid mesentery immediately below the superior hemorrhoidal artery at the level of the aortic bifurcation. The tissue separated from the superior hemorrhoidal artery contains the aortic plexus and, caudally, the presacral plexus and right and left hypogastric nerves.

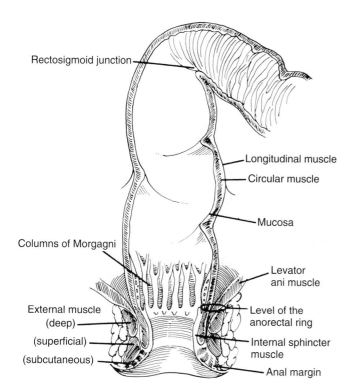

Rectosigmoid junction

Longitudinal muscle

Circular muscle

Mucosa

Columns of Morgagni

Levator
ani muscle

External muscle
(deep)

Level of the
anorectal ring

(superficial)

Internal sphincter
muscle

(subcutaneous)

Anal margin

FIGURE 140-7 The corrugated mucosa of the sigmoid colon gives way to the smooth mucosa of the rectum. Compared with Figure 140-6, the rectum has been "stretched" and the curves straightened. The layers of the rectal wall are also depicted.

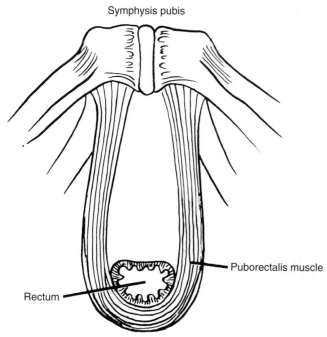

Symphysis pubis

Puborectalis muscle

Rectum

FIGURE 140-8 The puborectalis muscle from above. The puborectalis muscle lies adjacent to the anorectal junction laterally and swings around to encircle the sphincter posteriorly.

Pelvic Dissection. The arch of the superior hemorrhoidal artery is followed forward toward the rectum, which through strong upward traction is oriented in an anteroposterior direction. Again, with use of the forceps or scissors, the tissue behind the superior hemorrhoidal artery is pushed down, and once across the promontory, the retrorectal space is easily entered (Figure 140-9, C). With use of the scissors, this space is developed sharply down to about S3 and then down and forward to the rectosacral fascia at the level of S4. If easily seen, the rectosacral fascia is then sharply incised. If not, the posterior dissection is carried laterally with sweeping hand motions that loosen the perirectal areolar tissue. Sharp transection of the rectosacral fascia then allows safe dissection to the level of the levator raphe (Figure 140-9, D). By using this technique to enter the pelvis behind the rectum, the hypogastric nerves and the hypogastric plexus are protected throughout their course. There is no anatomic or physiologic benefit to be gained by pursuing an *intramesenteric* dissection.[13]

Lateral Mobilization. The peritoneum on both sides of the rectum is incised so the incisions meet in the midline over the rectum in the retrovesical or vaginal pouch (Figure 140-9, E). Sweeping hand motions, posteriorly and laterally, are then made on each side of the rectum, loosening and elevating the perirectal tissue. There are no nerves or vessels in this plane, because they lie on the side wall near the ureters. By elevating the rectum out of the pelvis, the lateral ligaments can be better identified.

Anterior Dissection. After incision of the peritoneum over the retrovesical or retrovaginal pouch, sharp dissection is carried posteriorly toward the rectum, thus exposing the Denonvilliers fascia (Figure 140-9, F to H). There are three potential planes of dissection of the low rectum anteriorly.[16] The close rectal plane lies immediately on the rectal musculature, but inside the fascia propria of the rectum. Anterior to this space is the mesorectal plane that leaves the fascia propria on the rectum and may be less bloody and more discernible than close dissection. Typically the mesorectal plane is used for dissection in benign disease as it minimizes risks of autonomic nerve damage. The extra mesorectal plane is anterior to Denonvilliers fascia, which stays immediately on and exposes the seminal vesicles and prostate. The risk of damage to the cavernous nerve plexus is theoretically highest in this plane. For malignant disease, Denonvilliers fascia is not entered until well below the level of the seminal vesicles or at about the midvaginal level. The dissection proceeds sharply between the rectum and Denonvilliers fascia to the level of the lower prostate or midvagina. For anteriorly located tumors, it may be appropriate to continue the dissection in the extra mesorectal plane entirely to ensure negative margins. The periprostatic plexus is adjacent to this dissection, but its fibers are sent to the genitals and prostate *above* the Denonvilliers fascia; they should therefore be protected by staying close to the rectum.

Division of Lateral Stalks (Ligaments). Only after anterior and posterior dissections are complete can the lateral ligaments be adequately defined and accurately divided (Figure 140-9, I). This is because traction of the rectum will not tent the ligaments if the posterior and anterior rectal attachments are present. The ligaments are defined through finger dissection. The thumb is placed anteriorly between the rectum and Denonvilliers fascia and is swept around and down toward the index finger, which has been positioned posteriorly underneath the lateral structures. A pinching motion thus defines the ligaments bilaterally. The ligaments are then divided and ligated close to the rectum in benign disease and laterally in malignant disease. If the superior hemorrhoidal artery is small, there is a higher chance that significant bleeding will occur from branches of the middle hemorrhoidal artery in the lateral ligaments. The pelvic plexus of nerves is quite lateral, being adjacent to the pelvic side walls, so that even relatively wide division of the lateral ligaments should not result in nerve damage. Problems do arise when the levators are excised radically, because fibers from the pelvic plexus run adjacent to the superior surface of the levator ani. Intersphincteric proctectomy in patients with benign disease,

however, preserves the pelvic plexus. After this dissection is completed, using a hand-sewn or stapled low anterior anastomosis, ileoanal or coloanal anastomosis, or intersphincteric proctectomy, bladder and sexual function should be normal.

Summary of Rectal Mobilization. A nerve-preserving, relatively bloodless, rapid, and safe mobilization of the rectum can be accomplished if (1) the retrorectal space is sharply developed just behind the superior hemorrhoidal artery, (2) the rectosacral ligament is sharply incised, (3) the anterior dissection is carried out deep to Denonvilliers fascia, and (4) anterior and posterior dissections are completed before the lateral ligaments are defined and ligated.

ANAL CANAL

The anal region is the most caudal portion of the alimentary canal and is divided into two regions: the cephalad anal canal and the caudal anal margin lying outside the

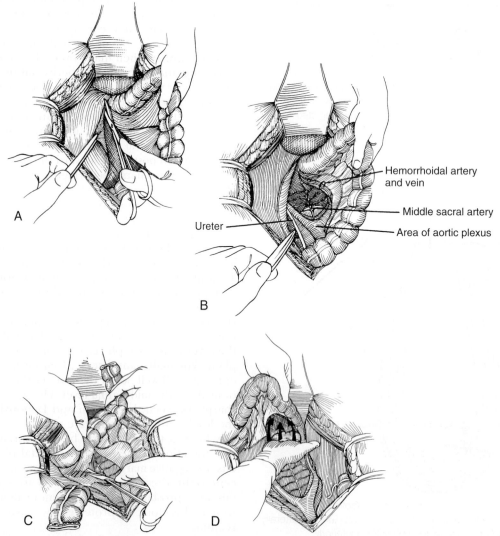

FIGURE 140-9 A, Pelvic dissection. The peritoneum of the mesosigmoid is incised on the left by retracting the sigmoid colon firmly out of the pelvis. **B,** The ureter is easily visualized at this point. The mesenteric "window" (underneath the tented superior hemorrhoidal artery and vein) is made carefully, in benign disease, so as not to disturb the aortic plexus. **C,** Pelvic dissection. Access to the presacral (retrorectal) space is achieved by pulling the sigmoid colon up and forward using sharp dissection. **D,** Careful finger dissection frees the rectum posteriorly to the level of Waldeyer fascia. *Arrows,* Motion of the hand used to loosen the lateral peritoneum and perirectal tissue.

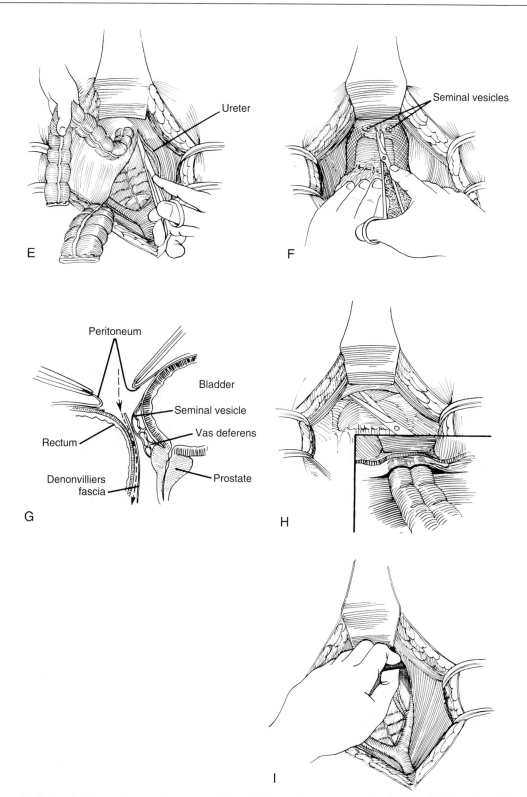

FIGURE 140-9, cont'd **E,** The right ureter is usually now seen beneath the peritoneum. The peritoneal incisions meet in the depths of the pouch of Douglas. **F,** The peritoneum is incised. **G** and **H,** Denonvilliers fascia is pierced with the scissors, allowing access to a bloodless plane posterior to the seminal vesicles (vagina) but anterior to the rectum. This plane is developed with the fingers to the level of the midprostate (or midvagina). **I,** After the lateral peritoneal fascia and lateral rectal tissue are loosened down to the level of the lateral stalks, the stalks themselves are loosened by lifting motions of the dissecting hand. Stalks are defined by pinching motions, and if feasible, they are ligated bilaterally.

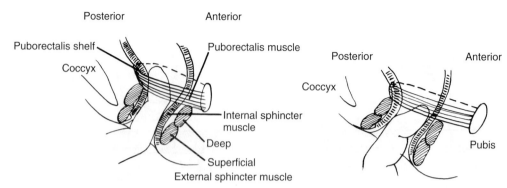

FIGURE 140-10 The anorectal ring is composed of the puborectalis muscle and the deepest portion of the external anal sphincter. The ring is most easily palpated *posteriorly* as the puborectalis "shelf."

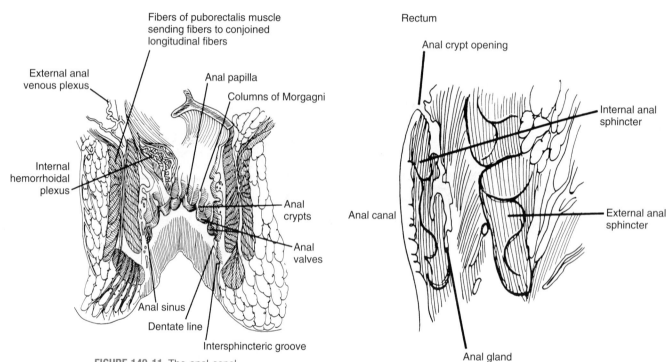

FIGURE 140-11 The anal canal.

FIGURE 140-12 An anal gland connected to an anal pit.

anal verge. This distinction is important because pathology in these two locations is often treated very differently. The anal canal begins at the anorectal junction and ends at the anal verge. The average length of the anal canal is 4 cm (range, 3 to 5 cm) and tends to be shorter in women than in men.[17] The anorectal junction is formed by the puborectalis muscle that forms a sling around the lowermost part of the rectum producing an acute angulation.[18] This angulation must be remembered when performing a digital or proctoscopic examination (Figure 140-10). It lies 2 to 3 cm in front of and slightly below the tip of the coccyx. The puborectalis fibers blend with the striated muscle of the external anal sphincter, whereas the internal anal sphincter is a continuation of the circular muscle coat of the rectum. The two sphincters form a funnel that constitutes the anal canal and at the distalmost point there is a palpable defect between the two muscles called the intersphincteric groove, which corresponds to the anal verge. This groove

can be identified visually as the part of the anal canal remaining closed when the buttocks are gently retracted. Outside of the anal verge lies the anal margin, also referred to as the perianal skin, which is of variable size but commonly encompasses a radius of 5 cm. The portion of the anal margin that overlies the external anal sphincter is pigmented in color. Lateral relations of the anal canal are the ischiorectal fossae and, anteriorly, it is related to the urethra in men and the lower vagina in women.[17]

Anal Canal Epithelium

The epithelium starts as a continuation of the rectal mucosa cranially and ends as squamous epithelium of skin (Figure 140-11). Approximately 2 cm cranial to the anal verge is the pectinate or dentate line. This line joins the anal valves and is located at the junction of the middle and distal thirds of the internal anal sphincter (IAS). Anal glands empty into small pockets above the

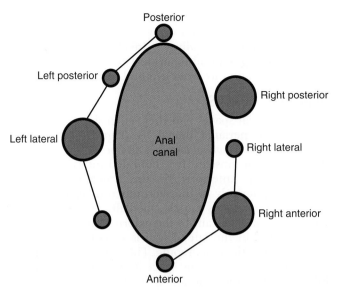

FIGURE 140-13 The positions of the three major (and five minor) arterial branches often identifiable at the level of the anorectal ring. This distribution is identical to the location of the major and minor internal hemorrhoidal groups.

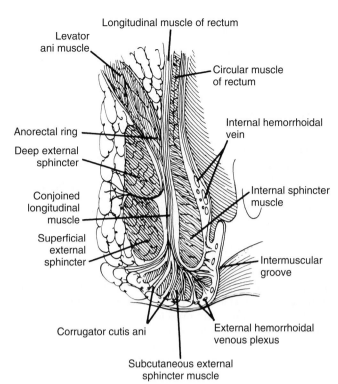

FIGURE 140-14 The voluntary and involuntary muscles of the anal canal.

valves called *anal crypts* (Figure 140-12). These glands number between 4 and 10, traverse the mucosa, and end in the submucosa, IAS, or intersphincteric plane. It is from these glands that perianal abscesses and fistulas arise.

Above the anal valves lie 12 to 14 columns of Morgagni. The mucosa in this region consists of several layers of cuboidal cells, which blend at varying distances from the anal verge to a single layer of columnar cells, characteristic of rectal mucosa. This is also called the *anal transitional zone* and extends for 1.5 to 2 cm.[19] It contains endocrine cells similar to the rectal mucosa above and melanin-containing cells from the anal canal below.[20] The junction of the columnar rectal mucosa and the anal transitional zone is irregular, with tongues of intervening columnar mucosa. These tongues may reach all the way down to the dentate line.[21]

The anal cushions lie above the dentate line. They appear at three primary positions—left lateral, right anterior, and right posterior (3 o'clock, 7 o'clock, and 11 o'clock, respectively) (Figure 140-13). Intermediate minor groups have also been described; these cushions consist of dilated submucosal hemorrhoidal venous plexus. These are fed by direct arteriovenous channels, which account for the bright red blood in hemorrhoidal bleeding. They are supported by Treitz muscle, which receives contributions from the IAS and the conjoined longitudinal muscle. Stretching and disruption of these ligaments cause them to prolapse into the anal canal, thus becoming "hemorrhoids"; this is one of the main theories of the cause of prolapse. Rubber band ligation, sclerotherapy, and infrared coagulation are used to attempt to place the anal cushions back into their original positions.

Caudal to the dentate line is a modified squamous epithelium devoid of hair and glands containing multiple somatic nerve endings. Grossly, this appears smooth,

thin, and stretched.[1] It changes to typical squamous epithelium with hair and glands at the anal verge. This is the reason why hidradenitis suppurativa does not extend into the anal canal and may be excised without anal stenosis.

Musculature of the Anal Canal

Internal Anal Sphincter. The IAS is about 2.5 to 4 cm long and 0.5 cm thick (Figure 140-14). It is the continuation of the circular muscle of the rectum and ends as a thickened edge 1 to 1.5 cm caudal to the dentate line.[1] This can be palpable as a distinct rounded edge slightly cranial to the external anal sphincter (EAS). When the anal canal is stretched with a bivalve retractor, the tip of the finger can be rolled over the distal edge to identify the intersphincteric groove. This landmark is important for perianal sepsis and when performing a lateral internal sphincterotomy.

Conjoined Longitudinal Muscle. The outer longitudinal muscle of the rectum thins out considerably below the rectum.[22] It joins some fibers from the puborectalis muscle and descends as a thin band in the space between the internal and external sphincters. The muscle terminates as a fan of fibers, which traverse the subcutaneous part of the EAS to form a supporting network around the hemorrhoidal venous plexus. Other fibers terminate in the perianal dermis and are called the *corrugator cutis ani.*[23]

External Anal Sphincter. This is a complex of striated muscle that envelops the entire length of the IAS and extends slightly beyond. This elliptical muscle is continuous with the puborectalis superiorly, and the two tend to

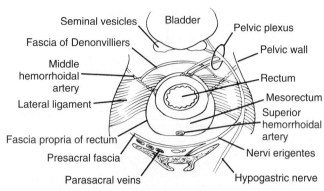

FIGURE 140-15 The pelvis viewed from above showing the major fascial, neural, and arterial structures.

act in concert. However, the nerve supplies to the puborectalis muscle and the EAS are different (Figure 140-15). Posteriorly, the muscle has a continuous attachment from the puborectalis, sacrococcygeal raphe, coccyx, and skin. Anteriorly, the muscle is attached in a similar manner to the puborectalis, transverse perineal muscle, and skin.[23] Whether the puborectalis muscle and EAS should be considered as one anatomic muscle group is the subject of continuing controversy. Perhaps the best evidence that the two are of the same striated muscle complex is provided by Wood.[9]

Perineal Body. This is the bulbous central portion of the perineum where the external sphincter, bulbospongiosus, and superficial and deep transverse perineal muscles meet. These insertions form crucial support for the perineum and vagina. Anterior sphincter repairs for fecal incontinence invariably involve the reconstruction of this structure.

PELVIC FLOOR

The pelvic floor is formed by two symmetric sets of muscles that interlink in the midline as a raphe. It functions as an inferior support for the abdominal and pelvic viscera, through which the gastrointestinal and genitourinary tracts traverse. The levator ani consists of three muscles that form the posterior portion of the diaphragm (Figure 140-16). The ileococcygeus originates from the ischial spine and obturator fascia to insert on S4, S5, and the anococcygeal raphe. The pubococcygeus originates from the obturator fascia and pubis and passes posteriorly, caudally, and medially, where fibers from both sides decussate (see Figure 140-8). The puborectalis arises next to the pubococcygeus from the pubis and proceeds posteriorly alongside the anorectal junction. Fibers from either side merge to form a sling behind the rectum at the anorectal junction. The anorectal ring that results is important, because division almost inevitably results in fecal incontinence.

The rectococcygeus that is present bilaterally attaches the rectum to the coccyx and is involuntary. This is in contrast to the coccygeus muscle, which is voluntary and arises from S5 and the coccyx. The superficial and deep transverse perineal muscles arise from the pubis and ischium, respectively. They insert into the perineal body

and serve to fix this central tendon. In men, these muscles merge with the external urinary sphincter and allow voluntary control of voiding.[23] Identification of these muscles during abdominoperineal resection guides the anterior dissection to avoid urethral injury.

PARAANAL SPACES

These potential spaces and their extensions are important sites of perianal infections (Figures 140-17 and 140-18).[5] The *ischiorectal fossa* has an apex at the origin of the levator ani muscles. It is bounded inferiorly by the perianal skin, anteriorly by the transversus perinei muscles, posteriorly by the sacrotuberous ligament and the gluteus maximus muscle, medially by the EAS and levator ani, and laterally by the external obturator fascia. Running within the lateral wall is Alcock canal, which curves around the ischial spine. This contains the pudendal nerve and vessels. The space itself is filled with large lobulated fat, the inferior hemorrhoidal vessels and nerves, and the scrotal or labial vessels.

The *perianal space* surrounds the anal verge and is continuous with the ischiorectal space laterally; therefore, infection from this space can spread into the latter. It contains the most caudal part of the EAS, the inferior hemorrhoidal vessels, and the external hemorrhoidal plexus. It also extends up into the intersphincteric space. The space itself is bound tightly by the corrugator cutis ani. Because of this, a thrombosis of the hemorrhoidal vessels here results in an exquisitely tender perianal hematoma.

The *intersphincteric space* is a potential space between the EAS and IAS that is continuous inferiorly with the perianal space. This is a common site of fistulas and abscesses, which are cryptoglandular in origin. If this space is infected without pointing through the perianal space, it can be drained transanally by dividing the IAS. This procedure reduces the amount of anal sphincter that needs to be cut. At the same time, postoperative pain is less, because the IAS has less pain fibers compared with the perianal skin.

The *postanal space* is divided into a superficial and deep space by the anococcygeal ligament (Figure 140-19). The superficial space is bounded caudally by the perianal skin, whereas the deep space is limited cranially by the anococcygeal raphe and the levator ani. It communicates anteriorly with the ischiorectal fossa and is responsible for the connections in "horse-shoe" abscesses. Failure to recognize this may lead to inadequate drainage and persistent sepsis.

VASCULATURE

The three main arterial trunks that provide blood supply to the rectum are the superior, middle, and inferior hemorrhoidal arteries, which are also referred to as *rectal arteries* (Figure 140-20; see Figure 140-13). The *superior hemorrhoidal artery* is in continuity with the inferior mesenteric artery (IMA) and proceeds down into the mesorectum. At the level of S3, it bifurcates into right and left branches. Each of these further divides into an anterior branch and a posterior branch, which reach the level of the columns of Morgagni.[24] The *middle hemorrhoidal artery* has classically been described as passing through the

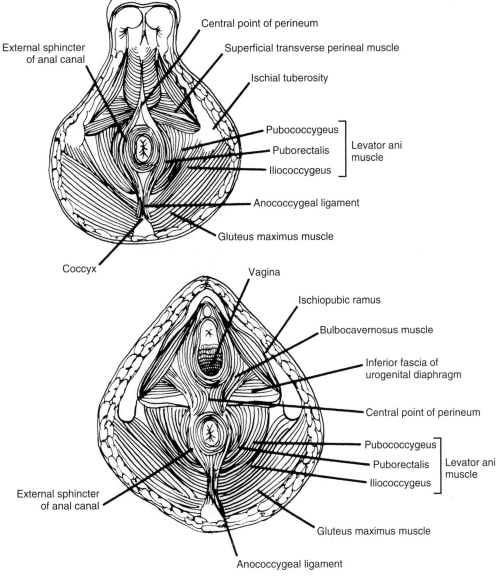

FIGURE 140-16 The levator ani muscles in men and women.

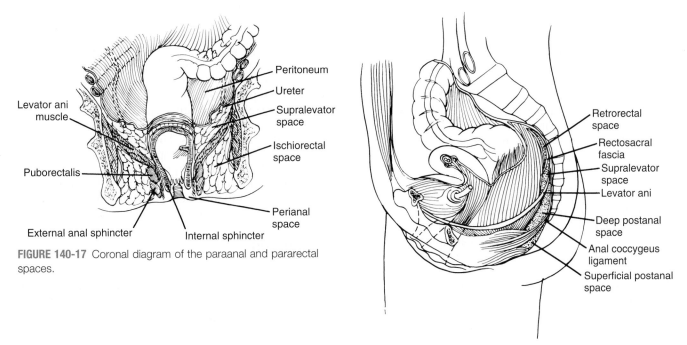

FIGURE 140-17 Coronal diagram of the paraanal and pararectal spaces.

FIGURE 140-18 Lateral diagram of the posterior pararectal spaces.

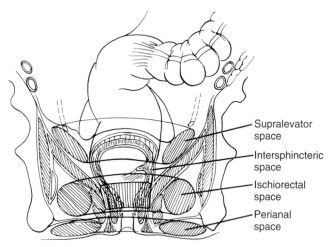

FIGURE 140-19 Coronal diagram of the pararectal and paraanal spaces illustrating how an abscess can track posteriorly from one lateral space to gain access to the contralateral space.

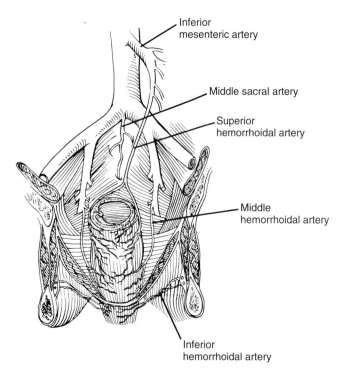

FIGURE 140-20 The vasculature of the rectum and anal canal. If present, the middle hemorrhoidal artery is small and lies immediately on top of the levator ani musculature and *not* in the lateral rectal stalks.

lateral ligaments of the rectum.[25] However, cadaver studies suggest that this occurs rarely and that the location of the middle artery is actually caudad and anterior to the lateral stalks. In addition, the middle hemorrhoidal artery has been described as being unilateral 40% of the time.[14] Although it is controversial whether this structure really exists and how often it is identifiable, it is generally agreed that the middle hemorrhoidal artery is not constantly present. The size of the middle

hemorrhoidal artery is usually inversely proportional to the size of the superior hemorrhoidal artery.

The *inferior hemorrhoidal artery* is a branch of the pudendal artery, which in turn derives from the internal iliac artery. It enters the EAS bilaterally and proceeds cephalad along the submucosa of the anal canal. The inconsistent *median sacral artery* can be infrequently encountered during the posterior mobilization of the sacrum. It originates at approximately 1.5 cm above the aortic bifurcation; descends along L4 and L5, the sacrum, and the coccyx; and terminates in branches that supply the rectal wall and pararectal tissues. An extensive intramural anastomotic network connects the three main branches.[9] It is therefore not surprising that even after sacrifice of the superior and middle hemorrhoidal arteries, necrosis of the rectum is infrequent.

The venous supply of the rectum follows the arterial routes, and there is free anastomosis between all venous channels.[26] In particular, the superior hemorrhoidal vein becomes a tributary of the portal circulation, whereas the middle and inferior veins drain into the systemic circulation.

Similarly, lymphatic channels course with the vessels (Figure 140-21). The upper two-thirds of the rectum drain into the inferior mesenteric nodes, whereas the inferior third drains into the internal iliac nodes. Importantly, lymphatic spread below the level of a rectal carcinoma commonly occurs only if extensive involvement of proximally draining lymphatic and venous channels has occurred.[27]

The arterial supply of the anus is derived from branches from the superior rectal artery, the inferior rectal branch of the pudendal artery and branches of the median sacral artery. The venous drainage of the anal canal is divided into two patterns based on the dentate line. The upper anal canal and internal anal sphincter drains via the terminal branches of the superior rectal vein into the inferior mesenteric vein and portal system. The lower anal canal and external anal sphincter drain via the inferior rectal vein into the pudendal vein passing to the internal iliac vein. The lymphatic drainage of the upper anal canal and internal anal sphincter drains upward into the submucosal and intramural lymphatics of the rectum that then drain to perirectal nodes of the mesorectum. The lower anal canal and external anal sphincter lymphatics drain downward via perianal plexuses into vessels that drain into the external inguinal lymph nodes. The lymphatics of the puborectalis drain into the internal iliac nodes. Therefore, typical squamous tumors of the anal canal will spread first to the inguinal nodes, mandating careful groin examination. It must be noted that there is considerable variation in the lymphatic drainage and that there are numerous connections between lymphatics at various levels of the anal canal.

INNERVATION

Rectum

Sympathetic stimulation produces relaxation of the rectal smooth musculature and contraction of the IAS (Figure 140-22). Conversely, *parasympathetic stimulation* results in contraction of the rectal wall and relaxation of the IAS.

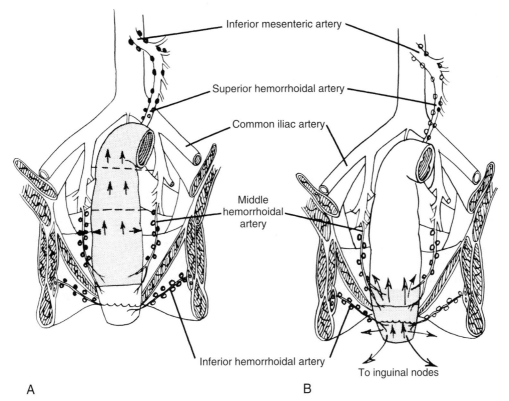

A   B

FIGURE 140-21 The lymphatic drainage of the rectum and anal canal. The "watershed" is the dentate line; tumors above this line may shed cells into the internal iliac and inferior mesenteric nodal chain **(A)**, whereas tumors below this line may shed cells into the inguinal lymph node chain **(B)**.

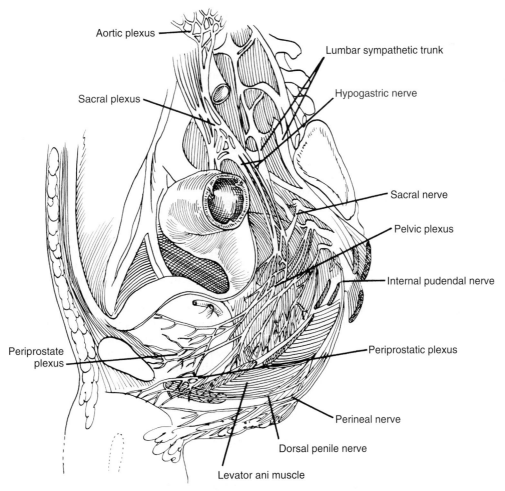

FIGURE 140-22 The innervation of the rectum, anal canal, and anterior structures. The sympathetic hypogastric nerves, together with the parasympathetic nerves arising from S2–4, join in the pelvic plexus.

The *sympathetic* nerve supply originates from L1-3, from which lumbar sympathetic fibers contribute to the aortic plexus. Some fibers of this plexus descend to form the presacral plexus caudally, whereas others join the inferior mesenteric plexus and follow the course of the respective artery. The *hypogastric nerves* originate from the hypogastric plexus above the aortic bifurcation and can be encountered approximately 2 cm medial to the ureters bilaterally. They generally lie close to the lateral pelvic walls, where they end in the *pelvic autonomic nerve plexus.*

The *parasympathetic* innervation of the rectum derives from the splanchnic branches of the sacral nerves, also referred to as *nervi erigentes*, which emerge from the sacral foramina at the levels of S2, S3, and S4. These fibers join with the sympathetic fibers in the presacral plexus. The third sacral nerve appears to be the largest when examined in the cadaver.[12] The hypogastric nerve and the sacral splanchnic nerve join on the pelvic side wall to form the *pelvic autonomic nerve plexus.* The pelvic plexus provides fibers to the rectum through the lateral stalks. There is experimental evidence that the nerve branches from the pelvic plexuses are constantly present in the lateral stalks.[28] A subdivision of the pelvic plexus with potential clinical implication is the periprostatic plexus, adjacent to the prostate and the rectum, which supplies sympathetic and parasympathetic fibers through anterolateral connections. Traditionally, the termination of these fibers has been said to occur above Denonvilliers fascia.[29] Conversely, it has been shown that the neurovascular bundle is not a discrete structure that lies beneath Denonvilliers fascia but rather a neural network that intermingles with the fascia itself and extends toward the midline.[30] At the apex and base of the prostate, the nerve fibers are particularly closely related to the anterior rectum, where they may be injured. This finding would be consistent with the occurrence of sexual and urologic dysfunction despite a properly performed "nerve-sparing" operation. There are four key zones where injury to nerves commonly occur during rectal mobilization.[16] In the abdomen, the sympathetic hypogastric plexus may be damaged during ligation of the inferior mesenteric artery, particularly if done flush with the aorta. When entering the mesorectal space posteriorly at the pelvic brim, the hypogastric plexus bilaterally lie just behind the fascia propria in loose areolar tissue and can be damaged if not recognized. Lower in the pelvis during lateral dissection, excessive traction on the lateral ligaments or performing a radical iliac lymphadenectomy may damage the pelvic plexus, which gives mixed sympathetic and parasympathetic dysfunction. Finally, deep anterolateral dissection in front of Denonvilliers fascia on the seminal vesicles and prostate risks injury to the periprostatic cavernous plexus to the bladder and penis. Erection of the penis is controlled by parasympathetic input (sympathetic input does inhibit vasoconstriction, thereby increasing vascular engorgement), whereas sympathetic inflow causes emission and parasympathetic inflow causes ejaculation. The pattern of sexual dysfunction gives a clue to the anatomic site of injury.[29]

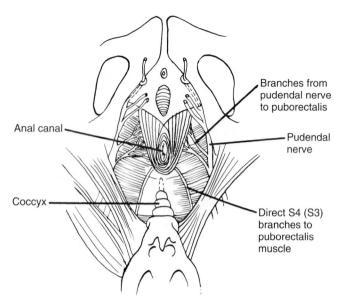

FIGURE 140-23 Innervation of the puborectalis muscle and other muscles of the levator plate.

Anal Canal

The IAS is tonically contracted through a combination of excitatory and inhibitory control mediated by sympathetic and parasympathetic nerves, respectively.[9] The former are postganglionic fibers that travel with the hypogastric nerve bilaterally (L5), whereas the latter are derived from the sacral nerves (S2, S3, and S4). Distention of the rectal wall results in relaxation of the IAS through the rectoanal inhibitory reflex (RAIR) (see later).

The EAS (Figure 140-23) is innervated by the pudendal nerve bilaterally, which originates from S2–3. The nerve supply to the levator ani originates from S2, S3, and S4. Branches of the pudendal nerve from below and direct pelvic branches of S3 and S4 supply the puborectalis muscle.

Sensation

There are multiple ganglion cells distributed throughout the rectum in three plexuses: Auerbach myenteric, deep submucous, and superficial (Figure 140-24).[22] Intraepithelial receptors, however, are rare.[31] The absence of receptors in the rectal mucosa may explain why the rectum is insensitive to painful stimuli. It is, however, sensitive to distention, although the exact mechanism of this is unclear. It has been postulated to be due to rectal wall stretch, reflex contraction, or stimulation of the mesentery. Sensation is present, and fecal continence is maintained after proctectomy. In addition, normal neorectal-anal reflexes are demonstrated after the ileal pouch–anal anastomosis.[32-35] These patients feel fullness in the pouch and are able to discriminate flatus from feces, suggesting that these receptors are outside the rectum, probably in the pelvic floor.

These sensations are carried in the parasympathetic nerves to S2, S3, and S4. Rectal sensation is abolished by parasympathetic blocks.[36]

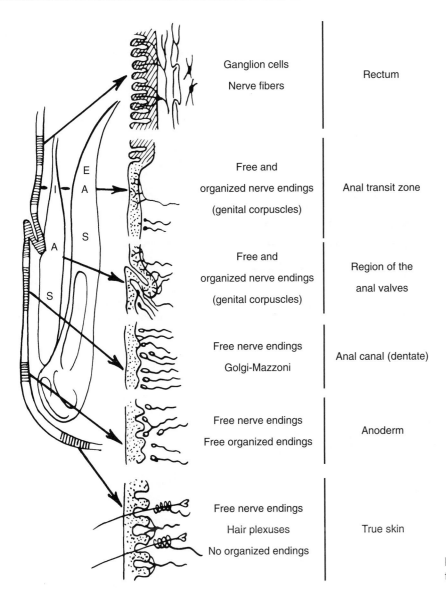

Ganglion cells

Nerve fibers

Rectum

Free and
organized nerve endings
(genital corpuscles)

Anal transit zone

Free and
organized nerve endings
(genital corpuscles)

Region of the
anal valves

Free nerve endings
Golgi-Mazzoni

Anal canal (dentate)

Free nerve endings
Free organized endings

Anoderm

Free nerve endings
Hair plexuses
No organized endings

True skin

FIGURE 140-24 Distribution of sensory nerves in the anorectum.

Free nerve endings can be observed about 1.5 cm above the anal valves to the anal verge. Meissner corpuscles, Krause bulbs, Golgi-Mazzoni corpuscles, and genital corpuscles respond to touch, cold, pressure, and friction, respectively.[31,37] These sensations are carried by the somatic nerves through the inferior hemorrhoidal branch of the pudendal nerve.

APPLIED PHYSIOLOGY OF THE RECTUM AND ANUS

CONTINENCE, DEFECATION, AND FUNCTIONAL DISTURBANCES

Fecal continence is the result of a complex combination of conscious and unconscious control, including, among other factors, a competent and closed anal sphincter acting synergistically with a coordinated pelvic floor, normal anorectal sensation and sampling reflex, adequate rectal capacity and compliance, and normal rectal

and anal canal motility.[38] Fecal incontinence occurs whenever anal pressures are lower than those in the rectum.[33]

ANAL CANAL HIGH-PRESSURE ZONE

This zone is maintained by the tonic contraction of the IAS (Figures 140-25 and 140-26). Mean intra–anal canal resting pressure is approximately 90 cm H_2O.[5] The IAS contributes about 75% of that pressure. In addition, the striated EAS contributes to the voluntary component, and the sum of the two muscles acting together produces the maximum squeeze pressure. The anal canal shortens during straining to defecate and lengthens when squeezed.[39] Moreover, resting pressures and squeeze pressures are lower in men than in women and lower in older persons.[40]

Resting pressures are distributed unequally around the circumference of the anal canal because of the anatomic arrangement of the anal sphincter and pubococcygeus muscles (Figure 140-27). Posteriorly, the resting

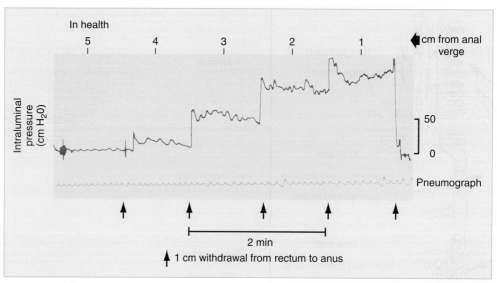

FIGURE 140-25 Perfused single-channel recording of resting anal canal pressure. At 5 cm from the anal verge, the intrarectal pressure is 5 mm Hg. Stepwise withdrawal of the probe shows the highest resting pressure to be 1 to 2 mm proximal to the anal verge.

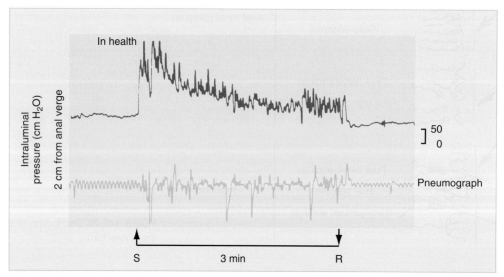

FIGURE 140-26 Anal canal squeeze pressure, in one quadrant, recorded by an indwelling perfused probe positioned 2 cm proximal to the anal verge. The overall duration of elevated pressure was 3 minutes, but the highest incremental pressure was recorded for less than 1 minute.

pressure is highest proximally and lowest near the anal verge.[41] Division of the IAS in the presence of a normal EAS weakens tone but does not entirely abolish it.

EAS tone is maintained during the day and is present, although reduced, during sleep.[42] Coughing and the Valsalva maneuver increase EAS activity.[39,42] With the exception of the cricopharyngeus and paraspinous muscles, the EAS and the levator complex are the only striated muscles that maintain a constant tonus. This tone is mediated by a low sacral reflex. Straining at defecation, however, usually renders the EAS electrically silent.

Squeeze Pressure

Squeeze pressure is generated by contraction of the EAS and the puborectalis muscle; intra–anal canal pressures are increased more than two times greater than resting levels during maximum effort.[42]

Squeeze pressures are also distributed unequally around the anal canal; in the proximal anal canal, they are highest posteriorly and lowest anteriorly.[41] In the mid–anal canal, squeeze pressures are distributed equally. In the distal anal canal, squeeze pressures are highest anteriorly and lowest posteriorly.

The maximum squeeze pressure elevation lasts for less than 1 minute, because the sphincter fatigues rapidly after that time (see Figure 140-26).[42,43] Because squeeze efforts briefly generate high pressure, the squeeze mechanism likely acts effectively only to prevent leakage on the presentation of enteric content to the proximal canal at inconvenient times. Squeeze pressure therefore is probably not responsible for maintaining fecal continence from hour to hour. A mechanism that does provide continence is the pressure differential between the rectum (6 cm H_2O) and the anal canal (90 cm H_2O).

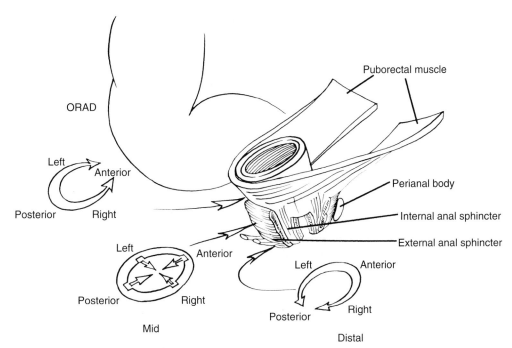

FIGURE 140-27 The anatomy of the anorectum might explain radial variations in resting pressure. The puborectalis muscle swings around behind the anal canal at its most proximal limit; posterior resting pressures are thus higher than anterior resting pressures. In the distal anal canal, radial pressures are lowest posteriorly and highest anteriorly.

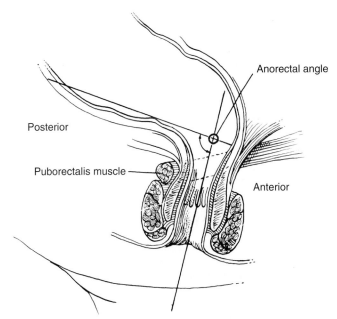

FIGURE 140-28 The angulation between the rectum and anal canal. This angle is formed by the anteriorly directed pull of the puborectalis muscle and is measured at the intersection of a line drawn through the center of the anal canal and a line drawn along the posterior wall of the rectum.

ANORECTAL ANGLE

Another mechanism that helps to maintain hour-to-hour fecal continence, particularly of solid content, is the configuration of the pelvic floor, formed predominantly by the anteriorly directed pull of the puborectalis muscle as it envelops the anorectum at the level of the anorectal ring (Figure 140-28). The result of these anatomic relationships is the *anorectal angle*. Barkel et al found that the mean $\pm$ SD angle was 102 ± 18 degrees at rest in the left lateral position.[44] Standing changed the angle slightly, but sitting widened the angle significantly to 119 ± 17 degrees. Sphincter squeeze, a maneuver that augments anorectal continence, and the Valsalva maneuver, which stresses continence, sharpened the angle to 81 ± 19 and 87 ± 23 degrees, respectively ($P < 0.05$, in the lying position). It has been found that if the angle is normal (puborectalis muscle is competent) but the sphincter is inadequate, continence of solid stool is usually maintained.[45] The puborectalis muscle has also the property of continuous resting electrical activity, even during sleep.

The angulation between the rectum and anal canal must be overcome to evacuate solid enteric content. This is accomplished by squatting; the angle is straightened to greater than 110 degrees by flexing the hips 90 degrees. Straightening of the anorectal angle is augmented by straining, which usually causes the puborectalis muscle and EAS to become electronically silent, although this does not always occur.[39] With the angle overcome, content passes into the anal canal.

In a novel experiment, Finlay et al investigated movements of the pelvic floor during the expulsion of air and liquid.[46] They found that the expulsion of air was achieved by sharpening the anorectal angle and by increasing anal canal and intrarectal pressures. Conversely, the expulsion of liquids was achieved by widening the anorectal angle, decreasing anal canal pressure, and increasing intrarectal pressure.

RECTAL COMPLIANCE, TONE, AND CAPACITY

A compliant rectum allows continence to be preserved, because the relationship of lower pressures in the rectum

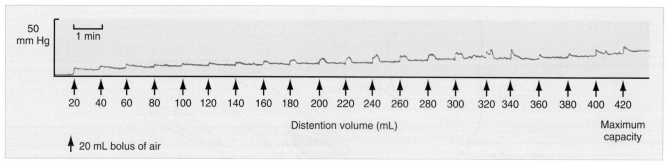

FIGURE 140-29 Effect of distention of an intrarectal balloon on rectal motility. Rectal accommodation ensures little rise in intraluminal pressure even at 420 mL of inflation.

and higher pressures in the anal canal is preserved (Figure 140-29). The volume of first sensation in the rectum varies from 11 to 68 mL, urgency normally develops after distention with about 200 mL, and the maximum tolerated volume varies from 220 to 510 mL.[47] The mean rectal compliance thus varies from 4 to 14 mL/cm H$_2$O. The rectum further adapts to filling and responds to rectal distention with a reflex increase in compliance. This phenomenon has been called *receptive relaxation*, and it allows the rectum to accommodate up to 300 mL without marked change in intraluminal pressure. Volumes higher than this result in a rise in pressure until tolerance is approached. This is associated with an urge to defecate.[48]

ANORECTAL SENSATION

As already described, anorectal sensory receptors reside in either the rectum or pelvic muscles. Flatus generates less pressure than do solids.[36] The ability to perceive different intrarectal pressures may help differentiate rectal contents. Sensory perception has also been found in the proximal anal canal mucosa.[49] Rectal wall contraction results in simultaneous distention of the upper anal canal. This sets off the rectoanal sphincter contractile response (Figure 140-30), where there is a transient rise in resting pressure of the distal anal canal. This is followed almost immediately by the rectoanal inhibitory response, where there is a transient relaxation of the internal sphincter in the proximal anal canal that results in decreased resting pressure. This transient relaxation is thought to allow recognition of rectal contents by the proximal anal mucosa and is called the *sampling reflex* (Figure 140-31). Sampling has been shown to occur between 4 and 10 times per hour in ambulatory manometric studies of healthy individuals.[50] This reflex is not the sole factor responsible for continence as it is absent after ileoanal anastomosis when continence can still be maintained. Continence is also unaffected when local anesthetic agents are applied to the anal mucosa.

MOTILITY OF THE RECTUM

Contemporary physiologic studies describe three types of rectal contractions: (1) simple contractions that occur at 5 to 10 cycles/min, (2) slower contractions that occur at about 3 cycles/min with amplitudes of up to 100 cm H$_2$O, and (3) slow propagated contractions that occur infrequently with high amplitude.[51] In addition, runs of

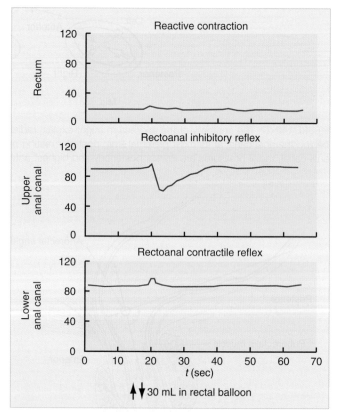

FIGURE 140-30 The rectoanal sphincter inhibitory response is composed of three parts: (1) reactive rectal muscular contraction, (2) relaxation of the internal anal sphincter with decreased resting anal canal pressure, and (3) contraction of the external sphincter. The decrease in resting pressure lasts approximately 20 sec and always returns to baseline.

powerful phasic contractions of more than 50 mm Hg that occur at 2 to 3 cycles/min and last 3 to 10 seconds have been described. These have a periodicity of about 92 minutes in the day and 56 minutes in the night.[52] They have been called *rectal motor complexes*, and they occur more regularly and frequently during sleep. They are disrupted after meals for periods ranging from 150 to 180 minutes. Rectal motor complexes are always accompanied by a rise in the mean anal canal pressure and contractile activity. It is postulated that the former keeps the rectum empty and the latter helps to keep

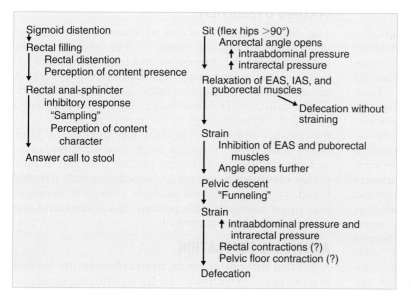

FIGURE 140-31 Sequence of defecation.

the anal canal closed, thus maintaining a greater anal canal pressure relative to rectal pressure and preserving continence.[53,54]

ANAL CANAL MOTILITY

The anal canal has a unique motility pattern that consists of slow waves and ultraslow waves. *Slow waves* are small oscillations at 10 to 20 cycles/min and an amplitude of 5 to 25 cm H_2O superimposed on the resting tone. These manifest a gradient with the anal canal with the frequency highest distally and result in the tendency to propel the contents proximally into the rectum.[17] The anal canal is kept empty, thus maintaining continence.

Ultraslow waves are found only in 40% of normal subjects. These have an amplitude of 30 to 100 cm H_2O, a duration of about 33 seconds, and a frequency of 3 cycles/min.[39] An association of ultraslow waves with high resting pressures of chronic anal fissures has been found.

STOOL VOLUME AND CONSISTENCY

Normally, between three stools per day to three stools per week are passed. In addition, there is a wide variation in consistency. Extreme changes in consistency can stress the continence mechanism. For example, liquid stools introduced rapidly into the rectum can overcome the continence mechanisms even in healthy individuals. It is therefore not surprising that volunteers have found it easier to pass large deformable stools than small hard pellets.[55] Semisolids are also more completely evacuated than are solid or liquid stools.[21] Therefore, it is logical that manipulation of stool consistency and volume is the first line in the management of fecal incontinence.

It is intuitive to imagine that large amounts of liquid that all at once flood into the rectum cannot be easily retained. Patients with incontinence and liquid stools usually benefit from bulking agents or dietary measures aimed at increasing the stool consistency, regardless of any other concurrent disorder in the anorectal function. However, there is evidence that increased stool consistency might not be necessarily associated with better

function. Ambroze at al showed that a semisolid stool is, not surprisingly, more thoroughly expelled than liquid stools; however, semisolid stools are also more easily evacuated than a solid fecal bolus.[21]

NORMAL PHYSIOLOGY OF DEFECATION

Sigmoid mass movement contractions are probably triggered by a volume threshold phenomenon (see Figure 140-31). This propels the enteric contents into the rectum. Receptors in the rectum or in the pelvic floor then sense the stretching of the rectum. At the same time, the rectoanal inhibitory reflex is initiated by intermittent, progressive rectal distention. There is concurrent external sphincter contraction that prevents stool leakage. The nature of the rectal contents is sensed by the upper anal canal, the *sampling reflex*. A conscious decision can now be made to evacuate, and the sitting position is adopted. This straightens the anorectal angle. Straining will increase the intraabdominal and intrarectal pressures and result in a coordinated reflex relaxation of the internal and external sphincters, as well as the puborectalis.

With further straining, the puborectalis relaxes further and the pelvic floor descends, creating a funnel with the outlet at the top of the anal canal. This allows the vector of pressure that is created by straining to expel the bolus through the anal canal. Defecation then proceeds either continuously or after straining. This pattern is usually the result of social habit.

The closing reflex initiates the completion of evacuation. The external sphincter and puborectalis contract transiently to restore the anorectal angle. The anal canal is finally closed by the restoration of internal sphincter tone.

Defecation can be deferred by voluntarily contracting the external sphincter and puborectalis. This pulls the perineum up and closes the funnel, causing the contents in the upper canal to be returned to the rectum. Passive accommodation then keeps rectal pressures low. The urge to defecate is then suppressed by cortical pathways.

FECAL INCONTINENCE

The Rome criteria (uniform clinical and diagnostic requirements) provide an encompassing definition of fecal incontinence based on symptoms: continuous or recurrent uncontrolled passage of fecal material (>10 mL) for at least 1 month in an individual.[56] Traumatic fecal incontinence usually results from an obstetric tear of the sphincter apparatus, which has been seen in up to 50% of patients after primarily sutured episiotomies. Other causes of this type of fecal incontinence include sphincter injury after anorectal procedures such as fistulotomy and hemorrhoidectomy and direct trauma to the sphincter. Anorectal manometry (ARM) typically shows a pronounced deficit in squeeze pressure, whereas the resting pressure is usually less affected. This represents the subset of patients who benefit the most from a sphincter repair; the success rate reaches 80%.[57,58] *Idiopathic fecal incontinence* results from damage to the innervation of the pelvic floor and, in particular, of the sphincteric musculature.[59,60] It can be related to excessive traction on the pudendal nerve during vaginal delivery or in patients with chronic constipation, straining, and long-standing rectal prolapse. Female gender and menopause are typically associated with this type of disorder. In this case, ARM shows a decreased resting pressure in addition to decreased squeeze pressure. Pudendal nerve terminal motor latency (PNTML) is helpful in delineating the activity of the pudendal nerve and sometimes can provide useful information on the neurogenic component of fecal incontinence.[60,61] Use of sacral nerve simulation in the treatment of idiopathic fecal incontinence has given new evidence in the etiology of this condition. Although stimulation of sacral nerves will cause contraction of the external anal sphincter, increasing anal tone, improvements in continence following stimulation of the posterior tibial nerve that persist following a course of treatment suggest a further pathway in the success of nerve simulation.[62] Experiments from animal models suggest that pudendal nerve injury results in reduced cortical awareness, leading to incontinence, and that stimulation of the sacral nerves may result in cerebral cortex sensory recruitment, leading to neuronal regeneration and improvement in continence.[63,64]

CONSTIPATION

According to the Rome II criteria, "Constipation has previously been defined by three methods: (1) symptoms, in descending order of frequency—straining, hard stools or scybala, unproductive calls ('want to but can't'), infrequent stools, incomplete evacuation...; (2) parameters of defecation outside the 95th percentile, e.g., <3 bowel movements per week..., daily stool weight <35 g/day)...or straining >25% of the time...; and (3) physiological measures such as prolonged whole gut transit or colonic transit, as determined by radio-opaque markers."[65]

The pathogenesis of constipation can be grouped into two main mechanisms: slow colonic transit and pelvic floor dysfunction. Guidelines from the American Gastroenterological Association suggest that outlet obstruction, anismus, pelvic floor dyssynergy, and paradoxical contraction of the pelvic musculature should be considered as particular forms of constipation.

COLONIC DYSMOTILITY

This disorder typically occurs in women in the absence of any obvious organic cause.[66-68] The patients usually report a history of infrequent and troublesome defecation, sometimes occurring less than once per week. A history of prolonged, unsuccessful use of a variety of laxatives is common. Different causes have been postulated to include abnormalities in the myenteric plexus or in the number and type of neurotransmitters in the large bowel, a decreased response to cholinergic stimulation, and a particular psychological profile. A variant of idiopathic constipation occurs in association with irritable bowel syndrome. In these patients, periods of constipation often alternate with periods of diarrhea and the colonic transit time is normal.

ABNORMAL DEFECATION

Abnormal defecation results from failure of the striated muscles of the pelvic floor to relax on straining (anismus, pelvic floor dyssynergia), failure of the internal sphincter to relax on rectal distention (Hirschsprung disease), laxity of the pelvic floor (descending perineum syndrome), rectal intussusception (occult rectal prolapse), complete rectal prolapse (procidentia), anterior rectal herniation (rectocele), posterior rectal herniation, and deficient or ignored rectal sensation. Of these, only Hirschsprung disease is well characterized pathophysiologically and the role of surgery is clearly defined; the aganglionic segment of rectum is removed (or bypassed), and a normal pattern of defecation is restored with a pull-through operation.

ANISMUS

The clinical findings in patients with anismus include an inability to initiate defecation, incomplete evacuation, a history of manual disimpaction, the assumption of contorted postures for defecation, laxative and enema abuse, leakage, and rectal "pain."

It has been proposed that the cause of symptoms in patients with anismus is failure of the puborectalis and EAS to relax during defecation straining.[69] This results in a failure of the anorectal angle to straighten during defecation. In some patients with anismus, these muscles not only fail to relax during defecation but also paradoxically contract, and many patients are unable to defecate a fluid-filled balloon.[69] However, studies of defecation using plugs, catheters, balloons, or radiology are artificial, and findings of paradoxical contraction may be due to conscious or unconscious restraint by the patient. Findings consistent with paradoxical contraction have been noted in healthy control subjects as well as in patients who are constipated.[39,70] In one study, there was no correlation between electromyographic evidence of anismus and the ability of the patient to evacuate the rectum or the symptoms of obstructed defecation.[71] Others have demonstrated that patients who evacuate poorly on proctography often do not strain sufficiently to raise their intrarectal pressure enough to defecate.[72] However, of the patients with manometric and electrophysiologic evidence of anismus, there may be a subgroup who do experience paradoxical contraction outside the anorectal laboratory.[73] Twenty percent of

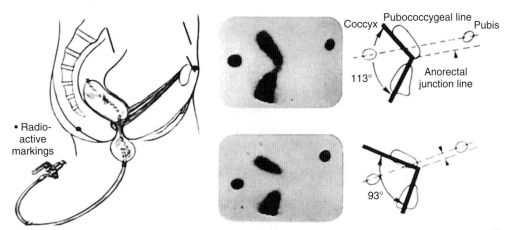

FIGURE 140-32 Scintigraphic imaging of the movements of the anorectal angle. *Left,* Balloon device in place filled with ^{99m}Tc-labeled water. Radioactive markers lie over the pubis and coccyx. *Right,* Scintigraphic image of the anorectal angle at rest *(top)* and during squeeze *(bottom).* To the right are diagrams of the same images. During squeeze, the angle narrows to 93 degrees, and the anorectal junction (the level of the pelvic floor) ascends.

patients with electrophysiologic evidence of anismus also demonstrated paradoxical contraction when studied with ambulatory electrophysiologic equipment.[69]

TEST OF COLONIC AND ANORECTAL FUNCTION

A variety of different tests have been introduced since the 1980s to diagnose anorectal disorders. Few studies have been conducted in the attempt to more precisely delineate the specific applicability of these tests. The American Gastroenterological Association published a position statement on anorectal testing techniques, suggesting indications for such testing.[56] In addition, the uniform clinical and diagnostic requirements of the Rome criteria have been proposed to enhance accuracy in nosologic definitions.[65]

ANORECTAL MANOMETRY

The measurement of the pressures in the anal canal can be carried out in many different ways: with water-perfused catheters or microtransducers and balloons filled with air or water. Four- or six-channel catheters are generally used to analyze the anal canal resting pressure and squeeze pressures at various levels of the anal canal. The resulting pressure profile can be plotted into a specific computer program to reconstruct a symmetry map of anal canal pressures, a technique referred to as *vector-manometry.* Balloons are used to test the presence of RAIR and the filling volumes. Three basic volumes are generally tested. The first detectable sensation is referred to as *rectal sensory threshold.* Further inflation of the balloon causes the perception of the need to defecate, referred to as *urgency* threshold. Last, the volume necessary to cause discomfort is recorded as the *maximum tolerable volume.* No single technique has proved to be superior to the others, and values can vary according to the different techniques used and the individual examiner. Therefore, it is essential to compare results with control values generated at the testing institution. In some institutions, ARM is preferentially complemented by the *balloon expulsion test,* which assesses the motor function and coordination of the anorectal pelvic floor muscles with the possible

addition of scaled weights to the balloon to enhance the simulated defecation. A variant of the balloon expulsion test is *scintigraphic balloon topography* (Figure 140-32), which allows measurement of the anorectal angle by filling a balloon with radiolabeled water.[44]

Suggested clinical indications for ARM are (1) fecal incontinence, (2) pelvic floor dysfunction, (3) Hirschsprung disease (ARM reveals the absence of RAIR), and (4) anatomic defects of the anal sphincter when anal ultrasonography is not available.

DEFECOGRAPHY (EVACUATION PROCTOGRAPHY)

The evacuation process can be investigated by filling the rectum with contrast material, which is then expelled under fluoroscopic observation (Figures 140-33 and 140-34).[74] The main disadvantages of this technique are a disproportionate incidence of abnormal findings in normal volunteers and a wide interobserver variability. However, defecography is useful in depicting the rectal lumen at rest and during the discharge of the contrast material. Guidelines recommend the optimal use of defecography when pelvic floor dysfunction (inappropriate contraction of the puborectalis muscle) and an enterocele or rectocele are suspected. *Scintigraphic evacuation* can be considered as an alternative of defecography; it uses artificial stools that contain a radioisotope.[75] This technique probably does not provide any additional information compared with defecography and lacks the capability to define the anorectal anatomy, but does quantify evacuation efficiency. More recently, the technique of dynamic magnetic resonance imaging (MRI) defecography has been introduced allowing rapid evaluation of pelvic floor disorders by visualizing all intrapelvic compartments in a single examination procedure. The technique involves dynamic visualization of rectal evacuation with fast-sequence MRI examination of the pelvis and may be advantageous in diagnosing complex, combined pelvic floor disorders such as rectal prolapse coexisting with an enterocele.[76] A disadvantage of MRI defecography is that patients perform the evaluation supine; however, there is evidence that the relative

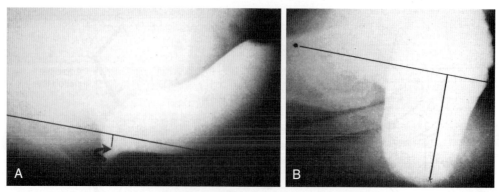

FIGURE 140-33 Defecating proctogram. **A,** Normal position of the rectum, anorectal angle, and anal canal. **B,** Gross perineal descent. (From Barthram CT, Makiev PHG: Radiology and the pelvic floor. In Henry MM, Swash M, editors: *Coloproctology and the pelvic floor: Pathophysiology and management.* London, 1985, Butterworth. Used with permission.)

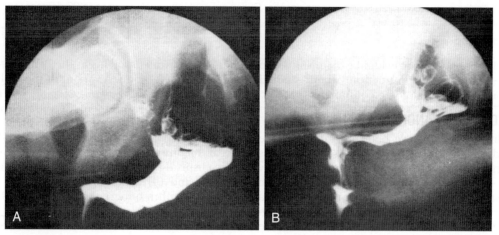

FIGURE 140-34 Series of defecating proctograms illustrating failure of the anorectal angle to widen in response to straining (anismus). (From Bartolo DCC: Pelvic floor disorders. In Schrock TR, editor: *Perspectives in colon and rectal surgery,* Vol. 1. St Louis, 1988, Quality Medical Publishing. Used with permission.)

dynamics of intrapelvic organs may be unaffected by changes in gravity.[77] With all measurements of defecography, clinical correlation is important as the techniques in general have been criticized as being oversensitive as diagnostic methods, detecting clinically irrelevant, minor defects.[78]

ELECTROMYOGRAPHY

This can be performed with needle or surface electrodes. It is operator dependent, causes patient discomfort, and carries a potential risk for infection. Although there remains a specific role for surface electromyography in the evaluation of sphincter function for pelvic floor–retraining techniques, this procedure has been largely replaced by endoanal ultrasonography.

ENDORECTAL ULTRASONOGRAPHY

Endorectal ultrasonography (EUS) has become increasingly important in the diagnostic assessment of the rectum. Although used on occasion to evaluate inflammatory bowel disease or recurrent cancer, EUS is mainly used to preoperatively stage primary rectal neoplasms.[79] It can help to assess the depth of the tumor (T stage) and the involvement of the perirectal lymph nodes (N

stage). Diagnostic information derived from EUS can be utilized to select local excision instead of formal surgical resection, or to plan for preoperative radiation or neoadjuvant treatment. Frequencies vary from 5.5 to 10 MHz, although most prefer a 7.0-MHz transducer.

A subdivision of the endosonographic anatomy of the rectal wall into five main layers is generally accepted. The depth of tumor penetration has been accordingly classified as uT_1 (ultrasound stage T1) for a tumor within the submucosa, uT_2 for a tumor invading the muscularis propria, uT_3 for invasion through the muscularis propria and into the perirectal fat, and uT_4 for invasion into an adjacent structure.

The accuracy of EUS for T staging reported in the last 15 years ranges between 84% and 95%, whereas the lymph node (N) staging accuracy ranges between 61% and 88%.[80,81] EUS-guided lymph node biopsy is also technically feasible in approximately 83% of patients and can improve diagnostic accuracy.[82] Errors in T staging are most frequently attributable to (1) angulation of the probe with respect to the tumor orientation, (2) prior radiation treatment, (3) large tumors protruding into the lumen, and (4) location of the tumor close to the anal canal or at one of the Houston valves. Overstaging

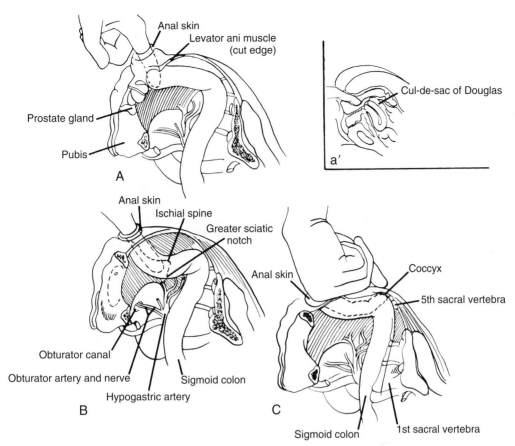

FIGURE 140-35 Relationships of the rectum palpable to the examining finger. Anteriorly, the prostate **(A)** and vagina and uterus **(a′)** are easily palpated. Laterally, the ischial spine, pelvic side wall, and levator plate **(B)** are palpable. Posteriorly, the coccyx and presacral space **(C)** can be palpated readily.

can result from inflammation and edema around the tumor, which typically occurs after biopsy. Understaging is simply an error. The N stage is determined by consideration of the size of the node, ratio between longitudinal and lateral diameters, echogenicity patterns, inhomogeneity, and regularity of lymph node contour. These are less than optimal criteria in case of microscopic tumor involvement and help to explain the lesser degree of accuracy in N compared with T staging. Despite this limitation, EUS remains the most accurate diagnostic modality, when compared to either MRI or CT, for both T and N stages.[83,84] Recently, high resolution MRI has been found to have vastly improved staging accuracy compared to standard MRI and may become an increasingly important modality for accurately determining the preoperative stage of rectal cancers.[85]

NERVE STIMULATION

The measurement of the PNTML has been successfully used to differentiate fecal incontinence caused by pudendal nerve injury versus sphincter injury. This test is carried out by placing electrodes inside the anal canal to measure conduction of the pudendal nerve when it reaches the pelvic rim. This study is controversial, but there is increasing evidence suggesting that PNTML can predict outcomes in patients undergoing sphincter repair for fecal incontinence.

DIGITAL EXAMINATION

The normal structures that can be palpated in digital examination per anus are shown in Figure 140-35. Essentially, they include the lining of the rectum and anal canal, extrarectal pelvic structures, the pelvic floor, and the anal sphincter. Normally palpable extrarectal structures include the bony confines of the pelvis, the uterus, and the prostate. Occasionally, the sigmoid colon or the ovary may be palpable. It is possible to digitally examine the rectum to a distance of about 12 cm from the anal verge in most patients. For a detailed discussion of the evaluation and management of constipation and fecal incontinence, see Chapters 141, 144, and 145.

REFERENCES

1. Goligher J: *Surgery of the anus, rectum and colon,* ed 5. London, 1984, Bailliere Tindall.
2. Heald RJ, Moran BJ: Embryology and anatomy of the rectum. *Semin Surg Oncol* 15:66, 1998.
3. ACPGBI. Guidelines for the management of colorectal cancer. 2007.
4. Lopez-Kostner F, Lavery IC, Hool GR, et al: Total mesorectal excision is not necessary for cancers of the upper rectum. *Surgery* 124:612; discussion 617, 1998.
5. Goldberg S, Gordon P, Nivatvongs S: *Essentials of anorectal surgery.* Philadelphia, 1980, Lippincott.
6. Hancock BD: The internal sphincter and anal fissure. *Br J Surg* 64:92, 1977.

7. Northover JM: The dissection in anterior resection for rectal cancer. *Int J Colorectal Dis* 4:134, 1989.

8. Steele RJ: Anterior resection with total mesorectal excision. *J R Coll Surg Edinb* 44:40, 1999.

9. Wood B: Anatomy of the anal sphinters and pelvic floor. In Henry M, Swash M, editors: *Coloproctology and the pelvic floor.* London, 1985, Butterworth. p 3.

10. Enker WE: Potency, cure, and local control in the operative treatment of rectal cancer. *Arch Surg* 127:1396; discussion 1402, 1992.

11. Crapp AR, Cuthbertson AM: William Waldeyer and the rectosacral fascia. *Surg Gynecol Obstet* 138:252, 1974.

12. Havenga K, DeRuiter MC, Enker WE, et al: Anatomical basis of autonomic nerve-preserving total mesorectal excision for rectal cancer. *Br J Surg* 83:384, 1996.

13. Fazio VW, Fletcher J, Montague D: Prospective study of the effect of resection of the rectum on male sexual function. *World J Surg* 4:149, 1980.

14. Nano M, Levi AC, Borghi F, et al: Observations on surgical anatomy for rectal cancer surgery. *Hepatogastroenterology* 45:717, 1998.

15. Quirke P, Steele R, Monson J, et al: Effect of the plane of surgery achieved on local recurrence in patients with operable rectal cancer: A prospective study using data from the MRC CR07 and NCIC-CTG CO16 randomised clinical trial. *Lancet* 373:821, 2009.

16. Lindsey I, Guy RJ, Warren BF, Mortensen NJ: Anatomy of Denonvilliers' fascia and pelvic nerves, impotence, and implications for the colorectal surgeon. *Br J Surg* 87:1288, 2000.

17. Hancock BD: Measurement of anal pressure and motility. *Gut* 17:645, 1976.

18. Milligan ETC, Morgan CN: Surgical anatomy of the anal canal: With special reference to anorectal fistulae. *Lancet* 2:1150, 1934.

19. Fenger C: The anal transitional zone. Location and extent. *Acta Pathol Microbiol Scand A* 87A:379, 1979.

20. Fenger C, Lyon H: Endocrine cells and melanin-containing cells in the anal canal epithelium. *Histochem J* 14:631, 1982.

21. Ambroze WL Jr, Pemberton JH, Dozois RR, et al: The histological pattern and pathological involvement of the anal transition zone in patients with ulcerative colitis. *Gastroenterology* 104:514, 1993.

22. Aldridge RT, Campbell PE: Ganglion cell distribution in the normal rectum and anal canal. A basis for the diagnosis of Hirschsprung's disease by anorectal biopsy. *J Pediatr Surg* 3:475, 1968.

23. Gordon P, Nivatvongs S: Surgical anatomy. In Nivatvongs S, Gordon P, editors: *Principles and practice of surgery for the colon, rectum and anus.* New York, 2007, Informa Healthcare.

24. Foster ME, Lancaster JB, Leaper DJ: Leakage of low rectal anastomosis. An anatomic explanation? *Dis Colon Rectum* 27:157, 1984.

25. Sato K, Sato T: The vascular and neuronal composition of the lateral ligament of the rectum and the rectosacral fascia. *Surg Radiol Anat* 13:17, 1991.

26. Thomson WH: The nature of haemorrhoids. *Br J Surg* 62:542, 1975.

27. Quer EA, Dahlin DC, Mayo CW: Retrograde intramural spread of carcinoma of the rectum and rectosigmoid: A microscopic study. *Surg Gynecol Obstet* 96:24, 1953.

28. Rutegard J, Sandzen B, Stenling R, et al: Lateral rectal ligaments contain important nerves. *Br J Surg* 84:1544, 1997.

29. Kellow JE, Gill RC, Wingate DL: Modulation of human upper gastrointestinal motility by rectal distension. *Gut* 28:864, 1987.

30. Kourambas J, Angus DG, Hosking P, et al: A histological study of Denonvilliers' fascia and its relationship to the neurovascular bundle. *Br J Urol* 82:408, 1998.

31. Duthie HL, Gairns FW: Sensory nerve-endings and sensation in the anal region of man. *Br J Surg* 47:585, 1960.

32. Beart RW Jr, Dozois RR, Wolff BG, et al: Mechanisms of rectal continence. Lessons from the ileoanal procedure. *Am J Surg* 149:31, 1985.

33. Ferrara A, Pemberton JH, Hanson RB: Preservation of continence after ileoanal anastomosis by the coordination of ileal pouch and anal canal motor activity. *Am J Surg* 163:83; discussion 88, 1992.

34. Lane RH, Parks AG: Function of the anal sphincters following colo-anal anastomosis. *Br J Surg* 64:596, 1977.

35. Sagar PM, Holdsworth PJ, Johnston D: Correlation between laboratory findings and clinical outcome after restorative proctocolectomy: Serial studies in 20 patients with end-to-end pouch-anal anastomosis. *Br J Surg* 78:67, 1991.

36. Goligher JC, Hughes ES: Sensibility of the rectum and colon. Its role in the mechanism of anal continence. *Lancet* 1:543, 1951.

37. Schuster M: Motor action of rectum and anal sphincters in continence and defecation. In American Society of Physiology: *Handbook of physiology. Section 6: Alimentary canal,* Vol. 4, Washington DC, 1968, p 2121.

38. Pemberton JH, Kelly KA: Achieving enteric continence: Principles and applications. *Mayo Clin Proc* 61:586, 1986.

39. Kerreman R: *Morphological and physiological aspects of anal canal continence and defecation.* Brussels, 1969, Arsica Ultgavin.

40. McHugh SM, Diamant NE: Anal canal pressure profile: A reappraisal as determined by rapid pullthrough technique. *Gut* 28:1234, 1987.

41. Taylor BM, Beart RW Jr, Phillips SF: Longitudinal and radial variations of pressure in the human anal sphincter. *Gastroenterology* 86:693, 1984.

42. Floyd WF, Walls EW: Electromyography of the sphincter ani externus in man. *J Physiol* 122:599, 1953.

43. Phillips SF, Edwards DA: Some aspects of anal continence and defaecation. *Gut* 6:396, 1965.

44. Barkel DC, Pemberton JH, Pezim ME, et al: Scintigraphic assessment of the anorectal angle in health and after ileal pouch-anal anastomosis. *Ann Surg* 208:42, 1988.

45. Varma KK, Stephens D: Neuromuscular reflexes of rectal continence. *Aust N Z J Surg* 41:263, 1972.

46. Finlay IG, Carter K, McLeod I: A comparison of intrarectal infusion of gas and mass on anorectal angle and anal canal pressure. *Br J Surg* 73:1025, 1986.

47. Rasmussen OO: Anorectal function. *Dis Colon Rectum* 37:386, 1994.

48. O'Connell PR, Pemberton JH, Kelly KA: Motor function of the ileal J pouch and its relation to clinical outcome after ileal pouch-anal anastomosis. *World J Surg* 11:735, 1987.

49. Parks AG: Royal Society of Medicine, Section of Proctology; Meeting 27 November 1974. President's Address. Anorectal incontinence. *Proc R Soc Med* 68:681, 1975.

50. Miller R, Bartolo DC, Cervero F, et al: Anorectal temperature sensation: A comparison of normal and incontinent patients. *Br J Surg* 74:511, 1987.

51. Scharli AF, Kiesewetter WB: Defecation and continence: Some new concepts. *Dis Colon Rectum* 13:81, 1970.

52. Kumar D, Waldron D, Williams NS, et al: Prolonged anorectal manometry and external anal sphincter electromyography in ambulant human subjects. *Dig Dis Sci* 35:641, 1990.

53. Bell AM, Pemberton JH, Hanson RB, et al: Variations in muscle tone of the human rectum: Recordings with an electromechanical barostat. *Am J Physiol* 260:G17, 1991.

54. Ferrara A, Pemberton JH, Levin KE, et al: Relationship between anal canal tone and rectal motor activity. *Dis Colon Rectum* 36:337, 1993.

55. Bannister JJ, Davison P, Timms JM, et al: Effect of stool size and consistency on defecation. *Gut* 28:1246, 1987.

56. Barnett JL, Hasler WL, Camilleri M: American Gastroenterological Association medical position statement on anorectal testing techniques. American Gastroenterological Association. *Gastroenterology* 116:732, 1999.

57. Engel AF, Kamm MA, Sultan AH, et al: Anterior anal sphincter repair in patients with obstetric trauma. *Br J Surg* 81:1231, 1994.

58. Londono-Schimmer EE, Garcia-Duperly R, Nicholls RJ, et al: Overlapping anal sphincter repair for faecal incontinence due to sphincter trauma: Five year follow-up functional results. *Int J Colorectal Dis* 9:110, 1994.

59. Swash M: Faecal incontinence. *BMJ* 307:636, 1993.

60. Swash M, Snooks S: Electromyography in pelvic floor disorders. In Henry M, Swash M, editors: *Coloproctology and the pelvic floor.* London, 1985, Butterworth. p 88.

61. Lubowski DZ, Swash M, Nicholls RJ, et al: Increase in pudendal nerve terminal motor latency with defaecation straining. *Br J Surg* 75:1095, 1988.

62. de la Portilla F, Rada R, Vega J, et al: Evaluation of the use of posterior tibial nerve stimulation for the treatment of fecal incontinence: Preliminary results of a prospective study. *Dis Colon Rectum* 52:1427, 2009.

63. Malaguti S, Spinelli M, Giardiello G, et al: Neurophysiological evidence may predict the outcome of sacral neuromodulation. *J Urol* 170:2323, 2003.

64. Peirce C, Healy CF, O'Herlihy C, et al: Reduced somatosensory cortical activation in experimental models of neuropathic fecal incontinence. *Dis Colon Rectum* 52:1417, 2009.

65. Drossman DA: *Rome III: The functional gastrointestinal disorders.* McLean, Va, 2000, Degnon Associates, p 382.

66. Bassotti G, Chiarioni G, Imbimbo BP, et al: Impaired colonic motor response to cholinergic stimulation in patients with severe chronic idiopathic (slow transit type) constipation. *Dig Dis Sci* 38:1040, 1993.

67. Dolk A, Broden G, Holmstrom B, et al: Slow transit chronic constipation (Arbuthnot Lane's disease). An immunohistochemical study of neuropeptide-containing nerves in resected specimens from the large bowel. *Int J Colorectal Dis* 5:181, 1990.

68. Krishnamurthy S, Schuffler MD, Rohrmann CA, et al: Severe idiopathic constipation is associated with a distinctive abnormality of the colonic myenteric plexus. *Gastroenterology* 88:26, 1985.

69. Preston DM, Lennard-Jones JE: Anismus in chronic constipation. *Dig Dis Sci* 30:413, 1985.

70. Jones PN, Lubowski DZ, Swash M, et al: Is paradoxical contraction of puborectalis muscle of functional importance? *Dis Colon Rectum* 30:667, 1987.

71. Miller R, Duthie GS, Bartolo DC, et al: Anismus in patients with normal and slow transit constipation. *Br J Surg* 78:690, 1991.

72. Roberts JP, Womack NR, Hallan RI, et al: Evidence from dynamic integrated proctography to redefine anismus. *Br J Surg* 79:1213, 1992.

73. Duthie GS, Bartolo DC: Anismus: The cause of constipation? Results of investigation and treatment. *World J Surg* 16:831, 1992.

74. Mahieu P, Pringot J, Bodart P: Defecography: I. Description of a new procedure and results in normal patients. *Gastrointest Radiol* 9:247, 1984.

75. O'Connell PR, Kelly KA, Brown ML: Scintigraphic assessment of neorectal motor function. *J Nucl Med* 27:460, 1986.

76. Rentsch M, Paetzel C, Lenhart M, et al: Dynamic magnetic resonance imaging defecography: A diagnostic alternative in the assessment of pelvic floor disorders in proctology. *Dis Colon Rectum* 44:999, 2001.

77. Lienemann A, Anthuber C, Baron A, et al: Dynamic MR colpocystorectography assessing pelvic-floor descent. *Eur Radiol* 7:1309, 1997.

78. Kelvin FM, Maglinte DD, Benson JT: Evacuation proctography (defecography): An aid to the investigation of pelvic floor disorders. *Obstet Gynecol* 83:307, 1994.

79. Orrom WJ, Wong WD, Rothenberger DA, et al: Endorectal ultrasound in the preoperative staging of rectal tumors. A learning experience. *Dis Colon Rectum* 33:654, 1990.

80. Kumar A, Scholefield JH: Endosonography of the anal canal and rectum. *World J Surg* 24:208, 2000.

81. Saclarides TJ: Endorectal ultrasound. *Surg Clin North Am* 78:237, 1998.

82. Gleeson FC, Clain JE, Papachristou GI, et al: Prospective assessment of EUS criteria for lymphadenopathy associated with rectal cancer. *Gastrointest Endosc* 69:896, 2009.

83. Bipat S, Glas AS, Slors FJ, et al: Rectal cancer: Local staging and assessment of lymph node involvement with endoluminal US, CT, and MR imaging—a meta-analysis. *Radiology* 232:773, 2004.

84. Harewood GC, Wiersema MJ, Nelson H, et al: A prospective, blinded assessment of the impact of preoperative staging on the management of rectal cancer. *Gastroenterology* 123:24, 2002.

85. Taylor FG, Quirke P, Heald RJ, et al: Preoperative high-resolution magnetic resonance imaging can identify good prognosis stage I, II and III rectal cancer best managed by surgery alone: Aprospective, multicenter, European study. *Ann Surg* 253:711, 2011.

Physiology of the Colon and Its Measurement

Adil E. Bharucha | Michael Camilleri

The human colon serves to absorb water and electrolytes, store intraluminal contents until elimination is socially convenient, and salvage nutrients after bacterial metabolism of carbohydrates that have not been absorbed in the small intestine. These functions are dependent on the colon's ability to control the distal progression of contents; in healthy adults, colonic transit normally requires several hours to almost 3 days for completion. There are differences in colonic structure and function even among mammals[1]; unless otherwise stated, this chapter will focus on the physiology of colonic function in humans. Although the colon is regarded as a single organ, there are regional differences between the right and left colon, indicated in Table 141-1. The right and left colon are derived from the embryologic midgut and hindgut, respectively and hind gut, and the junction is located just proximal to the splenic flexure.

ANATOMY

In adult cadavers, the colon is approximately 1.5 m long. The musculature in the colonic wall is composed of outer longitudinal and inner circular layers. From the cecum to the rectosigmoid junction, the longitudinal layer is organized in three thick bands, the taeniae, with a thin layer of longitudinal muscle in between these bands.[2] At the rectosigmoid junction, the three taeniae broaden to form a uniformly thick layer throughout the rectum. In the anal canal, the longitudinal muscle layer merges with the external anal sphincter while the circular muscle layer extends into the internal anal sphincter. Other than humans, only primates, horses, guinea pigs, and rabbits have taeniae coli[3]; the taeniae coli are thought to function as suspension cables on which the circular muscle arcs are suspended, facilitating efficient contraction of the circular muscle. Thus, a 17% contraction of circular muscle reduces the luminal diameter of the colon by two-thirds.[4] If the longitudinal muscles were arranged concentrically, an identical contraction of circular muscle would reduce luminal diameter by only one-third. Whether or not longitudinal and circular muscles contract synchronously during peristalsis is controversial.

The colon is suspended from the posterior abdominal wall by a mesentery. The mesentery is relatively narrow, restricting mobility of the cecum, ascending and descending colon. Around the transverse and sigmoid colon, the mesentery is broader, permitting considerable movement and contributing to the tendency in some individuals to have a pendulous transverse colon. This also partly contributes to the fluctuations associated with looping of the colonoscope during examination.

The colon is innervated by extrinsic and intrinsic nerves.[1] The extrinsic input includes sympathetic and parasympathetic components. In several species including primates, the vagus nerve innervates the proximal colon. The parasympathetic input to the distal colon is derived from the sacral (S2-4) segments of the spinal cord via the pelvic plexus. After entering the colon, these fibers form the ascending colonic nerves, traveling orad in the plane of the myenteric plexus to supply a variable portion of the left colon. The sympathetic fibers originate in the paravertebral "chain" ganglion, segments from the T12 to L4 levels of the spinal cord, and are conveyed to the colon via arterial arcades of the superior and inferior mesenteric vessels. The sympathetic nervous system provides excitatory input to the sphincters and a tonic inhibitory input to nonsphincteric muscle. Norepinephrine is the major neurotransmitter released by sympathetic nerves throughout the small and large intestine. The intrinsic or intramural nerves are organized into myenteric and submucous plexuses and the interstitial cells of Cajal (ICCs). The myenteric plexus and interstitial cells are primarily responsible for controlling motility; the submucous plexus regulates mucosal absorption. The extrinsic nerves modulate the intrinsic neural activity. For example, the sympathetic nervous system exerts a tonic inhibitory input on colonic motor function, primarily via stimulation of α_2-adrenergic receptors, which hyperpolarize cholinergic neurons in the myenteric plexus. Thus, the α_2-agonist clonidine decreases colonic tone, whereas the α_2-antagonist yohimbine increases colonic tone in humans[5]; clonidine also enhances mucosal absorption of fluid and salt.

FUNCTIONS

REGIONAL HETEROGENEITY IN COLONIC FUNCTION

Although the colon is regarded as a single organ, there are regional differences in normal motor function and mucosal absorption: the right colon functions primarily as a reservoir for mixing and storage processes, the left colon as a conduit, and the rectum and anal canal enable defecation and continence. The ileocolonic sphincter regulates the intermittent aborad transfer of ileal contents into the colon, mainly after meals. The rate of delivery of liquids into the proximal colon can influence colonic transit. Thus, a liquid marker injected directly into the proximal colon is emptied more rapidly than after oral ingestion of the same marker.[6] There is evidence for adaptation in these regional functions. Within 6 months after a right hemicolectomy, isotope movement

TABLE 141-1 Comparison of Right and Left Colon		
Feature	Right Colon	Left Colon
Embryologic origin	Midgut	Hindgut
Blood supply	Superior mesenteric vessels	Inferior mesenteric vessels
Extrinsic nerve supply		
Parasympathetic	Vagus	Pelvic nerves from sacral S2-4 segments
Sympathetic	Superior mesenteric ganglion	Inferior mesenteric ganglion
Function	Mixing and storage	Conduit

from the small to the large bowel normalizes in response to the augmented storage capacity in the residual transverse and descending colon.[7] In humans, the ileocolonic sphincter plays only a minor role in regulating ileocolonic transit.

COLONIC FLUID AND ELECTROLYTE TRANSPORT

Under basal conditions, the healthy colon receives approximately 1500 mL of chyme over 24 hours, absorbing all but 100 mL of fluid and 1 mEq of sodium and chloride, which are lost in the feces.[8] Colonic absorptive capacity can increase to 5 to 6 L and 800 to 1000 mEq of sodium and chloride daily when challenged by larger fluid loads entering the cecum, as long as there is a slow infusion rate, that is, 1 to 2 mL/min. In addition to the ascending and transverse colon, the rectosigmoid may also participate in this compensatory absorptive response.[9] For 25 years, secretory and absorptive processes were believed to be segregated to crypt and surface epithelial cells, respectively. It is now recognized that absorptive mechanisms are constitutively expressed in crypt epithelial cells; secretion is regulated by one or more neurohumoral agonists released from lamina propria cells, including myofibroblasts.[10]

When the colon is perfused with a plasma-like solution, water, sodium and chloride are absorbed while potassium and bicarbonate are secreted into the colon.[11] Absorption of sodium and secretion of bicarbonate in the colon are active processes occurring against an electrochemical gradient. There are several different active (transcellular) processes for absorbing sodium, and these show considerable segmental heterogeneity in the human colon. The regional differentiation of colonic mucosal absorption is also demonstrated by regional effects of glucocorticoids and mineralocorticoids on sodium and water fluxes. For example, in the *distal* colon, epithelial Na^+, K^+-ATPase is activated by mineralocorticoids.[12] On the other hand, the Na^+/H^+ exchange is activated in *proximal* colonic epithelium by the mineralocorticoid aldosterone.[13] Specific channels are involved in water transport across surfaces and epithelia. These water channels, or aquaporins (AQPs), are a diverse family of proteins, of which AQP8 is expressed preferen-

tially in colonic epithelium and small intestinal villus tip cells.

Potassium is absorbed and secreted by active processes; it is unclear if chloride is absorbed by an active process. In contrast to the small intestine, glucose and amino acids are not absorbed in the colon.

Colonic conservation of sodium is vital to fluid and electrolyte balance, particularly during dehydration, when it is enhanced by aldosterone.[14] Patients with ileostomies are susceptible to dehydration, particularly when placed on a low sodium diet or during an intercurrent illness. In addition to glucocorticoids and mineralocorticoids (aldosterone), other factors enhancing active sodium transport include somatostatin, α_2-adrenergic agents, and short-chain fatty acids (SCFAs). Clonidine mimics the effects of adrenergic innervation by stimulating α_2-receptors on colonocytes. In contrast, stimulation of mucosal muscarinic cholinergic receptors inhibits active NaCl absorption and stimulates active chloride secretion. Somatostatin, a peptide released by submucosal and myenteric nerves, also has potent antisecretory effects.

COLONIC METABOLISM

In the proximal colon, bacteria ferment organic carbohydrates to SCFAs, predominantly acetate, propionate, and butyrate.[15] There is a low, normal rate of SCFA production from "malabsorbed" (up to 10% of ingested) carbohydrates; diets high in fiber, beans, resistant starches, and complex carbohydrates increase the production of SCFA. SCFA are rapidly absorbed from the colon, augment sodium, chloride, and water absorption and constitute the preferred metabolic fuel for colonocytes. SCFA may also serve to regulate proliferation, differentiation, gene expression, immune function, and wound healing in the colon.

COLONIC MICROFLORA

The human intestinal tract contains a large variety of microorganisms, of which bacteria are the most dominant and diverse. This microbiome, which is composed of at least 10^{14} bacteria and dominated by anaerobic bacteria, is more than 100 times larger than the human genome.[16] Three bacterial divisions, the Firmicutes (gram-positive), Bacteroidetes (gram-negative), and Actinobacteria (gram-positive), dominate the adult human gut microbiota. Among other multifaceted effects, microflora can affect gastrointestinal motility by releasing bacterial substances or end products of bacterial fermentation (e.g., SCFA), affecting intestinal neuroendocrine factors, and by modulating immunity.[17] Our understanding of these effects is largely derived from germ-free animals. For example, germ-free rats have delayed gastric emptying and intestinal transit and megacecum; anaerobic organisms primarily mediate the effects of bacteria on gastrointestinal sensorimotor functions. Although small intestinal bacterial overgrowth is a recognized complication of intestinal motility disorders (e.g., intestinal pseudoobstruction, scleroderma, radiation enteropathy), more recently, it has been suggested that small intestinal bacterial overgrowth may also contribute to symptoms of irritable bowel syndrome (IBS).[18,19]

COLONIC MOTILITY

Assessment of Colonic Motor Function

Colonic Transit

Radiopaque Marker Methods. Since the original description by Hinton et al, there have been several refinements to the radiopaque marker technique for measuring colonic transit.[20] A widely used approach is to give a capsule containing 24 radiopaque markers on days 1, 2, and 3 and count remaining markers on a plain abdominal radiograph on days 4 and 7.[21] With this technique, a total of 68 or fewer markers remaining in the colon is normal, whereas more than 68 markers indicates slow transit (Figure 141-1).[21]

Scintigraphic Techniques. Colonic transit can also be assessed by scintigraphy (Figure 141-2).[20] To avoid dispersion of the radiolabel during passage through the gastrointestinal tract, the isotope is delivered into the colon by orocecal intubation or a delayed-release capsule. The delayed-release capsule contains activated charcoal or polystyrene pellets radiolabeled with ^{99m}Tc or ^{111}In and covered with a single coating of a pH-sensitive polymer, methacrylate. The capsule dissolves at a pH between 7.2 and 7.4, generally within the distal ileum, releasing the radioisotope within the ascending colon. The colonic distribution of radioisotope on scans taken 4, 24, and 48 hours after administration of the capsule is highly sensitive and specific for identifying rapid or slow colonic transit. The proportion of counts in each of four colonic regions of interest (i.e., ascending, transverse, descending, and rectosigmoid colon) and stool is multiplied by a specific weighting factor that ranges from 1 (for the ascending colon) to 5 (for stool), respectively. The aggregate of these products (proportion of counts × weighting factor), provides the geometric center of overall colonic transit. A low geometric center implies that most radiolabel is close to the cecum while a high geometric center implies that most radiolabel is close to stool.

pH-Pressure Capsule. Colonic transit can also be recorded by an ingested capsule that measures pH, pressure, and temperature as it traverses the gastrointestinal (GI) tract. The pH rises abruptly (by >2 units) when the capsule exits the stomach and drops rapidly (by >1 unit) when it crosses the ileocecal valve. In the largest studies to date, overall agreement between capsule and radiopaque markers for characterizing colonic transit was 87%.[22,23] Although the capsule can also assess gastric emptying and small intestinal transit, its sensitivity for detecting delayed gastric emptying (i.e., gastroparesis), as defined by gastric emptying measured by scintigraphy at 4 hours, is limited (i.e., 44%).[24]

In summary, allowing for differences in particle size, all three techniques probably provide comparable assessments of colonic transit. Scintigraphy and radiopaque

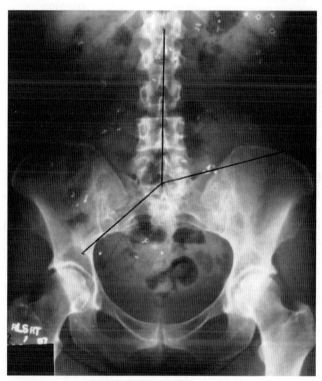

FIGURE 141-1 Abdominal radiograph demonstrating radiopaque markers and lines used to demarcate markers in the left, right, and sigmoid colon/rectum.

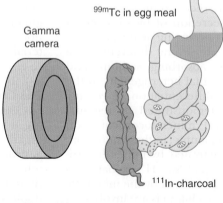

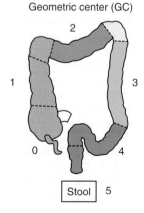

FIGURE 141-2 Scintigraphic assessment of gastrointestinal transit. **A,** Gastric emptying and small intestinal transit are assessed with ^{99m}Tc-labeled polystyrene pellets, whereas ^{111}In-labeled charcoal in delayed-release capsules measures colonic transit. **B,** Proportion of ^{111}In counts in each of four colonic regions of interest and stool is multiplied by the appropriate weighting factor, ranging from 1 to 5.

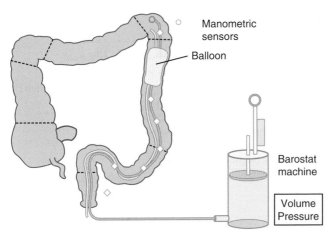

FIGURE 141-3 Barostat-manometric assembly positioned in the descending colon with polyethylene balloon in apposition with colonic mucosa.

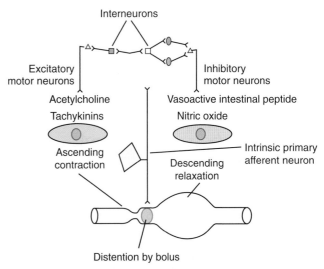

FIGURE 141-4 Schematic representation of major neurotransmitters mediating peristaltic reflex. Mechanical distention activates sensory neurons while interneurons transmit messages between sensory and motor neurons.

marker techniques entail similar total body radiation exposure, that is, 0.08 rad for the radioactive capsule and for each abdominal radiograph. Scintigraphy is a useful research tool that allows more thorough assessment of regional colonic functions.

Recording Techniques. Colonic motor activity can be assessed by recording electrical signals or variations in luminal pressure by pressure transducers, either water-perfused or solid-state, or a balloon controlled by a barostat.[25,26] There are several limitations to recording colonic motor activity in humans. Intraluminal colonic recording devices can only be positioned using flexible colonoscopy, per-oral, or per-nasal intubation techniques. Cleansing of the rectosigmoid and occasionally the entire colon is necessary to facilitate placement and accurate recording. Cleansing can accelerate colonic transit, but does not, with the exception of more frequent high-amplitude propagated contractions (HAPCs), fundamentally alter motor activity.[27]

Recording myoelectric activity with serosal, mucosal, or intraluminal electrodes is fraught with technical difficulties and has fallen out of favor. Currently, few centers use manometry to record colonic motor activity in clinical practice. Although manometry is reasonably reliable for identifying the colonic motor response to a meal (see Colonic Motor Function in Health, later) or to a stimulatory agent such as neostigmine or bisacodyl, intraluminal pressure changes may not necessarily reflect colonic contractions. Moreover, it can be challenging to assess propagation because of the distance, typically 10 cm, between manometric sensors. In contrast to manometry, barostat assessments by an infinitely compliant polyethylene balloon continuously apposed to the colonic mucosa can identify colonic contraction and relaxation (Figure 141-3). The barostat is a rigid piston within a cylinder that can adjust either the pressure or volume within the bag using a servomechanism. When the balloon is inflated to a low constant pressure, colonic contraction is accompanied by expulsion of air from the balloon into the barostat. Conversely, when the colon relaxes, the balloon volume increases to maintain a constant pressure. The advantages of the barostatic balloon over

manometry are greater sensitivity for recording contractions that do not occlude the lumen, particularly when the colonic diameter is greater than 5.6 cm.[28] Moreover, a barostat can record changes in baseline balloon volume and phasic fluctuations, colonic relaxation, and colonic pressure-volume relationships. Thus, the barostat is primarily a research tool that has been introduced into clinical practice in selected centers.

Peristalsis

Distention of a viscus evokes the peristaltic reflex, characterized by coordinated contraction of the orad segment and relaxation of the distal gut, facilitating propulsion. The neural pathways and neurotransmitters mediating this reflex are depicted in Figure 141-4. In the human colon, the principal excitatory neurotransmitter is acetylcholine, whereas in vitro studies suggest that nitric oxide and adenosine triphosphatase are inhibitory neurotransmitters in the human colon.

Cellular Basis for Motility. Contraction of smooth muscle results from interactions between smooth muscle, the ICCs, the intrinsic or enteric nervous system, and the extrinsic nervous system. ICCs are the pacemaker cells, responsible for generating slow wave activity that drives smooth muscle contraction. ICCs also amplify neuronal input, act as mechanotransducers, and regulate smooth muscle membrane potential. They are located in two networks, one in the myenteric plexus region and the other in the submucosa. They are also found interspersed in longitudinal and circular muscle layers (Figure 141-5). The three basic electrical events recorded from human colonic circular smooth muscle in vitro are[29] (1) slow wave activity with a frequency of 2 to 4 contractions/min, originating along the submucous plexus border of the circular muscle layer; (2) membrane potential oscillations (MPOs), with a frequency of about 18 contractions/min, originating in the myenteric plexus border of the circular muscle; and (3) action potentials superimposed on slow waves and MPOs.

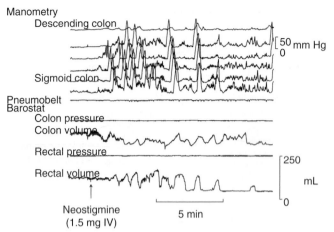

FIGURE 141-5 High-amplitude propagated contractions induced by neostigmine. (From Law NM, Bharucha AE, Undale AS, et al: Cholinergic stimulation enhances colonic motor activity, transit, and sensitivity in humans. *Am J Physiol Gastrointest Liver Physiol* 281:G1228, 2001.)

Slow waves and MPOs summate in the central region of circular muscle, producing a complex pattern of activity that regulates contractile amplitude and frequency. The predominant contractile rhythm recorded from the human colon in vitro and in vivo corresponds to the slow wave frequency of 2 to 4 per minute. Repolarization of membrane potential during slow waves results in opening of L-type calcium channels and, when a firing threshold is reached, action potentials. The result is Ca^{2+} influx through L-type Ca^{2+} channels initiating smooth muscle contraction. L-type Ca^{2+} channels are blocked by nifedipine. In the presence of nifedipine, smooth muscle contraction is inhibited and action potentials are absent. Tonic contractions are generated by continuous action potentials. In contrast to regular cyclical contractile activity in the stomach and small intestine, colonic motility is markedly irregular. This irregularity is partly attributable to the variable frequency and duration of action potentials, but is not well understood.

Colonic Motor Function in Health

In contrast to the canine colon, contractile activity in the human colon is not cyclical. Colonic motor activity may vary from no activity or quiescence, isolated contractions, bursts of contractions, or propagated contractions. Irregular phasic activity constitutes a major proportion of colonic motor activity and probably serves to segment and mix intraluminal contents. Combined assessments of motor activity and transit in the cleansed colon of healthy subjects reveal that transit is associated with nonpropagated and propagated contractions; propagated contractions propel contents over longer distances than nonpropagated contractions.[30] However, only one-third of propagated contractions are accompanied by propulsion of colonic contents. Propagated contractions are subclassified as low (5 to 40 mm Hg) or high amplitude (HAPCs, >75 mm Hg). In ambulatory, prolonged colonic manometry studies, HAPCs occur on an average of six times per day, originate predominantly in the cecum/ascending colon, and migrate over a variable distance.

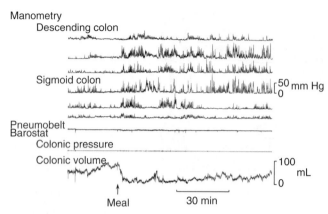

FIGURE 141-6 Colonic motor response to a 1000-kcal meal. Note the increased phasic pressure activity recorded by manometric sensors and reduction in barostat balloon volume maintained at constant pressure, indicating increased tone.

These HAPCs are probably responsible for mass movement of colonic contents. HAPCs occur more frequently after awakening and after meals and may account for the urge to defecate in healthy subjects and in patients with IBS (see Figure 141-5). The mechanisms that underlie HAPCs are poorly understood. In addition to occurring spontaneously, HAPCs can be induced by luminal distention, by the parenteral administration of the cholinesterase inhibitor neostigmine or by intraluminal stimuli, that is, glycerol, bisacodyl, and oleic acid.

Eating is accompanied by a brisk increase in tone and phasic activity throughout the colon (Figure 141-6).[31] Because this response is preserved even after a gastrectomy, the term "colonic motor response to eating" is preferred to "gastrocolonic reflex." The response may begin within a few seconds after eating and last, to a varying degree, for up to 2½ hours. A biphasic response with early (first 60 minutes) and late (120 and 150 minutes) components has also been described.[32] Meal composition and caloric content both influence the response. A mixed meal containing more than 500 kcal predictably elicits a response. Gastric distention and chemical stimulation by nutrients elicit comparable responses; lipids are the most potent stimuli, whereas amino acids appear to inhibit the response.[33]

The precise mechanisms mediating the response are uncertain, but neural and hormonal mechanisms have been implicated. It is conceivable that different mechanisms regulate the early and late components.[34] The early, particularly the immediate, component is likely to be neurally mediated. The later component temporally coincides with arrival of chyme into the ileum and may be mediated by humoral factors such as peptide YY, neuropeptide Y, and neurotensin released from the ileal mucosa. Although serum levels of gastrin and cholecystokinin rise after a meal, intravenous cholecystokinin actually induces colonic relaxation.[35] Atropine, naloxone, and the 5-hydroxytryptamine type 3 receptor (5-HT₃) antagonist ondansetron inhibit the response, indicating that cholinergic, opiate, and serotoninergic 5-HT₃ receptors may be involved in mediating the response.[36] There is also evidence to suggest that efferent vagal fibers contribute to the colonic motor response in primates.[37]

The colon relaxes during sleep, after intraluminal administration of SCFAs or glycerol, during balloon distention of the rectum, and in response to parenterally administered pharmacologic agents. In addition to the α_2-adrenergic agonist clonidine, morphine, and atropine; the 5-HT$_{1a}$ agonist buspirone[27]; and the 5-HT$_{1D}$ agonist sumatriptan all reduce colonic tone in humans.[38-40] Rectal distention by a balloon to subnoxious levels induces colonic relaxation in humans.[41] Colocolonic reflexes mediated via local nervous pathways through the prevertebral ganglia and independent of central nervous system activity have been well characterized in animal preparations.[42] This propensity for colonic relaxation, particularly that induced by sympathetic stimulation and opiates, may be relevant to the pathophysiology of acute colonic dilation or pseudoobstruction.[43] Colonic relaxation induced by rectal distention may explain left-sided colonic transit delays in patients with obstructed defecation because restoration of normal defecation tends to restore colonic motility to normal.[44]

There are regional and age-related differences in the biomechanical properties of the colon.[4] These biomechanical properties can be assessed by stress-strain relationships in vitro and by the pressure-volume relationships during balloon distention by a barostat in vivo. In ex vivo and in vivo studies, stiffness declines from the rectum to the transverse colon. These observations are probably relevant to the segmental heterogeneity in function depicted in Table 141-1 and to the pathophysiology of diverticulosis, as discussed later. Thus, the compliant ascending and transverse colon are ideally suited to function as a reservoir. Conversely, the descending and sigmoid colonic segments are suited to function as conduits, tend to have lower compliances, and are the primary sites of diverticula because intraluminal pressures are transmitted to weak points in the colonic wall.

DEFECATION

In health, rectal distention evokes the desire to defecate and reflex relaxation of the internal anal sphincter (Figure 141-7). If social circumstances are conducive, defecation is accomplished by adoption of a suitable posture and contraction of the diaphragm and abdominal muscles to raise intraabdominal pressure. Concomitant relaxation of the puborectalis and external anal sphincter, both striated muscles, enables widening of the anorectal angle by 15 degrees or more, reduction of pressure within the anal canal, and perineal descent. Appropriate coordination between abdominal contraction and pelvic floor relaxation is crucial to normal fecal expulsion. In addition, there is evidence to suggest that these somatic processes are integrated with visceral components such as colonic HAPCs during defecation.

COLONIC SENSATION

Healthy individuals, for the most part, do not perceive physiologic processes within the gut except for the sensation of fullness and the desire to defecate. Over the past few years, it has been proposed that symptoms associated with functional gastrointestinal disorders are partly related to enhanced sensory perception.[45] Visceral

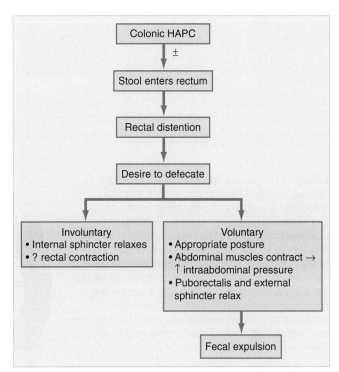

FIGURE 141-7 Schematic representation of events preceding defecation. *HAPC,* High-amplitude propagated contractions.

sensation is perceived in peripheral receptors and conveyed centrally by a three-neuron chain (Figure 141-8).[46] Although visceral afferents can respond to one or more stimulus modality (e.g., tension, temperature, osmolarity), mechanoreceptors are particularly important in the context of functional gastrointestinal diseases. Mucosal mechanoreceptors respond to mucosal pinching or stroking, whereas serosal mechanoreceptors respond to movement or strong distention of a viscus. Visceral perception is characterized by discriminative (localizing, precise) and affective motivational (diffuse, emotional) aspects, which are conveyed by discrete mechanisms, demonstrated in Table 141-2.

The predominant afferent fibers are rapidly conducting myelinated Aδ fibers and slowly conducting unmyelinated C fibers. The Aδ fibers convey the sensation of first pain, which is well localized and lasts as long as the stimulus. The C fibers convey the "second" pain, which is diffuse, lasts longer than the duration of the stimulus, and is associated with the affective-motivational aspects of pain. In the spinal cord, visceral afferents project centrally via spinothalamic, spinoreticular tracts and a nociceptive dorsal column. The spinothalamic tracts project to the medial and lateral thalamic nuclei, which are associated with affective-motivational and discriminative aspects of pain, respectively. These thalamic nuclei project to the cortical areas indicated in Table 141-2. Descending (chiefly serotonergic and adrenergic) pathways originating in the frontal cortex, hypothalamus, and brainstem reticular formation inhibit spinal cord dorsal horn neurons, thereby reducing pain perception.

In humans, colonic (and rectal) perception is assessed during balloon distention. The rate and pattern of balloon distention are important parameters. Perception

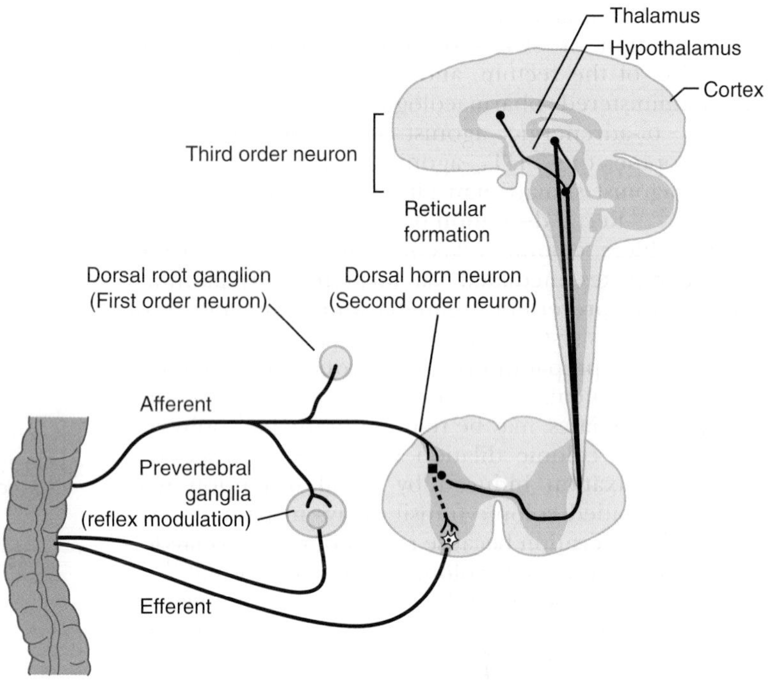

FIGURE 141-8 Visceral sensory pathways include reflexes mediated through prevertebral and other autonomic ganglia and a three-order neuron chain that ultimately projects to supraspinal centers. Convergence of visceral and somatic afferents at the dorsal horn explains referral of visceral discomfort to the body surface. Third-order neurons originating in the thalamus project to the cerebral cortex; those from the reticular formation project to the thalamus and hypothalamus. (From Camilleri M, Saslow SB, Bharucha AE: Gastrointestinal sensation: Mechanisms and relation to functional gastrointestinal disorders. *Gastroenterol Clin North Am* 25:247, 1996.)

TABLE 141-2 Visceral Afferent Pathways

Functions	Discriminative	Affective-Motivational
Afferent fibers	Rapidly conducting Aδ fibers	Unmyelinated C fibers
Thalamic nuclei	Lateral	Medial
Cortical area	Somatosensory cortex	Frontal, parietal, and limbic regions

is assessed by asking subjects to indicate when they perceive a given sensation, that is, first threshold, desire to defecate, or discomfort. To avoid bias resulting from gradually increasing stimuli, the distending stimuli can be randomized. The contractile response is more pronounced during fast than during slow distention. It is conceivable that this partly explains why rapid rectal distention is more likely than slow distention to be perceived in healthy subjects and to evoke visceral hypersensitivity in IBS.[47,48]

An alternative method involves asking patients to rate the intensity of perception during balloon distentions of standardized intensity delivered in random order.[49] Perceptual intensity is recorded on separate visual analogue scales for gas, desire to defecate, and discomfort. With this technique, subjective perceptual ratings are proportional to the intensity of the stimulus. Moreover, this technique is responsive to alterations in visceral perception induced by psychological stress and relaxation, by the α_2-agonist and antagonist clonidine and yohimbine, respectively, and by the cholinesterase inhibitor neostigmine.

In humans, balloon distention of the left colon evokes abdominal discomfort in the midline or left iliac fossa. The rectum is more sensitive than the colon and can distinguish between flatus and feces. Rectal distention induces rectal or sacral discomfort, akin to the desire to defecate or urgency. The anal canal is exquisitely sensitive, with sensitivity to touch, pain, and temperature comparable to the dorsum of the hand.

PERTURBATIONS OF COLONIC PHYSIOLOGY IN DISEASE STATES

The following are examples of illnesses that derange colonic physiology.

Constipation

Constipation may result from alterations of colonic transit and pelvic floor function; an algorithmic approach for the management of constipation includes tests of both physiologic processes (Figure 141-9). Colonic transit is frequently delayed in patients with obstructed defecation, which should be considered in all patients with delayed colonic transit. Patients with normal-transit constipation usually respond to dietary fiber supplementation[50]; those with slow-transit constipation frequently require judiciously administered laxatives, and pelvic floor retraining is necessary to reverse pelvic floor dysfunction in patients with obstructed defecation. Colonic motor assessments should be considered in patients with medically refractory chronic constipation, particularly when surgery (i.e., total colectomy with ileorectostomy) is considered. Intraluminal measurements are useful for confirming or excluding severe colonic motor dysfunction, manifest as a reduction in the number of colonic HAPCs and/or a reduced colonic motor response to eating.[51] In patients who have the most severe dysfunction, responses to a stimulant such as bisacodyl or neostigmine are also blunted (i.e., colonic inertia). The primary reason to consider colonic motility testing is that contrary to conventional concepts, which suggest that

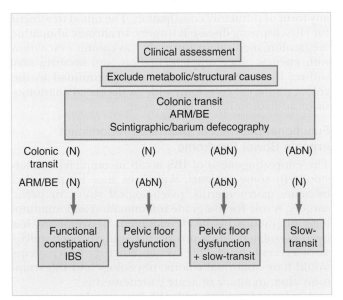

FIGURE 141-9 Diagnostic tests in management of constipated patients in clinical practice. Note that these simple tests permit categorization of patients and choice of therapy. *AbN,* Abnormal; *ARM,* anorectal manometry; *BE,* balloon expulsion; *IBS,* irritable bowel syndrome; *N,* normal.

colonic transit is a useful surrogate marker for colonic motor function, barostat assessments of colonic tone reveal reduced fasting colonic tone and/or postprandial colonic tonic responses in many patients with normal transit and normal motor responses in many patients with isolated slow-transit constipation.[52] Moreover, some patients with chronic constipation, particularly those with constipation-predominant IBS, have increased colonic motor activity, especially in the sigmoid colon.[52,53] Increased sigmoid colonic phasic pressure activity ("spastic colon") has been implicated to retard colonic transit in chronic constipation.[54,55] Detailed histopathologic studies with special stains reveal a marked loss of nerves and ICCs throughout the colon in slow-transit constipation and megacolon (Figure 141-10).[56] Rarely, constipation may be the presenting manifestation of a generalized gastrointestinal motility disorder resulting from a paraneoplastic syndrome (e.g., resulting from small cell carcinoma of the lung).[57]

Obstructed Defecation

Patients with obstructive defecation strain excessively to overcome the functional obstruction caused by inadequate relaxation of the external anal sphincter and/or puborectalis muscle sling.[58] The distinction between these two components, that is, puborectalis and external anal sphincter, is often blurred by the term *anismus* to describe pelvic floor dyssynergia. Symptoms that are suggestive, but not necessarily specific, of obstructed defecation include frequent straining, a sensation of incomplete evacuation, dyschezia, and digital evacuation of feces. The physical examination may reveal high resting anal sphincter tone, failure of puborectalis relaxation and/or perineal descent during simulated defecation, or anatomic abnormalities such as anal fissure or rectocele. The latter may occur alone or may be accompanied by pelvic

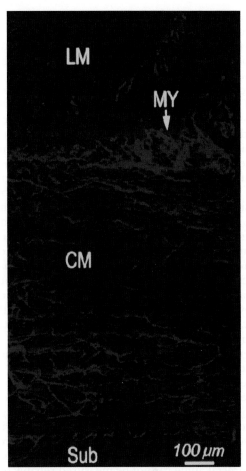

FIGURE 141-10 Distribution of interstitial cells of Cajal (ICCs) as demonstrated by c-Kit-positive immunoreactivity, shown in *red,* in the normal human sigmoid colon. Sections were cut parallel to the longitudinal muscle layer for both panels. *CM,* Circular muscle; *LM,* longitudinal muscle; *MY,* myenteric plexus region; *Sub,* submucosal border. (From He CL, Burgart L, Wang L, et al: Decreased interstitial cell of Cajal volume in patients with slow-transit constipation. *Gastroenterology* 118:14, 2000.)

BOX 141-1 Diagnostic Tests for Obstructed Defecation (During Simulated Defecation)

ANORECTAL MANOMETRY/ANAL SPHINCTER ELECTROMYOGRAPHY (EMG)
Failure of anal canal pressure/EMG activity to decline

BALLOON EXPULSION
Inability to expel rectal balloon within established norms for weight to facilitate expulsion

BARIUM/SCINTIGRAPHIC DEFECOGRAPHY
Increase in rectoanal angle by <15°
Perineal descent by <1 cm or >4 cm

floor laxity and organ prolapse (descending perineum syndrome). The clinical impression can be corroborated by objective assessments of pelvic floor function, beginning with anal manometry and a rectal balloon expulsion test (Box 141-1). With anal manometry or sphincter electromyography, paradoxical sphincter contraction or anismus can be observed in up to 20% of healthy subjects with no symptoms of obstructed defecation; this underscores the importance of considering clinical features in diagnosing obstructed defecation. The rectal balloon expulsion test, performed by measuring the time required to expel, or external traction required to facilitate expulsion of a rectal balloon filled with water or air, is a useful, highly sensitive (89%), and specific (84%) test for evacuation disorders.[59] The balloon expulsion test is a useful screening test but does not define the mechanism of disordered defecation nor does a normal balloon expulsion study always exclude a functional defecation disorder.[60] Anal manometry and an abnormal balloon expulsion test suffice to confirm the diagnosis of an evacuation disorder in most patients with typical symptoms and reduced perineal descent (i.e., <1 cm) at clinical examination. However, if the results of anal manometry and the rectal balloon expulsion test are discrepant, or conflict with the clinical impression, then evaluation of rectal and pelvic floor motion during attempted defecation by barium or magnetic resonance (MR) defecography, may be necessary to clarify the diagnosis. Defecography can detect structural abnormalities (rectocele, enterocele, rectal prolapse) and assess functional parameters (anorectal angle at rest and during straining, perineal descent, anal diameter, indentation of the puborectalis, in the posterior aspect of the rectoanal junction, degree of rectal emptying).[61,62] The diagnostic value of defecography has been questioned primarily because normal ranges for quantified measures are inadequately defined and because some parameters such as the anorectal angle cannot be measured reliably because of anatomic variations in rectal contour and location, for example, in the presence of perianal discomfort. Magnetic resonance imaging (MRI) is the only imaging modality that can visualize both anal sphincter anatomy and global pelvic floor motion (anterior, middle, and posterior compartments) in real time without radiation exposure. Dynamic MRI depicts the heterogeneity in functional defecation disorders and may be useful for clarifying the diagnosis in selected patients.[63,64] Patients with obstructed defecation may also have delayed left colonic transit, attributable to obstruction of luminal contents by retained stool, colonic motor dysfunction unrelated to obstructed defecation, rectocolonic inhibition, or decreased colonic motor response to a meal. The latter is reversible after biofeedback therapy.[44]

Acute Colonic Pseudoobstruction (Ogilvie Syndrome)

In *acute megacolon* (Ogilvie syndrome), colonic dilation is attributed to a sympathetically mediated reflex response to a number of serious medical or surgical conditions in elderly patients.[43] Cholinesterase inhibitors such as neostigmine enhance colonic contractility, reducing colonic distention in patients with acute colonic pseudoobstruction by increasing the availability of acetylcholine in the myenteric plexus and neuromuscular junction.[65]

Chronic Megacolon

Chronic megacolon may be congenital (due to Hirschsprung disease) or may represent the end stage of any form of refractory constipation. The initial treatment for Hirschsprung disease is surgery. In chronic idiopathic megacolon, medical measures such as colonic evacuation with enemas, fiber supplementation, and laxatives may suffice; if severe motor dysfunction is confined to the colon, a subtotal colectomy with an ileorectal anastomosis or an ileostomy may be necessary.

Functional Diarrhea or Diarrhea-Predominant Irritable Bowel Syndrome

The etiopathogenesis of IBS is still incompletely understood. In some patients, symptoms may be preceded by acute gastroenteritis, psychological stress, or pelvic surgery. A role for low-grade inflammation and immunologic alterations in the development of symptoms has been postulated.[66] In a prospective study, hypochondriasis or a recent stressful life event predicted which patients would have abnormal colonic physiology and IBS symptoms after an attack of acute gastroenteritis.[67]

A subset of patients with IBS have accelerated proximal colonic transit,[68] more frequent HAPCs,[69] and an exaggerated colonic motor response to eating. These result in postprandial abdominal discomfort and urgency to defecate in some patients with diarrhea-predominant IBS. Other studies have shown that approximately 50% of patients with diarrhea-predominant IBS have rectal hypersensitivity or project sensation to a wider cutaneous area during balloon distention. Although the significance of visceral hypersensitivity during balloon distention to symptoms in patients with IBS is unclear,[70] visceral hypersensitivity has been associated with abdominal pain and bloating.[71] However, rectal hypersensitivity does not accurately predict the response to therapy. Because bile acids can induce colonic secretion and propulsive contractions and increase epithelial permeability, bile acid malabsorption may contribute to diarrhea after cholecystectomy and in patients with idiopathic bile acid malabsorption.[72,73] Small intestinal bacterial overgrowth, as detected by breath hydrogen testing, has also been implicated as a cause for IBS. However, using a standard definition of bacterial overgrowth (i.e., ≥10^5 colonic organisms/mL in jejunal cultures), only 4% of IBS patients and asymptomatic controls had small intestinal bacterial overgrowth.[74] Of unclear significance, a higher proportion of IBS patients than controls (43% vs. 12%) had mildly increased bacterial counts (≥5×10^3/mL). Controlled studies suggest that a short course of antibiotics (e.g., rifaximin) may be beneficial in patients with IBS.[75] The therapeutic benefit was modest (e.g., 40.2% of the rifaximin group versus 30.3% of placebo reported adequate relief of bloating at 3 months after a 2-week course of treatment. However, the data have been replicated in two phase III randomized controlled studies.[76] Further studies evaluating the long-term risk-benefit ratio of repeating antibiotic therapy need to be evaluated.

Other Diarrheal Illnesses

In carcinoid syndrome, there is accelerated small intestinal transit and increased jejunal secretion. However, there is also evidence for altered colonic physiology. Increased delivery of contents to the colon is compounded by reduced capacitance in the ascending colon and an exaggerated colonic motor response to eating, causing rapid proximal colonic emptying.[77] 5-HT$_3$ antagonists, such as ondansetron and alosetron, reduce the colonic tonic response to eating and the rate of emptying, respectively, suggesting that 5-HT$_3$ receptors may partly mediate the motor dysfunction in these patients.[36]

Disturbances in motility and NaCl absorption have been described in patients with *ulcerative colitis*. Patients with active proctitis have a stiff, noncompliant rectum, which may explain the enhanced sensation of urgency prior to defecation.[78]

Diarrhea after *ileal resection* less than 100 cm is induced by the secretory effects of bile acids, associated with mild steatorrhea (<20 g/day) and responsive to cholestyramine (4 to 6 g/day).[79] After more extensive ileal resection (>100 cm) steatorrhea is severe (>20 g fat/day) and attributable to fat maldigestion and malabsorption secondary to low jejunal concentrations of bile acids. Cholestyramine will not ameliorate and may aggravate diarrhea in these patients.

Clonidine ameliorates the diarrhea related to *diabetic neuropathy* by restoring the α_2-mediated sympathetic "brake," that is, promoting intestinal and colonic absorption of NaCl and inhibiting motility.[80]

Diverticulosis

Considerations relevant to the pathophysiology of diverticulosis include the orientation of taeniae coli, the course taken by perforating arteries supplying the colonic wall, and changes in the biomechanical properties of the colon that accompany diverticulosis. Colonic diverticula are mucosal pouches that are pushed out between arcs of circular muscle at weak points, that is, where arteries pierce the muscularis propria in the spaces between the mesenteric taenia and the two antimesenteric taeniae. Thus diverticula do not occur where the taeniae fuse to form a longitudinal muscle layer surrounding the rectum.[81]

Thickening of the colonic circular and longitudinal muscle layers, partly because of elastin deposition with shortening of taeniae coli, may narrow the colonic lumen in diverticulosis. Recent studies also reveal colonic motor disturbances (i.e., more propulsive activity, more 2- to 3-cycle/min regular, phasic, nonpropagated activity), and heightened perception of colonic distention in patients with uncomplicated, symptomatic diverticulosis.[82] Thus, it is conceivable that increased motor activity, particularly rhythmic contractions, may lead to mucosal outpouching and formation of diverticula, particularly when the colon is less compliant and/or narrower, for example, in the sigmoid colon or in the presence of long-standing disorders of defecation. These motor disturbances may be partly attributable to cholinergic hypersensitivity.[83] It has been speculated that a low-residue diet with diminished fecal bulk predisposes to colonic luminal narrowing and ultimately diverticulosis. However, there is no direct evidence to corroborate a cause-and-effect relationship between lack of dietary fiber and luminal narrowing or elastin deposition in the taeniae coli.

IMPLICATIONS OF COLONIC PHYSIOLOGY FOR SURGICAL PRACTICE

These physiologic concepts have considerable implications on colorectal surgical practice. For example, it is crucial to treat pelvic floor dysfunction in patients with severe constipation before considering colectomy in those with delayed colonic transit. A colectomy with ileorectostomy is the preferred procedure for patients with intractable constipation and adequate anal sphincter function.[84] Assessment of gastric and small intestinal transit or motor activity may permit recognition of patients with generalized gut dysmotility disorders in whom long-term success rates after a colectomy for constipation are lower than in patients with selective colonic dysmotility. Left-sided colectomy may result in postoperative colonic transit delays in the unresected segment; this likely represents parasympathetic denervation, because ascending intramural fibers travel in retrograde manner from the pelvis to the ascending colon. The sigmoid colon and rectum are also supplied by descending fibers that run along the inferior mesenteric artery. These nerves may be disrupted during a low anterior resection, leaving a denervated segment that may be short or long depending on whether the dissection line includes the origin of the inferior mesenteric artery.[85] A long denervated segment is more likely to be associated with nonpropagated colonic pressure waves and delayed colonic transit than a short denervated segment. In addition to colonic denervation, a low anterior resection may also damage the anal sphincter and reduce rectal compliance[86]; in contrast to anal sphincter injury, rectal compliance may recover with time.[87] Physiologic assessments confirm clinical observations suggesting that colonic motor function recovers more rapidly after laparoscopic-assisted compared to open sigmoid colectomy.[88]

Surgeons should also be aware of the fluid absorptive capacity of the colon and its importance in fluid and electrolyte homeostasis. The retention of a segment of colon can make an enormous difference to the postoperative management of short bowel syndrome after massive resection for mesenteric vascular thrombosis or Crohn disease.

Motor disorders of the colon may be manifest with colonic dilation; not all dilation is secondary to obstruction and, in the presence of comorbidity or electrolyte imbalance, megacolon should be considered early, particularly because it can be treated medically or endoscopically without resorting to resection.

Finally, the colorectal surgeon, like the gastroenterologist, will encounter many patients in his or her practice in whom the diagnosis is functional diarrhea, constipation, or fecal retention. These patients deserve a compassionate, careful appraisal and advice on how to restore normal colonic physiology. Avoidance of unnecessary colonic or other surgery is the best course of management ... primum non nocere.

ACKNOWLEDGMENT

This study was supported in part by USPHS NIH Grants R01 HD41129 (AEB), R01 DK68055 (AEB), R01 DK 67071 (MC) from the National Institutes of Health.

REFERENCES

1. Christensen J: *Colonic motility.* Vol 1. Bethesda, 1989, American Physiological Society.
2. Fraser ID, Condon RE, Schulte WJ, et al: Longitudinal muscle of muscularis externa in human and nonhuman primate colon. *Arch Surg* 116:61, 1981.
3. Pace J: The anatomy of the haustra of the human colon. *Proc R Soc Med* 61:934, 1968.
4. Whiteway J, Morson BC: Pathology of the ageing—diverticular disease. *Clin Gastroenterol* 14:829, 1985.
5. Bharucha AE, Camilleri M, Zinsmeister AR, et al: Adrenergic modulation of human colonic motor and sensory function. *Am J Physiol* 273:G997, 1997.
6. Proano M, Camilleri M, Phillips SF, et al: Unprepared human colon does not discriminate between solids and liquids. *Am J Physiol* 260:G13, 1991.
7. Fich A, Steadman CJ, Phillips SF, et al: Ileocolonic transit does not change after right hemicolectomy. *Gastroenterology* 103:794, 1992.
8. Phillips SF, Giller J: The contribution of the colon to electrolyte and water conservation in man. *J Lab Clin Med* 81:733, 1973.
9. Hammer J, Phillips SF: Fluid loading of the human colon: Effects on segmental transit and stool composition. *Gastroenterology* 105:988, 1993.
10. Singh SK, Binder HJ, Boron WF, Geibel JP: Fluid absorption in isolated perfused colonic crypts [see comments]. *J Clin Invest* 96:2373, 1995.
11. Sandle GI: Salt and water absorption in the human colon: A modern appraisal. *Gut* 43:294, 1998.
12. Binder HJ, McGlone F, Sandle GI: Effects of corticosteroid hormones on the electrophysiology of rat distal colon: Implications for Na$^+$ and K$^+$ transport. *J Physiol* 410:425, 1989.
13. Cho JH, Musch MW, Bookstein CM, et al: Aldosterone stimulates intestinal Na$^+$ absorption in rats by increasing NHE3 expression of the proximal colon. *Am J Physiol* 274:C586, 1998.
14. Binder H, Sandle G: *Electrolyte transport in the mammalian colon,* Vol 2, ed 3. New York, 1994, Raven Press.
15. Cook SI, Sellin JH: Review article: Short chain fatty acids in health and disease. *Aliment Pharmacol Ther* 12:499, 1998.
16. Dethlefsen L, McFall-Ngai M, Relman DA: An ecological and evolutionary perspective on human-microbe mutualism and disease. *Nature* 449:811, 2007.
17. Barbara G, Stanghellini V, Brandi G, et al: Interactions between commensal bacteria and gut sensorimotor function in health and disease. *Am J Gastroenterol* 100:2560, 2005.
18. Pimentel M: An evidence-based treatment algorithm for IBS based on a bacterial/SIBO hypothesis: Part 2. *Am J Gastroenterol* 105:1227, 2010.
19. Pimentel M: Evaluating a bacterial hypothesis in IBS using a modification of Koch's postulates: Part 1. *Am J Gastroenterol* 105:718, 2010.
20. von der Ohe M, Camilleri M: Measurement of small bowel and colonic transit: Indications and methods. *Mayo Clin Proc* 67:1169, 1992.
21. Metcalf AM, Phillips SF, Zinsmeister AR, et al: Simplified assessment of segmental colonic transit. *Gastroenterology* 92:40, 1987.
22. Rao SS, Kuo B, McCallum RW, et al: Investigation of colonic and whole gut transit with wireless motility capsule and radioopaque markers in constipation. *Clin Gastroenterol Hepatol* 2009.
23. Camilleri M, Thorne NK, Ringel R, et al: Wireless pH-motility capsule for colonic transit: Prospective comparison with radiopaque markers in chronic constipation. *Neurogastroenterol Motil* 22:874, 2010.
24. Kuo B, McCallum RW, Koch KL, et al: Comparison of gastric emptying of a nondigestible capsule to a radio-labelled meal in healthy and gastroparetic subjects. *Alimentary Pharmacology & Therapeutics* 27:186, 2008.
25. Bassotti G, Iantorno G, Fiorella S, et al: Colonic motility in man: Features in normal subjects and in patients with chronic idiopathic constipation (Review). *Am J Gastroenterol* 94:1760, 1999.
26. Camilleri M, Ford M: Review article: Colonic sensorimotor physiology in health, and its alteration in constipation and diarrhoeal disorders (Review). *Aliment Pharmacol Ther* 12:287, 1998.
27. Lemann M, Flourie B, Picon L, et al: Motor activity recorded in the unprepared colon of healthy humans [see comments]. *Gut* 37:649, 1995.

28. von der Ohe M, Hanson R, Camilleri M: Comparison of simultaneous recordings of human colonic contractions by manometry and a barostat. *Neurogastroenterol Motil* 6:213, 1994.
29. Rae MG, Fleming N, McGregor DB, et al: Control of motility patterns in the human colonic circular muscle layer by pacemaker activity. *J Physiol* 510:309, 1998.
30. Cook I, Furukawa Y, Panagopoulos V, et al: Relationships between spatial patterns of colonic pressure and individual movements of content. *Am J Physiol* 278:G329, 2000.
31. Ford MJ, Camilleri M, Wiste JA, et al Differences in colonic tone and phasic response to a meal in the transverse and sigmoid human colon. *Gut* 37:264, 1995.
32. Narducci F, Bassotti G, Granata MT, et al: Colonic motility and gastric emptying in patients with irritable bowel syndrome. Effect of pretreatment with octylonium bromide. *Dig Dis Sci* 31:241, 1986.
33. Wiley J, Tatum D, Keinath R, et al Participation of gastric mechanoreceptors and intestinal chemoreceptors in the gastrocolonic response. *Gastroenterology* 94:1144, 1988.
34. Snape WJ Jr, Wright SH, Battle WM, et al: The gastrocolic response: Evidence for a neural mechanism. *Gastroenterology* 77:1235, 1979.
35. Coffin B, Fossati S, Flourie B, et al: Regional effects of cholecystokinin octapeptide on colonic phasic and tonic motility in healthy humans. *Am J Physiol* 276:G767, 1999.
36. von der Ohe MR, Camilleri M, Kvols LK: A 5HT3 antagonist corrects the postprandial colonic hypertonic response in carcinoid diarrhea. *Gastroenterology* 106:1184, 1994.
37. Dapoigny M, Cowles VE, Zhu YR, et al: Vagal influence on colonic motor activity in conscious nonhuman primates. *Am J Physiol* 262:G231, 1992.
38. Steadman CJ, Phillips SF, Camilleri M, et al: Control of muscle tone in the human colon. *Gut* 33:541, 1992.
39. Coulie B, Tack J, Gevers A, et al: Influence of the sumatriptan-induced colonic relaxation on the perception of colonic distention in man. *Gastroenterology* 112:A715, 1997.
40. Coulie B, Tack J, Vos R, Janssens J: Influence of the 5-HT1A agonist buspirone on rectal tone and the perception of rectal distention in man. *Gastroenterology* 114:G3046, 1998.
41. Law N-M, Bharucha A: Phasic rectal distention induces colonic relaxation in humans. *Gastroenterology* 114:G3233, 1998.
42. Kreulen DL, Szurszewski JH: Reflex pathways in the abdominal prevertebral ganglia: Evidence for a colo-colonic inhibitory reflex. *J Physiol* 295:21, 1979.
43. Phillips S: *Megacolon,* ed 1. New York, 1991, Raven Press.
44. Mollen RM, Salvioli B, Camilleri M, et al: The effects of biofeedback on rectal sensation and distal colonic motility in patients with disorders of rectal evacuation: Evidence of an inhibitory rectocolonic reflex in humans? *Am J Gastroenterol* 94:751, 1999.
45. Mertz H, Naliboff B, Munakata J, et al: Altered rectal perception is a biological marker of patients with irritable bowel syndrome [published erratum appears in Gastroenterology 1997 Sep;113(3):1054]. *Gastroenterology* 109:40, 1995.
46. Camilleri M, Saslow SB, Bharucha AE: Gastrointestinal sensation. Mechanisms and relation to functional gastrointestinal disorders. *Gastroenterol Clin North Am* 25:247, 1996.
47. Bharucha AE, Hubmayr RD, Ferber IJ, et al: Viscoelastic properties of the human colon. *Am J Physiol Gastrointest Liver Physiol* 281:G459, 2001.
48. Corsetti M, Cesana B, Bhoori S, et al: Rectal hypersensitivity to distention in patients with irritable bowel syndrome: Role of distention rate. *Clin Gastroenterol Hepatol* 2:49, 2004.
49. Ford MJ, Camilleri M, Zinsmeister AR, et al: Psychosensory modulation of colonic sensation in the human transverse and sigmoid colon. *Gastroenterology* 109:1772, 1995.
50. Voderholzer WA, Schatke W, Muhldorfer BE, et al: Clinical response to dietary fiber treatment of chronic constipation. *Am J Gastroenterol* 92:95, 1997.
51. O'Brien MD, Camilleri M, von der Ohe MR, et al: Motility and tone of the left colon in constipation: A role in clinical practice? *Am J Gastroenterol* 91:2532, 1996.
52. Ravi K, Bharucha AE, Camilleri M, et al: Phenotypic variation of colonic motor functions in chronic constipation. *Gastroenterology* 138:89, 2010.
53. Hasler WL, Saad RJ, Rao SS, et al: Heightened colon motor activity measured by a wireless capsule in patients with constipation: Relation to colon transit and IBS. *Am J Physiol Gastrointest Liver Physiol* 297:G1107, 2009.

54. Chaudhary NA, Truelove SC: Human colonic motility: A comparative study of normal subjects, patients with ulcerative colitis, and patients with the irritable colon syndrome I: Resting patterns of motility. *Gastroenterology* 40:1, 1961.

55. Connell AM: The motility of the pelvic colon. Part II: Paradoxical motility in diarrhea and constipation. *Gut* 3:342, 1962.

56. Lyford GL, He CL, Soffer E, et al: Pan-colonic decrease in interstitial cells of Cajal in patients with slow transit constipation [see comment]. *Gut* 51:496, 2002.

57. Jun S, Dimyan M, Jones KD, et al: Obstipation as a paraneoplastic presentation of small cell lung cancer: Case report and literature review. *Neurogastroenterol Motil* 17:16, 2005.

58. Bharucha AE: Obstructed defecation: Don't strain in vain [editorial comment]. *Am J Gastroenterol* 93:1019, 1998.

59. Minguez M, Herreros B, Sanchiz V, et al: Predictive value of the balloon expulsion test for excluding the diagnosis of pelvic floor dyssynergia in constipation. *Gastroenterology* 126:57, 2004.

60. Rao SS, Mudipalli RS, Stessman M, Zimmerman B: Investigation of the utility of colorectal function tests and Rome II criteria in dyssynergic defecation (anismus). *Neurogastroenterol Motil* 16:589, 2004.

61. Ekberg O, Mahiew PHG, Bartram CI, et al: Defecography: Dynamic radiological imaging in proctology. *Gastroenterol Internat* 3:93, 1990.

62. Shorvon PJ, McHugh S, Diamant NE, et al: Defecography in normal volunteers: Results and implications. *Gut* 30:1737, 1989.

63. Bharucha AE, Fletcher JG, Seide B, et al: Phenotypic variation in functional disorders of defecation. *Gastroenterology* 128:1199, 2005.

64. Karlbom U, Pahlman L, Nilsson S, et al: Relationships between defecographic findings, rectal emptying, and colonic transit time in constipated patients. *Gut* 36:907, 1995.

65. Ponec RJ, Saunders MD, Kimmey MB: Neostigmine for the treatment of acute colonic pseudo-obstruction [see comments]. *N Engl J Med* 341:137, 1999.

66. Ohman L, Simren M: Pathogenesis of IBS: Role of inflammation, immunity and neuroimmune interactions. *Nat Rev Gastroenterol Hepatol* 7:163, 2010.

67. Spiller RC: Postinfectious irritable bowel syndrome. *Gastroenterology* 124:1662, 2003.

68. Vassallo M, Camilleri M, Phillips SF, et al: Transit through the proximal colon influences stool weight in the irritable bowel syndrome. *Gastroenterology* 102:102, 1992.

69. McKee DP, Quigley EM: Intestinal motility in irritable bowel syndrome: Is IBS a motility disorder? Part 1. Definition of IBS and colonic motility. *Dig Dis Sci* 38:1761, 1993.

70. Whitehead WE, Palsson OS: Is rectal pain sensitivity a biological marker for irritable bowel syndrome? Psychological influences on pain perception. *Gastroenterology* 115:1263, 1998.

71. Posserud I, Syrous A, Lindstrom L, et al: Altered rectal perception in irritable bowel syndrome is associated with symptom severity. *Gastroenterology* 133:1113, 2007.

72. Odunsi-Shiyanbade ST, Camilleri M, McKinzie S, et al: Effects of chenodeoxycholate and a bile acid sequestrant, colesevelam, on intestinal transit and bowel function. *Clin Gastroenterol Hepatol* 8:159, 2010.

73. Wedlake L, A'Hern R, Russell D, et al: Systematic review: The prevalence of idiopathic bile acid malabsorption as diagnosed by SeHCAT scanning in patients with diarrhoea-predominant irritable bowel syndrome. *Aliment Pharmacol Ther* 30:707, 2009.

74. Posserud I, Stotzer P-O, Bjornsson ES, et al: Small intestinal bacterial overgrowth in patients with irritable bowel syndrome. *Gut* 56:802, 2007.

75. Pimentel M, Park S, Mirocha J, et al: The effect of a nonabsorbed oral antibiotic (rifaximin) on the symptoms of the irritable bowel syndrome: A randomized trial [Summary for patients in Ann Intern Med. 2006 Oct 17;145(8):I24; PMID: 17043334]. *Ann Intern Med* 145:557, 2006.

76. Pimentel M, Lembo A, Chey WD, et al: Rifaximin treatment for 2 weeks provides acute and sustained relief over 12 weeks of IBS symptoms in non-constipated irritable bowel syndrome: Results from 2 North American phase 3 trials (Target 1 and Target 2). *Gastroenterology* 138:S64, 2010.

77. von der Ohe MR, Camilleri M, Kvols LK, et al: Motor dysfunction of the small bowel and colon in patients with the carcinoid syndrome and diarrhea [published erratum appears in N Engl J Med 1993 Nov 18;329(21):1592]. *N Engl J Med* 329:1073, 1993.

78. Farthing MJ, Lennard-jones JE: Sensibility of the rectum to distension and the anorectal distension reflex in ulcerative colitis. *Gut* 19:64, 1978.

79. Hofmann AF, Poley JR: Role of bile acid malabsorption in pathogenesis of diarrhea and steatorrhea in patients with ileal resection. I: Response to cholestyramine or replacement of dietary long chain triglyceride by medium chain triglyceride. *Gastroenterology* 62:918, 1972.

80. Fedorak RN, Field M, Chang EB: Treatment of diabetic diarrhea with clonidine. *Ann Intern Med* 102:197, 1985.

81. Painter N, Truelove S, Ardran E, et al: Segmentation and the localisation of intraluminal pressures in the human colon with special reference to the pathogenesis of colonic diverticula. *Gastroenterology* 49:169, 1965.

82. Bassotti G, Battaglia E, De Roberto G, et al: Alteration in Colonic Motility and Relationship to Pain in Colonic Diverticulosis. *Clin Gastroenterol Hepatol.* 3:248, 2005.

83. Golder M, Burleigh DE, Belai A, et al: Smooth muscle cholinergic denervation hypersensitivity in diverticular disease [see comment]. *Lancet* 361:1945, 2003.

84. Nyam DC, Pemberton JH, Ilstrup DM, et al: Long-term results of surgery for chronic constipation [published erratum appears in Dis Colon Rectum 1997 May;40(5):529]. *Dis Colon Rectum* 40:273, 1997.

85. Koda K, Saito N, Seike K, et al: Denervation of the neorectum as a potential cause of defecatory disorder following low anterior resection for rectal cancer. *Diseases of the Colon & Rectum* 48:210, 2005.

86. Batignani G, Monaci I, Ficari F, Tonelli F: What affects continence after anterior resection of the rectum? *Dis Colon Rectum* 34:329, 1991.

87. Williamson ME, Lewis WG, Finan PJ, et al: Recovery of physiologic and clinical function after low anterior resection of the rectum for carcinoma: Myth or reality? *Dis Colon Rectum* 38:411, 1995.

88. Kasparek MS, Muller MH, Glatzle J, et al: Postoperative colonic motility in patients following laparoscopic-assisted and open sigmoid colectomy. *J Gastrointest Surg* 7:1073, 2003.

Diagnosis of Colon, Rectal, and Anal Disease

Julie K. Marosky Thacker

The appropriate treatment of diseases of the colon, rectum, and anus relies on a correct diagnosis. A correct diagnosis is built on three pillars: history, physical examination, and investigation. Taking a good, accurate, and targeted history; performing a careful and revealing physical examination; and choosing the right investigations require skill and acumen. Diagnostic skills are sometimes less valued with the plethora of imaging and investigative tests available. However, the thoughtful examination and the ability to employ only directed testing proves timely and cost-effective. We need to ask the right questions of our patients, to know what to look for on examination and how to look for it, and how to choose only tests that will make a difference. This chapter discusses the principles of diagnosis of colorectal and anal disease, and does so under the broad headings of history, examination, and investigation.

HISTORY

GENERAL PRINCIPLES

The history of a patient with colon, rectal, or anal disease can be the key to the diagnosis. When the patient describes symptoms, the likely site and nature of the problem direct the remainder of the history. Keeping an open mind is important though, as a patient may use diagnostic terminology in a lay application and misguide the investigation. For example, "hemorrhoids" could mean rectal prolapse, an abscess, or a fissure. Basic history-taking skills are important and are refined by a mental differential diagnosis that impels specific questions. The astute clinician should inquire about the patient's bowel habits, typical diet, and use of medications. Apart from the history of the presenting complaint, it is important to document comorbid diseases, medication use that includes over-the-counter drugs, drug allergies and intolerances, past operations, and family history of related diseases or colorectal cancer (CRC). Anal disorders in particular may be sexually transmitted and a sexual history is necessary. After a thorough interview, the differential diagnosis should be fairly well established. Examination and investigation can therefore be planned to confirm or exclude some of the possible diagnoses and to exclude other common complicating conditions.

SYMPTOMS

Bleeding

Rectal bleeding can be categorized as typical outlet bleeding, suspicious bleeding, or hemorrhage. *Outlet bleeding* is bright red, seen only on the toilet paper or in the water, and not associated with any risk factors for colorectal neoplasia (e.g., past history or family history for colorectal neoplasia). *Suspicious bleeding* includes dark blood, blood associated with mucus, blood on or in the stool, and blood associated with either a personal or familial risk or a change in bowel habits. *Hemorrhage* is an acute, large-volume blood loss; this is discussed in detail in Chapter 152.

Outlet bleeding is usually associated with an obvious anal cause. The history provides important clues. If the bleeding is associated with pain, suspect fissure, or excoriation. If it is painless, consider internal hemorrhoids or brim irritation. Suspicious rectal bleeding has a wider differential diagnosis than outlet bleeding. Internal hemorrhoids are still a likely cause, but rectal mucosal prolapse, occult full-thickness rectal procidentia, and even solitary rectal ulcer may present in this way. Constipation, difficult defecation, and rectal pain can be highly suggestive of one or all of these conditions.

Anorectal Pain, Itching, and Swelling

Anal pain is a common symptom in Western societies, because the modern Western diets' effect on bowel function places a strain on the anal canal. The pattern of the pain is usually highly suggestive of the cause. Burning pain after a bowel movement that lasts for 30 minutes to 2 hours, often accompanied by traces of blood, suggests an anal fissure. The pain can be quite severe and is sometimes traced to an episode of diarrhea or constipation. Alternatively, burning pain may be a result of perianal excoriation, which can also bleed if the perianal skin becomes ulcerated. A history of itching, mild incontinence, seepage, or an anastomosis that involves the anus suggests that excoriation may be present. A pressure-type pain associated with a tender lump could be either a thrombosed external hemorrhoid or a perianal abscess. Hemorrhoid pain is of sudden onset, usually occurring after an episode of difficult defecation. Acutely thrombosed hemorrhoids can be suspected when there is a history of a reduction in pain accompanied by bleeding independent of bowel motions. Abscess pain is more insidious, with slowly but relentlessly increasing severity.

Itching, or pruritus ani, has a wide differential diagnosis list. Clues in the history include the timing of the pruritus, its relationship to food and clothing, the use of specific soaps, and its response to topical medications. Patients who are obsessed with cleanliness are prone to damaging the perianal skin, as are those who are unable to keep their perianal skin clean. Frequent stooling, especially when the stool is liquid, is also a risk factor for pruritus. In the absence of specific causes, nonspecific pruritus can be diagnosed.

Nonpainful lumps include skin tags, fibrous anal polyps, or a large rectocele. Anal swellings that are reducible may be prolapsing internal hemorrhoids or full-thickness rectal prolapse.

A patient with rectal pain carries a complex differential diagnosis of poorly defined conditions. The interview needs to include questions regarding the pattern and nature of the pain. A constant, gradually worsening pain may indicate a tumor or an abscess; both should be palpable or visible on imaging or proctoscopy. A pressure-like pain that worsens on sitting is likely to be levator syndrome. Sharp, fleeting pains like electrical shocks are suggestive of proctalgia fugax. Constant anterior pain in a man may suggest prostatitis, whereas painful defecation in the absence of anal problems may imply a solitary rectal ulcer. Tenesmus is a type of rectal pain best described as a feeling of intense rectal contraction that is associated with rectal mucosal inflammation; it is typically associated with acute proctitis or a low-lying rectal tumor.

Abdominal Pain and Distention

Abdominal pain is a common symptom that has a vast differential diagnosis. This differential diagnosis can be considerably focused by analyzing the pain according to its timing, nature, pattern, site, and context. Sharp, steady pain is likely to be a result of some infectious process or a tumor, whereas colicky pain or intermittently crampy (pain that builds to a crescendo, then eases, and then builds again) is caused by either obstruction or spasm. When a constant pain is made worse by breathing or moving, infection, causing peritoneal irritation, is likely. Pain associated with diarrhea may be caused by colitis, irritable bowel, diverticulitis, or a stenosing tumor. When painful diarrhea is bloody, colitis is more likely. Pain associated with abdominal distention and reduction in bowel movements may be caused by a large bowel obstruction. Sudden-onset pain indicates an acute event (e.g., perforation, volvulus); gradually increasing pain is more likely caused by contained sepsis or tumor. Colonic pain may be felt anywhere in the abdomen, chest, back, or pelvis. Pain from an infectious process is generally felt near the site of the sepsis. Pain from spasm of the sigmoid colon is commonly felt in the lower abdomen. Patient age, gender, and past history guide the differential diagnosis of abdominal pain. For example, colon cancers are more common in elderly patients, and colitis is more typical in the young.

Abdominal distention may be a sign of colonic distention. If it is associated with pain, the distention is likely to be the result of a mechanical obstruction. If there is no pain, there may be a colonic ileus (i.e., pseudoobstruction). Distal small bowel obstruction may also produce considerable distention but is more often associated with nausea and vomiting.

Constipation

The word *constipation* has many definitions, and patients may imply different things by its use. Constipation may be used to describe small stools, hard stools, large stools, stools that are difficult to pass, stools that come infrequently, or stools that are incompletely passed. The range of normal stool frequency is three times per day to three times per week. There is no need to have a stool every day to be normal, but understanding what a patient considers normal or identifies as a change in bowel habits needs to be elicited by interview.

Small, hard stools are usually a result of lack of fiber. "Pebbles" may come from inside diverticula. Hard stools have been in the colon too long and have become inspissated. Infrequent stools may be caused by a lack of bulk in the diet or decreased colonic peristalsis because of one of a number of causes (see Chapter 145). A full history of medications and coexisting diseases may reveal the cause.

Serious constipation, with stools passed once a week or less often, is usually a result of either colonic inertia or rectal outlet obstruction. Patients with colonic inertia usually do not feel the urge to defecate. As time passes, they become more uncomfortable and distended. They may try to strain and pass stool, but this is usually unsuccessful. Often, these patients use laxatives to initiate bowel movements. Contrarily, with rectal outlet obstruction, stool reaches the rectum and is sensed but cannot be passed. Affected persons classically report difficult defecation as their main symptom, but they may experience abdominal cramps caused by colonic contractions. They commonly spend prolonged periods on the toilet straining to pass stool and often need to use their finger or some other instrument to push on the perineum or into the anus to help evacuate the stool. The most common causes of rectal outlet obstruction are a nonrelaxing puborectalis and rectal mucosal prolapse. Some patients may develop secondary colonic inertia after years of rectal outlet obstruction. In these cases, the history and the clinical presentation may be confusing.

A feeling of incomplete defecation may be the result of truly inefficient evacuation of stool. It may, however, be caused by a rectal tumor or redundant rectal mucosa as occurs in occult rectal prolapse. Incomplete defecation differs slightly from frequently repeated calls to stool. If a patient appears to completely evacuate but then is called to stool again soon, this suggests either stool stacking (fragmentation) or a rectocele. Stool stacking is common after a proctosigmoidectomy, which interrupts the normal defecation mechanism. The collection of stool in a rectocele can be sensed and is often associated with a feeling of perineal fullness or bulge. The use of a finger to splint the vagina or perineum to aid defecation is characteristic of persons with a symptomatic rectocele.

Diarrhea

Many causes of diarrhea exist; some are disorders of the small bowel, and others involve the large intestine. An analysis similar to that presented for abdominal pain may be helpful. Constant diarrhea is usually caused by an infectious or inflammatory process in either the small or large bowel. Endoscopy of the colon usually excludes a colonic cause or establishes the diagnosis. Postprandial diarrhea usually suggests some form of malabsorptive illness (e.g., celiac disease, lactose intolerance) but may also reflect short bowel syndrome. Intermittent diarrhea associated with abdominal cramps is a common variant of irritable bowel syndrome. Diarrhea with blood implies some variant of colitis such as infectious, ischemic, ulcerative, or Crohn disease. Sometimes blood associated with diarrhea is secondary to internal hemorrhoids or anal fissure/irritation. Diarrhea associated with abdominal pain may indicate ischemic colitis if it is of abrupt onset or an inflammatory colitis if it is chronic. The extent of disease in colitis can somewhat be predicted by the presence of diarrhea; generally patients with distal colitis or proctitis have formed stool, whereas pancolitis leads to diarrhea. A history of a trip abroad or the ingestion of questionable food raises the possibility of infectious diarrhea. The sensation of impending loss of control or the urgent need to use the lavatory is usually associated with rectal inflammation or strong muscular contractions characteristic of irritable bowel syndrome. Sometimes the well-meaning patient reports diarrhea when he or she actually has urgency.

Urgency and Incontinence

Urgency of stool is a sensation of impending defecation (see Chapters 144 to 146). It is associated with increased sensitivity of the rectal mucosa because of inflammation (e.g., proctitis) or an increased pressure of stool (e.g., irritable bowel syndrome). Intermittent urgency is more likely a result of irritable bowel syndrome, whereas constant urgency, especially in association with rectal bleeding, signifies proctitis.

Fecal incontinence, covered in Chapter 144, can be defined as an inability to defer passage of stool to a socially acceptable time and place. The history is crucial to making an initial diagnosis as to the cause of incontinence. A history of trauma or irradiation to the anal sphincter mechanism suggests sphincter damage. Classically, this is caused by obstetric trauma but may be secondary to surgical injury or other physical damage. Neurologic diseases may also contribute to or cause incontinence, whereas concomitant chronic bowel disease (e.g., inflammatory bowel disease, irritable bowel syndrome) is also important to document. *Urge incontinence,* defined as an inability to control the urge to defecate, implies external sphincter dysfunction, whereas the loss of control of stool unrelated to an urge (i.e., seepage) implicates the internal sphincter. Involuntary loss of stool without rectal sensation of fullness suggests fecal impaction with overflow of liquid waste.

EXAMINATION

GENERAL PRINCIPLES

Examination is primarily directed to the region of the body responsible for the presenting problem, but someone not seen in the past year should undergo a more generalized physical examination. Along with a general survey and recording of vital signs, this procedure typically includes an examination of the eyes, mouth and pharynx, thorax and lungs, heart, peripheral vascular system, gross neurologic function, and mental status. Patients examined for colorectal symptoms should have a digital rectal examination. An abdominal examination is required and is conducted with the patient supine. Particular attention to scars, deformities, distention, and

masses will detail this examination from the xiphoid to the pubis. Auscultation characterizes the quality of the bowel sounds and identifies any bruits. Percussion helps differentiate among distended bowel, ascites, and solid masses and identifies hepatomegaly or splenomegaly. Palpation of all four abdominal quadrants should identify abnormal masses that are evaluated for size, mobility, and pulsation. Last, the groins and all incisions should be palpated for hernias. Inguinal adenopathy may be very important in the evaluation of anorectal disorders and should always be interrogated.

Patients with a disease of the colon, rectum, or anus bear the burden of embarrassment in addition to concerns about their symptoms, likely diagnosis, and prognosis. A professional attitude, consideration to covering sensitive areas, and a minimal number of observers in the room are appreciated. A nurse should be present during the examination and ideally should be of the same gender as the patient. Gentleness in examination is paramount to minimizing discomfort, especially when performing anal examinations. Maximum information can be gleaned only if the patient is able to tolerate the examination and relax. Anoscopy allows visual evaluation of anal complaints, and proctosigmoidoscopy is similarly important if rectal symptoms predominate. Occasionally a vaginal or scrotal complaint will be interpreted as an anorectal problem. Being prepared to perform a genitourinary examination is essential.

POSITION

Most patients undergo anorectal examination in the prone jackknife or left lateral decubitus position (Figure 142-1). The former position provides the examiner with

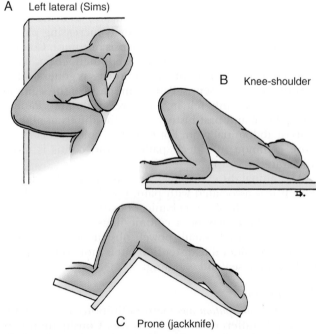

FIGURE 142-1 Positions of patient for anorectal examination. **A,** Left lateral (Sims) position. **B,** Knee-shoulder position. **C,** Prone (jackknife) position using proctoscopy table. (**A** to **C** from Hill GJ II: *Outpatient surgery,* ed 2. Philadelphia, 1980, Saunders.)

the greatest comfort, whereas the latter is easiest for the patient.

The prone jackknife position requires a special examination table that can be flexed to 90 degrees and tilted head-down. The patient kneels on a shallow ledge that is height adjusted to allow comfortable hip flexion and lowers his or her clothing and undergarments while shielded from direct view by a sheet held between the patient and examiner. The patient then lays his or her chest flat on the table, and the table is tilted to bring the anoperineum into clear vision after adjustment of the sheet. This position allows the rectum to fill with air while the liquid and solid luminal contents dependently settle into the rectosigmoid region.

If a specialized table is unavailable, colonoscopy is planned, or the patient is more easily positioned from prior abdominal examination, a left lateral decubitus position is recommended. With the patient covered with a sheet and lying in the left lateral decubitus (Sims) position, the hips and knees are flexed, and the patient's hips are positioned on the edge of the table. The head, knees, and feet are situated opposite the examiner, angling the patient's body across the table. The anoperineum is then undraped to allow isolated exposure of the examination area.

Lithotomy position allows for an excellent examination of the vagina, rectovaginal fascia, and perineal body. However, anal inspection in lithotomy can be more difficult than with the patient in prone or decubitus.

INSPECTION AND PALPATION

Examination of the perineum and anus must be systematic, incorporating both inspection and palpation, and the patient should be informed of all maneuvers before they occur to minimize anxiety, discomfort, and the potential for harm. The physician and assistant should position themselves on opposite sides of the patient and then gently separate the buttocks, with the examiner leaving his or her dominant hand free. The sacrococcygeal region is first surveyed to exclude pilonidal disease. The skin overlying the ischioanal fossae is then inspected for abnormalities that include excoriation, maceration, ulceration, drainage sites, lesions, and masses. The perianum is observed for external hemorrhoids, skin tags, scarring, and deformity. Last, retraction allows inspection of the anal verge and distal canal for a fissure, ulcer, and prolapsing anal papillae or internal hemorrhoids. If rectal procidentia is suspected, the patient is asked to perform the Valsalva maneuver while the examiner watches for prolapsing mucosa or rectal wall. The position of the anus and quality of the perineal body, including descent of these structures, should be consciously noted when a woman is inspected, especially when the presenting complaint is seepage, urgency, or incontinence.

Palpation of the perineum is performed next. This tactic may elicit tenderness and detect fluctuance or induration suggestive of an abscess. Fistula tracts can be felt as they course from an external os toward the anal canal. After palpation of the skin overlying the external sphincter, an anal wink is elicited by drawing a finger quickly across the sphincter while applying light

pressure. A well-lubricated finger is then gently and slowly inserted into the anal canal to assess sphincter tone. As the pad of the finger passes along the anoderm above the intersphincteric groove, the canal should feel smooth and nonulcerated. The examiner might encounter scarring or stricturing at this level; pain may preclude further examination except under anesthesia. The dentate line can be appreciated as the mucosa transitions into more irregular tissue. Hypertrophied anal papillae and masses can be best appreciated by slowly rotating the digit around the circumference of the canal. Internal hemorrhoids are rarely palpable unless they are hypertrophied due to chronic prolapse. Before the examination continues above the anorectal ring, the patient is asked to squeeze around the examining finger to assess external sphincter and puborectalis function. The thumb of the examining hand should be placed into the posterior vaginal fourchette to permit bidigital appreciation of an anterior anal sphincter defect. For patients who complain of nonspecific pelvic pain, the puborectalis and levators should be firmly palpated bilaterally and the coccyx bimanually manipulated, while the patient is asked whether the various maneuvers reproduce his or her presenting pain.

The distal rectum is examined last, beginning with palpation of the prostate or cervix through the anterior rectal wall; laxity of the rectal wall with significant anterior bulging is suggestive of a symptomatic rectocele. Bidigital examination of the rectovaginal septum often allows the identification of an enterocele that is palpable with straining. Like the anal canal, the rectum is circumferentially palpated to exclude tenderness, induration, polyps, and masses. The velvety soft texture of a large, sessile villous adenoma can be easily missed if the examiner is unaware of the subtle mucosal changes associated with these lesions. Any neoplasms that are encountered should be characterized according to size, position, and location relative to the anorectal ring to assist in planning the appropriate operative approach. In addition, palpation of the tumor for firmness, mobility, and ulceration that predict wall invasion and palpation of the posterior rectal wall for retrorectal lymph nodes that suggest local nodal metastases are pivotal for accurate clinical staging.

EXAMINATION OF SPECIFIC COMPLAINTS

Anorectal Pain and Swelling

Examination of the painful anus must be done gently, duly warning the patient of what can be expected. Typically, a patient with a fissure has a "shy" anus that resists distraction. However, the fissure, or its external component, usually can be seen with the use of gentle pressure to pull the anus slightly open. An acute fissure has no tags or rolled edges; these are signs of chronicity. If the principal complaint is that of mild pain or itching, specific causes of pruritus should be sought, such as infections, infestations, dermatitis, allergies, and mucus leakage caused by prolapsing hemorrhoids or rectal mucosa. Examination of the perianal skin may show minor excoriations that can be quite tender or the whitish appearance of lichenified skin that has been subjected to chronic wetness and irritation. Bowen disease may appear as asymmetrical patches of discolored skin, whereas a reddish hue is more suggestive of Paget disease and must be excluded by biopsy in any patient with unremitting pruritus and discolored perianal skin. Last, painful perianal ulcerations in the appropriate setting may be caused by herpes simplex infection, and a swab sample should be taken for culture.

A thrombosed external hemorrhoid is a swelling at the anal verge and may be small or involve nearly half of the anal circumference. A bluish tinge is usually visible as the clot shines through the skin. The skin over acutely thrombosed hemorrhoids is tight with edema and appears smooth. As days pass, the edema tends to disappear and the skin starts to wrinkle, whereas the clot occasionally erodes through the skin. An abscess is typically visible as a localized swelling in the perianal or ischioanal area. Fluctuance, erythema, tenderness, and sporadic skin discoloration may or may not be present because the deeper the sepsis, the less obvious are the signs. For instance, a deep postanal space abscess classically presents with pain and toxicity but a normal-appearing anal area. Examination under anesthesia and needle aspiration of the postanal or perianal space is the best method of diagnosis.

Although a painful perianal lump is usually a thrombosed external hemorrhoid or an abscess, nonpainful lumps may include skin tags, fibrous anal polyps, or a large rectocele. Anal swellings that are reducible may be prolapsing internal hemorrhoids or full-thickness rectal prolapse. Perianal condylomata are usually obvious, but anoscopy is necessary to exclude intraanal condylomata or prominent hemorrhoids.

Rectal pain can be poorly defined and difficult to treat. Again, taking a detailed history leads the direction of the necessary examination. Tumors and abscesses causing constant or gradually worsening pain should be palpable or visible on proctoscopy or imaging. Digital rectal examination may reveal an asymmetrically tender levator muscle in levator syndrome. The prostate is usually tender on digital rectal examination when prostatitis is causing constant anterior rectal pain. Although a digital examination is limited to the length of the examining finger, it is usually adequate to diagnose or exclude a mass lesion or sepsis in or around the lower rectum. Regardless, when a patient who complains of anal or rectal pain cannot be adequately examined or when the examination reveals no abnormalities, examination under anesthesia is warranted.

Bleeding

Perineal excoriation, anal fissure, internal hemorrhoids, or a low-lying neoplasm can cause outlet rectal bleeding. Excoriation and fissures can be identified through simple inspection of the perineal skin and anal verge. Inspection of the perianum may reveal grade III or IV internal hemorrhoids, especially if the hemorrhoids remain prolapsed after an enema. Although they are occasionally associated with external skin tags, internal hemorrhoids are rarely palpable unless they are hypertrophied because of chronic prolapse. Instead, symptomatic internal hemorrhoids are best diagnosed with anoscopy and appear as bulging mucosal cushions, often with prominent veins or

arteries that tend to lie anteriorly and posterolaterally on both sides of the anal canal. Chronically prolapsing internal hemorrhoids develop a whitish-gray lining termed *pseudoepitheliomatous hyperplasia.*

Suspicious rectal bleeding has a wider differential diagnosis than outlet bleeding. Internal hemorrhoids are still a likely cause, so anoscopy is important. Rectal mucosal prolapse, occult full-thickness rectal procidentia, and even solitary rectal ulcer may present in this way. Proctoscopy may show erythematous, redundant rectal folds that descend into the anus with a Valsalva maneuver. Suspicious bleeding may also herald neoplasia, and evaluation of the proximal colon is required. It is always important to recall that rectal bleeding is never normal and invariably requires further investigation because it should never be assumed that the cause is "merely" hemorrhoids.

Urgency and Incontinence

Examination of the anus and rectum confirms the diagnosis suggested by the history. The sensation of the perianal skin and the wink reflex of the corrugator cutis ani muscle can be tested with a light touch. This simple maneuver provides useful information about the innervation of the external sphincter. Perianal scarring suggests previous trauma, and a sphincter defect is usually visible or palpable. The thickness of the perineum in women provides a clue to sphincter bulk. A thorough clinical evaluation of the incontinent patient is discussed in Chapter 144.

Constipation

Once the diagnosis of an outlet obstruction is suspected on the basis of the history, examination can often suggest which of the common causes contributes. The ability of the puborectalis to relax while bearing down can be assessed during a digital examination. At the same time, laxity of the rectal mucosa or tendency of the rectal wall to prolapse can be noted. Similarly, a digital examination can exclude an anal stricture or a rectocele. If a rectocele is present, it will be noted as an anterior defect in the rectal wall, bulging into the perineum. Rectoceles are often asymptomatic; the mere presence of a rectocele does not mandate treatment.

Examination of the anus may reveal a rectocele in women, or a megarectum may be identified. Careful inspection can expose prolapse of the rectal mucosa during a Valsalva maneuver, or, occasionally, the pelvic floor fails to relax when the patient bears down.

INVESTIGATION

BLOOD AND STOOL TESTING

Routine blood and stool tests are helpful in the evaluation of some disorders of the large bowel and anus. Occasional abnormalities in blood levels directly cause a malady; some are signs that are associated with the disease that causes symptoms and others are the result of the disorder itself. For instance, serum electrolyte abnormalities can affect bowel frequency with few other systemic manifestations. Alternately, altered thyroid-stimulating hormone levels may identify the cause of intestinal symptoms related to thyroid dysfunction. Contrarily, a bleeding colorectal neoplasm may be the cause of a microcytic, hypochromic anemia. Infectious and neoplastic abnormalities of the colon and rectum are also investigated by stool and blood studies.

Stool tests for ova, parasites, and other pathogens may diagnose infectious colitides. Examples of common pathogens include *Giardia* and *Clostridium.* Giardiasis, acquired from contaminated water, is more likely found in the younger outpatient population. *Clostridium difficile* colitis, however, has a particularly high prevalence in the older, institutionalized, or hospitalized population; the stool of any patient with colitis after antibiotic use should be tested for the *C. difficile* antigen. An evaluation of new-onset diarrhea will also include fecal leukocytes, a stool culture, and tests specific for *Shigella* and *Salmonella.*

Stool assays are used to screen for large bowel neoplasms. Although the fecal occult blood test (FOBT) is a CRC screening tool that has been shown to reduce CRC mortality, it is a relatively insensitive and nonspecific marker. Compared to colonoscopy, FOBT detected only 66% of CRC. Even less sensitive to adenoma, FOBT detected only 20% of advanced adenomas. Stool studies are also significantly less sensitive at detecting right-sided lesions than at detecting left-sided lesions.[1] New stool assay panels of selected DNA alterations (i.e., K-*ras, p53, APC,* BAT-26, "long" DNA) are feasible potential screening tools and are endorsed as such by the American Cancer Society, the U.S. Multi-Society Task Force, and the American College of Gastroenterology.[2] However, fecal immunochemical testing, and fecal DNA assays are not considered vigorously enough studied to be promoted by the U.S. Preventive Services Task Force.[3]

Serum and urine tests are also used in the evaluation of CRC. Selected DNA alterations (i.e., K-*ras, p53, APC,* BAT-26, and "long" DNA) are sloughed with colonocyte turnover. Multitargeted DNA-based stool testing for these alterations is four times more sensitive than guaiac tests (52% compared to 13%) and just as specific at screening for invasive CRC.[4] As of this writing, none has been accepted as a screening tool,[2] although several are being studied.[5,6] For newly diagnosed and recurrent adenocarcinoma of the colon or rectum, serum carcinoembryonic antigen (CEA), a glycoprotein found in the cell membrane of CRCs, is the CRC tumor marker most often used. CEA enters the circulation and can be detected by radioimmunoassay in some patients with CRC. In a review of studies using CEA, Hundt et al describe a sensitivity of 43% to 69% for detection of CRC using CEA; sensitivity, however, was clearly higher in patients with higher stage cancer.[7] Comparative preoperative and postoperative CEA levels help in detection of postoperative disease recrudescence and recurrence.

Although colonoscopy, discussed in Colonoscopy, later, is considered the gold standard for CRC screening, several less invasive screening modalities exist. A common test is guaiac-based FOBT. Despite onerous dietary restrictions and collection processes, FOBT has been used widely for more than 30 years. The low cost of FOBT does not compensate for the spot-test low sensitivity, low specificity, and inconvenience, but FOBT is the only noninvasive screening test shown, as of this writing, to decrease mortality from CRC. Sensitivity of FOBT is slightly higher with serial examinations; however, newer stool studies, applying innovative DNA testing, promise to greatly improve noninvasive CRC screening. The future of cancer diagnostics will be molecular biomarkers. Although no such tests have been proven to be sensitive enough, specific enough, or cost-effective as of this writing, their development branches from the ongoing biomarker studies and are well reviewed by Søreide et al.[8]

Blood testing for gene abnormalities is used to define particular forms of inherited CRC, such as familial adenomatous polyposis (FAP) and hereditary nonpolyposis colorectal cancer (HNPCC). Although a specific adenomatous polyposis coli *(APC)* gene mutation is identified in approximately 80% of FAP families, the mismatch repair germline mutation is demonstrated only in approximately 50% of families meeting HNPCC criteria.[9] Because of heterogeneity of the mutations of mismatch genes, tests for the disease-causing mutation is first sought in a family member clinically known to have the disease. Once a mutation is found in the index case, other family members can be tested with approximately 100% accuracy, as all affected family members would have the same mutation. A negative result on genetic testing only rules out FAP or HNPCC if an affected family member has an identified mutation. Lynch et al offer an approach to the management of hereditary colorectal cancer using Lynch syndrome as a model.[9]

ENDOSCOPY

Evaluation of the distal gastrointestinal tract is possible by different modes of endoscopy. Depending on the patient complaint and clinical setting, the practitioner may choose anoscopy, rigid proctoscopy, flexible proctosigmoidoscopy, or full colonoscopy. Cappell and Friedel offer a comprehensive discussion of the role and findings of endoscopy; the following sections cover the general indications and techniques of endoscopy.[10]

Anoscopy

Inspection of the anal canal is best performed with an anoscope. Various types of anoscopes are manufactured but are described on the basis of size and whether they are disposable, lighted, and bivalved, slotted, or beveled (Figure 142-2). Regardless of the type of instrument that is used, digital examination should always precede insertion of the anoscope. Telling the patient each step of the planned procedure, the examiner gently applies the well-lubricated anoscope against the anus. Constant gradual pressure allows the scope to pass into the canal. If resistance is encountered because of increased sphincter tone, the patient is asked to strain. This will involuntarily relax the sphincter and allow passage of the anoscope. Continued difficulties are suggestive of anal stenosis, mandating the use of a smaller-caliber anoscope, or of anal pathology that necessitates examination under anesthesia. Once the anoscope is appropriately inserted, it is used to circumferentially inspect the anal canal and distalmost rectum. The scope is partially withdrawn in each quadrant to allow visualization of all mucosa.

Rigid Proctosigmoidoscopy

Historically, rigid proctosigmoidoscopy was used for routine visualization of the rectum and distal sigmoid colon. Rigid endoscopy remains the procedure of choice for evaluation and treatment of distal rectal lesions. In addition to allowing visualization without advanced equipment, rigid proctoscopy provides a much more accurate localization of rectal pathology compared to flexible endoscopy. Patients with rectal tumors at the University of California at Los Angeles were studied from 2001 to 2006, comparing localization of disease between rigid and flexible endoscopy. Twenty-five percent of patients had a therapy algorithm change based on the results of rigid proctoscopy compared to flexible. Interestingly, flexible endoscopy underestimates the distance between the anus and distal tumors, but tends to overestimate the distance between the anus and middle or upper rectal lesions.[11]

The rigid instruments are 25 cm long and have a diameter of 11, 15, or 19 mm (Figure 142-3). The smaller instruments are used in patients with strictures, whereas the larger proctosigmoidoscopes enable the evacuation

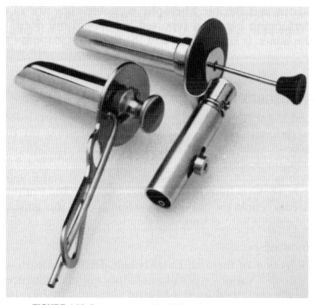

FIGURE 142-2 Large modified Hirschman anoscopes.

of stool or blood and the treatment of larger polyps. The scope is inserted after anoscopy has been completed and is passed similarly to the anoscope. After the rigid proctosigmoidoscope has passed through the sphincters while typically directed toward the umbilicus, the obturator is removed, and the scope is advanced under direct visualization. Luminal contents that obscure adequate inspection are aspirated or swabbed as the examination progresses, but close mucosal examination is best performed during scope withdrawal. If stool obscures significant segments of mucosa, the procedure is halted until an enema is delivered to clear the lower bowel.

Although the direction of rigid proctosigmoidoscope passage must be individualized, the general route is directed posteriorly along the sacral hollow, around the inferior (left posterior), middle (right anterior), and upper (left posterior) valves of Houston. The rectosigmoid junction will come into view after the proctosigmoidoscope has been inserted 17 to 19 cm. At this point, further insertion will cause many patients to experience crampy visceral pain that resolves with instrument withdrawal. The angulated rectosigmoid may appear as a blinded end to the rectum with no visible rectum. Gentle manipulation to the left and then to the right will often open the sigmoid lumen to inspection. Moderate air insufflation facilitates the procedure, but excessive use is painful and interferes with the examination. Examination is performed during withdrawal while sweeping the scope around to allow careful inspection of all mucosal surfaces, flattening the rectal valves to survey their cephalad components.

Biopsy samples are obtained posteriorly along the folds of the valves if possible to minimize the risk of perforation. Small lesions can be fulgurated, and larger polyps can be excised with a snare. Anterior biopsies above the middle rectal valve are especially prone to intraperitoneal perforation because this area is situated above the peritoneal reflection; perforation complicates 0.005% to 0.01% of rigid procedures.[12] Perforation by the tip of the scope occurs at areas of angulation, bowel wall weakness, and intestinal fixation. Bleeding after biopsy with the larger forceps or snare rarely occurs and usually spontaneously ceases. In the event that hemorrhage persists, a small artery is usually implicated, but it can be controlled by a combination of pressure and coagulation.

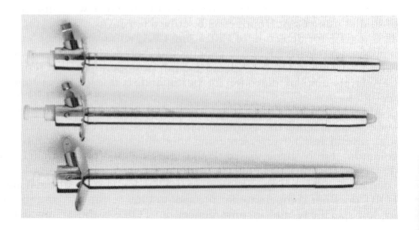

FIGURE 142-3 Large-, medium-, and small-diameter Welch-Allyn rigid sigmoidoscopes.

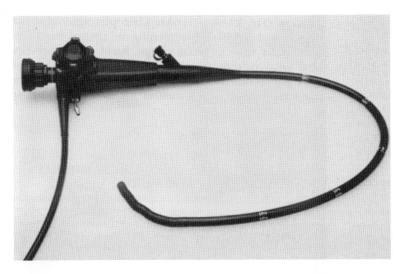

FIGURE 142-4 Pentax 65-cm flexible fiberoptic sigmoidoscope.

Flexible Proctosigmoidoscopy

In many units, flexible proctosigmoidoscopy has replaced rigid examination for most clinical indications, with the exception of those mentioned earlier. This shift in practice is because the length, flexibility, magnification, and optics of the newer instruments make flexible proctosigmoidoscopy better tolerated and more sensitive in detecting distal large bowel lesions while allowing greater length of intestine to be inspected (Figure 142-4). After at least one hypertonic sodium phosphate enema, the scope is inserted into the rectum, and air insufflation is used to open the ampulla. The scope is advanced to the rectosigmoid, where the lumen can be difficult to visualize. Passage through this area requires a combination of torque and in–out motion to avoid loop formation that causes discomfort, precluding further examination. Through a straightened sigmoid colon, the flexible instrument is advanced with care taken to avoid intubation of wide-mouthed diverticula. Patience is required to allow segmental spasms to resolve. The descending colon can usually be negotiated with ease but occasionally requires the assistant to splint the abdominal wall to avoid looping. In most patients, the flexible proctosigmoidoscope can be inserted to at least 50 cm but should be halted earlier if the patient becomes too uncomfortable.

Biopsy samples are obtained from haustral folds, but electrocoagulation should be avoided because of the risk of explosion. Alternatively, polyps can be "cold biopsied" or snared when the risk of hemorrhage is small. If a polyp is better treated with electrocautery, exceeds 1 cm in size, or appears adenomatous on biopsy, complete colonoscopy is recommended to safely remove the lesion and to exclude synchronous neoplasms. Perforation occurs in 0.01% of patients, whereas other complications such as infection transmission and bleeding are quite rare.[12]

Colonoscopy

Colonoscopy is essential in the diagnosis of several benign and any malignant diseases of the colon and rectum. Routinely used in the asymptomatic patient as screening for early neoplasms, colonoscopy is an important diagnostic tool in adenomatous, bleeding, and inflammatory conditions.

In the acutely bleeding patient, emergent colonoscopy can identify the bleeding source in 60% to 97% of patients with moderate or severe lower gastrointestinal hemorrhage. Endoscopic management of lower gastrointestinal hemorrhage can be achieved in most cases with coagulation, injection, and occlusion devices, with only 25% of acute lower gastrointestinal bleeding requiring operative intervention.[13]

For screening or nonemergent diagnostic colonoscopy, the patient is usually prepared with clear liquids and aboral gut lavage with polyethylene glycol or sodium phosphate during the 12 to 24 hours before examination. Prophylactic antibiotic therapy against bacteremia and endocarditis is not warranted for lower gastrointestinal procedures, as of the Consensus Statement of the American Heart Association in 2007.[14] Although colonoscopy can sometimes be safely and comfortably performed without medication, most individuals prefer to receive a sedative, analgesic, or both. Regardless, monitoring of blood pressure, pulse, and oxygen saturation is necessary in all instances because cardiopulmonary adverse effects complicate 2% of all colonoscopies.[15]

The technique of colonoscopy is beyond the scope of this chapter, but the procedure is performed in a manner similar to flexible proctosigmoidoscopy. Cold biopsy, brushing, and cytologic washing are used for diagnostic colonoscopy in appropriate individuals. Moreover, the therapeutic endoscopist's armamentarium must include competency with hot biopsy and snare polypectomy. Expert endoscopists possess further experience with hydrostatic balloon dilation for short benign strictures and endoscopically dispatched stents used to palliate selected malignant obstructions.

The risks of colonoscopy include diagnostic and therapeutic perforation, as well as hemorrhage related to polypectomy or splenic injury. A review of more than 10,000 scopes performed over 10 years was completed at the Mayo Clinic. Twenty perforations (0.19%) occurred during colonoscopy; 65% of these occurred in the sigmoid colon. This larger review confirms previously reported iatrogenic perforation rates of 0.09% to 0.3%.[15] Increased risks include female gender, diagnostic or therapeutic electrocoagulation, and colitis or obstruction symptoms of any etiology. A 15-year retrospective review of colonoscopy complications more recently showed similar incidence and patient profiles with a 0.12% risk of perforation, 74% being sigmoid.[16] Patients with perforation but no peritoneal signs can be safely managed with careful monitoring. For this complication carrying 25% mortality, a low threshold for proceeding to operative intervention is recommended. In a review of 180 such perforations, 165 were managed operatively at the Mayo Clinic.[17]

Intestinal hemorrhage complicates up to 4% of colonoscopies with rates being dependent on the interventions performed. A review of colonoscopy complications in Canada reported bleeding after biopsy at 0.04% and after polypectomy at 0.86%.[18] Immediate bleeding usually follows inadequate control of an artery during polypectomy, whereas delayed bleeding results from subsequent clot retraction and dislodgment 1 to 2 weeks after polypectomy. Delayed hemorrhage occurs more commonly with hot biopsy than with snare polypectomy and on the right side of the colon than on the left side. Immediate hemorrhage or moderate delayed bleeding usually can be controlled by endoscopic techniques, whereas severe delayed bleeding may require assistance from the interventional radiologist. Surgical intervention is necessary only when these other modalities fail or the hemorrhage is life-threatening.

RADIOLOGIC TESTS

Plain Films

Plain film radiography of the abdomen and pelvis requires interpretation of varying radiolucency that is characteristic of the different structures (Figure 142-5). This differentiation depends on the gas (intestine), water (fat, muscle, hollow organs, solid organs), and calcium (bones, calculi, nodes, thrombi, plaques) content of the structures. Normally, the stomach contains at least some gas, whereas a fair amount is distributed throughout the large bowel, especially the hindgut portion. In the healthy ambulatory adult, the small intestine occupies the center of the peritoneal cavity and contains little or no gas, but bedridden adults often demonstrate considerable amounts of small bowel gas without any causative abdominal pathology. The large bowel usually frames the abdomen, and parts of colon sometimes contain semisolid feces mixed with bubbles of gas that create a distinctive speckled shadow; these speckled fecal shadows are not seen in the small intestine. Abnormalities in the usual character and pattern of radiolucencies should alert the physician to potential intraabdominal disease processes.

Plain radiographs of the abdomen offer little to the experienced clinician performing a thoughtful examination. This was shown in an emergency medicine study in the Netherlands. Over 1000 patients were evaluated for abdominal pain. All of the patients underwent plain film and a confirmatory study, either CT or ultrasound. The plain films changed the diagnosis and plan in 117

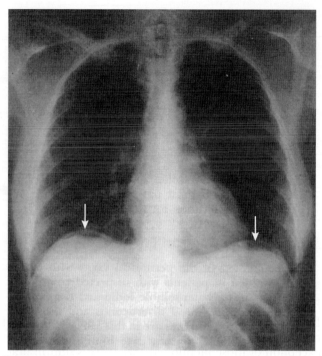

FIGURE 142-5 Erect chest film showing free air in the abdomen under the diaphragm *(arrows)*. (Courtesy Ruedi F. Thoeni, MD.)

patients, just over 10%, but only 39% of the 117 proved to be the correct diagnosis on confirmatory examination. The authors' conclusion was that the plain films did not significantly change the diagnosis from the clinical examination alone. They did report some increased sensitivity diagnosing small bowel obstruction with plain radiograph versus clinical examination.[19]

Colonic Transit Study

Chapter 141 thoroughly discusses the indications for and interpretation of a colonic transit study. Briefly, the test was initially designed as a method to measure whole and segmental gut transit with radiopaque markers and serial plain radiographs. Alternatively, radioisotopes that emit gamma radiation can be used, but this method is more time-consuming.

Single-Contrast Barium Enema

As alluded to earlier, soft tissue differentiation is limited on plain radiography by subtle differences in radiolucency. A radiopaque agent can enhance the interpretation of these studies by outlining the large bowel and its mucosa (Figure 142-6). A liquid that contains low concentrations of barium sulfate has been used for nearly a century to visualize the colon and rectum and to demonstrate its configuration. The bowel must be viewed in different projections, and subtle abnormalities are discernible only when the beam is passing tangential to the bowel edge. Otherwise, lesions are visible only if they are large enough to displace enough barium that the beam absorption is significantly reduced. Compression of the bowel and postevacuation films can somewhat compensate for this limitation, but the results are still less than desirable. Nearly one-third of filling defects seen on single-contrast barium enema are found to represent

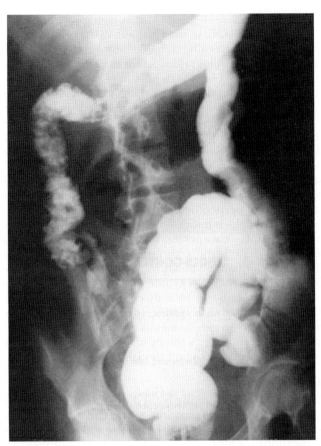

FIGURE 142-6 Single-contrast barium enema demonstrating Crohn disease involving right colon and distal ileum (oblique view). (Courtesy Henry I. Goldberg, MD.)

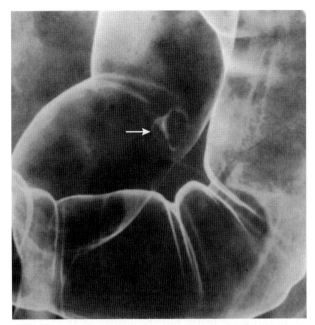

FIGURE 142-7 Double-contrast barium enema showing a colonic polyp *(arrow)*. (Courtesy Ruedi F. Thoeni, MD.)

mere artifacts when colonoscopy is subsequently performed. Similarly, a large number of lesions are missed by the technique, especially smaller (<1 cm) polyps.[20] Good bowel preparation is pivotal to an accurate examination because retained residue and stool reduce the specificity of the study. The procedure is still used routinely for patients who would have difficulty with colonoscopy or double-contrast barium enema, such as the aged, seriously ill, and disabled persons. Moreover, a single-contrast barium enema is the procedure of choice for the evaluation of fistulas and the exclusion of obstruction, assuming that concomitant perforation is unlikely. Perforation is the most common (0.01%) complication associated with barium enema, and it usually occurs when there is weakness of the bowel wall secondary to the underlying disease, traumatic insertion of the enema tip, overinflation of the rectal balloon, or excessive hydrostatic pressure associated with the study. Unfortunately, perforation and barium peritonitis confer a high mortality rate because barium concretions that contain small foci of viable bacteria are dispersed through the peritoneal cavity and cannot be adequately cleared.

Double-Contrast Barium Enema

The double-contrast barium enema was designed to overcome some of the shortcomings associated with the single-contrast study, such as identification of small polyps and diagnosis of colitis (Figure 142-7). Even more than the earlier-generation single-contrast study, the double-contrast barium enema relies on good bowel preparation to clear all stool and residue. A combination of dietary manipulation, oral hydration, cathartics, and optional enemas is recommended. The procedure is performed in a relatively standard manner in which barium is run into the transverse colon and the bowel is then distended with air. The patient is rolled into various positions so gravity and palpation can manipulate the barium column around the entirety of the large bowel that is continuously distended with air. Multiple spot and overhead films are generated and collected to create a composite evaluation of the adherence of the contrast agent to the large bowel.

Few clinicians will argue that double-contrast barium enema is simpler, safer, and less expensive than colonoscopy. However, even under ideal conditions with interpretation by experienced radiologists, the double-contrast barium enema is inferior to colonoscopy for the detection of CRC and polyps. Historically, the sensitivity of the procedure for detecting polyps smaller than 5 mm was poor, improving with polyps of 5 to 9 mm, and best for polyps larger than 1 cm. According to a literature review, the sensitivity for these larger polyps is approximately 80% and the specificity is approximately 95%.[21] Although the overall sensitivity of a double-contrast study for the detection of CRCs ranges from 80% to 100%, nearly one-fourth of the rectosigmoid carcinomas will be missed. The combination of sigmoidoscopy with double-contrast barium enema overcomes some of the deficiencies but adds costs and risks to screening.[22]

As part of the National Polyp Study, a prospective, blinded trial studied the relative accuracy of double-contrast barium enema compared with colonoscopy in 580 patients.[22] The sensitivity for the detection of advanced (>1 cm) adenomas of the contrast study and colonoscopy was 46% and 100%, respectively. The investigators concluded that colonoscopy detects many more adenomas than double-contrast barium enema and that the combination of the two studies adds little to the use of colonoscopy alone.

The benefits and limitations associated with imaging and endoscopy continue to fuel the debate over the best screening test, but, despite its long-standing acceptance in the available algorithm of CRC screening, double-contrast barium enema has fallen from favor among radiologists. For the radiographic evaluation of the colon, CT colonography is preferred.[23] Support of this is further discussed in Computed Tomography Enterography, later.

Water-Soluble Contrast Enema

A water-soluble contrast enema with Gastrografin or Urografin is favored over a barium study when the risk of perforation is at all likely because the water-soluble compounds will not cause the peritonitis mentioned earlier. Instead, the water-soluble agents are absorbed so that no peritoneal reaction ensues. The low viscosity of the agents makes them more likely than barium to identify fistulas and anastomotic leaks, but the clarity of the images is compromised, because these hypertonic, water-soluble compounds quickly become diluted. This hypertonicity feature can also be therapeutic, because diarrhea usually occurs after the study, which may be helpful in patients with pseudoobstruction. However, for the same reason, the agent can be detrimental in persons with obstruction because rare perforation might result from the massive amounts of fluid that can be drawn into the closed segment of bowel proximal to the obstructing lesion. In addition, dehydration might result in some individuals but is unlikely when small (<500 mL) volumes of contrast material are used.

Contrast Fistulography

Contrast fistulograms may provide valuable information and alter the treatment of select patients. Anal fistulas are rarely assessed with fistulography, but the modality can be useful for persons with chronic complex fistulas and suspected extrasphincteric fistulas. More

often magnetic resonance (MR) imaging or endorectal ultrasound (ERUS) is used to best discern anal fistula anatomy.[24] Conversely, reliable information can be gleaned from fistulography performed for an enterocutaneous fistula. The test is usually part of a group of investigations and should be performed before any other imaging examinations because retained barium can obscure the fistulography results. A small Foley catheter is inserted as deep as possible into the tract, and the balloon is inflated to secure the position of the catheter, seal the tract against reflux of contrast medium, and allow opacification of the entire proximal tract. Water-soluble contrast material should be used, and spot films are obtained perpendicular to the fistula tract.

Vaginography is indicated when a rectovaginal or colovaginal fistula is suspected and a water-soluble enema failed to identify the communication. The test is performed in a manner similar to fistulography with a large Foley catheter used to occlude the vaginal introitus. Cystograms uncommonly identify enterovesical or colovesical fistulas. Instead, a bladder deformity is often seen, which suggests an extrinsic mass or inflammatory process that often accompanies the fistula. Again, MR and ERUS are more sensitive imaging modalities.

Defecography

Evacuation proctography is used to study the dynamics of voluntary rectal evacuation, and techniques vary considerably. Chapters 144 and 146 thoroughly discusses the indications for and interpretation of defecography.

Endoluminal Ultrasound

Without radiation exposure, ERUS provides excellent evaluation of the distal colon, rectum, and anal canal. Rivaled only by MR with endorectal coil, ERUS shows details of anorectal anatomy, benign disorders, and malignant tumors (Figure 142-8).

Typically performed after an enema preparation, rigid, 10-MHz endoscopy using endoluminal contact for structure definition is used to evaluate fecal incontinence, rectal cancers, and perianal inflammatory

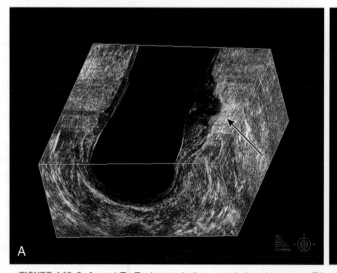
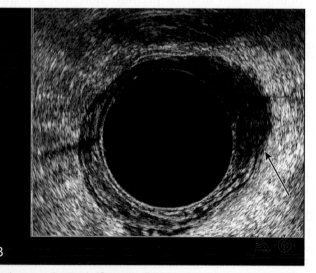

FIGURE 142-8 **A** and **B,** Endorectal ultrasound showing stage T3 rectal cancer *(arrows).* (Courtesy B-K Medical, Herlev, Denmark.)

conditions. Evaluation of ill-defined anal pain and anal cancers are also indications. Obstetric injuries to the sphincters, occult and complex fistula tracts, and perianal Crohn disease additionally are clarified by ultrasound examination.

ERUS is also used for rectal and anal cancer staging. The examination is performed with either a rigid or flexible probe and stages all cancers with more than 70% accuracy compared to surgical specimen. Ultrasound is the least accurate for bulky T4 tumors, and nearly 20% of all tumors may be overstaged. But as an available modality used to guide preoperative neoadjuvant therapies, ultrasound is considered as accurate as MR, while providing the surgeon with essential information for eventual operative planning regarding tumor location. Specifically regarding involvement of the sphincter, rigid endorectal ultrasound has been shown to have 100% sensitivity, a negative predictive value of 100%, a specificity of 87%, and a positive predictive value of 53%.[25] The flexible endoluminal ultrasound allows for evaluation of low colon cancers and higher rectal tumors than the rigid transducer probe. By this flexible probe technique, the iliac nodal basin is also evaluated. Biopsy of tumors and suspicious nodes is possible through a side port on either the rigid or flexible probe.

Computed Tomographic Scanning

CT scanning is useful in the diagnosis of benign and malignant diseases of the colon, rectum, and anus (Figure 142-9). Its role in the diagnosis and management of diverticulitis is unparalleled because it identifies extraluminal disease and features of severe inflammation (e.g., extraluminal gas and contrast, abscess) that predict or define a complicated disease course. Inflammatory bowel diseases are associated with nonspecific findings such as bowel wall thickening on CT scanning, but again, extraluminal disease can be visualized. Right lower quadrant masses in Crohn disease, for instance, caused by terminal ileal inflammation can be readily distinguished from abscesses related to perforated disease. Last, the role of

CT in the diagnosis and treatment of complex anoperineal sepsis is evolving as experience grows but is typically disappointing because the levators are not well defined and sphincter resolution is poor.

Although conventional CT scanning is insensitive for the diagnosis of intraluminal CRCs, it is still useful in evaluation of the patient with a known malignancy because it can demonstrate extracolonic spread to adjacent and remote organs. This knowledge might significantly alter the planned clinical and operative management of the primary lesion. CT scanning is indicated in the postoperative surveillance and identification of suspected disease recurrence (see later).

Computed Tomographic Enterography

CT enterography and CT colonography (also called "virtual colonoscopy") provide an effective means of imaging the bowel. The procedure requires adequate bowel preparation and low-dose, high-resolution helical CT imaging. The patient is initially placed in the supine position, and a barium enema tip is placed transanally to allow inflation of the large bowel with air or carbon dioxide to maximum patient tolerance. After adequate distention is ensured with a localizing CT scout, a helical CT scan of the abdomen and pelvis is performed. The procedure is then repeated in the prone position.

This less-invasive approach to bowel evaluation provides information about the entire bowel, particularly sensitive for inflammatory abnormalities and larger cancers. Crohn disease and rare tumors of the small bowel may be found with this modality (Figure 142-10). Used for CRC screening, CT colonography has the advantages of no sedation or recovery time. Only low-dose radiation exposure is required for this test, which can also provide three-dimensional reconstructions of the bowel and any observed abnormalities.

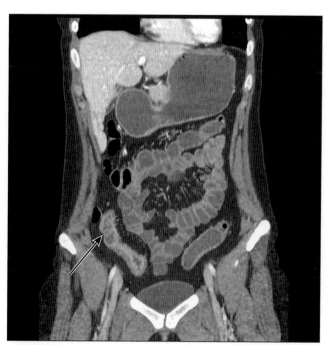

FIGURE 142-10 Crohn disease of the terminal ileum *(arrow)* as seen on CT enterography.

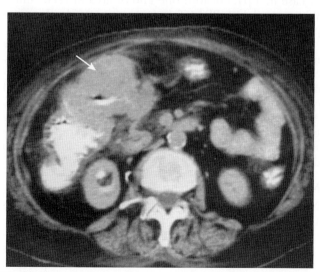

FIGURE 142-9 Abdominal CT scan showing carcinoma of hepatic flexure of the colon *(arrow)*. (Courtesy Ruedi F. Thoeni, MD.)

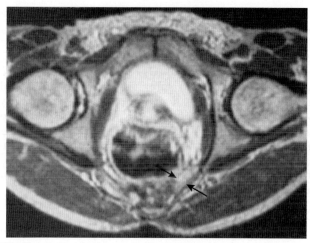

FIGURE 142-11 MR imaging of pelvis demonstrating recurrent carcinoma *(arrows)* after anterior resection of rectal adenocarcinoma. (Courtesy Ruedi F. Thoeni, MD.)

Similar to the challenge of adopting fecal immuno-chemical testing or DNA marker screening tools, CT colonography lacks decades of evidence to prove itself. Accepted as "the leading imaging technique for colorectal cancer screening" by the expert panel creating the Appropriateness Criteria for the Department of Quality and Safety of the American College of Radiology, CT colonography has the other advantage of finding extra-colonic pathology in 27% to 69% of those scanned.[3,26] The one indication without controversy is the recommended use of CT colonography for completion screening in patients having an incomplete colonoscopy.[27]

Magnetic Resonance Imaging

MR imaging is one of the more recent modalities used to study structural and functional disorders of the anus, rectum, colon, and surrounding structures (Figure 142-11). The examination is typically used to focus on an area of abnormality rather than to survey the entire abdomen and pelvis, like CT scanning. Usually, T1- and T2-weighted images are obtained in the axial plane with coronal, oblique, and sagittal planes selected when necessary to view a particular area of interest. Gradient-echo images depict flowing blood and make lesions more distinct, whereas chemical shift images determine the fat content of a lesion. Similar to contrast-enhanced CT scans, gadolinium-based contrast agents are used intravenously to demonstrate vascularity and enhance lesion patterns. In addition, various radiofrequency coils can be used depending on the anatomic structure that is to be imaged. External and internal coils that are relevant to imaging in this area include the body, surface (abdomen- or pelvis-phased multicoils), and endorectal coils. In general, higher resolution is seen with the smaller viewing fields because the dedicated coils are placed closer to the region of interest and this increases the signal-to-noise ratio.

MR imaging is used in the diagnosis of benign colorectal conditions. MR imaging more accurately delineates structural defects of pelvic floor disorders and of anal fistulous disease than does plain film or CT.[24] In addition,

MR imaging is more useful than digital examination in the diagnosis and differentiation of ischioanal and peri-rectal abscesses.[28] MR imaging is also commonly used in the diagnosis of malignant colorectal disease. Staging of rectal cancer by MR is used to guide neoadjuvant therapy and allows for accurate restaging preoperatively.[29] This modality is also efficacious in the evaluation of metastatic liver disease and recurrent rectal cancer, especially when adjacent organ or bony invasion is suspected. The MERCURY trial, from 11 colorectal units in four European countries, helped define the importance of MR in the preoperative evaluation of rectal cancer by showing the near perfect accuracy with which MR predicts resectability of rectal cancer.[30]

Magnetic Resonance Enterography

MR enterography is emerging as an alternative to CT enterography in younger Crohn disease patients who face a lifetime of surveillance for their disease. Limiting radiation exposure in this group of inflammatory bowel disease patients is important.

Positron Emission Tomography

Just as MR can provide a three-dimensional image through reconstruction, emission imaging allows for a three-dimensional representation of distribution to be created. If a single-photon emission is studied, such as technetium or thallium, a single-photon emission CT test is possible. The details of tests such as a single-photon emission CT are discussed with nuclear medicine imaging.

Positron emission tomography (PET) using [17]F-fluorodeoxyglucose is indicated in the evaluation of patients with known or suspected recurrent CRC. Because PET images can help differentiate postoperative changes from recurrent or residual tumor, this modality can be useful in the early postoperative period. [17]F-Fluorodeoxyglucose-PET can be used as a screening tool, although prohibitive costs and restricted availability have led to limited indications including evaluation of increased CEA levels without an obvious tumor recurrence or preoperatively for the exclusion of widespread disease in a patient with one known area of recurrence. Where available, PET-CT fusion tests provide the most powerful integrated images (Figure 142-12).[31]

In addition to evaluating malignant disease, PET is useful in the diagnosis and management of inflammatory bowel disease. Spier and Lapp at the University of Wisconsin have presented a literature review and two small case series demonstrating disease as studied by PET. Anecdotally, the changes seen on PET before and during treatment correlate to responsiveness of therapy.[32-34] The standardized uptake value (SUV) by PET correlates to disease severity and also helps with localization.[35]

Nuclear Medicine Imaging

Nuclear medicine imaging uses various radioisotopes (e.g., ^{131}I, ^{111}In, ^{99m}Tc) that are bound to a variety of materials and cells, including monoclonal antibodies, leukocytes, and erythrocytes (Figure 142-13). After intravenous injection or ingestion of the radiolabeled compounds, the patient is imaged with a gamma camera designed for the 140-MeV energy at one or several time points. This

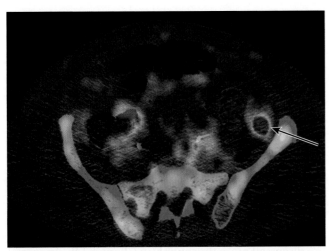

FIGURE 142-12 Left pelvic tumor *(arrow)* seen by PET-CT adjacent to the descending colon at the level of the iliac spine, which was found after normal colonoscopy and examination in a patient with a history of colorectal cancer and a rising carcinoembryonic antigen level.

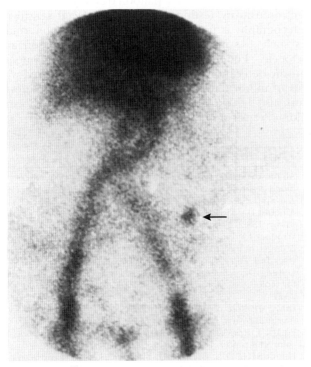

FIGURE 142-13 ⁹⁹ᵐTc red blood cell scan showing abnormal activity in area of sigmoid colon *(arrow)* 10 minutes after injection. Lesion subsequently proved to be a bleeding diverticulum. (Courtesy Barry L. Engelstad, MD.)

modality can be used to evaluate a variety of disease processes, including the detection of metastatic cancer, the identification of bowel infection or inflammation, the localization of intestinal hemorrhage, and the measurement of colonic transit. These uses are discussed elsewhere in detail, but their use in the diagnosis of disease deserves brief comment.

Radionuclide imaging of colon malignancies must be interpreted in conjunction with review of findings from physical examination and other investigative studies. The reported sensitivities of monoclonal antibody staging of CRC varies from 65% to 86%, with specificities for the detection of primary, metastatic, and recurrent disease ranging from 77% to 92%.[36] Thus, this principal contribution of the modality in the management of CRC lies in its ability to target potential sites of occult tumor and confirm the absence of distant metastases in persons with disease amenable to resection. At this time, clinicians would not base treatment solely on the outcome of a nuclear medicine scan.

Radiolabeled white blood cell scans can reliably contribute to the evaluation of a postoperative patient who develops fever and in the assessment of inflammatory bowel disease.[37] Similarly, radionuclide-based colonic transit assessment may contribute to an improved understanding of normal and abnormal colonic motility and might assist in the management of disorders such as idiopathic constipation, fecal incontinence, and megarectum.

For many surgeons, the most common indication for radionuclide imaging involves the management of intestinal hemorrhage. Most early series reported sensitivities of more than 90% for the detection of bleeding with radionuclide scans. Because this sensitivity was higher than that reported with angiography, it was recommended that a radionuclide study be performed before arteriography to identify a source of bleeding. The implication was a negative scan would dismiss the usefulness of emergent angiogram. However, several reports have produced compelling data (radionuclide scan sensitivity of 20% to 46%) that contradict this practice.[38] In addition to the difficulty of diagnosing bleeding that spontaneously stops in 85% of cases, there are the challenges of choosing the best study in usually older patients with comorbidities and an ongoing resuscitation.

Discussing the roles and limitations of scintigraphy in acute lower gastrointestinal bleeding, a recent review promotes scintigraphy as a safe and appropriate study with particularly relevant prognostic information for the patient with a high risk of rebleeding. They offer an updated algorithm and the details of a successful use of ⁹⁹ᵐTc-labeled red blood cell scan by detailing the applications leading to sensitivities greater than 90% and specificity near 100%.[39]

Intestinal transit can be measured using a radiolabeled nonabsorbable marker in solid food. Chapter 141 thoroughly discusses the particulars of this method.

Mesenteric Angiography

Mesenteric angiography may be performed by specially trained vascular surgeons or interventional radiologists and is commonly used to identify the source of intestinal hemorrhage and to determine acute arterial occlusion of the main visceral trunks (Figure 142-14). The application of mesenteric angiography specific to colorectal bleeding is briefly covered here. The important role of mesenteric angiography in the management of lower intestinal hemorrhage is as a diagnostic and possibly interventional tool. The key to successful localization of bleeding is early, prompt arteriography in the face of active, massive bleeding. The timing is crucial because angiography best

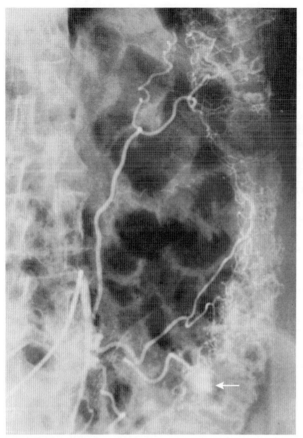

FIGURE 142-14 Selective inferior mesenteric arteriogram demonstrating bleeding site in sigmoid colon *(arrow).* (Courtesy Ernest J. Ring, MD.)

identifies the site of bleeding when the bleeding occurs at a rate exceeding 0.5 mL/min. Aggressive pharmacologic techniques with systemic heparinization, selective intraarterial vasodilators, and thrombolytic agents have been used to prolong or reactivate bleeding in an attempt to improve the diagnostic yield.

Even though the yield of bleeding site localization by angiography in acute lower gastrointestinal bleeding is low relative to the reported complications, if selective embolization is possible, clear benefits exist. Although it is well known that successful injection or embolization of an acute lower gastrointestinal bleed can be life-saving, the low yield of localization by angiography can be limiting. A well-studied, less-invasive alternative for localization is CT angiography, during which an arterial phase CT can localize acute bleeding with up to 88.5% accuracy.[40] Kennedy et al. reported on more than 4 years of reviewed CT angiographies for acute lower gastrointestinal bleeding. None of the patients with negative CT angiographies went on to have bleeding localized by angiography. The sensitivity (79%) and specificity (95%) led to an accuracy of 91% for localization by CT angiography with angiographic confirmation. They concluded that CT angiography is a useful, accurate, and safe step of the algorithm toward mesenteric angiography and surgery for acute lower gastrointestinal bleeding.[41]

Arteriography is the procedure of choice for the diagnosis of acute mesenteric ischemia. MR arteriography and CT arteriography are sensitive for diagnosis and carry less risk than arteriography, but these alternatives lack therapeutic options. Flush abdominal aortography with anteroposterior and lateral projections may visualize the main vascular trunks, but selective angiography, especially with digital subtraction, defines the artery and its branches. Moreover, this latter modality can differentiate among the three principal causes of acute ischemia and allows medical or mechanical revascularization without laparotomy in some instances. Chronic mesenteric ischemia, however, is better evaluated with noninvasive procedures such as abdominal duplex ultrasonography, laser Doppler flow analysis, and MR imaging.

Tests of Pelvic Floor Function

The diagnosis and treatment of pelvic floor dysfunction are discussed more thoroughly in Chapter 146. Anorectal manometry quantifies the luminal pressures in the anus and rectum to provide a direct measure of internal and external sphincter function. Microballoon systems, water-perfused catheters, or solid-state transducers can be used to measure these pressures, but each laboratory should establish its own standards. Balloon distention or mucosal electrosensitivity testing can evaluate rectal sensitivity. Defecography is used to diagnose anatomic abnormalities such as symptomatic internal intussusception and rectocele. Pudendal nerve damage can accompany chronic defecation disorders and is best elucidated with tests of motor and sensory conduction. Colonic inertia must also be excluded in these patients, and normal colonic transit should be documented.

REFERENCES

1. Ahlquist DA, Sargent DJ, Loprinzi CL, et al: Stool DNA and occult blood testing for screen detection of colorectal neoplasia. *Ann Intern Med* 149:441, W81, 2008.
2. Ahlquist DA: Molecular detection of colorectal neoplasia. *Gastroenterology* 138:2127, 2010.
3. Whitlock EP, Lin JS, Liles E, et al: Screening for colorectal cancer: A targeted, updated systematic review for the U.S. Preventive Services Task Force. *Ann Intern Med* 149:638, 2008.
4. Ouyang DL, Chen JJ, Getzenberg RH, et al: Noninvasive testing for colorectal cancer: A review. *Am J Gastroenterol* 100:1393, 2005.
5. Duffy MJ: Role of tumor markers in patients with solid cancers: A critical review. *Eur J Intern Med* 18:175, 2007.
6. Potack J, Itzkowitz SH: Practical advances in stool screening for colorectal cancer. *J Natl Compr Canc Netw* 8:81, 2010.
7. Hundt S, Haug U, Brenner H: Blood markers for early detection of colorectal cancer: A systematic review. *Cancer Epidemiol Biomarkers Prev* 16:1935, 2007.
8. Søreide K, Nedrebo BS, Knapp JC, et al: Evolving molecular classification by genomic and proteomic biomarkers in colorectal cancer: Potential implications for the surgical oncologist. *Surg Oncol* 18:31, 2009.
9. Lynch HT, Lynch JF, Attard TA: Diagnosis and management of hereditary colorectal cancer syndromes: Lynch syndrome as a model. *CMAJ* 181:273, 2009.
10. Cappell MS, Friedel D: The role of sigmoidoscopy and colonoscopy in the diagnosis and management of lower gastrointestinal disorders: Endoscopic findings, therapy, and complications. *Med Clin North Am* 86:1253, 2002.
11. Schoellhammer HF, Gregorian AC, Sarkisyan GG, et al: How important is rigid proctosigmoidoscopy in localizing rectal cancer? *Am J Surg* 196:904; discussion 908, 2008.
12. Nelson RL, Abcarian H, Prasad ML: Iatrogenic perforation of the colon and rectum. *Dis Colon Rectum* 25:305, 1982.

13. Lee J, Costantini TW, Coimbra R: Acute lower GI bleeding for the acute care surgeon: Current diagnosis and management. *Scand J Surg* 98:135, 2009.

14. Wilson W, Taubert KA, Gewitz M, et al: Prevention of infective endocarditis: Guidelines from the American Heart Association: A guideline from the American Heart Association Rheumatic Fever, Endocarditis, and Kawasaki Disease Committee, Council on Cardiovascular Disease in the Young, and the Council on Clinical Cardiology, Council on Cardiovascular Surgery and Anesthesia, and the Quality of Care and Outcomes Research Interdisciplinary Working Group. *Circulation* 116:1736, 2007.

15. Eckardt VF, Kanzler G, Schmitt T, et al: Complications and adverse effects of colonoscopy with selective sedation. *Gastrointest Endosc* 49:560, 1999.

16. Luning TH, Keemers-Gels ME, Barendregt WB, et al: Colonoscopic perforations: A review of 30,366 patients. *Surg Endosc* 21:994, 2007.

17. Iqbal CW, Cullinane DC, Schiller HJ, et al: Surgical management and outcomes of 165 colonoscopic perforations from a single institution. *Arch Surg* 143:701; discussion 706, 2008.

18. Singh H, Penfold RB, DeCoster C, et al: Colonoscopy and its complications across a Canadian regional health authority. *Gastrointest Endosc* 69:665, 2009.

19. van Randen A, Lameris W, Luitse JS, et al: The role of plain radiographs in patients with acute abdominal pain at the ED. *Am J Emerg Med* 29:582, 2011.

20. Rex DK, Johnson DA, Lieberman DA, et al: Colorectal cancer prevention 2000: Screening recommendations of the American College of Gastroenterology. American College of Gastroenterology. *Am J Gastroenterol* 95:868, 2000.

21. Ott DJ: Accuracy of double-contrast barium enema in diagnosing colorectal polyps and cancer. *Semin Roentgenol* 35:333, 2000.

22. Winawer SJ, Stewart ET, Zauber AG, et al: A comparison of colonoscopy and double-contrast barium enema for surveillance after polypectomy. National Polyp Study Work Group. *N Engl J Med* 342:1766, 2000.

23. Stevenson G: Colon imaging in radiology departments in 2008: Goodbye to the routine double contrast barium enema. *Can Assoc Radiol J* 59:174, 2008.

24. Buchanan GN, Halligan S, Bartram CI, et al: Clinical examination, endosonography, and MR imaging in preoperative assessment of fistula in ano: Comparison with outcome-based reference standard. *Radiology* 233:674, 2004.

25. Assenat E, Thezenas S, Samalin E, et al: The value of endoscopic rectal ultrasound in predicting the lateral clearance and outcome in patients with lower-third rectal adenocarcinoma. *Endoscopy* 39:309, 2007.

26. Yee J, Rosen MP, Blake MA, et al: ACR Appropriateness Criteria on colorectal cancer screening. *J Am Coll Radiol* 7:670, 2010.

27. Neerincx M, Terhaar sive Droste JS, Mulder CJ, et al: Colonic work-up after incomplete colonoscopy: Significant new findings during follow-up. *Endoscopy* 42:730, 2010.

28. Maruyama R, Noguchi T, Takano M, et al: Usefulness of magnetic resonance imaging for diagnosing deep anorectal abscesses. *Dis Colon Rectum* 43:S2, 2000.

29. Beets-Tan RG, Lettinga T, Beets GL: Pre-operative imaging of rectal cancer and its impact on surgical performance and treatment outcome. *Eur J Surg Oncol* 31:681, 2005.

30. MERCURY Study Group: Diagnostic accuracy of preoperative magnetic resonance imaging in predicting curative resection of rectal cancer: Prospective observational study. *BMJ* 333:779, 2006.

31. Delbeke D, Martin WH: PET and PET-CT for evaluation of colorectal carcinoma. *Semin Nucl Med* 34:209, 2004.

32. Spier BJ, Perlman SB, Jaskowiak CJ, et al: PET/CT in the evaluation of inflammatory bowel disease: Studies in patients before and after treatment. *Mol Imaging Biol* 12:85, 2010.

33. Spier BJ, Perlman SB, Reichelderfer M: FDG-PET in inflammatory bowel disease. *Q J Nucl Med Mol Imaging* 53:64, 2009.

34. Lapp RT, Spier BJ, Perlman SB, et al: Clinical utility of positron emission tomography/computed tomography in inflammatory bowel disease. *Mol Imaging Biol* 13:573, 2011.

35. Groshar D, Bernstine H, Stern D, et al: PET/CT enterography in Crohn disease: Correlation of disease activity on CT enterography with 18F-FDG uptake. *J Nucl Med* 51:1009, 2010.

36. Berlin JW, Gore RM, Yaghmai V, et al: Staging of colorectal cancer. *Semin Roentgenol* 35:370, 2000.

37. Li DJ, Middleton SJ, Wraight EP: 99Tcm and 111In leucocyte scintigraphy in inflammatory bowel disease. *Nucl Med Commun* 13:867, 1992.

38. Ogunbiyi OA, Fleshman JW: The limitations and disadvantages of radionucleotide scintigraphy. *Semin Colon Rectal Surg* 8, 1997.

39. Currie GM, Kiat H, Wheat JM: Scintigraphic evaluation of acute lower gastrointestinal hemorrhage: Current status and future directions. *J Clin Gastroenterol* 45:92, 2011.

40. Yoon W, Jeong YY, Shin SS, et al: Acute massive gastrointestinal bleeding: Detection and localization with arterial phase multidetector row helical CT. *Radiology* 239:160, 2006.

41. Kennedy DW, Laing CJ, Tseng LH, et al: Detection of active gastrointestinal hemorrhage with CT angiography: A 4(1/2)-year retrospective review. *J Vasc Interv Radiol* 21:848, 2010.

Ultrasonographic Diagnosis of Anorectal Disease

Dimitra G. Theodoropoulos | W. Douglas Wong[†]

Endorectal ultrasound (ERUS) is the diagnostic procedure of choice in the evaluation of many anorectal disorders. It is a valuable tool in the local staging of rectal and anal cancer and has an important role in surveillance for local recurrence. ERUS is used in the diagnosis of benign mucosal lesions, extrarectal masses, anal incontinence, fistula-in-ano, and anorectal abscesses. It can be performed by the surgeon in the office setting, providing information essential for treatment decisions. This chapter focuses on the role of ERUS in the evaluation of benign and malignant conditions of the rectum and anus.

TECHNIQUE

ERUS requires minimal patient preparation with two enemas the morning of the examination. The test is well tolerated, without need for sedation. Patients are preferably examined in the left lateral decubitus position. For rectal cancer staging, we perform a digital rectal examination (DRE) to determine the location of the tumor and its relation to the anorectal ring. We then evaluate the rectum using a 20-mm-wide rigid proctoscope (ElectroSurgical Instrument Company) to document the morphologic characteristics of the lesion (size, distance from the anal verge, location on the rectal wall, and appearance) and to ensure that a complete sonographic evaluation can be performed. At this time residual stool, mucus, and enema effluent are removed to avoid image artifacts.

It is important to advance the proctoscope proximal to the lesion, to facilitate complete imaging of the lesion from its most proximal to its most distal extent. The examination is complete only when the entire length of the tumor is imaged, because the findings at the lower end of the tumor may differ markedly proximally. Moreover, positive lymph nodes, when present, are most commonly found in the mesorectum proximal to the lesion. Blind insertion of the ultrasound probe into the rectum may distort the lesion, miss proximal areas of the tumor and surrounding mesorectum, and cause discomfort to the patient.

At Memorial Sloan-Kettering Cancer Center (MSKCC) we use a Brüel & Kjaer 2101 Hawk scanner with an 1850

rotating endosonic probe and a 10-MHz 6004 transducer (Figure 143-1). We also use a 2050 probe with capability for 10-, 12-, or 16-MHz (multifrequency transducer). The 10-MHz transducer with a focal length of 1 to 4 cm is the one most commonly used, providing superior near-image clarity and excellent visualization of the perirectal tissues. A 7-MHz transducer, which provides a focal length of 2 to 5 cm, may be used if there is a need to evaluate deeper structures. A 90-degree scanning plane is rotated at four to six cycles per second to provide a 360-degree radial scan of the rectum and surrounding structures. We use the rigid ultrasound probe because we find it provides better maneuverability and optimizes the image. However, a rigid probe cannot evaluate areas more than 12 to 15 cm from the anal verge. Flexible endosonoscopes are also available. Steele et al compared the two probes, with results suggesting a more reliable learning curve for the rigid devices and less accuracy of the flexible devices for visualizing depth of invasion.[1]

Once the proctoscope is advanced above the tumor, the ultrasound probe is lubricated and inserted gently through the proctoscope, allowing the transducer to be advanced above the cancer. The proctoscope is then pulled back and the balloon over the ultrasound crystal is instilled with fluid. The amount of fluid is estimated based on the luminal diameter from the proctoscopy, patient discomfort, and ability to pass the balloon beyond the lesion. For the 1850 probe, 30 to 60 mL is used on average, whereas the 2050 probe usually requires between 90 and 120 mL. It is important to make sure no air bubbles are present, to minimize acoustic impedance.

The key to the procedure is to keep the probe centered in the lumen of the rectum. Scanning is best conducted from proximal to distal. The probe and attached proctoscope are slowly withdrawn together, assessing the mesorectum for evidence of nodal metastases and the tumor for depth of penetration. Optimal evaluation often requires several passes back and forth across a lesion or a suspected lymph node. Measurements of lymph nodes' size and tumor dimensions are made, including any radial extension of tumor into the perirectal fat.

Endoanal ultrasound (EAUS) is used to evaluate disease in the anal canal. In the case of malignancy, the mesorectum needs to be evaluated with the balloon for nodal metastases. Then, a fluid-filled, hard, translucent plastic cap is used instead of the balloon for the EAUS. The ultrasound transducer is inserted into the anal canal without a proctoscope.

Ultrasonographic evaluation of the anorectum is based on real-time imaging. We routinely videotape all examinations and have found this to be helpful in the review of difficult cases. Spot images may be saved,

[†]Deceased. Doug Wong agreed to take on this chapter when he was extremely ill. He passed away shortly after its completion. I was hesitant to ask Doug to do this, but he enthusiastically wished to proceed and did so in his typical way, on time with no fuss. Doug's "baby" was endorectal ultrasound and he was the recognized expert in the field. We are honored that he felt his contribution to be such an important task at a very difficult time in his life. American surgery lost a fine scholar, teacher, and surgeon ~~and his colleagues~~ and I lost a dear and trusted friend.

—John H. Pemberton

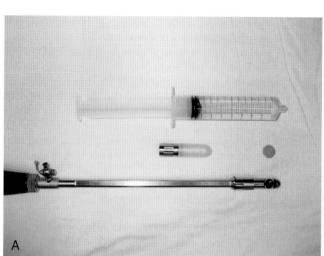

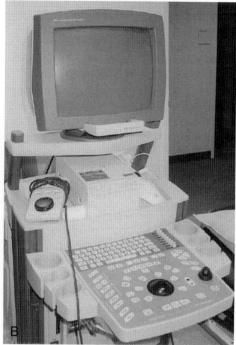

FIGURE 143-1 **A,** Brüel and Kjaer rotating endosonic probe with a 10-MHz 6004 transducer, with balloon and hard cap shown. **B,** Brüel and Kjaer Hawk 2102 unit. (**A** and **B** courtesy Brüel and Kjaer, Inc, Naerum, Denmark.)

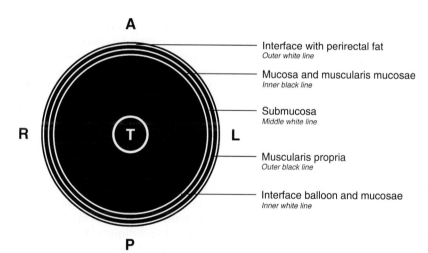

FIGURE 143-2 Five-layer anatomic model for interpretation of endorectal ultrasonographic scans. Three hyperechoic *(white)* layers and two hypoechoic *(black)* layers can be visualized. *A,* Anterior; *L,* left; *P,* posterior; *R,* right; *T,* transducer.

copied, and printed. These are useful for documentation and for the followup of suspicious areas.

NORMAL ENDORECTAL ULTRASOUND ANATOMY

The five-layer model for ERUS anatomy was proposed by Beynon et al in 1986 and is the one used today. Beynon et al demonstrated that the proposed five ultrasonic layers correspond to the anatomy of the rectal wall by correlating in vitro ultrasound scanning and sequential microdissection of the normal layers of the rectum from operative specimens.[2]

In this model, the first and innermost line encountered is hyperechoic (white), representing the interface between the fluid-filled balloon and the mucosa. Next is the first hypoechoic (black) line, which represents the mucosa and the muscularis mucosae. The middle hyperechoic (white) line represents the submucosa. The next hypoechoic line correlates to the muscularis propria. The third and outermost hyperechoic line represents the interface between the muscularis propria and the perirectal fat (Figure 143-2). Occasionally, a seven-layer model may be visualized in which the muscularis propria is observed as two black rings separated by a white ring. In this case, the inner circular and outer longitudinal layers of the muscularis propria appear as two distinct hypoechoic (black) layers, separated by a hyperechoic interface. In addition to the rectal wall, the mesorectum, urinary bladder, cul-de-sac and its contents, seminal vesicles, prostate, uterus, vagina, and cervix are visualized

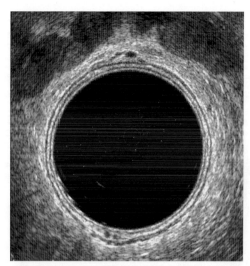

FIGURE 143-3 Normal rectal wall. Three hyperechoic *(white)* and two hypoechoic *(black)* layers are clearly visualized in the ultrasonographic image of the normal rectal wall. The seminal vesicles are seen anteriorly as bilateral hypoechoic structures.

with ERUS. Figure 143-3 depicts the ultrasonographic appearance of the normal rectal wall.

RECTAL CANCER

IMAGING MODALITIES IN THE LOCAL STAGING OF RECTAL CANCER

Accurate preoperative staging is necessary to determine the prognosis and select the optimal treatment, in terms of cure and quality of life, for patients with rectal cancer. Knowledge of the depth of rectal wall invasion and perirectal lymph node involvement is essential to select early cancers amenable to local excision and to identify locally advanced cancers that are best treated with neoadjuvant chemoradiotherapy. DRE, ERUS, computed tomography (CT), and magnetic resonance imaging (MRI) have been applied in the local staging of rectal cancer.

Digital Rectal Examination

DRE by an experienced surgeon is an important part of the evaluation of the patient and may predict pathologic stage, particularly for advanced tumors. However, DRE is subjective, cannot assess tumors in the proximal third of the rectum, and is unreliable in staging early lesions. Studies demonstrate the low accuracy of DRE compared to ERUS and MRI in the assessment of depth of wall invasion and nodal involvement.[3,4] DRE should rarely be used alone in the local staging of rectal cancer.

Computed Tomography Scan

CT is routinely used in the preoperative staging of rectal cancer and is particularly useful in detecting contiguous organ involvement and distant metastases. Its accuracy in local staging, however, is low, and less than that of the ERUS.[5,6] Kulinna et al found the multislice CT to be superior to ERUS in the local staging of rectal cancer in a study of 92 patients.[7] However, recent studies continue to demonstrate overall poor performance even with the

multidetector-row CT, and lower accuracy compared to phased-array MRI in the preoperative assessment of the circumferential rectal margin in patients with rectal cancer.[8,9]

Magnetic Resonance Imaging

MRI is gaining popularity in the local staging of rectal cancer, specifically in assessing the circumferential rectal margin. MRI with conventional body coils has poor overall performance compared to ERUS.[4] The use of endorectal coil improves the diagnostic accuracy of the test to a range comparable to that of ERUS in assessing the T stage (81%) and the presence of lymph node metastasis (63%).[10,11] Limitations of the endorectal coil are the long examination time (between 60 and 75 minutes), its relatively small field of view, and its large diameter, which often prevents the evaluation of bulky rectal tumors.[12,13] For these reasons the use of the endorectal coil has largely been abandoned.

The phased-array coil MRI is currently the preferred technique for the staging of rectal cancer; an arrangement of multiple external coils (without an endorectal probe) and fast T2-weighted spin-echo sequences are used to obtain high spatial resolution images with a large field of view, to include the entire mesorectum. The value of phased-array coil MRI was demonstrated in the MERCURY study, a landmark in the field of rectal cancer; this was the first prospective multicenter, multidisciplinary study to assess the accuracy and reproducibility of MRI in predicting the circumferential resection margin and thus the potential for curative resection in patients with rectal cancer.[14] The proximity of the cancer to within 1 mm of the fascia propria and the radial margin in the surgical specimen are strong predictors of recurrence and survival in patients undergoing radical resection. The results of the study indicated that in patients in whom MRI predicts that a clear circumferential resection margin is achievable by the surgeon, 94% will have a clear margin on histology. A potentially affected margin on MRI identifies the patients that will most likely benefit from neoadjuvant chemoradiation. The limitations of the phased-array coil MRI are the need for training in the acquisition techniques and the interpretation of the images, the long examination time (up to 45 minutes), movement-related artifacts, and its low accuracy in predicting nodal involvement.[15,16]

Comparing Computed Tomography, Magnetic Resonance Imaging, and Endorectal Ultrasound

Compared to MRI and CT, ERUS is more readily available, portable, and less expensive. It requires the least amount of time (average of 15 minutes) and causes minimal patient discomfort. In addition, ERUS is performed by the surgeon, who can direct the examination with specific operative considerations in mind, in the preoperative setting as well as during postoperative surveillance. Over the past 30 years, ERUS has become a valuable tool in the local staging of rectal cancer. Table 143-1 cites studies that have evaluated the diagnostic accuracy of ERUS, alone or in comparison with other modalities. In the hands of experienced clinicians, the accuracy of ERUS is reported to be as high as 95% in

TABLE 143-1 Accuracy of Endorectal Ultrasound in the Staging of Rectal Cancer

Authors	Year	No. of patients	Accuracy (%)	Sensitivity (%)	Specificity (%)	Positive Predictive Value (%)	Negative Predictive Value (%)	Overstaging (%)	Understaging (%)
Beynon[17]	1989	100 (T)	93 (T)	99 (T)	91 (T)	97 (T)	95 (T)	5 (T)	2 (T)
		95 (N)	83 (N)	88 (N)	79 (N)	78 (N)	89 (N)	11 (N)	2 (N)
Hildebrandt et al[18]	1990	113	79 (N)	72 (N)	83 (N)	72 (N)	83 (N)	11 (N)	11 (N)
Orrom et al[19]	1990	77 (T)	75 (T)	ND (T)	ND (T)	ND	ND	22 (T)	3 (T)
		61 (N)	82 (N)	62 (N)	88 (N)	ND	ND	ND (N)	ND (N)
Herzog et al[6]	1993	87 (T)	91 (T)	98 (T)	75 (T)	89 (T)	95 (T)	10 (T)	1 (T)
		111 (N)	80 (N)	89 (N)	73 (N)	71 (N)	90 (N)	15 (N)	5 (N)
Rafaelsen et al[3]	1994	107 (T)	89 (T)	96 (T)	77 (T)	88 (T)	91 (T)	8 (T)	3 (T)
		53 (N)	70 (N)	58 (N)	76 (N)	58 (N)	76 (N)	15 (N)	15 (N)
Sailer et al[20]	1997	162	78 (T)	97 (T)	80 (T)	83 (T)	97 (T)	19 (T)	3 (T)
Akasu et al[21]	1997	152	82 (T)	ND (T)	ND (T)	ND (T)	ND (T)	11 (T)	7 (T)
			77 (N)	79 (N)	75 (N)	78 (N)	76 (N)	12 (N)	11 (N)
Kim et al[10]	1999	89 (T)	81 (T)	ND (T)	ND (T)	ND (T)	ND (T)	10 (T)	9 (T)
		85 (N)	64 (N)	53 (N)	75 (N)	71 (N)	59 (N)	12 (N)	25 (N)
Hunerbein et al[12]	2000	30	83 (T)	ND	ND	ND	ND	4 (T)	12 (T)
			80 (N)					0 (N)	5 (N)
Kwok et al[22]	2000	2915 (T)	87 (T)	93 (T)	78 (T)	87 (T)	87 (T)	11 (T)	5 (T)
		2032 (N)	74 (N)	71 (N)	76 (N)	69 (N)	78 (N)	ND (N)	ND (N)
Garcia-Aguilar et al[23]	2002	545 (T)	69 (T)	ND (T)	ND (T)	72 (T)	93 (T)	18 (T)	13 (T)
		238 (N)	64 (N)	33 (N)	82 (N)	52 (N)	68 (N)	11 (N)	25 (N)
Marusch et al[24]	2002	422	63 (T)	83 (T)	70 (T)	ND	ND	24 (T)	13 (T)
Zammit et al[25]	2005	117 (2 groups)	76 (T)	ND (T)	ND (T)	ND (T)	ND (T)	11/15 (T)	21/5 (N)
			74 (N)	40/71 (N)	82/81 (N)	57/77 (N)	70/76 (N)	11/10 (N)	22/13 (N)
Kim et al[26]	2006	86	69 (T)	92 (T)	ND (T)	74 (T)	ND (T)	ND	ND
			56 (N)	56 (N)	57 (N)	53 (N)	57 (N)		
Ptok et al[27]	2006	3501	66 (T)	75 (T3)	ND	ND	ND	ND	ND
Skandarajah et al[28]	2006	2718	82 (T)	ND	ND	ND	ND	ND	ND
			73 (N)						
Landmann et al[29]	2007	134	70 (N)	ND	76 (N)	ND	ND	16 (N)	14 (N)
Badger et al[30]	2007	95	72 (T)	96 (T3)	33 (T3)	70 (T3)	86 (T3)	24 (T)	4 (T)
			69 (N)	73 (N)	62 (N)	74 (N)	60 (N)	16 (N)	15 (N)

N, Nodal disease; *ND*, not done; *T*, tumor.

assessing the T stage and 80% in assessing the N stage of rectal cancer.[3,6,10-12,17-30]

Two metaanalyses have compared the ERUS, MRI, and CT for staging of rectal cancer. In 2000, Kwok et al published a systematic review of 83 studies conducted between 1980 and 1998, with data on 4897 patients.[22] The analysis indicated that ERUS had the best performance in assessing depth of invasion, compared to MRI and CT. For assessment of nodal status, the performance of ERUS and MRI was similar, and better than that of CT. Bipat et al published a metaanalysis of 90 articles written between 1985 and 2002, in order to compare ERUS, CT, and MRI in rectal cancer staging.[31] ERUS and MRI had similar sensitivity in detecting T2 stage; however, ERUS had significantly higher specificity (86% vs. 69%). For evaluating perirectal tissue invasion (T3 stage), the sensitivity of ERUS (90%) was significantly higher than that of CT (79%) and MRI (82%); specificities were comparable. Sensitivity and specificity for adjacent organ invasion (T4 stage) were similar between the three modalities. The analysis showed no difference in performance between ERUS, CT, or MRI in the assessment of lymph node involvement.

Specificity, Sensitivity, and Accuracy of Endorectal Ultrasound

The technique involved in ERUS is highly operator dependent, with a significant learning curve. This was demonstrated by Orrom et al, who evaluated 77 patients with rectal cancer staged by ERUS and assessed the accuracy of the examination over three time periods.[19] In the first time period, examinations were performed by several clinicians, including nonsurgical staff. The accuracy of ERUS for determining the T stage during this period was only 58%, with 37% of lesions overstaged and 4% understaged. In the second and third time periods, all examinations were performed by one surgeon, and the use of a rigid proctoscope for the introduction of the ERUS probe was instituted. Accuracy of assessment during the second time period increased to 77%, with 20% overstaging and 3% understaging. In the third time period, all scans were interpreted according to the five-layer model of ERUS anatomy. Accuracy increased to 95%, with only 5% overstaging and no understaging. The accuracy for determining N stage also improved from 71% for the first period to 88% for the second and third periods.

In 2002, Garcia-Aguilar et al published the largest single-institution study to date, based on 10 years of ERUS experience at the University of Minnesota.[23] The study included 545 patients with rectal cancer staged with ERUS and treated with surgery without neoadjuvant chemoradiotherapy (307 were treated with local excision and 238 with radical surgery). Three board-certified, experienced colorectal surgeons performed 97% of the examinations. The overall accuracy of ERUS in assessing T stage was 69%, with 18% overstaging and 13% understaging. The accuracy of ERUS in diagnosing nodal disease was 64%, based on data from the 238 patients treated with radical surgery. The authors hypothesized that the study underestimated the overall accuracy of ERUS as a consequence of the exclusion of patients with locally advanced cancers who underwent neoadjuvant treatment. ERUS was most accurate in detecting benign villous adenomas. The stage-specific accuracy was 87% for T0, 47% for T1, 68% for T2, 70% for T3, and 50% for T4 tumors. The distance of the tumor from the anal verge did not influence the accuracy of the examination. In addition to the T stage of the tumor, the only other independent factor affecting the accuracy of the test was the surgeon performing the ERUS.

Currently, ERUS is widely used in the local staging of rectal cancer in the United States.[32] MRI is another valuable tool especially in distinguishing patients at risk for locally advanced disease (i.e., positive circumferential margin), who may benefit from preoperative chemoradiation. The two modalities should be considered complementary rather than mutually exclusive in the evaluation of patients with rectal cancer for treatment and operative planning.

Endorectal Ultrasound Assessment of Depth of Invasion

In 1985, Hildebrandt and Feifel introduced the ultrasonographic staging of rectal cancer as a modification of the TNM staging system (Table 143-2).[33] The prefix *u* denotes ultrasound staging, as opposed to the prefix *p*, which denotes pathologic staging. Sonographically, a rectal cancer appears as a hypoechoic mass that causes disruption of the layers of the rectal wall.

uT0 Lesions. Lesions staged as uT0 are noninvasive and confined to the rectal mucosa. Benign villous adenomas are uT0 lesions. On ERUS imaging, the mucosal layer is expanded but the middle white line (submucosa) remains intact. The middle white line is the key to determining whether a lesion is benign (Figure 143-4). Benign lesions accurately identified by ERUS may be treated with local excision in the submucosal plane. ERUS is reliable in distinguishing benign lesions, with accuracy ranging from 87%[23] to 96%.[34] Biopsies of villous tumors may miss foci of malignancy as a result of sampling error. However, ERUS can detect a malignant focus within a villous adenoma.[35] Worrell et al performed a metaanalysis on the data for 258 biopsy-negative rectal adenomas from five studies.[36] Focal carcinoma was detected in 24% of these tumors on histopathology. ERUS correctly established a diagnosis of cancer in 81% of these cases, thus decreasing the misdiagnosis rate from 24% to 5%. ERUS should be routinely used in the preoperative workup of rectal villous adenomas.

uT1 Lesions. A uT1 lesion is an early cancer that invades the mucosa and submucosa but not the muscularis propria. The ERUS finding is an irregular middle white line (submucosa) without alteration of the outer black line (muscularis propria) (Figure 143-5). Irregularities of the middle white line are seen as a thickening or stippling but must not constitute a distinct break. If a break is seen in the submucosa, the muscularis propria has been invaded and the tumor is a T2 lesion. Garcia-Aguilar et al reported staging accuracy of 47% in the subgroup of 105 patients with T1 tumors.[23] Kwok et al reported a 96% accuracy rate for T1 lesions.[22]

Accurate staging of uT1 lesions is important, because select uT1 lesions are amenable to local therapy. However, lymph node involvement occurs in up to 20% of T1 rectal cancers.[37-39] ERUS may identify this subgroup of patients with uT1 tumors and metastatic lymph nodes, for whom local therapy is contraindicated. In the setting of favorable tumor characteristics and very careful patient

TABLE 143-2 Ultrasound Staging Classification (uTNM) for Rectal Cancer

Classification	Criteria
uT0	Noninvasive lesion confined to the mucosa
uT1	Tumor confined to the submucosa
uT2	Tumor invades into but not through the muscularis propria, remains confined to the rectal wall
uT3	Tumor penetrates through the entire thickness of the rectum and invades the perirectal fat
uT4	Tumor invades an adjacent organ/structure
uN0	No evidence of lymph node metastasis (no definable lymph nodes by ultrasound)
uN1	Evidence of lymph node metastasis (ultrasonographically apparent lymph nodes)

uTNM, Ultrasonographic staging of tumor, node, and metastasis.

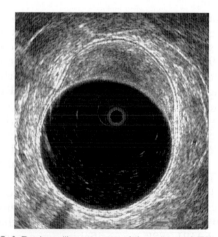

FIGURE 143-4 Benign villous tumor of the rectum (uT0). The *middle white line* is intact around the entire breadth of the tumor, indicating that the submucosa is not involved. (From Wong WD, Orrom WJ, Jensen LL: Preoperative staging of rectal cancer with endorectal ultrasonography. *Perspect Colon Rectal Surg* 3:315, 1990.)

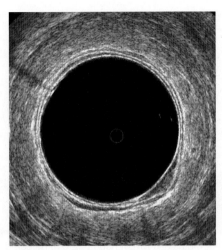

FIGURE 143-5 A uT1 lesion. There is invasion into the submucosa, and although the *middle white line* is not disrupted, it is thickened and irregular. The muscularis propria *(outer black line)* is not expanded, and the *outer white line* is intact.

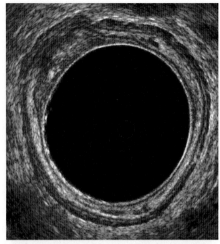

FIGURE 143-6 A uT2 lesion. The submucosa *(middle white line)* is disrupted, and there is expansion/invasion of the muscularis propria *(outer black line)*. The *outer white line* (perirectal fat) is intact, demonstrating that the tumor is confined to the bowel wall.

selection, local resection with negative margins can lead to low recurrence, and excellent quality of life.[39-41] We approach these patients with curative intent. Use of adjuvant chemoradiotherapy is based on the pathology of the excised tumor.

uT2 Lesions. A uT2 cancer disrupts the middle white line and invades the second hypoechoic layer (muscularis propria) but remains confined to the rectal wall. Characteristically there is expansion of the muscularis propria, but the interface between the muscularis propria and perirectal fat (outermost white line) remains intact. The expansion of the muscularis propria may be variable, depending on the degree of invasion. "Early" uT2 lesions may just penetrate the muscularis propria with minimal expansion of this layer. A distinct break in the middle white line must be identified. "Deep" uT2 lesions have a significant degree of expansion of the muscularis propria that may also appear as "scalloping," but they do not invade the perirectal fat. There is a significant tendency to overstage deep T2 lesions as T3 because of their "scalloped" appearance. Figure 143-6 shows an example of a uT2 lesion.

Accuracy of ERUS in detecting T2 stage is in the range of 68%.[23] Lymph node metastases occur in up to 29% of patients with T2 tumors.[38,42] Local recurrence rates of T2 tumors treated with local surgery alone have been reported as high as 47%, with survival rates as low as 65%.[40,43] We recommend radical surgery (either a sphincter-sparing resection or abdominoperineal resection) for patients who are acceptable surgical candidates and for whom there is a curative intent. Local therapy is reserved for patients with uT2 tumors who are poor-risk surgical candidates, those approached with palliative intent, or those who require an abdominoperineal resection but refuse a permanent colostomy despite appropriate counseling. When local therapy is used for the treatment of uT2 lesions, postoperative chemoradiation treatment is recommended to lower the risk of local recurrence.[44] The American College of Surgeons Oncology Group (ACOSOG) Z6041 phase II trial is currently

underway investigating the efficacy of neoadjuvant chemoradiotherapy and local excision for uT2N0 rectal cancers.

uT3 Lesions. A uT3 lesion is a locally advanced cancer that penetrates through the full thickness of the rectal wall and invades into the perirectal fat. Contiguous structures are not involved. The ERUS findings are a disruption of the outer white line, with extension (like a thumbprint) of the tumor into the perirectal fat. Figure 143-7 shows an example of a uT3 lesion.

The accuracy of ERUS in detecting T3 stage has been reported to be as high as 81%.[6,23] Early superficial uT3 lesions can be difficult to distinguish from deep uT2 lesions. Deep uT3 lesions with extensive invasion into the perirectal fat are readily recognized and reliably staged. Patients with uT3 lesions are candidates for neoadjuvant chemoradiotherapy, followed by surgery. Local therapy is not appropriate treatment for uT3 lesions because lymph node metastases may occur in up to 66%[45] of tumors, and local surgery carries a high rate of local recurrence, even with the addition of adjuvant therapy.[46]

uT4 Lesions. uT4 cancers are locally advanced tumors that invade into adjacent structures such as the bladder, uterus, cervix, vagina, prostate, or seminal vesicles. These tumors are clinically fixed. Sonographically, there is loss of the normal hyperechoic plane between the tumor and the adjacent organ. Specifically, Denonvilliers fascia, which normally appears as a hyperechoic interface between the rectal wall and prostate gland in men, becomes obscured by a uT4 tumor with prostatic invasion. Similarly, obliteration of the distinct hyperechoic plane between the rectum and vagina in women is characteristically seen with a uT4 rectal tumor invading the posterior vaginal wall. Figure 143-8 shows an example of a uT4 rectal cancer invading the posterior vaginal wall.

The treatment of uT4 tumors requires neoadjuvant chemoradiotherapy and in-continuity organ resection for potential cure. However, uT4 rectal cancers are resectable for cure in fewer than half of the cases. The use of preoperative chemoradiotherapy can shrink the

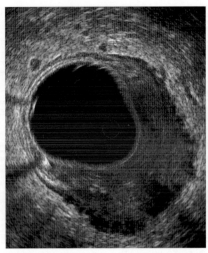

FIGURE 143-7 A uT3 lesion. The interface between the muscularis propria and perirectal fat (outer white line) is irregular and interrupted, indicating extension of tumor into the perirectal fat.

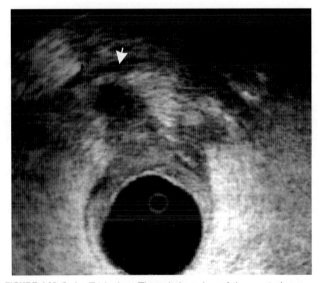

FIGURE 143-8 A uT4 lesion. There is invasion of the posterior vaginal wall (arrow).

tumor, allowing for increased resectability and decreased local recurrence rates. Intraoperative radiation therapy is used in some specialized centers; when used in combination with preoperative radiation, this appears to improve local control in T4 rectal cancers.[47]

Nodal Involvement

ERUS is used to detect potentially malignant mesorectal lymph nodes in patients with rectal cancer. Undetectable or benign-appearing lymph nodes are classified as uN0. Malignant-appearing lymph nodes are classified as uN1. Normal, nonenlarged lymph nodes are generally not seen with ultrasound. Inflamed, enlarged lymph nodes appear hyperechoic, with ill-defined borders, as most of the sound energy is reflected if the lymphatic structure remains unchanged. Metastatic lymph nodes that have been replaced by tumor reflect less sound energy and appear hypoechoic, with an echogenicity resembling that

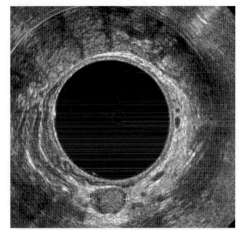

FIGURE 143-9 Metastatic lymph node (1.2 cm) detected with endorectal ultrasound.

of the primary tumor.[18] ERUS cannot detect lymph nodes with micrometastases, however, because these do not significantly alter the sound-reflecting characteristics of lymph node tissue. Malignant lymph nodes tend to be round rather than oval, have discrete borders, and are most commonly found in the mesorectum adjacent or proximal to the primary tumor.[48] Distal lymphatic spread in rectal cancer is unusual without the involvement of proximal lymphatics. Figure 143-9 depicts an example of a metastatic lymph node detected on ERUS.

Nodal size alone is not an accurate predictor of metastatic disease. Sunouchi et al studied hypoechoic lesions larger than 5 mm, and found that 20% were tumor deposits and 68% were metastatic lymph nodes.[49] In a study by Akasu et al, 50% of lymph nodes measuring 3 to 5 mm harbored metastases.[21] Sunouchi et al also described a "small-spot sign" for lesions of the mesorectum measuring 1 to 3 mm and suggested that small hypoechoic spots may correlate with tumor deposits or massive lymphovascular invasion histologically. The finding of small spots may indicate a high risk of hematogenous metastasis and local recurrence.[50] We consider lymph nodes seen on ERUS as potentially positive if they are larger than 3 mm in diameter, round, hypoechoic, and in an appropriate location.

The accuracy of ERUS for nodal staging is lower than that for T staging; accuracy has been reported to be between 64%[23] and 83%.[17] Overstaging is the major error in the diagnosis of lymph node metastases using ERUS. False-positive results may occur as a result of inflammatory lymph nodes. Also, the cross-sectional appearance of blood vessels in the perirectal fat may be confused with positive lymph nodes. Careful, repeated scanning of the area in question can demonstrate the sonographic continuity of hypoechoic vessels over a distance greater than the cross-sectional diameter, thus distinguishing them from hypoechoic lymph nodes. Another criterion is that blood vessels branch or extend longitudinally. Additionally, it may be difficult to differentiate the appearance of islands of tumor outside the bowel wall from that of involved nodes. Demonstrating continuity with the main tumor is helpful in making this distinction.

False-negative results (understaging) are also a problem. This is partially because of the presence of lymph node micrometastases, which current ERUS technology cannot detect. Moreover, involved lymph nodes may be missed when they lie beyond the imaging range of the ultrasound transducer. This is particularly true for nodes in the proximal mesorectum, above the reach of the rigid probe.

Landmann et al evaluated the ability of ERUS to identify or exclude lymph node metastasis in early (T1 and T2) rectal cancers and thereby select patients appropriate for local therapy.[29] The study cohort was 134 patients with rectal cancer evaluated with ERUS at MSKCC and treated with radical resection without neoadjuvant therapy. The overall accuracy of ERUS nodal staging was 70%, with a 16% false-positive rate and a 14% false-negative rate. Early rectal lesions were more likely to have small nodal deposits not detected by ERUS. This correlated with the relationship noted in the study between nodal staging accuracy and T stage: less than 50% accuracy for pT1 lesions, but more than 80% accuracy for pT3 lesions. The findings of this study may explain the relatively high rates of recurrence seen after local excision, and reinforce the need for better preoperative selection of node-negative patients, possibly through molecular profiling.[51]

Proposed Modification of the Endorectal Ultrasound Staging System

We have modified the uTNM classification into a treatment-oriented staging system to address clinical considerations for each stage (Table 143-3). In this system, uTw lesions include uT0 and uT1 tumors, which are amenable to local excision. The second group, uTy, consists of uT2 and select superficial uT3 lesions; the recommended treatment for this group is radical surgery without neoadjuvant therapy. The third group, uTz, includes deep uT3 and uT4 lesions, which are best treated with neoadjuvant therapy followed by radical resection. The stratification of rectal tumors into groups amenable to specific treatment plans constitutes the major advantage of this modified system. We are currently using this system at MSKCC, along with the uTNM classification, to stage our rectal cancer patients.

TABLE 143-3 Proposed Modified Endorectal Ultrasound Staging System (uTNM) for Rectal Cancer

Classification	Criteria
uTw: uT0/uT1	Amenable to local excision
uTy: uT2/superficial uT3	Recommend radical surgery
uTz: Deep uT3/any uT4	Recommend neoadjuvant treatment followed by radical surgery
uN1: probable or definite	Recommend neoadjuvant treatment
uNx: equivocal	Base treatment on T stage and pathologic features

uTNM, Ultrasonographic staging of tumor, node, and metastasis.

Limitations of Endorectal Ultrasound

The ERUS technique is highly operator dependent and requires experience in accurate interpretation of the results, with a significant learning curve.[19] Overall staging accuracy improves with adequate training and experience, optimal technique, and high-quality equipment. Overstaging of the depth of wall invasion has been reported in the range of 11%[22] to 18%.[23] Understaging occurs less frequently, with rates between 5%[22] and 13%[23] (see Table 143-1). Understaging is significantly more serious than overstaging because it may result in inadequate management; with overstaging potentially more aggressive management is advised than might be required. Overstaging depth of invasion may result from inflammation at the deep edge of the tumor, preoperative radiation, hemorrhage in the rectal wall following biopsy, or a tendency of the observer to fear understaging depth of invasion. ERUS tends to understage disease in the setting of stenotic, near-obstructing tumors; examination may not be possible or complete in the setting of lesions that cannot accommodate passage of the probe.

The accuracy of ERUS after a biopsy may differ based on the time interval from the biopsy. A study reported rates of T-stage accuracy as low as 53% if ERUS was done 3 weeks after biopsy. This is related mostly to overstaging. The study indicated that the best accuracy was obtained if the ERUS was done before the biopsy; the second best option was for ERUS to be done the first week after a biopsy.[52]

The impact of the tumor distance from the anal verge on the accuracy of ERUS staging has been controversial. A few small studies have reported higher accuracy for proximal compared to distal tumors, attributed to difficulties in achieving uniform contact between the water balloon and the rectal wall and to suboptimal delineation of the rectal wall layers immediately above the anorectal ring. However, Garcia-Aguilar et al in their study found that the distance from the anal verge had no impact on the staging accuracy of ERUS.[23]

Overstaging of lymph node involvement occurs between 5%[17] and 15%[6] of the time. This is a result of the presence of inflammatory lymph nodes, blood vessels, or tumor deposits in the mesorectum. Understaging occurs between 2%[17] and 25%[10] of the time, and is partially caused by the inability of ERUS to detect lymph node micrometastases.

It is particularly important to recognize factors that affect the accuracy of ERUS and may lead to misinterpretation of ultrasound images.[53] For example, if the ultrasound probe is not at a 90-degree angle with the area of interest, balloon–wall separation may occur, mimicking a (nonexistent) rectal lesion. Poor bowel preparation or retained air can produce shadowing artifacts. Finally, cautery burns from endoscopic biopsies or excisions may alter the image and significantly affect the accuracy of sonographic assessment.

Endorectal Ultrasound Restaging After Neoadjuvant Therapy

Neoadjuvant chemoradiotherapy is used to treat locally advanced rectal cancers, producing a complete pathologic response in up to 33% of cases.[54,55] Radiation causes inflammation, edema, and fibrosis and obscures differentiation of the layers of the rectal wall, making sonographic distinction between residual tumor and radiation-induced changes difficult. Reevaluation of rectal tumors with ERUS after neoadjuvant chemoradiotherapy is inaccurate, with high rates of overstaging.[56]

ERUS after chemoradiotherapy appears to be least accurate in patients with visual and sonographic evidence of response, and studies indicate that the misinterpretation correlates with the downstaging of the tumor.[57] It has been suggested that, after radiation therapy, the ERUS no longer stages the tumor but rather the fibrosis that takes its place.[58]

Unfortunately, all conventional imaging modalities (ERUS, CT, MRI) are unreliable in the detection of complete response following neoadjuvant treatment and cannot identify a subgroup of patients who might safely avoid radical surgery.[56,59] It is possible that advances in technology will enhance the restaging accuracy of MRI.[60] Positron emission tomography scan also shows promise in the restaging of rectal cancer after neoadjuvant chemoradiotherapy.[61]

Endorectal Ultrasound for Postoperative Followup

Local recurrence rates of rectal cancer have decreased significantly over the last decade, with the use of improved surgical technique and combined-modality therapy. Local recurrence rates for early rectal cancers after radical surgery are 3% for T1 cancers and 6% for T2 cancers.[39,40] The rate increases to 28% after local excision.[40] Greenberg et al reported a local recurrence rate of 18% for T2 cancers treated with local excision and adjuvant chemoradiotherapy.[44] Locally advanced rectal cancers treated with combined-modality therapy and total mesorectal excision have local recurrence rates as low as 6%.[62]

Early detection of recurrence is important, as well as challenging. Surveillance programs should focus on detection of resectable anastomotic and locoregional failures, in addition to treatable systemic metastases and metachronous colonic tumors. ERUS has been used to follow patients after local excision or low anterior resection for rectal cancer. Transvaginal ultrasound may be performed in female patients after abdominoperineal resection. ERUS is also used to follow patients after chemoradiation therapy for anal canal carcinomas. After surgery, the excision site appears as a pattern of mixed echogenicity, replacing the normal five-layer image. Anastomotic staples typically appear as a circumferential line of small, local hyperechoic foci, without shadowing.[63]

It is recommended that a "baseline" ultrasound be performed approximately 3 months after surgery, with future comparisons at 3- to 4-month intervals. A good baseline examination is useful in documenting postoperative scarring and evaluating possible changes over time. Serial ultrasound evaluations may identify and confirm suspicious areas, which may then be biopsied via a transrectal, ultrasound-guided approach.[64] Locally recurrent cancer that is advanced and detected by digital and endoscopic examination has hypoechoic ultrasonographic appearance similar to primary rectal cancers.

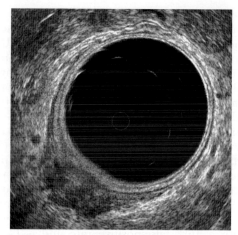

FIGURE 143-10 Locally recurrent rectal cancer. There is a hypoechoic mass in the extrarectal tissues, and the inner rectal wall appears normal. Sigmoidoscopy revealed normal rectal mucosa.

Tumor recurrence is often first identified outside the rectal wall, in an area adjacent to the anastomosis. Extrarectal recurrent tumor often appears on ERUS as a circumscribed, hypoechoic lesion in the paraanastomotic extrarectal tissues, with all or a portion of the rectal wall intact on the luminal aspect. Furthermore, ERUS may identify metastatic lymph nodes that develop in the mesorectum after local excision of a rectal cancer. Figure 143-10 is an example of a locally recurrent tumor detected by ERUS.

ERUS detects local recurrence at an earlier and asymptomatic stage, compared to other surveillance methods.[63,65] The impact of earlier diagnosis of local recurrences in patient survival has not been documented because of the lack of large, prospective, randomized trials; however, metaanalyses have established that overall survival is significantly improved for patients in the more intensive programs of followup.[66,67] Aggressive surveillance seems reasonable for patients who may be candidates for salvage treatment.[68] ERUS followup is particularly useful for patients treated with local therapies for early rectal cancers, because early diagnosis of tumor recurrence is critical if curative salvage surgery is to be considered.

Although the optimal interval for repeat followup examinations has not been determined, and the cost-effectiveness of followup ERUS has not been assessed, ERUS is recognized as an important test for postoperative followup. Certainly, ERUS should not be considered the sole constituent of any surveillance program; rather, ERUS should complement clinical examination, proctoscopy, and serum carcinoembryonic antigen levels as part of a comprehensive rectal cancer surveillance strategy. At MSKCC, we perform ultrasound examinations every 4 months for the first 3 years after local excision for rectal cancer and every 6 months for the next 3 to 5 years.

Three-Dimensional Endorectal Ultrasound

Three-dimensional ERUS provides high-resolution multiplanar images, which can then be rotated, tilted, and sliced to allow the operator to visualize the lesion at different angles, and measure accurately distance, area, angle, and volume. The three-dimensional view resembles closely the original anatomy and has the potential to improve the examiner's understanding of spatial relations between the tumor and anatomic structures and to increase the diagnostic accuracy of ERUS.[69] Volume render mode is a special feature that analyzes information inside three-dimensional data volume and reconstructs information inside the cube, thus enhancing the visualization of pathologic and anatomic structures.[70]

The three-dimensional ERUS has been shown in small studies to have similar or superior accuracy to standard ERUS.[12,26,71] Three-dimensional ERUS has also been evaluated in the staging of obstructive, stenotic rectal cancers[72] and the diagnosis of locally recurrent rectal cancer,[73] and anal cancer,[74] with promising results.

ENDOANAL ULTRASOUND: ENDOSONOGRAPHY OF THE ANAL CANAL

EAUS is the diagnostic test of choice for the evaluation of the anal sphincter anatomy and the identification of sphincter defects associated with fecal incontinence. It has particular value in the diagnosis of complex perianal fistulas. Furthermore, EAUS is used in the staging and followup of anal neoplasms.

The equipment used is the same as the equipment used for ERUS, with a minor modification. A translucent plastic cap (Brüel & Kjaer WA0453) is placed over the transducer and is filled with water, which provides the acoustic medium. A pinhole in the apex of the plastic cap allows for removal of the air bubbles through displacement with water. The technique for EAUS is similar to that for ERUS. Patients should be reassured that this examination will be no more uncomfortable than a DRE. The patient is examined in the left lateral decubitus position. Inspection of the perineum and digital examination precede EAUS assessment. The probe is lubricated with water-soluble jelly and gently inserted into the anus to the level of the upper anal canal. The entire length of the anal canal is evaluated while the probe is withdrawn slowly.

NORMAL ENDOANAL ULTRASOUND ANATOMY

The anatomy of the anal canal is imaged sonographically at three levels (upper, mid, and distal anal canal).[75] Figure 143-11 shows the upper anal canal. The puborectalis muscle is an important landmark for the upper anal canal and is seen as a horseshoe-shaped white structure (hyperechoic striated muscle) that forms the lateral and posterior portions of the upper anal canal.

In the midanal canal, the internal anal sphincter appears as a complete dark band around the probe (hypoechoic smooth muscle), surrounded by the hyperechoic external anal sphincter. A hyperechoic ring is seen between the transducer and the internal sphincter, representing subepithelial, hemorrhoidal, and submucosal tissues. Figure 143-12 shows the midanal canal. The internal anal sphincter is most prominent at the level of the midanal canal. The perineal body in women is usually measured at this level. With the ultrasound probe in place, the index finger of the examiner's right

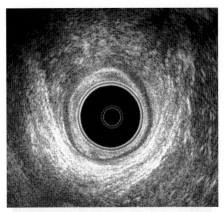

FIGURE 143-11 Upper anal canal. The puborectalis muscle is seen as a horseshoe-shaped hyperechoic structure and is an important landmark for the upper anal canal.

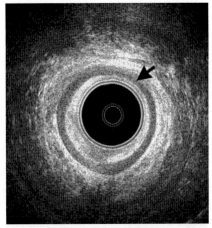

FIGURE 143-12 Midanal canal. The internal anal sphincter appears hypoechoic *(arrow)* and is surrounded by the hyperechoic external anal sphincter.

hand is simultaneously inserted into the vagina. As Figure 143-13 illustrates, the distance between the ultrasound reflection of the finger and the inner aspect of the internal sphincter may be measured; the distance corresponds to the perineal body. Normal values for perineal body thickness (PBT) are approximately 10 to 15 mm. Measurement of the perineal body is useful in evaluation of women with incontinence from anterior sphincter defects and pelvic floor disorders.[76]

In the distal anal canal (Figure 143-14), the internal anal sphincter is not seen. Only the hyperechoic external anal sphincter and surrounding soft tissues are visualized.

ANAL SPHINCTER DEFECTS AND FECAL INCONTINENCE

EAUS is a valuable tool in the workup of fecal incontinence, detecting anatomic anal sphincter defects and identifying patients who would benefit from surgery. Causes of sphincter defects include obstetric injury, perianal trauma, anorectal surgery, and congenital abnormalities.

Obstetric injury to the anal sphincter is the most common cause of incontinence in young women. Most

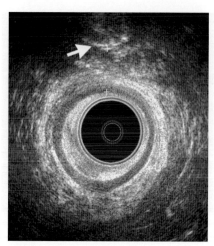

FIGURE 143-13 Perineal body measurement. The distance between the hyperechoic reflection of the examiner's finger *(arrow)* and the inner aspect of the internal sphincter is measured.

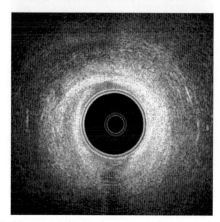

FIGURE 143-14 Distal anal canal. The internal anal sphincter is not seen, and only the hyperechoic external anal sphincter and surrounding soft tissues are visualized.

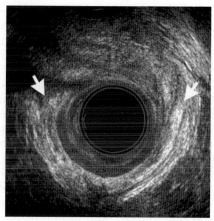

FIGURE 143-15 Anterior anal sphincter defect in a woman with incontinence. The distance between the two *arrows* represents an anterior defect in both the internal and external anal sphincters.

patients will have had primary repair of a fourth-degree tear at the time of vaginal delivery, with subsequent fecal incontinence. However, occult sphincter defects have been reported to be common after vaginal delivery, with an incidence as high as 30% in primiparous women.[77,78] Patients may develop delayed symptoms of incontinence several years following an unrecognized sphincter injury.[79] As the peak incidence of fecal incontinence among women occurs in the fifth and sixth decades, the effects of aging, menopause, and progression of a neuropathy all may contribute to sphincter weakness in the long-term. It appears that nerve damage is cumulative, whereas direct sphincter damage most likely occurs on first delivery.

Defects in the external anal sphincter muscle usually appear sonographically as hypoechoic defects, although some may be hyperechoic or may demonstrate mixed echogenicity. In the case of complete sphincter disruption, the ends of both internal and external sphincter muscles are widely separated and bridged by scar tissue. In many patients, complete sphincter disruption is not seen; rather, significant attenuation of the sphincter

muscle is present anteriorly, suggestive of a significant deficit. PBT measurement can help to identify anterior sphincter defects.[76] Normal values for PBT are approximately 10 to 15 mm. Values less than 10 mm are considered abnormal; a PBT of 10 to 12 mm was associated with a sphincter defect in one-third of the patients in a study, whereas patients with a PBT of 12 mm or more were unlikely to harbor a defect.[76] The detection of anterior sphincter defects on EAUS may be improved by gentle pressure on the posterior vaginal wall either with a gloved finger or a balloon.[80]

The importance of EAUS in the diagnostic evaluation of fecal incontinence has been demonstrated in several studies.[81] Other anorectal physiologic tests, such as anorectal manometry and electromyography, are complementary.[82,83] Women with symptoms of fecal incontinence and history of vaginal deliveries should be evaluated with EAUS for an anatomic sphincter defect that may account for the incontinence and be amenable to surgical repair.[84] EAUS is well tolerated, produces minimal discomfort, and provides high-resolution images of both the external and the internal sphincter. EAUS identifies sphincter injuries with a very high degree of accuracy when these injuries are present; however, it has a false-positive rate up to 25%. This can be improved by limiting the evaluation of the anal canal to the most distal 1.5 cm of the anal canal.[85] Figure 143-15 depicts an anterior internal and external anal sphincter defect.

Other causes of anal sphincter defects are perianal trauma and anorectal surgery. Major blunt and penetrating perineal trauma often involves the anal sphincter. Fecal diversion is often required, in addition to debridement, in the case of major soft-tissue perineal injuries. After the injuries have healed, EAUS may be used to assess the remaining anatomy and to determine whether reconstructive surgery is necessary before stomal closure. Fecal incontinence may also occur after anorectal surgery. Most of the time this is transient, but occasionally it persists, warranting evaluation. EAUS has been used to evaluate potential sphincter defects associated with postoperative fecal incontinence following hemorrhoidectomy, lateral internal sphincterotomy,[86,87] or

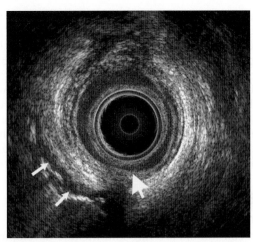

FIGURE 143-16 Fistula-in-ano. The fistula tract appears hypoechoic *(small arrows)*. The internal opening was identified in the midline posteriorly *(large arrow)*.

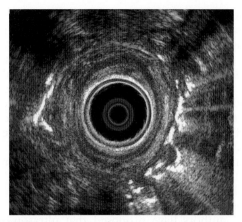

FIGURE 143-17 Fistula-in-ano. Hydrogen peroxide injected into the external orifice of the fistula appears brightly hyperechoic and outlines the fistulous tract.

sphincteroplasty.[88] EAUS has also been used in the evaluation of anterior rectoceles in women.[89]

PERIANAL SEPSIS AND FISTULA-IN-ANO

The diagnosis of a perianal abscess is usually made by clinical examination and requires only proper recognition and prompt drainage. However, sometimes an abscess is strongly suspected by history but is not readily evident on physical examination. EAUS may be used intraoperatively or in the office to localize an obscure abscess and aid in planning the appropriate incision for drainage.[90] Such an example is an intersphincteric abscess, which is often difficult to diagnose clinically but may be suspected because of a history of severe anal pain. Abscesses appear on EAUS as hypoechoic areas, often surrounded by a hyperechoic border.

EAUS may be applied in the evaluation of complex and recurrent fistula-in-ano with high accuracy. It has been shown to be valuable in detecting horseshoe extension and identifying the internal opening.[91] EAUS can anatomically delineate the fistula tract in relation to the anal sphincters. Sonographically, fistula tracts are generally hypoechoic defects and can be followed for direction and extent. Examination should include ultrasound scanning of the anal canal, as well as the distal rectum, to search for high blind tracts. Proposed ultrasonographic criteria for identification of the internal opening include a rootlike budding, formed by the intersphincteric tract, that contacts the internal sphincter; a rootlike budding with an internal sphincter defect; and a subepithelial breech connecting to the intersphincteric tract through an internal sphincter defect.[92] Figure 143-16 is an example of a fistula-in-ano demonstrated with EAUS.

EAUS has been shown to be accurate for determining the fistula anatomy in patients with perianal Crohn disease and useful in guiding their management.[93,94] A study comparing EAUS, pouchography, and CT in the evaluation of patients with dysfunctional ileoanal pouches and inconclusive clinical and endoscopic examinations suggested higher sensitivity of EAUS in the detection of anastomotic leaks and peripouch sepsis.[95]

A variety of techniques are used alone or in conjunction with EAUS in the identification of complex fistulous tracts. These include careful probing; fistulography; and injection with methylene blue dye, milk, hydrogen peroxide, or contrast agents such as Levovist.[96] Hydrogen peroxide injection is used along with EAUS to enhance the imaging of complex and recurrent anal fistulas.[97,98] The release of oxygen accentuates the fistula tract, which shows as a brightly hyperechoic image on the sonogram. Figure 143-17 is an example of a fistula-in-ano visualized on EAUS with hydrogen peroxide enhancement.

RECTOVAGINAL FISTULA

EAUS can be used in the diagnosis of a suspected rectovaginal fistula (RVF) when clinical examination fails to identify a communication.[99] Furthermore, EAUS is valuable in the preoperative workup of patients with RVF. Tsang et al reviewed the experience of the Minnesota Group with RVF repair.[100] EAUS or anal manometry was used preoperatively to detect sphincter defects. If a defect was found, then endorectal advancement flap was more likely to fail and overlapping sphincteroplasty was more likely to be successful, although this difference did not reach statistical significance. The authors proposed that all patients with RVF undergo preoperative evaluation for occult sphincter defects. This becomes especially important if the patient has symptoms of fecal incontinence or if the cause of the RVF is obstetric trauma.

ANAL CANAL NEOPLASMS

EAUS delineates the anal canal anatomy well and has an important role in the evaluation of benign and malignant anal neoplasms. Lesions of the anal canal appear as hypoechoic areas on EAUS, and the size and extent of lesions can be detailed. Tissue confirmation may be obtained with ultrasound-directed needle biopsies, if needed. Benign neoplasms such as lipomas and leiomyomas can be visualized with EAUS, and their relationship to other structures of the anal canal can be defined.

Squamous cell or epidermoid carcinoma is the most common malignancy of the anal canal. EAUS is effective in the initial evaluation and followup of patients with squamous cell carcinoma of the anal canal.[101] Because this cancer is primarily treated with combined chemoradiotherapy, an accurate method of staging the tumor and assessing response to treatment is essential.

EAUS complements the DRE in determining actual size and circumferential involvement of anal canal tumors. EAUS staging (uTNM) of anal canal cancers corresponds to TNM staging (Table 143-4). EAUS accurately measures the greatest diameter of the tumor, which is the basis of T staging for anal canal cancer. Furthermore, EAUS can demonstrate the extent of sphincter muscle involvement. ERUS should always be performed to assess the mesorectum for metastatic lymph nodes. Figure 143-18 depicts an EAUS image of a squamous cell carcinoma of the anal canal.

Some authors have proposed that ultrasound-based staging systems for cancers of the anal canal include depth of tumor invasion. Tarantino and Bernstein proposed a modified endoscopic staging system that emphasized depth of penetration over size of the tumor and used it to distinguish early lesions that might be amenable to less-aggressive treatment.[102] In this system, a uT1 tumor is confined to the submucosa; a uT2a lesion invades only the internal anal sphincter; a uT2b lesion penetrates into the external anal sphincter; a uT3 lesion invades through the sphincter complex into the perianal tissues; and a uT4 lesion invades adjacent structures. Giovannini et al proposed a different ultrasound staging system, where a uT2 lesion is defined as involving the internal sphincter and a uT3 lesion is defined as invading the external sphincter; this system was shown in a prospective, multicenter study to be superior to clinical staging in predicting local recurrence and patient survival.[103]

EAUS is useful in detecting residual tumor as well as early local recurrence after treatment.[104,105] Currently, EAUS is part of most surveillance programs for anal cancer. The small percentage of these patients who fail chemoradiotherapy may undergo abdominoperineal resection for salvage, with a reasonable chance for cure.[106]

MISCELLANEOUS ANORECTAL CONDITIONS

Retrorectal Tumors

Retrorectal tumors are rare and include developmental cysts, teratomas, chordomas, meningoceles, and miscellaneous neurologic and osseous tumors. CT and MRI are the best imaging modalities for identifying these tumors and their relationships to adjacent anatomic structures, such as the sacral nerves. However, ERUS is useful in assessing possible involvement of the rectal wall and may help in planning the appropriate surgical approach. Figure 143-19 shows an ultrasound image of a retrorectal tumor.

Solitary Rectal Ulcer Syndrome and Colitis Cystica Profunda

ERUS can be used in the evaluation of patients with solitary rectal ulcer syndrome or colitis cystica profunda. These conditions are uncommon, but it is important that they are accurately recognized and not mistaken for malignancy. The endoscopic appearance of a solitary rectal ulcer ranges from that of a typical ulcer with a fibrinous central depression to that of a polypoid lesion. It is always located on the anterior aspect of the rectum, 4 to 12 cm from the anal verge. The fold with the ulcer is thought to represent the lead point of an intussusception into the anal canal. Chronic, repeated straining or prolapse of this lead point result in ischemia and ulceration. Pathologic evaluation reveals obliteration of the lamina propria by fibrosis. In the case of

Table 143-4 Ultrasound Staging Classification (uTNM) for Anal Canal Cancer

Classification	Criteria
uT1	Maximal diameter <2 cm
uT2	Maximal diameter 2-5 cm
uT3	Maximal diameter >5 cm
uT4	Adjacent organ invasion
uN0	No evidence of lymph node metastasis
uN1	Evidence of lymph node metastasis

uTNM, Ultrasonographic staging of tumor, node, and metastasis.

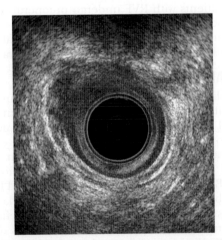

FIGURE 143-18 Squamous cell carcinoma of the anus. The lesion measured 2.4 cm in maximal diameter, indicating a uT2 anal canal tumor involving both internal and external anal sphincters.

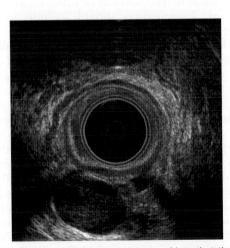

FIGURE 143-19 Retrorectal/presacral tumor. Note that the rectal wall is not involved on the basis of ultrasound assessment.

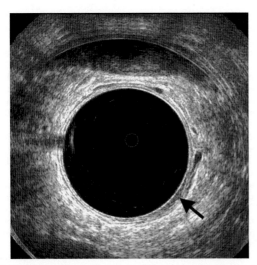

FIGURE 143-20 Solitary rectal ulcer syndrome. There is thickening of the mucosa and irregularity of the submucosa (arrow).

colitis cystica profunda, pathologic examination reveals mucin-containing glands misplaced in the submucosa and lined with normal colonic epithelium.

Sonographically, a solitary rectal ulcer appears as an area of thickened submucosa. The submucosa appears hyperechoic in patients with solitary rectal ulcer because of fibrosis. In contrast, in patients with colitis cystica profunda, the submucosa appears hypoechoic as a result of mucus-filled cysts.[107] Figure 143-20 is an example of a solitary rectal ulcer identified on ERUS.

SUMMARY

ERUS has proved to be a valuable tool in the diagnosis and management of many anorectal disorders. The accuracy of examination is operator dependent and improves with experience. ERUS is valuable in the preoperative local staging of rectal and anal canal cancers. Moreover, it has an important role in surveillance after treatment of rectal and anal cancers. ERUS is the diagnostic test of choice for evaluation of fecal incontinence and can be used in the diagnosis of several other benign anorectal conditions. The use of endorectal ultrasonography by surgeons has contributed greatly to the understanding and management of anorectal disease.

SUGGESTED READINGS

Barabouti DG, Wong WD: Clinical Staging of Rectal Cancer. *Semin Colon Rectal Surg* 16:104, 2005.

De Anda EH, Suk-Hawn L, Finne CO, et al: Endorectal ultrasound in the follow-up of rectal cancer patients treated by local excision or radical surgery. *Dis Colon Rectum* 47:818, 2004.

Kruskal JB, Kane RA, Morrin MM: Peroxide-enhanced anal endosonography: Technique, image interpretation, and clinical applications. *Radiographics* 21:S173, 2001.

Landmann RG, Wong WD, Hoepfl J, et al: Limitations of early rectal cancer nodal staging may explain failure after local excision. *Dis Colon Rectum* 50:1520, 2007.

Schaffzin DM, Wong WD: Surgeon-performed ultrasound: Endorectal ultrasound. *Surg Clin North Am.* 84:1127, 2004.

Skandarajah AR, Tjandra JJ: Preoperative loco-regional imaging in rectal cancer. *Aust N Z J Surg* 76:497, 2006.

REFERENCES

1. Steele SR, Martin MJ, Place RJ: Flexible endorectal ultrasound for predicting pathologic stage of rectal cancers. *Am J Surg* 184:126, 2002.
2. Beynon J, Foy DM, Temple LN, et al: The endosonic appearances of normal colon and rectum. *Dis Colon Rectum* 28:810, 1986.
3. Rafaelsen SR, Kronberg O, Fenger C: Digital rectal examination and transrectal ultrasonography in staging of rectal cancer. *Acta Radiol* 35:300, 1994.
4. Starck M, Bohe M, Fork FT, et al: Endoluminal ultrasound and low-field magnetic resonance imaging are superior to clinical examination in the preoperative staging of rectal cancer. *Eur J Surg* 161:841, 1995.
5. Goldman S, Arvidsson H, Norming U, et al: Transrectal ultrasound and computed tomography in preoperative staging of lower rectal adenocarcinoma. *Gastrointest Radiol* 16:259, 1991.
6. Herzog U, Von Flue M, Tondelli P, et al: How accurate is endorectal ultrasound in the preoperative staging of rectal cancer? *Dis Colon Rectum* 36:127, 1993.
7. Kulinna C, Scheidler J, Strauss T, et al: Local staging of rectal cancer: Assessment with double-contrast multislice computed tomography and transrectal ultrasound. *J Comput Assist Tomogr* 28:123, 2004.
8. Vliegen R, Dresen R, Beets G, et al: The accuracy of multidetector-row CT for the assessment of tumor invasion of the mesorectal fascia in primary rectal cancer. *Abdom Imaging* 33:604, 2008.
9. Maizlin Z, Brown J, Tiwari P, et al: Can CT replace MRI in preoperative assessment of the circumferential resection margin in rectal cancer? *Dis Colon Rectum* 53:308, 2010.
10. Kim NK, Kim MJ, Yun SH, et al: Comparative study of transrectal ultrasonography, pelvic computerized tomography, and magnetic resonance imaging in preoperative staging of rectal cancer. *Dis Colon Rectum* 42:770, 1999.
11. Kim NK, Kim MJ, Park JK, et al: Preoperative staging of rectal cancer with MRI: Accuracy and clinical usefulness. *Ann Surg Oncol* 7:732, 2000.
12. Hunerbein M, Pegios W, Rau B, et al: Prospective comparison of endorectal ultrasound, three-dimensional endorectal ultrasound, and endorectal MRI in the preoperative evaluation of rectal tumors: Preliminary results. *Surg Endosc* 14:1005, 2000.
13. Matsuoka H, Masaki T, Sugiyama M, et al: Gadolinium-enhanced endorectal coil and air enema magnetic resonance imaging as a useful tool in the preoperative examination of patients with rectal carcinoma. *Hepatogastroenterology* 51:131, 2004.
14. Mercury Study Group: Diagnostic accuracy of preoperative magnetic resonance imaging in predicting curative resection of rectal cancer: Prospective observational study. *BMJ* 333:779, 2006.
15. Taylor FG, Swift RI, Blomqvist L, et al: A systematic approach to the interpretation of preoperative staging MRI for rectal cancer. *AJR Am J Roentgenol* 191:1827, 2008.
16. Lahaye MJ, Engelen SM, Kessels AG, et al: USPIO-enhanced MR imaging for nodal staging in patients with primary rectal cancer: Predictive criteria. *Radiology* 246:804, 2008.
17. Beynon J: An evaluation of the role of rectal endosonography in rectal cancer. *Ann R Coll Surg Engl* 71:131, 1989.
18. Hildebrandt U, Klein T, Feifel G, et al: Endosonography of para-rectal lymph nodes: In vitro and in vivo evaluation. *Dis Colon Rectum* 33:863, 1990.
19. Orrom WJ, Wong WD, Rothenberger DA, et al: Endorectal ultrasound in the preoperative staging of rectal tumors: A learning experience. *Dis Colon Rectum* 33:654, 1990.
20. Sailer M, Leppert R, Bussen D, et al: Influence of tumor position on accuracy of endorectal ultrasound staging. *Dis Colon Rectum* 40:1180, 1997.
21. Akasu T, Sugihara K, Moriya Y, et al: Limitations and pitfalls of transrectal ultrasonography for staging of rectal cancer. *Dis Colon Rectum* 40:S10-S15, 1997.
22. Kwok H, Bissett IP, Hill GL: Preoperative staging of rectal cancer. *Int J Colorectal Dis* 15:9, 2000.

23. Garcia-Aguilar J, Pollack J, Lee S-K, et al: Accuracy of endorectal ultrasonography in preoperative staging of rectal tumors. *Dis Colon Rectum* 45:10, 2002.

24. Marusch F, Koch A, Schmidt U, et al: Routine use of transrectal ultrasound in rectal carcinoma: Results of a prospective multi-center study. *Endoscopy* 34:385, 2002.

25. Zammit M, Jenkins T, Urie A, et al: A technically difficult endorectal ultrasound is more likely to be inaccurate. *Colorectal Dis* 7:486, 2005.

26. Kim JC, Kim HC, Yu SC, et al: Efficacy of 3-dimensional endorectal ultrasonography compared with conventional ultrasonography and computed tomography in preoperative rectal cancer staging. *Am J Surg* 192:89, 2006.

27. Ptok H, Marusch F, Meyer F, et al: Feasibility and accuracy of TRUS in the pre-treatment staging for rectal carcinoma in general practice. *Eur J Surg Oncol* 32:420, 2006.

28. Skandarajah AR, Tjandra JJ: Preoperative loco-regional imaging in rectal cancer. *Aust N Z J Surg* 76:497, 2006.

29. Landmann RG, Wong WD, Hoepfl J, et al: Limitations of early rectal cancer nodal staging may explain failure after local excision. *Dis Colon Rectum* 50:1520, 2007.

30. Badger SA, Devlin PB, Neilly PJ, et al: Preoperative staging of rectal carcinoma by endorectal ultrasound: Is there a learning curve? *Int J Colorectal Dis* 22:1261, 2007.

31. Bipat S, Glas AS, Slors FJ, et al: Rectal cancer: Local staging and assessment of lymph node involvement with endoluminal US, CT, and MR imaging—a meta-analysis. *Radiology* 232:773, 2004.

32. Augestad KM, Lindsetmo RO, Stulberg J, et al: International pre-operative rectal cancer management: Staging, neoadjuvant treatment, and impact of multidisciplinary teams. *World J Surg* 34:2689, 2010.

33. Hildebrandt U, Feifel G: Preoperative staging of rectal cancer by intrarectal ultrasound. *Dis Colon Rectum* 28:42, 1985.

34. Pikarsky A, Wexner S, Lebensart P, et al: The use of rectal ultra-sound for the correct diagnosis and treatment of rectal villous tumors. *Am J Surg* 179:261, 2000.

35. Adams WJ, Wong WD: Endorectal ultrasonic detection of malig-nancy within rectal villous lesions. *Dis Colon Rectum* 38:1093, 1995.

36. Worrell S, Horvath K, Blakemore T, et al: Endorectal ultrasound detection of focal carcinoma within rectal adenomas. *Am J Surg* 187:625, 2004.

37. Okabe S, Shia J, Wong WD, et al: Lymph node metastasis in T1 adenocarcinoma of the colon and rectum. *J Gastrointest Surg* 8:1032, 2004.

38. Rasheed S, Bowley DM, Aziz O, et al: Can depth of tumour inva-sion predict lymph node positivity in patients undergoing resec-tion for early rectal cancer? A comparative study between T1 and T2 cancers. *Colorectal Dis* 10:231, 2008.

39. Nash GM, Weiser MR, Guillem JG, et al: Long-term survival after transanal excision of T1 rectal cancer. *Dis Colon Rectum* 52:577, 2009.

40. Mellgren A, Sirivongs P, Rothenberger DA, et al: Is local excision adequate therapy for early rectal cancer? *Dis Colon Rectum* 43:1064, 2000.

41. Hazard LJ, Shrieve DC, Sklow B, et al: Local excision vs. radical resection in T1-2 rectal carcinoma: Results of a study from the Surveillance, Epidemiology, and End Results (SEER) registry data. *Gastrointest Cancer Res* 3:105, 2009.

42. Kajiwara Y, Ueno H, Hashiguchi Y, et al: Risk factors of nodal involvement in T2 colorectal cancer. *Dis Colon Rectum* 53:1393, 2010.

43. Paty PB, Nash GM, Wong WD, et al: Long-term results of local excision for rectal cancer. *Ann Surg* 236:522, 2002.

44. Greenberg JA, Shibata D, Herndon JE 2nd, et al: Local excision of distal rectal cancer: An update of Cancer and Leukemia Group B 8984. *Dis Colon Rectum* 51:1185, 2008.

45. Sitzler PJ, Seow-Choen F, Ho YH, et al: Lymph node involvement and tumor depth in rectal cancers: An analysis of 805 patients. *Dis Colon Rectum* 40:1472, 1997.

46. Wagman R, Minsky BD, Cohen AM, et al: Conservative manage-ment of rectal cancer with local excision and postoperative adju-vant therapy. *Int J Radiat Oncol Biol Phys* 44:841, 1999.

47. Harrison LB, Minsky BD, Enker WE: High-dose-rate intraopera-tive radiation therapy (HDR-IORT) as part of the management strategy for locally advanced primary and recurrent rectal cancer. *Int J Radiat Oncol Biol Phys* 42:325, 1998.

48. Rafaelsen SR, Kronborg O, Fenger C: Echo pattern of lymph nodes in colorectal cancer: An in vitro study. *Br J Radiol* 65:218, 1992.

49. Sunouchi K, Sakaguchi M, Higuchi Y, et al: Limitation of endorec-tal ultrasonography: What does a low lesion more than 5 mm in size correspond to histologically? *Dis Colon Rectum* 41:761, 1998.

50. Sunouchi K, Sakaguchi M, Higuchi Y, et al: Small spot sign of rectal carcinoma by endorectal ultrasonography: Histologic rela-tion and clinical impact on postoperative recurrence. *Dis Colon Rectum* 41:649, 1998.

51. Kammula US, Kuntz EJ, Francone TD, et al: Molecular co-expression of the c-Met oncogene and hepatocyte growth factor in primary colon cancer predicts tumor stage and clinical outcome. *Cancer Lett* 248:219, 2007.

52. Goertz RS, Fein M, Sailer M: Impact of biopsy on the accuracy of endorectal ultrasound staging of rectal tumors. *Dis Colon Rectum* 51:1125, 2008.

53. Kruskal JB, Kane RA, Sentovich SM, et al: Pitfalls and sources of error in staging rectal cancer with endorectal US. *Radiographics* 17:609, 1997.

54. Mehta VK, Poen J, Ford J, et al: Radiotherapy, concomitant pro-tracted-venous-infusion 5-fluorouracil, and surgery for ultrasound-staged T3 or T4 rectal cancer. *Dis Colon Rectum* 44:52, 2001.

55. Guillem JG, Chessin DB, Cohen AM, et al: Long-term oncologic outcome following preoperative combined modality therapy and total mesorectal excision of locally advanced rectal cancer. *Ann Surg* 241:829, discussion 836, 2005.

56. Huh JW, Park YA, Jung EJ, et al: Accuracy of endorectal ultraso-nography and computed tomography for restaging rectal cancer after preoperative chemoradiation. *J Am Coll Surg* 207:7, 2008.

57. Rau B, Hunerbein M, Barth C, et al: Accuracy of endorectal ultra-sound after preoperative radiochemotherapy in locally advanced rectal cancer. *Surg Endosc* 13:980, 1999.

58. Gavioli M, Bagni A, Piccagli I, et al: Usefulness of endorectal ultrasound after preoperative radiotherapy in rectal cancer: Com-parison between sonographic and histopathologic changes. *Dis Colon Rectum* 43:1075, 2000.

59. Suppiah A, Hunter IA, Cowley J, et al: Magnetic resonance imaging accuracy in assessing tumour down-staging following chemoradiation in rectal cancer. *Colorectal Dis* 11:249, 2009.

60. Engelen SM, Beets-Tan RG, Beets GL, et al: MRI after chemora-diotherapy of rectal cancer: A useful tool to select patients for local excision. *Dis Colon Rectum* 53:979, 2010.

61. Capirci C, Rubello D, Pasini F, et al: The role of dual-time com-bined 18-fluorodeoxyglucose positron emission tomography and computed tomography in the staging and restaging workup of locally advanced rectal cancer, treated with preoperative chemo-radiation therapy and radical surgery. *Int J Radiat Oncol Biol Phys* 74:1461, 2009.

62. Sauer R, Becker H, Hohenberger W, et al: Preoperative versus postoperative chemoradiotherapy for rectal cancer. *N Engl J Med* 351:1731, 2004.

63. De Anda EH, Suk-Hawn L, Finne CO, et al: Endorectal ultrasound in the follow-up of rectal cancer patients treated by local excision or radical surgery. *Dis Colon Rectum* 47:818, 2004.

64. Morken JJ, Baxter NN, Madoff RD, et al: Endorectal ultrasound-directed biopsy: A useful technique to detect local recurrence of rectal cancer. *Int J Colorectal Dis* 21:258, 2006.

65. Lohnert MS, Doniec JM, Henne-Bruns D: Effectiveness of endo-luminal sonography in the identification of occult local rectal cancer recurrences. *Dis Colon Rectum* 43:483, 2000.

66. Tjandra JJ, Chan MK: Follow-up after curative resection of colorec-tal cancer: A meta-analysis. *Dis Colon Rectum* 50:1783, 2007.

67. Jeffery GM, Hickey BE, Hider P: Follow-up strategies for patients treated for non-metastatic colorectal cancer. *Cochrane Database Syst Rev* 1:CD002200, 2007.

68. Jimenez RE, Shoup M, Cohen AM, et al: Contemporary outcomes of total pelvic exenteration in the treatment of colorectal cancer. *Dis Colon Rectum* 46:1619, 2003.

69. Santoro GA, Gizzi G, Pellegrini L, et al: The value of high-resolution three-dimensional endorectal ultrasonography in the management of submucosal invasive rectal tumors. *Dis Colon Rectum* 52:1837, 2009.

70. Santoro GA, Fortling B: The advantages of volume rendering in three-dimensional endosonography of the anorectum. *Dis Colon Rectum* 50:359, 2007.

71. Giovannini M, Bories E, Pesenti C, et al: Three-dimensional endorectal ultrasound using a new freehand software program: Results in 35 patients with rectal cancer. *Endoscopy* 38:339, 2006.

72. Hunerbein M, Below C, Schlag PM: Three-dimensional endorectal ultrasonography for staging of obstructing rectal cancer. *Dis Colon Rectum* 39:636, 1996.

73. Hunerbein M, Dohmoto M, Haensch W, et al: Evaluation and biopsy of recurrent rectal cancer using three-dimensional endosonography. *Dis Colon Rectum* 39:1373, 1996.

74. Christensen AF, Nielsen MB, Svendsen LB, et al: Three-dimensional anal endosonography may improve detection of recurrent anal cancer. *Dis Colon Rectum* 49:1527, 2006.

75. Tjandra JJ, Milsom JW, Stolfi VM, et al: Endoluminal ultrasound defines anatomy of the anal canal and pelvic floor. *Dis Colon Rectum* 35:465, 1992.

76. Oberwalder M, Thaler K, Baig MK, et al: Anal ultrasound and endosonographic measurement of perineal body thickness: A new evaluation for fecal incontinence in females. *Surg Endosc* 18:650, 2004.

77. Johnson JK, Lindow SW, Duthie GS: The prevalence of occult obstetric anal sphincter injury following childbirth—literature review. *J Matern Fetal Neonatal Med* 20:547, 2007.

78. Oberwalder M, Connor J, Wexner SD: Meta-analysis to determine the incidence of obstetric anal sphincter damage. *Br J Surg* 90:1333, 2003.

79. Oberwalder M, Dinnewitzer A, Wexner SD, et al: The association between late-onset fecal incontinence and obstetric anal sphincter defects. *Arch Surg* 139:429, 2004.

80. Titi MA, Jenkins JT, Urie A, et al: Perineum compression during EAUS enhances visualization of anterior anal sphincter defects. *Colorectal Dis* 11:625, 2009.

81. Sajid MS, Khatri K, Siddiqui MR, et al: Endo-anal ultrasound versus endo-anal magnetic resonance imaging for the depiction of external anal sphincter pathology in patients with faecal incontinence: A systematic review. *Magy Seb* 63:9, 2010.

82. Titi MA, Jenkins JT, Urie A, et al: Correlation between anal manometry and endosonography in females with faecal incontinence. *Colorectal Dis* 10:131, 2008.

83. Pinsk I, Brown J, Phang PT: Assessment of sonographic quality of anal sphincter muscles in patients with faecal incontinence. *Colorectal Dis* 11:933, 2009.

84. Liberman H, Faria J, Ternent CA, et al: A prospective evaluation of the value of anorectal physiology in the management of fecal incontinence. *Dis Colon Rectum* 44:1567, 2001.

85. Sentovich SM, Wong WD, Blatchford GJ: Accuracy and reliability of transanal ultrasound for anterior anal sphincter injury. *Dis Colon Rectum* 41:1000, 1998.

86. Tjandra JJ, Han WR, Ooi BS, et al: Faecal incontinence after lateral internal sphincterotomy is often associated with coexisting occult sphincter defects: A study using endoanal ultrasonography. *Aust N Z J Surg* 71:598, 2001.

87. Garcia-Aguilar J, Belmonte Montes C, Perez JJ, et al: Incontinence after lateral internal sphincterotomy: Anatomic and functional evaluation. *Dis Colon Rectum* 41:423, 1998.

88. Ternent CA, Shashidharan M, Blatchford GJ, et al: Transanal ultrasound and anorectal physiology findings affecting continence after sphincteroplasty. *Dis Colon Rectum* 40:462, 1997.

89. Regadas FS, Murad-Regadas SM, Wexner SD, et al: Anorectal three-dimensional endosonography and anal manometry in assessing anterior rectocele in women: A new pathogenesis concept and the basic surgical principle. *Colorectal Dis* 9:80, 2007.

90. Subasinghe D, Samarasekera DN: Comparison of preoperative endoanal ultrasonography with intraoperative findings for fistula in ano. *World J Surg* 34:1123, 2010.

91. Toyonaga T, Tanaka M, Song JF, et al: Comparison of accuracy of physical examination and endoanal ultrasonography for preoperative assessment in patients with acute and chronic anal fistula. *Tech Coloproctol* 12:217, 2008.

92. Cho DY: Endosonographic criteria for an internal opening of fistula-in-ano. *Dis Colon Rectum* 42:515, 1999.

93. Schwartz DA, Pemberton JH, Sandborn WJ, et al: A comparison of endoscopic ultrasound, magnetic resonance imaging, and exam under anesthesia for evaluation of Crohn's perianal fistulas. *Gastroenterology* 121:1064, 2001.

94. Spradlin NM, Wise PE, Herline AJ, et al: A randomized prospective trial of endoscopic ultrasound to guide combination medical and surgical treatment for Crohn's perianal fistulas. *Am J Gastroenterol* 103:2527, 2008.

95. Solomon MJ, McLeod RS, O'Connor BI, et al: Assessment of peripouch inflammation after ileoanal anastomosis using endoluminal ultrasonography. *Dis Colon Rectum* 38:182, 1995.

96. Chew SS, Yang JL, Newstead GL, et al: Anal fistula: Levovist-enhanced endoanal ultrasound—a pilot study. *Dis Colon Rectum* 46:377, 2003.

97. Kim Y, Park YJ: Three-dimensional endoanal ultrasonographic assessment of an anal fistula with and without H(2)O(2) enhancement. *World J Gastroenterol* 15:4810, 2009.

98. Kruskal JB, Kane RA, Morrin MM: Peroxide-enhanced anal endosonography: Technique, image interpretation, and clinical applications. *Radiographics* 21:S173, 2001.

99. Baig MK, Zhao RH, Yuen CH, et al: Simple rectovaginal fistulas. *Int J Colorectal Dis* 15:323, 2000.

100. Tsang CB, Madoff RD, Wong WD, et al: Anal sphincter integrity and function influences outcome in rectovaginal fistula repair. *Dis Colon Rectum* 41:1141, 1998.

101. Drudi FM, Raffetto N, De Rubeis M, et al: TRUS staging and follow-up in patients with anal canal cancer. *Radiol Med* 106:329, 2003.

102. Tarantino D, Bernstein MA: Endoanal ultrasound in the staging and management of squamous-cell carcinoma of the anal canal: Potential implications of a new ultrasound staging system. *Dis Colon Rectum* 45:16, 2002.

103. Giovannini M, Bardou VJ, Barclay R, et al: Anal carcinoma: Prognostic value of endorectal ultrasound (ERUS)—results of a prospective multicenter study. *Endoscopy* 33:231, 2001.

104. Martellucci J, Naldini G, Colosimo C, et al: Accuracy of endoanal ultrasound in the follow-up assessment for squamous cell carcinoma of the anal canal treated with radiochemotherapy. *Surg Endosc* 23:1054, 2009.

105. Christensen AF, Nyhuus B, Nielsen MB: Interobserver and intraobserver variation of two-dimensional and three-dimensional anal endosonography in the evaluation of recurrent anal cancer. *Dis Colon Rectum* 52:484, 2009.

106. Akbari RP, Paty PB, Guillem JG, et al: Oncologic outcomes of salvage surgery for epidermoid carcinoma of the anus initially managed with combined modality therapy. *Dis Colon Rectum* 47:1136, 2004.

107. Petritsch W, Hinterleitner TA, Aichbichler B, et al: Endosonography in colitis cystica profunda and solitary rectal ulcer syndrome. *Gastrointest Endosc* 44:746, 1996.

CHAPTER

144

Diagnosis and Management of Fecal Incontinence

Susan C. Parker | Robert D. Madoff

Fecal incontinence is the inability to defer the passage of feces until a desired time and place. Although incontinence of gas, liquid, or solid stool is not a life-threatening disorder, it can dramatically affect an individual's lifestyle and lead to social isolation. Fortunately, most incontinence is amenable to medical or surgical therapy.[1]

The prevalence of fecal incontinence depends on the definition used and the population under study. Community prevalence has been estimated to range from 0.5% to 11%.[2] A Wisconsin telephone survey reported that 2.2% of the general population experienced fecal incontinence of varying degrees.[3] The prevalence increases to 13.4% in outpatients seeing their primary care physicians and 26% in outpatients seeing their gastroenterologist.[4] The highest rates of incontinence are seen in institutionalized individuals; a survey of 18,000 Wisconsin nursing home residents found that 47% of them had fecal incontinence.[5]

EVALUATION

The causes of fecal incontinence are divided into factors that alter anorectal anatomy (trauma, surgery), overwhelm physiologic control mechanisms (diarrhea, secretory tumors, fecal impaction), or interfere with neurologic function (diabetes, spinal cord injury, pudendal nerve injury). In many cases, a combination of factors leads to incontinence (Box 144-1). For example, incontinence associated with rectal prolapse is due to excessive physical stretching of both the anal sphincter and pudendal nerves. Similarly, diminished sphincter strength associated with aging can unmask a previously well-compensated obstetric sphincter injury.

Initial evaluation of the incontinent patient is performed in the physician's office and requires only careful elicitation of pertinent history and performance of a directed physical examination. However, although the initial evaluation can indicate the probable cause of incontinence in many patients, further testing is used to confirm the initial clinical impression. Pudendal nerve injury is not in and of itself visible, and sphincter injury due to surgery or childbirth can be undetectable on later examination after healing has occurred. Laboratory evaluation is also used to quantify the severity of the physiologic deficit, identify specific anatomic abnormalities, and elucidate the causes of incontinence when the diagnosis is obscure or there are multiple abnormalities.

HISTORY

Fecal incontinence is embarrassing, and many patients are reluctant to discuss their condition or even identify it by name. Accordingly, one of the first steps in evaluating the incontinent patient may be getting the patient to admit to the problem. Many patients present with complaints of "diarrhea," which on close questioning turns out to be involuntary loss of normal stool. It is also common for a patient to complain of the sudden onset of fecal incontinence and, on careful questioning, reveal that a change in stool consistency preceded the onset of incontinence. Certain risk factors or associated conditions should alert the physician to the presence of fecal incontinence: anal trauma or surgery[6]; vaginal deliveries,[7] especially multiple, difficult, or traumatic ones; pelvic radiation[8,9]; diabetes mellitus, especially with neuropathy; chronic diarrheal states; congenital conditions,[10] such as imperforate anus and spina bifida; urinary incontinence; or complaints of rectal prolapse or anal protrusion.[11,12]

The extent of incontinence should also be quantified. The key components of severity assessment include the nature of the material being lost (flatus, liquid stool, or solid stool), the frequency of loss, and the need to wear a pad. Although it is agreed that solid stool incontinence reflects a greater degree of physiologic impairment than incontinence for liquid stool only, it is noteworthy that patients perceive liquid stool incontinence to be more of a problem because it is more difficult to manage. Numerous scoring systems have been proposed for the evaluation of incontinence, but none have achieved universal acceptance to date.[13] However, the Fecal Incontinence Severity Index (FISI) is being used increasingly as its

BOX 144-1 Causes of Fecal Incontinence

NORMAL PELVIC FLOOR
Diarrheal states
    Infectious diarrhea
    Inflammatory bowel disease
    Short gut syndrome
    Laxative abuse
    Radiation enteritis
Overflow
    Impaction
    Encopresis
    Rectal neoplasms
Neurologic conditions
    Congenital anomalies (e.g., myelomeningocele)
    Multiple sclerosis
    Dementia, strokes, tabes dorsalis
    Neuropathy (e.g., diabetes)
    Neoplasms of brain, spinal cord, cauda equina

ABNORMAL PELVIC FLOOR
Congenital anorectal malformation
Trauma
Accidental injury (e.g., impalement, pelvic fracture)
Anorectal surgery
Obstetric injury
Aging

PELVIC FLOOR DENERVATION (IDIOPATHIC NEUROGENIC INCONTINENCE)
Vaginal delivery
Chronic straining at stool
Rectal prolapse
Descending perineum syndrome

From Madoff RD, Williams JG, Caushaj PF: Fecal incontinence. *N Engl J Med* 326:1002, 1992.

scores were derived from both patient- and colorectal surgeon–based weighting of severity.[14]

Quality-of-life assessment is a critical component to the evaluation of fecal incontinence and the success of its management. The concept itself is obvious, but quantification has proved to be difficult. General scales such as the Short Form–36 (SF-36) have not proved to be sufficiently sensitive to reflect real changes in patient status. Several incontinence scales combine a subjective quality-of-life assessment with a quantitative severity score to produce a single global incontinence score, an approach that, despite providing a single score per patient, combines two distinctly separate variables.[15] A validated fecal incontinence–specific quality-of-life score (FIQL) has been developed and is now enjoying widespread use.[16]

PHYSICAL EXAMINATION

Physical examination of the patient with fecal incontinence begins with external examination of the perianal area. Profuse incontinence, particularly of liquid stool, can lead to excoriation of the surrounding perianal skin. The perianal area should be inspected for scars from previous trauma, episiotomies, or anal surgery. The "keyhole deformity" is a groove in the anal canal, most commonly seen in the posterior midline, caused by a

sphincterotomy, fissurectomy, or fistulotomy, that permits seepage of stool or mucus. The female patient with an obstetric injury may have a thin perineal body, an associated rectovaginal fistula, or a cloaca due to loss of the distal portion of the rectovaginal septum and perineal body.

The patient with rectal prolapse may have a visibly patulous anus or one that gapes with traction. The prolapse itself, with its characteristic concentric folds, can be demonstrated by asking the patient to bear down, optimally while seated on a commode. Rectal mucosal prolapse, characterized by radial folds, can cause mucus seepage and staining but is not a cause of more severe incontinence.

The anocutaneous reflex is a test of perianal sensation that is elicited by stroking the perineal skin and observing an anal "wink" due to sphincter contraction. This spinal reflex has its afferent and efferent pathways in the pudendal nerve and is abolished if S4 is transected.

The findings to note on digital examination are the tone of the anal canal, the strength of the squeeze, and whether it seems symmetric. A strong contraction of the gluteal muscles should not be confused with contraction of the external anal sphincter muscle. Voluntary contraction of the external anal sphincter normally fatigues to a basal level within 3 minutes. A more rapid fatigue may be elicited in the incontinent patient.[17] Puborectalis function is evaluated separately from the external anal sphincter. This muscle forms a sling at the top of the anal canal that the examining finger can hook around posteriorly. Contraction of the muscle lifts the examining finger or is felt as a generalized tightening at the top of the anal canal. Fecal impaction leading to overflow incontinence should be evident on the initial digital examination. If there is a history of obstetric trauma, the examiner should palpate for a rectal vaginal fistula along with assessment of the perineal body width. Obstetric tears usually occur in the anterior midline, leaving a thin perineal body because of retraction of the sphincter muscle posterolaterally. A rectocele is present if there is a weakness in the rectovaginal septum that allows a digit placed in the rectum to push into the vagina. If a large rectocele is present, the posterior wall of the vagina can be pushed out the introitus.

The anoscope is used to look for prolapsing hemorrhoids, scarring in the anal canal from previous surgery, internal fistula openings, and mucosal inflammation. Any patient under evaluation for fecal incontinence should undergo a flexible sigmoidoscopy to exclude proctitis, cancer, or a benign secretory tumor such as a large rectal villous adenoma. A full colonic or small bowel evaluation is not usually necessary unless there is a history of diarrhea in addition to incontinence.

LABORATORY ASSESSMENT

In the majority of patients, the history and physical examination determine the cause of fecal incontinence. For the patient with a minor degree of fecal incontinence, medical management is instituted and further testing can be deferred. For most patients, testing at an anorectal physiology laboratory documents the degree of dysfunction, fully determines anatomic defects, and better directs the treatment plan.[18-20] Relevant tests include anal manometry, pudendal nerve latency testing or more advanced electrodiagnostics, endoanal ultrasound, and defecography or peritoneography and dynamic magnetic resonance imaging.

Manometry

Anal manometry determines anal canal pressure to provide an assessment of internal and external anal sphincter function. The entire length of the anal canal is evaluated, using either a "station" or continuous pull-through technique, and any one of a number of available catheters (e.g., water perfused, microballoon, and solid state). Despite the lack of methodologic standardization, the essential measurements are resting pressure, squeeze pressure, and rectoanal inhibitory reflex. The internal anal sphincter tone supplies 55% to 85% of the resting pressure,[21] and accordingly, manometric resting pressure, whether expressed as a maximum or mean, is an indication of internal anal sphincter function. Squeeze pressure reflects external anal sphincter function but, because it is under voluntary control, requires a cooperative patient to be accurate. Both resting and squeeze pressures are higher and sphincter length is longer in males than in females and pressures decrease with age.[22,23]

Rectal sensation is determined by inflating a rectal balloon with air and recording the volume of first sensation, sensation of fullness (urge to defecate), and maximum tolerated volume. Abnormal rectal sensation can lead to incontinence in two ways. Hyperacute sensation is seen when proctitis is present, typically because of inflammation or radiation therapy. Under these circumstances, the rectum is unable to tolerate an adequate volume of stool, and reservoir function is lost. Conversely, dulled sensation, as is seen in megarectum and some neurogenic disorders, leads to overflow incontinence.

The rectoanal inhibitory reflex is a decrease in resting pressure that occurs in response to rectal distention (accomplished in the laboratory by inflation of a rectal balloon). It is absent in Hirschsprung disease and immediately after rectal resection with coloanal anastomosis, and it can be difficult to detect in the presence of a megarectum or when resting pressures are very low. The rectoanal inhibitory reflex has been postulated to permit anal "sampling" of rectal contents to determine the appropriate sphincter response, such as expelling gas or withholding feces.[21] The exact nature of this sampling, however, has yet to be determined.

Pudendal Nerve Terminal Motor Latency

The pudendal nerve provides motor innervation to the external anal sphincter and sensory innervation to the perineum. Pudendal nerve injury is caused by traction on the nerve during straining (as seen during childbirth or prolonged efforts at defecation), and it results in denervation and subsequent reinnervation of the external anal sphincter and pelvic floor musculature. This reinnervation can be documented with needle electromyography (EMG), which demonstrates polyphasic motor unit action potentials and an increase in fiber density.[24] However, because the examination is uncomfortable, needle EMG is not widely used. Additional

useful tests include the pudendo-anal and anal reflex (or anal "wink"). The levels of the sacral cord involved in sacral reflexes are S2-S4. The pudendo-anal reflex is elicited by stimulating the dorsal nerve of the penis or clitoris. The pudendo-anal reflex is absent or delayed in many patients with fecal incontinence. The absence of an anal wink can also indicate injury, but it is more unreliable.[25]

Pudendal nerve integrity is now most commonly assessed by determination of pudendal nerve terminal motor latency (PNTML). PNTML is measured using the finger-mounted St. Mark's electrode (St. Mark's Pudendal Electrode), which stimulates the pudendal nerve at the level of the ischial spine and records the conduction time to the sphincter.[26] Prolonged conduction times are indicative of pudendal neuropathy, which is caused by traction injury to the nerve from vaginal childbirth, prolonged straining, rectal prolapse, or excessive perineal descent.[26] The test is affected by the skill of the examiner and body habitus of the patient; therefore, the significance of an undetectable PNTML is uncertain. Furthermore, because the test evaluates the function of the fastest remaining nerve fiber, incomplete nerve injuries can be missed with this technique. Indeed, fiber density but not pudendal nerve latency correlate with clinical and manometric variables in patients with fecal incontinence.[27] Some investigators have found an abnormal PNTML to be highly predictive of failure after sphincteroplasty,[28,29] but many others have observed no such correlation.[30,31]

Endoanal Ultrasound

Sphincter mapping helps the surgeon by confirming the presence of a sphincter defect and localizing the site and severity of the defect (Figure 144-1). The preferred method for sphincter mapping is endoanal ultrasound, optimally using a 360-degree rotating transducer probe that images through a plastic cap. The usual finding after an obstetric injury is an anterior (between rectum and vagina) disruption of the anal sphincters. Other common findings are disruptions of the internal anal sphincter after hemorrhoidectomy or sphincterotomy and disruptions of both sphincter muscles after fistulotomy or trauma. Endoanal ultrasound, in conjunction with manometry, can be particularly useful when evaluating trauma patients for continence before reversing a diverting stoma, because the degree of anal sphincter injury can be difficult to determine at the time of the initial trauma. Sphincter mapping is also described using MRI, but its use is limited and MRI may be less accurate at detection of internal anal sphincter defects.[32]

Defecography

Defecography, also termed evacuation proctography, is a dynamic study of rectal emptying. The rectum is filled with thick barium paste, which the patient is asked to evacuate under videofluoroscopy. Defecography is useful for evaluation of suspected rectal prolapse, including both internal intussusception and true procidentia. Patients with severe incontinence may be unable to hold the contrast agent without involuntary leakage, a finding that confirms the presence of a severe functional deficit.

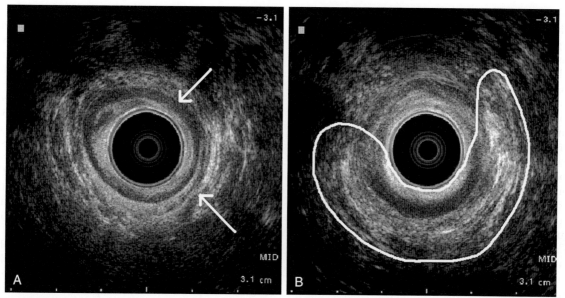

FIGURE 144-1 Endoanal ultrasound. **A,** Normal sphincter, mid-anal canal: the *arrow* at 1 o'clock indicates the internal anal sphincter, and the *arrow* at 4 o'clock points to the external anal sphincter. **B,** Disruption of anterior internal and external anal sphincter muscles with posterior retraction of muscles. The *line* indicates retracted muscle.

Defecography is also useful in demonstrating associated pelvic floor pathology that may be seen in the incontinent patient. The failure of appropriate pelvic floor relaxation is well visualized on defecography along with the degree to which flow of contrast is impeded. Although this is more often of significance in the evaluation of constipation, defecography can be helpful to identify a patient with overflow incontinence or incontinence because of a poorly emptying rectocele, especially if the patient also has sphincter dysfunction. Visualization of other associated pathology, such as enteroceles and pelvic floor hernias, can be optimized by the addition of a vaginal, small bowel, or peritoneal contrast agent.[33]

Dynamic Magnetic Resonance Imaging
Dynamic MRI has been utilized on a limited basis for the evaluation of pelvic floor disorders. A major drawback of this technique is that image acquisition occurs with the patient supine rather than sitting, thus not in the normal position assumed during defecation.[34] There is only limited reported experience with open MRI scanners that permit evacuation with the patient seated upon a commode.[35]

Benefits and Limitations of Physiology Testing for Incontinence
Over the years, many surgeons have argued that anorectal physiology tests add little to the "educated finger" in the evaluation of the incontinent patient. It is true that much can be learned by a careful physical examination and equally true that physiologic findings do not necessarily correlate with clinical status, but we believe that the appropriate use of anorectal physiology testing does improve the care of the incontinent patient. An early branch point in the algorithm for incontinence therapy is the presence or absence of a sphincter defect. Sphincter defects may be clinically obvious, or they may be subtle and difficult to detect. Anal ultrasonography

provides a rapid and definitive answer. Anal manometry provides an objective assessment of internal and external sphincter function, even if there is an underlying broad range of normal. Mild unilateral pudendal neuropathy may not accurately predict functional failure after sphincteroplasty, but the presence of severe bilateral neuropathy may help surgeons pick the best therapy for a given patient, or at least counsel the patient regarding a diminished likelihood of success. In short, we believe that careful and complete patient evaluation leads to accurate categorization, appropriate treatment, and optimized outcome.

TREATMENT

MEDICAL THERAPY
Because fecal incontinence can be exacerbated by abnormal bowel function, initial treatment efforts should be directed at correction of any associated underlying pathology. Severe diarrhea can overcome even a normal sphincter mechanism, and even mild chronic diarrheal states can be sufficient to tip a marginally compensated individual with abnormal sphincter function into frank clinical incontinence. Incontinent patients with loose stool should be evaluated for a cause of their diarrhea, including infection, malabsorption syndromes, and, in particular, occult inflammatory bowel disease. Irritable bowel syndrome is an important related entity. Although this disorder alone is not a cause of incontinence, it is widely prevalent and often complicates the management of patients with incontinence due to other disorders.

Management of the incontinent patient depends on the severity of his or her symptoms. Mild incontinence is usually best treated by conservative medical management. Food intolerance causing malabsorption can contribute significantly to symptoms, and patients should be alerted to this possibility. The classic example of this phenomenon is occult lactose intolerance, which can lead to liquid stool and excessive flatulence with consequent urgency and diminished bowel control.

Because solid stool is easier to control than liquid and because liquid stool incontinence is more distressing to patients than solid, all efforts should be made to optimize stool consistency. This goal is often best achieved by the consumption of adequate quantities of dietary fiber. Although 30 g/day of dietary fiber is most commonly quoted as the therapeutic goal, many patients find this level unachievable, and for most, 20 to 25 g/day is a reasonable target. Patients are able to best reach this goal with appropriate dietary counseling and the use of a stool bulking supplement such as psyllium or methylcellulose. Increased dietary fiber and supplemental psyllium should be gradually instituted to diminish the side effects of bloating and increased flatulence.

Patients with mild to moderate incontinence frequently improve with antidiarrheal medicines such as loperamide or diphenoxylate with atropine. Loperamide is related to haloperidol and decreases intestinal motility and secretion. Diphenoxylate with atropine has a mode of action similar to that of other related narcotics, such as morphine. Of these, only loperamide is a sphincter agonist that can increase sphincter pressure.[36] These drugs are often best used prophylactically when patients can predictably expect difficulty, such as at bedtime for patients with nocturnal incontinence and before leaving the home for patients with limited ability to defer evacuation. Patients with mild seepage may also benefit from several simple ancillary measures, including tap water irrigation of the rectum after bowel movements using a bulb syringe, use of a small absorbent cotton wick placed adjacent to the anal orifice, and regular application of a barrier cream to the perianal skin.

BIOFEEDBACK

Although Kegel exercises have been a popular approach to the incontinent patient, especially in the postpartum period, results for patients with significant incontinence are unimpressive. One reason for this may be that patients attempting to strengthen their pelvic floors may or may not be exercising the muscles they intend to exercise. In addition, because fecal incontinence is often related to several physiologic abnormalities, it is reasonable to suspect that addressing voluntary sphincter contraction alone may not improve a problem that is multifactorial in origin.

Biofeedback describes a class of techniques that use monitoring devices to provide information regarding a physiologic function so an individual may voluntarily alter or control that function. In the case of the anorectum, patients attempting to activate their sphincter mechanisms receive feedback confirming the extent to which muscle contraction is actually occurring.

Although initially popularized using the Schuster three-balloon system,[37] most centers now use either electromyographic or standard anal manometric approaches. Sensory training is variably provided, either to improve rectal sensation or to increase maximally tolerated rectal volume. Some stress the importance of coordinating appropriate sphincter contraction to rectal sensation.[37,38]

However, the physiologic mechanism by which biofeedback exerts its effect is uncertain. Although much biofeedback training is directed at improving voluntary sphincter contraction, successful results appear to correlate more with improved sensation[38,39] than improved motor function.[40,41]

Incontinent patients are candidates for biofeedback if they are adequately motivated and intellectually capable of following instructions. It is commonly held that they should have some ability to contract their anal sphincter and at least some rectal sensation, but these latter qualifications are vague and poorly substantiated in the literature. The cause of incontinence does not appear to affect the outcome of therapy, although patients with keyhole deformities do poorly because of continued stool leakage through the anatomic defect.[40]

A systematic review of biofeedback and pelvic floor exercises for treating fecal incontinence in adults identified 46 studies involving 1364 patients.[42] Nearly half (49%) of patients were reported cured, and 72% improved or cured. However, only 8 of the 46 studies reviewed included a control group, and the majority of individual reports are subject to criticism because of small patient numbers, short followup periods, heterogeneous patient groups, poor quantification of incontinence severity, and the addition of concurrent therapy (e.g., dietary counseling) and physician encouragement, each of which may alone lead to clinical improvement. Indeed, a randomized controlled trial called the efficacy of biofeedback into question as it showed no benefit when biofeedback was added to standard medical care (advice from a nurse specialist) or standard care plus sphincter exercises.[43] However, a more recent randomized controlled trial showed that biofeedback was more effective than pelvic floor exercises alone for treating fecal incontinence.[44]

Despite some caveats, most experts continue to believe that biofeedback is an effective treatment option for patients with fecal incontinence. Indeed, there are few contraindications to a trial of biofeedback, and the technique is painless and risk free. It plays a particularly important role in the treatment of patients with minor degrees of incontinence in whom no anatomic sphincter defect is present and for whom surgery is therefore not indicated. Biofeedback has also been shown to be useful to improve the function of patients with suboptimal results after sphincteroplasty.[45]

SURGERY

Surgical procedures for fecal incontinence vary considerably depending on the clinical situation. Traumatic sphincter disruptions are repaired. Should sphincter repair not be indicated or fail, novel procedures including insertion of an artificial anal sphincter, placement of a sacral nerve stimulator, or injection of sphincter-bulking agents are options. For patients with persisting refractory incontinence, fecal diversion remains an excellent choice.

Sphincter Reconstruction

Direct sphincter (Figure 144-2) repair can be performed in the acute setting in the presence of an isolated and

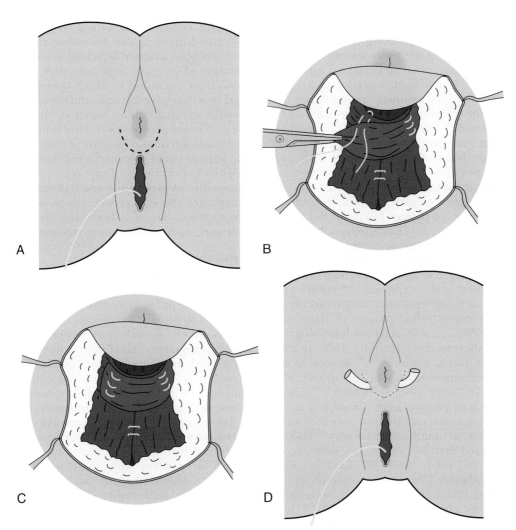

FIGURE 144-2 Sphincteroplasty. **A,** With the patient in the prone jackknife position, a curvilinear incision is made. Inferior rectal nerves cross the ischiorectal fossa posterolaterally. **B,** Anterior levatorplasty is performed, and overlapping sphincter repair is then initiated. **C,** Sphincter repair is completed. **D,** The incision is closed, with drains in place (optional), and V-Y plasty is done to restore the perineal body. (From Baxter NN, Madoff RD: Motility disorders. In Souba WW, Fink MJ, Jurkovich GJ, et al, editors: *ACS surgery: Principles and practice.* New York, 2005, WebMD.)

easily definable sphincter disruption; this scenario most often occurs in the delivery room after obstetric injury. These injuries are typically repaired with simple sphincter apposition, but up to 70% of women have persisting sphincter defects and 50% persisting incontinence after repair in this setting.[46] Nonoperative traumatic injuries can often be treated in a similar fashion; however, when severe associated pelvic injuries are present, when the patient is unstable, or when long-standing local contamination is present, debridement with the placement of a diverting stoma plus planned delayed sphincter repair is a better option. Delayed sphincter repair is also required to treat unrecognized sphincter injuries, failed primary repairs, and incontinence after fistulotomy. In each of these cases, definitive surgery should be delayed 3 to 6 months until all local inflammation has resolved.

Patients undergoing elective sphincter repair should have a complete mechanical bowel preparation preoperatively. The operation is best performed with the patient in the prone jackknife position with the buttocks taped apart. General or regional anesthesia may be used.

For anterior defects, a curved circumanal incision is performed along the perineal body and extended laterally over the ischiorectal fossae. A flap of anoderm and, proximally, rectal mucosa is raised along the length of the anal canal anteriorly. Next, the external anal sphincter is mobilized from the vagina anteriorly and laterally until the retracted scarred ends can be easily overlapped to form the repair. Posterior dissection of the sphincter muscle should not extend beyond the midlateral line to avoid potential injury to the pudendal nerves, which enter the sphincter posterolaterally. Proximal dissection continues until a proximal nonscarred plane is reached or the inferior fibers of the puborectalis are encountered as they run anteriorly to the pubis.

The midline scar is divided but not excised to minimize the risk of suture pull-through. The buttock tapes are released. Many surgeons perform an anterior levatoroplasty in an effort to lengthen the functional high-pressure zone. Some also advocate reefing of the rectovaginal septum to provide additional anterior support. The divided sphincter is then overlapped to create a "snug" wrap, and this is secured with a series of interrupted 2-0 polydioxanone or polyglycolic acid horizontal mattress sutures. Most surgeons perform a "mass" overlap of the combined internal and external sphincter muscles. Others advocate individual dissection and repair of the internal and external sphincter muscles, but the hypothetical superiority of this approach remains to be clinically demonstrated.[28] The skin is loosely closed in a T-shaped configuration, vertically in the anterior aspect to provide adequate length for the perineal body and transversely in the posterior aspect adjacent to the anal verge. No covering stoma is raised.

Results of incontinence surgery vary with definitions of success and closeness of patient followup. For many years, the reported results after overlapping sphinctero-plasty were remarkably consistent: approximately 60% to 75% of patients achieved a "good to excellent" surgical outcome, which in practice entailed perfect or near-perfect control of solid stool, occasional difficulties with control of liquid stool, and episodic "minor" accidents such as seepage or uncontrolled passage of flatus. An additional 15% to 20% of patients achieved lesser degrees of improvement, whereas the remaining 15% to 20% were unchanged or, rarely, worse.[28,30,47,48] Recent series, however, have raised questions about the quality and durability of results following sphincteroplasty.[49-52] Karoui et al found that 49% of patients were completely conti-nent 3 months after sphincteroplasty, but only 28% were completely continent 40 months after surgery.[52] Halver-son and Hull reported that 54% of patients were incon-tinent to liquid or solid stool 69 months after sphincteroplasty, and only 14% were completely conti-nent.[50] Malouf et al found that no patients were fully continent 77 months after sphincteroplasty; 84% had fecal urgency and 79% had passive soiling.[49] At the Uni-versity of Minnesota, we assessed long-term results in 191 consecutive patients after sphincteroplasty. At the 10-year followup, just 6% were completely continent, 57% were incontinent of solid stool, and 16% were incontinent of gas only. Results worsened significantly between 3 and 10 years after the procedure.[52]

Salvage Therapy: Postanal Repair and Anal Encirclement

There are a number of options available as salvage therapy for incontinent patients who have failed or are not candidates for standard therapy. The Parks postanal repair was initially devised as an operation for patients with intact but poorly functioning sphincters.[53] The pro-cedure, a posterior plication of the levator ani and exter-nal sphincter, is performed via an intersphincteric dissection. Although once popular in the United Kingdom, the operation never gained widespread accep-tance in North America and is performed relatively infre-quently. Long-term results from St. Mark's Hospital showed that 26% of patients were continent to stool at a median followup of 6 years.[54] However, despite imperfect continence, the majority of patients were improved from baseline.

Anal encirclement in a variety of forms has been used to treat fecal incontinence. The simplest form of this operation, using silver wire, was described by Thiersch in the 19th century.[55] Despite a trend toward the use of softer and more pliable encircling materials, the opera-tion has been plagued by a high local complication rate because of erosion and infection. In 1952, Pickrell devised an operation in which the anal canal was encir-cled by a transposed gracilis muscle whose neurovascular bundle was maintained intact in the proximal thigh.[56] Pickrell's operation was attractive both because it avoided foreign material and because it created a sphincter that the patient could voluntarily contract (by abducting the thighs). Unfortunately, functional results were generally poor with this procedure, and it never gained widespread acceptance. Several modifications of gluteus maximus transposition have also been described, with highly vari-able functional results being reported.[57-59]

Dynamic Myoplasty

Interest in gracilis transposition was renewed with the introduction of electrical stimulation by means of an implantable pulse generator.[60] Electrical stimulation is used first to convert the gracilis from predominantly type 2 ("fast-twitch," fatigable) to predominantly type 1 ("slow-twitch," fatigue-resistant) muscle fibers. The stimulator is then used to maintain tonic contraction of the trans-posed muscle, thereby providing continuous sphincter function. Defecation is effected by switching off the stim-ulator with a hand-held programmer.

Baeten et al[61] reported a continence rate of 73% in 52 patients who underwent dynamic gracioplasty for refrac-tory fecal incontinence. The success rate was highest (92%) in patients with sphincter trauma (including obstetric, operative, and accidental) and lowest in patients with anal atresia (50%). Similar success rates were documented in two multicenter trials of dynamic gracioplasty, but both also documented a prohibitively high rate of operative morbidity.[62,63] Because of this high morbidity rate, dynamic gracioplasty has not been approved for use in the United States, and its use world-wide is limited to a small number of specialty centers.

Artificial Anal Sphincter

The artificial anal sphincter (Figure 144-3) provides an alternative option for patients with severe refractory fecal incontinence. Compared with dynamic gracioplasty, it offers the advantages of simplicity, placement in a single operation, and use of the device 6 weeks after placement without the need for muscle conditioning.

The artificial anal sphincter in use is a modification of an artificial urinary sphincter (AMS 800). It is an implant-able device composed of a silicone elastomer that main-tains continence via a fluid-filled cuff that surrounds and compresses the anal canal. The patient controls the device via a pump placed in the scrotum or labia. Squeez-ing the pump 9 to 12 times forces the fluid from the cuff into a reservoir balloon, which is implanted in the space of Retzius. This deflates the cuff and opens the anal canal, allowing the passage of stool. The cuff then auto-matically slowly reinflates and occludes the anal canal, providing continence until defecation is again desired.

The implantation of an artificial anal sphincter for fecal incontinence was first reported by Christiansen and Lorentzen in 1987.[64] Reported results reflect the early

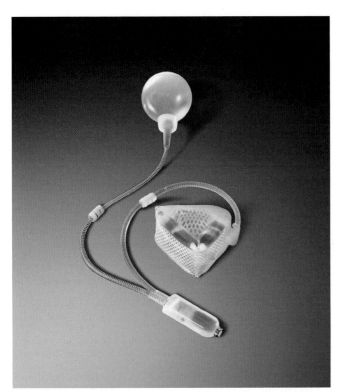

FIGURE 144-3 Acticon neosphincter. (Courtesy American Medical Systems, Inc, Minnetonka, Minn. www.americanmedicalsystems. com)

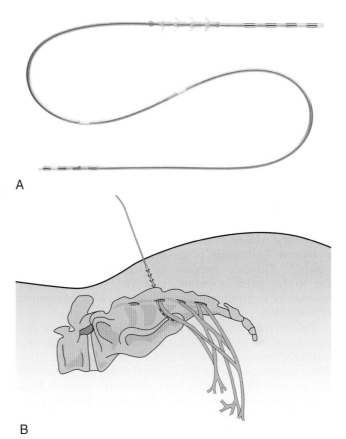

A

B

FIGURE 144-4 Sacral nerve stimulation (SNS). **A,** A lead containing four electrodes is used for SNS. **B,** The sacral foramina are identified; in most cases, S3 is the optimal choice for stimulation. The quadripolar lead is shown in position. (**A** copyright Medtronics, Inc; **B** from Baxter NN, Madoff RD: Motility disorders. In Souba WW, Fink MJ, Jurkovich GJ, et al, editors: *ACS surgery: Principles and practice,* New York, 2005, WebMD.)

use of the modified urinary sphincter (AMS 800) and the later use of a similar device (Acticon neosphincter) with additional modifications for use around the anal canal.[65-67] Wong et al performed a multicenter prospective trial of the Acticon neosphincter in 115 patients.[68] Forty-six percent of implanted patients required revisional surgery, frequently because of infectious complications. Forty-one percent of patients required device explantation; 17% of these were able to be reimplanted. Eighty-five percent of patients who retained their device had a successful outcome, but intention-to-treat success was only 53%. There is some evidence that results improve with surgical experience,[69] but the long-term explantation rate is 40% or greater.[65,70,71] A multicenter study using a specific antibiotic regimen decreased the infection rate of 25%, experienced in the initial multicenter trial, to 9%.[72] Despite several single-center series that have reported successful results in the majority of patients[69,73,74] a systematic review concluded that implantation of the artificial anal sphincter was "of uncertain benefit."[75]

SACRAL NERVE STIMULATION

Novel Surgical Techniques. Sacral nerve stimulation (SNS) represents a novel alternative approach to the management of fecal incontinence (Figure 144-4). The technique, like the artificial anal sphincter, was initially devised for urinary incontinence. Electrodes are placed percutaneously via the sacral foramina under local anesthesia with or without sedation. Because the sacral nerves also contribute fibers to the nerves of the lower extremity, it is not surprising that their stimulation leads to the

contraction of both the pelvic floor and various leg and foot muscles. It is important that the sacral foramen selected provides maximal pelvic floor and minimal lower extremity stimulation. In clinical practice, this site is most often S3. Once the optimal site has been selected, patients undergo a test period of stimulation with an external pulse generator. If function has improved adequately at the end of the test period, implantation of the permanent leads and pulse generator is performed.[76]

The clinical use of sacral nerve stimulation was pioneered by Matzel et al[77] in Erlangen. In a subsequent prospective multicenter trial of 34 patients, dramatic decreases in incontinent events were documented at 12 and 24 months, as well as improvements in pad use, ability to postpone defecation, and quality of life.[78] In a more recent prospective trial of 120 patients who underwent SNS, 83% of patients achieved a 50% reduction in incontinent events at 12 months, including 41% who became fully continent. These results appeared durable for at least 3 years.[79]

The mechanism of improvement after sacral nerve stimulation remains unknown. Although reported results have been variable, there has been no consistent effect demonstrated on anal tone or squeeze strength. Other possible alternatives include a decrease in gastrointestinal transit, decrease in rectal contractility, altered rectal sensation, and improved coordination of sensorimotor function. Lundby et al recently demonstrated focal brain activation in response to SNS in patients immediately and 2 weeks following institution of stimulation.[80] SNS has recently become FDA approved and is quickly becoming a first line intervention for patients with fecal incontinence.

Injectable Biomaterials. Several recent studies have investigated the role of injectable biomaterials in the management of fecal incontinence.[81,82] Injected materials have included autologous fat, cross-linked collagen, silicone Bioplastique, and carbon-coated beads. Graf et al performed a randomized, double-blind, sham-controlled trial of intraanal injection of dextranomer in stabilized hyaluronic acid (DSHA) for fecal incontinence.[83] Fifty-two percent of treated patients met the study's primary endpoint (a 50% decrease in the number of incontinent episodes) versus 31% of controls ($P = 0.0089$).

Potential advantages of injection therapy include simplicity and the ability to offer treatment in an outpatient setting. A successful result can require repeated injections, and migration of the injected material is reported. Manometric pressures are not significantly altered. Additional controlled trials with long-term followup are needed. One bioinjectable has recently been released for the indication of fecal incontinece and may become an important first line therapy as experience widens.

A Final Option: Fecal Diversion

Despite the broad range of therapies available to the incontinent patient, there inevitably remains a subgroup of patients who fail therapy or simply are not candidates for major reconstructive surgery. In most cases, unmanageable anal incontinence can be converted to a manageable situation by the creation of a stoma, most often a sigmoid colostomy. Although many patients shy from this approach, the loss of body image is generally more than compensated for by the gain in control, self-esteem, and freedom of action. Although available data are quite limited, one questionnaire study of patients who underwent colostomy for fecal incontinence documented marked improvement in subjective quality of life assessment after surgery.[84] Counseling by an enterostomal therapist and discussion with other ostomates are invaluable resources in assisting the patient to make an appropriate and informed choice regarding stoma creation. Furthermore, because patient satisfaction is critically dependent on the quality of the stoma provided, preoperative stoma site selection and careful attention to the technical details of stoma creation are mandatory.

CONCLUSION

Fecal incontinence is a clinically important disorder whose impact on the individual can range from distressing to devastating. An orderly approach to patient history and physical examination will lead to the diagnosis and its cause in the majority of patients. Patients with mild incontinence often improve with medical therapy. Those with more severe symptoms or an uncertain cause or who are medically refractory should undergo formal physiologic evaluation to optimize their treatment. Most of these patients are successfully treated using biofeedback or standard surgical approaches. For those for whom these strategies fail, novel theraputic approaches with what are now investigational techniques will increasingly become an option in the future.

REFERENCES

1. Madoff RD, Parker SC, Varma MG, et al: Faecal incontinence in adults. *Lancet* 364:621, 2004. A general overview of the diagnosis and management of fecal incontinence.
2. Nelson R: Epidemiology and incidence of anal incontinence: Magnitude of the problem. *Semin Colon Rectal Surg* 8:80, 1997.
3. Nelson R, Norton N, Cautley E, et al: Community-based prevalence of anal incontinence. *JAMA* 274:559, 1995.
4. Johanson JF, Lafferty J: Epidemiology of fecal incontinence: The silent affliction. *Am J Gastroenterol* 91:33, 1996.
5. Nelson R, Furner S, Jesudason V: Fecal incontinence in Wisconsin nursing homes: Prevalence and associations. *Dis Colon Rectum* 41:1226, 1998.
6. Garcia-Aguilar J, Belmonte Montes C, Perez JJ, et al: Incontinence after lateral internal sphincterotomy: Anatomic and functional evaluation. *Dis Colon Rectum* 41:423, 1998.
7. Sultan AH, Kamm MA, Hudson CN, et al: Anal-sphincter disruption during vaginal delivery. *N Engl J Med* 329:1905, 1993.
8. Montana GS, Fowler WC: Carcinoma of the cervix: Analysis of bladder and rectal radiation dose and complications. *Int J Radiat Oncol Biol Phys* 16:95, 1989.
9. Kimose HH, Fischer L, Spjeldnaes N, et al: Late radiation injury of the colon and rectum. Surgical management and outcome. *Dis Colon Rectum* 32:684, 1989.
10. Pena A: Anorectal malformations. *Semin Pediatr Surg* 4:35, 1995.
11. Williams JG, Wong WD, Jensen J, et al: Incontinence and rectal prolapse: A prospective manometric study. *Dis Colon Rectum* 34:209, 1991.
12. Madoff RD, Williams JG, Wong WD, et al: Long-term functional results of colon resection and rectopexy for overt rectal prolapse. *Am J Gastroenterol* 87:101, 1992.
13. Baxter NN, Rothenberger DA, Lowry AC: Measuring fecal incontinence. *Dis Colon Rectum* 46:1591, 2003.
14. Rockwood TH, Church JM, Fleshman JW, et al: Patient and surgeon ranking of the severity of symptoms associated with fecal incontinence: The fecal incontinence severity index. *Dis Colon Rectum* 42:1525, 1999.
15. Shelton AA, Madoff RD: Defining anal incontinence: Establishing a uniform continence scale. *Seminars in Colon & Rectal Surgery* 8:54, 1997.
16. Rockwood TH, Church JM, Fleshman JW, et al: Fecal Incontinence Quality of Life Scale: Quality of life instrument for patients with fecal incontinence. *Dis Colon Rectum* 43:9, 2000.
17. Marcello PW, Barrett RC, Coller JA, et al: Fatigue rate index as a new measurement of external sphincter function. *Dis Colon Rectum* 41:336, 1998.
18. Rao SS, Patel RS: How useful are manometric tests of anorectal function in the management of defecation disorders? *Am J Gastroenterol* 92:469, 1997.
19. Falk PM, Blatchford GJ, Cali RL, et al: Transanal ultrasound and manometry in the evaluation of fecal incontinence. *Dis Colon Rectum* 37:468, 1994.
20. Farouk R, Bartolo DC: The clinical contribution of integrated laboratory and ambulatory anorectal physiology assessment in faecal incontinence. *Int J Colorectal Dis* 8:60, 1993.
21. Henry M, Swash M, editors: *Coloproctology and the pelvic floor*, ed 2. Oxford, 1992, Butterworth Heinemann.
22. Read NW, Harford WV, Schmulen AC, et al: A clinical study of patients with fecal incontinence and diarrhea. *Gastroenterology* 76:747, 1979.
23. Matheson DM, Keighley MR: Manometric evaluation of rectal prolapse and faecal incontinence. *Gut* 22:126, 1981.

24. Neill ME, Swash M: Increased motor unit fibre density in the external anal sphincter muscle in ano-rectal incontinence: A single fibre EMG study. *J Neurol Neurosurg Psychiatry* 43:343, 1980.

25. Fowler CJ: Pelvic floor neurophysiology. *Methods Clin Neurophysiol* 2:1, 1991.

26. Laurberg S, Swash M, Snooks SJ, et al: Neurologic cause of idiopathic incontinence. *Arch Neurol* 45:1250, 1988.

27. Osterberg A, Graf W, Edebol Eeg-Olofsson K, et al: Results of neurophysiologic evaluation in fecal incontinence. *Dis Colon Rectum* 43:1256, 2000.

28. Gilliland R, Altomare DF, Moreira H Jr, et al: Pudendal neuropathy is predictive of failure following anterior overlapping sphincteroplasty. *Dis Colon Rectum* 41:1516, 1998.

29. Sangwan YP, Coller JA, Barrett RC, et al: Unilateral pudendal neuropathy. Impact on outcome of anal sphincter repair. *Dis Colon Rectum* 39:686, 1996.

30. Engel AF, Kamm MA, Sultan AH, et al: Anterior anal sphincter repair in patients with obstetric trauma. *Br J Surg* 81:1231, 1994.

31. Karakousis CP, Cheng C, Udobi K, et al: Abdominoinguinal incision in adenocarcinoma of the sigmoid or cecum: Report of two cases. *Dis Colon Rectum* 41:1322, 1998.

32. Malouf AJ, Williams AB, Halligan S, et al: Prospective assessment of accuracy of endoanal MR imaging and endosonography in patients with fecal incontinence. *AJR Am J Roentgenol* 175:741, 2000.

33. Bremmer S, Mellgren A, Holmstrom B, et al: Peritoneocele and enterocele. Formation and transformation during rectal evacuation as studied by means of defaeco-peritoneography. *Acta Radiol* 39:167, 1998.

34. Dann EW: Magnetic resonance defecography: An evaluation of obstructed defecation and pelvic floor weakness. *Semin Ultrasound CT MR* 29:414, 2008.

35. Fiaschetti V, Squillaci E, Pastorelli D, et al: Dynamic MRI defecography with an open-configuration, low-field, tilting MR system in patient with pelvic floor disorders (Abstract). *Radiol Med* 116:620, 2011.

36. Buie W: Nonoperative medical management of fecal incontinence. *Semin Colon Rectal Surg* 8:73, 1997.

37. Engel BT, Nikoomanesh P, Schuster MM: Operant conditioning of rectosphincteric responses in the treatment of fecal incontinence. *N Engl J Med* 290:646, 1974.

38. Reboa G, Frascio M, Zanolla R, et al: Biofeedback training to obtain continence in permanent colostomy. Experience of two centers. *Dis Colon Rectum* 28:419, 1985.

39. Miner PB, Donnelly TC, Read NW: Investigation of mode of action of biofeedback in treatment of fecal incontinence. *Dig Dis Sci* 35:1291, 1990.

40. MacLeod JH: Management of anal incontinence by biofeedback. *Gastroenterology* 93:291, 1987.

41. Wald A: Biofeedback therapy for fecal incontinence. *Ann Intern Med* 95:146, 1981.

42. Norton C, Kamm MA: Anal sphincter biofeedback and pelvic floor exercises for faecal incontinence in adults—a systematic review. *Aliment Pharmacol Ther* 15:1147, 2001.

43. Norton C, Chelvanayagam S, Wilson-Barnett J, et al: Randomized controlled trial of biofeedback for fecal incontinence. *Gastroenterology* 125:1320, 2003.

44. Heymen S, Scarlett Y, Jones K, et al: Randomized controlled trial shows biofeedback to be superior to pelvic floor exercises for fecal incontinence. *Dis Colon Rectum* 52:1730, 2009.

45. Jensen LL, Lowry AC: Biofeedback improves functional outcome after sphincteroplasty. *Dis Colon Rectum* 40:197, 1997.

46. Zetterstrom J, Lopez A, Holmstrom B, et al: Obstetric sphincter tears and anal incontinence: An observational follow-up study. *Acta Obstet Gynecol Scand* 82:921, 2003.

47. Fleshman JW, Dreznik Z, Fry RD, et al: Anal sphincter repair for obstetric injury: Manometric evaluation of functional results. *Dis Colon Rectum* 34:1061, 1991.

48. Buie WD, Lowry AC, Rothenberger DA, et al: Clinical rather than laboratory assessment predicts continence after anterior sphincteroplasty. *Dis Colon Rectum* 44:1255, 2001.

49. Malouf AJ, Norton CS, Engel AF, et al: Long-term results of overlapping anterior anal-sphincter repair for obstetric trauma. *Lancet* 355:260, 2000.

50. Halverson AL, Hull TL: Long-term outcome of overlapping anal sphincter repair. *Dis Colon Rectum* 45:345, 2002.

51. Karoui S, Leroi AM, Koning E, et al: Results of sphincteroplasty in 86 patients with anal incontinence. *Dis Colon Rectum* 43:813, 2000.

52. Bravo Gutierrez A, Madoff RD, Lowry AC, et al: Long-term results of anterior sphincteroplasty. *Dis Colon Rectum* 47:727; discussion 731, 2004.

53. Oliveira L, Pfeifer J, Wexner SD: Physiological and clinical outcome of anterior sphincteroplasty. *Br J Surg* 83:502, 1996.

54. Setti Carraro P, Kamm MA, Nicholls RJ: Long-term results of postanal repair for neurogenic faecal incontinence. *Br J Surg* 81:140, 1994.

55. Thiersch C: Carl Thiersch, 1822-1895. Concerning prolapse of the rectum with special emphasis on the operation by Thiersch [classic article]. *Dis Colon Rectum* 31:154, 1988.

56. Pickrell KL, Broadbent TR, Masters FW, et al: Construction of a rectal sphincter and restoration of anal continence by transplanting the gracilis muscle: A report of four cases in children. *Ann Surg* 135:853, 1952.

57. Pearl RK, Prasad ML, Nelson RL, et al: Bilateral gluteus maximus transposition for anal incontinence. *Dis Colon Rectum* 34:478, 1991.

58. Christiansen J, Hansen CR, Rasmussen O: Bilateral gluteus maximus transposition for anal incontinence. *Br J Surg* 82:903, 1995.

59. Devesa JM, Madrid JM, Gallego BR, et al: Bilateral gluteoplasty for fecal incontinence. *Dis Colon Rectum* 40:883, 1997.

60. Baeten C, Spaans F, Fluks A: An implanted neuromuscular stimulator for fecal continence following previously implanted gracilis muscle: Report of a case. *Dis Colon Rectum* 31:134, 1988.

61. Baeten GM, Geerdes BP, Adang EM, et al: Anal dynamic graciloplasty in the treatment of intractable fecal incontinence. *N Engl J Med* 332:1600, 1995.

62. Madoff RD, Rosen HR, Baeten CG, et al: Safety and efficacy of dynamic muscle plasty for anal incontinence: Lessons from a prospective, multicenter trial. *Gastroenterology* 116:549, 1999.

63. Baeten CG, Bailey HR, Bakka A, et al: Safety and efficacy of dynamic graciloplasty for fecal incontinence: Report of a prospective, multicenter trial. Dynamic Gracioplasty Therapy Study Group. *Dis Colon Rectum* 43:743, 2000.

64. Christiansen J, Lorentzen M: Implantation of artificial sphincter for anal incontinence. *Lancet* 2:244, 1987.

65. Christiansen J, Rasmussen OO, Lindorff-Larsen K: Long-term results of artificial anal sphincter implantation for severe anal incontinence. *Ann Surg* 230:45, 1999.

66. Lehur PA, Glemain P, Bruley des Varannes S, et al: Outcome of patients with an implanted artificial anal sphincter for severe faecal incontinence. A single institution report. *Int J Colorectal Dis* 13:88, 1998.

67. Wong WD, Jensen LL, Bartolo DC, et al: Artificial anal sphincter. *Dis Colon Rectum* 39:1345, 1996.

68. Wong WD, Congliosi SM, Spencer MP, et al: The safety and efficacy of the artificial bowel sphincter for fecal incontinence: Results from a multicenter cohort study. *Dis Colon Rectum* 45:1139, 2002.

69. Michot F, Costaglioli B, Leroi AM, et al: Artificial anal sphincter in severe fecal incontinence: Outcome of prospective experience with 37 patients in one institution. *Ann Surg* 237:52, 2003.

70. Parker SC, Spencer MP, Madoff RD, et al: Artificial bowel sphincter: Long-term experience at a single institution. *Dis Colon Rectum* 46:722, 2003.

71. Ortiz H, Armendariz P, DeMiguel M, et al: Complications and functional outcome following artificial anal sphincter implantation. *Br J Surg* 89:877, 2002.

72. Parker SC, Nogueras JJ, Kaiser AM, et al: Use of standardized prophylactic antibiotic regimen (SPAR) decreases Acticon (r) neosphincter complications (Abstract). *Dis Colon Rectum (In Press)*.

73. Devesa JM, Rey A, Hervas PL, et al: Artificial anal sphincter: Complications and functional results of a large personal series. *Dis Colon Rectum* 45:1154, 2002.

74. Lehur PA, Roig JV, Duinslaeger M: Artificial anal sphincter: Prospective clinical and manometric evaluation. *Dis Colon Rectum* 43:1100, 2000.

75. Mundy L, Merlin TL, Maddern GJ, et al: Systematic review of safety and effectiveness of an artificial bowel sphincter for faecal incontinence. *Br J Surg* 91:665, 2004.

76. Hetzer FH: Fifteen years of sacral nerve stimulation: From an open procedure to a minimally invasive technique. *Colorectal Dis* 13:1, 2011.

77. Matzel KE, Stadelmaier U, Hohenfellner M, et al: Electrical stimulation of sacral spinal nerves for treatment of faecal incontinence. *Lancet* 346:1124, 1995.

78. Matzel KE, Kamm MA, Stosser M, et al: Sacral spinal nerve stimulation for faecal incontinence: Multicentre study. *Lancet* 363:1270, 2004.

79. Wexner SD, Coller JA, Devroede G, et al: Sacral nerve stimulation for fecal incontinence: Results of a 120-patient prospective multicenter study. *Ann Surg* 251:441, 2010.

80. Lundby L, Moller A, Buntzen S, et al: Relief of fecal incontinence by sacral nerve stimulation linked to focal brain activation. *Dis Colon Rectum* 54:318, 2011.

81. Kumar D, Benson MJ, Bland JE: Glutaraldehyde cross-linked collagen in the treatment of faecal incontinence. *Br J Surg* 85:978, 1998.

82. Kenefick NJ, Vaizey CJ, Malouf AJ, et al: Injectable silicone biomaterial for faecal incontinence due to internal anal sphincter dysfunction. *Gut* 51:225, 2002.

83. Graf W, Mellgren A, Matzel KE, et al: Efficacy of dextranomer in stabilised hyaluronic acid for treatment of faecal incontinence: A randomised, sham-controlled trial. *Lancet* 377:997, 2011.

84. Norton C: Patients' views of a colostomy for faecal incontinence. *Neurourol Urodyn* 22:403, 2003.

Surgical Treatment of Constipation

David J. Maron | Steven D. Wexner

Constipation is one of the most frequently experienced gastrointestinal complaints and one of the most common indications for medical consultation.[1] It is estimated that more than 4 million patients in North America suffer from constipation, and laxatives are prescribed for 2 million individuals annually at a cost of more than $800 million.[2,3] In the United States, more than 90,000 patients are hospitalized each year for constipation-related problems.[4] Constipation is more prevalent in persons of lower socioeconomic background,[4,5] females,[6] and the elderly.[4]

The definition of constipation includes both subjective and objective aspects. In addition to decreased frequency of defecation, patients may present complaining of incomplete or difficult evacuation, abdominal or rectal pain, hard stools, decreased stool bulk or caliber, straining for evacuation, nausea, bloating, and tenesmus. Whitehead et al[7] proposed that at least two of the following need to be present in a patient who has not used laxatives for at least 12 months: (1) straining during more than 25% of bowel movements; (2) feeling of incomplete evacuation after more than 25% of bowel movements; (3) hard stool on more than 25% of bowel movements; and (4) bowel movement frequency of less than two per week with or without symptoms of constipation. Agachan et al[8] proposed a scoring system that includes frequency of bowel movements, painful evacuation, incomplete evacuation, abdominal pain, length of time per attempts, assistance for defecation, unsuccessful attempts for evacuation per 24 hours, and duration of constipation. After evaluating more than 230 patients, the authors concluded that a score of 15 or greater represents constipation.[8] Numerous subsequent studies have validated and proven the clinical value of this Cleveland Clinic Florida (CCF) scoring system. The Rome III criteria define constipation as two or more of the following abnormalities occurring for 3 months (with onset of symptoms more than 6 months prior to diagnosis): (1) less than three bowel movements per week, (2) sensation of incomplete evacuation, (3) feeling of anorectal obstruction, (4) hard or lumpy stool, (5) need for straining, or (6) need of manual disimpaction or support of the pelvic floor.[9]

ETIOLOGY

Numerous diseases can cause constipation. Therefore, before attributing constipation to functional or idiopathic reasons, other diagnoses (Box 145-1) must be excluded.

EVALUATION

HISTORY AND PHYSICAL EXAMINATION

The significant and critical information obtained from a highly detailed clinical history is mandatory. Surveys to measure constipation have been created. Agachan et al developed a scoring system of constipation to evaluate patients' improvement following medical or surgical treatment (Box 145-2).[8] Thorough abdominal and perineal examinations must be undertaken, with an inspection of the anal region, including a digital examination, anoscopy, and a rigid or flexible sigmoidoscopy. The abdominal examination should identify any masses, distention, scars, or tenderness. A digital examination can exclude distal obstructive causes of constipation and detect the presence of any hard stool in the rectum. This latter finding may be common in patients who present with irritable bowel syndrome, inadequate fiber intake, or adequate fiber intake with suboptimal fluid ingestion.

DIAGNOSTIC STUDIES

Barium Enema and Colonoscopy

No patient who complains of constipation should be considered to have a functional cause until mechanical and extracolonic causes are excluded. Therefore, sigmoidoscopy or proctoscopy should be supplemented by a double-contrast barium enema. Although colonoscopy is a better means of excluding neoplasia, it may be technically challenging because of the redundancy associated with constipation. Alternatively, a barium enema gives the physician a view of the anatomic configuration of the colon, including its size and length.[10] Both constipated and nonconstipated persons can present with large, dilated colons (megacolon) and dolichocolon (Figure 145-1).

CLINICAL APPROACH

Before beginning invasive and potentially expensive physiologic testing, all anatomic and extracolonic causes of constipation must be excluded. Therefore, after the initial office evaluation and air-contrast barium enema, the aim of the general evaluation should be to exclude all of the extracolonic entities listed in Box 145-1. After such exclusion, a 6-month course of fiber supplementation, dietary measures, and exercise should eliminate patients who have inadequate fiber or water intake as the

---

BOX 145-1 **Classification of Constipation**

CONGENITAL
Hirschsprung disease

ACQUIRED
Chagas disease

MECHANICAL (OBSTRUCTIVE)
Neoplasia
Adhesions
Hernia
Volvulus
Endometriosis
Severe sigmoid diverticulitis
Anal stenosis

FUNCTIONAL
Inadequate fiber intake
Irritable bowel syndrome

IDIOPATHIC
Colonic
Inertia
Dolichocolon

Pelvic
Intussusception/rectal prolapse
Rectocele
Sigmoidocele
Descending perineum
Paradoxical puborectalis contraction
Perineal hernia

EXTRAINTESTINAL
Pharmacologic
Analgesics
Anesthetics
Anticholinergics
Anticonvulsants
Antidepressants
Antiparkinsonian agents
Antacids
Barium sulfate
Diuretics
Ganglionic blockers
Iron
Hypotensives

Laxative abuse
Metallic intoxication (arsenic, lead, phosphorus)
Monoamine oxidase inhibitors
Opiates
Paralytic agents
Parasympatholytics
Phenothiazines
Psychotherapeutic

Metabolic and Endocrine
Amyloidosis
Diabetes
Hypercalcemia
Hyperparathyroidism
Hypokalemia
Hypopituitarism
Hypothyroidism
Pheochromocytoma
Porphyria
Pregnancy
Scleroderma
Uremia

NEUROGENIC
Peripheral
Autonomic neuropathy
von Recklinghausen disease
Multiple endocrine neoplasia 2b

Spinal
Cauda equina tumor
Iatrogenic
Meningocele
Multiple sclerosis
Paraplegia
Resection of nervi erigentes
Shy-Drager syndrome
Tabes dorsalis
Trauma

Central
Parkinson disease
Stroke
Tumors

---

source for their constipation.[11] The patient should strive to develop regular bowel habits and try to have a bowel movement in the morning or after meals to take advantage of the gastrocolic reflex. The prompt discontinuation of any stimulant laxative is generally advised, because the earlier-mentioned measures should suffice. If laxatives must be prescribed, stool softeners and lubricants are the preferred choices (Box 145-3).

The failure of such measures should prompt physiologic investigation. In our department, constipated patients typically undergo a colonic transit time study, manometry, defecography, and anal electromyography (EMG). The distinction between colonic inertia and a pelvic outlet obstruction syndrome is crucial, because it has a direct influence on therapy.

PHYSIOLOGY LABORATORY

Colonic Transit

Colonic motility studies have demonstrated that electric activity occurs in the colon as rhythmic or sporadic nonpropagating bursts and sporadic propagating bursts (mass movements) that occur approximately six times per day.[12] Colonic motility is modulated by parasympathetic and sympathetic innervation as well as gastrointestinal hormones such as gastrin, serotonin, vasoactive intestinal peptide, and substance P, and by a number of local colon reflexes.

The measurement of colonic transit through the ingestion of radiopaque markers has been used and often modified since 1981.[13-16] In its most "user-friendly" form, the test includes the ingestion of a single capsule

BOX 145-2 Constipation Scoring System (Minimum Score 0, Maximum Score 30)

Symptom	Score
FREQUENCY OF BOWEL MOVEMENTS	
1-2 times per 1-2 days	0
2 times per week	1
Once per week	2
Less than once per week	3
Less than once per month	4
DIFFICULTY: PAIN EVACUATION EFFORT	
Never	0
Rarely	1
Sometimes	2
Usually	3
Always	4
COMPLETENESS: FEELING INCOMPLETE EVACUATION	
Never	0
Rarely	1
Sometimes	2
Usually	3
Always	4
ABDOMINAL PAIN	
Never	0
Rarely	1
Sometimes	2
Usually	3
Always	4
TIME: MINUTES IN LAVATORY PER ATTEMPT	
<5	0
5 to 10	1
10 to 20	2
20 to 30	3
>30	4
ASSISTANCE: TYPE OF ASSISTANCE	
Without assistance	0
Stimulant laxatives	1
Digital assistance or enemas	2
FAILURE: UNSUCCESSFUL ATTEMPTS FOR EVACUATION PER 24 HOURS	
Never	0
1 to 3	1
3 to 6	2
6 to 9	3
>9	4
HISTORY: DURATION OF CONSTIPATION (YEARS)	
<1	0
1 to 5	1
5 to 10	2
10 to 20	3
>20	4

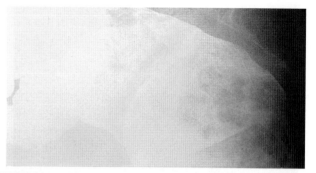

FIGURE 145-1 Barium enema of a patient with chronic constipation. Typical findings of megacolon include a very elongated and redundant colon.

BOX 145-3 General Classification of Laxatives

Bulk-forming agents
  Dietary
  Synthetic or processed
  Methylcellulose
  Polycarbophil
  Psyllium
Lubricants
  Mineral oil
Emollients
  Docusate (calcium, sodium, or potassium)
Saline laxatives (osmotic agents)
  Magnesium-containing compounds (citrate, hydroxide, sulfate)
  Sodium phosphate
  Lactulose
  Lactinol
  Sorbitol
Stimulant (irritant)
  Bisacodyl
  Senna
  Phenolphthalein
  Danthron
  Casanthranol
  Castor oil
  Cascara

From Wexner SD, Bartolo DCC: *Constipation: Etiology, evaluation, and management.* Oxford, Butterworth-Heinemann, 1995, p 141.

containing 24 radiopaque markers (Sitzmarks) followed by radiographs taken on the fifth day after the capsule ingestion. All laxatives, enemas, and suppositories must be discontinued prior to the examination. The diagnosis of colonic inertia is made if 20% or more of the markers are found to be diffusely scattered throughout the colon by the fifth day (Figure 145-2).[17] Pelvic retention of the markers is consistent with the diagnosis of outlet obstruction.

Advantages of this method to determine colonic transit are simplicity, reproducibility, and low cost. Nam et al[18] studied a group of 51 patients with chronic idiopathic constipation, each of whom underwent a colonic transit study on two separate occasions. Patients were divided into three groups: colonic inertia, anismus, and chronic idiopathic constipation. In 35 patients (69%), the results were equal between the two studies, and in 16 patients (31%), the results were disparate (gamma correlation coefficient [CC] = 0.53, $P < 0.01$). When the tests were repeated within 1 year, the CC was 0.38 ($P < 0.05$), whereas for periods of more than 1 year, the CC was 0.79 ($P < 0.01$). The authors concluded that colonic transit

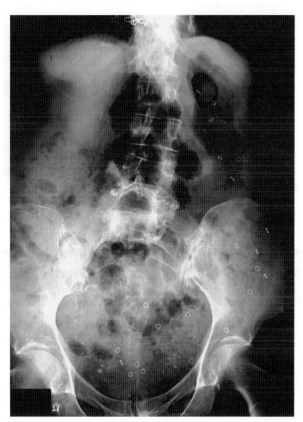

FIGURE 145-2 The radiograph shows the markers distributed diffusely throughout the colon on the fifth postingestion day. The diagnostic finding is consistent with colonic inertia.

studies are reproducible, despite the duration between tests. In an attempt to study segmental colonic transit, some authors have used different types of markers administered on successive days with plain abdominal films taken either serially[13,15] or on a single day.[16] Because there is no evidence that segmental colonic resection is an appropriate option in the treatment of colonic inertia, however, the determination of segmental transit does not justify the increased complexity of this approach.

Scintigraphy can also be applied to the measurement of colonic transit. A method of delivery by orocecal intubation was devised to avoid dispersion of the radiolabeled material ([111]Indium-diethylenetriamine pentaacetic acid [In-DTPA]) during its passage through the stomach and small intestine.[19] The need for orocecal intubation, however, is eliminated when labeled pellets are incorporated into a gelatin capsule coated with a methacrylate polymer[20] or activated charcoal.[21] Images can be obtained at three time points: 28, 52, and 60 hours after ingestion.[22] Disadvantages of this method include less-than-ideal image resolution and the difficult interpretation of the anatomy of the colon.

Small Bowel Transit

Studies indicate that there may be a subset of constipated patients in whom orocecal transit time is delayed.[23] When surgical treatment for constipation is being planned, measurement of small bowel transit is important to distinguish between isolated colonic inertia and panenteric

inertia. The first group of patients is known to benefit from colectomy; the second group may remain constipated even after colectomy.[24]

The breath hydrogen test was first described in 1975 by Bond et al[25] to measure orocecal transit time. This test is based on the principle that the bacterial metabolism in the colon produces hydrogen. Hydrogen is insoluble in water and highly diffusible; therefore, it is promptly absorbed by the intestinal mucosa, transported to the lungs, and then exhaled. An expiratory breath specimen is measured by means of a gas chromatograph analyzer after the patient ingests a dose of 10 g of lactulose diluted in 100 mL of water; breath samples are taken every 10 minutes for a minimum of 2 hours. The time between the ingestion of the lactulose and the first breath hydrogen peak should represent the time of arrival of the substrate to the colon. This test can be altered by smoking or exercise,[26] as well as by small bowel bacterial overgrowth.

A standard meal labeled with technetium-99m diethylenetriamine pentaacetic acid (^{99m}Tc-DTPA) can also be used to measure gastric emptying and small bowel transit; other radioisotopes may also be used (iodine, indium). The patient must ingest the meal after an overnight fast, and a gamma camera is used to obtain the images until the meal arrives in the cecum. The actual small bowel transit is determined as the time between 10% gastric emptying and the appearance of scintigraphic activity in the cecum. Apart from the exposure to radiation generated by this examination, the major disadvantage of this method is the difficulty in identifying cecal filling because of the overlap of small bowel loops. Bonapace et al[27] evaluated 73 patients with chronic constipation using whole-gut transit scintigraphy. Nineteen percent of patients were found to have delayed gastric emptying, and 7% had delayed small bowel transit time.

The detection of plasma sulfapyridine after the ingestion of sulfasalazine has also been described and corresponds to orocecal transit.[28] This technique has not been widely accepted because of its complexity and cost and the requirement for a nuclear camera. The use of a barium-labeled test meal to assess small bowel transit is not recommended because alterations in small bowel physiology can be caused by barium; moreover, radiation exposure can be significant.

Manometry

Anorectal manometry measures intraanal and intrarectal pressures by means of a transanally inserted catheter. Measurements can be taken in either a stationary pull-through or a motorized continuous withdrawal technique. We use a water-perfused catheter and measure pressures at 1-cm increments, in a proximal-to-distal orientation. With this method, one can establish the anal canal length (high pressure zone), resting and squeeze pressures, and rectal capacity volume to first sensation. Most important in constipated patients, one can elicit the rectoanal inhibitory reflex (RAIR). Because of the diversity of methods used in performing anorectal manometry, normal values do not always coincide among institutions; however, these parameters should remain identical within the same laboratory.[29]

Despite these pressure variations, the absence of the RAIR is abnormal. The lack of this reflex in patients with chronic constipation may suggest Hirschsprung disease. In addition, the same absence is noted in patients with Chagas disease and should be suspected in patients from endemic countries. An abnormal reflex may also be encountered in patients with dermatomyositis or scleroderma and after any coloanal or ileoanal anastomosis[30]; elicitation of the RAIR is qualitative and not quantitative.

Defecography

Defecography is a method to assess simulated evacuation under direct real-time fluoroscopic visualization.[31-34] The rectum is filled with a radiopaque material similar in consistency to stool, and the patient is seated on a water-filled commode. The evacuation process is then observed under fluoroscopic guidance. Radiographs and videos are taken during four distinct activities: at rest, during squeeze, while pushing, and after evacuation. The radiographs allow the measurement of the anorectal angle, perineal descent, and puborectalis length. Because the study is dynamic, one of the criticisms is the reproducibility of the test. Pfeifer et al,[35] however, confirmed an 83% accuracy rate for the examination when four independent observers used the same definition for each of the pathologic findings.

Under normal circumstances, the rectum is emptied during straining within 8 to 12 seconds, depending on the viscosity of the contrast medium.[35] Even though the examination may disclose multiple abnormalities such as rectoceles and sigmoidoceles, intussusception, or perineal descent, one should be cautious to not attribute clinical significance to normal anatomic variants.[36] Jorge et al[37] found that because defecography had the ability to detect associated abnormalities, it was superior to anal EMG in the diagnosis of nonrelaxing puborectalis syndrome.

The failure to eliminate rectal contents during defecography may not be a result of obstructed defecation but rather of the patient's inhibition to evacuate in the presence of an audience. To overcome potentially false-positive results, other methods have been devised, such as attempting the evacuation of a balloon from the rectum.[38-40] Radioactive isotopes can also be used to quantitatively assess evacuation.[41] The introduction of a radiolabeled artificial stool into the rectum is followed by the capture of images with a standard gamma camera, and the percentage of emptying is calculated using an equation. Even though this test provides good qualitative information about the percentage of rectal content evacuated, the low resolution of scintigraphic defecography does not permit the detection of abnormalities such as intussusception, mucosal prolapse, or many rectoceles.

Recently, dynamic pelvic magnetic resonance (MR) imaging has been used to diagnose pelvic floor disorders.[42-44] Matsuoka et al[42] compared MR defecography with conventional videoproctography. Although all 22 patients preferred MR defecography to videoproctography because of greater comfort, MR defecography was inferior in detecting rectoceles, rectoanal intussusception, and perineal descent. The authors concluded that the routine use of MR defecography in the evaluation of constipated patients could not be justified by the high cost of the test. Elshazly et al[44] evaluated 40 patients with obstructed defecation with MR defecography, and found that the results altered the management in more than 50% of the patients.

Electromyography and Pudendal Nerve Terminal Motor Latency

EMG and pudendal nerve terminal motor latency (PNTML) are the only methods available to analyze the neurologic status of the striated component of the anal sphincter muscles and its neural supply, respectively. This examination is based on the concept of the motor unit,[45] which consists of an anterior horn cell, its axon and axonal branches, motor end plates, and muscle fibers innervated by that cell. The examination is undertaken with the patient in the left lateral decubitus position, using concentric needle EMG to study the four quadrants of the external anal sphincter during rest, squeeze, cough, and simulated defecation. A disposable anal plug electrode may also be used for anal EMG. This technique has the advantage of being less invasive; however, it is not as accurate as the needle examination. The electrical activity of the muscular action potentials is recorded and analyzed by means of a computer-assisted system (Nicolet Viking II EMG System).

The number of muscle fibers in the anal sphincter innervated by each axon is small as a result of its continuously contracted activity. In a normal anal EMG, continuous electrical activity may be seen even at rest,[46] with an increase in activity during squeezing and coughing; electrical activity should return to its resting pattern during evacuation. In the evaluation of constipation, EMG can help diagnose paradoxical puborectalis contraction (PPC), and can be used as a tool in treatment of this condition.[47,48]

The PNTML technique was described by Kiff and Swash in 1984.[49] It can be measured with an electrode mounted on the examiner's finger and introduced into the rectum. The examiner's index finger is positioned so that the electrode is brought into contact with one of the ischial spines. The time between the application of the electric stimulus and the external sphincter contraction is called the *terminal motor latency of the pudendal nerve.* Initially, in small series, some authors argued for a correlation between the chronic straining encountered in constipated patients and abnormally prolonged PNTML.[50-52] Significantly larger series, however, have not substantiated this theoretical correlation between increased perineal descent and pudendal neuropathy.[53]

Regarding the sensory components of the anal canal, two techniques have been described: temperature sensation[54] and mucosal electrosensitivity.[55] The first consists of a water-perfused thermode to assess the thermal sensitivity of the anorectum. Even though the ability to discriminate temperature has been implicated in fecal continence, no studies show any aberration in constipation. For the assessment of mucosal electrosensitivity, a specially constructed probe that generates constant current is applied to the upper anal canal. The stimulus is increased until the patient feels a tingling sensation, which is recorded as the threshold of sensation. The use of rectal electrosensitivity in constipation[56] is based on the fact that rectal sensation may be decreased in these patients, although this observation may be a result of damage to sensory innervation of the surrounding muscles or of feces that prevent optimal mucosal contact.[57]

Minnesota Multiphasic Personality Inventory Assessment

The Minnesota Multiphasic Personality Inventory (MMPI) assessment was created in 1943 by Hathaway and McKinley.[58] It has been used to compare the psychological function of patient populations with different medical diagnoses. It describes how effectively the individual is functioning on an interpersonal and intrapersonal level. The test consists of 550 questions, which must be answered on a "true or false" basis. All scale scores are based on a mean of 50 and a standard deviation of 10, whereas two standard deviations from the mean is indicative of psychopathology.[59] When Devroede et al[60] compared constipated women and women with arthritis, they found a "conversion V" pattern on the MMPI of the constipated patients, a pattern indicating the presence of a somatization defense structure for dealing with psychological distress.

Heymen et al[61] used the MMPI to analyze three groups of patients who complained of constipation, fecal incontinence, and rectal pain. They found that constipated patients showed an elevation in the hypochondriasis, depression, and hysteria scales, which are referred to as the *neurotic triad*.[60] This indicates that these subgroups of patients use somatization as a defense mechanism, which is a good prognostic factor for psychotherapy. For these reasons, constipated patients who are candidates for colectomy should undergo the MMPI assessment before surgery, as they may benefit from perioperative psychotherapy and/or psychotropic medications.

INTERPRETATION OF RESULTS

The aim of the diagnostic evaluation is to determine whether the patient who presents with constipation has any objective abnormalities. As previously mentioned, the initial strategy should therefore be to exclude extracolonic and structural disorders with a barium enema or colonoscopy. If no cause for constipation is identified, a colonic transit study should be performed. If transit is normal, an assessment of the pelvic floor should be undertaken with defecography and EMG. Recurrent volvulus, Hirschsprung or Chagas disease, and systemic sclerosis must be excluded in patients who present with megabowel.

After completing the diagnostic evaluation, functional constipation can be categorized as follows:
1. Colonic causes—colonic inertia, idiopathic megabowel, adult Hirschsprung disease
2. Pelvic outlet obstruction—pelvic floor dysfunction, PPC, combined pelvic floor dysfunction and PPC
3. Combined colonic inertia with pelvic outlet obstruction
4. Normal transit constipation (usually as a result of irritable bowel syndrome)

TREATMENT

SURGICAL APPROACH

Colonic Inertia

Patients with abnormal transit and normal pelvic floor physiology who do not respond to conservative therapy are candidates for surgery. Surgical management for clinically intractable constipation was first attempted more than a century ago.[62,63] Three surgical techniques have been described to treat colonic inertia: subtotal colectomy with ileorectal anastomosis (IRA), ileosigmoid anastomosis, and cecorectal anastomosis (CRA). Many series have been reported, with variable results (Table 145-1). Despite early suboptimal results, the development and availability of anorectal physiologic testing have made better results possible during the past two decades. Subtotal colectomy with IRA has been established as the current procedure of choice for the treatment of colonic inertia. Pikarsky et al[64] assessed by telephone interview a group of 30 patients who underwent IRA at a minimum of a 5-year followup. All 30 patients rated their outcome as excellent, although during this period, six patients (20%) required hospitalization for small bowel obstruction, of whom three (10%) required laparotomy. In this series, two patients (6%) still required assisted bowel movements, one patient used laxatives, and two patients needed antidiarrheals to control frequency. FitzHarris et al[65] reported on 75 patients who underwent IRA. Sixtyone patients (81%) were at least somewhat pleased with their bowel movement frequency; however, 31 (41%) had persistent abdominal pain and 16 (21%) reported incontinence. The results appear to persist in long-term followup.[66,67] At a median followup of 11 years, Hassan et al[66] found that 85% of patients were satisfied with their bowel function.

Subtotal colectomy with CRA has the theoretical advantage of retaining the ileocecal valve to improve the absorption of water. Patients who undergo this procedure, however, may suffer from persistent cecal dilation.[68] Most series reporting results of CRA have been small. Yoshioka and Keighley[69] compared results of five patients who underwent CRA with 34 patients who underwent IRA and found no difference in the success rate. Sarli et al[70] reported the results of 26 patients. At 1-year followup, the mean number of bowel movements per day was 1.7, and all 26 patients were satisfied with the results of their surgery. Marchesi et al[71] reported results of 29 patients who underwent CRA, and found results similar to published results of patients who underwent IRA.

Because some patients may experience diarrhea or frequent bowel movements after subtotal colectomy with IRA, some authors have proposed segmental colectomy to avoid these unwanted side effects. The results of these procedures, however, have been less impressive, with an overall success rate of less than 70%. In addition, up to half of patients will develop megabowel of the remaining colon.

The use of laparoscopic surgery for diseases of the colon and rectum began in the early 1990s and has now become the standard of care in some disease states. Several authors have reported on the use of laparoscopy

TABLE 145-1 Results of Subtotal Colectomy for Constipation

Authors, Year	No. of Patients (% Female)	Mean Age (years)	Followup (years)	Barium Enema	Biopsy	NO MEGACOLON n	Success Rate (%)	MEGACOLON n	Success Rate (%)
Watkins, 1966[63]	3‡ (100)	43	0.7	Yes	Yes	—	—	3	100
Lane and Todd, 1977[129]	3‡ (33)	46	2.2	Yes	Yes*	—	—	3	33
Smith et al, 1977[130]	1‡ (100)	18	3	Yes	Yes	—	—	1	100
McCready et al, 1979[131]	6‡ (65)	32	2.4	Yes*	Yes*	—	—	6	100
Hughes et al, 1981[132]	17‡ (94)	35	—	Yes	Yes	10	80	7	100
Belliveau et al, 1982[133]	9‡	—	5.4	Yes*	—	—	—	7	78
Klatt, 1983[134]	9§ (100)	39	2.1	Yes	—	3	100	6	100
Gilbert et al, 1984[135]	6‡ (86)	36	0.7	Yes	—	—	—	6	100
Keighley and Shouler, 1984[111]	10‡ (100)	27	—	Yes	—	10	90	—	—
Preston et al, 1984[136]	8‡ (100)	26	5.7	Yes	Yes	8	63	—	—
Krishnamurthy et al, 1985[137]	12‡ (100)	33	—	—	—	12	100	—	—
Todd, 1985[68]	16‡	—	—	—	—	16	88	—	—
Barnes et al, 1986[138]	6‡ (43)	38	5	Yes	Yes	—	—	6	67
Roe et al, 1986[55]	7‡	—	0.7	Yes	Yes	7	71	—	—
Beck et al, 1989[139]	14‡ (100)	41	1.2	Yes	Yes*	14	100	—	—
Gasslander et al, 1987[140]	6‡ (86)	37	2	Yes	Yes*	6	100	—	—
Leon et al, 1987[141]	13‡ (100)	31	2.6	Yes*	Yes	13	77	—	—
Walsh et al, 1987[142]	19‡ (86)	—	3.2	Yes*	Yes*	17	65	2	50
Akervall et al, 1988[143]	12‡ (100)	39	3.4	Yes	—	12	66	—	—
Kamm et al, 1988[114]	33‡ (100)	34	2	Yes	Yes	33	50	—	—
Vasilevsky et al, 1988[144]	51‡ (94)	45	4	Yes	—	24	71	14	93
Yoshioka et al, 1989[69]	40† (98)	35	3	Yes	Yes	32	58‖	8	58¶
Zenilman et al, 1989[145]	12‡ (100)	35	2	Yes*	Yes*	12	100	—	—
Coremans, 1990[146]	11‡ (100)	46	3.8	Yes	Yes	10	60	1	100
Kuijpers, 1990[147]	12‡	42	—	—	—	12	50	—	—
Stabile et al, 1991[148]	11‡ (64)	43	7	Yes	—	—	—	11	100
Tajana et al, 1990[149]	7‡	—	—	Yes	—	5	100	2	100
Pemberton et al, 1991[150]	38‡ (84)	40	—	Yes	—	38	100	—	—
Wexner et al, 1991[151]	16‡ (92)	45	1.2	Yes	Yes	16	94	—	—
Mahendrarajah et al, 1994[152]	9‡ (100)	38	1.3	—	—	9	88	—	—
Stewart et al, 1994[153]	1‡	11	2	—	—	—	—	1	100
Takahashi et al, 1994[154]	38‡	—	3	Yes	Yes	37	97	—	—
Piccirillo et al, 1995[155]	54‡ (78)	49	2.2	Yes	Yes	54	94	—	—
Redmond et al, 1995[156]	34‡ (92)	43	7.5	Yes	—	34	90**,††	13	—
Lubowski et al, 1996[157]	59‡ (55)	42.3	3.6	—	Yes*	—	35	—	96
Nyam et al, 1997[158]	74‡ (68)	43	5	Yes*	—	—	72	—	96
Bernini et al, 1998[159]	106‡ (98)	41	6.5	Yes	—	106	74	—	—
Pikarsky et al, 2001[64]	30‡ (21)	—	9.8	—	—	30	100	—	—
Fan and Wang, 2000[160]	24 (79)	37	1.9	Yes	—	24	87.5	—	—
Sarli et al, 2001[161]	26‖	40	1	—	—	10	100	—	—
Verne et al, 2002[162]	13‡	22.9	—	Yes	Yes	13	92	—	—
FitzHarris et al, 2003[65]	75	—	3.9	—	—	75	92	—	—
Glia et al, 2004[24]	14	46	5	Yes	Yes*	14	100	—	—
Thaler et al, 2005[163]	17 (100)	47	4.8	—	—	17	100**	—	—
Hassan et al, 2006[66]	110 (95)	40	11	Yes*	Yes*	104	98	—	—
Zutshi, et al, 2007[67]	69 (97)	38	11	—	—	69	77	—	—

Adapted from Pfeifer J, Agachon F, Wexner SD: Surgery for constipation: A review. *Dis Colon Rectum* 39:444, 1996.
*Not all patients.
†Thirty-four ileosigmoid anastomoses, five cecorectal anastomoses, and one ileorectal anastomosis.
‡Ileorectal or ileosigmoid anastomosis.
§Ileosigmoid anastomosis.
‖Cecorectal anastomosis.
¶Overall success.
**For colonic inertia.
††For gastrointestinal disease.

in the treatment of colonic inertia.[72-77] Ho et al[73] compared seven patients who underwent laparoscopic-assisted colectomy with 17 patients who underwent open colectomy. Operative time was significantly longer in the laparoscopic group, but functional outcome was equal in both groups. Complications and length of stay were also equal in both groups; however, patients who underwent open surgery were less satisfied with the cosmetic outcome. Other authors have reported functional outcomes which are similar to reported outcomes for open colectomy.

Regardless of the type of surgery selected to treat constipation, patients must understand the risks. In addition to the standard risks such as anastomotic leak and postoperative bowel obstruction, problems specific to colectomy for constipation also exist. Specifically, although frequency of bowel movements will probably improve, bloating, pain, nausea, and other constitutional symptoms may persist or even worsen. Furthermore, patients without these symptoms preoperatively may develop them following surgery. No patient should undergo colectomy for constipation without understanding that the operation will not help ameliorate these associated symptoms. In addition, patients must also be aware of the possible need for a stoma at any time following surgery.[78,79] Patients with unrealistic psychological expectations, no matter how well suited by physiologic testing for surgery, are not surgical candidates.

In patients who wish to avoid resectional surgery, another option is the use of antegrade colonic enemas. This procedure involves the creation of an appendicostomy or a tubularized cecal conduit through which the patient delivers water enemas (up to 2 L/day). This procedure was first described in pediatric patients and for the use of fecal incontinence, but has since also been used in constipation.[80] Worsoe et al[81] evaluated 41 patients who underwent the antegrade colonic enema procedure and found that after a followup of 3 years, 61% were satisfied or very satisfied with the result. Other authors have found similar results; however, a fair number of patients may develop leakage at the stoma site or stomal stenosis leading to failure.[82,83]

Pelvic Outlet Obstruction

Sigmoidocele may account for symptoms of obstructed defecation, particularly in patients who have previously undergone hysterectomy. The mechanism of pelvic outlet obstruction is believed to be caused by collapse of the rectal wall as a result of extrinsic compression of the hernia contents and stasis of the sigmoid loop. Jorge et al[84] defined the classification system for sigmoidoceles based on the degree of descent of the lowest portion of the sigmoid: first degree, above the pubococcygeal line; second degree, below the pubococcygeal line and above the ischiococcygeal line; and third degree, below the ischiococcygeal line (Figure 145-3). First- and second-degree sigmoidoceles may represent normal anatomic variants, although a nonemptying sigmoidocele can be the cause of sensation of incomplete evacuation. Patients with first- and second-degree sigmoidocele can be treated conservatively with biofeedback therapy, whereas third-degree sigmoidoceles may benefit from operative therapy.

Jorge et al[84] reported their experiences with patients who had first-degree ($n = 9$), second degree ($n = 7$), and third-degree ($n = 8$) sigmoidocele. Impaired rectal emptying was present in 16 patients (67%). Five of eight patients with third-degree sigmoidocele underwent colonic resection with or without rectopexy, whereas the other three patients were managed conservatively. One of seven patients with second-degree sigmoidocele underwent colectomy, and the other six were managed conservatively, as were all nine patients with first-degree sigmoidocele. Posttreatment improvement was noted in all patients who underwent resection, but in only six (33%) of 18 patients treated conservatively. Furthermore, the clinical significance of third-degree sigmoidocele is supported by the fact that all five of the patients with third-degree sigmoidocele who underwent colonic resection reported symptomatic improvement at a mean followup period of 23 months.

Rectocele is a protrusion of the rectal wall into the vagina during defecation. It may be commonly seen in healthy women,[85] but is also associated with multiparity,[86] obstetric damage, and the presence of PPC.[87] Rectoceles can be classified as high level (usually caused by stretching or disruption of the upper third of the vaginal wall and the cardinal and uterosacral ligaments), mid level (usually caused by loss of pelvic floor support secondary to parturition), or low level (usually the consequence of perineal body defects).

The clinical significance of rectoceles is uncertain. Rectoceles may cause mild to severe anorectal symptoms, such as perineal pressure, the sensation of a pouch in the vagina, or incomplete evacuation requiring rectal or vaginal digitation.[36] In our institution, patients are chosen for surgery according to the size of the rectocele (>2 cm), the inability to empty the rectocele at defecography, and the use of digitation or perineal support to empty the rectum (Figure 145-4). Rectoceles can be repaired via a transvaginal[88,89] or transrectal[90-92] approach. Overall success rates range from 65% to 100%.

Rectal intussusception is an infolding of the rectum into but not beyond the anal verge. Although rectal intussusception is a common finding in defecography (Figure 145-5), it is not usually the cause of constipation. Treatment should consist of adequate fiber intake and the use of enemas or laxatives to assist in evacuation, as well as biofeedback. Surgical repair, including rectopexy, has had poor long-term results.[93,94] Choi et al[95] compared patients with large rectal intussusception treated with conservative dietary therapy, biofeedback, or surgery. Although 60% reported subjective improvement following surgery, half of these patients developed new symptoms such as rectal bleeding or pain, incomplete evacuation, or liquid stools. In addition, biofeedback showed a significant improvement in number of bowel movements per week when compared with a high-fiber dietary regimen alone.

In 1998, Longo introduced a new technique to surgically treat obstructed defecation, the stapled transanal rectal resection (STARR). The STARR procedure is intended to resect any internally prolapsed rectum, anatomically to correct a rectocele (if present), and to reestablish continuity of the rectal wall, with restoration of

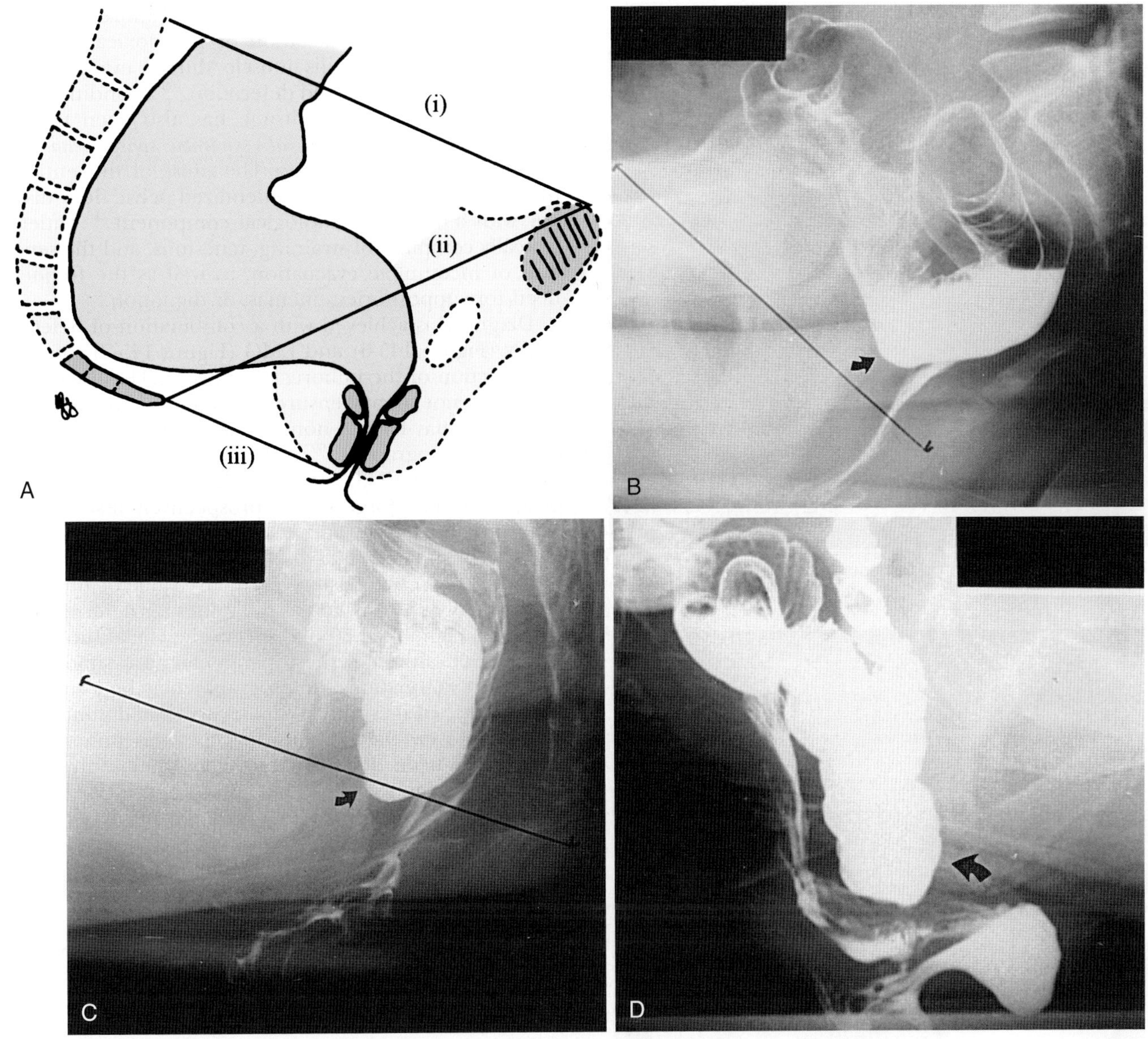

FIGURE 145-3 A, Schematic of the three degrees of sigmoidocele: pubosacral line (i), pubococcygeal line (ii), and ischiococcygeal line (iii). **B,** First-degree sigmoidocele is the descent of the lowest portion of the sigmoid to above the pubococcygeal line. **C,** The second-degree is below the pubococcygeal line but above the ischiococcygeal line. **D,** The third-degree is below the ischiococcygeal line.

normal anatomy, reduced rectal volume, and normal compliance. It involves the use of a circular stapler fired twice, plicating both the anterior and posterior rectal walls.

Boccasanta et al[96] evaluated 90 patients who underwent the STARR procedure. After 1 year of followup, 81 patients were satisfied and only four had poor results. The most common complications observed were urgency (17.8%), incontinence to flatus (8.9%), urinary retention space (5.5%), bleeding space (4.4%), and anal stenosis (3.3%). Ommer et al[97] reported good results and a significant reduction in constipation scores at a mean followup of 19 months in 14 consecutive patients. A retrospective study that evaluated 123 patients who underwent the STARR procedure was performed by Gagliardi et al[98] At a median followup of 17 months, 65% percent

of patients reported subjective improvement. Recurrence of rectocele, however, was 29%, recurrence of internal intussusception was 28%, and reoperation was required in 19% of patients. Other authors have reported similar results.[99-101]

Sacral nerve stimulation (SNS) has also been used for the treatment of constipation. The mechanism of action on the pelvic floor muscles and colorectal transit time is not entirely clear. The effects of SNS on chronic constipation were observed in patients with simultaneous urinary incontinence.[102] Ganio et al[103] reported benefits in patients with difficulty in rectal emptying and incomplete evacuation, independent of bowel frequency. Ten patients underwent placement of sacral nerve stimulators. The authors found significant reduction in difficulty of evacuation, number of unsuccessful visits to the toilet,

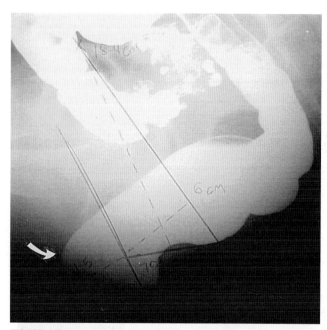

FIGURE 145-4 A nonemptying anterior rectocele is shown (arrow).

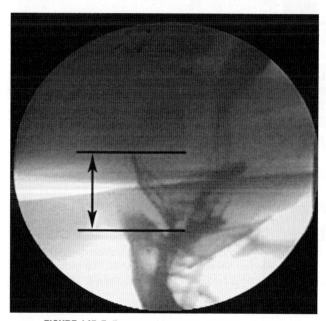

FIGURE 145-5 Rectoanal intussusception is shown.

and the time necessary to evacuate. All these improvements disappeared after removal of the electrodes. However, Kenefick et al[104] included patients with slow bowel frequency and straining, and found a significant improvement in frequency of bowel movements and quality of life. The results of these studies suggest application of SNS and improvement of symptoms for these two different types of constipation. Success rates among other series range from 42% to 95%.[105-108]

Paradoxical Puborectalis Contraction

The normal evacuatory mechanism includes the voluntary relaxation of the external anal sphincter and the pelvic floor muscles, thus increasing the anorectal angle. However, failure of relaxation or paradoxical contraction of the puborectalis muscle during evacuation is responsible for obstructed defecation,[109] a condition that is termed *PPC*. This syndrome has also been termed *anismus, nonrelaxing puborectalis syndrome, spastic pelvic floor syndrome*, and *rectal dyschezia*. The cause of this entity is unclear and may involve a generalized pelvic floor disorder with a strong psychological component.[110] Patients typically complain of straining, tenesmus, and the sensation of incomplete evacuation, as well as the frequent need for suppositories, enemas, or digitation.

Diagnosis is achieved with a combination of defecography (Figure 145-6) and EMG (Figure 145-7) to assess the function of the puborectalis muscle. The use of one test does not always ensure a diagnosis (the patients' inhibition may lead to nonrelaxation of the pelvic floor during defecography),[109] and pain may have the same effect during EMG,[111] both of which will lead to false-positive results. Jorge et al[37] prospectively assessed the role of defecography and EMG in the diagnosis of PPC in 112 constipated patients. In this series, EMG had a sensitivity of 67%, a positive predictive value of 70%, and a specificity of 83%, whereas the values for defecography were 70%, 66%, and 80%, respectively. The authors concluded that although these parameters are suboptimal for both examinations, defecography may be a superior test because of its ability to detect associated abnormalities. Moreover, the inability to relax the puborectalis muscle has been demonstrated in normal control subjects[112]; the diagnosis of PPC, therefore, must be consistent with the clinical findings and the results of more than one physiologic test.

Because of the intense psychological component in PPC, the treatment of choice for these patients is pelvic floor retraining with biofeedback. The success rate for this modality of treatment applied to PPC ranges from 29% to 100% depending on the series and the techniques that are used (Table 145-2). Attempts have been made to treat PPC through surgical division of the puborectalis muscle. Independent of the site of division on the muscle, either posteriorly or laterally, symptoms of obstructed defecation did not improve and adverse results including fecal incontinence occurred in a high number of patients.[113,114]

PELVIC FLOOR RETRAINING AND BIOFEEDBACK

Biofeedback is based on the concept that patients can be taught to recognize bodily functions of which they were not previously aware. Achieving control of such functions can be translated into visual or aural stimuli by means of different electronic devices. Electrical and hydrostatic information is displayed in such a way that patients can better understand the contraction and relaxation process. Both pressure-based (manometry) and electrical signal-based (EMG) systems have been used.[115-118] Heymen et al[119] performed a metaanalysis and found that the mean success rate of pressure-based biofeedback was 78%, whereas the success rate for EMG feedback was only 70%. In addition, there was no significant difference between the success rates using either intraanal sensors

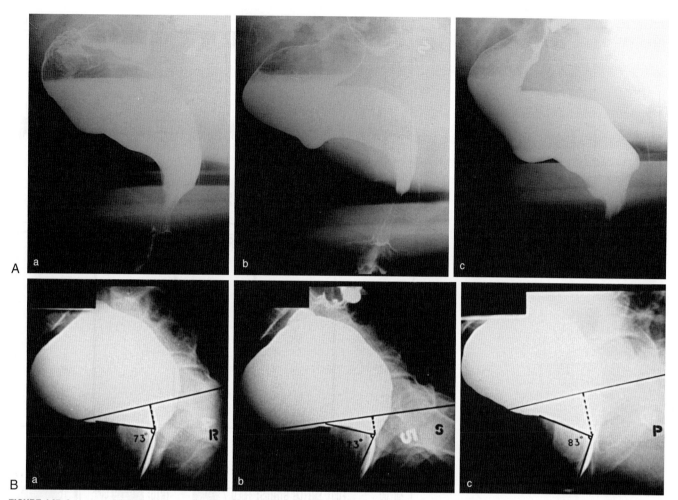

FIGURE 145-6 **A,** Normal cinedefecogram sequence at rest (a), squeeze (b), and attempted evacuation (c). **B,** Cinedefecogram shows paradoxical puborectalis contraction at rest (a), squeeze (b), and attempted evacuation (c). By contrasting these cinedefecograms, it can be seen that a normal sequence includes shortening of the anal canal and flattening of the anorectal angle with evacuation of barium contents. In comparison, paradoxical puborectalis contraction includes maintenance of the length of the closed anal canal and the anorectal angle or, in some instances, accentuation of these features by an even longer, more closed anal canal and an even more acute anorectal angle.

or perianal EMG sensors. These modalities also have been combined with rectal sensation training,[117,118] in which patients with a poor recognition of the rectal urge were taught to perceive progressively decreasing volumes of distention. In addition to these methods, portable units are available for use at home, allowing training in a friendly, familiar environment.[116,120-122]

Biofeedback training consists of three to ten 1-hour-long sessions under the supervision of a biofeedback therapist. The patients are also instructed to keep a daily record of bowel movements, medications, and the use of enemas, laxatives, or digitation. The training is done on an outpatient basis, with the patient dressed and seated on a chair after insertion of the anal plug. Patients are taught to recognize three events: rest, push, and squeeze. The push exercises are done only under supervision during the biofeedback session, whereas the squeeze and rest exercises (Kegel maneuvers) should be practiced at home as well. Discharge conditions include the

demonstration of control of pelvic floor musculature as shown with EMG, a reduction in the use of cathartics, and objective resolution of constipation as indicated in a bowel habit diary. Gilliland et al[123] reviewed the outcome of 194 patients who underwent biofeedback therapy; success rates were 29% for patients who self-discharged from therapy versus 63% for patients who were discharged by the therapist ($P < 0.0001$). In this multivariate analysis, which included duration of symptoms, age, gender, and multiple other variables, the self-discharge rate was the only predictor of successful outcome. The results of biofeedback are dependent both on the expectations of the patient and the expertise of the therapist. Currently, a multicenter prospective, randomized trial is underway to assess the placebo effect of biofeedback.

For the subset of patients who do not benefit from biofeedback, the use of *Clostridium botulinum* type A (BTX-A) in the treatment of PPC has been reported.[124-127] This potent neurotoxin causes paralysis of muscles

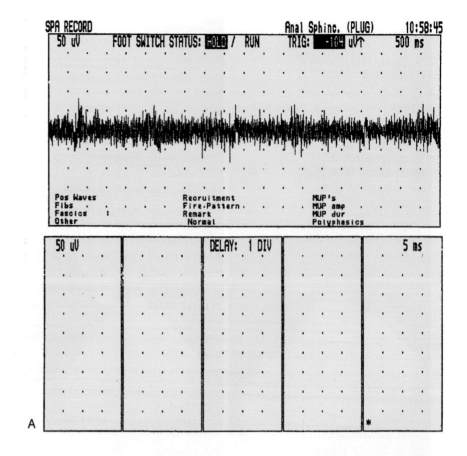

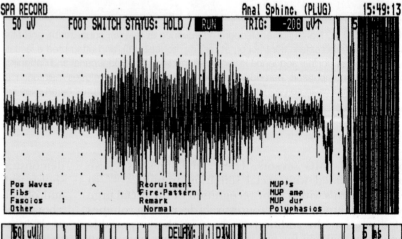

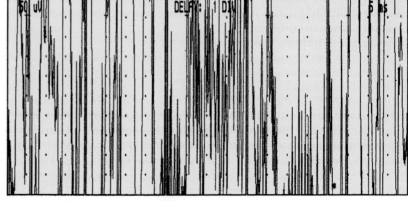

FIGURE 145-7 A, Normal electromyography during attempted evacuation is compared with paradoxical puborectalis contraction **(B).** **B,** Paradoxical increase in the recruitment of the external anal sphincter muscle and puborectalis is noted during attempted evacuation. The normal study shows appropriate external anal sphincter and puborectalis relaxation.

TABLE 145-2 Success of Biofeedback for Pelvic Floor Dysfunction

Authors, Year	No. of Patients	Mean Age or Range (years)	Diagnosis	Method of Treatment	Success Rate (%)
Wald et al, 1987[117]	9	6-15	PPC	Manometry	67
Bleijenberg and Kuijpers, 1987[164]	10	19-48	PPC	EMG	70
Keren et al, 1988[115]	12	8.3	PPC	Manometry	100
Loening-Baucke, 1990[165]	22	5-16	Encopresis	EMG	77
Loening-Baucke, 1991[166]	38	6-15	Encopresis	EMG	37
Lestar et al, 1991[121]	16	42	PPC	Manometry/balloon	44
Kawimbe et al, 1991[120]	15	45	PPC	EMG	87
Dahl et al, 1991[167]	14	6-60	PPC	EMG/balloon	93
Turnbull and Ritvo, 1992[116]	7	29-42	PPC	Manometry	71
Wexner et al, 1992[122]	18	67	PPC	EMG	89
Benninga et al, 1993[168]	29	5-16	Encopresis	Manometry	55
Bleijenberg et al, 1994[169]	11	35	PPC	EMG	73
Papachrysostomou et al, 1994[170]	22	42	PPC	EMG/balloon	86
Cox et al, 1994[171]	13	7	Encopresis	EMG	90
Siproudhis et al, 1995[172]	27	46	PPC	Manometry/balloon	52
Gilliland et al, 1997[123]	194	71	PPC	EMG	29
Karlbom et al, 1997[173]	29	46	PPC	EMG/balloon	43
Glia et al, 1997[174]	26	55	PPC	EMG/balloon	58
Wiesel et al, 2000[175]	13	38	PPC	EMG/balloon	38
Lau et al, 2000[176]	108	66	PPC	EMG	55
Battaglia et al, 2004[177]	24	27-54	PPC	EMG	50
Chiarioni et al, 2006[178]	54	33	PPC	EMG	90
Heymen et al, 2007[179]	30	50	PPC	EMG	70
Rao et al, 2010[180]	26	48	PPC	EMG	50

EMG, Electromyography; *PPC,* paradoxical puborectalis contraction.

through presynaptic inhibition of acetylcholine release. Joo et al[125] treated a group of four patients diagnosed with intractable constipation caused by PPC with BTX-A injections for a maximum of three sessions during a 3-month period. Under EMG guidance, the BTX-A was injected into the left and right sides of the puborectalis muscle. All patients were relieved of constipation between 2 and 4 days after BTX-A injection without any local or systemic side effects. However, 3 months after BTX-A injection, two of the four patients experienced symptomatic recurrence. Maria et al[126] recently reported improvement in 13 of 15 patients treated with injection of 25 units of BTX-A. Improvement, however, was maintained for a mean of only 5 months, requiring reinjection of the toxin.

CONCLUSIONS

Although only a small group of patients may benefit from surgical intervention, the evaluation of these patients must be extensive to ensure both the inclusion of appropriate candidates as well as the exclusion of inappropriate candidates.[128] In addition, the psychological status of these patients requires thorough assessment and often requires treatment. Through careful testing and selection, satisfactory results can be obtained in more than 90% of patients. Patients must understand, however, that although bowel frequency will improve and dependence on laxatives will be eliminated or significantly reduced, other symptoms, such as abdominal bloating and pain,

may persist, develop anew, or become exacerbated. Patients must also realize that they may eventually require a stoma.

REFERENCES

1. Sonnenberg A, Koch TR: Physician visits in the United States for constipation: 1958 to 1986. *Dig Dis Sci* 34:606, 1989.
2. Faigel DO: A clinical approach to constipation. *Clin Cornerstone* 4:11, 2002.
3. Lembo A, Camilleri M: Chronic constipation. *N Engl J Med* 349:1360, 2003.
4. Sonnenberg A, Koch TR: Epidemiology of constipation in the United States. *Dis Colon Rectum* 32:1, 1989.
5. Sandler RS, Jordan MC, Shelton BJ: Demographic and dietary determinants of constipation in the US population. *Am J Public Health* 80:185, 1990.
6. Everhart JE, Go VL, Johannes RS, et al: A longitudinal survey of self-reported bowel habits in the United States. *Dig Dis Sci* 34:1153, 1989.
7. Whitehead WE, Chaussade S, Corazziari E, et al: Report of an international workshop on management of constipation. *Gastroenterol Int* 4:99, 1991.
8. Agachan F, Chen T, Pfeifer J, et al: A constipation scoring system to simplify evaluation and management of constipated patients. *Dis Colon Rectum* 39:681, 1996.
9. Longstreth GF, Thompson WG, Chey WD, et al: Functional bowel disorders. *Gastroenterology* 130:1480, 2006.
10. Patriquin H, Martelli H, Devroede G: Barium enema in chronic constipation: Is it meaningful? *Gastroenterology* 75:619, 1978.
11. Burkitt DP, Walker AR, Painter NS: Effect of dietary fibre on stools and the transit-times, and its role in the causation of disease. *Lancet* 2:1408, 1972.
12. Bassotti G, Gaburri M, Imbimbo BP, et al: Colonic mass movements in idiopathic chronic constipation. *Gut* 29:1173, 1988.

13. Arhan P, Devroede G, Jehannin B, et al: Segmental colonic transit time. *Dis Colon Rectum* 24:625, 1981.
14. Bouchoucha M, Devroede G, Arhan P, et al: What is the meaning of colorectal transit time measurement? *Dis Colon Rectum* 35:773, 1992.
15. Chaussade S, Roche H, Khyari A, et al: [Measurement of colonic transit time: Description and validation of a new method]. *Gastroenterol Clin Biol* 10:385, 1986.
16. Metcalf AM, Phillips SF, Zinsmeister AR, et al: Simplified assessment of segmental colonic transit. *Gastroenterology* 92:40, 1987.
17. Hinton JM, Lennard-Jones JE, Young AC: A new method for studying gut transit times using radiopaque markers. *Gut* 10:842, 1969.
18. Nam YS, Pikarsky AJ, Wexner SD, et al: Reproducibility of colonic transit study in patients with chronic constipation. *Dis Colon Rectum* 44:86, 2001.
19. Krevsky B, Malmud LS, D'Ercole F, et al: Colonic transit scintigraphy. A physiologic approach to the quantitative measurement of colonic transit in humans. *Gastroenterology* 91:1102, 1986.
20. Proano M, Camilleri M, Phillips SF, et al: Unprepared human colon does not discriminate between solids and liquids. *Am J Physiol* 260, G13G, 1991.
21. Cheng KY, Tsai SC, Lin WY: Gallium-67 activated charcoal: A new method for preparation of radioactive capsules for colonic transit study. *Eur J Nucl Med Mol Imaging* 30:907, 2003.
22. Notghi A, Hutchinson R, Kumar D, et al: Simplified method for the measurement of segmental colonic transit time. *Gut* 35:976, 1994.
23. Cann PA, Read NW, Brown C, et al: Irritable bowel syndrome: Relationship of disorders in the transit of a single solid meal to symptom patterns. *Gut* 24:405, 1983.
24. Glia A, Akerlund JE, Lindberg G: Outcome of colectomy for slow-transit constipation in relation to presence of small-bowel dysmotility. *Dis Colon Rectum* 47:96, 2004.
25. Bond JH Jr, Levitt MD, Prentiss R: Investigation of small bowel transit time in man utilizing pulmonary hydrogen (H2) measurements. *J Lab Clin Med* 85:546, 1975.
26. Thompson DG, Binfield P, De Belder A, et al: Extra intestinal influences on exhaled breath hydrogen measurements during the investigation of gastrointestinal disease. *Gut* 26:1349, 1985.
27. Bonapace ES, Maurer AH, Davidoff S, et al: Whole gut transit scintigraphy in the clinical evaluation of patients with upper and lower gastrointestinal symptoms. *Am J Gastroenterol* 95:2838, 2000.
28. Kellow JE, Borody TJ, Phillips SF, et al: Sulfapyridine appearance in plasma after salicylazosulfapyridine. Another simple measure of intestinal transit. *Gastroenterology* 91:396, 1986.
29. Mavrantonis C, Wexner SD: A clinical approach to fecal incontinence. *J Clin Gastroenterol* 27:108, 1998.
30. Le Blanc I, Michot F, Duparc F, et al: [Anorectal manometry and ileo-anal anastomosis: Pre- and postoperative manometric comparison]. *Ann Chir* 48:183, 1994.
31. Bartolo DC, Bartram CI, Ekberg O, et al: Symposium. Proctography. *Int J Colorectal Dis* 3:67, 1988.
32. Jorge JM, Habr-Gama A, Wexner SD: Clinical applications and techniques of cinedefecography. *Am J Surg* 182:93, 2001.
33. Kuijpers HC, Strijk SP: Diagnosis of disturbances of continence and defecation. *Dis Colon Rectum* 27:658, 1984.
34. Mahieu P, Pringot J, Bodart P: Defecography: I. Description of a new procedure and results in normal patients. *Gastrointest Radiol* 9:247, 1984.
35. Pfeifer J, Oliveira L, Park UC, et al: Are interpretations of video defecographies reliable and reproducible? *Int J Colorectal Dis* 12:67, 1997.
36. Bartram CI, Turnbull GK, Lennard-Jones JE: Evacuation proctography: An investigation of rectal expulsion in 20 subjects without defecatory disturbance. *Gastrointest Radiol* 13:72, 1988.
37. Jorge JM, Wexner SD, Ger GC, et al: Cinedefecography and electromyography in the diagnosis of nonrelaxing puborectalis syndrome. *Dis Colon Rectum* 36:668, 1993.
38. Fleshman JW, Dreznik Z, Cohen E, et al: Balloon expulsion test facilitates diagnosis of pelvic floor outlet obstruction due to nonrelaxing puborectalis muscle. *Dis Colon Rectum* 35:1019, 1992.
39. Minguez M, Herreros B, Sanchiz V, et al: Predictive value of the balloon expulsion test for excluding the diagnosis of pelvic floor dyssynergia in constipation. *Gastroenterology* 126:57, 2004.
40. Wexner SD, Jorge JM: Colorectal physiological tests: Use or abuse of technology? *Eur J Surg* 160:167, 1994.

41. Pezim M, Pemberton J, Phillips S: The immobile perineum: Pathophysiologic implications in severe constipation. *Dig Dis Sci* 32:924, 1987.
42. Matsuoka H, Wexner SD, Desai MB, et al: A comparison between dynamic pelvic magnetic resonance imaging and videoproctography in patients with constipation. *Dis Colon Rectum* 44:571, 2001.
43. Roos JE, Weishaupt D, Wildermuth S, et al: Experience of 4 years with open MR defecography: Pictorial review of anorectal anatomy and disease. *Radiographics* 22:817, 2002.
44. Elshazly WG, El Nekady Ael A, Hassan H: Role of dynamic magnetic resonance imaging in management of obstructed defecation case series. *Int J Surg* 8:274, 2010.
45. Hutchinson R, Mostafa AB, Grant EA, et al: Scintigraphic defecography: Quantitative and dynamic assessment of anorectal function. *Dis Colon Rectum* 36:1132, 1993.
46. Sherrington CS: Notes on the arrangement of some motor fibres in the lumbo-sacral plexus. *J Physiol* 13:621, 1892.
47. Preston DM, Lennard-Jones JE: Anismus in chronic constipation. *Dig Dis Sci* 30:413, 1985.
48. Yeh CY, Pikarsky A, Wexner SD, et al: Electromyographic findings of paradoxical puborectalis contraction correlate poorly with cinedefecography. *Tech Coloproctol* 7:77, 2003.
49. Kiff ES, Swash M: Slowed conduction in the pudendal nerves in idiopathic (neurogenic) faecal incontinence. *Br J Surg* 71:614, 1984.
50. Ger GC, Wexner SD, Jorge JM, et al: Anorectal manometry in the diagnosis of paradoxical puborectalis syndrome. *Dis Colon Rectum* 36:816, 1993.
51. Jones PN, Lubowski DZ, Swash M, et al: Is paradoxical contraction of puborectalis muscle of functional importance? *Dis Colon Rectum* 30:667, 1987.
52. Snooks SJ, Barnes PR, Swash M, et al: Damage to the innervation of the pelvic floor musculature in chronic constipation. *Gastroenterology* 89:977, 1985.
53. Kiff ES, Barnes PR, Swash M: Evidence of pudendal neuropathy in patients with perineal descent and chronic straining at stool. *Gut* 25:1279, 1984.
54. Miller R, Bartolo DC, Cervero F, et al: Anorectal temperature sensation: A comparison of normal and incontinent patients. *Br J Surg* 74:511, 1987.
55. Roe AM, Bartolo DC, Mortensen NJ: New method for assessment of anal sensation in various anorectal disorders. *Br J Surg* 73:310, 1986.
56. Kamm MA, Lennard-Jones JE: Rectal mucosal electrosensory testing—evidence for a rectal sensory neuropathy in idiopathic constipation. *Dis Colon Rectum* 33:419, 1990.
57. Meagher AP, Kennedy ML, Lubowski DZ: Rectal mucosal electrosensitivity—what is being tested? *Int J Colorectal Dis* 11:29, 1996.
58. Hathaway SR, McKinley JC: *The Minnesota Multiphasic Personality Inventory*. Minneapolis, 1943, University of Minnesota Press.
59. Dahlstrom W, Welsh G, Dahlstrom L: *An MMPI Handbook, Volume 1: Clinical Interpretation*. Minneapolis, 1972, University of Minnesota Press.
60. Devroede G, Girard G, Bouchoucha M, et al: Idiopathic constipation by colonic dysfunction. Relationship with personality and anxiety. *Dig Dis Sci* 34:1428, 1989.
61. Heymen S, Wexner SD, Gulledge AD: MMPI assessment of patients with functional bowel disorders. *Dis Colon Rectum* 36:593, 1993.
62. Lane WA: Remarks on the results of the operative treatment of chronic constipation. *Br Med J* 1:126, 1908.
63. Watkins GL: Operative treatment of acquired megacolon in adults. *Arch Surg* 93:620, 1966.
64. Pikarsky AJ, Singh JJ, Weiss EG, et al: Long-term follow-up of patients undergoing colectomy for colonic inertia. *Dis Colon Rectum* 44:179, 2001.
65. FitzHarris GP, Garcia-Aguilar J, Parker SC, et al: Quality of life after subtotal colectomy for slow-transit constipation: Both quality and quantity count. *Dis Colon Rectum* 46:433, 2003.
66. Hassan I, Pemberton JH, Young-Fadok TM, et al: Ileorectal anastomosis for slow transit constipation: Long-term functional and quality of life results. *J Gastrointest Surg* 10:1330; discussion 1336, 2006.
67. Zutshi M, Hull TL, Trzcinski R, et al: Surgery for slow transit constipation: Are we helping patients? *Int J Colorectal Dis* 22:265, 2007.

68. Todd IP: Constipation: Results of surgical treatment. *Br J Surg* 72:S12, 1985.

69. Yoshioka K, Keighley MR: Clinical results of colectomy for severe constipation. *Br J Surg* 76:600, 1989.

70. Sarli L, Costi R, Iusco D, et al: Long-term results of subtotal colectomy with antiperistaltic cecoproctostomy. *Surg Today* 33:823, 2003.

71. Marchesi F, Sarli L, Percalli L, et al: Subtotal colectomy with anti-peristaltic cecorectal anastomosis in the treatment of slow-transit constipation: Long-term impact on quality of life. *World J Surg* 31:1658, 2007.

72. Athanasakis H, Tsiaoussis J, Vassilakis JS, et al: Laparoscopically assisted subtotal colectomy for slow-transit constipation. *Surg Endosc* 15:1090, 2001.

73. Ho YH, Tan M, Eu KW, et al: Laparoscopic-assisted compared with open total colectomy in treating slow transit constipation. *Aust N Z J Surg* 67:562, 1997.

74. Schiedeck TH, Schwandner O, Bruch HP: [Laparoscopic therapy of chronic constipation]. *Zentralbl Chir* 124:818, 1999.

75. Hsiao KC, Jao SW, Wu CC, et al: Hand-assisted laparoscopic total colectomy for slow transit constipation. *Int J Colorectal Dis* 23:419, 2008.

76. Iannelli A, Fabiani P, Mouiel J, et al: Laparoscopic subtotal colectomy with cecorectal anastomosis for slow-transit constipation. *Surg Endosc* 20:171, 2006.

77. Sample C, Gupta R, Bamehriz F, et al: Laparoscopic subtotal colectomy for colonic inertia. *J Gastrointest Surg* 9:803, 2005.

78. Scarpa M, Barollo M, Keighley MR: Ileostomy for constipation: Long-term postoperative outcome. *Colorectal Dis* 7:224, 2005.

79. El-Tawil AM: Reasons for creation of permanent ileostomy for the management of idiopathic chronic constipation. *J Gastroenterol Hepatol* 19:844, 2004.

80. Hill J, Stott S, MacLennan I: Antegrade enemas for the treatment of severe idiopathic constipation. *Br J Surg* 81:1490, 1994.

81. Worsoe J, Christensen P, Krogh K, et al: Long-term results of antegrade colonic enema in adult patients: Assessment of functional results. *Dis Colon Rectum* 51:1523, 2008.

82. Gerharz EW, Vik V, Webb G, et al: The value of the MACE (Malone antegrade colonic enema) procedure in adult patients. *J Am Coll Surg* 185:544, 1997.

83. Rongen MJ, van der Hoop AG, Baeten CG: Cecal access for antegrade colon enemas in medically refractory slow-transit constipation: A prospective study. *Dis Colon Rectum* 44:1644, 2001.

84. Jorge JM, Yang YK, Wexner SD: Incidence and clinical significance of sigmoidoceles as determined by a new classification system. *Dis Colon Rectum* 37:1112, 1994.

85. Shorvon PJ, McHugh S, Diamant NE, et al: Defecography in normal volunteers: Results and implications. *Gut* 30:1737, 1989.

86. Sehapayak S: Transrectal repair of rectocele: An extended armamentarium of colorectal surgeons. A report of 355 cases. *Dis Colon Rectum* 28:422, 1985.

87. Johansson C, Nilsson BY, Holmstrom B, et al: Association between rectocele and paradoxical sphincter response. *Dis Colon Rectum* 35:503, 1992.

88. Mellgren A, Anzén B, Nilsson BY, et al: Results of rectocele repair. A prospective study. *Dis Colon Rectum* 38:7, 1995.

89. Rao GN, Carr ND, Beynon J, et al: Endorectal repair of rectocele revisited. *Br J Surg* 84:1034, 1997.

90. Janssen LW, van Dijke CF: Selection criteria for anterior rectal wall repair in symptomatic rectocele and anterior rectal wall prolapse. *Dis Colon Rectum* 37:1100, 1994.

91. Sullivan ES, Leaverton GH, Hardwick CE: Transrectal perineal repair: An adjunct to improved function after anorectal surgery. *Dis Colon Rectum* 11:106, 1968.

92. Tjandra JJ, Ooi BS, Tang CL, et al: Transanal repair of rectocele corrects obstructed defecation if it is not associated with anismus. *Dis Colon Rectum* 42:1544, 1999.

93. Bartolo DC, Roe AM, Virjee J, et al: Evacuation proctography in obstructed defaecation and rectal intussusception. *Br J Surg* 72(Suppl):S111, 1985.

94. Christiansen J, Zhu BW, Rasmussen OO, et al: Internal rectal intussusception: Results of surgical repair. *Dis Colon Rectum* 35:1026; discussion 1028, 1992.

95. Choi YS, Kim SH, Kim JS, et al: Outcome and management of patients with large rectoanal intussusception. *Am J Gastroenterol* 96:740, 2001.

96. Boccasanta P, Venturi M, Stuto A, et al: Stapled transanal rectal resection for outlet obstruction: A prospective, multicenter trial. *Dis Colon Rectum* 47:1285; discussion 1296, 2004.

97. Ommer A, Albrecht K, Wenger F, et al: Stapled transanal rectal resection (STARR): A new option in the treatment of obstructive defecation syndrome. *Langenbecks Arch Surg* 391:32, 2006.

98. Gagliardi G, Pescatore M, Altomare DF, et al: Results, outcome predictors, and complications after stapled transanal rectal resection for obstructed defecation. *Dis Colon Rectum* 51:186; discussion 195, 2008.

99. Dodi G, Pietroletti R, Milito G, et al: Bleeding, incontinence, pain and constipation after STARR transanal double stapling rectotomy for obstructed defecation. *Tech Coloproctol* 7:148, 2003.

100. Pescatori M, Boffi F, Russo A, et al: Complications and recurrence after excision of rectal internal mucosal prolapse for obstructed defaecation. *Int J Colorectal Dis* 21:160, 2006.

101. Wolff K, Marti L, Beutner U, et al: Functional outcome and quality of life after stapled transanal rectal resection for obstructed defecation syndrome. *Dis Colon Rectum* 53:881, 2010.

102. Kollner TG, Schnee C, Gershenzon J, et al: The sesquiterpene hydrocarbons of maize (Zea mays) form five groups with distinct developmental and organ-specific distributions. *Phytochemistry* 65:1895, 2004.

103. Ganio E, Masin A, Ratto C, et al: Short-term sacral nerve stimulation for functional anorectal and urinary disturbances: Results in 40 patients: Evaluation of a new option for anorectal functional disorders. *Dis Colon Rectum* 44:1261, 2001.

104. Kenefick NJ, Nicholls RJ, Cohen RG, et al: Permanent sacral nerve stimulation for treatment of idiopathic constipation. *Br J Surg* 89:882, 2002.

105. Holzer B, Rosen HR, Novi G, et al: Sacral nerve stimulation in patients with severe constipation. *Dis Colon Rectum* 51:524; discussion 529, 2008.

106. Kamm MA, Dudding TC, Melenhorst J, et al: Sacral nerve stimulation for intractable constipation. *Gut* 59:333, 2010.

107. Kenefick NJ: Sacral nerve neuromodulation for the treatment of lower bowel motility disorders. *Ann R Coll Surg Engl* 88:617, 2006.

108. Malouf AJ, Wiesel PH, Nicholls T, et al: Short-term effects of sacral nerve stimulation for idiopathic slow transit constipation. *World J Surg* 26:166, 2002.

109. Kuijpers HC, Bleijenberg G, de Morree H: The spastic pelvic floor syndrome. Large bowel outlet obstruction caused by pelvic floor dysfunction: A radiological study. *Int J Colorectal Dis* 1:44, 1986.

110. Miller R, Duthie GS, Bartolo DC, et al: Anismus in patients with normal and slow transit constipation. *Br J Surg* 78:690, 1991.

111. Keighley MR, Shouler P: Outlet syndrome: Is there a surgical option? *J R Soc Med* 77:559, 1984.

112. Womack NR, Williams NS, Holmfield JH, et al: New method for the dynamic assessment of anorectal function in constipation. *Br J Surg* 72:994, 1985.

113. Barnes PR, Hawley PR, Preston DM, et al: Experience of posterior division of the puborectalis muscle in the management of chronic constipation. *Br J Surg* 72:475, 1985.

114. Kamm MA, Hawley PR, Lennard-Jones JE: Lateral division of the puborectalis muscle in the management of severe constipation. *Br J Surg* 75:661, 1988.

115. Keren S, Wagner Y, Heldenberg D, et al: Studies of manometric abnormalities of the rectoanal region during defecation in constipated and soiling children: Modification through biofeedback therapy. *Am J Gastroenterol* 83:827, 1988.

116. Turnbull GK, Ritvo PG: Anal sphincter biofeedback relaxation treatment for women with intractable constipation symptoms. *Dis Colon Rectum* 35:530, 1992.

117. Wald A, Chandra R, Gabel S, et al: Evaluation of biofeedback in childhood encopresis. *J Pediatr Gastroenterol Nutr* 6:554, 1987.

118. Weber J, Ducrotte P, Touchais JY, et al: Biofeedback training for constipation in adults and children. *Dis Colon Rectum* 30:844, 1987.

119. Heymen S, Jones KR, Scarlett Y, et al: Biofeedback treatment of constipation: A critical review. *Dis Colon Rectum* 46:1208, 2003.

120. Kawimbe BM, Papachrysostomou M, Binnie NR, et al: Outlet obstruction constipation (anismus) managed by biofeedback. *Gut* 32:1175, 1991.

121. Lestar B, Penninckx F, Kerremans R: Biofeedback defaecation training for anismus. *Int J Colorectal Dis* 6:202, 1991.

122. Wexner SD, Cheape JD, Jorge JM, et al: Prospective assessment of biofeedback for the treatment of paradoxical puborectalis contraction. *Dis Colon Rectum* 35:145, 1992.

123. Gilliland R, Heymen S, Altomare DF, et al: Outcome and predictors of success of biofeedback for constipation. *Br J Surg* 84:1123, 1997.

124. Hallan RI, Williams NS, Melling J, et al: Treatment of anismus in intractable constipation with botulinum A toxin. *Lancet* 2:714, 1988.

125. Joo JS, Agachan F, Wolff B, et al: Initial North American experience with botulinum toxin type A for treatment of anismus. *Dis Colon Rectum* 39:1107, 1996.

126. Maria G, Brisinda G, Bentivoglio AR, et al: Botulinum toxin in the treatment of outlet obstruction constipation caused by puborectalis syndrome. *Dis Colon Rectum* 43:376, 2000.

127. Shafik A, El-Sibai O: Botulin toxin in the treatment of nonrelaxing puborectalis syndrome. *Dig Surg* 15:347, 1998.

128. Pfeifer J, Agachan F, Wexner SD: Surgery for constipation: A review. *Dis Colon Rectum* 39:444, 1996.

129. Lane RH, Todd IP: Idiopathic megacolon: A review of 42 cases. *Br J Surg* 64:307, 1977.

130. Smith B, Grace RH, Todd IP: Organic constipation in adults. *Br J Surg* 64:313, 1977.

131. McCready RA, Beart RW Jr: The surgical treatment of incapacitating constipation associated with idiopathic megacolon. *Mayo Clin Proc* 54:779, 1979.

132. Hughes ES, McDermott FT, Johnson WR, et al: Surgery for constipation. *Aust N Z J Surg* 51:144, 1981.

133. Belliveau P, Goldberg SM, Rothenberger DA, et al: Idiopathic acquired megacolon: The value of subtotal colectomy. *Dis Colon Rectum* 25:118, 1982.

134. Klatt GR: Role of subtotal colectomy in the treatment of incapacitating constipation. *Am J Surg* 145:623, 1983.

135. Gilbert KP, Lewis FG, Billingham RP, et al: Surgical treatment of constipation. *West J Med* 140:569, 1984.

136. Preston DM, Hawley PR, Lennard-Jones JE, et al: Results of colectomy for severe idiopathic constipation in women (Arbuthnot Lane's disease). *Br J Surg* 71:547, 1984.

137. Krishnamurthy S, Schuffler MD, Rohrmann CA, et al: Severe idiopathic constipation is associated with a distinctive abnormality of the colonic myenteric plexus. *Gastroenterology* 88:26, 1985.

138. Barnes PR, Lennard-Jones JE, Hawley PR, et al: Hirschsprung's disease and idiopathic megacolon in adults and adolescents. *Gut* 27:534, 1986.

139. Beck DE, Fazio VW, Jagelman DG, et al: Surgical management of colonic inertia. *South Med J* 82:305, 1989.

140. Gasslander T, Larsson J, Wetterfors J: Experience of surgical treatment for chronic idiopathic constipation. *Acta Chir Scand* 153:553, 1987.

141. Leon SH, Krishnamurthy S, Schuffler MD: Subtotal colectomy for severe idiopathic constipation. A follow-up study of 13 patients. *Dig Dis Sci* 32:1249, 1987.

142. Walsh PV, Peebles-Brown DA, Watkinson G: Colectomy for slow transit constipation. *Ann R Coll Surg Engl* 69:71, 1987.

143. Akervall S, Fasth S, Nordgren S, et al: The functional results after colectomy and ileorectal anastomosis for severe constipation (Arbuthnot Lane's disease) as related to rectal sensory function. *Int J Colorectal Dis* 3:96, 1988.

144. Vasilevsky CA, Nemer FD, Balcos EG, et al: Is subtotal colectomy a viable option in the management of chronic constipation? *Dis Colon Rectum* 31:679, 1988.

145. Zenilman ME, Dunnegan DL, Soper NJ, et al: Successful surgical treatment of idiopathic colonic dysmotility. The role of preoperative evaluation of coloanal motor function. *Arch Surg* 124:947, 1989.

146. Coremans GE: Surgical aspects of severe chronic non-Hirschsprung constipation. *Hepatogastroenterology* 37:588, 1990.

147. Kuijpers HC: Application of the colorectal laboratory in diagnosis and treatment of functional constipation. *Dis Colon Rectum* 33:35, 1990.

148. Stabile G, Kamm MA, Hawley PR, et al: Colectomy for idiopathic megarectum and megacolon. *Gut* 32:1538, 1991.

149. Tajana A, Mori G, Micheletto G: Current status of surgery for severe idiopathic constipation. *Coloproctology* 6:340, 1990.

150. Pemberton JH, Rath DM, Ilstrup DM: Evaluation and surgical treatment of severe chronic constipation. *Ann Surg* 214:403; discussion 411, 1991.

151. Wexner SD, Daniel N, Jagelman DG: Colectomy for constipation: Physiologic investigation is the key to success. *Dis Colon Rectum* 34:851, 1991.

152. Mahendrarajah K, Van der Schaaf AA, Lovegrove FT, et al: Surgery for severe constipation: The use of radioisotope transit scan and barium evacuation proctography in patient selection. *Aust N Z J Surg* 64:183, 1994.

153. Stewart J, Kumar D, Keighley MR: Results of anal or low rectal anastomosis and pouch construction for megarectum and megacolon. *Br J Surg* 81:1051, 1994.

154. Takahashi T, Fitzgerald SD, Pemberton JH: Evaluation and treatment of constipation. *Rev Gastroenterol Mex* 59:133, 1994.

155. Piccirillo MF, Reissman P, Wexner SD: Colectomy as treatment for constipation in selected patients. *Br J Surg* 82:898, 1995.

156. Redmond JM, Smith GW, Barofsky I, et al: Physiological tests to predict long-term outcome of total abdominal colectomy for intractable constipation. *Am J Gastroenterol* 90:748, 1995.

157. Lubowski DZ, Chen FC, Kennedy ML, et al: Results of colectomy for severe slow transit constipation. *Dis Colon Rectum* 39:23, 1996.

158. Nyam DC, Pemberton JH, Ilstrup DM, et al: Long-term results of surgery for chronic constipation. *Dis Colon Rectum* 40:273, 1997.

159. Bernini A, Madoff RD, Lowry AC, et al: Should patients with combined colonic inertia and nonrelaxing pelvic floor undergo subtotal colectomy? *Dis Colon Rectum* 41:1363, 1998.

160. Fan CW, Wang JY: Subtotal colectomy for colonic inertia. *Int Surg* 85:309, 2000.

161. Sarli L, Costi R, Sarli D, et al: Pilot study of subtotal colectomy with antiperistaltic cecoproctostomy for the treatment of chronic slow-transit constipation. *Dis Colon Rectum* 44:1514, 2001.

162. Verne GN, Hocking MP, Davis RH, et al: Long-term response to subtotal colectomy in colonic inertia. *J Gastrointest Surg* 6:738, 2002.

163. Thaler K, Dinnewitzer A, Oberwalder M, et al: Quality of life after colectomy for colonic inertia. *Tech Coloproctol* 9:133, 2005.

164. Bleijenberg G, Kuijpers HC: Treatment of the spastic pelvic floor syndrome with biofeedback. *Dis Colon Rectum* 30:108, 1987.

165. Loening-Baucke V: Modulation of abnormal defecation dynamics by biofeedback treatment in chronically constipated children with encopresis. *J Pediatr* 116:214, 1990.

166. Loening-Baucke V: Persistence of chronic constipation in children after biofeedback treatment. *Dig Dis Sci* 36:153, 1991.

167. Dahl J, Lindquist BL, Tysk C, et al: Behavioral medicine treatment in chronic constipation with paradoxical anal sphincter contraction. *Dis Colon Rectum* 34:769, 1991.

168. Benninga MA, Buller HA, Taminiau JA: Biofeedback training in chronic constipation. *Arch Dis Child* 68:126, 1993.

169. Bleijenberg G, Kuijpers HC: Biofeedback treatment of constipation: A comparison of two methods. *Am J Gastroenterol* 89:1021, 1994.

170. Papachrysostomou M, Smith AN: Effects of biofeedback on obstructive defecation–reconditioning of the defecation reflex? *Gut* 35:252, 1994.

171. Cox DJ, Sutphen J, Borowitz S, et al: Simple electromyographic biofeedback treatment for chronic pediatric constipation/encopresis: Preliminary report. *Biofeedback Self Regul* 19:41, 1994.

172. Siproudhis L, Dautrème S, Ropert A, et al: Anismus and biofeedback: Who benefits? *Eur J Gastroenterol Hepatol* 7:547, 1995.

173. Karlbom U, Hallden M, Eeg-Olofsson KE, et al: Results of biofeedback in constipated patients: A prospective study. *Dis Colon Rectum* 40:1149, 1997.

174. Glia A, Gylin M, Gullberg K, et al: Biofeedback retraining in patients with functional constipation and paradoxical puborectalis contraction: Comparison of anal manometry and sphincter electromyography for feedback. *Dis Colon Rectum* 40:889, 1997.

175. Wiesel PH, Norton C, Roy AJ, et al: Gut focused behavioural treatment (biofeedback) for constipation and faecal incontinence in multiple sclerosis. *J Neurol Neurosurg Psychiatry* 69:240, 2000.

176. Lau CW, Heymen S, Alabaz O, et al: Prognostic significance of rectocele, intussusception, and abnormal perineal descent in biofeedback treatment for constipated patients with paradoxical puborectalis contraction. *Dis Colon Rectum* 43:478, 2000.

177. Battaglia E, Serra AM, Buonafede G, et al: Long-term study on the effects of visual biofeedback and muscle training as a therapeutic

modality in pelvic floor dyssynergia and slow-transit constipation. *Dis Colon Rectum* 47:90, 2004.

178. Chiarioni G, Whitehead WE, Pezza V, et al: Biofeedback is superior to laxatives for normal transit constipation due to pelvic floor dyssynergia. *Gastroenterology* 130:657, 2006.

179. Heymen S, Scarlett Y, Jones K, et al: Randomized, controlled trial shows biofeedback to be superior to alternative treatments for patients with pelvic floor dyssynergia-type constipation. *Dis Colon Rectum* 50:428, 2007.

180. Rao SS, Valestin J, Brown CK, et al: Long-term efficacy of biofeedback therapy for dyssynergic defecation: Randomized controlled trial. *Am J Gastroenterol* 105:890, 2010.

Pelvic Floor Dysfunction

Tracy Hull | Adele Burgess

Pelvic floor dysfunction encompasses a constellation of disorders that includes pelvic organ prolapse, dysfunctional bowel and/or bladder evacuation, and chronic pain. In the United States, it has been reported that almost 24% of women have at least one pelvic floor disorder and the incidence increases with age, obesity, and parity.[1,2] The exact prevalence of the great majority of pelvic floor disorders is unknown, because of underreporting and the lack of consistent definitions. For urinary incontinence, reported rates range from 9% to 22%.[3,4] For fecal incontinence in the general population, reported rates range from 2% to 24%[5,6] and for pelvic organ prolapse, the lack of universally accepted definition means that the true prevalence is unknown. Each pelvic floor disorder has a high propensity to coexist with others. This makes multispecialty evaluation and care mandatory, as isolated evaluation can lead to the diagnosis and management of one component of what is a multisystem process.

EVALUATION

Evaluation of pelvic floor dysfunction requires a multidisciplinary approach from colorectal, gynecologic, radiologic, and urologic teams. As with any evaluation, this begins with a careful history and physical examination.

HISTORY

The history should include details of presenting symptoms, onset, duration, frequency, severity, and any exacerbating or relieving factors. A complete past medical, obstetric (including current pregnancy status), and surgical history should be obtained. Current medication regimens should be documented. The pattern of bowel function needs to be documented in detail including frequency of evacuation, length of time spent for each evacuation, straining at stool, rectal pain, posturing and digitations, and the trend of any problems over time. Stool consistency influences the severity of incontinence and constipation and can be graded using the Bristol Stool Scale (Figure 146-1).[7] The use of scoring systems can add to the clinical history and include the Cleveland Clinic Continence (Wexner) score or Cleveland Clinic Constipation score, American Society of Colon and Rectal Surgeons (ASCRS) Fecal Incontinence score, ASCRS Fecal Incontinence Quality of Life score, St. Mark's Incontinence score and many others.[8]

Patients presenting with constipation can have a multitude of symptoms. The Rome III criteria defining constipation are shown in Box 146-1. Broadly speaking, constipation can be associated with slow transit, normal transit, or evacuatory dysfunction. For patients presenting with constipation, the investigations that are required should be guided by the symptoms described. Those with recent change in bowel habit or bleeding should be considered for a colonoscopy.

In patients presenting with fecal incontinence, the type should be delineated: "passive" incontinence—involuntary defecation without awareness, or "urge" incontinence—the inability to defer stool in spite of active attempts to retain bowel contents. Passive incontinence is felt by some to correlate with internal anal sphincter (IAS) dysfunction.[9] However, we believe it correlates with sphincter dysfunction or lack of sensation. Urge incontinence seems to result from an inability of the rectum to store stool. This can be from a sudden overwhelming bolus of stool or a rectum that is not compliant and will not hold the stool. Patients can have a combination of both problems and a careful history is needed to differentiate what is occurring during defecation. Most patients with severe fecal incontinence will require an endoanal ultrasound to define the sphincter muscle anatomy and physiological testing to define function.

One of the most important issues to define while taking a history from this group of patients is to learn exactly why the patient is seeking help and how much their problem is affecting their quality of life. The answer to these questions will help direct therapy choices.

EXAMINATION

A general examination, including documenting body mass index (BMI), should be undertaken to detect any systemic disease that may be contributing to the patient's symptoms. An abdominal examination including documenting previous surgical scars should also be carried out.

Simple inspection of the perineal area can be very enlightening. Inspect for scarring, excoriation, erythema, soiling, anal sphincter shape, the bulk of the perineal body, any skin tags or signs of inflammatory bowel disease, flattening of the perineum, hemorrhoids, or overt rectal prolapse. Next ask the patient to strain and assess for pelvic floor descent and for prolapse (although this is often best exhibited by having the patient take an enema and then evacuate on the toilet or commode). Vaginal examination and digital anal examination, both at rest and with strain, should be completed. Digital assessment should note any obvious anal pathology such as a mass, sphincter tone (at rest and squeeze), and muscle mass and any palpable sphincter defects. Stool load and consistency should also be documented. Levator ani and puborectalis muscles can also be assessed. It is important to differentiate sphincter contraction from puborectalis movement. Proctoscopy and sigmoidoscopy should be performed to help exclude neoplasia or undiagnosed inflammatory conditions and may also identify solitary rectal ulcers, hemorrhoids, and fissures.

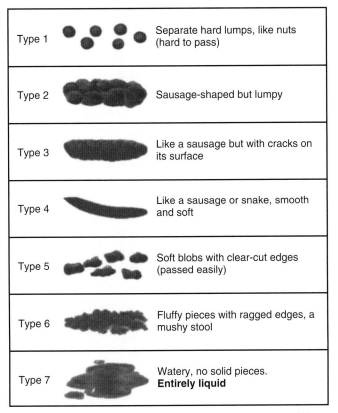

Type 1		Separate hard lumps, like nuts (hard to pass)
Type 2		Sausage-shaped but lumpy
Type 3		Like a sausage but with cracks on its surface
Type 4		Like a sausage or snake, smooth and soft
Type 5		Soft blobs with clear-cut edges (passed easily)
Type 6		Fluffy pieces with ragged edges, a mushy stool
Type 7		Watery, no solid pieces. **Entirely liquid**

FIGURE 146-1 Bristol Stool Chart. (From Lewis SJ, Heaton KW: Stool form scale as a useful guide to intestinal transit time. *Scand J Gastroenterol* 32:920, 1997.)

BOX 146-1 Rome III Diagnostic Criteria for Functional Constipation

SYMPTOMS ≥3 MONTHS; ONSET ≥6 MONTHS PRIOR TO DIAGNOSIS

Straining*
Lumpy or hard stools*
Sensation of incomplete evacuation*
Sensation of anorectal obstruction/blockage*
Manual maneuvers to facilitate defecation*
<3 defecations/week
Loose stools rarely present without the use of laxatives
Insufficient criteria for irritable bowel syndrome (constipation subtype)

Based on Longstreth GF, Thompson WG, Chey WD, et al: Functional bowel disorders. *Gastroenterology* 130:1480, 2006.
*≥25% of defecations.

INVESTIGATIONS

Pregnancy testing is considered for all women of child-bearing age before any invasive testing is carried out. Basic blood tests including thyroid studies and calcium levels help evaluate for metabolic etiology of bowel disorders. Colonoscopy and gastrointestinal contrast studies should be considered to rule out functional etiologies, inflammatory bowel disease, and malignancy. Stool microscopy and cultures can be considered for patients with diarrhea. Other testing for patients with diarrhea include colonoscopy with cold biopsies to rule out microcytic colitis along with other testing by a gastroenterologist to eliminate celiac and other diseases.

Anorectal Manometry

There are a variety of catheters and systems that are used to perform anal manometry. The available catheters are either water perfused, microballoon, or solid state. The technique to carry out the evaluation is either a "station" or continuous pull-through. Because of the lack of methodologic standardization, normal ranges vary between laboratories. Parameters most frequently measured are resting, squeeze, and strain anal pressure; rectoanal inhibitory reflex; rectal sensation and compliance; and the balloon expulsion tests. The resting pressure reflects the internal sphincter function, as this muscle contributes between 55% and 85% of resting pressure,[10] and the squeeze pressure reflects external sphincter function. Rectal sensation can be recorded by using a balloon inserted into the rectum and recording the volume of first sensation as the balloon is filled (rectal sensory threshold), sensation of fullness (urge to defecate, called first urge), and maximum tolerated volume (how much volume can be placed into the balloon where the patient feels they can stand no more). Rectal sensation can be altered by pathologies such as inflammation or radiation therapy, which decrease tolerated volumes. Increased tolerable volumes can be found in disorders such as megarectum or neurogenic abnormalities. Rectal sensory threshold has been shown to be valuable for determining whether biofeedback will be successful.[11]

The rectoanal inhibitory reflex (RAIR) is normally elicited by inflating a balloon in the rectum while measuring anal manometry. Normally a rapid rectal distention will lead to a brief increase in anal tone followed by a reflex IAS relaxation. This reflex is absent in Hirschsprung disease and immediately following colo-anal anastomosis. In the presence of a megarectum, a greater volume of rectal distension is required to elicit the reflex and this can lead to false-negative results.

Nonrelaxation of the puborectalis muscle (paradoxical contraction) during straining can be detected during anal physiology testing. Figure 146-2 shows the peak pressure generated by the levator muscles with squeeze, but when asked to strain there is no activity (no muscle contraction: see arrows). Figure 146-3 shows the normal levator muscle activity with squeeze, but when asked to strain (to simulate defecation) there is levator muscle activity shown at the arrows, which corresponds to inappropriate contraction of the muscle. This inappropriate contraction can obstruct defecation.

The balloon expulsion test is usually carried out using a 50-mL water-filled balloon and provides a simple baseline test for defecation. If the patient can expel the balloon in less than 1 minute, then it is less likely that dysfunction exists, although the test has been reported to have a sensitivity of about 90%.[12]

Pudendal Nerve Terminal Latency

Pudendal nerve terminal latency (PNTL) is measured with a finger-mounted St. Mark's electrode, which stimulates the pudendal nerve at the level of the ischial spine and records the conduction time to the sphincter.[13]

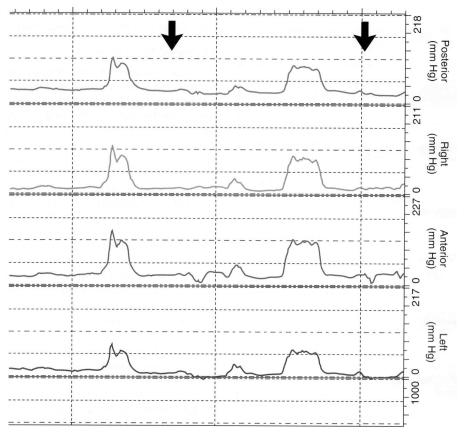

FIGURE 146-2 Normal levator activity. Increased pressures with squeeze but no activity with strain *(arrow)*. (With permission from Cleveland Clinic.)

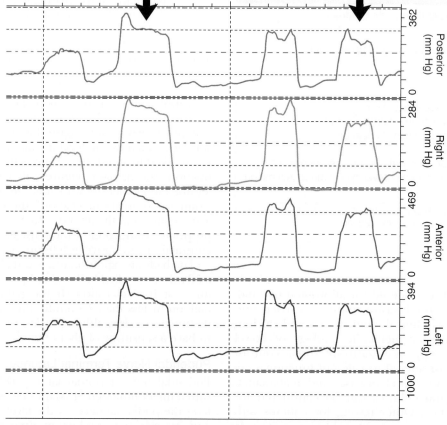

FIGURE 146-3 Levator activity with paradoxical contraction when the patient is asked to strain *(arrow)*. (With permission from Cleveland Clinic.)

Normal PNTL is less than 2.2 milliseconds and prolongation is intended to reflect nerve damage. The value of PNTL has been questioned, and the significance of an undetectable PNTL is uncertain. Furthermore, the test evaluates the function of the fastest remaining nerve fiber, and therefore incomplete nerve injuries can be missed with this technique. Some investigators have found an abnormal PNTL to be highly predictive of failure after sphincteroplasty[14] but others have observed no such correlation.[15]

Endoanal Ultrasound

Two-dimensional (2D) endoanal ultrasound (EUS) is now the preferred choice to image the anatomy of the sphincter complex. There is a high correlation between EUS findings and those found intraoperatively and histologically.[16] Assessment can be made of the external and internal anal sphincters, their length, thickness, and any asymmetry and sphincter defects. Several studies have been carried out on normal subjects to delineate the normal anatomy.[17-19]

The anal canal is divided into three levels on ultrasound: the upper level is defined by the presence of the puborectalis muscle; the middle canal has both external and internal sphincter muscles; and in the lower canal usually only the most distal portion of the external sphincter muscle is seen. On ultrasound, highly reflective tissues give a white hyperechoic image and poorly reflective tissues are hypoechoic and appear black. Thus, the internal sphincter, which contains a large degree of water, allows the waves to easily go through it and appears black.

The length of the anal canal varies from an average of 25 mm for women to 33 mm for men.[20] Age and gender changes the anatomy of the anal sphincters. The normal IAS is between 2 to 3 mm thick, but tends to become thicker with age[19] and the normal external anal sphincter (EAS) is between 7 to 9 mm thick and becomes thinner with age.[21] Sphincter injuries found on ultrasound have been reported to correlate well with manometric findings, with EAS defects accompanied by lower anal squeeze pressures and IAS defects associated with lower resting pressures.[16]

Additionally, the sonographer needs to be aware of gender-specific differences to avoid inaccurate interpretation of images. Sultan et al noted that in women the anterior part of the external anal sphincter is shorter and slopes downward. This can lead to the incorrect diagnosis of an anterior sphincter defect where one does not exist because demonstrating a complete ring of the EAS in one plane can be difficult.[21] The anococcygeal ligament appears as a hypoechoic triangular structure posteriorly and can be confused as a sphincter defect in this location in both men and women.

Three-dimensional (3D) EUS has become more widely available in recent years and uses computer software to reconstruct standard ultrasound images into a 3D image. Studies using 3D EUS are limited, but Gold et al carried out 3D reconstructions in 20 controls and 24 patients suffering fecal incontinence with sphincter injuries seen on regular EUS. 3D EUS was able to demonstrate the radial angle of the IAS or EAS defect better than with

standard EUS.[20] The sensitivity of detecting both internal and external sphincter defects is comparable between the 2D and 3D studies, but intraobserver variation is decreased and diagnosis is increased with the 3D imaging.[22]

Magnetic Resonance Imaging

MRI can be used for static studies to assess anatomy, and dynamic studies are used to assess pelvic floor function. Looking at anal sphincter anatomy, MRI is felt to be an excellent tool. A number of studies have compared the accuracy of EUS and MRI in detecting sphincter injuries and the results have been varied because of heterogeneous patient populations and varied expertise. Overall it appears that MRI is as accurate as EUS in delineating anal sphincter anatomy in experienced hands.[23,24]

Another use of MRI is looking at defecating function. Dynamic MRI (or MRI proctography) is now being used to investigate evacuatory dysfunction and allows pelvic motion to be studied in real time. It has the advantage of negating the need for pelvic radiation and can demonstrate peritoneoceles, cystoceles, perineal decent and prolapse, and allows measurement of the anorectal angle to assess for paradoxical contraction of the puborectalis muscle. Disadvantages of MRI include the cost and availability, and also the need for the patient to defecate in a supine position rather then seated as in traditional defecography (Figures 146-4 and 146-5).

Defecography

Defecography is a dynamic test preformed by instilling contrast into the rectum (and occasionally orally and per vagina and/or bladder) and taking video and still films at rest, during strain, and during the act of defecation. The patient is seated on a special commode which is

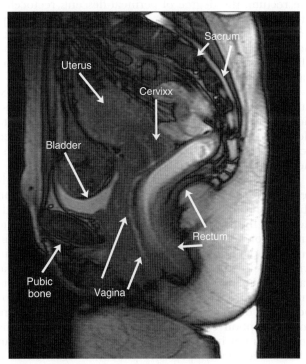

FIGURE 146-4 Normal dynamic MRI. (With permission from Cleveland Clinic.)

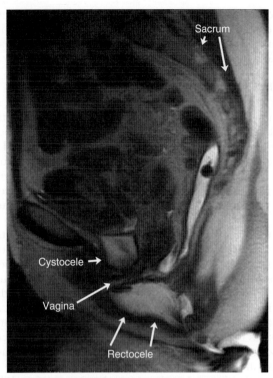

FIGURE 146-5 Dynamic MRI showing a rectocele and cystocele. (With permission from Cleveland Clinic.)

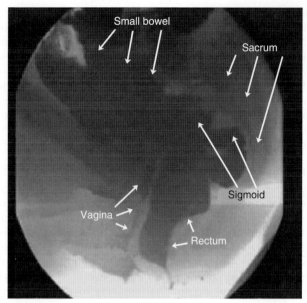

FIGURE 146-6 Defecogram showing normal anatomy. (With permission from Cleveland Clinic.)

behind a screen. The radiographs can be taken through the screen for this study while the patient performs the aforementioned acts of defecation. Measurements can include the anorectal angle (the angle between the longitudinal axis of the anal canal and the posterior wall of the lower part of the rectum), the ability to fully empty the rectum, the degree of perineal descent, rectoceles, enteroceles, sigmoidoceles, anismus, and intussusception. There is a large amount of overlap in the findings between what is considered normal and abnormal, and all findings need to be considered in the setting of clinical symptoms (Figure 146-6).

Nonrelaxation of the Puborectalis (Anismus). Nonrelaxation of the puborectalis muscle is a paradoxical contraction of the pelvic floor muscles as the patient is trying to defecate. On defecography, this is shown as impaired rectal evacuation, a fixed anorectal angle, and a prominent puborectalis indentation.[25]

Intussusception. Intussusception can be commonly seen on proctography although there is no consensus on the classification and the clinical relevance is hotly debated. Intussusception begins as an infolding of the anterior or posterior rectal wall and can progress to circumferential infolding. The intussusception can remain within the rectum (rectorectal) or extend into the anal canal (rectoanal). In symptomatic patients, it is speculated that the invaginated bowel leads to narrowing or occlusion of the lumen and this obstructs defecation. Intussusception can be seen in up to 80% of healthy volunteers but it tends to be less severe/extensive than what is seen in symptomatic patients.[26] Agachan et al reviewed 744 patients (60% with constipation; 16.5%, incontinence) and found that 12.6% of patients had

intussusception (defined as those extending into or through the anal canal), 25.7% of patients had a rectocele, 11% a sigmoidocele, and 30% of patients had a combination of findings.[27]

Rectocele. Rectoceles are the most common finding on defecography.[27] They may be associated with rectovaginal septum damage, which allows the anterior rectum to bulge into the posterior wall of the vagina. Rectoceles are reported to be significant only if they are greater than 3 cm or require digitation to empty.[28] Halligan and Bartram showed a correlation between the clinical need to vaginally digitate and trapping of contrast within the rectocele during defecation on defecography[29] (Figure 146-7).

Enterocele/Sigmoidocele. A protrusion of the peritoneum between the rectum and into the vagina containing small bowel is termed an enterocele. If the protrusion of the peritoneum is into the anterior rectal wall, it is a pouch of Douglas hernia or sigmoidocele. To detect an enterocele during defecography, some radiologists prefer a delayed late evacuation phase. Another method involves asking the patient to maximally strain as long as possible and look for the herniation in a dynamic setting. Enteroceles and sigmoidoceles are classified by the position of the lowest loop of bowel during maximal strain on defecography. A first degree is defined as when the bowel sits above the pubococcygeal line, a second degree is where bowel is below the pubococcygeal line but is still above the ischiococcygeal line, and with a third degree, the lowest loop of bowel is below the ischiococcygeal line[30] (Figures 146-8 and 146-9).

Transit Studies

Colonic transit time can be measured by the use of ingested radiopaque markers. There are many protocols used to perform the study, but all essentially evaluate the number of markers that remain on simple abdominal radiographs 5 to 7 days after marker ingestion. Other

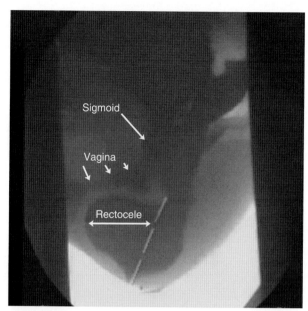

FIGURE 146-7 Defecogram demonstrating a rectocele. (With permission from Cleveland Clinic.)

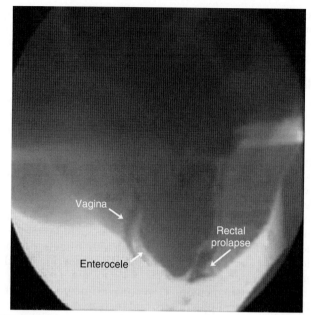

FIGURE 146-9 Defecogram demonstrating an enterocele and rectal prolapse. (With permission from Cleveland Clinic.)

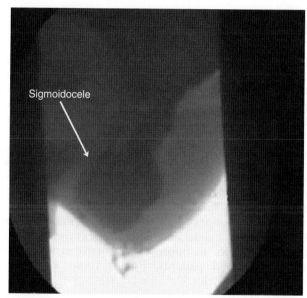

FIGURE 146-8 Defecogram demonstrating a sigmoidocele. (With permission from Cleveland Clinic.)

methods to measure colonic motility involve nuclear medicine specialists following orally ingested radioactive food through the digestive tract. Both methods are used successfully to diagnose slow-transit constipation. Patients with pelvic floor dysfunction can have coexisting slow-transit constipation, and some authors have noted a normalization in the transit time with correction of outflow problems.

MANAGEMENT OF PELVIC FLOOR DISORDERS

The management of fecal incontinence, rectal prolapse, and constipation are discussed elsewhere (Chapters 144,

145, and 148). Discussed next are management options for other etiologies of pelvic floor dysfunction.

NONRELAXATION OF THE PUBORECTALIS (ANISMUS, PARADOXICAL CONTRACTION OF THE PUBORECTALIS, PUBORECTALIS SYNDROME)

As discussed earlier, in normal individuals the puborectalis is contracted "at rest" and maintains the anorectal angle. With defecation, the external sphincter and the puborectalis muscle relax and evacuation occurs. In the case of paradoxical nonrelaxation, the muscle does not relax and maintains or increases the anorectal angle when straining to expel stool. Patients are then trying to defecate against an obstructed outlet and experience increased straining, incomplete evacuation, or may need to put a finger through the anus into the rectum to digitally remove stool and complete rectal evacuation. Conservative management of this problem includes a high fiber diet, adequate hydration, regular physical activity, enemas, and laxatives. Retraining the puborectalis to relax with straining through biofeedback has been used for this problem. Studies utilizing biofeedback therapy have yielded conflicting results with efficacy rates that ranged from 35% to 80%.[31-33] Studies have, however, shown that biofeedback is superior to laxatives, sham treatments, or alternative therapies and no studies have shown a negative outcome associated with biofeedback. Therefore this is often used as a safe second-line treatment when conservative therapy has failed.[34] Recently, a study reported that type A botulinum toxin injected into the puborectalis muscle under ultrasound guidance had superior short-term results compared with biofeedback for the obstructed symptoms associated with the paradoxical muscle contraction.[33,35]

Published results of partial division of the puborectalis muscle have shown mixed results. Studies in the 1960s[36]

reported excellent results after partial division of the puborectalis muscle. However, more recent results of this technique have been disappointing, and this operation has fallen out of favor.[37]

RECTOCELE

A rectocele is a defect of the rectovaginal septum allowing herniation of the anterior rectum into the vagina or surrounding perineal area. Rectoceles are common and seen in 80% of nulliparous, asymptomatic women undergoing defecography.[38] In patients who are constipated, it has been demonstrated that only 10% to 20% of rectoceles are clinically significant as the cause of symptoms.[39] As mentioned earlier, rectoceles are considered symptomatic only if they are greater than 3 cm or require digitation to empty.[28] The digitation can include stabilization of the posterior vaginal wall with fingers during defecation, or similarly stabilization of the perineal body or anterior perianal skin.

Medical management of rectoceles includes a high-fiber diet, fiber supplements, and increased water intake. Surgically, rectocele repair can be undertaken transvaginally, transrectally, or transperineally, with the transvaginal approach favored by gynecologists. All three techniques involve the rebuilding of tissue between the rectum and vagina. Two separate randomized trials have shown that the transanal approach has a significantly higher failure rate compared with the transvaginal approach. This is highlighted by the 2010 Cochrane review, which states for posterior vaginal wall prolapse: "The vaginal approach was associated with a lower rate of recurrent rectocele or enterocele, or both, than the transanal approach (relative risk, 0.24; 95% confidence interval, 0.09 to 0.64); although there was a higher blood loss and postoperative narcotic use."[40] Regardless of the approach, success rates are high—70% to 90% for improvement in defecation and 60% to 70% for elimination of the need to digitiate.[41-44]

ENTEROCELE

Enteroceles occur when the peritoneum elongates and opens the potential space in the pouch of Douglas between the anterior rectal wall and posterior vaginal wall. This allows small bowel to herniate into the lower pelvic cavity, which may then lead to mechanical obstruction of defecation by the bowel compressing the rectum with straining. Enterocele repair can be performed either transvaginally or transabdominally. The approach is often dictated by other procedures that will be performed at the same operation to address pelvic floor problems. Traditional techniques involve obliterating the pouch of Douglas. More recently, techniques that reestablish the pericervical ring have been trialed. There are few long-term studies of enterocele repair. Raz et al[45] reported an 82% cure rate in 49 patients who underwent simple enterocele repair. Overall, the enterocele recurrence rate appears to be approximately 10% in most series. The degree that the repair of the enterocele contributes to the clinical improvement of the patient's symptoms is difficult to assess as the procedure is usually preformed concurrently with other prolapse repairs.

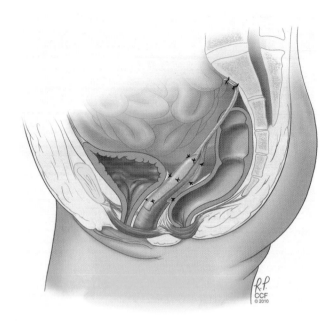

FIGURE 146-10 Sacral colpopexy using mesh to support vagina. (With permission from Cleveland Clinic.)

SIGMOIDOCELE

A sigmoidocele is similar to an enterocele, but it is the sigmoid that protrudes between the distal rectum and vagina, and not the small bowel. Sigmoidoceles are identified on 4% to 5% of defecography studies for obstructed constipation.[46] The surgical procedure for correcting a sigmoidocele is determined by severity of constipation, degree of prolapse, any coexisting incontinence, and the amount of sigmoid redundancy. Surgical approaches include sigmoid resection, sigmoidopexy alone, or obliteration of the cul-de-sac. The current favored procedure is sigmoid resection with obliteration of the potential space. Figure 146-10 shows mesh used for a sacral colpopexy to support the vagina. This also obliterates the cul-de-sac. Sigmoidopexy or resection have been shown to improve obstructive symptoms in carefully selected patients, usually those with third-degree sigmoidoceles.[46]

RECTOANAL INTUSSUSCEPTION (INTERNAL PROLAPSE)

Internal prolapse is a full-thickness intussusception of the rectal wall without protrusion beyond the anal canal, demonstrated on defecography.[30] It has been found in 31% to 40% of patients undergoing defecography for obstructed defecation.[47] Choi et al found, however, that the risk of full-thickness rectal prolapse developing in patients medically treated for large intussusception is very small (3.8%).[48] They also found that biofeedback was beneficial in improving symptoms of both constipation and incontinence in these patients and suggested that biofeedback should be considered as the initial therapy of choice for large internal intussusceptions. Failing conservative management, surgical intervention for internal intussusception includes the Delorme procedure, stapled transanal rectal resection (STARR), rectopexy, and resection rectopexy. The Delorme procedure has been reported to have good functional outcomes in well-selected patients that have the primary symptoms of constipation associated with their intussusception and no symptoms of incontinence or diarrhea.[49] STARR has reported initial results that appear to be excellent, with 100% rates of improvement.[50] However, there have also been reports of significant complications including hemorrhage, pain, early recurrence symptoms,[51] and rectovaginal fistula. The results of surgical rectopexy for the treatment of internal prolapse are conflicting, with a number of these studies reporting persistence or worsening of constipation and difficulty in evacuating postoperatively.[52] The addition of resection improves results in most reports, with symptomatic improvement found between 53% and 80% in selected groups.[53] Recently Collinson et al have published their 12-month followup results for 75 patients with internal rectal prolapse treated with laparoscopy and noted that laparoscopic ventral rectopexy for internal rectal prolapse improves symptoms of obstructed defecation and fecal incontinence in the short term and appears to have very good results thus far.[54]

CONCLUSION

Pelvic floor disorders are complex and are overall poorly understood. A careful history and examination is essential. This initial step allows clarification of symptoms and physical findings and allows tailored investigational planning. The results of testing then can assist in planning therapy. Not all patients will be surgical candidates; however, a thoughtful workup may increase the likelihood of symptomatic improvement after surgery.

REFERENCES

1. Nygaard I, Barber MD, Burgio Kl, et al: Prevalence of symptomatic pelvic floor disorders in U.S. women. *JAMA* 300:1311, 2008.
2. MacLennan AH, Taylor AW, Wilson DH, et al: The prevalence of pelvic floor disorders and their relationship to gender, age, parity and mode of delivery. *BJOG* 107:1460, 2000.
3. Shamliyan T, Wyman J, Bliss DZ, et al: Prevention of urinary and fecal incontinence in adults. *Evid Rep Technol Assess* 161:1, 2007.
4. Hunskaar S, Lose G, Skyes D, et al: The prevalence of urinary incontinence in women in four European countries. *BJU Int* 93:324, 2004.
5. Nelson R, Norton N, Cautley E, et al: Community-based prevalence of anal incontinence. *JAMA* 274:559, 1995.
6. Varma A, Gunn J, Gardiner A, et al: Obstetric anal sphincter injury: Prospective evaluation of incidence. *Dis Colon Rectum* 42:1537, 1999.
7. Lewis SJ, Heaton KW: Stool form scale as a useful guide to intestinal transit time. *Scand J Gastroenterol* 32:920, 1997.
8. Wang JY, Varma MG: Measures for fecal incontinence, constipation, and associated quality of life. *Semin Colon Rectal Surg* 21:22, 2010.
9. Engel AF, Kamm MA, Bartram CI, et al: Relationship of symptoms in faecal incontinence to specific sphincter abnormalities. *Int J Colorectal Dis* 10:124, 2008.
10. In: Henry M, Swash M, editors: *Coloproctology and the pelvic floor*, ed 2. Oxford, 1992, Butterworth-Heinemann.
11. Barnett JL, Hasler WL, Camilleri M, et al; American Gastroenterological Association: Medical position statement on anorectal testing techniques. *Gastroenterology* 116:732, 1999.
12. Minguez M, Herreros B, Sanchiz V, et al: Predictive value of the balloon expulsion test for excluding the diagnosis of pelvic floor dyssynergia in constipation. *Gastroenterology* 126:57, 2004.
13. Laurberg S, Swash M, Snooks SJ, et al: Neurologic cause of idiopathic incontinence. *Arch Neurol* 45:1250, 1988.
14. Barisic G, Krivokapic Z, Markovic V, et al: The role of overlapping sphincteroplasty in traumatic fecal incontinence. *Acta Chir Iugosl* 47:37, 2000.
15. Buie WD, Lowry AC, Rothenberger DA, et al: Clinical rather than laboratory assessment predicts continence after anterior sphincteroplasty. *Dis Colon Rectum* 44:1255, 2001.
16. Sultan AH, Kamm MA, Bartram CI, et al: Anal sphincter trauma during instrument delivery. *Int J Gynaecol Obstet* 43:263, 1993.
17. Nielsen MB, Hauge C, Rasmussen OO, et al: Anal sphincter size measured by endosonography in healthy volunteers. Effect of age, sex, and parity. *Acta Radiol* 33:453, 1992.
18. Sultan AH, Nicholls RJ, Kamm MA, et al: Anal endosonography and correlation with in vitro and in vivo anatomy. *Br J Surg* 80:508, 1993.
19. Burnett SJ, Bartram CI: Endosonographic variations in the normal internal anal sphincter. *Int J Colorectal Dis* 6:2, 1991.
20. Gold DM, Bartram CI, Halligan S, et al: Three-dimensional endoanal sonography in assessing anal canal injury. *Br J Surg* 86:365, 1999.
21. Sultan AH, Kamm MA, Hudson CN, et al: Endosonography of the anal sphincters: Normal anatomy and comparison with manometry. *Clin Radiol* 49:368, 1994.
22. Christensen AF, Nyhuus B, Nielsen MB, et al: Three-dimensional anal endosonography may improve diagnostic confidence of detecting damage to the anal sphincter complex. *Br J Radiol* 78:308, 2005.
23. Rociu E, Stoker J, Eijkemans MJ, et al: Fecal incontinence: Endoanal US versus endoanal MR imaging. *Radiology* 212:453, 1999.
24. Malouf AJ, Williams AB, Halligan S, et al: Prospective assessment of accuracy of endoanal MR imaging and endosonography in patients with fecal incontinence. *AJR Am J Roentgenol* 175:741, 2000.
25. Halligan S, Malouf A, Bartram C, et al: Predictive value of impaired evacuation at proctography in diagnosing anismus. *AJR Am J Roentgenol* 177:633, 2001.
26. Pomerri F, Zuliani M, Mazza C, et al: Defecographic measurements of rectal intussusception and prolapse in patients and in asymptomatic subjects. *Am J Roentgenol* 176:641, 2001.
27. Agachan F, Pfeifer J, Wexner SD: Defecography and proctography: Results of 744 patients. *Dis Colon Rectum* 39:899, 1996.
28. Halligan S, Bartram CI: The radiological investigation of constipation. *Clin Radiol* 50:429, 1995.
29. Halligan S, Bartram CI: Is digitation associated with proctographic abnormality? *Int J Colorectal Dis* 11:167, 1996.
30. Lowry AC, Simmang CL, Boulos P, et al: Consensus statement of definitions for anorectal physiology and rectal cancer. Conference on Definitions for Anorectal Physiology and Rectal Cancer, Washington, D.C., May 1, 1999.
31. Park UC, Choi SK, Piccirillo MF, et al: Patterns of anismus and the relation to biofeedback therapy. *Dis Colon Rectum* 39:768, 1996.
32. Gilliland R, Heymen S, Altomare DF, et al: Outcome and predictors of success of biofeedback for constipation. *Br J Surg* 84:1123, 1997.
33. Farid M, El Monem HA, Omar W, et al: Comparative study between biofeedback retraining and botulinum neurotoxin in the treatment of anismus patients. *Int J Colorectal Dis* 24:115, 2009.
34. Rao SS, Seaton K, Miller M, et al: Randomized controlled trial of biofeedback, sham feedback, and standard therapy for dyssynergic defecation. *Clin Gastroenterol Hepatol* 5:331, 2007.
35. Maria G, Cadeddu F, Brandara F, et al: Experience with type A botulinum toxin for treatment of outlet-type constipation. *Am J Gastroenterol* 101:2570, 2006.
36. Wallace WC, Madden WM: Experience with partial resection of the puborectalis muscle. *Dis Colon Rectum* 12:196, 1969.
37. Kamm MA, Hawely PR, Lennard-Jones JE: Lateral division of puborectalis muscle in the management of severe constipation. *Br J Surg* 75:661, 1988.
38. Mellgren A, Anzén B, Nilsson B-Y, et al: Results of rectocele repair: A prospective study. *Dis Colon Rectum* 38:764, 1995.
39. Ting K-H, Mangel E, Eilbl-Eibesfeldt B: Is the volume retained after defecation a valuable parameter at defecography? *Dis Colon Rectum* 35:762, 1992.
40. Maher C, Baessler K: Surgical management of posterior vaginal wall prolapse: An evidence-based literature review. *Int Urogynecol J Pelvic Floor Dysfunct.* 17:84, 2006.
41. Yamana T, Takahashi T, Iwadare J: Clinical and physiologic outcomes after transvaginal rectocele repair. *Dis Colon Rectum.* 49:661, 2006.

42. Paraiso MF, Barber MD, Muir TW, et al: Rectocele repair: A randomized trial of three surgical techniques including graft augmentation. *Am J Obstet Gynecol* 95:1762, 2006.

43. Van Dam JH, Huisman WM, Hop WCJ, et al: Fecal continence after rectocele repair: A prospective study. *Int J Colorectal Dis* 15:54, 2000.

44. Cohen SM, Wexner SD, Binderow R, et al: Prospective, randomized endoscopic-blinded trial comparing pre-colonoscopy bowel cleansing methods. *Dis Colon Rectum* 37:689, 1994.

45. Raz S, Nitti VW, Bregg KJ: Transvaginal repair of enterocele. *J Urol* 149:724, 1999.

46. Jorge JM, Yang YK, Wexner SD: Incidence and clinical significance of sigmoidoceles as determined by a new classification system. *Dis Colon Rectum.* 37:1112, 1994.

47. Mellgren A, Bremmer S, Johansson C, et al: Defecography. Results of investigations in 2816 patients. *Dis Colon Rectum* 37:1133, 1994.

48. Choi JS, Hwang YH, Salum MR, et al: Outcome and management of patients with large rectoanal intussusception. *Am J Gastroenterol* 96:740, 2001.

49. Sielezneff I, Malouf A, Cesari J, et al: Selection criteria for internal rectal prolapse repair by Delorme's transrectal excision. *Dis Col Rectum* 42:367, 1991.

50. Boccasanta P, Venturi M, Salamina G, et al: New trends in the surgical treatment of outlet obstruction: Clinical and functional results of two novel transanal stapled techniques from randomised contolled trial. *Int Colorectal Dis* 9:359, 2004.

51. Dodi G, Pietroletti R, Milito G, et al: Bleeding, incontinence, pain and constipation after STARR transanal double stapled rectotomy for obstructed defecation. *Tech Coloproctol* 7:148, 2003.

52. Shultz I, Mellgren A, Dolk A, et al: Long term results and functional outcome after Ripstein rectopexy. *Dis Colon Rectum* 49:1136, 2006.

53. Tsiaoussis J, Chrysos E, Athanasakis E, et al: Rectoanal intussusception: Presentation of the disorder and late results of resection rectopexy. *Dis Colon Rectum* 48:838, 2005.

54. Collinson R, Wijffels N, Cunningham C, et al: Laparoscopic ventral rectopexy for internal rectal prolapse: Short-term functional results. *Colorectal Dis* 12:97, 2010.

Rectovaginal and Rectourethral Fistulas

Jill C. Buckley | Patricia L. Roberts

RECTOVAGINAL FISTULAS

Rectovaginal fistulas are epithelial-lined communications between the rectum and vagina. Although they are relatively uncommon, accounting for approximately 5% of all anorectal fistulas, they may cause significant physical symptoms in addition to adversely affecting intimate relationships and sexual function. The operative approach to such fistulas depends on a variety of factors, including the size, location, condition of the surrounding tissues, and association with concomitant disease, such as inflammatory bowel disease. The lack of a uniformly successful surgical repair is a source of great frustration to both patients and surgeons.

ETIOLOGY

The most common cause of a rectovaginal fistula is obstetric trauma. A prolonged second stage of labor with ischemic necrosis of the rectovaginal septum may contribute to development of a fistula. Other risk factors include a high forceps delivery, shoulder dystocia, midline episiotomy, and third- or fourth-degree perineal laceration.[1] In one series in the United States, rectovaginal fistula after vaginal delivery occurred in 25 women out of 20,050 vaginal deliveries.[2] Although fistulas after prolonged labor are rare in developed countries, they are still a relatively frequent occurrence in undeveloped countries.[3] Obstetric fistula affect up to 3.5 million women in Africa and Asia, with up to 130,000 new cases occurring each year.[4] The backlog of unrepaired cases is believed to approach 1 million in such areas as northern Nigeria alone.[3,5] The primary cause of such fistulas is obstructed labor; women who develop such fistulas have been in labor often for 3 to 4 days without prompt access to appropriate health care facilities. After delivery (often associated with a stillborn fetus), the necrotic septal tissue sloughs, with a resultant fistula. For every death from obstructed labor, it is estimated that there are 1.8 women with obstetric fistula (including uretero-, urethra-, vesicovaginal, rectovaginal, or some combination thereof).[6] For every 100 obstetric fistulas encountered, 74% are vesicovaginal, 21% are vesicovaginal and rectovaginal, and 5% are rectovaginal alone. The social consequences for women with fistulas were significant with high rates of divorce, separation, and abandonment.

Fistulizing Crohn disease, a transmural inflammatory disease of the bowel, is associated with rectovaginal fistula in more than 10% of women with the disease.[7] The incidence of Crohn rectovaginal fistula is more common in patients with Crohn colitis. Ulcerative colitis is rarely associated with rectovaginal fistula. Other autoimmune diseases, such as Behçet disease, may also be associated with rectovaginal fistulas.

Anorectal suppurative disease, including abscesses in the rectovaginal septum and anterior horseshoe abscesses, may be associated with rectovaginal fistulas. Diverticulitis is more commonly associated with a colovaginal (not rectovaginal) fistula and occurs almost exclusively in women who have undergone a prior hysterectomy. Other infectious etiologies include tuberculosis, lymphogranuloma venereum, human immunodeficiency virus, and cytomegalovirus.

Rectovaginal fistulas can occur as a postoperative complication after a variety of rectal, vaginal, and pelvic operations, including hysterectomy, low anterior resection with stapled anastomosis, ileal pouch–anal anastomosis, the procedure for prolapse and hemorrhoids (PPH), and the stapled transanal rectal resection (STARR) procedure. Urogynecologic procedures using transvaginal, perineal, or pelvic mesh placement for pelvic organ prolapse may result in rectovaginal fistula. Anastomotic vaginal fistula is a manifestation of anastomotic leakage and occurs in up to 13% of women after low anterior resection for rectal cancer. Risk factors include low anastomosis and preoperative radiotherapy.[8] Early pouch-vaginal fistulas in women undergoing the ileoanal pouch procedure are a manifestation of anastomotic leakage, pelvic sepsis, ischemia, or tension on the anastomosis, whereas late fistulas are more commonly caused by unsuspected Crohn disease.[9]

Rectovaginal fistulas are also associated with malignant disease of the cervix, rectum, uterus, or vagina and may be a manifestation of recurrent disease but may also occur after radiation therapy. Although radiation delivery techniques have improved, the incidence of rectovaginal fistulas was as high as 18% in one series of patients who received external beam radiotherapy in addition to interstitial brachytherapy for advanced gynecologic malignancy.[10]

Less common causes of rectovaginal fistulas include congenital fistulas, fecal impaction, long-standing pessary usage, sexual assault, and ergotamine suppository usage.

DIAGNOSIS, CLASSIFICATION AND CLINICAL EVALUATION

PRESENTATION

The chief presenting complaint of women with a rectovaginal fistula is the passage of stool or air per vagina. On occasion, foul-smelling vaginal discharge with recurrent vaginitis or urinary tract infections may be the presenting complaint. In women with rectovaginal fistulas from an obstetric injury, the incidence of incontinence is close to 50%.[11] The true incidence of incontinence is difficult to determine because passage of air and stool through the vagina may be interpreted as fecal incontinence. Associated symptoms, such as diarrhea, abdominal pain, or mucous discharge, are suggestive of inflammatory bowel disease and should be investigated accordingly. Although many women will seek medical attention immediately, it is not uncommon for some patients to delay evaluation because of social embarrassment, the desire to have more children, or the belief that such symptoms "are to be expected" after childbirth.

Although rectovaginal fistulas occur anywhere along the rectovaginal septum, they most commonly arise from the region of the dentate line and communicate with the posterior vaginal fornix. Fistulas distal to the dentate line are more appropriately termed *anovaginal fistulas* but common usage terms all such fistulas as *rectovaginal fistulas.*

Fistulas are classified in addition as low, mid, or high. In *low fistulas,* the opening is near the posterior vaginal fourchette; in *high fistulas,* the opening is behind or near the cervix; and *mid rectovaginal fistulas* are midway between the two. From a practical standpoint, fistulas may be classified as those palpable on digital examination and within view of an anoscope or those that are not. Simple fistulas arise from obstetric trauma or infection and are relatively small, whereas complex fistulas are caused by inflammatory bowel disease, irradiation, cancer, or failed prior repairs. Complex fistulas may also result from complications of surgery such as after low anterior anastomosis (as a consequence of anastomotic leak) or after hysterectomy (as a result of unrecognized injury to the rectum).

Some authors have suggested a classification scheme based not on the location of the fistula but on the underlying cause, because this may provide the best tool for the treating physician as it assesses the integrity of the surrounding tissues and the overall medical condition of the patient.[12]

EXAMINATION AND DIAGNOSIS

The initial approach to rectovaginal fistula is not only to identify the fistula but also to assess the surrounding tissues particularly with respect to any inflammatory change. Associated abscesses require drainage and, at times, seton placement. In addition, the entire rectovaginal septum should be assessed; patients with an obvious sphincter defect require both repair of the sphincter for improvement of continence and also to bring healthy tissue into the repair. Patients with significant scarring, stenosis, and tissue defects may require tissue transfer techniques to maximize the chance of success with repair.

Low rectovaginal fistulas are easily visualized and palpated on examination. A dimple is palpated in the anterior midline on digital rectal examination and confirmed on anoscopic or speculum examination. This method results in confirmation of the fistula in most low fistulas, and other diagnostic modalities are rarely needed. A probe can generally be passed quite easily through a short tract into the vagina. Examination with one finger in the rectum and one in the vagina assists in assessing the surrounding tissues and the bulk (usually quite attenuated) of the rectovaginal septum. The size and location

of the fistula are noted. An attenuated or absent perineal body and anterior sphincter defect are often noted in patients with previous obstetric injury.

If a fistula is not seen on initial examination but is suspected on clinical grounds, a variety of other maneuvers may be performed to diagnose the fistula. Limited barium enema examination with a lateral view may be performed. It is important to visualize the distal rectum and anal canal because the balloon of the catheter may obscure a fistula. Alternatively, a tampon may be placed in the vagina and a dilute methylene blue enema instilled in the rectum, with care not to contaminate the string of the tampon. The presence of methylene blue on the tampon confirms the fistula is present and open. Another method is to examine the patient in the lithotomy position. Water is placed in the vagina, and air is insufflated into the rectum with a sigmoidoscope. The presence of air bubbles in the vagina indicates a fistula. Imaging studies, such as transrectal ultrasound with use of hydrogen peroxide, vaginography, and magnetic resonance imaging (MRI), may also demonstrate a rectovaginal fistula; however, information from such studies must then be transformed into in vivo identification of the fistula in the affected patient. Imaging studies are more useful in patients with mid- or high fistulas, especially patients with colovaginal or enterovaginal fistulas. Low rectovaginal fistulas are generally straightforward to demonstrate on physical examination.

It is essential to assess the anatomy and function of the sphincter muscles, especially in patients who have a rectovaginal fistula resulting from obstetric injury. In one study of primiparous women who had undergone a vaginal delivery alone,[13] 28% had a sphincter defect on ultrasound examination 6 weeks after delivery. One study suggested a 100% incidence of sphincter injuries on endoanal ultrasound in patients who sustained a rectovaginal fistula after vaginal delivery.[14] Furthermore, in one series of 52 women who had a rectovaginal fistula from obstetric injury,[11] 50% had preoperative incontinence. If available, preoperative studies, including ultrasound and anal manometry with pudendal nerve terminal motor latency studies, are helpful in evaluating patients with associated incontinence. A poorer outcome of repair has been associated with prolonged pudendal nerve terminal motor latency, although this has been questioned recently.[15]

TREATMENT OPTIONS

Although the mainstay of treatment for the majority of rectovaginal fistulas is surgery, there are a few exceptions. On occasion, patients with small fistulas and minimal symptoms choose to pursue bowel management. A small number of fistulas may close spontaneously after obstetric trauma in the immediate postpartum period. Hyperbaric oxygen has been reported to be associated with successful healing in small series of patients with rectovaginal fistulas from obstetric trauma.[16]

Medical therapy, particularly immunomodulation, has played an increasing role in the management of rectovaginal fistulas in patients with Crohn disease. Although the initial trial utilizing infliximab in 1999 showed short-term healing in 56% to 68% of abdominal and perianal fistulas, no rectovaginal fistulas were included.[17] Subsequently, the ACCENT II trial looked at 25 women with Crohn rectovaginal fistulas.[18] With infliximab, 60.7% healed initially, but long-term closure (at 14 weeks) was significantly lower, with a closure rate of 44.8%. Compared with other fistulas, the rate of healing with infliximab with rectovaginal fistulas is substantially less, and it has been suggested that this may be due to the relatively thin, nonmuscular, and poorly vascularized rectovaginal septum.[19] Use of MRI has shown that although fistulas have apparent healing, they may actually simply become less symptomatic with less drainage as tracks persist on radiographic studies. Furthermore, closure of the fistulas was associated with the development of an abscess in 10% of patients, presumably because the external opening heals over before the tract has healed.[17] Poritz et al have suggested that use of infliximab does not avoid the need for surgery in more than 70% of patients; however, such patients may be rendered relatively asymptomatic and have reasonable quality of life before requiring surgical intervention.[20] Infliximab and other immunomodulators are increasingly used as an adjunct to surgery. In a review of 65 women with Crohn disease and rectovaginal fistula, use of immunomodulators such as infliximab or adalimumab in addition to 6-mercaptopurine or azathioprine within 3 months prior to surgery was associated with successful healing ($P = 0.009$).[21] Biologics such as infliximab are commonly used in combination with surgery for Crohn rectovaginal fistulas and appear to improve outcome.

SURGICAL OPTIONS FOR R-V FISTULAS

A number of surgical options are available for patients with rectovaginal fistulas (Box 147-1). Local repairs are performed through a rectal, vaginal, or perineal approach and may be augmented with tissue transfer, such as gracilis and bulbocavernosus muscle, if the surrounding tissues are deficient or unsatisfactory. High rectovaginal fistulas or those associated with previous surgery or radiation therapy generally require an abdominal approach. Local repairs and abdominal repairs can be performed with fecal diversion, and fecal diversion may also be used, in selected patients, as the sole treatment for rectovaginal fistula. The choice of repair depends on a variety of factors, including the presence of associated incontinence, the size and location of the fistula, the degree of complexity of the fistula, and the status of the surrounding tissues.

All procedures for rectovaginal fistula repair have a significant failure rate; many reported series measure ultimate success rates and not initial success rates. Although fistula closure is ultimately achieved, a number of patients require more than one operation. Cigarette smoking is increasingly recognized as a predictor for adverse outcome and recurrent fistula.[21,22] Preoperative discussion should focus on the anticipated results, and at times abnormally high patient expectations need to be adjusted. Furthermore, quality of life and assessment of dyspareunia and sexual dysfunction after rectovaginal fistula surgery have not been rigorously evaluated in the majority of studies.

BOX 147-1 Treatment Options for Rectovaginal Fistulas

LOCAL REPAIR
Transanal approach
  Advancement flap
  Advancement sleeve flap
Vaginal approach
  Advancement flap
Perineal approach
  Sphincteroplasty
  Perineoproctotomy and layered closure
  Episioproctotomy
  Fistulotomy
Other
  Collagen fistula plug with button
  Injection of fibrin sealant
  Repair with interposition of bioprosthetics
  Purse-string closure

ABDOMINAL PROCEDURES
Low anterior resection
Coloanal anastomosis
Onlay patch anastomosis
Abdominoperineal resection
Fecal diversion

TISSUE TRANSPOSITION
Bulbocavernosus
Gluteus maximus
Gracilis
Pudendal thigh
Sartorius

OTHER
Hyperbaric oxygen
Infliximab or other biologics (for Crohn rectovaginal fistulas)

TIMING OF SURGERY

The timing of when to perform a repair for a rectovaginal fistula caused by obstetric trauma remains controversial. There is no level I evidence comparing immediate repair with secondary repair, particularly with respect to immediate outcome and long-term outcome and continence. If recognized at the time of delivery, initial repair is performed at the time of the delivery by the obstetrician.

In general, surgery may be performed for rectovaginal fistulas as long as the surrounding tissues are soft and pliable. The convention, particularly for fistulas of obstetric origin, has been to wait approximately 3 months, to maximize the condition of the surrounding tissues and also since a small percentage of fistulas close spontaneously in the immediate postpartum period. Data from series of patients with rectovaginal fistulas who have undergone MRI have challenged this dogma, because obstetric fistulas have short tracts and little associated inflammatory change on MRI compared with perianal fistulas.[23]

For patients whose previous repair has failed, a waiting period of 3 to 6 months has been advocated that permits some healing of the surrounding tissues and often decreases the size of the recurrent fistula.[24]

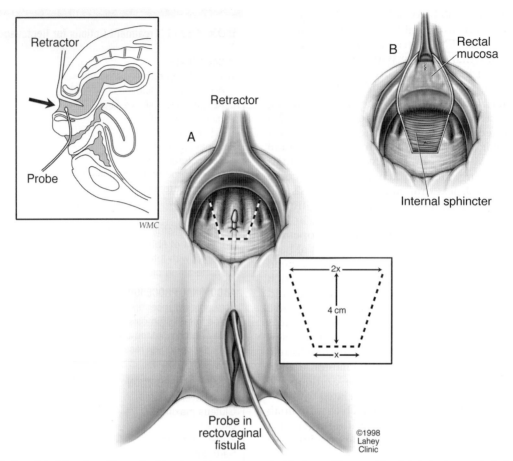

FIGURE 147-1 Endorectal sliding flap. The patient is placed in the prone jackknife position, and the fistula is demonstrated *(inset, arrow)*. **A,** The flap should extend for at least 4 cm, and the base should be at least two times the width of the apex. **B,** The flap should include mucosa and submucosa in addition to a portion of the internal sphincter muscle.

Waiting for 3 to 6 months may also give both surgeon and patient a much needed reprieve from further surgical intervention.

LOCAL REPAIR

Sliding Flap Repair

The sliding flap repair for the treatment of patients with rectovaginal fistulas was first reported by Noble[25] in 1902. He advocated splitting the rectovaginal septum, dissecting the lower end of the rectum from the vagina, and drawing the anterior wall down through and external to the anus. Since that time, many modifications of the sliding flap technique have been proposed. In 1948, Laird[26] described the use of a flap of mucosa, submucosa, and some fibers of the internal sphincter. Kodner et al[27] advocated the use of a flap similar to the Laird technique. Other authors[28] have advocated the use of a flap of mucosa, submucosa, and the full thickness of the internal sphincter. Incorporating part of the internal sphincter is generally necessary to ensure the flap is of adequate thickness. Regardless of the thickness of the flap used, the procedure is generally used for patients with simple low fistulas who have not had previous repairs. Patients with rectovaginal fistula from obstetric injuries (without an associated sphincter defect) and patients with Crohn rectovaginal fistulas without associated proctitis are good candidates for sliding flap repair.

The Operation. Patients undergo a full mechanical and antibiotic bowel preparation the day before surgery. This practice may be reexamined in view of accumulating evidence that mechanical bowel preparation is probably unnecessary and does not reduce infectious complications after elective bowel resection. The patient is placed in the prone jackknife position, with the buttocks taped apart and the anal canal and fistula tract exposed (Figure 147-1). A urinary catheter is placed. The intersphincteric groove is infiltrated with a combination of saline solution and epinephrine. Adequate exposure and lighting are key; a headlight and use of a Lone Star retractor to efface the anal canal is helpful.

A trapezoidal flap composed of mucosa, submucosa, and a portion of the internal sphincter is raised. The base of the flap should be at least twice the width of the apex, and mobilization should be continued for at least 4 cm. Before the flap is advanced, the internal sphincter is mobilized and approximated over the fistula. The flap is then advanced down the anal canal and secured with absorbable sutures. If the patient is incontinent or has a sphincter defect, a concomitant sphincteroplasty is performed. Patients are observed overnight if a sliding flap has been performed. A longer hospitalization

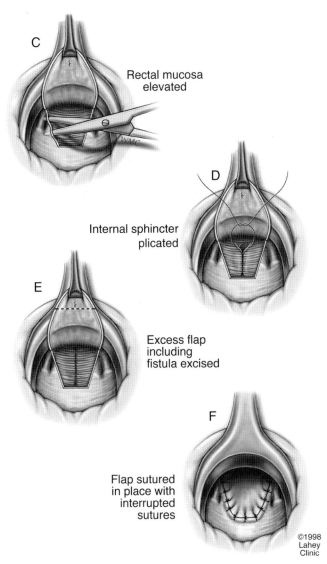

C, Rectal mucosa elevated

D, Internal sphincter plicated

E, Excess flap including fistula excised

F, Flap sutured in place with interrupted sutures

©1998 Lahey Clinic

FIGURE 147-1, cont'd C, The flap is raised, and dissection is performed laterally to permit a tension-free closure. **D,** The internal sphincter muscle is plicated over the area of the fistula. **E,** Excess flap, including the site of the internal opening of the fistula, is trimmed. **F,** The flap is secured with absorbable sutures. (Copyright 1998, Lahey Clinic, Burlington, Mass.)

period is generally required if concomitant sphincteroplasty is performed. Vaginal intercourse is avoided for 6 to 8 weeks.

Other modifications in flap construction have been reported. Ozuner et al[29] recommended a curvilinear flap incorporating mucosa, submucosa, and internal sphincter to avoid ischemia at the angled corners. Advancement of the entire rectal wall has been advocated for treatment of rectovaginal fistulas associated with Crohn disease with extensive scarring of the anal canal and multiple fistula tracts.[30,31] The influence of the technical nuances of flap construction including the thickness of the flap on the outcome of repair has not been determined.

Potential advantages of a sliding flap include the fact that no perineal wound is created and therefore pain is minimized, no sphincter (other than the internal sphincter if this is used for the flap) is cut, other procedures such as a concomitant sphincter repair can be performed, a diverting stoma is not necessary, and deformities such as a keyhole deformity, which may occur from fistulotomy, are avoided.

Outcomes. The success rate varies considerably, from 29% to 100%,[11,27,28,32-43] and is probably in part related to the heterogeneity of the patient groups in addition to variations in surgical technique. Common causes of flap failure include ischemia of the flap and hematoma and/or the development of infection under the flap. A variety of factors most likely account for the differing success rates after sliding flap repair, including the number of previous repairs, whether the initial or ultimate success rate was reported, the presence of a concomitant sphincter defect, and the cause of the rectovaginal fistula. If a patient has had one[35] or two[28] previous rectovaginal fistula repairs, the success rate with a sliding flap repair decreases significantly; therefore, a sliding flap repair should generally not be considered in a patient whose previous repairs have failed. Sphincter function should be assessed and concomitant significant sphincter defects at the time of sliding flap. The success rate for patients undergoing flap repair and sphincteroplasty with or without levatorplasty was significantly higher than the success rate for patients who underwent flap repair only (80% vs. 41%; $P < 0.02$).[11] As a result, some surgeons have advocated that anal ultrasonography and manometry be performed to detect occult sphincter defects in patients undergoing repair of rectovaginal fistulas; sphincter defects, however, in the majority of cases, can be determined by a thorough history and physical examination and then confirmed on manometry and ultrasound.[14] The underlying cause of the fistula may also determine the success of a flap repair. Patients with obstetric injuries as the cause of the rectovaginal fistula have a better outcome than patients with inflammatory bowel disease.

Transvaginal Techniques of Local Repair. A transvaginal approach for sliding flap may also be used to repair rectovaginal fistulas. Although a transvaginal approach addresses the fistula from the lower pressure vaginal side, not the higher pressure rectal side, this technique allows for good exposure and, as with transrectal advancement flap, the ability to perform a concomitant sphincteroplasty if needed. The patient undergoes similar preoperative preparation and the procedure is performed in the lithotomy position. An incision is made in the posterior vaginal wall by the introitus, and the flap is raised in a similar manner on the vaginal side and advanced. As with a rectal flap, the flap should be wide enough to ensure good blood supply and mobility. This approach may have an advantage in selected patients, especially patients with Crohn disease, because nondiseased, pliable vaginal tissue is used to form the flap, and there is little manipulation or dissection in the diseased rectum. Using this technique, Bauer et al[44] reported cure of the rectovaginal fistulas in 12 of 13 women with Crohn disease, with mean followup time of 50 months. Plication of the levator muscles was believed to be crucial to the repair. A transvaginal flap may also be useful in patients with pouch-vaginal fistulas after ileoanal pouch construction, obviating the need for a potentially difficult transanal approach.

ANOCUTANEOUS FLAP TECHNIQUE

There is a limited experience with use of anocutaneous flaps, raising anoderm and perianal skin and advancing this into the anal canal.[45] This technique may be used for very distal fistulas but has limited application because of the lack of adequate perineal skin between the rectum and vagina in most patients with rectovaginal fistulas.

Advancement Sleeve Flap

It is estimated that a rectovaginal fistula will develop in up to 10% of women with Crohn disease. These fistulas can be difficult to treat. For patients with associated severe anorectal and colonic disease, proctocolectomy with ileostomy is the best option. In selected patients with Crohn disease and a normal rectum, a local procedure can be considered. Although a sliding flap may be performed in selected patients, for patients with anal canal ulceration, a normal rectum, and rectovaginal fistula, an advancement sleeve flap may be performed (Figure 147-2). Using this technique in 13 patients with Crohn and a rectovaginal fistula in addition to other complex fistulas, a successful outcome was achieved in 8 patients. An additional modification was reported by Schouten et al,[46] who employed either a posterior "Kraske" approach or an abdominal approach in 8 women with persistent low rectovaginal fistula, with overall healing in 75%. No patient had dyspareunia, which may be an advantage to this technique compared to tissue interposition techniques, which may be associated with higher risks of dyspareunia.[47] The advancement sleeve flap is a good option for patients with persistent fistulas despite other local procedures, and patients in whom the only other option is fecal diversion or proctectomy.

Transperineal Repair

The two most commonly performed transperineal repairs include transperineal repair with layered closure with fistula repair (Figure 147-3) and perineoproctotomy (which essentially converts the fistula to a full-thickness laceration) followed by layered repair (Figure 147-4).[48] No study has directly compared the results of local repairs and reported series are generally small.

Transperineal Repair with Layered Closure. This procedure essentially involves an overlapping sphincteroplasty and is one of the most common operations performed for rectovaginal fistula. It may be performed as the sole procedure or combined with sliding flap repair. It corrects any underlying sphincter defect in addition to providing good muscle bulk to interpose in the rectovaginal septum. It is indicated for simple rectovaginal fistulas with an associated sphincter defect. The fistula is identified. After injection of saline with epinephrine to facilitate the dissection, a curvilinear incision is made in the perineum around the anus, and the edges of the external and internal sphincter muscles are identified and mobilized. Scar tissue is usually left in place on the muscle and not debrided. Care is taken to preserve the pudendal nerves that enter posterolaterally; however, a significant sphincter injury usually causes retraction of the nerves to

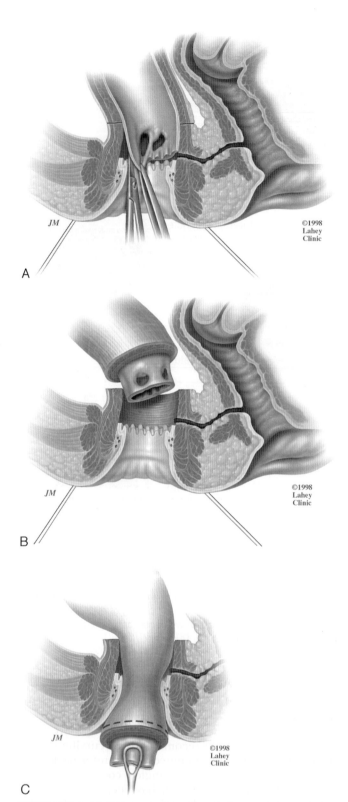

FIGURE 147-2 Advancement sleeve flap. **A,** Commencing at the level of the dentate line, a circumferential dissection of mucosa and submucosa is performed, thus excising the ulcerated areas of the anal canal. **B,** The dissection is continued cephalad and into the supralevator space, completing rectal mobilization. **C,** The fistula can then be cored out and closed, and the distal cuff (*dotted line*) of the rectum is trimmed and secured to the anoderm. (Copyright 1998, Lahey Clinic, Burlington, Mass.)

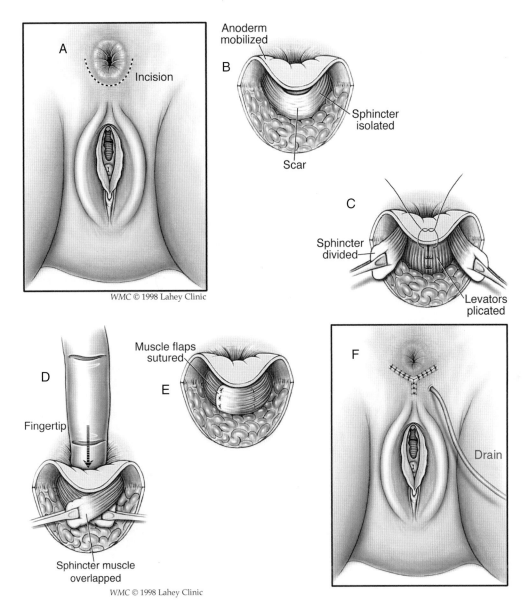

FIGURE 147-3 Overlapping sphincteroplasty. **A,** The patient is placed in the prone jackknife position, and a curvilinear incision is made approximately 180 degrees around the anus. **B,** Dissection is carried out medial to the ischiorectal fat, and the external sphincter is identified. **C,** Dissection is carried up to the level of the levatores, which are plicated. **D,** If sufficient muscle is present, an overlapping sphincter repair is performed. If not, simple apposition of the sphincter muscle is performed. **E,** The completed repair. **F,** The perineal body is reconstructed, and the wound is secured in a Y configuration. A drain may be placed. (Copyright 1998, Lahey Clinic, Burlington, Mass.)

a more posterior location and, therefore, injury is usually easily avoided. In the course of the dissection, the fistula is identified, and the dissection is carried cephalad, separating the rectum and vagina for several centimeters until soft pliable tissue is reached. It is important to adequately separate the rectum and vagina at the site of the fistula and to extend the dissection cephalad for 1 to 2 cm. The levator muscles are identified and plicated, which adds to the muscle bulk and appears to provide better results from a continence standpoint.[11,49] The perineal skin may be either closed loosely or left open. The vaginal mucosa is left open for drainage.

Sphincteroplasty for rectovaginal fistula is associated with success rates of 65% to 100%.[11,24,28,32,34,35] All reported

series of this technique are small, including 7 to 35 patients from single institutions.

Perineoproctotomy with Layered Closure. In this procedure, the fistula is converted to a fourth-degree perineal laceration. The tract is then excised, and the vagina, sphincter muscles, and rectal mucosa are identified, mobilized, and repaired in layers. Excellent results have been reported in several series.[36,50,51] Mazier et al[36] reported a success rate of 100% in 38 patients who underwent perineoproctectomy.

Episioproctotomy and Cloacal Defects. Patients with cloacal defects represent a severe form of obstetric trauma with essentially no perineal body, a shortened rectovaginal septum, and a retracted anal sphincter.

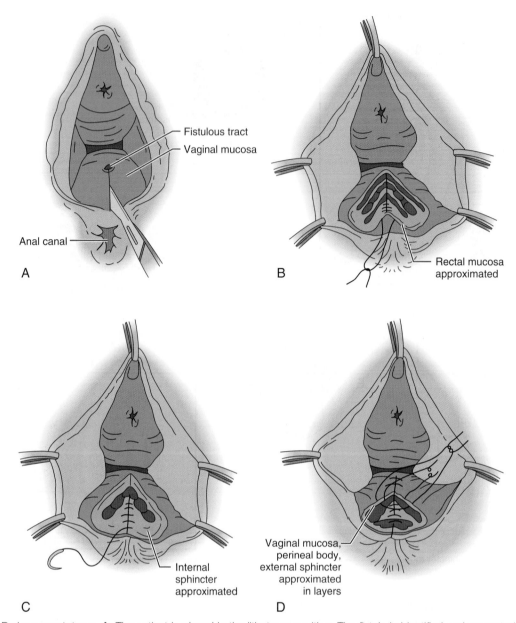

Fistulous tract
Vaginal mucosa
Anal canal

A

Rectal mucosa
approximated

B

Internal
sphincter
approximated

C

Vaginal mucosa,
perineal body,
external sphincter
approximated
in layers

D

FIGURE 147-4 Perineo-proctotomy. **A,** The patient is placed in the lithotomy position. The fistula is identified and converted into a full-thickness laceration. **B,** The layers are dissected out and repaired, first repairing the rectal mucosa. **C,** The repair continues, approximating the internal sphincter. **D,** The external sphincter is identified and repaired. Many patients will not have a discernible plane between the internal and external sphincter, and the internal and external sphincter may be repaired together. The vaginal mucosa is approximated.

Repair is carried out by developing the plane between the anorectal and vaginal epithelium and identifying the sphincter muscle on either side which is mobilized and subsequently approximated.[52,53] The procedure may also be combined with an anoplasty. Kaiser[53] reported 12 patients with a cloacal defect and treated with such a technique with X-flap anoplasty. Nine patients healed and 3 had a persistent rectovaginal fistula, and in 2 of them it closed spontaneously. One patient subsequently required a bulbocavernosus flap.

Fistulotomy

Simple fistulotomy for the treatment of patients with rectovaginal fistula is mentioned only to be avoided because of the risk of significant incontinence from transection of the internal and external sphincter. In a small series[54] of eight patients who underwent this procedure, all patients had postoperative incontinence and required a second procedure.

Autologous Fibrin Glue

Autologous fibrin tissue adhesive initially appeared to have some success in the treatment of patients with rectovaginal fistulas and is used for selective anal fistulas, particularly those with a long tract. The advantage of fibrin glue for treatment of fistulas is that it can be done as a minimally invasive technique without significant complications. However, the technique has, with the exception of one series, a high failure rate because the tract is characteristically too short to hold the glue for any length of time.[55-57] Modifications in the technique including closure of the internal opening and use of intraadhesive antibiotics have not improved the outcome.[58]

Fibrin glue has also been used as an adjunct with other procedures such as endorectal advancement flap. In one series,[41] fibrin glue was combined with an endorectal advancement flap in 12 patients; the failure rate was 50%, which was not significantly different than patients who had endorectal advancement flap alone. Despite initial enthusiasm, the technique is generally not used for rectovaginal fistulas.

Collagen Fistula Plug/Rectovaginal Fistula Button

Despite initial reports of good success with collagen fistula plugs for cryptoglandular fistulas, use of this plug for rectovaginal or pouch-vaginal fistulas has been associated with a high failure rate because of early dislodgement of the plug from the short tract. The plug has subsequently been modified with a button to potentially obviate this problem. The button fistula plug was used in 12 patients with a rectovaginal fistula ($n = 5$) or pouch-vaginal fistula ($n = 7$).[59] Ultimately, 7 of the 20 plugs that were inserted were successful, resulting in an overall success rate of 58%. The success rate with repeated plug insertion was only 12.5%, with all failures due to dislodgement of the plug. The fistula plug is associated with low morbidity and is an option in patients with rectovaginal fistulas without an associated sphincter defect or associated incontinence.

Bioprosthetics

Bioprosthetic mesh has been used as an interposition graft to repair rectovaginal fistulas. In a group of 27 women with rectovaginal fistulas who underwent advancement flap and placement of an interposition graft of bioprosthetic material, there were 5 recurrences (19%).[60] The recurrence rate was lower than women who underwent advancement flap repair without mesh (34%); the study was not randomized and the heterogeneous nature of the patients in addition to selection bias makes it difficult to make conclusions on these data. Another small prospective nonrandomized study of mesh for closure of rectovaginal fistulas where the fistula was excised and the mesh was placed transvaginally in 21 patients resulted in a success rate of 75%.[61]

MISCELLANEOUS REPAIRS

A variety of other repairs have been described for treatment of rectovaginal fistula, particularly in those patients without sphincter damage. A series of 39 patients who underwent transvaginal purse-string repair of rectovaginal fistula reported successful healing in 100%. No pre- or postoperative continence scores were provided and all patients had fistulas of obstetric origin.[62]

TISSUE INTERPOSITION PROCEDURES

Tissue interposition for the treatment of patients with rectovaginal fistula is intended to interpose normal well-vascularized healthy tissue between suture lines. Although

several types of tissues have been used, such as the gracilis, sartorius, and gluteus maximus muscles, the most commonly used are the bulbocavernosus muscle and gracilis muscle. This technique was first described by Martius[63] in 1928 and was originally used for the repair of vesicovaginal fistulas; however, it is also useful for radiation-induced rectovaginal fistulas, large obstetric fistulas, those for which previous repairs have failed, and selected pouch-vaginal fistulas after restorative proctocolectomy. Details of the procedure are outlined in Figure 147-5. Since the description by Martius,[63] Elkins et al[64] have shown that the bulbocavernosus muscle itself does not need to be included in the graft because the labial adipose tissue has excellent blood supply, thus decreasing the morbidity of using the bulbocavernosus muscle and reducing the operative time. Using this technique for complex fistulas, Pinedo and Phillips reported healing in 6 of 8 patients.[65] Modifications in surgical technique have been outlined by Hoskins et al,[66] who used a full-thickness island graft from the labia majora, and Symmonds and Hill,[67] who used a full-thickness graft from labia minora and majora. Boronow[68] reported a success rate of 84% in 25 women with rectovaginal fistulas. McNevin et al reported 16 patients who underwent Martius flap for complex rectovaginal fistula. The etiology of the fistula was obstetric ($n = 9$), cryptoglandular ($n = 5$), and Crohn disease ($n = 2$).[47] There was one recurrent fistula and one patient had a labial wound complication. Five patients had dyspareunia (31%), whereas only one had complained of dyspareunia preoperatively. Dyspareunia, infrequently reported as an outcome variable, is a potential concern with the procedure.[43] An additional concern is the patient's self-perception of the appearance of the graft site in addition to decreased sensation or numbness of the graft site. A small series of eight women who underwent Martius interposition were queried about the cosmetic appearance of the site and two believed it was identical to the preoperative appearance, two believed there were minimal changes, one believed the appearance was markedly different from the opposite side, and three patients had not examined the area. One patient complained of dyspareunia, three had intermittent discomfort in the harvest site, and five patients had decreased sensation and numbness at the harvest site.[69]

The gracilis muscle is also used for interposition. The gracilis is mobilized and brought through a tunnel with care to preserve the neurovascular bundle. There are five series of 4 to 17 patients with rectovaginal and pouch-vaginal fistulas with an overall healing rate per patient of 50% to 92% and a healing rate per procedure of 47% to 85%.[70-74] Despite healing of the fistula in the majority of patients, quality of life and sexual function remained altered, with only 4 of 7 patients who were sexually active after surgery and 25% of patients reporting dyspareunia.[70]

ABDOMINAL PROCEDURES

Complex fistulas, particularly those secondary to radiation therapy or previous pelvic surgery, are generally not suitable for a local repair. Fistulas may occur after operations that involve anterior rectal mobilization and

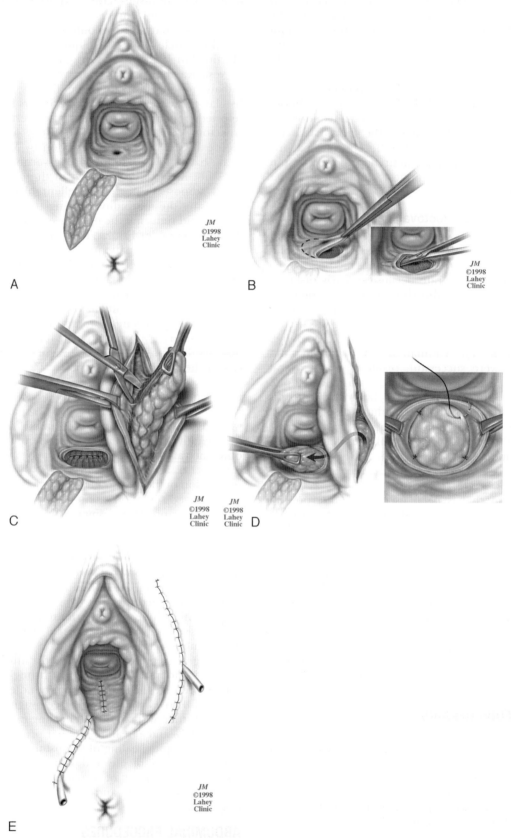

FIGURE 147-5 Bulbocavernosus (Martius) flap. **A,** The patient is placed in the lithotomy position, and a mediolateral episiotomy incision is made. **B,** The vaginal side of the fistula is mobilized and excised. The rectal side of the fistula is closed. **C,** Along the opposite labia majora, an incision is made and the bulbocavernosus muscle and labial fat pad are mobilized. **D,** The bulbocavernosus muscle and labial fat pad are brought through a subcutaneous tunnel and secured to the previously closed rectal side of the fistula *(inset).* **E,** The vaginal defect is closed, and the incisions are closed. Drainage is effected with a Penrose or closed-suction drain. (Copyright 1998, Lahey Clinic, Burlington, Mass.)

mobilization of the rectovaginal septum, such as low anterior resection, coloanal anastomosis, and ileal pouch–anal anastomosis. After colorectal procedures, such fistulas commonly arise from dehiscence of the anastomosis, with subsequent tracking into the vagina. Previous hysterectomy appears to predispose the patient to this complication, presumably because of the difficulty with adhesions between the anterior rectal wall and vaginal cuff.[75] Although rectovaginal fistula is reported after both hand-sewn and double-stapled anastomosis, the double-staple technique seems to be implicated in most cases, presumably because most low anastomoses are stapled and not hand-sewn. Anastomotic leakage with a resultant rectovaginal fistula may also result from a colonic J-pouch or coloplasty. Gynecologic surgery, such as hysterectomy, rectocele repair, and vaginal vault prolapse suspension, may also be complicated by rectovaginal fistula. In one series,[76] rectovaginal fistulas occurred in 1.2% of women undergoing repair of vaginal vault prolapse. These fistulas tend to be higher than obstetric fistulas and have surrounding tissues that are abnormal and poorly vascularized. Abdominal procedures permit excision of abnormal tissue, with interposition of well-vascularized normal tissue to correct the fistula. Preservation of the sphincter is possible with such procedures as coloanal anastomosis and onlay patch anastomosis.

Coloanal Anastomosis

Patients with radiation proctitis and rectovaginal fistula may be treated by resection and coloanal sleeve anastomosis as first reported by Parks et al.[77] The technique involves proximal loop diversion, rectal resection below the level of the fistula, and mobilization of the left colon. Although Parks et al described a distal mucosectomy followed by a coloanal anastomosis, a double-staple technique (as is used for the ileoanal pouch procedure) may also be used, and a colonic J-pouch may be added to improve neorectal function. If available, omentum is interposed between the anastomosis and the vagina. Using the coloanal anastomosis, Cooke and Wellsted[78] reported a 93% success rate in 55 patients. A modification of the coloanal technique has been reported by Simonsen et al,[79] who used the anterior rectal wall to construct a neovagina. The authors reported no operative deaths and no recurrent fistulas in 19 patients.

Onlay Patch Anastomosis

Bricker and Johnston[80] described an alternative approach for radiation-induced rectovaginal fistulas and particularly fistulas that involve large portions of the vagina. Although several modifications of the procedure have been described, the procedure involves mobilization of the rectosigmoid and exposure of the fistula. After transection of the rectosigmoid, an end stoma is formed. Subsequently, the distal rectosigmoid is rotated down, and the open end is anastomosed to the debrided edges of the fistula opening in the rectum. After healing has been confirmed with radiographic studies, the proximal sigmoid is sutured in end-to-side fashion to the loop in the rectosigmoid. The advantage of this procedure is that posterior rectal mobilization and entry into the presacral space are not necessary; however, it is still a technically difficult procedure, and a disadvantage is that a portion of the diseased rectum is left in place for the anastomosis. Using this technique, Bricker and Johnston[80] reported excellent or satisfactory results in 19 of 20 patients. The procedure is rarely performed in clinical practice.

Role of Diversion

For a patient with a rectovaginal fistula who is a poor medical risk and cannot tolerate major surgery, simple fecal diversion with either a loop ileostomy or colostomy may provide good symptomatic relief and return to a reasonable quality of life.

Fecal diversion also has a role in patients who have undergone repair of complex fistulas by coloanal anastomosis or Bricker onlay patch anastomosis. Patients who have Crohn disease and patients whose multiple previous local repairs have failed may also benefit from fecal diversion as an adjunct to primary repair or as a primary procedure.

SUMMARY

The optimal treatment for patients with rectovaginal fistulas depends on a number of factors, including the site of the fistula, the cause of the fistula, surgical expertise, and the presence of an associated sphincter defect and incontinence. With thorough preoperative evaluation, consideration of optimal treatment options, and meticulous surgical technique, a successful repair is achieved in the majority of patients. Quality of life following repair of rectovaginal fistula and sexual function are infrequently reported but there is increasing evidence that despite successful repair, postoperative quality of life and sexual activity remain significantly altered.

RECTOURETHRAL FISTULAS

Rectourethral fistulas (RUFs) are rare and may occur from either congenital or acquired causes. Congenital fistulas are often associated with other anorectal abnormalities, whereas acquired fistulas may result from trauma, previous surgery, Crohn disease, infection, malignancy, and/or radiation. Historically, RUFs occurred after such procedures as an open simple prostatectomy, transurethral prostatectomy (TURP), perineal prostatectomy, and perineal biopsy of the prostate. However, over the past two decades, the detection and treatment of prostate cancer has exponentially increased and now represents the primary cause of RUF with patients undergoing primary or salvage high-dose brachytherapy, external beam therapy (EBRT), cryotherapy, and radical prostatectomy by either an open or laparoscopic/robotic approach.[81-83] Not only has the incidence of RUF increased with more prostate cancer therapy occurring but the complexity and difficulty of the RUF has shifted dramatically. Before 1997, radiation-induced RUF accounted for only 3.8% of all RUFs. Since 1998, the incidence of radiation-induced RUF is 49.6% and growing, reflecting the widespread utilization of radiation therapy for the treatment of prostate cancer.[82,84] There has been a shift from predominantly small surgical fistulas with relatively healthy surrounding tissue to more complex fistulas associated with substantial tissue defect, severe fibrosis, unhealthy radiated tissue, and concurrent urethral strictures. The emergence of large, complex radiated RUFs has mandated a change in surgical technique away from simple fistula closure to patch graft urethral reconstruction with interposition muscle flap or complete prostatectomy. The diagnosis and approach to such fistulas are discussed, and further details are available in the references at the end of the chapter.[84,85]

INCIDENCE

Rectal injury is a well-recognized complication of prostate surgery, with RUF occurring in 0.5% to 3.0% of contemporary series.[81,86-89] Patients undergoing ablative brachytherapy, EBRT, or cryotherapy have a reported incidence of 0.2% to 3% for primary therapy and 7% to 9% for combined or salvage therapy.[90-96] RUF development (3.7%) also occurs in patients who undergo rectal biopsy after primary ablative therapy.[97]

PRESENTATION AND EVALUATION

The clinical presentation is generally straightforward, with most patients complaining of passage of urine per rectum, fecaluria, and pneumaturia. Patients who develop fistulas after brachytherapy or cryotherapy may initially complain of severe pain. An examination under anesthesia, retrograde urethrography, voiding cystourethrography, urethrocystoscopy, and digital rectal examination help define the location, size, and extent of the fistula as well as determine if a coexisting urethral stricture or bladder neck contracture is present. Anoscopy and either flexible sigmoidoscopy or colonoscopy identify the rectal opening and assess the anal sphincter and the rectum for evidence of intrinsic rectal disease such as inflammatory bowel disease or radiation proctitis.

ASSESSMENT AND TECHNIQUE

There are a number of surgical procedures for repair of rectourethral fistulas. Determining the optimal repair must take into account the complexity of the fistulas, the status of the surrounding tissues, the size of the defect, and prior radiation therapy. Delaying surgery for 3 months with both urinary and fecal diversion remains the mainstay in RUF management to allow for an attempt at spontaneous resolution, resolve acute infections, decrease inflammation, and optimize tissue for future reconstruction. In the case of a small surgically induced fistula, in a patient who has not had previous radiation, repair without fecal diversion can be considered. In patients with complex fistulas (size >2 cm, radiated/ablated, prior failed repair, concomitant pelvic abscess) that will require a patch graft and muscle interposition, fecal diversion is mandatory. In the presence of an intact anal sphincter and a compliant functional rectum, our preference is a temporary loop ileostomy, ideally performed laparoscopically, for its ease of creation and reversal. A temporary loop ileostomy prevents rectal wall distention and pressure during healing, and minimizes infection, which is critical for successful complex fistula closure. Additionally, it permits mobilization of the colon for colonic advancement if a proctectomy and coloanal anastomosis are required.[84] Large fistula defects require interposition of additional tissue, and the gracilis muscle

is ideally suited for this technique. The gracilis has been used extensively in colorectal surgery for construction of a neosphincter around the anus, for treatment of unhealed wounds after proctectomy for cancer or Crohn disease, for complex rectovaginal fistulas, and for rectourethral fistulas.

Complex, large radiated RUF currently represents more than 50% of all RUFs and will continue to increase with the widespread use of high-dose, combined, and salvage radiation therapy for prostate cancer and other pelvic malignancies. Radiated RUF represents one of the most challenging operative cases because of the inaccessible fibrotic space, with adherent planes creating a challenging dissection and closure of the fistula. The largest series reported 74 patients with RUF comparing nonradiated and radiated/ablation-induced RUF using a single technique.[84] All RUFs were repaired via an anterior perineal anal sphincter–preserving approach with an interposition muscle flap. Selective use of a buccal mucosal patch (BMG) for urethral closure was used in complex RUFs when the urethra was not able to be primarily closed (Figure 147-6). Seventy-four patients with RUFs were repaired with an anterior perineal approach and muscle interposition flap; 36 nonradiated and 38 radiated/ablation-induced RUFs were compared. Concurrent urethral strictures were present in 11% of nonradiated and 29% of radiated/ablated RUFs. At a mean followup of 20 months, 100% of nonradiated RUFs were closed with one procedure, whereas 84% of radiated/ablated RUFs were closed in a single stage. In the nonradiated RUF group, 35 of 36 patients (97%) had reversal of the fecal diversion without anal stenosis and with normal bowel function, whereas 1 patient remained diverted because of a devastating rectal injury. Sixty-nine percent of the radiated/ablated RUF patients had bowel continuity reestablished, whereas 31% required permanent fecal diversion. The anterior perineal approach with muscle interposition and selective use of BMG onlay is considered the optimal approach for successful closure of all RUFs, avoiding cystoprostatectomy and permanent urinary and fecal diversion.

Additional techniques used for repair of surgically induced RUFs are the York-Mason posterior transanosphincteric approach and endorectal sliding flap. The York-Mason procedure utilizes a prone jackknife position followed by posterior midline division of the sphincteric muscles for exposure and closure of the RUF. High fistula closure rates have been reported with this approach (85% to 100%).[98,99] The advantage of relatively unscarred tissue planes must be balanced against the risk of causing anal dysfunction and an inability to repair large, complex RUFs that cannot be closed primarily. Low, simple fistulas may also be repaired by an endorectal sliding flap. The main advantage of such a repair is minimal morbidity and quick recovery, whereas the main disadvantage of this procedure is that the high-pressure urethral side is not addressed and a period of prolonged catheter drainage is needed. Using such an approach, initial closure was achieved in 8 (67%) of 12 patients.[100]

Patients with rectourethral fistulas represent a heterogeneous group and consideration for treatment needs to address both rectal and urinary function. During the past

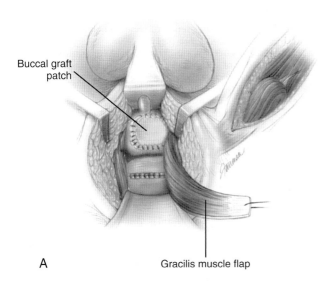

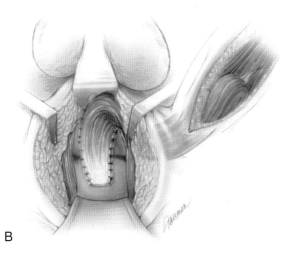

FIGURE 147-6 A, Gracilis muscle interposition flap with buccal mucosal patch closure of urethra. **B,** Gracilis muscle flap coverage and support of buccal graft and periurethral tissue (Used with permission from Vanni A, Buckley JC, Zinman LN: Management of surgical and radiation induced rectourethral fistulas with an interposition muscle flap and selective buccal mucosal onlay graft. *J Urol* 184:2400, 2010.)

decade, there has been a shift from small fistulas to more complex fistulas associated with substantial tissue defect, fibrotic radiated tissue, and concomitant urethral strictures, mandating modifications in the surgical technique and the use of tissue interposition and fecal diversion in a majority of cases.

REFERENCES

1. Goldaber KG, Wendel PJ, McIntire DD, et al: Postpartum perineal morbidity after fourth-degree perineal repair. *Am J Obstet Gynecol* 168:489, 1993.
2. Venkatesh KS, Ramanujam PS, Larson DM, et al: Anorectal complications of vaginal delivery. *Dis Colon Rectum* 32:1039, 1989.
3. Donnay F, Weil L: Obstetric fistula: The international response: *Lancet* 363:71, 2004.
4. Browning A, Allsworth JE, Wall LL: The relationship between female genital cutting and obstetric fistulae. *Obstet Gynecol* 115:578, 2010.
5. Kelly J: Outreach programmes for obstetric fistulae. *J Obstet Gynecol* 24:117, 2004.
6. Abou Zahr C: Global burden of maternal death and disability. *Br Med Bull* 67:1, 2003.
7. Radcliffe AG, Ritchie JK, Hawley PR, et al: Anovaginal and rectovaginal fistulas in Crohn's disease. *Dis Colon Rectum* 31:94, 1998.
8. Matthiessen P, Hansson L, Sjodahl R, et al: Anastomotic-vaginal fistula (AVF) after anterior resection of the rectum for cancer—occurrence and risk factors. *Colorectal Dis* 12:351, 2010.
9. Heriot AG, Tekkis PP, Smith JJ, et al: Management and outcome of pouch-vaginal fistulas following restorative proctocolectomy. *Dis Colon Rectum* 48:451, 2005.
10. Kasibhatia M, Clough RW, Montana GS, et al: Predictors of severe gastrointestinal toxicity after external beam radiotherapy and interstitial brachytherapy for advanced or recurrent gynecologic malignancies. *Int J Radiat Oncol Biol Phys* 65:398, 2006.
11. Tsang CB, Madoff RD, Wong WD, et al: Anal sphincter integrity and function influences outcome in rectovaginal fistula repair. *Dis Colon Rectum* 41:1141, 1998.
12. Saclarides TJ: Rectovaginal fistula. *Surg Clin North Am* 82:1261, 2002.
13. Sultan AH, Kamm MA, Hudson CN, et al: Anal-sphincter disruption during vaginal delivery. *N Engl J Med* 329:1905, 1993.
14. Yee LF, Birnbaum EH, Read TE, et al: Use of endoanal ultrasound in patients with rectovaginal fistulas. *Dis Colon Rectum* 42:1057, 1999.
15. Goetz LH, Lowry AC: Overlapping sphincteroplasty: Is it the standard of care? *Clin Colon Rectal Surg* 18:22, 2005.
16. Dohgomori H, Arikawa K, Nobori M, et al: Hyperbaric oxygenation for rectovaginal fistula: A report of two cases. *J Obstet Gynaecol Res* 25:343, 1999.
17. Present DH, Rutgeerts P, Targan S, et al: Infliximab for the treatment of fistulas in patients with Crohn's disease. *N Engl J Med* 340:1398, 1999.
18. Sands BE, Blank MA, Patel K, et al: Long-term treatment of rectovaginal fistulas in Crohn's disease: Response to infliximab in the ACCENT II study. *Clin Gastroenterol Hepatol* 2:912, 2004.
19. Andreani SM, Dang HH, Grondona P, et al: Rectovaginal fistula in Crohn's disease. *Dis Colon Rectum* 50:2215, 2007.
20. Poritz LS, Rowe WA, Koltun WA: Remicade does not abolish the need for surgery in fistulizing Crohn's disease. *Dis Colon Rectum* 45:771, 2002.
21. El-Gazzaz G, Hull T, Mignanelli E, et al: Analysis of function and predictors of failure in women undergoing repair of Crohn's related rectovaginal fistula. *J Gastrointest Surg* 14:824, 2010.
22. Pinto RA, Peterson RV, Shawki S, et al: Are there predictors of outcome following rectovaginal fistula repair? *Dis Colon Rectum* 53:1240, 2010.
23. Stoker J, Rociu E, Schouten WR, et al: Anovaginal and rectovaginal fistulas: Endoluminal sonography versus endoluminal MR imaging. *AJR Am J Roentgenol* 178:737, 2002.
24. Halverson AL, Hull TL, Fazio VW, et al: Repair of recurrent rectovaginal fistulas. *Surgery* 130:753, 2001.
25. Noble GH: A new operation for complete laceration of the perineum designed for the purpose of eliminating danger of infection from the rectum. *Trans Am Gynecol Soc* 27:357, 1902.
26. Laird DR: Procedures used in treatment of complicated fistulas. *Am J Surg* 76:701, 1948.
27. Kodner IJ, Mazor A, Shemesh EI, et al: Endorectal advancement flap repair of rectovaginal and other complicated anorectal fistulas. *Surgery* 114:682, 1993.
28. Lowry AC, Thorson AG, Rothenberger DA, et al: Repair of simple rectovaginal fistulas: Influence of previous repairs. *Dis Colon Rectum* 31:676, 1988.
29. Ozuner G, Hull TL, Cartmill J, et al: Long-term analysis of the use of transanal rectal advancement flaps for complicated anorectal/vaginal fistulas. *Dis Colon Rectum* 39:10, 1996.
30. Hull TL, Fazio VW: Surgical approaches to low anovaginal fistula in Crohn's disease. *Am J Surg* 173:95, 1997.
31. Marchesa P, Hull TL, Fazio VW: Advancement sleeve flaps for treatment of severe perianal Crohn's disease. *Br J Surg* 85:1695, 1998.

32. Wise WE Jr, Aquilar PS, Padmanabhan A, et al: Surgical treatment of low rectovaginal fistulas. *Dis Colon Rectum* 34:271, 1991.

33. Khanduja KS, Yamashita HJ, Wise WE Jr, et al: Delayed repair of obstetric injuries of the anorectum and vagina: A stratified surgical approach. *Dis Colon Rectum* 37:344, 1994.

34. Athanasiadis S, Oladeinde I, Kuprian A, et al: Endorectal advancement flap-plasty vs. transperineal closure in surgical treatment of rectovaginal fistulas: A prospective long-term study of 88 patients. *Chirurg* 66:493, 1995.

35. MacRae HM, McLeod RS, Cohen Z, et al: Treatment of rectovaginal fistula that has failed previous repair attempts. *Dis Colon Rectum* 38:921, 1995.

36. Mazier WP, Senagore AJ, Schiesel EC: Operative repair of anovaginal and rectovaginal fistulas. *Dis Colon Rectum* 38:4, 1995.

37. Watson SJ, Phillips RK: Non-inflammatory rectovaginal fistula. *Br J Surg* 82:1641, 1995.

38. Joo JS, Weiss EG, Nogueras JJ, et al: Endorectal advancement flap in perianal Crohn's disease. *Am Surg* 64:147, 1998.

39. Hyman N: Endoanal advancement flap repair for complex anorectal fistulas. *Am J Surg* 178:337, 1999.

40. Baig MK, Zhao RH, Yuen CH, et al: Simple rectovaginal fistulas. *Int J Colorectal Dis* 15:323, 2000.

41. Mizrahi N, Wexner DS, Zmora O, et al: Endorectal advancement flap: Are there predictors of failure? *Dis Colon Rectum* 45:1616, 2002.

42. Sonoda T, Hull T, Piedmonte MR, et al: Outcomes of primary repair of anorectal and rectovaginal fistulas using the endorectal advancement flap. *Dis Colon Rectum* 45:1622, 2002.

43. Zimmerman DD, Gosselink MP, Briel JW, et al: The outcome of transanal advancement flap repair of rectovaginal fistulas is not improved by an additional labial fat flap transposition. *Techn Coloproctol* 6:37, 2002.

44. Bauer JJ, Sher ME, Jaffin H, et al: Transvaginal approach for repair of rectovaginal fistulae complicating Crohn's disease. *Ann Surg* 213:151, 1991.

45. Hesterberg R, Schmidt WU, Muller F, et al: Treatment of anovaginal fistulas with an anocutaneous flap in patients with Crohn's disease. *Int J Colorectal Dis* 8:51, 1993.

46. Schouten WR, Oom DMJ: Rectal sleeve advancement for the treatment of persistent rectovaginal fistulas. *Tech Coloproctol* 13:289, 2009.

47. McNevin MS, Lee PY, Bax TW: Martius flap: Ad adjunct for repair of complex, low rectovaginal fistula. *Am J Surg* 193:597, 2007.

48. Lowry AC, Hoexter B: Benign anorectal: Rectovaginal fistulas. In Wolff BG, Fleshman JW, Beck DE, et al, editors: *The ASCRS Textbook of colon and rectal surgery.* 2007, Springer, p 215.

49. Stricker JM, Schoetz DJ, Jr, Coller JA, et al: Surgical correction of anal incontinence. *Dis Colon Rectum* 31:533, 1988.

50. Pepe F, Panella M, Arikan S, et al: Low rectovaginal fistulas. *Aust N Z J Obstet Gynecol* 27:61, 1987.

51. Tancer ML, Lasser D, Rosenblum N: Rectovaginal fistula or perineal and anal sphincter disruption, or both, after vaginal delivery. *Surg Gynecol Obstet* 171:43, 1990.

52. Hull TL, Bartus C, Bast J, et al: Success of episioproctotomy for cloaca and rectovaginal fistula. *Dis Colon Rectum* 50:97, 2006.

53. Kaiser AM: Cloaca-like deformity with faecal incontinence after severe obstetric injury—technique and functional outcome of ano-vaginal and perineal reconstruction with X-flaps and sphincteroplasty. *Colorectal Dis* 10:827, 2008.

54. Belt RL: Repair of anorectal vaginal fistula utilizing segmental advancement of the internal sphincter muscle. *Dis Colon Rectum* 12:99, 1969.

55. Abel ME, Chiu YS, Russell TR, et al: Autologous fibrin glue in the treatment of rectovaginal and complex fistulas. *Dis Colon Rectum* 36:447, 1993.

56. Cintron JR, Park JJ, Orsay CP, et al: Repair of fistulas-in-ano using autologous fibrin tissue adhesive. *Dis Colon Rectum* 42:607, 1999.

57. Venkatesh KS, Ramanujam P: Fibrin glue application in the treatment of recurrent fistulas. *Dis Colon Rectum* 42:1136, 1999.

58. Singer M, Cintron J, Nelson R, et al: Treatment of fistulas-in-ano with fibrin sealant in combination with intra-adhesive antibiotics and/or surgical closure of the internal fistula opening. *Dis Colon Rectum* 48:799, 2005.

59. Gonsalves S, Sagar P, Lengyel J, et al: Assessment of the efficacy of the rectovaginal button fistula plug for the treatment of ileal pouch-vaginal and rectovaginal fistulas. *Dis Colon Rectum* 52:1877, 2009.

60. Ellis CN: Outcomes after repair of rectovaginal fistulas using bioprosthetics. *Dis Colon Rectum* 52:1084, 2008.

61. Schwandner O, Fuerst A, Kunstreich K, et al: Innovative technique for the closure of rectovaginal fistula using Surgisis mesh. *Tech Coloproctol* 13:135, 2009.

62. Rahman MS, Al-Suleiman SA, El-Yahia AR, et al: Surgical treatment of rectovaginal fistula of obstetric origin: A review of 15 years' experience in a teaching hospital. *J Obstet Gynaecol* 23:607, 2003.

63. Martius H: Die operative Wiederherstellung der vollkommen fehlenden Harnröhre und des Schliessmuskels derselben. *Zentralbl Gynäk* 52:480, 1928.

64. Elkins TE, DeLancey JOL, McGuire EJ: The use of modified Martius graft as an adjunctive technique in vesicovaginal and rectovaginal fistula repair. *Obstet Gynecol* 75:727, 1990.

65. Pinedo G, Phillips R: Labial fat pad grafts (modified Martius graft) in complex perianal fistulas. *Ann R Coll Surg Engl* 80:410, 1998.

66. Hoskins WJ, Park RC, Long R, et al: Repair of urinary tract fistulas with bulbocavernosus myocutaneous flaps. *Obstet Gynecol* 63:588, 1984.

67. Symmonds RE, Hill LM: Loss of the urethra: A report on 50 patients. *Am J Obstet Gynecol* 130:130, 1978.

68. Boronow RC: Repair of the radiation-induced vaginal fistula utilizing the Martius technique. *World J Surg* 10:237, 1986.

69. Petrou SP, Jones J, Parra RO: Martius flap harvest site: Patient self-perception. *J Urol* 167:2098, 2001.

70. Lefevre JH, Bretagnol F, Maggiori L: Operative results and quality of life after gracilis muscle transposition for recurrent rectovaginal fistula. *Dis Colon Rectum* 52:1290, 2009.

71. Ruis J, Nessim A, Nogueras JJ, et al: Gracilis transposition in complicated perianal fistula and unhealed perineal wounds in Crohn's disease. *Eur J Surg* 166:218, 2000.

72. Zmora O, Tulchinsky H, Gur E, et al: Gracilis muscle transposition for fistulas between the rectum and urethra or vagina. *Dis Colon Rectum* 49:1316, 2006.

73. Furst A, Schmidbauer C, Swol-Ben J, et al. Gracilis transposition for repair of recurrent anovaginal and rectovaginal fistulas in Crohn's disease. *Int J Colorect Dis* 23:349, 2008.

74. Wexner SD, Ruiz DE, Genua J, et al: Gracilis muscle interposition for the treatment of rectourethral, rectovaginal, and pouch-vaginal fistulas. Results in 53 patients. *Ann Surg* 248:39, 2008.

75. Fleshner PR, Schoetz DJ Jr, Roberts PL, et al: Anastomotic-vaginal fistula after colorectal surgery. *Dis Colon Rectum* 35:938, 1992.

76. Penalver M, Mekki Y, Lafferty H, et al: Should sacrospinous ligament fixation for the management of pelvic support defects be part of a residency program procedure? The University of Miami experience. *Am J Obstet Gynecol* 178:326, 1998.

77. Parks AG, Allen CL, Frank JD, et al: A method of treating post-irradiation rectovaginal fistulas. *Br J Surg* 65:417, 1978.

78. Cooke SA, Wellsted MD: The radiation-damaged rectum: Resection with coloanal anastomosis using the endoanal technique. *World J Surg* 10:220, 1986.

79. Simonsen OS, Sobrado CW, Bochinni SF, et al: Rectal neovagina: Simonsen's technique for large rectovaginal fistula repair. *Dis Colon Rectum* 41:658, 1998.

80. Bricker EM, Johnston WD: Repair of postirradiation rectovaginal fistula and stricture. *Surg Gynecol Obstet* 148:499, 1979.

81. McLaren RH, Barrett DM, Zincke H: Rectal injury occurring at radical retropubic prostatectomy for prostate cancer: Etiology and treatment. *Urology* 41:401, 1993.

82. Lane BR, Stein DE, Remzi GH, et al: Management of radiotherapy induced rectourethral fistulas following external radiation or permanent brachytherapy for the treatment of prostate cancer. *J Urol* 175:1382, 2006.

83. Chrouser KL, Leibovich BC, Sweat SD, et al: Urinary fistula following external radiation or permanent brachytherapy for the treatment of prostate cancer. *J Urol* 173:1953, 2005.

84. Vanni A, Buckley JC, Zinman LN: Management of surgical and radiation induced rectourethral fistulas with an interposition muscle flap and selective buccal mucosal onlay graft. *J Urol* 184:2400, 2010.

85. Zinman L: The management of the complex recto-urethral fistula. *BJU Int* 94:1212, 2004.

86. Harpster LE, Rommel MF, Sieber PR, et al: The incidence and management of rectal injury associated with radical prostatectomy in a community-based urology practice. *J Urol* 154:1435, 1995.

87. Yee DS, Ornstein DK: Repair of rectal injury during robotic-assisted laparoscopic prostatectomy. *Urology* 72:428, 2008.

88. Martin-Marquina Aspiunza A, Zudaire Bergera JJ, Sanchez Zalabardo D, et al: Radical proctectomy. The Surgical complications. *Actas Urol Esp* 23:5, 1999.

89. Thomas C, Jones J, Jager W, et al. Incidence, clinical symptoms and management of rectourethral fistulas after radical prostatectomy. *J Urol* 183:608, 2010.

90. Grado GL, Larson TR, Balch CS, et al: Actuarial disease-free survival after prostate cancer brachytherapy using interactive techniques with biplane ultrasound and fluoroscopic guidance. *Int J Radiat Oncol Biol Phys* 42:289, 1989.

91. Theodorescu D, Gillenwater JY, Koutrouyelis PG: Prostato-uretral rectal fistulas after prostate brachytherapy. *Cancer* 89:2085, 2000.

92. Zacharakis E, Ahmed HU, Ishaq A, et al: The feasibility and safety of high intensity focused ultrasound as salvage therapy for recurrent prostate cancer following eternal beam radiotherapy. *BJU Int.* 102:786, 2008.

93. Stone NN, Stock RG: Complications following permanent prostate brachytherapy. *Eur Urol* 41:427, 2002.

94. Nguyen PL, D'Amico AV, Lee AK, et al: Patient selection, cancer control and complications after salvage local therapy for postradiation prostate-specific antigen failure: A systemic review of the literature. *Cancer* 110:1417, 2007.

95. Pisters LL, Rewcastle JC, Donnelly BJ, et al: Salvage prostate cryoablations: Initial results from the cryo on-line data registry. *J Urol* 180;559, 2008.

96. Ahmed HU, Ishaq A, Zacharakis E, et al: Rectal fistulae after salvage high-intensity focused ultrasound for recurrent prostate cancer after combined brachytherapy and external beam radiotherapy. *BJU Int* 103:321, 2009.

97. Dinges S, Deger S, Koswig S, et al: High-dose rate interstitial with external beam irradiation for localized prostate cancer-results of a prospective trial. *Radiother Oncol* 48:197, 1998.

98. Dal Moror F, Mancini M, Pinto F, et al: Successful repair of iatrogenic rectourinary fistulas using the posterior sagittal transrectal approach (York-Mason): 15 year experience. *World J Surg* 30:107, 2006.

99. Renschler TD, Middleton RG: Thirty years of experience with York-Mason repair of rectourinary fistulas. *J Urol* 170:1222, 2003.

100. Garafalo TE, Delaney CP, Jones SM, et al: Rectal advancement flap repair of rectourethral fistula: A twenty-year experience. *Dis Colon Rectum* 46:762, 2003.

Complete Rectal Prolapse

Vivek Chaudhry | Herand Abcarian

Complete rectal prolapse or procidentia is a circumferential, full-thickness descent of the rectum (and maybe the sigmoid colon). Classically, eversion of the rectum is externally visible. The spectrum of associated disorders linked with the putative pathophysiology of rectal prolapse includes lesser degrees of "hidden" prolapse, internal intussusception, and solitary rectal ulcer syndrome. True rectal prolapse should be distinguished from rectal mucosal prolapse and hemorrhoidal disease. On examination, the former has thick, concentric, circumferential folds while the latter has radial folds often shaped like a three-pointed star (Figures 148-1 and 148-2).

HISTORICAL PERSPECTIVE

Rectal prolapse has been described for centuries. In the Ebers Papyrus, the ancient Egyptians described honey-containing suppositories, laxatives, and enemas in the treatment of rectal prolapse. The ancient Greeks used the method of hanging a patient by the heels and shaking to reduce a prolapse. Rectal prolapse was recognized as an intussusception of the colon in the 18th century. Moschocowitz identified rectal prolapse as a sliding perineal hernia on identifying a deep cul-de-sac in affected patients. The evolution of surgery for rectal prolapse is replete with small studies, short followups, and numerous variations of technique.[1]

PATHOPHYSIOLOGY

The anatomic defect of complete rectal prolapse is relatively easy to describe. The pathophysiology, however, has been more difficult to define. The development of rectal prolapse occurs over a period of years, making it difficult to identify a specific cause. It is unclear whether the intussusception of the rectum is the main responsible factor or the result of some other anatomic or physiologic defect. Several findings have been associated with rectal prolapse. These include weak levator ani and anal sphincter muscles, a redundant rectosigmoid colon, a deep cul-de-sac, and loss of fixation of the rectum to the sacrum.

Regardless, the prevailing theory is one of distal intussusception of the rectum. Numerous diseases have been linked to rectal prolapse including connective tissue disorders, pelvic outlet obstruction, pelvic floor laxity, spina bifida, multiple sclerosis, cystic fibrosis, anorexia and bulimia nervosa, and excess straining or Valsalva maneuver. A history of mental illness has been linked to

rectal prolapse, with a fourfold higher rate in that population.

Straining at stool is often associated with rectal prolapse. A history of constipation is seen in up to 67% of patients and diarrhea in 15%. Paradoxically, incontinence is reported to be present in up to 70% of patients with rectal prolapse. Women are six times more likely than men to develop rectal prolapse. There is also a different age distribution in women and men, with men presenting in their twenties and thirties while women present more commonly after the sixth decade. Most patients who require surgery for rectal prolapse are elderly.

PHYSICAL EXAMINATION

The typical patient with complete rectal prolapse will present with a history of bleeding and a "bulge" in the anal region after bowel movements. The rectum is often obvious on inspection. Occasionally, the prolapse may become evident only when asking the patient to squat or strain on a toilet. An evaluation of resting anal tone and squeeze pressures is important in the workup. Identification of other concomitant pelvic floor defects including rectocele, cystocele, vaginal prolapse, and enterocele is important and may influence the operative approach.

DIAGNOSIS AND TESTING

Patients with a history of incontinence associated with rectal prolapse should be evaluated with anal manometry, ultrasonography, and pudendal nerve terminal motor latency to document baseline anorectal anatomy and function prior to repair.[2] Plain radiographs of the sacrum are useful to identify patients with occult spina bifida. Cinedefecography can be useful to diagnose "hidden" rectal prolapse or internal intussusception for patients in whom the rectum is not visible externally. Colonoscopy is essential to rule out synchronous or causative neoplasm prior to a planned surgical repair.

Colonic transit time should be evaluated with marker studies for patients with a history of constipation and rectal prolapse. This subgroup of patients may benefit from an abdominal approach with resection, as rectopexy alone typically worsens the constipation.[3]

If a perineal approach is planned and associated urinary or uterine prolapse is seen, intravenous pylogram will help identify the course of the ureters, which may travel quite low in the pelvis. Combined repair of enterocele, cystocele, and rectal prolapse has been described.

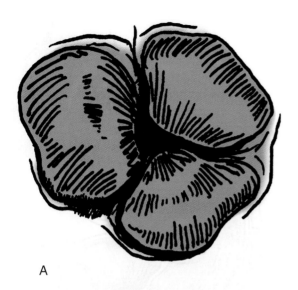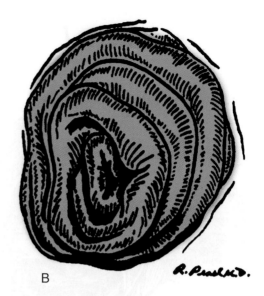

FIGURE 148-1 Prolapsing hemorrhoids **(A)** and complete rectal prolapse **(B).**

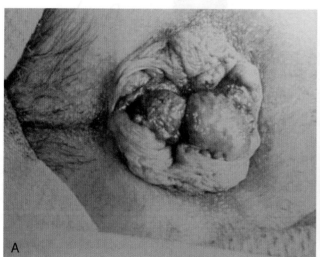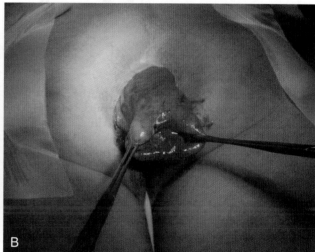

FIGURE 148-2 Prolapsing hemorrhoids **(A)** and rectal prolapse **(B).**

TREATMENT

ACUTE MANAGEMENT OF RECTAL PROLAPSE

The treatment of acute complete rectal prolapse involves early reduction. Often, especially in the mentally ill in whom persistent straining or Valsalva has contributed to the prolapse, the rectum will immediately reprolapse. Gentle constant pressure is often successful in reducing the prolapse and if the rectum continues to prolapse after reduction, taping the buttocks together may help temporarily.

If the prolapse has been neglected or unrecognized for a prolonged period, it may not easily reduce. Unless the rectum is frankly nonviable or necrotic, a few techniques may help return the bowel to its anatomic position. Sedation, placing the patient in the Trendelenburg position, and placement of salt or sugar topically can

decrease the edema of the prolapse and assist reduction.[4] Injection of hyaluronidase has also been described in the acute situation. These maneuvers can often be done at the bedside, but may need to be done in an operating room setting in certain cases, especially in uncooperative patients.

If the incarcerated rectum cannot be reduced, or if there is evidence of ischemic compromise, then operative resection, typically a perineal proctosigmoidectomy is indicated.

SURGICAL TREATMENT OF RECTAL PROLAPSE

A surgical intervention is nearly always necessary to correct rectal prolapse. The "perfect" treatment should offer safe, complete, and durable resolution of the anatomic and physiologic problems.[5] The current treatment modalities all have a recurrence rate, albeit the recurrence rate is low and decreasing. The search for the best

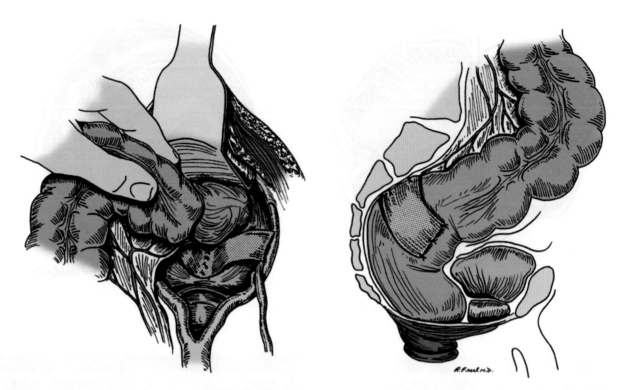

FIGURE 148-3 Rectopexy (Ripstein procedure).

surgical treatment of rectal prolapse spawned a multitude of approaches beginning in the 19th century. More than 100 different procedures or modifications have been described in the medical literature. In fact, newer innovations continue to appear in the literature.[6-10] The spectrum of current operative techniques includes both abdominal and perineal procedures. The laparoscopic approach has gained popularity, as surgeons have become comfortable operating on the colon laparoscopically.[11-15] Generally, patients who can tolerate laparotomy should be offered an abdominal approach to correct their prolapse, while elderly or debilitated patients are better managed with a perineal procedure. The exception may be young men who may prefer to accept the higher risk of recurrence of their prolapse with a perineal procedure to the increased risk of impotence or infertility with an abdominal procedure.

As is generally accepted at this time, all patients receive a mechanical bowel preparation the day prior to surgery, perioperative antibiotics, and prophylaxis against deep venous thrombosis.

Abdominal Approaches

General anesthesia is usually employed, but regional anesthesia has also been successfully used. Patients are placed in low dorsal lithotomy position for all laparoscopic or open laparotomy procedures. For laparoscopic approaches, the patients' arms are tucked at the side. Furthermore, it is important to place the patient on a torso-sized beanbag with which to cradle the body, as it will be tilted into a steep Trendelenburg position. This will help prevent the patient from sliding on the operative table.

Rectopexy. The various modifications of the technique described by Ripstein[16-22] all have in common a posterior mobilization of the rectum to the level of the coccyx. Ripstein's approach was to wrap a 5-cm-wide nonabsorbable polytetrafluoroethylene (Teflon) mesh around the anterior rectum, then suture it to the presacral fascia on the sides of the rectum 5 cm below the sacral promontory. The Well modification (Figure 148-3) places the Ivalon sponge posteriorly, leaving a 2-cm gap anteriorly to allow for rectal compliance. Successful rectopexy has been described simply using nonabsorbable suture or metal staples to fix the rectum to the sacrum and thus re-creating the normal rectal angulation. Recently it has been suggested that mobilization of the rectum itself is sufficient to produce enough fibrotic scar to fix the bowel to the sacral curvature.[19] Patients with constipation preoperatively will have worsening of their symptoms with rectopexy alone, because it results in acute angulation of the rectosigmoid by allowing the sigmoid colon to fall anteriorly into the pelvis. Speakman et al have reported that division of the lateral stalls will allow for better rectal mobilization and fixation and prevent recurrence but at a cost of worsening constipation.[21]

Resection. Anterior resection of the colon and rectum is familiar to most general, laparoscopic, and colorectal surgeons. This may partially explain the popularity of this approach. Through a low midline or transverse incision or laparoscopically, the rectum is mobilized to the level of the coccyx to produce fibrotic fixation to the sacrum upon healing. Next, the redundant sigmoid colon and rectum are resected and reanastomosed. The anastomosis should be at the level of the sacral promontory. The

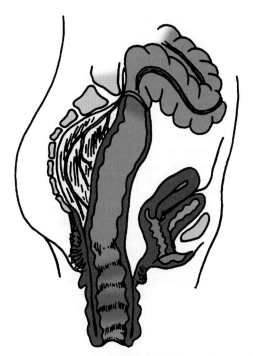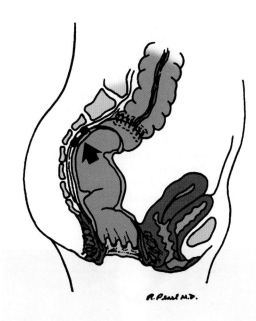

FIGURE 148-4 Sigmoid resection plus rectopexy (Fuykwan procedure).

splenic flexure should not be mobilized as lack of left upper quadrant fixation may theoretically contribute to recurrence of the prolapse. Resection procedures tend to alleviate preoperative constipation symptoms.

Resection-Rectopexy. The technique of resection plus rectopexy combines the benefits and risks of both procedures. Resection-rectopexy has the advantage of removing excess bowel and restoring the normal rectal angulation (Figure 148-4). There are reports that this approach improves symptoms of both incontinence and constipation.[23]

Laparoscopy. The laparoscopic approach to rectal prolapse has gained popularity as surgeons have obtained expertise at laparoscopic colon surgery in general and as safety concerns have abated.[12-15,24] Proponents describe a lower perioperative morbidity than open procedures.[15] The key steps of the operation should be comparable to the open technique.

Randomized, controlled trials by Solomon et al[14,15,25] comparing laparoscopic and open rectopexy showed both a lower cost and improved clinical outcome with the laparoscopic technique. The low recurrence and lack of deterioration of functional outcome were durable with long-term followup.[25] A recent metaanalysis of published studies comparing the two surgical modalities showed no difference in morbidity, mortality, or functional results, though an earlier Cochrane Review showed fewer complications with laparoscopic rectopexy compared to open rectopexy.[26,27]

Larger randomized studies are awaited to investigate and compare the outcomes of the different techniques for the treatment of rectal prolapse. Laparoscopic resection and resection-rectopexy can be performed with or without hand assistance. The resected colon can be removed from the abdomen either through a hand port or through an extension of a port incision.

Perineal Approaches

Many general surgeons shy away from perineal approaches to complete rectal prolapse because of a lack of training in and understanding of the anorectal anatomy and physiology. Nevertheless, many patients will not tolerate laparotomy or laparoscopy. These patients are better served with the approach of perineal proctosigmoidectomy (Altemeier), anorectal mucosectomy with muscular plication (Delorme procedure), or anal encirclement (Thiersch). Furthermore, recurrence rates in some series approach those described in abdominal treatments of rectal prolapse. Given that most patients with rectal prolapse are elderly women (many with multiple comorbidities) and young men (who may fear the risk of sexual dysfunction with injury of the hypogastric nerves and nervi erigentes during an abdominal approach), some argue that perineal procedures are the preferred operations for most patients with procidentia.

The various perineal procedures can be performed either in the lithotomy position, or preferably in the prone jack-knife position. Regional anesthesia is typically used, but some patients may require general anesthesia. A self-retaining–type retractor (e.g., Lone Star) helps with exposure (Figure 148-5).

Perineal Proctosigmoidectomy. Altemeier popularized the technique of resecting the prolapsed bowel directly.[28,29] The Prasad modification is the only surgical approach to correct each of the anatomic defects associated with rectal prolapse.[28] The first step is to completely prolapse the redundant rectum by gently pulling on the rectal wall. The dentate line will be easily visible on the everted rectum (see Figure 148-5). A dilute epinephrine solution is injected 1 to 2 cm proximal to the dentate line in the prolapsed rectal wall. Next, the rectal wall is incised full thickness, circumferentially, with electrocautery at the level of the injection. The vascular supply to the prolapsed rectum and sigmoid is then carefully ligated. Nonabsorbable suture is used to fix the nonprolapsing bowel to the presacrococcygeal fascia reproducing the normal posterior fixation of the rectum. The widely open pelvic floor is closed with a posterior levatorplasty. This recreates the normal anorectal angulation. The excess bowel is resected and a coloanal anastomosis is performed. The anastomosis can be hand-sewn with absorbable suture or stapled by any of a number of stapling techniques.

Anorectal Mucosectomy With Muscular Plication (Delorme). The Delorme procedure first described in 1900 continues to be employed in selected situations. The advantage of the procedure is that no bowel resection and anastomosis are needed.[10,30,31]

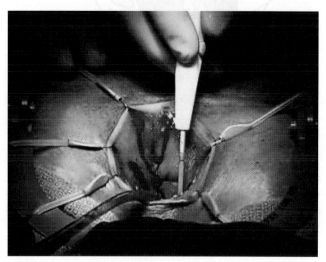

FIGURE 148-5 Lone Star retractor and incision for Delorme or perineal proctectomy.

Once the bowel is completely prolapsed, a dilute epinephrine solution is injected in the submucosal plane (Figure 148-6). The mucosa is circumferentially incised 1 cm proximal to the dentate line with electrocautery. The incision is deepened only to the level of the submucosa. The muscular layers are left intact. The mucosa is then stripped off the rectal wall musculature, continuing proximally to the apex of the redundant bowel (Figure 148-7). The mucosal sleeve is then excised. Longitudinal plicating sutures are placed along the length of the rectal wall musculature approximately 1 cm apart. The sutures are tied once all six to eight rows have been placed. Next, the proximal mucosal edge is resutured to the initial mucosal incision with absorbable sutures.

A modification utilizing a double purse-string suture and a circular stapler has been described.[7] The Delorme procedure can be combined with posterior levatorplasty[10] in an attempt to improve continence (Figure 148-8).

Anal Encirclement (Thiersch). Some surgeons have stated that anal encirclement[32,33] is a procedure that should be relegated to historical interest only. However, for the bedridden patient with short life expectancy, multiple comorbidities, and possible dementia or Alzheimer disease and those who may not tolerate even a perineal resection of rectal prolapse, the Thiersch technique can still be useful. It may also have a place after failure of the perineal procedures. This simple procedure can be performed quickly, with very low morbidity.

Two perianal skin incisions 180 degrees apart and lateral to the midline are made. The incisions are connected with a tunnel through the ischiorectal fossa. A strip of polypropylene mesh 1.5 cm wide is placed around the deep external sphincter. The mesh is passed around the anus from one incision to the second and then back to the first to completely encircle the anus (Figure 148-9). The mesh is tightened and sutured to

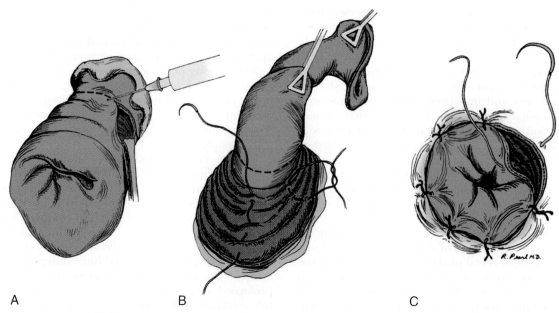

A   B   C

FIGURE 148-6 A to **C,** Anorectal mucosectomy and plication (Delorme procedure).

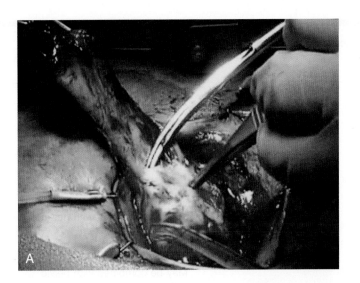

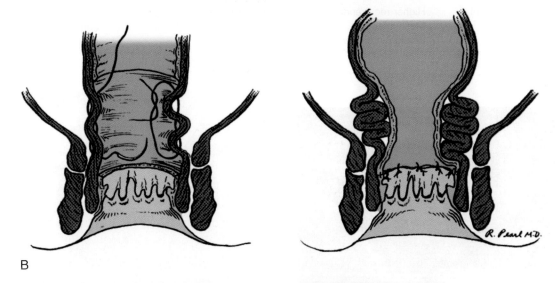

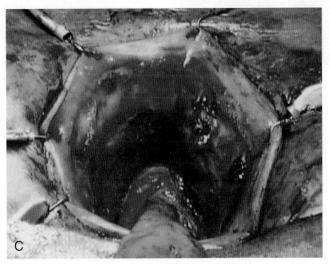

FIGURE 148-7 The Delorme procedure. Mucosal stripping **(A)**, illustration of muscular plication and mucosal anastomosis **(B)**, and after mucosal stripping and prior to plication **(C)**.

TABLE 148-1 Common Procedures for Rectal Prolapse

Procedure	Major Risks	Major Benefits	Best for
Rectopexy	Higher operative risk Presacral bleeding Pelvic abscess	Lower recurrence rate	Young, healthy patient without redundant sigmoid or constipation
Resection-rectopexy	Higher operative risk Anastomotic leak Presacral bleeding Pelvic abscess	Lower recurrence Correction of constipation	Young, healthy patient with redundant sigmoid and constipation
Perineal Proctosigmoidectomy and levatorplasty (Altmeier)	Higher recurrence Technique unfamiliar to many surgeons	Lower operative risk Correction of incontinence May be combined with pelvic floor reconstruction	Older patient with comorbidities and long-segment rectal prolapse
Rectal mucosectomy with muscular plication (Delorme)	Higher recurrence Technique unfamiliar	Lower operative risk Correction of incontinence May be combined with pelvic floor reconstruction	Older patient with comorbidities and short-segment rectal prolapse
Anal encirclement (Thiersch)	Higher recurrence Mesh infection Erosion into bowel	Lower operative risk	Elderly patient with comorbidities and short life expectancy

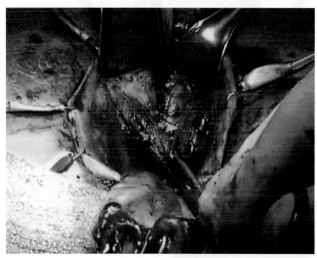

FIGURE 148-8 Delorme procedure combined with posterior levatorplasty.

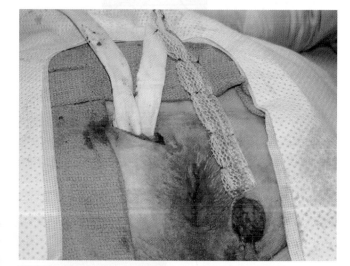

FIGURE 148-9 Thiersch encirclement. Note the two incisions 180 degrees apart and the already placed Penrose drain encircling the anus that will be used to pull the mesh around.

itself allowing an anal diameter only large enough to admit one finger in the anus. The risks of the procedure include erosion of the mesh into the rectum, infection of the mesh, recurrence of the prolapse, and impaction secondary to tight encirclement.

RESULTS AND PATIENT SELECTION

Proponents of abdominal rectopexy in its various forms claim lower recurrence rates (0% to 5%) than perineal procedures (10% to 15%). Surgeons with a preference for perineal proctosigmoidectomy and Delorme procedure point to their relative safety and ease of reoperation in the event of recurrence. Most likely, each clinical situation will favor one approach from the other

(Table 148-1). As such, proficiency in each approach is necessary.

Caution must be employed if a perineal approach is contemplated for recurrent rectal prolapse previously treated with an abdominal resection or, alternatively, if an abdominal resection is planned after a perineal resection. Unless the prior anastomotic line is resected there is a risk of ischemia, and necrosis of the intervening bowel between the two anastomoses can occur.[34]

RECURRENT RECTAL PROLAPSE

There are very few reports specifically addressing recurrent rectal prolapse. Most are single institution retrospective studies with relatively few patients and short followup.

Recurrent rectal prolapse has been reported to range from 0% to 60%[35,36] but is more commonly seen between 10% and 20% of patients after a mean time of 3 years.[37] In general, abdominal procedures (rectopexy/resection-rectopexy) have a lower recurrence rate compared with perineal procedures (Delorme, Altemeier, anal encirclement). Early recurrences (within 1 year) are often due to technical factors. Many of the early recurrences after abdominal procedures were due to failure of mesh fixation in the Ripstein operation, a procedure that is now seldom used in the United States. Failure to adequately re-create the anorectal angle during levatorplasty, improper suture rectopexy, and incomplete removal of the redundant sigmoid are the technical reasons for recurrence after perineal proctosigmoidectomy. Age alone is unrelated to recurrence, though as mentioned earlier, it is a factor in the decision algorithm (see Table 148-1).

Surgery for primary prolapse or recurrent rectal prolapse is performed using similar techniques. In a case-matched study of 27 patients with recurrent and primary rectal prolapse, Pikarsky et al found no difference in morbidity, hospital stay, and recurrence rate (15% vs. 11%). Perineal proctosigmoidectomy (14/27) and resection-rectopexy (8/27) were the most common procedures performed in the recurrent group.[35]

In a retrospective study of 78 patients with recurrent rectal prolapse with a mean followup of 9 months, Steele et al found more re-recurrences (19/51) after redo perineal proctosigmoidectomy compared with a repeat abdominal procedure (4/27).[37]

The choice of procedure depends on the degree of prolapse, comorbid factors, type of previous operation, bowel function, and surgeon experience. Younger patients with full-thickness prolapse are preferably treated with abdominal rectopexy. Constipation patients do better after resection-rectopexy. Older patients with multiple comorbidities are best treated with perineal proctosigmoidectomy with levatorplasty (large or complete full-thickness prolapse) or Delorme procedure (mucosal or small full-thickness prolapse). Anal encirclement is reserved for the moribund patient.

It is of utmost importance to remember that a patient who is treated with perineal proctectomy after failed anterior resection or, alternately, anterior resection after failed perineal proctectomy will develop ischemia and sloughing of the intervening rectum between the two anastomoses unless the previous anastomosis is resected or the superior hemorrhoidal artery was preserved during the abdominal procedure.[34]

Laparoscopic repair of recurrent rectal prolapse has been reported but should only be considered by the expert surgeon.[38]

ROBOTIC RECTOPEXY

Robotic surgery is gaining in popularity in many surgical specialties, especially urology, gynecology, and colon and rectal surgery. Compared with laparoscopy, the advantages of three-dimensional imaging, camera and instrument stability, ergonomic positioning of the operating surgeon, and wrist-like movement of the robotic instruments allow for ease of dissection and suturing in the pelvis.

A few small case series of robotic-assisted rectopexy have been published. Despite the superior technology of the robot, no advantage has been shown over open or laparoscopic surgery for rectal prolapse. The operating time and cost are increased with the robotic approach.[39] Additionally, one small study showed a higher recurrence after robotic rectopexy compared with open and laparoscopic procedure.[40]

Robotic surgery for rectal prolapse has not shown added benefit at this time though an improvement in instrumentation, technology, and expertise may change this opinion.

REFERENCES

1. Madiba TE, Baig MK, Wexner SD: Surgical management of rectal prolapse. *Arch Surg* 140:63, 2005.
2. Dvorkin LS, Chan CL, Knowles CH, et al: Anal sphincter morphology in patients with full-thickness rectal prolapse. *Dis Colon Rectum* 47:198, 2004.
3. Eu KW, Seow-Choen F: Functional problems in adult rectal prolapse and controversies in surgical treatment. *Br J Surg* 84:904, 1997.
4. Coburn WM 3rd, Russell MA, Hofstetter WL: Sucrose as an aid to manual reduction of incarcerated rectal prolapse. *Ann Emerg Med* 30:347, 1997.
5. Azimuddin K, Khubchandani IT, Rosen L, et al: Rectal prolapse: A search for the "best" operation. *Am Surg* 67:622, 2001.
6. Hayashi S, Masuda H, Hayashi I, et al: Simple technique for repair of complete rectal prolapse using a circular stapler with Thiersch procedure. *Eur J Surg* 168:124, 2002.
7. Schutz G: Extracorporal resection of the rectum in the treatment of complete rectal prolapse using a circular stapling device. *Dig Surg* 28:274; discussion 277, 2001.
8. Yamana T, Iwadare J: Mucosal plication (Gant-Miwa procedure) with anal encircling for rectal prolapse—a review of the Japanese experience. *Dis Colon Rectum* 46:S94, 2003.
9. Solomon MJ, Eyers AA: Laparoscopic rectopexy using mesh fixation with a spiked chromium staple. *Dis Colon Rectum* 39:279, 1996.
10. Lechaux JP, Lechaux D, Perez M: Results of Delorme's procedure for rectal prolapse. Advantages of a modified technique. *Dis Colon Rectum* 38:301, 1995.
11. Boccasanta P, Venturi M, Reitano MC, et al: Laparotomic vs. laparoscopic rectopexy in complete rectal prolapse. *Dig Surg* 16:415, 1999.
12. Bruch HP, Herold A, Schiedeck T, et al: Laparoscopic surgery for rectal prolapse and outlet obstruction. *Dis Colon Rectum* 42:1189; discussion 1194, 1999.
13. Madbouly KM, Senagore AJ, Delaney CP, et al: Clinically based management of rectal prolapse. *Surg Endosc* 17:99, 2003.
14. Salkeld G, Bagia M, Solomon M: Economic impact of laparoscopic versus open abdominal rectopexy. *Br J Surg* 91:1188, 2004.
15. Solomon MJ, Young CJ, Eyers AA, et al: Randomized clinical trial of laparoscopic versus open abdominal rectopexy for rectal prolapse. *Br J Surg* 89:35, 2002.
16. Duthie GS, Bartolo DC: Abdominal rectopexy for rectal prolapse: A comparison of techniques. *Br J Surg* 79:107, 1992.
17. Loygue J, Nordlinger B, Cunci O, et al: Rectopexy to the promontory for the treatment of rectal prolapse. Report of 257 cases. *Dis Colon Rectum* 27:356, 1984.
18. Madden MV, Kamm MA, Nicholls RJ, et al: Abdominal rectopexy for complete prolapse: Prospective study evaluating changes in symptoms and anorectal function. *Dis Colon Rectum* 35:48, 1992.
19. Nelson R, Spitz J, Pearl RK, et al: What role does full rectal mobilization alone play in the treatment of rectal prolapse? *Tech Coloproctol* 5:33, 2001.
20. McCue JL, Thomson JP: Clinical and functional results of abdominal rectopexy for complete rectal prolapse. *Br J Surg* 78:921, 1991.
21. Speakman CT, Madden MV, Nicholls RJ, et al: Lateral ligament division during rectopexy causes constipation but prevents

recurrence: Results of a prospective randomized study. *Br J Surg* 78:1431, 1991.

22. Yoshioka K, Heyen F, Keighley MR: Functional results after posterior abdominal rectopexy for rectal prolapse. *Dis Colon Rectum* 32:835, 1989.

23. Madoff RD, Williams JG, Wong WD, et al: Long-term functional results of colon resection and rectopexy for overt rectal prolapse. *Am J Gastroenterol* 87:101, 1992.

24. Boccasanta P, Rosati R, Venturi M, et al: Comparison of laparoscopic rectopexy with open technique in the treatment of complete rectal prolapse: Clinical and functional results. *Surg Laparosc Endosc* 8:460, 1998.

25. Byrne CM, Smith SR, Solomon MJ, et al: Long-term functional outcomes after laparoscopic and open rectopexy for the treatment of rectal prolapse. *Dis Colon Rectum* 51:1597, 2008.

26. Sajid M, Siddiqui M, Baig M: Open versus laparoscopic repair of full thickness rectal prolapse: A re-meta-analysis. *Colorectal Dis* 2009 Apr 13 [Epub ahead of print].

27. Tou S, Brown SR, Malik AI, et al: Surgery for complete rectal prolapse in adults. *Cochrane Database Syst Rev* CD001758, 2008.

28. Prasad ML, Pearl RK, Abcarian H, et al: Perineal proctectomy, posterior rectopexy, and postanal levator repair for the treatment of rectal prolapse. *Dis Colon Rectum* 29:547, 1986.

29. Kimmins MH, Evetts BK, Isler J, et al: The Altemeier repair: Outpatient treatment of rectal prolapse. *Dis Colon Rectum* 44:565, 2001.

30. Oliver GC, Vachon D, Eisenstat TE, et al: Delorme's procedure for complete rectal prolapse in severely debilitated patients. An analysis of 41 cases. *Dis Colon Rectum* 37:461, 1994.

31. Tsunoda A, Yasuda N, Yokoyama N, et al: Delorme's procedure for rectal prolapse: Clinical and physiological analysis. *Dis Colon Rectum* 46:1260, 2003.

32. Poole GV Jr, Pennell TC, Myers RT, et al: Modified Thiersch operation for rectal prolapse. Technique and results. *Am Surg* 51:226, 1985.

33. Sainio AP, Halme LE, Husa AI: Anal encirclement with polypropylene mesh for rectal prolapse and incontinence. *Dis Colon Rectum* 34:905, 1991.

34. Fengler SA, Pearl RK, Prasad ML, et al: Management of recurrent rectal prolapse. *Dis Colon Rectum* 40:832, 1997.

35. Pikarsky AJ, Joo JS, Wexner SD, et al: Recurrent rectal prolapse: What is the next good option? *Dis Colon Rectum* 43:1273, 2000.

36. Hool GR, Hull TL, Fazio VW: Surgical treatment of recurrent complete rectal prolapse: A thirty-year experience. *Dis Colon Rectum* 40:270, 1997.

37. Steele SR, Goetz LH, Minami S, et al: Management of recurrent rectal prolapse: Surgical approach influences outcome. *Dis Colon Rectum* 49:440, 2006.

38. Tsugawa K, Sue K, Koyanagi N, et al: Laparoscopic rectopexy for recurrent rectal prolapse: A safe and simple procedure without a mesh prosthesis. *Hepato-gastroenterology* 49:1549, 2002.

39. Heemskerk J, de Hoog DE, van Gemert WG, et al: Robot-assisted vs. conventional laparoscopic rectopexy for rectal prolapse: A comparative study on costs and time. *Dis Colon Rectum* 50:1825, 2007.

40. de Hoog DE, Heemskerk J, Nieman FH, et al: Recurrence and functional results after open versus conventional laparoscopic versus robot-assisted laparoscopic rectopexy for rectal prolapse: A case-control study. *Int J Colorectal Dis* 24:1201, 2009.

Pilonidal Disease

Debra H. Ford | H. Randolph Bailey

Pilonidal disease (PD) is a common condition that affects many patients. In the United States, approximately 70,000 patients are diagnosed with this chronic disease yearly. Since its first description in the early 1800s,[1,2] pilonidal disease and its treatment have been the subject of debate and controversy. It is believed to be an acquired infectious process leading to high rates of morbidity. This condition often results in discomfort and inconvenience. Patients are often prevented from working or attending school for extended periods. Although pilonidal disease has been described in other parts of the body, such as the hands, umbilicus, axillae, and external genitalia,[3] this discussion focuses on the disease as it affects the gluteal cleft or sacrococcygeal region.

Sacrococcygeal pilonidal disease occurs predominantly in young males at a ratio of 3:1.[4,5] The estimated incidence is 26 cases per 100,000 people.[5] The peak incidence is between 15 and 24 years of age. Symptoms rarely present before 15 years of age or after the age of 40.[3] The disease is most common in whites; however, all ethnic groups may develop the condition.[6] Other factors associated with the development of pilonidal disease are obesity, increased sweating activity, and local trauma.[7]

ETIOLOGY

The term *pilonidal* is derived from the Latin words for hair (pilas) and nest (nidus).[7] The pathogenesis of pilonidal disease has been the subject of debate. Approaches to the treatment of pilonidal disease have closely paralleled the theories of its development. For many years, the cause of pilonidal disease was thought to be congenital. However, the current prevailing explanation is that of an acquired condition caused by hair invading the skin at the natal cleft.[7] Although true pilonidal cysts have been reported, such cysts are quite rare. The majority of surgeons treat the disease as an acquired condition. Patey and Scarff,[6] with additional evidence from Bascom,[8] have provided a plausible explanation in support of the acquired theory.

The *acquired theory* emphasizes the role that hair plays in the development of pilonidal disease. Bascom's histologic studies demonstrate a sequence of stages in the development of this condition (Figure 149-1).[8] He describes a folliculitis that leads to the development of small subdermal abscesses that increase in size to form a larger abscess cavity. He also explains that hair is drawn into the pilonidal cavity through the suction effect of gluteal movement. Other factors believed to contribute to the creation of pilonidal disease are related to the condition of the gluteal cleft, including a catch basin effect, an anaerobic environment in the cleft, the depth of the gluteal cleft, and gluteal cleft friction.[8]

Over the years, because of confusion as to the etiology of pilonidal disease, surgeons have approached this condition in various ways, from the most conservative treatments to extensive resectional and plastic surgical procedures.

PATHOLOGY

Pilonidal disease is essentially a foreign-body reaction. Histopathology demonstrates foreign-body giant cells associated with hair shafts within a background of chronic granulation tissue lining the abscess cavities and sinus tracts.[7] Midline pits are lined with squamous epithelium. Although 1% of the tracts associated with these pits may be completely lined with squamous epithelium, most are lined with only granulation tissue.[3] Because the tract is not lined with epithelium, it should correctly be referred to as a sinus, not a cyst. Hair, in the form of broken hair shafts, is found in the cavities at least 50% of the time (Figure 149-2). Typical pilonidal cavities do not contain epidermis, sweat glands, or hair follicles. The tracts usually extend cephalad and lateral from the midline pits. Pilonidal tracts have, however, been described as extending toward the anus and being misdiagnosed as fistula-in-ano in as many as 7% of cases.[3]

CLINICAL PRESENTATION

The prevalence of pilonidal disease is not known. However, patients most commonly are in their mid- to late 20s and have symptoms for 4 to 5 years at initial presentation. PD is a common condition that can present in one of three ways: acute abscess, sinus tract, or complex disease with chronic recurring abscesses and extensive branching sinus tracts.[7] Patients may present to the surgeon with findings of asymptomatic small midline pits in the gluteal cleft (which may contain hair) or as an obvious, painful abscess (Figure 149-3). After surgical or spontaneous drainage, chronic PD may result. The presentation that is most distressing and challenging for the surgeon is recurrent disease or an unhealed wound after prior surgical treatment.

The patient with a pilonidal abscess typically presents with a history of increasing pain and the eventual development of a tender fluctuant mass in the sacrococcygeal area, often situated slightly off the midline and cephalad to the midline pits. Cellulitis of the surrounding skin, as well as fever and leukocytosis, is occasionally present. An acute abscess is the presenting finding in approximately 50% of patients with pilonidal disease.[3] A chronic sinus tract may develop after the abscess cavity resolves. These

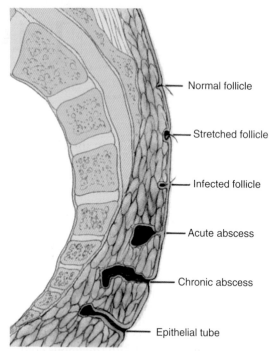

FIGURE 149-1 Pathogenesis of pilonidal abscess and sinus. (From Bascom J: Pilonidal disease: Origin from follicles of hairs and results of follicle removal as treatment. *Surgery* 87:567, 1980; redrawn from Nivatvongs S: Pilonidal disease. In Gordon PH, Nivatvongs S, editors: *Principles and practice of surgery for the colon, rectum, and anus,* ed 2, St. Louis, 1999, Quality Medical, p 288.)

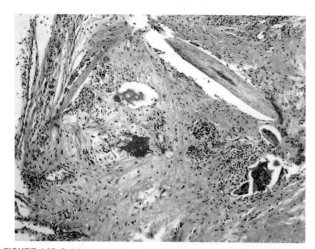

FIGURE 149-2 Histopathology: hair follicle with foreign-body giant cell reaction in a pilonidal cyst.

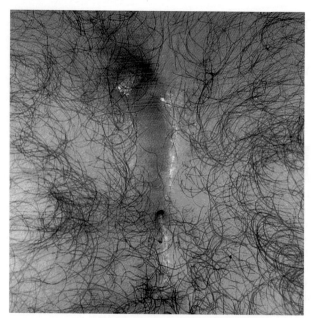

FIGURE 149-3 Sacrococcygeal pilonidal abscess and midline pit.

BOX 149-1 Differential Diagnosis for Pilonidal Disease

Furuncle
Hidradenitis suppurativa
Fistula-in-ano
Perianal abscess
Crohn disease
Sacral osteomyelitis with draining sinus
Syphilis
Actinomycosis

---

chronic sinus tracts may be branching. Most patients with chronic pilonidal disease have pain, intermittent discharge, or both. They may present with recurrent bouts of infection. On physical examination, there may be evidence of past drainage with or without cellulitis and induration. The midline pit or pits are usually present, and hair may be seen protruding from the orifice. These pits are usually located 4 to 8 cm from the anus.[5] The differential diagnosis of sacrococcygeal pilonidal disease includes furuncle, hidradenitis suppurativa, fistula-in-ano, perianal abscess, sacral osteomyelitis with draining sinus, syphilis, tuberculosis, and actinomycosis (Box 149-1).

TREATMENT

Surgical management of pilonidal disease depends on the clinical presentation (Table 149-1). Treatment options range from nonoperative modalities, simple incision and drainage of abscesses, to wide excision with extensive reconstructive procedures for complex disease. Many operations have been proposed for the definitive management of pilonidal disease. These treatment options have paralleled the theories of pilonidal development. During the period when widespread acceptance of the congenital theory prevailed, procedures were described that completely removed all tissue down to the sacral fascia.[9] These operations were done under general anesthesia and resulted in lengthy inpatient hospitalization. These aggressive operations produced large wounds that in many instances failed to heal properly and were the source of prolonged disability and discomfort.

Acceptance of the acquired theory has led to a "less is best" approach.[4,6] Current emphasis is placed on the elimination of factors that favor pilonidal development.

TABLE 149-1 Pilonidal Disease: Treatment Options

Medical Treatment	Surgical Treatment
Shaving	Incision and drainage alone
Laser depilation	Midline follicle excision and lateral drainage
Phenol injection	Incision and drainage with marsupialization
Fibrin glue injection	Excision with or without primary closure
Antibiotics	Excision with plastic surgical flap closures

In caring for patients with PD, the surgeon should strive for complete wound healing with minimal patient disability, a low recurrence rate, and early return to activities of daily living. Contemporary management of pilonidal disease is frequently performed in an ambulatory setting.

ACUTE PILONIDAL ABSCESS

An acute pilonidal abscess usually presents as a painful fluctuant mass located in the midline or lateral to the midline at the intergluteal cleft. Immediate incision and drainage provide prompt relief of symptoms. Although anaerobic and aerobic bacteria have been cultured from these abscess cavities, antibiotics are not required in the management of most cases of pilonidal abscess.[10] Drainage may be performed in the emergency department or in the office using local anesthesia. A large abscess may require drainage in the operating room using intravenous sedation or general anesthesia. Because the abscess and the surrounding edema often obscure the midline sinus (the source of the abscess), performing a definitive procedure may need to be delayed until the edema subsides.

Technique of Drainage

Essentially all operations for pilonidal disease are best performed in the prone jack-knife position with the buttocks taped apart for better exposure. After preparation of the skin and infiltration with local anesthesia containing epinephrine, the hair of the gluteal area is clipped and a cruciate lateral or midline incision is made over the abscess cavity that is large enough to allow for adequate drainage. Bascom favors a linear incision off the midline.[11] All debris and hair should be removed from the cavity if possible. Electrocautery usually suffices for hemostasis. On occasion, temporary light packing may be required. The patient is instructed to take warm tub baths at least twice daily and to return weekly for wound care and hair removal. After simple incision and drainage, healing may take as long as 4 to 10 weeks.[3]

Of the patients who have simple incision and drainage, approximately 40% to 60% will heal without further need for intervention.[12] Several reports have favored immediate unroofing of tracts during the initial drainage of the pilonidal abscess.[3,13] If the midline pits can be identified, a probe is inserted through the orifice into the cavity. The abscess cavity and associated tracts are unroofed with cautery. The cavity is debrided, and wound edges are loosely packed apart to facilitate drainage and healing of the wound. Hair remaining in an inadequately drained abscess cavity is the major factor for persistence or recurrence of the abscess. The hair surrounding the edges of the wound should be shaved or clipped.[4] Laser depilation has been described as a useful adjunct to management of pilonidal disease after unroofing of tracts. Laser removal of hair has also been described as a definitive nonoperative treatment. There are, however, no randomized controlled trials to support this treatment approach.[14]

CHRONIC PILONIDAL DISEASE

The progression to chronic pilonidal disease is expected in 40% to 60% of patients after incision and drainage.[3,5,15] In addition, 10% to 15% of patients with chronic pilonidal disease will have a recurrence of symptoms after healing. Because of this high rate of continued or recurrent disease, Bascom[8,11] has suggested that incision and drainage be followed by a definitive surgical procedure.

As mentioned previously, the midline pits, which are the origin of pilonidal disease, lead into a cavity lined with granulation tissue. The removal of all involved tissue is unnecessary. There is no clear consensus as to the preferred definitive treatment; however, acceptance of the acquired theory of origin has led to more operations with a minimalist approach and a strong emphasis on meticulous postoperative wound care. The treatment options usually fit into one of the following categories: conservative, nonresectional approach[9]; midline follicle excision and lateral drainage[2,11,16]; incision and curettage with minimal excision followed by marsupialization or saucerization of the wound[5,9,17]; and excision with or without primary closure.[18]

It is desirable to select an approach that can be carried out in an ambulatory setting with minimal patient inconvenience and disability. The role of antibiotics is not clear; there have been reports that have suggested antibiotics directed at anaerobic bacteria may improve healing rates.[10]

Conservative, Nonresectional Approach

The treatment for pilonidal sinus depends on the complexity of the pilonidal sinus or sinuses. The treatment can be nonoperative or operative. Armstrong and Barcia[9] advocated nonexcisional therapy consisting of meticulous hair control by shaving, good perineal hygiene, and limited lateral incision and drainage of abscesses. There have been reports describing the instillation of liquid or crystalline phenol into the pits.[5,19] Healing rates have been reported from 59% to 95% in an average of 40 days.[19,20] The injection is followed by hair control and strict hygiene. The use of phenol causes an intense inflammatory reaction that destroys the lining. This method can be painful and may require hospitalization for pain control. Fibrin glue has also been used as an adjunct in the treatment of chronic or recurrent sinuses.[21,22] Laser depilation of the natal cleft is now commonly available. Odili et al[23] have reported 14 patients with recurrent pilonidal disease, all of whom were successfully healed by laser hair removal.

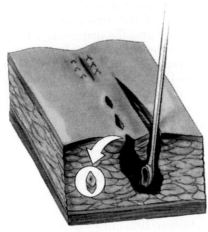

FIGURE 149-4 Treatment of pilonidal abscess by lateral incision into the abscess with curetting of granulation tissues and excision of midline pits. (From Bascom J: Pilonidal disease: Origin from follicles of hairs and results of follicle removal as treatment. *Surgery* 87:567, 1980; redrawn from Nivatvongs S: Pilonidal disease. In Gordon PH, Nivatvongs S, editors: *Principles and practice of surgery for the colon, rectum, and anus,* ed 2, St. Louis, 1999, Quality Medical, p 293.)

Technique of Midline Follicle Excision and Lateral Drainage

Although midline follicle excision and lateral drainage has been popularized by Bascom,[8] a similar technique was originally described by Lord and Millar in 1965.[2,16,24,25] The patient is reexamined in an outpatient setting approximately 5 days after drainage of the abscess when the edema and induration from the abscess have subsided. After the patient's gluteal cleft region is infiltrated with local anesthesia and shaved, a long, laterally placed incision is made over the previously drained cavity. The cavity is wiped clean with gauze or curetted and left open. The midline epithelium-lined pits are excised, leaving small wounds. These midline wounds are primarily closed with fine suture material (Figure 149-4). The patient is instructed to keep the wound clean and to return for weekly visits for shaving and debridement, if necessary, until the wound has healed. Bascom[11] reported a 15% recurrence rate with minimal disability and healing within 3 weeks. However, other surgeons have had mixed success with this approach.[26]

Technique of Incision and Curettage With Marsupialization or Saucerization

The technique of incision and curettage with marsupialization or saucerization is simply the laying open of tracts with minimal excision followed by either marsupialization or saucerization of the wound edges.[14,27-29] This is an approach favored by many surgeons. The patient is prepared in the ambulatory setting. Local anesthesia with or without intravenous sedation is appropriate; rarely is general anesthesia needed. A probe is introduced into the midline pit or pits, and all primary and secondary tracts are opened (Figure 149-5, *A*). Some surgeons instill methylene blue into the sinus opening prior to laying open tracts to better outline all involved areas. There is

some evidence in the literature that this may decrease the long-term risk of recurrence,[30] but the staining of the tissues may also obscure some small tracts. The resulting small open cavity is cleared of debris and hair, usually with a curette. The wound edges are beveled or saucerized to create a skin-level opening that is larger than the base of the cavity (Figure 149-5, *B*). The edges and base of the cavity are not disturbed except for the curettage. This allows for adequate drainage and prevents premature healing of the edges of the wound. Marsupialization involves a similar technique, except that the skin edge is not saucerized but rather sutured to the lateral wall of the cavity. Recurrence rates with this procedure have ranged from 1% to 19%, with healing time averaging 34 days.[4,31] It has been the authors' experience that suturing the skin edges to the wound does not consistently result in primary healing. Patients also seem to complain of more pain after marsupialization than after saucerization.

Technique of Excision With or Without Closure

Surgical procedures that involve the radical bloc excision of the pilonidal cavity with primary closure or secondary healing of the wound are, unfortunately, still performed frequently.[32] Because pilonidal disease does not involve a true cyst, there is little justification for removal of the entire cavity. Wide excision of all affected pilonidal tissue down to the sacral fascia is unnecessary for treatment of this disease and has resulted in a high rate of unhealed wounds and prolonged morbidity (Figure 149-6). In the extremely rare case where the chronic cavity may be lined with epithelium, the entire cavity may have to be excised.

It is difficult to interpret the literature with regard to recurrence rates after such excision. The extent of excision is usually unclear. In those situations where wide excision down to the sacral fascia with primary closure is performed, recurrence rates have been reported as high as 38%.[18] Reports have suggested that limited excision encompassing only the involved cavity followed by primary closure is a reasonable option for definitive treatment.[18,33,34] Primary healing is reported to occur within 2 weeks in 90% of cases.[3] Recurrence rates of 2% to 20% have been reported.[18] Failure of healing after primary closure is about 12%, and the incidence of wound infection varies among reports.[4,8] Evidence supports poor healing after primary closure in patients who are smokers and in patients who are obese.[35] As mentioned, total excision is usually not required to control chronic pilonidal disease. Although the concept of excision and primary closure is appealing and parallels the approaches that surgeons take to most other problems, the high rate of recurrence and the significant pain experienced because of the sutures make this approach low on the list of desirable treatment choices.

Postoperative wound care after either wide excision or unroofing and saucerization requires diligent attention to gluteal hygiene to reduce the incidence of secondary hair (i.e., scalp hair) from invading the healing wound. Local hair is shaved at weekly office visits. The patient is instructed to take warm tub baths twice a day. Dry gauze or wet-to-dry dressings are used to prevent premature

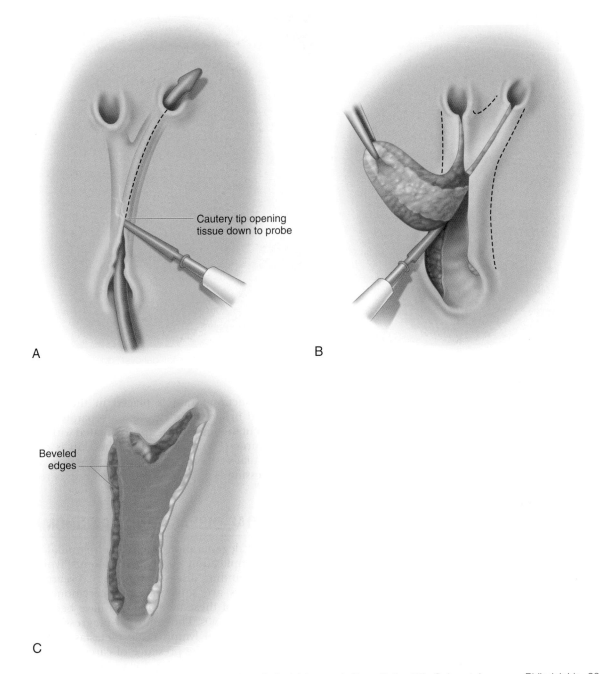

A

B

C

FIGURE 149-5 Technique of unroofing and saucerization of pilonidal wound. (From Bailey HR: *Colorectal surgery*. Philadelphia, 2012, Elsevier.)

healing and to minimize granulation tissue in the open wound. The use of a Water-Pik[36] or hand-held shower-head will aid in debriding the cavity. It is well documented that without careful follow-up even the best operation will have a poor result.

Recently, negative pressure (vacuum) dressings, which promote granulation, have been suggested as an alternative to open packing.[37,38] Negative pressure has beneficial effects on wounds. It has been shown to increase local blood flow, upregulate cell proliferation, decrease bacterial count, and facilitate wound granulation.[39] Following excision of the pilonidal disease, the vacuum dressing is applied. It has the advantage of decreasing the incidence

of primary failure or infection while promoting accelerated healing and decreasing the frequency of dressing changes.[37,38] This approach, however, is typically not necessary when a "minimal" excision is performed.

RECURRENT OR UNHEALED PILONIDAL DISEASE

Complex pilonidal disease includes patients with chronic draining sinuses, multiple recurrences, and nonhealing wounds. Recurrence rates following primary surgical treatment of pilonidal sinuses range from 3% to 40%.[4] Most recurrences respond to reoperation using one of the earlier-mentioned techniques. The patient with the unhealed chronic wound after multiple attempts at

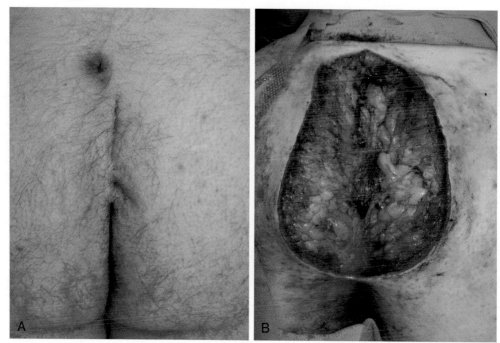

FIGURE 149-6 Recurrent pilonidal sinus shown in **A** and large wound created by excision of the "pilonidal cyst" down to the sacral fascia **(B)**.

eradication of disease usually presents with significant tissue loss. These situations are probably best treated by excision, debridement, and closure with myocutaneous or cutaneous flaps.[11,40-42] Many procedures have been described, including Z-plasty,[43] V-Y fasciocutaneous flap,[43,44] rhomboid excision and Limberg flaps,[43-45] gluteal myocutaneous flaps,[43] advancement flaps[46] (Karydakis operation),[46] and the cleft lift (closure) procedure (Figure 149-7).[47-49] These procedures have a recurrence rate in the range of 2% to 11%. However, these flap procedures carry significant morbidity and often require hospitalization. They should be reserved for highly complex pilonidal disease.

Technique of Cleft Lift

The cleft lift or closure operation as described by Bascom takes into account the problems of a healing wound in the midline with its associated negative factors, such as a deep cleft in an anaerobic environment. Therefore, the goal of the cleft closure technique is to place the final incision lateral to the midline and to flatten the gluteal cleft. The cleft lift procedure is performed in an ambulatory setting in the prone jackknife position. The buttocks are held together and the area of contact is marked (Figure 149-7, *A*). The buttocks are then taped apart (Figure 149-7, *B*). The gluteal cleft region and buttocks are shaved, prepped, and generously infiltrated with 1% lidocaine containing 1:100,000 epinephrine. An incision is made above the top of the cleft, which then crosses the midline at an acute angle at the top of the unhealed wound. The lower end of the incision points to the anus. The unhealed wound is excised in a triangular shape (Figure 149-7, *C*). A skin flap is then created out to the marked line (Figure 149-7, *D*). The tapes are then released. The skin flap is positioned to overlie the edges of the wound on the opposite side. Excess skin is excised.

A closed-suction drain is placed in the subcutaneous tissue and brought out through a separate stab wound. The subcutaneous tissue is approximated with 3-0 absorbable sutures (Figure 149-7, *E*). The skin is closed in a subcuticular fashion, and adhesive strips are applied. A light dressing is applied. Recurrence rate is reported at 3.3%.[47-49]

PILONIDAL DISEASE AND CARCINOMA

Malignant degeneration of chronic pilonidal wounds is a rare complication.[25,50,51] Such patients typically have had long-standing disease, averaging 23 years' duration. Most tumors are squamous cell carcinoma. Approximately 80% of these malignancies have been described in men in their 50s. The tumors are aggressive and locally invasive. Inguinal lymph node metastasis is present in 14% of patients. The presence of carcinoma in a pilonidal wound *is* an indication for wide en bloc excision of the mass including the sacral fascia. Flap techniques are usually required to close the defect. Recurrence rates have been reported at 38%. With a mean followup time of 28 months, 20% of all patients died as a result of the neoplasm.[50] Local recurrence rates seem to be lower when radiation therapy is added to surgical resection. There also appears to be some advantage to adding chemotherapy to the treatment regimen.[50]

SUMMARY

Sacrococcygeal pilonidal disease is a potentially disabling disease that is often made worse by overly aggressive treatment. Understanding the pathophysiology helps the surgeon manage the problem with less destructive techniques. Treating pilonidal disease as an abscess with a feeding sinus tract instead of as a "cyst" allows treatment

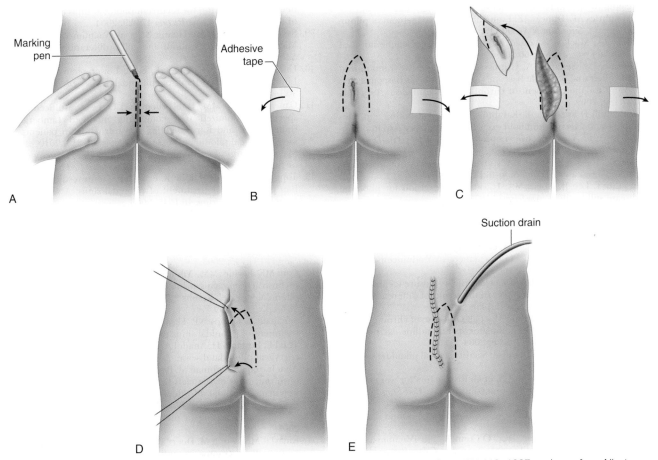

FIGURE 149-7 Cleft closure technique. (From Bascom J: Repeat pilonidal operations. *Am J Surg* 154:118, 1987; redrawn from Nivatvongs S: Pilonidal disease. In Gordon PH, Nivatvongs S, editors: *Principles and practice of surgery for the colon, rectum, and anus*, ed 2, St. Louis, 1999, Quality Medical, p 299.)

approaches that can be performed with satisfactory results, often on an ambulatory basis. Chronic pilonidal disease may require very complex reconstructive procedure to cure the disease.

REFERENCES

1. Anderson AW: Hair extracted from an ulcer. *Boston Med Surg J* 36:74, 1847.
2. Edwards MH: Pilonidal sinus: A five-year appraisal of the Millar-Lord treatment. *Br J Surg* 64:867, 1977.
3. Allen-Mersh TG: Pilonidal sinus: Finding the right track for treatment. *Br J Surg* 77:123, 1990.
4. Velasco AL, Dunlap WW: Pilonidal disease and hidradenitis. *Surg Clin N Am* 9:689, 2009.
5. Sondenaa K, Nesvik I, Anderson E, et al: Patient characteristics and symptoms in chronic pilonidal sinus disease. *Int J Colorectal Dis* 10:39, 1995.
6. Patey D, Scarff RW: The hair of the pilonidal sinus. *Lancet* 268:772, 1955.
7. Bendewald FP, Cima RR: Pilonidal disease. *Clin Colon Rectal Surg* 20:86, 2007.
8. Bascom J: Pilonidal disease: Origin from follicles of hairs and results of follicle removal as treatment. *Surgery* 87:567, 1980.
9. Armstrong JH, Barcia PJ: Pilonidal sinus disease: The conservative approach. *Arch Surg* 129:914, 1994.
10. Marks J, Harding KG, Hughes LE, et al: Pilonidal sinus excision: Healing by open granulation. *Br J Surg* 72:637, 1985.
11. Bascom JU: Pilonidal disease: Long-term results of follicle removal. *Dis Colon Rectum* 26:800, 1983.
12. Jensen SL, Harling H: Prognosis after simple incision and drainage for a first-episode acute pilonidal abscess. *Br J Surg* 75:60, 1988.
13. Kepenekci I, Demirkan A, Celasin H, et al: Unroofing and curettage for the treatment of acute and chronic pilonidal disease. *World J Surg* 34:153, 2010.
14. Oram Y, Kahraman F, Karincaoglu Y, et al: Evaluation of 60 patients with pilonidal sinus treated with laser epilation after surgery. *Dermatol Surg* 36:88, 2010.
15. Vahedian J, Nabavizadeh F, Nakhaee N, et al: Comparison between drainage and curettage in the treatment of acute pilonidal abscess. *Saudi Med J* 26:553, 2005.
16. Lord P, Millar D: Pilonidal sinus: A simple treatment. *Br J Surg* 52:298, 1965.
17. Solla JA, Rothenberger DA: Chronic pilonidal disease: An assessment of 150 cases. *Dis Colon Rectum* 33:758, 1990.
18. Sondennaa IN, Anderson E, Soriede JA: Recurrent pilonidal sinus after excision with closed or open treatment: Final result of a randomised trial. *Eur J Surg* 162:237, 1996.
19. Dogru O, Camci C, Aygen E, et al: Pilonidal sinus treated with crystallized phenol: An eight-year experience. *Dis Colon Rectum* 47:1934, 2004.
20. Hegge HG, Vos GA, Patka P, et al: Treatment of complicated or infected pilonidal sinus disease by local application of phenol. *Surgery* 102:52, 1987.
21. Saleem MI, Al-Hashemy AM: Management of pilonidal sinus using fibrin glue: A new concept and preliminary experience. *Colorectal Dis* 7:319, 2005.
22. Greenberg R, Kashtan H, Skornik Y, et al: Treatment of pilonidal sinus disease using fibrin glue as a sealant. *Tech Coloproctol* 8:95, 2004.

23. Odili J, Gault D: Laser depilation of the natal cleft—an aid to healing the pilonidal sinus. *Ann R Coll Surg Engl* 84:29, 2002.

24. Humphries AE, Duncan JE: Evaluation and management of pilonidal disease. *Surg Clin N Am* 90:113, 2010.

25. Davis KA, Mock CN, Versaci A, et al: Malignant degeneration of pilonidal cysts. *Am Surg* 60:200, 1994.

26. Nordon IM, Senapati A, Cripps NP: A prospective randomized controlled trial of simple Bascom's technique versus Bascom's cleft closure for the treatment of chronic pilonidal disease. *Am J Surg* 197:189, 2009.

27. Karakayali F, Karagulle E, Karabulut Z, et al: Unroofing and marsupialization versus rhomboid excision and Limberg flap in pilonidal disease: A prospective, randomized, clinical trial. *Dis Colon Rectum* 52:496, 2009.

28. Lee SL, Tejirian T, Abbas MA: Current management of adolescent pilonidal disease. *J Pediatr Surg* 43:1124, 2008.

29. Tejiran T, Lee JJ, Abbas MA: Is wide local excision for pilonidal disease still justified. *Am Surg* 73:1075, 2007.

30. Doll D, Novotny A, Rothe R, et al: Methylene blue halves the long-term recurrence rate in acute pilonidal sinus disease. *Int J Colorect Dis* 23:181, 2008.

31. Eryilmaz R, Okan I, Coskun A, et al: Surgical treatment of complicated pilonidal sinus with a fasciocutaneous V-Y advancement flap. *Dis Colon Rectum* 52:2036, 2009.

32. Petersen S, Koch R, Stelzner S, et al: Primary closure techniques in chronic pilonidal sinus: A survey of the results of different surgical approaches. *Dis Colon Rectum* 45:1458, 2002.

33. Tocch A, Mazzoni G, Bonomi M, et al: Outcome of chronic pilonidal disease treatment after ambulatory plain midline excision and primary suture. *Am J Surg* 196:28, 2008.

34. Lee PJ, Raniga S, Biyani DK, et al: Sacrococcygeal pilonidal disease. *Colorectal Dis* 10:639, 2008.

35. Al-Khayat H, Sadeq A, Groof A, et al: Risk factors for wound complications in pilonidal sinus procedures. *J Am Coll Surg* 205:439, 2007.

36. Hoexter B: Use of Water-Pik lavage in pilonidal wound care. *Dis Colon Rectum* 19:470, 1976.

37. McGuinness JG, Winter DC, O'Connell PR: Vacuum-assisted closure of a complex pilonidal sinus. *Dis Colon Rectum* 46:274, 2003.

38. Lynch JB, Laing AJ, Regan PJ: Vacuum-assisted closure therapy: A new treatment option for recurrent pilonidal sinus disease: Report of three cases. *Dis Colon Rectum* 47:929, 2004.

39. Saxena V, Hwang CW, Huang S, et al: Vacuum-assisted closure: Microdeformation of wounds and cell proliferation. *Plast Reconstr Surg* 114:1086, 2004.

40. Unalp HR, Derici H, Kamer E, et al: Lower recurrence rate for Limberg versus V-Y flap for pilonidal sinus. *Dis Colon Rectum* 50:1436, 2007.

41. Can MF, Sevinc MM, Hancerliogullari O, et al: Multicenter prospective randomized trial comparing modified Limberg flap transposition and Karydakis flap reconstruction in patients with sacrococcygeal pilonidal disease. *Am J Surg* 200:318, 2010.

42. Mahdy T: Surgical treatment of pilonidal disease: Primary closure or flap reconstruction after excision. *Dis Colon Rect* 51:1816, 2008.

43. Topgul K, Ozdemir E, Kilic K, et al: Long-term results of Limberg flap procedure for treatment of pilonidal sinus: A report of 200 cases. *Dis Colon Rectum* 46:1545, 2003.

44. Daphan C, Tekelioglu MH, Sayilgan C, et al: Limberg flap repair for pilonidal disease. *Dis Colon Rectum* 47:233, 2004.

45. Eryilmaz R, Sahin M, Alimoglu O, et al: Surgical treatment of sacrococcygeal pilonidal sinus with the Limberg transposition flap. *Surgery* 134:745, 2003.

46. Can MF, Sevinc MM, Yilmaz N: Comparison of Karydakis flap reconstruction versus primary midline closure in sacrococcygeal pilonidal disease: Results of 200 military service members. *Surg Today* 39:580, 2009.

47. Senapati A, Cripps NP, Flashman K, et al: Cleft closure for the treatment of pilonidal sinus disease. *Colorectal Dis* 13:333, 2011.

48. Tezel E, Bostanci H, Anadol AZ, et al. Cleft lip procedure for sacrococcygeal pilonidal disease. *Dis Colon Rectum* 52:135, 2009.

49. Abdelrazeq AS, Rahman M, Botterill ID, et al: Short term and long-term outcomes of the cleft lift procedure in the management of non acute pilonidal disorders. *Dis Colon Rectum* 51:1100, 2008.

50. de Bree E, Zoetmulder FA, Christodoulakis M, et al: Treatment of malignancy arising in pilonidal disease. *Ann Surg Oncol* 8:60, 2001.

51. Kulaylat MN, Gong M, Doerr RJ: Multimodality treatment of squamous cell carcinoma complicating pilonidal disease. *Am Surg* 62:922, 1996.

Traumatic Colorectal Injuries, Foreign Bodies, and Anal Wounds

Susan Galandiuk | Jason Smith | Adrian Billeter | Jeffrey Jorden

COLORECTAL TRAUMA

The management of injuries to the colon and in particular to the rectum may create problems for general and trauma surgeons who are not completely familiar with the advanced concepts and techniques that are associated with anorectal physiology and reconstruction. Similarly, even the most skillful colorectal surgeon may be presented with major problems in the overall management of diseases associated with the colorectum in the multiple trauma scenario. The purpose of this chapter is to describe the treatment of injuries to the colon, rectum, and anus, in which the best skills of both the trauma surgeon and the colorectal surgeon will be brought to bear in managing an individual patient.

The history of colon trauma is old, with at least one reference to it in the Old Testament (2 Samuel 20:9-10). Colorectal trauma was nearly uniformly fatal during the American Civil War, but the mortality rate began to decline during World War I. During World War II, the mortality rate declined again to about 25% to 30% as a result of the availability of blood transfusion and the standard practice of fecal diversion. Patient transportation during the Korean and Vietnam wars, as well as the continued refinement of resuscitation and the judicious individualization of colorectal wounds, also increased survival rates. Currently, the mortality rate is about 3% in the civilian scenario but depends on blunt injuries versus penetration.[1] In the United States, trauma is the major cause of death in people younger than 40 years and accounts for nearly 150,000 deaths a year. Trauma-related deaths have a tripartite distribution. There are *immediate deaths* that occur soon after injury and before hospital transport and, typically, are associated with major neurologic and cardiovascular injury. There are *early deaths* that occur at and about the time of transfer to the hospital and within a few hours after injury because of major hemorrhage, such as hemorrhage in the chest and abdomen, and because of severe blood loss from multiple, less specific injuries. Finally, there are deaths that occur *secondary to infection*, beginning toward the end of the first week of hospitalization and continuing well into the second and third months after injury. Infection, overt sepsis, and multiorgan failure are special problems in colonic injury because of the bacterial contamination that frequently coexists with hemorrhagic shock. In civilian practice in the United States, a gunshot wound to the colon is the most common cause of penetrating injury, with stab wounds being second, and shotgun wounds being third.[2] Blunt trauma occasionally causes colorectal trauma and presents special diagnostic problems.[3]

Table 150-1 provides a summary of selected studies from the past 38 years and lists the collective causes of penetrating and blunt colonic injury. With the increasing use of therapeutic endoscopy that is often performed by non-surgeons, iatrogenic or unintentional perforation of the colon has become a special problem that deserves separate comment in terms of overall management (see Iatrogenic Injury, later). The frequency of iatrogenic injury, especially in tertiary centers, is vastly underestimated.

Colonic injury, when combined with other injuries such as to parenchymal organs (i.e., liver, pancreas, spleen), is especially important in contributing to the second part of the "two-hit" hypothesis (i.e., bacterial contamination combined with hemorrhagic shock). It, therefore, has a substantial influence on survival rate and an even greater effect on infectious morbidity rates. Table 150-2 provides a summary of associated injuries for gunshot wounds to the colon, which again emphasizes the influence of the small bowel, liver, stomach, major vessels, and pancreas.[4-7]

The major factor in the assessment of patients with colorectal injuries, which is discussed in detail in Principles of Operative Management, later, depends on the severity of injury. Table 150-3 provides a grading system for both intraabdominal colon and rectal injuries that is current and helpful in recognizing the severity of the injury and in determining preferred therapy.[8,9]

All of these factors contribute significantly to the possibility of infectious complications and, in turn, are closely related to the likelihood of late death.[10] For example, there is a steady increase in infectious complications that parallel the number of units of blood transfused during a laparotomy for colon injury, rising to as much as 60% when more than 10 units of blood have been transfused. Similarly, and not surprisingly, the risk of infection approaches 100% when more than five organs have been injured, but the risk is only half that when four or fewer organs have been injured. Patient age also has a substantial effect on the infectious complications rate. Patients younger than 30 years have only a 12% to 15% infection rate, whereas those older than 30 years have an infection rate that exceeds 40%.

ASSESSMENT OF THE ABDOMEN IN TRAUMA

Although complete discussion of the initial evaluation and resuscitation of the trauma patient is beyond the scope of this discussion, special emphasis must be placed on the evaluation of the abdomen. As a general surgeon,

TABLE 150-1 Collected Causes of Penetrating Colonic Injuries

	Flint et al[45]	Samhouri et al[46]	Bartizal et al[47]	Wiener et al[4]	Kirkpatrick and Rajpal[2]	Steele and Blaisdell[8]	Thomson et al[9]	Stone and Fabian[15]	Jacobsen et al[5]	Totals
Gunshot	101	124	279	99	124	76	35	220	42	1100
Stab	13	18	111	27	31	37	30	37	9	312
Blunt trauma	21	6	16	20	2	10	3	4	—	82
Shotgun	7	—	9	17	8	4	3	7	7	62
Iatrogenic		2	—	10	—	—	—	—	—	12
Foreign bodies	—	—	—	8	—	7	—	—	—	15

From Galandiuk S: Injuries to the colon and rectum. In Keighley MRB, Williams NS, editors: *Surgery of the anus, rectum and colon*, ed 3. London, 2010, Elsevier.

TABLE 150-2 Distribution of Associated Injuries in Gunshot Wounds to the Colon

	Wiener et al[4]	Thompson et al[6]	Matolo and Wolfman[7]	Jacobsen et al[5]
Stomach	11	16	4	10
Duodenum	5	8	—	5
Small bowel	39	39	26	26
Gallbladder	5	7	1	3
Pancreas	3	9	—	6
Liver	8	32	7	11
Spleen	3	15	6	4
Kidneys	7	—	5	9
Bladder	4	—	2	1
Vascular	6	6	11	34
Diaphragm	3	—	5	9
			9	10

From Galandiuk S: Injuries to the colon and rectum. In Keighley MRB, Williams NS, editors: *Surgery of the anus, rectum and colon*, ed 3. London, 2010, Elsevier.

the evaluation of the abdomen for injury or pathology is paramount, particularly when dealing with a possible colorectal injury. Detecting the presence of an acute abdomen is of much higher precedent than actually detecting the specific injury. Most, if not all, traumatic intraabdominal pathology is best treated in the operating suite, and making the correct decision rapidly (with often incomplete information) is vital to the survival of these patients.

The abdominal cavity itself often extends high under the ribs because of diaphragmatic excursion; thus penetrating injuries to the thorax may often involve intraabdominal organs. Evaluation of the abdomen begins first with the careful examination of the patient for contusions, ecchymosis, or penetrating injuries. Careful log-rolling of the patient must be performed to exclude the back as a source for intraabdominal pathology. Auscultation of the abdomen in the trauma resuscitation room or emergency department is often futile given the loud, often chaotic environment associated with these locations; however, careful palpation of the abdomen can often detect other focal or generalized tenderness even

TABLE 150-3 Gradation of Injuries to Colon and Rectum

Injured Structure	Grade	Characteristics of Injury	AIS-05 Score
Colon	1	Contusion or hematoma; partial-thickness laceration	2
	2	Small (<50% of circumference) laceration	3
	3	Large (>50% of circumference) laceration	3
	4	Transection	4
	5	Transection with tissue loss; devascularized segment	4
Rectosigmoid and rectum	1	Contusion or hematoma; partial-thickness laceration	2
	2	Small (<50% of circumference) laceration	3
	3	Large (>50% of circumference)	4
	4	Full-thickness laceration with perineal extension	5
	5	Devascularized segment	5

Modified from the Abbreviated Injury Scale (AIS) 2005—update 2008. Association for the Advancement of Automotive Medicine, Barrington, Ill. *AIS-05*, Abbreviated Injury Scale Score, 2005 version.

in intubated patients. Guarding, rebound, and peritoneal signs on percussion are often harbingers of significant intraabdominal injuries.

If intraabdominal injury is likely, a broad-spectrum, safe antibiotic should be administered with one of the first liters of intravenous fluid. We continue to believe that the scenario of trauma with shock and resuscitation is ideal for the use of very large doses of antibiotics and their continuous infusion.[11,12]

As part of the care of the trauma patient, an evaluation of pelvic fractures is important, particularly when discussing colorectal injuries. Aside from an anteroposterior pelvic radiograph, it is important to examine the perineal area to determine the presence of ecchymosis, bony protuberances due to pelvic fracture, traction injuries, and/or penetrating injuries not assessed on abdominal evaluation.[13] Every trauma patient evaluated must undergo a digital rectal examination (DRE), particularly if pelvic fracture is suspected. Inability to palpate the prostate on DRE necessitates a retrograde urethrogram prior to Foley catheter insertion. Gross blood on DRE, as well as bony shards or rectal tears, are indicative of a complicated pelvic fracture with rectal laceration. Depending on patient stability, if a pelvic fracture is present, stabilization with an appropriate external fixator or ad hoc stabilization device (such as a military anti-shock trouser [MAST]) should be accomplished.[13]

Computed tomographic (CT) scanning remains the gold standard for evaluating the abdominal cavity in the hemodynamically stable patient. However, the evaluation of the abdomen in the unconscious or hemodynamically unstable patient represents a serious problem for clinicians.[14]

Although resuscitation and the initial assessment are ongoing, the insertion of a nasogastric tube, by nose or mouth, will permit the detection of blood within the stomach, as well as decompress the patient in preparation for an anesthetic. Any penetrating wound below the level of the nipples must be considered a possible intraabdominal injury.[15]

The evaluation of the abdomen in the unconscious patient continues to represent a serious problem. Evaluation by ultrasound examination or CT scanning is now the norm. Ultrasound examination, when carried out by the examining surgeon, is a most efficient, inexpensive, and reliable aid to patient care.[16,17] Ultrasound and the focused abdominal ultrasound for trauma (FAST) have replaced diagnostic peritoneal lavage (DPL) in most trauma centers.[18-20] Focused abdominal ultrasound includes evaluation of the pericardium, right and left upper quadrants, and pelvis. Skills in ultrasound evaluation of the acute abdomen have become as important as laparoscopy to the contemporarily trained general surgeon. Needless to say, FAST should always be performed by the operating surgeon. If FAST and/or CT are equivocal, then DPL, which has been a reliable procedure for nearly three decades, is performed under direct vision. If no gross blood is encountered, lavage of the peritoneal cavity with saline is performed. DPL is considered positive and indicative of intraabdominal injury if the effluent contains more than 100,000 red blood cells/mm³ or more than 500 white blood cells/mm³, with a hematocrit value of more than 2, or in the presence of bile, bacteria, and vegetable or fecal matter.

The overall priorities of trauma care are important and are dealt with elsewhere.

SPECIAL DIAGNOSTIC PROBLEMS

Colorectal injury associated with *blunt trauma* is especially treacherous and is uncommon enough to worry even the most experienced trauma surgeons. It represents only about 1 in 30 such injuries, and the diagnosis is then often made only at the time of laparotomy for other injuries. The diagnosis will often not have been made, and the surgeon will have to be alert intraoperatively to take appropriate measures. Reported data regarding these injuries are suspect in the sense that diagnosis is often delayed and then involves the treatment of a late-recognized colon perforation, as opposed to the more frequently and promptly diagnosed penetrating trauma.[21]

The diagnostic capabilities of abdominal CT for intraabdominal injuries, particularly bowel injuries, are influenced by early versus late generations of CT scanners, oral contrast ingestion, and types of abdominal injury. Recent generations of multidetector-row CTs (MRCT) are capable of scanning patients in a shorter period of time while producing clearer images with artifact suppression.[14] Overall, improved technology produces a higher quality of CT images, allowing for higher quality multiplanar and three-dimensional reformation. Oral contrast can improve the quality of the CT images. Oral contrast outlines small intramural or mesenteric hematomas. In addition, extravasation of oral contrast localizes the area of bowel rupture. However, ingestion of oral contrast increases time spent in the emergency department, decreases bowel motility, and increases the risk of vomiting and aspiration. Studies have shown that intravenous contrast-enhanced CT is sufficient to detect nearly 75% of intraabdominal injuries in these patients.[21]

Small bowel and colorectal injuries are difficult to diagnose because they have few pathognomonic CT findings. Bowel disruption or contrast extravasation confirms bowel or mesenteric injuries; however, these findings are exceedingly rare. Typical CT findings are bowel wall thickening, mesenteric infiltration, and free intraperitoneal fluid. Findings on CT of free abdominal fluid in the abscess of solid organ injury, in particular, should alert the clinician to remain suspicious of a bowel injury. A negative CT scan does not obviate the need for further monitoring though, because signs and symptoms of bowel and mesenteric injuries may take up to 24 to 72 hours to manifest. In adults who are able to cooperate and give a reliable physical examination, there is no need for admission for further monitoring. In the obtunded patient, serial abdominal monitoring is a necessity despite the absence of CT findings.

There is a 1% incidence of hollow viscus injury with blunt trauma and approximately a 0.3% incidence of colon or rectal injury.[3] No diagnostic test or combination of findings reliably excludes colon injury. Diagnosis is often made at the time of laparotomy for other injuries. The presence of colonic injury at laparotomy is associated with an increased risk of complications but not necessarily mortality.[3]

The proposed mechanisms of colon injury during blunt abdominal trauma are several. This injury is most commonly thought to occur secondary to direct compression between the blunt object and the vertebral column or bony pelvis. This compression produces a tearing or lacerating effect. A second mechanism of injury is thought to involve sudden deceleration, producing bowel-mesenteric disruption and subsequent devascularization. This makes the transverse and sigmoid colon most vulnerable during sudden deceleration injuries because these segments, to some degree, are on a mesenteric stalk.[22]

A further opportunity for diagnostic error regarding injury to the large bowel is the failure to carry out a careful, well-illuminated, and detailed perineal examination in the often unstable multitrauma victim. Lacerations of the perineum or rectum must be presumed to be associated with open pelvic fractures. Shards of bone associated with some pelvic fractures can readily lacerate all pelvic structures, including major blood vessels. The careful examination of the perineum and the rectum, including an examination for occult blood, is important in this scenario and can be difficult. There is no substitute for a specific examination by a person who is knowledgeable of and especially suspicious of the bizarre ramifications of perineal lacerations and pelvic fractures; a detailed note or drawing in the chart is often helpful. A standard of care often includes the use of sigmoidoscopy, but this can be technically difficult in the trauma patient. Triple-contrast CT scanning with intravenous, peroral, and rectal contrast medium can identify many rectal extraperitoneal injuries, particularly with the availability of newer multislice-detector CT scanners (MDCT) in emergency departments throughout much of the world.[23]

Diagnostic dilemmas occur in several typical scenarios, most commonly when a retroperitoneal portion of the colon has been injured and the patient presents with few anterior peritoneal signs, no pneumoperitoneum, and symptoms that may be masked by other overt manifestations of trauma or by treatment. Opening of the peritoneal reflection usually discloses the true nature of the problem.

PRINCIPLES OF OPERATIVE MANAGEMENT

The operative management of traumatic colorectal injuries can be divided into two distinct methodologies often adopted because of the hemodynamic stability and injury status of the patient. First is the damage control approach to colorectal injuries and second is the definitive repair and treatment of these injuries.

DAMAGE CONTROL AND COLORECTAL INJURIES

Little in surgery has changed more in the past 20 years than the popularization and adoption of damage control techniques in the management of traumatic injuries. Stone et al[24] are credited with introducing the technique of abbreviated laparotomy in 1985. They rapidly terminated the surgical procedure at the onset of coagulopathy by employing packing for nonsurgical bleeding, along with selective ligation of vessels and rapid bowel resection without anastomosis or stoma formation. Definitive surgery was performed after correction of physiologic derangements, including coagulopathy. Compared with 1 of 14 patients who survived after being treated with the traditional approach, 11 of 17 patients survived after abbreviated laparotomy. To describe such truncated surgery for trauma patients with massive hemorrhage and shock, acidosis, and hypothermia, the term *damage control* was coined in 1993 by Rotondo et al.[25]

The term *damage control* originates from the United States Navy and refers to the ability of a ship to absorb damage while maintaining mission integrity. Damage to the ship's hull is rapidly assessed, and adequate repairs are performed to allow the ship to return to the controlled environment of port. The intraoperative detection of coagulopathy represents an absolute indication for damage control surgery. However, the decision may be made too late, because it can be difficult to control nonsurgical hemorrhage by packing once coagulopathy has become manifest. Therefore, it would be ideal to predict the patients who are close to a state of coagulopathy early after admission. In 2001, Asensio et al proposed the following criteria after extensive literature review: pH of 7.2 or less, intraoperative temperature less than 34 °C, blood replacement greater than 4 L, and total intraoperative fluid replacement greater than 10 L.[25,26] Damage control has three separate components: (1) abbreviated resuscitative surgery for rapid control of hemorrhage and intestinal contamination, followed by temporary abdominal wall closure; (2) ongoing core rewarming, correction of coagulopathy and hemodynamics in the intensive care unit; and (3) scheduled reexploration for definitive management of injuries and abdominal wall closure.[27]

Control of the site of primary hemorrhage and stabilization of the patient take priority to treating colorectal injuries. Injury to the colon is seldom the cause of exanguinating hemorrhage. However, resectional debridement or stapling of the injured colon to limit or avoid peritoneal contamination early in the procedure is often prudent. Judicious use of intraabdominal packing to control hemorrhage is an integral part of damage control philosophy, but care must be taken when placing packs so as not to injure the colon or rectum while working in haste.

DEFINITIVE REPAIR AND MANAGEMENT

If the abdomen is the site of injury, our preferred approach for virtually all patients with such severe trauma is through a midline abdominal incision that can be extended in either direction depending on the nature of the intraoperative findings. The laparoscopic approach to major abdominal injury is still evolving, as are the requisite skills for minimal access surgery among younger surgeons; selected applications in experienced laparoscopic hands may become more acceptable. The burden of proof of overlooked injury is obviously substantial. We emphasize the need to stabilize the patient intraoperatively and to control or ameliorate ongoing blood loss. When that is accomplished, one is ready to turn attention

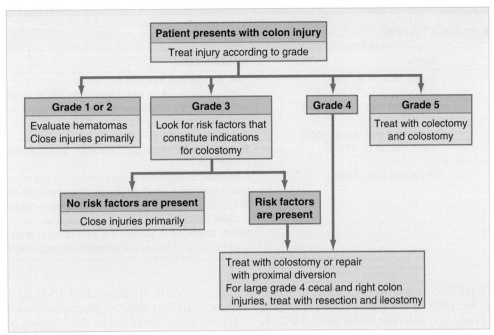

FIGURE 150-1 Algorithm outlining the treatment of colon injury. (From Lucas CE, Ledgerwood AM: Injuries to the stomach, duodenum, pancreas, small bowel, colon, and rectum. In Souba WW, Fink MP, Jurkovich GJ, editors: *ACS surgery principles and practice*. New York, 2005, Decker Publishing.)

to the possibly injured colon. A system of grading colon injuries is especially helpful to the surgeon (who is not often in this situation) in making a wise choice regarding options, ranging from primary repair to occasional resection and anastomosis, with or without protective proximal stoma. Just as the surgeon must begin to make that determination, he or she must constantly be alert to the stability of the patient and the patient's capacity to tolerate a preferred method of repair. The choices may include rapid stapling and discarding of a section of colon in a patient with a massive liver injury and multiple transfusions who is being packed to control a major hepatic parenchymal hemorrhage. The stapled ends are simply dropped back into the abdomen and more definitive care completed when the now more stable patient is returned to the operating theatre in 24 to 48 hours. The other end of the spectrum is represented by a stable patient who has an isolated injury of the lower sigmoid and is an excellent candidate for excision of the injured segment and primary repair in the best of circumstances.

In general, options for the treatment of colon injury include (1) proximal diversion and repair, (2) exteriorization of the wound itself as a colostomy, (3) simple suture of even lengthy colon lacerations, and (4) resection and anastomosis. The latter should be applied only with special thought.[28,29] The patient with injuries requiring resection often has associated injuries and, therefore, is seldom a candidate for an extensive and complex operation and may be better suited for resection and temporary diversion. On the other hand, if contamination is not extensive, the patient is hemodynamically stable, and a well-vascularized colon is available, then resection and anastomosis may be suitable. The algorithm (Figure 150-1)[10] is especially helpful to a surgeon who is unfamiliar with the treatment of colonic

injury. It is clear that many tangential and even penetrating wounds of the colon can be dealt with safely by primary suture in a stable patient. Even longitudinal tears can be repaired safely. A recent metaanalysis of currently published randomized trials favors primary repair over fecal diversion for penetrating injuries of the colon.[30] The method of anastomosis following colon resection for penetrating trauma does not seem to affect the incidence of abdominal complications.[31] Demetriades et al, in a prospective, nonrandomized multicenter trial, found no differences in complications among 297 patients with colonic injuries requiring resection and anastomosis by method of repair or anatomic location of injury. The authors excluded those who died within 72 hours of admission and all injuries in their study that were destructive based on the assessment of the treating surgeon (thus, requiring resection and anastomosis). The authors found no differences in complication rate between primary repair group and diversion group. Instead, they found that complications were associated with other factors, such as gross contamination, transfusion of greater than 4 units of packed red blood cells (PRBCs), and single-agent antibiotic prophylaxis across their entire population. (We do not agree with their indictment of single agent antibiotic use [Table 150-4].) The overall abdominal complication rate was 24%.

CONSIDERATION IN MILITARY INJURIES

The overall management of military trauma has been radically revised in the light of our now 10-year war in the Middle East. The principles still apply, particularly in the context of body armor and truncal protection.[32] Selectivity has also been helped by CT scanning, which, however, can be misleading.[23] Steele et al[33] reviewed the

TABLE 150-4 Antibiotic Priorities

Factor	Source	Recommendation
Timing	Richardson et al, 1987[1]	First intravenous infusion solution
Duration		Single dose to 24 hr when favorable; never longer than 5 d
Doses	Livingston and Wang, 1993[12]	Very large if a cephalosporin is chosen and/or hemorrhage and transfusion are significant
Route	Livingston and Wang, 1993[12]	Parenteral; continuous infusion may be better
	Galandiuk et al, 1997[48]	Special role for prolonged antibiotic beads in wound if closed and high risk
Drug preferences	Price and Polk, 1999[42]	Cefotetan or ceftriaxone; aztreonam for gram-negative coverage
		Metronidazole if overt evidence of established anaerobic infection
		Seldom: clindamycin/amikacin/tobramycin-gentamicin only for rare allergy and/or positive culture scenarios
Cost control issues		Safest antibiotic is always the best choice; drugs that require monitoring of levels are prohibitively expensive

treatment of 175 patients requiring treatment of colon injuries between the 2003 to 2004 period of Operation Iraqi Freedom. Primary repair was undertaken in 53%, the leak rate was 10%, and the overall mortality was 17.7%. Of the patients, 37% were U.S. or coalition forces and the remainder were local nationals. Mean injury severity score (ISS) and abbreviated injury score (AIS) were similar among different regions of the colon. Stomas were more frequently performed for rectal or anal sphincter injuries than colonic injuries, and for left-sided versus right-sided or transverse injuries. Leaks after primary repair were equally distributed throughout the colon. Although the leak rate was higher in the primary repair group, there was no difference in rates of sepsis or mortality among groups on multivariate analysis. Only ISS >15 was associated with an increase in sepsis, whereas only rectal or transverse colon injuries were associated with an increase in mortality.[34] Additionally, a 2009 Cochrane database review demonstrated that not only was primary repair safe but may be advantageous when compared with diversion, particularly when applied to penetrating injuries to the colon.[35]

ANORECTAL INJURY

Injuries to the intraperitoneal rectum are diagnosed and treated similarly to colonic injuries. Injuries to the extraperitoneal rectum may be much more difficult to diagnose. Injuries that are not diagnosed promptly or treated appropriately by postinjury day 1 usually become apparent by virtue of pelvic, perineal, or systemic signs of infection. The introduction of appropriate systemic antibiotics is justified by the suspicion that an anorectal injury exists. Diagnosis is preferably confirmed by an examination (even under anesthesia), rigid sigmoidoscopy, water-soluble contrast study of the rectum, or triple-contrast CT scanning. Sigmoidoscopy should be performed if there is blood within the rectum on digital examination or if there is evidence of a bladder or urethral injury, blood within the vagina, severe pelvic fracture, or bullet trajectory above the midthigh and below the pelvic rim.[36] If a rectal injury is suspected, the patient should be positioned in stirrups so there is free access to the perineum. In general, if such an injury has been complicated by delayed diagnosis, then diversion is preferred, complemented by the removal of palpable rectal fecal material, rectal "washout," and drainage of the presacral space. The efficacy of rectal washout has not been demonstrated prospectively.[37] Rectal washout can be performed via sterilized ventilator tubing inserted transanally after anal canal dilation. A large Foley catheter (e.g., 24 French) can be inserted into the distal rectum, and irrigation is performed until the effluent is clear.[38] Saline is most frequently used, often with a final irrigation of povidone-iodine.

Contrary to common attitudes among trauma surgeons, the promptly diagnosed anorectal injury is often best treated by a definitive early repair, assuming the patient is otherwise stable. This in particular applies to lacerations of the anal sphincter. Obviously, if the patient is badly hurt or in shock or the diagnosis is delayed, diversion becomes part of the care plan. The operating surgeon must be particularly careful that drainage of the area does not produce further sphincter injury. It requires the best of the trauma surgeon's overall assessment and the colorectal surgeon's anatomic expertise to optimize results in these often challenging wounds.

OTHER TYPES OF COLONIC TRAUMA

IATROGENIC INJURY

Colonoscopic perforation is remarkably infrequent, and even then, it is clear that many patients tolerate delayed diagnosis and conservative management.[39,40] Failure to consider the possibility of perforation is never acceptable, and when a patient has developed any evidence of instability, abdominal pain, tenderness, or pneumoperitoneum after a colonoscopic procedure, perforation should be assumed. Unlike the large bowel injury that occurs with trauma, colonoscopic laceration of the colon usually occurs in a mechanically clean bowel. Patients whose signs and symptoms immediately ameliorate with intestinal rest, systemic antibiotics, and volume resuscitation can often be treated conservatively without surgery. Patients who have continued tachycardia, fever, and leukocytosis and who do not respond to the measures of intestinal rest, systemic antibiotics, and resuscitation require surgery with simple repair of the perforation. If the perforation occurs at a site of extensive gross disease, then resection may be in order, and the surgeon can use his or her best judgment as to whether primary anastomosis, with or without a protecting colostomy, is warranted.

Another situation warranting immediate surgery is that associated with the extravasation of barium during the course of radiologic study of the alimentary tract. Barium is especially likely to promote and accentuate peritonitis associated with bacterial contamination. The mortality rate for barium peritonitis is extremely high.[41]

FOREIGN BODIES

Anorectal foreign bodies often pose a challenging diagnostic and management dilemma that begins with the initial evaluation in the emergency department and continues through the postoperative period. General surgeons are often called on to treat these patients since they are often reluctant to seek medical attention from a known physician and/or present to emergency department after a significant delay. Because of the wide variety of objects and the variable trauma that can be caused to the local tissues of the rectum and distal colon, a systematic approach to the diagnosis and management of the retained rectal foreign body is essential. Even after extraction, rectal foreign bodies may be associated with delayed perforation or significant bleeding from the rectum.

Although retained rectal foreign bodies have been reported in patients of all ages, genders, and ethnicities, more than two-thirds of patients are men in their 30s and 40s, and patients as old as 90 years have been reported. There is little critical evidence to guide the clinician in caring for these patients. The American Association for the Surgery of Trauma (AAST) colorectal organ injury scale is generally appropriate. Despite the potential for severe injury, most rectal injuries from foreign bodies result in grade I or grade II injuries.

Care of rectal injuries is guided by the degree of injury as evidenced by the percentage circumference, extent and nature of any hematoma, degree of ischemia of the rectum, and, finally, whether or not perforation/extension into the perineum or peritoneal cavity exists. However, special attention should be paid to possible sexual assault or body packing as in drug trafficking. Involuntary nonsexual foreign bodies are generally found in the elderly, children, or the mentally ill, such as retained thermometers, enema tips, aluminum foil wrapping from pill containers, and orally ingested objects of all sorts.

The first step in the evaluation and management of a patient with a rectal foreign body is to determine whether or not a perforation occurred. When a perforation is suspected, it should be determined as soon as possible whether the patient is stable or unstable. Hypotension, tachycardia, severe abdomen or pelvic pain, and fevers are indicative of a perforation. If there is free air or obvious peritonitis indicating a perforation, then the patient needs immediate resuscitation with an intravenous, broad-spectrum antibiotic and surgical exploration. If the patient appears stable and has normal vital signs but a perforation is suspected, a CT scan often helps determine if there has been a rectal perforation, especially for perforations below the peritoneal reflection. Rectal wall thickening, mesorectal/retroperitoneal air, fluid collections, and fat stranding are all indications of a full-thickness injury and should be explored operatively.

The most important factor in successful extraction is patient relaxation. This can be achieved with a perianal nerve block, a spinal anesthetic, or either of these in combination with intravenous conscious sedation. All of these techniques allow the patient to relax, decrease anal sphincter spasm, and improve visualization and exposure. Only after the patient has been appropriately sedated and anesthetized should attempts be made to remove the object. The high lithotomy position facilitates removal of most objects and has the added benefit of allowing for downward abdominal pressure to aid in extraction. A digital rectal examination should be performed to assess the feasibility of removal transanally. If the foreign body can be easily palpated, it is amenable to transanal extraction. After successful removal of a foreign body, the mucosa of the colon and rectum needs to be examined via rigid proctosigmoidoscopy. A repeat plain film of the abdomen is often warranted to ensure that no perforation took place during the extraction process.

If transanal extraction does not work via regional anesthesia, then general anesthesia and/or deep sedation may facilitate removal. However, if after general anesthesia the foreign body cannot be removed from below, then a laparotomy is indicated. In the absence of a perforation, initial attempts should be made to push the object distally into the rectum. If unsuccessful, a simple colotomy and removal of the foreign object is needed with primary repair, and often no diversion is needed. Colonic diversion should be reserved for patients with frank peritonitis and hemodynamic instability, perforation with extensive fecal contamination, or significant colonic ischemia. Surgeon judgment at the time of laparotomy is paramount in deciding on which course of action to take. The most serious complication of a rectal foreign body is perforation. Major complications from rectal foreign bodies are rare but can be life-threatening if missed. Bleeding from lacerations in the rectal mucosa is generally self-limited but can, on occasion, require repeat surgery and suture ligation. Traumatic disruption of the anal sphincter can result in mild to severe fecal incontinence, depending on the degree of the injury. Attempts for surgical correction of any sphincter injury should be delayed until adequate time has passed to evaluate any resultant defect and clinical symptoms.

POSTOPERATIVE COMPLICATIONS FOR ALL COLORECTAL TRAUMA

Complications that may follow colorectal injury encompass the surgeon's entire repertoire. Bacterial contamination, if accentuated by diagnostic delay, hemorrhage, transfusion, or other major organ damage, are overriding concerns once the ABCs of trauma care have been

TABLE 150-5 Lessons Regarding Colostomy Closure in the Trauma Patient

Issues	Comment
Timing	Despite preferences, little differences in morbidity rate can be attributed to early versus later closure.
Preoperative contrast study of distal bowel	Assuming the patient is well physically and no lesions were detected at first operation.
Management of the stoma site	Delayed primary or secondary closure often never occurred. Closure with prolonged local antibiotic instillation is very safe.
Home health care followup	Home care leads to uniform prolongation of wound closure and increases in cost.

From Pokorny RM, Heniford T, Allen JW, et al: Limited utility of preoperative studies in preparation for colostomy closure. Am Surg 65:338, 1999.

established. Infection is both the most frequent and the most dangerous problem.[42] The specter of multisystem organ failure and its supportive and definitive care are always the first priority. If the patient does not thrive after treatment, the surgeon must reassess the patient and must be certain that an error in diagnosis or treatment has not occurred. In general, mechanical treatment (drainage and diversion) is far better than reliance on medications and organ system support.

Colostomy is a special complication of several of the therapeutic options in colorectal trauma.[43] In a comparison of outcomes—morbidity and mortality—as well as cost, the closing of a stoma must always be considered. We examined our practices and provide some highlights of that experience in Table 150-5. Colostomy closure requires as much mental preparation for the surgeon as it does technical expertise. The practice in many respected residency programs of assigning "simple" colostomy closure to junior staff is a case in point. Furthermore, choosing a time to perform the closure has become especially contentious in this cost-obsessed era. Surely, if the stoma is complementary (i.e., to a primary repair or for exteriorization of an injury), then early closure is feasible. Although that might safely and wisely be performed within 8 weeks, the stoma constructed as part of the care of a rectal laceration produced by a major pelvic fracture or for a complicated sphincter repair secondary to a straddle injury should permit structural and functional healing for 90 days or more and may well be in order before the closure of a stoma. It should not be forgotten that one of the most common complications after blunt or penetrating colonic trauma is development of pneumonia, which may significantly affect mortality. The incidence of intraabdominal abscess formation ranges from approximately 8% to 12%[3,44] but may be even higher with multiple other injuries probably in the colon.

Psychologically, the surgeon who plans a colostomy closure of a Hartmann-style stoma must also be ready to perform a major laparotomy, and the patient should be prepared as well. Our practice has been to either perform this within 2 weeks or delay it for 90 days, with a hope of minimizing technical issues and errors.

REFERENCES

1. Richardson JD, Polk HC Jr, Flint LM, editors: *Trauma: Clinical care and pathophysiology*, Chicago, 1987, Year Book.
2. Kirkpatrick JR, Rajpal SG: The injured colon: Therapeutic considerations. Am J Surg 129:187, 1975.
3. Williams MD, Watts D, Fakhry S: Colon injury after blunt abdominal trauma: Results of the EAST multi-institutional hollow viscus injury study. J Trauma 55:906, 2003.
4. Wiener I, Rojas P, Wolma FJ: Traumatic colonic perforation. Ars J Surg 142:717, 1981.
5. Jacobsen LE, Gomez GA, Brodie TA: Primary repair of 58 consecutive penetrating injuries: Should colostomy be abandoned? Am Surg 63:170, 1997.
6. Thompson JF, Moore EE, Moore JB: Comparison of penetrating injuries of the right and left colon. Ann Surg 193:414, 1981.
7. Matolo NM, Wolfman EF Jr: Primary repair of colonic injuries: A clinical evaluation. J Trauma 17:554, 1977.
8. Steele M, Blaisdell FW: Treatment of colon injuries. J Trauma 17:557, 1977.
9. Thomson SR, Baker A, Baker LW: Prospective audit of multiple penetrating injuries to the colon: Further support for primary closure. J R Coll Surg Edinb 41:20, 1996.
10. Galandiuk S: Injuries to the colon and rectum. In Keighley MRB, Williams NS, editors: Surgery of the anus, rectum and colon, ed 2. London, 1999, Saunders, p 2227.
11. Livingston DH, Malangoni MA: Increasing antibiotic dose decreases polymicrobial infection after hemorrhagic shock. Surg Gynecol Obstet 176:418, 1993.
12. Livingston DH, Wang MT: Continuous infusion of cefazolin is superior to intermittent dosing in decreasing infection after hemorrhagic shock. Am J Surg 165:203, 1993.
13. Flint L, Cryer HG: Pelvic fracture: The last 50 years. J Trauma 69:483, 2010.
14. Aotri M, Hanson JM, Grinblat L, et al: Surgically important bowel and/or mesenteric injury in blunt trauma: Accuracy of multidetector CT for evaluation. Radiology 249:524, 2008.
15. Stone HH, Fabian TC: Management of perforating colon trauma. Ann Surg 190:430, 1979.
16. Fernandez L, McKenney MG, McKenney KL, et al: Ultrasound in blunt abdominal trauma. J Trauma 45:841, 1998.
17. Rozycki GS, Ballard RB, Feliciano DV, et al: Surgeon-performed ultrasound for the assessment of truncal injuries: Lessons learned from 1540 patients. Ann Surg 228:557, 1998.
18. Carrillo EH, Platz A, Miller FB, et al: Non-operative management of blunt hepatic trauma. Br J Surg 85:461, 1998.
19. Arrillaga A, Graham R, York JW: Increased efficiency and cost-effectiveness in the evaluation of the blunt abdominal trauma patient with the use of ultrasound. Am Surg 65:31, 1999.
20. Rozycki GS, Feliciano DV, Schmidt JA, et al: The role of surgeon-performed ultrasound in patients with possible cardiac wounds. Ann Surg 223:737, 1996.
21. Carrillo EH, Somberg LB, Ceballos CE, et al: Blunt traumatic injuries to the colon and rectum. J Am Coll Surg 183:548, 1996.
22. Ricciardi R, Paterson CA, Islam W, et al: Independent predictors of morbidity and mortality in blunt colon trauma. Am Surg 70:75, 2004.
23. Velmahos GC, Constantinou C, Tillou A, et al: Abdominal computed tomographic scan for patients with gunshot wounds to the abdomen selected for nonoperative management. J Trauma 59:1155, 2005.
24. Stone HH, Strom PR, Mullins RJ: Management of the major coagulopathy with onset during laparotomy. Ann Surg 197:532, 1983.
25. Rotondo MF, Schwab CW, McGonigal MD, et al: Damage control—an approach for improved survival in exsanguinating abdominal injury. J Trauma 35:375, 1993.

26. Asensio JA, McDuffie L, Petrone P, et al: Reliable variables in the exsanguinated patient which indicate damage control and predict outcome. *Am J Surg* 182:743, 2001.
27. Miller PR, Chang MC, Hoth JJ, et al: Colonic resection in the setting of damage control laparotomy: Is delayed anastomosis safe? *Am Surg* 76:606, 2007.
28. Miller PR, Fabian TC, Croce MA, et al: Improving outcomes following penetrating colon wounds: Application of a clinical pathway. *Ann Surg* 235:775, 2002.
29. Kashuk JL, Cothren CC, Moore EE, et al: Primary repair of civilian colon injuries is safe in the damage control scenario. *Surgery* 42:663, 2009.
30. Singer MA, Nelson RL: Primary repair of penetrating colon injuries: A systematic review. *Dis Colon Rectum* 45:1579, 2002.
31. Demetriades D, Murray JA, Chan LS, et al: Handsewn versus stapled anastomosis in penetrating colon injuries requiring resection: A multicenter study. *J Trauma* 52:117, 2002.
32. Vertrees A, Wakefield M, Pickett C, et al: Outcomes of primary repair and primary anastomosis in war-related colon injuries. *J Trauma* 66:1286, 2009.
33. Steele SR, Wolcott KE, Mullenix PS, et al: Colon and rectal injuries during Operation Iraqi Freedom: Are there any changing trends in management or outcome? *Dis Colon Rectum* 50:870, 2007.
34. Cho SD, Kiraly LN, Flaherty SF, et al: Management of colonic injuries in the combat theater. *Dis Colon Rectum* 53:728, 2010.
35. Guenaga KKFG, Matos D, Wille-Jorgensen P: Mechanical bowel preparation for elective colorectal surgery (Review). *The Cochrane Collaboration* 1, 2009.
36. Vitale GC, Richardson JD, Flint LM: Successful management of injuries to the extraperitoneal rectum. *Am Surg* 49:159, 1983.
37. Hargraves MB, Magnotti LJ, Fischer PE, et al: Injury location dictates utility of digital rectal examination and rigid sigmoidoscopy in the evaluation of penetrating rectal trauma. *Am Surg* 75:1069, 2009.
38. Jacobs LM, Plaisler BR: An efficient system for controlled distal colorectal irrigation. *J Am Coll Surg* 178:305, 1994.
39. Iqbal CW, Cullinane DC, Schiller HJ, et al: Surgical management and outcomes of 165 colonoscopic perforations from a single institution. *Arch Surg* 143:701, 2008.
40. Arora G, Mannalithara A, Singh G, et al: Risk of perforation from a colonoscopy in adults: A large population-based study. *Gastrointest Endosc* 69:654, 2009.
41. Grobmeyer AJ III, Kerlan RA, Peterson CM, et al: Barium peritonitis. *Am Surg* 50:116, 1984.
42. Price SA, Polk HC Jr: Prophylactic and therapeutic use of antibiotics in pelvic surgery (Review). *J Surg Oncol* 71:261, 1999.
43. Pokorny RM, Heniford T, Allen JW, et al: Limited utility of preoperative studies in preparation for colostomy closure. *Am Surg* 65:338, 1999.
44. O'Neill PA, Kirton OC, Dresner LS, et al: Analysis of 162 colon injuries in patients with penetrating abdominal trauma: Concomitant stomach injury results in a higher rate of infection. *J Trauma* 56:304, 2004.
45. Flint LM, Vitale GC, Richardson JD, et al: The injured colon: Relationships of management to complications. *Ann Surg* 193:619, 1981.
46. Samhouri F, Grodskinsky C, Fox T Jr: The management of colonic and rectal injuries. *Dis Colon Rectum* 21:426, 1978.
47. Bartizal JF, Body DR, Folk FA, et al: A critical review of management of 392 colonic and rectal injuries. *Dis Colon Rectum* 17:313, 1974.
48. Galanduik S, Wrightson WR, Young S, et al: Absorbable, delayed antibiotic beads reduce surgical wound infections. *Am Surg* 63:831, 1997.

Colonic Intussusception and Volvulus

Jason F. Hall | David J. Schoetz, Jr.

INTUSSUSCEPTION

Intussusception is defined as the telescoping of a proximal segment of intestine (intussusceptum) into a distal segment of intestine (intussuscipiens). Intussusceptions are classified into three general categories: *enteric* (small bowel into small bowel), *ileocolic* (small bowel into colon), and *colonic* (colon into colon). This disease entity is the most common cause of bowel obstruction in children. Only 5% to 10% of intussusceptions occur in adults, and it is a rare cause (1% to 5%) of adult bowel obstruction.[1,2] Intussusceptions characteristically produce ephemeral signs and symptoms. Although the diagnosis is sometimes difficult, modern cross-sectional imaging is often helpful in confirming the diagnosis.[3,4]

PATHOPHYSIOLOGY

Adult intussusception is thought to originate from pathologic lesions in the wall or lumen of the bowel that produce an alteration in peristaltic activity. This area can then serve as a lead point that permits one segment to invaginate into the next.[5,6] Compromise of the mesentery of the invaginated segment impairs venous outflow leading to bowel wall edema, entrapment of the bowel, and subsequent intestinal obstruction. In adult patients there is a demonstrable pathologic process acting as a lead point in 80% to 90% of patients. Potential causes include benign and malignant tumors of the small and large bowel, inflammatory lesions, appendiceal disease, and Meckel diverticulum.

PRESENTATION AND DIAGNOSIS

The presentation of intussusception can be quite variable. The classic triad of intestinal mass, bloody diarrhea, and crampy abdominal pain that is commonly identified in children is seldom observed in adults. Presenting symptoms in adults are those of partial mechanical bowel obstruction including crampy abdominal pain, nausea, vomiting, and diarrhea. Subacute or recurrent acute attacks are common.[7]

Because patients frequently present with symptoms of partial bowel obstruction, plain films are often employed in the initial evaluation. These may suggest evidence of mechanical obstruction but do not usually confirm the diagnosis. Barium contrast radiography may demonstrate "cup-shaped" or "coil-springed" appearances in patients with ileocolic or colonic disease.[8]

Computed tomography (CT) scanning is considered the most accurate method to confirm the diagnosis of intussusception. Accuracy rates range from 50% to 100%.[2,9,10] CT signs of intussusception include a "target' sign or a sausage-like soft tissue mass. Mesenteric vessels that appear within the lumen of the colon are also diagnostic of intussusception (Figure 151-1).[6]

TREATMENT

All adults who have been demonstrated to have intussusception should be offered operative resection of the involved bowel because of the high likelihood of a tumor, either benign or malignant. This approach is radically different from the treatment of intussusception in children, which relies primarily on reduction with air or barium enema. In adults in whom the condition spontaneously resolves, elective resection should be advised after appropriate investigation of the gastrointestinal tract. Urgent surgical resection may be necessary in the acute setting because of bowel ischemia or due to nonresolution of the obstructive episode. Nonviability mandates resection with primary anastomosis in most instances. Attempts to reduce the nonviable bowel risks intraoperative rupture and contamination of the peritoneal cavity with both succus entericus and tumor cells. It also increases the risk of subsequent anastomotic complications.[2,6,10]

Debate continues as to whether intraoperative reduction should be attempted in patients with a preoperative diagnosis of a benign lesion. This controversy balances concerns over operative rupture against the resection of excessive bowel length. In this situation the intussusception may be gently reduced, followed by a limited resection.[8] In patients with multiple small intestinal polyps (Peutz-Jeghers syndrome) limited resection can be combined with snare polypectomy.[11] Patients with colonic intussusception can most often be treated successfully with subtotal (or limited) colectomy because involvement of the descending colon and sigmoid is rare. If the lead point is in the left colon and preoperative mechanical bowel preparation cannot be achieved, resection with end colostomy and Hartmann closure of the rectum or on-table lavage with primary anastomosis should be considered.[12]

VOLVULUS

Volvulus is derived from the Latin word *volvere*, which means "to twist upon." In the colon, it refers to a condition in which the colon is twisted on its mesentery causing acute, subacute, or chronic colonic obstruction. Patients with colonic volvulus typically have a long and mobile colon that can rotate around a fixed mesenteric base.

Colonic volvulus presents with symptoms of crampy abdominal pain, distention, diminished stool output, and nausea and vomiting. Progression to constant abdominal pain implies the development of ischemia within the affected segment of colon because of compromise of the mesenteric vasculature. Many patients with colonic volvulus describe symptomatic episodes that resolve spontaneously, often with an associated explosive

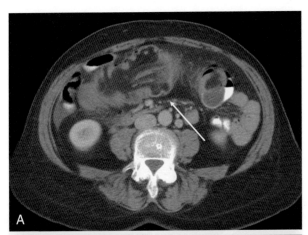

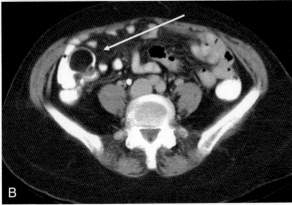

FIGURE 151-1 A, Abdominal CT scan demonstrating the typical "target sign" in a patient with ileocolic intussusception. **B,** Abdominal CT scan showing an ileocolic intussusception with a lipoma as the lead point.

bowel movement or passage of gas. Physical findings typically include tympany, abnormal bowel sounds, and abdominal wall tenderness.

SIGMOID VOLVULUS

Etiology and Pathophysiology

The first known description of a sigmoid volvulus appears in the Ebers Papyrus dating to 1550 BC.[13] Even in antiquity, reduction of the twist in the mesentery was known to be an important step in management. Hippocrates employed air insufflation and a long suppository to reduce the twisted bowel.[14]

Worldwide, sigmoid volvulus represents the leading cause of large bowel obstruction, accounting for 20% to 30% of the cases of intestinal obstruction.[15,16] In the United States, the sigmoid colon is the most common site of volvulus and sigmoid volvulus is the second commonest cause of large bowel obstruction following colon cancer. Sigmoid volvulus is endemic in Africa, India, Pakistan, Middle East, and Eastern Europe. The observed geographic variation in incidence is thought to be due to a much higher consumption of high-fiber diets in the latter locations.[17] High-fiber diets are thought to lengthen the colon, with resulting elongation of the sigmoid

mesentery. A genetic predisposition has also been identified within certain families and tribes.[18,19]

The sentinel predisposing factor for sigmoid volvulus is the presence of a long mesentery with a narrow base.[20] The sigmoid colon can then rotate at least 180 degrees in a clockwise direction around its vascular pedicle. This process results in a closed-loop obstruction of the sigmoid colon and possibly a second closed-loop obstruction of the proximal colon if the ileocecal valve is competent. Intestinal ischemia and necrosis may occur as a result of significant luminal distention and venous or arterial occlusion in the sigmoid mesentery.

The average age of patients with sigmoid volvulus in the United States is in the 60s and 70s, whereas patients in endemic areas tend to be younger. The two sexes are equally affected in English-speaking countries, but males predominate in other parts of the world. There is a higher prevalence of neuropsychiatric disorders in patients from Western countries with sigmoid volvulus. In a collected series of 244 patients, Ballantyne[17] found that 32.4% of patients were admitted from mental institutions and 12.7% were admitted from nursing homes. In addition, sigmoid volvulus is more common in patients with conditions associated with a redundant sigmoid colon such as Chagas disease, Parkinson disease, chronic neurologic disorders, diabetes, chronic constipation, laxative abuse, high-altitude, and previous surgery involving mobilization of the sigmoid colon.

Sigmoid volvulus is the second most common cause of intestinal obstruction (following adhesions) in pregnant women. A redundant sigmoid colon is prone to torsion as the uterus grows out of the pelvis during the second and third trimester. A high index of suspicion is needed in this patient population as symptoms of nausea, vomiting, and abdominal pain can often be incorrectly attributed to pregnancy. Urgent surgical intervention is often required because of the risk to both the mother and fetus.

Diagnosis

Sigmoid volvulus can often be diagnosed with plain radiographs of the abdomen. The classic plain radiographic sign of a sigmoid volvulus is a loop of sigmoid under the left diaphragm. This is sometimes described as the "coffee bean" sign (Figure 151-2).[21] This sign has a sensitivity of 75% and specificity of 100%.[21] Lower gastrointestinal contrast radiography can be obtained to confirm the diagnosis. The classic finding is a "bird's beak" deformity or mucosal spiral pattern at the site of the volvulus (Figure 151-3). Contrast radiography may also be therapeutic and temporarily reduce the volvulus. CT scans of the abdomen are commonly used to diagnose colonic volvulus. Cross-sectional imaging usually demonstrates a "whorl sign," that is, mesenteric fat with engorged vessels that converge toward the center. Dilated ahaustral segments of colon can be observed proximal to the site of obstruction (Figure 151-4).[22]

Treatment

Nonoperative. Endoscopic reduction of sigmoid volvulus should be attempted in patients without evidence of bowel necrosis or perforation. Rigid sigmoidoscopy can

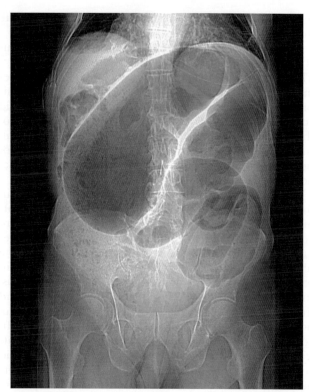

FIGURE 151-2 Plain abdominal radiograph of a sigmoid volvulus with a massively distended loop of colon under the left hemidiaphragm. The colon is the shape of a coffee bean.

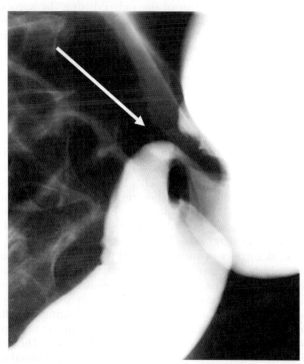

FIGURE 151-3 Barium enema of sigmoid volvulus demonstrating the classic "bird's beak" at the point of the twist.

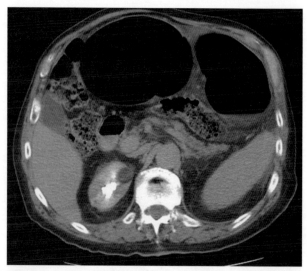

FIGURE 151-4 CT scan of a sigmoid volvulus showing dilated ahaustral segments of colon proximal to the site of obstruction.

be easily performed with minimal air insufflation in the emergency department. This modality allows for direct visualization of the rectal mucosa to exclude the presence of tissue necrosis and a distal neoplastic lesion. The sigmoidoscope can usually be gently passed through the narrowed edematous twisted point of obstruction to reduce the volvulus. A well-lubricated large-diameter rectal tube (no. 30 to 36 French) is then inserted through the sigmoidoscope across the twisted segment and secured to the skin for several days to maintain colonic decompression. An abdominal radiograph should be obtained following endoscopic detorsion to confirm resolution of the volvulus. A reported success rate of 59% was noted in a series of 352 consecutive patients with sigmoid volvulus.[20]

Alternatively, flexible endoscopy using minimal air insufflation and manipulation has been used to permit inspection of the mucosa at and proximal to the point of obstruction; again, a rectal tube is left in place in patients with viable bowel. At the time of flexible endoscopy, a blunt-ended guidewire can be inserted under direct visualization proximal to the volvulus and a rectal tube passed over the guidewire following removal of the endoscope.

Once the sigmoid colon has been detorsed, a number of alternatives to resection have been described. These include percutaneous endoscopic colostomy and endoscopic T-fastener fixation.[22-24] Although these techniques are intriguing, they have been primarily applied in high-risk patients and have not been adopted for most patients.

Operative. After initial reduction by sigmoidoscopy, recurrence of sigmoid volvulus is common. Such a high recurrence rate justifies an elective prophylactic sigmoid resection *during the same hospitalization* except in high-risk surgical candidates.[22,23] After the colon has been detorsed, a mechanical bowel preparation can be administered and a primary anastomosis performed. Laparoscopic resection can be attempted in patients managed conservatively with adequate colonic decompression.

Laparoscopic resection will only be successful in selected patients as colonic distention may preclude adequate visualization for the performance of a safe laparoscopic operation.[24]

Failure to successfully reduce the volvulus endoscopically or clinical evidence of compromised bowel mandates emergent celiotomy. Resection of gangrenous bowel is required; furthermore, the utility of nonresectional surgery is of questionable value in patients with viable colon.[25] A number of reviews have demonstrated a higher mortality rate (25% to 50%) in patients who undergo colostomies in comparison to patients who undergo primary anastomosis (8% to 13%).[26]

Single-stage resection with or without on-table lavage and primary anastomosis may be considered.[27] Some centers have reported mortality rates less than 5% in patients treated with primary anastomosis without bowel preparation.[28,29] As is always the case, there is no substitute for sound surgical judgment. The decision to perform an anastomosis should be governed by the patient's hemodynamic status, the quality of the tissues, and their ability to tolerate the consequences of an anastomotic leak.

ILEOSIGMOID KNOT

Ileosigmoid knotting is an unusual clinical entity in which a loop of ileum wraps around the base of a redundant sigmoid loop, causing a double obstruction of both the colon and the small bowel. The incidence of this disorder in the general population is not well known but ileosigmoid knotting is comparatively more common in the Middle East, Africa, and India.[30] Necrotic intestine is encountered in up to 80% of patients; therefore, prompt resuscitation and surgical decompression are of paramount importance.[31]

The etiology of ileosigmoid knotting is not known. There are a number of predisposing factors including a hypermobile small bowel with an elongated mesentery. A short, redundant, omega-shaped sigmoid also contributes to this phenomenon. High-fiber diets followed by a period of fasting are common historical associations.

Attempts at endoscopic reduction of the volvulus are always unsuccessful, and this diagnosis should be considered in the subgroup of patients in whom endoscopic decompression is not possible. Resection of the involved small bowel is added to whatever procedure is dictated by the condition of the sigmoid. Outcomes following surgical intervention for ileosigmoid knotting depend on the viability of the involved bowel at the time of operation. Mortality following surgical intervention for ileosigmoid knotting complicated by necrosis ranges from 20% to 100%[32] whereas it is only 6% to 8%[33] in patients who do not have gangrenous bowel. These facts emphasize the importance of prompt surgical management.

CECAL VOLVULUS

Etiology and Pathophysiology

In the United States, volvulus of the cecum represents 25% to 40% of cases of colonic volvulus but only accounts for 1% of all intestinal obstructions.[34] In the final stages of normal gastrointestinal embryologic development, the

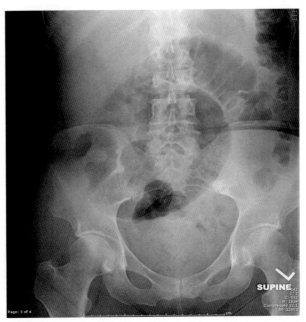

FIGURE 151-5 Abdominal plain film of a patient with cecal volvulus that demonstrates a kidney-shaped colon in the ileocecal region.

right colon rotates in a counterclockwise direction from the left side of the abdomen. Simultaneously, the right colon mesentery becomes fixed to the retroperitoneum. Persons with a lack of retroperitoneal fixation of the right colon are predisposed to axial rotation of the ileocolic junction, resulting in a cecal volvulus. Cadaveric dissections estimate that between 11% and 22% of adults have a sufficiently mobile right colon to allow for development of a cecal volvulus. Predisposing epidemiologic factors are similar to those discussed for sigmoid volvulus and include a history of chronic constipation, obstructing colon lesions, melioration, use of cathartics, pregnancy, and previous abdominal surgery. Cecal volvulus occurs more commonly in females and has been reported in all age groups, with an average age of presentation in the fourth decade.

The term *cecal volvulus* is misleading as this process is often not limited to the cecum alone but usually involves the terminal ileum, ileocecal valve, cecum, and ascending colon. The clinical presentation of cecal volvulus mimics that of small bowel obstruction. Typically, plain abdominal radiographs reveal a dilated kidney bean–shaped ileocecal region with associated proximal small bowel dilation (Figure 151-5). Abdominal CT scans are increasingly used in the evaluation of patients with abdominal pain. There are several CT signs associated with cecal volvulus. These included the "whirl" and "coffee bean" signs (Figure 151-6). The whirl sign refers to engorged mesenteric vessels pointing toward a collapsed cecum. The coffee bean sign refers to an axial view of a dilated cecum with an associated air–fluid level.[35]

A variant of cecal volvulus termed *cecal bascule* is a condition in which a mobile cecum folds interiorly and superiorly over a fixed ascending colon without rotation on the vascular pedicle. This entity is not a true volvulus because axial rotation of the intestine is not associated

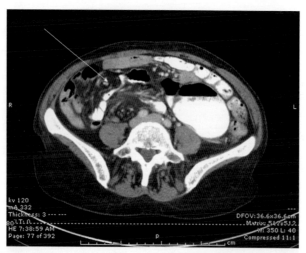

FIGURE 151-6 Abdominal CT of a patient with cecal volvulus that demonstrates the "whirl" sign. The *arrow* points to engorged and swirling mesenteric vessels.

with twisting of the associated mesentery and blood vessels. Although local ischemia and infarction have been reported, vascular embarrassment occurs less frequently. Radiographic investigation with barium enema is useful in diagnosing a cecal bascule, which accounts for 10% of instances of cecal volvulus.[36]

Treatment

Nonoperative. Nonoperative treatment of cecal volvulus with endoscopy is much less successful than in patients with sigmoid volvulus. Colonoscopy is usually reported to be successful in less than 30% of patients.[37] Colonoscopy is potentially dangerous because the procedure insufflates gas into the obstructed segment and may precipitate ischemic changes by increasing the intraluminal pressure. Contrast enemas are often useful in establishing a diagnosis of cecal volvulus as well as ruling out a distal partially obstructing colon lesion that may have predisposed to cecal distention. Attempts at reduction using barium insufflation pressure enemas are contraindicated and potentially dangerous.

Operative. Cecal volvulus is usually treated with surgical intervention. A number of approaches have been described for patients who have viable bowel: detorsion alone, detorsion with fixation, detorsion with cecostomy, and segmental resection all have been advocated. Resection of the involved bowel is required for ischemic or perforated colon, usually with a primary ileocolonic anastomosis. Cecal bascule can be managed with primary resection and anastomosis or cecopexy.

Outcomes Following Treatment

Surgical resection is associated with a recurrence rate of nearly zero compared with approximately 30% to 40% for cecopexy or detorsion alone. Cecopexy involves suturing the right colon to the lateral peritoneal surface. This procedure is risky because the cecum is typically distended and sutures may lacerate the thin-walled intestine or pull-through and fail to secure the cecum in proper position. Recurrence rates following cecostomy

range from 0% to 33%. Postoperative management of a cecostomy tube is associated with a high incidence of abdominal wall and wound complications, as well as a persistent fecal fistula in up to 50% of patients.[38,39] Furthermore, cecostomy tube placement is not an option in the presence of nonviable bowel. As a result, our preference has been to perform a resection and primary anastomosis in most patients with cecal volvulus. As is the case with all other types of volvulus, prompt surgical intervention is of primary importance as operative mortality rates are substantially higher in the presence of intestinal gangrene or perforation.

TRANSVERSE COLON AND SPLENIC FLEXURE VOLVULUS

Etiology and Pathophysiology

Volvulus of the transverse colon or splenic flexure is rare. The broad mesenteric attachment of the transverse colon combined with fixation at the hepatic and splenic flexures precludes rotation of the transverse colon in most patients. The incidence of transverse colon volvulus increases in patients with chronic constipation, distal obstructing lesions, previous abdominal surgery, pregnancy, and hypermobile colonic flexures. Additional risk factors include mental retardation, cerebral palsy, and Hirschsprung disease.[39] Anatomic variants such as absent gastrocolic, lienocolic, and phrenocolic ligaments can also lead to the development of transverse colon volvulus.

Clinical presentation is, again, as outlined earlier and cannot be distinguished from other causes of large bowel obstruction. However, vomiting is thought to be an earlier symptom due to twisting of the transverse mesocolon and compression of the duodenojejunal junction.

Treatment

Nonoperative. Plain abdominal radiographs typically show nonspecific colonic dilation and are frequently misread as a sigmoid volvulus because of the variable position of the transverse colon. As a result, patients are frequently colonoscoped with no clear transition point evident in the sigmoid colon. Under these circumstances, further attempts to identify a transition point should be terminated and a contrast enema study obtained. Although successful colonoscopic decompression has been previously described, there is a risk of excessive insufflation resulting in increased cecal distention and vascular compromise.

Operative. Confirmation of transverse colon or splenic flexure colon volvulus by abdominal CT scan or contrast enema study is generally followed by surgical intervention. Resection of the involved segment is usually required, with primary anastomosis when possible. This can be accomplished with either an extended right hemicolectomy, partial left colectomy, or segmental transverse colectomy. Subtotal colectomy with ileocolonic anastomosis is an attractive single-stage option in the unprepared bowel if the sigmoid colon is not long and tortuous. A technique of fixation without resection has been described in which the redundant transverse colon is sutured to the ascending and descending colon.[40]

Outcomes Following Treatment

Given the rarity of both transverse and splenic flexure volvulus, limited data are available regarding long-term results following the various surgical interventions. Anderson et al[41] reported a 75% recurrence rate in patients treated with colopexy alone. As a result, our bias has been to perform either an extended right hemicolectomy or subtotal colectomy with ileocolonic anastomosis.

REFERENCES

1. Zubaidi A, Al-Saif F, Silverman R: Adult intussusception: A retrospective review. *Dis Colon Rectum* 49:1546, 2006.
2. Azar T, Berger DL: Adult intussusception. *Ann Surg* 226:134, 1997.
3. Boudiaf M, Soyer P, Terem C, et al: CT evaluation of small bowel obstruction. *Radiographics* 21:613, 2001.
4. Beattie GC, Peters RT, Guy S, et al: Computed tomography in the assessment of suspected large bowel obstruction. *Austr N Z J Surg* 77:160, 2007.
5. Haas EM, Etter EL, Ellis S, et al: Adult intussusception. *Am J Surg* 186:75, 2003.
6. Begos DG, Sandor A, Modlin IM: The diagnosis and management of adult intussusception. *Am J Surg* 173:88, 1997.
7. Weilbacher D, Bolin JA, Hearn D, et al: Intussusception in adults: Review of 160 cases. *Am J Surg* 121:531, 1971.
8. Marinis A, Yiallourou A, Samanides L, et al: Intussusception of the bowel in adults: A review. *World J Gastroenterol* 15:407, 2009.
9. Takeuchi K, Tsuzuki Y, Ando T, et al: The diagnosis and treatment of adult intussusception. *J Clin Gastroenterol* 36:18, 2003.
10. Farrokh D, Saadaoui H, Hainaux B: Contribution of imaging in intestinal intussusception in the adult. Apropos of a case of ileocolic intussusception secondary to cecal lipoma. *Ann Radiol* 39:213, 1996.
11. Knowles MC, Fishman EK, Kuhlman JE, et al: Transient intussusception in Crohn disease: CT evaluation. *Radiology* 170:814, 1989.
12. Murray JJ, Schoetz DJ Jr, Coller JA, et al: Intraoperative colonic lavage and primary anastomosis in nonelective colon resection. *Dis Colon Rectum* 34:527, 1991.
13. Kuzu MA, Aslar AK, Soran A, et al: Emergent resection for acute sigmoid volvulus: Results of 106 consecutive cases. *Dis Colon Rectum* 45:1085, 2002.
14. Larkin JO, Thekiso TB, Waldron R, et al: Recurrent sigmoid volvulus—early resection may obviate later emergency surgery and reduce morbidity and mortality. *Ann R Coll Surg Engl* 91:205, 2009.
15. Pahlman L, Enblad P, Rudberg C, et al: Volvulus of the colon. *Acta Chir Scand* 155:53, 1989.
16. Öncü M, Piskin B, Calik A, et al: Volvulus of the sigmoid colon. *S Afr J Surg* 29:48, 1991.
17. Ballantyne GH: Review of sigmoid volvulus: Clinical patterns and pathogenesis. *Dis Colon Rectum* 25:823, 1982.
18. Northeast AD, Dennison AR, Lee EG: Sigmoid volvulus: New thoughts on the epidemiology. *Dis Colon Rectum* 27:260, 1984.
19. Schagen van Leeuwen JH: Sigmoid volvulus in a West African population. *Dis Colon Rectum* 28:712, 1985.
20. Atamanalp SS, Yildirgan MI, Bazoglu M, et al: Sigmoid colon volvulus in children: Review of 19 cases. *Pediatr Surg Int* 20:492, 2004.
21. Raveenthrian V, Madiba TE, Atamanalp SS, et al: Volvulus of the sigmoid colon. *Colorectal Dis* 12:e1, 2010.
22. Tsai MS, Lin MT, Chang KJ, et al: Optimal interval from decompression to semi-elective operation in sigmoid volvulus. *Hepatogastroenterology* 53:354, 2006.
23. Alam MK, Fahim F, Al-Akeely MH, et al: Surgical management of colonic volvulus during same hospital admission. *Saudi Med J* 29:1438, 2008.
24. Fleshman JL: Laparoscopic management of colonic volvulus. *Semin Colon Rectal Surg* 10:154, 1999.
25. Bagarani M, Conde AS, Longo R, et al: Sigmoid volvulus in west Africa: A prospective study on surgical treatments. *Dis Colon Rectum* 36:186, 1993.
26. Madiba TE, Thompson SR: The management of sigmoid volvulus. *J R Coll Edinb* 45:74, 2000.
27. Sule AZ, Misauno M, Opaluwa AS, et al: One stage procedure in the management of acute sigmoid volvulus without colonic lavage. *Surgeon* 5:268, 2007.
28. Raveenthiran V: Restorative resection of unprepared left colon in gangrenous versus viable sigmoid volvulus. *Int J Colorectal Dis* 19:258, 2004.
29. De U, Ghosh S: Single stage primary anastomosis without colonic lavage for left-sided colonic obstruction due to acute sigmoid volvulus: A prospective study of one hundred and ninety-seven cases. *Austr N Z J Surg* 73:390, 2003.
30. Mallick IH, Winslet MC: Ileosigmoid Knotting. *Colorectal Disease* 6, 220, 2004.
31. Alver O, Oren D, Apaydin B, et al: Internal herniation concurrent with ileosigmoid knotting or sigmoid volvulus: Presentation of 12 patients. *Surgery* 137:372, 2005.
32. Hsu ML: Ileosigmoid knot. *J R Coll Surg Edinb* 24:28, 1979.
33. Barnett WO, Petro AB, Williamson JW: A current appraisal of problems with gangrenous bowel. *Ann Surg* 183:653, 1976.
34. Rabinovici R, Simansky DA, Kaplan O, et al: Cecal volvulus. *Dis Colon Rectum* 33:765, 1990.
35. Consorti ET, Liu TH: Diagnosis and treatment of caecal volvulus. *Postgrad Med J* 81:772, 2005.
36. Ballantyne GH, Brandner MD, Beart RW Jr, et al: Volvulus of the colon: Incidence and mortality. *Ann Surg* 202:83, 1985.
37. Renzulli P, Maurer CA, Netzer P, et al: Preoperative colonoscopic derotation is beneficial in acute colonic volvulus. *Dig Surg* 19:223, 2002.
38. Benacci JC, Wolff BG: Cecostomy: Therapeutic indications and results. *Dis Colon Rectum* 38:530, 1995.
39. Asabe K, Ushijima H, Bepu R, et al: A case of transverse colon volvulus in a child and a review of the literature in Japan. *J Pediatr Surg* 37:1626, 2002.
40. Mortensen NJ, Hoffman G: Volvulus of the transverse colon. *Postgrad Med J* 55:54, 1979.
41. Anderson JR, Lee D, Taylor TV, et al: Volvulus of the transverse colon. *Br J Surg* 68:179, 1981.

Colonic Bleeding and Ischemia

Sarah Y. Boostrom | Thomas C. Bower | Scott J. Boley |

Ronald Kaleya

Lower gastrointestinal bleeding is defined as bleeding that occurs distal to the ligament of Treitz. It can be subdivided, however, into small bowel and colonic bleeding for diagnostic and therapeutic purposes. Colonic bleeding, whether acute hemorrhage or chronic, is associated with frequent hospital and clinic visits and admissions, thus resulting in considerable cost to society.[1] Patients typically complain of hematochezia or blood clots per rectum. Modalities of evaluation include endoscopy, nuclear medicine examinations, and angiography. The diagnostic approach used in patients with evidence of lower gastrointestinal bleeding varies with age, presence or absence of active bleeding, and the severity of hemodynamic compromise (Figure 152-1). All patients with lower gastrointestinal blood loss should have at the very least an evaluation of their coagulation profile. Further evaluation is dependent on the rate of blood loss. Imaging, including computed tomography or magnetic resonance angiography, may prove beneficial in diagnosing colonic bleeding as well. An operation with intraoperative endoscopy and subsequent resection may be required, however, in the instance that all other modalities of endoscopy and imaging remain negative.

Although colonic bleeding is a relatively common clinical condition, predictors of morbidity, mortality, and recurrence of bleeding are not well defined. Scoring systems have been attempted by clinicians in order to provide a predictive framework for the diagnosis and management of patients presenting with acute or chronic lower gastrointestinal bleeding. The most recent validation of colonic bleeding by Strate et al reviewed 275 patients and identified predictors of severe bleeding to include heart rate 100 or more beats per minute, systolic blood pressure 115 mm Hg or less, syncope, nontender abdominal examination, rectal bleeding in the first 4 hours of evaluation, aspirin use, and more than two comorbid conditions. Patients were stratified into groups determined by predictors of severe bleeding. Following stratification, the risk of severe bleeding in each category was determined and correlated with clinical outcomes. Predictive scoring models such as this may improve the immediate triage of bleeding patients and allow for a more efficient, standardized approach to lower gastrointestinal bleeding.[2]

Lower gastrointestinal bleeding may be due to multiple factors, including diverticulosis, carcinoma, ischemic colitis, infectious colitis, inflammatory bowel disease, vascular ectasias, and postpolypectomy. The American College of Gastroenterology Bleeding Registry reported that patients with colonic bleeding were more likely to be male, more likely to use alcohol and tobacco, and were more likely to be on aspirin or other nonsteroidal antiinflammatory agents.[3] The most common etiology of lower intestinal bleeding overall is carcinoma; however, the most common symptomatic etiology is diverticulosis.[4-6] Historically reported, the most common etiology in patients older than age 60 years were vascular lesions; however, a recent epidemiology report by Strate in 2005 revealed that this trend may be changing and vascular lesions may prove to be less common.[7,8] In 1982, Mulliken classified vascular lesions into vascular tumors, the majority being congenital, and vascular malformations, those usually acquired over time.[9] In 1996, the International Society for the Study of Vascular Anomalies approved this classification system to establish a common language for the many different medical specialists who are involved in the management of these lesions.

The first section of this chapter will focus on colonic bleeding due to various vascular ectasia and include varying clinical aspects, pathophysiology, and management algorithms. The second section will discuss colon ischemia.

VASCULAR ECTASIAS

Vascular ectasias of the colon, synonymous with angiodysplasia, arteriovenous malformation, and angioectasia, are by far the most common vascular lesions found in the colon and are the most frequent cause of recurrent lower intestinal bleeding after age 60 years.[10] They arise from age-related degeneration of previously normal colonic blood vessels. They are predominantly located in the cecum or ascending colon, are typically multiple in number, and are less than 5 mm in diameter. Multiple series suggest that up to 89% of vascular ectasias of the colon are located in the right colon.[11] Once symptomatic, they are usually diagnosed using colonoscopy or angiography. Other less common vascular lesions of the colon may be congenital or related to other syndromes or diagnoses (Box 152-1).

INCIDENCE AND PATHOPHYSIOLOGY

The prevalence of vascular ectasias in the general population is not known, largely because of the fact that most patients remain asymptomatic. However, a recent report of three prospective studies revealed that in asymptomatic adults undergoing routine screening colonoscopy, the incidence of vascular ectasia was 0.8% (8 of 964 patients).[12] It is estimated that up to 6% of the population older than age 50 years have some form of a colonic vascular lesion.[13] There is no sex predilection for the development and the majority of symptomatic patients are older than age 50 years.

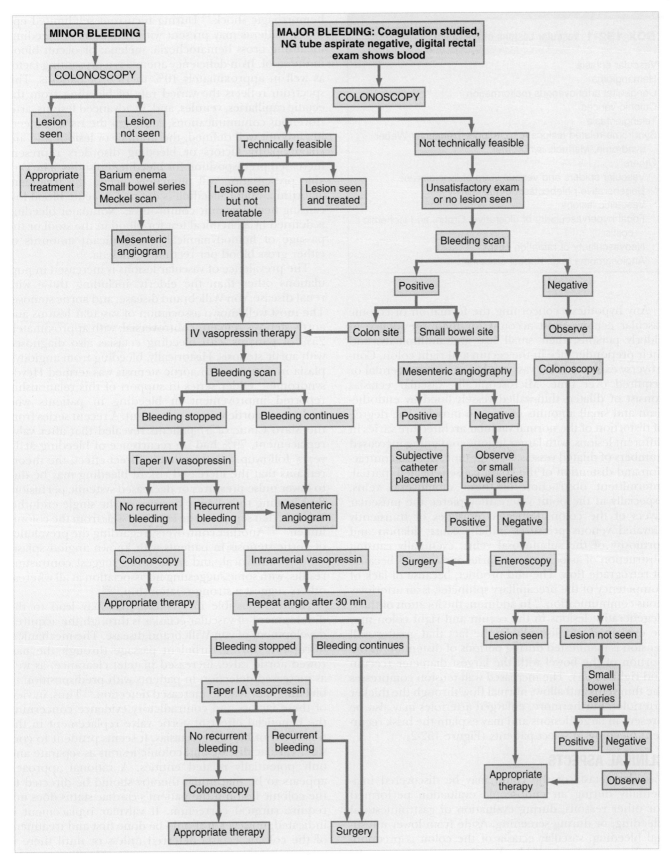

FIGURE 152-1 Diagnostic algorithm for lower intestinal bleeding. *IA,* Intraarterial; *IV,* intravenous; *NG,* nasogastric.

Any hypothesis concerning the formation of colonic vascular ectasias must account for their prevalence in elderly persons, their small size and multiplicity, and their preponderance in the cecum and right colon. Controversy exists whether vascular lesions are congenital or acquired over time. Microscopically, vascular ectasias consist of dilated thin-walled vessels lined by endothelium and small amounts of smooth muscle. The degree of distortion of the normal vascular architecture varies in different lesions, with larger lesions containing increased numbers of dilated vessels.[7,14] Over time, normal contraction and distention of the colon cause repeated, partial, intermittent obstruction of these submucosal veins, especially at the point where they pierce the muscular layers of the colon. Repeated episodes of transiently elevated venous pressures initially cause dilation and tortuosity of the submucosal veins, eventually causing obstruction of associated capillaries and venules because of retrograde flow. The end product, because of lack of competency of the precapillary sphincter, is an arteriovenous communication.[15] In addition, the location of these degenerative lesions in the cecum and right colon may be explained simplistically by the fact that greater wall tension is manifested during periods of distention in the portion of the bowel with the largest diameter (cecum and right colon). The increased wall tension compresses the thin veins and allows normal flow through the thicker arterioles. Furthermore, enlarged arterioles may also be present in larger lesions and may explain the brisk recurrent bleeding in select patients (Figure 152-2).

CLINICAL ASPECTS

Vascular ectasia of the colon may be discovered incidentally during an endoscopic evaluation performed for other reasons, during evaluation of gastrointestinal bleeding, or during screening. Aside from lower intestinal bleeding, vascular ectasia of the colon is predominantly asymptomatic. If bleeding does occur, it is usually recurrent and self-limiting. In fact, in greater than 90% of patients, the bleeding stops spontaneously. However, approximately 15% of patients present with massive hemorrhage, and even less frequently, some present with hemorrhagic shock.[16] During recurrent self-limited episodes, patients may present with variations of bleeding, including gross hematochezia, melena, or occult blood in the stool. Iron-deficiency anemia is a presenting factor as well in approximately 10% to 15% of patients. This spectrum reflects the varied rate of bleeding from the ectatic capillaries, venules, and, in advanced lesions, arteriovenous communications. Although the risks of bleeding are not well defined, the number of lesions and any coagulopathy factors or bleeding disorders represent increased predisposition for bleeding episodes. The variable presentation will ultimately dictate the treatment algorithm. Major bleeding is defined as acute blood loss causing hemodynamic compromise. Nonmajor bleeding is defined by a chemical test for blood in the stool or the passage of hemodynamically insignificant amounts of either gross blood per rectum or melena.

The prevalence of vascular lesions is increased in populations other than the elderly, including those with renal disease, von Willebrand disease, and aortic stenosis. The most well-known association of vascular lesions and aortic stenosis remains controversial, with approximately 25% of patients with bleeding ectasias also diagnosed with aortic stenosis. Historically, bleeding from angiodysplasia in patients with aortic stenosis was termed Heyde syndrome.[17] Older series in support of this relationship reported improvement in bleeding in patients who underwent aortic valve replacement. A recent series from the Mayo Clinic of 57 patients revealed that after valve replacement, 79% had no recurrence of bleeding at 15 years' followup.[18] Rather than a direct effect, the theory remains that the increased risk of bleeding may be due to lower pulse pressures or decreased systemic perfusion, thus leading to ischemic necrosis of the single endothelial layer that separates the ectatic vessels from the colonic lumen.[19,20] Another controversy regarding the prevalence of aortic stenosis in patients with known angiodysplasia remains equivocal, and small series suggest contrasting results, with some suggesting no association at all whereas others suggest a strong relationship.[21,22]

Another possible mechanism that may lead to the development of vascular ectasias is through the acquired development of von Willebrand disease. The mechanical disruption during turbulent passage through the narrowed aortic valve, increased platelet clearance, as well as increased detection in patients with predisposition to bleeding may lead to increased detection.[23] Thus, in view of these factors and contradictory evidence concerning the beneficial effect of aortic valve replacement in the treatment of bleeding ectasias, it seems prudent to consider cardiac disease and colonic lesions as separate and only potentially related entities. A rational approach appears to be that initial therapy should be directed to the colonic lesion if the patient's cardiac status does not require surgical correction. If valvular replacement is indicated, however, it should be done first and treatment of the colonic ectasia deferred unless or until there is continuing or recurrent postoperative bleeding.

DIAGNOSIS

Vascular ectasias of the colon are usually diagnosed with endoscopy, specifically colonoscopy. The vascular lesions

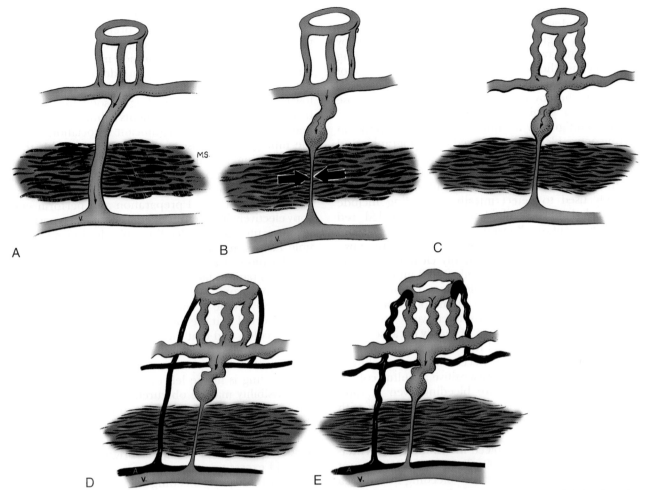

FIGURE 152-2 Diagrammatic illustration of a proposed concept of the development of cecal vascular ectasia. **A,** Normal state of a vein perforating the muscular layers. **B,** With muscular contraction or increased intraluminal pressure, the vein is partially obstructed. **C,** After repeated episodes over a period of many years, the submucosal vein becomes dilated and tortuous. **D,** Later, the veins and venules draining into the abnormal submucosal vein become similarly involved. **E,** Ultimately, the capillary ring becomes dilated, the precapillary sphincter becomes incompetent, and a small arteriovenous communication is present through the ectasia. (From Boley SJ, Sammartano RJ, Adams A, et al: On the nature and etiology of vascular ectasias of the colon: Degenerative lesions of aging. *Gastroenterology* 72:650, 1977, with permission.)

have a characteristic finding of a small flat red lesion with ectatic vessels radiating from the central lesion. The sensitivity of colonoscopic detection of vascular ectasias is estimated to be greater than 80%.[24] Adequate bowel prep as well as visualization around haustral folds is necessary to identify these small lesions. In select cases of occult bleeding, endoscopic means are unable to diagnose vascular lesions. Radiographic imaging or even surgery may be required for diagnosis and, ultimately, treatment.

A nasogastric tube should be inserted in order to exclude an upper gastrointestinal etiology. Bloody aspirate from the nasogastric tube indicates an upper gastrointestinal source, whereas the absence of blood and the presence of bile in the aspirate exclude bleeding proximal to the ligament of Treitz. A clear, nonbilious aspirate is, however, an indication for upper endoscopy in actively bleeding patients because there may be a lesion distal to a closed pylorus. Digital rectal examination and possibly rigid proctosigmoidoscopic examination are prudent in order to exclude anorectal or distal sigmoid pathology.

TREATMENT

Once a colonic vascular ectasia has been identified, management consists of control of the acute hemorrhage followed by definitive treatment of the lesion itself. Major changes in management have occurred since the original descriptions of vascular ectasia and include the increasing roles of therapeutic angiography and endoscopy. In addition, treatment of vascular ectasias depends on multiple factors and varies depending on presenting patient factors, patient clinical status, and available resources.

In past years, definitive treatment of vascular lesions of the colon consisted of some form of colonic resection. Endoscopic therapeutic options were limited. Today, however, use of the argon laser, endoscopic sclerosis, monopolar and bipolar electrocoagulation, and the heater probe for various vascular lesions of the colon, as well as upper gastrointestinal tract, are well described. In institutions where physicians experienced in endoscopic surgery are available, a greater number of patients can be managed endoscopically, and resection is often reserved for patients whose bleeding cannot be stopped or in whom endoscopic treatment is unsuccessful.

Historically, rigid sigmoidoscopy was followed by abdominal scintigraphy, if available, in actively bleeding patients because the latter would allow for localization of the bleeding site or, alternatively, confirm the cessation of bleeding, thereby enabling the clinician to choose colonoscopy or angiography as the next diagnostic modality. Scintigraphy is noninvasive, more sensitive in detecting active bleeding compared to angiography, and capable of identifying bleeding over a 24-hour period.[25] However, it remains less precise and is unable to treat once the lesion is identified. Two radionuclides once commonly used to detect intestinal bleeding include 99mTc-labeled sulfur colloid and 99mTc-labeled red blood cells (RBCs). Previously, 99mTc-sulfur colloid scanning was considered the more sensitive of these two techniques and, because it is rapidly cleared from the circulation (plasma half-life of only 2 to 3 minutes), the best agent for detecting active bleeding. Although it was thought to be less sensitive than sulfur colloid scanning, 99mTc-RBC scanning was considered very useful for detecting intermittent bleeding, primarily because of the 24-hour half-life of Tc-labeled RBCs. It now appears that only 99mTc-RBC labeling is necessary because clinical studies have found that it is as sensitive as sulfur colloid and can reliably detect active bleeding even at rates below 0.1 mL/min.[26] Unlike sulfur colloid scanning, with RBC scintigraphy, serial studies can be obtained for up to 36 hours after a single injection of the radionuclide, thus detecting lesions that bleed intermittently. Furthermore, unlike sulfur colloid, 99mTc-labeled RBCs are not cleared by the liver and spleen, so bleeding in the area of these organs, which is often obscured with sulfur colloid, can be visualized. In contrast to older algorithms, scintigraphy is impractical today and not routinely used. Generally, colonoscopy is performed and continues to increase in diagnostic and therapeutic purposes regarding gastrointestinal bleeding. It should be noted that the patient should be actively resuscitated and hemodynamically stable prior to endoscopy.

Control of Acute Hemorrhage

Management of colonic bleeding follows a similar algorithm regardless of the etiology. Massive hemorrhage is followed by immediate patient assessment and resuscitation. In most patients, acute hemorrhage can be controlled by nonoperative means, and an emergency operation, with its increased morbidity and mortality rates, can be avoided. Patient assessment and resuscitation are followed by the placement of a nasogastric tube in order to rapidly rule out an upper gastrointestinal source. Following the exclusion of an upper gastrointestinal source, endoscopy of the colon is the initial diagnostic and possibly therapeutic examination of choice. In fact, the practice parameters from the American College of Gastroenterology recommend colonoscopy as the initial examination in patients acutely bleeding from a lower gastrointestinal source.[27] Factors related to colonoscopic evaluation including bowel preparation, timing, and success vary. Although a bowel preparation in a massively bleeding patient is unreasonable and endoscopy is

warranted immediately, no data exist regarding recurrence of bleeding related to preparation in patients whose bleeding has ceased. Also, given that blood acts as a cathartic, a full bowel preparation may not prove necessary in the emergent setting. In addition, there are no data regarding the optimum timing of colonoscopy following an acute colonic bleeding episode. In fact, a series from the Mayo Clinic of patients admitted for colonic hemorrhage found no significant association between the timing of colonoscopy after admission with that of encountering bleeding.[28] Thus, in those patients who have bled and spontaneously stopped, urgent colonoscopy does not seem advantageous, and so it is reasonable to administer a bowel preparation and perform endoscopy electively. The results of endoscopy when performed for an acute colonic bleeding episode depend on multiple factors, including the experience of the endoscopist, location of the lesion, magnitude of the bleeding, as well as patient factors such as preexisting coagulopathy. Colonoscopic success ranges in the literature from 69% to 80%. One of the largest clinical series by Rossini et al reported that the most common site of bleeding was the left colon and that the most commonly encountered lesions included carcinomas and diverticula.[29-31] The majority of endoscopists are able to differentiate whether the bleeding is in the left or right colon. The endoscopist's visibility may be obscured by clotted blood within the colon; thus the ability to diagnose vascular lesions of the colon may be limited. Also, vascular lesions may be mimicked by other lesions, including those of inflammatory, neoplastic, and iatrogenic origin. Thus, it is crucial to avoid excess trauma and suction artifact during colonoscopy for actively bleeding colonic vascular lesions. In patients in whom colonoscopy has been successful and an actively bleeding ectasia or fresh mucosal thrombus (i.e., a sentinel clot) has been identified, transendoscopic ablation of the lesion is an effective mode of therapy. The approach of endoscopic treatment depends on the endoscopist, the location of the lesion, as well as the size of the lesion. It is important to recognize that the right colon is thin walled and more prone to perforation than other areas of the colon. Although a variety of treatments are available for use with endoscopy, coagulation with either heater probe or Nd:YAG laser is the treatment of choice and remains the most commonly used mode of therapy for actively bleeding vascular lesions. Other methods of endoscopic treatment include mechanical devices such as clips and bands, injectable agents, and other forms of electrocoagulation. Although banding is more useful in gastric or small bowel lesions and not as common for colonic lesions, reports have described the utilization of endoclips selectively for the management of colonic vascular lesions.[32] Injection of sclerosing agents and argon plasma coagulation are reportedly safe and successful modalities used to treat vascular lesions of the colon through high-frequency energy and ionized gas.[33,34] Submucosal saline injections may prevent perforation by lifting the lesion. However, perforation can happen, with an occurrence of approximately 2% of patients treated with endoscopic coagulation.[35]

In following the American College of Gastroenterology practice parameters, angiography should be used following unsuccessful endoscopy or in the setting of ongoing bleeding. It should also be mentioned that the practice parameters emphasize that there is no role for barium enema in the evaluation of acute, severe colonic bleeding.[27] Angiography can be diagnostic as well as therapeutic. In the majority of cases, active bleeding can be at least temporarily stopped by the transcatheter infusion of vasopressin. A selective superior mesenteric arteriogram is the initial study performed because 50% to 80% of all lower gastrointestinal bleeding occurs in the vascular arcade perfused by the superior mesenteric artery (SMA). Selective inferior mesenteric artery (IMA) and celiac axis (CA) studies are performed in that order if the initial superior mesenteric arteriogram does not identify the lesion. Flush aortography is of no use in identifying bleeding lesions and is not performed. In patients who undergo angiography because colonoscopy was unsuccessful or not technically feasible, injection of intraarterial vasopressin, or selective embolization with gels or cellulose materials may be performed in order to obtain hemostasis in patients in whom extravasation is demonstrated. The intravenous route for vasopressin appears to be as effective as the intraarterial route when the bleeding is in the left colon; however, intraarterial administration has been more successful when the bleeding is from the right colon. The results of arteriography are slightly worse than those of endoscopy and range in the literature from 40% to 78%. Given the necessity for the administration of contrast, arterial access puncture, and use of the vasoconstrictor vasopressin and embolizing material, complications including renal toxicity, arterial injury with bleeding, and ischemia lend a higher complication rate to arteriography when compared to endoscopy. The less optimal results and higher complication rate for angiography support the algorithm for endoscopic attempts prior to angiography.[36-38] Mesenteric arteriography may be productive both in patients with active bleeding and in those who have stopped bleeding. Extravasation of contrast material is the angiographic hallmark of active hemorrhage and can be seen with bleeding rates as low as 0.5 mL/min.[39] Although angiography is more sensitive in detecting diverticular bleeding, extravasation is less common in patients bleeding from vascular ectasias because the bleeding is usually episodic. There are three major angiographic signs of ectasia (Figure 152-3). The earliest sign to develop in the evolution of an ectasia, and hence the one most frequently seen, is a densely opacified, dilated, tortuous, slowly emptying intramural vein that reflects ectatic changes in the submucosal veins. This sign is present in more than 90% of patients with ectasias. A vascular tuft, present in 70% to 80% of patients, represents a more advanced lesion and corresponds to extension of the degenerative process to mucosal venules. An early-filling vein is a sign of even more advanced changes and reflects an arteriovenous communication through a dilated arteriolar/capillary/venular unit. It is a late sign, present in only 60% to 70% of patients. All three angiographic signs are present in more than half of patients with bleeding ectasias. Intraluminal extravasation of contrast material alone is inadequate to diagnose an ectasia, but when seen in conjunction with at least one of the three signs of ectasia, it is indicative of a ruptured mucosal lesion.

In patients with negative endoscopy and angiography in whom the bleeding is significant, operative intervention is warranted. Indications for operative intervention include hemodynamic instability, ongoing transfusion requirements, and persistent hemorrhage not responsive to other methods of treatment. Intraoperative endoscopy remains an option and attempts should be made at identifying the bleeding site. Other methods of intraoperative identification maneuvers include isolating segments of colon and performing colotomies or temporary midtransverse colostomy for identification of a left versus right colonic bleed. However, subtotal colectomy may be required. In patients who have bled and in whom an ectasia of the right colon has been identified by either colonoscopy or angiography, right hemicolectomy remains the treatment of choice if the bleeding is unable to be stopped by endoscopic and angiographic modalities or the size or number of lesions is not amenable to endoscopic or angiographic treatment. The operation entails removing the right colon. It is important that the entire right colon is excised to ensure that no ectasias remain. In addition, because up to 80% of bleeding ectasias are located in the right side of the colon, the risk of leaving the left colon in situ is far outweighed by the increased morbidity and mortality rates for subtotal colectomy.[40] Occasionally, vascular lesions may be oversewn; however, the risk of rebleeding is increased. Directed segmental resection is preferable over blind segmental resection or total colectomy and portrays a lower morbidity and mortality rate. However, subtotal colectomy may be necessary in patients with persistent colonic bleeding and normal colonoscopy and selective angiograms.

Minor Bleeding

Asymptomatic patients or patients with occult blood loss will typically not require the resuscitative efforts of those patients with massive hemorrhage and hemodynamic instability. Evaluation of patients with minor bleeding consists of full colonoscopic examination. Flexible sigmoidoscopy is inadequate as most vascular lesions are located in the right colon. If colonoscopy is negative, esophagogastroduodenoscopy is performed followed by double-contrast radiography of the upper gastrointestinal tract. If these studies are repeatedly normal but occult or slow bleeding continues, small bowel enteroscopy, scintigraphy, or mesenteric angiography may at times be helpful.[41,42] Arteriography, when performed in patients whose bleeding has stopped, is used primarily to diagnose tumor neovascularity or vascular lesions, many of which have characteristic angiographic findings, thereby permitting them to be identified in the absence of extravasation. Another modality of choice used in patients with nonemergent colonic bleeding includes that of nuclear medicine scans. In contrast to arteriography, in which the rate of bleeding necessary to detect bleeding is approximately 1 to 1.5 mL/min, bleeding rates as minimal as 0.1 to 0.4 mL/min may be detectable with nuclear scans. In a number of clinical series, the likelihood of a positive scan performed in the evaluation of acute lower gastrointestinal bleeding ranges from 26% to 72%.[43-45]

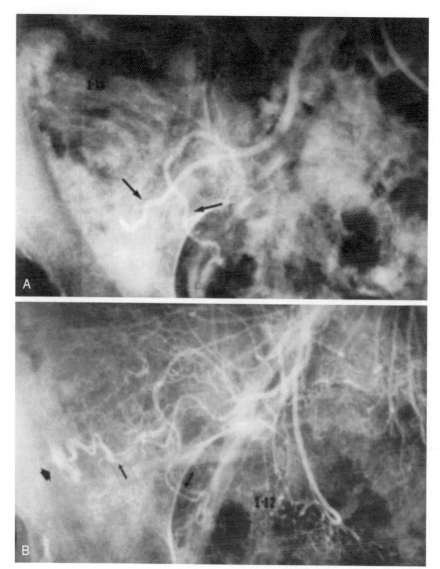

FIGURE 152-3 A, Superior mesenteric arteriogram from a patient with vascular ectasias showing only two densely opacified, slowly emptying, dilated, tortuous cecal veins *(arrows)* at 14 seconds. Note the late visualization of the ileocolic vein after other veins have cleared. **B,** Arterial phase from the same arteriogram showing an avascular tuft *(large wide arrow)* and two early-filling veins *(small arrows)* at 6 seconds. (From Boley SJ, Sprayregen S, Sammartano RJ, et al: The pathophysiologic basis for the angiographic signs of vascular ectasias of the colon. *Radiology* 125:615, 1977, with permission.)

Occasionally, an initially negative 99mTc-RBC study, performed because it was not clinically apparent whether the bleeding had stopped, may reveal extravasation during serial scanning and localize a lesion that bleeds intermittently. Patients with recurrent or persistent major bleeding for which no site of hemorrhage is found may require exploratory laparotomy with attempts at intraoperative localization with endoscopy in order to avoid blind resection of part or all of the colon.

In patients with occult gastrointestinal bleeding or iron-deficiency anemia, endoscopy may reveal evidence of angiodysplasia. However, whether the angiodysplasia is the source of the occult bleeding is unknown in lesions that are not actively bleeding. However, generally angiodysplasia is more likely the etiology in patients with chronic, ongoing occult bleeding, multiple lesions within the colon, or a bleeding diathesis. Thus, if vascular lesions are found on endoscopy in a patient with occult bleeding, treatment should be performed. Distinguishing bleeding vascular lesions from diverticular bleeding, which is more common, may prove difficult in some instances especially because both pathologic entities are present in the same age group.[46] However, specific clinical entities are useful in distinguishing the two diagnoses. For example, bleeding is likely related to a vascular lesion rather than diverticula if the bleeding is venous in origin, there are multiple recurrent episodes of significant bleeding, or the patient has a medical condition associated with angiodysplasia, including renal disease or aortic stenosis as described previously.[47] It should be mentioned that patients with occult gastrointestinal bleeding and medical comorbidities that may exacerbate bleeding have reportedly been managed with hormonal therapy consisting of estrogen, angiogenesis inhibitors, and octreotide or somatostatin.[48-53] However, results are equivocal and data remain limited.

OUTCOMES

Because of the low incidence as well as variable presentation of colonic vascular lesions, reporting success of treatment modalities remains a challenge. Furthermore, reports of colonic vascular lesions are limited. A recent prospective study of 100 patients with colonic vascular lesions, who were treated with argon plasma coagulation, reported cessation of major bleeding with stable hemoglobin values in 85 patients over a mean followup of 20 months. One patient in this study required surgical intervention for continued bleeding.[54] Rebleeding rates following successful endoscopic therapy range from 14% to 53% at 3 years and have been shown to increase with further followup.[55,56] In addition, new lesions over time may develop and prove to be the causative factor for recurrent bleeding. However, endoscopic treatment is preferred over immediate surgical intervention because of the lower morbidity and mortality associated with endoscopic treatment. Furthermore, rebleeding may be treated endoscopically as well.

OTHER VASCULAR LESIONS

As shown in Box 152-1, other vascular lesions that affect the colon may be unrelated to any other clinical process or may be a component of a syndrome or a systemic disease.

HEMANGIOMAS

The second most common vascular lesion of the colon is the hemangioma. Colonic hemangiomas may occur as solitary lesions, as multiple lesions, or as a part of a diffuse gastrointestinal (GI) or multisystem angiomatoses such as blue rubber bleb nevus, Klippel-Trénaunay-Sturge-Weber, Maffucci, and Proteus syndromes. Hemangiomas are usually not present at birth; however, they do have a propensity to proliferate during the first few years of life. Contrasting the constant growth of vascular ectasia due to vessel dilation, hemangiomas may exhibit involution and regression. Hemangiomas may be broadly classified as cavernous, capillary, or mixed.

Clinically, bleeding from colonic hemangiomas is usually slow and produces occult blood loss with anemia or melena. They are usually found in young adults with a long history of episodic and painless rectal bleeding. Hematochezia is less common, except in the case of large cavernous hemangiomas of the rectum, which can cause massive hemorrhage. The diagnosis is best established by colonoscopy. In the presence of gastrointestinal bleeding, hemangiomas of the skin or mucous membranes should suggest the possibility of associated bowel lesions. They can also invade adjacent structures.

Most hemangiomas are small and range from a few millimeters to 2 cm. Larger lesions do occur, however, especially in the rectum. Pathologically, hemangiomas are well circumscribed but not encapsulated. Grossly, cavernous hemangiomas appear as polypoid or mound-like reddish-purple lesions of the mucosa. Sectioning of the lesion reveals numerous dilated, irregular blood-filled spaces within the mucosa and submucosa, sometimes extending through the muscular wall to the serosal surface. The vascular channels are lined by flat endothelial cells with flat or plump nuclei. Their walls do not contain smooth muscle fibers but are composed of fibrous tissue of various thickness (Figure 152-4). Capillary hemangiomas are plaque or mound-like reddish-purple lesions composed of a proliferation of fine, closely packed, newly formed capillaries separated by very little edematous stroma. The endothelial lining cells are large, usually hypertrophic, and in some areas may form solid cords or nodules with ill-defined capillary spaces. There is little or no pleomorphism or hyperchromasia.

Treatment of hemangiomas is typically delayed by several years because of error in diagnosis as well as failed treatment of other pathology, most commonly hemorrhoids. Small hemangiomas that are either solitary or few in number can be treated by colonoscopic laser coagulation. Large or multiple lesions usually require resection of either the hemangioma alone or the involved segment

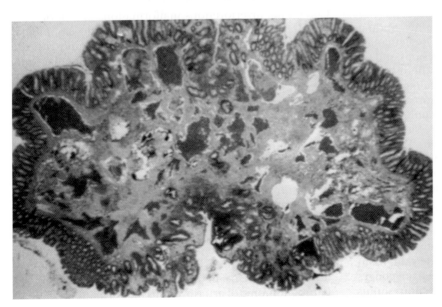

FIGURE 152-4 Polypoid cavernous hemangioma located in the submucosa with focal extension into the mucosa. Note the large, irregular vascular channels with fibrous walls of various thickness (hematoxylin-eosin stain, ×20). (From Boley SJ, Brandt LJ, Mitsudo S: Vascular lesions of the colon. *Adv Intern Med* 29:301, 1984.)

of colon. The hemangioma can either be palpated directly or be revealed by transilluminating the bowel wall with an operative endoscope. The affected area can be resected, which can frequently be accomplished without opening the bowel.

Cavernous Hemangiomas of the Rectum

A distinct form of colonic hemangioma is a cavernous hemangioma of the rectum. These lesions are not usually associated with other gastrointestinal hemangiomas; however, they are typically extensive, with involvement of the entire rectum, portions of the rectosigmoid, and perirectal tissues. They can cause massive, sometimes uncontrollable, hemorrhage, often early in life. Historically, diagnosis was by plain film, revealing multiple phleboliths in cavernous lakes, or barium enema, revealing narrowing and rigidity of the rectal lumen. Today, however, the diagnosis is obtained more often with computed tomography (CT) or magnetic resonance imaging (MRI). Colonoscopy may be both diagnostic and potentially therapeutic. Endoscopically, elevated nodules or vascular congestion causing a plum-red coloration is seen. Ulcers and signs of proctitis may be evident as well. A variety of thermal treatment modalities may be used endoscopically to ablate the lesion; however, treatment of transmural lesions must be avoided. Endoscopic measures as well as angiography may not be successful and typically serve as temporizing measures. Ultimately, the massive bleeding often necessitates excision of the rectum. Although sphincter sparing is ideal, involvement of perirectal tissues may not allow for this.

COLONIC AND EXTRACOLONIC INVOLVEMENT

Diffuse Intestinal Hemangiomatosis

This condition is characterized by numerous, as many as 50 to 100, lesions involving the stomach, small bowel, and colon. Bleeding or anemia generally leads to the diagnosis in childhood. Hemangiomas of the skin or soft tissues of the head and neck are frequently present. Continuous slow, but pernicious, bleeding requiring transfusions or intussusception led by one of the lesions may necessitate surgical intervention. The diagnosis may be made by endoscopy and barium studies; angiographic findings can be normal despite numerous lesions. The hemangiomas are similar in appearance to solitary lesions and are generally cavernous, although some have the histologic appearance of hemangioendotheliomas (benign lesions in children). At surgery, all identifiable lesions should be excised either through enterotomies or by limited bowel resections. Transillumination and compression of the bowel wall are helpful in finding small lesions. When they are multiple, the colon can be opened along a taenia and then intussuscepted on itself. Each hemangioma can be ligated with a surgical clip or polyglycolic acid sutures. Unfortunately, repeated operations may be necessary to control blood loss.

Universal (miliary) hemangiomatosis is usually fatal in infancy. It is, fortunately, a rare condition in which there are hundreds of hemangiomas involving the skin, brain, lungs, and abdominal viscera. Death results from congestive heart failure secondary to large arteriovenous shunts,

or it may be due to local effects of the lesions. Colonic lesions are rarely of significance.

Blue Rubber Bleb Nevus Syndrome (Cutaneous and Intestinal Cavernous Hemangiomas)

In 1860, Gascoyen reported an association between cutaneous vascular nevi, intestinal lesions, and GI bleeding. Bean later coined the term blue rubber bleb syndrome and distinguished it from other cutaneous vascular lesions. A familial history is infrequent, although a few cases of transmission in an autosomal dominant pattern have been reported. Blue rubber bleb nevus syndrome is a rare disease associated with multiple rubbery cavernous hemangiomas on the skin and gastrointestinal tract mucosa which tend to bleed easily. The lesions in this syndrome are distinctive. They vary in size from 0.1 to 5.0 cm, are blue and raised, and have a wrinkled surface. The hemangiomas may be single or innumerable and are usually found on the trunk, extremities, and face, but not on mucous membranes. They increase in size and number with advancing age yet do not undergo malignant transformation.[57] They may be present in any portion of the gastrointestinal tract but are most common in the small bowel. In the colon, they occur more commonly on the left side and in the rectum and are located in the submucosa. Microscopically, they are cavernous hemangiomas composed of clusters of dilated capillary spaces lined by cuboidal or flattened endothelium with connective tissue stroma. They are best detected by endoscopy. Treatment is indicated when the gastrointestinal hemangiomas lead to complications such as severe anemia or massive bleeding. The main goal is to abolish the hemangiomas, thus preventing further bleeding. Resection of the involved segment of bowel is recommended for recurrent hemorrhage; although endoscopic coagulation remains an option, transmural injury of the bowel wall and risk of perforation remains a concern.

LESS COMMON VASCULAR LESIONS

Congenital Arteriovenous Malformations

Congenital arteriovenous malformations are embryonic growth defects and are considered to be developmental anomalies. Although they are found mainly in the extremities, they occur anywhere in the vascular tree. In the colon, they may be small, similar to ectasias, or they may involve a long segment of bowel. The more extensive lesions are most often seen in the rectum and sigmoid.

Histologically, arteriovenous malformations are persistent communications between arteries and veins located primarily in the submucosa. Characteristically, there is arterialization of the veins: tortuosity, dilation, and thick walls with smooth muscle hypertrophy and intimal thickening and sclerosis (Figure 152-5). In long-standing arteriovenous malformations, the arteries are dilated with atrophic and sclerotic degeneration.

Angiography is the primary means of diagnosis. Early-filling veins in small lesions and extensive dilation of arteries and veins in large lesions (Figure 152-6) are pathognomonic of arteriovenous malformations. Patients

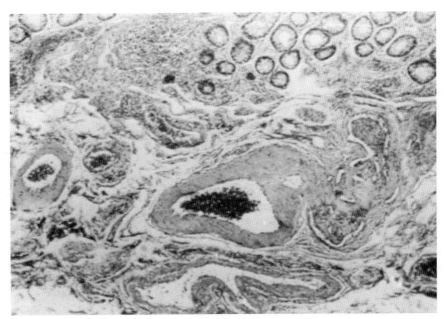

FIGURE 152-5 Arteriovenous malformation characterized by tortuous veins with sclerotic intima, hypertrophied smooth muscle, and thick-walled sclerotic arteries (hematoxylin-eosin stain, ×100). (From Boley SJ, Brandt LJ, Mitsudo S: Vascular lesions of the colon. *Adv Intern Med* 29:301, 1984.)

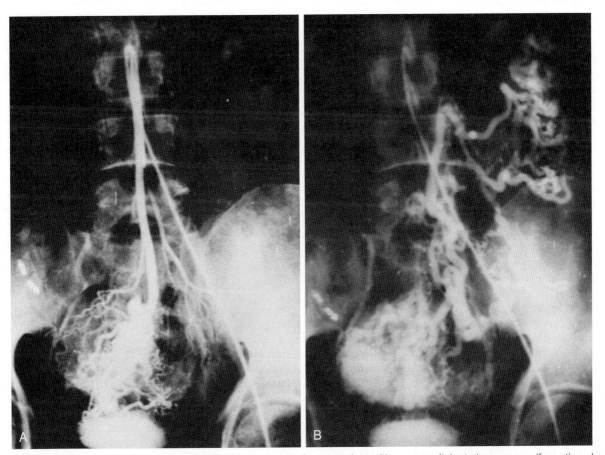

FIGURE 152-6 A, Arterial phase of an inferior mesenteric arteriogram from a patient with a congenital arteriovenous malformation showing multiple dilated arteries going to a large segment of the rectosigmoid. **B,** Venous phase of the same arteriogram showing dilated tortuous vessels to the same segment, as well as to other more proximal areas. (From Boley SJ, Brandt LJ, Mitsudo S: Vascular lesions of the colon. *Adv Intern Med* 29:301, 1984.)

with significant bleeding should undergo resection of the involved segment of colon.

Colonic Varices

Varices of the colon are very rare but may be a cause of hematochezia or melena. In most cases, the varices are located in the rectosigmoid; they are found progressively less often in the more proximal portion of the colon. The most common cause of colonic varices is portal hypertension, with congenital anomalies, mesenteric venous obstruction, congestive heart failure, and pancreatitis accounting for the other causes. Why varices form so rarely in the colon and why they bleed are unclear. Varices are easily diagnosed by proctosigmoidoscopy, colonoscopy, or angiography and may even be seen on conventional barium studies of the colon. Therapy consists of segmental colonic resection, portocaval shunting, or local ligation or sclerosis.

Telangiectasia

Telangiectases are small vascular lesions found on cutaneous, mucocutaneous, and mucosal surfaces throughout the body. Grossly and at endoscopy, they are millet seed sized and appear as cherry-red spots, vascular spiders, smooth hillocks, or lesions resembling ectasias. They may be hereditary or acquired and have been described in association with many disorders (e.g., chronic renal failure, progressive systemic sclerosis, von Willebrand disease, CREST syndrome [calcinosis cutis, Raynaud phenomenon, esophageal dysfunction, sclerodactyly, and telangiectasia]) but are best known as part of Osler-Weber-Rendu disease, or hereditary hemorrhagic telangiectasia.

Hereditary hemorrhagic telangiectasia is a familial disorder characterized by telangiectases of the skin and mucous membranes and recurrent GI bleeding. Lesions are frequently noticed in the first few years of life, and recurrent epistaxis in childhood is characteristic of the disease. By the age of 10 years, about half of patients will have had some bleeding, but severe hemorrhage is unusual before 30 years of age and has a peak incidence from 50 to 60 years. In almost all patients, bleeding is manifested as melena, whereas epistaxis and hematemesis are less frequent. Bleeding may be quite severe, and patients commonly receive more than 50 transfusions in a lifetime. A family history of disease has been reported in 80% of patients with the disorder, but less commonly in those with bleeding, especially when the bleeding occurs later in life.

Telangiectases are almost always present on the lips, oral and nasopharyngeal membranes, tongue, or hand, and lack of involvement of these sites casts suspicion on the diagnosis. Lesions on the lips are more common in patients with GI bleeding than in those without. Telangiectases occur in the colon but are far more common in the stomach and small bowel. Upper gastrointestinal lesions are more apt to cause significant bleeding.

Telangiectases are not demonstrable on barium enema examination but are easily seen on endoscopy. Occasionally, in the presence of severe anemia and blood loss, they transiently become less visible, but with blood replacement they again increase in prominence. Findings on

angiography are usually normal, but it may demonstrate arteriovenous communications or small clusters of abnormal vessels.

Pathologically, the major changes involve the capillaries and venules, but arterioles may also be affected. The lesions consist of irregular, ectatic, tortuous, blood-filled spaces lined by a delicate single layer of endothelial cells and supported by a fine layer of fibrous connective tissue. No elastic lamina or muscular tissue is present in these vessels. The arterioles show some intimal proliferation and often have thrombi in them, suggestive of vascular stasis, but the most conspicuous findings are in the venules. In contrast to those in vascular ectasia, these venules are abnormally thick and have very prominent, well-developed longitudinal muscles. Apparently, these abnormal venules play a major role in regulating blood flow to the telangiectases.

Many treatments have been recommended, including oral and parenteral estrogen therapy and multiple resections of involved bowel. Endoscopic electrosurgery or laser coagulation appears to be most promising and may be performed during active bleeding or before any bleeding episodes. Although endoscopic therapy has diminished the need for resecting bowel in some cases, long-term followup studies are needed to evaluate the ultimate course of patients so treated.

Klippel-Trénaunay-Weber Syndrome

Originally described by Klippel and Trénaunay in 1900, this syndrome is characterized by unilateral congenital lesions of the lower extremities, including (1) cutaneous hemangiomas, usually of the flat, diffuse capillary type; (2) varicose veins dating from childhood; and (3) soft tissue hypertrophy and bony elongation. Involvement of the colon is uncommon and poorly defined, but when lower gastrointestinal involvement does occur, the rectum or rectosigmoid is generally affected.[58]

The cause of the syndrome has been variably ascribed to congenital arteriovenous fistulas or to aplasia, hypoplasia, dysplasia, atresia, or obstruction of the deep venous system. Rectal lesions usually cause bleeding during childhood and have been described by some as being cavernous hemangiomas or varicosities of the rectal veins.[59] Computed tomography scanning and ultrasonography were found helpful in determining the extent of colonic and other visceral disease.[60] Major rectal or bladder bleeding has occurred in a few children, with one reported death. Ligation of bleeding hemorrhoids or sclerosis of rectal veins is often temporarily effective, but proctectomy may be necessary in some patients.

COLONIC ISCHEMIA

Before 1950, colonic ischemia (CI) was considered synonymous with colonic infarction or gangrene. Since that time, CI has become recognized as one of the more common disorders of the colon in elderly persons and the most common form of ischemic injury of the GI tract. CI is used to describe a general pathophysiologic process that leads to varied clinical outcomes. The spectrum includes (1) reversible ischemic colopathy (submucosal or intramucosal hemorrhage), (2) reversible or transient

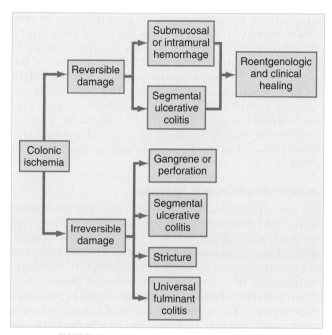

FIGURE 152-7 End results of colonic ischemia.

ischemic colitis, (3) chronic ischemic ulcerative colitis, (4) ischemic colonic stricture, (5) colonic gangrene, and (6) fulminant universal colitis (Figure 152-7).

COLONIC CIRCULATION

The colon is normally protected from ischemia by its abundant collateral circulation. Communications between the CA, SMA, IMA, and iliac artery beds are numerous. Collateral flow around small arterial branches is made possible by the multiple arcades within the colonic mesentery, and SMA or IMA occlusions are bypassed via the arch of Riolan, the central anastomotic artery, and the marginal artery of Drummond. In addition, within the bowel wall there is a network of communicating submucosal vessels that can maintain the viability of short segments of the colon when the extramural arterial supply has been compromised.

The colon has inherently lower blood flow than the small intestine does and is therefore more sensitive to injury during acute reductions in blood flow. Moreover, experimental studies have shown that functional motor activity of the colon is accompanied by decreased blood flow. In contrast, blood flow to the small intestine increases markedly during periods of increased peristalsis and digestion. In addition, the pronounced effect of straining on systemic arterial and venous pressure in constipated versus normal patients provides indirect evidence that constipation may accentuate the adverse circulatory effects of defecation. Geber[61] postulated that "the combination of normally low blood flow and decreased blood flow during functional activity would seem to make the colon (1) rather unique among all areas of the body where increased motor activity is usually accompanied by an increased blood flow and (2) more susceptible to pathology." Other factors that decrease colonic blood flow include changes in the environment, digestion, and emotionally stressful situations.

Experiments evaluating the hypothalamic influence on GI blood flow in the awake cat model suggest that "of the entire GI tract, the colon blood flow is most affected by autonomic stimulation."[62]

PATHOPHYSIOLOGY OF COLONIC ISCHEMIA

What ultimately triggers the episode of CI remains conjectural in most instances. Whether it is increased demand by colonic tissue superimposed on already marginal blood flow or whether the flow itself is acutely diminished has not been determined. However, because CI is a disease of the elderly, an association with degenerative changes of the mesenteric vasculature has been postulated. Histologically, narrowing of small arteries, arterioles, and veins is evident in colons resected for nonocclusive CI. Autopsy studies have also shown abnormal musculature in the wall of the superior rectal artery in the elderly population, which confirms an age-related alteration in the mesenteric vasculature.[63] In addition, postmortem angiographic studies have revealed an age-related tortuosity of the longer colonic arteries that may cause increased resistance to colonic blood flow, thus predisposing the patient to ischemia.[64]

Despite this suggestive evidence for a vascular or autonomic cause of CI, most cases have no identifiable cause. These spontaneous episodes are thought to be the result of local nonocclusive ischemia in association with small vessel disease. Colonic blood flow can be further compromised by alterations in systemic perfusion. The inadequate systemic perfusion accompanying congestive heart failure, digitalis toxicity, or arrhythmias is a rare cause of CI. Many other conditions, spontaneous or iatrogenic, have been associated with CI, although a direct cause-and-effect relationship has not been established (Box 152-2). Two specific and well-recognized exceptions include the development of CI proximal to a potentially obstructing stricture—carcinoma or diverticulitis—and after aortic reconstruction.

DEMOGRAPHICS

The diagnosis of CI is usually made after the period of ischemia has passed and blood flow to the affected segment of colon has returned to normal. Many cases of transient or reversible ischemia are probably missed because the condition resolves before medical attention is sought or because a barium enema or colonoscopy is not performed early in the course of the disease. In addition, many cases of CI are misdiagnosed as infectious colitis or inflammatory bowel disease. Thus, to date, no study has provided an accurate determination of the incidence of CI.

Although historically data were lacking regarding the incidence of CI, recent data have been published on this topic. A research database of insurance claims involving 19 individual states reported an incidence rate in the general population of approximately 7.2 per 100,000 person-years. This study also reported evidence of CI occurring across all age groups, thus challenging the historic thought that CI is only a disease of the elderly.[65] A similar metaanalysis revealed that the incidence of CI in the general population ranges from 4.5 to 44 cases per 100,000 person-years.[66]

Several retrospective reviews of older clinical material have revealed many cases of CI that were either undiagnosed or misdiagnosed because the various clinical manifestations of this disorder were not recognized. Using the modern clinical, roentgenologic, and pathologic criteria for the diagnosis of CI, two retrospective reviews of 154 patients in whom colitis was identified after the age of 50 revealed that approximately 75% of the patients had probable or definite CI. In half of these patients, inflammatory bowel disease had been erroneously diagnosed.[67,68]

CI affecting young individuals has been recognized more frequently in case reports or small series. Causes in the younger population include vasculitis (especially systemic lupus erythematosus),[69] medications (estrogens, danazol,[70] vasopressin,[71] gold,[72] psychotropic drugs[73]), sickle cell anemia,[74] coagulopathies (thrombotic thrombocytopenic purpura,[75] protein C and protein S deficiency,[76] antithrombin III deficiency[77]), competitive long-distance running,[78] and cocaine abuse.[79] It should also be mentioned that distal obstructing lesions of the colon, including carcinoma, stricture, and fecal impaction, may also raise intracolonic pressure, thus reducing colonic flow.[80] It is imperative that such obstructions be excluded from the differential.

CLINICAL MANIFESTATIONS

Symptoms

CI is usually manifested as a sudden onset of mild, crampy abdominal pain, usually localized to the lower left quadrant. Less commonly the pain is severe, or conversely, in other patients the description of pain can be elicited only retrospectively, if at all. An urgent desire to defecate frequently accompanies the pain and is followed, within 24 hours, by the passage of either bright red or maroon blood in the stool. The bleeding is not vigorous, and blood loss requiring transfusion is so rare that it should suggest an alternative diagnosis. Physical examination may reveal mild to severe abdominal tenderness elicited in the location of the involved segment of bowel.

Distribution of Colonic Ischemia

Any part of the bowel may be affected, but the splenic flexure and descending and sigmoid colon are the most common sites (Figure 152-8). No region is spared, although some regions are affected more than others. A recent retrospective series of 313 patients with histologic confirmation of colonic ischemia revealed that segmental involvement is common and involvement of the entire colon is rare.[81] The segmental nature of colonic ischemia is due to the vascular anatomy, specifically the SMA, the IMA, and the superior hemorrhoidal artery. Although specific causes, when identified, tend to affect defined areas of the colon, no prognostic implications can be derived from the distribution of the disease. Nonocclusive ischemic injuries generally involve watershed areas of the colon, which are regions susceptible to ischemic injury because of their location between two different main vascular pedicles. These watershed regions include the splenic flexure and the junction of the sigmoid and rectum. The rectum is very rarely involved because of its abundant dual blood supply from both the splanchnic and systemic arcades. Recently, series have revealed worse outcomes and increased mortality for patients with isolated right-sided colonic ischemia, likely because of the fact that most patients with right-sided ischemia do not have bloody diarrhea and present with main complaint of abdominal pain. Patients noted to have right-sided-only ischemia also more commonly have atrial fibrillation, coronary artery disease, and chronic kidney disease.[82,83] Typically, the length of bowel affected varies with the cause. For example, atheromatous emboli result in short segment changes, and nonocclusive injuries usually involve much longer portions of the colon. Depending on the severity and duration of the ischemic insult, fever or leukocytosis may develop. There is generally no acidemia, hypotension, or septic shock. In more severe ischemia, signs of peritonitis may develop.

Natural History of Colonic Ischemia

Despite similarities in the initial manifestation of most episodes of CI, the outcome cannot be predicted at its onset unless the initial physical findings indicate an unequivocal intraabdominal catastrophe. The ultimate course of an ischemic insult depends on many factors, including (1) the cause (i.e., occlusive or nonocclusive), (2) the caliber of an occluded vessel, (3) the duration and degree of ischemia, (4) the rapidity of onset of the ischemia, (5) the condition of the collateral circulation, (6) the metabolic requirements of the affected bowel, (7) the presence and virulence of the bowel flora, and

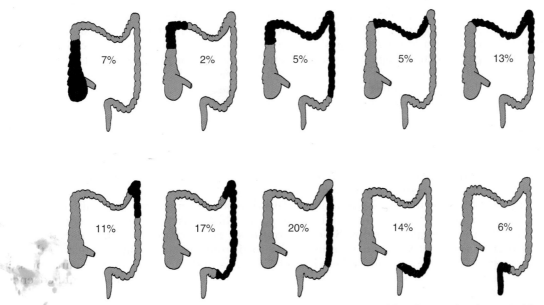

FIGURE 152-8 Distribution and length of involvement in 250 cases of colonic ischemia. More frequent involvement of the left half of the colon is apparent.

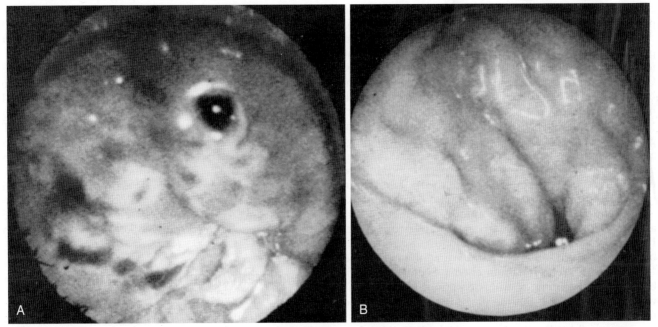

FIGURE 152-9 **A,** Endoscopic appearance of the colon during the initial evaluation of a patient with colonic ischemia. The dark nodular mass is a submucosal hemorrhage below which are ulcerations where other areas of hemorrhage have broken down. **B,** A followup study 3 weeks later demonstrates complete healing of the colonic mucosa. (From Littman L, Boley SJ, Schwartz S: Sigmoidoscopic diagnosis of reversible vascular occlusion of the colon. *Dis Colon Rectum* 6:142, 1963, with permission.)

(8) the presence of associated conditions, such as colonic distention.

Most commonly, symptoms subside within 24 to 48 hours, and clinical, roentgenographic, and endoscopic evidence of healing is seen within 2 weeks (Figure 152-9). More severe, but still reversible, ischemic damage may take 1 to 6 months to resolve. The majority of patients with reversible disease exhibit only colonic hemorrhage or edema, whereas transient colitis develops in about a third. At times, with more severe yet reversible ischemia,

the entire mucosa may slough as a tube. In half of patients with CI, the ischemic damage is too severe to heal, and irreversible disease ultimately develops. In approximately two-thirds of these patients, CI follows a more protracted course and develops into either chronic segmental ulcerative colitis or ischemic stricture. In the remaining third, signs and symptoms of an intraabdominal catastrophe develop, such as gangrene with or without perforation, and become obvious within hours of the initial manifestation.

Patients in whom CI develops as a complication of shock, congestive heart failure, myocardial infarction, or severe dehydration have a particularly poor prognosis. These are typically elderly patients taking digitalis preparations, which may act as potent splanchnic vasoconstrictors and exacerbate the already compromised colonic perfusion. In one series, these factors were present in a fourth of patients with CI, and 12 of 13 patients who were initially seen in shock died.[84]

Because the outcome of an episode of CI cannot usually be predicted, patients must be examined serially for evidence of peritonitis, rising temperature, elevation of the white blood cell count, or worsening symptoms. In patients with diarrhea or bleeding that persists beyond the first 10 to 14 days, perforation or, less frequently, a protein-wasting enteropathy generally develops. Strictures may develop over a period of weeks to months and may be asymptomatic or produce progressive bowel obstruction. Some of the asymptomatic strictures resolve spontaneously over a span of many months.

Diagnosis

Early and appropriate diagnosis of CI depends on serial radiographic or colonoscopic evaluation, or both, of the colon, as well as repeated clinical evaluations of the patient. More severe cases of CI may be difficult to distinguish from acute mesenteric ischemia, whereas patients with less severe cases may have findings similar to those with acute or chronic idiopathic ulcerative colitis, Crohn colitis, infectious colitis, or diverticulitis. A combination of radiographic, colonoscopic, and clinical findings may be necessary to establish the diagnosis of CI.

In a patient with suspected CI, if abdominal radiographs are nonspecific, sigmoidoscopy is unrevealing, and there are no signs of peritonitis, a gentle barium enema or colonoscopy should be performed in the unprepared bowel within 48 hours of the onset of symptoms. The most characteristic finding on barium enema is "thumbprinting" or "pseudotumors" (Figure 152-10) and on colonoscopy is hemorrhagic nodules or bullae. Hemorrhagic nodules seen at colonoscopy represent bleeding into the submucosa and are equivalent to the "thumbprints" seen on barium enema. Segmental distribution of these findings, with or without ulceration, is very suggestive of CI, but the diagnosis of CI cannot be made conclusively on the basis of a single study. In fact, persistence of the thumbprints suggests a diagnosis other than CI, such as lymphoma or amyloidosis.

Repeated radiographic or endoscopic examination of the colon together with observation of the clinical course is necessary to confirm the diagnosis. Segmental colitis associated with a tumor or other potentially or partially obstructing lesions is also characteristic of ischemic disease. The radiographic findings of universal colonic involvement, loss of haustrations, or pseudopolyposis are more typical of chronic idiopathic ulcerative colitis, whereas the presence of skip lesions, linear ulcerations, or fistulas suggests Crohn colitis.

It is imperative to perform the diagnostic study early in the course of the disease because the thumbprinting disappears within days as the submucosal hemorrhages are either resorbed or evacuated into the colon when the overlying mucosa ulcerates and sloughs. Barium enema or colonoscopy performed 1 week after the initial study should reflect the evolution of the disease, either by return to normal or by replacement of the thumbprints with a segmental ulcerative colitis pattern.

If colonoscopy is chosen as the initial study, caution is indicated. Distention of the bowel with air to a pressure greater than 30 mm Hg diminishes colonic blood flow, shunts blood from the mucosa to the serosa, and causes a progressive decrease in the arteriovenous oxygen difference.[85] If intraluminal pressure exceeds 30 mm Hg during routine endoscopic examination of the colon, colonoscopy can potentially induce or exacerbate CI. This risk can be minimized by insufflation with carbon dioxide, which increases colonic blood flow at similar pressures. Furthermore, carbon dioxide is rapidly absorbed from the colon, thus decreasing the duration of distention and elevation of intraluminal pressure.[86]

Biopsies of nodules or bullae identified endoscopically early in the course of CI reveal submucosal hemorrhage, whereas biopsies of the surrounding mucosa usually show nonspecific inflammatory changes.[87] Histologic evidence of mucosal infarction, though rare, is pathognomonic for ischemia. Angiography seldom shows significant occlusions or other abnormalities and is not indicated in patients suspected of having CI. Computed tomography may show thickening of the bowel wall, but this finding is not specific for CI.

Current preoperative diagnostic tools may also include CT angiography. CT angiography allows imaging of the aorta and its branches in axial, coronal, and sagittal planes and is able to identify developed meandering mesenteric artery. If patients are unable to tolerate CT angiography, however, MR angiography is performed in select circumstances. These imaging modalities are particularly helpful when the distinction between chronic and acute mesenteric ischemia cannot be made and when only the ascending colon is involved, thus emphasizing the need to exclude SMA occlusion. A cardiac evaluation, excluding a source of embolic disease, is also necessary.

MANAGEMENT OF COLONIC ISCHEMIA

General Principles

Once the diagnosis of CI has been established and the physical examination does not suggest intestinal gangrene or perforation, the patient is treated expectantly. Parenteral fluids are administered, and the bowel is placed at rest. Historically, antibiotics have been administered with the thought that antibiotics reduce the severity of bowel ischemia. Although most treating physicians continue to administer antibiotics providing coverage against colonic flora, data are lacking and the utility of antibiotics and their efficacy are not proven.[88] Cardiac function is optimized to ensure adequate systemic perfusion. Medications that cause mesenteric vasoconstriction (e.g., digitalis and vasopressors) should be withdrawn if possible. Urine output is monitored and maintained with parenteral isotonic fluids. If the colon appears distended, either clinically or radiographically, it can be decompressed with a rectal tube, with or without gentle saline

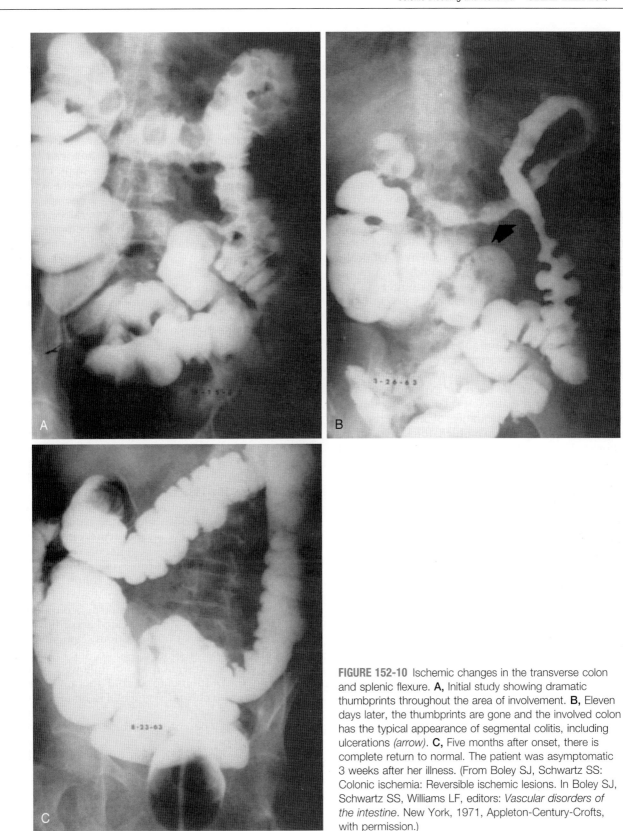

FIGURE 152-10 Ischemic changes in the transverse colon and splenic flexure. **A,** Initial study showing dramatic thumbprints throughout the area of involvement. **B,** Eleven days later, the thumbprints are gone and the involved colon has the typical appearance of segmental colitis, including ulcerations *(arrow)*. **C,** Five months after onset, there is complete return to normal. The patient was asymptomatic 3 weeks after her illness. (From Boley SJ, Schwartz SS: Colonic ischemia: Reversible ischemic lesions. In Boley SJ, Schwartz SS, Williams LF, editors: *Vascular disorders of the intestine.* New York, 1971, Appleton-Century-Crofts, with permission.)

irrigation. Contrary to their efficacy in ulcerative colitis, parenteral corticosteroids are contraindicated because they increase the possibility of perforation and secondary infection. Appropriate management of patients seen during or soon after the ischemic episode requires serial radiographic or endoscopic evaluation of the colon and continued monitoring of the patient.

Determination of the white blood cell count, hemoglobin, and hematocrit should be repeated frequently during the acute episode. Though rarely needed, blood products should be administered according to the patient's requirements. Serum potassium and magnesium levels must be monitored because the levels of these electrolytes may be disturbed by the associated diarrhea and tissue necrosis. Systemic levels of lactate dehydrogenase, creatine phosphokinase, aspartate aminotransferase, and alanine aminotransferase may reflect the degree of bowel necrosis, but these serum markers are neither sensitive nor specific for CI. Patients with significant diarrhea are started on parenteral nutrition early. It should be mentioned, however, that prior to initiating parenteral nutrition, an albumin level should be obtained as hypoalbuminemia has been shown to worsen clinical outcomes in patients with colonic ischemia. Narcotics should be withheld until it is clear that an intraabdominal catastrophe is not present and that the patient is clinically improving. Cathartics are contraindicated. No attempt should be made to prepare the bowel for surgery in the acute phase because such preparation may precipitate a perforation.

Increasing abdominal tenderness, guarding, rebound tenderness, rising temperature, and paralytic ileus during the period of observation suggest colonic infarction. These signs, though not distinct indicators of transmural CI or infarction, dictate the need for expedient laparotomy for resection of the affected segment of colon. At laparotomy, the serosal appearance of infarcted colon ranges from wet tissue paper to mottled, thickened, aperistaltic bowel. The resected specimen should be opened in the operating suite and examined for mucosal injury, and if the margins are involved, additional colon should be removed until the margins appear grossly normal.

Management of Reversible Lesions

In the mildest cases of CI, in which the signs and symptoms of illness disappear within 24 to 48 hours, submucosal and intramural hemorrhages are resorbed, and there is complete clinical and radiographic resolution within 1 to 2 weeks, no further therapy is indicated. More severe ischemic insults result in necrosis of the overlying mucosa with ulceration and inflammation and the subsequent development of segmental ulcerative colitis. Various amounts of mucosa may slough, which may ultimately heal over a period of several months. Patients with such protracted healing may be clinically asymptomatic, even in the presence of persistent radiographic or endoscopic evidence of disease. These asymptomatic patients are placed on a high-residue diet, and frequent followup evaluations are performed to confirm complete healing or the development of a stricture or persistent colitis. Recurrent episodes of sepsis in asymptomatic patients with unhealed areas of segmental colitis are generally caused by the diseased segment of bowel and are an indication for elective resection.

Management of Irreversible Lesions

Perforation usually develops in patients with persistent diarrhea, rectal bleeding, protein-losing enteropathy, or recurrent sepsis for more than 10 to 14 days. Hence, early resection is indicated to prevent this complication. Despite a normal serosal appearance, there may be extensive mucosal injury, and the extent of resection should be guided by the distribution of disease as seen on preoperative studies rather than by the appearance of the serosal surface of the colon at the time of surgery. As in all resections for CI, the specimen must be opened at the time of surgery to ensure normal mucosa at the margins. If at the time of surgery the segmental ulcerative colitis is found to involve the rectum, a mucous fistula or Hartmann procedure with an end colostomy should be performed. The mucous fistula can be fashioned through diseased bowel, and in some cases, this segment will heal sufficiently to allow subsequent restoration of bowel continuity. Local steroid enemas may be helpful in this setting; however, parenteral steroids are, again, contraindicated. Simultaneous proctocolectomy is rarely indicated except in the case of CI after abdominal aortic replacement.

In instances in which the patient has suffered a concurrent or recent myocardial infarction or if the patient has major medical contraindications to surgery, a trial of prolonged parenteral nutrition with concomitant intravenous antibiotic therapy may be considered as an alternative, albeit less optimal, method of management.

MANAGEMENT OF LATE MANIFESTATIONS OF COLONIC ISCHEMIA

CI may not be accompanied by clinical symptoms during the acute insult but may still produce chronic segmental colitis. This form of CI may frequently be misdiagnosed if not seen during the acute episode. Barium enema studies may show a segmental colitis pattern, a stricture simulating a carcinoma, or even an area of pseudopolyposis (Figure 152-11). The clinical course at this stage of disease is often indistinguishable from that of other causes of colitis or stenosis unless the patient has been observed from the time of the acute episode. Crypt abscesses and pseudopolyposis, generally considered histologically diagnostic of chronic idiopathic ulcerative colitis, can also be seen in ischemic colitis. Regardless, the de novo occurrence of a segmental area of colitis or stricture in an elderly patient should be considered to most likely be ischemic and be treated accordingly.

The natural history of noninfectious segmental colitis in the elderly is that of ischemic colitis; the involvement remains localized, resection is not followed by recurrence, and the response to steroid therapy is usually poor. Patients with chronic segmental ischemic colitis are initially managed symptomatically. Local steroid enemas may be helpful, but parenteral steroids should be avoided. In patients whose symptoms cannot be controlled by medication, segmental resection of the diseased bowel should be performed.

MANAGEMENT OF ISCHEMIC STRICTURES

Stenosis or stricture of the colon may develop in patients with asymptomatic segmental ulcerative colitis (Figure 152-12). Strictures that produce no symptoms should be observed, and some of them will return to normal over a 12- to 24-month period with no further therapy. If, however, symptoms of obstruction develop, segmental resection is required. Endoscopic dilation of chronic colonic strictures as a result of ischemia is generally not recommended and data are lacking.

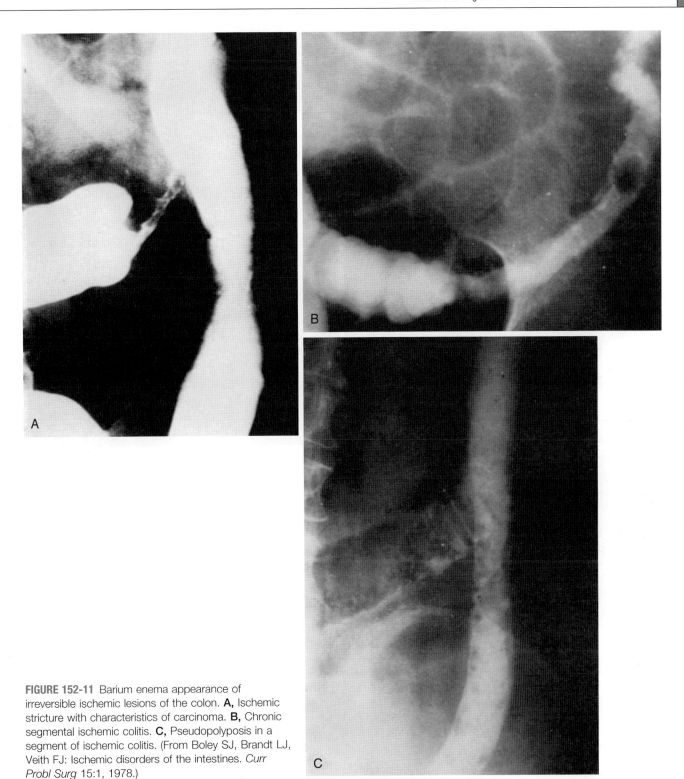

FIGURE 152-11 Barium enema appearance of irreversible ischemic lesions of the colon. **A,** Ischemic stricture with characteristics of carcinoma. **B,** Chronic segmental ischemic colitis. **C,** Pseudopolyposis in a segment of ischemic colitis. (From Boley SJ, Brandt LJ, Veith FJ: Ischemic disorders of the intestines. *Curr Probl Surg* 15:1, 1978.)

Management of Specific Clinical Problems

Colonic Ischemia Complicating Abdominal Aortic Surgery. Mesenteric vascular reconstruction is not indicated in most cases of CI, but it may be required to prevent CI during and after aortic reconstruction. After elective aneurysmectomy, colonoscopic evidence of CI develops in 3% to 7% of patients.[89,90] The incidence of CI after repair of ruptured aortic aneurysms has been reported to be as high as 60%.[91] Although clinical evidence of this complication occurs in only 1% to 2% of patients, when it does occur, it is responsible for approximately 10% of the deaths that take place after aortic replacement.[92]

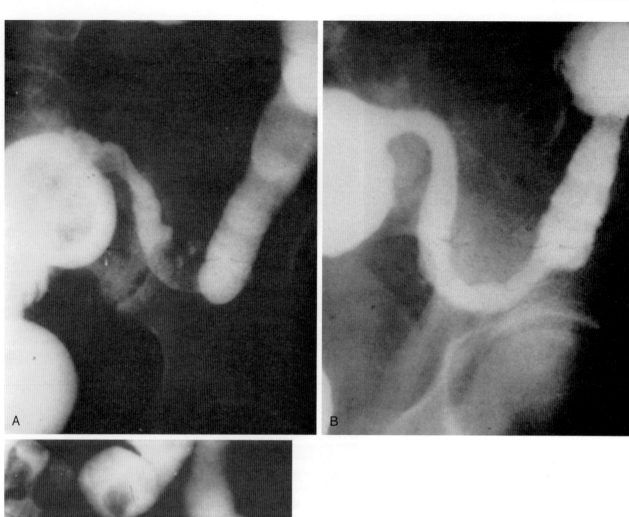

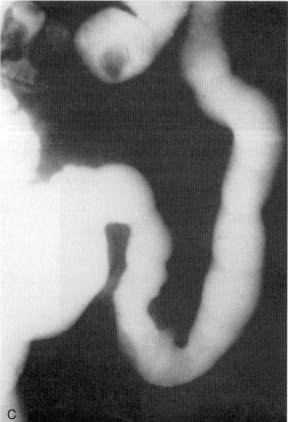

FIGURE 152-12 A, Ischemic stricture of the sigmoid colon. **B,** Eighteen months later, the stricture is still obvious. **C,** Two years after the initial study, the colon has almost returned to normal. (From Boley SJ, Brandt LJ, Veith FJ: Ischemic disorders of the intestines. *Curr Probl Surg* 15:1, 1978.)

Factors that contribute to the occurrence of postoperative CI include rupture of the aneurysm, hypotension, operative trauma to the colon, hypoxemia, arrhythmias, prolonged cross-clamp time, and improper management of the IMA during aneurysmectomy. It also should be mentioned that endovascular repair is now an option for straightforward infrarenal abdominal aortic aneurysms in the elderly. However, open repair is typically performed in younger patients and is required for juxtarenal or suprarenal aortic aneurysms. Thus, if a transperitoneal approach is used to expose the aorta and renal arteries, the IMA and adjacent soft tissues require ligation and division. A small percentage of patients will have an important mesenteric collateral artery running in this pedicle. Should it be necessary to divide these tissues and sacrifice such a collateral, the surgeon must be certain that there is adequate flow to the colon.

The most important aspect of management of CI after aortic surgery is its prevention. Collateral blood flow to the left colon after occlusion of the IMA comes from the SMA via the arch of Riolan ("the meandering artery") or the marginal artery of Drummond and from the internal iliac arteries via the middle and inferior hemorrhoidal arteries. If these collateral pathways are intact, postoperative CI can be minimized. Therefore, aortography is essential before aortic reconstruction. Aortography is advised to determine the patency of the CA, SMA, IMA, and internal iliac artery. The presence of a meandering artery does not, in and of itself, allow safe ligation of the IMA because blood flow in the meandering artery frequently originates from the IMA and reconstitutes an obstructed SMA. Ligation of the IMA in the latter circumstance can be catastrophic and result in infarction of the small and large bowel (Figure 152-13). Ligation of the IMA is safe only when it has been confirmed angiographically that blood flows in the meandering artery from the SMA to the IMA. Reimplantation of the IMA and revascularization of the SMA are therefore required in instances in which the SMA is occluded or tightly stenosed and the IMA provides inflow to the meandering artery (Figure 152-14).

Occlusion of both hypogastric arteries on the preoperative arteriogram indicates that rectal blood flow is dependent on collateral flow from the IMA or from the SMA via the meandering artery. In this circumstance, reconstitution of flow to one or both hypogastric arteries is desirable at the time of aneurysmectomy (Figure 152-15).

At surgery, cross-clamp time should be minimized, and hypotension must be avoided. If a meandering artery is identified, it should be carefully preserved. Because the serosal appearance of the colon is not a reliable indicator of collateral blood flow, several methods have been suggested to determine the need for IMA reimplantation. Stump pressure greater than 40 mmHg in the transected IMA or a mean IMA stump pressure–to–mean systemic blood pressure ratio greater than 0.40 indicates adequate collateral circulation and can be reliably used to avoid IMA reimplantation.[93] The presence of Doppler ultrasound flow signals at the base of the mesentery and at the serosal surface of the colon with temporary occlusion of IMA inflow also suggests that the IMA can be

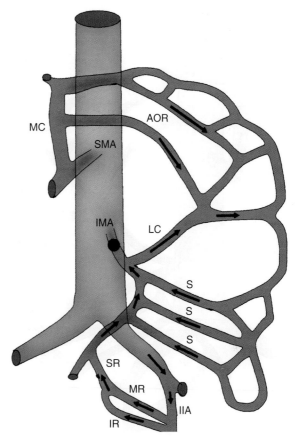

FIGURE 152-13 Collateral blood flow to the colon from the marginal artery, arch of Riolan, and internal iliac artery via the inferior and middle rectal arteries to an occluded IMA. *AOR*, Arch of Riolan; *IIA*, internal iliac artery; *IMA*, inferior mesenteric artery; *IR*, inferior rectal artery; *LC*, left colic artery; *MC*, middle colic artery; *MR*, middle rectal artery; *S*, sigmoid arteries; *SMA*, superior mesenteric artery; *SR*, superior rectal artery.

ligated safely without reimplantation. However, in the presence of superior mesenteric and internal iliac artery disease, the risk of colonic ischemia is increased, and surgeons should have a low threshold to reimplant the IMA. Alternatively, interposition grafts to the internal iliac arteries or reconstruction of the SMA can be performed. If the SMA is occluded, the SMA can be reimplanted on the graft; however, this is only feasible if aneurysms of the perivisceral or pararenal aorta are repaired. The simplest method of reconstructing the SMA is via a short bypass taken from the body of the aortic graft to the SMA with a lateral anastomosis end-to-side. The second alternative is to place a bypass graft from one of the limbs in a C-shaped fashion, so that even though blood flow originates retrograde toward the SMA, the C-shape allows it to be antegrade vis-à-vis the SMA.

The difficulty in accurately assessing CI after surgery and the significant mortality rates associated with its occurrence mandate that postoperative colonoscopy be performed in high-risk patients. Patients at high risk for the development of postoperative CI after aortic reconstruction are those with ruptured abdominal aortic aneurysms, prolonged cross-clamping time, a patent IMA on

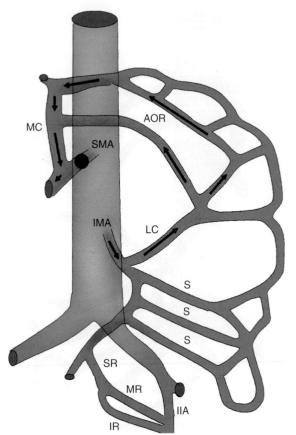

FIGURE 152-14 Collateral blood flow from the IMA via the marginal artery and arch of Riolan to an occluded SMA. *AOR*, Arch of Riolan; *IIA*, internal iliac artery; *IMA*, inferior mesenteric artery; *IR*, inferior rectal artery; *LC*, left colic artery; *MC*, middle colic artery; *MR*, middle rectal artery; *S*, sigmoid arteries; *SMA*, superior mesenteric artery; *SR*, superior rectal artery.

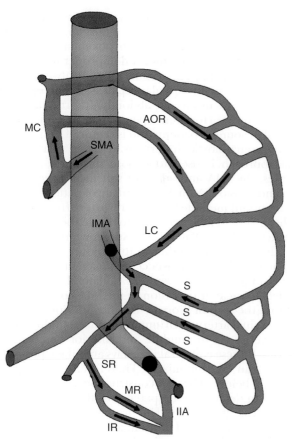

FIGURE 152-15 The entire rectal blood flow is dependent on collateral flow after occlusion of both internal iliac arteries. In this figure, the IMA is also occluded, so rectal blood flow is dependent on collateral flow from the SMA via the arch of Riolan and the marginal artery and then via the superior rectal vessel to the middle and inferior rectal arteries. *AOR*, Arch of Riolan; *IIA*, internal iliac artery; *IMA*, inferior mesenteric artery; *IR*, inferior rectal artery; *LC*, left colic artery; *MC*, middle colic artery; *MR*, middle rectal artery; *S*, sigmoid arteries; *SMA*, superior mesenteric artery; *SR*, superior rectal artery.

preoperative aortography, nonpulsatile flow in the hypogastric arteries at surgery, and postoperative diarrhea. In these cases, colonoscopy is routinely performed within 2 to 3 days of the operation, and if CI is identified, therapy is begun before major complications develop. Clinical symptoms or signs that would suggest postoperative colonic ischemia following aortic surgery include unexplained fever, a slowly worsening metabolic acidosis, increase in fluid requirements, a widening of the A-aO$_2$ gradient, or rarely thrombocytopenia. Moreover, most patients who undergo open abdominal aortic reconstruction are ready to give up retained fluid acquired during operation, usually within 40 to 72 hours after operation. Thus, in the absence of worsening renal function or infection, the need for fluid or retention of fluid at this point is another harbinger of possible colonic ischemia. Clinical deterioration indicating progression of the ischemic insult to transmural necrosis necessitates reoperation. These patients should undergo resection and colostomy. Primary anastomosis is contraindicated because of potential contamination of the aortic prosthesis in the event of an anastomotic leak. If the rectum is involved, it must also be resected. Every effort should be made to protect the aortic graft from contamination; as such, the retroperitoneum overlying the graft should be reperitonealized with local tissues or omentum.

Fulminating Universal Colitis. A rare fulminating form of CI involving all or most of the colon and rectum has been identified in a few patients. These patients experience the sudden onset of a toxic universal colitis. Bleeding, fever, severe diarrhea, and abdominal pain and tenderness, often with signs of peritonitis, have been noted. The clinical course is rapidly progressive. Management of this condition is similar to that for other forms of fulminating colitis. Total abdominal colectomy with an ileostomy is generally required. A second-stage proctectomy has been necessary in some patients within 1 month of the original surgery. The histologic appearance of the resected colon is a combination of ischemic changes, severe ulcerating colitis, and necrosis.

Lesions Mimicking Colon Carcinoma. Ischemic colitis can be accompanied by lesions that appear, on barium enema and colonoscopy, to be colon carcinoma. Colonoscopy may be able to distinguish malignant lesions from those resulting from ischemic cicatrization and is advisable when an annular lesion is identified on barium enema. Treatment is local resection with immediate restoration of bowel continuity.

Colitis Associated With Colon Carcinoma. Acute colitis in patients with carcinoma of the colon has been recognized for many years.[94] The colitis is usually, but not always, proximal to the tumor and occurs with and without clinical obstruction. It is of ischemic origin and has the radiologic and endoscopic appearance of ischemic colitis. Clinically, patients may have symptoms of CI or symptoms related to the primary cancer (i.e., crampy pain of a chronic nature, bleeding, or acute colonic obstruction). In most cases, however, the predominant complaints are related to the ischemic episode—sudden onset of mild to moderate abdominal pain, fever, bloody diarrhea, and abdominal tenderness.

It is imperative for both the radiologist and surgeon to be aware of the frequent association of CI and colon cancer. The radiologist must be careful to exclude cancer in every case of CI, and for the surgeon, it is vital to examine any colon resected for cancer to exclude the presence of an ischemic process in the area of the anastomosis because involvement may lead to stricture or a leak.

REFERENCES

1. Zuckerman GR, Prakash C: Acute lower intestinal bleeding. Part I: Clinical presentation and diagnosis. *Gastrointest Endosc* 48:606, 1998.
2. Strate LL, Saltzman JR, Ookubo R, et al: Validation of a clinical prediction rule for severe acute lower intestinal bleeding. *Am J Gastroenterol* 100:1821, 2005.
3. Peura DA, Gudmundson J, Siepman N, et al: Proton pump inhibitors: Effective first-line treatment for management of dyspepsia. *Dig Dis Sci* 52:983, 2007.
4. Longstreth GF: Epidemiology and outcome of patients hospitalized with acute lower gastrointestinal hemorrhage: A population-based study. *Am J Gastroenterol* 92:419, 1997.
5. Gostout CJ, Wang KK, Ahlquist DA, et al: Acute gastrointestinal bleeding. Experience of a specialized management team. *J Clin Gastroenterol* 14:260, 1992.
6. Gayer C, Chino A, Lucas C, et al: Acute lower gastrointestinal bleeding in 1,112 patients admitted to an urban emergency medical center. *Surgery* 146:600; discussion 606, 2009.
7. Boley SJ, DiBiase A, Brandt LJ, et al: Lower intestinal bleeding in the elderly. *American Journal of Surgery* 137:57, 1979.
8. Strate LL: Lower GI bleeding: Epidemiology and diagnosis. *Gastroenterol Clin North Am* 34:643, 2005.
9. Mulliken JB, Glowacki J, Hemangiomas and vascular malformations in infants and children: A classification based on endothelial characteristics. *Plast Reconstruct Surg* 69:412, 1982.
10. Boley SJ, Sammartano R, Adams A, et al: On the nature and etiology of vascular ectasias of the colon. Degenerative lesions of aging. *Gastroenterology* 72:650, 1977.
11. Danesh BJ, Spiliadis C, Williams CB, et al: Angiodysplasia—an uncommon cause of colonic bleeding: Colonoscopic evaluation of 1,050 patients with rectal bleeding and anaemia. *Int J Colorectal Dis* 2:218, 1987.
12. Foutch PG, Rex DK, Lieberman DA: Prevalence and natural history of colonic angiodysplasia among healthy asymptomatic people. *The Am J Gastroenterol* 90:564, 1995.
13. Heer M, Sulser H, Hany A: Angiodysplasia of the colon: An expression of occlusive vascular disease. *Hepatogastroenterology* 34:127, 1987.
14. Mitsudo SM, Boley SJ, Brandt LJ, et al: Vascular ectasias of the right colon in the elderly: A distinct pathologic entity. *Hum Pathol* 10:585, 1979.
15. Semba T, Fujii Y: Relationship between venous flow and colonic peristalsis. *Jpn J Physiol* 20:408, 1976.
16. Cappell MS, Gupta A: Changing epidemiology of gastrointestinal angiodysplasia with increasing recognition of clinically milder cases: Angiodysplasia tends to produce mild chronic gastrointestinal bleeding in a study of 47 consecutive patients admitted from 1980-1989. *Am J Gastroenterol* 87:201, 1992.
17. Heyde EC: Gastrointestinal bleeding in aortic stenosis (Letter). *N Engl J Med* 259:196, 1958.
18. Thompson JL, 3rd, Schaff HV, et al: Risk of recurrent gastrointestinal bleeding after aortic valve replacement in patients with Heyde syndrome. *J Thorac Cardiovascu Surg* Epub Aug 22, 2011.
19. Cappell MS, Lebwohl O: Cessation of recurrent bleeding from gastrointestinal angiodysplasias after aortic valve replacement. *Ann Intern Med* 105:54, 1986.
20. Scheffer SM, Leatherman LL: Resolution of Heyde's syndrome of aortic stenosis and gastrointestinal bleeding after aortic valve replacement. *Ann Thorac Surg* 42:477, 1986.
21. Bhutani MS, Gupta SC, Markert RJ, et al: A prospective controlled evaluation of endoscopic detection of angiodysplasia and its association with aortic valve disease. *Gastrointest Endosc* 42:398, 1995.
22. Batur P, Stewart WJ, Isaacson JH: Increased prevalence of aortic stenosis in patients with arteriovenous malformations of the gastrointestinal tract in Heyde syndrome. *Arch Intern Med* 163:1821, 2003.
23. Warkentin TE, Moore JC, Anand SS, et al: Gastrointestinal bleeding, angiodysplasia, cardiovascular disease, and acquired von Willebrand syndrome. *Transfusion Med Rev* 17:272, 2003.
24. Richter JM, Hedberg SE, Athanasoulis CA, et al: Angiodysplasia: Clinical presentation and colonoscopic diagnosis. *Dig Dis Sci* 29:481, 1984.
25. Winzelberg GG, Froelich JW, McKusick KA, et al: Scintigraphic detection of gastrointestinal bleeding: A review of current methods. *Am J Gastroenterol* 78:324, 1983.
26. Smith R, Copely DJ, Bolen FH: 99mTc RBC scintigraphy: Correlation of gastrointestinal bleeding rates with scintigraphic findings. *AJR Am J Roentgenol* 148:869, 1987.
27. Zuccaro G Jr: Management of the adult patient with acute lower gastrointestinal bleeding. American College of Gastroenterology, Practice Parameters Committee. *The American Journal of Gastroenterology* 93:1202, 1998.
28. Smoot RL, Gostout CJ, Rajan E, et al: Is early colonoscopy after admission for acute diverticular bleeding needed? *Am J Gastroenterol* 98:1996, 2003.
29. Rossini FP, Ferrari A, Spandre M, et al: Emergency colonoscopy. *World J Surg* 13:190, 1989.
30. Caos A, Benner KG, Manier J, et al: Colonoscopy after Golytely preparation in acute rectal bleeding. *J Clin Gastroenterol* 8:46, 1986.
31. Forde KA: Colonoscopy in acute rectal bleeding. *Gastrointest Endosc* 27:219, 1981.
32. Pishvaian AC, Lewis JH: Use of endoclips to obliterate a colonic arteriovenous malformation before cauterization. *Gastrointest Endosc* 63:865, 2006.
33. Bemvenuti GA, Julich MM: Ethanolamine injection for sclerotherapy of angiodysplasia of the colon. *Endoscopy* 30:564, 1998.
34. Vargo JJ: Clinical applications of the argon plasma coagulator. *Gastrointest Endosc* 59:81, 2004.
35. Naveau S, Aubert A, Poynard T, et al: Long-term results of treatment of vascular malformations of the gastrointestinal tract by neodymium YAG laser photocoagulation. *Dig Dis Sci* 35:821, 1990.
36. Leitman IM, Paull DE, Shires GT 3rd: Evaluation and management of massive lower gastrointestinal hemorrhage. *Ann Surg* 209:175, 1989.
37. Browder W, Cerise EJ, Litwin MS: Impact of emergency angiography in massive lower gastrointestinal bleeding. *Ann Surg* 204:530, 1986.
38. Koval G, Benner KG, Rösch J, et al: Aggressive angiographic diagnosis in acute lower gastrointestinal hemorrhage. *Dig Dis Sci* 32:248, 1987.
39. Nusbaum, M, Baum S: Radiographic demonstration of unknown sites of gastrointestinal bleeding. *Surg Forum* 14:374, 1963.
40. Reinus JF, Brandt LJ: Vascular ectasias and diverticulosis. Common causes of lower intestinal bleeding. *Gastroenterol Clin North Am* 23:1, 1994.
41. Lewis BS, Waye JD: Chronic gastrointestinal bleeding of obscure origin: Role of small bowel enteroscopy. *Gastroenterology* 94:1117, 1988.
42. Schmidt KG, Rasmussen JW, Grove O, et al: The use of indium-111-labelled platelets for scintigraphic localization of gastrointestinal bleeding, with special reference to occult bleeding. *Scand J Gastroenterol* 21:407, 1986.
43. Hunter JM, Pezim ME: Limited value of technetium 99m-labeled red cell scintigraphy in localization of lower intestinal bleeding. *Am J Surg* 159:504, 1990.

44. McKusick KA, Froelich J, Callahan RJ, et al: 99mTc red blood cells for detection of gastrointestinal bleeding: Experience with 80 patients. *AJR Am J Roentgenol* 137:1113, 1981.

45. Nicholson ML, Neoptolemos JP, Sharp JF, et al: Localization of lower gastrointestinal bleeding using in vivo technetium-99m-labelled red blood cell scintigraphy. *Br J Surg* 76:358, 1989.

46. Mudhar HS, Balsitis M: Colonic angiodysplasia and true diverticula: Is there an association? *Histopathology* 46:81, 2005.

47. Sharma R, Gorbien MJ: Angiodysplasia and lower gastrointestinal tract bleeding in elderly patients. *Arch Intern Med* 155:807, 1995.

48. Junquera F, Feu F, Papo M, et al: A multicenter, randomized, clinical trial of hormonal therapy in the prevention of rebleeding from gastrointestinal angiodysplasia. *Gastroenterology* 121:1073, 2001.

49. Lewis BS, Salomon P, Rivera-MacMurray S, et al: Does hormonal therapy have any benefit for bleeding angiodysplasia? *J Clin Gastroenterol* 15:99, 1992.

50. Mimidis K, Kaliontzidou M, Tzimas T, et al: Thalidomide for treatment of bleeding angiodysplasias during hemodialysis. *Renal Failure* 30:1040, 2008.

51. Alberto SF, Felix J, de Deus J: Thalidomide for the treatment of severe intestinal bleeding. *Endoscopy* 40:788; author reply 789, 2008.

52. Blich M, Fruchter O, Edelstein S, et al: Somatostatin therapy ameliorates chronic and refractory gastrointestinal bleeding caused by diffuse angiodysplasia in a patient on anticoagulation therapy. *Scand J Gastroenterol* 38:801, 2003.

53. Junquera F, Saperas E, Videla S, et al: Long-term efficacy of octreotide in the prevention of recurrent bleeding from gastrointestinal angiodysplasia. *Am J Gastroenterol* 102:254, 2007.

54. Olmos JA, Marcolongo M, Pogorelsky V, et al: Long-term outcome of argon plasma ablation therapy for bleeding in 100 consecutive patients with colonic angiodysplasia. *Dis Colon Rectum* 49:1507, 2006.

55. Roberts PL, Schoetz DJ Jr, Coller JA: Vascular ectasia. Diagnosis and treatment by colonoscopy. *Am Surg* 54:56, 1988.

56. Gostout CJ, Bowyer BA, Ahlquist DA, et al: Mucosal vascular malformations of the gastrointestinal tract: Clinical observations and results of endoscopic neodymium: yttrium-aluminum-garnet laser therapy. *Mayo Clin Proc* 63:993, 1988.

57. Wong SH, Lau WY: Blue rubber-bleb nevus syndrome. *Dis Colon Rectum* 25:371, 1982.

58. Ghahremani CG, Kangarloo H, Volberg F, et al: Diffuse cavernous hemangioma of the colon in Klippel-Trénaunay syndrome. *Radiology* 118:673, 1976.

59. Servelle M, Bastin R, Loygue J, et al: Hematuria and rectal bleeding in the child with Klippel and Trénaunay syndrome. *Ann Surg* 183:418, 1976.

60. Jafri SZH, Bree RL, Glazer GM: Computed tomography and ultrasound findings in Klippel-Trénaunay syndrome. *J Comput Asst Tomogr* 7:457, 1983.

61. Geber WF: Quantitative measurements of blood flow in various areas of the small and large bowel. *Am J Physiol* 198:985, 1960.

62. Delaney JP, Leonard AS: Hypothalamic influence on gastrointestinal blood flow in the awake cat. *Fed Proc* 29:260, 1970.

63. Quirke P, Campbell I, Talbot IC: Ischaemic proctitis and adventitial fibromuscular dysplasia of the superior rectal artery. *Br J Surg* 71:33, 1984.

64. Binns JC, Issacson P: Age-related changes in the colonic blood supply: Their relevance to ischemic colitis. *Gut* 19:384, 1978.

65. Cole JA, Cook SF, Sands BE, et al: Occurrence of colon ischemia in relation to irritable bowel syndrome. *Am J Gastroenterol* 99:486, 2004.

66. Higgins PD, Davis KJ, Laine L: Systematic review: The epidemiology of ischaemic colitis. *Aliment Pharmacol Ther* 19:729, 2004.

67. Brandt LJ, Boley SJ, Goldberg L, et al: Colitis in the elderly. *Am J Gastroenterol* 76:239, 1981.

68. Wright HG: Ulcerating colitis in the elderly: Epidemiological and clinical study of an in-patient hospital population [thesis]. Yale University, 1970.

69. Tedesco FJ, Volpicelli NA, Moore FS: Estrogen- and progesterone-associated colitis: A disorder with clinical and endoscopic features mimicking Crohn's colitis. *Gastrointest Endosc* 28:247, 1982.

70. Miyata T, Tamechika Y, Torisu M: Ischemic colitis in a 33-year-old woman on danazol treatment for endometriosis. *Am J Gastroenterol* 83:1420, 1988.

71. Schmitt W, Wagner-Thiessen E, Lux G: Ischaemic colitis in a patient treated with Glypressin for bleeding oesophageal varices. *Hepatogastroenterology* 34:134, 1987.

72. Wright A, Benfield GF, Felix-Davies D: Ischaemic colitis and immune complexes during gold therapy for rheumatoid arthritis. *Ann Rheum Dis* 43:495, 1984.

73. Gollock JM, Thompson JP: Ischaemic colitis associated with psychotropic drugs. *Postgrad Med J* 26:449, 1984.

74. Gage TP, Gagnier JM: Ischemic colitis complicating sickle cell crisis. *Gastroenterology* 84:171, 1983.

75. Dubois A, Lyonnet P, Cohendy R, et al: Ischemic colitis as a manifestation of Moschkowitz's syndrome. *Ann Gastroentrol Hepatol* 25:19, 1989.

76. Blanc P, Bories P, Donadio D, et al: Colite ischemique et thromboses veineuses recidivante par deficit familial en proteine S [letter]. *Gastroenterol Clin Biol* 13:945, 1989.

77. Knot E, Tencate J, Bruin T, et al: Antithrombin III metabolism in two colitis patients with acquired antithrombin III deficiency. *Gastroenterology* 89:421, 1985.

78. Heer M, Repond F, Hany A, et al: Acute ischemic colitis in a female long distance runner. *Gut* 28:896, 1987.

79. Fishel R, Hamamoto G, Barbul A, et al: Cocaine colitis: Is this a new syndrome? *Dis Colon Rectum* 28:264, 1985.

80. Walker AM, Bohn RL, Cali C, et al: Risk factors for colon ischemia. *Am J Gastroenterol* 99:1333, 2004.

81. Brandt LJ, Feuerstadt P, Blaszka MC: Anatomic patterns, patient characteristics, and clinical outcomes in ischemic colitis: A study of 313 cases supported by histology. *Am J Gastroenterol* 105:2245; quiz 2253, 2010.

82. Sotiriadis J, Brandt LJ, Behin DS, et al: Ischemic colitis has a worse prognosis when isolated to the right side of the colon. *Am J Gastroenterol* 102:2247, 2007.

83. Guttorson NL, Bubrick MP: Mortality from colonic ischemia. *Dis Colon Rectum* 32:469, 1989.

84. Boley SJ, Agrawal GP, Warren AR, et al: Pathophysiological effects of bowel distension on intestinal blood flow. *Am J Surg* 117:226, 1969.

85. Kozarek RA, Ernest DL, Silverman ME: Air pressure–induced colon injury during diagnostic colonoscopy. *Gastroenterology* 78:7, 1980.

86. Brandt LJ, Boley SJ, Sammartano RJ: Carbon dioxide and room air insufflation of the colon. *Gastrointest Endosc* 32:324, 1986.

87. Boley SJ, Brandt LJ, Veith FJ: Ischemic disorders of the intestine. *Curr Probl Surg* 15:1, 1978.

88. Díaz Nieto R, Varcada M, Ogunbiyi OA, et al: Systematic review on the treatment of ischaemic colitis. *Colorectal Dis* 13:744, 2011.

89. Ernst CB, Hagihara PF, Daugherty ME, et al: Ischemic colitis incidence following abdominal aortic reconstruction: A prospective study. *Surgery* 80:417, 1976.

90. Zelenock GB, Strodel WE, Knol JA, et al: A prospective study of clinically and endoscopically documented colonic ischemia in 100 patients undergoing aortic reconstructive surgery with aggressive and direct pelvic revascularization: Comparison with historic controls. *Surgery* 106:771, 1989.

91. Hagihara PF, Ernst CB, Griffen WB: Incidence of ischemic colitis following abdominal aortic reconstruction. *Surg Gynecol Obstet* 149:571, 1979.

92. Kim MW, Hundahl SA, Dang CR, et al: Ischemic colitis following aortic aneurysmectomy. *Am J Surg* 145:392, 1983.

93. Ernst CB, Hagihara PF, Daugherty ME, et al: Inferior mesenteric artery stump pressure: A reliable index for safe IMA ligation during abdominal aortic aneurysmectomy. *Ann Surg* 187:641, 1978.

94. Teitjen GW, Markowitz AM: Colitis proximal to obstructing colonic carcinoma. *Arch Surg* 110:1133, 1975.

Diverticular Disease

Jeffrey Cohen | John Welch | Paul Joyner | Kristy Thurston

Diverticular disease of the colon refers to a spectrum of clinical scenarios that can vary from an asymptomatic state to life-threatening peritonitis. This chapter gives a clinical overview of the pathophysiology, diagnosis, and clinical management of a wide variety of complications of the disorder.

PATHOPHYSIOLOGY AND EPIDEMIOLOGY

Colonic diverticulosis refers to the presence of 0.5- to 1-cm saccular outpouchings termed *diverticula*. Anatomically, diverticula are situated between the single mesenteric taenia and one of the antimesenteric taeniae (Figure 153-1). Virtually all patients with diverticulosis have sigmoid involvement (95%), although other segments may be affected as well. About 5% have cecal diverticula.

At least two factors account for formation of diverticula: weak areas in the colonic wall, and a pressure differential between the colonic lumen and the serosa. Diverticula may form in response to development of localized high-pressure zones or segments in the colon and hence the term *segmentation* has been coined (Figure 153-2).[1] Typically they are "pseudodiverticula," with a thin-wall component of a flattened mucosa and submucosa and an attenuated or absent muscularis propria. Diverticula are essentially herniations through the muscular wall of the colon. In addition, there may be gross thickening of the less compliant colonic wall and derangement of the collagen fibers. Increased elastin content in the taeniae may cause shortening of the taeniae, which in turn leads to corrugation of the circular muscle. A defect in cholinergic innervation of the colon has been identified in patients with diverticulosis.

Ten percent to 20% of patients with diverticula develop symptoms from them. Inflammation of one or more diverticula (diverticulitis) sometimes develops, with spread of infection into adjacent or, less commonly, distant sites. The diverticular wall may be devitalized, because of mechanical trauma from fecaliths or from high intracolonic pressures in the presence of an overgrowth of bacteria. Perforation of a diverticulum may be facilitated by commonly ingested nonsteroidal antiinflammatory drugs (NSAIDs) such as low-dose aspirin.[2] Smoking, corticosteroids, obesity,[3] and physical inactivity[4] have also been associated with diverticular complications. "Diverticular colitis" has occurred in the presence of diverticular disease, even in the absence of inflammation of the diverticula themselves. Diverticula can bleed as well, since they occur at sites where intramural vessels penetrate the colonic wall.

Diverticular disease is an affliction that reached prominence in the 20th century. The incidence of diverticulosis increases linearly with age after age 20 years, and hospitalized patients tend to be elderly. The prevalence of diverticulosis approaches 50% in Western adults older than age 60 years. In the United States, the annual age-related admissions for acute diverticulitis increased from 120,500 in 1998 to 151,900 in 2005 (a 26% increase).[5] In England, there was an increase in national admissions from 0.56 to 1.20 per 1000 population/year between 1996 and 2006.[6] The sexes tend to be affected similarly; however, males are affected more frequently under the age of 40 years, whereas females predominate after age 40.[7] Patients of lower economic status with diverticulitis are more likely to present emergently with multiple comorbid conditions.[8] Epidemiologic studies suggest that fiber-deficient diets in the Western world lead to the development of smaller, firmer bowel movements, as well as higher pressures within the sigmoid colon, with areas of segmentation. In areas where high-fiber diets are common (rural Africa), diverticulosis is unusual.

Myoelectric studies of patients with symptomatic diverticular disease show an abnormal slow-wave pattern that returns to normal when they ingest bran. Asymptomatic patients with diverticulosis have unchanged motility patterns after eating bran. Dietary supplementation with fiber increases stool weight, decreases intraluminal pressure, and alters transit time. However, firm evidence is lacking that ingestion of a high-fiber diet actually slows the progression of established diverticulosis or the risk of complications.

DIAGNOSTIC MODALITIES

A number of modalities are available to make the diagnosis of diverticular disease. In the noninflamed colon, diverticula are easily recognized during colonoscopy, although the presence of numerous diverticula can make visualization of the colonic lumen more confusing (Figure 153-3). Radiating folds enter the colonic lumen and by lessening colonic peristalsis, administration of glucagon facilitates identification of the lumen. In the case of active diverticulitis, colonoscopy is generally not indicated because there is risk of converting a minor site of intestinal perforation into a free perforation (Table 153-1). The lumen may also be narrowed by edema and spasm, and the procedure is apt to be painful with fixation of the bowel wall. Little air should be insufflated. The value of the test is limited as well by the fact that diverticulitis is usually extraluminal. In the case of a chronic stricture, it may be quite difficult to enter the area of disease and even to differentiate it from cancer (see later).

Computed tomography (CT) scanning has become the most useful modality for the evaluation of acute

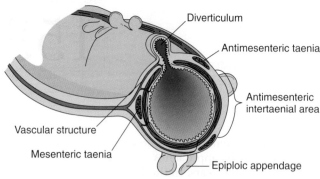

FIGURE 153-1 Anatomy of the colon that contains diverticula.

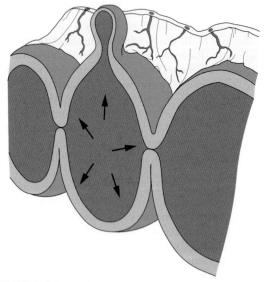

FIGURE 153-2 Schematic representation of the process of segmentation in the colon.

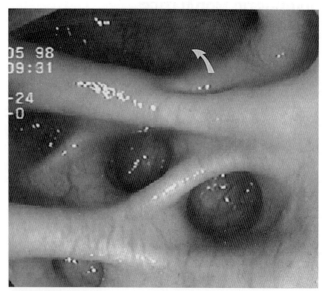

FIGURE 153-3 Multiple sigmoid diverticula seen with the colonoscope. The lumen is seen in the upper portion of the photograph *(arrow)*.

TABLE 153-1 Diagnostic Tools for Acute Diverticulitis

Type of Study	Advantages	Disadvantages
Barium enema	Inexpensive, widely available	Potential for extravasation
CT scan	Extramural detail, abdominal evaluation, therapeutic potential	No mucosal detail
Endoscopy	Mucosal evaluation, ability to biopsy	Perforation, inability to completely evaluate

diverticulitis in hospitalized patients. It defines not only the nature of the process involving the colon (Figure 153-4) but extracolonic changes as well, such as fluid collections, abscesses, extraluminal air, or fistulas. The sensitivity is as high as 97% (Box 153-1).[9] Diseases in other organs such as the ovaries or appendix can also be evaluated.

Appropriate candidates for CT scans are patients with suspected abscess, with deteriorating clinical status despite standard medical treatment, or with suspected complicated diverticulitis. In the uncommon event that findings are unclear, a contrast enema is useful.[10] Helical CT with colonic contrast alone has been suggested to avoid the risks, costs, and delays of oral and intravenous contrast administration. CT scanning may result in more appropriate patient care and allow cost savings.

Experience with magnetic resonance imaging (MRI) is limited, but the technique has high sensitivity and specificity for acute diverticulitis. Furthermore, the technique does not expose patients to radiation.[11]

Contrast studies are still useful in the elective setting (following resolution of the acute process), by showing mucosal details and the anatomic distribution of diverticula (Figure 153-5), or in the uncommon instance when CT findings are unclear. They also help differentiate carcinoma from diverticulitis.[10] The technique is of relatively low cost and is widely available. Contrast studies should be used judiciously in the acute setting because of the risk of iatrogenic perforation. The enema should be done under low pressure with visualization of the involved sigmoid only. In the case of a suspected localized perforation, a water-soluble agent such as Gastrografin should be used because of the deleterious effects of stool and barium in the peritoneal cavity. Water-soluble agents are less reactive in the peritoneal cavity and will be absorbed over time.

CLINICAL FEATURES

UNCOMPLICATED DIVERTICULITIS

The classic signs and symptoms of uncomplicated acute sigmoid diverticulitis are fever, left lower quadrant abdominal pain, irregular bowel habits, and variable urinary symptoms. Patients may complain of diarrhea or of constipation with rectal urgency. The abdomen is maximally typically tender in the left lower quadrant with some rebound tenderness. Plain abdominal films are of

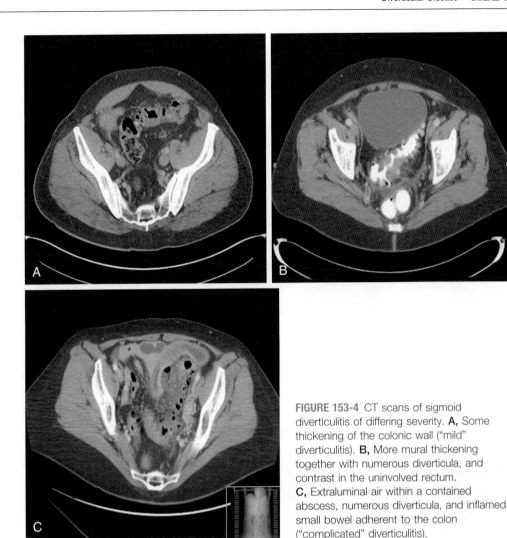

FIGURE 153-4 CT scans of sigmoid diverticulitis of differing severity. **A,** Some thickening of the colonic wall ("mild" diverticulitis). **B,** More mural thickening together with numerous diverticula, and contrast in the uninvolved rectum. **C,** Extraluminal air within a contained abscess, numerous diverticula, and inflamed small bowel adherent to the colon ("complicated" diverticulitis).

BOX 153-1 CT Criteria for Diagnosing Diverticulitis

Presence of sigmoid diverticula
Inflammatory infiltration of pericolonic fat
Thickened colonic wall (>4 mm)
Fluid and/or contrast collection within thickened colonic wall
Pelvic abscess associated with inflamed sigmoid colon
Extrapelvic abscess and/or peritonitis associated with inflamed sigmoid
Fistula formation (especially sigmoidovesical)

From Neff CC, van Sonnenberg E: CT of diverticulitis: Diagnosis and treatment. *Radiol Clin North Am* 27:744, 1989.

---

limited value. The white blood cell count is frequently elevated with a left shift, and the urinalysis is normal. Usually the erythrocyte sedimentation rate is elevated. Patients with uncomplicated diverticulitis are managed either on an outpatient basis or in the hospital, depending on the severity of the attack, with antibiotics and a liquid diet or intravenous fluids. Such attacks may recur after variable time periods, and the frequency of such recurrences weighs in the decision whether to treat patients medically or surgically.

DISEASES CONFUSED WITH DIVERTICULITIS

Diverticulitis and colon cancer are common disorders that may coexist. Differentiating a perforated cancer from diverticulitis or detecting a sigmoid carcinoma amid numerous diverticula may be difficult. Because a perforated cancer will ordinarily require early operation, an effort should be made to establish the correct diagnosis.

CT scanning can be a valuable early test. The patient should receive oral and rectal contrast if possible to increase sensitivity. Certain signs are suggestive of diverticulitis, including (1) localized thickening of the colonic wall; (2) the presence of diverticula; (3) inflammation of the adjacent pericolic fat; and (4) a possible associated fluid collection or abscess. Despite these signs, making the correct diagnosis sometimes is difficult using CT alone.

If contrast studies are chosen, water-soluble contrast is limited to the left colon. Several signs suggest diverticulitis rather than carcinoma, including (1) a gradual rather than abrupt transition from normal to diseased colon; (2) intact mucosa in the abnormal segment; (3) a long involved segment (>6 cm) (Figure 153-6); and (4) an intramural mass deforming the colon with intact

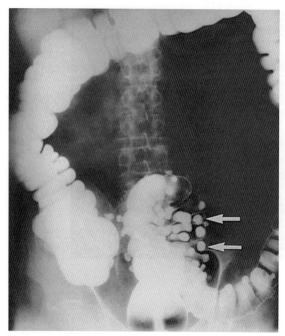

FIGURE 153-5 View from a barium enema showing sigmoid diverticulosis *(arrows)*. (From Oliveira L, Werner SO: Abdominal pain and diverticulosis. In Welch JP, Cohen JL, Sardella WV, et al, editors: *Diverticular disease: Management of the difficult surgical case.* Philadelphia, 1998, Lippincott Williams & Wilkins, p 39.)

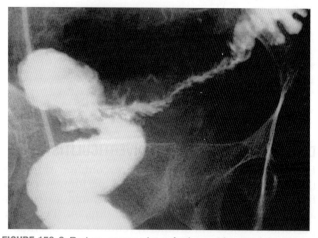

FIGURE 153-6 Barium enema view of a long stricture of the colon. (From Morgenstern L: "Malignant" diverticulitis. In Welch JP, Cohen JL, Sardella WV, et al, editors: *Diverticular disease: Management of the difficult surgical case.* Philadelphia, 1998, Lippincott Williams & Wilkins, p 184.)

mucosa. The greater the number of diverticula, the more difficult it is to detect a neoplasm lying within them; thus, most incorrect diagnoses are false negatives. Other radiologic tests such as ultrasound (endoluminal or transabdominal) or nuclear imaging are of limited value.

Does endoscopy play a role? If rectal bleeding has occurred, the risk of neoplasm is increased and the procedure should be done if possible. Unfortunately, endoscopy can be difficult because of narrowing or spasm of the colon. A risk of worsening a site of local perforation exists as well. If the diseased segment cannot be completely traversed, a neoplasm cannot be ruled out and

operative exploration may be necessary. Colonoscopy is facilitated if associated inflammation is allowed to subside (a useful approach if acute diverticulitis appears more likely than a neoplasm) over a period of 4 to 6 weeks.

Usually diverticulitis and Crohn colitis can be differentiated, except in a few difficult cases. "Red flags" suggesting the possibility of Crohn disease include rectal bleeding, perianal inflammation, unusual fistulas, extraintestinal signs, multiple operations, or postoperative complications. Patients with diverticulitis tend to be older and to have more localized pain. Ongoing diarrhea is suggestive of inflammatory bowel disease. Differential radiologic findings also exist (e.g., presence vs. absence of transverse fissures, or short vs. long paracolic tracts). Histologic features suggesting a Crohn disease type of reaction in a localized segment of diverticulitis should not be given undue weight if diverticulitis is suspected as the primary disease. However, the finding of noncaseating epithelioid granulomas along with deep-fissuring ulcers is virtually pathognomonic of Crohn disease.

Occasional patients with diverticula develop a unique inflammatory pattern in the sigmoid colon that has been termed diverticular colitis. Unlike classic diverticulitis, where the mucosa is spared, diverticular colitis is associated with varying forms of mucosal inflammation, and the diverticular orifices themselves are spared. Patients may develop abdominal pain, diarrhea, or rectal bleeding, and at times the clinical picture can mimic that of ulcerative colitis or Crohn disease. However, improvement usually follows intake of a high-fiber diet and antibiotics, and other portions of the bowel are not involved. The etiology appears to be multifactorial.

Individuals hospitalized in the intensive care unit following cardiovascular or aortic surgery occasionally develop abdominal catastrophes attributed to the colon; ischemic colitis is characteristic in this setting, rather than complicated diverticulitis. Patients with ischemic colitis and diverticulitis complain of abdominal pain, but rectal bleeding is more characteristic of ischemia. An abdominal mass suggests a diverticular phlegmon or abscess rather than ischemia. Endoscopy is the most accurate way to differentiate the two disorders.

Patients with diverticulosis may develop abdominal pain resembling that of diverticulitis.[12] The term *painful diverticulosis* has been coined to describe episodes of abdominal pain and irregular bowel habits. This condition and another source of abdominal pain, the irritable bowel syndrome (IBS), are managed with a high-fiber diet and increased fluid intake, as well as antispasmodics. Patients with IBS have a higher incidence of diverticulosis, and the two conditions may be connected.[13] Other illnesses that can be confused with diverticulitis include appendicitis, pelvic inflammatory disease, and pyelonephritis.

COMPLICATED DIVERTICULAR DISEASE

Included under this designation are a number of complications of diverticular disease that challenge the clinical acumen, judgment, and technical abilities of the surgeon. These include obstruction, abscess or fistula formation, free perforation, and bleeding (Figure 153-7).

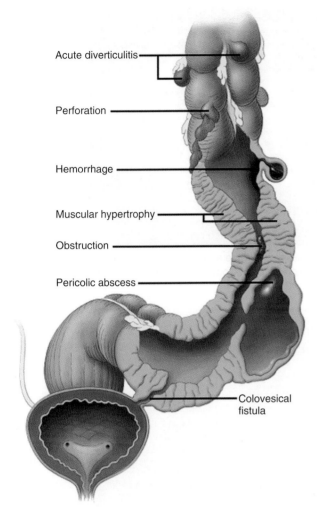

FIGURE 153-7 Complications of diverticular disease. (Redrawn from Zollinger RW, Zollinger RM: Diverticular disease of the colon. *Adv Surg* 5:255, 1971.)

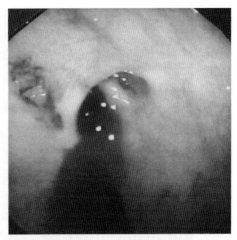

FIGURE 153-8 Colonoscopic view of an actively bleeding diverticulum.

Subacute (Persistent) Diverticulitis

Inflammation accompanying phlegmonous acute diverticulitis usually resolves with bowel rest and antibiotic therapy.[14] However, occasional patients develop a persistent form of inflammation following the onset of diverticulitis that fails to respond to standard treatment. Characteristically an abscess is not present but the patient does have persistent pain, a low-grade fever, possible urinary symptoms, and failure to thrive. An abdominal mass may be present. Some patients have few symptoms such as vague pelvic discomfort. Because of the varied clinical presentation, definitive surgical treatment is often delayed, and the irritable bowel syndrome must be ruled out.

Because the inflammation is persistent rather than episodic or brief, the colon tends to thicken with development of fibrosis. Patients will often develop chronic symptoms of partial large bowel obstruction. Attempts should be made in these patients to prepare the bowel for a one-stage resection and anastomosis, as the obstruction is rarely complete.

Diverticular Hemorrhage

Diverticulosis is the most common cause of lower gastrointestinal bleeding of colonic origin (30% to 50%), followed by inflammatory bowel disease, neoplasia (polyps and cancer), coagulopathy, benign anorectal disease, and arteriovenous malformations. Disorders proximal to the ligament of Treitz cause 10% to 15% of rectal bleeds, and small bowel disease accounts for 3% to 5%.

Patients with diverticular bleeding tend to be elderly males[7] with diseases such as hypertension or atherosclerosis. Hospitalizations for this complication will likely increase in the future. Anticoagulation and diabetes mellitus are also associated with diverticular hemorrhage.[15] The bleeding likely is caused by a ruptured vas rectum that has undergone intimal proliferation and has been damaged by traumatic factors within the diverticulum or the lumen of the colon.[16] In half the cases, bleeding originates in the right colon, despite the fact that diverticula are situated much more commonly in the sigmoid. Regular use of NSAIDs may potentiate bleeding from diverticula.

Most diverticular bleeds are self-limited. Monitoring is per standard protocol, with its intensity based on the severity of the bleeding and the patient risk. Transfusions may be needed, especially in patients with anemia or heart disease. Colonoscopy can then be performed (Figure 153-8). There are a few reports of aggressive colonoscopy within hours of hospitalization (following an oral purge). Just as with an upper gastrointestinal bleed, endoscopists can use epinephrine injections or coagulation at the site of the diverticular bleed, and the colon can be tattooed to facilitate surgical recognition of the bleeding site. There are also reports of endoscopic band ligation and of endoclip usage on the protruding vessels in bleeding diverticula. Mechanical clips have the theoretic advantage of marking the bleeding site.[17]

Only 3% to 5% of patients with diverticular bleeding have massive bleeding.[15] Hypotensive patients need aggressive resuscitation followed by computed tomographic angiography (CTA) or arteriography (Figure 153-9). Operative exploration is the only alternative if the blood pressure cannot be maintained. For some patients

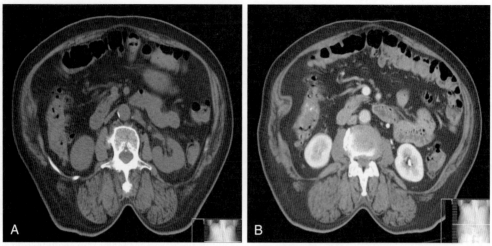

FIGURE 153-9 **A,** Noncontrast phase of abdominal CTA, revealing multiple diverticula in the ascending colon. **B,** Contrast phase of abdominal CTA, with extravasation from bleeding diverticulum in ascending colon. *CTA,* Computed tomographic angiography.

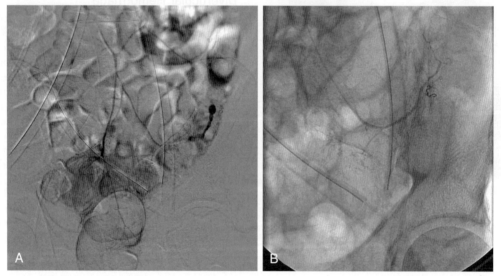

FIGURE 153-10 **A,** Selective angiographic view, showing active extravasation from perforating branch of the left colic artery at junction of sigmoid and descending colon. **B,** View post superselective embolization shows intact marginal artery and complete occlusion of bleeding vessel with microcoils.

who can be stabilized, angiographic approaches provide both a sensitive diagnostic and capable therapeutic avenue. To this end, contrast studies with oral or rectal contrast should be avoided, as they interfere with the ability to perform accurate angiography. In the event of a positive arteriogram, vasopressin and more recent angioembolization techniques have been used successfully (Figure 153-10). Certain situations may call for a "provocative" angiogram using agents such as urokinase, heparin, or tolazoline to promote localization by inducing bleeding. There have been reports of cessation of all bleeding with barium enema in patients who have failed both endoscopic and angiographic therapies.[18]

Pericolic Abscess

An inflammatory mass adjacent to the colon may develop into an abscess, the most common complication of acute diverticulitis, occurring in 10% to 68% of patients. It begins as a small abscess in the sigmoid mesentery and may remain localized by adherence of omentum and adjacent viscera. The collection may also enlarge and extend to more distant sites such as the pelvis. Retroperitoneal abscesses may extend into extraabdominal areas such as the hip, groin, flank, or leg.

Abscesses cause fever and chills, and a tender mass may be felt on abdominal, rectal, or vaginal examination. Leukocytosis is characteristic.

When an abscess is suspected, a CT scan is the imaging test of choice, because the study delineates the size and the location of the collection and the feasibility of CT-guided aspiration or drainage.

Fistula

Some abscesses complicating diverticulitis lead to the formation of fistulas by rupturing into adjacent viscera. The most common (50% to 65%) are colovesical fistulas.

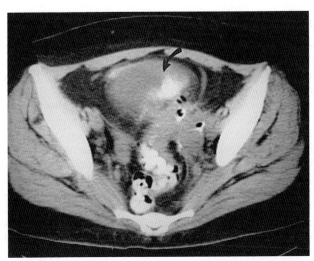

FIGURE 153-11 In this patient who had a sigmoidovesical fistula, rectal contrast was administered and contrast filling of the bladder is present *(arrow)*. (From Markowitz SK, Kirejczyk W: Radiologic evaluation of diverticular disease of the small and large intestines. In Welch JP, Cohen JL, Sardella WV, et al, editors: *Diverticular disease: Management of the difficult surgical case.* Philadelphia, 1998, Lippincott Williams & Wilkins, p 119.)

These develop more frequently in males because of the protective effects of the uterus in women. Symptoms caused by the fistula are usually urologic, including recurrent urinary tract infections, pneumaturia, and fecaluria. The most sensitive diagnostic test is a CT scan with contrast agent that shows a thickened bladder wall, thickening of the bowel adjacent to the bladder, an abscess or extraluminal mass, an opacified fistula, air in the bladder, and rarely oral contrast in the bladder (Figure 153-11). Cystoscopy may show bullous edema or erythema at the site of the fistula.

Most colovaginal fistulas occur in women with diverticular disease who have undergone a hysterectomy. The fistula occurs at the site of contact of the inflamed colon with the vaginal cuff (Figure 153-12). Vaginal discharge is the most frequent complaint. CT scans with contrast are of significant diagnostic value. Vaginography using a Foley catheter is a highly sensitive test as well.

Colocutaneous fistulas rarely occur spontaneously and should raise the suspicion of Crohn disease. They tend to complicate a previous operation for diverticulitis.

The diagnosis of Crohn disease should be ruled out in all patients with fistulas.

Generalized Peritonitis

Generalized peritonitis complicates only 1% to 2% of cases of acute diverticulitis, when an abscess ruptures or when the surrounding tissues are unable to wall off an open rent in a diverticulum. Immunocompromised patients taking steroids are at particular risk of developing the latter complication. In the Hinchey classification of the pathologic stages of perforated diverticulitis, free perforation of a localized peridiverticular abscess site into the peritoneal cavity with purulent peritonitis is termed *stage III,* and diffuse feculent peritonitis is *stage IV* (Figure 153-13). Patients usually present with rather severe abdominal pain, but pain and tenderness may be

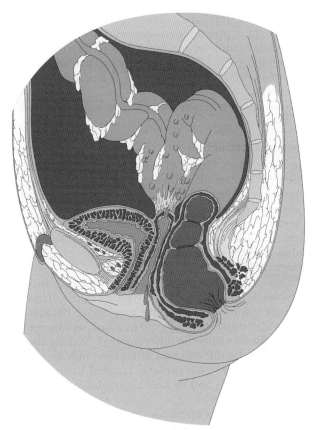

FIGURE 153-12 Depiction of a colovaginal fistula caused by diverticulitis. The fistula is occurring at the site of the vaginal cuff.

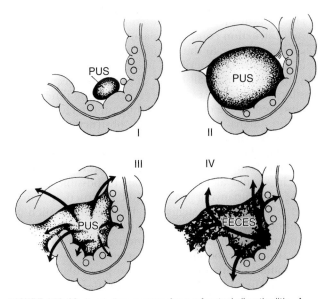

FIGURE 153-13 A grading system for perforated diverticulitis. A localized pericolic abscess (I); a larger mesenteric abscess spreading toward the pelvis (II); a free perforation causing purulent peritonitis (III); fecal peritonitis caused by free perforation (IV). (From Hinchey EJ, Schaal PG, Richards GK: Treatment of perforated diverticulitis of the colon. *Adv Surg* 12:89, 1978.)

limited to the left lower quadrant. Plain films may or may not show pneumoperitoneum. Early CT scanning allows visualization of small amounts of free air or fluid, suggesting free perforation. Use of a barium contrast enema for diagnosis is dangerous if free perforation is suspected.

These patients require urgent operative intervention (see later).

Intestinal Obstruction

One in 10 cases (10%) of large bowel obstruction are caused by diverticular disease. The usual mechanisms include circumferential colonic thickening and fibrosis, as well as marked angulation of the pelvic colon, with adherence to the pelvic side wall. Stricturing of the colon develops as a result of recurrent attacks of diverticulitis (symptomatic or subclinical) or of persistent inflammation.

Patients complain of chronic constipation and narrowed stools. The obstruction is typically partial in nature, although complete obstruction may occur. Because carcinoma is a much more frequent cause of obstruction, the two diseases must be differentiated. Making this distinction may be difficult and, therefore, may be an indication for surgery (see earlier). Limited barium studies (see Figure 153-6) and flexible sigmoidoscopy are useful diagnostic adjuncts.

Although 10% of operations carried out for diverticular disease involve intestinal obstruction, the risk of acute high-grade obstruction is only in the range of 3% in patients with acute diverticulitis. In the latter group, edema of the colon contributes to the mechanical obstruction; some resolution may occur following administration of antibiotics along with bowel rest. If distention of the colon is marked, there is risk of cecal perforation, and the cecal diameter is monitored with periodic abdominal films and physical examinations.

The clinical picture may be confusing if acute small bowel obstruction complicates acute diverticulitis. Small bowel may adhere to the point of colonic inflammation or to the walls of a pericolic abscess. Fistula formation into the adherent small bowel should raise suspicion of possible Crohn disease. The presence of one illness may be obscured by the other depending on the clinical presentation. Signs of small bowel obstruction can be obscured by symptomatic diverticulitis, or conversely, the patient may be suspected of having small bowel obstruction alone. Symptoms such as diarrhea or lower abdominal pain should alert the clinician to possible colonic disease accompanying small bowel obstruction. Small bowel obstruction is suggested by symptoms such as periumbilical crampy pain, vomiting, and abdominal distention, as well as physical findings of dehydration, tachycardia, and abdominal tenderness.

Abdominal films or CT scans are particularly useful tests in making the differentiation. Contrast material can also be administered per rectum to determine if there is a stricture of the colon. Small bowel studies following oral barium are less desirable, because the colon may be obscured by contrast and any operation is complicated by considerable barium within the bowel.

UNUSUAL PROBLEMS

Diverticulitis of the Right Colon

The incidence of right-sided diverticulitis appears to be related to the number of diverticula. Thus the highest incidence comes from areas in Asia where the disorder is most common. The natural history of this disease appears to be mild and self-limited in most cases, responding to medical therapy,[19,20] as opposed to left-sided diverticulitis that more frequently requires emergent surgery. Acute appendicitis is usually suspected because of similar symptoms of right lower quadrant pain and tenderness, emesis, fever, and leukocytosis. This disorder should be considered in patients who have undergone appendectomy or when cecal diverticulosis has been detected previously. In Japan, patients have been managed nonsurgically, despite recurrent attacks.[20] The appropriate diagnosis can be made with CT scans, although the differentiation from appendicitis or carcinoma may still be difficult.

A useful classification scheme for cecal diverticular disease has been proposed by Thorsen and Ternent,[21] as follows:
Grade I is a discrete, inflamed diverticulum.
Grade II represents a simple cecal wall mass.
Grade III refers to a localized abscess or fistula.
Grade IV is associated with peritonitis (purulent or feculent).
Grades III and IV cecal diverticulitis can be easily mistaken for a perforated adenocarcinoma.

If an operation is done, nonresection or diverticulectomy can be applied to grade I and possibly grade II lesions. If the degree of inflammation is minimal, nonresectional treatment is favored with antibiotic therapy (and incidental appendectomy if the cecum at the base of the appendix is uninvolved). If perforated carcinoma is suspected (grade III to IV lesions), colectomy is recommended; anastomosis is reserved for the stable patient with limited contamination.

Giant Diverticula

Rarely a diverticulum can increase to a large size (as much as 40 cm), termed a *giant diverticulum*, or less commonly a giant air cyst, solitary gas cyst, or pneumocyst of the colon. Some have speculated that growth occurs because of a ball-valve mechanism that is a result of fecal material intermittently occluding the neck of the diverticulum and trapping air within it.

Most patients are asymptomatic or present with chronic symptoms such as mild abdominal pain or bloating; rarely, acute complications such as perforation or torsion develop. Classically a soft, somewhat mobile, mass is palpable; this is seen as a solitary gas-filled cyst in plain films of the abdomen. The cyst and its relation to the colon are apparent with a barium enema or CT scan (Figure 153-14). The contrast studies are useful in differentiating other causes of gas-filled masses such as an intraabdominal abscess or a duplication of the colon. The diverticulum tends to adhere to adjacent structures such as the bladder or small bowel. Once discovered, the diverticulum should be resected in most patients along

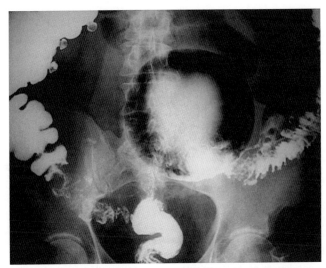

FIGURE 153-14 Barium enema view showing a giant diverticulum arising from the sigmoid colon. (From de Oliveira NC, Welch JP: Giant diverticula of the colon. In Welch JP, Cohen JL, Sardella WV, et al, editors: *Diverticular disease: Management of the difficult surgical case.* Philadelphia, 1998, Lippincott Williams & Wilkins, p 414.)

with the adjacent sigmoid colon. Recurrence is not seen following this procedure. Diverticulectomy alone can lead to formation of a colocutaneous fistula.

The Immunocompromised Patient

Increasing numbers of immunocompromised patients (alcoholics, diabetics, transplant recipients, or patients receiving chemotherapy or steroids) are being hospitalized with diverticulitis. Because of a predisposition to infection in these patients, they are at risk of complications.[22] Patients with adult polycystic kidney disease may be at particular risk.

Of interest, immunocompromised patients do not have a higher risk of developing diverticulitis from asymptomatic diverticulosis. However, once diverticulitis develops, it is typically more complex and severe in the immunosuppressed individual.[23] Corticosteroids serve to mask symptoms and signs of peritonitis in these patients because of their known antiinflammatory effects. As a consequence, definitive treatment may be delayed and the mortality increased. Surgical mortality has been reported in the range of 40% to 50%.[24]

If diverticulitis is suspected, the clinician should be particularly observant. Toxic granulations are a "red flag" for a septic process. If the patient is receiving high doses of steroids, few physical findings should be expected. Contrast-enhanced CT scans provide important information about perisigmoidal inflammatory changes and possible free perforation in the presence of an "unimpressive" physical examination. We recommend early operative intervention in these patients because of the difficult nature of their clinical course and the potential lethality of their disease. In the emergent setting, colonic anastomosis should be avoided and wound closure should be used sparingly.

Diverticulitis in the Young

Autopsy studies suggest that only 6% to 9% of patients younger than age 40 years have colonic diverticular disease. Young patients diagnosed with diverticulitis are usually obese men, perhaps because of underdiagnosis of the disease in women of reproductive age. Diverticulitis may be missed in men as well, because it may not be suspected by the treating clinician. The theory that younger patients may have more virulent forms of diverticulitis is countered by significant numbers of undiagnosed patients who are never hospitalized. Because young patients do not tend to have comorbid illnesses (unlike elderly patients), those hospitalized have advanced diverticulitis.

An aggressive surgical approach has been advocated for diverticulitis occurring in young patients. Support for this approach is predicated on the impression that young patients experience a more aggressive variant of the disease, as well as an increased rate and severity of recurrence. The higher operative rate following the first presentation of these patients is more likely because of the mistaken diagnosis of appendicitis than to an increased virulence of the initial presentation. Although the patients who develop a recurrence may be more likely to require surgery than the general population, there does not appear to be an increased rate of recurrence. Furthermore, young patients who develop a recurrence generally undergo an elective procedure and do not require a staged resection. For these reasons, diverticulitis in young patients does not need to be distinguished from and treated separately from the disease in the general population.[25]

Recurrent Diverticulitis Following Resection

Following a colectomy for diverticulitis, recurrent diverticulitis may be seen 1% to 10 % of the time.[26] This process can be confused with ischemic colitis, Crohn disease, and carcinoma (see Postresection Diverticulitis, later).

Atypical Presentations

Inflammatory diseases originating in bowel such as diverticulitis, Crohn disease, or appendicitis can be accompanied by unusual systemic manifestations or complications. The atypical presentations of diverticulitis are summarized in Table 153-2 and can be classified as either intraabdominal or extraabdominal. Immunosuppressed patients are at increased risk of developing these complications.

Intraabdominal fistulas usually are colovesical, colocutaneous, or colovaginal but may be coloureteral, colorenal, colouterine, colovenous (involving the mesenteric veins), or colobiliary. Pylephlebitis developing as a complication of diverticulitis can lead to a pyogenic liver abscess. Adnexal masses managed surgically by a gynecologist can prove to be a diverticular phlegmon or abscess.

Pyoderma gangrenosum may complicate diverticulitis. Arthritis may also be seen. Distant abscesses have been seen in the brain. Retroperitoneal perforations can manifest in a number of ways. Fistulous communication to

TABLE 153-2 Unusual Extraabdominal Presentations of Diverticulitis

Type of Presentation	Specific Manifestation
Dermatologic	Pyoderma gangrenosum
Urinary	Ureteral obstruction, coloureteral fistula
Soft tissue	Thigh abscess, necrotizing fasciitis
Orthopedic	Osteomyelitis
Gynecologic	Colouterine fistula, ovarian tumor/abscess
Genital	Epididymitis, pneumoscrotum
Neurologic	Coloepidural fistula
Vascular	Femoral vein thrombosis, mesenteric vein thrombosis, pylephlebitis, colovenous fistula
Perineal	Fournier gangrene, complex anal fistula

From Polk HC, Tuckson WB, Miller FB: The atypical presentations of diverticulitis. In Welch JP, Cohen JL, Sardella WV, et al, editors: *Diverticular disease: Management of the difficult surgical case.* Philadelphia, 1998, Lippincott Williams & Wilkins, p 385.

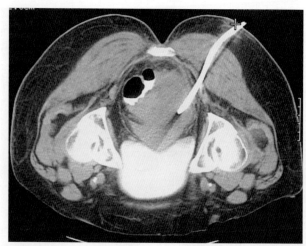

FIGURE 153-15 CT view of patient with a large pelvic abscess secondary to acute diverticulitis. A drainage catheter introduced via the transgluteal approach is seen within the cavity.

the thigh, genitalia, or knee can lead to cellulitis or abscesses in these locations. The usual portals include the psoas muscle, the femoral canal, the obturator foramen, or the sacrosciatic notch. Escape of air into the mediastinum can lead to pneumomediastinum and even subcutaneous emphysema in the neck.

MEDICAL MANAGEMENT

The medical therapy of diverticular disease depends greatly on the severity of the clinical presentation. In its mildest form, symptomatic diverticulosis may be manifested solely by left lower quadrant discomfort. In the absence of signs of infection, empiric therapy can be initiated and directed toward the treatment of a colonic motility problem. The initiation of a high-fiber diet has been demonstrated to have a beneficial effect on patients with symptomatic diverticulosis. Increased fiber probably decreases intestinal transit time, lessening the deleterious effects of constipation, including the development of diverticular complications. Nonabsorbable antibiotics are useful in symptomatic patients and alternative treatments such as probiotics and mesalazine have been proposed, but definitive data are lacking.[27]

Patients who present with localized abdominal pain and tenderness but without systemic signs of toxicity are usually managed successfully on an outpatient basis. A liquid or low-residue diet is initiated along with oral antibiotic therapy directed at the bacterial flora of the gut. For mild cases of diverticulitis, we tend to prescribe oral trimethoprim-sulfamethoxazole or ciprofloxacin in conjunction with metronidazole. Unfortunately, it may be difficult for patients to tolerate the combination of trimethoprim-sulfamethoxazole and metronidazole when they may already be experiencing some degree of gastrointestinal upset. Within several days, the patient's symptoms usually begin to resolve and antibiotic therapy is continued for a 7- to 10-day period. If a patient has not been previously diagnosed with diverticulitis, an elective evaluation of the colon is performed once the clinical symptoms have resolved.

Patients who present with a more advanced form of acute diverticulitis generally require admission to the hospital. The disease may be manifested by high fevers, lower abdominal peritonitis, and dehydration secondary to nausea or vomiting. Bowel rest is initiated with intravenous hydration and antibiotic therapy. Although cost-effective treatment for these more serious infections may still include triple-antibiotic therapy with ampicillin, gentamicin, and metronidazole, newer combinations of third-generation cephalosporins with metronidazole or even single-drug therapy such as ampicillin/sulbactam may be preferable in certain hospitals or regions. Furthermore, if the patient improves clinically and can tolerate oral intake, intravenous antibiotic therapy can be completed, and the patient can be discharged to home on oral antibiotics.

For most patients presenting with acute diverticulitis severe enough to require hospitalization, early evaluation with CT imaging is extremely beneficial (see Figure 153-4). Not only does CT scanning confirm the diagnosis, but it also reliably assesses the degree of surrounding inflammation. Although this information can assist in predicting the treatment course for the patient, the ability to detect diverticular abscesses can also lead to further therapeutic benefit. Percutaneous drainage of diverticular abscesses is now routinely performed in the treatment of complicated diverticular disease. The ability to drain these abscesses percutaneously, either under CT or ultrasound guidance, has led to more elective, single-stage resections.

Small pericolic abscesses (<5 cm) generally resolve with bowel rest and intravenous antibiotics and are amenable to resection of the diseased segment en bloc with the abscess. Larger abscesses should be drained percutaneously, provided several caveats are followed (Figure 153-15). The abscess cavity should be well defined, localized, and have a safe access route, either via an abdominal approach or transgluteally (Figure 153-16). Deep pelvic abscesses can be difficult to drain.[28] Furthermore, pneumoperitoneum and gross feculent peritonitis are contraindications to this approach.

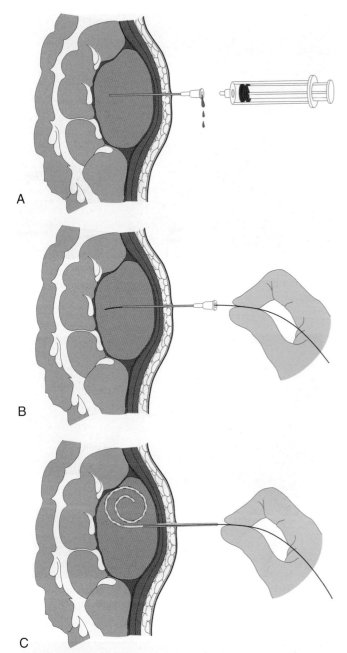

FIGURE 153-16 Schematic views of percutaneous drainage of paracolic abscess using CT. (Redrawn from Keighley RB, Williams NS, editors: *Surgery of the anus, rectum, and colon,* ed 3. Philadelphia, 2007, Saunders.)

The timing of surgery following percutaneous drainage depends on factors such as the patient's response to drainage, the degree of surrounding inflammation on CT scan, and the nutritional status. If patient improvement is rapid following drainage of a single abscess and minimal surrounding inflammation is seen on CT scan, an operation may be performed during the same admission. Alternatively, if the CT demonstrates significant surrounding inflammation or the patient is otherwise debilitated, a more prudent course is to delay surgery for 4 to 6 weeks.

SURGICAL MANAGEMENT

ELECTIVE RESECTION

It has been estimated that 20% of patients with acute diverticulitis ultimately require surgery. Although many of these patients develop a complication necessitating emergency operative intervention, there remain several indications for elective surgical intervention.

Following an episode of acute diverticulitis, recurrent attacks requiring readmission to the hospital occur in 20% to 40% of patients. Complication rates related to diverticulitis increase with subsequent attacks, exceeding 50% after two episodes. Because of the natural history of the disease, the most common indication for elective surgery in diverticular disease is recurrent episodes of acute diverticulitis interfering with the quality of the patient's daily living. The actual number of attacks warranting elective resection has been somewhat controversial. Latest guidelines recommend that elective resection should be done on a case-by-case basis, depending on the patient's age and medical condition, the frequency and severity of the attacks, and the presence of symptoms after the acute attack.[23,29,30] Other indications for elective sigmoid resection are fistula formation and previous percutaneous drainage of a diverticular abscess. Although some evidence exists that percutaneous drainage of an abscess does not mandate followup surgery, most surgeons believe that this complication is serious enough to warrant definitive surgical treatment.

Given the difficulty in distinguishing the symptoms of recurrent diverticulitis from other sources of abdominal pain, especially irritable bowel syndrome, some objective evidence of diverticulitis should be present before recommending surgery. This is most commonly obtained with a CT scan, although signs of acute diverticulitis, such as sinus tracts or extraluminal barium, can be seen in contrast studies. Even when operated on for proven diverticulitis, the patient should be cautioned regarding the possibility that not all of the abdominal symptoms will resolve following surgery.

Patients undergoing elective diverticular resection receive a mechanical and antibiotic bowel prep. Placing the patient in the lithotomy position allows access to the anus for performing a stapled anastomosis. Furthermore, should difficulty arise in identifying the ureter, this position allows for intraoperative urologic manipulations. For elective resections, preoperative placement of ureteral stents is unnecessary and adds cost to the procedure. Should an unexpected inflammatory mass be found and ureteral identification and preservation be difficult, stents can be placed intraoperatively. Ureteral stents clearly save time during the difficult operation, although placement of the stents has never been shown to reduce the rate of ureteral injury.

At the time of operation, the abnormally thickened and diseased sigmoid colon should be resected. Although this may involve only a small portion of the sigmoid colon, the distal point of resection must extend to the rectosigmoid junction. This can be identified by the loss of the taeniae coli. Failure to resect the distal sigmoid colon increases the incidence of recurrent diverticulitis

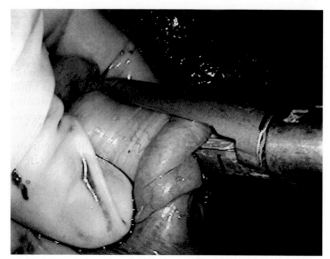

FIGURE 153-17 Hand-assisted laparoscopic surgery demonstrating transection of rectosigmoid colon with an endoscopic stapler.

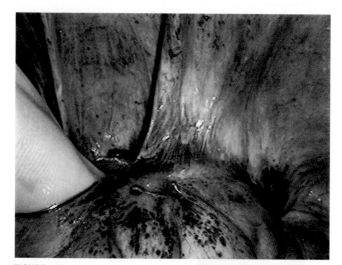

FIGURE 153-18 Inflamed sigmoid colon stuck to the left pelvic side wall. Separation is facilitated using hand-assisted laparoscopic surgery.

from 6% to between 13% and 23% (see later). The extent of proximal resection is not as important but should always be performed through soft, healthy-appearing bowel. Mobilization of the splenic flexure is performed if there is concern regarding anastomotic tension. Often mobilization of the rectum from the pre-sacral space will obviate the need for splenic flexure mobilization.

In the past decade, laparoscopic approaches to uncomplicated and complicated diverticular disease have become increasingly routine.[31] Laparoscopic procedures result in decreased postoperative pain, hospital length of stay, surgical site infections, bleeding, and ileus when compared to open operations, leading to an earlier return of normal patient function.[32,33] Hand-assisted laparoscopic surgery (HALS) facilitates minimally invasive operations for complicated diverticular disease (Figure 153-17).[34] The opportunity for the surgeon to preserve tactile sense facilitates dissection of the chronically inflamed sigmoid colon and shortens operative time and the learning curve. HALS has had its greatest impact in separating the colon from the left pelvic side wall and in resecting the thickened sigmoid mesentery (Figure 153-18). The use of the surgeon's hand (usually non-dominant) also simplifies maneuvers such as control of bleeding, manipulation of staplers into position, or occlusion of the bowel during testing of a low-stapled anastomosis (Figure 153-19). HALS for sigmoid diverticular disease leads to shorter operative times and lower conversion rates than purely laparoscopic procedures.[35]

Diverticular fistulas can usually be treated on an elective basis, because they tend to develop slowly and rarely lead to sepsis with patient instability. Most of these fistulas presumably develop from the sigmoid colon to the bladder or vagina after a diverticular abscess has developed (Figure 153-20). Once other etiologies have been excluded, treatment involves disconnection of the fistula with resection of the diseased sigmoid colon. It is not necessary to repair the defect in either the bladder or vagina, although a bladder repair is usually performed with an omental flap interposition between the colonic

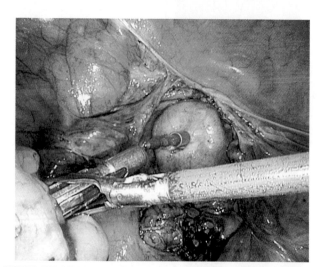

FIGURE 153-19 Manipulating the rectum and left colon in preparation for a stapled low anterior anastomosis.

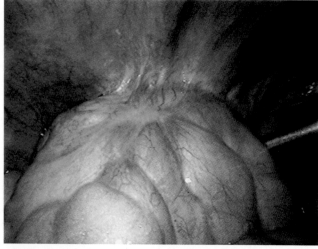

FIGURE 153-20 Appearance of a colovesical fistula. There is fusion of the chronically inflamed sigmoid colon to the urinary bladder.

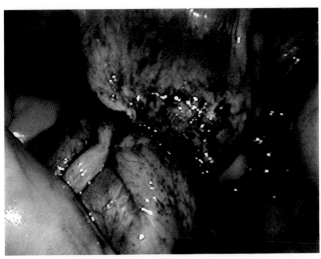

FIGURE 153-21 Hand-assisted laparoscopic surgical approach to a colovesical fistula. The surgeon's finger is encompassing the fistula prior to division.

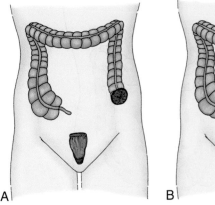
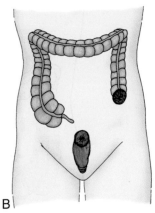

A   B

FIGURE 153-22 A, The Hartmann procedure is commonly done for patients who have perforated diverticulitis without a bowel prep. **B,** If the distal bowel reaches the abdominal wall, a mucous fistula is constructed. (From Gordon PH: Diverticular disease of the colon. In Gordon PN, Nivatvongs S, editors: *Principles and practice of surgery for the colon, rectum, and anus.* St. Louis, 1992, Quality Medical, p 766.)

anastomosis and the bladder. Postoperatively, the bladder is routinely drained for 5 to 7 days, although this time interval can be shortened if a voiding cystogram is obtained.

There are several technical aspects to division of the diverticular fistula that facilitate the dissection and increase the safety of the procedure. It is beneficial to divide the proximal bowel early in the operation and to identify the ureter at the pelvic brim. If a phlegmon is present, dissection distal to the fistula at the level of the proximal rectum can facilitate isolation of the fistulous segment. Finally, the fistula can be "pinched" between the surgeon's fingers, allowing safe separation of the fused organs and minimizing injury to the bladder or ureter. If performed laparoscopically, this maneuver is made significantly easier by using hand assistance (Figure 153-21). In a series of 36 HALS performed for colovesical fistulas, 75% were successfully completed without the need for conversion.[36] With increased experience over a 6-year period, the conversion rate decreased to lower than 15%.

In most patients, primary anastomosis can be performed safely because the degree and extent of the surrounding acute inflammation are minimal. The surgeon's experience appears to be a variable in the success of this procedure, with the goal of avoiding the need for temporary diversion.

EMERGENCY SURGERY

Many patients with diverticular disease develop a surgical emergency as their first presentation. Generalized peritonitis, free perforation, and high-grade obstruction all require urgent surgical intervention, and bleeding may also occasionally lead to an emergency operative procedure.

Historically, surgery for diverticular disease was performed in stages. By the 1980s, however, it had become clear that leaving the diseased colon in place while merely diverting the fecal stream (three-stage resection) was associated with unacceptably high morbidity and

mortality rates. Removing the septic focus at the time of the initial operative intervention decreased mortality from up to 30% to less than 10%. In a national survey of emergent surgery for diverticular disease in the United Kingdom from 1996 to 2007, the 30-day in-hospital mortality was 15%.[37] Today the three-stage resection is of historical interest only, and is not recommended.

When operating on unprepped bowel in the case of perforation, generalized peritonitis, or obstruction, the most difficult decision relates to restoration of intestinal continuity. Systemic issues such as hemodynamic instability, malnutrition, or coagulopathy are of paramount concern and may preclude any consideration of performing an intestinal anastomosis. Otherwise, the degree of peritoneal contamination at the time of surgery reliably predicts the safety of performing a primary anastomosis versus resection with diversion. The classification system devised by Hinchey et al attempts to describe the degree of inflammation associated with complicated diverticular disease (see Figure 153-13), but it does not account for patient comorbidities. Resection with primary anastomosis (one stage) appears to be safe for Hinchey I and II stages, whereas we favor resection and diversion in (1) most cases of widespread purulent peritonitis (Hinchey stage III) and in (2) all instances of feculent peritonitis (Hinchey stage IV). Controversy exists, however, and there are reports of successful resection and primary anastomosis for stage III and IV cases employing extensive abdominal lavage and on-table colonic lavage.[38-42]

The Hartmann procedure is the most widely practiced two-stage operation for the treatment of diverticulitis. First described by the French surgeon Henri Hartmann in 1921 as an alternative for the treatment of carcinoma of the rectosigmoid, it involves resection of the sigmoid colon with proximal diversion and oversewing of the distal stump (Figure 153-22, *A*). Alternatively, the distal segment may be exteriorized (as a mucus fistula) to facilitate subsequent restoration of intestinal continuity (Figure 153-22, *B*). However, the latter procedure usually is not feasible for diverticulitis, because resection of the

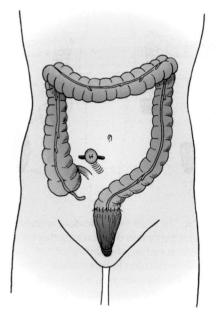

FIGURE 153-23 An alternative to the Hartmann procedure, including sigmoid resection, primary anastomosis, and proximal diverting loop ileostomy.

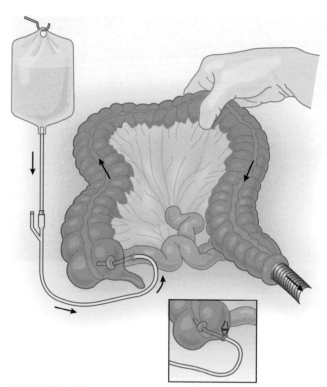

FIGURE 153-24 Technique of on-table lavage. The Foley catheter is introduced through the base of the appendix. If the appendix has been removed, the catheter can be placed through an enterotomy in the ileum or a cecotomy. Corrugated plastic tubing introduced into the colon is passed off the table into canisters. (From Ross HM, Roberts PL: Role of on-table lavage for complicated diverticular disease. *Semin Colon Rectal Surg* 11:219, 2000.)

involved segment does not leave enough length to reach the anterior abdominal wall. The operative mortality of performing a Hartmann procedure for perforated diverticulitis ranges from 0% to 15%. A disadvantage of this approach is that a second major procedure with attendant risks is needed to restore intestinal continuity.

The timing of the second operation to reverse the colostomy after the Hartmann procedure is of some importance. Most surgeons recommend waiting at least 3 months to allow for postoperative inflammation to resolve. In a review of more than 6000 possible Hartmann reversals, the mean reversal rate was only 44%.[43] The quality of life of these patients is clearly improved following the reversal.[44] The second operation can be technically difficult, leading to an anastomotic leak rate of 1% (laparoscopic) to 5% (laparotomy).[43]

An alternative procedure attempts to reduce the difficulties of reversing the Hartmann procedure. At the time of initial resection, a primary anastomosis is performed with creation of a proximal diverting loop ileostomy (Figure 153-23).[45] This is a much easier stoma to reverse, and the procedure avoids reoperation in the pelvis. A recently described "damage control" procedure includes peritoneal lavage, limited bowel resection, abdominal vacuum-assisted closure, and scheduled second look with possible anastomosis.[46]

OBSTRUCTION

Obstruction is the indication for surgery in approximately 10% of patients requiring operation for symptomatic diverticular disease. Only rarely, however, is emergency surgery required because of a high-grade obstruction, placing the patient at risk for cecal perforation. Typically, patients experience repeated bouts of acute diverticulitis that heal with progressive scarring. This leads to mild obstructive symptoms including pain, bloating, and chronic constipation.

When a patient presents with complete obstruction and develops proximal colonic dilation, urgent surgery is required to prevent the life-threatening complication of perforation. In this setting it is difficult, if not impossible, to perform an adequate preoperative mechanical preparation. Because proximal fecal loading has been demonstrated to impair anastomotic healing, this situation has generally mandated a staged resection such as a Hartmann procedure, with delayed restoration of bowel continuity. Alternatively, an anastomosis can be performed with proximal diversion by a loop ileostomy. If a diverticular stricture cannot be reliably diagnosed preoperatively, a wide mesenteric resection must be performed in case the obstruction is secondary to sigmoid carcinoma.

In the absence of hemodynamic instability or a perforation with feculent peritonitis, on-table colonic lavage can be used to prepare the bowel intraoperatively for a primary anastomosis. The technique was first described by Muir in 1968 and refined by Radcliffe. Following intestinal resection, both flexures are mobilized, an appendectomy is performed, and an appendicostomy tube is placed through the base of the appendix. Corrugated tubing is inserted into the end of the colon proximal to the resection and secured with a Dacron tape (Figure 153-24). Three to 6 L of saline are used to wash out any feculent material from the colon. This technique has significant morbidity but appears safe for patients with obstruction who are hemodynamically stable during the operation.

BLEEDING

Lower gastrointestinal bleeding occurs in approximately 20% of patients with diverticulosis, of whom 5% experience severe hemorrhage. Although bleeding spontaneously ceases in 80% to 90% of patients, the risk of rebleeding approaches 25%. For this reason, a rapid evaluation of the patient should take place even while the patient is being resuscitated in the emergency department.

Because 10% of all lower gastrointestinal bleeding ultimately arises from a gastroduodenal source, a nasogastric tube should be placed early in the evaluation. Furthermore, proctoscopy must be performed to confirm that the source of bleeding is not from the rectum or anal canal. CT angiography is a newer modality that is promising.[47,48] Bleeding rates need to be at least 0.5 mL/min for a detectable bleed to be localized. Continued developments in CT technology should improve the sensitivity. CT angiography is technically less demanding and faster to obtain than angiography in the acute setting. Angiography has the ability to be both diagnostic and therapeutic. Superselective embolization can be performed safely, obviating the need for operation in more than 80% of patients (see Figure 153-10). Postembolization ischemia is rare, but carries a high morbidity rate as well as an increased anastomotic leakage rate at the site, should surgery become necessary.[49] Even without direct intervention, localization improves operative mortality from 50% to 10%.

Every attempt should be made to localize the source of bleeding preoperatively, because the mortality rate of emergency subtotal colectomy ranges from 10% to 50%. Although nuclear imaging scans can detect bleeding at rates as low as 0.1 mL/min, they sacrifice accuracy for sensitivity. This is made evident by miss rates of 25% when an operation is performed solely based on localization by bleeding scan.

An alternative approach for localizing a colonic source utilizes colonoscopy. Advocates of emergency colonoscopy during the initial period of presumed ongoing bleeding point to the high rate of localization (two-thirds of cases)[17] while incurring low complication rates. The examination is facilitated by either rapid whole-gut lavage via a nasogastric tube or, alternatively, the use of cleansing enemas combined with frequent, aggressive pulsatile irrigations during the colonoscopy procedure. Additional arguments for this approach point to the potential therapeutic benefit of colonoscopy and its cost-effective advantage when compared with arteriography.

Admittedly, emergency colonoscopy in a patient with ongoing bleeding is a difficult technical exercise, even for the experienced endoscopist. Furthermore, hemodynamic instability limits the ability to sedate patients well for colonoscopy, thereby increasing the difficulty of the examination. Given these considerations, a more reasonable, safe approach is to stabilize the patient first and then perform early colonoscopy after a rapid gut lavage with polyethylene glycol. Only if the patient presenting

with lower gastrointestinal bleeding cannot be easily stabilized should other diagnostic modalities be used first. The diagnostic accuracy of early colonoscopy for lower gastrointestinal bleeding has been reported to be 40% to 90%. Although the varied results depend to a large degree on the timing of the procedure, the criteria for diagnosis also play a role. Findings at colonoscopy that help support a definitive source include an actively bleeding site, isolated fresh blood in one segment of the colon only, or adherent clot to a "lesion."

Should emergency surgery be necessary without the benefit of preoperative localization, intraoperative colonoscopy can be performed to assist in identifying the bleeding site. If a localized site of bleeding is not found within the colon, an emergency subtotal colectomy should be performed. The mortality rate in this setting is equal to that of a blind segmental resection but with a much lower rebleeding rate. If a localized site of bleeding is not found intraoperatively, maneuvers such as multiple colotomies or a transverse colostomy should be discouraged—they only increase the complication rate without controlling the source of bleeding.

POSTRESECTION DIVERTICULITIS

Recurrent diverticulitis following resection is uncommon, occurring in 1% to 10% of patients. Given the unusual nature of this situation, a complete evaluation should be performed to eliminate other potential causes. Symptoms of irritable bowel syndrome frequently overlap those of diverticular disease, with the exception of fever and leukocytosis. Other conditions such as Crohn disease, carcinoma, and ischemic colitis may be confused with acute diverticulitis. Previous pathology specimens should be reviewed with the differential diagnosis in mind.

The most likely explanation for the development of recurrent disease is an incomplete resection at the time of the initial operation. Although the inflammatory process frequently involves only a small portion of the sigmoid colon, a complete sigmoidectomy needs to be performed. The distal point of resection should be through soft, pliable bowel at the rectosigmoid junction. This area is identified by the convergence of the taeniae coli into a confluent sheet of longitudinal muscle surrounding the rectum. In a series of 501 patients undergoing a resection for diverticular disease, recurrent diverticulitis developed in 12.5% in whom the sigmoid colon was used as the distal resection margin. This contrasts to a 6.7% recurrence rate when the anastomosis was performed to the rectum.[26]

Although the routine use of ureteral stents is unnecessary for diverticular resections, they can be beneficial when operating for recurrent disease, because fibrosis may make the resection particularly difficult. Typically the inflammatory process involves the left pelvic side wall that has been dissected previously. The preoperative placement of a left ureteral stent may not prevent injury in this setting, but it can facilitate the dissection and allow for rapid identification of an injury should it occur.

As with the initial operation, reoperative surgery should commence by dissection through noninflamed tissue with early identification of the left ureter. Splenic flexure mobilization becomes mandatory, and often the anastomosis will be to the transverse colon. Most important, the previous anastomosis must be resected and the new anastomosis must incorporate the noninflamed rectum.[50]

SUGGESTED READINGS

Etzione DA, Mack TM, Beart RW Jr, et al: Diverticulitis in the United States: 1998-2005. Changing patterns of disease and treatment. *Ann Surg* 249:210, 2009.

Rafferty J, Shellito P, Hyman NH, et al: Practice parameters for sigmoid diverticulitis. *Dis Colon Rectum* 49:939, 2006.

Welch JP, Cohen JL, Sardella WV, et al, editors: *Diverticular disease: Management of the difficult surgical case.* Philadelphia, 1998, Lippincott Williams & Wilkins.

REFERENCES

1. Painter NS: The cause of diverticular disease of the colon, its symptoms and its complications. *J R Coll Surg Edinb* 30:118, 1985.
2. Laine L, Smith R, Min K, et al: Systematic review: The lower gastrointestinal adverse effects of non-steroidal anti-inflammatory drugs. *Aliment Pharmacol Ther* 24:751, 2006.
3. Strate LL, Liu YL, Aldoori WH, et al: Obesity increases the risks of diverticulitis and diverticular bleeding. *Gastroenterology* 136:115, 2009.
4. Strate LL, Liu YL, Aldoori WH, et al: Physical activity decreases diverticular complications. *Am J Gastroenterol* 104:1221, 2009.
5. Etzione DA, Mack TM, Beart RW Jr, et al: Diverticulitis in the United States: 1998-2005. Changing patterns of disease and treatment. *Ann Surg* 249:210, 2009.
6. Jeyarajah S, Faiz O, Bottle A, et al: Diverticular disease hospital admissions are increasing, with poor outcomes in the elderly and emergency admissions. *Aliment Pharmacol Ther* 30:1171, 2009.
7. McConnell EJ, Tessier DJ, Wolff BG: Population-based incidence of complicated diverticular disease of the sigmoid colon based on gender and age. *Dis Colon Rectum* 46:1110, 2003.
8. Csikesz NH, Singla A, Simons JP, et al: The impact of socioeconomic status on presentation and treatment of diverticular disease. *J Gastrointest Surg* 13:1993, 2009.
9. Kircher MF, Rhea JT, Kihiczak D, et al: Frequency, sensitivity, and specificity of individual signs of diverticulitis on thin-section helical CT with colonic contrast material: Experience with 312 cases. *AJR Am J Roentgenol* 178:1313, 2002.
10. Ambrosetti P, Jenny A, Becker C, et al: Acute left colonic diverticulitis—compared performance of computed tomography and water-soluble contrast enema: Prospective evaluation of 420 patients. *Dis Colon Rectum* 43:1363, 2000.
11. Heverhagen JT, Sitter H, Zielke A, et al: Prospective evaluation of the value of magnetic resonance imaging in suspected acute sigmoid diverticulitis. *Dis Colon Rectum* 51:1810, 2008.
12. Oliveira L, Wexner SD: Abdominal pain and diverticulosis. In Welch JP, Cohen JL, Sardella WV, et al, editors: *Diverticular disease: Management of the difficult surgical case.* Philadelphia, 1998, Lippincott Williams & Wilkins, p 33.
13. Jung HK, Choung RS, Locke GR, et al: Diarrhea-predominant irritable bowel syndrome is associated with diverticular disease: A population-based study. *Am J Gastroenterol* 105:652, 2010.
14. Holmer C, Lehmann KS, Engelmann S, et al: Microscopic findings in sigmoid diverticulitis: Changes after conservative therapy. *J Gastrointest Surg* 14:812, 2010.
15. Lewis M: Bleeding colonic diverticula. *J Clin Gastroenterol* 42:1156, 2008.
16. Jansen A, Harenberg S, Grenda U, et al: Risk factors for colonic diverticular bleeding: A Westernized community based hospital study. *World J Gastroenterol* 15:457, 2009.
17. Pilchos C, Bobotis E: Role of endoscopy in the management of acute diverticular bleeding. *World J Gastroenterol* 14:1981, 2008.
18. Iwamoto J, Mizokami Y, Shimokobe K, et al: Therapeutic barium enema for bleeding colonic diverticula: Four case series and review of the literature. *World J Gastroenterol* 14:6413, 2008.
19. Park HC, Chang MY, Lee BH: Nonoperative management of right colonic diverticulitis using radiologic evaluation. *Colorectal Dis* 12:105, 2010.
20. Komuta K, Yamanaka S, Okada K, et al: Toward therapeutic guidelines for patients with acute right colonic diverticulitis. *Am J Surg* 187:233, 2004.
21. Thorsen AG, Ternent CA: Cecal diverticulitis. In Welch JP, Cohen JL, Sardella WV, et al, editors: *Diverticular disease: Management of the difficult surgical case.* Philadelphia, 1998, Lippincott Williams & Wilkins, p 433.
22. Yoo PS, Garg R, Salamone LF, et al: Medical comorbidities predict the need for colectomy for complicated and recurrent diverticulitis. *Am J Surg* 196:710, 2008.
23. Klarenbeek BR, Samuels M, van der Wal MA, et al: Indications for elective sigmoid resection in diverticular disease. *Ann Surg* 251:670, 2010.
24. Coccolini F, Caatena F, DiSaverio S, et al: Colonic perforation after renal transplantation: Risk factor analysis. *Transplant Proc* 41:1189, 2009.
25. Guzzo J, Hyman N: Diverticulitis in young patients: Is resection after a single attack always warranted? *Dis Colon Rectum* 47:1187, 2004.
26. Benn PL, Wolff BC, Ilstrup DM: Level of anastomosis and recurrent colonic diverticulitis. *Am J Surg* 151:269, 1986.
27. Rocco A, Compare D, Caruso F, et al: Treatment options for uncomplicated diverticular disease of the colon. *J Clin Gastroenterol* 43:803, 2009.
28. Harisinghani MG, Gervais DA, Maher MM, et al: Transgluteal approach for percutaneous drainage of deep pelvic abscesses: One hundred fifty-four cases. *Radiology* 228:701, 2003.
29. Rafferty J, Shellito P, Hyman NH, et al: Practice parameters for sigmoid diverticulitis. *Dis Colon Rectum* 49:939, 2006.
30. Stocchi L: Current indications and role of surgery in the management of sigmoid diverticulitis. *World J Gastroenterol* 21:804, 2010.
31. Martel G, Bouchard A, Soto CM, et al: Laparoscopic colectomy for complex diverticular diseases: A justifiable choice? *Surg Endosc* 24:2273, 2010.
32. Russ AJ, Obma KL, Rajamanickam V, et al: Laparoscopy improves short-term outcomes after surgery for diverticular disease. *Gastroenterology* 138:2267, 2010.
33. Siddiqui MRS, Sajid MS, Qureshi E, et al: Elective laparoscopic sigmoid resection for diverticular disease has fewer complications than conventional surgery: A meta-analysis. *Am J Surg* 200:144, 2010.
34. Loungnarath R, Fleshman JW: Hand-assisted laparoscopic colectomy techniques. *Semin Laparoscop Surg* 10:219, 2003.
35. Lee SW, Yoo J, Dujovny N, et al: Laparoscopic vs. hand-assisted sigmoidectomy for diverticulitis. *Dis Colon Rectum* 49:464, 2006.
36. Bartus CM, Lipoff T, Shahbaz Sarwar CM, et al: Colovesical fistula is not a contraindication to elective laparoscopic colectomy. *Dis Colon Rectum* 48:233, 2005.
37. Faiz O, Warusavitarne J, Bottle A, et al: Nonelective excisional colorectal surgery in English National Health Service Trusts: A study of outcomes from hospital episode statistics data between 1996 and 2007. *J Am Coll Surg* 210:390, 2010.
38. Regenet N, Teuch JJ, Pessaux P, et al: Intraoperative colonic lavage with primary anastomosis vs. Hartmann's procedure for perforated diverticular disease of the colon: A consecutive study. *Hepatogastroenterology* 49:664, 2002.
39. Bretagnol F, Pautrar K, Mor C, et al: Emergency laparoscopic management of perforated sigmoid diverticulitis: A promising alternative to more radical procedures. *J Am Coll Surg* 206:654, 2008.
40. Myers E, Hurley M, O'Sullivan GC, et al: Laparoscopic peritoneal lavage for generalized peritonitis due to perforated diverticulitis. *Br J Surg* 95:97, 2008.
41. Stumpf MJ, Vinces FY, Edwards J, et al: Is primary anastomosis safe in the surgical management of complications of acute diverticulitis? *Am Surg* 73:787, 2007.
42. Toorenvliet BR, Swank H, Schoones JW, et al: Laparoscopic peritoneal lavage for perforated colonic diverticulitis: A systematic review. *Colorectal Dis* 12:862, 2009.
43. Van der Wall BJ, Diaaisma WA, Schouten ES, et al: Conventional and laparoscopic reversal of the Hartmann procedure: A review of literature. *J Gastrointest Surg* 14:743, 2010.

44. Vermeulen J, Gosselink MP, Busschbach JJV, et al: Avoiding or reversing Hartmann's procedure provides improved quality of life after perforated diverticulitis. *J Gastrointest Surg* 14:651, 2010.

45. Sakai Y, Nelson H, Larson D, et al: Temporary transverse colostomy versus loop ileostomy in diversion. *Arch Surg* 136:338, 2001.

46. Parathoner A, Klaus A, Muhlmann G, et al: Damage control with abdominal vacuum therapy (VAC) to manage perforated diverticulitis with advanced generalized peritonitis—a proof of concept. *Int J Colorect Dis* 25:767, 2010.

47. Hizawa K, Miura N, Matsumoto T, et al: Colonic diverticular bleeding: Precise localization and successful management by a combination of CT angiography and interventional radiology. *Abdom Imaging* 34:777, 2009.

48. Chua AE, Ridley LJ: Diagnostic accuracy of CT angiography in acute gastrointestinal bleeding. *J Med Imaging Radiat Oncol* 52:333, 2008.

49. Tan KK, Wong D, Sim R: Superselective embolization for lower gastrointestinal hemorrhage: An institutional review over 7 years. *World J Surg* 32:2707, 2008.

50. Thaler K, Baig MK, Berho M, et al: Determinants of recurrence after sigmoid resection for uncomplicated diverticulitis. *Dis Colon Rectum* 46:385, 2003.

Hemorrhoids

Theodor Asgeirsson | Anthony Senagore

There are few diseases more chronicled in human history than symptomatic hemorrhoidal disease. References occur in ancient texts dating back to Babylonian, Egyptian, Greek, and Hebrew cultures.[1,2] Included in many of these writings are multiple recommended treatment regimens, including anal dilation, topical ointments, and the intimidating red hot poker.[3,4] Although few people have died of hemorrhoidal disease, many patients wish they had, particularly after therapy, and this fact led to the beatification of St. Fiachre, the patron saint of gardeners and hemorrhoidal sufferers.[5] It is hoped this discussion will guide the practitioner in a more humane approach to hemorrhoidal disease, with the emphasis on cost-effectiveness with minimal morbidity and mortality.

ANATOMY AND ETIOLOGY

The hemorrhoidal cushions appear predictably in the right anterior, right posterior, and left lateral positions, although there may be intervening secondary hemorrhoidal complexes that blur this classic anatomy.[6] The blood supply is similarly constant, deriving from the superior rectal artery, a branch of the inferior mesenteric; the middle rectal arteries arising from the internal iliac arteries; and the inferior rectal arteries arising from the pudendal arteries. The venous drainage transitions from the portal venous system above the level of the dentate line to the systemic venous system below this level.[6]

It was originally reported that the vascular cushions from the termination of the vascular supply within the anal canal contributed to the maintenance of anal continence.[6] Hemorrhoidal disease occurs as the result of abnormalities within the connective tissue of these cushions, producing bleeding with or without prolapse of the hemorrhoidal tissue.[7] This can occur as the result of excessive straining, chronic constipation, or low-fiber dietary intake.[8] A clear understanding of the pathophysiology is important when considering therapeutic interventions. At the earlier stages of disease progression, when the major manifestation is transudation of blood through thin-walled, damaged veins and/or arterioles, ablation of the vessels should be adequate. Conversely, in late stages of the disease, when there is significant disruption of the mucosal suspensory ligament, a technique requires fixation of the mucosa to the underlying muscular wall for effective therapy.[9] Internal anal sphincter dysfunction may play a role, and a number of investigators have demonstrated increased internal anal sphincter tone in patients with hemorrhoidal disease.[10-12] In reality, probably a combination of all of these factors is important for the ultimate development of large prolapsing hemorrhoidal disease.

The standard classification for hemorrhoidal diseases[13] is as follows:
- Grade I = bleeding
- Grade II = protrusion with spontaneous reduction
- Grade III = protrusion requiring manual reduction
- Grade IV = irreducible protrusion of hemorrhoidal tissue

Although this staging system tends to correlate with patients' symptoms, it is unclear that it can be completely relied on when making therapeutic decisions. As outlined later, it is important to consider the relative role of internal hemorrhoidal tissue, prolapsing anoderm, and external skin tagging when choosing a modality for complete resolution of all of the patient's symptoms.[7]

CLINICAL EVALUATION

Bleeding, protrusion, and pain are among the most common symptoms associated with hemorrhoidal disease. While many patients associate anorectal complaints with hemorrhoids only one third are found to have significant hemorrhoidal disease.[14] Hemorrhoidal bleeding typically results in bright red blood either on the toilet paper or actually into the commode after bowel movements, generally painless in nature. More vigorous bleeding can occur, however, as the hemorrhoids enlarge and particularly in advanced stages when a portion of the complex is fixed externally, allowing the blood to drip or spurt into the commode. Usually, prompt reduction of the protruding mass causes this symptom to abate. Acute thromboses of internal or external hemorrhoids are usually associated with severe pain in association with a palpable perianal mass. These patients are generally quite uncomfortable, and the diagnosis is immediately obvious on clinical examination.

Examination of the patient with hematochezia, although tailored by the age of the patient, should include sufficient investigations to rule out a proximal source of bleeding such as inflammatory bowel disease and neoplasia. Hemorrhoids should not be dismissed as the cause of iron-deficiency anemia as this is an uncommon occurrence.

We prefer to examine the patient in the left lateral position with the knees drawn up toward the chest as high as possible. This approach allows relative patient comfort and the ability to clearly inspect the perianal skin and perform anoscopy and proctosigmoidoscopy. A careful digital examination of the anal canal and distal rectum should be performed to include the prostate in men. An anoscope is essential to clearly inspect the hemorrhoidal tissue and anal canal. The three common locations for hemorrhoids should be inspected, and the size, friability, and ease of prolapse of these areas should be recorded. Next, the degree of hemorrhoidal prolapse can be ascertained quite accurately by asking the patient to strain on the toilet. Following this, the decision regarding the need for more proximal colorectal evaluation should be considered, although rigid proctoscopy would be the minimum in all patients. After the hemorrhoids are appropriately graded, a discussion can be enjoined with the patient regarding treatment options.

NONEXCISIONAL OPTIONS

Most patients evaluated for hematochezia that ultimately proves to be hemorrhoidal in origin can be managed with fiber supplementation and a variety of available anal ointments. Although it is not clearly proven that constipation is causal, it appears of practical utility to improve bowel function and thereby reduce hemorrhoidal complaints in most early-stage patients. Similarly, the ointments available, although homeopathic, may minimize ongoing trauma to the hemorrhoidal cushions and similarly reduce symptoms. The remaining nonoperative and operative interventions should be reserved for patients with advanced hemorrhoidal disease who are unresponsive to conservative medical management.

SCLEROTHERAPY

Sclerotherapy of symptomatic internal hemorrhoidal disease was first advocated by Mitchell in 1871 and has enjoyed significant experience.[13] The purpose of sclerotherapy is ultimately to scar the submucosa, resulting in atrophy of the tissue injected and scarification with fixation of the hemorrhoidal complex within its normal location in the anal canal. A variety of solutions have been advocated, although it appears that sodium morrhuate and sodium tetradecyl sulfate predominate currently. This modality is most effective in situations with minimal enlargement of hemorrhoidal complexes where the primary complaint is bright red rectal bleeding.

The procedure is performed with the patient in the left lateral decubitus position. An anoscope is inserted to clearly identify the symptomatic complex and a 25-gauge spinal needle is used to instill the sclerosant into the submucosal space (Figure 154-1). The syringe should be aspirated before injection to avoid a direct intravascular injection. Typically 1 to 2 mL of sclerosant is adequate. The surgeon can inject as many locations as desired because the procedure is essentially painless. It is important, however, not to circumferentially inject the anal canal because this may induce stricture formation.

BIPOLAR DIATHERMY

Bipolar diathermy employs electrical current to coagulate the hemorrhoidal tissue, including the mucosa and submucosa.[15,16] The machine generates a 2-second pulse of energy to accomplish the treatment. Once again, this approach is applicable for small bleeding hemorrhoids and probably has no greater efficacy than does sclerosing.

Other variations on the use of energy to destroy internal hemorrhoids includes infrared coagulation and Ultroid (direct-current) therapy.[16,17] Infrared coagulation employs a tungsten halogen lamp that generates heat energy generally for a 1.5-second period resulting in destruction of the mucosa and submucosa at the application site (Figure 154-2). The depth of penetration of this injury is usually 3 mm. Conversely, the Ultroid uses electrical current that is applied for up to 10 minutes per complex treated. Ultimately, all of these modalities are a

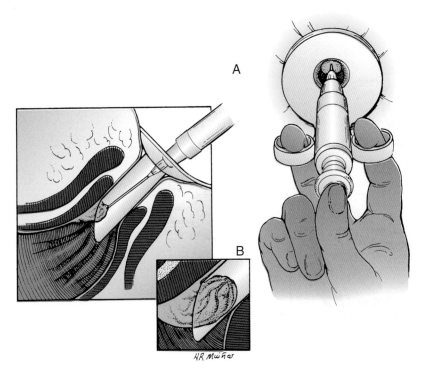

HR Muñas

FIGURE 154-1 A, Injection of internal hemorrhoid. **B,** Postinjection striations.

variation on the theme of local tissue destruction and fixation of the hemorrhoidal tissue at the appropriate level. There is probably no advantage of one technique over the other; however, sclerotherapy offers an advantage to the physician since minimal instrumentation is required.

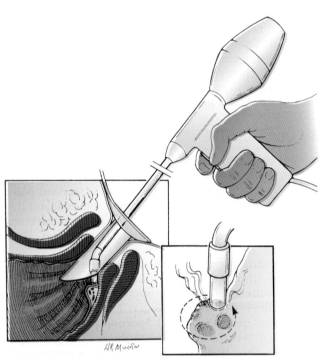

FIGURE 154-2 Infrared coagulation. *Left,* Coagulator inserted through a Hirschman anoscope. *Right,* Coagulation points.

HEMORRHOIDAL LIGATION WITH RUBBER BANDS

Barron was the first to describe hemorrhoidal banding using rubber bands in 1963.[18] Since this original description, there have been a number of reports that have documented the significant efficacy banding offers for the management of most patients with grades II and III internal hemorrhoids.[19-23] The procedure is generally well tolerated without the need for prescription analgesia if the band is placed above the level of the dentate line. The technique is demonstrated in Figure 154-3. It is important to ask patients if they experience any pain during placement of the bander, before deployment of the band. If they have pain before placement of the bander, it will worsen after deployment. Discomfort immediately after band placement may be reduced by the injection of a local anesthetic agent; however, this does not appear to be a long-lasting benefit.[24] Banding does carry the rare but frequently fatal complication of post-banding sepsis, which is heralded by the symptoms of increasing rectal pain, fever, and inability to void.[25-28] It is essential to treat these symptoms early and aggressively with early antibiotic treatment coupled with aggressive surgical drainage.[28]

Bayer et al reported a series of 2934 patients with 79% of patients achieving complete relief of symptoms following a single session of banding at only one or two locations.[19] Using this approach, patients required multiple sessions for control of symptoms (two sessions, 32%; three sessions, 17%; four sessions, 25%; and five or more sessions, 20%). Although the multiple sessions required are a negative aspect of this technique, only 2.1% of patients required excisional hemorrhoidectomy. It may

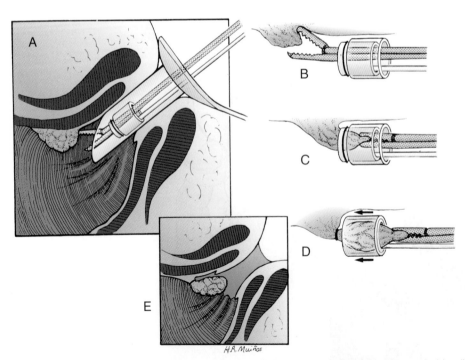

FIGURE 154-3 **A,** Ligator in a Hirschman anoscope. **B,** Internal hemorrhoid being grasped. **C,** Internal hemorrhoid pulled up into drum. **D,** O-ring applied to internal hemorrhoid. **E,** Appearance of hemorrhoid after ligation.

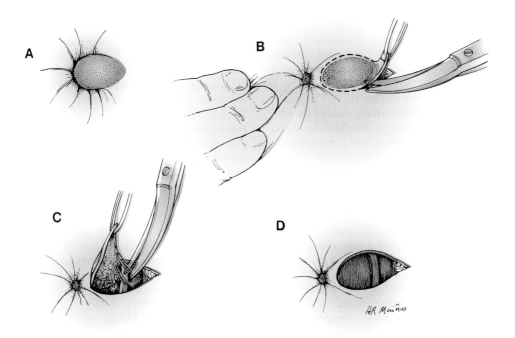

FIGURE 154-4 A, Thrombosed external hemorrhoid in the right lateral quadrant. **B,** Allis clamp applied to apex of thrombosis and elliptical incision made. **C,** Thrombosis dissected free of sphincter. **D,** Appearance of wound after thrombectomy.

be possible to achieve a similar outcome with a shorter duration of therapy, albeit at the expense of greater post-treatment pain, by banding all symptomatic hemorrhoidal sites at the initial visit.[29,30] Banding techniques appear to be durable after initial control of symptoms, with 69% of patients maintaining long-term relief and only 7.5% ultimately requiring excisional hemorrhoidectomy.[23] This method is cost effective in treating grade II hemorrhoids as shown by McKenzie et al in a randomized controlled trial comparing banding to stapled hemorrhoidopexy (SH). The mean cost for SH was £1483 greater than rubber band ligation (95% confidence interval [CI] = 1339 to 1676) and there was no evidence of statistical difference in quality of life-years despite higher recurrence rates for banding (odds ratio [OR] = 0.18, 95% CI = 0.03 to 0.86) at 12 months.[31]

EXCISIONAL HEMORRHOIDECTOMY

The decision to proceed to excisional hemorrhoidectomy requires a mutual decision by the physician and patient that medical and nonexcisional options have either failed or are not appropriate. The usual clinical symptoms that lead to surgical excision are frequent prolapsing of the internal hemorrhoids that result in discomfort and anal seepage. Alternatively, the thickened and prolapsing internal/external hemorrhoidal complexes may make anal hygiene difficult for the patient and may make excision preferable. The final indication for excisional hemorrhoidectomy, although debatable, is the development of acutely thrombosed and gangrenous internal hemorrhoids. Surgical excision of acutely thrombosed external hemorrhoids may also be warranted, primarily for more rapid pain relief and avoidance of a residual skin tag. These external thromboses are usually easily managed in the office setting with local anesthesia and complete excision with or without skin closure (Figure 154-4).

Options for excisional hemorrhoidectomy include the following techniques: Milligan-Morgan hemorrhoidectomy; Ferguson closed hemorrhoidectomy; Whitehead hemorrhoidectomy; and the more recently described SH. The procedures are usually performed in the operating theater after minimal preoperative preparation of the bowel. The use of lasers for excisional hemorrhoidectomy offers no advantage and in fact causes delayed healing, increased pain, and increased cost.[32] Anesthetic selection is usually left to the anesthesiologist and patient; however, local anesthesia supplemented by the administration of intravenous narcotics and propofol is highly effective and short-acting. The use of spinal anesthesia, although effective, may increase the risk of postoperative urinary retention partially because of a higher intraoperative administration of intravenous fluids.

The Milligan-Morgan hemorrhoidectomy, which is widely practiced in Europe, was originally described in 1937, and its efficacy has been documented in many series subsequently.[33-35] This technique includes resection of the entire enlarged internal hemorrhoid complex, ligation of the arterial pedicle, and preservation of the intervening anoderm.[32] The distal anoderm and external skin are left open to minimize the risk of infection in the wounds. Results from this technique have shown this to be a safe and effective means for managing advanced hemorrhoidal disease.[32] However, the fact that the external wounds are left open for delayed healing can be a cause of considerable discomfort and prolonged morbidity after this procedure. The closed Ferguson hemorrhoidectomy was proposed as an alternative to the Milligan-Morgan technique and enjoys a similar large body of evidence regarding its safety and efficacy.[36-39] This technique employs an hourglass-shaped (centered at the midportion of the anoderm) excision of the entire internal/external hemorrhoidal complex, preservation of the internal and external anal sphincters, and primary closure of the entire wound. Occasionally, it is necessary to undermine flaps of anoderm and perianal skin to allow removal of intermediate hemorrhoidal tissue while preserving the bridges of anoderm between pedicles. This technical adjustment avoids postoperative strictures.

The Whitehead hemorrhoidectomy, described in 1882, was devised to eradicate the enlarged internal hemorrhoidal tissue in a circumferential fashion and to relocate the prolapsed dentate line that is often a component of prolapsing hemorrhoids.[40] Although this technique enjoyed a long period of widespread application, it was subsequently largely abandoned because of the high rates of mucosal ectropion and anal stricture.[41-44] The technique has enjoyed renewed support, with several authors documenting minimal stricture rates and no occurrences of mucosal ectropion.[41-46] Despite these promising reports, the Whitehead procedure is technically demanding because of the need to accurately identify the dentate line and relocate it to its proper location.

INSTRUMENTATION FOR EXCISIONAL HEMORRHOIDECTOMY

The specific techniques for excisional hemorrhoidectomy were reviewed earlier, and this section discusses the relative benefits of scalpel and the available energy-delivering excisional tools. Cold scalpel or scissor excision has long been the mainstay of surgical hemorrhoidectomy, and the data on outcomes are well validated. Over the past 10 to 15 years, a variety of new devices have been advocated for hemorrhoidectomy. These energy-based cutting devices have been devised to allow simultaneous tissue division and coagulation. The main advantage proposed for these devices is provision of hemostasis without need for suture ligation and therefore reduction in postoperative pain. However, these benefits must be interpreted in the context of the significant cost of acquisition of the devices as compared to the low cost of a disposable scalpel blade.

The first energy cutting tool applied to hemorrhoidectomy is standard monopolar electrocautery. The tool has been reported widely for the two dominant types of hemorrhoidectomy. Surgeons using this tool have also employed various degrees of wound closure by suture, ranging from pedicle ligation only to complete wound closure.[47-49] Despite the value of hemostasis, the thermal spread leaves patients with significant postoperative pain compared to SH. The STOPP trial study group compared diathermy hemorrhoidectomy to stapled hemorrhoidopexy in a randomized clinical trial for grade III and IV hemorrhoids. Hemorrhoidal prolapse was corrected equally by either operation at 1 year but total pain scores were significantly higher in the first 14 days using diathermy (daily: 25.2 vs. 36.8, $P = 0.002$; peak: 41.7 vs. 61.1,

$P < 0.001$).[50] Similar findings were reported by Thaha et al looking at grade II, III, and IV hemorrhoids, but the superiority of diathermal excision was related to prolapse control at 1 year ($P = 0.087$).[51]

Laser technology has been evaluated both as a means of cutting hemorrhoidal tissue and as a technique for ablation. Zahir et al evaluated the role of the Nd-YAG laser for excision and coagulation of residual tissue and reported a reduction in postoperative pain and a greater percentage of patients returning to work at 1 week.[52] Alternatively, we found delayed wound healing, increased cost, and increased pain scores with Nd-YAG hemorrhoidectomy compared with scalpel excision.[32] Hodgson and Morgan evaluated a series of patients with second- and third-degree hemorrhoids managed by CO_2 excision, with only one patient readmitted for postoperative hemorrhage.[53] The data suggest that either Nd-YAG or CO_2 laser excision may be performed; however, it is not clear that the added expense or benefits are superior to scalpel or scissor excision.[54]

A bipolar cautery device capable of simultaneous tissue division and blood vessel coagulation is the LigaSure. This device has been compared to monopolar diathermy hemorrhoidectomy, with most of the data suggesting reductions in operative time and early postoperative pain.[55,56] Chung and Wu compared a sutureless LigaSure technique to the standard closed Ferguson hemorrhoidectomy and confirmed a reduction in operative time and pain reduction during the first 48 hours.[55] However, there were no significant differences in wound complications or time to full recovery. Fareed et al found improvement in pain over 2 weeks compared to the Ferguson hemorrhoidectomy in addition to shorter hospital stay and shorter time to achieve complete wound healing (4.4 ± 0.7 vs. 6.4 ± 1.0 weeks; $P = 0.001$). Postoperative manometric testing and squeeze pressures were significantly decreased in the Ferguson group at the 6-week followup.[57] Similarly, a comparison of LigaSure to a standard Milligan-Morgan hemorrhoidectomy confirmed reduction in operating time and early postoperative pain.[56] A metaanalysis from 2008 compared hemorrhoidectomy with Ligasure to conventional excisional techniques and found similar cure rates but shorter operative time, decreased pain, wound healing time, and time off from work were all in favor of the Ligasure excision for hemorrhoidal disease.[58]

A competing technology is the Harmonic Scalpel, which relies on a rapidly reciprocating blade to generate heat for coagulation and tissue transection. The largest reported experience was provided by Armstrong et al with 500 consecutive excisional hemorrhoidectomies.[59] They reported a low postoperative hemorrhage rate (0.6%). The overall postoperative complication rates were low, with urinary retention in 2%, fissure in 1%, and abscess/fistula in 0.8%. Several subsequent prospective, randomized comparisons of diathermy to Harmonic Scalpel failed to confirm any advantages between the two tools.[60-62] A randomized controlled trial by Abo-hashem et al compared bipolar electrocautery hemorrhoidectomy to Harmonic Scalpel and found favorable results in regard to pain scores and return to work but complications were similar, except for urine retention, which was significantly less frequent in the Harmonic Scalpel group (9.4% vs. 34.4%, P < 0.05). Followup was 6 weeks.[63]

Probably the best guidance on this topic is the study by Chung et al, who evaluated scissor/Milligan-Morgan, Harmonic Scalpel, and bipolar scissors for hemorrhoidectomy: Harmonic Scalpel demonstrated superior early pain scores to scissor; however, the long-term recovery was similar between the groups.[64] Therefore, the cumulative data suggest that patient benefits are modest for any of the energy-delivering techniques and the cost differential is significant.

PROCEDURE FOR PROLAPSING HEMORRHOIDS

Another option for advanced hemorrhoidal disease is a nonexcisional hemorrhoidectomy or pexy procedure referred to as the procedure for prolapsing hemorrhoids (PPHs) or SH.[65] The technique (Figure 154-5) uses a circular, transanally placed purse-string suture placed 4 cm proximally from the dentate line and within the enlarged internal hemorrhoids. A 31-mm stapler is then placed transanally to perform a circumferential excision of rectal mucosa just rostral to the hemorrhoidal columns. The procedure provides for a repositioning of both the anoderm and hemorrhoidal columns to the appropriate locations within the anal canal and fixation of these structures via the rectal staple line.

Since the introduction of the PPH technique, there have been a large number of prospective randomized trials comparing this approach to excisional hemorrhoidectomy.[66-70] Most of the data support the concept that PPH is associated with a lesser degree of early postoperative pain and a general reduction in the duration of pain after surgery.[66-70] A multicenter trial comparing PPH to Ferguson closed hemorrhoidectomy confirmed similar benefits and reported a reduction in the need for early reoperation for complications in the PPH group.[71] Most recently, several metaanalyses have been published comparing PPH to the Ferguson closed hemorrhoidectomy and the Milligan-Morgan open hemorrhoidectomy. There was significant heterogenicity of trials and followup was short but publications concluded that PPH is associated with less pain and reduced operative time and hospital stay in addition to earlier return to normal activity. Complications did not differ but the rate of recurrence appears to be higher in PPH.[72,73] Two analyses have looked at long-term outcomes after SH. A Cochrane systematic review looked at all randomized controlled trials from 1998 to 2006 comparing SH to conventional excisional hemorrhoidectomy. SH patients were significantly more likely to have recurrent hemorrhoids in long-term followup than those receiving conventional hemorrhoidectomy (seven trials, 537 patients; OR = 3.85; 95% CI = 1.47 to 10.07; P = 0.006). In trials where there was followup of 1 year or more, SH was associated higher recurrence rates (five trials, 417 patients; OR = 3.60; 95% CI = 1.24 to 10.49; P = 0.02). A significantly higher proportion of patients with SH complained of the symptom of prolapse (eight studies, 798 patients; OR = 2.96; 95% CI = 1.33 to 6.58; P = 0.008).

Followup longer than 1 year yielded similar results. Nonsignificant trends in favor of SH were seen in pain, pruritus ani, and fecal urgency. All other clinical parameters showed trends favoring SH.[74] Giordano et al looked at long-term outcome for PPH in a separate analysis looking at all randomized controlled trials that had followup of 1 year or longer comparing PPH to conventional hemorrhoidectomy. Fifteen articles met their inclusion criteria, for a total of 1201 patients. Outcomes at 1 year showed a significantly higher rate of prolapse recurrence in the PPH group (14 studies, 1063 patients; OR = 5.5; P < 0.001) and patients were likely to undergo further treatment to correct recurrent prolapses compared with conventional hemorrhoidectomy (10 studies, 824 patients; OR = 1.9; P < 0.002) and concluded rightly that it is a matter of discretion whether to accept a higher recurrence rate to take advantage of the short-term benefits of PPH, but as pointed out in the Cochrane review patients need to be educated about the pros and cons of techniques available.[75] The final publication took into account the cost and found that because of shorter operative time and hospital stay, the cost of the stapling gun was offset and the techniques did not differ.[76] Similar findings have been published comparing Ligasure to PPH.[77]

Although the bulk of the data supports the safety of this new technique, there have been several reports of complications. Early complications after 150 consecutive SHs by Bove et al were 6.6%: 5 bleeding, 4 acute urinary retention, 1 external hemorrhoid thrombosis, and 1 hematoma of the rectal wall. Late complications were 10%: 5 fecal urgency (improved after 6 months), 6 moderate asymptomatic strictures, and 4 persistent skin tags. Recurrences were 5.1% and all were in grade III and IV patients and occurred within the first 24 months.[78] Festen et al have shown that recurrences can be successfully treated with redo PPH as more than 90% of their recurrences treated with redo PPH achieved prolapse reduction.[79] In a retrospective review, Jongen et al looked at reoperations for 1233 patients undergoing SH over a 10-year time frame. Reoperation rate was 10%, with the majority stapler-related, recurrent/persistent hemorrhoidal symptoms, or other anorectal issues not addressed by the circular SH procedure. No life-threatening complications occurred, and the need for both early and late reoperations decreased significantly over time (P < 0.05).[80] Case reports have been published on severe pelvic sepsis after SH. Van Wensen et al reported a case requiring exploratory laparotomy with presacral drainage and diverting ileostomy. On reoperation, a digital examination revealed a dorsolateral rectal perforation. It is unclear in their publication whether this was at the staple line or not.[81] Martellucci et al reported a double rectal perforation after SH. The more distal perforation was related to a staple line dehiscence, and they theorized that the more proximal perforation at the rectosigmoid junction may have been related to a sigmoidocele trapped in the stapler during the initial operation.[82] Molloy and Kingsmore reported a case of severe pelvic sepsis, likely resulting from an inadvertent rectal injury.[83] Cheetham et al also raised concern over persistent severe anorectal pain as a possible sequela of PPH.[84]

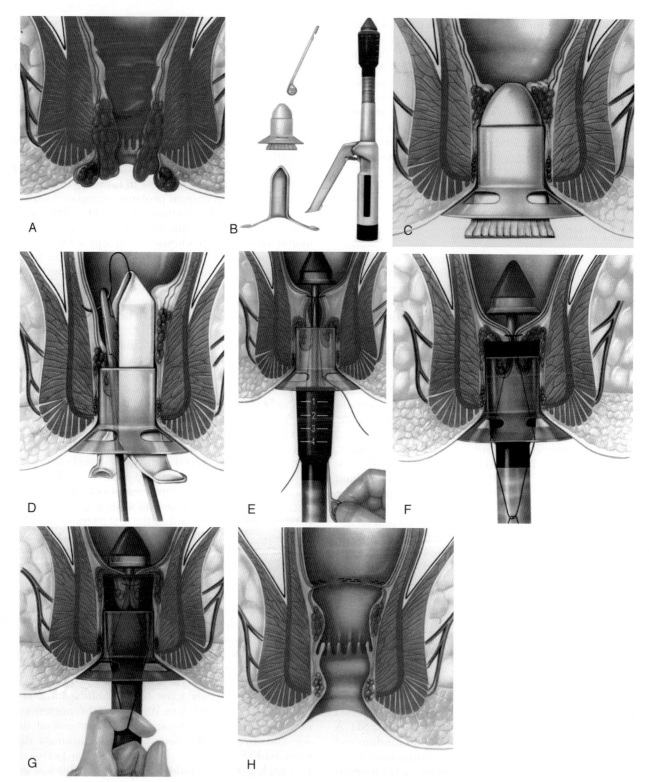

FIGURE 154-5 **A** and **B,** Identification of the internal hemorrhoidal complexes and the instrumentation used for a stapled hemorrhoidectomy are shown. **C** and **D,** A purse-string suture is accurately placed 4 cm above the dentate line by the use of an anoscope. **E** to **G,** The purse string is tied securely around the rod of the stapling anvil, which allows the hemorrhoidal tissue to be pulled into the barrel of the stapler head. **H,** The stapler is closed, fired, and held in place for 20 to 30 seconds. The staple line should be inspected and any bleeding sites suture-ligated.

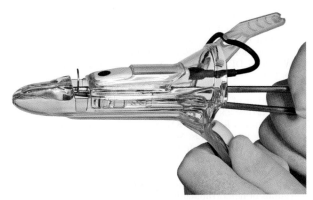

FIGURE 154-6 Image of device for transanal hemorrhoidal dearterialization (THD). A Doppler incorporated in device is used to locate terminal branches of the hemorrhoidal arteries. Once localized, the arteries are suture-ligated. A hemorrhoidopexy can be performed for prolapse repair with a running absorbable suture above the dentate line. This repair atrophies the hemorrhoidal cushions and restores prolapsed tissue to its anatomic position.

HEMORRHOIDAL ARTERIAL LIGATION

A new technique that is gaining popularity is Doppler-guided hemorrhoidal artery ligation, or transanal hemorrhoidal dearterialization (THD). The guided reduction in arterial blood flow can be coupled with a mucosopexy when there is significant prolapse—so that this aspect can be corrected and venous outflow improved. This technique was first described by Morinaga et al in 1995 and is based on closure of the hemorrhoidal blood flow that feeds the hemorrhoidal plexus via the terminal branches of the superior rectal artery.[85] A specifically designed proctoscope is used coupled with a Doppler transducer. At the distal end, there is a small window that allows suturing of the rectal mucosa 2 to 3 cm above the dentate line (Figure 154-6). The reduction of blood flow is thought to lead to shrinkage of the hemorrhoidal complex. In addition, a mucosopexy can be performed that lifts up the prolapsing tissue into its normal anatomic position. Giordano et al published an extensive review of the current evidence on THD, looking specifically at safety and effectiveness of the technique. Sixteen of the 17 articles that met inclusion criteria were observational studies, and the study quality ranged from low to very low. The majority of patients treated had grade II or III disease. Of the 1996 patients who were involved in these studies, the most common early postoperative event was postoperative pain (18.5%). Residual protrusion, bleeding, and fever were complications documented with an incidence higher than 3%. When the studies with a followup of 1 year or more were analyzed (6/17 publications), the incidence of prolapse was 10.8%, bleeding 9.7%, and pain on defecation 8.7%.[86]

POSTOPERATIVE MANAGEMENT AFTER HEMORRHOID SURGERY

Regardless of the excisional technique used for treatment of advanced hemorrhoidal disease, the key to effective patient management is avoidance of postoperative complications. Pain is the most frequent complication and is the most feared sequela of the procedure from the patient's perspective. A variety of analgesic regimens have been recommended, usually consisting of a combination of oral and parenteral narcotics.[87-91] The use of local infiltration of bupivacaine into the wounds and perianal skin has been variably successful in long-term pain reduction.[92,93] Conversely, ketorolac has demonstrated considerable efficacy in managing posthemorrhoidectomy pain.[94] The use of alternative administration routes for narcotics either by patch or subcutaneous pump have been successful in controlling pain; however, the management of these routes of administration can be risky in the outpatient setting because of the risk of narcotic-induced respiratory depression. The most appropriate regimen following outpatient hemorrhoidectomy appears to be intraoperative use of ketorolac, sufficient doses of oral narcotic analgesics for home administration, and supplementation of the narcotics by an oral nonsteroidal antiinflammatory drug (NSAID). Two recent publications have supported the use of nifedipine with lidocaine ointment and glyceryl trinitrate (GTN) ointment for posthemorrhoidectomy pain. Reducing the internal sphincter spasm may contribute to the effectiveness of this therapy. Of 69 patients randomized to receive 0.2% GTN or placebo, the patients in the GTN group experienced significantly less postoperative pain on days 1, 3, and 7 ($P < 0.05$), used less analgesics, and had improved wound healing compared to placebo at 3 weeks from a diathermy Ferguson hemorrhoidectomy.[95,96] Joshi et al looked at evidence-based management of pain after hemorrhoidectomy surgery in a systemic review in 2010. The findings revealed that local anesthetic infiltration as a sole technique or with general or regional anesthetic should be recommended in addition to a combination of NSAID, paracetamol, and opiates. Other medications that are recommended as analgesic adjuncts may include laxatives and oral metronidazole started before surgery.[97]

Urinary retention is a frequent postoperative problem following hemorrhoidectomy, ranging in incidence from 1% to 52%.[98-101] A variety of strategies have been used to treat the problem, including parasympathomimetics, α-adrenergic blocking agents, and sitz baths.[98,102] The best approach, however, seems to be a strategy of prevention that includes limiting perioperative fluid administration to 250 mL, an anesthetic approach that avoids use of spinal anesthesia, avoidance of anal packing, and an aggressive oral analgesic regimen.[103]

Early postoperative bleeding (<24 hours) occurs in approximately 1% of cases and represents a technical error requiring return to the operating theater for resuturing of the offending wound.[104] Delayed hemorrhage occurs in 0.5% to 4% of cases of excisional hemorrhoidectomy at 5 to 10 days postoperatively.[105-107] The etiology has been held to be early separation of the ligated pedicle before adequate thrombosis in the feeding artery can occur.[108] The bleeding in this scenario is usually significant and requires some method for control of ongoing hemorrhage. Options include return to the operating theater for suture ligation or tamponade at the bedside by Foley catheter or anal packing.[108-110] The subsequent outcome after control of secondary hemorrhage is generally good, with virtually no risk of recurrent bleeding. It may be helpful to irrigate out the distal colorectum with posthemorrhage enemas or at the time of intraoperative control of bleeding to avoid confusion when the residual clots pass per anum.

CONCLUSION

The management of symptomatic hemorrhoidal disease should be directed at the symptom complex of the individual patient. Most of these patients can be successfully treated by improving bowel function, correcting constipation, and using any of a variety of anal ointments. For persistent symptoms, either injection or banding of the internal hemorrhoids is predictably successful. Only a few patients should require excisional hemorrhoidectomy by any of the described techniques. Circular SH and transanal hemorrhoidal dearterialization with or without mucosopexy may prove to be an effective, less painful technique to manage grade III hemorrhoids.

REFERENCES

1. Holley CJ: History of hemorrhoidal surgery. *South Med J* 39:536, 1946.
2. Madoff RD: Biblical management of anorectal disease. Presented at the Midwest Society of Colon and Rectal Surgeons. March, 1991, Brechenridge, Colorado.
3. Dirckx JH: The biblical plague of "hemorrhoids". An outbreak of bilharziasis. *Am J Dermatopathol* 7:341, 1985.
4. Maimonides M, Rosner F, Munter S [trans]: *Treatise on hemorrhoids.* Philadelphia, 1969, JB Lippincott.
5. Rachochot JE, Petourand CH, Riovoire JO: Saint Fiacre: The healer of hemorrhoids and patron saint of proctology. *Am J Proctol* 22:175, 1971.
6. Thomson WH: The nature of haemorrhoids. *Br J Surg* 62:542, 1975.
7. Morgado PJ, et al: Histoclinical basis for a new classification of hemorrhoidal disease. *Dis Colon Rectum* 31:474, 1988.
8. Burkitt DP, Graham-Steward CW: Hemorrhoid-postulated pathogenesis and proposed prevention. *Postgrad Med J* 51:631, 1975.
9. Haas PA, Fox TA Jr, Haas GP: The pathogenesis of hemorrhoids. *Dis Colon Rectum* 27:442, 1984.
10. Arabi Y, Alexander Williams J, Keighley MR: Anal pressures in hemorrhoids and anal fissure. *Am J Surg* 134:608, 1977.
11. Hancock BD: Internal sphincter and the nature of haemorrhoids. *Gut* 18:651, 1977.
12. Arscia SD: *Morphological and physiological aspects of anal continence and defecation.* Brussels, 1969, Presses Academiquues Europeenes, p 150.
13. Goligher J: Haemorrhoids or piles. In *Surgery of the anus, rectum and colon.* London, 1984, Balliere Tindall, p 98.
14. Benyon J: *Endorectal and anal sonography in surgery of the colon, rectum and anus.* Philadelphia, 1995, Saunders.
15. Dennison A, Whiston RJ, Rooney S, et al: A randomized comparison of infrared photocoagulation with bipolar diathermy for the outpatient treatment of hemorrhoids. *Dis Colon Rectum* 33:32, 1990.
16. Hinton CP, Morris DL: A randomized trial comparing direct current therapy and bipolar diathermy in the outpatient treatment of third-degree hemorrhoids. *Dis Colon Rectum* 33:931, 1990.
17. Zinberg SS, Stern DH, Furman DS, et al: A personal experience in comparing three nonoperative techniques for treating internal hemorrhoids. *Am J Gastroenterol* 84:488, 1989.
18. Barron J: Office ligation of internal hemorrhoids. *Am J Surg* 105:563, 1963.
19. Bayer I, Myslovaty B, Picovsky BM: Rubber band ligation of hemorrhoids. Convenient and economic treatment. *J Clin Gastroenterol* 23:50, 1996.
20. Marshman D, Huber PJ Jr, Timmerman W, et al: Hemorrhoidal ligation. A review of efficacy. *Dis Colon Rectum* 32:369, 1989.
21. Oueidat DM, Jurjus AR: Management of hemorrhoids by rubber band ligation. *J Med Liban* 42:11, 1994.
22. Wrobleski DE: Rubber band ligation of hemorrhoids. *R I Med* 78:172, 1995.
23. Wrobleski DE, Corman ML, Veidenheimer MC, et al: Long-term evaluation of rubber ring ligation in hemorrhoidal disease. *Dis Colon Rectum* 23:478, 1980.
24. Alemdaroglu K. Ulualp KM: Single session ligation treatment of bleeding hemorrhoids. *Surg Gynecol Obstet* 177:62, 1993.
25. Clay LD 3rd, White JJ Jr, Davidson JT, et al: Early recognition and successful management of pelvic cellulitis following hemorrhoidal banding. *Dis Colon Rectum* 29:579, 1986.
26. Quevedo-Bonilla G, Farkas AM, Abcarian H, et al: Septic complications of hemorrhoidal banding. *Arch Surg* 123:650, 1988.
27. Russell TR, Donohue JH: Hemorrhoidal banding. A warning. *Dis Colon Rectum* 28:291, 1985.
28. Scarpa FJ, Hillis W, Sabetta JR: Pelvis cellulitis: A life-threatening complication of hemorrhoidal banding. *Surgery* 103:383, 1988.
29. Lau WY, Chow HP, Poon GP, et al: Rubber band ligation of three primary hemorrhoids in a single session. A safe and effective procedure. *Dis Colon Rectum* 25:336, 1982.
30. Lee HH, Spencer RJ, Beart RW Jr: Multiple hemorrhoidal bandings in a single session. *Dis Colon Rectum* 37:37, 1994.
31. McKenzie L, de Verteuil R, Cook J, et al: Economic evaluation of the treatment of grade II haemorrhoids: A comparison of stapled haemorrhoidopexy and rubber band ligation. *Colorectal Dis* 12:587, 2010.
32. Senagore A, Mazier WP, Luchtefeld MA, et al: Treatment of advanced hemorrhoidal disease: A prospective, randomized comparison of cold scalpel vs. contact Nd:YAG laser. *Dis Colon Rectum* 36:1042, 1993.
33. Duhamel J, Romand-Heurer Y: Technische Bensonderheiten bei der Hamorrhoidektomie nach Milligan and Morgan. *Coloproctology* 4:265, 1980.
34. Milligan ET, Morgan CN, Lond LE: Surgical anatomy of anal canal, and the operative treatment of hemorrhoids. *Lancet* 2:1119, 1937.
35. Tajana A: Hemorrhoidectomy according to Milligan-Morgan: ligature and excision technique. *Int Surg* 74:158, 1989.
36. Ferguson JA, Heaton JR: Closed hemorrhoidectomy. *Dis Colon Rectum* 2:176, 1959.
37. Ganchrow MI, Mazier WP, Friend WG, et al: Hemorrhoidectomy revisited—computer analysis of 2,038 cases. *Dis Colon Rectum* 14:128, 1971.
38. McConnell JC, Khubchandani IT: Long-term follow-up of closed hemorrhoidectomy. *Dis Colon Rectum* 26:797, 1983.
39. Muldoon JP: The completely closed hemorrhoidectomy: a reliable and trusted friend for 25 years. *Dis Colon Rectum* 24:211, 1981.
40. Whitehead W: The surgical treatment of haemorrhoids. *Br Med J* 1:148, 1882.
41. Andrews E: Disastrous results following Whitehead's operation and the so-called American operation. *Columbus Med J* 15:97, 1895.
42. Andrews E: Some of the evils caused by Whitehead's operation and by its modification, the American operation. *Trans Illinois Med Soc* 1895, p 433.
43. Khubchandani M: Results of Whitehead operation. *Dis Colon Rectum* 27:730, 1984.
44. Rand AA: The sliding skin-flap graft operation for hemorrhoids: A modification of the Whitehead procedure. *Dis Colon Rectum* 12:265, 1969.
45. Bonello JC: Who's afraid of the dentate line? The Whitehead hemorrhoidectomy. *Am J Surg* 156:182, 1988.
46. Wolff BG, Culp CE: The Whitehead hemorrhoidectomy. An unjustly maligned procedure. *Dis Colon Rectum* 31:587, 1988.
47. Andrews BT, Layer GT, Jackson BT, et al: Randomized trial comparing diathermy hemorrhoidectomy with the scissor dissection Milligan-Morgan operation. *Dis Colon Rectum* 36:580, 1993.
48. Ibrahim S, Tsang C, Lee YL, et al: Prospective, randomized trial comparing pain and complications between diathermy and scissors for closed hemorrhoidectomy. *Dis Colon Rectum* 41:1418, 1998.
49. Quah HM, Seow-Choen F: Prospective, randomized trial comparing diathermy excision and diathermy coagulation for symptomatic, prolapsed hemorrhoids. *Dis Colon Rectum* 47:367, 2004.

50. Nystrom PO, Qvist N, Raahave D, et al: Randomized clinical trial of symptom control after stapled anopexy or diathermy excision for haemorrhoid prolapse. *Br J Surg* 97:167, 2010.

51. Thaha MA, Campbell KL, Kazmi SA, et al: Prospective randomized multi-centre trial comparing the clinical efficacy, safety and patient acceptability of circular stapled anopexy with closed diathermy haemorrhoidectomy. *Gut* 58:668, 2009.

52. Zahir KS, Edwards RE, Vecchia A, et al: Use of the Nd-YAG laser improves quality of life and economic factors in the treatment of hemorrhoids. *Conn Med* 64:199, 2000.

53. Hodgson WJ, Morgan J: Ambulatory hemorrhoidectomy with CO_2 laser. *Dis Colon Rectum* 38:1265, 1995.

54. Leff EI: Hemorrhoidectomy—laser vs. nonlaser: outpatient surgical experience. *Dis Colon Rectum* 35:743, 1992.

55. Chung YC, Wu HJ: Clinical experience of sutureless closed hemorrhoidectomy. *Dis Colon Rectum* 46:87, 2003.

56. Franklin EJ, Seetharam S, Lowney J, et al: Randomized clinical trial of Ligasure vs conventional diathermy in hemorrhoidectomy. *Dis Colon Rectum* 46:1380, 2003.

57. Fareed M, El-Awady S, Abd-El Monaem H, et al: Randomized trial comparing Ligasure to closed Ferguson hemorrhoidectomy. *Tech Coloproctol* 13:243, 2009.

58. Milito G, Cadeddu F, Muzi MG, et al: Haemorrhoidectomy with Ligasure vs conventional excisional techniques: Meta-analysis of randomized controlled trials. *Colorectal Dis* 12:85, 2010.

59. Armstrong DN, Frankum C, Schertzer ME, et al: Harmonic Scalpel hemorrhoidectomy: Five hundred consecutive cases. *Dis Colon Rectum* 45:354, 2002.

60. Armstrong DN, Ambroze WL, Schertzer ME, et al: Harmonic Scalpel vs. electrocautery hemorrhoidectomy: A prospective evaluation. *Dis Colon Rectum* 44:558, 2001.

61. Khan S, Pawlak SE, Eggenberger JC, et al: Surgical treatment of hemorrhoids: Prospective, randomized trial comparing closed excisional hemorrhoidectomy and the Harmonic Scalpel technique of excisional hemorrhoidectomy. *Dis Colon Rectum* 44:845, 2001.

62. Tan JJ, Seow-Choen F: Prospective, randomized trial comparing diathermy and Harmonic Scalpel hemorrhoidectomy. *Dis Colon Rectum* 44:677, 2001.

63. Abo-hashem AA, Sarhan A, Aly AM: Harmonic Scalpel compared with bipolar electro-cautery hemorrhoidectomy: A randomized controlled trial. *Int J Surg* 8:243, 2010.

64. Chung CC, Ha JP, Tai YP, et al: Double-blind, randomized trial comparing Harmonic Scalpel hemorrhoidectomy, bipolar scissors hemorrhoidectomy, and scissors excision: Ligation technique. *Dis Colon Rectum* 45:789, 2002.

65. Kohlstadt CM, Weber J, Prohm P: [Stapler hemorrhoidectomy. A new alternative to conventional methods]. *Zentralbl Chir* 124:238, 1999.

66. Boccasanta P, Venturi M, Orio A, et al: Circular hemorrhoidectomy in advanced hemorrhoidal disease. *Hepatogastroenterology* 45:969, 1998.

67. Khalil KH, O'Bichere A, Sellu D: Randomized clinical trial of sutured versus stapled closed haemorrhoidectomy. *Br J Surg* 87:1352, 2000.

68. Mehigan BJ, Monson JR, Hartley JE: Stapling procedure for haemorrhoids versus Milligan-Morgan haemorrhoidectomy: Randomized controlled trial. *Lancet* 355:782, 2000.

69. Rowsell M, Bello M, Hemingway DM: Circumferential mucosectomy (stapled haemorrhoidectomy) versus conventional haemorrhoidectomy: randomized controlled trial. *Lancet* 355:779, 2000.

70. Ganio E, Altomare DF, Gabrielli F, et al: Prospective randomized multicentre trial comparing stapled with open haemorrhoidectomy. *Br J Surg* 88:669, 2001.

71. Sengore AJ, Singer M, Abcarian H, et al: Procedure for Prolapse and Hemmorrhoids (PPH) Multicenter Study Group. A prospective, randomized, controlled multicenter trial comparing stapled hemorrhoidopexy and Ferguson hemorrhoidectomy: Perioperative and one-year results. *Dis Colon Rectum* 47:1824, 2004.

72. Madiba TE, Esterhuizen TM, Thomson SR: Procedure for prolapsed haemorrhoids versus excisional haemorrhoidectomy—a systematic review and meta-analysis. *S Afr Med J* 99:43, 2009.

73. Laughlan K, Jayne DG, Jackson D, et al: Stapled haemorrhoidopexy compared to Milligan-Morgan and Ferguson haemorrhoidectomy: A systematic review. *Int J Colorectal Dis* 24:335, 2009.

74. Jayaraman S, Colquhoun PH, Malthaner RA: Stapled versus conventional surgery for hemorrhoids. *Cochrance Database Syst Rev* CD005393, 2006.

75. Giordano P, Gravante G, Sorge R, et al: Long-term outcomes of stapled hemorrhoidopexy vs conventional hemorrhoidectomy: A meta-analysis of randomized controlled *trials*. *Arch Surg* 144:266, 2009.

76. Burch J, Epstein D, Sari AB, et al: Stapled haemorrhoidopexy for the treatment of haemorrhoids: A systematic review. *Colorectal Dis* 11:233; discussion 243, 2009.

77. Sakr MF, Moussa MM: LigaSure hemorrhoidectomy versus stapled hemorrhoidopexy: A prospective, randomized clinical trial. *Dis Colon Rectum* 53:1161, 2010.

78. Bove A, Bongarzoni G, Palone G, et al: Effective treatment of haemorrhoids: Early complication and late results after 150 consecutive stapled haemorrhoidectomies. *Ann Ital Chir* 80:299, 2009.

79. Festen S, van Geloven AA, Gerhards MF: Redo procedure for prolapse and haemorrhoids (PPH) for persistent and recurrent prolapse after PPH. *Dig Surg* 26:418, 2009.

80. Jongen J, Eberstein A, Bock JU, et al: Complications, recurrences, early and late reoperations after stapled haemorrhoidopexy: Lessons learned from 1,233 cases. *Langenbecks Arch Surg* 395:1049, 2010.

81. Van Wensen RJ, van Leuken MH, Bosscha K: Pelvis sepsis after stapled hemorrhoidopexy. *World J Gastroenterol* 14:5924, 2008.

82. Martellucci J, Papi F, Tanzini G: Double rectal perforation after stapled haemorrhoidectomy. *Int J Colorectal Dis* 24:1113, 2009.

83. Molloy RG, Kingsmore D: Life threatening pelvic sepsis after stapled haemorrhoidectomy. *Lancet* 355:810, 2000.

84. Cheetham MJ, Mortensen NJ, Nystrom PO, et al: Persistent pain and faecal urgency after stapled haemorrhoidectomy. *Lancet* 356:730, 2000.

85. Morinaga K, Hasuda K, Ikeda T: A novel therapy for internal hemorrhoids: Ligation of the hemorrhoidal artery with newly devised instrument (Moricorn) in conjunction with a Doppler flowmeter. *Am J Gastroenterol* 90:610, 1995.

86. Giordano P, Overton J, Madeddu F, et al: Transanal hemorrhoidal dearterialization: A systematic review. *Dis Colon Rectum* 52:1665, 2009.

87. Goldstein ET, Williamson PR, Larach SW: Subcutaneous morphine pump for postoperative hemorrhoidectomy pain management. *Dis Colon Rectum* 36:439, 1993.

88. Kilbride M, Morse M, Senagore A: Transdermal fentanyl improves management of postoperative hemorrhoidectomy pain. *Dis Colon Rectum* 37:1070, 1994.

89. Kilbride MJ, Senagore AJ, Morse M: Improving patient safety with transdermal-fentanyl for post-hemorrhoidectomy pain. *Dis Colon Rectum* 38:104, 1995.

90. Kuo RJ: Epidural morphine for post-hemorrhoidectomy analgesia. *Dis Colon Rectum* 27:529, 1984.

91. O'Donovan S, Ferrara A, Larach S, et al: Intraoperative use of Toradol facilitates outpatient hemorrhoidectomy. *Dis Colon Rectum* 37:793, 1994.

92. Chesterm JF, Stanford BJ, Gazet JC: Analgesic benefit of locally injected bupivacaine after hemorrhoidectomy. *Dis Colon Rectum* 33:487, 1990.

93. Hussein MK, Taha AM, Haddad FF, et al: Bupivacaine local injection in anorectal surgery. *Int Surg* 83:56, 1998.

94. Bleday R, Pena JP, Rothenberger DA, et al: Symptomatic hemorrhoids: Current incidence and complications of operative therapy. *Dis Colon Rectum* 35:477, 1992.

95. Perrotti P, Dominici P, Grossi E, et al: Topical nifedipine with lidocaine ointment versus active control for pain after hemorrhoidectomy: Results of a multicentre, prospective, randomized, double-blind study. *Can J Surg* 53:17, 2010.

96. Karanlik H, Akturk R, Camlica H, et al: The effect of glyceryl trinitrate ointment on posthemorrhoidectomy pain and wound healing: Results of a randomized double-blind, placebo-controlled study. *Dis Colon Rectum* 52:280, 2009.

97. Joshi GP, Neugebauer EA: Evidence-based management of pain after haemorrhoidectomy surgery. *Br J Surg* 97:1155, 2010.

98. Hoff SD, Bailey HR, Butts DR, et al: Ambulatory surgical hemorrhoidectomy—a solution to postoperative urinary retention? *Dis Colon Rectum* 37:1242, 1994.

99. Leventhal A. Pfau A: Pharmacologic management of postoperative overdistention of the bladder. *Surg Gynecol Obstet* 146:347, 1978.

100. Petros JG, Bradley TM: Factors influencing postoperative urinary retention in patients undergoing surgery for benign anorectal disease. *Am J Surg* 159:374, 1990.

101. Tammela T, Kontturi M, Lukkarinen O: Postoperative urinary retention. I. Incidence and predisposing factors. *Scand J Urol Nephrol* 20:197, 1986.

102. Shafik A: Role of warm water bath in inducing micturition in postoperative urinary retention after anorectal operations. *Urol Int* 50:213, 1993.

103. Corman ML: Complications in hemorrhoid and fissure surgery. In Ferrari BT, Ray JE, Gathright JB, editors: *Complications of colon and rectal surgery: Prevention and management.* Philadelphia, 1985, Saunders, p 91.

104. Kilbourne NJ: Internal haemorrhoids: Comparative value of treatment by operative and by injection methods: A survey of 62,910 cases. *Ann Surg* 99:600, 1934.

105. Gabriel WB: Hemorrhoids. In *The Principles and Practice of Rectal Surgery,* ed 5, Springfield Ill, 1964, Charles C Thomas, p 110.

106. Milsom JW: Hemorrhoidal disease. In Wexner SD, Beck DE, editors: *Fundamentals of anorectal surgery.* New York, 1992, McGraw-Hill, p 192.

107. Salvati EP, Eisenstat TE: Hemorrhoidal disease. In Zuidema GD, Condon RE, editors: *Shackelford's surgery of the alimentary tract.* Philadelphia, 1991, Saunders, p 294.

108. Rosen L, Sipe P, Stasik JJ, et al: Outcome of delayed hemorrhage following surgical hemorrhoidectomy. *Dis Colon Rectum* 36:743, 1993.

109. Basso L, Pescatori M: Outcome of delayed hemorrhage following surgical hemorrhoidectomy. *Dis Colon Rectum* 37:288, 1994.

110. Cirocco WC, Golub RW: Local epinephrine injection as treatment for delayed hemorrhage after hemorrhoidectomy. *Surgery* 117:235, 1995.

Fissure-in-Ano

Clifford L. Simmang | Harry T. Papaconstantinou | Philip J. Huber, Jr.

Anal fissure (fissure-in-ano) is a common condition that usually presents as anal pain or bleeding with defecation. Bleeding is usually scant, bright red, and found on the tissue when cleansing after a bowel movement. Anal fissure is described as a linear defect, or laceration, in the anoderm, located between the dentate line and the anal verge. An acute fissure is a simple laceration, whereas a chronic anal fissure is an ulceration with built-up scarred edges and exposed internal anal sphincter muscle fibers at its base. Additional findings may include a perianal skin tag at the external margin of the fissure and a hypertrophied papilla at the dentate line. Chronic fissure is defined by these three findings—visible muscle, a skin tag (sentinel tag), and hypertrophied papilla (Figure 155-1). Importantly, acute and chronic anal fissures are almost always located in the midline with the posterior location predominating (women, 90%; men, 99%). Fissures located off the midline are usually associated with more serious systemic diseases such as Crohn disease and immunodeficiency syndromes (Figure 155-2).

ETIOLOGY

Trauma to the anal canal, because of passing hard stools, is probably the most frequent cause of fissure-in-ano. Loose watery stools may also be associated with the development of anal fissures. Preexisting anal canal irritation has been postulated to lead to fissure. Scarring, stricture, and stenosis, from prior anal injury or surgery, are recognized conditions that predispose to fissure formation.[1] Because fissures occur most often in the posterior midline, various structural theories have been proposed as causes,[2-4] the most compelling of which is the vascular anatomy of the internal sphincter.

In 1989, Klosterhalfen et al[5] reported on anatomic dissections that detailed the blood supply of the inferior hemorrhoidal artery. In the majority of cadaver specimens (85%), the posterior commissure of the anal canal was not directly perfused except by end arterioles. Branching from the sphincteric arterioles occurred at right angles to the parent vessels and coursed perpendicularly through the circular fibers of the internal sphincter. These anatomic findings established the possibility of decreased mucosal perfusion, particularly in the posterior midline. Furthermore, sphincter spasm and hypertonicity, which is common in this disease, may further decrease blood flow posteriorly. Schouten et al[6,7] have shown increased anal canal pressures correlated with decreased mucosal blood flow as measured by laser Doppler flowmetry. Reports of normal anal maximal resting pressure are highly variable, ranging from 60 to 100 cm H_2O in females and slightly higher in males;

however, the measurement is defined as the maximal pressure recorded at rest.[8] The higher pressures seen in patients with anal fissures will produce a sawtooth pattern on manometry tracings. This vascular-anal resting pressure hypothesis has prompted trials aimed at improving blood flow and lowering anal canal resting pressures. Whether sphincter hypertonia is a cause or effect is unknown.

The most common systemic conditions that are associated with atypical anal fissure/anal ulcer are Crohn disease and acquired immunodeficiency syndrome. Both of these conditions lead to an immunocompromised patient. Atypical features include fissures off the true midline, shaggy large defects with undermined edges, and granulation tissue in the base. Actual cavitation of the internal sphincter is another ominous clue to the presence of systemic disease. In the immunocompromised patient, a fissure or an ulcer and a concomitant mass should raise the question of malignancy. Lymphoma, leukemic ulcer, and anal canal epithelial tumors are often associated with surface defects. There are subtle changes, which distinguish these conditions from uncomplicated acute or chronic anal fissure.

Infections also cause fissure-in-ano. Syphilis and tuberculosis were seen frequently in the United States over the last century but are currently uncommon causes of anal fissure. Today, sexually transmitted diseases and infections associated with immunocompromised conditions may be the cause of anal fissure and include chancroid, herpes simplex virus, and cytomegalovirus. Herpes simplex infection manifests as multiple superficial ulcers and vesicles, while syphilitic ulcers are purulent and have a granular base. The treatments for these disease processes are different, and therefore, it is important to recognize the differences between anal canal fissures and atypical anal canal ulcers (see Figure 155-2).

DIAGNOSIS

A tearing or burning discomfort during defecation is by far the most common symptom of anal fissure. Bleeding is usually only detected on the toilet paper. The pain associated with anal fissure lasts for minutes to hours, and in patients with a chronic fissure, it is most often described as profound anal "tightness" or "spasm." Examination must be carefully performed; the pain caused by an aggressive examination of an anal fissure is not easily forgotten. Simple spreading of the buttocks to gently roll open the anal verge will usually demonstrate the fissure (Figure 155-3). Endoscopy, which must be performed as part of the complete evaluation of patients with fissure, should be postponed; a more complete anorectal examination can be better accomplished when the

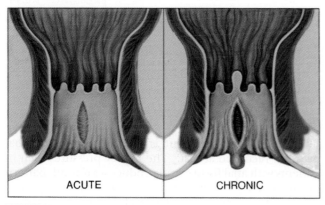

FIGURE 155-1 Acute and chronic fissure. (Modified from Hicks TC, Ray JE: Rectal and perianal complaints. In Polk HC Jr, Stone HH, Gardner B, editors: *Basic surgery*, ed 3. Norwalk, Conn, 1987, Appleton-Century-Crofts, p 455.)

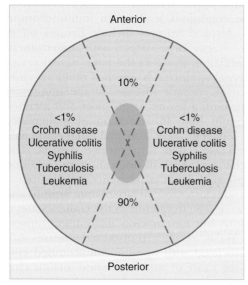

FIGURE 155-2 Diagram of the location of typical fissures and atypical fissures where a systemic illness should be suspected.

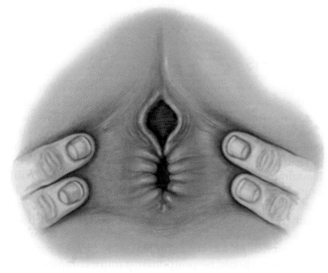

FIGURE 155-3 Inspection of fissure.

fissure is healed. Importantly, topical anesthetics do not facilitate pain-free examinations.

Atypical-appearing fissures require more intensive inquiry. Symptoms of inflammatory bowel disease should be sought. Sexual activity and drug history should likewise be documented. High-risk behavior for human immunodeficiency virus infection necessitates screening and may explain the presence of the atypical fissure. Syphilitic ulcers can be diagnosed with dark-field, wet prep microscopy. Tuberculous ulcer, although commonly superinfected, will show acid-fast bacilli on staining. The critical issue in patients with atypical-appearing fissures is a high index of suspicion. If an atypical fissure is treated the same way as a typical fissure, a large nonhealing wound could result.

Most diagnostic tests will not be tolerated as office procedures. Examination under anesthesia permits a thorough evaluation of the anus and rectum. Cultures, biopsies, and possible therapeutic interventions can be safely and carefully performed with anesthesia. Indeed, patients embrace the opportunity to have a pain-free evaluation under anesthesia.

NONSURGICAL MANAGEMENT

CONSERVATIVE

The first-line therapy for patients with simple, acute fissure-in-ano includes warm-water sitz baths and stool-bulking agents. Warm-water soaks likely relieve anal discomfort by muscle relaxation, which lowers anal canal pressures; however, results from prospective studies are contradictory.[9] Nevertheless, heat provides dramatic relief to most patients with acute and chronic fissure-in-ano, and should be used in all patients. Stool-bulking agents, such as psyllium, bran, and fiber, draw water into the stool, changing its consistency, and therefore, prevent the formation of hard stool that causes sustained trauma to the anal canal. Furthermore, bran has been shown to be effective in preventing recurrence of acute anal fissure.[10] Topical creams and steroids are of limited utility and not routinely recommended as management options, because these modalities do not address the underlying problem. These conservative, nonsurgical measures successfully heal 90% of acute anal fissures, but only 40% of chronic fissures. Chronic anal fissures are managed with medications that provide a "chemical sphincterotomy," and are described later.

NITROGLYCERIN

It has been suggested that poor posterior anal canal blood flow and generalized hypertonia of the internal anal sphincter are causes of anal fissures. Therefore, improvement in the blood supply and sphincter relaxation should facilitate healing. Nitric oxide is a potent smooth muscle relaxant and promotes vasodilation. Topical nitroglycerin is a nitric oxide donor that is absorbed transcutaneously, and when applied to the anus, has been shown to reduce anal canal pressure.[11] Indeed, nitroglycerin has become an important adjuvant treatment option in patients with fissures that do not heal with stool-bulking agents and local heat therapy.[12,13] A recent metaanalysis of randomized controlled trials comparing nitroglycerin ointment to placebo for the treatment of anal fissures has shown that nitroglycerin is significantly more effective than placebo in primary healing of anal fissure (46% vs. 33%, $P < 0.0001$).[14] In fact, several independent studies have demonstrated the therapeutic efficacy of nitroglycerin paste in 60% to 75% of patients with anal fissures.[15-20]

The dosage and strength of the nitroglycerin have varied from study to study, but there is some correlation between dose and degree of sphincter relaxation.[21] Application of 200 to 500 mg of 0.2% nitroglycerin paste (about the size of a pea) to the anus is performed at least twice daily. It is important to inform patients that either they should use a Q-tip, or a glove should be worn, to protect against absorption of the nitroglycerin through the skin on the finger. The ointment should be protected from exposure to air and light because nitroglycerin paste is volatile and will deactivate. Pain relief is nearly immediate (5 minutes) and lasts for up to 12 hours.[12,15,16] Headache is a significant side effect and limits the amount of paste that can be applied. With this therapy, healing of the fissure takes 4 to 6 weeks. Patients with fissures that fail to heal often have persistently elevated anal canal pressures despite the use of nitroglycerin. Recurrent disease after initial healing can be successfully re-treated.[15,16] Other adverse effects such as orthostatic hypotension, syncopal attacks, and tachyphylaxis are well described and may limit the use of this treatment modality; they are uncommon.[21-23]

NIFEDIPINE AND DILTIAZEM

Alternatives to nitroglycerin ointment that can produce a similar "chemical sphincterotomy" effect include topical application of calcium channel blockers (nifedipine and diltiazem) and botulinum toxin A injection. Topical nifedipine has been shown to reduce resting anal sphincter pressures, and heal significantly more chronic anal fissures than control (95% vs. 16%; $P < 0.001$).[24] These positive effects were achieved with no significant side effects of this medication. Other calcium channel blockers, such as topical 2% diltiazem, have been shown to be as effective as nitroglycerin in the treatment of chronic anal fissures.[25,26] In fact, topical diltiazem heals between 48% and 75% of fissures that have failed to heal with nitroglycerin alone.[27,28] This class of drug may ultimately supersede nitroglycerin in the treatment of chronic anal fissure because it is equally effective in treating chronic anal fissures and has a superior side-effect profile. Oral calcium channel blockers have been used but have a lower rate of healing than topical application with a higher rate of side effects, primarily headaches.[29,30] Two new topical smooth muscle relaxants, indoramin and minoxidil, were tested in randomized controlled trials, and neither were effective in healing anal fissure.[29]

BOTOX

Another alternative is botulinum toxin A, an exotoxin produced by the bacterium *Clostridium botulinum* that causes paralysis of skeletal muscle by preventing the presynaptic release of acetylcholine. Botulinum toxin A has been shown to be efficacious in the treatment of chronic anal fissure. In one study, 73% of anal fissures were healed at 8 weeks, with no recurrences at a mean of 16 months followup.[31] Results of a randomized double-blind placebo-controlled trial comparing botulinum toxin A injection to topical nitroglycerin ointment showed that at 8 weeks anal fissures were healed in 96% of patients injected with neurotoxin and 60% of those treated with nitroglycerin.[32] There was no recurrence in either group at a mean followup of 15 months.[33] The optimal dose and injection site of botulinum toxin A for the treatment of chronic anal fissures are unclear. There are no data to determine the optimal dose and anywhere from 10 to 100 units have been reported. A report of 50 units of botulinum toxin A has shown to be well tolerated.[33] Healing of posterior anal fissures are accelerated in patients injected with neurotoxin in the anterior anus when compared to posterior injection.[34] Although initial studies reported injections into the external anal sphincter, recent studies have performed intersphincteric injections or injection into the internal sphincter with excellent results, with healing rates of 60% to 80%.[30,32,35] Complications of this form of treatment are infrequent and include transient incontinence to flatus in 18%[30] and stool in 5%[30] and perianal hematoma. Although botulinum toxin A injection has been supported as a first-line therapy for the treatment of chronic anal fissures, cost and convenience issues argue for its second-line use after failure of topical agents. The topical calcium channel blockers nifedipine and diltiazem have become the initial first-line treatment. Although compounding is required, they are cheap, convenient, and widely available with an excellent, low side-effect profile.

SURGICAL THERAPY

Lateral internal anal partial sphincterotomy (LIS) (Figure 155-4) is reserved for chronic anal fissures that fail nonsurgical management, and this technique requires the surgeon to be familiar with anal canal anatomy. The strategy of operative sphincterotomy is to divide the hypertonic portion of the internal anal sphincter muscle to reduce anal canal pressure and facilitate healing of the anal fissure. This procedure was originally described by Eisenhammer in 1951 as a midline posterior incision through the fissure.[3] However, subsequent studies noted problems with wound healing and the formation of a "keyhole" deformity to the anus.[2] "Keyhole" deformities are a persistent groove in the midline following sphincter division that may result in a significant degree of anal seepage or incontinence. Subsequent modifications to this procedure included repositioning the incision to the right or left lateral position, which has effectively eliminated the complication of this deformity.[4] Notaras is credited with introducing the "closed" sphincterotomy that is performed through a stab incision at the intersphincteric groove (Figure 155-5) rather than an "open" exposure of the internal sphincter.[36] This closed technique can be done in the office setting with local anesthetic using either a small anoscope or a finger in the anal canal to guide division of a portion of the sphincter.

Lateral internal sphincterotomy has produced excellent results for the treatment of chronic anal fissure, with

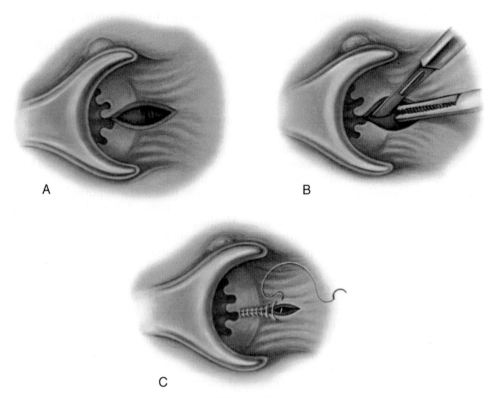

FIGURE 155-4 Lateral internal anal sphincterotomy. **A,** Internal anal sphincter visible through incision. **B,** Lateral division of internal anal sphincter. **C,** Wound closure. (Modified from Storer EH, Goldberg SM, Nivatvongs S: Colon, rectum and anus. In Schwartz SI, editor: *Principles of surgery*, ed 4. New York, 1984, McGraw-Hill, p 1169.)

an 85% to 100% healing rate and very low incidence of persistent or early relapse (Table 155-1).[37-45] There has been a low, but persistent, complication rate for soiling (1% to 22%) and incontinence to flatus (0% to 28%) and stool (0% to 11%). Comparing open versus closed techniques has not shown any differences of significance in postoperative pain, treatment success, complication of incontinence, or overall outcome. The length of internal sphincterotomy has been evaluated in a combined analysis. In terms of healing and incontinence, division of the sphincter limited to the length of the fissure was compared to a longer division beyond the fissure to the level of the dentate line.[45] The longer sphincterotomy was associated with a significantly lower risk of treatment failure, with no difference in postoperative incontinence rates as measured by the Wexner score.[45] Some degree of transient incontinence may be experienced by the patient in the early postoperative period, but this usually improves with time.[44] To further lower incontinence rates, a calibrated sphincterotomy has been performed. A fissure apex sphincterotomy was performed and extended using a calibrated sound to 30-mm base aperture. In three small series, this technique showed similar healing, with lower rates of incontinence compared to standard apex sphincterotomy.[46-48] Therefore, given the low but persistent rate of incontinence with lateral internal sphincterotomy, this operation should be performed in select patients who have failed nonsurgical therapy. Absence of preoperative continence problems and meticulous surgical techniques are necessary to achieve good results.

Other surgical procedures for the management of chronic anal fissures exist, but are performed less frequently. Fissurectomy is the excision of the anal fissure and is still performed today. This procedure results in a defect in the anoderm that can be covered with a rotation or advancement flap to avoid a keyhole deformity and address a coincidental stricture or anal stenosis.[49] Advancement flap without fissurectomy is attractive as theoretically there should be less risk of incontinence. One series showed a trend to better healing in the flap group; however, the recurrence rate was higher.[50] Surgical adjuncts to surgery to improve outcome have included anal papilla excision. Satisfaction was higher in those who had their papilla excised.[51] In another study, 39 patients were randomized to have the anal wound dressed open to avoid infection or sutured shut to hasten healing.[52] Wound problems occurred more often in the open group (4/17) compared to the sutured group (1/22). Healing occurred twice as fast in the sutured group.[52]

Dilation of the anal canal by finger insertion technique has fallen out of favor and should be discouraged because this procedure stretches the anal canal in an uncontrolled fashion resulting in unacceptable levels of postoperative incontinence. Furthermore, a recent metaanalysis showed that anal dilation resulted in significantly greater persistence of disease than sphincterotomy.[53] Retractors and balloon-tipped dilating catheters have been used for dilation in the treatment of chronic anal fissures.[54-57] These more controlled dilation procedures have been reported to be as efficacious as lateral internal sphincterotomy.

TABLE 155-1 Impaired Anal Incontinence After Lateral Internal Sphincterotomy

Authors, Year	No. of Patients	Healed (%)	Recurrence/ Persistence (%)	Impaired Anal Continence (%)		
				Soiling	*Flatus*	*Stool*
Hoffman and Goligher, 1970[37]	99	97	3	1.0	6.1	7.1
Notaras, 1971[38]	82	100	0	1.4	2.7	5.5
Rudd, 1975[39]	200	99.5	0.5	0	0	0
Boulos and Araujo, 1984[40]	23	100	0	0	17.9	NA
Pernikoff et al, 1994[41]	500	97	3	4	3	1
Garcia-Aguilar et al, 1996[42]	549	89	11	22	28	8
Hananel and Gordon, 1997[43]	312	99	1	1	1	1
Nyam and Pemberton, 1999[44]	487	96	4	8	6	1

NA, Not available.

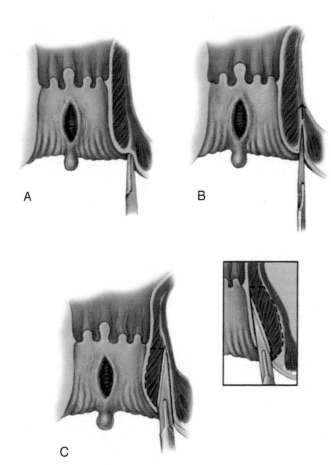

FIGURE 155-5 Blind lateral subcutaneous internal anal sphincterotomy. **A,** Hemostat demonstrating intersphincteric groove. **B,** Insertion of scalpel between internal and external sphincters. **C,** Sphincter division by inward motion of the scalpel. *Inset,* Original Notaras technique showing outward motion of scalpel. (Modified from Notaras MJ: The treatment of anal fissure by lateral subcutaneous internal sphincterotomy: A technique and results. *Br J Surg* 58:96, 1971.)

In a recent study, patients with symptomatic chronic anal fissure were randomly assigned to pneumatic balloon dilation or LIS with anal ultrasonography and anal manometry performed before and 6 months after surgery. Anal continence, scored by using a validated continence grading scale, was evaluated preoperatively at 1 and 6 weeks and at 12 and 24 months.[58] Twenty-four patients (11 males; mean age, 42 ± 8.2 years) underwent pneumatic balloon dilation and 25 patients (10 males; mean age, 44 ± 7.3 years) underwent lateral internal sphincterotomy. Fissure healing rates were 83.3% in the pneumatic balloon dilation and 92% in the lateral internal sphincterotomy group. Recurrent anal fissure was observed in one patient (4%) after lateral internal sphincterotomy. At anal manometry, mean resting pressure decrements obtained after pneumatic balloon dilation and lateral internal sphincterotomy were 30.5% and 34.3%, respectively. After pneumatic balloon dilation, anal ultrasonography did not show any significant sphincter damage. At 24-month followup, the incidence of incontinence, irrespective of severity, was zero in the pneumatic balloon dilation group and 16% in the lateral internal sphincterotomy group ($P < 0.0001$).[58] Calibrated balloon dilation may provide a method that is safe and as efficacious as sphincterotomy. As with lateral internal sphincterotomy, pneumatic balloon dilation generates a high anal fissure healing rate but with a statistically significant reduction in postoperative anal incontinence.

CONCLUSION

Most acute anal fissures will heal with conservative measures, while chronic anal fissures may respond to medical therapies, or injection of botulinum toxin. Patients with persistent fissures should be considered for lateral partial internal sphincterotomy. Our approach is outlined in the algorithm (Figure 155-6). The gratitude from a patient successfully treated after suffering with a painful anal fissure may be more immense than that from the cure of a cancer patient.

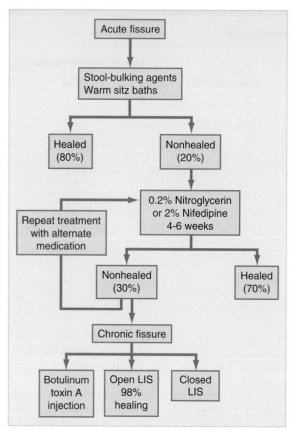

FIGURE 155-6 Algorithm for therapeutic options in decision making for managing anal fissures. *LIS,* Lateral internal sphincterotomy.

REFERENCES

1. Oh C: The role of internal sphincterotomy. *Mt Sinai J Med* 49:484, 1982.
2. Abcarian H: Surgical correction of chronic anal fissure: Results of lateral internal sphincterotomy vs. fissurectomy–midline sphincterotomy. *Dis Colon Rectum* 23:31, 1980.
3. Eisenhammer S: The surgical correction of chronic internal anal (sphincteric) contracture. *S Afr Med J* 25:486, 1951.
4. Eisenhammer S: The evaluation of the internal anal sphincterotomy operation with special reference to anal fissure. *Surg Gynecol Obstet* 109:583, 1959.
5. Klosterhalfen B, Vogel P, Rixen H, et al: Topography of the inferior rectal artery: A possible cause of chronic, primary fissure. *Dis Colon Rectum* 32:43, 1989.
6. Schouten WR, Briel JW, Auwerda JJD: Relationship between anal pressure and anodermal blood flow—the vascular pathogenesis of anal fissure. *Dis Colon Rectum* 37:664, 1994.
7. Schouten WR, Briel JW, Auwerda JJA, et al: Ischaemic nature of anal fissure. *Br J Surg* 83:63, 1996.
8. Lowry AC, Simmang CL, Boulos P, et al: Consensus statement of definitions of anorectal physiology and rectal cancer: Report of the Tripartite Consensus Conference on definitions for anorectal physiology and rectal cancer, Washington D.C., May 1999. *Dis Colon Rectum* 44:915, 2001.
9. Stein BL: Nitroglycerin and other nonoperative therapies for anal fissure. *Semin Colon Rectal Surg* 8:24, 1997.
10. Jensen SL: Maintenance therapy with unprocessed bran in the prevention of acute anal fissure recurrence. *J R Soc Med* 80:296, 1987.
11. Loder PB, Kamm MA, Nicholls RJ, et al: "Reversible chemical sphincterotomy" by local application of glyceryl trinitrate. *Br J Surg* 81:1386, 1994.
12. Gorfine SR: Treatment of benign anal disease with topical nitroglycerin. *Dis Colon Rectum* 38:453, 1995.
13. Watson SJ, Kamm MA, Nicholls RJ, et al: Topical glyceryl trinitrate in the treatment of chronic anal fissure. *Br J Surg* 83:771, 1996.
14. Nelson R: A systematic review of medical therapy for anal fissure. *Dis Colon Rectum* 47:422, 2004.
15. Lund JN, Scholefield JH: A randomized, prospective, double-blind, placebo-controlled trial of glyceryl trinitrate ointment in treatment of anal fissure. *Lancet* 349:11, 1997.
16. Scholefield JH, Lund JN: A nonsurgical approach to chronic anal fissure hospital practice. *Hosp Pract* 32:181, 1997.
17. Kenny SE, Irvine T, Driver CP, et al: Double blind randomized controlled trial of topical glyceryl trinitrate in anal fissure. *Arch Dis Child* 85:404, 2001.
18. Oettle GJ: Glyceryl trinitrate vs. sphincterotomy for treatment of chronic fissure-in-ano: A randomized, controlled trial. *Dis Colon Rectum* 40:1318, 1997.
19. Were AJ, Palamba HW, Bilgen EJ, et al: Isosorbide dinitrate in the treatment of anal fissure: A randomised, prospective, double blind, placebo-controlled trial. *Eur J Surg* 167:382, 2001.
20. Sonmez K, Demirogullari B, Ekingen G, et al: Randomized, placebo-controlled treatment of anal fissure by lidocaine, EMLA, and GTN in children. *J Pediatr Surg* 37:1313, 2002.
21. Watson SJ, Kamm MA, Nicholls RJ, et al: Topical glyceryl trinitrate in the treatment of chronic anal fissure. *Br J Surg* 83:771, 1996.
22. Richard CS, Gregoire R, Plewes EA, et al: Internal sphincterotomy is superior to topical nitroglycerine in the treatment of chronic anal fissure: Results of a randomized, controlled trial by the Canadian Colorectal Surgical Trials Group. *Dis Colon Rectum* 43:1048, 2000.
23. Altomere DF, Rinaldi M, Milito G, et al: Glyceryl trinitrate for chronic anal fissure—Healing or headache? Results of a multicenter, randomized, placebo-controlled, double-blind trial. *Dis Colon Rectum* 43:174, 2000.
24. Perrotti P, Bove A, Antropoli C, et al: Topical nifedipine with lidocaine ointment versus active control for treatment of chronic anal fissure: Results of a prospective, randomized, double-blind study. *Dis Colon Rectum* 45:1468, 2002.
25. Kocher HM, Steward M, Leather AJM, et al: Randomized clinical trial assessing the side-effects of glyceryl trinitrate and diltiazem hydrochloride in the treatment of chronic anal fissure. *Br J Surg* 89:413, 2002.
26. Bielecki K, Kolodziejczak M: A prospective randomized trial of diltiazem and glyceryl trinitrate ointment in the treatment of chronic anal fissure. *Colorectal Dis* 5:256, 2003.
27. DasGupta R, Franklin I, Pitt J, et al: Successful treatment of chronic anal fissure with diltiazem gel. *Colorectal Dis* 4:20, 2002.
28. Griffin N, Acheson AG, Jonas M, et al: The role of topical diltiazem in the treatment of chronic anal fissures that have failed glyceryl trinitrate therapy. *Colorectal Dis* 4:430, 2002.
29. Nelson RL, Thomas K, Morgan J, et al: Non surgical therapy for anal fissure. *Cochrane Database Syst Rev* 2:CD003431, 2012.
30. Perry WB, Dykes SL, Buie WD, et al: Practice parameters for the management of anal fissures (3rd revision). *Dis Colon Rectum* 2010; 53:1110.
31. Maria G, Cassetta E, Gui D, et al: A comparison of injections of botulinum toxin and saline for the treatment of chronic anal fissure. *N Engl J Med* 338:217, 1998.
32. Brisinda G, Maria G, Bentivoglio AR, et al: A comparison of injections of botulinum toxin and topical nitroglycerine ointment for the treatment of chronic anal fissure. *N Engl J Med* 341:65, 1999.
33. Brisinda G, Albanese A, Cadeddu F, et al: Botulinum neurotoxin to treat chronic anal fissure: Results of a randomized "Botox vs. Dysport" controlled trial. *Aliment Pharmacol Ther* 19:695, 2004.
34. Maria G, Brisinda G, Bentivoglio AR, et al: Influence of botulinum toxin site of injections on healing rate in patients with chronic anal fissure. *Am J Surg* 179:46, 2000.
35. Lindsey I, Jones OM, Cunningham C, et al: Botulinum toxin as second-line therapy for chronic anal fissure failing 0.2 percent glyceryl trinitrate. *Dis Colon Rectum* 46:361, 2003.
36. Notaras MJ: Lateral subcutaneous sphincterotomy for anal fissure—a new technique. *Proc R Soc Med* 62:713, 1969.
37. Hoffman DC, Goligher JC: Lateral subcutaneous internal sphincterotomy in the treatment of anal fissure. *BMJ* 3:673, 1970.
38. Notaras MJ: The treatment of anal fissure by lateral subcutaneous internal sphincterotomy—a technique and results. *Br J Surg* 58:96, 1971.

39. Rudd WW: Lateral subcutaneous internal sphincterotomy for chronic anal fissure, an outpatient procedure. *Dis Colon Rectum* 18:319, 1975.

40. Boulos PB, Araujo JG: Adequate internal sphincterotomy for chronic anal fissure: Subcutaneous or open technique? *Br J Surg* 71:360, 1984.

41. Pernikoff BJ, Eisenstat TE, Rubin RJ, et al: Reappraisal of partial lateral internal sphincterotomy. *Dis Colon Rectum* 37:1291, 1994.

42. Garcia-Aguilar J, Belmonte C, Wong WD, et al: Open vs. closed sphincterotomy for chronic anal fissure: Long-term results. *Dis Colon Rectum* 39:440, 1996.

43. Hananel N, Gordon PH: Lateral internal sphincterotomy for fissure-in-ano—revisited. *Dis Colon Rectum* 40:597, 1997.

44. Nyam DC, Pemberton JH: Long-term results of lateral internal sphincterotomy for chronic anal fissure with particular reference to incidence of fecal incontinence. *Dis Colon Rectum* 42:1306, 1999.

45. Nelson RL: Operative procedures for fissure in ano (Review). *Cochrane Library* 1:1, 2010.

46. Cho DY: Controlled lateral sphincterotomy for chronic anal fissure. *Dis Colon Rectum* 48:1037, 2005.

47. Rosa G, Lolli P, Piccinelli D, et al: Calibrated lateral internal sphincterotomy for chronic anal fissure. *Tech Coloproctol* 9:127, 2005.

48. Mentes BB, Guner MK, Leventoglu S, et al: Fine-tuning of the extent of lateral internal sphincterotomy: Spasm-controlled vs. up to the fissure apex. *Dis Colon Rectum* 51:128, 2008.

49. Arnell T, Stamos MJ: Sphincterotomy for anal fissure. *Semin Colon Rectal Surg* 8:24, 1997.

50. Leong AF, Seow-Choen F: Lateral sphincterotomy compared with anal advancement flap for chronic anal fissure. *Dis Colon Rectum* 38:69, 1995.

51. Gupta PJ, Kalaskar S: Removal of hypertrophied anal papillae and fibrous anal polyps increases patient's satisfaction after anal fissure surgery. *Tech Coloproctol* 2003;7:155.

52. Aysan E, Aren A, Ayar E: Lateral internal sphincterotomy incision: Suture or not? A prospective randomized controlled trial. *Am Surg* 187:291, 2004.

53. Nelson RL: Meta-analysis of operative techniques for fissure-in-ano. *Dis Colon Rectum* 42:1424, 1999.

54. Sohn N, Eisenberg MM, Weinstein MA, et al: Precise anorectal sphincter dilation—its role in therapy of anal fissures. *Dis Colon Rectum* 35:322, 1992.

55. Marby M, Alesander-Williams J, Buchmann P, et al: A randomized controlled trial to compare anal dilatation with lateral subcutaneous sphincterotomy for anal fissure. *Dis Colon Rectum* 22:308, 1979.

56. Oliver DW, Booth MW, Kernick VF, et al: Patient satisfaction and symptom relief after anal dilatation. *Int J Colorectal Dis* 13:228, 1998.

57. Saad AM, Omer A: Surgical treatment of chronic fissure-in-ano: A prospective randomized study. *East Afr Med J* 69:107, 1992.

58. Renzi A, Izzo D, Di Sarno G, et al: Clinical, manometric and ultrasonographic results of pneumatic balloon dilatation vs. lateral internal sphincterotomy for chronic anal fissure: A prospective, randomized, controlled trial. *Dis Colon Rectum* 51:121, 2008.

CHAPTER

156

Anal Sepsis and Fistula

Lucas A. Julien | Jennifer S. Beaty | Alan G. Thorson

Anorectal suppurative disease may manifest itself in an acute or a chronic setting. Anal sepsis (abscess) represents the acute manifestation, and anal fistula represents the chronic form of the suppurative process. In its simplest form, an anal fistula represents a communication between an internal opening in the anal canal and an external opening through which an abscess has drained. A fistula and abscess may coexist or be associated with atypical internal openings and multiple tracts that result in a complex suppurative process.

ETIOLOGY

Foreign bodies, malignancy, trauma, tuberculosis, actinomycosis, leukemia, postoperative infection, inflammatory bowel disease, and simple skin infections have *long* been associated with anal sepsis. Recently, an association between anal abscess-fistula and history of concurrent or recent cigarette smoking has been demonstrated.[1] This association diminishes as the history of cigarette smoking grows more remote. Most anal sepsis, however, is related to an infection of the anal glands and ducts. Fecal bacterial plugging of the ducts leads to obstruction and subsequent abscess formation. This process represents the cryptoglandular theory of anal sepsis. Robinson,[2] Seow,[3] and their associates have suggested that the description of the anal glands by Chiari in 1878 and the subsequent histologic studies of Parks in 1961 contributed to the acceptance of the cryptoglandular theory as the most common cause for anal sepsis.

CLASSIFICATION

ANORECTAL ABSCESSES

Anorectal abscesses are classified according to the perirectal space involved in the suppurative process; these include the perianal, ischiorectal, intersphincteric, submucosal, deep postanal, and supralevator spaces (Figure 156-1). A given suppurative process may involve multiple perirectal spaces. For example, the classic "horseshoe" abscess originates in an infected gland in the posterior midline extending through the intersphincteric and deep postanal spaces to one or both of the ischiorectal spaces. A condition known as "floating anus" may occur with circumanal spread of intersphincteric, supralevator, or ischiorectal collections.

It is difficult to accurately assess the incidence of various abscesses because of the numerous classifications and referral patterns reflected in large series.[4-8] However, perianal abscesses account for the largest number in most series (Table 156-1).

ANAL FISTULA

Historically, anal fistulas have been classified in many different ways. However, the Parks classification introduced in 1976 is the most comprehensive and widely used. It is derived from the cryptoglandular hypothesis and has therapeutic implications. Parks classified fistulas into four main subgroups according to the course taken by the main tract: intersphincteric, transsphincteric, suprasphincteric, or extrasphincteric.[9] Each category can be further subclassified based on associated secondary tracts and other anatomic details (Figure 156-2). As with abscesses, the incidence of various fistulas is difficult to quantify. Overall, however, intersphincteric fistulas seem to predominate (Table 156-2).

DIAGNOSIS

ANORECTAL ABSCESS

History

Symptoms common to all abscesses include the slow, gradual onset of pain, increasing in intensity to the sensation of pressure and fullness. This is a constant, nonrelieving sensation. These symptoms should always lead to the consideration of an abscess even in the absence of obvious physical findings (hidden abscesses). Approximately 20% to 33% of all patients will report a history of a previous episode of anorectal sepsis.[8,13]

Physical Examination

The physical findings associated with anorectal abscesses vary depending on the anatomic location of the abscess. The presence of pus in any of the perianal and perirectal spaces may be confirmed with needle aspiration. An examination under general anesthesia may be necessary to confirm the diagnosis.

PERIANAL ABSCESS

Localized swelling, hyperemia, induration or fluctuance, and tenderness are present adjacent to the anus. A purulent discharge may be present if spontaneous drainage has occurred. Although there usually are no systemic symptoms, the patient may have fever or malaise or be acutely ill.

ISCHIORECTAL ABSCESS

Although small collections may present with discrete localized swelling, more commonly there is a large, erythematous, and indurated mass in the buttock. Large volumes of purulent material may accumulate in the ischiorectal space. Fever and leukocytosis are common but not always present. A large ischiorectal abscess

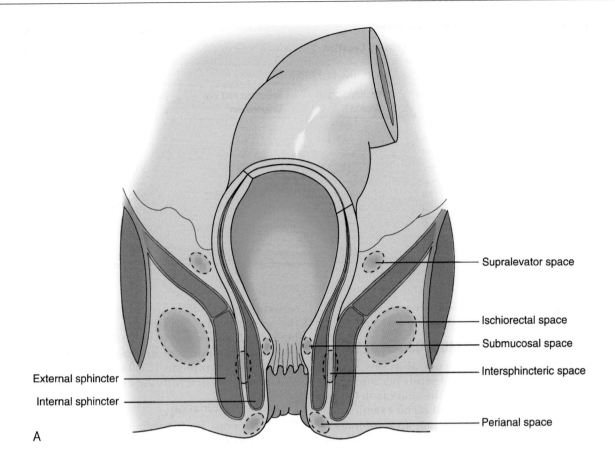

External sphincter

Internal sphincter

A

Supralevator space

Ischiorectal space

Submucosal space

Intersphincteric space

Perianal space

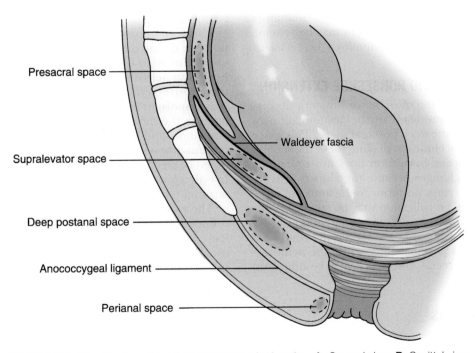

Presacral space

Supralevator space

Deep postanal space

Anococcygeal ligament

Perianal space

Waldeyer fascia

B

FIGURE 156-1 Classification of anorectal abscesses by location. **A,** Coronal view. **B,** Sagittal view.

TABLE 156-1 Incidence of Anorectal Abscess by Location

Abscess Locations	NO. OF PATIENTS					TOTAL	
	McElwain et al[4]	Scoma et al[7]	Vasilevsky and Gordon[8]	Schouten and van Vroonhoven[6]	Ramanujam et al[5]	No. of Patients	%
Perianal	456	174	20	—	437	1087	44.8
Submucosal	3	—	—	—	—	3	0.1
Intermuscular	541	30	—	—	59	630	26
Intersphincteric	—	—	18	28	219	265	11
Transsphincteric	—	—	—	30	—	30	1.2
Ischiorectal	—	14	63	—	233	310	12.8
Supralevator	—	9	2	—	75	86	3.6
Retrorectal	—	5	—	—	—	5	0.2
Unclassified	—	—	—	8	—	8	0.3
Total	1000	232	103	66	1023	2424	100

frequently represents a horseshoe extension (see later). A source in the posterior midline should be sought.

INTERSPHINCTERIC AND SUBMUCOUS ABSCESS

The intersphincteric and submucous abscesses usually present with no visible evidence of sepsis because these "hidden abscesses" are confined to the anal canal. Owing to the patient's discomfort, a digital rectal examination is not always possible. In this situation, an examination under general anesthesia is warranted to identify the abscess.

SUPRALEVATOR ABSCESS

Supralevator abscess may occur as an upward extension of a collection in the distal anal canal, usually an intersphincteric abscess, or as a true pelvic abscess secondary to intraabdominal or pelvic pathology. Possibilities include appendicitis, diverticulitis, pelvic inflammatory disease, or ruptured viscus. The patient may be systemically ill. A pelvic mass may be identified by rectal or vaginal examination.

POSTANAL ABSCESS AND HORSESHOE EXTENSION

Transsphincteric extension of an intersphincteric abscess in the posterior midline leads to the accumulation of purulent material in the deep postanal space. This space is difficult to evaluate clinically, making these the second type of hidden abscess. Inspection does not reveal any inflammatory skin changes because the abscess is deep. There may be tenderness posterior to the anus but anterior to the coccyx. The collection may be apparent only by needle aspiration or with an examination under general anesthesia. A horseshoe abscess is the result of a direct extension of a postanal abscess into the ischiorectal space (see Ischiorectal Abscess). It may be unilateral or bilateral.

ANORECTAL FISTULAS

History

Most patients with a fistula-in-ano have a previous history of anorectal suppuration. The patient usually presents with complaints of intermittent or persistent purulent or serosanguineous drainage from an external opening in the perianal area. Symptoms classically consist of a buildup of pain, slight fever, and pain on defecation followed by mucopurulent drainage and abatement of the pain. Pruritic symptoms may be present because of skin irritation associated with the chronic discharge.

Physical Examination

Fistula tracts are fibrous inflammatory tubes with a diameter of 3 to 7 mm. They are lined with infected granulation tissue. Many fistulas may be palpated during a careful digital rectal examination. Essential points that should be obtained from a clinical examination were described nearly 100 years ago by Goodsall and Miles[14]; they include the identification of the external and internal openings, the course of the primary and any secondary tracts, and an assessment for the presence of an underlying complicating disease.

Using an anoscope, systematic inspection and palpation can define most of these characteristics. The gentle use of a number of malleable anorectal probes and crypt hooks can help delineate the fistula by attempting to pass these instruments via the internal or external opening. It is important not to force the passage of the probe because the development of false tracts can complicate evaluation and management. Secondary tracts may be present when induration is palpated or asymmetry is noted between the right and left sides of the anorectum. In only a few cases will the use of sophisticated diagnostic imaging techniques be required.

The external opening is identified as a small pit surrounded by scar or granulation tissue. Active seropurulent drainage may be present. Intersphincteric tracts usually open externally close to the anal verge; transsphincteric and other complicated tracts open farther away. Occasionally, the external opening may be localized inside the anal canal or at the distal end of a fissure. Several external openings may be present because of multiple complex fistula tracts; this condition is known as "watering-pot perineum."

The internal opening may be felt as an indurated nodule, most often at the dentate line. This is consistent with the cryptoglandular theory of anorectal sepsis. The

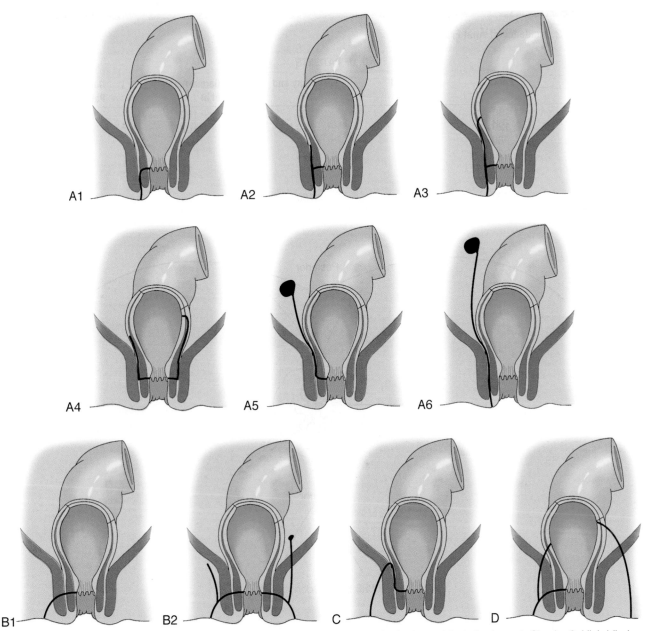

FIGURE 156-2 Classification of anal fistulas. **A,** Intersphincteric: The tract remains in the intersphincteric plane. *1,* Simple. *2,* High blind tract. There is a high extension of the fistula between the internal sphincter and the longitudinal muscle of the upper anal canal. *3,* High tract with rectal opening. *4,* High intersphincteric fistula without a perineal opening. There may or may not be a rectal opening. *5,* High intersphincteric fistula with a pelvic extension. The infection spreads up to reach the true pelvic cavity lying above the levator musculature. *6,* Intersphincteric fistula secondary to pelvic disease. This fistula results from the spread of pelvic collections via the intersphincteric plane. This does not represent a true anal fistula because its origin is outside the anal area. There is no opening at the dentate line. **B,** Transsphincteric: The fistula tract passes from the intersphincteric plane through the external sphincter muscle. *1,* Uncomplicated. *2,* High blind tract. The upper tract extension may go to the apex of the ischiorectal fossa or extend higher through the levator musculature into the pelvic cavity. **C,** Suprasphincteric: There is an upward extension of the fistula tract in the intersphincteric plane. The tract then passes above the level of the puborectalis muscle and continues downward through the ischiorectal fossa to the perianal area. **D,** Extrasphincteric: There is a tract that passes from the skin of the perineum through the ischiorectal fossa and the levator muscles before entering the rectal wall. This fistula may be a consequence of an extension of a transsphincteric fistula or secondary to trauma, anorectal disease, or pelvic inflammation.

use of saline, milk, dye, or dilute hydrogen peroxide as an injection into the external fistula opening has been made in an attempt to localize the internal opening. An enlarged papilla may be noted at this site. Because most of the anal glands are located in the posterior midline,

it is not surprising that 61% to 69% of internal openings can be traced to this location.[3]

The Goodsall rule may be helpful in locating the internal opening. This rule states that an external opening anterior to an imaginary transverse anal line in the

TABLE 156-2 Incidence of Anal Fistulas

| | NO. OF PATIENTS | | | | TOTAL | |
Fistula Type	Parks et al[9]	Marks and Ritchie[10]	Vasilevsky and Gordon[11]	Garcia-Aguilar et al[12]	No. of Patients	%
Intersphincteric	180	428	67	180	855	49.5
Transsphincteric	120	167	83	108	478	27.7
Suprasphincteric	80	24	3	6	113	6.5
Extrasphincteric	20	24	0	6	50	2.9
Miscellaneous or nonclassified	—	150	7	75	232	13.4
Total	*400*	*793*	*160*	*375*	*1728*	*100*

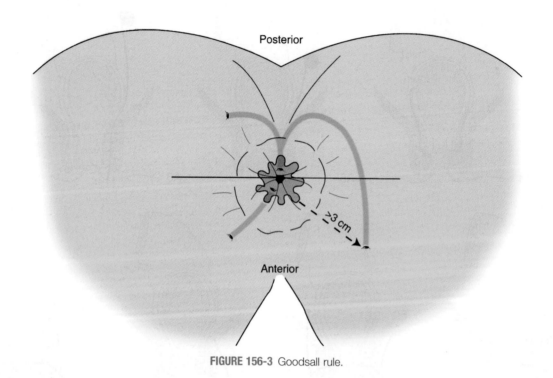

FIGURE 156-3 Goodsall rule.

coronal plane most likely communicates with an internal opening lying at the end of a radial line drawn to the nearest crypt at the dentate line. If the external opening is posterior to this line, the internal opening will most likely be located in the posterior midline with the tract following a curved route to reach its source. Exceptions to this rule include anterior openings more than 3 cm from the anal verge and the presence of multiple external openings. In these cases, the internal opening will most likely be in the posterior midline (Figure 156-3). However, the predictive accuracy of Goodsall rule has been challenged, especially with anterior external openings[15] or when Crohn disease or carcinoma is present.[16]

SPECIAL STUDIES

Sigmoidoscopy and Colonoscopy

Sigmoidoscopy should be performed in all patients with anorectal fistulas. The presence of associated pathology

such as neoplasms, inflammatory bowel disease, or associated secondary tracts in the rectum must be sought. Such findings may dictate the need for full colonoscopic evaluation.

Fistulography

Fistulography may be warranted in patients with recurrent fistulas or when a prior procedure has failed to identify the internal opening. With this technique, the external opening is cannulated with a small-caliber tube and contrast material is injected under minimal pressure while films are taken in several projections. Fistulography may be useful in identifying unsuspected pathology, planning surgical management, and demonstrating anatomic relationships. However, a study by Kuijpers and Schulpen[17] found fistulography to be unreliable compared with operative findings. They observed a prohibitively high incidence of false-positive results that could lead to unnecessary and harmful surgical exploration.

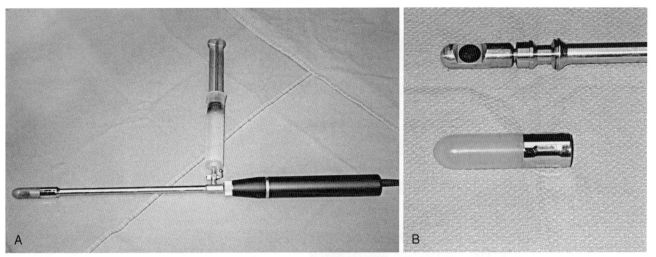

FIGURE 156-4 **A,** Transanal ultrasound probe (type 1850; Brüel and Kjaer, Naerum, Denmark). **B,** The rotating transducer is covered by a hard plastic sonolucent cone, which is then filled with water to provide an acoustic interphase.

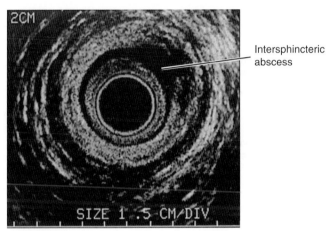

Intersphincteric abscess

FIGURE 156-5 Intersphincteric abscess as seen with the use of transanal ultrasound.

Anorectal Ultrasonography

Transanal ultrasound can delineate the muscular anatomy of the anal sphincters in relation to an abscess or a fistula. Most commonly, ultrasonographic examination of the anal canal is performed with the use of a 360-degree rotating probe using a 7- , 10-, or 13-MHz transducer with a water-filled sonolucent plastic cone over the transducer (Figure 156-4). Fistula tracts and abscesses appear as hypoechoic defects within the muscular elements of the anal canal (Figure 156-5). The internal opening is not distinctly identified. Although generally accurate in the localization of abscesses and fistula tracts, primary superficial, extrasphincteric, and suprasphincteric tracts or secondary supralevator or infralevator tracts may be missed.[18] The use of hydrogen peroxide injected into fistulas as an image enhancer has been shown to be safe, effective, and sometimes helpful in the detection of these complex fistulas (Figure 156-6).[19] Additionally, three-dimensional endoanal ultrasonography is now reliable and accurate in the diagnosis of fistula-in-ano with or without hydrogen peroxide enhancement.[20]

The use of a linear 7-MHz ultrasound device instead of a radial probe has been described and may carry the advantages of greater focal depth, improved ischiorectal and supralevator visualization, multiplanar views of complex fistulas, and less need for echo-enhancing injection.[21] Finally, it has been shown that vaginal endosonography may increase the diagnostic yield of perianal sepsis in 25% of patients and may obviate the need for uncomfortable digital or endoanal ultrasound examinations in those patients with hidden abscesses or anal stenosis.[22]

Magnetic Resonance Imaging

Another accurate method of imaging anal fistula disease is magnetic resonance imaging (MRI). A majority of anal fistulas have a single simple fistula track that is easily identified during surgery. However, 5% to 15% of complex fistulas are often associated with recurrent fistulas and fistulas associated with underlying Crohn disease. MRI has shown to be helpful, especially in these complex fistulas in identification of fistulous tracks, secondary extensions, and internal openings.[23] In a study by Beets-Tan et al, preoperative MRI had a sensitivity and specificity of 100% and 86%, respectively, in identification of fistula tracks. Additionally, the study found a 96% sensitivity and 90% specificity for preoperative MR detection of internal fistula openings.[23] MRI is particularly useful in the evaluation of complex fistulous disease. Combining MRI with endoanal ultrasonography and an examination under anesthesia may enhance the accuracy of these tests in determining fistula anatomy.[24]

Computed Tomography

The use of computed tomography (CT) in the evaluation of anal fistulas is limited because of poor visualization of the levators and sphincter complex. The role of CT in anal sepsis and fistula is thus limited to the assessment of associated pelvic pathology in patients with supralevator abscesses and in patients with some complex anal fistulas.

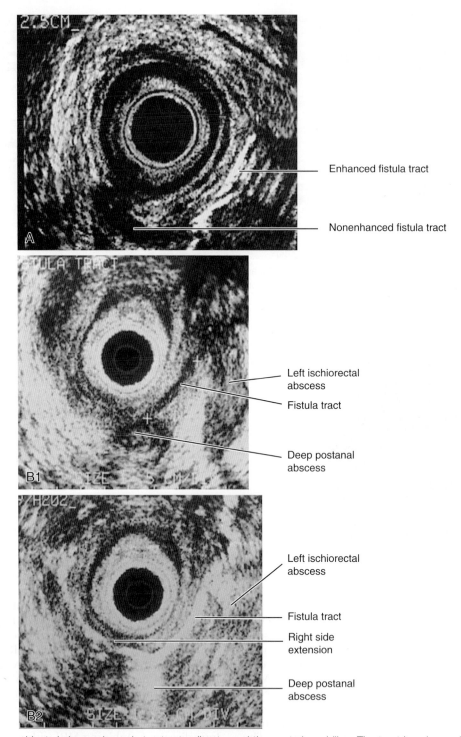

Enhanced fistula tract

Nonenhanced fistula tract

Left ischiorectal abscess

Fistula tract

Deep postanal abscess

Left ischiorectal abscess

Fistula tract

Right side extension

Deep postanal abscess

FIGURE 156-6 A, Transsphincteric hypoechogenic tract extending toward the posterior midline. The tract is enhanced as hydrogen peroxide is injected into the external opening. **B,** Complex fistula tract and collections as seen without *(1)* and with *(2)* hydrogen peroxide enhancement. Hydrogen peroxide enhancement allowed for a more precise delineation of the tracts in addition to a right-sided extension of the tract.

Anorectal Manometry

Anorectal manometry is an objective method for studying the contribution of the anorectal sphincter to the physiologic process of defecation. Manometry can assist in identifying patients at the greatest risk for postoperative incontinence. Surgical management can be tailored accordingly, improving clinical and functional outcome.

The selective use of anorectal manometry is especially warranted in patients with suspected sphincter impairment; patients suspected of needing substantial portions of the external sphincter divided for fistula cure; and women with a history of multiparity, forceps delivery, third-degree perineal tear, high birthweight, or prolonged second stage of labor.[16] Patients with lower

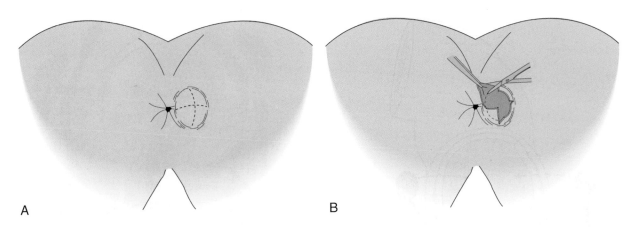

FIGURE 156-7 A, Cruciate incision made over the most tender or fluctuant area. **B,** The skin edges are excised.

preoperative resting pressures have significantly poorer continence control following surgery for intersphincteric fistula when compared prospectively to patients with normal preoperative resting pressures.[25]

Fistuloscopy

Anorectal fistuloscopy using flexible ureteroscopes has been described.[26] This is a potentially useful intraoperative technique used to identify primary fistula openings, multiple or complex tracts, and iatrogenic tracts. Modified flexible ureteroscopes are in the early developmental stages. We look forward to their evolution because they represent a novel diagnostic and therapeutic tool that may significantly improve the outcomes of complex fistula diagnosis and treatment.

TREATMENT

ANORECTAL ABSCESS

The treatment of anorectal abscesses should be considered a surgical emergency, with early drainage the mainstay of treatment. There is no place for conservative management. Treatment delay may result in chronic infection and tissue destruction with fibrosis and long-term impairment of function. The condition of the patient and the type of abscess usually determine whether drainage can be performed in the office or emergency department or in the operating room. Antibiotics should be used as adjunctive therapy in special circumstances only; these include patients with valvular heart disease, immunosuppression, extensive associated cellulitis, and diabetes.

Anorectal abscesses associated with gut-derived organisms are more likely to be associated with an underlying fistula than are abscesses associated with skin-derived organisms.[27] However, the positive predictive value for this association has been found to be quite low; therefore, cultures are rarely indicated.[28]

Perianal Abscess

Simple perianal abscesses can almost always be drained as an office or outpatient procedure, usually under local anesthesia. A cruciate incision is made over the most tender or fluctuant point as close to the anal verge as possible. If a fistula develops, the external opening will be close to the verge, so a fistulotomy would require division of the least amount of muscle. The skin edges are usually excised to avoid early coaptation, which could seal the cavity prematurely and lead to recurrence (Figure 156-7).

After all loculations are broken, packing is not required; packing contributes to significant discomfort and does not allow for free drainage of the abscess cavity. Continued drainage of large cavities may be achieved with the use of a 3- to 5-mm de Pezzer or similar catheter left in situ until drainage subsides. This technique may be used in a number of different abscesses but is not suitable for use in cases of submucous or intersphincteric abscess.

Ischiorectal Abscess

After horseshoe extension is excluded by ensuring that the deep postanal space is not involved, unilateral ischiorectal abscesses may be drained through a single incision or several counterincisions over the area of maximal swelling, pain, and fluctuance but as close to the anal verge as possible. Here, too, a de Pezzer catheter may be used to enhance the drainage of large cavities.

Intersphincteric Abscess

An intersphincteric abscess is drained by laying open the internal sphincter (sphincterotomy) overlying the cavity. By definition, a fistulotomy is performed by destruction of the inciting anal gland. For hemostasis, adequate drainage, and faster healing, the edges of the wound may be marsupialized.

Submucosal Abscess

Submucosal abscesses are drained internally by incising the mucosa over the abscess. The edges of the wound may be marsupialized. No packing or drainage catheter is indicated.

Supralevator Abscess

Anatomic localization of the septic origin is of paramount importance in the management of supralevator collections. Collections that result from abdominopelvic

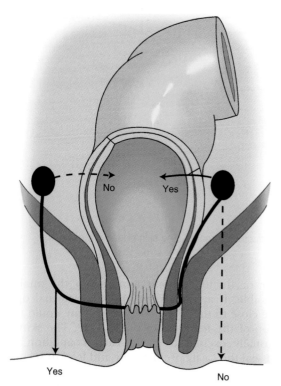

FIGURE 156-8 Appropriate type of drainage of supralevator abscesses depending on the course taken by the fistula tract.

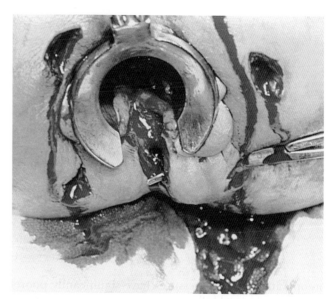

FIGURE 156-9 Drainage of a postanal abscess with horseshoe extension. The postanal space has been laid open as described by Hanley. Secondary incisions are placed in the skin overlying the ischiorectal space.

disease may be drained transrectally or transabdominally. Overall management depends on the underlying pathology. Supralevator collections that result from an upward extension of an intersphincteric abscess should be drained transrectally. Transperineal drainage through the ischiorectal fossae could result in a suprasphincteric fistula. Supralevator collections that result from the cephalad extension of a transsphincteric fistula or an ischiorectal collection should be drained transperineally through the ischioanal fossae. If erroneously drained transrectally, the result will be an extrasphincteric fistula. Transperineal drainage of this type of collection will likely result in a transsphincteric fistula that is relatively easy to manage (Figure 156-8).

Postanal Abscess and Horseshoe Extension

Hanley first described the conservative surgical approach to a horseshoe abscess that preserved function and anatomy.[29] The abscess in the postanal space is drained by a deep posterior midline incision. All of the muscles attached to the coccyx, the superficial external sphincter, and the lower edge of the internal sphincter are divided. When the suppurative process extends to the ischiorectal spaces as a horseshoe, one or multiple secondary incisions are placed in the skin overlying the ischiorectal space. These may be connected to each other with soft drains to allow for continuous drainage. We favor a modification of Hanley's technique in which the posterior midline incision consists of only a partial distal internal sphincterotomy to include a fistulotomy with destruction of the anal gland at the dentate line. The external sphincter and the muscular attachments to the coccyx are not divided. This allows for faster healing while maintaining

adequate drainage (Figure 156-9). Counterincisions and drains are used for horseshoe extensions as previously described.

Primary Versus Delayed Fistulotomy

The use of primary fistulotomy when draining an abscess remains controversial. Issues surrounding this controversy include the ability to localize an internal opening at the time of an acute septic event and the effect of primary fistulotomy on recurrence and continence. Does the type of abscess affect the risk of recurrent fistula? Is it cost-effective to take a patient for whom an outpatient procedure is performed under local anesthesia to the operating room for a thorough examination under general anesthesia and a primary fistulotomy in the hope of avoiding a second procedure for a fistula that might develop if only simple drainage were performed?

A one-stage procedure theoretically destroys the cryptoglandular source of sepsis, decreasing the incidence of fistula formation. However, internal openings may not always be found. Attempts to define a primary opening in the setting of an acute infection may be a hazardous undertaking. Not all abscesses lead to fistulas; hence, some patients would undergo an unnecessary procedure that puts them at risk for incontinence.

The reported incidence of recurrent abscess and subsequent development of anorectal fistula varies considerably. Scoma et al[7] found that 66% of 232 patients developed a fistula or recurrent abscess after incision and drainage alone. Vasilevsky and Gordon[8] found that 11% of 83 patients developed recurrent abscess and 37% developed a fistula after incision and drainage. They noted that the greatest risk of recurrence was in patients who had ischiorectal abscesses, an observation we have also made. The subset of patients with no previous episode of anorectal suppuration had a lower incidence of recurrence. Both authors advocated incision and drainage alone for acute abscesses, reserving fistulotomy as a secondary procedure in patients with recurrence.

In contrast, several authors favor a policy of immediate fistulotomy in the treatment of anorectal abscesses. In a series of almost 800 cases, Eisenhammer[30] described a nearly 100% cure rate obtained with a single operation. McElwain et al[4] reported on the outcome of 1000 cases of primary fistulotomy for anorectal abscesses, including intersphincteric and postanal abscesses. The recurrence rate was 3.6%, and the disturbance of continence rate was 3.2%. This approach is further supported by a randomized, prospective trial of 200 patients. Oliver et al demonstrated that drainage with fistulotomy was safe (incontinence 6% at 1 year) and effective (recurrence 5% at 1 year) when compared with drainage alone (0% incontinence and 29% recurrence).[31] Ultimately, this approach requires the consistent finding of an internal opening to perform fistulotomy. In general, internal openings can be identified in 34% to 88% of acute abscesses.[5,32]

In summary, a percentage of patients who have drainage alone for the treatment of anal abscess develop a recurrent abscess or subsequent fistula. A primary fistulotomy in this setting may decrease this risk but at the expense of a small increase in the risk for disturbances of continence. Primary fistulotomy should be considered in patients who have a history of previous anorectal sepsis or who present with an ischiorectal abscess with an internal opening that is readily apparent. This controversy has no impact in dealing with postanal abscesses with horseshoe extensions or intersphincteric abscesses. In these cases, a fistulotomy is performed when the sphincterotomy is the primary drainage technique.

ANORECTAL FISTULAS

Once diagnosed, patients with anorectal fistulas should undergo surgical treatment. Anorectal fistulas rarely heal spontaneously. Untreated patients frequently develop chronic abscess formation and complex fistula tracts. Surgical treatment for most anorectal fistulas is best accomplished in the operating room, with good lighting and appropriate instrumentation. The patient is positioned in prone jackknife position with the buttocks taped apart. General, regional, or local anesthesia with intravenous sedation should be selected on the basis of individual patient characteristics. The three basic surgical techniques for the treatment of anorectal fistulas are fistulotomy, use of a seton, and endorectal advancement flaps. The use of fistulectomy is not recommended except when it is necessary to provide histologic material.

Fistulotomy

Most anorectal fistulas may be adequately treated by the classic laying-open technique or fistulotomy. Recurrence rates are low, and risks for continence disturbances are minimal.[3] A fistulotomy is accomplished by passing a fistula probe via the external opening, along the tract, and through the internal opening. With the probe in place, the relationship of the fistulous tract to the external sphincter muscle can be determined. If the tract lies distal to the majority of the external muscle, then cautery is used to lay it open. Secondary tracts should be drained

through the fistulotomy incision after all tracts have been curetted. Marsupialization with a running continuous absorbable suture is associated with faster healing.

In patients with otherwise normal continence, the perianal skin, anal epithelium, a portion of the internal anal sphincter, and a few fibers of subcutaneous external sphincter may be divided with minimal risk of incontinence. However, in women with anterior fistulas, such a fistulotomy is associated with an unacceptably high risk of incontinence because of the intrinsic thin nature of the sphincter mechanism in this area. Therefore, sphincter-preserving techniques should be used in the treatment of anterior fistulas in women.

Recently, a method termed the LIFT procedure or "ligation of the intersphincteric fistula tract" has become popular. This is a novel sphincter-preserving method for fistula closure that involves making an incision in the intersphincteric groove, dissection between the sphincter muscles, and identification of the fistula tract. The fistula probe is left in situ during this time to facilitate identification of the tract. The fistula tract is then dissected free and the probe removed. Next, the fistula tract is divided and ligated. The internal opening is closed with absorbable suture and the external opening curetted and left open to drain. Initial retrospective studies show this procedure has a success rate similar to other sphincter-preserving procedures, between 57% and 82%.[33,34]

Seton Management

The word *seton* is derived from the Latin word *seta*, meaning "bristle." It refers to any foreign material that can be inserted into the fistula tract to encircle the sphincter muscles. These materials may include silk, Penrose drains, Silastic vessel loops, rubber bands, nylon or polypropylene, and braided steel wire. Setons are placed by securing the selected material to the end of a fistula probe after the probe has been passed through the internal opening (Figure 156-10).

Setons are useful in the management of complex anorectal fistulas where there is an appreciable risk of incontinence or poor healing; such cases include patients with Crohn disease, immunocompromised and incontinent patients, patients with chronic diarrheal states, and anterior fistulas in women. Complete healing of selected anorectal fistulas has been reported solely with the use of long-term setons.[35]

Setons may be used for marking, draining, cutting, or staging. A marking seton is useful when it is difficult to determine the amount of muscle the fistula tract crosses. Encircling the tract with a seton allows the surgeon to assess the amount of muscle, particularly the puborectalis, once the patient is awake. If adequate muscle is present above the fistula tract, a fistulotomy may be performed without significant risk for incontinence.

A draining seton traverses a fistula tract to provide long-term drainage of a septic process. It may be used as a bridge to definitive surgical therapy or be left in place for long periods. Epithelialization of the tract prevents recurring abscesses. Long-term draining setons are tied loosely. They are particularly useful in the management of complex fistulas associated with Crohn disease. The

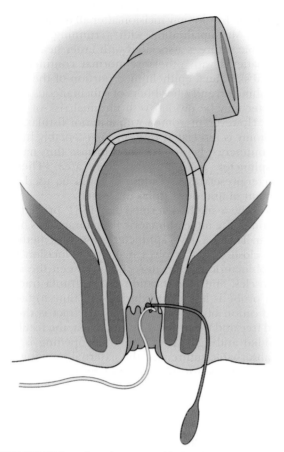

FIGURE 156-10 Insertion of a seton with the aid of a fistula probe.

combination of a draining seton and immunomodulation therapy with infliximab appears to improve outcomes while maintaining sphincter function in Crohn patients with complex anal fistulas.[36]

A cutting seton is used to gradually transect the striated sphincter muscle. This technique promotes fibrosis in the tissue surrounding the muscle encircled by the seton. At regular, 2-week intervals, the seton is progressively tightened, dividing the muscle by a process of ischemic necrosis. The cut edge of the divided muscle does not separate because of the fibrosis that forms during the time it takes to divide the muscle. The seton can be progressively tightened with silk ligatures. Alternatively, a hemorrhoid ligator may be used to progressively tighten the seton with rubber bands.

When a staging seton is used, the fistula tract is identified and only the most superficial portion is divided. The seton is placed through that portion of the fistula tract that traverses the sphincter, thus encircling the muscle. This portion of the tract is divided as a second procedure once adequate fibrosis occurs (usually 8 weeks). A "high" fistula may be converted to a "low" fistula by dividing only the proximal portion of the tract, leaving the distal tract encircled with a seton for division at a later date.

Whether to use a cutting seton or a staging seton with second-stage fistulotomy appears to be up to surgeon preference. In a study of 59 patients with high anal fistula, Garcia-Aguilar et al[37] showed no difference in fistula eradication, incontinence, and patient satisfaction between 12 patients treated with cutting setons and 47 treated with two-stage seton fistulotomy.

Anorectal Advancement Flaps

Advancement flaps consist of mucosa, submucosa, and part of the internal sphincter. The underlying fistula tract is debrided, and the internal opening is sutured at the level of the muscle. The edge of the elevated flap containing the internal opening is excised, and the flap is advanced and sutured over the internal defect (Figure 156-11).

Advancement flaps offer the advantage of a one-stage procedure, quicker healing, limited damage to the underlying sphincter, and minimal risk of anal canal deformity.[3] Several studies have reported good success, with few complications using anorectal advancement flaps in the treatment of both simple and complex fistulas.[38]

Fibrin Glue

The use of fibrin glue in the management of anorectal fistulas has been popularized. A prepared mixture of fibrinogen and thrombin is injected into the fistula tract after it has been curetted. The resulting coagulum plugs the fistula tract. This technique represents an alternative mode of treatment in complex cases for which standard treatment has failed. The complete healing rate in one series was 60% and included patients with Crohn disease and human immunodeficiency virus (HIV)–associated anal disease.[39] Sentovich performed a two-stage fistulotomy with injection of fibrin glue into the external opening after seton removal at the second operation, with 69% success in 48 patients.[40] Buchanan et al[41] found only a 14% complex fistula closure rate in 22 patients. Despite mixed results, fibrin glue remains a viable treatment option because of its safety, ease of application, and low risk of sphincter injury.

Fistula Plug

Recently, a cone-shaped fistula plug created from a bioabsorbable xenograft made of lyophilized porcine intestinal submucosa has become available for high transsphincteric fistulas. The material has an inherent resistance to infection, produces no foreign body or giant cell reaction, and becomes repopulated with host cell tissue during a period of 3 months. The fistula plug is inserted into the primary opening of the fistula and secured into place with one or two interrupted stitches. This intervention appears to be a safe option as it preserves anal function and is associated with a low morbidity. In prospective studies of complex fistula-in-ano, there was a moderate success rate of 35% to 87%.[42] Further randomized controlled trials studying objective parameters of fistula healing are needed to substantiate these findings.

POSTOPERATIVE CARE

In general, most anorectal surgery is performed as an outpatient procedure. Patients are instructed to consume

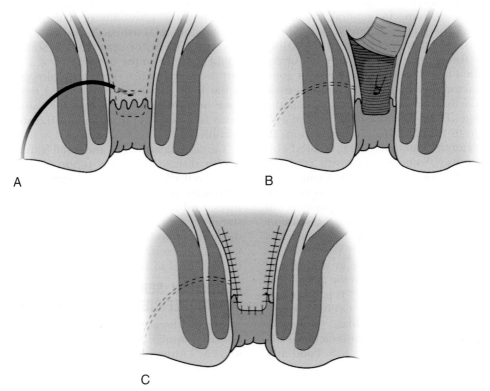

FIGURE 156-11 **A,** Anorectal advancement flap for closure of the internal opening in the treatment of perianal fistulas. The base of the flap should be wider than the apex. **B,** With the flap elevated, the internal opening is debrided and closed with a suture. **C,** The apex of the flap is advanced and sutured over the defect.

a high-fiber diet postoperatively. No bowel confinement regimen is required for the treatment of simple conditions. For complex procedures, bowel confinement has been recommended, but it is of questionable value.[43] Sitz baths are recommended for perianal hygiene and comfort. More complex procedures may require inpatient status for pain management and wound care. Wound healing after fistulotomy usually takes 4 to 8 weeks. Patients with an anorectal abscess should be followed closely after drainage for possible fistula development.

COMPLICATIONS

Complications after surgical intervention for anorectal suppurative disease are numerous and related to surgical technique. Urinary retention is the most common complication, occurring in up to 25% of patients.[44] Other complications include hemorrhage, acute external thrombosed hemorrhoids, cellulitis, fecal impaction, stricture, rectovaginal fistula, incontinence, and recurrence. Local wound problems and complications associated with anesthesia, such as hypotension, hypertension, and seizures, have also been reported. The issue of fistula recurrence after drainage of anorectal abscess has been discussed previously.

The rate of recurrent fistula after fistulotomy ranges from 0% to 18%,[45] although the true incidence is probably around 3% to 7%.[5,12] The primary causes of fistula recurrence relate to unrecognized internal openings and inadequate drainage of abscess cavities.[2] In a study of 375 patients, Garcia-Aguilar[12] found that recurrence was also associated with lateral location of internal openings and fistulas with horseshoe extension.

The rate of disorders of continence after fistulotomy ranges from 18% to 52%.[45] Factors associated with incontinence risk include the complexity of the fistula, female sex, division of a significant portion of the external sphincter, the use of two-stage seton or cutting seton fistulotomy (probably because of complexity of the fistula), and a history of prior fistula surgery.[12]

SPECIAL CONSIDERATIONS

CROHN DISEASE

Crohn disease manifests with perianal or rectal symptoms in approximately one-third of patients and is associated with a more aggressive natural history (see Chapters 159 and 161), with many due to anorectal sepsis and fistula.[46] Anorectal abscess in patients with Crohn disease should be treated with prompt drainage. Long-term catheter drainage has been found to be safe and effective and may be of benefit in preventing or delaying recurrence and the subsequent need for proctectomy.

The treatment of anorectal fistulas in patients with Crohn disease should be tailored to the specific situation encountered. Consideration should be given to the complexity of the fistula and the presence of active Crohn disease in the rectum. In general, treatment modalities should be conservative. Extensive procedures may increase the risk of incontinence and nonhealing wounds. A simple fistula in a patient with a normal rectum can be treated by primary fistulotomy with good outcome and satisfactory healing rates.[47] Complex fistulas in patients with active rectal Crohn disease remain a therapeutic challenge. These cases are better served with prolonged drainage to achieve long-term palliation. In selected cases, rectal advancement flaps may be used with good functional results.[48] Some patients with complex anorectal fistulas in the presence of anal Crohn may require diversion of the fecal stream for symptomatic relief. Ultimately, between 12% and 39% of patients will require proctectomy for progressive intestinal disease or intractable perianal disease.[49] Shinozaki et al, in a series of 39 patients, found that simultaneously performing a bowel resection for active Crohn disease at the time of drainage of perianal sepsis or draining seton placement led to better healing of the anal fistula.[50] It is theorized that control of the intraabdominal Crohn disease improves healing of perianal Crohn fistulas.

A monoclonal antibody to tumor necrosis factor (TNF-α) was approved in August 1998 by the U.S. Food and Drug Administration for the treatment of patients with fistulizing Crohn disease. Infliximab (Remicade) is a genetically constructed murine-human chimeric immunoglobulin. It neutralizes the biologic activity of TNF-α and inhibits binding to its receptors. A randomized trial in which infliximab was used in the management of patients with Crohn fistulas (perianal and abdominal) demonstrated a 62% clinical response (defined as >50% reduction from baseline in the number of draining fistulas) and a 46% complete closure of all fistulas compared with 26% and 13%, respectively, of patients in the placebo group.[51] However, the duration of response is short-lived. Repeat treatment or chronic use may be required for a long-term beneficial effect.

FISTULA IN INFANCY

Anal fistula in infancy occurs almost exclusively in otherwise healthy boys younger than 2 years of age. The cause of this condition appears to be a congenital abnormality of the anal glands with abnormally deep and thick crypts of Morgagni. These factors predispose the patients to cryptitis with abscess and fistula formation. Simple fistulotomy is recommended in this patient population with expected good results. A concomitant cryptotomy has been recommended by some to decrease the likelihood of recurrence. Nonoperative management is favored by those who believe that abscess and fistula are self-limited in this population. Opponents argue that such fistula disease is seldom time limited. They argue that the process is truly characterized by frequent intermittent relapse or a prolonged silent state with late recurrence requiring subsequent intervention.

MALIGNANT TRANSFORMATION IN CHRONIC ANAL FISTULA

Carcinoma arising in an anorectal fistula is a rare condition. Rosser[52] established the first association between adenocarcinoma and anal fistula. There is controversy regarding the possibility of malignancy arising from a benign anorectal fistula. A slow-growing cancer may not become evident for years, and in some cases the fistula could result from the breakdown of a neoplasm. To rule out the preexistence of even the slowest growing cancer, it has been arbitrarily determined that a fistula should have been present for at least 10 years before the diagnosis of carcinoma if malignant transformation is to be considered.

Carcinoma arising in anorectal fistulas in patients with Crohn disease has been reported; the estimated incidence is 0.7%.[53] Deep biopsy samples, careful histologic examination of atypical cells obtained from ductal structures, and a high index of suspicion in cases of long-standing anorectal fistulas may provide a clue to the diagnosis of underlying carcinoma. Resection with either wide local excision or abdominoperineal resection has the potential to result in cure.

ANORECTAL SEPSIS AND FISTULA IN HUMAN IMMUNODEFICIENCY VIRUS DISEASE

Anorectal disease is a prevalent problem in the HIV-positive population, with an estimated frequency of 6% to 34%.[54] Although there is concern in performing elective anorectal surgery in this population because of the fear of poor healing, symptomatic anorectal sepsis and fistula often require surgical management. Treatment should be tailored to the patient's severity of illness. The risk for disturbed wound healing increases as the preoperative CD4+ count decreases. The presence of an acquired immunodeficiency syndrome and a white blood cell count of less than $3000/mm^3$ are also associated with poor wound healing.[55] In the absence of these risk factors, fistulotomy for simple fistulas may be performed with expected good results. For complex fistulas and patients with risk factors for poor healing, the liberal use of draining setons is recommended for symptomatic relief.

ANORECTAL COMPLICATIONS IN PATIENTS WITH LEUKEMIA

Anorectal complications in patients with leukemia represent a rare but potentially life-threatening problem. The incidence of concomitant symptomatic anorectal disease and leukemia has been reported to be as high as 5.8%, with acute anorectal sepsis accounting for a majority of all cases.[56] The mortality rate for patients with acute perianal sepsis in this population has been reported to be from approximately 20%.[57] In general, surgical treatment of anorectal sepsis in uncontrolled acute leukemia has been avoided because of the fear that the septic process would spread and wound healing would be impaired. Historically, this led to a policy of combined radiation therapy and symptomatic care as primary treatment, with surgical management reserved for the drainage of an obviously fluctuant abscess. Symptomatic care consisted of sitz baths or warm compresses, stool softeners, analgesic agents, and broad-spectrum antibiotics. Additional precautionary measures included no rectal examinations, no instrumentation, and no enemas. However, reports indicate that surgical intervention in the form of incision and drainage appears to be safe in this patient population.[56]

REFERENCES

1. Cosman BC, Devaraj B: Recent smoking is a risk factor for anal abscess and fistula. *Dis Colon Rectum* 48:630, 2005.
2. Robinson AMJ, DeNobile JW: Anorectal abscess and fistula-in-ano. *J Natl Med Assoc* 80:1209, 1988.
3. Seow CF, Nicholls RJ: Anal fistula [see comments]. *Br J Surg* 79:197, 1992.
4. McElwain JW, MacLean MD, Alexander RM, et al: Anorectal problems: Experience with primary fistulectomy for anorectal abscess—a report of 1,000 cases. *Dis Colon Rectum* 18:646, 1975.
5. Ramanujam PS, Prasad ML, Abcarian H, et al: Perianal abscesses and fistulas: A study of 1023 patients. *Dis Colon Rectum* 27:593, 1984.
6. Schouten WR, van Vroonhoven TJ: Treatment of anorectal abscess with or without primary fistulectomy: Results of a prospective randomized trial. *Dis Colon Rectum* 34:60, 1991.
7. Scoma JA, Salvati EP, Rubin RJ: Incidence of fistulas subsequent to anal abscesses. *Dis Colon Rectum* 17:357, 1974.
8. Vasilevsky CA, Gordon PH: The incidence of recurrent abscesses or fistula-in-ano following anorectal suppuration. *Dis Colon Rectum* 27:126, 1984.
9. Parks AG, Gordon PH, Hardcastle JD: A classification of fistula-in-ano. *Br J Surg* 63:1, 1976.
10. Marks CG, Ritchie JK: Anal fistulas at St Mark's Hospital. *Br J Surg* 64:84, 1977.
11. Vasilevsky CA, Gordon PH: Results of treatment of fistula-in-ano. *Dis Colon Rectum* 28:225, 1985.
12. Garcia-Aguilar J, Belmonte C, Wong WD, et al: Anal fistula surgery: Factors associated with recurrence and incontinence. *Dis Colon Rectum* 39:723, 1996.
13. Buchan R, Grace RH: Anorectal suppuration: The results of treatment and the factors influencing the recurrence rate. *Br J Surg* 60:537, 1973.
14. Goodsall DH, Miles WE: *Diseases of the anus and rectum.* London, 1900, Longman and Green.
15. Cirocco WC, Reilly JC: Challenging the predictive accuracy of Goodsall's rule for anal fistulas. *Dis Colon Rectum* 35:537, 1992.
16. Fazio VW: Complex anal fistulae. *Gastroenterol Clin North Am* 16:93, 1987.
17. Kuijpers HC, Schulpen T: Fistulography for fistula-in-ano: Is it useful? *Dis Colon Rectum* 28:103, 1985.
18. Choen S, Burnett S, Bartram CI, et al: Comparison between anal endosonography and digital examination in the evaluation of anal fistulae. *Br J Surg* 78:445, 1991.
19. Buchanan GN, Bartram CI, Williams AB, et al: Value of hydrogen peroxide enhancement of three-dimensional endoanal ultrasound in fistula-in-ano. *Dis Colon Rectum* 48:141, 2005.
20. Kim Y, Park YJ: Three-dimensional endoanal ultrasonographic assessment of an anal fistula with and without H_2O_2 enhancement. *World J Gastroenterol* 15:4810, 2009.
21. Orsoni P, Barthet M, Portier F, et al: Prospective comparison of endosonography, magnetic resonance imaging and surgical findings in anorectal fistula and abscess complicating Crohn's disease. *Br J Surg* 86:360, 1999.
22. Poen AC, Felt-Bersma RJ, Cuesta MA, et al: Vaginal endosonography of the anal sphincter complex is important in the assessment of faecal incontinence and perianal sepsis. *Br J Surg* 85:359, 1998.
23. Beets-Tan RG, Beets GL, van der Hoop AG, et al: Preoperative MR imaging of anal fistulas: Does it really help the surgeon? *Radiology* 218:75, 2001.
24. Schwartz DA, Wiersema MJ, Dudiak KM, et al: A comparison of endoscopic ultrasound, magnetic resonance imaging, and exam under anesthesia for evaluation of Crohn's perianal fistulas. *Gastroenterology* 121:1064, 2001.
25. Chang SC, Lin JK: Change in anal continence after surgery for intersphincteral anal fistula: A functional and manometric study. *Int J Colorectal Dis* 18:111, 2003.
26. Johnson E, Gaw JU, Armstrong DN: Role of anorectal fistuloscopy in evaluating complex anorectal fistulas. *Dis Colon Rectum* 48:631, 2005.
27. Toyonaga T, Matsushima M, Tanaka Y, et al: Microbiological analysis and endoanal ultrasonography for diagnosis of anal fistula in acute anorectal sepsis. *Int J Colorectal Dis* 22:209, 2007.
28. Seow CF, Leong AF, Goh HS: Results of a policy of selective immediate fistulotomy for primary anal abscess. *Aust N Z J Surg* 63:485, 1993.
29. Hanley PH: Conservative surgical correction of horseshoe abscess fistula. *Dis Colon Rectum* 8:361, 1965.
30. Eisenhammer S: The final evaluation and classification of the surgical treatment of the primary anorectal cryptoglandular intermuscular (intersphincteric) fistulous abscess and fistula. *Dis Colon Rectum* 21:237, 1978.
31. Oliver I, Lacueva FJ, Perez-Vicente F, et al: Randomized clinical trial comparing simple drainage of anorectal abscess with and without fistula track treatment. *Int J Colorectal Dis* 18:107, 2003.
32. Fucini C: One-stage treatment of anal abscesses and fistulas: A clinical appraisal on the basis of two different classifications. *Int J Colorectal Dis* 6:12, 1991.
33. Shanwani A, Nor AM, Nil Amri N: Ligation of the intersphincteric fistula tract (LIFT): A sphincter-saving technique for fistula-in-ano. *Dis Colon Rectum* 53:39, 2010.
34. Bleier JIS, Moloo H, Goldberg SM: Ligation of the intersphincteric fistula tract: an effective new technique for complex fistulas. *Dis Colon Rectum* 53:43, 2010.
35. Lentner A, Wienert V: Long-term, indwelling setons for low transsphincteric and intersphincteric anal fistulas: Experience with 108 cases. *Dis Colon Rectum* 39:1097, 1996.
36. Topstad DR, Panaccione R, Heine JA, et al: Combined seton placement, infliximab infusion, and maintenance immunosuppressives improve healing rate in fistulizing anorectal Crohn's disease. *Dis Colon Rectum* 46:577, 2003.
37. Garcia-Aguilar J, Belmonte C, Wong DW, et al: Cutting seton versus two-stage seton fistulotomy in the surgical management of high anal fistula. *Br J Surg* 85:243, 1998.
38. Soltani A, Kaiser AM: Endorectal advancement flap for cryptoglandular or Crohn's fistula-in-ano. *Dis Colon Rectum* 53:486, 2010.
39. Abel ME, Chiu YS, Russell TR, et al: Autologous fibrin glue in the treatment of rectovaginal and complex fistulas. *Dis Colon Rectum* 36:447, 1993.
40. Sentovich SM: Fibrin glue for anal fistulas. *Dis Colon Rectum* 46:498, 2003.
41. Buchanan GN, Bartram CI, Phillips RK, et al: Efficacy of fibrin sealant in the management of complex anal fistula. *Dis Colon Rectum* 46:1167, 2003.
42. Garg P, Song J, Bhatia A, Kalia H, et al: The efficacy of anal fistula plug in fistula-in-ano: A systematic review. *Colorectal Dis* 12:965, 2010.
43. Nessim A, Wexner SD, Agachan F, et al: Is bowel confinement necessary after anorectal reconstructive surgery? A prospective, randomized, surgeon-blinded trial. *Dis Colon Rectum* 42:16, 1999.
44. Mazier WP: The treatment and care of anal fistulas: A study of 1,000 patients. *Dis Colon Rectum* 14:134, 1971.
45. Vasilevsky CA: Fistula-in-ano and abscess. In Beck DE, Wexner SD, editors: *Fundamentals of anorectal surgery.* London, 1998, WB Saunders, p 153.
46. Lewis RT, Maron DJ: Anorectal Crohn's disease. *Surg Clin North Am* 90:83, 2010.
47. Morrison JG, Gathright JBJ, Ray JE, et al: Surgical management of anorectal fistulas in Crohn's disease. *Dis Colon Rectum* 32:492, 1989.
48. Makowiec F, Jehle EC, Becker HD, et al: Clinical course after transanal advancement flap repair of perianal fistula in patients with Crohn's disease. *Br J Surg* 82:603, 1995.
49. Whiteford MH, Kilkenny J, Hyman N, et al. Practice parameters for the treatment of perianal abscess and fistula-in-ano (Revised). *Dis Colon Rectum* 48:1337, 2005.
50. Shinozaki M, Koganei K, Fukushima T: Simultaneous anus and bowel operation is preferable for anal fistula in Crohn's disease. *J Gastroenterol* 37:611, 2002.
51. Present DH, Rutgeerts PJ, Targan SR, et al: Infliximab for the treatment of fistulas in patients with Crohn's disease. *N Engl J Med* 340:1398, 1999.
52. Rosser C: The relation of fistula-in-ano to cancer of the anal canal. *Trans Am Proctol Soc* 65, 1934.
53. Ky A, Sohn N, Weinstein MA, et al: Carcinoma arising in anorectal fistulas of Crohn's disease. *Dis Colon Rectum* 41:992, 1998.

54. Consten EC, Slors FJ, Noten HJ, et al: Anorectal surgery in human immunodeficiency virus-infected patients: Clinical outcome in relation to immune status. *Dis Colon Rectum* 38:1169, 1995.

55. Nadal SR, Manzione CR, Galvao VM, et al: Healing after anal fistulotomy: Comparative study between HIV-positive and HIV-negative patients. *Dis Colon Rectum* 41:177, 1998.

56. Grewal H, Guillem JG, Quan SH, et al: Anorectal disease in neutropenic leukemic patients: Operative versus nonoperative management. *Dis Colon Rectum* 37:1095, 1994.

57. Büyükaşik Y, Ozcebe OI, Sayinalp N, et al: Perianal infections in patients with leukemia: Importance of the course of neutrophil count. *Dis Colon Rectum* 41:81, 1998.

Miscellaneous Disorders of the Rectum and Anus

David E. Beck

O ther chapters in this text have covered the more common anorectal conditions. A group of less common but still important conditions are discussed here. This summary of the disease process, evaluation, and management will prepare the reader to manage patients with these conditions.

STRICTURE

Nonmalignant stricture or stenosis of the anal canal is an uncommon but debilitating condition. Patients with this condition have anal pain, obstipation, and frequent bleeding. The scarred anal canal may also be sufficiently noncompliant to cause incontinence. Anal stenosis is most commonly (87%) caused by excessive excision of the anoderm during hemorrhoidectomy.[1] An improperly performed hemorrhoidectomy may also produce an ectropion (rectal mucosa in the distal anal canal), also referred to as a *Whitehead deformity* (if it is circumferential). Other causes of anal stenosis include recurrent anal fissure, chronic diarrhea, recurrent abscess and fistula requiring surgical treatment, anal Crohn disease, radiation, and excision of perianal skin lesions as in Paget or Bowen disease.[1,2]

The treatment of anal stenosis depends on its severity and position in the anal canal. High anal strictures that are covered entirely by mucosa are more difficult to treat than the low anal strictures at the level of the anoderm. Mild anal stenosis responds to more conservative therapy, whereas severe anal stenosis may require more extensive surgical procedures.

MEDICAL THERAPY

Medical therapy for anal stenosis combines bulking of the stool with dilation in the office or at home using the finger or calibrated rubber dilators and topical anesthetics. Dilation is an ideal treatment for patients with Crohn disease or high-risk patients with otherwise weakened external sphincters.[3]

The combination of repeated dilation and steroid suppositories may prevent early recurrence of the stenosis, but no well-controlled trials have been reported. Anal stenosis in elderly patients has been shown to cause megarectum. These patients are usually nursing home residents who require daily enemas for constipation.

SURGICAL THERAPY

The surgical treatment of anal stenosis includes lateral internal sphincterotomy, any one of a number of advancement flaps, and occasionally a colostomy. A lateral internal sphincterotomy has been suggested as a means of treating anal stenosis that is mild and low in the anal canal. Although the results have been adequate,

sphincterotomy does not treat an associated ectropion, and the procedure may have to be repeated.

Several varieties of flaps have been used to manage anal stenosis. Some, as described later, also address the problem of the ectropion. The flaps are formed with either mucosa or skin and include advancement, island, or rotational flaps.

Advancement Flaps

Advancement flaps advance mucosa or skin supported by muscle or subcutaneous fat.

The flap's blood supply comes from the adjacent intact lateral or inferior tissue. The mucosal advancement flap (Martin anoplasty) advances a pedicle of mucosa into the stenotic anal canal by way of an incision made through the stenotic area.[4] This posterior or lateral flap results in a posterior mucosal ectropion that prevents repeat stricturing. This technique is simple and safe but creates an ectropion with associated mucous discharge. This type of flap is best used for proximal anal canal stenosis.

A Y-V advancement flap moves perianal skin into the distal anal canal.[1] The vertical limb of the Y is inscribed on the anal canal at the level of the stenosis, and the V of the Y is drawn on the lateral perianal skin (Figure 157-1). The skin is incised, and the V-shaped flap of skin is freed laterally. The blood supply of the flap comes from adjacent or underlying subcutaneous tissue. The V is then introduced into the stenotic anal canal to close the wound as a V-shaped incision. This can be used unilaterally or bilaterally with good results. Because the base of the V is still attached to the buttock skin, the flap will not remain in the anal canal if the tension is too great and the stenosis will recur.

Island Flaps

An island flap differs from an advancement flap in that it entails a division of all adjacent mucocutaneous edges. The blood supply is derived solely from the inferior supporting tissue. The increased mobility of these flaps makes them especially useful to treat anal stenosis.[4,5] Following incision of the stenotic scar at the dentate line, a flap is created. The V-Y flap advances a V-shaped portion of skin into the anal canal. The V is drawn with the wide base at the dentate line and incised through the skin (Figure 157-2). The subcutaneous attachments in the lateral edges of the V are released to allow mobilization of the skin into the anal canal. The blood supply to the flap relies on perforating vessels in the subcutaneous fat. The skin is then closed behind the V at the external portion of the perineum to push the V into the anal canal and widen the stenotic area. This method may be used for the treatment of ectropion or low stenosis. However,

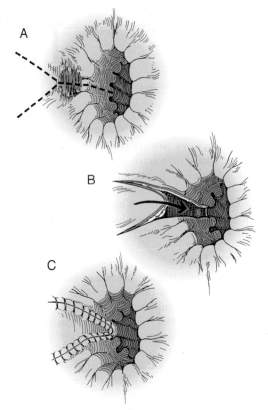

FIGURE 157-1 Y-V advancement flap. **A,** Y flap inscribed outside ectropion and stenosis. **B,** Ectropion excised, Y flap incised. **C,** Flap sutured with V closure. (From Fleshman JW: Fissure-in-ano and anal stenosis. In Beck DE, Wexner SD, editors: *Fundamentals of anorectal surgery*, ed 2. London, 1998, Saunders, p 209.)

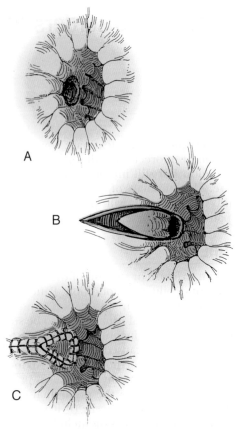

FIGURE 157-2 V-Y advancement flap. **A,** Lateral inverted V inscribed over ectropion or mucosal defect. **B,** Flap mobilized to preserve vasculature after stenosis is divided or ectropion is excised. **C,** Flap sutured in place with Y closure. (From Fleshman JW: Fissure-in-ano and anal stenosis. In Beck DE, Wexner SD, editors: *Fundamentals of anorectal surgery*, ed 2. London, 1998, Saunders, p 209.)

the flap does not advance a wide portion of skin into the scar. The benefit obtained with this flap is derived from soft pliable tissue inserted into the nonpliable scar. If more tissue is needed to allow the canal to dilate, this technique may be repeated on the opposite side of the anal canal.

Island flaps are frequently used for the treatment of anal stenosis.[5] The stenotic scar is first incised laterally at the dentate line (Figure 157-3). A *diamond-shaped island* of skin from the lateral perineum is inscribed to match the defect in the anal canal made by this incision. The flap is then mobilized from its lateral subcutaneous attachments and advanced into the incision made in the stenotic anal canal. This flap of skin will open the stenosis widely when the lateral corners of the diamond are sutured at the level of the stenosis. This flap allows advancement of maximal skin to the point of stenosis with minimal tension. A *U-shaped flap* as described by Pearl et al[6] is especially useful for patients with White-head deformity and ectropion. The U is a broader-based version of the V-Y advancement flap but allows the ectropion to be excised across a wide base and the inverted U to be advanced into the anal canal to fill the defect.

Christensen et al[7] proposed the "house" advancement pedicle flap. This flap is easy to construct, can cover as much as 25% of the anal circumference, and permits

primary closure of the donor site (Figure 157-4).[8] If additional coverage is needed, two, three, or even four flaps may be used.

S-Plasty (Rotational Flap)

The S-plasty is best used for the treatment of Bowen or Paget disease where a large amount of skin has to be excised and new skin rotated into the area. The S-plasty is a rotational flap that does not open a stricture as well as the previously described advancement flaps. It is used to provide a wide area of skin to cover a perineum that is entirely excised for disease. The base of the S is drawn on the lateral buttock, and the necessary tissue is excised (Figure 157-5). The skin and subcutaneous tissue in the S are rotated down to the mucosal incision and sutured in place. The opposite curve of the S is treated similarly on the other side of the anal canal. This shape provides for adequate blood supply and avoids tension; unilateral or bilateral S-flaps can be performed.

Advancement, rotational, or island flaps can be fashioned using local or regional anesthesia. Each type of flap has advantages, and proper selection produces good results.[2] Surgeons should therefore be experienced in all types, allowing individualized treatment. Rotation and advancement flap techniques require more mobilization

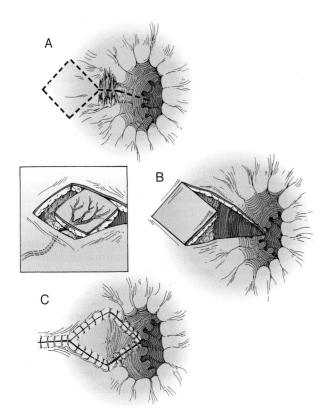

FIGURE 157-3 Diamond island flap. **A,** Stenosis incised in lateral midline and diamonds inscribed laterally to match defects. **B,** Diamond flap incised and advanced into anal canal. **C,** Flap secured with wide point at stenosis line. (From Fleshman JW: Fissure-in-ano and anal stenosis. In Beck DE, Wexner SD, editors: *Fundamentals of anorectal surgery*, ed 2. London, 1998, Saunders, p 209.)

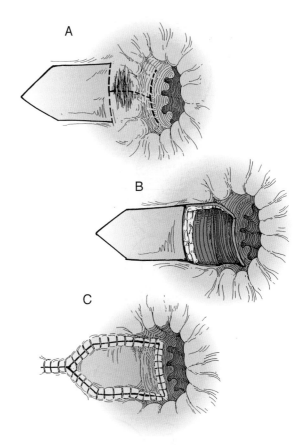

FIGURE 157-4 House advancement flap. **A,** House-shaped flap is created. **B,** The flap is advanced into the anal canal. **C,** The flap is sutured in place. (From Fleshman JW: Fissure-in-ano and anal stenosis. In Beck DE, Wexner SD, editors: *Fundamentals of anorectal surgery*, ed 2. London, 1998, Saunders, p 209.)

of tissue, more suture lines, and a complete bowel preparation. Flap anoplasty techniques are reserved for the most severe problems after conservative measures have failed. Complications of anoplasty include infection, failure of the anoplasty to correct the stenosis, and slough of the flap. These can usually be avoided with adequate preparation and adherence to good technique. In certain settings, a diverting stoma may be considered.

Patients with strictures secondary to Crohn disease, lymphogranuloma venereum, or syphilis usually respond best to repeated dilation.[3] Only rarely has anal stenosis secondary to inflammatory bowel disease been treated with anoplasty. The patients may require anoderm release incisions with repeated dilation. The use of an anoplasty is problematic as the underlying disease process is continuous and may affect the healing.

PRURITUS ANI

Pruritus ani is a symptom complex that consists of an intense itch and burning discomfort of the perianal skin. It has a multiplicity of causes, several of which may coexist. It is frequently associated with varying degrees of skin breakdown, weeping, maceration, lichenification, and superinfection. Pruritus ani may be refractory until the specific cause is identified, but many symptoms can

be successfully treated without determining a specific cause.[9]

HISTORY

A careful history often aids in identification of the cause of pruritus ani.[10] The history should include the onset of symptoms and their relationship to diet, medication, bowel evacuation, and anal hygiene practices. Pruritus may begin insidiously, with the patient complaining of the sensation of uneasiness or itching in the perianal region. Symptoms are more frequent in the evenings and summer months. As the area of involvement spreads and the intensity of itching increases, the patient reflexively begins scratching and clawing at the skin. This leads to further skin damage, excoriation, and potentially a secondary skin infection.

All medications should be identified and tabulated, as many can contribute to pruritus; special attention should be given to antibiotics, colchicine, quinidine, and topical medicines that contain corticosteroids, estrogens, or "-caine" drugs. Systemic illnesses, such as diabetes mellitus, chronic renal failure, or lymphoreticular diseases, such as polycythemia vera or Hodgkin disease, should be identified. The history should also elicit any symptoms of inflammatory bowel disease or acholic stools. Prior anorectal surgery may suggest deformed

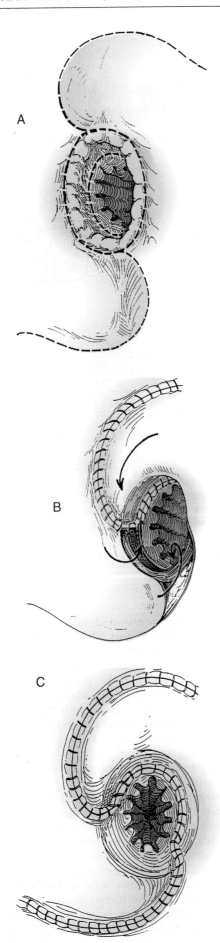

FIGURE 157-5 S-plasty. **A,** Perianal skin lesion requiring removal of large skin area. **B,** Area of perianal skin excised, with lateral curves incised onto buttocks. **C,** Curves of skin advanced into perianal defect and secured laterally to produce S-shaped closure of rotated flaps. (From Fleshman JW: Fissure-in-ano and anal stenosis. In Beck DE, Wexner SD, editors: *Fundamentals of anorectal surgery*, ed 2. London, 1998, Saunders, p 209.)

anorectal anatomy, which in turn can lead to poor continence. The physician should also document allergies or any generalized dermatoses such as psoriasis or seborrhea. A sexual history should include sexual orientation and specific practices, especially the practice of anal receptive intercourse. The immune status is also important, not only because of primary immunodeficient states or contracted states such as acquired immune deficiency syndrome but also in transplant recipients who are receiving immunosuppressive medications. A careful gynecologic and obstetric history should be obtained from female patients and should include contraceptive practices and any history of inflammatory or ulcerative lesions. A history of difficult vaginal deliveries or perineal trauma should increase the suspicion for anatomic or functional sphincter compromise; manometry and rectal ultrasonography can be helpful in selected cases. A brief psychological profile may be beneficial to identify any association between symptoms and social or financial stresses with which the patient may be confronted.

PHYSICAL EXAMINATION

After completing a detailed medical history, the clinician should perform a meticulous physical examination. Initially, the general dermatologic evaluation may isolate conditions such as psoriasis, seborrheic dermatitis, or fungal or other infections. The patient should come to the examining suite without bowel preparation and with instructions not to have applied any creams or ointments to the perianal area. After the patient is assisted into the prone jackknife position, the perianal region should be carefully inspected for signs of excessive moisture, soiling, excoriation, skin maceration (Figure 157-6), or any perianal dermatoses. Having the patient strain (Valsalva maneuver), allows evaluation for possible prolapsing hemorrhoidal tissue and a digital examination evaluates the consistency of the stool. All abnormalities should be carefully documented, including an assessment of the resting and squeeze sphincter strengths.

Next, the clinician can take any culture materials, biopsy samples, or scrapings that are thought necessary to make an appropriate clinical diagnosis. Suspicious skin lesions can be biopsied using a punch biopsy technique.[9] This technique involves the subdermal infiltration of a few milliliters of 1% lidocaine with epinephrine (1 : 200,000) under the biopsy site. A punch biopsy tool is driven into the area with a circular motion by swirling the punch between the thumb and index fingers. After the punch is 4 to 5 mm beneath the skin, it is gently raised and the resulting circular wedge of skin and subcutaneous tissue is excised with a fine scissors. Bleeding should be minimal, and simple pressure should

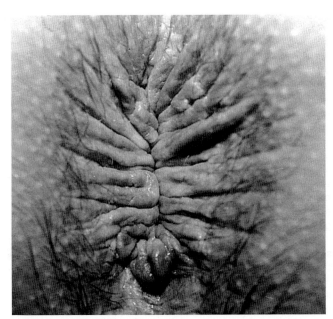

FIGURE 157-6 Pruritus ani. (From Hicks TC, Stamous MJ: Pruritus ani: Diagnosis and treatment. In Beck DE, Wexner SD, editors: *Fundamentals of anorectal surgery*, ed 2. London, 1998, Saunders, p 199.)

adequately effect hemostasis. A simple gauze dressing is all that is required. The punches are available in a number of sizes ranging in diameter from 1.0 mm to 1.0 cm. Disposable punches are very convenient. Two disposable enemas should then be administered to the patient, after which a careful sigmoidoscopy and anoscopy are performed. Evaluation for hemorrhoids, polyps, cancer, fistula, mucosal prolapse, stenosis, or evidence of previous surgery is documented. Sigmoidoscopy may be helpful to identify proctitis, inflammatory bowel disease, rectal lesions, or active infections. Pruritus ani may be associated with colorectal neoplasms at a disproportionately high rate,[9] particularly when the symptom is chronic. The examiner should take special precautions when evaluating patients who engage in anal receptive intercourse or who may be strong candidates for exposure to sexually transmitted diseases. The physician should decide on a case-by-case basis whether to perform pelvic examinations in female patients or to recommend pelvic examination be performed by a gynecologist.

PATHOPHYSIOLOGY

The perianal skin is richly supplied with sensory nerve endings that mediate a variety of sensations.[10] These sensations may be elicited by local irritation from excoriation, alkaline secretions, and various chemical irritants. The receptor apparatus for both itch and pain is located at the dermoepidermal junction of the skin and consists of a plexus of free nerve endings. Damage to cells in proximity to these nerve endings causes a release of diffusible mediators that may stimulate the receptors. Slow-conducting neurons transmit the itch sensation to the lateral spinothalamic tracts through synapses that connect with secondary fibers and send the sensation to the thalamus. It is questionable whether tertiary neurons relay the itch sensation to the cortex. Pain and itch are served by the same receptors and neural pathways, which explains the effectiveness of pain (scratching) in relieving itch.[9]

CAUSES

The cause of pruritus ani is appropriately categorized under the headings of idiopathic and secondary types. The specific etiologic factors responsible for the diagnosis of secondary pruritus ani are nearly encyclopedic, yet despite comprehensive evaluations, in more than one-half of patients with pruritus ani, the cause is categorized as idiopathic. The major contributors to secondary pruritus ani are listed in Table 157-1.

Personal Hygiene

Clinicians have long been aware of the irritant effect of feces on the perianal area, especially in cases of prolonged contact. In patients with continued fecal contamination, the use of bulking agents and an appropriate cleansing regimen often will alleviate symptoms. Another group of patients, known as the "overachiever group," have pruritus secondary to their personal hygiene practice of compulsively cleaning the perianal area. Their meticulous cleansing is usually associated with abrasive rubbing and the use of irritating alkaline soaps, which can result in chronic pruritus. Physicians have categorized this maneuver as the "polishing the anus syndrome." Symptoms often resolve immediately once patients adopt a less traumatic perianal hygiene program.

Anatomic Compromise

An estimated 25% of patients with pruritus ani have causative or contributory anorectal disorders.[9] Lesions such as anal fistula, fissure, skin tags, prolapsing anal papillae, or mucosal prolapse may lead to the seepage of fluid from the anal canal onto the perianal skin, which in turn leads to inflammation, ulcerations, and, if infected, suppuration. Surgical intervention to relieve pruritus has been extremely variable in results, so it is very important to be highly selective in choosing surgical candidates, preferably only after appropriate medical therapy has failed.[10]

Obese patients are predisposed to pruritus because their anatomy produces a persistently moist environment that may lead to difficulties in achieving appropriate personal hygiene. Patients with weak sphincter tone may have mucosal prolapse or fecal contamination of the perianal area, leading to pruritus. Wearing tight clothing (tight jeans, underwear, and girdles) or clothing that does not allow proper ventilation also predisposes to this trapped moisture syndrome.

Systemic Diseases

On occasion, systemic diseases may lead to generalized itching. These include cholestatic jaundice, chronic renal failure, diabetes, iron deficiency (with or without the presence of anemia), thyrotoxicosis, Hodgkin disease, and polycythemia vera.[9]

Diet

Dietary factors may represent the most significant cause of secondary pruritus ani. Diet may incite symptoms

TABLE 157-1 Major Causes of Pruritus Ani

Causes	Examples
Personal hygiene	Poor cleansing habits resulting in chronic exposure to residual irritating feces; conversely, overmeticulous cleansing with excessive rubbing and soap use
Diet	Consumption of large volumes of liquids; coffee (caffeinated and decaffeinated, coffee-containing products), chocolate, citrus, spicy foods, tea, beer, and foods high in milk content; vitamin A and D deficiencies, fat substitutes
Anatomic compromise	Obesity, deep anal clefts, excessive hair, tight-fitting clothing (tight clothing or clothing that impairs adequate ventilation), fistula, fissure, skin tags, prolapsing papilla, or mucosal prolapse
Systemic disease	Jaundice, diabetes mellitus, chronic renal failure, iron deficiency, thyrotoxicosis, myxedema, Hodgkin lymphoma, polycythemia vera
Gynecologic conditions	Pruritus vulvae, vaginal discharge (endocervicitis, vaginitis)
Neoplasms	Bowen disease, extramammary Paget disease, squamous cell carcinoma, cloacogenic carcinoma, anorectal polypoid lesions
Diarrheal states	Irritable bowel syndrome, Crohn disease, chronic ulcerative colitis
Radiation	Postirradiation changes
Psychogenic	Anxiety, neuroses, psychoses
Drugs	Quinidine; colchicine; antibiotics (tetracycline); intravenous hydrocortisone phosphate; ointments or creams that contain "-caine" drugs, and nonprescription medications for personal hygiene such as perfumed soaps and ointments that may contain alcohol, witch hazel, or other astringents
Dermatologic conditions	Psoriasis, seborrheic dermatitis, atopic dermatitis, lichen simplex and lichen sclerosis
Infections	Viruses: herpes simplex, cytomegalovirus, papillomavirus
	Bacteria: *Staphylococcus aureus*, erythrasma, mixed infections, syphilis
	Fungi: dermatophytosis, candidiasis
	Parasites: pinworms, scabies, pediculosis
Idiopathic	—

through three major pathways. First, it will affect the consistency of the stool, which in turn can lead to fecal soiling. Second, the components of the diet may lead to direct irritation secondary to their chemical composition. Third, if an excessive volume of liquid is consumed, it could directly lead to more watery stools and pruritus as a result of frequent contact irritation. Many food groups, such as coffee (caffeinated and decaffeinated), chocolate, citrus, spicy foods, tea, beer, and foods with a high milk content have been implicated in initiating or promoting symptoms. Patients with vitamin A and vitamin D deficiencies are also believed to be predisposed to pruritus ani.[10]

The majority of patients with diet-induced pruritus ani can relate the onset of their symptoms to the ingestion of coffee or dairy products. Coffee is an irritant that can elicit pruritus when it is ingested in any form (fresh, instant, decaffeinated, or when used as a flavor additive to other foods, such as ice cream). An apparent threshold for coffee drinkers usually varies between 2 and 4 cups per day. A similar threshold, noted in milk-drinking patients, arises at the ingestion of 6 to 10 oz daily.[9] Pruritus caused by chocolate, tea, and cola is believed to be related to the xanthine content of these substances. Olestra, a fat substitute, may result in pruritus ani secondary to fecal seepage induced by the nonabsorbed, oily food additive. The appearance of diet-induced pruritus is often symmetric.[10]

Gynecologic Conditions

Pruritus ani often can be attributed specifically to diseases of gynecologic origin. Pruritus vulvae may extend posteriorly to involve the anal skin and can often be attributed to vaginal discharge or urinary incontinence. Irritation secondary to vaginal discharge may also lead to pruritus as the result of endocervicitis, trichomonal vaginitis, or candidal vaginitis, which cause a leukorrhea that irritates the perianal skin. Physicians should be prepared to perform pelvic examinations and to obtain appropriate cultures and stains in this subset of patients. Pruritus ani can be reported in women during menopause independent of any identifiable local causes, probably secondary to estrogen deficiency.

Neoplasms

Perianal neoplasms can produce pruritus. Polypoid tumors of the anorectum may lead to soiling, which may be secondary to changes in the normal anatomy or mucous secretions, as seen in the case of villous lesions. Premalignant lesions such as squamous cell (Bowen disease) or adenocarcinoma-in-situ (Paget disease) can present as pruritus or may be found incidentally in an anorectal surgical specimen. Lesions are characteristically erythematous, indurated, and plaque-like. The treatment for these noninvasive lesions is wide local excision.

Squamous and basal cell carcinoma of the perianal region may also present as pruritus. The characteristic appearance is similar to that found elsewhere on the body. It is imperative that the clinician take a biopsy sample of any suspicious or nonresponding lesions of the perianal region.

Diarrheal States

Clinical and experimental data have shown that skin trauma secondary to moisture is one of the primary contributors to pruritus ani. Excessive moisture is seen in patients with colitis (Crohn, ulcerative, or nonspecific) and those who abuse laxatives or ingest an excessively high-fiber diet. Patients with dumping or malabsorption syndromes, such as lactose intolerance, are also predisposed to pruritus. In the diarrheal patient, not only is the stool a direct skin irritant, but also the frequent hygiene it necessitates leads to abrasive trauma.

Radiation

Radiation to the skin, as used in rectal or anal canal cancers, causes alterations in the normal cell cycle that induce erythema and edema, which may progress to sclerosis and fibrosis. If the injury progresses, a full-thickness radiation burn will lead to ulcerations. Patients complain of pain, burning, and itching due to perianal skin injury. In addition, radiation proctitis leads to diarrhea, which further exacerbates local perianal skin irritation. Radiodermatitis is difficult to treat; initially, the physician should closely inspect the anoderm and take a biopsy sample of all suspicious areas. Controlling pruritus is often difficult; treatment should include cleansing the anoderm with a mild emollient soap substitute such as Balneol and water. If these simple maneuvers fail to control symptoms, a short trial of topical hydrocortisone (1% to 2.5%) may be helpful.

Psychological Factors

The clinician should not underestimate the significance that psychological factors play in the cause of pruritus ani. Often, the patient with pruritus can relate its onset to anxiety. The "stress years" of midlife produce the largest patient population that complains of pruritus ani, perhaps suggesting more than a casual relationship with other etiologic factors.

Drugs

Several oral medications (see Table 157-1) have been implicated in eliciting pruritus ani through both contact irritation and increased leakage of fecal material from the anal opening. The application of certain topical ointments, creams, or cleansing agents may also elicit pruritus. Preparations containing the "-caines" are notorious for producing intense inflammation in some susceptible patients. Many over-the-counter hygiene products, such as scented soaps, deodorants, colored toilet tissues, and laundry detergents, contain chemicals that may cause increased skin sensitivity and irritation. These chemicals include formaldehyde, alcohol, perfumes, and astringents that elicit symptomatology by depriving the skin of its natural acidity. The increased use of anal wipes that contain alcohol or witch hazel may lead to excoriation if used frequently or if left in contact with the skin for a prolonged period. Because of this, many of the new personal cleansing tissues are free of alcohol and witch hazel. Patients must be assisted in their selection of appropriate nonirritating, atraumatic perianal cleansing products.

Dermatologic Conditions

A large proportion of cases of pruritus ani may be attributable to nonmalignant dermatologic lesions. Perianal psoriasis may be a cause of refractory pruritus ani. The clinician should carefully inspect the patient for the presence of characteristic psoriatic patches elsewhere on the body, such as the scalp, knees, elbows, or other bony prominences. A perianal lesion may be the first or the only psoriatic lesion and is usually found in the gluteal cleft spreading toward the sacrum. Although a perianal psoriatic lesion has a definitive border, it does not have the scaling of systemic psoriatic plaques. A multitude of treatment modalities exist for psoriasis, including local lubrication to prevent fissuring and to maintain flexibility of the skin, topical corticosteroids, coal tar applications, phototherapy (ultraviolet A light used in conjunction with the photosensitizing properties of psoralen compounds [PUVA]), methotrexate, and low-dose cyclosporine.[9]

Infections

Infectious agents must be considered in the differential diagnosis of secondary pruritus ani. The etiologic agents may be bacterial, viral, mycotic, or parasitic. Primary bacterial infections are an unusual occurrence, and when infectious agents can be documented, they are usually superimposed on preexisting perianal skin trauma. Pruritus secondary to infectious agents often has an asymmetric appearance around the anus.[9]

Parasitic infections with pinworms (*Enterobius vermicularis*) are the most common cause of perianal itching in children. The diagnosis can be made by microscopically evaluating perianal skin samples collected on cellulose tape. It is imperative that other family members be evaluated so they can be treated and recontamination does not occur. The symptoms usually occur in the evening, when these 6-mm-long parasites migrate to the perianal skin. *Scabies,* a contagious skin infestation due to the mite *Sarcoptes scabiei,* can elicit severe pruritus. Although usually found on the finger webs or sides of the fingers, these lesions can often be identified in the perianal region. The diagnosis of scabies can be confirmed by demonstrating the mite or its products, such as ova or feces, from scrapings prepared on a slide with one drop of 10% potassium hydroxide. Lesions appear initially as vesicles as the mite burrows its way into the stratum corneum. Treatment consists of the application of an appropriate scabicide such as Kwell lotion (Reed & Carnrick, Jersey City, NJ). The parasite *Pediculosis pubis* (crab or louse) can often be found grasping the base of a hair shaft and is noted to produce macular steel-gray spots, especially on the thighs and chest. With careful examination under magnification, this parasite strikingly resembles a crab. Management requires the treatment of all infected family members; appropriate delousing of all fomites such as clothes, bedding, and upholstery; and showering with an appropriate pediculicide such as permethrin.[9]

TREATMENT

Once the clinician has acquired a comprehensive history, performed a thorough examination, and obtained appropriate culture samples, scrapings, and biopsy samples, the primary cause for pruritus ani may be identified and appropriate therapy instituted.[11] Treatment may include

- Conservative dietary changes to identify offending agents or their symptomatic thresholds
- Appropriate medical therapy for infections, dermatoses, or systemic disorders
- Surgical intervention for the few anatomic deformities that contribute to pruritus
- Nonspecific therapy for most cases of pruritus with no identifiable etiology

Treating idiopathic pruritus requires a focused therapeutic approach, which includes clear instructions tempered with realistic expectations for a response and a consistent followup pattern. Instructions begin with appropriate perianal hygiene. These initial efforts are directed toward keeping the perianal skin dry, clear, and slightly acidic.[12] Any nonessential antibiotics should be discontinued, as should other irritants to the perianal area such as harsh toilet paper, soaps, and any personal hygiene products being applied to the area. The use of any topical steroid agents also should be discontinued initially because of harmful thinning of the perianal skin. Trauma incurred by scratching must be stopped, and for patients with severe symptoms, wearing white cotton gloves at bedtime may be necessary. An alternative to harsh toilet paper is small nonalcoholic towelettes, with appropriate drying of the perianal region with either a soft towel or a hair dryer. Substitute soap preparations such as Balneol are useful and can be applied with the fingertips or moist cotton balls. During the day and at bedtime, it may be helpful to apply a thin cotton pledget directly into the anal crease. The pledget should be small enough that the patient is not conscious of its presence. Dusting the pledget with baby powder (nonperfumed) or cornstarch may improve moisture control.

The patient should also be counseled on dietary changes. As mentioned earlier, food products such as coffee, teas, cola, chocolate, beer, and tomatoes have been identified as offending agents, but there appears to be a threshold at which these products elicit pruritus. For this reason, the patient should discontinue ingestion of these items and then slowly reinstate them into the diet in an attempt to isolate the offending agent. Once the offending agent, such as coffee, is identified, it may be possible to find the patient's threshold so that total abstinence from the produce is unnecessary. Any habit-forming cathartics should be discontinued, and a bulking agent (such as psyllium) should be taken instead to keep the stool soft, large, and nonirritating. The psyllium will decrease trauma to the anal canal and help maintain better perianal hygiene.

For continued uncontrolled leakage, rectal irrigation performed with a 4-oz bulb syringe and warm water is an acceptable adjunct. Daily sitz baths in warm water may also be helpful, but no chemicals should be added. In the unfortunate patient who has intractable pruritus ani, many therapies have been tried: injection of alcohol- or oil-soluble anesthetics, injection of methylene blue, tattooing of the perianal skin with mercuric sulfide, surgical undercutting, and radiation therapy, most of which have had unacceptable results.[9] These procedures have been associated with complications such as skin necrosis, local sepsis, and sloughing of the perianal skin. The use of sedation, tranquilizers, and biofeedback by well-trained practitioners may demonstrate some clinical benefit. Regardless of the treatment or initial success, intermittent recurrences of the disease are common. The patient should be instructed not to become despondent on relapse, but to reconsult the physician so that the appropriate therapeutic corrections can be made. If symptoms continue despite aggressive therapy and if appropriate changes in therapy fail to give relief, a second opinion from a dermatologist, gynecologist, or internist should be considered.

PAIN SYNDROMES

Pain syndromes of the pelvic, rectal, and perianal region are referred to by a variety of names: levator syndrome, levator spasm, proctalgia fugax, coccygodynia, and chronic idiopathic rectal pain. These terms describe a "wastebasket" of pain syndromes that are localized to the rectal area.[9] Each of these syndromes may describe a distinct entity or these pain syndromes may overlap.[13] Once organic causes have been excluded, the patient can present a therapeutic challenge.

Levator spasm is characterized by episodic pelvic or rectal pain caused by spasm in the levator ani muscles. Symptoms of this syndrome are variable and include complaints of pressure or discomfort and the feeling "like sitting on a ball." Left-sided involvement is more common, and the pain occasionally radiates into the gluteal region. The syndrome is more common in women and sometimes occurs after pelvic infections or surgery. The clinical finding in this group of patients is levator sling tenderness on transanal palpation.

Proctalgia fugax is described as brief and sometimes severe episodes of rectal pain similar to "having a knife inserted up the rectum." Patients are often awakened from sleep and have associated irritable bowel syndrome and constipation. The syndrome is more common in men, and there are no physical signs. It is theorized that the pain results from spasm of the rectal muscle wall. For the purpose of this discussion, proctalgia fugax is considered a variant of levator spasm.

Coccygodynia refers to a syndrome of rectal and perineal discomfort associated with coccygeal injury.[14] This is a rare cause of rectal pain. Tenderness is elicited by coccygeal motion in excess of that elicited by the levator muscle. True coccygodynia is a secondary condition of the coccyx and so is not a variant of this functional syndrome.

Multiple factors associated with these syndromes include irritable bowel syndrome, previous pelvic surgery, and disordered defecation syndromes. Occasionally, the rectal or pelvic pain does not match the classic descriptions, in which case it is labeled as *chronic idiopathic rectal pain.*

Evaluation of the patient with levator spasm, proctalgia fugax, and pelvic pain must include a methodical history and careful examination of the pelvic viscera to rule out an organic cause for the discomfort. Inspection, digital rectal examination, and sigmoidoscopy will reveal most common anorectal pathology. Diagnostic imaging may be helpful and includes computed tomographic (CT) scanning, magnetic resonance imaging (MRI), and endorectal ultrasonography to seek less obvious sources of rectal pain. The role for anorectal physiologic testing in these conditions is uncertain.[15] Finally, many patients with pelvic pain syndrome have a psychiatric illness.[16] The following overview of the organic and functional perineal pain syndromes will provide a framework for the evaluation and the results of treatments for this commonly encountered condition.

ANATOMIC CONSIDERATIONS

As previously stated, proctalgia fugax, levator spasm, and pelvic pain can involve overlapping presentations. Pain syndromes may involve any or all of the structures of the pelvis. Disorders of the following organs or organ systems can lead to the complaint of pelvic pain. A complete assessment should exclude each of these as potential causes. An integrated approach may be required and may necessitate orthopedic, neurosurgery, gynecology, and urology consultation.

Spine and Bony Pelvis

Primary and secondary diseases of the pelvic girdle and the lower axial skeleton may present as pelvic pain. Trauma, inflammatory conditions, or malignancy can affect these supporting structures. *Coccygodynia* refers to primary coccygeal injury that causes pain localized to the coccyx. Used in this specific fashion, the term denotes a coccyx that is tender to touch and movement.

Pelvic Musculature

The pelvic floor or pelvic diaphragm is composed of the levator ani muscles. The levator ani are striated muscles: the puborectalis, pubococcygeus, and iliococcygeus. Inferiorly, the external sphincter encircles both the anal canal and the internal sphincter. As is the case in all striated muscles, the levator ani are subject to sustained contractions that can produce local ischemia and pain. Most authors attribute the pain of levator spasm to spasm in this muscle group. The internal sphincter is smooth muscle and is located medial to the striated muscle of the external sphincter. Physiologic testing suggests hypertrophy of the internal anal sphincter as a possible cause of this pain syndrome.

Other Causes

Previous pelvic surgery can also produce pain in this region. Dissection of the pelvic floor during a low anterior resection of the rectum can produce mechanical trauma, which might result in pain in some patients, although the pain most likely is caused by an infection. Inflammatory conditions or malignancy of the prostate and seminal vesicles can be diagnosed in men by eliciting tenderness of these structures on digital rectal examination. In women, diseases of the vagina, uterus, fallopian tubes, or ovaries may present as pelvic pain. Careful inspection and bimanual examination of the female patient are critical to an accurate assessment of pelvic pain. Malignancy and inflammatory conditions of the lower alimentary tract may produce complaints of pain.

Nervous System

Any condition that affects the cauda equina, roots S-2 through S-4, and the pudendal nerve can cause pelvic pain. Degenerative disease of the spine, primary or metastatic disease of the spine, primary or metastatic tumors, cysts, and local trauma must all be considered. Other neurologic disease, such as multiple sclerosis or spastic neuropathy, can produce pain. Laxity of the pelvic floor may cause traction on the pelvic nerves, creating this type of pain syndrome. Specific physiologic testing, such as electromyography (EMG), anorectal manometry, and dynamic proctography, may be useful in the assessment of these conditions. Last, psychiatric illness is frequently associated with the complaint of pelvic pain. When indicated, competent psychiatric evaluation may be illuminating.

CAUSES OF PELVIC AND RECTAL PAIN

Considering the number of anatomic structures, there are many disease processes that cause pelvic and rectal pain. In some patients, no actual disease process can be identified. Box 157-1 describes a classification system that provides the clinician with a systematic approach to the diagnosis and management of pelvic pain syndromes.

Organic: Inflammatory Diseases That Affect the Pelvis and Anorectum

Common anorectal disorders that present as perineal or pelvic pain readily lend themselves to diagnosis; these include abscesses (cryptoglandular, intramuscular), fistulas, Crohn disease, and ulcerative proctitis. These conditions must be excluded as the source of pelvic pain.

In the male patient, chronic or acute prostatitis may present as rectal or pelvic pain. Urinary symptoms are often present and should be elicited in questioning. Digital rectal examination in men should always include careful prostatic palpation to exclude these conditions. Transrectal ultrasound may be helpful to diagnose pelvic pain, revealing pathology of the male reproductive organs. In women, tuboovarian infections, ectopic pregnancy, endometritis, and endometriosis are potential sources of pelvic pain. Bimanual pelvic examination with speculum visualization of the cervix will usually suffice to eliminate these concerns. Occasionally, ultrasonography or CT of the pelvic viscera is necessary to complete the evaluation.

Occasionally, complicated diverticular disease of the sigmoid colon or a pelvic appendicitis may present as pelvic pain. The history will generally direct the clinician to a more specific gastrointestinal workup. Contrast radiography, CT, and ultrasonography may assist in this determination.

Mechanical

Pelvirectal pain may be multifactorial. Causes include constipation or dyschezia, pudendal neuropathy, descending perineum syndrome, incomplete or internal rectal prolapse, rectal ulcer, and pelvic floor hernias. Other mechanical causes of pelvic and rectal pain are muscle spasm or inflammation of surrounding tissue. Anal fissures commonly cause perineal pain. Simple mechanical trauma due to straining can produce this

---

BOX 157-1 Classification of the Causes of Pelvic Pain

ORGANIC

Inflammatory diseases of the pelvis and anorectum
  Cryptoglandular abscess
  Fistula-in-ano
  Crohn disease
  Ulcerative colitis
  Radiation proctitis
  Endometriosis
  Infectious proctitis
  Prostatitis
  Tuboovarian abscess
  Endometritis
  Pelvic appendicitis
Ectopic pregnancy

MECHANICAL

Incomplete rectal prolapse
Descending perineum syndrome
Torsed ovary
Fissure
Pelvic surgery

NEOPLASTIC

Nonmalignant tumors
  Nerve
  Muscle

  Bone
  Endometriosis
Malignant tumors: primary and recurrent
  Rectum
  Prostate
  Ovary
  Uterus
  Bladder
  Nerve
  Muscle
  Bone
  Metastatic gastric

NEUROLOGIC

Multiple sclerosis
Peripheral neuritic/degenerative disease

ORTHOPEDIC

Coccygeal trauma–coccygodynia
Degenerative disease of the lumbosacral spine
Osteogenic tumors

FUNCTIONAL/IDIOPATHIC CAUSES

Levator spasm/proctalgia fugax
Depression
Chronic idiopathic rectal pain

---

condition. Pain of fissure can be exacerbated by an inflammatory response in internal sphincter spasm and secondary hypertrophy. Anorectal or pelvic surgery is a frequently associated factor in patients with this type of pelvic pain. The pain of pelvic surgery may be due to a perioperative inflammatory process, traumatic neuropathy, or fibrosis of the pelvic floor. After anorectal surgery, levator spasm and sphincter spasm frequently result in anorectal pain complaints. Fortunately, these complaints are often self-limited and resolve spontaneously with time.

Neoplastic

In a report by Oliver et al,[17] 12 of 102 patients with the diagnosis of levator spasm were subsequently found to have organic causes of their rectal pain. Two patients had pelvic recurrence of visceral cancer, and one patient had prostate cancer. This highlights the importance of considering malignant recurrence in patients presenting with complaints of pelvic pain and a known history of previous malignancy.

Nonmalignant tumors rarely cause levator spasm. Symptoms are related to their mass effect on adjacent structures. Neurogenic benign tumors (rhabdomyomas and leiomyomas), cysts, and endometriosis should be sought when preliminary tests are suggestive or when an obvious cause is lacking. Endometriosis produces pain via its ectopic growth pattern and subsequent sclerotic tissue reaction. The cyclic nature of the pain and bleeding should alert the clinician to consider this diagnosis. Although endometriosis is common, it is uncommon as a cause of isolated pelvic pain.

Both primary and recurrent pelvic malignant tumors can cause pain by direct extension and by involvement of the sensory pathways in this region. Most commonly, advanced rectal, prostate, ovarian, uterine, or bladder cancer is the cause of malignant pelvic pain syndromes. Occasionally, pelvic metastases from gastric carcinoma produce this syndrome. Less commonly, malignant bone, muscle, or nerve tumors are the cause. The chronic, progressive, and persistent nature of pain due to malignant disease suggests its consideration in the evaluation of this complaint. A history of pelvic organ malignancy should provoke a thorough search for recurrent disease in any patient who complains of pelvic or perineal pain.

Neurologic

Multiple sclerosis, peripheral neuritis, and degenerative conditions that affect the cauda equina may produce rectal pain. Degenerative disease of the lumbosacral spine not infrequently causes complaints of pain, although pain related to such disorders is more commonly noted in the buttock or thigh region. Radicular symptoms should prompt a search for a reversible neurologic process. Evaluation might necessitate CT, MRI, or EMG testing.

Orthopedic

The classic orthopedic condition associated with rectal pain is coccygodynia. Injury to the coccyx may result in degenerative joint disease, arachnoiditis, and/or secondary spasm of the muscles with insertion or origin on the coccyx. This diagnosis should be made only when direct manipulation of the coccyx results in painful complaints. Radiologic confirmation of coccygeal damage reinforces the diagnosis. Postacchini and Massobrio[18] argue that anatomic variations in coccygeal shape and configuration are responsible for a condition they term *idiopathic coccygodynia*. They advocate surgical coccygectomy, partial or complete, based on the radiologic configuration noted. Overall, the treatment of any form of coccygodynia by coccygectomy is a questionable practice. For all cases of coccygodynia not due to direct trauma, a thorough search for the precipitating cause will provide a rational approach to therapy.

Functional

Functional or idiopathic cases of rectal pain occur with disturbing frequency. A survey of American patients confirmed that between 8% and 19% of the population experiences functional rectal pain.[19] This study also demonstrated a great deal of overlap in patients who experience functional gastrointestinal symptoms. Interestingly, only 22.6% of patients with functional anorectal pain sought medical care. Although the syndrome of paroxysmal rectal pain is quite common, few patients will ever see a physician because of this complaint.

EVALUATION

The evaluation of the patient with pelvic pain begins with a thorough history. This is followed by inspection, palpation, and local endoscopy, which are the first steps in excluding organic causes. On palpation of the levator ani muscle group, palpation of the right levator ani reproduces the patient's discomfort exactly. Diagnostic tests such as transrectal ultrasound, anorectal manometry, cinedefecography, and EMG have all been used in the assessment of the patient with levator spasm and its variants with varying results.[16] The problem seems to be in correlation of the findings with the symptoms.

CT scanning and MRI are useful to rule out mass lesions that may cause rectal pain. Transrectal ultrasonography will further reveal tumors or abscesses of the anorectum. For patients in whom the specific pathology is elusive, however, specific anorectal physiologic testing has been performed to elucidate the cause of pain, but anorectal manometry, for example, has been found to have a low diagnostic yield for patients with levator spasm. There are studies, however, that report abnormalities in anal resting pressures in patients with rectal pain.[16]

Unlike manometry, EMG and nerve conduction study of the patient with rectal pain frequently show abnormalities. These abnormalities include paradoxical puborectalis contraction and prolonged pudendal nerve terminal motor latency on electrophysiologic testing. Unfortunately, these can also be found in patients with no symptoms.[16] Thus, it appears that this occurrence can be a cause of rectal pain in a subgroup of patients.

Cinedefecography can demonstrate dysfunction of pelvic floor musculature, although EMG is more sensitive for the diagnosis of paradoxical puborectalis contraction.[16] Cinedefecography can also show rectocele, increased perineal descent, and early rectovaginal intussusception. Because these radiologic findings can be detected in patients who are completely asymptomatic, some authors have questioned the clinical significance of these findings as far as providing clues for therapeutic intervention.

Despite the diagnostic tools available, the cause of levator spasm remains unknown or at least multifactorial. Most evidence points to actual spasm of the pelvic floor. The precise cause of the spasm is unknown, and most therapies are directed at relieving the spasm.

TREATMENT

When an organic cause of rectal pain is diagnosed, treatment is directed at that cause. For most patients, the cause of their discomfort remains unknown. First, these patients must be reassured that they do not have a malignancy. The next level of therapy is local massage. This entails massaging the levator sling with the examiner's index finger until the muscle feels relaxed. For patients with refractory symptoms, consideration may be given to adding a muscle relaxant or an oral analgesic. This treatment is combined with local heat provided by warm soaks in a tub, heating pads, or heat lamps.

In 1982, Sohn et al[20] introduced electrogalvanic muscle stimulation (EGS) for the treatment of levator spasm. Low-frequency oscillating electrical current applied to a muscle induces fasciculation and fatigue. The success of EGS is quite variable in the literature.[16,21]

Biofeedback may also benefit patients with levator spasm. When conservative management fails to relieve severe pain, biofeedback and EGS, other therapeutic alternatives, are available but are investigational. Pharmacologic agents that relax smooth muscle such as β-adrenergic agonists and calcium channel blockers have been demonstrated to decrease the frequency and intensity of pain in some patients with proctalgia fugax.[16] The results are preliminary, and more research will be required to evaluate the effectiveness of these forms of therapy. Local anesthetic steroid mixtures block the nerves that may have contributed to the spasm of the muscle. Botulinum toxin type A injected into the levator muscle to cause local paralysis has also been used with some success; however, further research is needed before more patients can be offered this form of therapy for the treatment of levator spasm. Finally, short-wave diathermy (available through physicians who are interested in physical medicine and rehabilitation) is an excellent approach for patients with levator spasm.

Importantly, anxiety and depression are common in patients with levator spasm. Regardless of whether this psychiatric state is a coexisting, separate illness or secondary to the chronic painful state engendered by the most extreme forms of levator spasm, expert psychiatric help may be mandatory. The clinician who treats a patient with levator spasm must be alert to the more serious signs of psychiatric illness. With this in mind, it is ill advised to prescribe antianxiety agents or narcotic analgesics for long periods. Although most patients do well with a conservative regimen, the few with serious psychological problems will be helped only with an appropriate referral to receive competent psychiatric care. The management of patients with levator spasm is summarized in Box 157-2.

> **BOX 157-2** Management of Levator Spasm and Its Variants
>
> **EVALUATION OF UNDERLYING CAUSE**
> History and physical examination
> Radiologic investigation where appropriate
>
> **CONSERVATIVE MEASURES**
> Local heat (tub soaks, diathermy)
> Stool softeners
> Short-term muscle relaxants, analgesics, antidepressants
>
> **REFRACTORY CASES**
> Levator massage
> Electrogalvanic stimulation
> Nerve blocks, steroid injection, local anesthetic, botulinum
> toxin type A injection (investigational)

SOLITARY RECTAL ULCER SYNDROME AND COLITIS CYSTICA PROFUNDA

Solitary rectal ulcer syndrome (SRUS) is an uncommon benign condition characterized by rectal bleeding, copious mucous discharge, anorectal pain, tenesmus, and feelings of obstructed defecation or incomplete evacuation which results in intense prolonged straining to defecate. This straining to defecate results in trauma and possibly ischemic ulceration of the anterior rectal wall. Occasionally, the straining results in anterior mucosal prolapse, rectal intussusception, or rectal procidentia. SRUS has its peak incidence in the 20s and 30s, with the female predominance emerging after the age of 30.[22] These symptoms lead to numerous daily trips to the toilet, many of which produce nothing more than frustration. Self-digitation to facilitate evacuation is a not uncommon practice.

SRUS is actually a misnomer because in many patients, no ulceration is present and occasionally multiple ulcerations are evident. When present, the typical solitary rectal ulcer ranges from 1 to 5 cm in size and is located on the anterior rectal wall 5 to 8 cm from the anal verge. These traumatic ulcers can be distinguished from malignant ulceration because they are punched out and shallow with a gray-white base and have a surrounding zone of edema or hyperemia without a thickened margin. A biopsy is performed to rule out rectal cancer because an SRUS can mimic rectal cancer in appearance. Often, there is granularity, friability, and localized proctitis. In general, up to 70% of solitary rectal ulcer lesions are located in the anterior rectum.[23,24] Some patients exhibit circumferential ulceration, particularly those with associated rectal prolapse or internal intussusception. The ulceration can also present as a fungating polypoid mass or nodules or as an area of serpiginous ulceration with intervening pseudopolyps. These lesions are far more difficult to differentiate from carcinoma or inflammatory bowel disease, and a biopsy is almost always necessary.

DIAGNOSIS

The diagnosis is almost invariably established by endoscopy and biopsy. This procedure also excludes benign and malignant neoplasms, localized areas of inflammatory bowel disease, radiation proctitis, and pseudomembranous colitis. Contrast enemas are occasionally useful in confirming other abnormalities, but the actual ulcer is identified in fewer than half.[25] A cinedefecogram is best used to document the presence of associated rectal intussusception and anterior rectal mucosal prolapse. It is occasionally necessary to document complete rectal prolapse in cases where the patient is unable to reproduce the prolapse in the office. The cinedefecogram can suggest the presence of nonrelaxing puborectalis syndrome if the anorectal angle remains acute during straining, but as was stated earlier, this finding can occur in asymptomatic subjects. Defecography can also demonstrate the extent of rectal emptying and perineal descent. The goal of physiologic studies of patients with SRUS has been to explain its cause and prominent symptoms of disordered evacuation. Paradoxical puborectalis and overt or internal rectal intussusception have been described. It should also be noted that internal intussusception is neither a necessary nor a sufficient condition for the development of SRUS, as patients can develop the syndrome without intussusception and not all patients with rectal intussusception develop SRUS. Despite these criticisms, it appears likely that in many cases, a causal relationship does exist between internal rectal intussusception and SRUS. Supporting this notion is the fact that surgical approaches designed to correct rectal intussusception are often beneficial in the treatment of the rectal ulceration.

The histologic features of solitary rectal ulcer and colitis cystica profunda are essentially the same and pathognomonic. Muscle fibers are seen streaming out into the lamina propria below and between glands (Figure 157-7). There is thickening of the muscularis mucosae, with intense fibrosis of the lamina propria. The epithelium is hyperplastic with a preponderance of sialomucins, as opposed to the usual sulfomucins. And most importantly, mucous glands are displaced deep within the submucosa and muscularis mucosae—hence, the name *colitis cystica profunda*. Rutter and Riddell[26] believed that the displaced glands represented the healing phase of a rectal ulcer. These displaced mucinous glands associated with ulceration make it imperative to differentiate this lesion from well-differentiated mucinous adenocarcinoma lest an unnecessary radical operation be performed. Cellular atypia, multilayering of the cystic glandular mucosa, intraglandular budding, and papillation, as well as a desmoplastic host stromal response, are features characteristic of carcinoma.

TREATMENT

Medical management should be attempted in all cases except for those patients with complete full-thickness rectal prolapse. Such treatment consists primarily of avoidance of straining and the use of bulking agents, stimulating suppositories, and enemas or laxatives to retrain the patient to achieve a regular bowel habit. With this approach, as many as 70% of patients were improved and showed healing of the ulcer.[27] Those patients with concomitant nonrelaxing puborectalis syndrome may benefit from biofeedback, as discussed earlier.

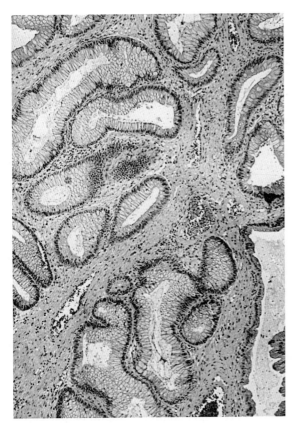

FIGURE 157-7 Colitic cystica profunda (micrograph, hematoxylin–eosin, ×100). (From Timmcke AE: Functional anorectal disorders. In Beck DE, Wexner SD, editors: *Fundamentals of anorectal surgery*, ed 2. London, 1998, Saunders, p 90.)

Local excision of the rectal ulcer is *not recommended* because this procedure does not address the responsible pathophysiology and because the lesions tend to recur. Surgery should be considered only in those patients refractory to persistent attempts at medical management. Surgery that is attempted to correct the results of a behavioral disorder is seldom successful, as evidenced by the large number of surgical procedures that have been used to treat SRUS (e.g., local excision, DeLorme procedure, Gant-Miwa procedure, and excision of anterior rectal mucosal prolapse). A DeLorme procedure can be very difficult to perform secondary to fibrosis. Furthermore, any surgery performed for rectoanal intussusception is fraught with the potential for resolution of the anatomic problem without any symptomatic improvement. Abdominal rectopexy and anterior resection have been successful in the treatment of patients with concomitant complete rectal prolapse, and these procedures have also had some success in treating patients with rectal intussusception and anterior mucosal prolapse.[28,29]

HIDRADENITIS SUPPURATIVA

Hidradenitis suppurativa (HS) is a chronic and often debilitating inflammatory disorder of the skin that involves apocrine gland–bearing tissue, notably in the axilla, groin, perineum, and perianal regions.[41] The disease usually exhibits a chronic course marked by recurrent suppurative events that result in chronic draining wounds. Recurrence after surgical treatment is common and reflects the aggressive nature of the disease.[30]

PATHOPHYSIOLOGY

Fundamentally, HS occurs secondary to a mechanical plugging or obstruction of the apocrine gland unit with keratotic debris, which leads to infection in the gland. Glandular obstruction leads to apocrine sweat retention, followed by suppuration secondary to bacterial proliferation. As the gland ruptures into the surrounding subcutaneous tissues, multiple small epithelial tracks develop. Ultimately, these tracks emerge on the epidermis as tiny pits. Left untreated, apocrine infections and the associated inflammatory responses result in thickening and fibrosis of the involved skin. In support of this proposed pathogenesis, HS has been experimentally induced by the application of occlusive tape to apocrine gland–bearing areas.[31]

HS presents clinically in a distribution strictly related to the distribution of apocrine glands, in the inguinal, axillary, and perianal regions. Because apocrine glands typically become activated with the onset of puberty, HS usually presents after puberty, with the highest incidence in the teens, 20s, and 30s.[32] Although HS most commonly occurs in the axillary region, the second most frequently affected area is the perianal region. Approximately 16% of all patients with HS have perianal involvement.[24] Overall, HS is more common in women and blacks; however, perianal HS has been reported to be twice as common in men than in women.[33]

The exact cause of HS remains unknown.[34] Histologic studies have not convincingly demonstrated significant differences in apocrine gland size or density between normal control subjects and patients with HS.[35] Because anatomic glandular differences do not account for susceptibility to HS, presumably HS occurs in patients with an increased propensity to apocrine duct occlusion. Factors predisposing to duct occlusion that have been implicated in HS include close shaving, poor personal hygiene, tight-fitting clothes, and the use of antiperspirants and depilatories.[36] Many different bacteria identified in association with HS include *Staphylococcus aureus*, *Streptococcus milleri*, and *Chlamydia trachomatis*.[37,38]

CLINICAL PRESENTATION

Patients with perianal HS typically present with complaints of pain and swelling. Early in the course of the disease, they will be found to have localized disease with tender, subcutaneous nodules in the perianal region or buttocks. Patients with a previous history of HS will demonstrate chronic inflammatory changes in the skin with findings of diffuse induration and multiple pits (Figure 157-8). Evidence of the disease should be sought in other body regions, including the axilla, groin, and perineum, to confirm the diagnosis and to ensure complete treatment of all disease.

Although frequently simple, the clinical presentation and management of perianal HS may be complicated by two factors. First, the presenting signs and symptoms are

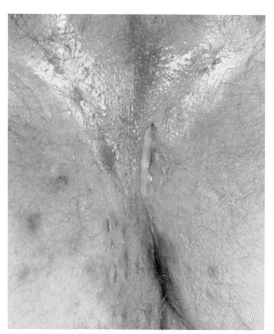

FIGURE 157-8 Hidradenitis suppurativa. (From Timmcke AE: Functional anorectal disorders. In Beck DE, Wexner SD, editors: *Fundamentals of anorectal surgery*, ed 2. London, 1998, Saunders, pp 90.)

often nonspecific. Second, perianal HS may coexist with other diseases, specifically Crohn disease and squamous cell carcinoma.

The clinical presentation of perianal HS can be readily confused with other perianal disorders, including lymphogranuloma venereum (diagnosed by positive titers for *C. trachomatis*), granuloma inguinale (diagnosed by staining of biopsy for Donovan bodies), tuberculosis of perianal skin (diagnosed by demonstration of acid-fast bacillus in biopsy specimens), and actinomycosis (diagnosed by culture of tissues or exudates or by the demonstration of sulfur granules). Finally, the suppurative disease and resulting fistula tracks from HS may be difficult to distinguish from those of complex cryptoglandular disease or isolated perianal Crohn disease.[36,38] In the absence of a clear history or physical evidence in support of cryptoglandular abscesses leading to fistula formation or other gastrointestinal manifestations of Crohn disease, HS can be differentiated from these diseases by examination for the origin of the fistula tracks. Although cryptoglandular fistulas arise at the level of the dentate line, Crohn disease typically originates cephalad and HS originates caudad to the dentate line.[39]

As well as confounding the diagnosis of perianal HS, Crohn disease can coexist with perianal HS. A series of 61 patients with perianal HS revealed that 38% also had Crohn disease.[40] Although this series is composed of selected patients, and probably overestimates the true coexistence of HS and Crohn disease, the two diseases should be considered when perianal HS is coupled with gastrointestinal symptoms or when tracks originate proximal to the dentate line.[39]

Squamous cell carcinoma has also been identified in association with perianal and perineal HS. Of 27 cases reported in the literature since 1958, all have involved perineal, perianal, or buttocks skin.[38,41-43] The incidence of squamous cell carcinoma in patients with perianal HS is not known, but these reported cases underscore the importance of early intervention to prevent chronic wounds and close observation to ensure early detection.

TREATMENT

Perianal HS presents a spectrum of disease, with regard to both severity and chronicity, ranging from single acute episodes of mild disease that require simple surgical drainage to recurrent aggressive disease that requires extensive excision and tissue coverage.

In its simplest form, perianal HS may present as a single painful inflamed nodule with or without a draining sinus track. The treatment of uncomplicated disease should be directed toward symptomatic relief with heat, improved hygiene, and drainage of any collections of purulence. Many systemic remedies have been prescribed, including antibiotics, isotretinoin,[44] and steroids; however, none of these have proved to be beneficial over drainage. Although antibiotics do not play a major role in the management of HS, associated cellulitis may at times indicate the use of antibiotics, with target organisms being those of skin flora, as discussed earlier. Oral erythromycin (500 mg four times daily) is recommended to treat the most commonly encountered organisms. In addition to drainage, emphasis should be placed on the prevention of recurrence. Specifically, patients should be counseled on factors that may predispose to apocrine gland occlusion, such as poor hygiene and the wearing of tight-fitting garments such as synthetic support stockings.

Chronic perianal HS often requires more aggressive treatment. Approaches include unroofing of tracks, incision and drainage, or limited excision and/or wide local excision. Unroofing of all sinus tracks with secondary healing has been reported as a successful treatment option for perianal HS.[39,45] This approach involves the opening and exposure of all involved tracks with preservation of the floor of the track to aid in closure by secondary intent. Because the floor of the track is an epithelialized surface, preservation of this surface allows quick and complete healing through rapid reepithelialization. With this approach, healing rates without recurrence as high as 100% have been reported.[39]

For extensive perianal disease, wide excision appears to be the most frequently used surgical approach.[46] Anderson and Dockerty reported on 117 cases of perianal HS, of which 64 were treated with wide local excision.[32] Two-thirds of the patients were successfully treated with a one-stage excision; the remaining third required multiple staged excisions. Of all patients available for followup, 21% had no further symptoms, 32% had mild symptoms but did not require further surgery, and 45% required further treatment, usually surgery. Another report included 43 patients with perianal HS treated in large part (72%) by wide local excision.[47] This aggressive treatment was considered more effective than unroofing or incision and drainage; however, 9 of 43 (21%) patients had a recurrence at the surgical site, and 12 of 43 (28%) had a flare of disease at another perianal site, for a combined perianal recurrence rate of 49%. These studies have established that even with wide surgical excision, recurrence can be expected.

Because of the pathophysiology of HS, the most appropriate therapy for severe disease should achieve ablation of involved and surrounding apocrine glands, removal of infected tissue, and establishment of a clean wound bed for optimal healing. Because aggressive wide local excision achieves all of these objectives, it should be considered the procedure of choice for severe chronic cases of perianal HS.

Just as the extent of resection remains controversial, so does the best strategy for wound management. For small and moderate wounds, primary closure (sometimes with flaps) can often be performed. For large wounds, options include split-thickness skin grafting and closure by delayed healing or secondary intent. Skin grafting offers the advantages of early wound coverage, rapid healing, and reduction in the pain and inconvenience of chronic open wounds.[38,48] This technique requires that the patient be motivated and able to comply with early postoperative wound care and avoid behavior detrimental to graft healing, including smoking, poor perianal hygiene, and direct pressure or trauma to the new graft. Healing by secondary intent eliminates the early risks of the grafting procedure and has been reported as satisfactory to patients. Wound healing can take 2 to 3 months, and the care of these large wounds is cumbersome.[9] For patients who cannot comply with early postoperative wound care, secondary healing may be the best option. However, because of more rapid wound healing and avoidance of chronic dressing changes, split-thickness skin grating is the preferred method of coverage of these large wounds in most patients.

The possibility of coexisting cancer must be considered, especially in cases where there is a mass lesion or chronic nonhealing component. Biopsies are indicated for all suspicious lesions. In cases complicated by squamous cell carcinoma, excision must provide margins wide enough for oncologic clearance. Because these are principally skin cancers, as such they will rarely if ever require abdominoperineal resection. In cases associated with severe perianal Crohn disease or in association with severe rectal Crohn involvement, wide excision may be combined with proctocolectomy. In general, standard guidelines for treatment of associated disorders should principally be followed, with complementary management of HS as indicated.

In summary, perianal HS is a chronic inflammatory condition of the skin that involves the infection of apocrine glands in the perianal region.[45] The disease causes chronic scarring with persistent sinus tracks. It can be confused with other inflammatory and infectious disorders and in rare cases can occur in association with other benign and malignant conditions such as Crohn disease and squamous cell carcinoma. Treatment should be tailored to the severity and chronicity of the presenting disease. Acute localized infections can be drained, and preventive measures are stressed. For intermediate lesions that are chronic but not severe, unroofing is preferred, yet for severe chronic disease, wide excision with grafting or delayed healing may be required. Despite aggressive surgical therapy, high recurrence rates can be anticipated.

REFERENCES

1. Fleshman JW: Fissure-in-ano and anal stenosis. In Beck DE, Wexner SD, editors: *Fundamentals of anorectal surgery*, ed 2. London, 1998, Saunders, p 209.
2. Brisinda G, Vanella S, Cadeddu F, et al: Surgical treatment of anal stenosis. *World J Gastroenterol* 15:1921, 2009.
3. Linares L, Moreira LF, Andrews H, et al: Natural history and treatment of anorectal strictures complicating Crohn's disease. *Br J Surg* 75:653, 1988.
4. Rosen L: Anoplasty. *Surg Clin North Am* 68:1441, 1988.
5. Kaldarde MV, Ricciardi R: Anal stenosis. *Surg Clin North America* 90:137, 2010.
6. Pearl RK, Hooks VH III, Abcarian H, et al: Island flap anoplasty for the treatment of anal stricture and mucosal ectropion. *Dis Colon Rectum* 33:581, 1990.
7. Christensen MA, Pitsch RM Jr, Cali RL, et al: "House" advancement pedicle flap for anal stenosis. *Dis Colon Rectum* 35:201, 1992.
8. Farid M, Youssef M, El Nakeeb A, et al: Comparative study of the house advancement flap, rhomboid flap, and Y-V anoplasty in treatment of anal stenosis: A prospective randomized study. *Dis Colon Rectum* 53:790, 2010.
9. Beck DE: Miscellaneous disorders of the colon, rectum and anus: Stricture, pruritus ani, proctalgia, colitis cystica profunda, solitary rectal ulcer, hidradenitis. In *Shackleford's surgery of the alimentary tract*, Vol 4, ed 6. Philadelphia, 2007, Saunders, p 2062.
10. Finne CO: Perianal dermatology and pruritis ani. In Wolff BG, Fleshman JW, Beck DE, et al, editors: *ASCRS textbook of colorectal surgery*. New York, 2007, Springer-Verlag, p 240.
11. Markel KW, Billingham RP: Pruritis ani: Etiology and management. *Surg Clin North Am* 90:125, 2010.
12. Siddiqp S, Vijay V, Ward M, et al: Pruritus ani. *Ann R Coll Surg* 90:457, 2008.
13. Wald A: Functional anorectal and pelvic pain. *Gastroenterol Clin North Am* 30:243, 2001.
14. Drossman DA, Li Z, Andruzzi E, et al: U.S. Householder Survey of functional gastrointestinal disorders: Prevalence, sociodemography, and health impact. *Dig Dis Sci* 38:1569, 1993.
15. Ger GC, Wexner SD, Jorge JMN, et al: Evaluation and treatment of chronic intractable rectal pain—a frustrating endeavor. *Dis Colon Rectum* 36:139, 1993.
16. Green S, Oliver GC: Proctalgia fugax, levator syndrome, and pelvic pain. In Beck DE, Wexner SD, editors: *Fundamentals of anorectal surgery*, ed 2. London, 1998, Saunders, p 254.
17. Oliver GC, Rubin RJ, Salvati EP, et al: Electrogalvanic stimulation in the treatment of levator syndrome. *Dis Colon Rectum* 28:662, 1985.
18. Postacchini F, Massobrio M: Idiopathic coccygodynia: Analysis of fifty-one operative cases and a radiographic study of the normal coccyx. *J Bone Joint Surg* 65:1116, 1983.
19. Douthwaite AH: Proctalgia fugax. *Br Med J* 2:164, 1962.
20. Sohn N, Weinstein MA, Robbins RD: The levator syndrome and its treatment with high-voltage electrogalvanic stimulation. *Am J Surg* 144:580, 1982.
21. Hull TL, Milsom JW, Church J, et al: Electrogalvanic stimulation for levator syndrome: How effective is it in the long-term? *Dis Colon Rectum* 36:731, 1993.
22. Timmcke AE: Functional anorectal disorders. In Beck DE, Wexner SD, editors: *Fundamentals of anorectal surgery*, ed 2. London, 1998, Saunders, p 90.
23. Keighley MRB, Shouler P: Clinical and manometric features of the solitary rectal ulcer syndrome. *Dis Colon Rectum* 27:507, 1984.
24. Madigan MR, Morson BC: Solitary ulcer of the rectum. *Gut* 10:871, 1969.
25. Mahieu PH: Barium enema and defaecography in the diagnosis and evaluation of solitary rectal ulcer syndrome. *Int J Colorectal Dis* 1:85, 1986.
26. Rutter KRP, Riddell RH: The solitary ulcer syndrome of the rectum. *Clin Gastroenterol* 4:505, 1975.
27. Brandt-Gradel V, Huibregste K, Tythat GNJ: Treatment of solitary rectal ulcer syndrome with high-fiber diet and abstention from straining at defecation. *Dig Dis Sci* 29:1005, 1984.

28. Marchal F, Bresler L, Brunaud L, et al: Solitary rectal ulcer syndrome: A series of 13 patients operated with a mean follow-up of 4.5 years. *Int J Colorectal Dis* 16:228, 2001.

29. Nicholls RJ, Simson JNL: Anteroposterior rectopexy in the treatment of solitary rectal ulcer syndrome without overt prolapse. *Br J Surg* 73:222, 1986.

30. Waters GS, Nelson H: Perianal hidradenitis suppurativa. In Beck DE, Wexner SD, editors: *Fundamentals of anorectal surgery,* ed 2. London, 1998, Saunders, p 233.

31. Shelley WB, Cahn MM: Pathogenesis of hidradenitis suppurativa in man: Experimental and histiologic observations. *Arch Dermatol* 72:562, 1955.

32. Anderson JJ, Dockerty MB: Perianal hidradenitis suppurativa. *Dis Colon Rectum* 1:23, 1958.

33. Jackman RJ, McQuarrie HB: Hidradenitis suppurativa: Its confusion with pilonidal disease and anal fistula. *Am J Surg* 77:349, 1949.

34. Slade DE, Powel BW, Mortimer PS: Hidradenitis suppurativa: Pathogenesis and management. *Br J Plast Surg* 6:451, 2003.

35. Morgan WP, Hughes LE: The distribution, size and density of the apocrine glands in hidradenitis suppurativa. *Br J Surg* 66:853, 1979.

36. Williams ST, Busby RC, DeMuth RJ, et al: Perineal hidradenitis suppurativa: Presentation of two unusual complications and a review [Review]. *Ann Plast Surg* 26:456, 1991.

37. Bendahan J, Paran H, Kolman S, et al: The possible role of *Chlamydia trachomatis* in perineal suppurative hidradenitis. *Eur J Surg* 158:213, 1992.

38. Highet AS, Warren RE, Weekes AJ: Bacteriology and antibiotic treatment of perineal suppurative hidradenitis. *Arch Dermatol* 124:1047, 1988.

39. Culp CE: Chronic hidradenitis suppurativa of the anal canal: A surgical skin disease. *Dis Colon Rectum* 26:669, 1983.

40. Church JM, Fazio VW, Lavery IC, et al: The differential diagnosis and comorbidity of hidradenitis suppurativa and perianal Crohn's disease. *Int J Colorectal Dis* 8:117, 1993.

41. Roy MK, Appleton MAC, Delicata RJ, et al: Probable association between hidradenitis suppurativa and Crohn's disease: Significance of epithelioid granuloma. *Br J Surg* 84:375, 1997.

42. Perez-Diaz D, Calvo-Serrano M, Martinez-Hijosa E, et al: Squamous cell carcinoma complicating perianal hidradenitis suppurativa. *Int J Colorectal Dis* 10:225, 1995.

43. Shukla VK, Hughes LE: A case of squamous cell carcinoma complicating hidradenitis suppurativa. *Eur J Surg Oncol* 21:106, 1995.

44. Brown CF, Gallup DG, Brown VM: Hidradenitis suppurativa of the anogenital region: Response to isotretinoin. *Am J Obstet Gynecol* 158:12, 1988.

45. Brown SC, Kazzazi N, Lord PH: Surgical treatment of perineal hidradenitis suppurativa with special reference to recognition of the perianal form. *Br J Surg* 73:978, 1986.

46. Bocchini SF, Habr-Gamma A, Kiss DR, et al: Gluteal and perineal hidradenitis suppurativa: Surgical treatment by wide excision. *Dis Colon Rectum* 46:944, 2003.

47. Wiltz O, Schoetz DJ Jr, Murray JJ, et al: Perianal hidradenitis suppurativa: The Lahey Clinic experience. *Dis Colon Rectum* 33:731, 1990.

48. Ramasastry SS, Conklin WT, Granick MS, et al: Surgical management of massive perianal hidradenitis suppurativa. *Ann Plast Surg* 5:218, 1985.

Colonoscopy

Eduardo A. Bonin | Todd H. Baron, Sr.

Colonoscopy, introduced in the 1970s, is one of the most commonly performed endoscopic procedures worldwide and is the preferred colorectal cancer (CRC) screening method in the United States.[1] Improvements in bowel preparations and colonoscopic techniques allow safer, more accurate, and comfortable examinations with higher completion rates and shorter procedure time.[2] Despite the development of newer imaging methods such as CT colonography, colonoscopy has advantages that include direct inspection of detailed mucosal architecture, targeted tissue sampling, and removal of lesions. Therapeutic colonoscopy allows curative and palliative management of benign and malignant colorectal diseases and is the primary method for evaluation and treatment of lower gastrointestinal bleeding.

INDICATIONS AND CONTRAINDICATIONS

Indications for colonoscopy are divided into screening, surveillance, diagnostic, and therapeutic.

The ultimate goal of screening is to reduce both the incidence and mortality of colorectal cancer within large population groups. Great effort has been made toward creating comprehensive screening guidelines that encompass colonoscopy and other less invasive screening modalities.[3] Recently a study encompassing 1,800,000 screening colonoscopies in Germany estimated that more than 15,000 CRC cases were prevented between 2003 and 2010 and they concluded that approximately 5000 CRC cases were prevented in 2010.[4] This study also found that removal of advanced adenomas at screening colonoscopy prevented 11% to 14% of otherwise expected CRC cases in 2010 among individuals aged 55 to 69 years.

Colonoscopy not only provides high-quality examination of the mucosa facilitating diagnosis of subtle lesions, but also establishes a tissue diagnosis, which is the gold standard for diagnosing inflammatory and neoplastic lesions. The highest yield indications for diagnostic colonoscopy are lower gastrointestinal bleeding, clinically significant acute and chronic diarrhea, lesions identified by CT colonography and barium enema, surveillance of patients with inflammatory bowel disease, and followup after polypectomy and cancer resection. Low-yield indications for diagnostic colonoscopy include abdominal pain and chronic constipation.

Contraindications to colonoscopy include poor clinical status and expressed unwillingness or noncompliance for undertaking the examination. Bowel preparation is also a limiting factor for patient cooperation, and the administration of bowel preparation may worsen conditions such as intravascular volume depletion and renal dysfunction. Relative contraindications include patients with acute diverticulitis and those who have just undergone an operation owing to the risk of perforation from manipulation and air insufflation during the exam.

The most common indication for therapeutic colonoscopy is polypectomy, and new colonoscopic techniques provide effective definitive and palliative treatment of early and advanced colorectal cancer. Several thermal and mechanical hemostatic endoscopic devices, historically adapted from upper endoscopy, facilitate ablation and coagulation of a variety of vascular lesions, including acutely bleeding vessels (Table 158-1).

PREPROCEDURAL PREPARATION

Patients undergoing colonoscopy should be informed of the risks, benefits, and alternatives of the procedure. Because of the potential complications of an interventional procedure, the presence of comorbidities and medication use should be carefully assessed. A careful preprocedure evaluation should be undertaken for detecting and correcting any metabolic, coagulation, or cardiopulmonary derangements in order to minimize the risk of complications. The use of electrocautery during therapeutic colonoscopy may interfere with pacemakers.[5,6]

COAGULATION DISORDERS AND USE OF ANTITHROMBOTIC AGENTS

Routine preprocedural laboratory testing for coagulopathy with prothrombin time, partial thromboplastin time, platelet count, and bleeding time, either alone or in combination, is not recommended.[7] Patients with a known history of alterations in coagulation because of the use of medications or underlying hematologic diseases should, however, be evaluated with a coagulation panel. The use of nonsteroidal antiinflammatory drugs (including aspirin) does not appear to increase the risk of clinical bleeding after polypectomy.[8]

However, the management of stronger antiplatelet agents (APAs) such as clopidogrel as well as antithrombotic medications (warfarin) differs.[9] Recommendations for management of antithrombotic agents (ATAs) are based on the type of medication, procedural bleeding risk and urgency, and the patient's risk of thrombotic events when the APA/ATA are withheld.[9] Procedures can be classified as low risk and high risk for bleeding. High-risk conditions for thromboembolic events are mechanical valves in the mitral position, atrial fibrillation associated with underlying valvular heart disease, and the presence of mechanical valves in patients with previous thromboembolic events. Low-risk conditions for thromboembolic events are deep venous thrombosis, paroxysmal or chronic atrial fibrillation without valvular heart disease, mechanical valve in the aortic position, and bioprosthetic valves. The management of patients

TABLE 158-1 Indications for Therapeutic Colonoscopy

Indication	Therapeutic Intervention
Malignant and benign colon obstruction (colorectal cancer/anastomotic stricture) Colonic pseudoobstruction	Endoscopic insertion of colonic stents and colonic decompression tubes/balloon dilation/argon plasma ablation/Nd:Yag laser ablation
Small/large, flat/elevated colonic adenomas	Endoscopic mucosal resection (submucosal dissection, piecemeal resection)/"hot biopsy" forceps polypectomy/snare polypectomy/endoscopic marking (tattooing)
Vascular lesions (ectasias/malformations, hemorrhoids)	Endoscopic injection (epinephrine)/bipolar or multipolar coagulation/argon plasma coagulation/Nd:Yag laser coagulation/endoscopic band ligation (rectal varices)*
Radiation proctopathy	Endoscopic injection/argon plasma coagulation/mono, multi- or bipolar coagulation/cryotherapy/Nd:Yag laser coagulation
Foreign body (toothpick, dental prosthesis)	Endoscopic foreign body retrieval using endoscopic graspers, polyp retrieval net
Gallstone ileus	Polyp retrieval net, electrohydraulic lithotripsy†
Acute colorectal bleeding (diverticular)	Endoscopic treatment of visible bleeding vessels using endoscopic injection (epinephrine)/bipolar or multipolar/argon plasma coagulation/endoscopic clip application

*Coelho-Prabhu N, Baron TH, Kamath PS: Endoscopic band ligation of rectal varices: A case series. *Endoscopy* 42:173, 2010.
†Zielinski MD, Ferreira LE, Baron TH: Successful endoscopic treatment of colonic gallstone ileus using electrohydraulic lithotripsy. *World J Gastroenterol* 16:1533, 2010.

with endovascular grafts should be individualized. Detailed recommendations on the use of APAs and ATAs in the periendoscopic period are available.[9]

ANTIBIOTIC PROPHYLAXIS

Recommendations for antibiotic prophylaxis are based on high-risk procedures for bacteremia in patients at risk for developing endocarditis. Colonoscopic procedures that are associated with high risk of bacteremia are endoscopic dilation and laser or argon plasma coagulation. Immunocompromised and neutropenic patients may benefit from antibiotic prophylaxis.[10] However, recent guidelines do not recommend routine antibiotic prophylaxis for patients undergoing endoscopic diagnostic or therapeutic gastrointestinal procedures for the prevention of infective endocarditis.[11] Patients undergoing continuous ambulatory peritoneal dialysis appear to benefit from antibiotic prophylaxis before colonoscopy.[12] Routine antibiotic prophylaxis is not recommended for diagnostic colonoscopy with or without polypectomy or in patients with pacemakers, implantable defibrillators, hip prosthesis, or a history of coronary revascularization.[11]

BOX 158-1 Predictors of Poor Bowel Preparation

Later colonoscopy starting time
Longer interval between completion of preparation and start of procedure*
Reported failure to follow preparation instructions
Inpatient status
Procedural indication of constipation
Use of tricyclic antidepressants
Male gender
Obesity†
History of cirrhosis, stroke, or dementia
? Diabetes

From Ness RM, Manam R, Hoen H, et al: Predictors of inadequate bowel preparation for colonoscopy. *Am J Gastroenterol* 96:1797, 2001.
*Siddiqui AA, Yang K, Spechler SJ, et al: Duration of the interval between the completion of bowel preparation and the start of colonoscopy predicts bowel-preparation quality. *Gastrointest Endosc* 69:700, 2009.
†Borg BB, Gupta NK, Zuckerman GR, et al: Impact of obesity on bowel preparation for colonoscopy. *Clin Gastroenterol Hepatol* 7:670, 2009.

BOX 158-2 Commonly Prescribed Products for Bowel Preparation for Colonoscopy

Whole gut lavage solutions (electrolyte lavage solution)
Polyethylene glycol (PEG)
Sulfate-free PEG (SF-PEG)
Low-volume PEG/PEG-3350 and bisacodyl delayed-release tablets
Aqueous sodium phosphate (NaP)*
Tablet sodium phosphate (NaP)*
Adjuncts to colonic cleansing before colonoscopy
Flavoring (cherry, citrus-berry, lemon-lime, orange, and pineapple)
Carbohydrate-electrolyte solutions
Enemas (tap water/sodium sulfate/bisacodyl/mineral oil)
Metoclopramide
Simethicone
Bisacodyl
Saline laxatives (sodium picosulfate/magnesium citrate)
Senna products

*Sodium phosphate was withdrawn from the market in Canada. In the United States, the only available formulation for NaP is tablets and they must be sold under prescription.

BOWEL PREPARATION

The adequacy of bowel preparation directly affects the quality of the colonoscopic examination because adequate visualization is required for safe navigation and for detecting polyps and mucosal abnormalities. Poor preparation occurs in up to 21% of patients,[13] increasing cost of care, rate of missed lesions, and complications such as bowel perforation (Box 158-1).

Purgatives are almost always required for adequate bowel preparation in adults,[14] either used by oral (antegrade) or anal route (retrograde). Orthograde peroral (also referred to as whole gut lavage) administration of bowel preparation is the preferred route in the absence of suspected intestinal obstruction. A wide variety of bowel preparation products and regimens are available for colonoscopy (Box 158-2). Because of the risk of renal injury, the use of sodium phosphate products has been restricted by the U.S. Food and Drug Administration (FDA). Sodium phosphate–based formulations should not be prescribed for children, elderly patients, patients with renal insufficiency, and those with hypertension who are receiving angiotensin-converting enzyme inhibitors or angiotensin-II receptor blockers.[15] Split dosage regimens consist of a PM/AM dosing regimen given at an interval of 6 to 8 hours and it seems to be preferred to single-dose regimens for optimal bowel cleansing.[16] Reduced-volume gut lavage regimens reduce the usual full 4-L dosing regimen to 2 L in order to improve tolerance and increase compliance. Afternoon procedures may require a different approach to improve preparation.[17] Oral bowel preparation can be administered in lower volumes to patients with diarrhea and are preferred in the presence of acute lower gastrointestinal bleeding. A suggested regimen for preparation in the setting of massive acute lower gastrointestinal bleeding is the administration of 1 L of polyethylene glycol (PEG) solution each 30 to 45 minutes per oral or nasogastric tube until a clear effluent is seen.[18]

Bowel preparations administered by the anal route using per rectal irrigations are reserved for patients who present with fecal impaction, those with excluded colonic segments, and for patients with known or suspected colonic obstruction. These regimens can also be combined with peroral magnesium citrate given the evening before the procedure as an alternative for individuals who cannot tolerate peroral administration of full-dose gut lavage.[19] Instillation of bisacodyl enemas may also be carried out through the colonoscope channel to allow bowel preparation when inadequate bowel preparation is encountered during the colonoscopy.[20] Electrocautery (including argon plasma coagulation) should be avoided in the setting of a poor preparation because of the potential for colonic explosion.[21]

METHODS FOR REDUCING DISCOMFORT DURING COLONOSCOPY

SEDATION

Sedation is used to increase patient cooperation during the examination and for reducing pain and discomfort. Moderate sedation (as defined by the American Society of Anesthesiologists [ASA]) is the most commonly reached sedation stage during colonoscopy because it facilitates patient cooperation while maintaining verbal and contact stimulation and maintaining airway protection, spontaneous ventilation, and adequate cardiovascular function. Current sedation techniques are associated with a high level of patient satisfaction and low risk of serious adverse effects.[22]

Moderate sedation using a benzodiazepine/opioid combination is administered for nearly three quarters of all colonoscopies performed in the United States.[23] Although generally safe, administration of these agents may produce deep sedation with resultant adverse events. Midazolam combined with either meperidine or fentanyl is the most common benzodiazepine/opioid sedation regimen.

Propofol (2,6-diisopropyl phenol) is the most common single agent used to achieve moderate/deep sedation because of its safety, efficacy, and faster recovery profiles.[24] Propofol may also be combined with low doses of opiates or benzodiazepines for a synergic effect, resulting in shorter procedure times (without changes in cognitive behavior after discharge) as compared to propofol alone.[25] Propofol-based sedation regimens have a narrow therapeutic effect with wide fluctuations in sedation stages during colonoscopy. To overcome these issues, patient-controlled sedation (PCS) has been used. Despite encouraging results,[26] further studies are needed to address PCS efficacy, safety, and economic viability. There is considerable debate between anesthesiologists and gastroenterologists about administering propofol during colonoscopy.[27]

Whereas the majority of patients undergoing colonoscopy have a preference for sedation, there are patients who are willing to have their examination performed without sedation. In one study, 27% of patients opted to begin the procedure without sedation and 80% were able to complete the exam without the need for sedation.[28] Advantages of unsedated colonoscopy include avoidance of sedation risk, reduced costs, and prompt return to daily activities. Based on these advantages, novel strategies to reduce colonic manipulation and distention have been proposed to lessen patient discomfort and need for sedation.

NOVEL STRATEGIES TO REDUCE COLONIC MANIPULATION AND DISTENTION

Newer colonoscopes with variable stiffness and smaller diameter have been used in an attempt to reduce bowel looping and stretching.[29] Other technologies such as magnetic endoscope imaging have not been shown to improve patient tolerance or reduce the need for sedation but seem to reduce sedation dosage.[30] In a recent randomized trial, the use of water instillation instead of air insufflation has been shown to significantly decrease maximum discomfort.[31] Colonoscopy using insufflation with carbon dioxide (CO_2) appears to be safe in patients without severe underlying pulmonary disease and has also been shown to reduce postprocedural pain and discomfort because of less bowel distention and gas accumulation compared with room air insufflation,[32] as well as to reduce pain and shorten procedural time.[33]

ADVANCED COLONOSCOPIC IMAGING MODALITIES

Since the introduction of the video colonoscope more than two decades ago, recent advances in colonoscopy imaging technology and mechanical design are changing the practice of colonoscopy toward a highly specialized examination capable of detecting microscopic mucosal changes in the colon. As current standard colonoscopes are incorporating higher imaging definition capabilities, up to 50% of patients undergoing high-resolution colonoscopy are being diagnosed with small polyps, which causes a significant increase in time and cost for obtaining mucosal biopsy sampling. Hence, optically enhanced

TABLE 158-2 Technologies to Enhance Neoplasia Detection

	Effective	Practical
For Detection of Flat Lesions		
Conventional chromoendoscopy	Yes	No
Narrow-banded imaging	Yes*	Yes[†]
High definition	Unknown	Yes
Autofluorescence	Yes	Unknown[¶]
For Exposure of Hidden Mucosa		
Cap-fitted endoscope	Yes	Yes
Third Eye Retroscope	Unknown	Unknown
Wide-angle optics	No	Yes

Adapted from Huh KC, Rex DK: Missed neoplasms and optimal colonoscopic withdrawal technique. In Waye JD, Rex DK, Williams CB, editors: *Colonoscopy principles and practice*, ed 2. Hoboken, NJ, 2009, Blackwell Publishing, p 560.

*Appears effective as a learning tool but not effective for high-level white-light adenoma detectors.

[†]More difficult than white light in large luminal diameter sections and when preparation is poor.

[¶]Limited number of studies; not currently adaptable to color chip charge-coupled device systems.

colonoscopic techniques are gaining importance as a potential tool to reliably diagnose small colorectal lesions while reducing the need for unnecessary biopsies and formal histologic assessment. The impact of such techniques on clinical practice is still under evaluation and dependent on economic and validation studies regarding its reproducibility, specificity, and sensitivity (Table 158-2).

OPTICAL TECHNIQUES FOR FACILITATING NEOPLASIA DETECTION

Chromoendoscopy and High-Definition Endoscopy

Chromoendoscopy was introduced to facilitate detection and characterization of gastrointestinal lesions. Chromoendoscopy is performed using contrast agents applied directly onto the mucosa or by using a special imaging modality. Although cumulative studies have shown that chromoscopy enhances detection of neoplastic colorectal lesions using conventional video colonoscopies,[34] the development of high-definition imaging technology (magnifying colonoscopy) provides a more detailed morphologic assessment. The adoption of both chromoscopy and high-definition imaging together allows classification of colorectal neoplastic lesions according to morphologic patterns of the glandular openings (pit patterns) that correspond to the transition from nonneoplastic to malignant neoplasia. Estimates and understanding of the relationship between serrated and nonpolypoid colorectal lesions with colorectal cancer have ensued. Novel imaging techniques such as virtual (or electronic) chromoscopy use optical contrast imaging for mucosal inspection and polyp detection and as a substitute for dye-based chromoscopy.[35] Virtual chromoscopy is an imaging modality designed for enhancing the mucosal surface or superficial capillaries network by applying different spectrals of light; however, it is not yet sufficiently standardized or validated for routine practice.[35] Autofluorescence

(light-induced fluorescence endoscopy [LIFE]) is another imaging technique that uses ultraviolet and short-wavelength light into tissue molecules resulting in the emission of fluorescence light and was developed for detecting mucosal tissue derangements associated with neoplastic changes. This technology thus far has been useful for detecting dysplastic lesions in long-standing chronic inflammatory bowel disease[36]; however, there are limitations for discriminating small colorectal lesions.[37,38] Another interesting imaging technique under evaluation is probe-based confocal laser endomicroscopy (pCLE), which allows in vivo imaging of tissue at micrometer resolution and is designed to be a substitute for histologic analysis. In a recent study, pCLE was compared to virtual chromoscopy for classification of colon polyps and pCLE was found to have a higher sensitivity with similar specificity[39]; however, larger series are needed to confirm these results.

With enhanced capability of morphologic assessment, these novel techniques might be capable of replacing histopathology for nondepressed, diminutive lesions but are not precise enough to detect adenomatous changes and neoplasia, which would obviate the need for biopsies and formal pathologic assessment.[40] Virtual chromoscopy and high-definition colonoscopy should be introduced into practice using standardized training programs in order to reduce intra- and interobserver variabilities so as to achieve adequate imaging interpretation.[41]

Auxiliary Devices for Decreasing the Rate of Missed Adenomas

The adenoma miss rate using standard colonoscopy is 22% for polyps of any size and is higher with smaller lesions. Studies analyzing polyp miss rates by tandem colonoscopy show that the miss rates of polyps measuring greater than or equal to 10 mm, 5 to 10 mm, and less than 5 mm are 2.1%, 13%, and 26%.[42] The most common causes of missed adenomas are more rapid colonoscope withdrawal times and adenomas located behind folds. To achieve better adenoma detection rates, there has been an effort from the industry and physicians to develop new techniques and modalities.

The Third Eye Retroscope (Avantis Medical Systems, Sunnyvale, Calif) is a disposable optic probe that is inserted into the working channel of a standard colonoscope allowing retroflex views that complement the forward view of the colonoscope during endoscope withdrawal.[43] The use of a cap-fitted colonoscope is another technique that has been proposed for increasing the detection of adenomas.[44] Wide-angle colonoscopes (using 170-degree optical lenses) have been compared to standard colonoscopes, and results were favorable regarding colonoscope withdrawal time[45] but conflicting in respect to improvement of adenoma detection rate.[45-47]

NEW TECHNOLOGIES FOR ASSESSING THE COLON

Novel technologies for assessing the colon include colon capsule endoscopy (CC) and endoscopes with unique propelling systems such as the Aer-O-scope (GI view, Ramat Gan, Israel) and the Invendoscope (Invendo Medical, Kissing, Germany). The Neoguide navigator endoscopy system (Neoguide Systems, San Jose, Calif) is a computerized device comprising an articulated endoscope with an external position sensor. The endoscope insertion is carried out by regulating the shape of its segments to assume the shape of the colon based on the three-dimensional navigation map.[48]

The PillCam Colon capsule (Given Imaging, Yokneam, Israel) was approved for research in 2006 with great appeal as a less invasive endoscopic procedure compared with conventional colonoscopy. A few studies have addressed its efficacy as compared to conventional colonoscopy.[49,50] However, improvements in colon capsule technology and examination technique are needed to increase sensitivity. Cost-effective analyses are also needed for CC use as a screening method in larger population groups. Other new devices and techniques for assessing the colon are being developed to improve cecal intubation rates. These include guidewire-assisted endoscopy using a small-diameter endoscope that fits into the colonoscope working channel[51] and dedicated overtubes such as the EndoEase (Sync Medical, Stoughton, Mass), USGI ShapeLock system (USGI, San Clemente, Calif), and Megachannel (Minos Medical, Irvine, Calif) that prevent loop formation in the left colon and facilitate procedure instrumentation.

THE DIFFICULT COLONOSCOPY

Approximately 6% of patients undergoing colonoscopy have their examination prematurely terminated because of technical difficulties unrelated to disease or bowel preparation.[52] Factors associated with a difficult colonoscopy include older patients, patients with low body mass index (<25), previous hysterectomy, diverticular disease, female gender, and history of constipation.[53] Management options for difficult colonoscopies include the use of pediatric colonoscopes and balloon enteroscopes to reach the cecum.[54,55] Barium enema or CT colonography are also options for difficult colonoscopies when the cecum is not reached.[56]

THERAPEUTIC COLONOSCOPY

ENDOSCOPIC RESECTION OF COLORECTAL ADENOMAS: ENDOSCOPIC POLYPECTOMY AND ENDOSCOPIC MUCOSAL RESECTION

Since the first colonoscopic polypectomy in 1969, endoscopic resection of colonic adenomas has evolved into complex procedures with the capability of removing large colorectal lesions that once would have been managed surgically. Currently, more than 80% of colon polyps (up to 1 cm in size) can be safely and successfully resected endoscopically. The ideal endoscopic resection technique must be the safest method to perform an en bloc (including both depth and lateral extensions) excision while preserving the removed tissue for pathologic analysis. Other technical principles should

include adequate hemostasis and protection of adjacent normal tissue. With the development of novel techniques and endoscopic instruments such as dedicated electrosurgical knives, it has been possible to perform complex resection techniques such as endoscopic submucosal dissection. Flat polyps are removed most commonly using endoscopic mucosal resection (EMR) techniques (Figure 158-1). Injection of various agents into the submucosal layer separates the mucosal layer from the muscular layer. Failure of the lesion to "lift" with injection (nonlifting sign) (Figure 158-2) suggests invasion of the submucosa in the setting of a polyp not previously biopsied or treated; however, it does not reliably predict deeper cancerous invasion.[56] Such lesions should not be resected using conventional EMR. Saline injection with or without epinephrine is commonly used, and hyaluronic acid and hydroxypropyl methylcellulose[57] have been advocated for resection of larger lesions because of its longer duration without diffusing. Endoscopic tattooing is another technique introduced for endoscopic marking of adenomas to facilitate surveillance of previously resected adenoma or for guiding surgical resection. It is performed by injecting sterile ink submucosally. Long-lasting inks are India ink, indocyanine green, and carbon-based ink (Spot, GI Supply, Camp Hill, Penna), the latter the only FDA-approved product for endoscopic tattooing.[58] One important technical aspect is to inject the ink at two to four sites on opposite walls to increase the likelihood of locating the lesion during surgery.[59]

Endoscopic polypectomy is a safe procedure. However, complications may occur as described later in this chapter. The polypectomy snare technique is used to encircle the base of pedunculated polyps to allow a clear margin of nonneoplastic tissue. Advances in polypectomy techniques have been toward safer use of electrocautery while avoiding bleeding and perforation. Cold snare technique refers to snare polypectomy without electrocautery, with the snare acting as a guillotine (Figure 158-3). This technique has been safely used for removal of sessile polyps less than 0.8 mm and is a substitute for hot biopsy forceps removal. Endoscopic snare technique has also been used as a standard procedure for endoscopic mucosal resection (EMR) of larger polypoid and flat lesions in virtually all colonic areas by using the piecemeal technique.[60]

Endoscopic submucosal dissection (ESD) is a recent adjuvant procedure for increasing the rate of complete and en bloc adenoma resection. It is especially useful for the resection of large, flat colorectal lesions. Of all emerging resection techniques, ESD is one that allows en bloc resection of large, flat adenomas and early colorectal cancers (Figure 158-4). ESD has been successfully used in Asian countries for more than 10 years to remove early upper gastrointestinal cancers and superficial colonic neoplastic lesions. However, it is technically more difficult and complex to perform with longer procedure times and higher complication rates (specifically, perforation) compared to standard EMR. In a recent case-control study using prospectively collected data of patients with superficial colorectal cancers, the outcomes of ESD and EMR were compared. Perforation occurred in 9 of 145 (6.2%) patients treated with ESD as compared

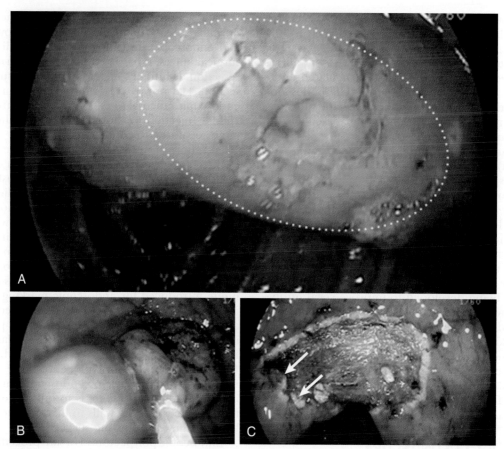

FIGURE 158-1 Endoscopic mucosal resection. **A,** Flat lesion after submucosal injection of saline. **B,** Snare encircling the lesion. **C,** Postpolypectomy site after piece-meal snare resection. Complementary snare resection of any remaining adenoma tissue *(white arrows)* is further undertaken to ensure macroscopic clearance.

to 3 of 228 (1.3%) patients treated with EMR. Delayed bleeding occurred in 1.4% and 3.1% (*P* = nonsignificant), respectively. All complications were successfully managed endoscopically.[61] In a recent metaanalysis evaluating resection of large flat colonic polyps by ESD,[62] en bloc resection was achieved in 85% of lesions, and clear vertical and lateral margins were achieved in 75%, as opposed to 7% and 34% en bloc success rates for conventional snare polypectomy. However, the complexity and time required to complete the resection and higher complication rates remain barriers to its adoption in Western countries. In Japan, current indications for ESD in superficial colorectal tumors are as follows: (1) lesions difficult to remove en bloc with a snare (e.g., nongranular laterally spreading tumors, type VI lesions (pit pattern), and large protruded-type lesions suspected to be carcinoma; (2) lesions with fibrosis; (3) sporadic localized lesions arising in the setting of chronic ulcerative colitis; and (4) local residual carcinoma after endoscopic mucosal resection.[63]

Other more aggressive techniques designed to remove deeper layers of the GI tract, such as endoluminal full-thickness resections, have been shown to be technically feasible in experimental studies.[64] This technique would be an option to avoid segmental colonic resection and anastomosis. However, it will probably only be suitable for treating early colonic cancer when there are efficient

minimally invasive techniques for staging and treating regional lymph node metastasis.

Indications for Resection of Adenomas

Indications for endoscopic adenoma resection are mostly based on colonoscopic morphologic evaluation.[65] Classification systems for endoscopic macroscopic evaluation of colorectal adenomas include the Paris classification, which is based on the superficial gross macroscopic appearance (Figure 158-5) and the pit pattern classification, which is based on a superficial microscopic groove pattern. Apart from diminutive polyps with hyperplastic appearance found in the left colon and rectum, every effort should be made to remove adenomatous or serrated lesions found at colonoscopy, especially those larger than 10 mm in diameter. From a technical standpoint, tumors larger than 20 mm in diameter (also called laterally spreading tumors [LSTs]) (Figure 158-6) that do not have gross endoscopic signs of submucosal invasion are amenable for endoscopic resection regardless of size.[66] LSTs are classified into two types according to their morphology: granular type (LST-G) and nongranular type (LST-NG) (see Figure 158-6). Most of these large adenomatous lesions can be cured by endoscopic piece-meal snare resection. However, LST-Gs with large whole nodular-type or type V pit pattern and LST-NGs with pseudodepression usually cannot be resected en bloc with

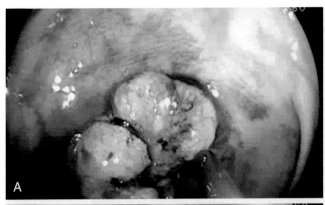

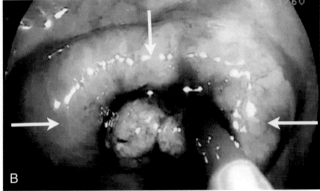

FIGURE 158-2 Nonlifting sign. **A,** Elevated lesion at sigmoid. **B,** Nonlifting sign after saline submucosal injection. *Arrows* show submucosal elevations surrounding the lesion. Surgical specimen confirmed submucosal invasion.

a snare and thus are better suited for ESD. The therapeutic strategy for choosing between endoscopic snare piecemeal resection and ESD for large LST lesions should be based on the macroscopic findings of their subtype and pit pattern finding.[61] Modern imaging and diagnostic modalities for evaluating the presence of metastatic lymph nodes in superficial adenomas, such as endoscopic ultrasound, do not seem to be advantageous relative to magnifying colonoscopy with chromoscopy, as observed in a Japanese study using prospectively collected data from 102 patients with superficial adenomas.[67]

The pedunculated polyp is separated from the submucosal layer by a tubular stalk, whereas the sessile polyp is directly contiguous to the submucosa (Figure 158-7). Pedunculated polyps with cancer limited to the submucosa and without evidence of unfavorable histologic factors such as poorly differentiated histology, vascular or lymphatic invasion, cancer at the resection margin, and incomplete resection are adequately treated with endoscopic resection.[68] Pedunculated polyps have a 0.3% risk of cancer recurrence or lymph node metastasis after complete endoscopic removal, whereas similar sessile polyps have a 4.8% risk.[69]

The single most important prognostic factor for adenomas with malignancy is the depth of submucosal invasion, which is assessed by histopathologic analysis. Invasion to deeper submucosal layers is associated with a 6% to 14% risk of lymph node metastasis (Table 158-3). The only precise method is a quantitative measure in micrometers (μm) of the depth of invasion, measured from the lower

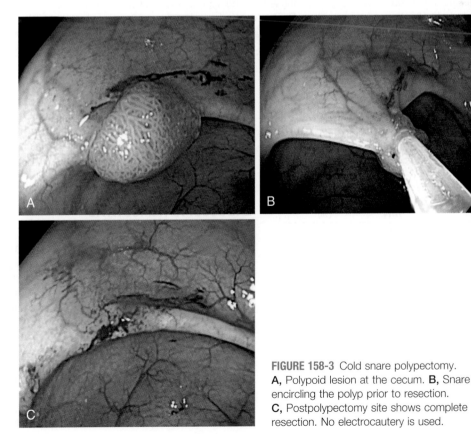

FIGURE 158-3 Cold snare polypectomy. **A,** Polypoid lesion at the cecum. **B,** Snare encircling the polyp prior to resection. **C,** Postpolypectomy site shows complete resection. No electrocautery is used.

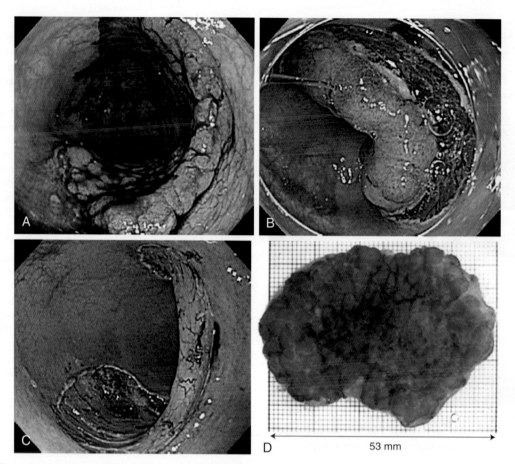

FIGURE 158-4 Example of colorectal ESD. **A,** The margins of the lesion were delineated by using chromoscopy with 0.4% indigo carmine dye spraying. **B,** After injection of glycerol, a circumferential incision in the mucosa was made by using a B-knife. Sodium hyaluronate acid solution was then injected at the submucosal layer to lift the lesion. The submucosal dissection was undertaken using an insulated tip (IT) knife. **C,** The operated site after the en bloc resection. **D,** The resected specimen was 53 mm in diameter. Histopathologic analysis revealed high-grade dysplasia, and the margins of the specimen were free of tumor. (Adapted from Saito Y, Uraoka T, Matsuda T, et al: Endoscopic treatment of large superficial colorectal tumors: A case series of 200 endoscopic submucosal dissections [with video]. *Gastrointest Endosc* 66:966, 2007.)

TABLE 158-3 Proportion of Nodal Metastases in Relation to the Depth of Invasion Into the Submucosa (sm) Presented in Three Groups*

		Presence of Lymph Node Metastasis	
		n/N	(%)
Depth of invasion	sm1	1/147	<1
	sm2	7/105	6
	sm3	10/71	14

Adapted from The Paris endoscopic classification of superficial neoplastic lesions: Esophagus, stomach, and colon: November 30 to December 1, 2002. *Gastrointest Endosc* 58:S3, 2003.
*Endoscopic series with pathology confirmation in Red Cross Hospital in Akita, Japan (323 in lesions type 0).

layer of the muscularis mucosae.[69] The risk of nodal metastasis is assumed to be low when the depth of invasion is less than a determined cutoff. Cutoff values for colorectal lesions are 1000 μm between sm1 and sm2 mucosal invasion, which means that when the lesion invades beyond 1000 μm, surgical resection should be considered (Figures 158-8 and 158-9). Other risk factors for invasive cancer in colorectal adenomas are lesions larger than 3 cm; depressed type, Paris classification; and type V, pit pattern classification. Patient age and the number and size of prior adenomas have also been described as prognostic factors.[70]

ENDOSCOPIC HEMOSTATIC AND ABLATION TECHNIQUES

Hemostatic and ablative devices used during colonoscopy include contact thermal devices (heater probe and multipolar electrocautery probes), noncontact thermal devices (argon plasma coagulator and laser), injection needles, and mechanical devices (band ligators, Endoclips, and detachable ligating loops) (Figure 158-10; see also Figure 158-7).[71] Hemostatic monopolar or bipolar forceps are novel alternatives for the treatment of gastrointestinal bleeding.[72,73] Hemostatic principles for the control of lower gastrointestinal bleeding (LGIB) are the same as used for upper gastrointestinal bleeding, though with a tendency to use less coagulation energy in order to avoid bowel perforation. In general, epinephrine

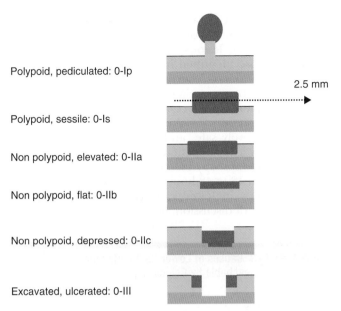

Polypoid, pediculated: 0-Ip

Polypoid, sessile: 0-Is   2.5 mm

Non polypoid, elevated: 0-IIa

Non polypoid, flat: 0-IIb

Non polypoid, depressed: 0-IIc

Excavated, ulcerated: 0-III

FIGURE 158-5 The Paris classification of superficial neoplastic lesions: polypoid type 0-I lesions are pedunculated or sessile. The elevation of sessile lesions above the surface of the mucosa is more than 2.5 mm. Nonpolypoid type 0-II lesions are slightly elevated, flat, or slightly depressed. The elevation of elevated lesions is less than 2.5 mm. Excavated or ulcerated type 0-III superficial neoplastic lesions do not occur in the colon. (Adapted from Lambert R, Kudo SE, Vieth M, et al: Pragmatic classification of superficial neoplastic colorectal lesions. *Gastrointest Endosc* 70:1182, 2009.)

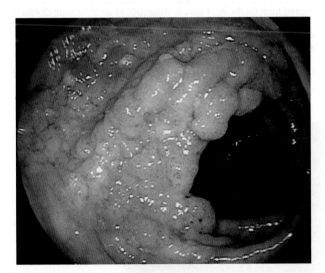

FIGURE 158-6 Lateral spreading tumor (LST) in the transverse colon, granular type.

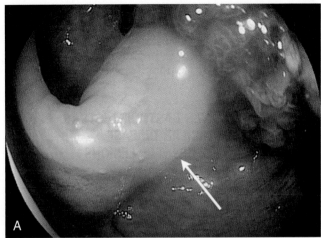

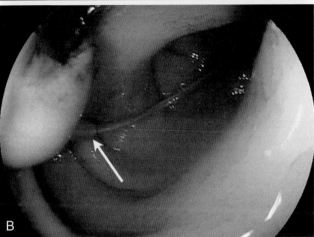

FIGURE 158-7 Endoscopic polypectomy using endoscopic detachable snare for preventing postpolypectomy bleeding. **A,** Pedunculated polypoid lesion with a large-bore stalk *(arrow)* at the sigmoid. **B,** Polypectomy site after resection. *Arrow* shows endoscopic detachable snare attached at the base of the lesion. Endoscopic resection was curative in this case.

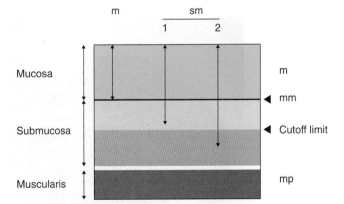

FIGURE 158-8 Depth of invasion into the submucosa in the columnar epithelium (colon and rectum) assessed in the specimen obtained after surgery. Depth of submucosal invasion is divided into two groups: superficial *(sm1)* and deep *(sm2)* with respect to a cutoff limit determined on a micrometric scale (1000 μm in the colon). (Adapted from The Paris endoscopic classification of superficial neoplastic lesions: Esophagus, stomach, and colon: November 30 to December 1, 2002. *Gastrointest Endosc* 58:S3, 2003.)

injection alone or in combination with thermal coagulation is commonly used for hemostasis of active bleeding, especially from postpolypectomy and diverticular hemorrhage (Figure 158-11). Preferred methods of thermal coagulation are bipolar or multipolar (heater probe) because of their limited depth of coagulation and are used to treat visible vessels or after cessation of active bleeding from vascular lesions, postpolypectomy sites, or colonic diverticula. Argon plasma coagulation can be used for treating superficial vascular lesions, such as vascular ectasias and chronic radiation proctopathy, the latter with sustained responses in 83% to 100% of patients.[74]

APPROACH TO LOWER GASTROINTESTINAL BLEEDING, DIVERTICULAR DISEASE, AND VASCULAR COLORECTAL LESIONS

Colonoscopy is valuable for treatment of acute LGIB for a variety of lesions (Box 158-3). Indeed, colonoscopy is now the most common intervention performed for

management of LGIB because of its diagnostic and therapeutic capabilities. Colonoscopic hemostasis techniques are used to treat lesions with stigmata of hemorrhage similar to those identified in the upper gastrointestinal tract as predictors of recurrent bleeding.[75]

Severe LGIB is associated with high morbidity and mortality in patients with comorbidities and in the setting of emergent surgery.[76] Colonoscopy has the advantages of being relatively safe, and can be performed at the bedside in critically ill patients.[77]

Urgent colonoscopy has been defined as being performed within 12 to 48 hours of admission.[76] The timing of colonoscopy in lower gastrointestinal bleeding has been a matter of discussion, because urgent colonoscopy

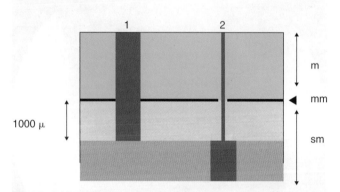

FIGURE 158-9 Depth of invasion of the submucosa in the columnar epithelium, assessed for the clinical relevance of endoscopic resection and for the risk of nodal metastases.* Group 1 *(m and sm1)*: endoscopic mucosal resection is possible. Group 2 *(sm2)*: surgical treatment is preferred. *The cutoff limit between sm1 and sm2 is 1000 μm. (Adapted from The Paris endoscopic classification of superficial neoplastic lesions: esophagus, stomach, and colon: November 30 to December 1, 2002. *Gastrointest Endosc* 58:S3, 2003.)

BOX 158-3 Causes of Lower Gastrointestinal Hemorrhage Reachable by Colonoscopy*

Diverticulosis[†]
Ischemic colitis
Vascular ectasia[†]
Hemorrhoids[†]
Neoplasia
Postpolypectomy[†]
Inflammatory bowel disease
Infectious colitis
Nonsteroidal antiinflammatory drug–induced colopathy
Radiation colopathy[†]
Aortoenteric fistula (sigmoid colon)
Dieulafoy's lesions[†]
Colorectal ulcerations
Rectal varices[†]

Adapted from Davila RE, Rajan E, Adler DG, et al; Standards of Practice Committee: ASGE Guideline: The role of endoscopy in the patient with lower-GI bleeding. *Gastrointest Endosc* 62:656, 2005.
*Meckel's diverticula and other small bowel sources were excluded.
[†]Lesions most likely to benefit from endoscopic treatment (colorectal ulcerations might benefit from endoscopic treatment when visible vessel is present).

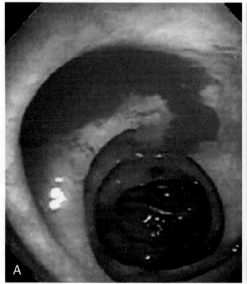
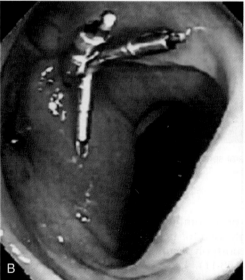

FIGURE 158-10 Endoscopic placement of clips for treatment of diverticular bleeding. **A,** Active bleeding seen. **B,** Hemostasis after Endoclip placement. (Courtesy Dr. Louis M. Wong Kee Song, Mayo Clinic, Rochester, Minn.)

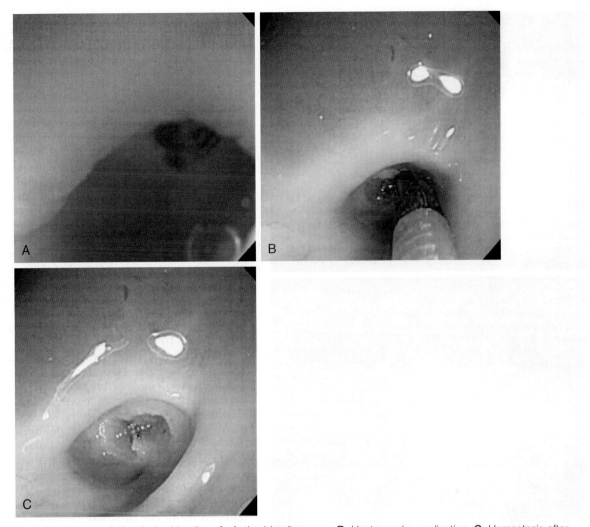

FIGURE 158-11 Coagulation therapy of diverticular bleeding. **A,** Active bleeding seen. **B,** Heater probe application. **C,** Hemostasis after treatment. (Courtesy Dr. Louis M. Wong Kee Song, Mayo Clinic, Rochester, Minn.)

may provide higher diagnostic yield[77] but does not seem to be advantageous for increasing the likelihood of diagnosing stigmata of hemorrhage in patients bleeding from diverticular disease.[78] To address this issue, a randomized study of 100 patients comparing urgent colonoscopy with angiography as a primary approach for severe LGIB has shown that colonoscopy identified a source of bleeding more often than angiography, though without differences in outcome.[79] Another randomized study comparing urgent versus elective colonoscopy has demonstrated that urgent colonoscopy in hospitalized patients with severe LGIB showed no evidence of improving clinical outcomes or lowering costs as compared to routine elective colonoscopy.[80] Urgent colonoscopy has some limitations in diagnostic yield and a definitive diagnosis can be made only when there is endoscopic evidence of active bleeding or stigmata of recent bleeding, which is present in only 20% to 25% of patients.

DIVERTICULAR BLEEDING

The most common cause of acute LGIB is colonic diverticular disease, which accounts for approximately 22% to 40% of cases.[81,82] Most of the clinical experience

regarding hemostatic procedures in the colon is derived from diverticular bleeding (excluding anorectal disorders). In a prospective study of 121 patients with severe hematochezia and diverticulosis,[83] urgent colonoscopy was performed within 6 to 12 hours after hospitalization or onset of hematochezia. Twenty-seven (22%) patients had definite signs of diverticular hemorrhage (active bleeding in 11, nonbleeding visible vessels in 6, and adherent clots in 10). The first 73 patients had colonoscopy only for diagnosis; 9 of these patients had recurrent diverticular bleeding and 6 underwent surgery. Of the subsequent 48 patients, 10 with definite diverticular hemorrhage were treated endoscopically by means of epinephrine injection, bipolar coagulation, or both, and none experienced recurrent bleeding or required surgery. In conclusion, colonoscopic treatment of such patients may prevent recurrent bleeding and decrease the need for surgery.

VASCULAR ECTASIAS

Vascular ectasias (also known as angiodysplasias and angioectasias) are red, flat lesions, usually from 5 to 20 mm in diameter, and account for 11% of LGIB.[82]

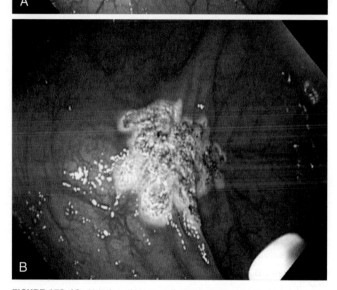

FIGURE 158-12 Ablation therapy of an angiodysplastic lesion using argon plasma coagulation (APC). **A,** Angiodysplastic lesion **B,** Ablated site after APC application. (Courtesy Dr. Louis M. Wong Kee Song, Mayo Clinic, Rochester, Minn.)

Vascular ectasias are predominantly located in the right side of the colon, may be multiple, and are incidentally found at colonoscopy in 2% of nonbleeding patients older than age 65 years.[84] Colonic arteriovenous malformation (AVM) is another vascular lesion that may be a cause of LGIB. Unlike small vascular ectasia or angiodysplasia, colonic AVMs tend to be solitary, large in size, and identified endoscopically as a flat or elevated bright red lesion.[84] Endoscopic application of argon plasma coagulation (APC) has become commonly used for the treatment of angiodysplastic lesions; however, treatment is not predictive of a lower rate of recurrence after an episode of acute bleeding (Figure 158-12).[85] Bipolar coagulation and heater probe have also been successfully used for bleeding colonic angiomas in 108 patients by the CURE hemostasis research group.[86] In their experience, 70% of patients had a good outcome with colonic coagulation, experiencing fewer bleeding episodes, requiring fewer blood transfusions, and maintenance of a higher hematocrit during followup.

COLONIC DECOMPRESSION TECHNIQUES AND PALLIATION FOR COLORECTAL CANCER

Acute colonic obstruction occurs more frequently in the left side of the colon and is the first presentation of colorectal cancer in 7% to 29% of patients.[87] Colorectal stent placement is an attractive technique for achieving colonic decompression of obstructed colorectal cancer because it combines nonoperative immediate colonic decompression and allows bowel preparation for an elective oncologic resection. Patients who benefit the most are high-risk surgical patients and candidates for laparoscopic resection. Colorectal stenting can be achieved with technical and clinical success rates of 92% to 94% and 88% to 91%, respectively, with a 0.6% to 1% mortality.[88] Emergency surgery is avoided in up to 94% of patients[89]; however, colonic perforation during stent placement is a concern because of the potential for peritoneal contamination and spreading of tumor cells. In a review designed to evaluate comparative studies reporting outcomes on colonic stenting and surgery, 451 patients with malignant colorectal obstruction were identified from 10 selected studies.[90] Stent insertion was attempted in 244 patients (54.1%) and was successful in 226 (92.6%). Patients undergoing colorectal stenting had a shorter length of hospital stay ($P < 0.001$), lower mortality ($P = 0.03$), and fewer medical complications ($P < 0.001$). In this latter study, when stents were used as a temporary measure before definitive surgery, long-term survival was not adversely influenced. In one prospective, randomized trial, self-expandable metal stents (SEMS) were placed as a bridge to surgery in acute left-sided malignant colonic obstruction.[91] SEMS placement allowed for subsequent laparoscopic resection with reduced incidence of stoma creation because of ability to perform a one-stage operation.

Benign colonic inflammatory and anastomotic strictures may be safely treated with serial colonoscopic dilations thus avoiding unnecessary surgery. Endoscopic dilation of strictures from Crohn disease within the reach of a colonoscope may have long-term efficacy for selected patients, especially after a second dilation session.[92] Dilation for anastomotic strictures from oncologic anterior rectal resection is also a valid option. In a retrospective study of 24 patients, dilation was successful in 90%, with a mean number of sessions of 2.3. There was no relationship between the number of dilation sessions and stricture recurrence.[93] Colorectal stents have been used as a decompressive procedure in selected patients with acute colorectal obstruction and benign colonic strictures such as anastomotic strictures, Crohn disease, radiation therapy, and diverticular disease. However, this technique is not yet accepted as a standard option for these patients, especially when uncovered (nonremovable) stents are used. Fully covered stents would be an interesting option for temporary colonic decompression for such patients; however, they are associated with unacceptably high migration rates.

Another nonsurgical technique to relieve acute colonic cancerous obstruction is transanal tube placement (Dennis colorectal tube),[94] which can be used as a bridge to surgery in more than 90% of patients.

However, this procedure has the disadvantage of being labor intensive and is less effective in allowing bowel preparation.[95] Transanal tube placement can also be used for colonic decompression before stent placement. No comparative studies have been performed comparing tube placement to stent placement or surgical decompression of obstructed colorectal tumors.

Colonoscopy has also been used as a temporary measure for decompression of colonic pseudoobstruction (Ogilvie syndrome).[96] Colonoscopy is usually indicated in patients without signs of perforation after a trial of conservative treatment including neostigmine if not contraindicated. The use of a decompressing tube significantly reduces recurrence of pseudoobstruction compared to colonic decompression alone. Technical success rates at the initial procedure, with or without tube placement, are 61% and 95%, respectively.[97] Clinical success after one or more procedures ranges from 73% to 88%. Complications of colonoscopic decompression occur in up to 3% of patients, including perforation in 2% and mortality in 1%. In refractory or recurrent pseudoobstruction, a percutaneous endoscopic colostomy has been used. Colonic volvulus occurs commonly at the sigmoid colon and the cecum. Nonoperative decompression with rectal tube placement has been reported to be successful in 78% of 575 patients with sigmoid volvulus (including 13 patients without endoscopic approach) with a mortality of 1%, a complication rate of 3%, and an early recurrence rate of 3%.[98] Elective surgical treatment is generally recommended after endoscopic detorsion of the bowel because of higher rates of recurrence. However, endoscopic reduction of sigmoid volvulus with subsequent percutaneous endoscopic sigmoidopexy has been described.[99] Colonoscopy is not recommended for treatment of cecal volvulus, and surgical management is the preferred option. As many as 7% of colorectal cancer patients will develop a complication during their treatment because of local tumor growth. Tumor compression occurring from postoperative local tumor recurrence and in stage IV disease treated nonoperatively with chemoirradiation can lead to colonic obstruction. Because the use of colonic stents is associated with a high risk of complications if left in place for more than 6 weeks, ablation techniques such as Nd:YAG laser or argon plasma coagulation with or without percutaneous cecostomy appear to be acceptable options in this difficult clinical scenario, although both require multiple sessions. Brachytherapy has been reported for palliation of rectal cancer and was recently used to relieve symptoms in a patient with obstruction at the hepatic flexure.[100]

COMPLICATIONS OF COLONOSCOPY

Complications from colonoscopy are related to sedation, bowel preparation, and bacterial translocation or may be patient or procedure related. These are rare in the setting of screening colonoscopy.[101] Colonoscopic polypectomy accounts for most reported complications seen in colonoscopy. It is associated with a 10% rate of complications, and three-quarters of these are of minor severity.[102] More than 90% of postpolypectomy complications can be managed nonoperatively. A recent U.S. study using the National Endoscopic Database comprising 21,375 patients reported an overall incidence of complications from colonoscopy of 2.01 per 1000 exams (95% CI, 1.46 to 2.71). A logistic regression analysis demonstrated an increased risk of complications associated with prior use of warfarin and performance of polypectomy with electrocautery.

Colonoscopy may result in colonic wall laceration and perforation from colonoscope maneuvering (mechanical) or from polyp removal. Colonic perforations should be sealed to avoid risk of fecal spillage. Small sealed-off contained perforations may be managed nonoperatively in selected cases. Surgical management options for colonic perforations are simple closure of the perforation or segmental colon resection with primary anastomosis with or without fecal diversion, the former usually indicated for perforations recognized within 24 hours. Overall mortality from colonoscopic perforation ranges from 2.9% to 25%.[103] Minimally invasive closure of perforations has evolved over the past decade. Laparoscopic repair is gaining preference over conventional surgery,[104] and endoscopic repair has been shown to be a viable option for treatment of perforations up to about 1 cm. A variety of endoscopic techniques for perforation closure have been described, including application of endoscopic clips[105] alone or combined with detachable endoscopic loops.[106] In a case series of 30 patients with colonic perforation (27 from therapeutic colonoscopy), conservative treatment using endoscopic clipping was attempted in 27 and failed in 2 patients.[107] A total of 5 patients underwent operative management and 25 patients were subsequently treated nonoperatively. The mean postoperative hospital stay for patients undergoing surgery was 12.2 days compared with 3.5 days for patients treated conservatively.

Postpolypectomy bleeding may occur immediately after polyp resection or delayed for an average of 6 days (range, 1 ± 14 days). Polyps larger than 17 mm, pedunculated polyps with a stalk diameter greater than 5 mm, sessile polyps, and malignant lesions of the colorectal region have higher risk for bleeding after endoscopic resection.[108] Immediate postpolypectomy bleeding may be prevented with the use of ancillary endoscopic techniques such as endoscopic clipping,[109] endoscopic epinephrine injection, or placement of detachable endoscopic loop on large polyp stalks prior to snare resection (see Figure 158-7).[110,111] Risk factors for delayed postpolypectomy bleeding are arterial systemic hypertension,[112] polyp size, and resuming anticoagulation treatment within 1 week following polypectomy.[113] Use of aspirin does not seem to be associated with increased risk.[114] Postpolypectomy bleeding can be successfully managed endoscopically in most cases and include use of endoscopic clips,[115] epinephrine injection, electrocoagulation, or a combination of detachable loop placement and endoscopic clipping.[116]

CONCLUSION

Colonoscopy was introduced in the 1970s and is one of the most commonly performed endoscopic procedures worldwide. Significant improvements have been made resulting in a safer and more accurate and comfortable examinations. The increasing importance of colonoscopy in clinical practice can be credited to its significant benefits in colorectal cancer prevention and treatment. Despite the development of other less invasive imaging modalities for colorectal screening, colonoscopy still has advantages such as direct inspection of detailed mucosal architecture and ability to obtain targeted mucosal tissue sampling. Colonoscopy is also becoming a more complex therapeutic procedure with increasing relevance in curative and palliative management of malignant and benign colorectal diseases. Colonoscopy is currently among the front-line methods for evaluating and treating acute lower gastrointestinal bleeding.

REFERENCES

1. Klabunde CN, Lanier D, Nadel MR, et al: Colorectal cancer screening by primary care physicians: Recommendations and practices, 2006-2007. *Am J Prev Med* 37:8, 2009.
2. Cappell MS, Abboud R: The impact of advances in instrumentation and techniques of colonoscopy from 1988 to 2008 on inpatient colonoscopy performance at a high volume endoscopy unit in the United States: Significantly shorter procedure time, higher completion rate, performance on sicker inpatients, and near disappearance of flexible sigmoidoscopy. *Dig Dis Sci* 55:3521, 2010.
3. Winawer SJ, Zauber AG, Fletcher RH, et al; US Multi-Society Task Force on Colorectal Cancer; American Cancer Society: Guidelines for colonoscopy surveillance after polypectomy: A consensus update by the US Multi-Society Task Force on Colorectal Cancer and the American Cancer Society. *Gastroenterology* 130:1872, 2006.
4. Brenner H, Hoffmeister M, Brenner G, et al: Expected reduction of colorectal cancer incidence within 8 years after introduction of the German screening colonoscopy programme: Estimates based on 1,875,708 screening colonoscopies. *Eur J Cancer* 45:2027, 2009.
5. Petersen BT, Hussain N, Marine JE, et al; Technology Assessment Committee: Endoscopy in patients with implanted electronic devices. *Gastrointest Endosc* 65:561, 2007.
6. American Society of Anesthesiologists Task Force on Perioperative Management of Patients with Cardiac Rhythm Management Devices: Practice advisory for the perioperative management of patients with cardiac rhythm management devices: Pacemakers and implantable cardioverter-defibrillators: A report by the American Society of Anesthesiologists Task Force on Perioperative Management of Patients with Cardiac Rhythm Management Devices. *Anesthesiology* 103:186, 2005.
7. ASGE Standards of Practice Committee, Levy MJ, Anderson MA, Baron TH, et al: Position statement on routine laboratory testing before endoscopic procedures. *Gastrointest Endosc* 68:827, 2008.
8. Hui AJ, Wong RM, Ching JY, et al: Risk of colonoscopic polypectomy bleeding with anticoagulants and antiplatelet agents: Analysis of 1657 cases. *Gastrointest Endosc* 59:44, 2004.
9. Zuckerman MJ, Hirota WK, Adler DG, et al: ASGE guideline: The management of low-molecular-weight heparin and nonaspirin antiplatelet agents for endoscopic procedures. Standards of Practice Committee of the American Society for Gastrointestinal Endoscopy. *Gastrointest Endosc* 61:189, 2005.
10. Allison MC, Sandoe JA, Tighe R, et al; Endoscopy Committee of the British Society of Gastroenterology: Antibiotic prophylaxis in gastrointestinal endoscopy. *Gut* 58:869, 2009.
11. ASGE Standards of Practice Committee, Banerjee S, Shen B, Baron TH, et al: Antibiotic prophylaxis for GI endoscopy. *Gastrointest Endosc* 67:791, 2008.
12. Yip T, Tse KC, Lam MF, et al: Risks and outcomes of peritonitis after flexible colonoscopy in CAPD patients. *Perit Dial Int* 27:560, 2007.
13. Ness RM, Manam R, Hoen H, et al: Predictors of inadequate bowel preparation for colonoscopy. *Am J Gastroenterol* 96:1797, 2001.
14. Burke CA, Church JM: Enhancing the quality of colonoscopy: The importance of bowel purgatives. *Gastrointest Endosc* 66:565, 2007.
15. Wexner SD, Beck DE, Baron TH, et al; American Society of Colon and Rectal Surgeons; American Society for Gastrointestinal Endoscopy; Society of American Gastrointestinal and Endoscopic Surgeons: A consensus document on bowel preparation before colonoscopy: Prepared by a task force from the American Society of Colon and Rectal Surgeons (ASCRS), the American Society for Gastrointestinal Endoscopy (ASGE), and the Society of American Gastrointestinal and Endoscopic Surgeons (SAGES). *Gastrointest Endosc* 63:894, 2006.
16. Cohen LB: Split dosing of bowel preparations for colonoscopy: An analysis of its efficacy, safety, and tolerability. *Gastrointest Endosc* 72:406, 2010.
17. Gurudu SR, Ratuapli S, Heigh R, et al: Quality of bowel cleansing for afternoon colonoscopy is influenced by time of administration. *Am J Gastroenterol* 105:2318, 2010.
18. American Society for Gastrointestinal Endoscopy Standards of Practice Committee ASGE Guideline: The role of endoscopy in the patient with lower-GI bleeding. *Gastrointest Endosc* 62:65, 2005.
19. Chang KJ, Erickson RA, Schandler S, et al: Per-rectal pulsed irrigation versus per-oral colonic lavage for colonoscopy preparation: A randomized, controlled trial. *Gastrointest Endosc* 37:444, 1991.
20. Sohn N, Weinstein MA: Management of the poorly prepared colonoscopy patient: Colonoscopic colon enemas as a preparation for colonoscopy. *Dis Colon Rectum* 51:462, 2008.
21. Ladas SD, Karamanolis G, Ben-Soussan E: Colonic gas explosion during therapeutic colonoscopy with electrocautery. *World J Gastroenterol* 13:5295, 2007.
22. McQuaid KR, Laine L: A systematic review and meta-analysis of randomized, controlled trials of moderate sedation for routine endoscopic procedures. *Gastrointest Endosc* 69:983, 2009.
23. Cohen LB, Wecsler JS, Gaetano JN, et al: Endoscopic sedation in the United States: Results from a nationwide survey. *Am J Gastroenterol* 101:967, 2006.
24. Singh H, Poluha W, Cheung M, et al: Propofol for sedation during colonoscopy. *Cochrane Database Syst Rev* CD006268, 2008.
25. Padmanabhan U, Leslie K, Eer AS, et al: Early cognitive impairment after sedation for colonoscopy: The effect of adding midazolam and/or fentanyl to propofol. *Anesth Analg* 109:1448, 2009.
26. Mandel JE, Lichtenstein GR, Metz DC, et al: A prospective, randomized, comparative trial evaluating respiratory depression during patient-controlled versus anesthesiologist-administered propofol-remifentanil sedation for elective colonoscopy. *Gastrointest Endosc* 72:112, 2010.
27. Standards of Practice Committee of the American Society for Gastrointestinal Endoscopy, Lichtenstein DR, Jagannath S, Baron TH, et al: Sedation and anesthesia in GI endoscopy. *Gastrointest Endosc* 68:815, 2008.
28. Petrini JL, Egan JV, Hahn WV: Unsedated colonoscopy: Patient characteristics and satisfaction in a community-based endoscopy unit. *Gastrointest Endosc* 69:567, 2009.
29. Othman MO, Bradley AG, Choudhary A, et al: Variable stiffness colonoscope versus regular adult colonoscope: meta-analysis of randomized controlled trials. *Endoscopy* 41:17, 2009.
30. Shah SG, Brooker JC, Thapar C, et al: Effect of magnetic endoscope imaging on patient tolerance and sedation requirements during colonoscopy: A randomized controlled trial. *Gastrointest Endosc* 55:832, 2002.
31. Leung FW, Harker JO, Jackson G, et al: A proof-of-principle, prospective, randomized, controlled trial demonstrating improved outcomes in scheduled unsedated colonoscopy by the water method. *Gastrointest Endosc* 72:693, 2010.
32. Dellon ES, Hawk JS, Grimm IS, et al: The use of carbon dioxide for insufflation during GI endoscopy: A systematic review. *Gastrointest Endosc* 69:843, 2009.
33. Yamano HO, Yoshikawa K, Kimura T, et al: Carbon dioxide insufflation for colonoscopy: Evaluation of gas volume, abdominal pain, examination time and transcutaneous partial CO_2 pressure. *J Gastroenterol* 45:1235, 2010.
34. Brown SR, Baraza W, Hurlstone P: Chromoscopy versus conventional endoscopy for the detection of polyps in the colon and rectum. *Cochrane Database Syst Rev* CD006439, 2007.
35. Pohl J, Ell C: Impact of virtual chromoendoscopy at colonoscopy: The final requiem for conventional histopathology? *Gastrointest Endosc* 69:723, 2009.

36. Matsumoto T, Nakamura S, Moriyama T, et al: Auto-fluorescence imaging colonoscopy for the detection of dysplastic lesions in ulcerative colitis: A pilot study. *Colorectal Dis* 12:e291, 2010.

37. Boparai KS, van den Broek FJ, van Eeden S, et al: Hyperplastic polyposis syndrome: A pilot study for the differentiation of polyps by using high-resolution endoscopy, autofluorescence imaging, and narrow-band imaging. *Gastrointest Endosc* 70:947, 2009.

38. Matsumoto T, Esaki M, Fujisawa R, et al: Chromoendoscopy, narrow-band imaging colonoscopy, and autofluorescence colonoscopy for detection of diminutive colorectal neoplasia in familial adenomatous polyposis. *Dis Colon Rectum* 52:1160, 2009.

39. Buchner AM, Shahid MW, Heckman MG, et al: Comparison of probe-based confocal laser endomicroscopy with virtual chromoendoscopy for classification of colon polyps. *Gastroenterology* 138:834, 2010.

40. Zanoni EC, Cutait R, Averbach M, et al: Magnifying colonoscopy: Interobserver agreement in the assessment of colonic pit patterns and its correlation with histopathological findings. *Int J Colorectal Dis* 22:1383, 2007.

41. Raghavendra M, Hewett DG, Rex DK: Differentiating adenomas from hyperplastic colorectal polyps: Narrow-band imaging can be learned in 20 minutes. *Gastrointest Endosc* 72:572, 2010.

42. van Rijn JC, Reitsma JB, Stoker J, et al: Polyp miss rate determined by tandem colonoscopy: A systematic review. *Am J Gastroenterol* 101:343, 2006.

43. DeMarco DC, Odstrcil E, Lara LF, et al: Impact of experience with a retrograde-viewing device on adenoma detection rates and withdrawal times during colonoscopy: The Third Eye Retroscope study group. *Gastrointest Endosc* 71:542, 2010.

44. Hewett DG, Rex DK: Cap-fitted colonoscopy: A randomized, tandem colonoscopy study of adenoma miss rates. *Gastrointest Endosc* 72:775, 2010.

45. Fatima H, Rex DK, Rothstein R, et al: Cecal insertion and withdrawal times with wide-angle versus standard colonoscopes: A randomized controlled trial. *Clin Gastroenterol Hepatol* 6:109, 2008.

46. Pellisé M, Fernández-Esparrach G, Cárdenas A, et al: Impact of wide-angle, high-definition endoscopy in the diagnosis of colorectal neoplasia: A randomized controlled trial. *Gastroenterology* 135:1062, 2008.

47. Tribonias G, Theodoropoulou A, Konstantinidis K, et al: Comparison of standard versus high-definition, wide-angle colonoscopy for polyp detection: A randomized controlled trial. *Colorectal Dis* 12:e260, 2010.

48. Gaglia A, Papanikolaou IS, Veltzke-Schlieker W: New endoscopy devices to improve population adherence to colorectal cancer prevention programs. *World J Gastrointest Endosc* 2:244, 2010.

49. Van Gossum A, Munoz-Navas M, Fernandez-Urien I, et al: Capsule endoscopy versus colonoscopy for the detection of polyps and cancer. *N Engl J Med* 361:264, 2009.

50. Gay G, Delvaux M, Frederic M, et al: Could the colonic capsule PillCam Colon be clinically useful for selecting patients who deserve a complete colonoscopy?: Results of clinical comparison with colonoscopy in the perspective of colorectal cancer screening. *Am J Gastroenterol* 105:1076, 2010.

51. Long G, Fritscher-Ravens A, Mosse CA, et al: The Cath-Cam: A new concept in colonoscopy. *Gastrointest Endosc* 64:997, 2006.

52. Anderson JC, Messina CR, Cohn W, et al: Factors predictive of difficult colonoscopy. *Gastrointest Endosc* 54:558, 2001.

53. Chung YW, Han DS, Yoo KS, et al: Patient factors predictive of pain and difficulty during sedation-free colonoscopy: A prospective study in Korea. *Dig Liver Dis* 39:872, 2007.

54. Teshima CW, Aktas H, Haringsma J, et al: Single-balloon-assisted colonoscopy in patients with previously failed colonoscopy. *Gastrointest Endosc* 71:1319, 2010.

55. Gay G, Delvaux M: Double-balloon colonoscopy after failed conventional colonoscopy: A pilot series with a new instrument. *Endoscopy* 39:788, 2007.

56. Kobayashi N, Saito Y, Sano Y, et al: Determining the treatment strategy for colorectal neoplastic lesions: Endoscopic assessment or the non-lifting sign for diagnosing invasion depth? *Endoscopy* 39:701, 2007.

57. Fujishiro M, Yahagi N, Kashimura K, et al: Comparison of various submucosal injections solutions for maintaining mucosal elevation for endoscopic submucosal dissection. *Endoscopy* 36:579, 2004.

58. ASGE Technology Committee, Kethu SR, Banerjee S, Desilets D, et al: Endoscopic tattooing. *Gastrointest Endosc* 72:681, 2010.

59. Fyock CJ, Draganov PV: Colonoscopic polypectomy and associated techniques. *World J Gastroenterol* 16:3630, 2010.

60. Oka S, Tanaka S, Kanao H, et al: Therapeutic strategy for colorectal laterally spreading tumor. *Dig Endosc* 21:S43, 2009.

61. Saito Y, Fukuzawa M, Matsuda T, et al: Clinical outcome of endoscopic submucosal dissection versus endoscopic mucosal resection of large colorectal tumors as determined by curative resection. *Surg Endosc* 24:343, 2010.

62. Puli SR, Kakugawa Y, Saito Y, et al: Successful complete cure en-bloc resection of large nonpedunculated colonic polyps by endoscopic submucosal dissection: A meta-analysis and systematic review. *Ann Surg Oncol* 16:2147, 2009.

63. Tanaka S, Oka S, Chayama K: Colorectal endoscopic submucosal dissection: Present status and future perspective, including its differentiation from endoscopic mucosal resection. *J Gastroenterol* 43:641, 2008.

64. von Renteln D, Schmidt A, Vassiliou MC, et al: Endoscopic full-thickness resection and defect closure in the colon. *Gastrointest Endosc* 71:1267, 2010.

65. Lambert R, Kudo SE, Vieth M, et al: Pragmatic classification of superficial neoplastic colorectal lesions. *Gastrointest Endosc* 70:1182, 2009.

66. Hurlstone DP, Sanders DS, Cross SS, et al: Colonoscopic resection of lateral spreading tumours: A prospective analysis of endoscopic mucosal resection. *Gut* 53:1334, 2004.

67. Fu KI, Kato S, Sano Y, et al: Staging of early colorectal cancers: Magnifying colonoscopy versus endoscopic ultrasonography for estimation of depth of invasion. *Dig Dis Sci* 53:1886, 2008.

68. Davila RE, Rajan E, Adler D, et al; ASGE: ASGE guideline: the role of endoscopy in the diagnosis, staging, and management of colorectal cancer. *Gastrointest Endosc* 61:1, 2005.

69. No authors listed. The Paris endoscopic classification of superficial neoplastic lesions: Esophagus, stomach, and colon: November 30 to December 1, 2002. *Gastrointest Endosc* 58:S3, 2003.

70. Martínez ME, Baron JA, Lieberman DA, et al: A pooled analysis of advanced colorectal neoplasia diagnoses after colonoscopic polypectomy. *Gastroenterology* 136:832, 2009.

71. ASGE Technology Committee, Conway JD, Adler DG, Diehl DL, et al: Endoscopic hemostatic devices. *Gastrointest Endosc* 69:987, 2009.

72. Coumaros D, Tsesmeli N: Active gastrointestinal bleeding: Use of hemostatic forceps beyond endoscopic submucosal dissection. *World J Gastroenterol* 16:2061, 2010.

73. Kataoka M, Kawai T, Yagi K, et al: Clinical evaluation of emergency endoscopic hemostasis with bipolar forceps in non-variceal upper gastrointestinal bleeding. *Dig Endosc* 22:151, 2010.

74. Johnston MJ, Robertson GM, Frizelle FA: Management of late complications of pelvic radiation in the rectum and anus: A review. *Dis Colon Rectum* 46:247, 2003.

75. Elta GH: Urgent colonoscopy for acute lower-GI bleeding. *Gastrointest Endosc* 59:402, 2004.

76. Ríos A, Montoya MJ, Rodríguez JM, et al: Severe acute lower gastrointestinal bleeding: Risk factors for morbidity and mortality. *Langenbecks Arch Surg* 392:165, 2007.

77. Lin CC, Lee YC, Lee H, et al: Bedside colonoscopy for critically ill patients with acute lower gastrointestinal bleeding. *Intensive Care Med* 31:743, 2005.

78. Smoot RL, Gostout CJ, Rajan E, et al: Is early colonoscopy after admission for acute diverticular bleeding needed? *Am J Gastroenterol* 98:1996, 2003 Sep.

79. Green BT, Rockey DC, Portwood G, et al: Urgent colonoscopy for evaluation and management of acute lower gastrointestinal hemorrhage: A randomized controlled trial. *Am J Gastroenterol* 100:2395, 2005.

80. Laine L, Shah A: Randomized trial of urgent vs. elective colonoscopy in patients hospitalized with lower GI bleeding. *Am J Gastroenterol* 105:2636, 2010.

81. Schuetz A, Jauch KW: Lower gastrointestinal bleeding: Therapeutic strategies, surgical techniques and results. *Langenbecks Arch Surg* 386:17, 2001.

82. Davila RE, Rajan E, Adler DG, et al; Standards of Practice Committee: ASGE Guideline: The role of endoscopy in the patient with lower-GI bleeding. *Gastrointest Endosc* 62:656, 2005.

83. Jensen DM, Machicado GA, Jutabha R, et al: Urgent colonoscopy for the diagnosis and treatment of severe diverticular hemorrhage. *N Engl J Med* 342:78, 2000.

84. Kim BK, Han HS, Lee SY, et al: Cecal polypoid arteriovenous malformations removed by endoscopic biopsy. *J Korean Med Sci* 24:342, 2009.

85. Saperas E, Videla S, Dot J, et al: Risk factors for recurrence of acute gastrointestinal bleeding from angiodysplasia. *Eur J Gastroenterol Hepatol* 21:1333, 2009.

86. Gay G, Delvaux M, Frederic M, et al: Could the colonic capsule PillCam Colon be clinically useful for selecting patients who deserve a complete colonoscopy?: Results of clinical comparison with colonoscopy in the perspective of colorectal cancer screening. *Am J Gastroenterol* 105:1076, 2010.

87. Smothers L, Hynan L, Fleming J, et al: Emergency surgery for colon carcinoma. *Dis Colon Rectum* 46:24, 2003.

88. Khot UP, Wenk Lang A, Murali K, Parker MC: Systematic review of the efficacy and safety of colorectal stents. *Br J Surg* 89:1096, 2002.

89. Sebastian S, Johnston S, Geoghegan T, et al: Pooled analysis of the efficacy and safety of self-expanding metal stenting in malignant colorectal obstruction. *Am J Gastroenterol* 99:2051, 2004.

90. Tilney HS, Lovegrove RE, Purkayastha S, et al: Comparison of colonic stenting and open surgery for malignant large bowel obstruction. *Surg Endosc* 21:225, 2007.

91. Cheung HY, Chung CC, Tsang WW, et al: Endolaparoscopic approach vs conventional open surgery in the treatment of obstructing left-sided colon cancer: A randomized controlled trial. *Arch Surg* 144:1127, 2009.

92. Stienecker K, Gleichmann D, Neumayer U, et al: Long-term results of endoscopic balloon dilatation of lower gastrointestinal tract strictures in Crohn's disease: A prospective study. *World J Gastroenterol* 15:2623, 2009.

93. Araujo SE, Costa AF: Efficacy and safety of endoscopic balloon dilation of benign anastomotic strictures after oncologic anterior rectal resection: Report on 24 cases. *Surg Laparosc Endosc Percutan Tech* 18:565, 2008.

94. Xu M, Zhong Y, Yao L, et al: Endoscopic decompression using a transanal drainage tube for acute obstruction of the rectum and left colon as a bridge to curative surgery. *Colorectal Dis* 11:405, 2009.

95. Dekovich AA: Endoscopic treatment of colonic obstruction. *Curr Opin Gastroenterol* 25:50, 2009.

96. ASGE Standards of Practice Committee, Harrison ME, Anderson MA, Appalaneni V, et al: The role of endoscopy in the management of patients with known and suspected colonic obstruction and pseudo-obstruction. *Gastrointest Endosc* 71:669, 2010.

97. Saunders MD: Acute colonic pseudo-obstruction. *Best Pract Res Clin Gastroenterol* 21:671, 2007.

98. Oren D, Atamanalp SS, Aydinli B, et al: An algorithm for the management of sigmoid colon volvulus and the safety of primary resection: Experience with 827 cases. *Dis Colon Rectum* 50:489, 2007.

99. Witherspoon P, Wright DM: Three-dimensional magnetic image guided percutaneous endoscopic sigmoidopexy for the treatment of recurrent sigmoid volvulus. *Colorectal Dis* 12:72, 2010.

100. Tam TY, Mukherjee S, Farrell T, et al: Endoscopic brachytherapy for obstructive colorectal cancer. *Brachytherapy* 8:313, 2009.

101. Ko CW, Riffle S, Michaels L, et al: Serious complications within 30 days of screening and surveillance colonoscopy are uncommon. *Clin Gastroenterol Hepatol* 8:166, 2010.

102. Heldwein W, Dollhopf M, Rösch T, et al; Munich Gastroenterology Group: The Munich Polypectomy Study (MUPS): Prospective analysis of complications and risk factors in 4000 colonic snare polypectomies. *Endoscopy* 37:1116, 2005.

103. Lüning TH, Keemers-Gels ME, Barendregt WB, et al: Colonoscopic perforations: A review of 30,366 patients. *Surg Endosc* 21:994, 2007.

104. Coimbra C, Bouffioux L, Kohnen L, et al: Laparoscopic repair of colonoscopic perforation: A new standard? *Surg Endosc* 25:1514, 2011.

105. Trecca A, Gaj F, Gagliardi G: Our experience with endoscopic repair of large colonoscopic perforations and review of the literature. *Tech Coloproctol* 12:315; discussion 322, 2008.

106. Katsinelos P, Chatzimavroudis G, Terzoudis S, et al: The endoloop-clips technique for closure of large iatrogenic colonic perforations. *Endoscopy* 42:343, 2010.

107. Magdeburg R, Collet P, Post S, et al: Endoclipping of iatrogenic colonic perforation to avoid surgery. *Surg Endosc* 22:1500, 2008.

108. Dobrowolski S, Dobosz M, Babicki A, et al: Blood supply of colorectal polyps correlates with risk of bleeding after colonoscopic polypectomy. *Gastrointest Endosc* 63:1004, 2006.

109. Luigiano C, Ferrara F, Ghersi S, et al: Endoclip-assisted resection of large pedunculated colorectal polyps: Technical aspects and outcome. *Dig Dis Sci* 55:1726, 2010.

110. Di Giorgio P, De Luca L, Calcagno G, et al: Detachable snare versus epinephrine injection in the prevention of postpolypectomy bleeding: A randomized and controlled study. *Endoscopy* 36:860, 2004.

111. Paspatis GA, Paraskeva K, Theodoropoulou A, et al: A prospective, randomized comparison of adrenaline injection in combination with detachable snare versus adrenaline injection alone in the prevention of postpolypectomy bleeding in large colonic polyps. *Am J Gastroenterol* 101:2805, 2006.

112. Watabe H, Yamaji Y, Okamoto M, et al: Risk assessment for delayed hemorrhagic complication of colonic polypectomy: Polyp-related factors and patient-related factors. *Gastrointest Endosc* 64:73, 2006.

113. Sawhney MS, Salfiti N, Nelson DB, et al: Risk factors for severe delayed postpolypectomy bleeding. *Endoscopy* 40:115, 2008.

114. Yousfi M, Gostout CJ, Baron TH, et al: Postpolypectomy lower gastrointestinal bleeding: Potential role of aspirin. *Am J Gastroenterol* 99:1785, 2004.

115. Parra-Blanco A, Kaminaga N, Kojima T, et al: Hemoclipping for postpolypectomy and postbiopsy colonic bleeding. *Gastrointest Endosc* 51:37, 2000.

116. Chou KC, Yen HH: Combined endoclip and endoloop treatment for delayed postpolypectomy hemorrhage. *Gastrointest Endosc* 72:218, 2010.

PART THREE

Inflammatory Diseases

Inflammatory Bowel Disease

Edward V. Loftus, Jr. | Robert R. Cima

ULCERATIVE COLITIS

EPIDEMIOLOGY AND ETIOPATHOGENESIS

Ulcerative colitis (UC) is an idiopathic inflammatory condition involving the mucosa of the colon and rectum. The adjusted incidence of UC in Olmsted County, Minnesota, was 8.8 cases per 100,000 person-years in the 1990s,[1] and 12.5 per 100,000 in 2001 to 2004.[2] The adjusted prevalence in the same location on January 1, 2005, was 266 cases per 100,000 persons.[2] If these figures are extrapolated to the national population of 308.7 million persons in 2010, then approximately 38,500 new cases of UC are diagnosed annually in the United States, and overall there are approximately 815,000 people with UC.[3]

UC is most likely caused by a complex interplay of genetic factors, immune dysregulation, and environmental factors, including alterations in the fecal microbiome.[3] Genetic susceptibility is likely, given the 5% to 15% prevalence of the disease occurring in families,[4-6] compared with a 0.25% occurrence in the general population.[1] Twin studies also suggest a genetic basis for UC (albeit weaker than what has been observed in Crohn disease)—the concordance for UC in monozygotic twins is 15% to 20% compared with a concordance of 0% to 5% in dizygotic twins.[7-9] The incidence of UC may be higher among Jews in a given geographic region compared to non-Jews[10]; furthermore, the familial risk of UC in Jews appears to be higher than in non-Jews.[11]

Well-established environmental influences on the risk of UC include cigarette smoking and a history of appendectomy.[2] Current cigarette smokers are significantly less likely than never smokers to develop UC, whereas former smokers are at increased risk.[12] The "protective effect" of smoking may be explained by nicotine, which exerts important changes in rectal blood flow, colonic mucus, and cytokine and eicosanoid production.[13] Appendectomy in childhood for appendicitis also appears to diminish the risk of UC, suggesting that removing the appendix might influence the mucosal immune system.[14] The role of dietary factors in UC remains controversial, but increased intake of total fat, polyunsaturated fatty acids, omega-6 fatty acids, and meat may be deleterious, whereas high vegetable intake may be protective.[15] An infectious cause of UC has been suggested, but no specific bacterial or viral agent has been isolated. However, specific pathogens such as cytomegalovirus or *Clostridium difficile* that result in acute colitis may trigger UC in susceptible hosts.[16,17] Historically, psychosomatic factors were thought to play a major role in the etiology of UC, but this hypothesis has been discarded for the most part. In certain patients with established UC, increased stress may result in disease exacerbation.[18]

Because immune dysregulation is suspected to play a major role in inflammatory bowel disease (IBD) etiopathogenesis, much effort is being made to understand the role of cytokines in IBD. Cytokines modulate the intestinal immune system. It is hypothesized that regulation of the immune response is a result of the balance between proinflammatory cytokines such as interleukin (IL)-1, tumor necrosis factor (TNF)-α, interferon (IFN)-γ, IL-6, IL-8, and IL-12, and antiinflammatory cytokines such as IL-1 receptor antagonist (IL-1RA), IL-4, IL-10, IL-11, and transforming growth factor (TGF)-β. Perturbations in this balance may result in a loss of gut homeostasis and uncontrolled bowel inflammation.[19]

Recent advances in the field of genetics, including genomewide association studies (GWAS) of large cohorts of patients, have resulted in the identification of more than 60 susceptibility loci for IBD, with roughly 40% of these associated with both UC and Crohn disease and approximately one-third associated with UC alone.[20] Some of the major histocompatibility complex (MHC) genes were the first to be linked with ulcerative colitis. Products of these genes play a role in modulating immune response to various antigens. The human leukocyte antigen (HLA) DRB1*0103 allele is associated with extensive and refractory disease and extraintestinal manifestations of IBD. Other putative susceptibility genes in UC include the receptor to IL-23, the IL-10 receptor, and several barrier function genes, including ECM1, HNF4A, CDH1, and LAMB1.[20]

TABLE 159-1 Characteristics of Crohn Colitis and Ulcerative Colitis

Features	Crohn Colitis*	Ulcerative Colitis*
MACROSCOPIC		
Thickened bowel wall	+++	+
Narrowing of bowel lumen	+++	+
Discontinuous disease	++	⊕
Rectal involvement	⊕	+++
Deep fissures and fistulas	++	⊕
Confluent linear ulcers	++	⊕
Perianal disease	++	⊕
MICROSCOPIC		
Transmural inflammation	+++	+
Submucosal infiltration	+++	+
Submucosal thickening, fibrosis	+++	⊕
Ulceration through mucosa	+++	++
Fissures	+++	+
Granulomas	++	⊕

*Features are characterized as being present consistently (+++), frequently (++), infrequently (+), or rarely (⊕).

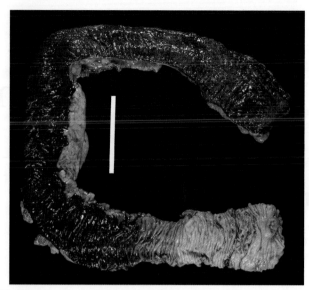

FIGURE 159-1 Chronic ulcerative colitis. Continuous involvement of the colon extending from the rectum to ascending colon. The mucosa is erythematous and atrophic in areas. No "skip areas" are present, and no deep linear ulcers are seen. (Courtesy Jason T. Lewis, MD.)

PATHOLOGIC FEATURES

In general, UC is present in the rectum and extends proximally to involve the remainder of the colon in a diffuse, continuous manner (Table 159-1). The disease process may end gradually or abruptly at any level within the colon. Approximately 10% to 20% of patients with extensive UC have mild mucosal inflammation of the terminal ileum, or "backwash ileitis." The extent of the disease may vary from proctitis (i.e., involvement of the rectum alone, 25% of patients in most population-based cohorts) to left-sided colonic involvement (distal to splenic flexure, 25%) to extensive colonic involvement (proximal to splenic flexure, 50%).[21]

On gross examination, the lesions of UC begin with erythema, granularity, mucosal edema, and loss of the normal vascular pattern (see Table 159-1).[22] Mucosal friability increases with activity, and this produces the bleeding that is seen with the disease. Ulcerations occur with moderate and severe UC. These may be superficial and smooth or ragged and undermined. Eventually, ulcers may replace the entire colonic mucosa. With ongoing chronic inflammation, marked narrowing, thickening, and rigidity of the bowel occur as the muscular coats are replaced by scar tissue (Figure 159-1). Polypoid masses or pseudopolyps, caused by hyperplasia of remaining small islands of mucosa and by the margins of ulcerations, may be present and may persist or recede as the inflammatory process becomes quiescent.

Microscopic examination of the inflamed colon shows distortion of crypt architecture and infiltration of the lamina propria not only with polymorphonuclear leukocytes but also basal plasma cells (see Table 159-1).[22] Distortion of the crypt architecture is a hallmark feature of chronic colitis. Microscopic crypt abscesses are common and penetrate just into the submucosa with the production of wide areas of ulceration of the overlying mucosa. Depletion of goblet cell mucin and superficial erosions are also commonly seen. There usually is an increase in

the number of Paneth cells in the colonic crypts distal to the hepatic flexure. Granulomas, which are often seen in Crohn disease, are extremely uncommon in UC.

CLINICAL COURSE

Like many chronic inflammatory conditions, UC is highly variable in severity, clinical course, and ultimate prognosis. In general, the severity of the disease correlates with the extent and severity of the changes in the bowel wall. UC has a peak incidence in the third and fourth decades of life—the median age at diagnosis in most series is in the early 30s.[3] The condition may be slightly more common among males, but data are conflicting.[3] After its onset, the disease may take one of several courses. In a few patients (<10%), UC may be fulminant, typically becoming its most severe in the first few months after diagnosis, often requiring surgery.[23] In most cases, UC becomes a chronic condition characterized by remissions and exacerbations.[24] Approximately 75% of patients have intermittent attacks of symptoms, with complete symptomatic remissions between attacks. Disease activity in the preceding year and the presence of systemic symptoms such as fever and weight loss appear to be the strongest predictors of UC relapse.[24] A few patients (<5%) are troubled by continuous symptoms without any remission. Up to 20% of patients have only one attack, with no subsequent symptoms.[24]

The most common symptoms of active UC are diarrhea and the passage of blood and mucus.[24] Unlike Crohn colitis, in which hematochezia may be absent, bloody diarrhea is the hallmark of UC. The amount of blood may vary from a small amount of bright red blood, which is mistaken for hemorrhoidal bleeding, to massive bleeding. The diarrhea may be minimal, or patients may have 10 to 20 bowel movements per day. Patients who complain of constipation usually have proctitis or

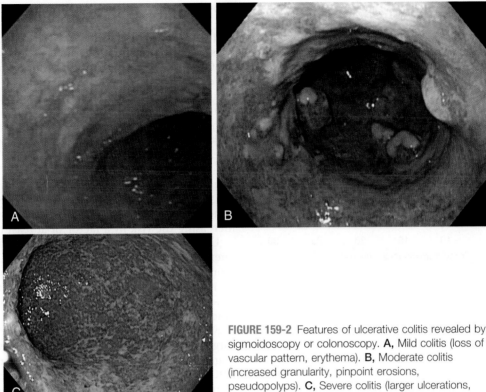

FIGURE 159-2 Features of ulcerative colitis revealed by sigmoidoscopy or colonoscopy. **A,** Mild colitis (loss of vascular pattern, erythema). **B,** Moderate colitis (increased granularity, pinpoint erosions, pseudopolyps). **C,** Severe colitis (larger ulcerations, spontaneous bleeding).

left-sided inflammation. These patients often have tenesmus and urgency but pass only a bloody mucous discharge, so it is important to inquire not only about the number of stools per day but also the number of trips to the bathroom.

In patients with acute severe colitis, abdominal pain is a frequent manifestation. It tends to be colicky. On examination of the abdomen, there may be tenderness over the colon, especially in the left lower quadrant. Large doses of corticosteroids may mask clinical signs in acute disease.

With milder forms of distal colitis, there may be only slight impairment of general health. In severe UC, systemic symptoms can be profound, and the patient may become rapidly debilitated and emaciated. Associated with these effects is fever; however, a temperature of more than 38° C is unusual, except in the rare fulminating type of colitis or in cases in which there is an intraabdominal perforation. Weight loss and anemia tend to occur in proportion to the severity of symptoms.

DIAGNOSIS

The diagnosis of UC should be suspected in patients with a history of bloody diarrhea in whom an infectious cause has been eliminated.[25] Flexible sigmoidoscopy and colonoscopy are the cornerstones of diagnosis. Colonoscopy with biopsies is more accurate than barium radiography, particularly for detecting mild colitis and determining extent. Colonoscopy with intubation of the ileocecal valve and examination of the terminal ileum allows an assessment for backwash ileitis or Crohn ileitis. Sigmoidoscopy or colonoscopy reveals the typical gross features

already described (Figure 159-2). Frequently, there also is a purulent exudate with bloody mucus, an adherent membrane, or both. With chronic inflammation, one can expect to find loss of haustral markings associated with narrowing of the lumen and shortening of the colon. Colonoscopy is generally the preferred endoscopic test, but sigmoidoscopy is useful as an office procedure requiring little preparation or in the case of a severely ill UC patient. To complete the gastrointestinal investigation, a small bowel imaging study (i.e., small bowel follow-through, enteroclysis, or computed tomographic enterography) should be performed to exclude the possibility of disease of the small bowel.

COLORECTAL CANCER AND DYSPLASIA

Patients with UC are at increased risk of colorectal cancer (CRC).[26,27] In well-designed studies of population-based cohorts, the relative risk of CRC in UC is two to eight times higher than that in the general population.[28] The two most important risk factors for cancer are the duration of the colitis and the extent of colonic involvement.

The incidence of CRC increases with the duration of the disease.[29] The incidence rate varies widely, and, in general, population-based studies yield lower cancer incidence rates than referral center–based or hospital-based studies. A metaanalysis pooling the results of 116 observational studies of CRC risk in UC involving more than 54,000 patients concluded that annual CRC incidence was 0.2% in the first decade of disease, 0.7% in the second decade, and 1.2% in the third decade (Figure 159-3).[30] Altogether, the cumulative risk of CRC was

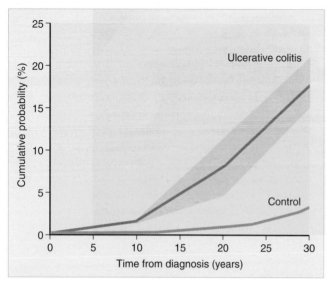

FIGURE 159-3 Cumulative risk of colorectal cancer in ulcerative colitis estimated from a metaanalysis of 116 studies. (Redrawn from Eaden JA, Abrams KR, Mayberry JF: The risk of colorectal cancer in ulcerative colitis: A meta-analysis. *Gut* 48:526, 2001.)

estimated to be 18% after 30 years of disease. Because the pooled analysis included referral center–based studies, the "real" absolute risk of CRC in UC may actually be lower than 18%.[30] Indeed, in several population-based cohort studies published after this metaanalysis, the risk of CRC is no higher than expected in the general population.[29,31,32] Whether variations in cancer incidence among population-based cohorts can be explained by differences in treatment policies (e.g., higher rates of 5-aminosalicylate use or higher colectomy rates) remains unclear.

The extent of the colitis is an important determinant of CRC risk in UC.[29] Patients with proctitis alone do not have a significantly increased risk of developing carcinoma relative to the background population.[28] Patients with pancolitis have the highest relative risk, and patients with left-sided colitis carry an intermediate risk.[28] Significant differences in CRC risk according to UC extent have been demonstrated both in referral center–based[26,27] and population-based studies.[28,33-35]

Whether age at onset of UC is a risk factor for CRC independent of duration of disease remains controversial.[29,30,36,37] Although some studies have suggested that childhood-onset UC has a higher risk of CRC, independent of duration,[36] at least one study has suggested that patients diagnosed in the sixth and seventh decades of life have a higher relative risk of CRC.[37]

Another controversial point is whether disease activity is a risk factor for colorectal neoplasia in UC.[38,39] Studies focusing on clinical activity (i.e., symptoms) could not demonstrate a relationship between disease activity and CRC.[40] Indeed, a common clinical scenario is the UC patient with clinically quiescent disease who is lost to followup and returns years later with a symptomatic malignancy. A study from St. Mark's Hospital, focusing on endoscopic and histologic activity (rather than symptoms), suggested that increased endoscopic activity was associated with a twofold increase in the risk of colorectal

neoplasia, whereas increased histologic activity increased the risk by a factor of five.[38]

Two additional risk factors warrant comment. The presence of concomitant primary sclerosing cholangitis (PSC) appears to be another important cancer risk factor.[41-43] It can be debated whether PSC is an independent risk factor or whether it is a marker for long-standing pancolitis. One study of newly diagnosed PSC patients with no history or symptoms of UC showed that the vast majority had subclinical pancolitis, and one patient already had low-grade dysplasia present.[44] Regardless of the mechanism for increased cancer risk, PSC-IBD patients are at high risk for CRC.[45] Family history of CRC (regardless of the family history of IBD) is another independent indicator of cancer risk in several studies, increasing the risk by a factor of at least two.[46,47]

Unlike sporadic CRC, which tends to occur more frequently within the left colon, cancers in UC patients are more evenly distributed throughout the colon.[48] There is a higher likelihood of synchronous tumors in UC-related CRC. These lesions are more likely to be mucinous and poorly differentiated. For these reasons, they may escape detection via colonoscopy or even at surgery. As a result, they tend to be discovered at a later stage. Another reason for the late detection of UC-related CRC is that the common symptoms of abdominal pain, change of bowel habit, bleeding, and mucous discharge are often attributed by both patient and physician to the underlying UC rather than to CRC.

Despite these differences in tumor characteristics, most recent studies show no significant differences between sporadic and UC-related CRC with respect to prognosis. The most recent study compared the prognosis of 241 UC patients with CRC diagnosed at the Mayo Clinic between 1976 and 1996 with the prognosis of a group of sporadic CRC patients matched on age at cancer diagnosis, gender, and cancer stage.[48] The 5-year survival in the UC-CRC group was 55%, compared to 53% in the sporadic CRC group.

In the past, prophylactic proctocolectomy was recommended for patients with long-standing disease, regardless of their disease activity, because of the risk of the development of cancer. However, with the availability of colonoscopy for surveillance of the entire colon and the recognition that premalignant changes on rectal biopsy were associated with CRC, the standard practice in the gastroenterology community is to recommend periodic colonoscopic surveillance in a search for premalignant lesions ("dysplasia") in the colonic epithelium. The objective of this course of action is to recognize dysplastic changes before the onset of carcinoma.

More than 25 years ago, the Inflammatory Bowel Disease–Dysplasia Morphology Study Group published a consensus report on the classification of colorectal dysplasia.[49] Histologic changes were classified as positive, negative, or indefinite for dysplasia. Definite dysplasia was further classified into low grade and high grade. There is reasonably good evidence that dysplastic change precedes frank carcinoma in most cases. Unfortunately, however, carcinoma may already be present when dysplastic changes are detected. It is also recognized that the pathologist may have difficulty deciding whether microscopic changes are due to the normal regenerative changes seen in UC or represent true dysplastic changes. Despite the availability of a standardized classification system for colorectal dysplasia for more than two decades, there remains considerable interobserver variability among pathologists for the finding of low-grade dysplasia.

Numerous professional societies have issued practice guidelines or consensus statements regarding the practice of surveillance colonoscopy in UC. A task force of the Crohn's and Colitis Foundation of America (CCFA), recommended surveillance colonoscopy every 1 to 2 years in patients with left-sided or extensive colitis with approximately 8 to 10 years of disease duration.[50] Patients with proctitis alone do not require surveillance, whereas patients with concomitant PSC should enter a surveillance program immediately regardless of UC duration. A medical position statement by the American Gastroenterological Association recommended a surveillance colonoscopy with extensive biopsies of all anatomic segments of colorectal mucosa a maximum of 8 years after onset of symptoms (regardless of extent), to be repeated every 1 to 3 years.[51]

The patient must be properly prepared for colonoscopy so that all of the mucosa can be visualized. The colonoscopy must be complete to the cecum, and the endoscopist must search for any suspicious plaque-like or nodular lesions. The CCFA consensus statement recommends that at least 33 random biopsies of the colon be obtained, typically in a four-quadrant fashion every 10 cm in the proximal colon and every 5 cm in the rectosigmoid.[49] At our institution, we obtain a total of 32 biopsies divided into four bottles (8 pieces from the cecum and ascending colon, 8 pieces from the transverse colon, 8 pieces from the descending colon and proximal sigmoid colon, and 8 pieces from the rectosigmoid). Visible lesions should be biopsied separately. Dysplasia may be present in grossly flat mucosa or may have a villous or nodular appearance. With accurate endoscopic and pathologic assessment of the mucosa, a reasonable course of management can be recommended to the patient.

Although there is broad consensus that patients with high-grade dysplasia should undergo immediate colectomy, there is no consensus on how to manage a finding of low-grade dysplasia.[50,51] Some recommend attempting to manage the disease medically and repeating colonoscopy and biopsy in 3 months. If there is no further dysplasia, the patient will undergo colonoscopy in 1 year. If low-grade dysplasia is again present, the patient will undergo repeat colonoscopy in 3 months, and if dysplasia is still present, serious consideration will be given to surgical intervention. However, others recommend colectomy for a finding of low-grade dysplasia, because several studies of patients with low-grade dysplasia have suggested that the actuarial rate of progression to high-grade dysplasia or cancer may be higher than 50% after 5 years.[52,53]

As the optical capabilities of endoscopes improve and our diagnostic awareness of dysplasia increases, we are beginning to understand that not all colorectal dysplasia in IBD is flat. Indeed, recent studies suggest that polypoid dysplasia is more common than flat dysplasia.[54]

Patients with "dysplasia-associated lesion or mass (DALM)" were once thought to be at a particularly high risk for synchronous or metachronous CRC. Blackstone et al reported that invasive carcinomas were present in 7 (28%) of 25 patients in whom mild dysplastic changes were found in so-called villous lesions.[55] However, more recent studies suggest that certain polypoid dysplastic lesions can be managed via endoscopic polypectomy.[56,57] If the lesion is well defined and amenable to endoscopic polypectomy, and if biopsies of the flat mucosa immediately surrounding the polypectomy site do not demonstrate dysplastic change, then these patients can be managed with close colonoscopic followup. For lesions that are not amenable to endoscopic polypectomy or have surrounding dysplasia, colectomy is recommended.

ACUTE SEVERE COLITIS

Although acute severe colitis is an uncommon form of UC, affecting approximately 15% of all patients with the disease, it can be life-threatening.[58] Fortunately, the mortality of acute severe colitis has dropped at referral centers over the past half-century from 30% to less than 5%, with increased recognition of the more toxic forms of the condition and with more intensive therapy.[59] Nevertheless, among those requiring hospitalization for acute severe colitis, approximately 30% require colectomy.[59] *Toxic megacolon*, the most fulminant form of acute colitis, is defined as a severe attack of colitis with total or segmental dilation of the colon (usually defined as a colonic diameter >5.5 cm on plain films). In a case series of 55 UC patients with toxic dilation, Jalan et al defined toxicity as the presence of any three of the following conditions: fever higher than 38.5° C, tachycardia (>120 beats/min), leukocytosis (>10,500 cells), and anemia (hemoglobin <60% of normal).[60] In addition, one of the following conditions must have been present: dehydration, mental changes, electrolyte disturbances, or hypotension. This degree of toxicity, coupled with clinical or radiographic evidence of colonic distention, completes the presentation of toxic megacolon.

Toxic megacolon can complicate long-standing UC or can occur in patients presenting with their first attack. Various precipitating factors for toxic megacolon have been identified, including antidiarrheal agents, opioid analgesics, barium enema, and electrolyte abnormalities (including hypokalemia). The cause is unknown but is thought to be due to a paralysis of the myenteric plexus, perhaps resulting from transmural inflammation occurring acutely.

Toxic dilation of the colon is generally considered the most serious complication of UC. The colon loses its ability to contract and becomes widely distended, resulting in a thinned wall in danger of perforation. The most common sites of perforation are around the peritoneal attachments of the splenic flexure and at the cecum.

The clinical presentation of toxic megacolon is dramatic. Patients may suddenly become acutely ill with rapid progression of symptoms that include fever, mental aberrations, tachycardia, tachypnea, and bloody diarrhea. Abdominal pain may be diffuse and severe but may be lacking, particularly in patients who are taking high-dose corticosteroids. Sigmoidoscopy may reveal changes typical of UC. Biopsies should be obtained, and the pathologist should be instructed to exclude the possibility of cytomegalovirus superinfection as a cause of the exacerbation.[17] A stool sample for *C. difficile* toxin should be obtained, as *C. difficile* toxin can be recovered from approximately 20% of patients with UC exacerbations, and treatment with metronidazole or vancomycin frequently results in improvement.[16] The diagnosis of toxic megacolon can usually be made on a plain radiograph of the abdomen, which shows dilation of the large bowel. Although colonoscopy appears to be surprisingly safe in "garden variety" acute severe colitis, it remains contraindicated in the patient with toxic megacolon.[61]

Patients who present with signs of localized or generalized peritonitis, radiographic evidence of perforation, or systemic instability should undergo immediate surgery. Otherwise, intensive medical management, consisting of high-dose parenteral steroids and intravenous (IV) fluids, should be initiated immediately. Patients tend to be dehydrated and may have electrolyte imbalances because of losses from vomiting and diarrhea. These imbalances must be corrected, and the patients who are anemic should undergo transfusion. Restriction of oral intake is initiated along with nasogastric suction to avoid further intestinal distention. Although randomized trials have not shown convincing benefit, broad-spectrum antibiotics are frequently administered in this setting because of the potential for bacteremia or microperforation.

The patient with toxic megacolon must be observed very closely with serial physical examinations every 2 to 4 hours and serial plain films of the abdomen daily. The timing of surgery in toxic megacolon remains controversial, with some authors advocating early colectomy (i.e., shortly after recognition of toxic megacolon) and others noting little or no mortality by treating with IV corticosteroids and antibiotics for up to 7 days in patients who appear to be improving. Most authors agree that patients who are not improving or are deteriorating need surgery urgently. Several studies indicate that the presence of more than eight stools daily, or a combination of elevated C-reactive protein (>4.5 mg/dL) and more than three stools daily, on the third hospital day predict colectomy in about 85%.[62,63] Close followup by both the medical and surgical teams, with open lines of communication between the two, is required.

MASSIVE HEMORRHAGE

Although rectal bleeding is a common symptom of UC, massive hemorrhage that necessitates rapid blood transfusion and emergency treatment is unusual, occurring in fewer than 5% of patients. Most frequently, it occurs in patients with acute severe colitis. The treatment of these patients is usually twofold. First, treatment of the UC necessitates the use of high-dose steroids and other supportive measures. Second, the bleeding must be treated expeditiously and any coagulation abnormality corrected. In most patients, hemorrhage subsides spontaneously. It is unusual that the bleeding originates from a discrete site. The indication for surgery is not arbitrary but must be individualized for each patient. Once the decision is made to operate, the standard procedure has

been proctocolectomy. However, this procedure, as previously mentioned, can be associated with higher mortality and morbidity rates than subtotal colectomy and it obviates the possibility of a reconstructive procedure in the future. Thus, in selected cases, one might consider a total abdominal colectomy, leaving a short rectal stump, sufficient to allow future reconstructive surgery. In most instances, this type of surgery controls the bleeding, although continuing massive hemorrhage can still occur in approximately 10% to 12% of patients.

CROHN (GRANULOMATOUS) COLITIS

EPIDEMIOLOGY AND ETIOPATHOGENESIS

Crohn disease is the other major subtype of idiopathic IBD. Crohn disease results in transmural, often granulomatous, inflammation that can occur anywhere in the gastrointestinal tract, and it has a propensity to cause intestinal fistulas and/or strictures. It is now well accepted that Crohn disease of the large and small intestine is one disease, but it is separate and distinct from UC. The incidence and prevalence of Crohn disease are similar to that of UC. The adjusted incidence of Crohn disease was approximately 6 cases per 100,000 person-years in the 1990s,[1] and 12.4 per 100,000 in 2001 to 2004.[2] The adjusted prevalence on January 1, 2005, was 214 cases per 100,000 persons.[2] Extrapolating these figures to the 2010 U.S. population suggests that about 38,000 patients are diagnosed annually and that there are approximately 660,000 people with Crohn disease.[2] As is the case with UC, Crohn disease appears to be more common in whites, especially Jews, less common in African Americans, and more frequent in populations of westernized cultures than those of Africans and Asians.[64] However, many studies suggest that these differences are narrowing over time. For example, one pediatric study from Atlanta suggested that Crohn disease was as common among African American children as among whites. Studies from Japan, South Korea, Singapore, and now India suggest that IBD is becoming more common in these areas, too.[64]

In contrast to UC, cigarette smoking is a risk factor for Crohn disease,[12] and patients with Crohn disease who smoke have a more severe clinical course (i.e., requiring more corticosteroids, immunosuppressive agents, and surgery) than those who do not.[13,65] Similar to UC, a family history of IBD is one of the strongest risk factors for Crohn disease identified.[5,6] Studies of twin registries suggest a strong genetic component in the pathogenesis of Crohn disease—approximately 50% of monozygotic twin pairs are concordant for the disease versus only 20% concordance among dizygotic twins.[7-9] The identification in 2001 of the *CARD15/NOD2* mutations provided the first definitive genetic link to the condition.[66-68] Up to 40% of Crohn disease patients carry at least one of three mutations in this gene, which appears to encode a protein important in the innate immune system (pattern recognition of muramyl dipeptide). As mentioned previously, multiple other susceptibility genes have been identified. These genes seem to fall under several categories: other pattern recognition receptors (TLR4, CARD9), autophagy genes (ATG16L1 and IGRM), Th17 lymphocyte differentiation (IL-23R, JAK2), barrier function genes (IBD5, DLG5), and genes important in adaptive immunity (HLA, TNFSF15).[69] The fact that these particular genes are linked to Crohn disease has provided clues to the etiopathogenesis, but it will take years to understand the functional implications of mutations in these genes.

Crohn disease primarily affects young individuals, with the median age at diagnosis being in the late 20s.[3] There may be a slight female predominance in Crohn disease, in contrast to the slight male predominance seen in UC. Approximately 40% to 50% of Crohn disease patients have both small bowel and colonic involvement, 20% have isolated small bowel (usually ileal) involvement, and one-third have colonic disease alone.[70] Disease in which the colon is primarily involved may occur more frequently in patients diagnosed at a somewhat older age.

The colon may be involved with Crohn disease in one of several ways. First, the colon alone may be the site of Crohn disease. The large bowel may be involved in its entirety, but more often there is segmental disease, with sparing of the rectum and part of the sigmoid. In addition to Crohn colitis, there may be involvement of the small bowel. This form of ileocolitis is the most common type of Crohn disease. The colon may become involved with Crohn disease only after surgery for ileitis, but this is not particularly common, because most recurrences appear proximal to the ileocolonic anastomosis. Finally, the colon may be involved indirectly via fistula formation from a loop of small bowel that is the site of the primary disease. In this case, most commonly there is no primary disease in the colon but only secondary inflammation from the disease in the small intestine.

PATHOLOGIC FEATURES

Crohn colitis typically involves all layers of the bowel wall as a transmural reaction (Figure 159-4). This transmural reaction may be noted grossly but is present in the early phases of the disease when only microscopic changes are noted.[22] Although the gross and microscopic features of Crohn disease are well established, there is no pathognomonic feature. The features of UC and Crohn disease are listed in Table 159-1. In approximately 10% to 15% of patients, it may be difficult to unequivocally differentiate Crohn disease from UC. The term *indeterminate colitis* has been used in these cases in which a definitive pathologic diagnosis cannot be made.[71]

On macroscopic examination, the bowel wall appears to be thickened, particularly in the submucosal layer (see Table 159-1).[22] There is a corresponding narrowing of the lumen. Edema, thickening, and overgrowth of the mesenteric fat encroaching on the serosal aspect of the bowel wall are extremely common in Crohn disease of both the small and large intestine (Figure 159-5). The serosa tends to be hyperemic, and there are chronic subserosal inflammatory changes with exudate production. Mesenteric lymphadenopathy may be present. The gross appearance of the mucosal surface varies depending on the extent and severity of the disease. The mucosa may appear to be normal except for hyperemia and edema, or there may be longitudinal ulcers that cause the mucosal surface to have a cobblestone appearance. The ulcers vary in depth but usually extend at least to

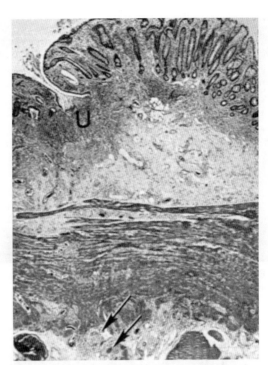

FIGURE 159-4 Crohn disease of the colon. Transmural involvement is present with mucosal ulceration *(U)*, edema of the entire bowel wall, and serosal noncaseating granulomas *(arrows)* (hematoxylin-eosin, ×25). (Courtesy Stanley Hamilton, MD, Department of Pathology, School of Medicine, Johns Hopkins University, Baltimore, Md.)

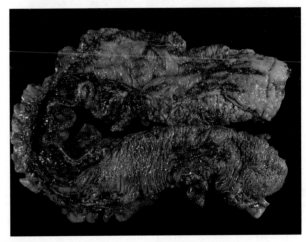

FIGURE 159-5 Crohn disease of the colon. A spectrum of inflammatory patterns are seen. "Skip areas" are present, characterized by ulceration with intervening areas of more normal-appearing colon. There is stricture formation within the transverse colon, and linear ulcerations are present distally. (Courtesy Jason T. Lewis, MD.)

the submucosa and often to the serosa (Figure 159-6). Because of this, frequently other loops of intestine adhere to the involved segment, and fistulas may occur. In addition, skip areas may be seen.

Microscopic changes include infiltration of inflammatory cells in all layers and marked submucosal and subserosal thickening and intramural fissures that can

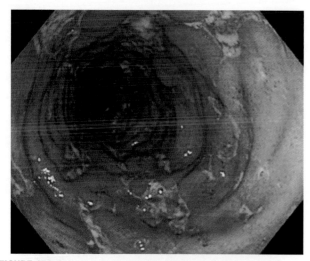

FIGURE 159-6 Endoscopic view of Crohn colitis with loss of vascular pattern, erythema, edema, and longitudinal ulcers.

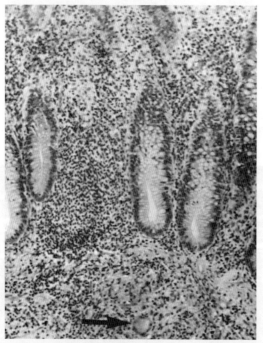

FIGURE 159-7 Crohn disease of the colon. A noncaseating granuloma with epithelioid macrophages and a multinucleated giant cell *(arrow)* is present in the submucosa (hematoxylin-eosin, ×160). (Courtesy Stanley Hamilton, MD, Department of Pathology, School of Medicine, Johns Hopkins University, Baltimore, Md.)

extend through to the mesenteric fat (see Table 159-1). Giant cells or epithelioid granulomas may occur either intramurally or within regional lymph nodes (Figure 159-7). Other histologic findings include transmural fibrosis, submucosal lymphangiectasia, chronic serositis when there has been no prior surgery, muscle wall thickening (more than twice that of normal), and segmental involvement.

CLINICAL FEATURES

Symptoms of Crohn colitis include diarrhea, midabdominal and lower abdominal crampy pain, malaise, and weight loss.[25] Other symptoms and clinical findings include fever, rectal bleeding, anemia, nausea, and vomiting. Occasionally, patients may present with symptoms suggestive of an acute abdomen. It is now recognized that toxic megacolon can complicate Crohn colitis as well as other forms of colitis. Extraintestinal manifestations are common, with musculoskeletal manifestations being the most frequent.

Clinically, Crohn colitis often has an extremely variable onset and course. Although diarrhea is a dominant feature of both UC and Crohn colitis, colonic bleeding is less common with Crohn disease.[25] However, massive bleeding from acute Crohn colitis can occur on occasion. Colonic sinuses, fistulas, and strictures are characteristic of Crohn colitis. However, these internal complications do not occur as frequently in colon disease as they do in terminal ileum disease.

Perianal Crohn disease is a frequent complication. It is an extremely troublesome problem and difficult to treat successfully. Population-based studies suggest that up to 40% of Crohn disease patients develop perianal involvement at some point during their clinical course.[72] The perianal lesions can precede the clinical appearance of the colitis by a variable number of years. Perianal Crohn disease has been classified into the following categories: skin lesions, anal canal lesions, fistulas, and hemorrhoids.[73] *Skin lesions* include maceration, erosion, ulceration, abscess formation, and skin tags. Because of the frequency of diarrhea in this disease, the skin around the anus may become macerated, leading to ulceration and subcutaneous abscess formation. Skin tags are frequent manifestations. They tend to be edematous and larger, thicker, and harder than those seen in patients without Crohn disease. *Anal canal lesions* include fissures, ulcers, and stenosis of the anal canal. The fissures tend to be deep and wide, with undermined edges. The fissures may be eccentrically placed in any position around the anus, in contrast to uncomplicated midline fissures in patients who do not have Crohn disease. *Fistulas* and *abscesses* are perhaps the most difficult of the perianal lesions to treat. They may arise from an infected anal gland, as in patients without Crohn disease. More commonly, however, they result from penetration by anal canal or rectal fissures or ulcers. The most superficial fistulas can be treated in a conventional manner, but more complex fistulas may have a high internal opening with multiple indirect tracts opening on the buttocks or scrotum. Fistulas tend to be chronic, indurated, and cyanotic, but despite their appearance, they are often painless. If the patient does complain of pain, one should suspect an abscess.

Rectovaginal fistulas can also complicate Crohn disease and tend to result from direct penetration of rectal wall fistulas into the vagina. They are a relatively frequent complication of severe perianal disease, with rates varying from 3.5% to 20%.[74-76] Quite frequently, these fistulas are asymptomatic, and no surgical intervention should be attempted. However, if the patient is symptomatic, surgery is indicated. Various local procedures have been described, but none are extremely successful. Some patients require proctectomy (see Chapters 147 and 161).

DIAGNOSIS OF CROHN COLITIS

Endoscopic evaluation of the colon and rectum is essential. Colonoscopy is particularly important to determine the extent of the disease and is more sensitive than radiographic examination. The often discontinuous nature of Crohn colitis can be seen better with the colonoscope than on barium enema. All patients who undergo surgery for Crohn disease, including those with presumed ileitis, should undergo a preoperative colonoscopy to fully determine the extent of the disease. The endoscopic appearance of Crohn colitis is usually quite different from that of UC. The rectum is spared in approximately 50% of patients with large bowel involvement. Depending on the extent and severity of the disease, there may be isolated aphthous ulcers with normal intervening mucosa, or there may be irregular mucosal thickening, congestion, edema, and a cobblestone appearance with deep linear ulcerations and fistulas. Pathognomonic histologic features of Crohn disease (i.e., granulomas) are present only infrequently.

Radiographic features characteristic of Crohn colitis are similar to those seen in terminal ileum disease. The radiographic features that substantiate the diagnosis of Crohn colitis include skip areas, longitudinal ulcerations, transverse fissures, eccentric involvement, pseudodiverticula, narrowing, strictures, pseudopolypoid changes, a cobblestone pattern, internal fistulas, sinus tracts, and intramural fistulas that extend parallel to the lumen of the thickened bowel (Figure 159-8). Any portion of the colon may be involved with Crohn colitis. The segment least frequently involved is the rectum. Skip areas must be sought carefully, because discontinuous involvement may be limited to one wall, may appear as a nodular filling defect, or may involve straightening and rigidity of a short segment of the colon. The combination of longitudinal ulcers, edematous mucosa, and transverse linear ulcers produces the cobblestone pattern previously described. Transverse linear ulcers may penetrate so deeply into the wall of the colon that they appear in contour as numerous long, thin spicules perpendicular to the long axis of the bowel or as a sinus tract. They may ultimately lead to small intramural abscesses or fistulas. A small bowel enema or enteroclysis should be included as part of the workup in patients with Crohn colitis to document the total extent of the disease.

CROHN COLITIS AND COLORECTAL CANCER

Crohn colitis has been recognized as a condition predisposing to the development of CRC. The risk of developing carcinoma in Crohn disease is not as well defined as in UC, with relative risks in well-designed population-based studies ranging from no increased risk[77-80] to a sixfold elevation.[81] Carcinoma may also occur in chronic perianal fistulas. Although the incidence of cancer in Crohn colitis is increased, it is still unclear how frequently these patients should be followed with surveillance colonoscopy and biopsies. Our recommendations for patients with Crohn colitis are similar to those for patients with chronic UC of similar extent (see earlier).

THERAPY OF ULCERATIVE COLITIS AND CROHN DISEASE

Although traditional drugs such as corticosteroids, sulfasalazine (Azulfidine), and 5-aminosalicylic acid (5-ASA) compounds are the mainstays of the medical

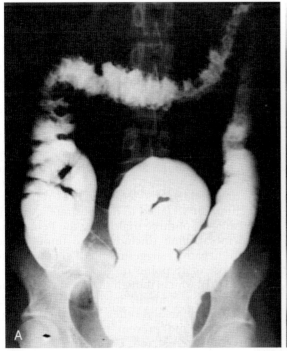
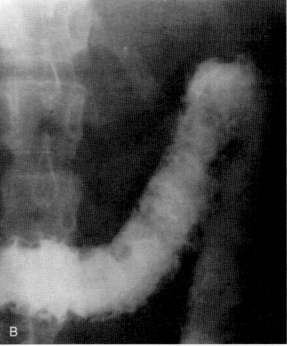

FIGURE 159-8 Granulomatous colitis. **A,** Barium enema showing segmented colonic narrowing and mucosal ulceration, especially of the proximal descending colon. **B,** Barium enema showing intramural fistulous tract of medial aspect of distal transverse colon.

management of IBD (especially UC), many other modalities and drugs are used, including antibiotics, the purine analogues azathioprine and 6-mercaptopurine, methotrexate, cyclosporine, and biologic agents such as anti-TNF-α agents and monoclonal antibodies to adhesion molecules.

SULFASALAZINE AND 5-AMINOSALICYLIC ACID COMPOUNDS

Sulfasalazine is composed of sulfapyridine linked to 5-ASA by an azo bond. It is poorly absorbed in the upper gastrointestinal tract and is degraded into its two components by colonic bacteria containing azoreductase. The 5-ASA moiety is the active antiinflammatory compound of sulfasalazine, whereas sulfapyridine acts only as the carrier for 5-ASA.[82] It is the sulfapyridine moiety to which many patients have side effects and allergic reactions. Various 5-ASA compounds have been developed and have been shown to be as effective as sulfasalazine but with reduced side effects. Olsalazine (Dipentum) is a 5-ASA dimer joined by an azo bond. Mesalamine, or 5-ASA alone, is commercially available in four delivery systems in the United States. Asacol is mesalamine coated with an acrylic-based resin, Eudragit S, which does not dissolve until the luminal pH rises to 7.0 or higher. In general, this agent is released in the terminal ileum and colon. Pentasa is an ethylcellulose-coated, controlled-release formulation of mesalamine. Approximately 20% to 30% of this agent is released and absorbed in the small bowel, with the remainder delivered to the colon. Lialda is mesalamine embedded within a multimatrix system of hydrophobic and lipophilic matrices enclosed in a pH-dependent coating (similar to the coating in Asacol). The hydrophilic matrix results in swelling and formation of a viscous gel mass which is thought to slow the diffusion of drug and result in sustained release throughout the colon. Apriso is a gelatin capsule containing microgranules of mesalamine embedded within a polymer matrix. Each microgranule is coated with a pH-dependent coating that dissolves when the luminal pH is above 6. Finally, balsalazide (Colazal) is a non-sulfa 5-ASA prodrug, containing 5-ASA and 4-aminobenzoyl-β-alanine joined by an azo bond. Free active 5-ASA is released in the colon similar to sulfasalazine and olsalazine. Mesalamine in enema formulation (Rowasa) is efficacious in mildly to moderately active left-sided UC and proctitis. Mesalamine suppositories (Canasa) are efficacious for active ulcerative proctitis.

Sulfasalazine and the 5-ASA compounds inhibit various products of the metabolism of arachidonic acid (e.g., prostaglandin G_2, leukotriene B_4, and thromboxane A_2)—all known to play a major role in the inflammatory process in the intestinal mucosa.[83] They also decrease the synthesis of other inflammatory cytokines (IL-1 and TNF-α) and inhibit the action of IFN.

Sulfasalazine

Sulfasalazine is the oldest and the least expensive 5-ASA compound in use. In a low dosage (1 to 2 g/day), it is used to maintain remission in patients with UC, whereas in a higher dosage (4 to 6 g/day), it can be used to treat active UC.[84] In Crohn disease, the efficacy of sulfasalazine is less clear and depends on the site of the disease. Because sulfasalazine is cleaved into its active compounds in the colon, its use is limited to Crohn disease with ileocolonic or colonic involvement.[85-87] It is of little known benefit in isolated small bowel disease. A recent meta-analysis of 5-ASA therapies in Crohn disease found a trend toward benefit of sulfasalazine over placebo for induction of remission of Crohn disease, but no evidence of benefit in maintaining remission.[85]

Adverse events following sulfasalazine therapy are common and include nausea, headaches, malaise, and vomiting.[88] These side effects can be minimized or prevented by initiation of therapy with a low starting dose (500 mg every 6 to 12 hours) and gradual increase in the dosage. Hypersensitivity reaction to sulfasalazine can cause rash, fever, hemolytic anemia, and hepatotoxicity. We typically coadminister folic acid 1 mg daily to prevent folate deficiency. The drug may cause a reversible but clinically significant azoospermia in men, so discontinuation of the drug should be considered in the family planning stage. This particular effect is not seen with the non-sulfa 5-ASA compounds.

Olsalazine

Olsalazine delivers intact 5-ASA to the terminal ileum, which is then cleaved by the colonic bacteria to free 5-ASA. Olsalazine has been shown to be of benefit in the maintenance of remission of patients with UC, although in a recent systematic review that excluded lower quality trials, it was not significantly better than placebo.[84] At higher doses, it may result in a watery secretory diarrhea.[88] No therapeutic benefit has been shown in patients with mild to moderate attacks of Crohn disease.[85]

Mesalamine

At a dosage of 2.4 to 4.8 g/day (usually given in three to four divided doses), mesalamine has been shown to be efficacious in patients for both induction and maintenance of remission of mildly to moderately active UC.[84] Mesalamine enemas at dosages of 1 to 4 g/day are effective in treating patients with distal UC, whereas patients with limited ulcerative proctitis can benefit from mesalamine suppositories at a dosage of 500 mg twice a day.[89]

The role of mesalamine for treatment of mildly to moderately active Crohn disease remains controversial. Although mesalamine at dosages between 3.2 and 4 g/day has been associated with clinical improvement or remission in mildly to moderately active Crohn disease,[90,91] other studies have failed to demonstrate a benefit.[92,93] A pooled analysis of three trials using the Pentasa formulation of mesalamine (including two unpublished trials that were negative) suggested that Pentasa resulted in a net decrease of 18 points on the Crohn Disease Activity Index (CDAI), which, though statistically significant, may not represent a clinically meaningful response.[93] The role of mesalamine and other 5-ASA therapies to maintain remission and prevent relapse in Crohn disease remains controversial, too. The most recent metaanalysis to examine the role of 5-ASA therapies in Crohn disease could not demonstrate that mesalamine provided any benefit in either inducing or maintaining remission.[85] A less rigorous per-protocol analysis of these trials suggested a modest benefit in maintaining remission, however.[85] Mesalamine does not carry an indication approved by the U.S. Food and Drug Administration (FDA) for the treatment of Crohn disease.

Potential adverse events from mesalamine therapy include headache, abdominal pain, nausea, and diarrhea.[88] Mesalamine can less commonly cause hypersensitivity colitis, pancreatitis, pleuritis, interstitial pneumonitis, interstitial nephritis, and hepatotoxicity.

Balsalazide

Balsalazide at a dosage of 6.75 g/day (in three divided doses) has been shown to be effective for the treatment of mildly to moderately active UC.[84] Adverse events include headache, abdominal pain, nausea, and diarrhea.[88] Rare reports of aggravation of colitis, pancreatitis, and hepatotoxicity have been described.

CORTICOSTEROIDS

The benefit of corticosteroid therapy for UC was first reported in a randomized trial by Truelove and Witts.[94] Corticosteroids still remain the cornerstone of medical treatment of moderately to severely active IBD. Their broad mechanism of action occurs through modification of gene expression, ultimately resulting in inhibition of proinflammatory cytokines; repression of phospholipase A, cyclooxygenase-2, and nitric oxide synthase; and inhibition of adhesion molecules.[83] The end result is reduction in leukocyte migration and inhibition of multiple inflammatory mediators.[83]

The initial treatment in patients with moderate to severe UC is prednisone at 40 to 60 mg daily. In severely ill, hospitalized patients, initial therapy consists of hydrocortisone 100 mg IV three times daily or its equivalent. Standard corticosteroids were found to be significantly better than placebo for induction of remission of UC in a recent metaanalysis.[95] Corticosteroids are also effective in the treatment of moderate to severe Crohn disease. In the National Cooperative Crohn's Disease Study, prednisone administered at dosages of 0.25 to 0.75 mg/kg/day to 85 patients with active Crohn disease resulted in remission in 60% of patients compared with a rate of only 30% in a placebo group.[86] A metaanalysis of placebo-controlled trials found that corticosteroids were more effective than placebo for inducing remission in Crohn disease, but because of significant heterogeneity across studies these results did not meet statistical significance.[95] Although corticosteroids are highly effective in the short term for inducing remission, only a few patients remain in remission off corticosteroids over the longer term.[96,97] Studies of population-based cohorts in the preimmunosuppressive era suggest that approximately one-third of patients receiving corticosteroids will be steroid dependent and about one-third will have required surgical resection at the end of 1 year.[96,97] These studies highlight the need for early and aggressive use of steroid-sparing medications in IBD patients whose disease is active enough to require corticosteroids.

The systemic side effects of conventional corticosteroids have led to the development of modified formulations that are more potent and more rapidly metabolized. Modified corticosteroids offer the promise of being as effective as traditional corticosteroids and have fewer systemic side effects. Similar to 5-ASA preparations, different packaging of these agents is available, which offers the possibility of drug delivery to the small bowel and the colon with minimum side effects. Oral delayed-release budesonide (Entocort EC) is the most notable of these new corticosteroids.[98] This controlled ileal release formulation is indicated for induction of remission in mildly to moderately active Crohn disease involving the ileum or right colon. In one head-to-head study, budesonide at 9 mg/day was more efficacious than mesalamine 4 g/day for this indication.[99] A metaanalysis found that budesonide was significantly better than placebo for inducing remission in Crohn disease, but it did not prevent relapse of Crohn disease.[95]

Topical corticosteroids may be of benefit in patients with either limited distal disease or with rectal involvement along with more proximal disease.[89] Corticosteroid enemas or foams can be used for the treatment of active disease, but no role in maintenance therapy has been proved.

ANTIBIOTICS

Multiple lines of evidence suggest that bacteria may play a role in the pathogenesis of IBD, perhaps because of an unusual response of the mucosal immune system to normal intestinal flora, or a breakdown in the intestinal defenses allowing microorganisms to invade the intestinal mucosa.[100] Some have even hypothesized that a specific bacteria such as *Mycobacterium avium* subspecies *paratuberculosis* may be responsible for Crohn disease, but this remains extremely controversial.[3]

In patients with UC, both IV and oral antibiotics have been studied in placebo-controlled trials. A wide variety of antibiotics and combinations thereof have been investigated. A recent pooled analysis of nine randomized placebo-controlled trials found a modest benefit for antibiotics over placebo for induction of remission of UC, although moderate heterogeneity across trials was noted.[101] At the present time, oral antibiotics are not routinely prescribed for UC; however, the results of this recent metaanalysis, and the wide heterogeneity across studies, suggest that additional studies need to be performed to better understand the role of oral antibiotics in mildly to moderately active UC.

Similarly, evidence for antibiotic use in Crohn disease from individual randomized, controlled trials is limited. As in the case of UC, a wide variety of antimicrobials and combinations have been employed. However, a metaanalysis of 10 placebo-controlled trials of antibiotics for induction of remission in Crohn disease demonstrated a modest benefit.[101] Interestingly, subgroup analyses of studies containing rifamycin derivatives or clofazimine appeared to show the most benefit.[101] A pooled analysis of three trials examining the role of antibiotics in maintaining Crohn disease remission also showed a significant benefit.[101] These results would be in keeping with the concept that IBD results from the interplay between the fecal microbiome and both innate and adaptive immunity of the gut.

IMMUNOSUPPRESSIVE AGENTS

Immunosuppressive agents such as azathioprine/6-mercaptopurine and methotrexate are being increasingly used to treat IBD patients who do not respond to first-line therapies or who are steroid dependent or steroid refractory. In general, the threshold to use these agents is lower in Crohn disease than in UC, likely a reflection of the relatively poor efficacy of first-line agents such as 5-ASA drugs in maintaining remission in Crohn disease. These drugs are thought to act by blocking the proliferation and activation of the T-helper lymphocytes, which play a major role in the inflammatory cascade through the production of various cytokines such as IL-1, IL-2, IL-6, IL-8, TNF-α, and IFN-γ.[83]

Azathioprine and 6-Mercaptopurine

Azathioprine (Imuran, Azasan) and 6-mercaptopurine (Purinethol) are thiopurine compounds used in the management of steroid-dependent IBD, steroid-refractory IBD, and fistulizing Crohn disease. They act either via inhibition of purine RNA synthesis and cell proliferation or via inhibition of natural killer cells and suppression of cytotoxic T-cell functions.[83] Azathioprine is a prodrug of 6-mercaptopurine, and both drugs are converted via several enzymatic steps to the 6-thioguanine nucleotides, which are thought to be the active metabolites. These mechanisms of action likely explain the 3- to 4-month delay in the onset of their clinical effectiveness. One of the inactivating enzymes in the metabolism of these agents, thiopurine methyltransferase (TPMT), has a trimodal distribution of activity in the population.[102] About 89% of patients have normal TPMT activity, 11% have intermediate activity, and 1 in 300 persons have minimal or no enzyme activity, such that normal doses of purine analogues can result in prolonged bone marrow suppression and fatal infectious complications. Many physicians routinely obtain a TPMT genotype or enzyme activity level prior to initiation of these agents to better predict a dosage that will not result in early leukopenia.

Azathioprine and 6-mercaptopurine are both used in the management of patients with active Crohn disease and UC who have not responded to systemic steroids.[103,104] In addition, both drugs have been successfully used as steroid-sparing agents in patients with IBD who are unable to be weaned from steroid therapy.[103,104] Although a previous Cochrane metaanalysis had found that azathioprine and 6-mercaptopurine were more effective than placebo for inducing remission in active Crohn disease,[105] a more recent pooled analysis using more rigorous endpoints could not demonstrate a statistically significant benefit.[106] These drugs also appear to be moderately effective for maintaining remission in Crohn disease.[106] Similarly, although previous systematic reviews of thiopurines for inducing remission in ulcerative colitis suggested modest benefit,[107,108] a more recent pooled analysis could not demonstrate this.[106] For IBD patients with normal TPMT levels, the typical dose of azathioprine is 2 to 2.5 mg/kg body weight daily and the dose of 6-mercaptopurine is 1 to 1.5 mg/kg body weight daily. The typical dose of these agents in those with intermediate TPMT levels is half that of patients with normal enzyme activity.

Unfortunately, observational studies suggest that 20% to 25% of IBD patients taking these agents need to discontinue them because of adverse events.[109] Among the side effects of azathioprine and 6-mercaptopurine are pancreatitis, which occurs in approximately 3% of patients, usually presents within the first 6 weeks of therapy, and resolves promptly when the drug is withdrawn.[110] Other adverse events include nausea, fatigue, and hepatotoxicity, all of which seem to be dose related. Other idiosyncratic reactions that can occur include fever, influenza-like symptoms, and abdominal pain. Patients on these agents should undergo monthly complete blood counts to monitor for leukopenia, and quarterly hepatic biochemistries to monitor for hepatotoxicity. Like all immunosuppressive agents, these drugs seem to be associated with an increased risk of non-Hodgkin lymphoma. A metaanalysis of observational studies suggested a three- to fourfold increased relative risk,[111] and a multicenter French study of almost 20,000 patients with IBD found that current thiopurine use was associated with a fivefold increased risk of lymphoma.[112] However, the absolute risk of lymphoma remains low (approximately 1 case per 1600 person-years or less), and decision analysis models suggest that the benefit far outweighs the risk in properly selected patients.[113]

Methotrexate

Methotrexate acts via inhibition of dihydrofolate reductase to impair DNA synthesis and reduce production of IL-1, IL-6, and TNF-α.[83] A multicenter, placebo-controlled trial with 141 patients with active Crohn disease confirmed that methotrexate at a dosage of 25 mg administered intramuscularly or subcutaneously once a week, over 16 weeks, allowed steroid tapering and maintenance of remission in 39% of patients treated compared with 19% in those receiving placebo.[114] A subsequent trial randomized Crohn disease patients with methotrexate-induced remission to continued methotrexate at 15 mg weekly or placebo.[115] Patients receiving methotrexate were significantly less likely to experience relapse (35%) compared to those receiving placebo (61%). A randomized trial of methotrexate in ulcerative colitis failed to demonstrate efficacy[116]; however, methotrexate was administered orally, not parenterally, and the dose may have been too low. At the present time, the routine use of methotrexate in steroid-dependent or steroid-refractory UC is not recommended.

Potential side effects of methotrexate include leukopenia, requiring monthly monitoring of the blood count, and hepatic fibrosis, necessitating monthly hepatic biochemistries. Patients with risk factors for fatty liver disease (e.g., obesity, diabetes mellitus, ethanol use) and those with persistent elevations in hepatic biochemistries should undergo percutaneous liver biopsy. Methotrexate-induced pneumonitis is occasionally encountered, so patients who develop cough or fever while on this agent should be investigated thoroughly.

Cyclosporine and Tacrolimus

Cyclosporine is a potent immunosuppressive drug that is used in organ transplantation as well as "rescue therapy" in patients with acute severe UC.[117] It blocks transcription of cytokines that activate T-helper lymphocytes, thus inhibiting the production and liberation of proinflammatory cytokines.[83] IV cyclosporine has been shown to be effective in the short term in patients with acute severe colitis.[118] The major problem with the drug is that although short-term improvement may be achieved, long-term maintenance with the oral form of the drug produces excessive side effects.[118] Side effects and toxicity of treatment with cyclosporine include electrolyte abnormalities, seizures, paresthesias, hypertrichosis, nephrotoxicity, hypertension, tremors, and headaches, which can occur in up to 60% of patients treated.[83] Fatal opportunistic infections have been reported with the use of this agent; therefore, the risks of cyclosporine therapy must be weighed against the benefits on a case-by-case basis.

INFLIXIMAB AND OTHER BIOLOGIC THERAPIES

It would not be an exaggeration to state that the availability of infliximab (Remicade), a chimeric monoclonal antibody to TNF-α, has significantly altered the way gastroenterologists treat steroid-dependent, steroid-refractory, and fistulizing Crohn disease. Randomized trials have established that infliximab is effective for inducing and maintaining remission of Crohn disease in patients who failed to respond to conventional therapy[119,120] and that the antibody significantly reduces the number of open, draining perianal and enterocutaneous fistulas and maintains this response.[121,122] Endoscopic studies suggest that infliximab is associated with a significant reduction in endoscopic activity of Crohn disease and in some cases is associated with complete mucosal healing.[123] Patients receiving infliximab on a regularly scheduled basis appear significantly less likely to require hospitalization and surgery.[124,125] Trials in patients with moderate to severe UC also demonstrated efficacy.[126] Infliximab is approved by the FDA for both Crohn disease and ulcerative colitis.

The typical starting dose of infliximab is an infusion of 5 mg/kg body weight over a 2- to 4-hour period. A three-dose induction is administered at 0, 2, and 6 weeks, and maintenance doses are administered every 8 weeks thereafter. The chimeric nature of the molecule results in immunogenicity, which may result in the formation of antibodies to infliximab. These antibodies are associated with infusion reactions and, more important, a loss of response to the drug over time.[127] For this reason, maintenance use (and not episodic use) of the drug is strongly recommended. Many physicians routinely coadminister a concomitant immunosuppressive such as azathioprine, 6-mercaptopurine, or methotrexate because there is considerable evidence that this will further reduce the risk of antibody formation.[128] Some physicians also administer corticosteroids as IV premedication to reduce antibody formation on the basis of a randomized trial.[129]

Adverse events following infliximab therapy have included serious (and sometimes fatal) infections including tuberculosis, histoplasmosis, coccidioidomycosis, listeriosis, and *Pneumocystis carinii* pneumonia.[129] Hepatotoxicity, worsening of congestive heart failure, serious hematologic events, demyelinating disorders (e.g., multiple sclerosis and optic neuritis), and

malignancies (lymphoma, lung malignancies) have been reported following the use of the drug. As with all immunosuppressive agents, the potential benefits of infliximab need to be weighed against the possible risks, but with proper selection of patients the risks appear manageable.[130]

If Crohn disease is a chronic, progressive, destructive illness, then intervention with more effective therapies may need to occur earlier in the disease course, before intestinal complications ensue. Along these lines, several trials have strongly suggested that greater benefit with these agents can be seen when given earlier in the disease course, and in combination with other medications such as immunosuppressive agents.[131,132]

Other anti-TNF-α agents have been studied in IBD. Etanercept (Enbrel) did not demonstrate efficacy in Crohn disease.[133] Adalimumab (Humira) is a fully human antibody to TNF-α that has demonstrated efficacy in Crohn disease (both induction and maintenance of remission) in several randomized trials.[134-136] This drug is administered at a dose of 40 mg subcutaneously every 2 weeks, after a loading dose of 160 mg followed 2 weeks later by 80 mg. An 8-week trial in patients with moderately to severely active ulcerative colitis showed modest benefit for inducing remission at the 160 mg/80 mg loading dose,[137] but the drug is not yet approved by the FDA for use in ulcerative colitis. Certolizumab pegol (formerly known as CDP870) is a humanized Fab TNF-α antibody fragment that has been "PEG-ylated" (i.e., attached to a polyethylene glycol [PEG] molecule) to improve the half-life of the drug. Most but not all randomized trials have demonstrated efficacy for this agent in Crohn disease with once-monthly subcutaneous dosing.[138-141] A metaanalysis of biologic therapies for IBD showed that anti-TNF-α antibodies as a group are more effective than placebo for inducing and maintaining remission in Crohn disease, and that infliximab is effective for inducing remission in moderately to severely active UC.[142]

The other biologic therapy currently approved by the FDA for Crohn disease is natalizumab (Tysabri), a monoclonal antibody to the adhesion molecule α$_4$ integrin.[143-145] Natalizumab was shown in the aforementioned metaanalysis to be effective in inducing remission of active Crohn disease.[142] Its use has been limited by the rare risk of progressive multifocal leukoencephalopathy, a serious neurologic complication caused by JC virus.

Agents that are currently being investigated for the treatment of IBD include vedolizumab (formerly known as MLN-02 or MLN0002), a humanized antibody to α$_4$/β$_7$ integrin, which may have more gut specificity than natalizumab[146,147]; and ustekinumab, a fully human antibody to the shared p40 subunit of IL-12 and IL-23.[148]

SURGICAL CONSIDERATIONS IN INFLAMMATORY BOWEL DISEASE

Surgical intervention in IBD patients is primarily reserved for patients with disease complications or for those who achieve symptom control on maximal medical therapy. Depending on the underlying disease, surgery may be curative for the intestinal manifestations of the disease, as in UC, or as an adjunct to medical therapy to control symptoms or to treat a disease complication, which is often the case in Crohn disease. Ideally there is frequent consultation between the patient's gastroenterologist and surgeon to ensure the timing and planned interventions are coordinated in the entire context of the patient's disease course and treatment plan. To assist the surgeon in operative decision making, there needs to be a clear understanding of the goals of the current medical therapy as well as possible future therapies as this might influence both the timing and choice of operation. In the following section, we briefly discuss the indications, surgical approaches, and reported outcomes of surgical intervention in UC and Crohn disease. We also discuss the role of laparoscopy in the surgical management of both diseases.

SURGICAL MANAGEMENT OF ULCERATIVE COLITIS

The surgical approach to patients with UC can be divided into two broad categories: emergent and elective surgical intervention. Indications for emergent intervention in UC include fulminant colitis, toxic megacolon, colonic perforation, and massive hemorrhage. Fortunately, with better understanding of the disease and improved medical treatments, these situations arise less frequently, but even today the risk of a fulminant UC flare is approximately 20% over the course of a patient's disease.[149] In emergent situations, the goal of the surgical procedure is to address a life-threatening clinical situation without precluding a future restorative procedure. In virtually all emergent UC cases, there is no role for performing a rectal dissection. This is time-consuming, increases the complexity of the surgery, and makes possible future ileal pouch reconstruction extremely difficult if not impossible. In a patient with known UC or indeterminate colitis who requires emergent operation to treat their colonic disease, the procedure of choice is the subtotal colectomy with end ileostomy. This procedure removes most of the diseased organ but leaves the rectum in situ and avoids any disturbance to the important dissection planes in the pelvis. This approach addresses the complication that prompted surgical intervention and also allows the patient to improve his or her overall health and nutritional status and to transition off medications such as corticosteroids. The patient can then proceed at a later date to a restorative or definitive operation without any deleterious impact on the functional outcomes. If the rectal disease does become troublesome, it can usually be managed with topical corticosteroids or mesalamine. Until recently, emergent subtotal colectomies were considered a contraindication to a laparoscopic approach. However, it has recently been shown to be equally effective and safe in an experienced surgeon's hands and to provide some patient benefits related to recovery.[150] The more common situation in the UC patient is to address electively the failure of medical therapy to control disease symptoms, long-term deleterious side effects of medications, or the development of intestinal dysplasia or cancer.

As discussed more fully in Chapter 160, the currently accepted surgical approaches to treating UC are total proctocolectomy with end ileostomy or total proctocolectomy with ileal pouch–anal anastomosis (IPAA). Both operations cure the patient of the intestinal manifestations of the disease. However, the IPAA avoids the requirement for a permanent ileostomy. Parks and Nicholls first described the IPAA procedure in 1978.[151] IPAA is an ideal operation for the treatment of UC in appropriately selected patients because it removes the entire diseased organ while simultaneously preserving the normal route for defecation.[152] Construction of the ileal pouch is the key to the success of this operation, since it provides an adequate fecal reservoir to allow voluntary defecation, albeit at a higher but manageable daily frequency than patients with a normal rectum. The decision to proceed with an operation other than IPAA for UC is based on individual patient circumstances or preexisting medical or physiologic conditions that are considered contraindications for this type of restorative procedure. Previously, "advanced age" (i.e., age >50 years) was considered a contraindication; however, a recent publication suggested that chronologic age itself should not be considered a contraindication because many older patients seem to have quite comparable surgical and functional outcomes relative to younger patients.[153] Details of the IPAA procedure are beyond the scope of this chapter and are discussed more fully in Chapter 160. Although each surgeon might have slightly different ways of performing the operation, the operation basically involves the following four steps:

1. Removal of the intraabdominal colon
2. Dissection and removal of the rectum, sparing the pelvic nerves and the anal sphincter mechanism
3. Construction of an ileal reservoir
4. Anastomosis of the ileal reservoir to the anal canal

Outcomes

Even though a large number of surgeons and institutions have reported their experience with the IPAA procedure, the functional results are quite similar.[154-159] Most patients report good to excellent function with their ileal pouch. In a Mayo Clinic series of more than 1300 IPAAs, the average number of daytime bowel movements at the time of discharge after closure of the ileostomy was six per day, and the average number of nocturnal bowel movements was one per night.[154,155] During the day, 79% of patients reported complete continence, 19% had occasional incontinence and 2% had frequent episodes of incontinence. During the night, 59% of patients had no incontinence whatsoever, whereas 49% reported occasional nocturnal incontinence. A followup report from this cohort who were followed for more than 15 years showed that pouch function is relatively stable over time, with no real significant decline in functional parameters, except for an increase in episodes for both day and nocturnal incontinence.[160] Although it would appear at first glance that these functional changes might result in a decline in satisfaction with the outcome of the surgery, the patients reported no such decline.

Quality of Life after IPAA. Although the functional results of the surgery are fairly well described and are consistent among the many reported series, the degree of improved patient of quality of life (QoL) is variable after IPAA.[161] In the majority of studies, patients report a high degree of satisfaction with the functional result from IPAA. Fazio et al have shown that the QoL after IPAA is comparable to the norms for the general healthy U.S. population.[162] Most QoL assessments of these patients are confounded by the differential impact on QoL of the removal of the diseased bowel with respect to overall health, the ability to discontinue medications, and the ability to voluntarily control stools. The literature contains conflicting reports on this point. Some authors report improved QoL after IPAA compared to end or continent ileostomy,[163-165] whereas others have shown that QoL improves no matter what procedure is performed and is probably due to eradication of the disease.[166-168] In a report using specific and generic QoL questionnaires and a survey instrument that estimated the monetary value for continuing disability related to the surgical procedure, they found that the patients with an IPAA had much better body image compared to patients with a Brooke or Kock ileostomy.[169] However, all patients assigned an equal monetary value to the disability associated with each operation. The IPAA patients actually reported altered bowel emptying function as more disabling than patients with stomas. In a recent report, the long-term followup (>10 years) demonstrated adjustment to living with IPAA was good with minimal restrictions to normal living, particularly in patients who had good pouch function.[170] Overall, UC patients who undergo IPAA seem to do very well after surgery and return to a good to excellent QoL. However, there is a strong correlation between a poor IPAA functional result and worse QoL.

Although there are a few technical issues related to the IPAA procedure that are still debated, such as hand-sewn versus double-stapled anastomosis, or the role of a temporary ileostomy, the most recent advance related to the procedure is the role of laparoscopic surgery (see also Chapter 178). As surgeons have become more familiar with laparoscopic colorectal surgery, and newer instrumentation has been developed specifically for complex laparoscopic colorectal surgery, an increasing number of institutions have reported their results with laparoscopic IPAA.[171,172] A number of different laparoscopic techniques have been described, including purely laparoscopic, a combined laparoscopic mini-laparotomy, or a hand-assisted laparoscopic technique. These reports presented small series of patients and have demonstrated fairly similar perioperative complication rates and short-term functional outcomes as compared to traditional open techniques. Although laparoscopic IPAA surgeries usually have longer operative times compared to open procedures, often there are other reported advantages, including decreased length of stay, decreased postoperative narcotic use, and improved cosmesis. A possible additional advantage of a laparoscopic approach to IPAA may be a reduction in postoperative complications. Fleming et al used the American College of Surgeons' National Surgical Quality Improvement Program data set to compare outcomes between open and laparoscopic IPAA.[173] They found that laparoscopic IPAA was associated with a significant decrease in both minor and major postoperative events. In the only reported long-term

matched case-control study of laparoscopic versus open IPAA, there were no long-term functional or QoL differences between the two surgical modalities.[174] Aside from the technical challenge associated with performing this complex procedure laparoscopically, there is no reason to believe that it is not equivalent to the traditional open surgery and that it might provide some substantial benefits to the patient.

SURGICAL MANAGEMENT OF CROHN DISEASE

Unlike UC, where surgery can be considered curative for the intestinal manifestations of the disease, surgery in Crohn disease is directed toward at relieving symptoms or complications of the disease. Elective surgery should be considered once maximal medical therapy has failed in controlling symptoms, to treat complications of the disease that prevent the initiation of medical therapy. Because Crohn disease can manifest itself anywhere along the intestinal tract, the location of disease and the indications requiring surgery are numerous. However, in the most general terms, surgical intervention for abdominal Crohn disease is directed at three areas: relief of obstruction, treatment of intestinal fistulas, or treatment of medically refractory disease. Less frequent indications for surgery include addressing free perforations and cancer. An essential component of treating Crohn disease patients is a close collaboration between the treating gastroenterologist and the surgeon. A thorough review of the patient's medical options and postoperative treatment options need to be considered during surgical planning. Finally, the performed surgery should always be directed at performing the minimal amount of surgery to resolve the problem. Given the recurring nature of Crohn disease, surgical resection of the intestine, especially the small intestine, needs to be minimized to avoid the possible complications related to short bowel syndrome.

As previously noted, the main indications for surgical intervention in the treatment of abdominal Crohn disease are relief of obstruction, treatment of intestinal fistulas, or treatment of medically refractory disease. These different indications seem to be influenced by the site of primary disease activity. In a review of patients who underwent surgery at the Cleveland Clinic, bowel obstruction and internal fistula or abscess tended to be the most common reasons for surgery in patients with small bowel disease. The indications for surgery in 127 patients with colonic disease were poor response to medical care (25%), internal fistula and abscess (23%), toxic megacolon (20%), perianal disease (19%), and intestinal obstruction (12%).[175] A detailed discussion of the specific indications and surgical treatment options for Crohn disease patients is presented in Chapter 161. Important to the discussion of the surgical treatment of abdominal Crohn disease is a consideration of the disease natural history after surgery. Surgery is not curative, with nearly 60% to 80% of patients developing endoscopic recurrence by 1 year after surgery, 10% to 20% experiencing clinical relapse, and 5% developing recurrence that requires repeat surgical intervention.[176,177] The impact of the standard use of immunosuppressives (azathioprine and 6-mercaptopurine) to reduce the need for surgery or recurrence after surgery is not clearly understood. In fact, there appears to be no significant impact on the need for repeat surgery in patients treated postoperatively with immunomodulators.[178] The role of the new biologic agents, such as infliximab, in slowing the progression of disease to the point that it would not require surgery, or reducing the incidence of recurrence after surgery, is not clear at this time. Large well-designed and well-powered clinical trials need to be performed to test the efficacy of these novel but expensive agents before they become routinely recommended as agents that can change the need for or prevent a clinical recurrence of the disease that requires surgery.[179]

Perianal (Perineal) Crohn Disease

Although abdominal complications of Crohn disease can be challenging to treat, the surgical decision making is often fairly straightforward; however, treatment of perianal Crohn disease can be quite difficult. The dreaded end result of unsuccessful treatment can lead to removal of the entire rectum and anus and the need for a permanent ostomy. As in treatment strategies for proximal intestinal Crohn disease, judicious surgery combined with maximal medical therapy with an eye toward symptomatic disease control as opposed to disease eradication should be the therapeutic goal. The incidence of perianal involvement has been reported to range from 13% to 43% of patients.[180,181] Although the manifestations of perianal Crohn disease are numerous, encompassing enlarged anal tags to complex abscesses and fistulas, the most difficult problem to manage is fistulas. Before embarking on treatment of perianal Crohn disease fistulas, it is important to ensure that any abscess that might be perpetuating the fistula is adequately drained. It is not uncommon to have both abscess and fistula occurring either simultaneously or close in time. As the complexity of the fistula tract increases, the higher is the likelihood of a persistent abscess.[182]

The most important component of treatment is evaluating the perineum and determining the anatomy of the fistula. Traditionally, an examination under anesthesia has been the mainstay of determining the perianal anatomy. However, advanced radiographic imaging modalities have demonstrated good success in determining the path of anal fistulas. In a study in which each patient had anal endoscopic ultrasound, pelvic magnetic resonance imaging (MRI), and surgical examination under anesthesia, the anal ultrasound was found to be more sensitive in determining the extent and course of anal fistulas than MRI and equivalent to surgical evaluation.[183]

Once the fistula tract is identified, primary surgical management should be directed at controlling any septic process associated with the fistula. Once any local sepsis is drained, a minimalist approach to further surgery should be considered. As discussed in greater detail in Chapters 156 and 161, liberal use of draining setons to maintain adequate drainage of the tract should be encouraged for all but the most superficial fistulas. Surgical drainage combined with maximal medical therapy including infliximab has dramatically improved treatment outcomes for this difficult problem. In a report by

Talbot et al, combined infliximab and surgery for complex perianal Crohn fistula disease resulted in complete resolution of the disease in 47% of patients and marked improvement in all of the remaining patients.[184] Essential to the successful treatment of perianal disease is bringing under control rectal and more proximal disease. Failure to control the rectal disease leads to a much higher rate of proctectomy and permanent ileostomy than in patients whose proximal and rectal disease is improved. If perianal disease continues and is symptomatic, proctectomy may be necessary. Before a proctectomy is performed, it is important that the patient be in optimal medical condition, because this operation is associated with relatively high morbidity rates. Preoperative measures to decrease local sepsis and improve healing should be undertaken, including improved control of local sepsis, maximal nutritional supplementation, and decreasing corticosteroid use if possible. To decrease local sepsis and improve the patient's overall medical condition, a staged procedure may be planned by performing an initial subtotal colectomy and ileostomy or ileostomy alone. Overall, the successful management of perianal Crohn disease, just as treatment of Crohn disease elsewhere in the intestine, requires close collaboration with the treating gastroenterologist to ensure that appropriate maximal medical therapy is being administered. Furthermore, a conservative surgical approach, to improve the patient's symptoms and not with the goal of eradicating the disease, should be employed.

QUALITY OF LIFE IN INFLAMMATORY BOWEL DISEASE

IBD is a chronic disease that profoundly impacts the patient's daily QoL. Many of the patients are diagnosed in their early adulthood, which means that they will require chronic medical attention, medication use, frequent surgeries, or live with the aftereffects of surgical treatment for the remainder of their lives. A patient's health-related QoL (HR-QoL) comprises three general domains: physical, social, and psychological.[185] Although many generic HR-QoL instruments exist that are useful for measurements across all diseases and medical intervention, they evaluate the three health domains in general terms. The most commonly used validated disease-specific QoL instrument for IBD patients is the Inflammatory Bowel Disease Questionnaire (IBDQ) developed by Guyatt, Irvine, and colleagues.[186,187]

Chronic medical conditions have been linked to increased psychological distress in numerous community and clinical studies.[188,189] Overall, patients with IBD demonstrate a higher degree of psychological distress compared to healthy controls.[190] Not surprisingly, the level of distress correlates with the level of disease activity.[190,191] Also, nearly all studies have shown that patients with Crohn disease have more psychological distress and, in general, worse QoL than patients with UC.[191] In a large population-based study in Sweden using both a generic HR-QoL instrument (the SF-36) and the IBDQ, the authors found that UC patients reported superior QoL in all dimensions of health-related and disease-specific QoL than did patients with Crohn disease.[192] The latter reported more anxiety and depression, which was directly related to the severity of their symptoms. Having an ileostomy in either the Crohn disease or UC patient groups was not associated with a negative impact on QoL. However, among UC patients with either an ileostomy or an IPAA, there was overall better QoL in those patients with an ileostomy, because of better physical function, emotional function, and fewer bowel-related symptoms. This finding differs from many other studies that have shown that patients with a properly functioning IPAA reported an HR-QoL comparable to the general public.[193] An important issue to consider when discussing QoL measurement in patients with IBD is the difficulty in comparing how the interaction of medical and surgical therapy affects QoL. For example, in Crohn disease surgical therapy often is reserved for patients who have progressive symptoms or complications in spite of medical therapy. In this setting, a comparison of patients with medically controlled disease to those who undergo surgery might demonstrate a negative impact on QoL because of surgery. However, the confounder is that those patients who underwent surgery were in general sicker or had a more chronic course of their disease. Similarly, it is difficult to compare UC patients on chronic medical management for UC to those who underwent surgery. Patients who are on chronic medical therapy even with good symptom control perceive themselves as having a chronic disease, whereas patients who have undergone surgery are cured of the intestinal manifestations of the disease but now have altered bowel function. In general, QoL assessments in both Crohn disease and UC patients have shown that the most important predictor of good or improved QoL is directly related to the severity of symptoms and the success of interventions that control patient symptoms.

SUMMARY

The inflammatory bowel diseases, which are broadly divided into Crohn disease and chronic ulcerative colitis, are notable for relapsing disease activity. In most cases, initial management is directed at symptom control using medical management. Current medical therapy includes a broad array of options including agents directed at local control of the inflammatory process, immunosuppressive agents, and monoclonal antibodies directed at specific inflammatory mediators. Surgical interventions in Crohn disease should be directed at controlling complications from the disease that are unresponsive to maximal medical therapy. Although surgery for UC can cure the intestinal manifestations of the disease, it often requires a staged approach associated with significant morbidity and change in lifestyle. For IBD patients, the most important contributor to a patient's QoL is controlling the disease symptoms. To achieve this goal, there needs to be a coordinated treatment approach between gastroenterologists and surgeons to ensure that complementary medical and surgical interventions are instituted directed at achieving long-term control of disease symptoms.

REFERENCES

1. Loftus CG, Loftus EV, Sandborn WJ, et al: Update on incidence and prevalence of Crohn's disease (CD) and ulcerative colitis (UC) in Olmsted County, Minnesota [Abstract]. *Gastroenterology* 124:A36, 2003.
2. Ingle SB, Loftus EV, Tremaine WJ, et al: Increasing incidence and prevalence of inflammatory bowel disease in Olmsted County, Minnesota, 2001-2004 [Abstract]. *Gastroenterology* 132:A19, 2007.
3. Loftus EV Jr: Clinical epidemiology of inflammatory bowel disease: Incidence, prevalence, and environmental influences. *Gastroenterology* 126:1504, 2004.
4. Monsen U, Brostrom O, Nordenvall B, et al: Prevalence of inflammatory bowel disease among relatives of patients with ulcerative colitis. *Scand J Gastroenterol* 22:214, 1987.
5. Monsen U, Bernell O, Johansson C, et al: Prevalence of inflammatory bowel disease among relatives of patients with Crohn's disease. *Scand J Gastroenterol* 26:302, 1991.
6. Orholm M, Munkholm P, Langholz E, et al: Familial occurrence of inflammatory bowel disease. *N Engl J Med* 324:84, 1991.
7. Thompson NP, Driscoll R, Pounder RE, et al: Genetics versus environment in inflammatory bowel disease: Results of a British twin study. *BMJ* 312:95, 1996.
8. Orholm M, Binder V, Sorensen TI, et al: Concordance of inflammatory bowel disease among Danish twins: Results of a nationwide study. *Scand J Gastroenterol* 35:1075, 2000.
9. Halfvarson J, Bodin L, Tysk C, et al: Inflammatory bowel disease in a Swedish twin cohort: A long-term follow-up of concordance and clinical characteristics. *Gastroenterology* 124:1767, 2003.
10. Mayberry JF, Judd D, Smart H, et al: Crohn's disease in Jewish people: An epidemiological study in southeast Wales. *Digestion* 35:237, 1986.
11. Yang H, McElree C, Roth MP, et al: Familial empirical risks for inflammatory bowel disease: Differences between Jews and non-Jews. *Gut* 34:517, 1993.
12. Mahid SS, Minor KS, Soto RE, et al: Smoking and inflammatory bowel disease: A meta-analysis. *Mayo Clin Proc* 81:1462, 2006.
13. Rubin DT, Hanauer SB: Smoking and inflammatory bowel disease. *Eur J Gastroenterol Hepatol* 12:855, 2000.
14. Koutroubakis IE, Vlachonikolis IG, Kouroumalis EA: Role of appendicitis and appendectomy in the pathogenesis of ulcerative colitis: A critical review. *Inflamm Bowel Dis* 8:277, 2002.
15. Hou JK, Abraham B, El-Serag H: Dietary intake and risk of developing inflammatory bowel disease: A systematic review of the literature. *Am J Gastroenterol* 106:563, 2011.
16. Goodhand JR, Alazawi W, Rampton DS: Systematic review: *Clostridium difficile* and inflammatory bowel disease. *Aliment Pharmacol Ther* 33:428, 2011.
17. Ayre K, Warren BF, Jeffery K, et al: The role of CMV in steroid-resistant ulcerative colitis: A systematic review. *J Crohn's Colitis* 3:141, 2009.
18. Maunder RG, Levenstein S: The role of stress in the development and clinical course of inflammatory bowel disease: Epidemiological evidence. *Curr Mol Med* 8:247, 2008.
19. Asquith M, Powrie F: An innately dangerous balancing act: Intestinal homeostasis, inflammation, and colitis-associated cancer. *J Exp Med* 207:1573, 2010.
20. Thompson AI, Lees CW: Genetics of ulcerative colitis. *Inflamm Bowel Dis* 17:831, 2011.
21. Loftus EV Jr, Silverstein MD, Sandborn WJ, et al: Ulcerative colitis in Olmsted County, Minnesota, 1940-1993: Incidence, prevalence, and survival. *Gut* 46:336, 2000.
22. Riddell RH: Pathology of idiopathic inflammatory bowel disease. In Sartor RB, Sandborn WJ, editors: *Kirsner's inflammatory bowel diseases*, ed 6. Edinburgh, 2004, WB Saunders, p 399.
23. Langholz E, Munkholm P, Davidsen M, et al: Colorectal cancer risk and mortality in patients with ulcerative colitis. *Gastroenterology* 103:1444, 1992.
24. Langholz E, Munkholm P, Davidsen M, et al: Course of ulcerative colitis: Analysis of changes in disease activity over years. *Gastroenterology* 107:3, 1994.
25. Sands BE: From symptom to diagnosis: Clinical distinctions among various forms of intestinal inflammation. *Gastroenterology* 126:1518, 2004.

26. Devroede GJ, Taylor WF, Sauer WG, et al: Cancer risk and life expectancy of children with ulcerative colitis. *N Engl J Med* 285:17, 1971.

27. Mir-Madjlessi SH, Farmer RG, Easley KA, et al: Colorectal and extracolonic malignancy in ulcerative colitis. *Cancer* 58:1569, 1986.

28. Ekbom A, Helmick C, Zack M, et al: Ulcerative colitis and colorectal cancer: A population-based study. *N Engl J Med* 323:1228, 1990.

29. Loftus EV: Epidemiology and risk factors for colorectal dysplasia and cancer in ulcerative colitis. *Gastroenterol Clin N Am* 35:517, 2006.

30. Eaden JA, Abrams KR, Mayberry JF: The risk of colorectal cancer in ulcerative colitis: A meta-analysis. *Gut* 48:526, 2001.

31. Winther KV, Jess T, Langholz E, et al: Long-term risk of cancer in ulcerative colitis: A population-based cohort study from Copenhagen County. *Clin Gastroenterol Hepatol* 2:1088, 2004.

32. Jess T, Loftus EV Jr, Velayos FS, et al: Risk of intestinal cancer in inflammatory bowel disease: A population-based study from Olmsted County, Minnesota. *Gastroenterology* 130:1039, 2006.

33. Brostrom O, Lofberg R, Nordenvall B, et al: The risk of colorectal cancer in ulcerative colitis: An epidemiologic study. *Scand J Gastroenterol* 22:1193, 1987.

34. Gilat T, Fireman Z, Grossman A, et al: Colorectal cancer in patients with ulcerative colitis: A population study in central Israel. *Gastroenterology* 94:870, 1988.

35. Karlen P, Lofberg R, Brostrom O, et al: Increased risk of cancer in ulcerative colitis: A population-based cohort study. *Am J Gastroenterol* 94:1047, 1999.

36. Langholz E, Munkholm P, Krasilnikoff PA, et al: Inflammatory bowel diseases with onset in childhood: Clinical features, morbidity, and mortality in a regional cohort. *Scand J Gastroenterol* 32:139, 1997.

37. Lashner BA, Silverstein MD, Hanauer SB: Hazard rates for dysplasia and cancer in ulcerative colitis: Results from a surveillance program. *Dig Dis Sci* 34:1536, 1989.

38. Rutter M, Saunders B, Wilkinson K, et al: Severity of inflammation is a risk factor for colorectal neoplasia in ulcerative colitis. *Gastroenterology* 126:451, 2004.

39. Rubin DT, Huo D, Rothe JA, et al: Increased inflammatory activity is an independent risk factor for dysplasia and colorectal cancer in ulcerative colitis: A case-control analysis with blinded prospective pathology review [Abstract]. *Gastroenterology* 130:A2, 2006.

40. Eaden J, Abrams K, Ekbom A, et al: Colorectal cancer prevention in ulcerative colitis: A case-control study. *Aliment Pharmacol Ther* 14:145, 2000.

41. Broome U, Lindberg G, Lofberg R: Primary sclerosing cholangitis in ulcerative colitis—a risk factor for the development of dysplasia and DNA aneuploidy? *Gastroenterology* 102:1877, 1992.

42. Kornfeld D, Ekbom A, Ihre T: Is there an excess risk for colorectal cancer in patients with ulcerative colitis and concomitant primary sclerosing cholangitis? A population-based study. *Gut* 41:522, 1997.

43. Jayaram H, Satsangi J, Chapman RW: Increased colorectal neoplasia in chronic ulcerative colitis complicated by primary sclerosing cholangitis: Fact or fiction? *Gut* 48:430, 2001.

44. Broome U, Lofberg R, Lundqvist K, et al: Subclinical time span of inflammatory bowel disease in patients with primary sclerosing cholangitis. *Dis Colon Rectum* 38:1301, 1995.

45. Loftus EV Jr, Harewood GC, Loftus CG, et al: PSC-IBD: A unique form of inflammatory bowel disease associated with primary sclerosing cholangitis. *Gut* 54:91, 2005.

46. Nuako KW, Ahlquist DA, Mahoney DW, et al: Familial predisposition for colorectal cancer in chronic ulcerative colitis: A case-control study. *Gastroenterology* 115:1079, 1998.

47. Askling J, Dickman PW, Karlen P, et al: Family history as a risk factor for colorectal cancer in inflammatory bowel disease. *Gastroenterology* 120:1356, 2001.

48. Delaunoit T, Limburg PJ, Goldberg RM, et al: Colorectal cancer prognosis among patients with inflammatory bowel disease. *Clin Gastroenterol Hepatol* 4:335, 2006.

49. Riddell RH, Goldman H, Ransohoff DF, et al: Dysplasia in inflammatory bowel disease: Standardized classification with provisional clinical applications. *Hum Pathol* 14:931, 1983.

50. Itzkowitz SH, Present DH, Crohn's and Colitis Foundation of America Colon Cancer in IBD Study Group: Consensus conference: Colorectal cancer screening and surveillance in inflammatory bowel disease. *Inflamm Bowel Dis* 11:314, 2005.

51. Farraye FA, Odze RD, Eaden J, et al: AGA medical position statement on the diagnosis and management of colorectal neoplasia in inflammatory bowel disease. *Gastroenterology* 138:738, 2010.

52. Ullman TA, Loftus EV Jr, Kakar S, et al: The fate of low-grade dysplasia in ulcerative colitis. *Am J Gastroenterol* 97:922, 2002.

53. Ullman T, Croog V, Harpaz N, et al: Progression of flat low-grade dysplasia to advanced neoplasia in patients with ulcerative colitis. *Gastroenterology* 125:1311, 2003.

54. Rutter MD, Saunders BP, Wilkinson KH, et al: Most dysplasia in ulcerative colitis is visible at colonoscopy. *Gastrointest Endosc* 60:334, 2004.

55. Blackstone MO, Riddell RH, Rogers BH, et al: Dysplasia-associated lesion or mass (DALM) detected by colonoscopy in long-standing ulcerative colitis: An indication for colectomy. *Gastroenterology* 80:366, 1981.

56. Odze RD, Farraye FA, Hecht JL, et al: Long-term follow-up after polypectomy treatment for adenoma-like dysplastic lesions in ulcerative colitis. *Clin Gastroenterol Hepatol* 2:534, 2004.

57. Kisiel JB, Loftus EV, Harmsen WS, et al: Outcome of sporadic adenomas and adenoma-like dysplasia in patients with ulcerative colitis undergoing polypectomy. *Inflamm Bowel Dis* 18:226, 2012.

58. Edwards FC, Truelove SC: The course and prognosis of ulcerative colitis. *Gut* 4:299, 1964.

59. Turner D, Walsh CM, Steinhart AH, et al: Response to corticosteroids in severe ulcerative colitis: A systematic review of the literature and a meta-regression. *Clin Gastroenterol Hepatol* 5:103, 2007.

60. Jalan KN, Sircus W, Card WI, et al: An experience of ulcerative colitis: I. Toxic dilation in 55 cases. *Gastroenterology* 57:68, 1969.

61. Modigliani R: Medical management of fulminant colitis. *Inflamm Bowel Dis* 8:129, 2002.

62. Travis SPL: Predicting outcome in severe ulcerative colitis. *Dig Liver Dis* 36:448, 2004.

63. Dunckley P, Jewell D: Management of acute severe colitis. *Best Pract Res Clin Gastroenterol* 17:89, 2003.

64. Thia KT, Loftus EV Jr, Sandborn WJ, et al: An update on the epidemiology of inflammatory bowel disease in Asia. *Am J Gastroenterol* 103:3167, 2008.

65. Johnson GJ, Cosnes J, Mansfield JC: Review article: Smoking cessation as primary therapy to modify the course of Crohn's disease. *Aliment Pharmacol Ther* 21:921, 2005.

66. Hugot JP, Chamaillard M, Zouali H, et al: Association of *NOD2* leucine-rich repeat variants with susceptibility to Crohn's disease. *Nature* 411:599, 2001.

67. Ogura Y, Bonen DK, Inohara N, et al: A frameshift mutation in *NOD2* associated with susceptibility to Crohn's disease. *Nature* 411:603, 2001.

68. Hampe J, Cuthbert A, Croucher PJ, et al: Association between insertion mutation in *NOD2* gene and Crohn's disease in German and British populations. *Lancet* 357:1925, 2001.

69. Van Limbergen J, Wilson DC, Satsangi J: The genetics of Crohn's disease. *Annu Rev Genomics Hum Genet* 10:89, 2009.

70. Loftus EV, Silverstein MD, Sandborn WJ, et al: Crohn's disease in Olmsted County, Minnesota, 1940-1993: Incidence, prevalence, and survival. *Gastroenterology* 114:1161, 1998.

71. Geboes K, Colombel JF, Greenstein A, et al: Indeterminate colitis: A review of the concept—what's in a name? *Inflamm Bowel Dis* 14:850, 2008.

72. Schwartz DA, Loftus EV Jr, Tremaine WJ, et al: The natural history of fistulizing Crohn's disease in Olmsted County, Minnesota. *Gastroenterology* 122:875, 2002.

73. Buchmann P, Alexander-Williams J: Classification of perianal Crohn's disease. *Clin Gastroenterol* 9:323, 1980.

74. Radcliffe AG, Ritchie JK, Hawley PR, et al: Anovaginal and rectovaginal fistulas in Crohn's disease. *Dis Colon Rectum* 31:94, 1988.

75. Scott NA, Nair A, Hughes LE: Anovaginal and rectovaginal fistula in patients with Crohn's disease. *Br J Surg* 79:1379, 1992.

76. Michelassi F, Melis M, Rubin M, et al: Surgical treatment of anorectal complications in Crohn's disease. *Surgery* 128:597, 2000.

77. Fireman Z, Grossman A, Lilos P, et al: Intestinal cancer in patients with Crohn's disease: A population study in central Israel. *Scand J Gastroenterol* 24:346, 1989.

78. Persson PG, Karlen P, Bernell O, et al: Crohn's disease and cancer: A population-based cohort study. *Gastroenterology* 107:1675, 1994.

79. Mellemkjaer L, Johansen C, Gridley G, et al: Crohn's disease and cancer risk (Denmark). *Cancer Causes Control* 11:145, 2000.

80. Jess T, Winther KV, Munkholm P, et al: Intestinal and extra-intestinal cancer in Crohn's disease: Follow-up of a population-based cohort in Copenhagen County, Denmark. *Aliment Pharmacol Ther* 19:287, 2004.

81. Ekbom A, Helmick C, Zack M, et al: Increased risk of large-bowel cancer in Crohn's disease with colonic involvement. *Lancet* 336:357, 1990.

82. Azad Khan AK, Piris J, Truelove SC: An experiment to determine the active therapeutic moiety of sulphasalazine. *Lancet* 2:892, 1977.

83. Mahadevan U, Sandborn WJ: Clinical pharmacology of inflammatory bowel disease therapy. In Sartor RB, Sandborn WJ, editors: *Kirsner's inflammatory bowel diseases*, ed 6. Edinburgh, 2004, WB Saunders, p 484.

84. Ford AC, Achkar JP, Khan KJ, et al: Efficacy of 5-aminosalicylates in ulcerative colitis: Systematic review and meta-analysis. *Am J Gastroenterol* 106:601, 2011.

85. Ford AC, Kane SV, Khan KJ, et al: Efficacy of 5-aminosalicylates in Crohn's disease: Systematic review and meta-analysis. *Am J Gastroenterol* 106:617, 2011.

86. Summers RW, Switz DM, Sessions JT Jr, et al: National Cooperative Crohn's Disease Study: Results of drug treatment. *Gastroenterology* 77:847, 1979.

87. Malchow H, Ewe K, Brandes JW, et al: European Cooperative Crohn's Disease Study (ECCDS): Results of drug treatment. *Gastroenterology* 86:249, 1984.

88. Loftus EV Jr, Kane SV, Bjorkman D: Systematic review: Short-term adverse effects of 5-aminosalicylic acid agents in the treatment of ulcerative colitis. *Aliment Pharmacol Ther* 19:179, 2004.

89. Regueiro M, Loftus EV Jr, Steinhart AH, et al: Medical management of left-sided ulcerative colitis and ulcerative proctitis: Critical evaluation of therapeutic trials. *Inflamm Bowel Dis* 12:979, 2006.

90. Singleton JW, Hanauer SB, Gitnick GL, et al: Mesalamine capsules for the treatment of active Crohn's disease: Results of a 16-week trial. Pentasa Crohn's Disease Study Group. *Gastroenterology* 104:1293, 1993.

91. Tremaine WJ, Schroeder KW, Harrison JM, et al: A randomized, double-blind, placebo-controlled trial of the oral mesalamine (5-ASA) preparation, Asacol, in the treatment of symptomatic Crohn's colitis and ileocolitis. *J Clin Gastroenterol* 19:278, 1994.

92. Singleton J: Second trial of mesalamine therapy in the treatment of active Crohn's disease. *Gastroenterology* 107:632, 1994.

93. Hanauer SB, Stromberg U: Oral Pentasa in the treatment of active Crohn's disease: A meta-analysis of double-blind, placebo-controlled trials. *Clin Gastroenterol Hepatol* 2:379, 2004.

94. Truelove SC, Witts LJ: Cortisone in ulcerative colitis: Final report on a therapeutic trial. *BMJ* 2:1041, 1955.

95. Ford AC, Bernstein CN, Khan KJ, et al: Glucocorticosteroid therapy in inflammatory bowel disease: Systematic review and meta-analysis. *Am J Gastroenterol* 106:590, 2011.

96. Munkholm P, Langholz E, Davidsen M, et al: Frequency of glucocorticoid resistance and dependency in Crohn's disease. *Gut* 35:360, 1994.

97. Faubion WA Jr, Loftus EV Jr, Harmsen WS, et al: The natural history of corticosteroid therapy for inflammatory bowel disease: A population-based study. *Gastroenterology* 121:255, 2001.

98. Kane SV, Schoenfeld P, Sandborn WJ, et al: The effectiveness of budesonide therapy for Crohn's disease. *Aliment Pharmacol Ther* 16:1509, 2002.

99. Thomsen OO, Cortot A, Jewell D, et al: A comparison of budesonide and mesalamine for active Crohn's disease. International Budesonide-Mesalamine Study Group. *N Engl J Med* 339:370, 1998.

100. Sartor RB: Therapeutic manipulation of the enteric microflora in inflammatory bowel diseases: Antibiotics, probiotics, and prebiotics. *Gastroenterology* 126:1620, 2004.

101. Khan KJ, Ullman TA, Ford AC, et al: Antibiotic therapy in inflammatory bowel disease: A systematic review and meta-analysis. *Am J Gastroenterol* 106:661, 2011.

102. Lennard L, Van Loon JA, Weinshilboum RM: Pharmacogenetics of acute azathioprine toxicity: Relationship to thiopurine methyltransferase genetic polymorphism. *Clin Pharmacol Ther* 46:149, 1989.

103. Hanauer SB: Medical therapy for ulcerative colitis. In Sartor RB, Sandborn WJ, editors: *Kirsner's inflammatory bowel diseases*, ed 6. Edinburgh, 2004, WB Saunders, p 503.

104. Sandborn WJ: Medical therapy for Crohn's disease. In Sartor RB, Sandborn WJ, editors: *Kirsner's inflammatory bowel diseases*, ed 6. Edinburgh, 2004, WB Saunders, p 531.

105. Prefontaine E, MacDonald JK, Sutherland LR: Azathioprine or 6-mercaptopurine for induction of remission in Crohn's disease. *Cochrane Database Syst Rev* 6:CD000545, 2010.

106. Khan KJ, Dubinsky MC, Ford AC, et al: Efficacy of immunosuppressive therapy for inflammatory bowel disease: A systematic review and meta-analysis. *Am J Gastroenterol* 106:630, 2011.

107. Leung Y, Panaccione R, Hemmelgarn B, et al: Exposing the weaknesses: A systematic review of azathioprine efficacy in ulcerative colitis. *Dig Dis Sci* 53:1455, 2008.

108. Gisbert JP, Linares PM, McNicholl AG, et al: Meta-analysis: The efficacy of azathioprine and mercaptopurine in ulcerative colitis. *Aliment Pharmacol Ther* 30:126, 2009.

109. Loftus CG, Loftus EV, Tremaine WJ, Sandborn WJ: The safety profile of azathioprine/6-mercaptopurine in the treatment of inflammatory bowel disease: A population-based study in Olmsted County, Minnesota [Abstract]. *Am J Gastroenterol* 98:S242, 2003.

110. Sturdevant RA, Singleton JW, Deren JL, et al: Azathioprine-related pancreatitis in patients with Crohn's disease. *Gastroenterology* 77:883, 1979.

111. Kandiel A, Fraser AG, Korelitz BI, et al: Increased risk of lymphoma among inflammatory bowel disease patients treated with azathioprine and 6-mercaptopurine. *Gut* 54:1121, 2005.

112. Beaugerie L, Brousse N, Bouvier AM, et al: Lymphoproliferative disorders in patients receiving thiopurines for inflammatory bowel disease: A prospective observational cohort study. *Lancet* 374:1617, 2009.

113. Lewis JD, Schwartz JS, Lichtenstein GR: Azathioprine for maintenance of remission in Crohn's disease: Benefits outweigh the risk of lymphoma. *Gastroenterology* 118:1018, 2000.

114. Feagan BG, Rochon J, Fedorak RN, et al: Methotrexate for the treatment of Crohn's disease. The North American Crohn's Study Group Investigators. *N Engl J Med* 332:292, 1995.

115. Feagan BG, Fedorak RN, Irvine EJ, et al: A comparison of methotrexate with placebo for the maintenance of remission in Crohn's disease. North American Crohn's Study Group Investigators. *N Engl J Med* 342:1627, 2000.

116. Oren R, Arber N, Odes S, et al: Methotrexate in chronic active ulcerative colitis: A double-blind, randomized, Israeli multicenter trial. *Gastroenterology* 110:1416, 1996.

117. Lichtiger S, Present DH, Kornbluth A, et al: Cyclosporine in severe ulcerative colitis refractory to steroid therapy. *N Engl J Med* 330:1841, 1994.

118. Shibolet O, Regushevskaya E, Brezis M, et al: Cyclosporine A for induction of remission in severe ulcerative colitis. *Cochrane Database Syst Rev* 1:CD004277, 2005.

119. Targan SR, Hanauer SB, van Deventer SJ, et al: A short-term study of chimeric monoclonal antibody cA2 to tumor necrosis factor alpha for Crohn's disease. Crohn's Disease cA2 Study Group. *N Engl J Med* 337:1029, 1997.

120. Hanauer SB, Feagan BG, Lichtenstein GR, et al: Maintenance infliximab for Crohn's disease: The ACCENT I randomised trial. *Lancet* 359:1541, 2002.

121. Present DH, Rutgeerts P, Targan S, et al: Infliximab for the treatment of fistulas in patients with Crohn's disease. *N Engl J Med* 340:1398, 1999.

122. Sands BE, Anderson FH, Bernstein CN, et al: Infliximab maintenance therapy for fistulizing Crohn's disease. *N Engl J Med* 350:876, 2004.

123. D'Haens G, Van Deventer S, Van Hogezand R, et al: Endoscopic and histological healing with infliximab anti-tumor necrosis factor antibodies in Crohn's disease: A European multicenter trial. *Gastroenterology* 116:1029, 1999.

124. Lichtenstein GR, Yan S, Bala M, et al: Remission in patients with Crohn's disease is associated with improvement in employment and quality of life and a decrease in hospitalizations and surgeries. *Am J Gastroenterol* 99:91, 2004.

125. Lichtenstein GR, Yan S, Bala M, et al: Infliximab maintenance treatment reduces hospitalizations, surgeries, and procedures in fistulizing Crohn's disease. *Gastroenterology* 128:862, 2005.

126. Rutgeerts P, Sandborn WJ, Feagan BG, et al: Infliximab for induction and maintenance therapy for ulcerative colitis. *N Engl J Med* 353:2462, 2005.

127. Baert F, Noman M, Vermeire S, et al: Influence of immunogenicity on the long-term efficacy of infliximab in Crohn's disease. *N Engl J Med* 348:601, 2003.

128. Farrell RJ, Alsahli M, Jeen YT, et al: Intravenous hydrocortisone premedication reduces antibodies to infliximab in Crohn's disease: A randomized controlled trial. *Gastroenterology* 124:917, 2003.

129. Reddy JG, Loftus EV Jr: Safety of infliximab and other biologic agents in the inflammatory bowel diseases. *Gastroenterol Clin N Am* 35:837, 2006.

130. Sandborn WJ, Loftus EV: Balancing the risks and benefits of infliximab in the treatment of inflammatory bowel disease. *Gut* 53:780, 2004.

131. D'Haens G, Baert F, van Assche G, et al: Early combined immunosuppression or conventional management in patients with newly diagnosed Crohn's disease: An open randomized trial. *Lancet* 371:660, 2008.

132. Colombel JF, Sandborn WJ, Reinisch W, et al: Infliximab, azathioprine, or combination therapy for Crohn's disease. *N Engl J Med* 362:1383, 2010.

133. Sandborn WJ, Hanauer SB, Katz S, et al: Etanercept for active Crohn's disease: A randomized, double-blind, placebo-controlled trial. *Gastroenterology* 121:1088, 2001.

134. Hanauer SB, Sandborn WJ, Rutgeerts P, et al: Human anti-tumor necrosis factor monoclonal antibody (adalimumab) in Crohn's disease: The CLASSIC-I trial. *Gastroenterology* 130:323, 2006.

135. Colombel JF, Sandborn WJ, Rutgeerts P, et al: Adalimumab for maintenance of clinical response and remission in patients with Crohn's disease: The CHARM trial. *Gastroenterology* 132:52, 2007.

136. Sandborn WJ, Rutgeerts P, Enns R, et al: Adalimumab induction therapy for Crohn disease previously treated with infliximab: A randomized trial. *Ann Intern Med* 146:829, 2007.

137. Reinisch W, Sandborn WJ, Hommes DW, et al. Adalimumab for induction of clinical remission in moderately to severely active ulcerative colitis: Results of a randomized controlled trial. *Gut* 60:780, 2011.

138. Schreiber S, Rutgeerts P, Fedorak RN, et al: A randomized, placebo-controlled trial of certolizumab pegol (CDP870) for treatment of Crohn's disease. *Gastroenterology* 129:807, 2005.

139. Schreiber S, Khaliq-Kareemi M, Lawrance IC, et al: Maintenance therapy with certolizumab pegol for Crohn's disease. *N Engl J Med* 357:239, 2007.

140. Sandborn WJ, Feagan BG, Stoinov S, et al: Certolizumab pegol for the treatment of Crohn's disease. *N Engl J Med* 357:228, 2007.

141. Sandborn W, Schreiber S, Feagan B, et al: Induction therapy with certolizumab pegol in patients with moderate to severe Crohn's disease: A placebo-controlled trial [Abstract]. *Am J Gastroenterol* 105:S419, 2010.

142. Ford AC, Sandborn WJ, Khan KJ, et al: Efficacy of biological therapies in inflammatory bowel disease: Systematic review and meta-analysis. *Am J Gastroenterol* 106:644, 2011.

143. Ghosh S, Goldin E, Gordon FH, et al; Natalizumab Pan-European Study Group: Natalizumab for active Crohn's disease. *N Engl J Med* 348:24, 2003.

144. Sandborn WJ, Colombel JF, Enns R, et al: Natalizumab induction and maintenance therapy for Crohn's disease. *N Engl J Med* 353:1912, 2005.

145. Targan SR, Feagan BG, Fedorak RN, et al: Natalizumab for the treatment of active Crohn's disease: Results of the ENCORE trial. *Gastroenterology* 132:1672, 2007.

146. Feagan BG, Greenberg GR, Wild G, et al: Treatment of ulcerative colitis with a humanized antibody to the $\alpha_4\beta_7$ integrin. *N Engl J Med* 352:2499, 2005.

147. Feagan BG, Greenberg GR, Wild G, et al: Treatment of active Crohn's disease with MLN0002, a humanized antibody to the $\alpha_4\beta_7$ integrin. *Clin Gastroenterol Hepatol* 6:1370, 2008.

148. Sandborn WJ, Feagan BG, Fedorak RN, et al: A randomized trial of ustekinumab, a human interleukin-12/23 monoclonal antibody, in patients with moderate-to-severe Crohn's disease. *Gastroenterology* 135:1130, 2008.

149. Van Assche G, Vermeire S, Rutgeerts P: Treatment of severe steroid refractory ulcerative colitis. *World J Gastroenterol* 14:5508, 2008.

150. Bell RL, Seymour NE: Laparoscopic treatment of fulminant ulcerative colitis. *Surg Endosc* 16:1778, 2002.

151. Parks AG, Nicholls RJ: Proctocolectomy without ileostomy for ulcerative colitis. *BMJ* 2:85, 1978.

152. Parks AG, Nicholls RJ, Belliveau P: Proctocolectomy with ileal reservoir and anal anastomosis. *Br J Surg* 67:533, 1980.

153. Chapman JR, Larson DW, Wolff BG, et al: Ileal pouch-anal anastomosis: Does age at the time of surgery affect outcome? *Arch Surg* 140:534, 2005.

154. Meagher AP, Farouk R, Dozois RR, et al: J ileal pouch–anal anastomosis for chronic ulcerative colitis: Complications and long-term outcome in 1310 patients. *Br J Surg* 85:800, 1998.

155. Farouk R, Pemberton JH, Wolff BG, et al: Functional outcomes after ileal pouch–anal anastomosis for chronic ulcerative colitis. *Ann Surg* 231:919, 2000.

156. Bullard KM, Madoff RD, Gemlo BT: Is ileoanal pouch function stable with time? Results of a prospective audit. *Dis Colon Rectum* 45:299, 2002.

157. Dayton MT, Larsen KP: Outcome of pouch-related complications after ileal pouch–anal anastomosis. *Am J Surg* 174:728, 1997.

158. Romanos J, Samarasekera DN, Stebbing JF, et al: Outcome of 200 restorative proctocolectomy operations: The John Radcliffe Hospital experience. *Br J Surg* 84:814, 1997.

159. Fazio VW, Ziv Y, Church JM, et al: Ileal pouch–anal anastomoses complications and function in 1005 patients. *Ann Surg* 222:120, 1995.

160. Hahnloser D, Pemberton JH, Wolff BG, et al: The effect of ageing on function and quality of life in ileal pouch patients: A single cohort experience of 409 patients with chronic ulcerative colitis. *Ann Surg* 240:615, 2004.

161. Berndtsson I, Oresland T: Quality of life before and after proctocolectomy and IPAA in patients with ulcerative proctocolitis—a prospective study. *Colorectal Dis* 5:173, 2003.

162. Fazio VW, O'Riordain MG, Lavery IC, et al: Long-term functional outcome and quality of life after stapled restorative proctocolectomy. *Ann Surg* 230:575, 1999.

163. Pezim ME, Nicholls RJ: Quality of life after restorative proctocolectomy with pelvic ileal reservoir. *Br J Surg* 72:31, 1985.

164. Pemberton JH, Phillips SF, Ready RR, et al: Quality of life after Brooke ileostomy and ileal pouch–anal anastomosis: Comparison of performance status. *Ann Surg* 209:620, 1989.

165. Kohler LW, Pemberton JH, Zinsmeister AR, et al: Quality of life after proctocolectomy: A comparison of Brooke ileostomy, Kock pouch, and ileal pouch–anal anastomosis. *Gastroenterology* 101:679, 1991.

166. McLeod RS, Churchill DN, Lock AM, et al: Quality of life of patients with ulcerative colitis preoperatively and postoperatively. *Gastroenterology* 101:1307, 1991.

167. Jimmo B, Hyman NH. Is ileal pouch–anal anastomosis really the procedure of choice for patients with ulcerative colitis? *Dis Colon Rectum* 41:41, 1998.

168. Weinryb RM, Gustavsson JP, Liljeqvist L, et al: A prospective study of the quality of life after pelvic pouch operation. *J Am Coll Surg* 180:589, 1995.

169. O'Bichere A, Wilkinson K, Rumbles S, et al: Functional outcome after restorative panproctocolectomy for ulcerative colitis decreases an otherwise enhanced quality of life. *Br J Surg* 87:802, 2000.

170. Berndtsson IE, Carlsson EK, Persson EI, et al: Long-term adjustment to living with an ileal pouch-anal anastomosis. *Dis Colon Rectum* 54:193, 2011.

171. Santoro E, Carlini M, Carboni F, et al: Laparoscopic total proctocolectomy with ileal J pouch–anal anastomosis. *Hepatogastroenterology* 46:894, 1999.

172. Young-Fadok TM, Dozois EJ, Sandborn WJ, et al: A case-matched study of laparoscopic proctocolectomy and ileal pouch–anal anastomosis (PC-IPAA) versus open PC-IPAA for ulcerative colitis (UC) [Abstract]. *Gastroenterology* 120:A452, 2001.

173. Fleming FJ, Francone TD, Kim MJ, et al: A laparoscopic approach does reduce short-term complications in patients undergoing ileal pouch-anal anastomosis. *Dis Colon Rectum* 54:176, 2011.

174. Larson DW, Dozois EJ, Piotrowicz K, et al: Laparoscopic-assisted versus open ileal pouch–anal anastomosis: Functional outcome in a case-matched series. *Dis Colon Rectum* 48:1845, 2005.

175. Farmer RG, Hawk WA, Turnbull RB Jr: Indications for surgery in Crohn's disease: Analysis of 500 cases. *Gastroenterology* 71:245, 1976.

176. Rutgeerts P, Geboes K, Vantrappen G, et al: Predictability of the postoperative course of Crohn's disease. *Gastroenterology* 99:956, 1990.

177. Sandborn WJ, Feagan BG, Hanauer SB, et al: A review of activity indices and efficacy endpoints for clinical trials of medical therapy in adults with Crohn's disease. *Gastroenterology* 122:512, 2002.

178. Cosnes J, Nion-Larmurier I, Beaugerie L, et al: Impact of the increasing use of immunosuppressants in Crohn's disease on the need for intestinal surgery. *Gut* 54:237, 2005.

179. Rutgeerts P: Strategies in the prevention of post-operative recurrence in Crohn's disease. *Best Pract Res Clin Gastroenterol* 17:63, 2003.

180. Lapidus A, Bernell O, Hellers G, et al: Clinical course of colorectal Crohn's disease: A 35-year follow-up study of 507 patients. *Gastroenterology* 114:1151, 1998.

181. Sandborn WJ, Fazio VW, Feagan BG, et al: American Gastroenterological Association Clinical Practice Committee: AGA technical review on perianal Crohn's disease. *Gastroenterology* 125:1508, 2003.

182. Scott HJ, Northover JM: Evaluation of surgery for perianal Crohn's fistulas. *Dis Colon Rectum* 39:1039, 1996.

183. Orsoni P, Barthet M, Portier F, et al: Prospective comparison of endosonography, magnetic resonance imaging, and surgical findings in anorectal fistula and abscess complicating Crohn's disease. *Br J Surg* 86:360, 1999.

184. Talbot C, Sagar PM, Johnston MJ, et al: Infliximab in the surgical management of complex fistulating anal Crohn's disease. *Colorectal Dis* 7:164, 2005.

185. Fallowfield L: *The quality of life: The missing measurement in health care*, London, 1990, Souvenier Press.

186. Guyatt G, Mitchell A, Irvine EJ, et al: A new measure of health status for clinical trials in inflammatory bowel disease. *Gastroenterology* 96:804, 1989.

187. Irvine EJ, Feagan B, Rochon J, et al: Quality of life: A valid and reliable measure of therapeutic efficacy in the treatment of inflammatory bowel disease. Canadian Crohn's Relapse Prevention Trial Study Group. *Gastroenterology* 106:287, 1994.

188. Hays RD, Marshall GN, Wang EY, et al: Four-year cross-lagged associations between physical and mental health in the Medical Outcomes Study. *J Consult Clin Psychol* 62:441, 1994.

189. Aneshensel CS, Frerichs RR, Huba GJ: Depression and physical illness: A multiwave, nonrecursive causal model. *J Health Social Behav* 25:350, 1984.

190. Drossman DA, Leserman J, Mitchell CM, et al: Health status and health care use in persons with inflammatory bowel disease: A national sample. *Dig Dis Sci* 36:1746, 1991.

191. Schwarz SP, Blanchard EB: Inflammatory bowel disease: A review of the psychological assessment and treatment literature. *Ann Behav Med* 12:95, 1990.

192. Nordin K, Pahlman L, Larsson K, et al: Health-related quality of life and psychological distress in a population-based sample of Swedish patients with inflammatory bowel disease. *Scand J Gastroenterol* 37:450, 2002.

193. Robb B, Pritts T, Gang G, et al: Quality of life in patients undergoing ileal pouch–anal anastomosis at the University of Cincinnati. *Am J Surg* 183:353, 2002.

Surgery for Inflammatory Bowel Disease: Chronic Ulcerative Colitis

Peter M. Sagar | John H. Pemberton

The optimal surgical procedure for most patients with chronic ulcerative colitis (CUC) is proctocolectomy with ileal pouch–anal anastomosis (IPAA). Patients with CUC need no longer live with the fear that their ultimate surgical fate is to be a permanent ileostomy with its attendant psychological, social, physical, and sexual problems. Indeed, IPAA confers a good quality of life. The principal aim of this chapter is to review the technical details of IPAA and the available choices of ileal pouch and ileoanal anastomosis, as well as the complications and their sequelae. Alternative procedures will also be discussed.

INDICATIONS FOR SURGERY

Indications for surgery can be divided into two major types: elective and emergency.

INDICATIONS FOR ELECTIVE SURGERY

Failure of Medical Therapy

Patients with CUC may require surgery either because they have failed to respond to medical therapy or because the complications of the medical therapy outweigh its benefits. CUC can cause debilitating symptoms and lead to a poor quality of life despite appropriate medical treatment. Persistent anemia, undernutrition, and protein-losing enteropathy should prompt consideration of surgical intervention. Close consultation between the patient, gastroenterologist, and surgeon is important. Delayed surgery for patients with acute severe ulcerative colitis is associated with an increased risk of postoperative complications.[1] Careful explanations of the long-term side effects and implications of medical therapy and the risks, benefits, goals, and alternatives of the surgical options need to be given. Patients who undergo definitive surgery for CUC have reduced direct medical costs in the 2 years after surgical recovery—surgical intervention is associated with long-term economic benefit.[2]

Presence of Cancer and Dysplasia

Cancer-complicating long-standing colitis is an obvious indication for surgery. Patients with ulcerative colitis for more than 10 to 15 years have a well-recognized increased risk for cancer. Those with sclerosing cholangitis as a complication of ulcerative colitis seem to have a particularly high incidence. Colonoscopic surveillance is recommended in patients with long-standing ulcerative colitis. The development of an obstructing lesion, dysplasia, or a dysplasia-associated lesion of the mucosa is an indication for surgery.

INDICATIONS FOR EMERGENCY SURGERY

Fulminant Colitis

Patients with a severe attack of ulcerative colitis should be resuscitated and treated medically. Deterioration of the patient's condition or failure to improve within 5 days is an indication for surgical intervention. In an ill patient, intervention should take the form of emergency total colectomy with preservation of the rectum and an end ileostomy. The rectal stump may be oversewn or brought up to the abdominal wall as a mucus fistula.

Toxic Megacolon

Toxic megacolon is a life-threatening condition. Although it may occur as an acute exacerbation of the disease, it is an initial manifestation in most patients. There is segmental or total dilation of the colon. Patients are very ill with high fever, abdominal pain and tenderness, tachycardia, and leukocytosis. Prompt resuscitation and medical therapy are essential, along with early recourse to resection.

Hemorrhage, Perforation, and Obstruction

Massive hemorrhage is uncommon and accounts for only up to 10% of emergency colectomies in patients with CUC. Perforation of the colon is a clear indication for surgery. If it occurs in the absence of megacolon, the possibility of Crohn disease should be raised. High doses of steroids mask the symptoms and signs. Strictures in patients with CUC are rare unless a carcinoma has developed.

ILEAL POUCH–ANAL ANASTOMOSIS

OVERVIEW OF THE OPERATION

The operation is usually performed in two stages.[3] First, the cecum, colon, and rectum are mobilized and removed. Care is taken to preserve the pelvic nerves. The ileum is preserved in its entirety. A reservoir (ileal pouch) is constructed from 30 to 44 cm of distal ileum and anastomosed to the anal canal at or just above the dentate line. IPAA can be performed with sutures or stapling instruments and with or without transanal rectal mucosectomy. A temporary ileostomy is used to protect the pouch and anastomosis. The ileostomy is closed 8 to 12 weeks later. IPAA removes all diseased tissue and yet maintains normal bowel function and fecal continence. As experience has been acquired with the procedure, the technique has been simplified, which has led to improved outcomes. Early readmission after IPAA is common, however, mainly because of subacute obstruction, dehydration, or surgical site infection. Quality of life in patients with a pelvic ileal reservoir is better than that of patients with Brooke ileostomies, continent Kock ileostomies, and medically treated colitis.[4,5]

LAPAROSCOPIC ILEAL POUCH–ANAL ANASTOMOSIS

Techniques for laparoscopic colectomy have been developed and now provide an adjunct to traditional operative modalities for colonic surgery. The use of these techniques has expanded, and they have been applied to the performance of IPAA. Laparoscopic surgery appeals to patients undergoing IPAA because they are generally young and hope to gain the potential benefit of reduced disability, more rapid recovery, and a better body image as a result of more cosmetic incisions. Most reports have consisted of relatively small series and have tended to avoid patients with a body mass index greater than 30, toxic megacolon, or treatment with high-dose steroids. The best laparoscopic technique to use, be it laparoscopically assisted[6] or hand assisted,[7] is presently the subject of much debate. Furthermore, single-incision laparoscopic techniques via a single 2.5-cm port have been described.[8]

OPERATIVE TECHNIQUE

The patient is placed in the dorsolithotomy position with Allen stirrups and minimal hip flexion (Figure 160-1). A 12-mm port is placed at the umbilicus, and pneumoperitoneum is initiated at 15 mm Hg. A 10-mm, 30-degree laparoscope is used throughout. Additional ports are placed at the lateral edge of the rectus sheath: a 12-mm port at the site of the temporary ileostomy, a 5-mm port

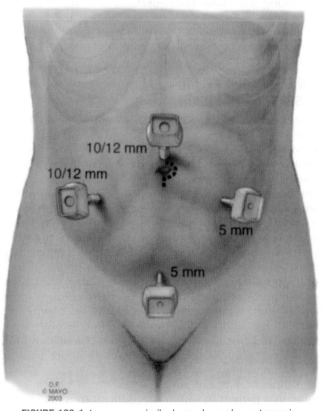

FIGURE 160-1 Laparoscopic ileal pouch–anal anastomosis.

at the lateral edge of the future Pfannenstiel incision, a 5-mm suprapubic port, and a 5-mm left upper quadrant port. With the patient in a steep reverse Trendelenburg position and rotated to the right, the dissection begins at the left lower quadrant. The colon is retracted with atraumatic graspers and mobilized with a Harmonic Scalpel up to the splenic flexure. The patient is then rotated to the left and the ascending colon is mobilized similarly. The omentum is retracted in a cephalad direction and mobilized from the colon, again with the harmonic scalpel. The transverse mesocolon is approached from either side and divided with the Harmonic Scalpel, and the major mesenteric vessels are ligated with clips. With the patient then in a steep Trendelenburg position, the presacral space is entered and the dissection continued to the pelvic floor while avoiding damage to the autonomic nerves and ureters. A 6-cm Pfannenstiel incision is used to complete the mobilization of the lower portion of the rectum, and the rectum is transected at the anorectal junction with a linear stapler. The ileal pouch is then constructed through the Pfannenstiel incision after securing the anvil of a circular stapler within the pouch with interrupted sutures. The IPAA is then constructed with a double-staple technique. A suitable loop of ileum is identified for the diverting loop ileostomy at the right midquadrant trocar site.

Alternatively, laparoscopic proctocolectomy can be accomplished with a hand-assisted technique. Here, a 7- to 8-cm Pfannenstiel or low midline incision is made at the start of the operation through which the hand port is placed. Two or three additional trocars are used, one 5 or 10 mm above the umbilicus (laparoscope), a 5-mm port in the epigastrium (for dissection), and a 12-mm trocar in the lower left quadrant (for dissection, stapling, and clipping). A randomized trial that compared 30 patients after hand-assisted laparoscopic IPAA with 30 patients after open IPAA by measuring postoperative recovery and quality of life in the 3 months after surgery found no difference between the two procedures in quality of life at 3 months after surgery. Operative times were longer in the laparoscopic group than in the open group (210 vs. 133 minutes, $P < 0.001$). No significant differences were found in morphine requirements, morbidity, or postoperative hospital stay between the two groups. However, postoperative stays were quite long in both groups, and 10% of patients required a reoperation. The median overall cost was 16,728 euros for the hand-assisted laparoscopic procedure and 13,406 euros for the open procedure.[9]

Laparoscopic IPAA is technically feasible and can be carried out within a reasonable time frame. In addition, it is safe. The operative technique will undoubtedly undergo modification, and operating times will decrease as laparoscopic surgeons become more experienced with the technique. One difficulty is precise division of the rectum at the appropriate level above the dentate line without resorting to the use of incisions as described earlier, that is, using a totally intracorporeal procedure. Current stapling devices do not permit a satisfactory intracorporeal single division of the anorectum without risking a skewed line of division or an anastomosis sited too high above the dentate line. Although alternative

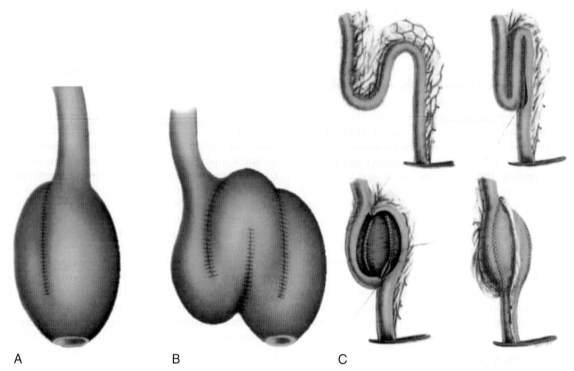

FIGURE 160-2 The three most commonly performed ileal pouch procedures. **A,** J pouch. **B,** W pouch. **C,** S pouch.

methods exist, such as a transanal method of everting the rectum that allows easier transection under visual control and a sufficiently low pouch-anal anastomosis, it is likely that the problem will only be solved with development of improved stapling devices. Concern about operative cost needs to be balanced with earlier return to work and economic benefit to the community. Furthermore, maintenance of the integrity of the abdominal wall may also benefit patients by reducing long-term disability, including the development of incisional hernias and late interventions for adhesions. Certainly, laparoscopic IPAA results in few adhesions to the abdominal wall and to gynecologic organs with or without the use of adhesional barriers.[10] Operative cost analysis alone should not condemn laparoscopic surgery.

The functional outcome after laparoscopically assisted IPAA is no different from that after conventional IPAA. In a case-control study of 16 patients after laparoscopic IPAA, questionnaires were completed to assess functional outcome, quality of life, body image, and cosmesis. No differences were found in functional outcome and quality of life. Satisfaction with the cosmetic result was significantly higher in the laparoscopic group than in the conventional group.[11] Similarly, a case-control study of 20 patients who had undergone laparoscopic IPAA versus 20 open cases found significantly longer operative times, quicker return of bowel function, and shorter length of stay in laparoscopic versus open cases. A case-matched series of 33 laparoscopically assisted and 33 open IPAA procedures reported a postoperative morbidity rate of 6% in the laparoscopic group versus 12% in the open group.[6] No differences were observed in functional outcome between the two groups, and quality of life was similar.

DESIGN OF THE ILEAL POUCH

The pelvic ileal reservoir may be constructed from two, three, or four limbs of distal ileum anastomosed in side-to-side fashion (Figure 160-2).[12] There is no agreement regarding the ideal configuration, and there is little difference in functional outcome among the available designs of pouch. However, some pouches are easier to construct than others, and the patient's body habitus may influence the choice of pouch.

THREE-LIMBED PELVIC ILEAL RESERVOIR—S POUCH

The S pouch was the first pelvic ileal reservoir to be described (see Figure 160-2).[13] It was a modification of the reservoir originally described by Kock for use as a continent ileostomy[14] and was constructed from 30 cm of distal ileum. A 25-cm segment was opened along the antimesenteric border and folded three times, and the adjacent edges were sutured together. The most distal 5 cm was not incorporated into the reservoir but rather acted as an efferent conduit or spout. Unlike the Kock reservoir, there was no inverted nipple valve. Self-catheterization was needed to empty the pouch in four of the original five patients, but this problem was largely overcome by reducing the length of the efferent spout and avoiding a long rectal muscular cuff. A long efferent limb (4 to 6 cm) would tend to impede evacuation because of acute angulation between the pouch and the efferent spout. The longer the limb, the more likely it was to angulate and hence obstruct.

Although it is not widely used, the S pouch is of value in a patient in whom it is difficult to mobilize the ileum sufficiently to allow the apex of a conventional two-limbed pelvic ileal reservoir to reach the anal canal without tension. In this situation, the most distal part of the ileum can usually be made to reach low enough in the pelvis to allow construction of a tension-free anastomosis.

There is no firm rule with regard to the length of ileum used to construct the S pouch or, indeed, any pouch. After the initial descriptions, most S pouches have been constructed from three limbs of 15 cm of ileum. If too large a pouch is made, however, there is a tendency for it to become distended and atonic. Although such pouches may be both capacious and compliant, the tone of the muscular wall may be low, which can lead to stasis and incomplete evacuation. Furthermore, the efferent spout possesses peristaltic activity that is independent of the body of the ileal reservoir, and this may further impede emptying. The S pouch can be constructed with no efferent spout. The distal end of the ileum is oversewn and an enterotomy made at the apex of the first and second loops at the most dependent part. The IPAA is constructed in side-to-end fashion between the most dependent part of the reservoir and the anal canal. Such construction permits spontaneous evacuation. Although the S pouch is usually hand-sutured, linear stapling instruments can be used with no increase in morbidity.

The efficiency of evacuation of S pouches is less than that of J- and W-pouches, and a small minority of patients still need to self-catheterize.[15] Self-catheterization is not popular with patients because it is messy, time-consuming, and unpleasant. Such pouches can be revised, particularly if the efferent limb is too long either because of the original construction or because the spout has lengthened with time after surgery. A small group of patients who have an efferent spout of only 1 cm at the time of surgery return with a 4- or 5-cm spout. Revision of the segment, without changing the configuration of the pouch, can restore satisfactory function.[16] Long efferent limbs may be shortened or excised, or the S pouch may be converted to a J pouch.[16] Resection of a long efferent limb and reanastomosis may be performed by means of a transanal approach, but the success rate is low. Revision usually requires complete mobilization of the reservoir and its efferent conduit by a transabdominal approach, which can be a challenge. The ileoanal anastomosis is taken down and the entire efferent spout excised. The IPAA is then reestablished. Most of the small number of patients who have undergone such revision surgery have been able to evacuate their reservoir spontaneously. Alternatively, the septum between the pouch and the efferent limb may be divided transanally with the linear stapler, or the efferent spout may be shortened by inserting a circular staple gun into the pouch and positioning it such that when the gun is closed, part of the efferent spout is trapped. When the gun is subsequently fired, the spout is shortened and the IPAA simultaneously re-created. Nevertheless, the difficulties of revision surgery on the IPAA must not be underestimated, and only about 50% of these patients will eventually have good function.[16]

TWO-LIMBED PELVIC ILEAL RESERVOIR—J POUCH

The two-limbed J-shaped reservoir was introduced by Utsunomiya et al[3] in 1980 (see Figure 160-2) and is now by far the most popular pouch. The J pouch is constructed from a long side-to-side anastomosis along the antimesenteric border of the ileum with the limbs arranged in an iso-antiperistaltic fashion. The apex of the ileal loop that reaches to the level of the anal canal without tension is chosen to form the most dependent part of the reservoir. Transillumination of the mesentery helps identify the vessel arcades. The ileocecal artery may be divided to increase the mobility of the ileal mesentery. Reach may be increased by making windows in the ileal mesentery and scoring the peritoneum over the mesentery, although this may predispose to the development of hematomas. The length of the two limbs is variable and depends partly on the amount of fat in the ileal mesentery and the distribution of the ileal arcades. There is no difference in functional outcome between J pouches constructed from two 10-cm limbs or two 20-cm limbs. The J-shaped reservoir is simple and quick to construct, particularly if linear stapling devices are used.

Despite the aforementioned maneuvers, difficulty may be experienced in allowing the apex of the ileal loop to reach down to the anal canal without tension. In this event, two further tactics are useful. First, an efferent limb may be constructed by division of the apex of the ileal loop. The two ileal limbs are then anastomosed in the usual iso-antiperistaltic fashion, with a 2-cm efferent spout emerging from the isoperistaltic limb (see Figure 160-2). This design facilitates greater length of the reservoir and reduces the possibility of tension on the IPAA. Alternatively, the ileal loop may be divided at a point proximal to the apex. An efferent spout is fashioned such that the ileal spout is positioned in an antiperistaltic manner, which may result in improved continence and reduced fecal leakage, although this might be outweighed by a tendency for the antiperistaltic efferent limb to impede evacuation. In practice, careful division of the ileocolic vessels will usually permit a tension-free anastomosis. Division of the visceral peritoneum on either side of the ileal mesentery allows the mesentery to stretch, but this can be risky because tension on the pouch as it is brought down to the anal canal may tear the terminal branches of the superior mesenteric arcades at the apex of the J, which are now unsupported by their protective mesentery. Generally, if the most dependent part of the pouch will reach to a level 5 to 6 cm below the upper border of the symphysis pubis, there is sufficient length to allow a tension-free anastomosis.

QUADRUPLICATED PELVIC ILEAL RESERVOIR—W POUCH

The quadruplicated or W pouch was introduced in 1985 in an attempt to answer the problems of incomplete evacuation of the S pouch and to improve the functional results obtained with the J pouch.[17] It was constructed from four 12-cm lengths of ileum that were sutured in a W arrangement. The IPAA was created in side-to-end fashion between the most dependent part of the reservoir and the top of the anal canal.

The spheroidal design gives the greatest volume for a given length of ileum, the pouch sits well within the confines of the pelvis, and the horizontal diameter of the

W pouch is similar to that of the normal rectal ampulla. One drawback, however, is that the bulky nature of this pouch can cause difficulty, especially in an obese male patient with a narrow pelvis. The design of the reservoir may be modified such that the distal two limbs are each 11 to 12 cm in length, whereas the more proximal two limbs are 9 to 10 cm long (see Figure 160-2). The reservoir is then effectively two J-shaped reservoirs anastomosed together but slightly offset. This arrangement allows the reservoir to sit more comfortably within the bony confines of the pelvis while maintaining its large capacity.

COMPARATIVE STUDIES OF POUCH DESIGN

There is an inverse relationship between the frequency of bowel movements and the volume of the reservoir. The volume of expansion, however, may be less in J pouches and W pouches than in S-shaped pouches, where outflow obstruction may lead to dilation of the reservoir.

A 2 × 2 prospective randomized trial that compared J and W pouches, as well as large and small pouches (2 × 20 vs. 2 × 10 cm and 4 × 10 vs. 4 × 15 cm), showed no statistically significant difference between the pouch designs; indeed, the smaller reservoirs in the study paradoxically seemed to offer slightly better functional outcome.[18] Improved results for the W pouch may be related to both the volume and the shape of the configuration. Studies of the influence of pouch design on function during the so-called maturation period after closure of the ileostomy have been conducted in a randomized setting in which 24 patients randomly assigned to J-pouch or W-pouch construction were studied at regular intervals in the 12 months after closure of the ileostomy. During the maturation period, the frequency of defecation decreased in both groups, but patients with a W reservoir had significantly lower values than did patients with a J reservoir. Similarly, both nighttime defecation and the use of antidiarrheal medication were significantly lower for patients with a W reservoir.[19]

Comparative studies have suggested that W pouches have some benefits over other designs of pouch in terms of capacity, compliance, and evacuation characteristics,[15] but prospective randomized studies have not shown a significant benefit in functional outcome.[20] Essentially, the few published prospective randomized studies that have compared the design of the ileal reservoir have failed to provide a convincing argument for surgeons to abandon the relatively quick and easy J pouch in favor of the W pouch, which tends to be hand-sutured and take much longer to construct than the stapled J pouch.

The J pouch has therefore become established as the most popular design of ileal reservoir.

FUNCTION OF THE ILEAL POUCH

POUCH COMPLIANCE AND CAPACITY

The maximum tolerated capacity of the normal rectum is 300 to 400 mL.[21] At these volumes, intrarectal pressure rarely exceeds 15 to 20 cm H_2O, and compliance (rate of increase in pressure per unit increase in volume) is

about 18 mL/cm H_2O. Compliance of the distal ileum is considerably lower, however, at 2 mL/cm H_2O.

In contrast to the ileum, the capacity and compliance of ileal pouches differ little from those of a normal rectum. One study of 23 patients found the maximum capacity to be 320 ± 36 mL with a compliance of 14.7 ± 1.4 mL/cm H_2O.[21]

Although low pouch compliance has been suggested as a possible cause of functional disturbance of ileal pouches, measurement of pouch compliance offers no influence on the clinical management of idiopathic pouch dysfunction.[22]

ILEAL MOTILITY

In terms of motor function, the principal difference between normal rectum and ileum is the response to distention. The rectum relaxes, whereas the ileum responds by contraction and forceful peristalsis. The rectum acts as a reservoir, whereas the ileum acts as a conduit.

Two types of motor waves are generated by the ileum— a low-amplitude (<10 mm Hg) phasic contraction of short duration (3 to 6 seconds) and a tonic contraction of longer duration (40 to 60 seconds) and large amplitude (>25 mm Hg). The frequency and amplitude of high-pressure waves increase after feeding and are abolished by evacuation. Tonic waves occur in response to ileal distention, and patients feel the need to evacuate. Both phasic and tonic waves are also seen in patients with Kock continent reservoirs, straight ileoanal anastomoses, and pelvic ileal reservoirs. Tonic waves are generated in response to distention, and the volume required to provoke these high-pressure contractions is significantly less in a single-lumen ileum (30 mL) than in three-limbed pouches (322 mL). The ileal reservoir therefore acts more like a capacitance organ with the ability to distend without contraction before a significant volume has amassed, whereas a single-lumen ileum constantly attempts to clear its contents.

Propulsive peristaltic waves are seen in a single-lumen ileum even when not distended. Although ileal reservoirs develop similar propulsive peristaltic waves, they occur only during distention of the reservoir when the filling pressure exceeds 20 cm H_2O. The frequency and amplitude of the peristaltic waves are proportional to the degree of distention. Measurement of myoelectrical activity confirms the motor findings, with uncoordinated activity being present in the ileal reservoir at rest. Myoelectrical spike activity becomes coordinated in the reservoir only in response to distention and produces coordinated propulsion.

As the pouch fills with effluent, high-pressure waves are produced. They are recognized by the patient as a desire to evacuate the pouch or as lower abdominal discomfort. They occur more frequently after meals and are largely abolished by evacuation of the pouch. The interval between onset of the high-pressure waves is directly related to the frequency of bowel action. Therefore, the volume of distention at which high-pressure waves occur is a major determinant of stool frequency. The *threshold volume* at which high-pressure waves occur is related to stool frequency: the larger the threshold volume, the lower the frequency of bowel movements.[21] An increase in pressure within the lumen of the pouch is associated with increased resting anal canal pressure and rate of contraction. The pressure gradient between the anal canal and pouch is less in incontinent patients, who have lower resting anal pressure, higher nocturnal pouch pressure, and larger-amplitude high-pressure waves in the pouch than continent pouch patients do. The pressure gradient in the neorectal canal is frequently reversed in incontinent patients. These patients have lower resting anal pressure during sleep, and this lower pressure, together with marked variations in mean anal canal pressure, leads to incontinence. In a small minority of patients, high-pressure waves may be generated within the ileal wall at low volumes of distention. The amplitude of these waves may exceed that of resting anal pressure and thus may lead to seepage or soilage of the perineum.

Continuous manometric recordings at spaced intervals throughout the jejunoileum have demonstrated the presence of large-amplitude waves that propagate rapidly throughout the jejunum of patients who have undergone IPAA. Such waves are normally confined to the distal ileum of healthy individuals. They have been shown to propel intestinal contents through canine ileum. These waves may be a manifestation of increased storage and distention of the distal ileum.

The presence of a pouch influences proximal gut transit. Although gastric emptying is similar in patients with pouches, patients with Brooke ileostomies, and controls, small bowel transit of radiolabeled material was significantly longer in patients with pouches than in controls or those with Brooke ileostomies.

The use of radiolabeled artificial stool has shown that as the ileal reservoir fills to its threshold volume and defecation is postponed, the pouch does not continue to distend, but rather there is retrograde reflux of up to 40% of the stool into the ileum immediately proximal to the reservoir. As this more proximal part of the ileum distends, high-pressure waves are generated that tend to propel the ileal contents back into the pouch. As the volume of distal ileal and pouch contents increases, the frequency and intensity of the high-pressure waves increase and will eventually produce abdominal discomfort and urgency of defecation.[21] Reflux of stool into the proximal ileum at the time of defecation does not appear to occur.

Irritable pouch syndrome (IPS) is a functional disorder in patients with an ileal pouch that presents with symptoms in the absence of structural abnormalities of the pouch. It resembles other functional disorders such as irritable bowel syndrome that are characterized by visceral hypersensitivity. Similarly, IPS is characterized by visceral hypersensitivity as evidenced by scores of sensation of gas, urge to defecate, and pain as measured by visual analogue scales.[23]

EFFICIENCY OF EVACUATION

The desire to evacuate the pouch occurs as it distends to the threshold volume. The time between one evacuation and the desire to evacuate again is influenced by a number of factors, such as capacity and compliance, the rate at which fecal contents reach the reservoir, and the completeness of evacuation. Most ileal reservoirs fail to empty as completely as normal rectum.[24] Nevertheless, studies with radiolabeled gel have shown that two-limbed pouches generally evacuated 60% to 70% of their contents. The rate of evacuation of ileal pouches is about 11 mL of stool per second. In the absence of pouch dysfunction, the intrinsic motility of the pouch is not directly responsible for evacuation. The frequency of bowel action is directly correlated with the efficiency of evacuation. Thus, pouches that evacuate most efficiently result in the lowest frequency of bowel action.[21] Similarly, the slower the reservoir fills to its threshold volume, the lower the frequency of bowel movements and the volume of stool produced each day. This is one of the most important determinants of the frequency of bowel action.[21] Therefore, factors that either hasten filling of the reservoir or impede emptying promote earlier onset of reservoir contractions and lead to a greater frequency of defecation.

POSTPRANDIAL POUCH TONE

Small intestinal motility is propagated into the ileal pouch, and this may influence pouch function. Both the tone of the pouch and motility have been shown to increase after a meal.[25] The extent to which pouch function is influenced by changes in pouch tone and motility induced by a meal has been studied with the electronic barostat. The electronic barostat is an ideal instrument to characterize not only the compliance and sensory characteristics of the pouch but also postprandial changes in pouch tone and motility. The electronic barostat used to distend the ileoanal pouch involves the use of a polyethylene bag tied to the end of a 19-French multilumen tube, and this catheter in turn is connected to the barostat. The barostat is able to induce distention at constant pressure (isobaric distention), and the pressure is kept constant by electronic feedback regulation of the air volume within the bag.[26] A functional study of 19 patients with ileal pouches and either high stool frequency ($n = 8$) or adequate stool frequency ($n = 11$) were studied in this way. This comparative study found similar pouch compliance and sensitivity between the two groups of patients but demonstrated that postprandial pouch tone was increased significantly in patients with high stool frequency.[27] Many patients report the urge to defecate directly after a meal. Not only is pouch tone increased after a meal, but the increase in pouch tone also appears to be related to pouch function—the postprandial increase in pouch tone is greater in patients with poor pouch function than in patients with adequate pouch function. Therefore, in the absence of differences in pouch compliance, sensitivity, and 24-hour stool volume, the postprandial meal response may have an important influence on pouch function. The increase in pouch tone depends on the state of filling of the pouch. When the pouch is full, an increase in tone will increase pouch pressure. This results in urgency. If the pouch is empty, an increase in tone will reduce pouch volume. Therefore, it will be full earlier and the frequency of stool evacuation will increase.[27] Although there is a significant correlation between postprandial pouch tone and pouch function, the correlation between pouch compliance and pouch function is less strong, thus implying that the clinical significance of postprandial pouch tone may be greater than that of pouch compliance in patients with ileal reservoirs. Reports of rupture of J reservoirs after the rapid consumption of high-calorie, high-fiber meals support this hypothesis and suggest that the meal response can lead to serious complications.

ECOLOGY OF THE POUCH

The bacterial flora of pouches, together with their products of metabolism, especially volatile fatty acids, may have an important influence on the function of pouches. Major differences have been observed between the ecology of three- and four-limbed pouches.[15] Significantly greater numbers of bacteroides and concentrations of acetic, propionic, butyric, and valeric acid are seen in the effluent from three-limbed pouches than in the effluent from four-limbed pouches. The absolute numbers of bacteroides and bifidobacteria, the ratio of anaerobes to aerobes, and the concentrations of volatile fatty acids are also greater in the effluent from patients with pouches than in the effluent from patients who have undergone conventional panproctocolectomy with ileostomy. The flora of ileal reservoirs therefore more closely resembles that of the colon than normal ileum. There appears to be no correlation between the proportion of stool retained after defecation and the number of anaerobic bacteria.

Volatile fatty acids may be beneficial to pouches. Within the colon, they are the major substrate, and butyrate promotes sodium and hence water absorption. Indeed, increased production of volatile fatty acids in experimental animals is associated with suppression of enteropathic bacteria.

FUNCTIONAL OUTCOME

The choice of reservoir design is largely a question of personal preference and occasionally operative restraints. The decision is usually a compromise between the smaller-capacity, but easily constructed, duplicated (J) pouch and the larger-capacity, but more time-consuming, three- or four-limbed pouches.

Frequency of bowel action correlates inversely with the capacity of the reservoir.[21] The best results should therefore be obtained in patients with the largest reservoirs. However, huge reservoirs are associated with impaired contractility and poor evacuation, and several authors have noticed an improvement in bowel frequency with a decrease in size of the reservoir.

Patients with a pouch pass about 600 to 700 mL of semiformed stool each day, which is about four times that of healthy controls with intact anorectums. Loperamide reduces intestinal motility and thus may improve intestinal absorption and reduce the volume of stool and the frequency of bowel action. Although dietary discretion and stool-bulking agents may decrease the urgency of defecation and perianal irritation by increasing stool consistency, these measures seem to have minimal effect on stool volume. Studies have shown little difference in the efficiency of evacuation of pouches according to the consistency of stool, which implies that measures to alter

the consistency of stool will have no influence on pouch function.[28]

The frequency of bowel action has been shown to be significantly less in patients with three-limbed pouches than in those with two-limbed pouches and significantly less in patients with four-limbed pouches than in those with either two- or three-limbed pouches.[17] However, the only prospective randomized trial that compared the functional results of duplicated (J) with quadruplicated (W) pouches failed to show any significant difference in the frequency of bowel action. Compliance of the pouch is closely related to capacity: the larger the pouch, the greater the compliance. The correlation between frequency of bowel action and compliance of the reservoir is not, however, as strong as the correlation with capacity of the pouch. Larger reservoirs have lower contractility, which may lead to stasis and progressive dilation, particularly in the presence of a long efferent limb with its potential to impede evacuation.

Function is maintained long-term with very little if any deterioration in terms of frequency of bowel movements, efficiency of evacuation, and fecal leakage as the years pass by.

The perfect pouch has not been described. The choice of pouch design depends on the characteristics of the patient and the surgeon's preference. The functional outcome varies little between the basic options, and most patients will find that they will have bowel action between four and seven times per 24 hours with perhaps one nocturnal evacuation. They will experience a normal urge to defecate and will be able to defer defecation and to discriminate between flatus and feces.

THE ILEOANAL ANASTOMOSIS

The method used to construct the IPAA is debatable, and there are two options:
1. Transanal mucosal resection with a hand-sutured anastomosis between the pouch and the internal anal sphincter fashioned at the level of the dentate line
2. Single- or double-stapled technique with construction of the IPAA at a slightly higher level.[29]

An advantage of transanal mucosectomy is that all diseased mucosa is removed with no possibility of symptoms from residual diseased mucosa. The risk of cancer developing in the persistent rectal mucosa is eliminated. Resting anal pressure falls after IPAA, irrespective of the surgical technique used.[30] However, significant recovery of anal sphincter function, with a rise in resting anal pressure, return of the rectoanal inhibitory reflex, and improvement in clinical outcome, is seen to occur for at least 12 months after stapled IPAA.[31] Similar recovery may or may not occur after transanal mucosectomy. Surgeons in favor of the double-stapled technique suggest that it is an easier operation, with improved functional outcome. This latter point is debatable, however, because most reports of studies in which comparisons have been made between the two operative techniques have not been randomized and have included historical controls, which have invariably been taken from the learning curve of the surgeon's experience. The few randomized trials and case-control studies published to date, though small in numbers, show no functional differences. However, a large retrospective review of 3109 patients that compared 474 patients with a hand-sewn anastomosis with 2635 patients with a stapled anastomosis of similar demographics suggested better outcomes in patients who had undergone a stapled IPAA. Anastomotic stricture, septic complications, and fecal seepage were all greater after hand-sewn anastomosis than after stapled IPAA.[32]

TRANSANAL MUCOSECTOMY

To preserve normal rectal sensation, it was long thought necessary to preserve a long muscular cuff of rectum. Preservation of a 10- to 12-cm rectal cuff denuded of its mucosa was very tedious and difficult, especially in the presence of severe disease, and it often required a combination of both abdominal and transanal dissection. Transanal mucosal resection required a long period of anal retraction, which was associated with significant functional impairment of the anal sphincter,[30] although this problem was minimized if the amount of anal retraction was reduced. Extensive rectal mucosectomy was also associated with a high incidence of postoperative pelvic sepsis in the form of cuff abscesses despite meticulous hemostasis and drainage of the cuff space. The realization that the sensation of rectal fullness and the need to evacuate were preserved in the absence of a rectum allowed the length of mucosal resection to be shortened significantly. Transanal mucosal resection is now carried out for a distance of only 3 to 4 cm and can be completed with minimal retraction on the anal sphincter, especially if a specifically designed ring retractor is used.

After the rectum has been fully mobilized to the pelvic floor, the surgeon moves to the perineum. With the patient in the modified Lloyd-Davies position, retraction hooks are placed circumferentially into the dentate line to splay the mucosa of the anal canal (Lone Star retractor; Lone Star Company, Texas). The submucosal plane is infiltrated with a solution of 1:100,000 epinephrine, and the mucosa is dissected off the underlying rectal wall with either scissors or diathermy. Dissection is continued to the level of the pelvic floor, at which point the muscularis is incised and the presacral space is entered. The rectum is fully divided at this level and the mucosectomy specimen retrieved through the anus. The pouch is then delivered into the pelvis and its apex brought down to the pelvic floor. An abdominal operator may insert four-quadrant sutures into the incised apex of the pouch, which in turn are passed to the perineal operator to complete the IPAA (Figure 160-3).

SINGLE- OR DOUBLE-STAPLED TECHNIQUE

This technique, in which either a purse-string suture is inserted into the anal stump or the anal stump is cross-stapled about 2 cm above the dentate line and a circular stapling device is inserted into the anal stump to perform the IPAA, has acquired wide popularity. The technical difficulties of transanal mucosal resection and hand-sutured IPAA are eliminated.

An early stimulus to the development of this procedure was the high incidence of nocturnal incontinence after mucosectomy and hand-sutured anastomosis. The anal transitional zone (ATZ) is richly innervated and

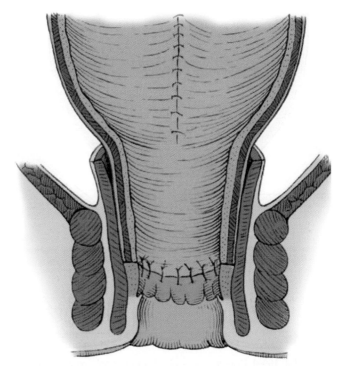

FIGURE 160-3 Ileal pouch–anal anastomosis with mucosal resection.

seems to be important in the discrimination between flatus and feces. Preservation of the ATZ improves anal sensation,[33] and several authors have demonstrated recovery of motor function of the anal sphincter.

The cecum, colon, and rectum are mobilized in the usual manner, with care taken to preserve the pelvic nerves. The rectum is mobilized fully to the pelvic floor and a small (35-mm) linear cross-stapler is maneuvered into the lower portion of the pelvis. When the surgeon is confident that the stapler is in the correct position, which is confirmed by measuring the distance above the dentate line by insertion of a digit, the linear stapler is closed and fired. This leaves a stapled anal stump with the ATZ intact. A circular stapling device is then inserted into the anal stump and the central trocar advanced through the cross-staple line. The detached head of the gun, positioned within the ileal pouch, is manipulated into line with the shaft of the circular gun. The gun is closed and fired, and the double-stapled IPAA is complete (Figure 160-4). Concern about the possibility of an anastomotic leak after stapling across a staple line (double-stapled technique) has led some surgeons to use a purse-string suture to close the anal stump around the shaft of the circular stapler (single-stapled technique).

The exact distance between the level of the ileoanal anastomosis and the dentate line may be critical in terms of functional outcome. A comparison of ileoanal anastomoses made at the dentate line, at the top of the anal columns of Morgagni, and at a level 1 cm above the columns showed the importance of this region in terms of fecal continence and fine control of defecation.[34] Construction of the ileoanal anastomosis at the dentate line was associated with a higher incidence of seepage and

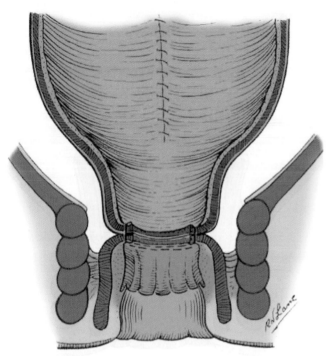

FIGURE 160-4 Double-stapled ileal pouch–anal anastomosis.

soilage than when the anastomosis was made at the top of the anal columns. If the anastomosis was made too far proximal, however, recurrence of disease was noted. It can be very difficult to accurately place the linear stapler, particularly if the patient is a thick-set male with a narrow pelvis. However, it remains surprising just how low the stapler can be placed, even in such large patients. Conversely, in a thin female with an accessible pelvis, the linear stapler may be positioned too low on the rectum such that the doughnuts of the stapling device may include part of the internal sphincter. To permit direct inspection of the upper border of the ATZ, the anorectum can be everted by fully mobilizing the rectum to the level of the upper anal canal. The rectum is then transected at midbody. Stay sutures are inserted into the lateral walls of the rectal stump and passed transanally to the perineal operator. Strong distal traction on the anorectum everts it through the anal canal and allows direct visualization of the ATZ and accurate placement of the cross-stapler. The residual rectal sleeve is then removed and the blind anal stump allowed back into the pelvis. The IPAA is then stapled into position in the usual manner.[35] This technique is more likely to result in a true IPAA than in an ileal pouch–rectostomy.

Despite full rectal mobilization, quite firm traction is required by the perineal operator to achieve complete eversion. Early reports of this technique suggested that the functional results of everted and noneverted ileoanal anastomoses were similar. However, measurements of anal sphincter function have shown increased pudendal nerve latency times and blunted electrosensation after double-stapled IPAA with anorectal eversion. This appears to result in some impairment in anal sensation and a greater tendency of patients to experience seepage than after conventional IPAA.

THE CRITICAL LEVEL OF THE ILEAL POUCH–ANAL ANASTOMOSIS

The precise relationship between the level of the ileoanal anastomosis and the dentate line may be critical in terms of recurrence of disease and objective measurements of pouch and anal function. Preservation of the ATZ may be associated with a potential for the development of proctitis, dysplasia, and cancer. The upper border of the ATZ is irregular, with fingers of ATZ interdigitating with true rectal columnar mucosa. The rectal tongues may extend all the way down to the dentate line. Ulcerative colitis has been shown to be present within the transitional area in 90% of specimens resected by conventional proctocolectomy.[36] Mucosal columnar epithelial cells may remain within the ATZ in up to 20% of patients after mucosectomy.[37] However, mucosectomy does not guarantee elimination of the disease. Indeed, the only reports to date of rectal cancer after restorative proctocolectomy have been in patients who had undergone mucosectomy with hand-sutured anastomoses and preservation of a rectal cuff. Most patients with a stapled IPAA will have inflammation at the margin of the staple line. The incidence of dysplasia in mucosal strippings from the anal stump was 2.5% in a series of 118 patients with ulcerative colitis.[38] A retrospective study of 254 patients who underwent restorative proctocolectomy for ulcerative colitis with a stapled IPAA revealed low-grade dysplasia in 8 patients (3.1%).[39] Neither high-grade dysplasia nor cancer was identified in the ATZ. However, biopsies of the ATZ taken 6 months later revealed dysplasia in 2 patients, in one of whom the initial diagnosis was chronic ulcerative colitis with concurrent colon cancer (T3, N0, M0), whereas the other patient had CUC with concurrent high-grade dysplasia. Both subsequently underwent completion mucosal resection. Although the incidence of low-grade dysplasia in the ATZ is low after restorative proctocolectomy with stapled IPAA[39] and it remains to be determined whether low-grade dysplasia always progresses to high-grade dysplasia and cancer, it is probably wiser to perform total mucosectomy with a hand-sutured IPAA in patients with a preoperative diagnosis of concurrent colon carcinoma or dysplasia.

Resting anal pressure falls after restorative proctocolectomy irrespective of surgical technique. Factors other than simple traction on the sphincter have been implicated. Submucosal dissection may result in inadvertent dissection of the inner circular muscle fibers, with consequent fibrosis. Similarly, the submucosal neurologic plexus may be partially disrupted and the autonomic nervous supply to the anal sphincter may be injured. Extrinsic sympathetic nerves reach the anorectum from two sources: the presacral nerves, which form two nerve trunks and run along the lateral pelvic walls, and the inferior mesenteric nerves, which form a periarterial plexus around the inferior mesenteric and later the superior rectal arteries. Although the presacral nerves can be easily identified at the pelvic brim and swept out of the operative field, their direct connections to the internal sphincter are at risk in the later stages of mobilization and division of the rectum. Division of the superior rectal artery and therefore the periarterial mesenteric nerves results in an immediate drop in resting anal pressure of about 20%.[40] Complete mobilization of the rectum and division at the anorectal junction also contribute to the fall in resting anal pressure. However, significant recovery in anal sphincter function, with a rise in resting anal pressure and improvement in clinical outcome, is seen to occur for at least 12 months after stapled restorative proctocolectomy.[31] Similar recovery has not been reported in patients after mucosectomy. Therefore, avoiding significant anal manipulation with the stapled technique provides better manometric results than transanal mucosectomy does.

Any potential benefit in terms of functional outcome achieved by preservation of the ATZ must be balanced against the potential need for intervention if symptomatic inflammation or malignancy develops. The majority of patients who undergo restorative proctocolectomy are young adults. They are likely to require good anal sphincter function for many years, but conversely, any residual rectal mucosa will potentially have that long to undergo malignant degeneration. This may be dealt with by reoperation consisting of transanal dissection of the residual mucosa, disconnection of the IPAA, resection of any rectal cuff, and reanastomosis.[41]

TWO-STAGE OR ONE-STAGE: USE OF A DIVERTING ILEOSTOMY

Pelvic sepsis is a highly feared complication of IPAA. Postoperative leakage from either the pouch or the pouch-anal anastomosis leads to a high rate of eventual failure and excision of the pouch.[16,42] Concern about sepsis has meant that most surgeons use a temporary diverting ileostomy as a matter of routine to divert the intestinal contents away from the pouch and anastomosis until they have healed.

The temporary ileostomy is itself a potential source of morbidity.[43] Intestinal obstruction, before and after closure of the stoma, is more common in patients with a temporary ileostomy than in patients whose IPAA is completed as a one-stage procedure. Inevitably, the stoma is located more proximal than with a conventional ileostomy and is therefore more commonly associated with dehydration secondary to high stomal losses. The stoma may also be associated with peristomal skin breakdown, retraction, stenosis, and prolapse.

Several centers have presented the outcome of one-stage IPAA.[44] These studies suggest that a one-stage procedure is safe. Selection of patients is critical, however. An acutely unwell malnourished colitic patient taking high-dose steroids is not a candidate for a one-stage procedure. If a surgeon opts for a one-stage operation, even when all factors are favorable, a heavy burden is assumed. The surgeon must have a low threshold to reoperate if signs suggestive of pelvic peritonitis develop. Patients who undergo this one-stage procedure should (1) not be taking high-dose steroids, (2) undergo an uneventful operation, and (3) be in good general health. The postoperative course is more difficult for patients because they must adapt to the ileal reservoir at the same time as recovering from their operation. A study of cost data available on 835 patients of whom the ileostomy had

been omitted in 120 (14%) suggested cost savings in the region of $2000 for the hospital.[45]

A number of precautions can be taken to minimize the risk for complications after one-stage IPAA. The distal ileum should be irrigated with a solution of antibiotics before construction of the pouch. Likewise, the anorectum should be irrigated before division of the rectum, and a 24-French urinary catheter should be placed in the pouch and brought out through the anal canal to allow drainage of accumulated blood, mucus, and other secretions in the postoperative period.

There have been no randomized trials of sufficient power to adequately address the question of the advantages and disadvantages of one-stage versus two-stage IPAA. Either way, hospital readmission after IPAA is common, with many centers reporting readmission rates of about 30%. With current trends toward enhanced recovery after intestinal surgery, a more intensive followup may be needed to prevent readmission of selected high-risk patients who might be effectively managed as outpatients.

Most centers perform the ileal pouch–anal anastomosis procedure with the use of a protective ileostomy, although reports continue to emerge of large series of patients operated on by one surgeon with relatively low complication rates. It is, however, important to remember that reports of a single surgeon's experience may not always be extrapolated beyond that surgeon's practice. Most surgeons in institutions where randomized controlled trials are being carried out to compare the ileal pouch procedure with and without a diverting stoma continue to believe that they would rather deal with the complications associated with the ileostomy and its subsequent closure rather than deal with the potentially catastrophic complications of pelvic sepsis and failure of the pouch that may occur in patients without a diverting stoma.

MANAGEMENT OF POUCH-SPECIFIC POSTOPERATIVE COMPLICATIONS

INVESTIGATION

Awareness of common postoperative problems and close liaison with radiologists are the keys to success. Radiologists need to be familiar with surgical technique and postoperative anatomy so that they can identify complications at CT, magnetic resonance imaging (MRI), and fluoroscopy. Leaks from the blind end of the pouch and the pouch-anal anastomosis that result in collections or abscesses may require ultrasonography- or CT-guided drainage. Precise and judicious catheter placement and management can help improve clinical outcomes and avoid excessive imaging. The venous system must be scrutinized for thrombi secondary to surgical manipulation and sepsis. Pouchitis may be recognized by the presence of a thickened enhancing pouch wall and associated inflammatory changes and lymphadenopathy. Fistulas secondary to chronic inflammation or infection may be seen at MR imaging, CT, or fluoroscopy. Strictures appear as areas of focal luminal narrowing with proximal dilation that can lead to obstruction. To avoid repeated exposure to radiation, MR imaging may be performed in patients who need to undergo frequent imaging.

POSTOPERATIVE HEMORRHAGE

The linear stapling devices used to construct J pouches are not hemostatic. If marked bleeding is noted at the time of construction of the pouch, the pouch should be inverted and the bleeding points under-run. A large Foley catheter can be passed into the pouch for irrigation. Most bleeding will promptly stop. Sometimes the anal sphincter will retain blood in the pouch and obscure hemorrhage. Persistent bleeding warrants examination under anesthesia. Frequently, a single point of bleeding may be identified and controlled with diathermy coagulation or under-running with a suture, but more often bleeding of this extent is secondary to a disrupted suture line either in the pouch or at the ileoanal anastomosis. Postoperative bleeding after IPAA is uncommon and it usually requires nonsurgical intervention. The largest published series that addressed this problem reported pouch bleeding in 47 (1.5%) of 3194 patients undergoing IPAA. Pouch endoscopy with clot evacuation and epinephrine enemas were successful in 96%.[46] If the bleeding is uncontrollable by the transanal approach, laparotomy is indicated. Intraabdominal bleeding that is not pouch related may be from one of three sites: the colonic bed, the lateral pelvic walls, particularly in the region of the lateral ligaments, and slipped ligatures from the mesenteric vessels.

If a defect in the ileoanal anastomosis is seen and no sepsis has occurred, the problem may be corrected by interrupted sutures. A significant hematoma developing within the walls of the pouch does not augur well and may be a prelude to a leak from the pouch. The patient should be treated with broad-spectrum antibiotics, careful observation, and laparotomy if indicated.

SMALL BOWEL OBSTRUCTION

Small bowel obstruction is the most common complication seen after IPAA. Most large studies report a combined incidence of between 15% and 40% after IPAA and closure of ileostomy. This rate is higher than that reported after construction of a Brooke ileostomy. A previous colectomy with avoidance of the use of a temporary ileostomy reduces but does not eliminate the problem. Most episodes respond to conservative management such as intestinal rest, nasogastric suction, and intravenous fluids. Failure to respond necessitates laparotomy. Most cases are due to adhesions. If adhesiolysis is indicated, care must be taken to prevent damage to the pouch that may otherwise go unrecognized and lead to pelvic sepsis. If laparotomy is undertaken in the interval before closure of the ileostomy, reversal of the stoma is appropriate as long as contrast studies have demonstrated satisfactory healing of the pouch and ileoanal anastomosis. Occasionally, the afferent limb to the pouch may be identified as the site of obstruction either by becoming stuck in the pelvis and creating a flap valve or by herniating behind the pouch. Once mobilized, it is wise to tack the limb to the abdominal wall to prevent recurrence.

INTRAABDOMINAL ABSCESS

Septic complications are the most common cause of IPAA failure. An intraabdominal abscess is usually the result of a defect in the pouch or a leak from the site of closure of the ileostomy. Patients have abdominal pain, diarrhea, localized or generalized peritonitis, and fever. A computed tomographic (CT) scan will confirm the presence of an abscess. Pelvic sepsis develops in up to 25% of patients and is likely to be secondary to pouch dehiscence or a defect in the ileoanal anastomosis. The risk for sepsis decreases as surgical experience increases.

Intraabdominal abscesses require drainage either percutaneously or surgically, together with broad-spectrum antibiotics. Immediate management of a pelvic abscess includes examination under anesthesia, catheterization of the pouch, and drainage of any collection of pus. Drainage of pus from above or even removal of the pouch may be required.

A pouchogram and examination under anesthesia will reveal whether a pelvic abscess is due to dehiscence of the ileoanal anastomosis or disruption of the pouch itself. A collection associated with dehiscence of the ileoanal anastomosis is best drained through the suture line because the incidence of pouch-vaginal fistula and fistula-in-ano is high if the collection is drained through the perineum or vaginal vault. A pelvic collection may discharge spontaneously through the IPAA with subsequent formation of a fistula or stricture. Fifty percent of patients with pelvic sepsis require laparotomy, and a secondary ileostomy may need to be created. Prompt treatment is essential if the pouch is to be saved. Pelvic sepsis results in a stiff, noncompliant reservoir. The ultimate functional result is likely to be poor, and these patients have a high rate (40%) of excision of the pouch.[42] In contrast, more than 90% of patients in whom no reoperation is required may expect a satisfactory outcome.[42]

ANASTOMOTIC CUFF ABSCESS

Sepsis in the space between the residual rectal muscle and the pouch, often accompanied by partial separation of the anastomosis, is associated with persistent anal pain, diarrhea, and fecal leakage. The clinical findings can be subtle, so a high index of suspicion is essential. Predisposing factors are a difficult mucosectomy with troublesome hemostasis and a long rectal cuff. The incidence of cuff abscess has decreased with the use of shorter rectal cuffs. A cuff abscess may be the result of an ascending infection from anastomotic disruption or a descending infection as a result of intraoperative contamination or a pelvic hematoma. A cuff abscess may drain through the IPAA and create a sinus or a fistula. A pouchogram with water-soluble contrast medium and examination under anesthesia should establish the diagnosis, and a CT scan will identify any associated collections in the pelvis. A sinus should be treated by curettage, whereas a fistula should be managed by fistulotomy, curettage of the fistula, insertion of a seton, or mucosal flap advancement. The fecal stream should be diverted or reversal of the stoma delayed. A high rate of ileal pouch salvage can be achieved after leaks associated with IPAA if management is individualized. Improved rates of salvage of ileal pouches over time are likely a reflection of increased experience with the management of complications. Late manifestation of anastomotic sinuses or fistulas months or years after the original operation are often subsequently found to be associated with Crohn disease.

STRICTURE AT THE ILEAL POUCH–ANAL ANASTOMOSIS

Stricture at the site of the IPAA has been reported in up to 38% of patients. It is persistent and severe in 16%.[47] Tension and ischemia are predisposing factors. Stricture is more likely to develop if there was dehiscence of the IPAA, with or without pelvic sepsis, or if a small-diameter (25 mm) stapling gun was used. Conversely, there is no significant association with the size of the stapler used at IPAA and long-term development of anastomotic stricture as long as stapler sizes are in the range of 28 to 29 mm or 31 to 33 mm.[48] If the pouch is placed under tension or if the sutures between the pouch and anus are placed haphazardly or break such that the anastomosis separates, the denuded anal sphincter is left exposed. Heavy scarring and a dense stricture result. A pouch that has been brought down under some tension is more likely to be associated with anastomotic stricture, probably because of ischemia or partial disruption of the anastomosis with healing by secondary intention and stenosis. Patients with an IPAA stricture usually have frequent watery stools and urgency of defecation associated with straining and a sensation of incomplete evacuation. The stricture generally responds to dilation with a digit in the clinic or Hegar dilators under a brief general anesthetic. A lumen that allows insertion of an index finger to the level of the distal interphalangeal joint is adequate. Self-dilation with a St. Marks dilator is useful. In the absence of pelvic sepsis, the anastomotic stricture is usually web-like after a stapled IPAA but long and narrow after mucosectomy and a hand-sewn anastomosis.[47] Pelvic sepsis leads to longer strictures that are less likely to yield to simple dilation. Refractory strictures are best treated by pouch advancement and a new ileoanal anastomosis.[49] The functional outcome of patients who have undergone successful treatment of their strictures is no different from that of other patients with pouches.

A study of 1884 pouch-anal anastomoses constructed at the Mayo Clinic between 1981 and 1996 was carried out to identify and define different types of strictures and the factors that influence their occurrence.[50] Strictures developed in 213 patients, 86% of which were nonfibrotic and 14% were fibrotic. A greater number of strictures were seen in patients who had undergone a hand-sewn anastomosis than in those with a stapled anastomosis. Intraoperative technical difficulties were noted in 13% of patients, with anastomotic tension being the most commonly described problem. Postoperative complications such as abscess, fistula, and pouch retraction occurred in 13% of cases and were primarily associated with fibrotic strictures. The time between construction of the IPAA and the appearance of nonfibrotic and fibrotic strictures was 9 and 6.2 months, respectively. Anal canal anastomotic dilation was successful in 95% of the nonfibrotic strictures but in only 45% of the fibrotic strictures, and the average number of dilations was 1.5 (range, 1 to 7). In the Mayo series, surgical procedures were

necessary in 12% of all strictures (mainly fibrotic). The surgical procedures included (1) excision of the strictured segment with advance of a flap of ileal mucosa over the excised area; this technique was used for segmental and short strictures that appeared as a fibrous ring, with the rest of the pouch remaining supple; (2) excision of the pouch and permanent ileostomy; almost all of these patients had other perianastomotic complications—abscess, fistula, pouch retraction; (3) disconnection with segmental excision of the fibrotic segment and reanastomosis of the pouch to the anus; and (4) repeated anal dilation with drainage of abscess, division of an obstructing bridge, or debridement and curettage of a fistula.[50] Unusually, strictures may develop within the body of the pouch usually as a result of a misdiagnosis of Crohn disease. Such strictures can be located with water-soluble contrast studies, negotiated with an endoscopically placed wire and subsequent balloon dilation.

SYMPTOMATIC PROCTITIS OR DYSPLASIA IN RESIDUAL RECTAL MUCOSA

Symptomatic proctitis may develop after double-stapled IPAA, especially if an excessively long anorectal stump has been left in situ. Foci of high-grade dysplasia may also be seen in surveillance biopsies of retained ATZ.[41] Although proctitis may respond to topical or oral steroids, some patients prove resistant.

The troublesome mucosa is mobilized via a perineal approach with submucosal infiltration of a solution of 1:100,000 epinephrine. Mucosal resection is performed from the level of the dentate line to the level of the stapled IPAA. The anastomosis is then dissected radially and circumferentially mobilized to allow delivery of the pouch to the level of the anal verge. A new IPAA is made with interrupted sutures.[41] Although this technique may seem to be an attractive option, the mucosal resection and mobilization of the IPAA are actually quite difficult because of extensive fibrosis and adhesions between the pouch and the sphincter. The lack of mobility of the pouch may prevent the construction of a tension-free anastomosis. In practice, it may be necessary to perform transabdominal mobilization of the pouch or sacrifice the anal canal altogether and create a permanent ileostomy.

ENTEROCUTANEOUS FISTULAS

Enterocutaneous fistulas typically occur after unrecognized injury to the small bowel, often at the time of closure of the abdominal wound or after closure of the ileostomy. Usually, they can be managed conservatively with total parenteral nutrition as long as there is no distal obstruction. If the fistula arises from the pouch itself, a prolonged period of diversion of the intestinal stream, excision of the fistula, or closure of the defect in the pouch will generally be successful. Persistence of a fistula suggests unresolved sepsis or Crohn disease.

POUCH-VAGINAL FISTULAS

Fistulas from the pouch to the vagina may be the result of sepsis and anastomotic dehiscence or may represent technical error. The use of stapling instruments places the posterior vaginal wall at risk. Fistulas may develop in patients with transmural inflammation, and deep ulceration of the pouch may occur in those with unsuspected Crohn disease. Fistulas related to technical error occur early, whereas disease-related fistulas tend to occur late.

Investigation involves pouchoscopy and a vaginal speculum examination with the instillation of either methylene blue or 1% hydrogen peroxide solution. Water-soluble contrast studies via the pouch or vagina may delineate the fistulous tract. Pouch biopsy and small bowel contrast studies are needed when Crohn disease is suspected. Fecal diversion should be established. A small low fistula may be managed by means of mucosal flap advancement via a transanal or transvaginal approach if no significant sepsis is present. Large high tracts, especially if stapled, require reconstruction or abandonment of the IPAA.

A retrospective review of 60 females with pouch-vaginal fistulas managed at the Cleveland Clinic found that the average time to pouch-vaginal fistula formation after IPAA was 21 months (range, 1 to 132 months).[51] Postoperative pelvic sepsis had occurred in 17 patients (28%). The primary treatment modality was local repair (77%), the majority of which took the form of an ileal advancement flap, redo restorative proctocolectomy (10%), and excision of the pouch (8%). Initial healing was achieved in 20 of 52 evaluable patients, and an additional 11 patients had a successful outcome, albeit with repeat procedures. The overall healing rate was 52% at a mean 50 months' followup. A delayed diagnosis of Crohn disease was eventually made in 24 patients, and the chance of success after an ileal advancement flap was significantly lower in patients with Crohn disease than in those without Crohn disease (25% vs. 48%, respectively).

The reported experience in the Cleveland Clinic mirrors that of other major centers—about half the patients with a pouch-vaginal fistula will eventually achieve a successful outcome, with a quarter of the patients having persistence of a fistula but with the pouch in situ and a further quarter of patients undergoing long-term diversion or pouch excision. The majority of patients with pouch-vaginal fistulas can be managed by local methods, and several key technical points should be stressed. Adequate drainage of any septal sepsis must be achieved preoperatively—usually with draining setons with or without antibiotics. Careful and thorough hemostasis must be achieved. Any concurrent stricture should be débrided or excised, and the repair should be free of any tension.

A transvaginal approach to a pouch-vaginal fistula allows direct access to the internal opening and permits closure without damage to the anal sphincter (Figure 160-5).[52] With the patient in the lithotomy position and the bladder catheterized, an inverted T-shaped incision is made along the midline longitudinal access of the posterior vaginal wall. With the horizontal limb located at the junction of the perineal skin and the posterior vaginal wall, the vagina is then dissected from the anal canal and ileal pouch, and two lateral flaps are created to expose the anterior wall of the pouch and the pouch-anal anastomosis. The internal opening of the fistula (pouch end) is then excised and the defect closed transversely with dissolvable sutures. The vaginal flaps are replaced and closed with dissolvable suture, and a vaginal pack is inserted to reduce the formation of hematoma by opposing the vaginal wall to the pouch and therefore reducing the dead space. Because the vagina has an excellent blood supply, creation of a full-thickness flap is technically straightforward. This technique avoids trauma to the anal sphincters and therefore reduces the risk for sphincter injury and subsequent fecal incontinence. Although there is no definite evidence that a diverting stoma reduces recurrence of a pouch-vaginal fistula, an argument can be made for its use in this situation first to give the patient some relief from symptoms and second

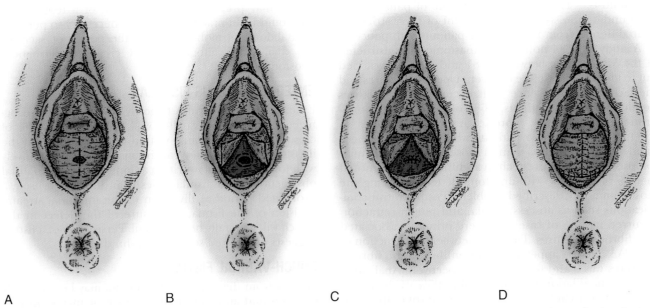

| A | B | C | D |

FIGURE 160-5 Transvaginal repair of a pouch-vaginal fistula. **A,** Incision site. **B,** Lateral flaps raised. **C,** Lateral opening excised and closed. **D,** Flaps replaced.

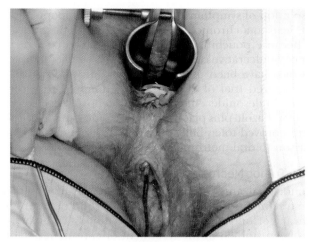

FIGURE 160-6 Button collagen plug to correct a pouch vaginal fistula greater than 7 mm in diameter.

to maximize the chance for success of the repair. This technique achieved success in 11 of 14 patients at St. Marks Hospital, London.[52]

The innovation of collagen plugs for the treatment of anal fistulas has been modified for use in pouch-vaginal fistulas (Figure 160-6). The regular plug was largely unsuccessful in such fistulas probably because of the relatively short track. The addition of a button secured on the pouch side of the fistula with dissolvable sutures and which passes spontaneously within 4 weeks leaving the collagen plug in situ to act as a scaffold to promote ingrowth of tissue has been associated with promising early results. Four of seven patients (57%) were successfully treated with MR confirmation of resolution.[53]

Functional Results After Perineal Complications

As noted earlier, there are a significant number of complications that involve the perineum after IPAA. Although the various complications can be minor, some lead to poor functional results or even loss of the pouch. A review of a registry of 628 patients from the Lahey Clinic identified 24.4% of patients in whom perineal complications had developed—anastomotic strictures, anastomotic separation, pouch fistulas, and pelvic sepsis. If the complications were addressed, the pouch failure rate was low (10%). Indeed, most of the pouch failures that occurred were the result of pouch fistulas, and in turn, most of these fistulas occurred in patients in whom the ultimate diagnosis was Crohn disease. The functional result in patients in whom the perineal complications were successfully dealt with were no different from those of control patients in whom no such complications developed.

POUCHITIS

The pelvic ileal reservoir may become nonspecifically inflamed—pouchitis. The incidence of pouchitis varies from 11% to 34%, depending on the diagnostic criteria used, and its frequency increases with time after surgery. The cause is unknown.

Pouchitis is associated with episodes of increased frequency of bowel action along with the passage of loose,

blood-stained stools usually accompanied by malaise, low-grade fever, and lower abdominal discomfort. Extraintestinal manifestations similar to those seen in colitis, such as erythema nodosum, uveitis, and arthritis, may occur at the same time as relapse of pouchitis. The mucosa is inflamed and extensively ulcerated, produces a copious exudate, and bleeds on contact. Biopsies reveal a marked acute inflammatory infiltrate with villous atrophy and crypt abscesses. Neutrophils migrate from the circulation to an inflamed pouch. A positive indium-labeled granulocyte scan together with increased 4-day fecal indium granulocyte excretion may help identify patients with pouchitis and allow assessment of response to treatment. A subgroup of patients are eventually found to have Crohn disease or an indeterminate form of colitis.[47]

The use of these descriptive diagnostic criteria is open to misinterpretation. There has been a tendency to set the threshold for each of the three components too high such that only patients with severe pouchitis are included. Therefore, more objective quantification of pouchitis is needed. A Pouchitis Disease Activity Index (PDAI) has been developed that quantitates clinical findings and the endoscopic and histologic features (Table 160-1).[54] It includes several clinical symptoms, not simply diarrhea, and expresses the endoscopic and histologic findings on a continuous scale rather than requiring minimum scores. Patients with pouchitis of mild or moderate severity can therefore be included in the diagnosis. The PDAI is significantly greater in patients with pouchitis than in patients without pouchitis, and it provides a simple, objective, and reproducible scoring system for pouchitis.

Pathogenesis of Pouchitis

The causes of pouchitis are not well understood. Previous expectations that the knowledge of inflammatory bowel diseases in general would be expanded by means of studies of pouchitis have not been achieved. A number of etiologic factors involved in the development of pouchitis have been suggested, such as mucosal ischemia, immune deficiency, stasis of pouch contents, bacterial imbalance, or a recurrent form of ulcerative colitis or a variation of Crohn disease. Certainly, the incidence of pouchitis is higher in patients with ulcerative colitis associated with primary sclerosing cholangitis and is very low in patients with familial adenomatous polyposis. Therefore, there may be a persistent predisposition to inflammation in patients with ulcerative colitis after IPAA, and this predisposition, with or without other factors, may result in pouchitis. Patients with extraintestinal manifestations of ulcerative colitis before IPAA had a tenfold increased risk for the development of pouchitis (48% vs. 4.6%, $P = 0.01$).[55] There is some evidence that dietary factors may play a role by modification of the ecology of the ileal pouch. A study that looked at interactions between nutritional factors, fecal and mucosal bacterial flora, and mucosal morphology in 21 patients with pouchitis versus 11 patients with healthy ileal pouches found no difference in mean nutrient intake, fecal bile acids, or microbial tissue biopsy cultures between the two groups, but there was a significantly higher

TABLE 160-1 Pouchitis Disease Activity Index

Criteria	Score
CLINICAL	
Stool frequency	
Usual postoperative BM	0
1-2 BM more than usual	1
3+ more than usual	2
Rectal bleeding	
None	0
Present daily	1
Fecal urgency or cramps	
None	0
Occasional	1
Usual	2
Fever	
Absent	0
Present	1
ENDOSCOPIC INFLAMMATION	
Edema	1
Granularity	1
Friability	1
Loss of vascular pattern	1
Mucous exudate	1
Ulceration	1
ACUTE HISTOLOGIC INFLAMMATION	
Leukocyte infiltration	
Mild	1
Moderate with crypt abscess	2
Severe with crypt abscess	3
Ulceration per low-power field (mean)	
<25%	1
25%-50%	2
>50%	3

From Sandborn WJ, Tremaine WJ, Batts KP, et al: Pouchitis after ileal pouch–anal anastomosis: A Pouchitis Disease Activity Index. *Mayo Clin Proc* 69:409, 1994.
BM, Bowel movement.
Note: Pouchitis is defined as a total score greater than 7 points.

concentration of anaerobes and aerobes in the feces of patients with pouchitis. Differences in the composition of the pouch microbial flora may be of key importance in the interaction with epithelial cells within the pouch mucosa and thus in the subsequent development of pouchitis.[56] Sulfate-reducing bacteria (a species of strict anaerobes) appear to exclusively colonize ileal pouches in patients with ulcerative colitis. There appears to be an increase in the ratio of strict to facultative anaerobes in ileal pouch patients with pouchitis as compared with those who have normal ileal pouches.[57]

Recent advances in molecular and cell biology have raised the possibility of a synergistic hypothesis that links interactions between epithelial metaplasia, changes in luminal bacteria (especially the sulfate-reducing bacteria), and altered mucosal immunity. Specifically, colonic metaplasia supports colonization by sulfate-reducing bacteria that produce hydrogen sulfide. This causes mucosal depletion and subsequent inflammation. Although in most cases antibiotics lead to bacterial clearance and

resolution of symptoms, immunogenetic subpopulations can lead to a chronic refractory variant of pouchitis.

Because pouchitis has been suggested to be a recurrence of ulcerative colitis in colonic-type mucosa, topical steroids have been used as a therapeutic alternative. A randomized trial of 26 patients randomized to receive either budesonide enema plus placebo tablets or oral metronidazole plus placebo enema found similar efficacy but improved tolerability of budesonide enemas in comparison to oral metronidazole.[58]

Anti–Tumor Necrosis Factor

Monoclonal antibodies have been successfully used in the treatment of fistulating perianal Crohn disease. The efficacy of one such monoclonal antibody (infliximab) has been studied in the treatment of chronic refractory pouchitis complicated by perianal fistulas after IPAA. An open study of seven patients with pouchitis complicated by fistulas in whom Crohn disease had been carefully excluded were treated with infliximab, 5 mg/kg at 0, 2, and 6 weeks. At the 10-week followup, six of the seven patients had a complete clinical response.[59]

Infliximab, the anti–tumor necrosis factor antibody, has demonstrated efficacy in the medical management of ulcerative colitis. Studies have shown that patients treated with infliximab before IPAA have an increased risk of postoperative pouch-related and infectious complications. Therefore, in patients who need an operation before 6 to 8 weeks have elapsed since their last dose of infliximab, it may be advisable to carry out a total colectomy with end ileostomy and preservation of the rectal stump as stage 1 with completion proctectomy and ileal pouch at a later date as stage 2.

The long-term efficacy of infliximab in patients with refractory pouch complications such as luminal inflammation or pouch fistulas was evaluated in 28 patients. Eighty-eight percent of patients with refractory luminal inflammation showed clinical response, whereas 86% of patients showed fistula response.[60]

Severe Pouchitis

Severe refractory pouchitis is rare, and when it occurs, other causes such as infection with cytomegalovirus or *Clostridium difficile* needs to be considered. Pouchitis induced by cytomegalovirus requires treatment with antiviral therapy such as ganciclovir. *C. difficile*–associated infection requires treatment with oral metronidazole or vancomycin.[61]

Morphologic Changes in Ileal Pouch Mucosa

A number of studies have demonstrated morphologic changes in the ileal pouch mucosa, including villous atrophy and crypt hyperplasia. The changes are classified as colonic metaplasia. It is not clear whether such changes represent long-term adaptation or response to inflammation. A study of 24 patients with no history of pouchitis, 31 patients with a history of pouchitis, and 8 patients in whom IPAA was carried out because of familial adenomatous polyposis found that the colonic metaplasia score was higher in patients with inflammation. The greater the colonic metaplasia score, the greater the inflammation score, and the authors concluded that colonic metaplasia is found primarily on a background of inflammation and therefore probably represents a reparative response.[62]

Inflammation proximal to the pouch has been described—pre-pouch ileitis (PPI). PPI was diagnosed in 34 (5.7%) of 742 patients who underwent pouchoscopy, all of whom had concurrent pouch inflammation. PPI did not, however, imply missed Crohn disease or predict an increased rate of pouch failure, at least in the short term.[63] Combination antibiotic therapy (ciprofloxacin 500 mg twice daily and metronidazole 400 mg twice daily for 28 days) appears to be effective in reducing the length of pre-pouch inflammation and in inducing symptomatic remission in most patients.

Treatment of Acute Pouchitis

Patients with pouchitis generally respond to metronidazole either orally or applied topically. The usual oral dose is 750 to 1500 mg/day for 7 to 14 days, and clinical improvement is generally prompt (within 3 days). A randomized, double-blind, placebo-controlled crossover trial in 13 patients has confirmed the long-held view of the efficacy of this form of treatment. The side effects of oral therapy are avoided by topical therapy, in which serum concentrations of metronidazole are very low. Patients who are unresponsive to metronidazole may respond to cyclic courses of three or four antibiotics given at weekly intervals, corticosteroids, ciprofloxacin, amoxicillin/clavulanic acid, erythromycin, tetracycline, allopurinol, sulfasalazine, or 5-aminosalicylic acid. Budesonide suppositories (1.5 mg/day) have also been shown to be efficacious. Frequent relapses of pouchitis require treatment with long-term, low-dose suppressive metronidazole therapy.

The fecal concentration of lactobacilli and bifidobacteria is significantly decreased in patients with pouchitis. A randomized, double-blind, placebo-controlled trial evaluated use of the probiotic VSL#3, which consists of eight bacterial strains, in the prevention of recurrence of pouchitis. In the treatment group, 17 of 20 patients were still in remission at 9 months, as compared with 0 of 20 patients treated with placebo. All patients who received VSL#3 relapsed within 4 months of concluding the treatment. The fecal concentrations of lactobacilli and bifidobacteria were significantly increased in the treatment group during the study but returned to baseline 1 month after completion of the study.[64] It remains unclear whether multiple bacterial strains are required to induce remission.

A Cochrane analysis of the treatment and prevention of pouchitis reviewed 11 randomized controlled trials that fulfilled the inclusion criteria with evaluation of 10 different pharmacologic agents. Ciprofloxacin was more effective at inducing remission in acute pouchitis than metronidazole, but neither rifaximin nor lactobacillus GG were more effective than placebo. VSL#3 was more effective than placebo in maintaining remission in chronic pouchitis and in preventing pouchitis.[65]

OTHER COMPLICATIONS

Polyps may develop within a pouch as in the rest of the small bowel. Inflammatory polyps may occur in up to 20% of patients with ulcerative colitis. Inflammatory fibroid polyps, though rare, may cause bleeding or obstruction. Such polyps may occasionally grow sufficiently to fill the lumen of the pouch and require resection with conversion to a permanent ileostomy.

There have been occasional reports of alopecia after IPAA. Indeed, one series reported a somewhat surprising incidence of 38% (in a series of 24 patients).[66] Fortunately, it is a temporary phenomenon, but female patients in particular should be warned. Treatment, if it occurs, is reassurance.

Lateral popliteal nerve palsy has been reported and is related to compression damage from pressure exerted by the leg supports after particularly long procedures. Anterior compartment syndrome of the lower limbs has similarly been reported after lengthy operations and may result in myonecrosis and footdrop unless fasciotomy is carried out. Careful positioning and adequate padding should eliminate these complications.

Distal small bowel obstruction can occur secondary to angulation or prolapse of the afferent limb at the pouch inlet. This afferent limb syndrome can be diagnosed by careful pouchoscopy and/or imaging and corrected by either balloon dilation of the afferent limb inlet, repeated as necessary, or resection of the angulated bowel. Surgical therapy appears to be more effective.[67] Ileal pouch prolapse is another rare complication with no obvious predisposing factors. A series of 3176 patients identified 11 patients in whom either full-thickness ($n = 7$) or mucosal ($n = 4$) prolapse developed. Although mucosal prolapse was found to respond to either stool bulking or a local perineal procedure, full-thickness prolapse required definitive surgery and was associated with the risk of pouch loss.[68]

Risk for Neoplasia

There are suggestions that the mucosa of ileal pouches may be at risk for the development of neoplasia. If true, the likelihood is that the incidence of such events is very low. In a series of 160 patients undergoing routine pouch surveillance with multiple biopsies and a mean length of followup of 8.4 years, only one patient was found to have low-grade dysplasia, but even this was not confirmed on further routine followup. The incidence of cancer after IPAA is very low, with only 19 reported cases of adenocarcinoma of the pouch or anal canal after this operation in the literature.[69] The majority of these cases have occurred either in the rectal stump or around the anastomosis, and in all but two cases the original pathologic specimen demonstrated either dysplasia or cancer. The performance of a stapled IPAA does not appear to be inferior to mucosectomy and hand-sewn anastomosis in oncologic outcome.

The widespread adoption of the use of stapled IPAA with preservation of the ATZ has raised questions about the need for long-term surveillance. The Cleveland Clinic group carried out a prospective evaluation with a minimum 10-year followup on 289 patients who were studied by serial ATZ biopsy. ATZ dysplasia developed in only 8 patients between 4 and 123 (median, 9) months after surgery. The dysplasia was high grade in 2 patients and low grade in 6 patients. No cancers developed in the

ATZ during the study period. This group recommended that in patients in whom there had been no dysplasia in the original proctocolectomy specimen and no other risk factors such as primary sclerosing cholangitis or a strong family history of colorectal cancer, a biopsy specimen should be taken from the ATZ at 1 year and then every 2 to 3 years thereafter. In patients in whom there was dysplasia in the original proctocolectomy specimen but no involvement of the lower two-thirds of the rectum, biopsy of the ATZ should be performed every year. In patients in whom there was either a carcinoma-complicating ulcerative colitis or dysplasia in the lower two-thirds of the rectum at the time of proctocolectomy, a stapled IPAA was not performed but rather transanal mucosectomy and a hand-sewn anastomosis; close followup at 6 months then yearly intervals is recommended for these patients. Even within this group, the option of a stapled IPAA would be offered to obese or elderly patients or those with low sphincter pressure, in whom mucosectomy and a hand-sewn anastomosis might not be easily feasible because of reach or concerns about poor pouch function. In patients in whom low-grade dysplasia is found on biopsy, repeat biopsy should be performed every 6 months for up to 3 years. If no further dysplasia is detected, annual biopsies would be required thereafter, but if persistent low-grade or, indeed, high-grade dysplasia is found on three consecutive samples, the patient should undergo mucosectomy and pouch advancement.[70] However, the finding of dysplasia early after surgery underscores the importance of early pouch surveillance.

Male Sexual Function

Most patients who undergo the IPAA procedure are young, sexually active, and concerned about their sexual function after pelvic surgery. Pelvic surgery may cause male sexual problems such as erectile dysfunction, absence of ejaculation, or retrograde ejaculation. Only a small percentage (2% to 4%) of male patients have severe sexual problems after surgery. Sexual function of males has been examined in a systematic manner by means of a validated scoring system, the International Index of Erectile Function (IIEF). The IIEF was used to study 122 males who underwent IPAA between 1995 and 2000, with comparison of results before and after IPAA. There was a statistically significant improvement in erectile function, sexual desire, intercourse satisfaction, and overall satisfaction, with patients having improved scores after surgery versus before surgery. The mean erectile function score was higher after surgery than before surgery. Overall psychometric sexual satisfaction and sexual quality of life were increased, most likely because of enhanced general health. This study would suggest that male patients undergoing IPAA may be counseled that their sexual function is likely to be retained after surgery.[71] The application of the laparoscopic approach to IPAA may be expected to be associated with improved sexual function and body image compared with open IPAA. A comparison of 100 laparoscopic and 189 open operations reported excellent body image and high cosmetic and quality-of-life scores regardless of operative approach. However, orgasmic function scores were lower in men who underwent laparoscopic IPAA compared with the open group.[72]

Female Reproductive Health

IPAA does not seem to affect menstrual function or gynecologic symptoms. Overall sexual satisfaction may be improved with surgery, although the ability to experience orgasm and the frequency of coitus are unchanged. There is an increase in dyspareunia after IPAA, and fertility is adversely affected, most likely because of pelvic adhesions. During pregnancy, there is a transient increase in the frequency of stools both by day and by night. Nocturnal incontinence increases, but this resolves after delivery. The ideal route of delivery has yet to be determined, but vaginal delivery is safe and does not appear to directly influence pouch function.[73]

Ileal Pouch–Anal Anastomosis and the Menstrual Cycle. The majority of women report no change in their menstrual cycle after IPAA. Any noted change in menses or related symptoms seem to be infrequent. A study of 46 women who had undergone IPAA with a followup of 28 months showed no change in menses in 68%, increased regularity in 26%, and dysmenorrhea in 15%.[74] A similar study of 21 women a mean of 38 months after IPAA noted dysmenorrhea in 10%; no patients identified changes in their cycle.[75]

Ileal Pouch–Anal Anastomosis and Female Sexual Function. Although most women report no change in overall sexual satisfaction, 16% to 50% reported an increase in satisfaction after IPAA.[76] Nine percent to 26% of women reported decreased overall satisfaction. IPAA does not seem to affect the ability to experience orgasm, with a similar frequency of orgasm before and after surgery (range, 67% to 86%).[74-76] An increase in the ability to attain orgasm was noted in 9% to 18% of patients, whereas 0% to 15% of patients reported decreased ability. Although the frequency of coitus remains unchanged or is increased after IPAA, 3% to 18% of women fear leakage of stool at the time of sexual intercourse. This concern is alleviated by emptying the pouch before intercourse. Preexistent dyspareunia may be exacerbated by surgery. In studies that included preoperative baseline data, the incidence of dyspareunia rose from 5% to 10% to as high as 15% to 22% after surgery.[77] This may be due to alterations in pelvic anatomy or the formation of adhesions after IPAA. Alternatively, because the most systematic physical reaction to sexual stimulation is an increase in vaginal vasocongestion, sexual dysfunction may be associated with autonomic pelvic nerve damage or partial devascularization of the vagina. This hypothesis may imply a possible advantage to a full close rectal dissection.

Ileal Pouch–Anal Anastomosis and Fertility. A number of studies (mostly characterized by small number of subjects attempting conception after surgery) suggest reduced fertility in women after IPAA. Two large studies that were methodologically sound have shown decreased postoperative fertility. A postal questionnaire of 300 women of reproductive age who underwent IPAA between 1983 and 2001 found that before IPAA, 48 (38%) of 127 patients were unsuccessful in their attempt to conceive after 1 year of unprotected intercourse, whereas after

IPAA, 76 (56%) of 135 patients were unsuccessful. The infertility rate was higher after surgery than before ($P < 0.001$). In a subgroup of 56 women who tried to get pregnant both before and after surgery, the infertility rate was higher after surgery than before (69% vs. 46%, $P = 0.005$). The use of an intraoperative blood transfusion was associated with a higher rate of infertility than in patients who did not have an intraoperative blood transfusion (54% vs. 21%, $P = 0.023$).[78] A Scandinavian study of 237 women compared the rate of preoperative fertility from the age of 15 until colectomy and the rate of postoperative fertility from 12 months after closure of ileostomy until data collection or menopause. There was a mild decrease in observed preoperative births (87% of expected, $P < 0.05$), whereas the incidence of postoperative births was only 35% of expected after IPAA ($P < 0.001$). Successful in vitro fertilization was excluded from the study.[79] This decrease in postoperative fertility has been attributed to probable tubal occlusion from adhesions, although the possibility that physicians and surgeons have recommended against conception after IPAA and the possibility of patient concerns about having children affected with ulcerative colitis may well play a role. Stool frequency and incontinence are not significantly affected by pregnancy or mode of delivery.

Mode of Delivery after Ileal Pouch–Anal Anastomosis. In theory, a vaginal delivery may increase the risk for pudendal nerve damage, injury to the anal sphincter complex, and loss of fecal continence in patients after IPAA as compared with cesarean section before the onset of labor. However, a postal questionnaire study that addressed this issue in 29 subjects who had undergone 49 deliveries found that there were 25 vaginal deliveries and 24 cesarean sections. A third of the subjects had disturbances in pouch function during pregnancy, almost exclusively during the third trimester, with an increase in stool frequency by day and by night and transient loss of nighttime control. There was no correlation between the mode of delivery and pouch complications or functional impairment. In particular, vaginal delivery was not shown to adversely affect pouch or anal function. Vaginal delivery after IPAA would appear to be safe, and the method of delivery should be dictated by obstetric or specific local perineal conditions.[80]

Age-Related Surgical Results and Functional Outcome

Although no age cutoff for patients undergoing IPAA has been defined, many surgeons would anecdotally suggest an upper age limit of 60 or 65 years. There is little evidence to support such a recommendation, and the relative infrequency of IPAA in older patients has made it difficult to assess outcomes of surgery according to age. The Cleveland Clinic carried out a prospective evaluation of the functional outcome and quality of life in 1895 patients who had undergone IPAA, with stratification of patients by age at the time of surgery into younger than 45 years, between 46 and 55 years, between 56 and 65 years, and older than 65 years. Functional outcome and quality of life were assessed at 1, 3, 5, and 10 years of followup. The study reported incontinence and nighttime seepage to be more common in older patients, and

there were minor differences in quality of life, health, energy, and happiness, with a slight benefit for those younger than 45 years. There were no differences in the level of happiness with surgery at 1, 3, 5, or 10 years of followup. At all times in the study, at least 95% of patients in each group would undergo their surgery again and would recommend IPAA to someone else with the same diagnosis.[81]

The effect of the aging process itself on functional outcome and the quality of life of patients with an ileal pouch was studied by the Mayo Clinic group, with the functional and quality-of-life outcomes of 409 patients being assessed at 5, 10, and 15 years. Over this time frame, there was little change in daytime stool frequency, whereas nighttime frequency increased from one stool to two stools per night. Incontinence to gas and stool increased from 1% to 10% during the day and from 2% to 24% at night over the 15-year period. After 15 years, more than 90% of patients were in the same job, and social activities, recreational sports, long-distance travel, and sexual activity all improved after surgery and did not show deterioration over time.[82]

REVISIONAL POUCH SURGERY

In a small subset of patients, the long-term functional result is poor. Although in many of these cases the problem may be related to recurrent episodes of pouchitis or postoperative pelvic sepsis, some patients may benefit from surgical intervention.

Patients who are being evaluated for pouch dysfunction months or years after the original operation should undergo a series of investigations, including inspection and palpation of the anastomosis, stool culture, pouchoscopy and multiple biopsies, water-soluble contrast enema, manometry of the anal sphincter and pouch, and a small bowel contrast study if Crohn disease is suspected. Mechanical causes of dysfunction may be identified, such as an excessively long efferent spout, a small pouch, a long mobile blind limb capable of obstructing outflow from the pouch, twisted pouches, or intussusception of bowel proximal to the pouch within the pouch. Problems specific to the IPAA included partial separation, residual disease after a double-stapled anastomosis, and a long stenosis.

Surgical Technique

With the patient in the synchronous (combined) position, the abdomen is opened through the previous laparotomy incision. Adhesiolysis is performed and the ileal pouch identified and dissected out with a combination of electrocautery and sharp dissection. In most cases, mobilization of the pouch can be achieved without major difficulty and without entering the lumen. Once the IPAA has been identified from above, attention is turned to the perineal dissection. Again, a combination of electrocautery and scissors dissection is used to dissect out the IPAA. Further transanal mucosectomy is performed if residual mucosa is identified. Great care is taken to identify and preserve the sphincter musculature. The IPAA is then disconnected and the pouch delivered out of the abdomen. The pouch is revised according to the nature of the problem, which may involve excision of a long efferent spout with or without sacrifice of the original pouch, excision of the original pouch with construction of a new pouch, excision of a long blind end, rotation of the pouch on its longitudinal axis, and excision of fistulous tracts with repair of the pouch. The new pouch is then anastomosed to the anal canal with four anchoring sutures placed into the walls of the pouch and the levator muscles and then a series of interrupted absorbable sutures placed between the pouch and the anal mucosa. The procedure should be covered with a diverting ileostomy in all cases. Intestinal continuity is restored 2 to 3 months later after a water-soluble contrast study has demonstrated satisfactory healing.

A series of 23 patients in whom disconnection, pouch revision, and reanastomosis were carried out has been reported.[83] Functional problems included impaired evacuation ($n = 15$), excessive frequency ($n = 4$), and fistulas ($n = 4$). At surgery, the functional problems were found to be due to a long efferent spout ($n = 9$), a redundant or perforated blind limb ($n = 6$), a twisted pouch ($n = 3$), or other causes ($n = 5$). The pouch was salvaged in 14 patients, and a new pouch was constructed in 9. The pouch-anal anastomosis was resutured in 22 patients and stapled in 1. Postoperative complications (all minor) occurred in 5 of 23 patients. Two patients underwent revision IPAA twice. At a median followup of 5 years (range, 1 to 10), 11 patients reported good to excellent function, 5 patients reported fair function, and 1 patient reported recurrent pouchitis. Revision surgery was unsuccessful in 6 of 23 patients (gross incontinence in 3, excessive bowel movements in 2, Crohn disease in 1), and they subsequently underwent pouch excision. Table 160-2 shows the results of studies of redo IPAA.[17,41,83-91]

A series of 63 reconstructive procedures were performed in 57 patients. The primary indication for reconstruction was a pouch-vaginal fistula in 21 patients, a long outlet in 14, pelvic sepsis in 14, IPAA stricture in 5,

---

TABLE 160-2 Disconnection, Pouch Revision, and Redo Ileal Pouch–Anal Anastomosis

Author	No. of Patients	Problem	Outcome
Liljeqvist[84]	7	Long spout	Good function in 5 patients, 2 failures
Pogglioli[85]	6	Twisted pouch (1)	Good function in 4 patients, pouch excised in 1,
		Afferent limb stricture (1)	and stoma not closed in 1
		Pouch-urethral fistula (1)	
		Pelvic sepsis (1)	
		Ischemic pouch (1)	
		Outflow obstruction (1)	
Nicholls[17]	6	Long spout	Good function in 4 patients, 2 self-catheterize
Fazio[41]	2	Residual disease, dysplasia	Good function in both patients after transanal advancement
Sagar[83]	23	Long spout (9)	Success in 17 patients
		Sepsis (4)	
		Blind limb (3)	
		Twisted pouch (3)	
		Revision of IPAA (3)	
		No pouch (1)	
Herbst[86]	16	Pouch outlet obstruction	Improved function in 12 patients
Fonkalsrud[87]	58	Elongated IPAA spout	Improved function in 93%
Baixauli[88]	100	Chronic leak (27)	5-year survival rate of pouch = 74%
		PV fistula (47)	
		Stricture (22)	
		Long spout (36)	
		Previous pouch excision (6)	
MacLean[89]	57	PV fistula (21)	Success in 89%
		Pelvic sepsis (14)	
		Long spout (14)	
		Stricture (5)	
		Perineal fistula (2)	
		Pouchitis (1)	
Remzi[90]	241	Fistula (67)	New pouch constructed in 71
		Leak (65)	Pouch salvages in 170
		Stricture (42)	Redo procedure associated with increased daytime and nighttime seepage
		Pouch dysfunction (40)	
		Pelvic abscess (25)	
Mathis[91]	51	Infectious/inflammatory (65%)	BM = 5 times a day, 1 time at night
		Mechanical difficulties (35%)	93% pouch survival at 1 yr
			89% pouch survival at 5 yr

IPPA, Ileal pouch–anal anastomosis; PV, pouch-vaginal.

pouch-perineal fistula in 2, and chronic pouchitis in 1 patient.[89] All patients received a covering loop ileostomy. Forty-two patients (73.7%) have a functioning pouch, whereas 7 (12.3%) have had their pouch excised and an ileostomy has not been closed in the other 8 (14.0%) patients. The functional results in the patients with a pouch in use were categorized as good, and this group of patients rated their physical and psychological health as good to excellent.

Good results can be obtained by experienced surgeons after abdominoperineal reconstruction for a failed IPAA. Selection of patients is important. The original pathology and current pouch biopsies should be reviewed by an experienced gastrointestinal pathologist and every effort made to rule out Crohn disease. Active sepsis must be controlled, and on occasion it may be necessary for the pouch to be made nonfunctional for a period before reconstructive surgery is attempted. A major commitment is required by both the patient and surgeon, but the effort is worthwhile when satisfactory function and quality of life are obtained.

Alternative Techniques for Pouch Salvage

A technique to treat and salvage an ileal pouch affected by chronic fistulating disease on a background of ulcerative colitis has been described and involves an abdominoperineal approach with transabdominal mobilization of the pouch to the level of the anastomosis and then perineal dissection to disconnect the anastomosis transanally (Figure 160-7). The pouch is delivered out of the abdomen and the pouch fistulous connections are excised. This part of the pouch is then closed and the pouch inverted through the cone formed by the J pouch anteriorly and the mesentery posteriorly. The formerly hidden part of the pouch then becomes the apparent one and vice versa. A 180-degree forward rotation with 180-degree axial rotation permits enough length to bring a new healthy part of the same pouch to the anus. The

pouch-anal anastomosis is constructed after any granulation and fibrotic tissue has been fully curetted and a mucosectomy has been performed to remove any residual mucosa distal to the previous anastomotic site. The anastomosis and pouch are protected with a temporary diverting ileostomy. This is a useful technique to perform before admitting defeat and excising the pouch so that the patient is left with a permanent ileostomy, although difficulties may result if there is insufficient mesenteric length remaining after pouch inversion and double rotation. Usually, however, the mesentery has elongated several months after the original IPAA has been formed, so length is not generally a problem. The technique permits excision of all inflamed tissue related to the fistulating disease, it permits diagnosis and closure of all fistula tracks, the anastomosis is constructed with a new healthy part of the pouch, and the inflamed bowel specimen excised from the pouch can be examined histologically and Crohn disease excluded.

A short small bowel mesentery can create difficulty with reach of the pouch to the pelvic floor at the time of the original IPAA. Indeed, this may account for a number of postoperative problems and pouch dysfunction. If such patients come to revision or redo surgery, it may prove technically impossible for the new pouch to reach down to the pelvic floor if the original pouch has had to be sacrificed because of sepsis or other problems. A technique to overcome this problem has been described in which a new 18-cm J pouch is formed with a jejunal segment (Figure 160-8). Selective division of axial vessels allows adequate length to form a jejunal pouch–anal anastomosis, and the small bowel distal to the pouch is then interposed between the proximal jejunum and the J pouch. This technique of jejunal J-pouch formation and small bowel interposition offers a useful alternative to definitive ileostomy or Kock pouch in patients undergoing salvage surgery after failed IPAA. Nevertheless, a continent ileostomy is a reasonable alternative for patients

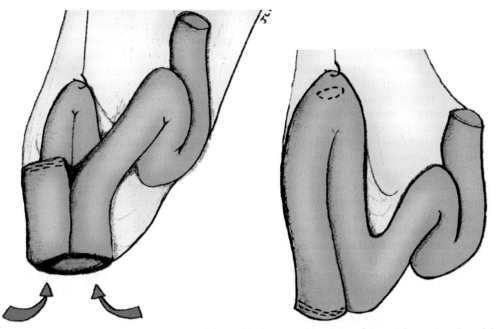

FIGURE 160-7 Inversion, 180-degree forward rotation, and then 180-degree axial rotation. See text for explanation of this maneuver.

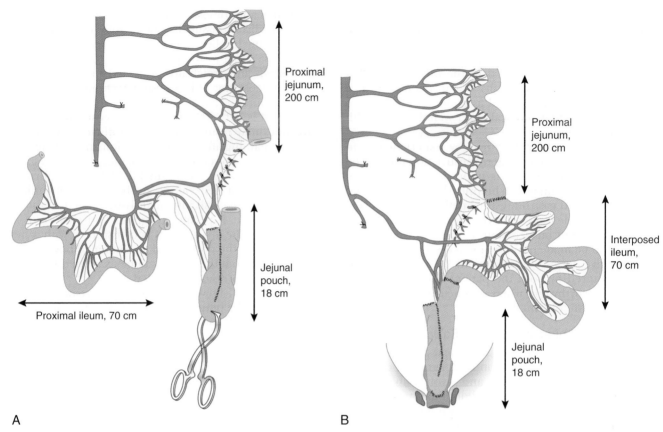

A   B

FIGURE 160-8 Salvage ileal pouch–anal anastomosis with a jejunal pouch and ileal interposition. **A,** Conceptual diagram of formation of a proximal jejunal J pouch with ileal interposition. **B,** Final appearance of the jejunal J pouch with ileal interposition.

with a failed IPAA. In a series of 64 patients in whom pelvic sepsis was the most common cause of ileal pouch failure, most of the patients were highly satisfied with their choice of continent ileostomy. There was a significant morbidity, however, with a 30-day complication rate of 31.3% and a long-term dysfunction rate of 50% and revision rate of 45%.[92]

QUANTIFICATION OF THE RISK FOR POUCH FAILURE

Although IPAA is an effective and safe surgical option for patients with ulcerative colitis and is associated with low perioperative mortality and acceptable functional results, there are marked variations in the characteristics of patients in whom the pouch procedure is ultimately shown to fail. For instance, a study from Birmingham, England, reported a failure rate of 12.7% as a result of pouch ischemia (19.3%), pelvic sepsis or fistula (35.5%), Crohn disease (12.9%), anastomotic stricture (16.1%), or pouchitis (16.1%),[93] whereas a series from Rochester, Minnesota, reported a failure rate of only 3.8% with the principal causes being anastomotic stricture (19%), pelvic sepsis or fistula (73%), and poor function (8%).[16] These and similar discrepancies together with the move into an era of public and professional accountability for clinical outcomes have led to a need for predictive indices to allow quantification of operative risk after IPAA that is based on the comorbid condition of the patient and the complexity of the procedure. The Cleveland Clinic Foundation (CCF) ileal pouch failure model is one such index.[94] Data on 23 preoperative, 7 intraoperative, and 10 postoperative risk factors were recorded from 1965 patients between 1983 and 2001. With ileal pouch failure as the primary endpoint, the CCF ileal pouch failure model was developed by means of parametric survival analysis and a 70% to 30% split-sample validation technique for model training and testing. This split-sample validation procedure was repeated 10,000 times to calculate standard errors and correct bias. Independent predictors of pouch survival were patient diagnosis, previous anal pathology, abnormal anal manometry, comorbidity, pouch-vaginal or pouch-perineal fistula, pelvic sepsis, anastomotic stricture, and anastomotic separation. The CCF ileal pouch failure model is to be commended because it was based on extensive preoperative, intraoperative, and postoperative data with good followup (median, 4.1 years). It is a simple additive scoring system with eight risk factors used to calculate the risk for pouch failure at a particular time interval after IPAA. It can be readily applied to surgical practice. Even more simply, the probability of the need for a permanent ileostomy after IPAA increases with age.

CROHN DISEASE

A recently completed metaanalysis of more than 8500 patients who have undergone IPAA over the last 20 years in 20 major centers around the United States suggested an overall failure rate of 6%. If only reports from the last 5 years are considered, however, the failure rate appears to have fallen to around 2%, probably as a result of selection of patients, more experience and better surgical techniques, and improved postoperative care. Today, the main contributor to failure appears to be Crohn disease or suspected Crohn disease–related complications. Crohn disease is an independent predictor of pouch failure.

Patients with Crohn disease have generally been excluded as candidates for IPAA. Clinical and histopathologic distinction between ulcerative colitis and Crohn disease can be difficult. The pouch failure rate in patients in whom IPAA has been carried out inadvertently and Crohn disease proved to be the ultimate diagnosis is about 50%.

Somewhat controversially, a number of authors have suggested that IPAA can indeed be used in selected patients with colorectal Crohn disease in whom proctocolectomy with permanent end ileostomy would be the only alternative. Rather than compare the results of IPAA in patients with Crohn disease against IPAA for other conditions such as ulcerative colitis and familial adenomatous polyposis, perhaps we should consider IPAA in Crohn disease just as a restorative operation in its own right. A French group reported the results of IPAA in 41 patients with Crohn disease limited to the large bowel, that is, with no past or present history of small bowel involvement or anal manifestations. At a median followup of about 2 years, 27% of patients had experienced Crohn disease–related complications—seven with pouchperineal fistulas treated surgically, two with extrasphincteric abscesses, and two with persistent anal ulceration with pouchitis and granulomas on pouch biopsy.[95] In a subset of 20 patients with followup greater than 10 years, 35% had experienced Crohn disease–related complications and in 2 patients the pouch was eventually excised. The authors concluded that such good long-term results justified the results of IPAA in selected patients. Technical complications after IPAA may be mislabeled as Crohn disease—such patients need to be carefully reevaluated because the prognosis and management will vary.

The disparity in outcome between previous studies of patients undergoing inadvertent IPAA for Crohn disease and the French group raised the question of whether the latter study population had suffered from indeterminate or even ulcerative colitis rather than Crohn disease. There were questions over the exact pathologic criteria used. It is well recognized that patients with indeterminate colitis, although it has a lower success rate than ulcerative colitis does, do much better than those suffering from Crohn disease. The situation may of course change with the advent of the era of monoclonal antibodies raised against tumor necrosis factor-α. Adalimumab seems to be well-tolerated and efficacious in treating Crohn disease of the pouch at least in open-labeled induction studies. The selection of future patients for IPAA may well change as we gain longer patient followup and are able to correlate clinical, endoscopic, and histologic features with outcome. Ultimately, it is for the patient to decide with appropriate and thorough counseling from the surgeon and physician.[95]

Investigations useful in the assessment of patients with dysfunction of the ileal pouch are shown in Table 160-3 and algorithms for the management of such patients are shown in Figure 160-9.

TABLE 160-3 Assessment of Dysfunction of the Ileal Pouch

CLINICAL EXAMINATION	Inspection	Fecal seepage
		External fistulas
		Anal fissures/abrasions
		Excoriation
		Mucosal prolapse
	Digital exam	Anastomotic stenosis
		Perianal induration
		Height of anastomosis above dentate line
ENDOSCOPY	Anoscopy	Cuffitis
		Mucosal prolapse
	Pouchoscopy	Mucosal inflammation
		Distensibility of pouch
		4-quadrant biopsies
	Fiberoptic	Pre-pouch inflammation
		Small bowel Crohn disease
	Examination under anesthesia	If too uncomfortable for the above
IMAGING	CT	Suspicion of pelvic sepsis
	MR	Assessment of fistulas
	Contrast	Structural abnormality of the pouch
		Small bowel Crohn disease
ANAL ASSESSMENT	Anal manometry	Fecal seepage/soilage

ALTERNATIVES TO ILEAL POUCH–ANAL ANASTOMOSIS

PANPROCTOCOLECTOMY WITH ILEOSTOMY

This procedure removes all diseased tissue and thus "cures" the disease. Gastrointestinal output is effectively managed by an ileostomy appliance. All patients are suitable candidates for the operation irrespective of age, size, and body shape. However, the fatter the patient, the more difficult it is to construct a stoma and the more likely the patient is to run into problems with the stoma. Rectal mobilization is carried out close to the rectum, the sympathetic nerves are protected at the sacral promontory, and the hypogastric plexus is protected in the pelvis. The perineal phase completes the dissection, and the intersphincteric plane is used to afford protection to the external anal sphincter and the puborectalis and levator muscles. Bladder paralysis and sexual dysfunction occur rarely with this approach. The perineal wound is small and can be closed relatively easily.

The downside of the operation is obvious. Patients are incontinent of gas and stool and must always wear an appliance. Some patients consider life with a stoma to be worse than the disease itself. The quality of life of patients with ileostomies seems to have improved little since the original description of Brooke ileostomy in 1952.

COLECTOMY WITH ILEORECTAL ANASTOMOSIS

Ileorectostomy removes most of the diseased colon but leaves the diseased rectum in situ. The operation avoids

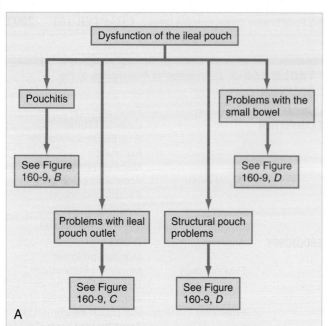

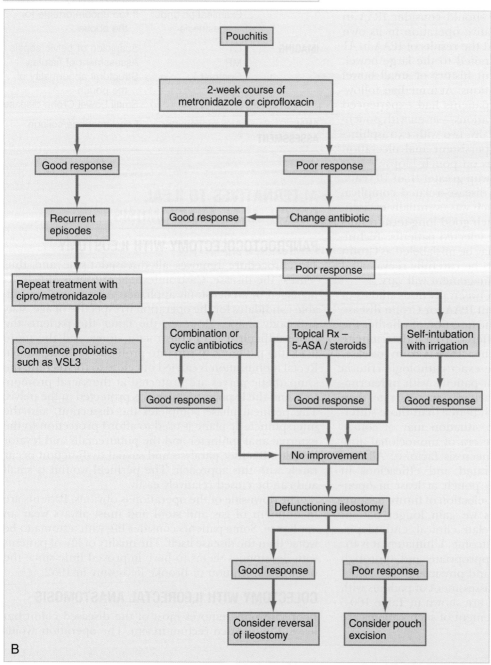

FIGURE 160-9 Algorithms for the investigation of dysfunction of the ileal pouch. **A,** Overall conceptual framework for pouch problems. Specific probelms are then dealth with in parts **A** to **D.**

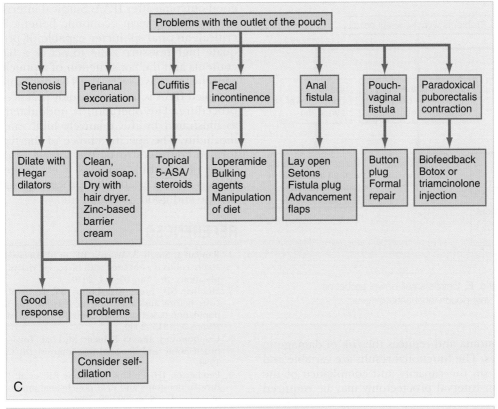

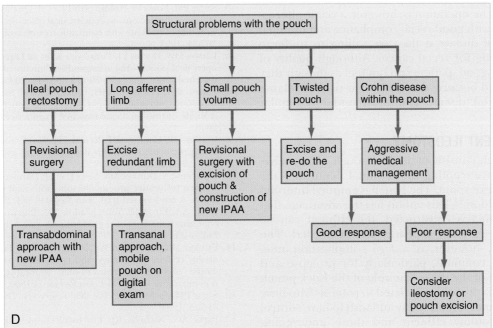

FIGURE 160-9—cont'd.

Continued

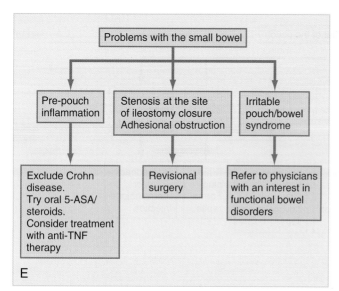

FIGURE 160-9, cont'd E, Details small bowel probelms encountered after ileal pouch–anal anastomosis.

the need for a stoma and reduces the risk of damage to the pelvic nerves. The functional results are variable and depend largely on the capacity and compliance of the residual rectum. Interval proctectomy may be required in up to 40%, and the risk for rectal cancer is about 15% after 30 years. The operation is, however, a viable alternative in patients with good rectal compliance and minimal quiescent rectal disease if they are willing to undergo regular screening for rectal cancer. Although quality of life is generally good, patients do not feel as though they have been cured because they are still at risk for relapse from their rectal disease and must undergo regular surveillance.

KOCK CONTINENT ILEOSTOMY

The Kock pouch consists of an ileal pouch with a valve, created by intussuscepting the terminal ileum into the pouch, and an exit spout. The pouch is emptied intermittently by intubation.[14] This option has the advantage that although a stoma is constructed, the effluent can be controlled. An external appliance is not needed. The main problem, however, is a *high* complication rate. Reoperation is common, particularly for prolapse and intussusception of the valve. The role of the Kock pouch is minor and it is probably restricted to patients who have undergone panproctocolectomy and wish to have control over their ileostomy effluent and those undergoing restorative proctocolectomy in whom the ileal reservoir cannot be safely brought down to the anal canal because of a short mesentery. Other patients should be discouraged.

CONCLUSION

The development of IPAA has led to significant advances in the surgical treatment of CUC. IPAA is safe and successful in about 95% to 98% of patients. The procedure is now increasingly performed laparoscopically. The vast majority of patients, if carefully selected, can expect a good outcome after IPAA. Surgical intervention is associated with long-term economic benefit. Two factors are critical: an anal sphincter capable of providing an adequate high-pressure zone to act as a barrier to pouch contents and the construction of a pouch with adequate capacity to act as a reservoir. The duplicated J pouch with a stapled IPAA is the most widely practiced variant of the procedure. The operation is undoubtedly complicated, as illustrated by the relatively high rates of associated morbidity. The specific choice of the type of IPAA performed continues to be the subject of debate, and the cause of pouchitis remains a challenge. Nevertheless, IPAA is now an established procedure that offers cure of disease and good quality of life.

REFERENCES

1. Randall J, Singh B, Warren BF, et al: Delayed surgery for acute severe colitis is associated with increased risk of postoperative complications. *Br J Surg* 97:404, 2010.
2. Holubar SD, Long KH, Loftus EV, Jr, et al: Long-term direct costs before and after proctocolectomy for ulcerative colitis: A population-based study in Olmsted County, Minnesota. *Dis Colon Rectum* 52:1815, 2009.
3. Utsunomiya J, Iwama T, Imajo M, et al: Total colectomy, mucosal proctectomy and ileo-anal anastomosis. *Dis Colon Rectum* 23:459, 1980.
4. Pemberton JH, Phillips SF, Ready RR, et al: Quality of life after Brooke ileostomy and ileal pouch–anal anastomosis. Comparison of status. *Ann Surg* 209:620, 1989.
5. Sagar PM, Lewis W, Holdsworth PJ, et al: Quality of life after restorative proctocolectomy with pelvic ileal reservoir compares favorably with that of patients with medically treated colitis. *Dis Colon Rectum* 36:584, 1993.
6. Larson DW, Dozois EJ, Piotrowicz K, et al: Laparoscopic assisted vs open ileal pouch–anal anastomosis: Functional outcome in a case matched series. *Dis Colon Rectum* 48:1845, 2005.
7. Larson DW, Pemberton JH, Cima RR, et al: Safety, feasibility, and short-term outcomes of laparoscopic ileal pouch–anal anastomosis: A single institutional case-matched experience. *Ann Surg* 243:667, 2006.
8. Geisler DP, Condon ET, Remzi FH: Single incision laparoscopic total proctocolectomy with ileopouch anal anastomosis. *Colorectal Dis* 12:941, 2010.
9. Maartense S, Dunker MS, Slors J, et al: Hand-assisted laparoscopic vs open restorative proctocolectomy with ileal pouch–anal anastomosis: A randomized trial. *Ann Surg* 240:984, 2004.
10. Indar AA, Efron JE, Young-Fadok TM: Laparoscopic ileal pouch–anal anastomosis reduces abdominal and pelvic adhesions. *Surg Endosc* 23:174, 2009.
11. Dunker MS, Bemelman WA, Slors JFM, et al: Functional outcome, quality of life, body image and cosmesis in patients after laparoscopic assisted and conventional restorative proctocolectomy: A comparative study. *Dis Colon Rectum* 44:1800, 2001.
12. Sagar PM, Taylor BA: Pelvic ileal reservoirs: The options. *Br J Surg* 81:325, 1994.
13. Parks AG, Nicholls RJ: Proctocolectomy without ileostomy for ulcerative colitis. *BMJ* 2:85, 1978.
14. Kock NG: Intra-abdominal "reservoir" in patients with permanent ileostomy. Preliminary observations on a procedure resulting in faecal "continence" in five ileostomy patients. *Arch Surg* 99:223, 1969.
15. Sagar PM, Holdsworth PJ, Godwin PGR, et al: Comparison of triplicated (S) and quadruplicated (W) pelvic ileal reservoirs. Studies on manovolumetry, fecal bacteriology, fecal volatile fatty acids, mucosal morphology and functional results. *Gastroenterology* 102:520, 1992.
16. Galandiuk S, Scott NA, Dozois RR, et al: Ileal pouch–anal anastomosis: Reoperation for pouch-related complications. *Ann Surg* 212:446, 1990.
17. Nicholls RJ, Lubowski DZ: Restorative proctocolectomy: The four loop (W) reservoir. *Br J Surg* 74:564, 1987.

18. Johnston D, Williamson ME, Lewis WG, et al: Prospective controlled trial of duplicated (J) versus quadruplicated (W) pelvic ileal reservoirs in restorative proctocolectomy for ulcerative colitis. *Gut* 39:242, 1996.

19. Selvaggi F, Giuliani A, Gallo C, et al: Randomized controlled trial to compare J pouch and W pouch configurations for ulcerative colitis in the maturation period. *Dis Colon Rectum* 43:615, 2000.

20. Keighley MRB, Yoshioka K, Kmiot W: A prospective randomized trial to compare the stapled double lumen pouch and the sutured quadruple pouch for restorative proctocolectomy. *Br J Surg* 75:1008, 1988.

21. O'Connell PR, Pemberton JH, Brown ML, et al: Determinants of stool frequency after ileal pouch–anal anastomosis. *Am J Surg* 153:157, 1987.

22. Maeda Y, Molina ME, Norton C, et al: The role of pouch compliance measurement in the management of pouch dysfunction. *Int J Colorectal Dis* 25:499, 2010.

23. Shen B, Achkar JP, Lashner BA, et al: Irritable pouch syndrome: A new category of diagnosis for symptomatic patients with ileal pouch-anal anastomosis. *Am J Gastroenterol* 97:972, 2002.

24. Nasmyth DG, Williams NS, Johnston D: Comparison of function of triplicated and duplicated pelvic ileal reservoirs after mucosal proctectomy and ileoanal anastomosis for ulcerative colitis and adenomatous polyposis. *Br J Surg* 73:361, 1986.

25. Mularczyk A, Contessini-Avesani E, Ceana B, et al: Local regulation of postprandial motor responses in ileal pouches. *Gut* 45:575, 1999.

26. Whitehead WE, Delvaux M: Standardisation of barostat procedures for testing smooth muscle tone and sensory thresholds in the gastrointestinal tract. *Dig Dis Sci* 42:223, 1997.

27. Steens J, Bemelman WA, Meijerink WJHJ, et al: Ileoanal pouch function is related to postprandial pouch tone. *Br J Surg* 88:1492, 2001.

28. Ambroze WL, Pemberton JH, Bell AM, et al: The effect of stool consistency on rectal and neorectal emptying. *Dis Colon Rectum* 34:1, 1990.

29. Kmiot WA, Keighley MR: Totally stapled abdominal restorative proctocolectomy. *Br J Surg* 79:961, 1989.

30. Johnston D, Holdsworth PJ, Nasmyth DG, et al: Preservation of the entire anal canal in conservative proctocolectomy for ulcerative colitis: A pilot study comparing end-to-end ileo-anal anastomosis without mucosal resection with mucosal proctectomy and endoanal anastomosis. *Br J Surg* 74:940, 1987.

31. Sagar PM, Holdsworth D, Johnston D: Correlation between laboratory findings and clinical outcome after restorative proctocolectomy: Serial studies in 20 patients after end to end pouch-anal anastomosis. *Br J Surg* 78:67, 1991.

32. Kirat HT, Remzi FH, Kiran RP, et al: Comparison of outcomes after hand-sewn versus stapled ileal pouch-anal anastomosis in 3,109 patients. *Surgery* 146:723, 2009.

33. Holdsworth PJ, Johnston D: Anal sensation after restorative proctocolectomy for ulcerative colitis. *Br J Surg* 75:993, 1988.

34. Martin LW, Torres AM, Fischer JE, et al: The critical level for preservation of continence in the ileoanal anastomosis. *J Pediatr Surg* 20:664, 1985.

35. Lewis WG, Holdsworth PJ, Sagar PM, et al: Effect of anorectal eversion during restorative proctocolectomy on anal sphincter function. *Br J Surg* 80:121, 1993.

36. Ambroze WL, Pemberton JH, Dozois RR, et al: The histologic pattern and pathologic involvement of the anal transition zone in patients with ulcerative colitis. *Gastroenterology* 104:514, 1993.

37. O'Connell PR, Pemberton JH, Weiland LH: Does rectal mucosa regenerate after ileoanal anastomosis? *Dis Colon Rectum* 30:1, 1987.

38. Tsunoda A, Talbot IC, Nicholls RJ: Incidence of dysplasia in the anorectal mucosa in patients having restorative proctocolectomy. *Br J Surg* 77:506, 1990.

39. Ziv Y, Fazio VW, Sirimarco MT, et al: Incidence, risk factors, and treatment of dysplasia in the anal transitional zone after ileal pouch–anal anastomosis. *Dis Colon Rectum* 37:1281, 1994.

40. Hallgren T, Fasth S, Delbro D, et al: Possible role of the autonomic nervous system in sphincter impairment after restorative proctocolectomy. *Br J Surg* 80:631, 1993.

41. Fazio VW, Tjandra JJ: Transanal mucosectomy: Ileal pouch advancement for anorectal dysplasia or inflammation after restorative proctocolectomy. *Dis Colon Rectum* 37:1008, 1994.

42. Scott NA, Dozois RR, Beart RW, et al: Postoperative intra-abdominal and pelvic sepsis complicating ileal pouch–anal anastomosis. *Int J Colorectal Dis* 3:149, 1988.

43. Feinberg SM, McLoed RS, Cohen Z: Complications of loop ileostomy. *Am J Surg* 153:102, 1987.

44. Sagar PM, Lewis WG, Holdsworth PJ, et al: One stage restorative proctocolectomy without temporary defunctioning ileostomy. *Dis Colon Rectum* 35:582, 1992.

45. Joyce MR, Kiran RP, Remzi FH, et al: In a select group of patients meeting strict clinical criteria and undergoing ileal pouch-anal anastomosis, the omission of a diverting ileostomy offers cost savings to the hospital. *Dis Colon Rectum* 53:905, 2010.

46. Lian L, Serclova Z, Fazio VW, et al: Clinical features and management of postoperative pouch bleeding after ileal pouch-anal anastomosis (IPAA). *J Gastrointest Surg* 12:1991, 2008.

47. Lewis WG, Kuzu A, Sagar PM, et al: Stricture at the pouch-anal anastomosis after restorative proctocolectomy. *Dis Colon Rectum* 37:120, 1994.

48. Kirat HT, Kiran RP, Lian L, et al: Influence of stapler size used at ileal pouch-anal anastomosis on anastomotic leak, stricture, long-term functional outcomes, and quality of life. *Am J Surg* 200:68, 2010.

49. Fazio VW, Tjandra JJ: Treatment of strictured ileal pouch–anal anastomosis by pouch advancement and neo-ileoanal anastomosis. *Br J Surg* 79:694, 1992.

50. Prudhomme M, Dozois RR, Godlewski G, et al: Anal canal strictures after ileal pouch–anal anastomosis. *Dis Colon Rectum* 46:20, 2003.

51. Shah N, Remzi F, Massmann A, et al: Management and treatment outcome of pouch-vaginal fistulas following restorative proctocolectomy. *Dis Colon Rectum* 46:911, 2003.

52. Burke D, van Laarhoven CJHM, Herbst F, et al: Transvaginal repair of pouch-vaginal fistulas. *Br J Surg* 88:241, 2001.

53. Gonsalves S, Sagar P, Lengyel J, et al: Assessment of the efficacy of the rectovaginal button fistula plug for the treatment of ileal pouch-vaginal and rectovaginal fistulas. *Dis Colon Rectum* 52:1877, 2009.

54. Sandborn WJ: Pouchitis following ileal pouch–anal anastomosis: Definition, pathogenesis and treatment. *Gastroenterology* 107:1856, 1994.

55. Hata K, Watanabe T, Shinozaki M, et al: Patients with extraintestinal manifestations have a higher risk of developing pouchitis in ulcerative colitis: Multivariate analysis. *Scand J Gastroenterol* 38:1055, 2003.

56. Kuisma J, Mentula S, Luukkonen P, et al: Factors associated with ileal mucosal morphology and inflammation in patients with ileal pouch–anal anastomosis for ulcerative colitis. *Dis Colon Rectum* 46:1476, 2003.

57. Smith FM, Coffey JC, Kell MR, et al: A characterisation of anaerobic colonization and associated mucosal adaptations in the undiseased ileal pouch. *Colorectal Dis* 7:563, 2005.

58. Sambuelli AI, Boerr L, Negreira S, et al: Budesonide enema in pouchitis—a double blind double dummy controlled trial. *Aliment Pharm Ther* 16:27, 2002.

59. Viscido A, Habib FI, Kohn A, et al: Infliximab in refractory pouchitis complicated by fistulae following ileo-anal anastomosis for ulcerative colitis. *Aliment Pharm Ther* 17:1263, 2003.

60. Ferrante M, D'Haens G, Dewit O, et al: Belgian IBD Research Group: Efficacy of infliximab in refractory pouchitis and Crohn's disease related complications of the pouch: A Belgian case series. *Inflamm Bowel Dis* 16:243, 2010.

61. Mann SD, Pitt JP, Springall RG, et al: *Clostridium difficile* infection—an unusual cause of refractory pouchitis: Report of a case. *Dis Colon Rectum* 46:267, 2003.

62. Fruin AB, El-Zammer O, Stucchi AF, et al: Colonic metaplasia in the ileal pouch is associated with inflammation and is not the result of long term adaptation. *J Gastrointest Surg* 7:246, 2003.

63. McLaughlin SD, Clark SK, Bell AJ, et al: Incidence and short-term implications of prepouch ileitis following restorative proctocolectomy with ileal pouch-anal anastomosis for ulcerative colitis. *Dis Colon Rectum* 52:879, 2009.

64. Gionchetti P, Rizzello F, Venturi A, et al: Oral bacteriotherapy as maintenance treatment in patients with chronic pouchitis: A double blind placebo-controlled trial. *Gastroenterology* 119:305, 2000.

65. Holubar SD, Cima RR, Sandborn WJ, et al: Treatment and prevention of pouchitis after ileal pouch-anal anastomosis for chronic ulcerative colitis. *Cochrane Database Syst Rev* CD001176, 2010.

66. Thompson JS: Alopecia after ileal pouch–anal anastomosis. *Dis Colon Rectum* 32:457, 1989.

67. Kirat HT, Kiran RP, Remzi FH, et al: Diagnosis and management of afferent limb syndrome in patients with ileal pouch-anal anastomosis. *Inflamm Bowel Dis* 17:1287, 2011.

68. Joyce MR, Fazio VW, Hull TT, et al: Ileal pouch prolapse: Prevalence, management, and outcomes. *J Gastrointest Surg* 14:993, 2010.

69. Lee SW, Sonoda T, Milsom J: Three cases of adenocarcinoma following restorative proctocolectomy with hand sewn anastomosis for ulcerative colitis: A review of reported cases in the literature. *Colorectal Dis* 7:591, 2005.

70. Remzi FH, Fazio VW, Delaney CP, et al: Dysplasia of the anal transitional zone after ileal pouch–anal anastomosis. Results of prospective evaluation after a minimum of ten years. *Dis Colon Rectum* 46:6, 2003.

71. Gorgun E, Remzi FH, Montague DK, et al: Male sexual function improves after ileal pouch anal anastomosis *Colorectal Dis* 7:545, 2005.

72. Larson DW, Davies MM, Dozois EJ, et al: Sexual function, body image, and quality of life after laparoscopic and open ileal pouch-anal anastomosis. *Dis Colon Rectum* 51:392, 2008.

73. Wax J, Pinette MG, Cartin A, et al: Female reproductive health after ileal pouch–anal anastomosis for ulcerative colitis. *Obstet Gynecol Surv* 58:270, 2003.

74. Metcalf AM, Dozois RR, Kelly KA: Sexual function in women after proctocolectomy. *Ann Surg* 204:624, 1986.

75. Oresland T, Palmblad S, Ellstrom M, et al: Gynecological and sexual function related to anatomical changes in the female pelvis after restorative proctocolectomy. *Int J Colorectal Dis* 9:77, 1994.

76. Damgaard B, Wettergren A, Kirkegaard P: Social and sexual function following ileal pouch–anal anastomosis. *Dis Colon Rectum* 38:286, 1995.

77. Counihan TC, Roberts PL, Schoetz DJ, et al: Fertility and gynaecologic function after ileal pouch–anal anastomosis. *Dis Colon Rectum* 37:1126, 1994.

78. Gorgun E, Remzi FH, Goldberg JM, et al: Fertility is reduced after restorative proctocolectomy with ileal pouch anal anastomosis. A study of 300 patients. *Surgery* 136:795, 2004.

79. Olsen KO, Joelsson M, Laurberg S, et al: Fertility after ileal pouch–anal anastomosis in women with ulcerative colitis. *Br J Surg* 86:493, 1999.

80. Ravid A, Richard CS, Spencer LM, et al: Pregnancy, delivery and pouch function after ileal pouch–anal anastomosis for ulcerative colitis. *Dis Colon Rectum* 45:1283, 2002.

81. Delany CP, Fazio VW, Remzi FH, et al: Prospective age-related analysis of surgical results, functional outcome, and quality of life after ileal pouch–anal anastomosis. *Ann Surg* 238:221, 2003.

82. Hahnloser D, Pemberton JH, Wolff BG, et al: The effect of ageing on function and quality of life in ileal pouch patients: A single cohort experience of 409 patients with chronic ulcerative colitis. *Ann Surg* 240:615, 2004.

83. Sagar PM, Dozois RR, Wolff BG, et al: Disconnection, pouch revision and reconnection of the ileal pouch anal anastomosis. *Br J Surg* 83:1401, 1996.

84. Liljeqvist L, Lindquist K: A reconstructive operation on malfunctioning S-shaped pelvic reservoirs. *Dis Colon Rectum* 28:506, 1985.

85. Pogglioli G, Marchetti F, Selleri S, et al: Redo pouches: Salvaging of failed ileal pouch–anal anastomoses. *Dis Colon Rectum* 36:492, 1993.

86. Herbst F, Sielezneff I, Nicholls RJ: Salvage surgery for ileal pouch outlet obstruction. *Br J Surg* 83:368, 1996.

87. Fonkalsrud E, Bustorff-Silva J: Reconstruction for chronic dysfunction of ileoanal pouches. *Ann Surg* 229:197, 1999.

88. Baixauli J, Delaney CP, Remzi FH, et al: Functional outcome and quality of life after repeat ileal pouch–anal anastomosis (IPAA) for septic and functional complications of ileo-anal surgery. *Br J Surg* 89:58, 2002.

89. MacLean AR, O'Connor B, Parkes R, et al: Reconstructive surgery for failed ileal pouch–anal anastomosis. A viable surgical option with acceptable results. *Dis Colon Rectum* 45:880, 2002.

90. Remzi FH, Fazio VW, Kirat HT, et al: Repeat pouch surgery by the abdominal approach safely salvages failed ileal pelvic pouch. *Inflamm Bowel Dis* 16:243, 2010.

91. Mathis KL, Dozois EJ, Larson DW, et al: Outcomes in patients with ulcerative colitis undergoing partial or complete reconstructive surgery for failing ileal pouch-anal anastomosis. *Ann Surg* 249:409, 2009.

92. Lian L, Fazio VW, Remzi FH, et al: Outcomes for patients undergoing continent ileostomy after a failed ileal pouch-anal anastomosis. *Dis Colon Rectum* 52:1409, 2009.

93. Korsgen S, Keighley MR: Causes of failure and life expectancy of the ileoanal pouch. *Int J Colorectal Dis* 12:4, 1997.

94. Fazio VW, Tekkis PP, Remzi FH, et al: Quantification of risk for pouch failure after ileal pouch anal anastomosis surgery. *Ann Surg* 238:605, 2003.

95. Regimbeau JM, Panis MD, Pocard M, et al: Long-term results of ileal pouch–anal anastomosis for colorectal Crohn's disease. *Dis Colon Rectum* 44:769, 2001.

Surgery for Inflammatory Bowel Disease: Crohn Disease

David W. Larson | Bruce G. Wolff

Crohn disease (CD) presents multiple surgical challenges and has done so since the first description of the disease by Penner and Crohn.[1] Although new biologic medications such as infliximab (Remicade) have changed the way CD is managed medically, underlying surgical principles remain unchanged.

The philosophy of bowel and sphincter preservation has been coupled with medical management in a combined approach; this has become central to the management of the disease. The historical concern that surgery is futile and leads to further complications has largely disappeared. Today, the options for management and treatment have expanded greatly, with improved medical therapy and new, more minimally invasive surgical techniques. Working in concert, the gastroenterologist and surgeon are helping to shape modern care with the patient's best interest in mind. From a purely technical perspective, the widespread adoption of laparoscopic resectional techniques is indeed the most important change in surgical management.

INDICATIONS FOR SURGERY

Between 70% and 90% of patients with CD will undergo an operation at some point during their lifetime.[2] It is an unpredictable and insidious disease, which affects patients in the prime of their lives. There is a bimodal distribution of incidence, with patients developing Crohn in their 20s and 30s, and others in their 60s and 70s. By far, the leading indication for operation is the failure of medical management. The most common complication leading to surgery is intestinal obstruction, which is rarely complete. Other surgical indications include fistula or abscess, gastrointestinal bleeding, and the rare cases of spontaneous perforation with peritonitis.[3] Unique indications for operative intervention include children who experience growth failure; these children will often benefit dramatically and rapidly from surgery, experiencing accelerated growth after resection. Toxic megacolon and fulminant colitis are fortunately unusual presentations. The ultimate choice to intervene surgically is one that is based on the informed discussion between the patient, surgeon, and gastroenterologist.

MEDICAL TREATMENT OF CROHN DISEASE

Crohn disease may present as one of three different subtypes: inflammatory, fibrotic, or fistulizing. It typically has a chronic relapsing course in which roughly 50% who are undergoing medical therapy are in clinical remission. Many patients present to the surgeon with the diagnosis of Crohn already made and on medical therapy. The current options for medical therapy are extensive and complex.

In the setting of mild to moderate disease, patients are often treated with 5-aminosalicylate products, including sulfasalazine, oral mesalamine (Pentasa, Asacol), and rectal mesalamine (Rowasa). For ileal, ileocolonic, and colonic disease, sulfasalazine as a 3- to 6-g daily divided dose is effective treatment.[4] Multiple trials from the United States and Europe have demonstrated its benefits over placebo, although it is less effective than steroids in inducing clinical remission.[4] Overall, sulfasalazine or mesalamine appear to provide minimal benefit for inducing remission, and both are less effective than oral corticosteroids for active Crohn disease. Controlled-release formulations of budesonide (9 mg/day) are effective for disease that is limited to the ileum and right colon.[4] Moreover, budesonide has been shown to be more effective than placebo or mesalamine, and equal in efficacy when compared to conventional oral corticosteroids in the treatment of mild to moderate ileal and right colonic disease. Antimicrobial agents in contrast have undergone multiple placebo-controlled trials, which have not demonstrated short- or long-term efficacy.[4] Based on these results, the role of antibiotic therapy in patients with Crohn disease as it relates to remission is not indicated.

For patients with moderate to severe disease, the use of steroids (40 to 60 mg of prednisone per day) can be utilized until symptoms resolve. Controlled trials have also demonstrated that azathioprine at doses of 2 to 3 mg/kg/day and 6-mercaptopurine at a dose of 1.5 mg/kg/day are effective for inducing remission and closing fistulas in patients with active Crohn disease. Additional medications such as methotrexate (25 mg/wk) have been found to be effective in steroid-dependent or refractory Crohn disease. The newest medication classes include the anti–tumor necrosis factor monoclonal antibodies, infliximab (Remicade; Centocor, Horsham, Penna, USA), adalimumab (Humira; Abbott Laboratories, Chicago, Ill, USA), and certolizumab pegol (Cimzia; UCB Inc., Symrna, Ga, USA). They are often efficacious in patients who have not responded to corticosteroids or other immunosuppressives. Infliximab, either alone or in combination with azathioprine, is more effective than azathioprine treatment alone in the treatment of moderate to severe Crohn disease that has failed first-line therapy. Dosing of infliximab includes a regimen of 5 mg/kg infusion at week 0, 2, and 6 followed by maintenance therapy.[4] A preliminary maintenance of remission study showed that infliximab 10 mg/kg administered intravenously every 8 weeks is effective.[4] This type of maintenance therapy not only is effective but also reduces the immunogenic consequences of infliximab given episodically. It is critical that assessment for tuberculosis exposure be performed before initial treatment with any biologic medication. Finally, other immunosuppressant therapies such as azathioprine 2 to 3 mg/kg/day and 6-mercaptopurine 1.5 mg/kg/day have demonstrated effectiveness in maintaining remission and are steroid sparing.[4]

In summary, initial treatment of mild to moderately active Crohn disease should consist of budesonide or oral corticosteroids. Patients with persistent symptoms may require oral corticosteroids, azathioprine or 6-mercaptopurine, methotrexate, infliximab, or surgical resection. Patients with more refractory disease may require treatment with azathioprine or 6-mercaptopurine and/or infliximab. Remission in patients with Crohn disease should be maintained with azathioprine or 6-mercaptopurine (these medications are also steroid sparing), methotrexate (also steroid sparing), or infliximab.[4]

PREOPERATIVE PREPARATION

The decision to operate is one made in the context of the patient's preoperative comorbidities. Nutritional status is often compromised by severe disease and longstanding poor nutrition. Total parenteral nutrition (TPN) is occasionally indicated in patients who are chronically ill. In a study of 395 malnourished patients, those who received 1 week of TPN had fewer noninfectious complications[5] than did those who did not receive TPN (43%).[6] It is currently debated whether medical therapy, specifically immunomodulators and biologic therapy, has an impact on surgical outcomes. A number of studies have been published with conflicting results. An older study, from our own institution in 2004, shows that early complications after elective bowel surgery were not associated with aggressive therapy.[7a] In a recent study from Appau et al,[7b] however, anastomotic complications were increased in the setting of biologic therapy, and temporary diversion should be considered in these patients. We recently updated our series and confirmed our original findings of no increased risk of complications after biologic therapy.[8] The findings of our series suggest that the risks of patients undergoing anastomosis after colectomy or small bowel resection for Crohn are not increased in the setting of biologic therapy.[8]

Patients who have been treated with steroids within the past 6 to 12 months are administered dexamethasone intravenously intraoperatively, and postoperatively to avoid adrenal crisis induced by the stress of surgery. In addition, standard intravenous antibiotics should be administered within 1 hour of the skin incision, as per protocol. We do not believe it is necessary to administer both preoperative and postoperative broad-spectrum antibiotics unless an infectious complication is present at the time of surgery. In addition, preoperative urethral stent placement is an important adjunct to surgical therapy in situations in which a large abdominal abscess or phlegmon is situated adjacent to the pelvic brim or sidewall.

OPERATIVE CONCERNS

Intraoperative assessment of what is to be the remaining bowel length is an important part of any surgical procedure in patients with CD. Not only does this allow assessment of nutritional viability but provides needed information for future discussions about additional surgical resections. The dreaded fear of short bowel syndrome, although real, has been significantly reduced with the addition of newer medications and more conservative operative approaches.

The mean length of the normal small bowel in healthy people is approximately 640 cm.[9] Important anatomic markers of resection such as the terminal 80 cm of ileum are important, as resection of this will lead to disruption of the enterohepatic circulation and subsequent diarrhea, as well as hyperoxaluria, and vitamin B_{12} malabsorption. In addition, surgeons must keep in mind that with greater resection length a greater degree of malabsorption of fat-soluble vitamins and lactose may occur. It is well known that resection of more than 50% of the small bowel almost always will produce malabsorption, and if 70% of the small bowel is resected, supplemental parenteral nutrition is nearly always required.

RECURRENCE

Possible predisposing factors for recurrence of Crohn disease are as follows: age and onset of disease, sex, site of disease (ileocolic having the highest risk), number of resections, smoking, symptomatic status at the time of surgery, length of small bowel resection, fistulizing versus obstructing forms of disease, proximal margin length, microscopic margin histology, strictureplasty, and number of sites of disease, as well as the presence of colonic-only disease, the presence of granulomas, blood transfusions, family history, and prophylactic treatment.[10,11] Several authors have reported that there may indeed be cofactors or stimulants in the luminal contents, which may induce early recurrence of Crohn disease at a preanastomotic site.[12,13] Cameron et al[12] have shown that patients who have a side-to-end ileocolonic anastomosis have recurrent involvement of the portion of ileum adjacent to the colon but not of the blind pouch distal to the anastomosis. Rutgeerts et al[14] have shown that proximal diversion above an ileocolonic anastomosis prevents recurrence at that anastomotic site, but with closure of the proximal ileostomy, recurrence, if it occurs at all will present promptly. From a medical therapy point of view, there is much conflicting evidence regarding the use of postoperative prophylaxis as some recent studies suggest limited utility in uncomplicated disease.[11] The need for further surgical resection varies widely from 15% to 45% at 3 years, 26% to 65% at 10 years, and 33% to 82% at 15 years.[15] Clearly patients undergoing an ileocolonic anastomosis face high rates of recurrence of 42% by 15 years.[16-18] Given these high rates of surgical reoperation, future study and intervention are needed in an attempt to minimize this recurrence risk. Despite studies such as our own, which showed a limited benefit of prophylactic medical therapy in terminal ileal disease,[11] it is likely that prophylactic treatment after surgical resection will remain an individualized recommendation.

ANASTOMOTIC TECHNIQUE

As with all bowel anastomosis, the principles of a successful anastomosis (no tension, good blood flow, and no contaminants) are followed in surgery for CD. Options include hand-sewn and the stapled anastomoses. It is helpful for surgeons to remember that when choosing a stapling device, there are 3.6- and 4.8-mm staple sizes. The largest staple length may be more appropriate for very thickened bowel. However, hemostasis may not be as good as that obtained with the 3.6-mm-length staple. Although resectional procedures can be performed in either manner, we have found that stapling strictureplasties can be difficult in fibrotic bowel. The technical question of whether a wide side-to-side anastomosis (illustrated in Figure 161-1), as opposed to an end-to-end, would reduce recurrence rates has been evaluated by a recent randomized trial—with the findings that no specific anastomotic type is better suited to reduce postoperative recurrence, although a stapled anastomosis can be accomplished faster.[19]

RESECTION MARGIN

The role that margins play in recurrence of CD is controversial as well. A long-term retrospective study by Krause et al[20] compared two groups of patients: one group with a "radical" resection of a group with more than 10 cm of disease-free margins incorporated into the resection versus less than 10 cm of uninvolved bowel. They found, after a 14-year followup, that patients with longer margins had a lower recurrence rate (31%) and a better quality of life than patients with a shorter margin (83%). A similar retrospective review[21] reported similar results; a margin of normal tissue of less than 4 cm was associated with a 10-fold higher recurrence. In contrast, a study by Raab[22] showed that the length of disease-free resection margins did not influence the risk of recurrence in both univariate and multivariate analyses in 353 patients undergoing a "curative" resection between 1969 and 1986. The only prospective study to address this issue compared patients undergoing ileocolic resection who were randomly assigned to one of two groups: (1) proximal margin of only 2 cm or (2) a proximal margin of 12 cm from the macroscopically involved disease.[23] There was no significant difference in recurrence rate in the 56 patients undergoing extended resection in contrast to the 75 patients undergoing limited resection, although the recurrence rate in the extended group was lower (18% vs. 25%).[23] These studies, along with several retrospective studies, have small numbers of patients and may harbor type II errors. This includes our own study, which did not show a significant difference between a proximal margin length of less than 5 cm versus a margin of 5 cm or more.[17] In general terms, however, the recommendation remains that a 2-cm disease-free margin is adequate and helps conserve bowel length.[24]

SITE-SPECIFIC CROHN DISEASE

COLONIC CROHN DISEASE

CD involving only the colon occurs in 10% of patients, as the majority of patients present with either small

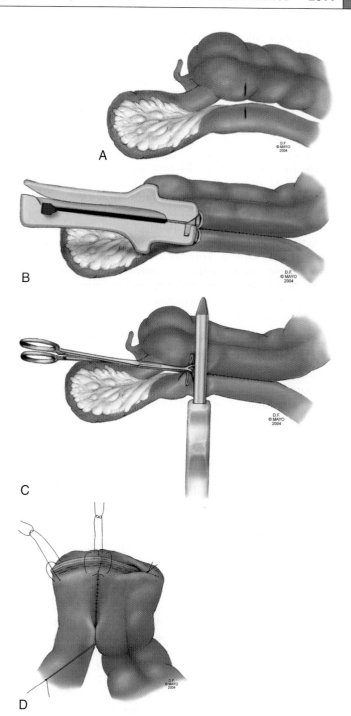

FIGURE 161-1 Line of resection for a right hemicolectomy done for cancer. **A,** 1-cm transverse incisions are made on the antimesenteric borders of the ileum and colon to begin a stapled anastomosis. **B,** The first of two staple firers need to create an anastomosis. **C,** The second of two staple firers needed for completion of a stapled anastomosis. **D,** Oversewing the staple line with interrupted suture.

bowel (30%) or ileocolonic (40%) disease. The selection of proper operation for colonic CD depends on multiple variables, including age, disease distribution, and extent of involvement, previous resections, rectal compliance, and adequacy of fecal continence. The three basic approaches—segmental resection, subtotal colectomy with ileorectostomy or ileosigmoidostomy, and proctocolectomy with Brooke ileostomy—are used to address the patient's individual needs.

The issue of retaining intestinal continuity is one that has been debated for years. Goligher[25] reported on 207 patients who underwent resection for colonic CD. He found that there was a significantly higher recurrence rate in those undergoing subtotal colectomy and ileorectal anastomosis than in those undergoing proctocolectomy and ileostomy. These observations have also been made in other series.[26] In our series of patients with colonic CD, there was a significantly lower risk of recurrence in the group of patients who underwent a total proctocolectomy versus any other procedure.[27] However, our followup series on the utility of segmental resection clearly showed that long-term intestinal continuity can be maintained with a conservative surgical approach.[28] Given these observations, segmental resection should be the primary surgical procedure, with an ostomy reserved for patients with extensive disease, prompting proctocolectomy.[24,28]

ILEAL POUCH–ANAL ANASTOMOSIS IN PATIENTS WITH CROHN DISEASE

Although ileal pouch-anal anastomosis (IPAA) can be performed in patients with Crohn disease, complication rates are high[29-31] and long-term success in terms of pouch retention is only about 50%.[32] In our institutional series[33] of 37 patients who developed Crohn disease subsequent to ileal pouch–anal anastomosis, 34 had manifestations of CD in the pouch and/or anal canal. Forty-five percent of these patients required diversion or pouch excision. Braveman et al found among their 32 patients with IPAA and CD that 93% had complications and 29% experienced pouch failure within 5 years of surgery.[29] Recently, our group reported pouch salvage rates with infliximab of 67% in patients with CD.[34] The most recent review by the Cleveland Clinic looked at more than 200 patients with Crohn disease and IPAA. The 10-year pouch retention rate was 71%. Within a highly selected patient group with long-standing disease and colonic CD only, the results and retention of IPAA are actually quite high, that is, 85% at 10 years.[32] In a series by Regimbeau et al,[35] only 35% of such highly selected patients experienced morbidity, with 10% experiencing failure. In 20 highly selected CD patients treated in the study by Melton et al, long-term pouch survival was observed at 85% at 10 years.[32] Given these results, IPAA may be considered for patients with CD limited to the colon, without evidence of anal canal involvement or small bowel disease.

LAPAROSCOPE-ASSISTED SURGERY FOR CROHN DISEASE

Minimally invasive techniques are ideally suited for patients with Crohn disease, and have been shown in both randomized and nonrandomized studies to demonstrate similar or improved morbidity and mortality compared with open resection.[36-43] Unfortunately, only approximately 6% of patients undergo a laparoscopic operation, with the remainder undergoing open operations.[43]

Although laparoscopy is less successful in patients with Crohn disease who have large fixed masses or multiple complex fistulas, it may still be technically possible. Laparoscopic surgery can be successfully used in recurrent ileocolonic disease with more than 75% of patients being potential candidates.[44] For the most common form of Crohn disease, four metaanalysis and systematic reviews have been published regarding laparoscopic versus open surgery for small bowel and ileocolonic Crohn disease.[45] Although the vast majority of these series are not randomized controlled trials, they show a decrease in postoperative length of stay, cost, and improved postoperative complication risk in laparoscopic patients. It is important to realize that these excellent results require the presence of experienced minimally invasive surgeons and systems to provide care for these CD patients.

In general terms, patients who underwent laparoscopic ileocolic resection for Crohn disease had a shorter time to resumption of diet, time to bowel function, and length of stay.[38] Milsom[36] et al found that recovery of pulmonary function returned earlier in the laparoscopic group, but time to first bowel movement and hospital stay were not significantly different. A most interesting finding by Bergamaschi et al[37] found not only shorter hospital stay but also a decreased rate of small bowel obstruction (35% in the open group vs. 11% in the laparoscopic group). Two published series from our own institution involving over 100 patients confirmed the benefits of laparoscopic surgery over open surgery. The largest series to date included 335 patients with a mean hospital stay of 5 days and overall complication rate of 13%. In addition to ileal colonic disease, new evidence exists that colonic Crohn disease may be addressed successfully utilizing a minimally invasive approach. In a recent study published in our institution, 92 patients were treated successfully for their colonic disease using a laparoscopic approach.[46] Nearly half the cases involved total colectomy, with 20% undergoing subtotal and 35% undergoing segmental colectomy.

SPECIFIC OPERATIONS

With improvements in medical therapy and acute care, emergency procedures for Crohn disease are thankfully uncommon. In patients with acutely perforated CD, depending on the degree of peritonitis,[47] either resection with primary anastomosis or diverting ileostomy or colostomy can be performed. Even though hemorrhage is rare, this can occasionally occur and all of the usual methods to localize bleeding points, including mesenteric arteriography, should be used. With localization of the disease and surgical resection, results are excellent.[48]

SMALL BOWEL

The three operative options that have been widely used for small bowel Crohn disease are bypass, resection, and strictureplasty. Bypass was commonly used in the decades of the 1950s and 1960s but is rarely used today, because a severely diseased segment of bowel left in place may cause continued symptoms (bacterial overgrowth), require treatment with steroids, and perhaps harbor a malignancy. Small bowel bypass might be useful in patients with an already shortened small bowel, or in

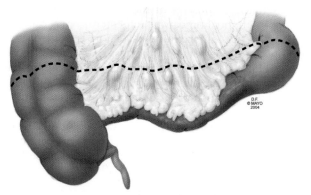

FIGURE 161-2 Ileocolonic Crohn.

patients with extensive strictures throughout the small bowel. Gastrojejunostomy is useful in gastroduodenal Crohn disease as an alternative to duodenal strictureplasty.

RESECTION

Resection and primary anastomosis are used in patients with fistulous disease of the small bowel, containing abscess, and with isolated stenotic lesions in patients in whom there is adequate bowel remaining. During exploration, bowel length should always be measured. Careful assessment of the extent of the disease is made. Typically, ileal Crohn disease will affect the distal 25 to 30 cm of terminal ileum and may continue into the cecum (Figure 161-2). This type of resection for isolated Crohn disease accounts for 80% to 90% of operations for Crohn disease. An end-to-end ileoascending colostomy can be hand-sutured or a wide-stapled side-to-side, functional end-to-end anastomosis can be performed with the linear stapler (see Figure 161-1), with equal chance of recurrence.[19]

STRICTUREPLASTY

Short areas of stenosing CD or multiple sites of disease lend themselves to strictureplasty. Frequently, a combination of resection and strictureplasty is the optimal choice and has become widely accepted. Strictureplasty plays a prominent role in the surgical management of small bowel Crohn disease. Isolated strictures under 10 cm in length are often considered best for strictureplasty (Figure 161-3). Our original experience with 35 patients, in whom 71 strictureplasties were performed, and who were followed for more than 3 years, found a symptomatic recurrence rate of 20%.[49] Two more reports of more than 1400 strictureplasties, followed for more than 7 years, reported reoperation rates of between 34% to 44% and symptomatic relief in more than 95% of patients.[50] A recent metaanalysis by Yamamoto et al reported the results of more than 1000 patients and 3000 strictureplasties[54]; they found that strictureplasty was both safe and effective and the majority of recurrences occurred at sites other than the strictureplasty site. The technique of strictureplasty is shown in Figure 161-3. It may be helpful to use a Baker tube, after making the initial transverse incision, to define proximal and distal strictures that may be subtle or undetected. This also provides a method to further decompress the small bowel. Importantly, biopsy

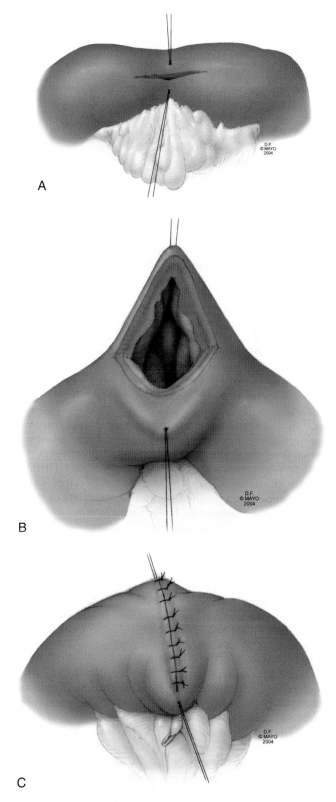

FIGURE 161-3 A, Longitudinal opening of a small bowel Crohn stricture. **B,** Preparing for a strictureplasty. **C,** Completing the anterior interrupted row of sutures for a strictureplasty.

of the wall of each strictureplasty will occasionally reveal an unsuspected adenocarcinoma.

COLONIC CROHN DISEASE

Preservation of intestinal continuity remains the primary goal in patients with CD of the colon.[24] For those patients with severe disease scattered throughout the colon, subtotal colectomy and ileorectostomy can be safely performed. Of the 42 patients who had this operation at the Mayo Clinic, 91% had improved health and quality of life after surgery, and 66% maintained an acceptable, functioning ileorectal anastomosis for at least 10 years.[51] In our hands, a side (of ileum) to end (of rectum) anastomosis has become a preferred technique. Some patients may have more limited colonic involvement, and in this situation a segmental colon resection with colo-colonic anastomosis is indicated. Eighty-six percent of these patients will remain stoma free over a 14-year followup.[28]

Strictureplasty has occasionally been used for colonic CD, but this may not be judicious as colonic strictures may harbor carcinomas, and recurrent CD in the colon is very common. Given the success of medical therapy, some argue that if the patient has mild rectal disease and minimal perianal involvement, then it is reasonable to leave a short segment of rectum and anal canal in place, but exclude it from the fecal stream. In this way, a patient with anorectal CD may respond to diversion and local treatment, with an opportunity for future reanastomosis.[52] In one study,[53] the long-term chances for closure of a temporary stoma were 75% when used for anastomotic protection, 79% after postoperative complications, but only 40% in patients with genital fistulas or rectal inflammation or stenosis. Rectal disease and perianal fistula were independent predictors of a low possibility of stoma closure during followup. Unfortunately, many patients have both severe colonic disease and mild to severe rectal disease with anorectal complications; these patients are best served with proctocolectomy and Brooke ileostomy.[54]

On those rare occasions when a patient presents with toxic megacolon from CD, colectomy with closure of the proximal rectum and end ileostomy is the procedure of choice.[24] This operation can be done expeditiously and leaves no anastomosis in the abdomen. A common concern remains the treatment of the distal rectal stump.[55] It is our practice to oversew the stump, or in severe cases, to exteriorize it as a mucus fistula. In extreme cases, when both the colon and the rectum are severely involved, proctocolectomy with permanent end ileostomy (Brooke ileostomy) may be required emergently.[56]

Crohn disease patients are at high risk for perianal wound complications after proctocolectomy. Among 32 patients with Crohn disease treated with proctocolectomy and primary closure at the Mayo Clinic, 50% had a healed perineum by 1 month after surgery, and 90% had healed by 1 year.[57] Persistent nonhealing of perineal wounds requires excision of the wound surface and secondary closure, skin grafts, a musculocutaneous flap, or some combination thereof.[58] To avoid the problem of a nonhealing wound, endorectal (intersphincteric) and sphincter-saving excisions rather than wide excision of the entire anorectum are useful. By using the

well-vascularized muscles of the anal canal, more rapid and complete healing can be expected.

The practice of proximal diversion is controversial. This operation may have its greatest role in patients who are extremely ill with CD of the colon. Proponents have reported improvement from fecal diversion.[59] In light of medical therapy such as infliximab, the future treatment of diseased segments and the ability to close existing stomas may indeed be improved. Future studies in this area will be needed. In the past, it has been commonly noted that once the stoma is reversed the disease flares again, requiring surgical treatment.[59]

ANORECTAL CROHN DISEASE

The surgical treatment of perianal Crohn disease is evolving. Management is customarily a combined approach, encompassing both aggressive medical and conservative surgical management.[60] Anorectal CD typically presents in three ways: ulceration, fistula, and stricture. Michelassi et al[61] observed that 23% of patients with Crohn disease manifested perineal fistulas, 18% stenosis, 16% abscesses, 9% rectovaginal fistulas, 5% incontinence, and 29% with a combination of problems. The cumulative incidence of perianal fistulas in Crohn disease has been estimated by two population-based studies. Hellers et al[62] reported a cumulative incidence of perianal fistulas of 23%. In a Mayo series, Schwartz et al[60] showed that the cumulative incidence of fistulizing Crohn disease in Olmsted County, Minnesota, between 1970 and 1993 was 38%. The lifetime risk for developing a fistula is 20% to 40%.[63,64] The key concept when operating on patients with anorectal Crohn disease is to be conservative. Wide excision of large amounts of tissue should not be performed. Currently, there are no controlled trials showing benefit to treating a CD fistula with antibiotics, azathioprine, or 6-mercaptopurine.[4] Two controlled trials, however, show that infliximab treatments at 0, 2, and 6 weeks are effective at reducing the number of draining fistulas in patients with Crohn disease.[4] This medical treatment in combination with appropriate surgical management (placement of setons, etc.) remains the most effective method to aid in the treatment of anorectal Crohn disease.

PERIANAL ABSCESS

The treatment of perianal abscess is prompt and adequate surgical drainage. Superficial abscesses require simple incision and drainage. Abscesses that are deep (supralevator or ischiorectal) should be drained using a mushroom catheter and/or a noncutting seton to provide adequate drainage with as little tissue trauma as possible (Figure 161-4).

FISTULAS

Fistula disease is common among CD patients. The surgical treatment of Crohn fistula most commonly involves using a noncutting seton.[65-69] A seton is a nonabsorbable suture (Penrose drain, or vessel loop) that is placed through the fistula tract (Figure 161-5). The purpose of the seton is to promote drainage and, thus, decrease the risk of recurrent abscess while aggressive medical therapy is being instituted. At the Mayo Clinic, 110 patients were

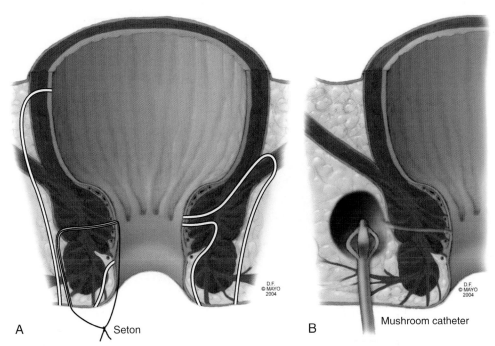

A   Seton

B   Mushroom catheter

FIGURE 161-4 **A,** Draining seton in place through a transsphincteric fistula. **B,** Perianal abscess treated with a Malecot catheter.

surgically treated for perianal Crohn fistulas with either seton or superficial fistulotomy and aggressive medical therapy. After a median followup of 3 years, 86% had complete healing or were asymptomatic.[70]

Others have studied similar patients. Among 27 patients with fistulizing CD, Scott and Northover[66] reported that 85% of patients treated with noncutting setons experienced fistula closure. A high recurrence rate, which may be as much as 40% after removing the seton,[71] lends legitimacy to our use of concomitant antibiotics, azathioprine, or 6-mercaptopurine and infliximab.[71] With the use of medications such as infliximab, long-term initial healing rates may be improved. We recently reported that infliximab along with seton placement led to the complete resolution of perianal fistulas in 68% of patients[72] and reduced the rate of recurrent abscess. In a comparative study by Regueiro et al, perianal fistulas were treated with infliximab alone versus combination infliximab plus seton placement. They found that initial response was improved with seton placement (100% vs. 82.6%), and that the combination had lower recurrence rates (44% vs. 79%), and longer time to recurrence (13.5 months vs. 3.6 months).[73]

In addition to medical and surgical therapy, there are additional device-related therapies. These therapies include fibrin glue and the fistula plug. Although the data are mixed, there are several studies worth mentioning. The first was a small randomized trial of fibrin glue versus conventional therapy.[74] In this study, fibrin glue was more effective for complex fistula and associated with higher patient satisfaction. A study by O'Connor reported that fistula plugs were both safe and resulted in improved healing in up to 80% of patients.[75] A recent prospective multicenter study showed mixed results: significant healing with fistulotomy in 87% of patients and only 32% healing with fibrin plugs.[76]

Although improvements in medical therapy and conservative surgical management of perianal CD may lead to healing, some patients will go on to proctectomy. In our own long-term series of patients with anorectal CD,[77] two groups emerged. The first suffered severe rectal involvement and proceeded to proctectomy very early in the disease process. The second group had more limited rectal disease and has been managed well with conservative treatment. Within this series, the cumulative probability of avoiding proctectomy was 92% at 10 years and 83% at 20 years.[77] In our more recent study of 110 patients treated surgically for perianal disease, the severity of proctitis, extent of fistulas and abscesses, and the presence of recurrent abscess all led to a higher incidence of failure.[70]

RECTOVAGINAL FISTULA

This is a particularly distressing complication of CD. About 2% of women with CD will develop a rectovaginal fistula (RVF). Luckily most fistulas are very low and have no associated symptoms. Surgical treatment is reserved for those patients with an unacceptable quality of life in whom medical treatment has failed. Unfortunately, the development of an RVF is a poor prognostic sign and may require proximal diversion to decrease local sepsis. In patients undergoing rectovaginal fistula repair, the disease should be quiescent and the rectum distensible. In general, for very low RVF (<15% of the sphincter involved) and normal sphincter function, simple fistulotomy is a viable option. However, some surgeons advocate use of an endorectal advancement flap as an alternative to fistulotomy, or noncutting setons in patients with a simple fistula who do not have active rectal inflammation.[78,79] An advancement flap involves creating a flap of tissue around the internal opening of a fistula and then moving healthy tissue over the excised area.[78] Joo

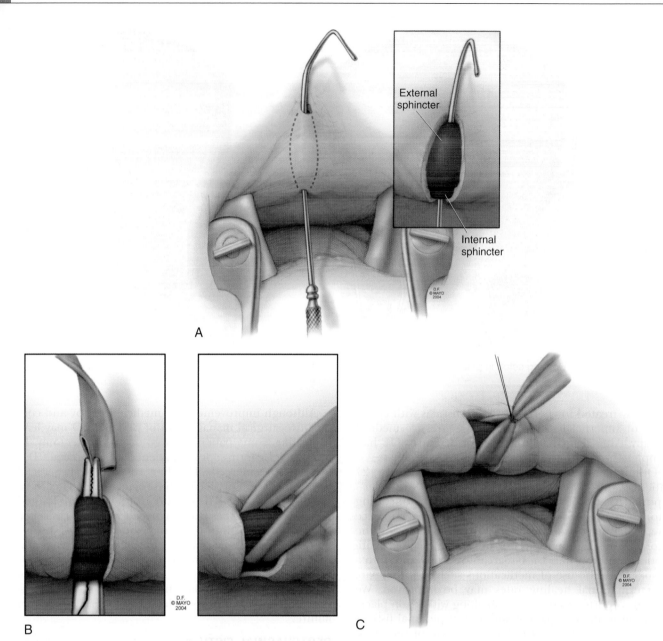

A

External
sphincter

Internal
sphincter

B

C

FIGURE 161-5 A, Probe through a perianal fistula with the internal sphincter exposed. **B,** Placement of a seton. **C,** Securing a seton in place.

et al[78] reported sustained closure in 74% of 26 patients with fistulizing CD treated with endorectal advancement flap. Hull and Fazio[80] reported that among 35 patients with an advancement flap for low rectovaginal fistulas, the initial healing rate was 54%, and the ultimate healing rate with repeat procedure was 68%, but few others have reported such good outcomes. Although these reported successes exist, in our experience this approach yields unpredictable results at best.

SUMMARY

Surgery for CD is both frustrating and rewarding. Surgeons must be familiar with a variety of techniques and options to adapt to the multitude of possible presentations of CD. Innovation, research, surgical technique,

and a combined approach will aid surgeons in conserving bowel length, preserving intestinal continuity, restoring patients to active lives, and most importantly, improving their quality of life.

REFERENCES

1. Penner A, Crohn B: Perianal fistulae as a complication of regional ileitis. *Ann Surg* 108:867, 1932.
2. Hurst RD, Cohen RD: The role of laparoscopy and strictureplasty in the management of inflammatory bowel disease. *Semin Gastrointest Dis* 11:10, 2000.
3. Andrews HA, Keighley MR, Alexander-Williams J, et al: Strategy for management of distal ileal Crohn's disease. *Br J Surg* 78:679, 1991.
4. Lichtenstein GR, Hanauer SB, Sandborn WJ: Management of Crohn's disease in adults. *Am J Gastroenterol* 104:465, 2009.

5. Perioperative total parenteral nutrition in surgical patients. The Veterans Affairs Total Parenteral Nutrition Cooperative Study Group. *N Engl J Med* 325:525, 1991.

6. Buzby GP, Knox LS, Crosby LO, et al: Study protocol: A randomized clinical trial of total parenteral nutrition in malnourished surgical patients. *Am J Clin Nutr* 47:366, 1988.

7a. Colombel JF, Sandborn WJ: Development of fistulae in ileo-anal pouch does not necessarily indicate Crohn's disease: Response. *Am J Gastroenterol* 99:2067, 2004.

7b. Appau KA, Fazio VW, Shen B, et al: Use of infliximab within 3 months of ileocolonic resection is associated with adverse postoperative outcomes in Crohn's patients. *J Gastrointest Surg* 12:1738, 2008.

8. Nasir BS, Dozois EJ, Cima RR, et al: Perioperative anti-tumor necrosis factor therapy does not increase the rate of early postoperative complications in Crohn's disease. *J Gastrointest Surg* 14:1859, 2010.

9. Slater G, Aufses AH Jr: Small bowel length in Crohn's disease. *Am J Gastroenterol* 86:1037, 1991.

10. Wolff BG: Factors determining recurrence following surgery for Crohn's disease. *World J Surg* 22:364, 1998.

11. Malireddy K, Larson DW, Sandborn WJ, et al: Recurrence and impact of postoperative prophylaxis in laparoscopically treated primary ileocolic Crohn's disease. *Arch Surg* 145:42, 2010.

12. Cameron JL, Hamilton SR, Coleman J, et al: Patterns of ileal recurrence in Crohn's disease. A prospective randomized study. *Ann Surg* 215:546, 1992.

13. D'Haens GR, Geboes K, Peeters M, et al: Early lesions of recurrent Crohn's disease caused by infusion of intestinal contents in excluded ileum. *Gastroenterology* 114:262, 1998.

14. Rutgeerts P, Goboes K, Peeters M, et al: Effect of faecal stream diversion on recurrence of Crohn's disease in the neoterminal ileum. *Lancet* 338:771, 1991.

15. Chardavoyne R, Flint GW, Pollack S, et al: Factors affecting recurrence following resection for Crohn's disease. *Dis Colon Rectum* 29:495, 1986.

16. Williams JG, Wong WD, Rothenberger DA, et al: Recurrence of Crohn's disease after resection. *Br J Surg* 78:10, 1991.

17. McLeod RS, Wolff BG, Steinhart AH, et al: Risk and significance of endoscopic/radiological evidence of recurrent Crohn's disease. *Gastroenterology* 113:1823, 1997.

18. Lock MR, Farmer RG, Fazio VW, et al: Recurrence and reoperation for Crohn's disease: The role of disease location in prognosis. *N Engl J Med* 304:1586, 1981.

19. McLeod RS, Wolff BG, Ross S, et al: Recurrence of Crohn's disease after ileocolic resection is not affected by anastomotic type: Results of a multicenter, randomized, controlled trial. *Dis Colon Rectum* 52:919, 2009.

20. Krause U, Ejerblad S, Bergman L: Crohn's disease. A long-term study of the clinical course in 186 patients. *Scand J Gastroenterol* 20:516, 1985.

21. Softley A, Myren J, Clamp SE, et al: Factors affecting recurrence after surgery for Crohn's disease. *Scand J Gastroenterol Suppl* 144:31, 1988.

22. Raab Y, Bergstrom R, Ejerblad S, et al: Factors influencing recurrence in Crohn's disease. An analysis of a consecutive series of 353 patients treated with primary surgery. *Dis Colon Rectum* 39:918, 1996.

23. Fazio VW, Marchetti F, Church M, et al: Effect of resection margins on the recurrence of Crohn's disease in the small bowel. A randomized controlled trial. *Ann Surg* 224:563, 1996.

24. Strong SA, Koltun WA, Hyman NH, et al: Practice parameters for the surgical management of Crohn's disease. *Dis Colon Rectum* 50:1735, 2007.

25. Goligher JC: The long-term results of excisional surgery for primary and recurrent Crohn's disease of the large intestine. *Dis Colon Rectum* 28:51, 1985.

26. Andrews HA, Lewis P, Allan RN: Prognosis after surgery for colonic Crohn's disease. *Br J Surg* 76:1184, 1989.

27. McLeod RS, Wolff BG, Steinhart AH, et al: Prophylactic mesalamine treatment decreases postoperative recurrence of Crohn's disease. *Gastroenterology* 109:404, 1995.

28. Prabhakar LP, Laramee C, Nelson H, et al: Avoiding a stoma: Role for segmental or abdominal colectomy in Crohn's colitis. *Dis Colon Rectum* 40:71, 1997.

29. Braveman JM, Schoetz DJ Jr, Marcello PW, et al: The fate of the ileal pouch in patients developing Crohn's disease. *Dis Colon Rectum* 47:1613, 2004.

30. Deutsch AA, McLeod RS, Cullen J, et al: Results of the pelvic-pouch procedure in patients with Crohn's disease. *Dis Colon Rectum* 34:475, 1991.

31. Hyman NH, Fazio VW, Tuckson WB, et al: Consequences of ileal pouch-anal anastomosis for Crohn's colitis. *Dis Colon Rectum* 34:653, 1991.

32. Melton GB, Fazio VW, Kiran RP, et al: Long-term outcomes with ileal pouch-anal anastomosis and Crohn's disease: Pouch retention and implications of delayed diagnosis. *Ann Surg* 248:608, 2008.

33. Sagar PM, Dozois RR, Wolff BG: Long-term results of ileal pouch-anal anastomosis in patients with Crohn's disease. *Dis Colon Rectum* 39:893, 1996.

34. Colombel JF, Ricart E, Loftus EV Jr, et al: Management of Crohn's disease of the ileoanal pouch with infliximab. *Am J Gastroenterol* 98:2239, 2003.

35. Regimbeau JM, Panis Y, Pocard M, et al: Long-term results of ileal pouch-anal anastomosis for colorectal Crohn's disease. *Dis Colon Rectum* 44:769, 2001.

36. Milsom JW, Hammerhofer KA, Bohm B, et al: Prospective, randomized trial comparing laparoscopic vs. conventional surgery for refractory ileocolic Crohn's disease. *Dis Colon Rectum* 44:1, 2001.

37. Bergamaschi R, Pessaux P, Arnaud JP: Comparison of conventional and laparoscopic ileocolic resection for Crohn's disease. *Dis Colon Rectum* 46:1129, 2003.

38. Duepree HJ, Senagore AJ, Delaney CP, et al: Advantages of laparoscopic resection for ileocecal Crohn's disease. *Dis Colon Rectum* 45:605, 2002.

39. Soop M, Larson DW, Malireddy K, et al: Safety, feasibility, and short-term outcomes of laparoscopically assisted primary ileocolic resection for Crohn's disease. *Surg Endosc* 23:1876, 2009.

40. Reissman P, Salky BA, Pfeifer J, et al: Laparoscopic surgery in the management of inflammatory bowel disease. *Am J Surg* 171:47, 1996.

41. Larson DW, Pemberton JH: Current concepts and controversies in surgery for IBD. *Gastroenterology* 126:1611, 2004.

42. Nguyen SQ, Teitelbaum E, Sabnis AA, et al: Laparoscopic resection for Crohn's disease: An experience with 335 cases. *Surg Endosc* 23:2380, 2009.

43. Lesperance K, Martin MJ, Lehmann R, et al: National trends and outcomes for the surgical therapy of ileocolonic Crohn's disease: A population-based analysis of laparoscopic vs. open approaches. *J Gastrointest Surg* 13:1251, 2009.

44. Holubar SD, Dozois EJ, Privitera A, et al: Laparoscopic surgery for recurrent ileocolic Crohn's disease. *Inflamm Bowel Dis* 16:1382, 2010.

45. Holubar SD, Wolff BG: Advances in surgical approaches to Crohn's disease: Minimally invasive surgery and biologic therapy. *Expert Rev Clin Immunol* 5:463, 2009.

46. Holubar SD, Dozois EJ, Privitera A, et al: Minimally invasive colectomy for Crohn's colitis: A single institution experience. *Inflamm Bowel Dis* 16:1940, 2010.

47. Voeller G, Britt L: Surgical management of perforated Crohn's disease. *Am J Surg* 56:100, 1990.

48. Cirocco WC, Reilly JC, Rusin LC: Life-threatening hemorrhage and exsanguination from Crohn's disease. Report of four cases. *Dis Colon Rectum* 38:85, 1995.

49. Spencer MP, Nelson H, Wolff BG, et al: Strictureplasty for obstructive Crohn's disease: The Mayo experience. *Mayo Clin Proc* 69:33, 1994.

50. Dietz DW, Laureti S, Strong SA, et al: Safety and longterm efficacy of strictureplasty in 314 patients with obstructing small bowel Crohn's disease. *J Am Coll Surg* 192:330; discussion 337, 2001.

51. Pastore RL, Wolff BG, Hodge D: Total abdominal colectomy and ileorectal anastomosis for inflammatory bowel disease. *Dis Colon Rectum* 40:1455, 1997.

52. Hashemi M, Novell JR, Lewis AA: Side-to-side stapled anastomosis may delay recurrence in Crohn's disease. *Dis Colon Rectum* 41:1293, 1998.

53. Post S, Herfarth C, Schumacher H, et al: Experience with ileostomy and colostomy in Crohn's disease. *Br J Surg* 82:1629, 1995.

54. Yamamoto T, Bain IM, Allan RN, et al: An audit of strictureplasty for small-bowel Crohn's disease. *Dis Colon Rectum* 42:797, 1999.

55. Carter FM, McLeod RS, Cohen Z: Subtotal colectomy for ulcerative colitis: Complications related to the rectal remnant. *Dis Colon Rectum* 34:1005, 1991.

56. Scammell BE, Andrews H, Allan RN, et al: Results of proctocolectomy for Crohn's disease. *Br J Surg* 74:671, 1987.

57. Waits JO, Dozois RR, Kelly KA: Primary closure and continuous irrigation of the perineal wound after proctectomy. *Mayo Clin Proc* 57:185, 1982.

58. Pezim ME, Wolff BG, Woods JE, et al: Closure of postproctectomy perineal sinus with gracilis muscle flaps. *Can J Surg* 30:212, 1987.

59. Winslet MC, Keighley MR: Fecal diversion for Crohn's disease of the colon. *Dis Colon Rectum* 23:99, 1991.

60. Schwartz DA, Pemberton JH, Sandborn WJ: Diagnosis and treatment of perianal fistulas in Crohn's disease. *Ann Intern Med* 135:906, 2001.

61. Michelassi F, Melis M, Rubin M, et al: Surgical treatment of anorectal complications in Crohn's disease. *Surgery* 128:597, 2000.

62. Hellers G, Bergstrand O, Ewerth S, et al: Occurrence and outcome after primary treatment of anal fistulae in Crohn's disease. *Gut* 21:525, 1980.

63. Rankin GB, Watts HD, Melnyk CS, et al: National Cooperative Crohn's Disease Study: Extraintestinal manifestations and perianal complications. *Gastroenterology* 77:914, 1979.

64. Schwartz DA, Loftus EV Jr, Tremaine WJ, et al: The natural history of fistulizing Crohn's disease in Olmsted County, Minnesota. *Gastroenterology* 122:875, 2002.

65. Sugita A, Koganei K, Harada H, et al: Surgery for Crohn's anal fistulas. *J Gastroenterol* 30:143, 1995.

66. Scott HJ, Northover JM: Evaluation of surgery for perianal Crohn's fistulas. *Dis Colon Rectum* 39:1039, 1996.

67. Takesue Y, Ohge H, Yokoyama T, et al: Long-term results of seton drainage on complex anal fistulae in patients with Crohn's disease. *J Gastroenterol* 37:912, 2002.

68. White RA, Eisenstat TE, Rubin RJ, et al: Seton management of complex anorectal fistulas in patients with Crohn's disease. *Dis Colon Rectum* 33:587, 1990.

69. Koganei K, Sugita A, Harada H, et al: Seton treatment for perianal Crohn's fistulas. *Surg Today* 25:32, 1995.

70. Gaw JLD, Pemberton J, Wolff B: Surgical management of Crohn's fistula-in-ano. *Colorectal Disease* 6:25, 2004.

71. Pearl RK, Andrews JR, Orsay CP, et al: Role of the seton in the management of anorectal fistulas. *Dis Colon Rectum* 36:573, 1993.

72. Ricart E, Panaccione R, Loftus EV, et al: Infliximab for Crohn's disease in clinical practice at the Mayo Clinic: The first 100 patients. *Am J Gastroenterol* 96:722, 2001.

73. Regueiro M, Mardini H: Treatment of perianal fistulizing Crohn's disease with infliximab alone or as an adjunct to exam under anesthesia with seton placement. *Inflamm Bowel Dis* 9:98, 2003.

74. Ogunbiyi OA, Fleshman JW: Place of laparoscopic surgery in Crohn's disease. *Baillieres Clin Gastroenterol* 12:157, 1998.

75. Bauer JJ, Harris MT, Grumbach NM, et al: Laparoscopic-assisted intestinal resection for Crohn's disease. Which patients are good candidates? *J Clin Gastroenterol* 23:44, 1996.

76. Hyman N, O'Brien S, Osler T: Outcomes after fistulotomy: Results of a prospective, multicenter regional study. *Dis Colon Rectum* 52:2022, 2009.

77. Wolff BG, Culp CE, Beart RW Jr, et al: Anorectal Crohn's disease. A long-term perspective. *Dis Colon Rectum* 28:709, 1985.

78. Joo JS, Weiss EG, Nogueras JJ, et al: Endorectal advancement flap in perianal Crohn's disease. *Am Surg* 64:147, 1998.

79. Makowiec F, Jehle EC, Starlinger M: Clinical course of perianal fistulas in Crohn's disease. *Gut* 37:696, 1995.

80. Hull TL, Fazio VW: Surgical approaches to low anovaginal fistula in Crohn's disease. *Am J Surg* 173:95, 1997.

Appendix

Matthew I. Goldblatt | Gordon L. Telford | James R. Wallace

ACUTE APPENDICITIS

Acute appendicitis is one of the most common causes of an abdominal emergency and accounts for approximately 1% of all surgical operations.[1] Although rare in infants, appendicitis becomes increasingly common throughout childhood and reaches its maximal incidence between the ages of 10 and 30 years. After 30 years of age, the incidence declines, but appendicitis can occur in individuals of any age. Among teenagers and young adults, the male-to-female ratio is about 3:2. After age 25 years, the ratio gradually declines until the sex ratio is equal by the mid-30s.

PATHOPHYSIOLOGY

The most commonly accepted theory of the pathogenesis of appendicitis is that it results from obstruction followed by infection.[2] The lumen of the appendix becomes obstructed by hyperplasia of submucosal lymphoid follicles, a fecalith, tumor, or other pathologic condition. Once the lumen of the appendix is obstructed, the sequence of events leading to acute appendicitis is probably as follows: Mucus accumulates within the lumen of the appendix, and pressure within the organ increases. Virulent bacteria convert the accumulated mucus into pus. Continued secretion combined with the relative inelasticity of the serosa leads to a further rise in pressure within the lumen. This results in obstruction of the lymphatic drainage, leading to edema of the appendix, diapedesis of bacteria, and the appearance of mucosal ulcers. At this stage, the disease is still localized to the appendix; therefore, the pain perceived by the patient is visceral and is localized to the epigastrium or periumbilical area.

Continued secretion into the lumen and increasing edema bring about a further rise in intraluminal and tissue pressure, resulting in venous obstruction and ischemia of the appendix. Bacteria spread into and through the wall of the appendix, and acute suppurative appendicitis ensues. Somatic pain occurs when the inflamed serosa of the appendix comes in contact with the parietal peritoneum and results in the classic shift of pain to the right lower quadrant.

As this pathologic process continues, venous and arterial thromboses occur in the wall of the appendix, resulting in gangrenous appendicitis. At this stage, small infarcts occur, permitting escape of bacteria and contamination of the peritoneal cavity. The final stage in the progression of acute appendicitis is perforation through a gangrenous infarct and the spilling of accumulated pus. Perforating appendicitis is now present, and morbidity and mortality increase.

SYMPTOMS

The symptomatic history in acute appendicitis may vary, but cardinal symptoms are usually present.[1,3] The history usually begins with abdominal pain often localized to the epigastrium or the periumbilical area, followed by anorexia and nausea. Vomiting, if it occurs, appears next. After a variable period, usually about 8 hours, the pain shifts to the right side and usually into the right lower quadrant. At the time of presentation, the duration of pain is less than 24 hours in 75% of patients.

Pain

The typical pain of acute appendicitis initially consists of diffuse, central, minimally severe visceral pain, which is followed by somatic pain that is more severe and usually well localized to the right lower quadrant. Failure to follow the classic visceral-somatic sequence is common in acute appendicitis, occurring in up to 45% of patients who are proved subsequently to have appendicitis. Atypical pain may be somatic and localized to the right lower quadrant from its initiation. Conversely, the pain may remain diffuse and may never become localized. In older patients, atypical pain patterns occur more frequently.

Patients with high retrocecal appendicitis may present with only diffuse pain in the right flank. Similarly, patients in whom the entire appendix is within the true pelvis may never experience somatic pain and, instead, may have tenesmus and vague discomfort in the suprapubic area.

Anorexia, Nausea, and Vomiting

Anorexia and nausea are present in almost all patients with acute appendicitis, but vomiting occurs in less than 50% of patients. The presence or absence of vomiting is not a criterion for the diagnosis of appendicitis. When vomiting does occur, it is usually not persistent, and most patients vomit only once or twice. If vomiting occurs, it occurs *after* the onset of pain with such regularity that if it precedes pain, the diagnosis of appendicitis should be questioned.

Constipation and Diarrhea

A history of the recent onset of constipation or diarrhea is not helpful in the diagnosis of appendicitis. A greater percentage of patients with appendicitis complain of constipation, but some give a history that defecation relieves the pain.

PHYSICAL EXAMINATION

Typical physical signs of acute appendicitis include localized tenderness in the right lower quadrant, muscle guarding, and rebound tenderness. Cutaneous hyperesthesia, right-sided pelvic tenderness on rectal examination, and the presence of a psoas or obturator sign occur less frequently and tend to be highly dependent on the examiner. Although often the temperature is normal, fever up to 38° C or higher may occur. In the usual case of acute, nonperforated appendicitis, higher fever occurs infrequently.

Tenderness and Muscle Guarding

On routine abdominal examination, an area of maximal tenderness often is elicited in the area of McBurney point, which is located two-thirds of the distance along a line from the umbilicus to the right anterior superior iliac spine. If the appendix is in a high retrocecal position or is entirely within the true pelvis, point tenderness and muscle rigidity might not be elicited. In high retrocecal appendicitis, tenderness may occur over a large area, and there may be no signs of muscle rigidity. In pelvic appendicitis, neither tenderness nor muscle guarding may be present. Both signs are often lacking or only minimally expressed in the aged population.

Signs of peritoneal inflammation or irritation in the right lower quadrant are also helpful in the diagnosis of acute appendicitis and can be demonstrated by many methods. Asking the patient to cough or bounce on the heels elicits this type of pain in 85% of patients. Rebound tenderness is elicited by the sudden release of abdominal palpation pressure. Rovsing sign—pain elicited in the right lower quadrant with palpation pressure in the left lower quadrant—is a sign of acute appendicitis. Muscle guarding, manifested as resistance to palpation, increases as the severity of inflammation of the parietal peritoneum increases. Initially, there is only voluntary guarding, but this is replaced by reflex involuntary rigidity.

Abdominal Mass

As the disease process progresses, it may be possible to palpate a tender mass in the right lower quadrant. Although the mass may be caused by an abscess, it can also result from adherence of the omentum and loops of intestine to an inflamed appendix. When appendicitis becomes advanced enough that there is a large, inflamed mass and the anterior abdominal wall is involved, the patient often avoids sudden movements that can cause pain.

Psoas Sign

The right hip is often kept in slight flexion to keep the iliopsoas muscle relaxed. Stretching the muscle by extension of the hip or further flexion against resistance can initiate a positive psoas sign, indicating irritation of the muscle by an inflamed appendix. A psoas sign is seldom seen in early appendicitis and can be elicited in patients without any pathologic condition (false positive).

Rectal Examination

Rectal examination, although essential in all patients with suspected appendicitis, is helpful in only a few of them. In patients with an uncomplicated appendicitis, the finger of the examiner cannot reach high enough to elicit pain on rectal examination.

If the appendix ruptures, the physical examination will change. If the infection is contained, a tender mass will often develop in the right lower quadrant, and the area of tenderness will now encompass the entire right lower quadrant. Involuntary guarding becomes evident and rebound tenderness more marked. The patient's temperature will be more like that seen with abscess formation and may rise to 39° C with a corresponding tachycardia.

If appendiceal rupture fails to localize, signs and symptoms of diffuse peritonitis will develop. Tenderness and guarding become generalized, the temperature remains higher than 38° C with spikes to 40° C, and the pulse rate increases to more than 100 beats/min.

LABORATORY TESTS

In the early diagnosis of acute appendicitis, laboratory tests are of little value. Up to one-third of patients, particularly older patients,[4] have a normal total leukocyte count with acute appendicitis,[1,5] and more than half have, at most, a mild elevation. Even when the total leukocyte count and the differential white blood cell (WBC) count are abnormal, the degree of abnormality does not correlate well with the degree of appendiceal inflammation.[6] Even when the total WBC count is normal, the differential WBC count often reveals a shift to the left with an increase in the percentage of polymorphonuclear neutrophils.[5] Less than 4% of patients with appendicitis have both a normal total WBC count and a normal differential count. Patients with a normal WBC count and normal C-reactive protein rarely have appendicitis.[7] The most important fact to remember when considering the diagnosis of appendicitis is that the clinical findings take precedence over the WBC count when they are at variance.

Urinalysis is helpful in the differential diagnosis of patients with lower abdominal pain only when it reveals significant numbers of red blood cells (RBCs), WBCs, or bacteria. Minimal numbers of RBCs, WBCs, and bacteria are seen in normal patients as well as in patients with appendicitis.

Patients with advanced appendicitis and abscess formation or generalized peritonitis may have abnormalities in liver function tests that mimic obstructive jaundice, biliary stasis, or other primary liver problems.

RADIOGRAPHIC EXAMINATION

With rare exceptions, plain roentgenologic examination of the abdomen is of little help in the differential diagnosis of acute appendicitis. The exceptions are when a fecalith is demonstrated (usually in the right lower quadrant) and when other diagnoses such as acute cholecystitis, perforating duodenal ulcer, perforating colon cancer, acute diverticulitis, and pyelonephritis are being excluded.

It is not unusual to see cecal distention or a sentinel loop of distended small intestine in the right lower quadrant in patients with acute appendicitis. In late appendicitis with perforation and abscess formation, a mass can often be demonstrated that is extrinsic to the cecum. There may be scoliosis to the right, lack of the right psoas shadow, lack of small bowel gas in the right lower quadrant with abundant gas elsewhere in the small bowel, and signs of edema of the abdominal wall. With late appendicitis and generalized peritonitis, there is an ileus pattern with generalized gas throughout the small and large intestine.

Barium enema (BE) examination was recommended in the past in young women in whom the diagnosis was still in question after hours of observation and in patients with a debilitating systemic disease, such as leukemia, in whom the operative risk is markedly increased.[8] The findings of significance on BE include lack of filling or partial filling of the appendix and an extrinsic pressure defect on the cecum (the "reverse 3" sign).[9] Computed tomography (CT) and ultrasonography (US) are now preferred to BE in these circumstances.

As demonstrated in many studies, an experienced radiologist is able to diagnose acute appendicitis using US with an accuracy greater than 90%.[10-12] Appendicitis is diagnosed if the maximal cross-sectional diameter of appendix exceeds 6 mm, if it is noncompressible, if an appendolith is present, or if a complex mass is demonstrated.[13] There are other criteria that are not universally agreed on, such as rigidity and nonmobility. Nonvisualization of the appendix is not a criterion for appendicitis. US can also be helpful in the diagnosis of perforated appendicitis with abscess formation. Studies that compared US and CT have demonstrated CT to be more accurate than US in the diagnosis of appendicitis in clinically equivocal cases.[3] Therefore, US should be used only when an experienced radiologist with an interest in appendicitis is available.

Although more expensive, CT has also been demonstrated to be of benefit in the diagnosis of acute appendicitis and has an accuracy greater than 94%.[14,15] The cost can be reduced with no significant loss in diagnostic accuracy by performing a limited, unenhanced CT.[16] Appendicitis is diagnosed when the appendix is thickened with a diameter greater than 6 mm; a phlegmon, fluid, or abscess is present; there is an appendolith; and there are inflammatory changes in the periappendiceal fat (streaking and poorly defined increased attenuation).[14,15] The presence of pericecal inflammation without the presence of an inflamed appendix or an appendolith without the presence of periappendiceal inflammation are both insufficient to diagnose acute appendicitis.

An important consideration for CT in the diagnosis of acute appendicitis is when to use it. In one study, CT scanning excluded appendicitis in almost half of the patients in the study and identified an alternative diagnosis in 51% of those patients. The authors stated that the routine use of CT in patients with suspected appendicitis avoids unnecessary appendectomies and unnecessary delays before surgical treatment and saves money.[17] In another institution, the routine use of CT scanning for the evaluation of suspected appendicitis has led to a decrease in the negative appendectomy rate from 23% to 1.7%.[18] CT is not indicated in patients with an unequivocal diagnosis of appendicitis or in patients with a low risk of the diagnosis. In menstruating women and any patient with an equivocal diagnosis, a CT scan is probably indicated. An added benefit of the use of CT is that an identified abscess can be percutaneously drained during the same procedure.[19]

ACUTE APPENDICITIS IN INFANTS AND YOUNG CHILDREN

The diagnosis of acute appendicitis is difficult in infants and young children for many reasons. The patient is unable to give an accurate history, and although appendicitis is infrequent, acute nonspecific abdominal pain is common in infants and children. Because of such factors, the diagnosis and treatment are often delayed, and complications develop.[20,21]

The clinical presentation of appendicitis in children can be quite similar to nonspecific gastroenteritis; thus, the suspicion of appendicitis often is not entertained until the appendix has ruptured and the child is obviously ill.[22] Two-thirds of young children with appendicitis have had symptoms for more than 3 days before appendectomy.[21] Because children often cannot give an accurate history of their pain, the physical examination and other aspects of the history must be relied on to make the diagnosis. Vomiting, fever, irritability, flexing of the thighs, and diarrhea are likely early complaints. Abdominal distention is the most consistent physical finding. Among the most common atypical findings in children with appendicitis are absence of fever, absence of Rovsing sign, normal or increased bowel sounds, and absence of rebound pain.[18] As in adults, the total leukocyte count is not a reliable test.

The incidence of perforation in infants younger than 1 year of age is almost 100%, and although it decreases with age, it is still 50% at 5 years of age. The mortality rate in this age group remains as high as 5%. In one series, nearly 40% of children with complicated appendicitis had been seen previously by a physician who failed to make the diagnosis of appendicitis.[21]

APPENDICITIS IN YOUNG WOMEN

Although the overall incidence of negative laparotomy in patients suspected of having appendicitis is as high as 20%, the incidence in women younger than 30 years of age is as high as 45%. Pain associated with ovulation; diseases of the ovaries, fallopian tubes, and uterus; and urinary tract infections (cystitis) account for most of the misdiagnoses. If a young woman has atypical pain, no muscular guarding in the right lower quadrant, and no fever, leukocytosis, or leftward shift in the differential WBC count, it is best to observe the patient with frequent reexaminations. If after several hours, the patient's signs and symptoms remain stable, it is appropriate to perform a CT scan.

APPENDICITIS DURING PREGNANCY

The risk of appendicitis during pregnancy is the same as it is in nonpregnant women of the same age; the incidence is 1 in 2000 pregnancies. Appendicitis occurs more frequently during the first two trimesters, and during this period the symptoms of appendicitis are similar to those seen in nonpregnant women.[23] Surgery should be performed during pregnancy when appendicitis is suspected, just as it would be in a nonpregnant woman. As in the nonpregnant patient, the effects of a laparotomy that produces no findings are minor, whereas the effects of ruptured appendicitis can be catastrophic. Recent studies indicate that there is no increase in morbidity and mortality with laparoscopic appendectomy versus open appendectomy for the patient or the fetus.[24]

During the third trimester of pregnancy, the cecum and appendix are displaced laterally and are rotated by the enlarged uterus. This results in localization of pain either more cephalad or laterally in the flank, leading to delay in diagnosis and an increased incidence of perforation. Factors such as displacement of the omentum by the uterus also impair localization of the inflamed appendix and result in diffuse peritonitis. In cases of uncomplicated appendicitis, the prognosis for the infant following appendectomy is directly related to the infant's birth weight. If peritonitis and sepsis ensue, infant mortality increases because of prematurity and the effects of sepsis.

The selection of imaging studies for the workup of suspected appendicitis during pregnancy is often controversial. The use of ionizing radiation on a developing fetus should always be avoided. Ultrasound and magnetic resonance imaging (MRI) have been shown to be both sensitive and specific in evaluating patients; however, their lack of immediate availability in most hospitals may delay diagnosis. The effects of radiation on the fetus are significantly decreased after the first trimester.[23]

Acute appendicitis can be confused with pyelitis and torsion of an ovarian cyst. However, death from appendicitis during pregnancy is mainly caused by a delay in diagnosis. In the final analysis, early appendectomy is the appropriate therapy in suspected appendicitis during all stages of pregnancy.[23]

APPENDICITIS IN THE ELDERLY POPULATION

Appendicitis has a much greater mortality rate among elderly persons when compared with young adults. The increased risk of mortality appears to result from both delay in seeking medical care and delay in making the diagnosis.[25] The presence of other diseases associated with aging contributes to mortality, but the major reason for the increased mortality of appendicitis in the aged is delay in treatment. Classic symptoms are present in elderly persons but are often less pronounced. Right lower quadrant pain localizes later and may be milder in elderly persons. On initial physical examination, the findings are often minimal, although right lower quadrant tenderness will eventually be present in most patients.[26]

Approximately 25% of elderly patients will have a ruptured appendix at the time of operation. Although other factors play a role, delay in seeking care and in making the diagnosis are the major reasons for perforation. Routine CT scanning appears to be reducing the delay in diagnosis often associated with appendicitis in the elderly.[26] It is imperative, therefore, that once the diagnosis of acute appendicitis is made, an urgent operation must be advised.

DIFFERENTIAL DIAGNOSIS

The differential diagnosis of abdominal pain is a stimulating exercise. When the classic symptoms of appendicitis are present, the diagnosis of appendicitis is usually easily made and is seldom missed. When the diagnosis is not obvious, knowledge of the differential diagnosis becomes important. Most of the entities in the differential diagnosis of appendicitis also require operative therapy or are usually not made worse by an exploratory laparotomy. Therefore, it is essential that one eliminate those diseases that do not require operative therapy and can be made worse by operation, such as pancreatitis, myocardial infarction, and basilar pneumonia.

The diseases in young children that are most frequently mistaken for acute appendicitis are gastroenteritis, mesenteric lymphadenitis, Meckel diverticulum, pyelitis, small intestinal intussusception, enteric duplication, and basilar pneumonia. In mesenteric lymphadenitis, an upper respiratory tract infection is often present or has recently subsided. Acute gastroenteritis is usually associated with crampy abdominal pain and watery diarrhea. Intestinal intussusception occurs most frequently in children younger than 2 years of age, an age at which appendicitis is uncommon. With intussusception, a sausage-shaped mass is frequently palpable in the right lower quadrant. The preferred diagnostic procedure is a gentle BE, which, in addition to making the diagnosis, usually reduces the intussusception.

In teenagers and young adults, the differential diagnosis is different in men and women. In young women, the differential diagnosis includes ruptured ectopic pregnancy, mittelschmerz, endometriosis, and salpingitis.[27] Chronic constipation also needs to be considered in young women. The symptoms that accompany the acute onset of regional enteritis can mimic acute appendicitis, but a history of cramps and diarrhea and the lack of an appropriate history for appendicitis are hints that the diagnosis is regional enteritis.

In young men, the potential list of differential diagnoses is smaller and includes the acute onset of regional enteritis, right-sided renal or ureteral calculus, torsion of the testes, and acute epididymitis.

In older patients, the differential diagnosis of acute appendicitis includes diverticulitis, a perforated peptic ulcer, acute cholecystitis, acute pancreatitis, intestinal obstruction, perforated cecal carcinoma, mesenteric vascular occlusion, rupturing aortic aneurysm, and the disease entities already mentioned for young adults.

TREATMENT

Preoperative Preparation

It is not necessary to rush a patient with a presumed diagnosis of acute appendicitis directly to the operating room. Retrospective reviews of operative delays of more than 12 hours do not negatively effect patient outcomes.[28] All patients, especially those with a presumed diagnosis of peritonitis, should be adequately prepared before being taken to the operating room. Selected patients with a palpable right lower quadrant mass, periappendiceal phlegmon, or abscess on imaging may be managed without operation.[29]

Intravenous fluid replacement should be initiated and the patient resuscitated as rapidly as possible, especially when peritonitis is suspected. Once the patient has a good urinary output, it can be assumed that resuscitation is complete. Nasogastric suction is especially helpful in patients with peritonitis and profound ileus. If the patient's body temperature is higher than 39° C, appropriate measures should be taken to reduce fever before beginning an operation.

A broad-spectrum antibiotic, such as cefoxitin or ertapenem, should be administered preoperatively to help control sepsis and to reduce the incidence of postoperative wound infections. If, at the time of operation, the patient has early appendicitis, antibiotic administration should be stopped after one postoperative dose. Antibiotics should be continued as clinically indicated in patients who have gangrenous or ruptured appendicitis with localized or generalized peritonitis.

Examination Under Anesthesia

After the induction of anesthesia, the patient's abdomen should be systematically palpated. Such an examination may, on occasion, demonstrate another pathologic condition to be the cause of the patient's symptoms, such as acute cholecystitis. It also may be possible to palpate an appendiceal mass that will confirm the suspected diagnosis.

Uncomplicated Appendicitis Without a Palpable Mass

In this circumstance, when the diagnosis of acute appendicitis has been made and there is no reason to suspect that the appendix has ruptured, an appendectomy should be performed. One recommended incision for a routine appendectomy is a transverse one (i.e., Rockey-Davis, Fowler–Weir Mitchell incisions). The incision is made in a transverse direction, 1 to 3 cm below the umbilicus, and is centered on the midclavicular line. The length of the incision should be approximately 1 cm longer than the breadth of the surgeon's hand. The aponeurosis and muscles of the abdominal wall are split or incised in the direction of their fibers (Figure 162-1). Exposure of the appendix through this incision is better when compared with that obtained through the classic McBurney incision, particularly in patients with a retrocecal appendix and in those who are obese.

The other recommended incision, the gridiron, or muscle-splitting one (McBurney incision), can be used. This is the most widely used incision in uncomplicated appendicitis. The skin incision is made through a point one-third of the way along a line from the anterosuperior spine of the ileum to the umbilicus. The incision is made obliquely, beginning inferiorly and medially, and extending laterally and superiorly. It should be 8 to 10 cm in length, with its most medial extent being the lateral edge of the rectus muscle. The aponeurosis and muscles of the abdominal wall are split or incised in the direction of their fibers in such a manner that the entire skin incision can be used for exposure. After entering the peritoneum, the appendix is found as described for the transverse incision. The exposure through a McBurney incision, especially for a retrocecal appendix, can be awkward unless the appendix lies immediately below the incision. If necessary, the incision can be extended medially, partially transecting the rectus sheath, but this maneuver is usually helpful only in a pelvic appendicitis.

If there is doubt about the diagnosis of acute appendicitis and an exploratory laparotomy is indicated, a vertical midline incision is more appropriate. An appendectomy can be performed with little difficulty through such an incision.

After the peritoneum is opened, the appendix is identified by following the anterior cecal taenia to the base of the appendix. The inflamed appendix is coaxed into the wound by gentle traction and the transection of adhesions, if present. If the appendix is retrocecal or retroperitoneal, or if the local inflammation and edema are intense, exposure is improved by dividing the lateral peritoneal reflection of the cecum. At the end of this maneuver, the cecum should lie within the wound and the appendix should be at the level of the anterior abdominal wall so that continuing vigorous retraction is unnecessary while removing the appendix (see Figure 162-1).

If the appendix is not adherent, its base can be identified easily because the entire appendix often pops into the operative field. If the appendix is adherent, however, its base may be difficult to recognize. Aids in recognition include the following:
1. All three taeniae lead to and end at the base of the appendix.
2. The ileocecal junction can usually be identified, just below which is the base of the appendix.

If the appendix does not come into the wound but the base has been identified, an Allis clamp can be placed around but not on the appendix for traction. An effort is made to deliver the tip of the appendix into the operative field. If the appendix is not adherent to surrounding tissues, traction on the Allis clamp is usually successful in delivering the appendix.

Once the appendix has been freed up, the mesoappendix is transected beginning at its free border, taking small bites of the mesoappendix between pairs of hemostats placed approximately 1 cm from and parallel to the appendix. This process should be repeated until the base of the appendix is reached. If exposure of a long, adherent appendix is difficult, the mesoappendix can be transected in a retrograde manner beginning at the base of the appendix.

There are three ways to handle the appendiceal stump: simple ligation, inversion, and a combination of ligation and inversion. Either simple ligation or inversion is acceptable and has a comparable incidence of complications. The combination of ligation and inversion is not recommended, because it does not reduce the risk of septic complications, but it does create conditions conducive to the development of an intramural abscess or mucocele. Also, the ligated and inverted appendiceal stump may later appear on a subsequent BE as a cecal "tumor" and be a source of diagnostic difficulties.[30]

Simple ligature of the appendiceal stump is accomplished by crushing the appendix at its base with a hemostat, then moving the hemostat and replacing it on the appendix just distal to the crushed line. A ligature of monofilament suture is placed in the groove caused by the crushing clamp and is tied tightly (Figure 162-2). The appendix is transected just proximal to the hemostat and removed. Inversion of an unligated stump using a Z-stitch

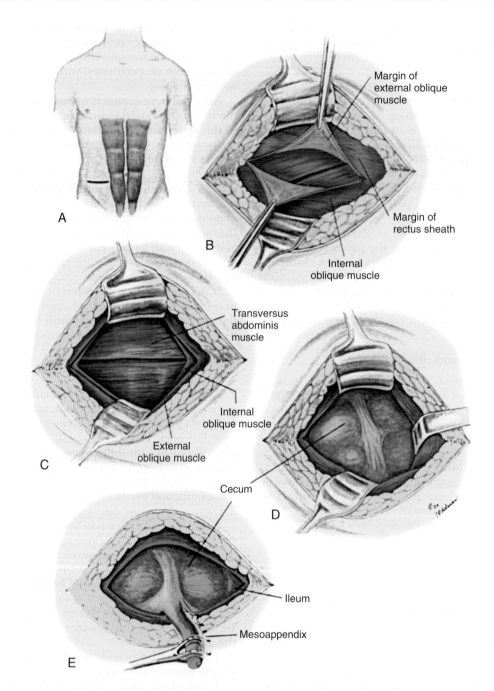

FIGURE 162-1 Steps in exposing the appendix for an appendectomy through a transverse incision. **A,** Placement of the skin incision. **B** and **C,** External and internal oblique and transversus abdominis muscles are divided in the direction of their fibers. **D,** After incision of the peritoneum, the cecum is exposed and the appendix is located by following the anterior cecal taenia inferiorly. **E,** The cecum is mobilized into the wound through incision of its lateral peritoneal reflections. (From Moody FG, Carey L, Jones RS, et al: *Surgical treatment of digestive diseases.* Chicago, 1986, Year Book.)

(Figure 162-3), rather than the more conventional purse-string suture, is preferred. The upper level of the Z-stitch is placed as a Lembert suture in the cecum, just distal to the base of the appendix. The suture is then brought around the base of the appendix and continued as a second Lembert suture beneath the base of the appendix. The appendix is then transected between clamps, the stump is inverted into the cecum, the proximal clamp is removed, and the ends of the Z-stitch are tied over the stump of the appendix. The appendiceal stump is not ligated. If the appendiceal stump is unsuitable for inversion because of edema, it should simply be ligated and not inverted.

Laparoscopic Appendectomy

Laparoscopic and minimal access surgery continues to expand in the field of general surgery, and diagnostic laparoscopy and laparoscopic appendectomy have become

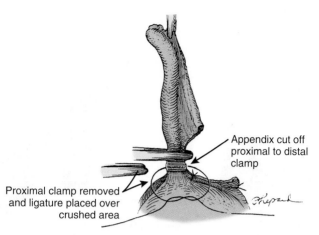

Appendix cut off
proximal to distal
clamp

Proximal clamp removed
and ligature placed over
crushed area

FIGURE 162-2 Ligation of the stump of the appendix in the groove formed by a crushing clamp. (From Partipilo AV: *Surgical technique and principles of operative surgery*, ed 4. Philadelphia, 1949, Lea & Febiger.)

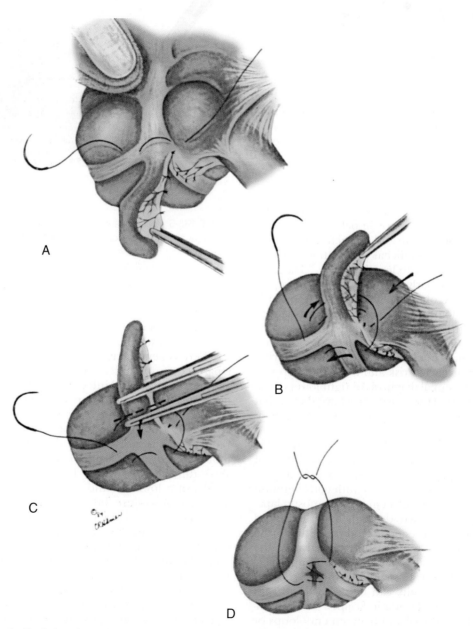

FIGURE 162-3 Use of a Z-stitch to invert the unligated appendiceal stump. **A,** Two bites of the suture are placed in the cecum 1 cm distal to the base of the appendix. **B,** The suture is then brought around the appendix medially and two additional bites are placed beneath the base of the appendix. **C,** The appendix is then transected. **D,** The stump of the appendix is inverted into the cecum and the clamp is removed as the suture is tightened. (From Adams JT: Z-stitch suture for inversion of the appendiceal stump. *Surg Gynecol Obstet* 127:1321, 1968.)

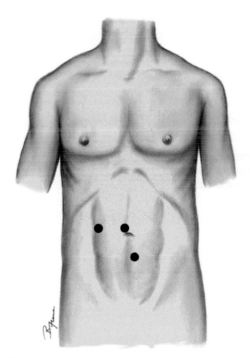

FIGURE 162-4 Trocar placement for laparoscopic appendectomy. Additional trocars can be placed in the right upper or left lower quadrants. (From Frantzides CT: *Laparoscopic and thoracoscopic surgery.* St Louis, 1994, Mosby Year Book, p 66.)

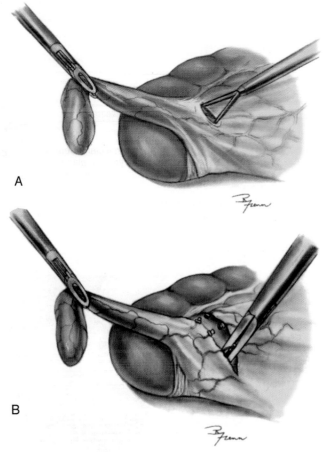

FIGURE 162-5 Technique for laparoscopic appendectomy. **A,** The appendix is grasped and retracted toward the pelvis, thus exposing the mesoappendix. **B,** The mesoappendix is divided using individually placed clips. (From Frantzides CT: *Laparoscopic and thoracoscopic surgery.* St Louis, 1994, Mosby Year Book, p 67.)

accepted procedures in many surgeons' practices. The early use of diagnostic laparoscopy in patients with right lower quadrant abdominal pain and suspected appendicitis reduces the risk of appendiceal perforation and the negative appendectomy rate to less than 10%.[31] Diagnostic laparoscopy is particularly useful in women of reproductive age and in the obese. In the former, frequently confounding gynecologic disorders can be well visualized to provide the diagnosis, and in the latter, laparoscopy can eliminate the morbidity risks of a large incision. Performing an appendectomy with a normal-appearing appendix has a relatively low risk and will remove appendicitis from the differential diagnosis of right lower quadrant pain in the future. However studies have shown that it is safe to not proceed with appendectomy if the appendix appears normal.[32,33]

Conversion of diagnostic laparoscopy to therapeutic laparoscopy is easily accomplished by the addition of other ports. Trocar placement for laparoscopic appendectomy is a matter of surgeon choice with consideration of the triangle rule for port placement. Diagnostic laparoscopy is usually performed through a periumbilical port, with a 10/11-mm port added midway between the umbilicus and pubis and a 5-mm port placed over the appendix or the right midlateral abdomen if appendectomy is performed (Figure 162-4). Once the diagnosis is confirmed, the mesoappendix can be taken down with either hemoclips or the Harmonic Scalpel. The appendix is amputated from the cecum between endoloops or with an endo-GIA stapler (Figure 162-5). The appendix can then be removed from the abdomen with a specimen pouch or withdrawn into the 10/11-mm port. Care

should be taken to prevent contact of the appendix or its contents with the wound edges.

There is general agreement that patients undergoing laparoscopic appendectomy have less postoperative pain, a lower rate of wound infection, a lower overall complication rate, a more rapid return to diet, a shorter hospital stay, a longer operative time, and more equipment charges in the operating room.[34-37] In contrast, a more rapid return to work and a lower complication rate are more controversial claims because prospective studies show differing results.[38,39] Laparoscopic appendectomy results in a lower wound infection rate compared with an open procedure but has a higher intraabdominal abscess rate if the appendix is perforated.[40] Relative contraindications to laparoscopic appendectomy include previous abdominal surgery precluding safe trocar placement, uncontrolled coagulopathy, and significant portal hypertension.

Laparoscopic appendectomy appears to be safe and efficacious. It provides a rapid diagnosis and a significant reduction in negative appendectomy rates in females of childbearing age with suspected appendicitis. Minimal access surgery reduces the morbidity risk in obese patients who require an appendectomy.

Perforated or Gangrenous Appendicitis With a Periappendiceal Mass

When a mass is detected by examination under anesthesia, a transverse incision is made over the most prominent portion of the mass. The muscles and aponeuroses are split along their lines of cleavage in gridiron fashion. After entering the peritoneal cavity, the wound should be packed immediately to prevent contamination of the abdominal cavity. As mentioned earlier, the mass may be made up of omentum and loops of small intestine adherent to the inflamed appendix, and an abscess may not be present. If feasible, an appendectomy is then performed; usually it will not be possible to invert the stump, so simple ligation is preferred.

It is not necessary to place a subfascial drain in a patient with a gangrenous appendix and minimal or no periappendiceal pus. If there is a periappendiceal abscess and the tissues are fixed so as to create a dead space, the cavity should be drained with one or more closed-suction drains brought out through a separate stab incision.

Before fascial closure, the right iliac fossa and the wound should be liberally irrigated. Muscles and aponeuroses should be closed with interrupted nonabsorbable sutures. The skin should be left open, to be closed with adhesive paper tapes on the fifth or sixth postoperative day. Parenteral antibiotics should be continued for 5 days after operation or until clinical signs indicate no infection.

Perforated Appendicitis With Localized Abscess Formation

If, at the time of initial physical examination, a well-localized periappendiceal mass is found and the patient's symptoms are improving, it is acceptable in healthy adults to initiate parenteral antibiotic treatment and to follow the patient expectantly.[41] This form of therapy is not appropriate in children, pregnant women, or elderly patients. In these groups, an emergency operation is indicated. In two-thirds of patients, expectant treatment of an appendiceal mass succeeds, and an interval appendectomy can be performed at a later date or can be avoided altogether.[29,41] In one-third of patients, symptoms do not subside and an emergency CT scan should be performed. If an abscess is identified on CT scan, an attempt should be made to drain the abscess percutaneously under CT or US guidance.[19] If not successful, the abscess should be drained surgically.

The skin incision for drainage of a periappendiceal abscess is made just medial to the crest of the ilium at the level of the abscess. Using a muscle-splitting technique, the lateral edge of the peritoneum is exposed and pushed medially so that the abscess is approached from its lateral aspect. Once the abscess is entered, a finger should be used to break up the loculations. If the appendix can be freed up without breaking down adhesions, an appendectomy should be performed. If an appendectomy is not performed, an interval appendectomy can be done 3 to 6 months after drainage from the abscess has ceased and the wound has completely healed.

After the wound has been thoroughly irrigated with normal saline, a closed-suction drain should be inserted into the abscess cavity and brought out through a separate stab wound in the flank. The muscles and aponeuroses are closed with interrupted nonabsorbable sutures, and the skin and subcutaneous tissues are packed open with saline-soaked gauze. The drain should be left in place until it is draining less than 50 mL/day and then advanced progressively until removed.

Systemic antibiotics should be continued for 5 days postoperatively or until signs of sepsis have cleared. A daily rectal examination should be done to detect pelvic abscess. The patient may be discharged from the hospital when there is no fever 48 hours after the discontinuation of antibiotic therapy.

Perforated Appendicitis With Diffuse Peritonitis

The major cause of mortality from appendicitis is generalized peritonitis. Therefore, immediate exploration is indicated in a patient with a diagnosis of acute appendicitis in whom the physical findings are consistent with diffuse peritonitis. If a perforated appendix and diffuse peritonitis are documented at operation, an appendectomy should be performed and the abdomen thoroughly irrigated. The use of drains in diffuse peritonitis is not recommended unless there are localized abscesses requiring drainage.[42] The wound and postoperative care should be handled as described in a patient with a periappendiceal abscess.

Normal Appendix When Appendicitis Is Suspected

If a patient undergoes exploratory laparotomy (especially through a right lower quadrant incision) for suspected acute appendicitis, and a normal appendix is subsequently found, a careful search for another pathologic condition should be made and an appendectomy performed. The abdomen should not be closed until the cause of the symptoms has been identified and treated or the surgeon is sure that no lesion requiring treatment is present. The normal appendix is *removed* to obviate diagnostic confusion in the future.

If the history and physical examination were appropriate for the diagnosis of acute appendicitis, it is not an error to perform an exploratory laparotomy and remove what appears to be a normal appendix. A policy of early surgical intervention on the basis of clinical suspicion has been demonstrated overall to reduce both the morbidity and mortality of acute appendicitis.

In the past, a negative appendectomy rate of 20% was acceptable.[43] Studies have suggested that rates of 10% to 15% and lower are feasible without an unacceptably high rate of perforated appendix.[44-46]

Complications

Postoperative complications occur in 5% of patients with an unperforated appendix but in more than 30% of patients with a gangrenous or perforated appendix. The most frequent complications after appendectomy are wound infection, intraabdominal abscess, fecal fistula, pylephlebitis, and intestinal obstruction.

Subcutaneous tissue infection is the most common complication after appendectomy. The organisms most frequently cultured are anaerobic *Bacteroides* species and the aerobes *Klebsiella, Enterobacter,* and *Escherichia coli.*[47] When early signs of wound infection (undue pain and edema) are present, the skin and subcutaneous tissue should be opened. The wound should be packed with saline-soaked gauze and reclosed with Steri-Strips in 4 to 5 days.

Pelvic, subphrenic, or other intraabdominal abscesses occur in up to 20% of patients with a gangrenous or perforated appendicitis. They are accompanied by recurrent fever, malaise, and anorexia of insidious onset. CT scanning is of great help in making the diagnosis of intraabdominal abscess. When an abscess is diagnosed, it should be drained either operatively or percutaneously.

Some fecal fistulas close spontaneously, provided that there is no anatomic reason for the fistula remaining open. Those that do not close spontaneously obviously require operation. Pylephlebitis, or portal pyemia, is characterized by jaundice, chills, and high fever. It is a serious illness that frequently leads to multiple liver abscesses. The infecting organism is usually *E. coli*. This complication has become rare with the routine use of antibiotics in complicated appendicitis. Although not frequent, true mechanical bowel obstruction may occur as a complication of acute appendicitis. As with any other mechanical small bowel obstruction, operative therapy is indicated.

CHRONIC AND RECURRENT APPENDICITIS

There are occasional patients who have had one or more attacks of what appears to be acute appendicitis. Between attacks, these patients are free of symptoms and the physical examination is normal. In such patients, if a fecalith is present on abdominal radiograph, if a BE demonstrates no filling of the appendix, or if repeated examinations during an attack provide evidence of recurrent appendicitis, elective appendectomy should be undertaken.[48] To sustain a diagnosis of chronic appendicitis, the resected appendix must demonstrate fibrosis in the appendiceal wall, partial to complete obstruction of the lumen, evidence of old mucosal ulceration and scarring, and infiltration of the wall of the appendix with chronic inflammatory cells.

MUCINOUS CYSTADENOMA AND CYSTADENOCARCINOMA

Distention of the lumen of the appendix by the mucus secreted by proliferating tumor cells can occur with both mucinous cystadenoma and cystadenocarcinoma. Because it is difficult to distinguish between benign and malignant tumors, a right hemicolectomy should be performed, since appendectomy is not curative in the usual circumstance. When there are numerous peritoneal implants of a mucinous-like substance, a diagnosis of pseudomyxoma peritonei is appropriate. Within these gelatinous masses are nests of tumor cells attached to the peritoneum.

TUMORS OF THE APPENDIX

Neoplasms of the appendix are rare. The two most frequently observed are carcinoid tumor and adenocarcinoma. The appendix is the most common site of carcinoid tumor, and carcinoid is the most common neoplasm of the appendix. It is found in approximately 0.1% of all surgically removed appendices. The only setting in which the diagnosis is suspected preoperatively is in the rare patient with symptoms of the carcinoid syndrome. This syndrome is characterized by flushing, diarrhea, and asthma-like symptoms. If a carcinoid tumor is in the mid- or distal appendix and is less than 1 cm in diameter, a simple appendectomy is adequate therapy. If the tumor is greater than 1 cm in diameter or is in the base of the appendix or if there is evidence of nodal metastases, a right hemicolectomy is recommended.[49]

Adenocarcinoma of the appendix may appear as either a well-differentiated mucus-producing tumor or as a poorly differentiated adenocarcinoma that appears as a solid mass. Both types of adenocarcinoma of the appendix have been reported to metastasize to regional lymph nodes, although malignant mucocele has been considered clinically to be less virulent. If an adenocarcinoma of the appendix is confined to the mucosa (carcinoma in situ), there is no difference in survival between simple appendectomy and appendectomy combined with right hemicolectomy. If the tumor is invasive, however, the prognosis is improved by right hemicolectomy, so the more extensive operation is recommended for most cases.[50]

REFERENCES

1. Lewis FR, Holcroft JW, Boey J, et al: Appendicitis: A critical review of diagnosis and treatment in 1,000 cases. *Arch Surg* 110:677, 1975.
2. Wangensteen OH, Dennis C: Experimental proof of obstructive origin of appendicitis in man. *Ann Surg* 110:629, 1939.
3. Pieper R, Kager L, Nasman P: Acute appendicitis: A clinical study of 1018 cases of emergency appendectomy. *Acta Chir Scand* 148:51, 1982.
4. Hubbell DS, Barton WK, Soloman OD: Leukocytosis in appendicitis in older patients. *JAMA* 175:139, 1961.
5. Bolton JP, Craven ER, Croft RJ, et al: An assessment of the value of the white cell count in the management of suspected acute appendicitis. *Br J Surg* 62:906, 1975.
6. Coleman C, Thompson JE, Bennion RS, et al: White blood cell count is a poor predictor of severity of disease in the diagnosis of appendicitis. *Am Surg* 68:983, 1998.
7. Sengupta A, Bax G, Paterson-Brown S: White cell count and C-reactive protein measurement in patients with possible appendicitis. *Ann R Coll Surg Engl* 91:113, 2009.
8. Rajagopalan AE, Mason JH, Kennedy M, et al: The value of the barium enema in the diagnosis of acute appendicitis. *Arch Surg* 112:531, 1977.
9. Jona JZ, Belin RP, Selke AC: Barium enema as a diagnostic aid in children with abdominal pain. *Surg Gynecol Obstet* 144:351, 1977.
10. Hayden CK, Kuchelmeister J, Lipscomb TS: Sonography of acute appendicitis in childhood: Perforation versus nonperforation. *J Ultrasound Med* 11:209, 1992.
11. Rioux M: Sonographic detection of the normal and abnormal appendix. *Am J Radiol* 158:773, 1992.
12. Sivit CJ, Newman KD, Boenning DA, et al: Appendicitis: Usefulness of US in diagnosis in a pediatric population. *Radiology* 185:549, 1992.
13. Yacoe ME, Jeffrey RB: Sonography of appendicitis and diverticulitis. *Radiol Clin North Am* 32:899, 1994.
14. Fuchs JR, Schlamberg JS, Shortsleeve MJ, et al: Impact of abdominal CT imaging on the management of appendicitis: An update. *J Surg Res* 106:131, 2002.
15. Holloway JA, Westerbuhr LM, Chain J, et al: Is appendiceal computed tomography in a community hospital useful? *Am J Surg* 186:682, 2003.

16. Malone AJ, Wolf CR, Malmed AS, et al: Diagnosis of acute appendicitis: Value of unenhanced CT. *Am J Radiol* 160:763, 1993.

17. Rao RM, Rhea JT, Novelline RA, et al: Effect of computed tomography of the appendix on treatment of patients and use of hospital resources. *N Engl J Med* 338:141, 1998.

18. Raja AS, Wright C, Sodickson AD, et al: Negative appendectomy rate in the era of CT: An 18-year perspective. *Radiology* 256:460, 2010.

19. Jamieson DH, Chait PG, Filler R: Interventional drainage of appendiceal abscesses in children. *Am J Radiol* 169:1619, 1997.

20. Becker T, Kharbanda A, Bachur R: Atypical clinical features of pediatric appendicitis. *Acad Emerg Med* 14:124, 2007.

21. Stone HH, Sanders SL, Martin JD: Perforated appendicitis in children. *Surgery* 69:673, 1971.

22. Graham JM, Pokorny WJ, Harberg FJ: Acute appendicitis in preschool age children. *Am J Surg* 139:247, 1980.

23. Gilo NB, Amini D, Landy HJ: Appendicitis and cholecystitis in pregnancy. *Clin Obstet Gynecol* 52:586, 2009.

24. Sadot E, Telem DA, Arora M, et al: Laparoscopy: A safe approach to appendicitis during pregnancy. *Surg Endosc* 24:383, 2010.

25. Owens BJ III, Hamit HF: Appendicitis in the elderly. *Ann Surg* 187:392, 1978.

26. Paranjape C, Dalia S, Pan J: Appendicitis in the elderly: A change in the laparoscopic era. *Surg Endosc* 21:777, 2007.

27. Bongard F, Landers DV, Lewis F: Differential diagnosis of appendicitis and pelvic inflammatory disease: A prospective analysis. *Am J Surg* 150:90, 1985.

28. Ingraham AM, Cohen ME, Bilimoria KY, et al: Effect of delay to operation on outcomes in adults with acute appendicitis. *Arch Surg* 145:886, 2010.

29. Andersson RE, Petzold MG: Nonsurgical treatment of appendiceal abscess or phlegmon: A systematic review and meta-analysis. *Ann Surg* 246:741, 2007.

30. Myllariemi H, Perttala Y, Peltokallio P: Tumor-like lesions of the cecum following inversion of the appendix. *Dig Dis* 19:547, 1974.

31. Karamanakos SN, Sdralis E, Panagiotopoulos S, et al: Laparoscopy in the emergency setting: A retrospective review of 540 patients with acute abdominal pain. *Surg Laparosc Endosc Percutan Tech* 20:119, 2010.

32. Barrat C, Catheline JM, Rizk N, et al: Does laparoscopy reduce the incidence of unnecessary appendicectomies? *Surg Laparosc Endosc* 9:27, 1999.

33. Moberg AC, Ahlberg G, Leijonmarck CE, et al: Diagnostic laparoscopy in 1043 patients with suspected acute appendicitis. *Eur J Surg* 164:833, 1998.

34. Guller U, Hervey S, Purves H, et al: Laparoscopic versus open appendectomy: Outcomes comparison based on a large administrative database. *Ann Surg* 239:43, 2004.

35. Sauerland S, Lefering R, Neugebauer EA: Laparoscopic versus open surgery for suspected appendicitis. *Cochrane Database Syst Rev* CD001546, 2002.

36. Chung RS, Rowland DY, Li P, et al: A meta-analysis of randomized controlled trials of laparoscopic versus conventional appendectomy. *Am J Surg* 177:250, 1999.

37. Garbutt JM, Soper NJ, Shannon WD, et al: Meta-analysis of randomized controlled trials comparing laparoscopic and open appendectomy. *Surg Laparosc Endosc* 9:17, 1999.

38. Sporn E, Petroski GF, Mancini GJ, et al: Laparoscopic appendectomy: Is it worth the cost? Trend analysis in the US from 2000 to 2005. *J Am Coll Surg* 208:179, 2009.

39. Kouhia ST, Heiskanen JT, Huttunen R, et al: Long-term follow-up of a randomized clinical trial of open versus laparoscopic appendicectomy. *Br J Surg* 97:1395, 2010.

40. Markides G, Subar D, Riyad K: Laparoscopic versus open appendectomy in adults with complicated appendicitis: Systematic review and meta-analysis. *World J Surg* 34:2026, 2010.

41. Vargas HI, Averbook A, Stamos MJ: Appendiceal mass: Conservative therapy followed by interval laparoscopic appendectomy. *Am Surg* 60:753, 1994.

42. Haller JA, Shaker IJ, Donahoo JS, et al: Peritoneal drainage versus non-drainage for generalized peritonitis from ruptured appendicitis in children. *Ann Surg* 177:595, 1973.

43. Cantrell JR, Stafford ES: The diminishing mortality from appendicitis. *Ann Surg* 141:749, 1995.

44. Colson M, Skinner KA, Dunnington G: High negative appendectomy rates are no longer acceptable. *Am J Surg* 174:723, 1997.

45. Hale DA, Molloy M, Pearl RH, et al: Appendectomy: A contemporary appraisal. *Ann Surg* 225:252, 1997.

46. Temple CL, Huchcroft SA, Temple WJ: The natural history of appendicitis in adults: A prospective study. *Ann Surg* 221:278, 1995.

47. Leigh DA, Simmons K, Norman E: Bacteria flora of the appendix fossa in appendicitis and postoperative wound infection. *J Clin Pathol* 27:997, 1974.

48. Lee AW, Bell RM, Griffen WO, et al: Recurrent appendiceal colic. *Surg Gynecol Obstet* 161:21, 1985.

49. Dent TL, Batsakis JG, Lindenauer SM: Carcinoid tumors of the appendix. *Surgery* 73:828, 1973.

50. Andersson A, Bergdahl L, Boquist L: Primary carcinoma of the appendix. *Ann Surg* 183:53, 1976.

PART FOUR

Neoplastic Disease

<table>
<tr><td>CHAPTER
163</td><td>## Colorectal Polyps and Polyposis Syndromes

Emily Steinhagen | José G. Guillem</td></tr>
</table>

POLYPS OF THE COLON AND RECTUM

The word polyp is derived from Latin and Greek words meaning "many feet" and is defined as a mass that protrudes into the lumen of the bowel. It is believed that most polyps originate as sessile lesions, defined grossly by a broad base without a stalk. Traction can lead to a pedunculated polyp with a stalk.

Several histologic types of colorectal polyps have been described and can be broadly classified into neoplastic and nonneoplastic based on their malignant potential (Table 163-1). The most common neoplastic polyp is the adenoma, which harbors malignant potential. Serrated polyps are another type of polyp that also have malignant potential. The most common nonneoplastic polyp of the colorectum is the hyperplastic polyp. Other nonneoplastic polyps include hamartomatous (such as those seen in juvenile polyposis syndrome [JPS] and Peutz-Jeghers syndrome [PJS]) and inflammatory polyps. Submucosal lesions that may resemble polyps include lymphoid polyps, lipomas, leiomyomas, neuromas, angiomas, and small carcinoids.

ADENOMATOUS POLYPS

Adenomatous polyps (adenomas) are benign neoplasms of the epithelium. Most are smooth in appearance and may be slightly redder in color than the surrounding mucosa. However, the surface may become nodular as they increase in size. Adenomas may be classified by shape as sessile or pedunculated. Size varies from 1 mm to several centimeters. The distribution of adenomas in the colon is as follows: cecum, 5%; ascending colon, 7%; hepatic flexure, 4%; transverse colon, 16%; splenic flexure, 6%; descending colon, 19%; sigmoid colon, 40%; and rectum, 3%.[1]

There are three histologic subtypes of adenoma: tubular (85% to 91%); villous (5% to 10%); and tubulovillous (1%) (Figure 163-1).[2] Tubular adenomas consist of at least 80% dysplastic tubules that are packed tightly and extend into normal-appearing lamina propria. Villous adenomas have at least 80% villous fronds that are made of a core lamina propria surrounded by adenomatous epithelium; these fronds are crypts that have elongated to at least twice the normal length. Tubulovillous adenomas are those polyps that have more than 20% tubular components and less than 80% villous components.

Microscopically, the nuclei of adenomatous cells are hyperchromatic. Cellular proliferation in adenomas differs from normal colonic epithelium in that it is not confined to the base of the crypts. Dysplasia in adenomas can be categorized as low or high grade. As dysplasia progresses, nuclear atypia, mitotic figures, and a loss of polarity become evident and tall columnar cells become mucin depleted with basally located, oval nuclei.

Adenomas are the most common type of colorectal polyps and are found in 23% to 58% of adults, and their incidence increases with age.[3] Adenomas are considered premalignant lesions that can grow in size, become increasingly dysplastic, and eventually develop into carcinoma. Most adenomatous polyps are asymptomatic and are discovered during screening or surveillance. However, symptoms may include rectal bleeding, a change in bowel habits, and nonspecific abdominal pain. Adenomas may occur sporadically or as part of one of the hereditary syndromes.

HYPERPLASTIC POLYPS

Hyperplastic polyps appear as pale, broadly based, flat, smooth nodules. Usually, they are less than 5 mm in size. Most occur in the rectosigmoid, and multiple hyperplastic polyps are often noted in one individual. They arise from faulty epithelial maturation and a failure of apoptosis.

Histologically, they are characterized by elongated, nonbranching mucosal crypts and hyperplasia without atypia (Figure 163-2). The main component is mature goblet cells. Hyperplastic polyps are generally considered to be nonmalignant, though adenomatous changes can occur. "Mixed" hyperplastic and adenomatous or serrated polyps can also occur. Serrated polyps are sometimes characterized as a type of hyperplastic polyp, and these do have malignant potential. When hyperplastic polyps occur as part of a polyposis syndrome, they are associated with an increased risk of malignancy.

SERRATED POLYPS

Serrated polyps (also called serrated adenomas) are a recently recognized type of polyp that has been

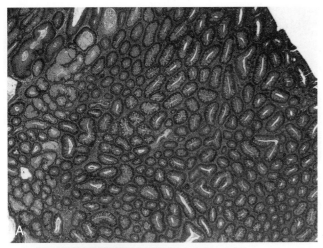

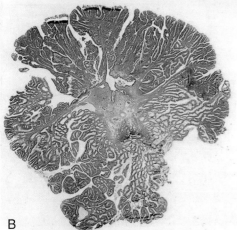

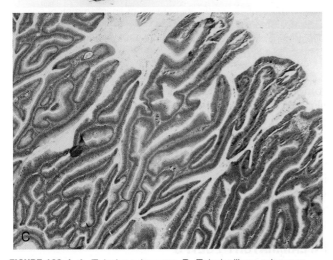

FIGURE 163-1 A, Tubular adenoma. **B,** Tubulovillous adenoma. **C,** Villous adenoma. (Courtesy Jinru Shia, MD, Department of Pathology, Memorial Sloan-Kettering Cancer Center, New York.)

TABLE 163-1 Histologic Classification of Colorectal Polyps

Neoplastic	Nonneoplastic
Adenomatous	Hyperplastic
Tubular	Hamartomas
Villous	Juvenile
Tubulovillous	Peutz-Jeghers
Serrated	Inflammatory
Traditional serrated	Submucosal lesions
Mixed	Lymphoid
Sessile serrated adenoma	Lipoma
Rare malignant lesions	Leiomyoma
Carcinoid	Neuroma
Melanoma	Angioma
Lymphoma	
Mesenchymal tumors	

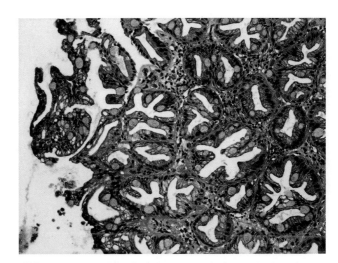

FIGURE 163-2 Microscopic appearance of a hyperplastic polyp. (Courtesy Jinru Shia, MD, Department of Pathology, Memorial Sloan-Kettering Cancer Center, New York.)

classified by various authors as a subset of adenomatous or hyperplastic polyps; other authors have suggested that hyperplastic polyps are a subtype of serrated polyps. They appear grossly similar to hyperplastic polyps as pale, small lesions. Their true incidence is not clear at this time.

Histologic characteristics of the serrated polyp are serrated, dilated crypts with branching at the base, enlarged hyperchromatic nuclei, and normally arranged, small basilar nuclei (Figure 163-3). Crypts may be oriented horizontally. Focal mucus overproduction is also characteristic.[4] There are varying degrees of atypia and dysplasia found in serrated polyps.[5] The proliferation zone that is found in the base of the crypt in normal colorectal mucosa may be found in the middle or upper portion of the crypt in a serrated polyp.[4]

Serrated polyps are further classified into traditional serrated polyps, mixed polyps, and sessile serrated adenomas.[6] Traditional serrated polyps can contain low- and high-grade dysplasia of the crypt surface epithelium, whereas the mixed polyps contain a combination of serrated architecture seen in hyperplastic polyps but with dysplasia characteristic of adenomas. Sessile serrated adenomas are characterized by morphology of both hyperplastic polyps and traditional serrated polyps. They grow larger than other serrated adenomas and display

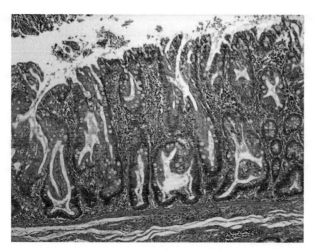

FIGURE 163-3 Microscopic appearance of a serrated polyp. (Courtesy Jinru Shia, MD, Department of Pathology, Memorial Sloan-Kettering Cancer Center, New York.)

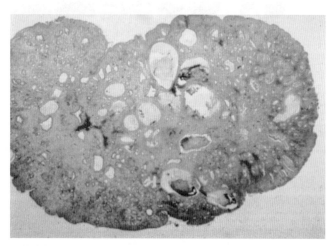

FIGURE 163-4 Microscopic appearance of a juvenile polyp. (Courtesy Stephen S. Sternberg, MD, and Satish Tickoo, MD, Department of Pathology, Memorial Sloan-Kettering Cancer Center, New York.)

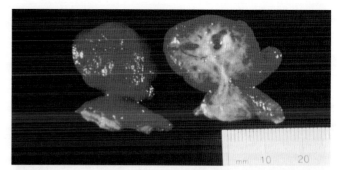

FIGURE 163-5 Gross appearance of a juvenile polyp. (Courtesy Stephen S. Sternberg, MD, and Satish Tickoo, MD, Department of Pathology, Memorial Sloan-Kettering Cancer Center, New York.)

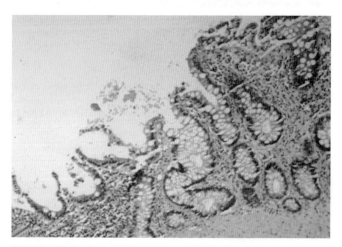

FIGURE 163-6 Microscopic appearance of an inflammatory polyp. (Courtesy Stephen S. Sternberg, MD, and Satish Tickoo, MD, Department of Pathology, Memorial Sloan-Kettering Cancer Center, New York.)

changes in the proliferative zone and dilation of crypts at the base, often with lateral extension parallel to muscularis mucosae, or herniation through it.[6] Serrated polyps may represent the neoplastic risk of serrated polyposis syndrome (SPS) when they appear as part of this syndrome.

HAMARTOMATOUS POLYPS

Hamartomatous polyps are localized overgrowths of normal, mature intestinal epithelial cells. On endoscopic evaluation, they appear round, pink, smooth, and pedunculated. They are usually lined with normal epithelium over a submucosal core that does not involve the muscularis mucosae. The pathogenesis is thought to be mucosal ulceration or inflammation that blocks colonic glands. This leads to proliferation and dilation of the glands, followed by the growth of granulation and connective tissue in the area. Histologic evaluation reveals cystic dilation of mucus-filled glands, prominent fibrous stroma, and rich vascularity (Figure 163-4).[7] They are

sometimes referred to as retention or juvenile polyps (Figure 163-5). It appears that sporadic hamartomatous polyps do not have any malignant potential unless they contain adenomatous components.[7]

Symptoms from hamartomatous polyps may include abdominal pain, bleeding from ulceration, diarrhea, intussusception, or transanal prolapse if the polyp is located in the rectum. Hamartomatous polyps may occur sporadically, but when more than three are present, a polyposis syndrome should be considered.

INFLAMMATORY POLYPS

Inflammatory polyps, also known as pseudopolyps, arise from mucosal ulceration and repair. They occur most frequently in the setting of chronic ulcerative colitis but are also seen in Crohn disease and other forms of colitis. Inflammatory polyps are uniform in width from the base to the head and consist of islands of inflamed regenerating mucosa surrounded by ulceration (Figure 163-6). Because of their etiology, they nearly always occur in multiples. Patients with inflammatory polyps usually require no treatment other than for the underlying colitis, but the possibility of neoplastic disease should be excluded.

TABLE 163-2 Summary of Gastrointestinal Polyposis Syndromes

Polyp Histology	Syndrome	Genetic Basis	Gene Locus
Adenomatous	FAP	Germline *APC* mutation	5q21
	AFAP	Germline *APC* mutation	5q21
	MAP	Biallelic germline *MUTYH* mutation	1p32.1-34.3
	Lynch syndrome	Germline MMR gene mutation	*MLH1*: 3p21
			MSH2: 2p16
			MSH6: 2p16
			PMS2: 7p22
	Familial CRC type X	Unknown	Unknown
Hyperplastic/serrated	Serrated polyposis syndrome	Unknown	Unknown
Hamartomatous	Juvenile polyposis syndrome	Germline *SMAD4* mutation	18q21.1
		Germline *BMPR1A* mutation	10q21-22
	Peutz-Jeghers syndrome	Germline *LKB1/STK11* mutation	19p13.3
	PTEN hamartoma tumor syndrome	Germline *PTEN* mutation	10q23.3
	Cronkhite-Canada syndrome	Unknown	N/A
Mixed	Hereditary mixed polyposis syndrome	Unknown Possibly *CRAC1*	15q14-22

AFAP, Attenuated familial adenomatous polyposis; *CRC*, colorectal cancer; *FAP*, familial adenomatous polyposis; *MAP*, MUTYH-associated polyposis; *MMR*, mismatch repair gene.

POLYPOSIS SYNDROMES

Gastrointestinal polyposis syndromes include a variety of entities that are characterized by the number and histologic type of colorectal polyps, as well as polyposis of the upper gastrointestinal tract and specific extraintestinal manifestations (Table 163-2). Adenomatous polyposis syndromes are characterized by adenomas of the gastrointestinal tract and include familial adenomatous polyposis (FAP), attenuated familial adenomatous polyposis (AFAP), MUTYH-associated polyposis (MAP), Lynch syndrome, and familial colorectal cancer type X (FCC X). HPS is characterized by hyperplastic, and sometimes serrated and adenomatous, polyps. Hamartomatous polyposis syndromes are characterized by gastrointestinal hamartomas, and include JPS, PJS, PTEN hamartoma syndromes (Cowden disease and Bannayan-Riley-Ruvalcaba syndrome), and Cronkhite-Canada syndrome. Hereditary mixed polyposis syndrome is characterized by both hamartomatous and adenomatous polyps of the gastrointestinal tract.

ADENOMATOUS POLYPOSIS SYNDROMES

FAMILIAL ADENOMATOUS POLYPOSIS

FAP is a dominantly inherited syndrome with an approximate occurrence of 1 in 10,000 live births. It is the second most common inherited colorectal cancer (CRC) syndrome. Though it is an autosomal dominant disease, expression may vary within kindred. FAP is characterized by hundreds to thousands of polyps throughout the colon as well as a variety of extracolonic manifestations (Figures 163-7 and 163-8). The median age for adenoma development in patients with FAP is 17 years. Untreated patients develop colorectal cancer at a median age of 40, and death occurs by age 44.[8]

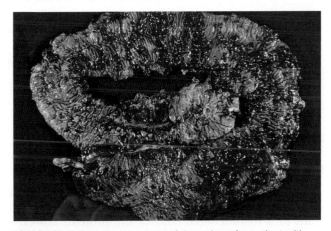

FIGURE 163-7 Gross appearance of the colon of a patient with familial adenomatous polyposis. (Courtesy Jinru Shia, MD, Department of Pathology, Memorial Sloan-Kettering Cancer Center, New York.)

Genetics

The *APC* gene is located on chromosome 5q21 and has many intracellular functions. One of the most well described is its role in the Wnt signaling pathway, in which the APC protein forms a complex with c-myc, GSK3, axin, and casein that allows the degradation of β-catenin. If β-catenin accumulates, it enters into the cell nucleus and induces transcription of cellular growth factors. Cell proliferation, enhanced cell-to-cell adhesion, and cell migration follow. Another function of APC is to stabilize microtubules, which are important for cell migration, and APC has a role in actin-based cell protrusion, motility, and polarity.[9] APC also has binding sites for cytoskeletal regulators and its loss can lead to missegregation of chromosomes during mitosis.[10]

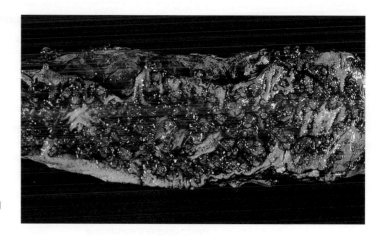

FIGURE 163-8 Close-up image of colonic mucosa in a specimen from a patient with familial adenomatous polyposis. (Courtesy Jinru Shia, MD, Department of Pathology, Memorial Sloan-Kettering Cancer Center, New York.)

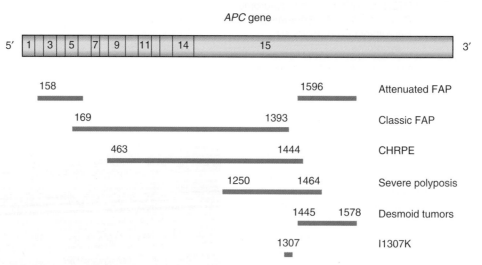

FIGURE 163-9 Genotype-phenotype correlations between the APC gene and familial adenomatous polyposis. *CHRPE,* Congenital hypertrophy of the retinal pigment epithelium; *FAP,* familial adenomatous polyposis. (From Jo WS, Chung DC: Genetics of hereditary colorectal cancer. *Semin Oncol* 32:11, 2005.)

The most frequent alteration in the APC protein is caused by a truncating mutation of the *APC* gene that leads to a dysfunctional copy of the protein. Missense mutations can also occur.[11] Mutations in the *APC* gene are an example of chromosomal instability, and this is often the first step in the genetic pathway leading to colorectal cancer. Chromosomal instability refers to changes in chromosome number and structure, leading to changes in amount, structure, and function of proteins. Mutations in the *APC* gene are the first step in the classic pathway for the development of colorectal cancer, or the adenoma-to-carcinoma sequence.

Germline mutations in one copy of the *APC* gene leave all cells open to a loss of heterozygosity if their second copy of *APC* is mutated or lost. When sporadic mutations of both copies of *APC* occur in a single cell, this is the first step in the sporadic adenoma-to-carcinoma sequence, and leads to the formation of adenomas. Patients with FAP already have one mutated copy of the *APC* gene in each of their cells, so this process is accelerated.

APC mutations are inherited in an autosomal dominant pattern and are highly penetrant. There are some correlations between a specific genotype and a phenotypic pattern. Although not exact, they sometimes allow for predictions about polyposis severity and the risk of extraintestinal manifestations (Figure 163-9). However, in some FAP families, there are variations in disease expression despite sharing the same genotype, so treatment decisions cannot be made based on genotype. These differences may be attributable to modifier genes, environmental influences, or other factors.

Diagnosis

Many patients with FAP present without symptoms, either because of a known family history leading to screening or during investigation of an unrelated complaint.[12] Some patients are referred for testing based on extracolonic manifestations such as extra teeth, osteomas, or congenital hypertrophy of the retinal pigment epithelium (CHRPE). Others present with symptoms from polyposis that may include bleeding, change in bowel habits, and abdominal pain.

The most common reason patients have not been screened is a lack of family history. Though most patients have a family history of FAP, between 10% and 30% will represent de novo mutations in the gene. When symptoms from polyposis occur, cancer is present in more than 60% of patients.[12]

A clinical diagnosis of FAP is made when at least 100 colonic adenomas are identified.[13] Smaller numbers of polyps may be present in younger patients. Extracolonic manifestations may also contribute to the diagnosis. The clinical diagnosis is confirmed with *APC* mutation testing. Typically, DNA from peripheral blood leukocytes of a clinically affected patient is sequenced. If a pathologic mutation is found, genetic testing is said to be informative in the family. Thereafter, unaffected family members can be screened to look for the same mutation.

Extracolonic Manifestations

Extracolonic manifestations reflect the systemic growth regulation disorder that afflicts patients with FAP.

CHRPE. Congenital hypertrophy of the retinal pigment epithelium is the most common extracolonic manifestation of FAP. It appears as well demarcated grey-brown round or oval lesions on the retinae of affected individuals. They are asymptomatic and have no malignant potential. CHRPE is present in approximately 60% of FAP patients and the presence of multiple or bilateral patches of these lesions is highly suggestive of FAP.[14] Isolated lesions can be present sporadically in individuals without FAP. In some cases, the presence of CHRPE can be used to identify affected individuals in an FAP family. Mutations between codons 543 and 1309 of the *APC* gene are associated with a high risk of CHRPE.[14]

Soft Tissue and Bone Tumors. Osteomas are benign, slow-growing neoplasms of the bone. The most common site for FAP patients is the skull and mandible, but they can occur in any part of the body. Size ranges from less than 1 mm to several centimeters. They may be detected on physical examination if they are large, or on dental radiographs. Osteomas are associated with a subtype of FAP known as Gardner syndrome and they may precede the development of gastrointestinal polyposis. Other manifestations of Gardner syndrome include epidermoid cysts, supernumerary teeth, and desmoids.

Subcutaneous, benign lesions such as epidermoid cysts, fibromas, and lipomas can occur up to 25 times more frequently in the FAP population than in age-matched non-FAP populations.[14] Epidermoid cysts are commonly diagnosed in the mid- to late teenage years, are often multiple, and occur in atypical locations such as the face, scalp, and extremities. Supernumerary teeth, dentigerous cysts, and secondary retention of teeth can all arise in FAP patients. Supernumerary teeth are usually present before age 10, and should be removed only if they impede the development of normal dentition. Dentigerous cysts develop from the epithelium of the enamel organ and develop before teeth erupt from the jaw. They can grow and occupy a significant portion of the jaw.

Thyroid. The estimated incidence of thyroid carcinoma (TC) is thought to be 1% to 2% in FAP patients; however, one small series reports an incidence of 12%.[15,16] As in sporadic TC, most cases are papillary, and the cribriform-morular variant is closely associated with FAP.[17] The female propensity for TC found in the general population is even more pronounced in the FAP population. The average age at diagnosis is 27 years, which is somewhat earlier than sporadic TC.[14] Most cases of TC present as a nodule in the thyroid gland. Confirmation

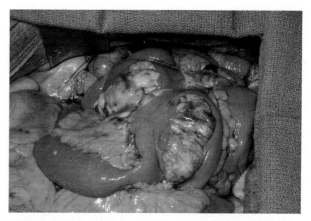

FIGURE 163-10 Intraabdominal desmoid. (Courtesy Ethan Kavit, Department of Medical Graphics, Memorial Sloan-Kettering Cancer Center, New York.)

is provided by fine-needle aspiration, but this is occasionally nondiagnostic, leading to diagnostic hemithyroidectomy. More often than in sporadic cases, FAP-associated TC is multifocal and regional lymph node involvement may occur. TC may present before other manifestations of FAP in approximately one-third of cases. Another one-third are diagnosed concurrently, and the remainder are known to have FAP at the time of TC diagnosis.[15] Therefore, FAP should be considered in patients presenting with the characteristic cribriform-morular variant of papillary TC, especially if they are younger than 30 and present with multifocal disease.[17,18] There may be a genotypic association with a mutation in exon 15, in the 5′ portion of the *APC* gene. This leads to an association with CHRPE, because the associated genotype is in the same region.[14,15]

Treatment may include total thyroidectomy, radioiodine administration, and thyroid-stimulating hormone suppression via synthetic thyroid hormone replacement. Surgeons operating on FAP patients with TC may perform a total thyroidectomy because of the high risk of multicentric disease.[15] There are currently no clear recommendations for thyroid screening in FAP patients. Neck palpation and ultrasound may be used.

Desmoids. Desmoids are slow-growing, benign mesenchymal tumors characterized by mature, highly differentiated fibroblasts and myofibroblasts with an abundant collagen matrix. It has been estimated that up to one-third of patients with FAP develop desmoids, and they are diagnosed at a rate of almost 1000 times that in the general population.[14,19] They do not metastasize but are locally aggressive, tend to infiltrate surrounding tissues, and have a high recurrence rate following surgical therapy. Desmoids can be fatal, related in large part to their aggressive local growth with compression of surrounding organs (intestine, ureter, and vessels), erosion of adjacent structures, and interference with surgical therapy. They represent the second most common cause of mortality in FAP patients, following colorectal cancer.[20]

In patients with FAP, up to 80% of desmoids are intraabdominal (Figure 163-10).[21] The remainder occur primarily in the abdominal wall, with a small minority in extraabdominal locations.[12] Early desmoids, which have been termed desmoid precursor lesions or desmoid reactions appear as flat, white plaques. These lesions can cause puckering of the small bowel mesentery and can lead to ischemic bands or bowel obstruction. Larger lesions tend to form nonencapsulated, lobulated masses. Desmoids can become massive and occupy a large portion of the abdomen or pelvis. Clinical presentation ranges from asymptomatic plaques or masses discovered incidentally on imaging or during prophylactic surgery to many nonspecific symptoms. Symptomatic desmoids may cause abdominal pain, bowel obstruction, ischemia, deep venous thrombosis from venous compression, sensory and motor deficits from nerve compression, ureteric obstruction, sepsis from enteric fistula, upper gastrointestinal hemorrhage, and ileo-anal pouch failure.

Surgical trauma is a major risk factor for the development of intraabdominal and abdominal wall desmoid tumors. Desmoids are found in the abdominal cavity at the time of first surgical intervention in 2% of patients.[22] The median interval between surgery and diagnosis of desmoid tumor is approximately 2 years.[14] Other risk factors for desmoid disease include female gender, the presence of other extraintestinal manifestations of FAP, and a family history of desmoids.[19] Mutations toward the 3′ end of the *APC* gene are associated with the development of desmoid tumors, but family history is a risk factor for the development of disease, independent of genotype.

Intraabdominal desmoid staging takes into account tumor size, symptoms, behavior, and presence of complications.[23] This can help in evaluating desmoids over time and determining treatment options. Stage I desmoids are asymptomatic and not growing. They are usually found incidentally at the time of surgery or CT scan performed for other reasons. Stage II tumors are symptomatic and 10 cm or less, but not growing. These tumors may require treatment because of symptoms. Stage III desmoids are symptomatic tumors that are 11 to 20 cm in size, or asymptomatic and slowly growing. Treatment may also be recommended for these large desmoid tumors. Finally, stage IV desmoids are symptomatic and more than 20 cm in size, display rapid growth, or cause significant complications. Tumors that cause life-threatening complications such as sepsis, free bowel perforation, or massive bleeding require urgent treatment. Other features of desmoids that are taken into account include their shape (mass, nodular, or flat), the number of tumors present, the location, whether they occur before or after operative intervention, and hormone receptor status. These can all help guide management.

Treatment of desmoids may be broadly categorized into nonsurgical and surgical approaches, although there is no singularly effective therapy. Because failure with one treatment does not preclude successful therapy with a different approach, clinicians may explore all options in resistant or recurrent cases. Both cytotoxic and noncytotoxic pharmacologic agents have been used with variable success in the treatment of desmoid tumors. Nonsteroidal antiinflammatory drugs (NSAIDs) such as sulindac and indomethacin are considered first-line therapy for desmoids. Antiestrogens, primarily tamoxifen and raloxifene, have been reported to produce response rates comparable to those of NSAIDs, but there are no randomized studies documenting their efficacy. NSAIDs and antiestrogens may be used in combination, with up to 77% response according to one report.[24] The most commonly used and apparently successful cytotoxic chemotherapy regimens in the treatment of desmoids are combinations of antisarcoma agents. Vinblastine and methotrexate regimens have demonstrated a response in 40% to 50% of patients.[21] Tyrosine kinase inhibitors such as imatinib have also been used. Overall, responses are most common in patients receiving regimens containing doxorubicin or other anthracyclines.[25] Toxicity is a major concern with cytotoxic therapy, which limits its use to extensive life-threatening disease that is resistant to other therapy, or when alternative approaches are contraindicated. In addition, in carefully selected cases, radiation therapy may provide acceptable local control following surgical resection and as primary therapy for unresectable tumors, but the benefit must be weighed against the risk of irradiating a large portion of the small bowel.[26]

Surgery for intraabdominal desmoids should be reserved for select cases of symptomatic disease given their often unresectable nature because of their common location in the root of the mesentery, and their high recurrence rates following resection. Often, the characteristic infiltrating growth pattern makes complete resection impossible without extensive small bowel resection. Local control rates following resection with positive and negative margins are reported as 41% and 72%, respectively.[27] The addition of postoperative radiation therapy, when clinically feasible, can improve local control to as high as 94% when negative pathologic margins are achieved. Bypass procedures are controversial but may be required to treat select cases of nonresolving bowel obstruction. Major complications have been reported in up to 50% of patients with intraabdominal desmoids treated with surgical resection. In addition, extensive resection may lead to short bowel syndrome and its associated difficult management. Another difficult issue associated with the surgical treatment of intraabdominal desmoids is the high recurrence rate. Abdominal wall desmoids may be treated with surgical resection, with margins of 2 cm. Reconstruction with prosthetic mesh or a myocutaneous flap may be required when large lesions are treated.

A reasonable approach to desmoids may be to begin with NSAIDs such as sulindac (150 mg twice per day) as first-line therapy. If the tumor does not respond or progresses following 6 or more months of therapy, an antiestrogen such as tamoxifen (starting at 30 mg per day, with a slow increase up to 120 mg per day) or raloxifene (60 mg twice a day) may be added. If the tumor responds, therapy can be gradually withdrawn over 6 months. Cytotoxic chemotherapy with a doxorubicin-based regimen should be reserved for extensive or life-threatening tumors that do not respond to noncytotoxic pharmacologic regimens and are not amenable to surgery. Surgery should be reserved for carefully selected localized desmoids of the limbs or abdominal wall or intraabdominal desmoids causing significant symptoms or complications.

TABLE 163-3 Modified Spigelman Classification for Staging Duodenal Polyposis in FAP Patients

	POINTS		
Variable	1	2	3
Polyp number	1-4	5-20	>20
Polyp size (mm)	1-4	5-10	>10
Histology	Tubular	Tubulovillous	Villous
Dysplasia	Low grade		High grade

From Spigelman AD, Williams CB, Talbot IC, et al: Upper gastrointestinal cancer in patients with familial adenomatous polyposis. *Lancet* 2:783, 1989.
FAP, Familial adenomatous polyposis.
Stage 0 (no polyps), 0 points; *stage I,* 1-4 points; *stage II,* 5-6 points; *stage III,* 7-8 points; *stage IV,* 9-12 points.

Upper Gastrointestinal Neoplasia. Upper gastrointestinal polyps in patients with FAP may be nonneoplastic, as is the case for most gastric polyps, or neoplastic, which is typical of duodenal or periampullary polyps. Gastric polyps are also called fundic gland polyps, and are benign hyperplastic-type polyps. However, they may be associated with an increased risk for adenomas. Cancer arising from gastric fundic polyps has been reported, but the risk is very low and most endoscopists do not remove all fundic gland polyps. When biopsied, many fundic gland polyps demonstrate dysplasia, and this risk increases with polyp size. Up to 10% of patients will also have gastric antral adenomas, and these are believed to confer a risk of gastric cancer.[12] Overall, FAP patients in Western nations appear to have lower rates of gastric cancer than Japanese and Korean patients.[28] Because of the risk of dysplasia and cancer, FAP patients are advised to undergo lifelong surveillance and biopsies with intervals varying based on number and histology of polyps.

Duodenal adenomas are found in more than 90% of patients with FAP. They can be staged according to the Spigelman staging system, which takes into account the number and size of polyps, histologic type, and dysplasia (Table 163-3).[29] Using these features, patients are stratified into a low-risk group (stages 0, I, and II) in whom screening endoscopy is recommended every 2 to 3 years, and a high-risk group (stages III and IV) in whom endoscopy with biopsy is recommended every 6 to 12 months. In addition, surgical intervention is justified in advanced duodenal polyposis (stage IV and select stage III).

Adenomas in the duodenum are thought to progress in a similar manner to colorectal polyps. Duodenal cancer risk in FAP patients is approximately 4%.[30] It is the second most common malignancy in FAP patients after CRC. There is no known relationship between the position of the mutation on the gene and duodenal cancer risk. However, it has been observed that duodenal cancer is associated with a lower colonic polyp burden.[30] Because many duodenal cancers present asymptomatically, and because prognosis for advanced lesions is poor, screening is important.

Surveillance is accomplished via endoscopy and biopsy. It is important to take numerous biopsy samples in order to accurately detect and stage disease.[30] The recurrence rate of adenomas is high after removal, but representative biopsies should be taken for evaluation. The use of capsule endoscopy for surveillance of the small bowel has been investigated in some trials. Capsule endoscopy is a noninvasive procedure that allows evaluation of small bowel mucosa beyond the reach of the usual endoscope. Although it can be used for diagnostic purposes, if therapeutic intervention is needed, traditional endoscopic or surgical techniques must be used. However, it is not adequate for assessing the duodenum because of rapid transit time and it can be difficult to estimate the size of polyps visualized in the study.[31]

Surgical therapy is reserved for patients at a high risk for cancer, including those with extensive duodenal polyposis, rapid polyp growth, villous lesions with high-grade dysplasia, and suspicious endoscopic features. In addition, patients with Spigelman IV polyposis have a high risk of harboring or developing duodenal cancer (reported as high as 36%), and surgical resection should be considered in these patients.[12] Operative intervention should be individualized, and alternatives include local excision, ampullectomy, pancreas-sparing duodenectomy, and pancreaticoduodenectomy. Local excision is a less attractive option because it has a high failure rate, it makes subsequent surgical resection difficult, and it is associated with a significant morbidity from postoperative duodenal leaks. Pancreaticoduodenectomy is indicated for cancer and large, rapidly growing adenomas with severe dysplasia and may be performed with acceptable morbidity and limited mortality.[12]

There is also an increased incidence of pancreatic tumors in the FAP population, ranging from adenocarcinoma, mucinous neoplasms, cystic neoplasms, and acinar cell and islet cell tumors. According to one study, the relative risk of pancreatic tumors in FAP patients is 4.5 compared with the general population.[14]

Hepatoblastoma. Hepatoblastoma is a malignant embryonal tumor of the liver. It usually occurs in children between 6 months and 3 years of age but can occur from birth to 16 years.[14] More than 50 cases of hepatoblastoma in FAP patients have been reported; the risk is 750 to 7500 times higher in children with a mutation compared with the general population. However, the absolute risk of hepatoblastoma in FAP patients is still less than 2%.[14]

The tumor presents with an abdominal mass that is usually asymptomatic but may lead to constipation, abdominal pain, vomiting, weight loss, anemia, and thrombocytopenia. An elevated α-fetoprotein (αFP) level is present in most cases. Some authors have suggested surveillance via serial αFP measurements and abdominal ultrasound every 3 months from age 1 month to 4 years.[32] One difficulty with this is that αFP is often elevated in normal newborns. Another complicating issue is that to identify individuals in need of screening, genetic testing would need to be performed in the first month of life. As of now, there is no consensus regarding screening for hepatoblastoma.

There is no specific genotype that has been associated with a higher risk of hepatoblastoma.[32] Hepatoblastoma is also related to genetic abnormalities other than FAP including Beckwith-Wiedemann syndrome, trisomy 18, and fetal alcohol syndrome. Treatment includes surgery and chemotherapy. Survival is approximately 75% and depends on the stage at which the tumor is diagnosed.[14]

Adrenal Adenoma. Adrenal adenomas are present in 7% to 13% of the FAP population.[14] Incidence is likely increasing as a result of detection on imaging performed for other reasons. The clinical presentation and biologic behavior of these incidentalomas seem to be the same as those found in the general population. The workup for these tumors is the same as in non-FAP patients; excess hormone production should be ruled out and they should be monitored for growth. Adrenal carcinomas are rare and only 6 have been reported in FAP patients.[14]

Brain Tumors. The association between primary brain tumors and colorectal polyposis has been labeled Turcot syndrome or the brain tumor polyposis (BTP) syndrome. This represents a heterogeneous group of disorders, including FAP and Lynch syndrome. The brain tumors are usually medulloblastomas, glioblastomas, or astrocytomas.

Medulloblastomas account for 80% of brain tumors diagnosed in the FAP population, but astrocytomas, glioblastomas, ependymomas, pineal blastomas, and gangliogliomas have also been described.[33] The absolute lifetime risk of brain tumor for FAP patients is seven times that of the normal population. For medulloblastoma, it is 90 times higher. However, the overall lifetime risk of a brain tumor in an FAP patient is still low at 1% to 2%.[14] Comparisons of pooled APC mutation data and FAP families with central nervous system tumors show a higher likelihood of medulloblastoma in patients with APC mutation between codons 697 and 1224.[33] There are no formal recommendations regarding screening for brain tumors in FAP patients.

Medulloblastomas are highly malignant and usually affect children under age 10, predating the appearance of colorectal manifestations of FAP. They usually occur in the midline cerebellum and present with symptoms of cerebellar dysfunction such as emesis, horizontal diplopia, ataxia, and headaches. Patients may also experience obstructive hydrocephalus. In FAP populations, there appears to be a preponderance of female cases, in contrast to the general population.[33] Treatment includes surgery, radiation, and chemotherapy. The 5-year survival rate is approximately 50% to 70%.[14]

Medical Management

Although chemoprevention is not recommended as a primary treatment for patients with multiple adenomatous polyps, it may serve as an adjunct to treatment in some patients.[34] The goal is to reduce the appearance of new polyps and possibly induce regression of existing ones. This may potentially delay the need for surgery and perhaps lengthen the time polyposis can be managed endoscopically. Sulindac has been shown to suppress the formation of adenomas and to induce regression of existing adenomas in adult patients with FAP, resulting in a 35% to 44% decrease in polyp burden.[35] The selective cyclooxygenase-2 inhibitor celecoxib was also found to reduce colorectal adenomas in up to 30% of adult FAP patients.[36] Small studies suggest similar results in children.[37] Though celecoxib may cause adenoma regression, it does not seem to prevent adenomas from

occurring.[38] In a large-scale trial of patients taking celecoxib with or without aspirin, 0.9% of patients experienced cardiovascular events when taking both drugs, and 0.5% when taking celecoxib without aspirin. The risk of cardiovascular events in patients taking NSAIDS was 1.0% and 0.4%, respectively.[39] NSAIDS have also been used postcolectomy with ileorectal anastomosis to decrease rectal polyp burden. There seems to be a slight decrease in polyp number with 6 months of use.[35] However, some authors have raised the possibility that resistance to therapy may occur over time and that the early results are not durable.[40] Early data concerning the omega-3 polyunsaturated fatty acid eicosapentaenoic acid (EPA) in adult FAP patients shows that it may decrease polyp number and size after 6 months of use, making it a target for further research.[41]

Surgical Management

Prophylactic proctocolectomy is recommended for patients with FAP, given the near 100% risk of early-onset CRC. Patients with FAP who present for surgical management may be stratified into two major groups: (1) asymptomatic members of a known FAP kindred with a mutation detected by screening and (2) symptomatic patients, of whom approximately 30% have no family history of FAP. Symptoms from FAP are attributed to CRC in up to 60% of cases. In asymptomatic patients, surveillance endoscopy may be continued when polyps are small (<6 mm) and there is no evidence of dysplasia or cancer. Risk-reducing surgery is commonly deferred until after the high school years in asymptomatic patients, because of patient and parental wishes. However, it should not usually be deferred beyond the early 20s because the risk of CRC is substantial in untreated patients. Registry data suggest that 7% of FAP patients develop colorectal cancer by age 21, and 95% by age 50.[13]

Surgical Options. Surgical options for patients with FAP include total proctocolectomy with end ileostomy, colectomy with ileorectal anastomosis (IRA), and total proctocolectomy with ileal pouch–anal anastomosis (IPAA). Another alternative, although rarely used, is total proctocolectomy with continent ileostomy (Kock pouch) (Table 163-4). The most important consideration in choosing an operation for FAP is its effectiveness for prophylaxis against the development of CRC. However, these procedures are often performed in asymptomatic, young patients who perceive the operation as preventive rather than therapeutic, so issues such as operative morbidity, functional results, and patient acceptability are important variables. Although IPAA meets the goals of surgical therapy in most patients, there remains a defined role for IRA and total proctocolectomy with end ileostomy in specific clinical scenarios.

A total proctocolectomy with either a continent ileostomy (Kock pouch) or end ileostomy eliminates the risk of subsequent development of CRC by removing all at-risk mucosa. However, the permanent ileostomy associated with these procedures is often unacceptable to young patients with FAP because of its perceived restriction on social, athletic, and sexual activities. Because the postoperative functional results in a patient with FAP are likely to be observed by family members in need of

TABLE 163-4 Surgical Options for Colorectal Polyposis in FAP Patients

Procedure	Indications	Advantages	Disadvantages
TPC	Cancer of lower rectum Anatomic limitations Patient preference	Eradicates all at-risk mucosa	Pelvic and perineal dissection (nerve injury, wound healing issues) Permanent Ileostomy
IRA	Rectal sparing	Improved function/continence Simpler operation (one stage, no stoma, no pelvic dissection)	Risk of rectal cancer Requires lifelong surveillance
IPAA	Rectal adenomas Poor compliance with followup	Eradicates all at-risk mucosa Acceptable function and continence	Pelvic dissection (nerve injury) Retained at-risk mucosa Requires lifelong surveillance

FAP, Familial adenomatous polyposis; *IPAA*, ileal pouch–anal anastomosis; *IRA*, ileorectal anastomosis; *TPC*, total proctocolectomy.

prophylactic surgery, poor functional outcome and patient dissatisfaction may deter at-risk family members from undergoing appropriate screening, surveillance, and surgical management. Total proctocolectomy without IPAA is appropriate for patients with a distal rectal cancer in whom a sphincter-preserving resection would be oncologically suboptimal. It is also indicated when IPAA is not technically feasible (secondary to desmoid disease and foreshortening of the small bowel mesentery, making it surgically impossible to bring the ileal pouch to the anus) or unlikely to lead to good function in patients with weak anal sphincters. It is also occasionally chosen by patients who perceive that their lifestyle would be compromised by the frequent bowel movements (five to six per day) sometimes associated with the IPAA procedure.

IRA with close postoperative followup and endoscopic ablation of rectal polyps is an option for patients with rectal sparing who are reliable and willing to undergo regular endoscopic surveillance of the rectum. It has been shown to result in excellent postoperative function. Most patients report two to four stools per day with excellent continence.[12] There are some reports of better and some of equal functional outcomes when compared with IPAA.[42,43] Following IRA, surveillance of the rectum is needed because of the risk of rectal cancer, and a potential need for secondary proctectomy. The long-term risk of developing cancer in the remaining rectum is estimated at 4% at 5 years and 25% at 20 years.[44] It is significantly higher if there are more than 20 rectal adenomas or 1000 colonic adenomas at the time of surgery, or if the *APC* mutation is at the 3′ end of codon 1250, or between codon 1250 and 1464.[34] A study that divided patients into three genotype groups predicting attenuated, intermediate, and severe polyposis based on the location of the mutation found that the cumulative risk of secondary proctectomy and rectal cancer rose with each of the groups as expected. However, even in the lowest-risk group, rectal cancers did occur and proctectomies were required.[45] Although the concept of using genotype-phenotype correlations to help guide the management of a specific patient is appealing and studies show promise for this approach, it is important to recognize that phenotypic expression varies even between members of the same family. At the current time, the surgical approach should be based on clinical (rather than genetic) grounds. Overall, up to 40% of IRA patients

require completion proctectomy because of diffuse polyposis, functional problems, or rectal cancer. However, this number appears to be decreasing as patient selection for IRA has become more stringent with time.[46]

IPAA consists of removing the entire colon and rectum to a point just above the levators and creating a pouch. It is indicated when the polyposis involves the rectum, though some consider it in all FAP patients. The procedure is commonly performed in two stages. Resection of the entire colon and rectum followed by an IPAA with a protecting loop ileostomy whenever possible is the first operation. The anastomosis in IPAA may be performed hand-sewn, with a mucosectomy to remove all at-risk rectal mucosa, or stapled with approximately 1 cm of anal transition zone mucosa left behind. When there are no polyps near the upper part of the anorectal ring, a stapled anastomosis can be performed. However, when polyps are noted, a mucosectomy from the dentate line approximately 5 cm cephalad is preferred. During the mucosectomy, care is taken to preserve the internal and external anal sphincters. A pouch (usually J-shaped, occasionally S-shaped) is constructed from the terminal ileum, which requires mobilization of the small bowel mesentery up to the level of the duodenum and uncinate process of the pancreas as well as mesenteric-lengthening maneuvers. An anastomosis is then performed. The second operation, performed 2 to 3 months later, consists of reversal of the ileostomy. Closure of the ileostomy is preceded by a water-soluble contrast enema to exclude pouch leaks and confirm sacralization of the pouch. Some perform IPAA as a one-stage operation, without a protective ileostomy. However, this approach is controversial because of the potential for an increase in clinically significant anastomotic leaks and pouch failure. The morbidity of the single-stage approach must be balanced against ileostomy-related complications from the two-stage procedure, which may lead to pouch failure and permanent ileostomy.

Postoperatively, IPAA patients report an average of five to six stools per day.[12] Continence is still excellent for most patients, but there is a higher risk of decreased control and limited functional outcome compared to IRA.[34] Patients may experience frequency, incontinence, nocturnal defecation, and urgency.

IPAA should eliminate any future risk of CRC. However, a stapled IPAA without mucosectomy leaves a small ring of at-risk rectal mucosa, even when performed close to the dentate line. Similarly, a hand-sewn IPAA with mucosectomy can leave small areas of rectal mucosa between the rectal cuff and serosa of the pouch, a location that is difficult to palpate and visualize endoscopically. The incidence of neoplasia at the ileoanal anastomosis has been reported to be as high as 15% after mucosectomy and hand-sewn anastomosis, and up to 30% with the double-staple technique.[34] The incidence of adenomas in the pouch is 42% at 7 years after pouch construction. Severe pouch polyposis may require pouchectomy in some patients. Consequently, lifetime surveillance of the ileal pouch is required.

As with IRA, IPAA can be performed as open surgery, with laparoscopic assistance, or as a completely laparoscopic procedure. The postoperative course of patients undergoing laparoscopic procedures is notable for earlier return to bowel function and resumption of diet and decreased or equivalent hospital stay. Postoperative pain and narcotic requirements are decreased.[47,48] With regard to long-term functional outcomes, matched cohorts have shown equivalent numbers of stool per 24-hour period and similar continence.[47,49] Studies of postoperative quality of life and cosmesis show no difference in long-term outcomes regardless of open or laparoscopic procedure.[50]

Issues That Modify Surgical Therapy. When CRC is present, cancer stage and location, presence of symptoms, overall patient status, and the extent and location of benign polyp disease are important considerations in planning the extent of surgical resection. If symptomatic incurable metastatic disease is diagnosed, a partial colectomy encompassing the colorectal cancer may suffice. However, if metastatic disease is resectable, a curative total colectomy with IRA should be performed in patients with colon cancer and limited rectal polyposis. Some suggest that patients with FAP and colon cancer can safely undergo IPAA, but it may be prudent to perform a colectomy and delay IPAA until after definitive pathologic and radiographic staging of the colon cancer and adjuvant treatment is completed, and after a period of recovery and observation. In addition, when unsuspected colon cancer is discovered on pathologic examination following IPAA, a period of observation may be warranted before ileostomy closure because adjuvant chemotherapy may worsen incontinence and increase the frequency of bowel movements. For upper rectal cancer in the setting of FAP, a staged rectal resection and subsequent IPAA may be considered. However, when the rectal cancer involves the anal sphincters, a total proctocolectomy with ileostomy is required.

A preoperative CT scan is helpful in the identification of desmoids, as they may influence the surgical approach. Patients with a personal or family history of desmoids are at particular risk and should have an IPAA as an initial procedure when technically feasible because future attempts at proctectomy may be impossible because of dense desmoid fibrosis. However, patients with extensive mesenteric desmoids at initial operation may be poor candidates for IPAA because a shortened mesentery may prohibit the terminal ileal pouch from reaching the anal canal. In addition, desmoids may

cause subsequent pouch-related complications such as ulceration, bleeding, or dysfunction from pressure effects. The presence of an intraabdominal desmoid tumor can preclude the formation of IPAA, either at the time of colectomy or for completion proctectomy after IRA.[21]

Another important consideration when choosing a surgical procedure is the potential effect on fertility in young women. Because of evidence that IPAA is associated with decreased fertility in ulcerative colitis patients, there has been some concern that this is also true after IPAA in FAP patients.[51,52] A population based study in Denmark, Finland, Sweden, and Norway showed that fertility was decreased after IPAA, though not to the same extent as it was for ulcerative colitis patients; notably, it was not decreased following IRA.[53] However, a recent study of women with FAP in the Netherlands came to a different conclusion: They found no change in fertility based on the type of surgery (IRA, IPAA, or total proctocolectomy with ileostomy), indication, or complications. The only factors that affected fertility were age at diagnosis and age at first surgical procedure.[54] Some authors suggest that it may be worthwhile to perform IRA as the initial surgery in young women desiring children, with a plan for completion proctectomy and IPAA at a later date, if and when indicated.[53]

Attenuated Familial Adenomatous Polyposis. Attenuated FAP (AFAP) is a subset of FAP characterized by fewer, more proximal colonic distribution and later onset of polyps and cancer compared to classic FAP.[55] In one study, the mean number of adenomas was 25 and the average age of colorectal cancer diagnosis was 55 years.[56] The average lifetime risk of colorectal cancer is 69%.[57]

There is some correlation between genotype and AFAP phenotype. Mutations in the 5′ end of the gene, exon 6, exon 9, and after codon 1580 in the 3′ end have all been linked to an attenuated phenotype. Mutations at the 3′ end and within exon 9 are associated with fewer adenomas, whereas those at the 5′ end result in a more variable phenotype and more severe upper intestinal manifestations.[55,58] However, some of the genotype-phenotype variability within AFAP may be related to interactions with other hereditary or environmental factors.[58] Approximately 40% of AFAP patients have a detectable genetic mutation, which is considerably lower than the detection rate in classic FAP.[56] It is possible that some of the patients who do not have a detectable APC mutation may turn out to have MAP on further genetic evaluation.[59]

Extracolonic manifestations include gastric fundic gland polyps, gastric adenomas, duodenal adenomas, and periampullary tumors.[58] The frequencies of these upper gastrointestinal manifestations vary by report.[56,57] CHRPE, desmoids, and osteomas have been reported but appear to be rare in these patients.[57] Cancer in the stomach and duodenum may also occur at increased rates in this population.[57]

Diagnosis of AFAP may be difficult because of the wide variability of the phenotype. In addition, screening with flexible sigmoidoscopy is inadequate, because a number of AFAP patients have colonic lesions located beyond the reach of a flexible sigmoidoscope. The variability of extracolonic manifestations can also be a challenge in identifying AFAP patients. However, the presence of gastric fundic glands or other common extracolonic features should prompt a more detailed history and physical examination.

Surgical options for the AFAP patient are similar to those with classic FAP if many polyps are present. In reliable patients with relatively few polyps, close endoscopic surveillance and colonoscopic polypectomy may be feasible. When surgery is indicated, many AFAP patients are suitable candidates for IRA because of the tendency for rectal sparing. Compared with classic FAP patients undergoing the same procedure, fewer AFAP patients who undergo IRA develop rectal polyps or require secondary proctectomy.[56,57]

MUTYH-ASSOCIATED POLYPOSIS

MUTYH-associated polyposis (MAP) is an autosomal recessive disorder associated with multiple adenomas and carcinomas of the colon and rectum. Various studies have shown biallelic *MUTYH* mutations in 30% of patients with 10 to 100 polyps and no *APC* mutation.[60]

Genetics

The base excision repair gene called mutY homologue (*MUTYH* or *MYH*) excises products of oxidative damage in DNA.[61] This gene is located on chromosome 1p34.3-32.1. Two missense mutations, Y179C and G396D, account for the majority of *MUTYH* mutations identified, but other mutations are found at varying rates in different populations.[62] Deletions and in-frame skipping of exons have also been described.[63] When the *MUTYH* gene is mutated, a specific somatic G:C to T:A transversion occurs in the *APC* gene and base excision repair fails to correct it.[64] If this occurs in all cells, a polyposis phenotype results. Mutations in the *MUTYH* gene also affect the *K-ras* gene in a similar fashion. Mutations in *K-ras* have been found in MAP patients with adenomas and carcinomas.[65]

A very important feature of MAP is that the inheritance is autosomal recessive and the syndrome has variable penetrance. Heterozygous individuals have not been shown to be at an increased risk of colorectal cancer. When a patient with adenomatous polyposis is *APC* mutation negative, *MUTYH* variants have been shown to be present 30 to 50% of the time.[60,66] At this time, there is no reported role of *MUTYH* in sporadic colorectal cancer.[61]

Diagnosis

The phenotype of MAP tends to be closer to an AFAP phenotype, with fewer polyps and a higher likelihood of proximal colorectal cancer.[67] The average age at diagnosis is 45 years, and most patients are symptomatic at presentation.[68] Cancer risk for MAP is estimated at 100% and usually occurs between the fourth and seventh decade.[68] Some MAP patients may also have hyperplastic or sessile serrated adenomas. However, there have been no cases of MAP in patients with hyperplastic polyps and without multiple adenomas.[65]

Extraintestinal manifestations of MAP are less well described than other hereditary CRC syndromes. Duodenal polyps are found in 17% to 25% of cases.[68] Gastric adenomas and fundic gland polyps are also described. Extraintestinal cancers have been found to occur at a rate double that of the general population, including breast, endometrial, ovarian, bladder, and skin malignancies.[68] Benign tumors of the skin and soft tissue, endometrium, and breast have all been described. Desmoids and osteomas do not seem to occur. Though there are patients with both MAP and CHRPE, this appears to be an incidental association.[68]

One study determined that immunohistochemical and histologic features could not be used to distinguish between cancers arising in patients with MAP and sporadic colorectal cancers. The MAP patients' tumors tended to be low grade, have mild levels of extraglandular necrosis, and be associated with synchronous polyps. Most, but not all, are microsatellite stable. Although no differences were found regarding depth of tumor invasion, there was a lower frequency of positive lymph nodes in the *MUTYH* mutation group. Tumors were more likely to be located in the proximal colon compared with sporadic colon cancers.[60]

Management

When the adenomatous polyp burden is low, MAP may be managed endoscopically. Surgery is indicated when polyps cannot be managed endoscopically, either due to size, number, or difficulties completing surveillance colonoscopies. Some authors recommend endoscopic surveillance, while others believe that the high rate of carcinoma is an indication for prophylactic surgery.[69,70] When undergoing surgery, colectomy and ileorectal anastomosis is the most common procedure. However, if there is significant rectal involvement, total proctocolectomy and IPAA can be performed.[66]

LYNCH SYNDROME AND FAMILIAL COLORECTAL CANCER TYPE X

Lynch syndrome is an autosomal dominant familial CRC syndrome characterized by familial clustering of early age-of-onset CRC (average age, 40 to 48 years), as well as a variety of other cancers. It is the most common familial colorectal cancer predisposing syndrome and accounts for 2% to 3% of all colorectal cancers.[21] The first description of this syndrome was by Aldred Warthin in 1913, who reported a kindred known as "Family G" with an increased incidence of colon, gastric, and endometrial cancer.[71] However, the significance of the familial clustering of these malignancies was not fully appreciated until 1966, when Henry Lynch et al reported two large families with the "cancer family syndrome."[72] Further observations led to the description of two patterns of disease presentation, termed Lynch syndrome I (CRC only) and Lynch syndrome II (CRC and associated malignancies).[73] Because of the subsequent difficulty in differentiating between these two patterns of disease, the term hereditary nonpolyposis colorectal cancer (HNPCC) was given to this syndrome. However, the HNPCC label is used variably to include patients who meet the Amsterdam II Criteria (Box 163-1) with or without a mismatch repair gene mutation. Currently, individuals who meet the Amsterdam II Criteria and have positive gene mutation testing are referred to as having the Lynch syndrome; those

---

BOX 163-1 Amsterdam II Criteria for Diagnosis of Lynch Syndrome

At least three relatives who have an HNPCC-associated cancer (colorectal, endometrial, ureter, renal pelvis, small bowel)
One is a first-degree relative of the other two
At least two generations are affected
At least one relative was diagnosed at ≤50 years of age
Familial adenomatous polyposis has been excluded

From Vasen HF, Mecklin JP, Khan PM, et al: The International Collaborative Group on Hereditary Non-Polyposis Colorectal Cancer. *Dis Colon Rectum* 34:424, 1991.
HNPCC, Hereditary nonpolyposis colorectal cancer.

BOX 163-2 Revised Bethesda Guidelines for Testing of Colorectal Tumors for Microsatellite Instability

Individuals who meet any of the following criteria:
Colorectal cancer diagnosed at ≤50 years of age
Two HNPCC-related cancers (synchronous or metachronous)
Colorectal cancer with MSI-H histology at ≤60 years of age
First-degree relative who has HNPCC-related cancer, one of the cancers diagnosed at ≤50 years of age
Colorectal cancer in two or more first- or second-degree relatives with HNPCC-related tumors

From Umar A, Boland CR, Terdiman JP, et al: Revised Bethesda Guidelines for hereditary nonpolyposis colorectal cancer (Lynch syndrome) and microsatellite instability. *J Natl Cancer Inst* 96:261, 2004.
HNPCC, Hereditary nonpolyposis colorectal cancer; *MSI-H,* microsatellite instability—high.

---

who meet the criteria and are gene mutation test negative are referred to as familial colorectal cancer type X.[74]

Genetics

The genetic etiology of cancer predisposition in patients with Lynch syndrome is a germline mutation in a mismatch repair (MMR) gene, which recognizes and repairs mismatched nucleotides during DNA replication. When the MMR genes function properly, DNA nucleotides that are mismatched during replication are excised and replaced with the correct base pairs. Patients with a mutation in the MMR gene lack appropriate repair of mismatched DNA and express the "mutator phenotype." Cancer develops in these patients because of a failure of repair of replication errors and ultimately dysfunction of tumor suppressor genes and oncogenes. A number of different types of MMR gene mutations have been described, including truncating, missense, and frameshift mutation.

The first two MMR genes to be identified were *MSH2* and *MLH1*. Each of these proteins forms a heterodimer with so-called minor partners, *MSH6* and *PMS2*. Other mismatch repair genes are rarely implicated in Lynch syndrome and are not usually evaluated. In contrast to the chromosomal abnormalities associated with the classic adenoma-to-carcinoma sequence, the genetic changes associated with MMR mutations are more subtle. Microsatellite instability (MSI) refers to changes in small, repetitive DNA sequences. These changes accumulate from the failure of mismatch repair near the coding regions of growth regulatory genes. In colorectal cancer, these include the tumor suppressor genes transforming growth factor-β receptor II and BAX, as well as other regulators of the cell cycle, apoptosis, and immune surveillance. The protein products of these genes then become nonfunctional.

Deficient MMR proteins can also be present in sporadic colorectal cancer cases. However, the defective function is a result of methylation that silences the gene, rather than a mutation in the gene. This is called the CpG island methylator phenotype (CIMP). MLH1 is the gene most likely to be affected in this way in sporadic cases of MSI-H colon cancer.

Microsatellite instability is of prognostic significance in colon cancer. Tumors can be characterized as microsatellite stable (MSS), as having low microsatellite instability (MSI-L), or as having high microsatellite instability

(MSI-H). Patients with MSI-H colorectal cancer have a better prognosis when compared to patients with microsatellite-stable tumors of similar stages.[75] The absence of MMR proteins may also predict decreased responsiveness to 5-fluorouracil–based chemotherapy.[76]

Diagnosis

The Amsterdam II Criteria suggest the presence of Lynch syndrome. These criteria include three individuals in a kindred with colorectal or HNPCC-associated cancer—one a first-degree relative of the other two, occurring in at least two generations, and one with a diagnosis at age 50 years or younger. Additionally, FAP or AFAP must be excluded. Another set of guidelines for selecting patients for testing for MSI is the Bethesda Guidelines, which are more inclusive (Box 163-2).[21] The syndrome should be suspected in a patient with multiple adenomatous polyps, an early-onset colorectal or other associated cancer, and an appropriate family history.

The phenotype in Lynch syndrome includes tumors that tend to be right sided, an increased incidence of synchronous and metachronous colorectal cancers, and tumors that occur at an earlier age compared to sporadic colorectal cancer; 60% of carriers will develop colorectal cancer before age 50.[78]

Histologic features of adenomas and cancers associated with Lynch syndrome include an increased risk of dysplasia, the presence of tumor-infiltrating lymphocytes, and a Crohn-like lymphocytic reaction.[79] Tumors tend to be poorly differentiated, contain an excess of mucin, and often have signet cell features.[80] Adenomas seem to be more aggressive than sporadic adenomas, with an average progression to carcinoma in 2 to 3 years.[80]

There are several options for testing patients for Lynch syndrome. When cancer tissue is available, testing may begin with immunohistochemical (IHC) staining for the loss of MMR proteins.[77] IHC staining uses antibodies to the MMR proteins produced by the MMR genes. A lack of staining for a particular protein indicates a possible mutation of that gene. Although the sensitivity and specificity of IHC testing is excellent when performed on cancer tissue, only 70% of adenomas will have abnormal IHC in patients with a known MMR mutation.[81,82] IHC testing can also be used to screen for Lynch syndrome in all early-age-of-onset (<50 years) colorectal cancer patients. This systematic approach has yielded positive results in 19% of patients, most of whom would not have been suspected of having Lynch syndrome based on family history or traditional histologic markers.[83]

An alternative and equally effective option to IHC testing is MSI testing.[84] Microsatellite instability refers to the expansion or contraction of areas of DNA that are composed of short, repeating sequences of nucleotides. MSI testing compares the length of microsatellites in tumor DNA to normal DNA from blood or normal tissue. There is up to 94% of concordance between MSI and IHC testing in colorectal cancer tissue.[75] However, only 58% of adenomatous polyps will demonstrate MSI in patients with known MMR mutations. In this population, 70% of adenomatous polyps will demonstrate the absence of the appropriate MMR protein on IHC analysis.[81] Because the yield for MSI and IHC testing is lower in adenomatous polyps than it is in cancer, gene sequencing should be performed on the patient who presents with multiple adenomatous polyps when Lynch syndrome is suspected. If the involved gene is known from another affected family member, or based on loss of a specific MMR protein detected on IHC, only that gene needs to be sequenced. Recently, targeted genetic approaches such as the single amplicon *MSH2* A636P mutation test in Ashkenazi Jewish patients with colorectal cancer have demonstrated how a rapid and inexpensive preoperative test can be effectively used in certain populations.[85]

Extracolonic Manifestations

Lynch syndrome results in the development of a variety of extracolonic cancers including those of the small bowel, ureter, renal pelvis, pancreas, biliary tract, endometrium, ovaries, and brain. Associations with breast and prostate cancer have also been suggested.

Urogenital Cancers. Women with Lynch syndrome have a significantly higher rate of gynecologic cancers than the average population. These cancers tend to occur in the fifth to sixth decade of life.[34] Endometrial cancer risk is 43%, and ovarian cancer risk is 9%.[21] The risk of development of endometrial cancer is higher in *MSH2* and *MSH6* carriers compared with *MLH1* mutation carriers.[21] The Bethesda Guidelines recommend testing for MSI in any patient who is diagnosed with endometrial cancer before age 45 in order to screen for Lynch syndrome.

Upper urinary tract urothelial cancer is part of the Lynch syndrome spectrum. Individuals have a 6% lifetime risk of developing these tumors, which is 22 times that of the general population.[86] The highest-risk group is the *MSH2* mutation carriers, with an incidence of 28% for men and 12% for women.[86]

Gastric Cancer. The incidence of gastric cancer in Lynch syndrome patients is between 30% and 70%, or a relative risk of 2.9 to 6.1 times higher than the general population depending on the type of mutation. *MSH6* mutation carriers seem to have a very low risk, and those with an *MSH2* mutation have a higher risk than *MLH1* mutation carriers.[87] The incidence seems to vary by geography and time. Gastric cancer seems to be a less prominent feature in Western countries, and its predominance has decreased since the syndrome was first described.

When it does occur, it tends to be of the intestinal type rather than the diffuse type. In a study of the Dutch Hereditary Cancer Registry, carcinomas occurred in the antrum (15%), corpus (9%), or cardia (23%); the remaining locations were not described.[87]

Breast Cancer. The inclusion of breast cancer as a feature of Lynch syndrome has been somewhat controversial. Some studies have found that breast cancer in known MMR carriers demonstrates a high level of MSI and that breast cancer occurred at an earlier age in Lynch syndrome patients.[88] Authors have therefore concluded that MMR deficiencies may accelerate tumor growth and development but are unlikely to be the initiating event.

Cancer Screening and Surveillance

Colonoscopic, rather than sigmoidoscopic, surveillance is strongly recommended for families with Lynch syndrome, as 70% to 80% of cancers are proximal to the splenic flexure.[89] A prospective trial showed that surveillance led to a reduction in the incidence of colorectal cancer, and another study showed decreased mortality associated with surveillance.[90,91] Colonoscopic surveillance should be performed every 1 to 2 years.[92]

Screening for gynecologic cancers may include regular gynecologic examination, transvaginal ultrasound, and endometrial aspiration biopsy starting at age 25.[21] Recommendations for urologic cancer screening include urinalysis once or twice per year, even though there are no data to support the efficacy of this approach.[86] Despite the low sensitivity of urine cytology of 29%, some authors recommend annual screening with urinalysis, cytology, and urine ultrasound.[86] Screening for hematuria with dipstick testing and microscopy has also been suggested. These tests are not invasive and are relatively inexpensive. Given the preponderance of urothelial cancer in *MSH2* carriers, some have chosen to offer more aggressive screening for urothelial cancers in this higher risk group.

Surgical Management

The goals of surgical therapy are to maximize life expectancy and maintain quality of life. There are four groups of Lynch syndrome patients to consider: patients who are at risk but do not have cancer or adenomas at the time of presentation, those with newly diagnosed adenomas, those with newly diagnosed cancer, and those who have undergone segmental colectomy for colorectal cancer in the past.

For a variety of reasons, prophylactic surgery is not performed as frequently in Lynch syndrome patients as it is in FAP patients. However, mathematical models do seem to suggest a survival advantage if prophylactic surgery is performed at an early age. One study demonstrated an increased life expectancy of up to 2.3 years in patients who underwent extended colectomy at a younger age, and another showed the greatest improvement if surgery is performed at 25 years of age, before cancer is diagnosed.[93,94] Prophylactic colectomy may be considered in highly selected situations. Some patients who do not have cancer will have adenomas; these can be managed endoscopically in most cases. When the number, size, or recurrence precludes polypectomy, surgery is indicated. It may also be indicated when colonoscopy is technically difficult or impossible, or when the patient expresses a strong preference for prophylactic surgery. Other considerations include the similarity of lifetime cancer risk between patients with *APC* and MMR gene mutations, and the fact that total abdominal colectomy with IRA produces less functional disturbance than the prophylactic procedure sometimes recommended for FAP (total abdominal proctocolectomy with IPAA).

Surgical options for the management of colorectal cancer in a Lynch syndrome patient include segmental resection or total colectomy. Because of the high rate of metachronous colorectal neoplasms in Lynch syndrome patients, total colectomy rather than segmental colectomy is the recommended surgical procedure in a patient presenting with a colorectal cancer.[21] In one study, Lynch syndrome patients who underwent partial colectomy had a high rate of metachronous high-risk adenomas (22%) and carcinomas (25%) compared with patients who underwent total colectomy (11% and 8%, respectively).[95] It is therefore not surprising that Lynch syndrome patients who undergo total colectomy at initial operation will require fewer abdominal surgeries when compared with those who undergo segmental colectomy.[89] Despite these considerations, there are no prospective trials to demonstrate an improvement in survival in patients who undergo a more extensive resection at the time of initial surgery. Segmental resection requires close periodic colonoscopy, whereas surveillance following total colectomy requires only flexible sigmoidoscopy. However, IRA does not eliminate the risk of cancer in the rectum, which is estimated at 3% to 12% over 6 to 12 years.[34]

When a female Lynch syndrome patient is undergoing colon surgery, prophylactic hysterectomy and oophorectomy may be offered at the same time because of the increased risk for gynecologic cancers in these patients.[96] This option may depend on the age of the patient and her desires regarding future childbearing.

Familial Colorectal Cancer Type X

Familial colorectal cancer type X (FCC X) patients may appear similar to Lynch syndrome patients since the family history will meet Amsterdam II Criteria. However, the major distinguishing feature from Lynch syndrome is that these patients do not have a detectable MMR mutation. In addition, they are more likely to have left-sided cancer as compared to Lynch syndrome patients, and a slightly older age at presentation (55 vs. 41 years).[97] Overall, FCC X tumors tend to be more well-differentiated, more often aneuploid, and less often mucinous compared with the MSI-H tumors in Lynch syndrome.[98]

Individuals with FCC X have a twofold risk of developing colorectal cancer when compared to the general population, but appear to be at lower risk compared with Lynch syndrome patients.[99] There are no specific guidelines for colonoscopic surveillance for FCC X patients, but it is reasonable to use the guidelines for Lynch syndrome patients in this population.[100]

In these cases, it is difficult to assess patients' risk of extraintestinal manifestations. The largest study to date found no statistically increased risk for other cancers.[99]

However, other studies have shown a potential for association with a variety of other tumors.[68]

Surgical treatment should be based on the phenotype of the patient and patient preference. Prophylactic surgery is only recommended when polyps cannot be managed endoscopically. There are no data on the risk of metachronous cancers, so it is not known if total colectomy would offer any benefit over segmental colectomy at the time of surgery for cancer.

SERRATED POLYPOSIS SYNDROME

SPS (formerly known as Hyperplastic Polyposis Syndrome) is the presence of multiple hyperplastic polyps spread throughout the colon and rectum. Many patients will have a mix of hyperplastic polyps, serrated adenomas, and mixed polyps. Adenomas are also reported in many patients.[101] The phenotype of patients with SPS varies, with wide variation in the number and distribution of polyps, from a median of 6 to 40.[102,103] Most patients are diagnosed in the fourth or fifth decade of life.[104]

The World Health Organization criteria for diagnosis of SPS include any one of the following:
1. The presence of five or more hyperplastic or serrated polyps proximal to the sigmoid colon, with two or more measuring at least 1 cm in diameter
2. Any number of polyps occurring proximal to the sigmoid colon in an individual with a first-degree relative with SPS
3. More than 20 hyperplastic or serrated polyps of any size located anywhere in the colon.[105]

Other authors have suggested that atypical serrated polyps be included in the total polyp count, that the total polyp count be cumulative, and that the threshold polyp count be higher.[106,107]

Patients with other genetic polyposis syndromes may have hyperplastic polyps and patients with SPS may harbor other types of polyps. The coincident diagnosis of Lynch syndrome or FCC X and HPS has led some authors to postulate that a subgroup of patients have both oncogenic pathways, that serrated polyps and hyperplastic polyps are part of the Lynch syndrome, or that some patients are misdiagnosed when they actually have SPS.[102] In MAP, hyperplastic and serrated polyps are also noted and some patients who have a known *MUTYH* gene mutation also fit the criteria for HPS.[65]

The genetic etiology of SPS is unknown at this time. SPS is associated with an increased risk of colorectal cancer. However, the magnitude of the risk is not completely defined. Studies show a 40% to 50% rate of colorectal cancer, and although some studies report a predominance of proximal lesions, others report a majority of distal lesions.[101,102] When cancer does occur, the tumors have been found to occur at an early age of onset, in multiplicity, and can be MSS, MSI-L, or MSI-H.[104] Changes found within sessile serrated polyps, such as *BRAF* mutations and methylation of CpG islands, are likely part of the serrated neoplasia pathway that functions in this syndrome. There also appears to be a strong family history of colorectal cancer in patients with hyperplastic polyposis.

The management of SPS depends on the phenotype. When possible, polyps can be managed endoscopically.

However, because of the risk of carcinoma, if the colon cannot be cleared endoscopically, surgery should be considered. This is especially true if serrated adenomas are seen on histologic evaluation. The appropriate surgical procedure will be determined by the phenotype. When SPS presents with carcinoma, colectomy with ileorectal anastomosis may be considered if polyps are present throughout the colon.

HAMARTOMATOUS POLYPOSIS SYNDROMES

Hamartomatous polyps are benign, localized overgrowths of mature epithelial cells. The hamartomatous polyp syndromes are rare entities that include JPS, PJS, and PTEN hamartoma tumor syndrome—which includes Cowden syndrome and Bannayan-Riley-Ruvalcaba syndrome.

JUVENILE POLYPOSIS SYNDROME

Juvenile polyps are the most common type of polyp encountered in the pediatric population.[108] Solitary hamartomatous polyps are generally located in the rectosigmoid area and are separate from JPS. In the solitary form, polyps occur at age 4 to 5 years, whereas in JPS, most polyps present later, with an average age of 18.5 years at diagnosis.[109] The incidence of JPS is 1 in 100,000 to 160,000.[108] The diagnosis of JPS is based on meeting one of three criteria: 3 to 10 hamartomatous polyps detected on colonoscopy; hamartomatous polyps detected outside of the colon; or any number of hamartomatous polyps in a patient with a family history of juvenile polyps.[108]

There are three major subtypes of JPS: juvenile polyposis coli, in which hamartomatous polyps are only in the colon; generalized juvenile polyposis, in which hamartomatous polyps can be found in the colon, stomach, and small bowel; and juvenile polyposis of infancy, which is characterized by diarrhea, protein-losing enteropathy, bleeding, and rectal prolapse, and is often fatal.

Hamartomatous polyps appear grossly as spherical or lobular. Most are pedunculated and have long stalks. Size can range up to 3 cm. Typically, the polyps are very vascular with a smooth and glistening surface. Large polyps may have an ulcerated surface from autoinfarction.

Presenting symptoms include rectal bleeding, anemia, abdominal pain, diarrhea, intussusception, obstruction, and polyp prolapse.[109] Heart defects, polydactyly, clubbing, intestinal malrotation, Meckel diverticulum, hydrocephalus, macrocephaly, hypertelorism, cleft lip, cleft palate, double renal pelvis and ureter, bifid uterus and vagina, undescended testes, and supernumerary teeth have all been described in JPS patients. These extraintestinal manifestations have been reported in approximately 11% to 20% of cases.[108]

Twenty-five to 50% of JPS patients have a positive family history.[108] The disease has an autosomal dominant pattern with variable penetrance. The genes associated with JPS, SMAD4, BMPR1A, and ENG, are part of the TGF-β family of proteins. SMAD4 is also associated with hereditary hemorrhagic telangiectasia (HHT). Therefore, a patient presenting with HHT and found to have hamartomatous polyps on further investigation is more likely to have an SMAD4 mutation.

Though sporadic hamartomatous polyps do not confer a cancer risk, individuals with JPS are at risk of developing adenomatous changes and then carcinoma in their polyps. The estimated risk of colorectal cancer is between 17% and 48%, occurring at a mean age of 34 to 43 years.[108] There is also an increased risk of intestinal, pancreatic, and gastric cancer in this syndrome.

At this time, there are no standardized screening guidelines for JPS. The most recent set of proposed guidelines suggests initiating screening colonoscopy at 15 to 18 years of age, and upper endoscopy at 25 years of age in asymptomatic patients. If the clinical and genetic workup is negative, screening should be continued every 1 to 2 years until age 35. If a mutation is detected, screening should continue until age 70.[110] However, these guidelines may be perceived as too stringent by others.

Indications for surgery in JPS are a large number of polyps that cannot be managed endoscopically, adenomatous change in one or more polyps, and severe symptoms including diarrhea, hypoproteinemia, and bleeding leading to anemia. Surgical options depend on distribution and number of polyps. Following surgery, endoscopic surveillance is essential.

PEUTZ-JEGHERS SYNDROME

PJS is a rare syndrome characterized by gastrointestinal tract hamartomatous polyps (usually <100) and mucocutaneous melanin pigmentation. The incidence is 1 in 150,000 to 1 in 200,000.[108] PJS is caused by a mutation in the tumor suppressor STK11 gene, known as LKB1, located on chromosome 19p13.3. It encodes a serine-threonine kinase that affects proteins essential in cell cycle arrest, apoptosis, and cellular energy levels. The diagnosis of PJS is made when one of the following is found: two or more histologically confirmed hamartomatous polyps, any number of hamartomatous polyps in an individual with a family history of PJS, characteristic mucocutaneous pigmentation in an individual with a family history of PJS, or hamartomatous polyps and mucocutaneous pigmentation. Twenty-five percent of PJS patients represent a de novo STK11 mutation, with no family history.[111] There are reports of overexpression of COX-2 in PJS polyps and cancers. Additionally, a few families with PJS have shown linkage to a different genetic locus, so there may be some genetic heterogeneity.[112]

The gastrointestinal polyps range in size from less than 1 mm to 4 cm in diameter. The most common site is the jejunum and the rest of the small bowel (60%), whereas colonic polyps are found in approximately half of all cases.[112] Gastric polyps are also frequent. Additionally, polyps outside the gastrointestinal tract including the nose, bronchi, renal pelvis, and biliary tree have all been described. The polyps are hamartomas, with hypertrophy or hyperplasia of smooth muscle in the intestinal wall. Normal epithelium usually covers the polyps, and mucus-filled cysts are common. The polyps of PJS are known to have frond-like elongated epithelium, cystic duct dilation that extends to the submucosa or muscularis propria, and smooth muscle that extends into the superficial epithelial layer in a pattern labeled arborization. Epithelial cell trapping, or pseudoinvasion, also occurs (Figure 163-11). Because of these features, when

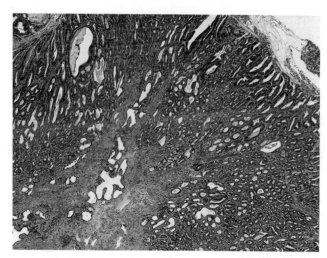

FIGURE 163-11 Microscopic appearance of a Peutz-Jeghers polyp. (Courtesy Jinru Shia, MD, Department of Pathology, Memorial Sloan-Kettering Cancer Center, New York.)

TABLE 163-5 Recommendations for Screening and Surveillance in Peutz-Jeghers Syndrome

Colon and rectum	Baseline colonoscopy at age 8
	If polyps detected, colonoscopy every 3 years until age 50
	If no polyps detected, repeat colonoscopy at age 18 and every 3 years after until age 50
	Continue surveillance at 1- to 2-year intervals after age 50
Small intestine	Baseline EGD at age 8
	If polyps detected, EGD every 3 years until age 50
	If no polyps detected, repeat EGD at age 18 and every 3 years after until age 50
	Continue surveillance at 1- to 2-year intervals after age 50
	Baseline video capsule endoscopy at age 8
	Repeat every 3 years
Genital tract	Annual testicular examination beginning at birth until 12 years
	Testicular ultrasound if abnormalities on examination
	Cervical smear with liquid-based cytology at age 25 years
	Repeat every 3 years
Breast	Monthly self-examination beginning at age 18
	Annual breast MRI from age 25 to 50
	Annual mammography beginning at age 50
General	Annual complete blood count and liver function tests
	Annual full physical examination

From Beggs AD, Latchford AR, Vasen HFA, et al: Peutz-Jeghers syndrome: A systematic review and recommendations for management. *Gut* 59:975, 2010.
EGD, Endoscopic gastroduodenoscopy.

malignancy is diagnosed in a Peutz-Jeghers polyp, cellular atypia or an elevated mitotic rate is noted.

The characteristic hypermelanotic macules of PJS are most frequently found in the perioral region, buccal mucosa, digits of the hands and feet, and perianal and genital regions. The most common sites are the vermilion border of the lips, which is noted in 95% of cases, followed by the buccal mucosa.[108] Mucocutaneous pigmentation usually appears in infancy. Macules vary in size. Pigmented spots tend to occur in the first few years of life, reach a maximal level in adolescence, and can fade after puberty.

The most common presentation of PJS is abdominal pain due to intussusception. Patients may also present with symptoms of obstruction from large polyps, anemia, hematochezia, or hematemesis. Biliary obstruction and gastric outlet obstruction are unusual presentations of PJS. Approximately one-third of patients will present in the first decade of life, and up to two-thirds by the third decade.[108]

Patients with PJS have an estimated risk of cancer ranging between 23% and 93%.[108,112] The average age of first detected malignancy is 43 years. The syndrome has been linked to adenocarcinoma of the esophagus, stomach, small intestine, and colon. Extraintestinal cancers of the thyroid, breast, lung, pancreas, gallbladder and biliary tree have all been described. In women, there is an increased risk of malignancies of the ovary and uterus and in men there is an increased risk of Sertoli cell tumor of the testis. It is not surprising that the major cause of death in PJS patients is malignancy.[113]

The role of PJS polyps in cancer remains controversial. It has been proposed that there is a hamartoma-adenoma-carcinoma pathway, whereas others believe that there is no malignant potential in PJS polyps.[112] Some PJS polyps have been shown to be polyclonal and possibly represent a form of mucosal prolapse caused by changes in cell polarity because of mutations in the *STK11* gene, rather than a true hamartoma. This would imply that cancer arises on a background of mucosal

instability.[112] Dysplasia and neoplasia in PJS polyps is extremely rare.

A surveillance regimen is important for all PJS patients. The Mallorca guidelines aim to detect polyps before they become symptomatic and detect cancer at an early stage (Table 163-5).[112] Surgical intervention in patients with PJS is indicated for symptomatic lesions, complications related to polyposis, polyps larger than 1.5 cm that are not able to be removed endoscopically, or cancer.[113] Aggressive endoscopic polypectomy may limit the need for operative intervention or increase the interval between surgical interventions, but it is not clear if polypectomy alters cancer risk.[112] The introduction of laparoscope-assisted endoscopic polyp clearance in PJS may further reduce morbidity and improve management of these patients. Indications for bowel resection include the detection of adenomatous changes in an incompletely removed polyp, as well as patients presenting with intussusception, obstruction, or gastrointestinal bleeding. Prophylactic colectomy is not recommended because of the relatively low incidence of CRC.

PTEN HAMARTOMA TUMOR SYNDROME

The *PTEN* hamartoma tumor syndrome includes both Cowden syndrome and Bannayan-Riley-Ruvalcaba syndrome. Both are associated with gene mutations on chromosome 10q23.3, and the differences between the syndromes are likely based on variable phenotypic expression. The *PTEN* gene is a tumor suppressor gene that acts as a negative regulator of the Akt/PKB signaling pathway, which regulates levels of phosphoinositol triphosphate. It is also involved in regulating cell cycle, apoptosis, and angiogenesis. Although intestinal polyps are important features of these syndromes, they are both characterized primarily by their extraintestinal manifestations. There is no strong evidence of an increased risk for colorectal cancer, but there is a risk of colon polyps. The polyps have the gross and histologic appearance of other hamartomatous polyps.

Cowden syndrome is an autosomal dominant syndrome with an incidence of 1 in 200,000.[108] Its characteristic features are benign hamartomas and malignant tumors of the breast, thyroid, uterus, brain, and mucocutaneous tissue. Hamartomatous polyps throughout the intestines are associated with Cowden syndrome in anywhere from 30% to 85% of cases.[108] Diagnosis is based on meeting pathognomonic, major, and minor criteria developed by the National Comprehensive Cancer Network (NCCN). Approximately 85% of Cowden syndrome patients are found to have germline mutations of the *PTEN* gene.[111]

Breast cancer rates in women with Cowden syndrome are between 30% to 50%; men are also at risk.[108] Benign breast conditions are also common in Cowden syndrome. Thyroid abnormalities including goiter, thyroglossal duct cysts, and thyroid cancer are an important feature of Cowden syndrome. Renal cell cancer has also been described.

Bannayan-Riley-Ruvalcaba syndrome is characterized by macrocephaly, developmental delays, pigmented speckling of the penis in men, and lipomas and hamartomas of the intestine. The incidence of gastrointestinal polyps is 45%.[108] There are no formal diagnostic criteria because this syndrome is so rare, and the cancer risk has not been elucidated. Most authors suggest considering individuals with Bannayan-Riley-Ruvalcaba syndrome at higher than average risk for malignancy, similar to Cowden syndrome. More than 60% of Bannayan-Riley-Ruvalcaba syndrome patients are found to have germline mutations of the *PTEN* gene.[111]

Guidelines for screening and surveillance of patients with *PTEN* mutations have been developed by the NCCN as surveillance is the cornerstone of management for these syndromes. They include breast cancer screening beginning at age 25 or younger, thyroid cancer screening starting at age 18, and endometrial cancer screening beginning at age 35. Renal cancer screening is also recommended. At this time, manifestations of PTEN hamartoma tumor syndrome are treated the same way as their sporadic counterparts.[114]

CRONKHITE-CANADA SYNDROME

Cronkhite-Canada syndrome is a rare acquired gastrointestinal polyposis syndrome characterized by hamartomatous polyps (similar to juvenile polyps) and other epidermal changes including dystrophic changes in the nails, alopecia, and cutaneous hyperpigmentation.[115] It involves tissues arising from the ectodermal germ cell layer but does not appear to be an inherited disorder.

The etiology of Cronkhite-Canada syndrome is unclear, although infection, toxins, nutritional deficiency, and psychological and physical stress all have been suspected as risk factors.

Patients typically present in the sixth decade of life with cutaneous or gastrointestinal manifestations. Symptoms including watery diarrhea associated with dysgeusia (alterations in taste), anemia and electrolyte disturbances that may be related to malabsorption, anorexia, weight loss, peripheral edema, and hypoproteinemia are characteristic. Cutaneous manifestations include alopecia, macular pigmentation, patchy vitiligo, and onychodystrophy and other nail changes, and skin hyperpigmentation.[109] Polyps are found throughout the gastrointestinal tract, with characteristic sparing of the esophagus. The most common site of gastrointestinal involvement is the stomach, although the small and large bowel are also affected.

Complications of Cronkhite-Canada syndrome are often severe and include mucosal ulceration, gastrointestinal bleeding, infection, and malnutrition. Severe intestinal polyposis can cause profound metabolic and electrolyte disturbances. In addition, intussusception and rectal prolapse have been described in these patients. There is also a cancer risk associated with the syndrome from the transition from hamartomatous polyps in the colon to adenomatous polyps, which then go on to develop dysplasia and eventually carcinoma.[109] Rates of colorectal cancer and gastric cancer seem to be increased.[111]

No formal recommendations exist regarding surveillance protocols, but because of the increased risk of cancer of the stomach, colon, and rectum, endoscopic surveillance has been advocated, as often as on a yearly basis.[115] Supportive care, with management of fluids, electrolytes, nutrition, and anemia, is an important consideration. Corticosteroids, antibiotics, anabolic steroids, cromolyn sodium, histamine receptor antagonists, and proton pump inhibitors have been used with variable success. Medical management is usually required for 6 to 12 months, and corticosteroids have been used successfully for disease recurrence.

Surgical management may be indicated if the stomach, colon, or rectum is the source of excessive bleeding, bowel obstruction, or cancer. However, case reports suggest that surgical management of Cronkhite-Canada syndrome may be associated with high perioperative morbidity.

HEREDITARY MIXED POLYPOSIS SYNDROME

Hereditary mixed polyposis syndrome (HMPS) is an autosomal dominant inherited polyposis syndrome characterized by colon polyps of varied histology, increased risk of CRC, and no extraintestinal manifestations. The colon lesions include hamartomas, adenomas, serrated polyps, and hyperplastic polyps. The hamartomas are similar to those seen in juvenile polyposis, and the adenomas may be tubular, villous, or flat.[109] Hyperplastic and serrated polyps with areas of dysplasia have also been described in patients with this syndrome. Hereditary mixed polyposis syndrome is associated with early-age-of-onset CRC. There is no evidence that patients with this syndrome are at increased risk for any other type of cancer.

The polyps in HMPS are spread evenly throughout the colon and usually number fewer than 15.[109] The colon appears to be the only affected organ system, with no extraintestinal manifestations yet described. Several kindred with HMPS have been the subject of genetic investigations. Linkage analysis of these families has implicated several candidate genes. *CRAC1*, on chromosome 15q14-22, has been noted to be altered in some HMPS families. Another family demonstrated a deletion at chromosome 15q21.1, where the tumor suppressor gene *THBS1* was felt to be the involved gene.[109]

Because phenotypic heterogeneity is common among the gastrointestinal polyposis syndromes, clinical distinction of the hereditary mixed polyposis syndrome from FAP, MAP, Lynch syndrome, JPS, and PJS may initially be difficult. However, patients with hereditary mixed polyposis syndrome do not display the characteristic extracolonic features of FAP and PJS, and patients with Lynch syndrome and MAP do not have hamartomatous polyps. It is more difficult to distinguish hereditary mixed polyposis syndrome from juvenile polyposis. However, pure adenomas are rare in juvenile polyposis. In addition, patients with juvenile polyposis usually have more extensive polyposis and tend to be diagnosed with polyps and cancer at an earlier age than patients with hereditary mixed polyposis syndrome.

Because of the rarity of this syndrome, definitive management recommendations have yet to be established. However, because polyps have been detected as early as 18 years of age and can develop within a 2-year interval, screening colonoscopy should begin at age 18 to 20 years and be repeated every 1 to 2 years. Total abdominal colectomy with ileorectal anastomosis is an option for selected individuals and should be the treatment of choice for patients who develop CRC. In these circumstances, close postoperative surveillance following surgery is mandatory because cancer may develop in the rectal remnant.

REFERENCES

1. Gillespie PE, Chambers TJ, Chan KW, et al: Colonic adenomas—a colonoscopy survey. *Gut* 20:240, 1979.
2. O'Brien MJ, Winawer SJ, Zauber AG, et al: The National Polyp Study: Patient and polyp characteristics associated with high-grade dysplasia in colorectal adenomas. *Gastroenterology* 98:371, 1990.
3. Heitman S, Ronksley P, Hilsden R, et al: Prevalence of adenomas and colorectal cancer in average risk individuals: A systematic review and meta-analysis. *Clin Gastroenter Hepatol* 7:1272, 2009.
4. Torlakovic E, Snover DC: Serrated adenomatous polyposis in humans. *Gastroenterology* 110:748, 1996.
5. Lu F-I, van Niekerk D, Owen D, et al: Longitudinal outcome study of sessile serrated adenomas of the colorectum: An increased risk for subsequent right-sided colorectal carcinoma. *Am J Surg Pathol* 34:927, 2010.
6. Bauer V, Papaconstantinou H: Management of serrated adenomas and hyperplastic polyps. *Clin Colon Rectal Surg* 21:273, 2008.
7. Mesiya S, Ancha H, Ancha H, et al: Sporadic colonic hamartomas in adults: A retrospective study. *Gastrointest Endosc* 62:886, 2005.
8. Bulow S: Results of national registration of familial adenomatous polyposis. *Gut* 52:742, 2003.
9. Okada K, Bartolini F, Deaconescu A, et al: Adenomatous polyposis coli protein nucleates actin assembly and synergizes with the formin mDia1. *J Cell Biol* 189:1087, 2010.
10. Aoki K, Taketo M: Adenomatous polyposis coli (APC): A multi-functional tumor suppressor gene. *J Cell Sci* 120:3327, 2007.
11. Obrador-Hevia A, Chin S-F, Gonzalez S, et al: Oncogenic KRAS is not necessary for Wnt signalling activation in APC-associated FAP adenomas. *J Pathol* 221:57, 2010.
12. Church J: Familial adenomatous polyposis. *Surg Oncol Clin North Am* 18:585, 2009.
13. Jasperson K, Tuohy T, Neklason D, et al: Hereditary and familial colon cancer. *Gastroenterology* 138:2044, 2010.
14. Groen E, Roos A, Muntinghe F, et al: Extra-intestinal manifestations of familial adenomatous polyposis. *Ann Surg Oncol* 15:2439, 2008.
15. Harb WJ, Sturgis EM: Differentiated thyroid cancer associated with intestinal polyposis syndromes: A review. *Head Neck* 31:1511, 2009.
16. Herraiz M, Barbesino G, Faquin W, et al: Prevalence of thyroid cancer in familial adenomatous polyposis syndrome and the role of screening ultrasound examinations. *Clin Gastroenterol Hepatol* 5:367, 2007.
17. Harach HR, Williams GT, Williams ED: Familial adenomatous polyposis associated thyroid carcinoma: A distinct type of follicular cell neoplasm. *Histopathology* 25:549, 1994.
18. Perrier ND, van Heerden JA, Goellner JR, et al: Thyroid cancer in patients with familial adenomatous polyposis. *World J Surg* 22:738; discussion 743, 1998.
19. Elayi E, Manilich E, Church J: Polishing the crystal ball: Knowing genotype improves ability to predict desmoid disease in patients with familial adenomatous polyposis. *Dis Colon Rectum* 52:1762, 2009.
20. de Campos FG, Perez RO, Imperiale AR, et al: Evaluating causes of death in familial adenomatous polyposis. *J Gastrointest Surg* 14:1943, 2010.
21. Guillem J, Wood W, Moley J, et al: ASCO/SSO review of current role of risk-reducing surgery in common hereditary cancer syndromes. *J Clin Oncol* 24:4642, 2006.
22. Sinha A, Gibbons D, Phillips R, et al: Surgical prophylaxis in familial adenomatous polyposis: Do pre-existing desmoids outside the abdominal cavity matter? *Fam Cancer* 9:407, 2010.
23. Church J, Berk T, Boman B, et al: Staging intra-abdominal desmoid tumors in familial adenomatous polyposis: A search for a uniform approach to a troubling disease. *Dis Colon Rectum* 48:1528, 2005.
24. Hansmann A, Adolph C, Vogel T, et al: High-dose tamoxifen and sulindac as first-line treatment for desmoid tumors. *Cancer* 100:612, 2004.
25. de Camargo VP, Keohan ML, D'Adamo DR, et al: Clinical outcomes of systemic therapy for patients with deep fibromatosis (desmoid tumor). *Cancer* 116:2258, 2010.
26. Micke O, Seegenschmiedt MH: Radiation therapy for aggressive fibromatosis (desmoid tumors): Results of a national Patterns of Care Study. *Int J Radiat Oncol Biol Phys* 61:882, 2005.
27. Nuyttens JJ, Rust PF, Thomas CR Jr, et al: Surgery versus radiation therapy for patients with aggressive fibromatosis or desmoid tumors: A comparative review of 22 articles. *Cancer* 88:1517, 2000.
28. Lynch HT, Snyder C, Davies JM, et al: FAP, gastric cancer, and genetic counseling featuring children and young adults: A family study and review. *Fam Cancer* 9:581, 2010.
29. Spigelman AD, Williams CB, Talbot IC, et al: Upper gastrointestinal cancer in patients with familial adenomatous polyposis. *Lancet* 2:783, 1989.
30. Latchford A, Neale K, Spigelman A, et al: Features of duodenal cancer in patients with familial adenomatous polyposis. *Clin Gastroenterol Hepatol* 7:659, 2009.
31. Gunther U, Bojarski C, Buhr HJ, et al: Capsule endoscopy in small-bowel surveillance of patients with hereditary polyposis syndromes. *Int J Colorectal Dis* 25:1377, 2010.
32. Aretz S, Koch A, Uhlhaas S, et al: Should children at risk for familial adenomatous polyposis be screened for hepatoblastoma and children with apparently sporadic hepatoblastoma be screened for APC germline mutations? *Pediatric Blood Cancer* 47:811, 2006.
33. Attard T, Giglio P, Koppula S, et al: Brain tumors in individuals with familial adenomatous polyposis: A cancer registry experience and pooled case report analysis. *Cancer* 109:761, 2007.

34. Smith KD, Rodriguez-Bigas MA: Role of surgery in familial adenomatous polyposis and hereditary nonpolyposis colorectal cancer (Lynch syndrome). *Surg Oncol Clin N Am* 18:705, 2009.

35. Giardiello FM, Hamilton SR, Krush AJ, et al: Treatment of colonic and rectal adenomas with sulindac in familial adenomatous polyposis. *N Engl J Med* 328:1313, 1993.

36. Steinbach G, Lynch PM, Phillips RK, et al: The effect of celecoxib, a cyclooxygenase-2 inhibitor, in familial adenomatous polyposis. *N Engl J Med* 342:1946, 2000.

37. Lynch P, Ayers G, Hawk E, et al: The safety and efficacy of celecoxib in children with familial adenomatous polyposis. *Am J Gastroenterol* 105:1437, 2010.

38. Giardiello FM, Yang VW, Hylind LM, et al: Primary chemoprevention of familial adenomatous polyposis with sulindac. *N Engl J Med* 346:1054, 2002.

39. Silverstein FE, Faich G, Goldstein JL, et al: Gastrointestinal toxicity with celecoxib vs nonsteroidal anti-inflammatory drugs for osteoarthritis and rheumatoid arthritis: The CLASS study: A randomized controlled trial. Celecoxib Long-term Arthritis Safety Study. *JAMA* 284:1247, 2000.

40. Cruz-Correa M, Hylind LM, Romans KE, et al: Long-term treatment with sulindac in familial adenomatous polyposis: A prospective cohort study. *Gastroenterology* 122:641, 2002.

41. West N, Clark S, Phillips RKS, et al: Eicosapentaenoic acid reduces rectal polyp number and size in familial adenomatous polyposis. *Gut* 59:918, 2010.

42. da Luz Moreira A, Church J, Burke C: The evolution of prophylactic colorectal surgery for familial adenomatous polyposis. *Dis Colon Rectum* 52:1481, 2009.

43. Aziz O, Athanasiou T, Fazio VW, et al: Meta-analysis of observational studies of ileorectal versus ileal pouch-anal anastomosis for familial adenomatous polyposis. *Br J Surg* 93:407, 2006.

44. Heiskanen I, Jrvinen HJ: Fate of the rectal stump after colectomy and ileorectal anastomosis for familial adenomatous polyposis. *Int J Colorectal Dis* 12:9, 1997.

45. Nieuwenhuis M, Blow S, Bjrk J, et al: Genotype predicting phenotype in familial adenomatous polyposis: A practical application to the choice of surgery. *Dis Colon Rectum* 52:1259, 2009.

46. Bulow S, Bulow C, Vasen H, et al: Colectomy and ileorectal anastomosis is still an option for selected patients with familial adenomatous polyposis. *Dis Colon Rectum* 51:1318, 2008.

47. El-Gazzaz GS, Kiran RP, Remzi FH, et al: Outcomes for case-matched laparoscopically assisted versus open restorative proctocolectomy. *Br J Surg* 96:522, 2009.

48. Fichera A, Silvestri M, Hurst R, et al: Laparoscopic restorative proctocolectomy with ileal pouch anal anastomosis: A comparative observational study on long-term functional results. *J Gastrointest Surg* 13:526, 2009.

49. Larson D, Dozois E, Piotrowicz K, et al: Laparoscopic-assisted vs. open ileal pouch-anal anastomosis: Functional outcome in a case-matched series. *Dis Colon Rectum* 48:1845, 2005.

50. Larson D, Davies M, Dozois E, et al: Sexual function, body image, and quality of life after laparoscopic and open ileal pouch-anal anastomosis. *Dis Colon Rectum* 51:392, 2008.

51. Lepist A, Sarna S, Tiitinen A, et al: Female fertility and childbirth after ileal pouch-anal anastomosis for ulcerative colitis. *Br J Surg* 94:478, 2007.

52. Waljee A, Waljee J, Morris AM, et al: Threefold increased risk of infertility: A meta-analysis of infertility after ileal pouch anal anastomosis in ulcerative colitis. *Gut* 55:1575, 2006.

53. Olsen KO, Juul S, Bulow S, et al: Female fecundity before and after operation for familial adenomatous polyposis. *Br J Surg* 90:227, 2003.

54. Nieuwenhuis MH, Douma KF, Bleiker EM, et al: Female fertility after colorectal surgery for familial adenomatous polyposis: A nationwide cross-sectional study. *Ann Surg* 252:341, 2010.

55. Soravia C, Berk T, Madlensky L, et al: Genotype-phenotype correlations in attenuated adenomatous polyposis coli. *Am J Hum Genet* 62:1290, 1998.

56. Knudsen AL, Bulow S, Tomlinson I, et al: Attenuated familial adenomatous polyposis (AFAP) results from an international collaborative study. *Colorectal Dis* 12:243, 2010.

57. Burt R, Leppert M, Slattery M, et al: Genetic testing and phenotype in a large kindred with attenuated familial adenomatous polyposis. *Gastroenterology* 127:444, 2004.

58. Hernegger GS, Moore HG, Guillem JG: Attenuated familial adenomatous polyposis: An evolving and poorly understood entity. *Dis Colon Rectum* 45:127; discussion 134, 2002.

59. Filipe B, Baltazar C, Albuquerque C, et al: APC or MUTYH mutations account for the majority of clinically well-characterized families with FAP and AFAP phenotype and patients with more than 30 adenomas. *Clin Genet* 76:242, 2009.

60. O'Shea AM, Cleary SP, Croitoru MA, et al: Pathological features of colorectal carcinomas in MYH-associated polyposis. *Histopathology* 53:184, 2008.

61. Markowitz SD, Bertagnolli MM: Molecular origins of cancer: Molecular basis of colorectal cancer. *N Engl J Med* 361:2449, 2009.

62. Sampson JR, Jones S, Dolwani S, et al: MutYH (MYH) and colorectal cancer. *Biochem Soc Trans* 33:679, 2005.

63. Fostira F, Papademitriou C, Efremidis A, et al: An in-frame exon-skipping MUTYH mutation is associated with early-onset colorectal cancer. *Dis Colon Rectum* 53:1197, 2010.

64. Gryfe R: Overview of colorectal cancer genetics. *Surg Oncol Clin N Am* 18:573, 2009.

65. Boparai K, Dekker E, Van Eeden S, et al: Hyperplastic polyps and sessile serrated adenomas as a phenotypic expression of MYH-associated polyposis. *Gastroenterology* 135:2014, 2008.

66. Dunlop MG, Farrington SM: MUTYH-associated polyposis and colorectal cancer. *Surg Oncol Clin N Am* 18:599, 2009.

67. Lubbe S, Di Bernardo M, Chandler I, et al: Clinical implications of the colorectal cancer risk associated with MUTYH mutation. *J Clin Oncol* 27:3975, 2009.

68. Vogt S, Jones N, Christian D, et al: Expanded extracolonic tumor spectrum in MUTYH-associated polyposis. *Gastroenterology* 137:1976, 2009.

69. Vasen HF, Moslein G, Alonso A, et al: Guidelines for the clinical management of familial adenomatous polyposis (FAP). *Gut* 57:704, 2008.

70. Leite JS, Isidro G, Martins M, et al: Is prophylactic colectomy indicated in patients with MYH-associated polyposis? *Colorectal Dis* 7:327, 2005.

71. Warthin A: Heredity with reference to carcinoma. *Arch Intern Med* 12:546, 1913.

72. Lynch HT, Shaw MW, Magnuson CW, et al: Hereditary factors in cancer. Study of two large midwestern kindreds. *Arch Intern Med* 117:206, 1966.

73. Vasen HF, Mecklin JP, Khan PM, et al: The International Collaborative Group on Hereditary Non-Polyposis Colorectal Cancer (ICG-HNPCC). *Dis Colon Rectum* 34:424, 1991.

74. Lindor N: Familial colorectal cancer type X: The other half of hereditary nonpolyposis colon cancer syndrome. *Surg Oncol Clin North Am* 18:637, 2009.

75. Hampel H: Point: Justification for Lynch syndrome screening among all patients with newly diagnosed colorectal cancer. *J Nat Comprehensive Cancer Net* 8:597, 2010.

76. Sargent DJ, Marsoni S, Monges G, et al: Defective mismatch repair as a predictive marker for lack of efficacy of fluorouracil-based adjuvant therapy in colon cancer. *J Clin Oncol* 28:3219, 2010.

77. Umar A, Boland CR, Terdiman JP, et al: Revised Bethesda Guidelines for hereditary nonpolyposis colorectal cancer (Lynch syndrome) and microsatellite instability. *J Nat Cancer Inst* 96:261, 2004.

78. Lynch P: The hMSH2 and hMLH1 genes in hereditary nonpolyposis colorectal cancer. *Surg Oncol Clin North Am* 18:611, 2009.

79. Meijer TWH, Hoogerbrugge N, Nagengast F, et al: In Lynch syndrome adenomas, loss of mismatch repair proteins is related to an enhanced lymphocytic response. *Histopathology* 55:414, 2009.

80. Drescher KM, Sharma P, Lynch HT: Current hypotheses on how microsatellite instability leads to enhanced survival of Lynch syndrome patients. *Clin Dev Immunol* 2010:170432, 2010.

81. Pino M, Mino-Kenudson M, Wildemore B, et al: Deficient DNA mismatch repair is common in Lynch syndrome-associated colorectal adenomas. *J Mole Diagnost* 11:238, 2009.

82. Recommendations from the EGAPP Working Group: Genetic testing strategies in newly diagnosed individuals with colorectal cancer aimed at reducing morbidity and mortality from Lynch syndrome in relatives. *Genet Med* 11:35, 2009.

83. Lee-Kong SA, Markowitz AJ, Glogowski E, et al: Prospective immunohistochemical analysis of primary colorectal cancers for loss of mismatch repair protein expression. *Clin Colorectal Cancer* 9:255, 2010.

84. Baudhuin LM, Burgart LJ, Leontovich O, et al: Use of microsatellite instability and immunohistochemistry testing for the identification of individuals at risk for Lynch syndrome. *Fam Cancer* 4:255, 2005.

85. Guillem JG, Glogowski E, Moore HG, et al: Single-amplicon MSH2 A636P mutation testing in Ashkenazi Jewish patients with colorectal cancer: Role in presurgical management. *Ann Surg* 245:560, 2007.

86. Acher P, Kiela G, Thomas K, et al: Towards a Rational Strategy for the Surveillance of Patients with Lynch Syndrome (Hereditary Non-Polyposis Colon Cancer) for Upper Tract Transitional Cell Carcinoma. *BJU Int* 106:300, 2010.

87. Capelle L, Van Grieken NCT, Lingsma H, et al: Risk and epidemiological time trends of gastric cancer in Lynch syndrome carriers in the Netherlands. *Gastroenterology* 138:487, 2010.

88. Walsh M, Buchanan D, Cummings M, et al: Lynch syndrome-associated breast cancers: Clinicopathologic characteristics of a case series from the colon cancer family registry. *Clin Cancer Res* 16:2214, 2010.

89. Natarajan N, Watson P, Silva-Lopez E, et al: Comparison of extended colectomy and limited resection in patients with Lynch syndrome. *Dis Colon Rectum* 53:77, 2010.

90. Vasen HFA, Abdirahman M, Brohet R, et al: One to 2-year surveillance intervals reduce risk of colorectal cancer in families with Lynch syndrome. *Gastroenterology* 138:2300, 2010.

91. de Jong AE, Hendriks YM, Kleibeuker JH, et al: Decrease in mortality in Lynch syndrome families because of surveillance. *Gastroenterology* 130:665, 2006.

92. Steinhagen E, Markowitz AJ, Guillem JG: How to manage a patient with multiple adenomatous polyps. *Surg Oncol Clin N Am* 19:711, 2010.

93. de Vos tot Nederveen Cappel WH, Buskens E, van Duijvendijk P, et al: Decision analysis in the surgical treatment of colorectal cancer due to a mismatch repair gene defect. *Gut* 52:1752, 2003.

94. Syngal S, Weeks JC, Schrag D, et al: Benefits of colonoscopic surveillance and prophylactic colectomy in patients with hereditary nonpolyposis colorectal cancer mutations. *Ann Intern Med* 129:787, 1998.

95. Kalady M, McGannon E, Vogel J, et al: Risk of colorectal adenoma and carcinoma after colectomy for colorectal cancer in patients meeting Amsterdam criteria. *Ann Surg* 252:507, 2010.

96. Boilesen AEB, Bisgaard M, Bernstein I: Risk of gynecologic cancers in Danish hereditary non-polyposis colorectal cancer families. *Acta Obstet Gynecol Scand* 87:1129, 2008.

97. Mueller-Koch Y, Vogelsang H, Kopp R, et al: Hereditary nonpolyposis colorectal cancer: Clinical and molecular evidence for a new entity of hereditary colorectal cancer. *Gut* 54:1733, 2005.

98. Valle L, Perea J, Carbonell P, et al: Clinicopathologic and pedigree differences in Amsterdam I-positive hereditary nonpolyposis colorectal cancer families according to tumor microsatellite instability status. *J Clin Oncol* 25:781, 2007.

99. Lindor N, Rabe K, Petersen G, et al: Lower cancer incidence in Amsterdam-I criteria families without mismatch repair deficiency: Familial colorectal cancer type X. *JAMA* 293:1979, 2005.

100. Rex D, Johnson D, Anderson J, et al: American College of Gastroenterology guidelines for colorectal cancer screening 2009 [corrected]. *Am J Gastroenterol* 104:739, 2009.

101. Buchanan D, Sweet K, Drini M, et al: Phenotypic diversity in patients with multiple serrated polyps: A genetics clinic study. *Int J Colorectal Dis* 25:703, 2010.

102. Jarrar A, Church J, Fay S, et al: Is the phenotype mixed or mistaken? Hereditary nonpolyposis colorectal cancer and hyperplastic polyposis syndrome. *Dis Colon Rectum* 52:1949, 2009.

103. Boparai K, Mathus-Vliegen EMH, Koornstra J, et al: Increased colorectal cancer risk during follow-up in patients with hyperplastic polyposis syndrome: A multicentre cohort study. *Gut* 59:1094, 2010.

104. Chow E, Lipton L, Lynch E, et al: Hyperplastic polyposis syndrome: Phenotypic presentations and the role of MBD4 and MYH. *Gastroenterology* 131:30, 2006.

105. Snover D, Ahnen DJ, Burt RW, et al: Serrated polyps of the colon and rectum and serrated polyposis. In Bosman FT, Carneiro F, et al, editors: *WHO cassication of tumours of the digestive system*, Lyon, 2010, IARC, p 160.

106. Higuchi T, Jass JR: My approach to serrated polyps of the colorectum. *J Clin Pathol* 57:682, 2004.

107. Hyman NH, Anderson P, Blasyk H: Hyperplastic polyposis and the risk of colorectal cancer. *Dis Colon Rectum* 47:2101, 2004.

108. Manfredi M: Hereditary hamartomatous polyposis syndromes: Understanding the disease risks as children reach adulthood. *Gastroenterol Hepatol* 6:185, 2010.

109. Calva D, Howe J: Hamartomatous polyposis syndromes. *Surg Clin North Am* 88:779, 2008.

110. Dunlop MG: Guidance on gastrointestinal surveillance for hereditary non-polyposis colorectal cancer, familial adenomatous polyposis, juvenile polyposis, and Peutz-Jeghers syndrome. *Gut* 51:V21, 2002.

111. Chen H-M, Fang J-Y: Genetics of the hamartomatous polyposis syndromes: A molecular review. *Int J Colorectal Dis* 24:865, 2009.

112. Beggs AD, Latchford AR, Vasen HFA, et al: Peutz-Jeghers syndrome: A systematic review and recommendations for management. *Gut* 59:975, 2010.

113. You YN, Wolff BG, Boardman LA, et al: Peutz-Jeghers syndrome: A study of long-term surgical morbidity and causes of mortality. *Fam Cancer* 9:609, 2010.

114. Hobert J, Eng C: PTEN hamartoma tumor syndrome: An overview. *Genet Med* 11:687, 2009.

115. Kao KT, Patel JK, Pampati V: Cronkhite-Canada syndrome: A case report and review of literature. *Gastroenterol Res Pract* 2009:619378, 2009.

Adenocarcinoma of the Colon and Rectum

Martin R. Weiser | Mitchell C. Posner | Leonard B. Saltz

Colorectal cancer remains one of the most dynamic fields in oncology, both in the laboratory and in the clinic. The molecular events associated with cellular transformation were reported more than 20 years ago, and mechanisms of carcinogenesis and tumor progression continue to be intensely studied. Molecularly based therapies are currently being used and may be the harbingers of more elegant, tumor-specific colorectal cancer therapy. Clinically, colorectal cancer is a diverse disease, requiring individually based treatment strategies. This chapter will review the most current data available regarding epidemiology, screening, diagnosis, staging, and multimodal treatment of colorectal cancer.

INCIDENCE AND EPIDEMIOLOGIC ASSOCIATIONS

Colorectal cancer ranks as the third most common malignancy in the United States (behind prostate and lung cancer in men, and breast and lung cancer in women), and is the second leading cause of cancer-related mortality. Approximately 143,000 patients are diagnosed with colorectal cancer each year, and 51,000 deaths are attributed to this disease.[1] The probability of colorectal cancer developing during a lifetime is approximately 6%. In contrast to the three previous decades, however, the overall incidence and mortality rate for colorectal cancer has declined for both men and women (Figure 164-1). Age-adjusted incidence and mortality rates are associated with race and ethnicity; however, the relationships are complex, influenced by social and economic confounding factors more so than tumor biology.[2]

Worldwide, more than 1 million patients are diagnosed with colorectal cancer, with more than 500,000 associated deaths.[3] The highest rates of colorectal carcinoma predominate in the more industrialized countries. Lower rates are found in Eastern Europe, Asia, Africa, and South America. Studies of Japanese migration to the United States, Asiatic Jewish migration to Israel, and Eastern European migration to Australia have shown that migrants acquire the high rates of colorectal cancers prevalent in their adopted countries. There is little question that environmental factors, most likely dietary, account for this rise in cancer rates.

Colon cancer is three times more common than rectal cancer. Interestingly, epidemiologic studies indicate a rising proportion of right-sided colon lesions. The proximal migration of colon cancer may relate to changing environmental factors; however, there is no doubt that increased screening results in detection of early lesions in an aging population.[4]

GENETIC PATHWAYS TO COLORECTAL CANCER

Cancer cells are characterized by uncontrolled growth, a capacity to avoid normal senescence and death, and the ability to invade and metastasize. Alterations in genes, oncogenes, and the tumor suppressor genes that normally control these functions result in cellular transformation. This is referred to as the adenoma-carcinoma cascade, and was first described in relation to colorectal cancer by Fearon and Vogelstein[5] more than 20 years ago.

There are at least two well-described genetic pathways leading to the development of colorectal adenocarcinoma. The chromosomal instability (CIN) pathway is the result of an accumulation of inactivated tumor suppressor genes and overactive protooncogenes. Tumors developing along this pathway are characterized by mutations of the APC, p53, and K-ras genes, allelic loss of 18q, and aneuploidy. The APC gene plays a pivotal role in tumorigenesis: 100% of familial adenomatous polyposis (FAP) patients, who carry this mutation, develop colorectal cancer if prophylactic surgery is not performed. Up to 80% of tumors develop along the CIN pathway.

The microsatellite instability (MIN) pathway is the other well-described genetic cascade implicated in the development of colorectal cancer. These tumors have aberrant DNA mismatch repair, a near-diploid karyotype, and lower levels of p53, SMAD4, and K-ras mutations but higher frequencies of BAX, TGF-BIIR, and BRAF mutations. Interestingly, these tumors generally arise proximal to the splenic flexure, and carry a better prognosis than those developing along the CIN pathway. Patients with Lynch syndrome develop malignancy along the MIN pathway, with mutation in DNA mismatch repair genes. This pathway is also referred to as the replication error (RER) pathway, and is responsible for approximately 20% of carcinomas.

In addition, excessive gene methylation has been termed the CpG island methylator phenotype (CIMP) and is believed to be fundamentally different from other colon cancers.[6] The existence of CIMP is controversial in that it is unclear whether CIMP simply reflects the far end of a continuous distribution of tumors with methylated genes, or if it is a unique subgroup of colorectal cancers with a distinct molecular etiology. Serrated polyps commonly display CIMP and V600E BRAF mutations. This finding suggests that CIMP colorectal cancers may arise from serrated polyps, which in turn may arise from a stem-like cell that is different from the stem-like cell of origin giving rise to colorectal cancers that develop from tubular adenomas. Aberrant DNA methylation in colorectal cancer is currently an active field of investigation.

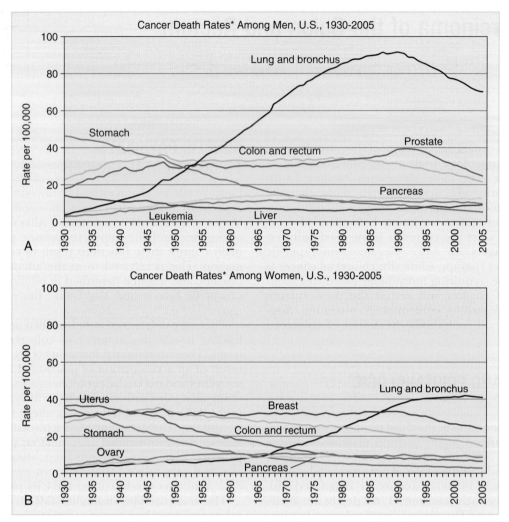

FIGURE 164-1 Cancer incidence and mortality trends over time in men (**A** and **C**) and women (**B** and **D**). *, Age-adjusted to the 2000 U.S. standard population. (From American Cancer Society, *Cancer Facts and Figures 2010*. www.cancer.org/Research/CancerFactsFigures/CancerFactsFigures/most-requested-tables-figures-1010.)

Not surprisingly, some tumors do not fall into any currently defined category, indicating that other genetic pathways exist.[7] Further study of molecular events will undoubtedly lead to a better understanding of multistep carcinogenesis, molecular staging, and tumor-specific therapy. Figure 164-2 outlines the genetic pathways of colorectal cancer and the potential prophylactic role for chemopreventive agents.

COLORECTAL CANCER RISK FACTORS

GENERAL
Clearly, the development of colorectal malignancy involves interplay between genetic and environmental influences. The most easily identified risk factors include age greater than 50, a personal or family history of colorectal cancer or adenoma, and a personal history of long-standing inflammatory bowel disease. Colorectal cancers that develop in individuals without hereditary links are referred to as "sporadic," and account for 75%

of all colorectal cancers. A potential genetic influence is identified in the remaining 25% of patients, including family history (15% to 20%); Lynch syndrome (5%); and FAP (<1%). Age is the most common risk factor. The incidence of colorectal cancer increases from the fourth to the eighth decade of life.[8] Most individuals present with disease after age 60, and only 10% of cancers occur in individuals younger than age 40. A personal history of colorectal polyps is also a significant risk factor; cancer can present within the polyp, or at another site in the colon. The risk of a polyp harboring invasive disease is related to the lesion's size, morphology, and histology. Polyps can be classified as tubular, villous, or tubulovillous. Large villous lesions are most likely to harbor malignancy, with about 50% of villous polyps larger than 2 cm containing cancer. Approximately 40% of patients are noted to have multiple adenomatous polyps, and these individuals are at highest risk for having or developing subsequent invasive cancer.[9] Not surprisingly, individuals previously diagnosed and treated for colorectal cancer are at significant risk for developing metachronous

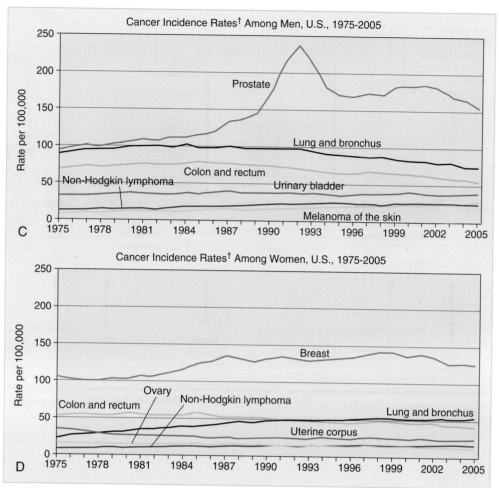

FIGURE 164-1, cont'd †, Age-adjusted to the 2000 U.S. standard population and adjusted for delays in reporting. (**C** and **D** from Surveillance, Epidemiology, and End Results Program, Delay-adjusted Incidence database: SEER Incidence Delay-adjusted Rates, 9 Registries, 1975-2005, National Cancer Institute, 2008.)

disease. Approximately 40% of patients treated for sporadic colorectal cancer will develop metachronous polyps, and at least 6% will develop a second colorectal cancer while under surveillance.[10]

INFLAMMATORY BOWEL DISEASE

Patients with inflammatory bowel disease (IBD) are at significantly increased risk for developing colorectal cancer; the risk is proportional to the extent and duration of disease. This has been extensively studied in ulcerative colitis patients, where the risk of cancer appears to begin after 8 to 10 years of disease and increases at a rate of about 0.5% to 1.0% per year. Institutional and population-based studies report the absolute risk to be 2% to 5% at 10 years, 8% to 10% at 20 years, and 20% to 30% at 30 years.[11] The risk is highest in patients with pancolitis (disease extending proximal to the splenic flexure), disease diagnosed at a young age, and colitis-associated sclerosing cholangitis. Cancer that occurs in patients with ulcerative colitis can arise in any portion of the large bowel, usually presents in the fourth decade of life, and appears to carry the same prognosis as colon cancer in general.[12] However, in these patients the disease often presents at a late stage because endoscopic

identification of a malignancy in the setting of active colitis is quite difficult. Because all currently available screening tests (including repetitive biopsies linking dysplasia and bowel mucosa transformation to cancer) are problematic, most patients with long-standing colitis will probably benefit at some point from prophylactic proctocolectomy. The risk of colorectal cancer is also increased in longstanding Crohn colitis, a fact that was underappreciated until recently. Currently it is believed that the cancer risk is equivalent in Crohn and ulcerative colitis patients who have disease of similar duration and extent.[13]

FAMILIAL ADENOMATOUS POLYPOSIS

Familial factors are associated with 25% of colorectal cancer cases. Individuals with a first-degree relative affected by colorectal cancer have twice the risk of developing the disease themselves. This risk is nearly threefold for individuals with two or more affected first-degree relatives. Not surprisingly, a positive family history is associated with younger age of diagnosis, and this finding implies a genetic predisposition.[14] The highest-risk patients are those carrying the genetic mutations associated with FAP and Lynch syndrome (Figure 164-3). Nearly 100% of individuals with FAP and 80% with

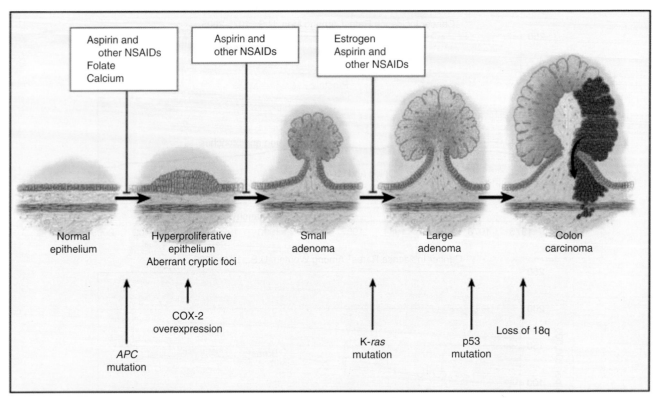

FIGURE 164-2 Colon carcinogenesis and the effects of chemopreventive agents. *NSAIDSs*, Nonsteroidal antiinflammatory drugs; *COX*, cyclooxygenase. (From Janne PA, Mayer RJ: Chemoprevention of colorectal cancer. *N Engl J Med* 342:1960, 2000.)

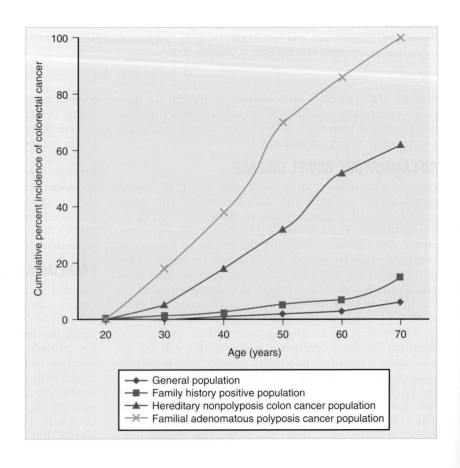

FIGURE 164-3 Colorectal cancer risk.

Lynch syndrome will develop colorectal cancer in their lifetime.

The FAP syndromes account for 1% of all colorectal cancers, and are characterized by early onset of hundreds to thousands of polyps throughout the colon. Adenomas typically begin to present early in the second decade of life, with cancer inevitably developing by the fourth or fifth decade if colectomy is not performed. These syndromes affect approximately 1:8000 to 10,000 persons; 10% to 20% of cases represent de novo mutations with no apparent family history. The disease is inherited as an autosomal dominant trait; therefore, 50% of offspring from an affected individual will develop polyposis coli. The gene that causes FAP (the adenomatous polyposis coli [APC] gene) resides on chromosome 5 (5q21). The most common genetic abnormality results in the generation of a premature stop codon, resulting in a truncated and nonfunctional protein.[15] This finding is the basis for a commonly used screening procedure in which the truncated protein is identified in vitro, thereby confirming the diagnosis.

In addition to colonic polyps, FAP patients commonly develop periampullary cancers, gastric fundic gland polyps, and intraabdominal desmoid tumors. After the colorectal cancer is eliminated by surgery, periampullary tumors are the most frequent cause of death among individuals with FAP.[16] A variant of FAP is Gardner syndrome, characterized by colorectal adenomas and extraintestinal manifestations including osteomas (mainly of the mandible and skull), soft tissue tumors (such as lipomas, fibromas, and epidermoid and sebaceous cysts), supernumerary teeth, desmoid tumors, mesenteric fibromatosis, and congenital hypertrophy of the retinal pigmentation epithelium (CHRPE). Turcot syndrome is another variant of FAP, in which colorectal adenomas are associated with brain tumors. Attenuated FAP syndrome is characterized by the development of fewer polyps, more likely in the right colon and arising later in life.[17] This can make clinical diagnosis of attenuated FAP versus Lynch syndrome quite difficult. The various FAP phenotypes appear to be related to the site of mutation on the *APC* gene.[17] For example, gene mutation in attenuated FAP is usually located more proximal or distal on the *APC* gene than it would be in the more common FAP syndrome.

LYNCH SYNDROME

Lynch syndrome is a familial disorder characterized by a high incidence of colon cancer without the excessive polyposis identified in classic FAP. Lynch syndrome accounts for 5% to 6% of colorectal cancers.[18] Its phenotypic features include early-onset colorectal cancer (a mean age of 46 years), synchronous or metachronous colorectal cancers (noted in 35% of cases), and a predominance of right-sided tumors.[19] There is also an association with early onset of adenocarcinoma of the ovary, pancreas, breast, bile duct, endometrium, stomach, genitourinary tract, and small bowel.[20] Lynch I syndrome refers to the cohort with colorectal cancer only, while Lynch II syndrome refers to the cohort of patients with colorectal cancer and other associated adenocarcinomas. Muir-Torre syndrome is a Lynch syndrome variant associated with sebaceous gland adenomas and carcinoma.

The molecular genetic marker reflecting Lynch syndrome is microsatellite instability, which is a consequence of mutations in DNA mismatch repair genes (*hMSH2*, *hMLH1*, *hPMS1*, and *hPMS2*). The diagnostic criteria for identifying individuals with Lynch syndrome were established in 1991 at a consensus conference in Amsterdam, to help identify and categorize patients with familial history of colorectal cancer.[19] These initial criteria, referred to as Amsterdam I Criteria, require the following: (1) three relatives with colorectal cancer, one being a first-degree relative of the other two; (2) two successive generations afflicted with colorectal cancer; and (3) one family member who developed colorectal cancer before age 50. Furthermore, FAP must be excluded, and all cancers verified pathologically. However, these criteria were found to underestimate Lynch syndrome in some family pedigrees.[18] Therefore the Amsterdam II Criteria, which included extracolonic tumors, was developed. Accepted Lynch syndrome–associated cancers include colorectal, endometrial, small bowel, ureteral, or renal pelvic cancers (Box 164-1). The term familial colorectal cancer type X is used when the Amsterdam criteria are met but there is no known DNA mismatch repair defect. These families appear to have a lower overall incidence of cancer and lower risk for noncolorectal cancers than families with documented DNA mismatch repair deficiency.[21] About 35% of patients meeting Amsterdam criteria do not have a DNA-mismatch-repair gene mutation.[22]

MISMATCH REPAIR

Some tumors demonstrating mismatch repair (MMR) deficiency do not show familial inheritance or genetic mutation. These sporadic MMR tumors are more likely associated with gene promoter hypermethylation. Tumors with MMR deficiency (both hereditary and sporadic) have a characteristic histologic appearance. Adenomas tend to have a villous component, with more dysplasia than is typically seen in sporadic cases. Cancers commonly have signet-ring histology marked by poor differentiation and inflammatory cell infiltrate.[18,23] In spite of the aggressive histologic appearance, stage-for-stage survival in colorectal cancer patients with MMR deficiency is better than that in patients with intact MMR.[20] Interestingly, colorectal neoplasms appear to

---

BOX 164-1 Amsterdam II Criteria

- At least three relatives with an HNPCC-associated cancer (colorectal, endometrium, small bowel, ureter, or renal pelvis). One affected relative should be a first-degree relative of the other two.
- At least two successive generations should be affected.
- At least one relative should have been diagnosed before age 50 years.
- Familial adenomatous polyposis should be excluded.

Tumors should be verified by pathologic examination.
HNPCC, Hereditary nonpolyposis colon cancer.

develop more rapidly in patients with Lynch syndrome, which affects their followup regimen.

OTHER GENETIC SYNDROMES

There are other genetic syndromes associated with an increased incidence of colorectal cancer, including Peutz-Jeghers and familial juvenile polyposis. These are autosomal dominant syndromes characterized by hamartomatous polyposis. The histology of intestinal hamartomas consists of an overgrowth of cells or tissues native to the area in which they normally occur.[24] The molecular mechanisms of these syndromes are currently being studied, and specific mutations have been described.

Peutz-Jeghers syndrome is characterized by multiple gastrointestinal hamartomatous polyps associated with mucocutaneous melanin pigmentation. Patients may present with impending obstruction, polyp intussusception, or anemia from gastrointestinal blood loss. The polyps are generally nonneoplastic, with a characteristic branching muscular framework, but they can contain carcinoma. Peutz-Jeghers patients are at increased risk for developing both gastrointestinal and extraintestinal malignancies such as pancreatic, breast, ovarian, testicular, and uterine carcinomas[25]; therefore, prophylactic colectomy is usually not indicated. Polyps are usually managed endoscopically, and surgery is reserved for lesions that are large, symptomatic, or have a neoplastic appearance.

Familial juvenile polyposis syndrome is characterized by multiple (often 50 to 200) juvenile polyps throughout the gastrointestinal tract, often associated with other congenital (including cardiac and genitourinary) anomalies. Patients may present in childhood with anemia caused by chronic gastrointestinal blood loss, crampy abdominal pain due to intussusception, a protein-losing enteropathy, or frank rectal bleeding. (Patients presenting with the often self-limited, solitary juvenile polyp are not included in this definition.) Individuals with this syndrome are at an increased risk for developing both upper and lower gastrointestinal cancers.[26] The polyps are generally controlled endoscopically; total abdominal colectomy with ileal pouch–anal anastomosis is reserved for patients who have large and numerous polyps or invasive malignancy.

RECENTLY IDENTIFIED RISK FACTORS

Recent research has identified additional genetic risk factors associated with colorectal cancer. A polymorphism in the *APC* gene is associated with development of colorectal neoplasms in descendants of Eastern European (Ashkenazi) Jews. This population is noted to have the highest colorectal cancer incidence of any Israeli ethnic group. Studies have reported that 6% of unselected Ashkenazi Jews and 28% of those with a family history of colorectal cancer carry an *APC* missense mutation (referred to as I 1307 K). These patients do not have the typical phenotype seen with FAP. Rather, the polymorphism creates a hypermutable region on the *APC* gene, which causes a predisposition to colorectal cancer.[27] This translates into a high frequency of synchronous cancer in patients with polyps: 13% of individuals carrying this

polymorphism and identified adenomatous polyps harbor an invasive cancer.[28,29] Another relatively new syndrome, involving mutation in the exon-excision-repair gene *MYH*, has also been described. Individuals carrying this mutation can present with either the FAP or Lynch syndrome phenotype.[30] Lastly, an association between hyperplastic polyposis, defined as more than 20 hyperplastic polyps (of at least 1 cm in size) in sites other than the rectosigmoid, and colorectal adenomas and carcinomas, has recently been identified.[31] These cancers are associated with methylation silencing of MMR genes and HPP1. Ultimately, further identification and characterization of the various molecular pathways of carcinogenesis may lead to tumor-specific therapy.

SUMMARY

There is no doubt that environmental factors play a critical role in the development of colorectal cancer.[32] However, the association between dietary and lifestyle factors and development of colorectal neoplasms is extraordinarily complex. The largest body of epidemiologic data is based on case-controlled studies limited by significant recall bias. Prospective cohort studies avoid limitations in patient recollection but may be inadequate, as the food frequency questionnaires are rarely validated. Clinical trials in which nutrient supplementations are given as interventions are similarly limited, because colorectal carcinogenesis has a relatively long latency (Table 164-1) (see also Chapter 163).

COLORECTAL CANCER SCREENING

The goals of screening asymptomatic patients are to identify and remove premalignant adenomatous polyps and identify early malignancies. Polyps most likely to contain invasive disease are sessile rather than pedunculated, villous rather than tubular, and large (>1.5 cm) rather than small. The National Polyp Study confirmed that colonoscopic polypectomy reduces colon cancer mortality. In this study, patients who underwent endoscopic removal of adenomas had a lower probability of developing colorectal cancer, compared with a reference group that did not have polyps removed, and with individuals in a population-based registry (Surveillance Epidemiology and End Results [SEER]), most of whom did not have polyps.[33] In essence, this study validated the colorectal adenoma-to-adenocarcinoma sequence and reinforced the importance of screening. When an

TABLE 164-1 Dietary and Lifestyle Risk Factors for Colon and Rectal Cancer

Likelihood of Association	Decreased Risk	Increased Risk
Probable	Physical activity, folate, vegetables	Obesity, smoking, red meat
Possible	Fruit, calcium, vitamin D, methionine	Alcohol, processed meat, heavily cooked meat, iron
Unknown	Fiber supplement	—

TABLE 164-2 Screening Guidelines for Average-Risk Individuals

Test	Internal (Beginning at Age 50 Yr)	Comment
FOBT and flexible sigmoidoscopy	FOBT annually and flexible sigmoidoscopy every 5 yr	Flexible sigmoidoscopy together with FOBT is preferred compared with FOBT or flexible sigmoidoscopy alone
		All positive tests should be followed up with colonoscopy
Flexible sigmoidoscopy	Every 5 yr	All positive tests should be followed up with colonoscopy
FOBTs	Annually	The recommended take-home multiple-sample method should be used
		All positive tests should be followed up with colonoscopy
Colonoscopy	Every 10 yr	Colonoscopy provides an opportunity to visualize, sample, and/or remove significant lesions
Double-contrast barium enema	Every 5 yr	All positive tests should be followed by colonoscopy

FOBT, Fecal occult blood test.

adenomatous polyp is detected, the entire large bowel should be visualized endoscopically because synchronous lesions are found 35% to 40% of the time.

The specifics of colorectal cancer screening rely on an understanding of patient risk (Tables 164-2 and 164-3). Asymptomatic, average-risk individuals are candidates for routine screening, whereas those at increased risk—as a result of a personal or family history of colorectal cancer or the presence of adenomas, inflammatory bowel disease, or a hereditary colon cancer syndrome—require more individualized screening and surveillance regimens.

AVERAGE-RISK SCREENING

Average-risk men and women should begin routine colorectal cancer screening at age 50 (see Table 164-2). Several options exist. The first includes stool occult blood testing annually and flexible sigmoidoscopy every 5 years. If a positive stool blood test is detected, the patient should undergo a complete colonoscopy to evaluate the entire colon. On screening sigmoidoscopy, single small lesions should be biopsied and additional treatment predicated on histology. If the lesion is an adenomatous polyp, colonoscopy should be performed to complete the polypectomy and assess the proximal colon for synchronous lesions. If the polyp is a benign hyperplastic polyp, no additional testing is necessary. However, if screening sigmoidoscopy reveals either a large polyp or multiple polyps, initial biopsy is not necessary and the patient should undergo complete colonoscopy with biopsy. The second option for screening the average-risk individual is complete colonoscopy, repeated at 10-year intervals if negative for neoplasia. (This is the preferred screening method.) The third and least common option includes double-contrast barium enema plus flexible sigmoidoscopy every 5 to 10 years. Any positive test should be followed up by a full colonoscopy.

HIGH-RISK SCREENING

High-risk individuals include those with personal history of adenomas or cancers, family history of adenocarcinoma or genetic syndromes, or predisposing medical conditions such as inflammatory bowel disease (see Table 164-3). Patients with a history of colorectal adenomas require increased surveillance for metachronous polyps or previously undetected small, synchronous polyps, which can occur in 15% of cases.[34] Based on the findings of the National Polyp Study, a repeat examination can be performed 3 years after polypectomy.[33] A shorter followup interval may be necessary after removal of multiple adenomas, excision of an adenoma with invasive cancer, incomplete or piecemeal removal of a large sessile adenoma, or suboptimal examination because of poor preparation. On the other hand, if the 3-year followup colonoscopy is clear, the surveillance interval can be increased to once every 5 years.[35]

PERSONAL HISTORY OF ADENOCARCINOMA

Patients with a personal history of colorectal cancer require increased surveillance for metachronous disease. In general, the first surveillance colonoscopy should be performed 1 year following cancer resection. If the colon was not fully evaluated preoperatively, the first colonoscopy should be performed within 3 months of surgery; if this first postresection colonoscopy is normal, the interval can be increased to once every 3 years. However, if additional disease is noted, more frequent examinations are warranted.

Patients with a family history of colorectal cancer or adenomas, including affected first-degree relatives, also require more aggressive surveillance. These individuals should undergo screening colonoscopy beginning at 40 years of age or earlier, that is, when they are 10 years younger than the affected family members were at age of initial diagnosis.

INFLAMMATORY BOWEL DISEASE

Patients with long-standing inflammatory bowel disease are at increased risk of colorectal cancer and should undergo routine surveillance. The cancer risk in chronic Crohn disease appears to be the same as that in ulcerative colitis; therefore, these patients should be examined similarly. In patients with pancolitis (typically defined as disease extending proximal to the splenic flexure) surveillance colonoscopy should begin after 8 years of symptoms. Surveillance can begin later in patients with left-sided colitis: generally after 12 to 15 years of disease. Colonoscopy should be performed every 1 to

TABLE 164-3 Screening Guidelines for High-Risk Individuals

Risk Category	Age to Begin	Recommendation	Comment
INCREASED RISK			
Patient with a single small (<1 cm) adenoma	3-6 yr after the initial polypectomy	Colonoscopy	If examination is normal, they can thereafter be screened as per average-risk guidelines
Patient with a large (>1 cm) adenoma, multiple adenomas, or adenomas with high-grade dysplasia or villous change	Within 3 yr after the initial polypectomy	Colonoscopy	If normal, repeat examination in 3 yr; if normal then, the patient can thereafter be screened as per average-risk guidelines
Personal history of curative-intent resection of colorectal cancer	Within 1 yr after cancer resection	Colonoscopy	If normal, repeat examination in 3 yr; if normal then, repeat examination every 5 yr
Either colorectal cancer or adenomatous polyps, in any first-degree relative before age 60 yr, or in ≥2 first-degree relatives at any age (if not a hereditary syndrome)	Age 40 yr, or 10 yr before the youngest case in the immediate family	Colonoscopy	Every 5-10 yr Colorectal cancer in relatives more distant than first-degree does not increase risk substantially above the average-risk group
HIGH RISK			
Family history of familial adenomatous polyposis (FAP)	Puberty	Early surveillance with endoscopy, and counseling to consider genetic testing	If the genetic test is positive, colectomy is indicated These patients are best referred to a center with experience in the management of FAP
Family history of HNPCC	Age 21 yr	Colonoscopy and counseling to consider genetic testing	If the genetic test is positive or if the patient has not had genetic testing, every 1-2 yr until 40 yr of age, then annually These patients are best referred to a center with experience in the management of HNPCC
Inflammatory bowel disease Chronic ulcerative colitis Crohn disease	Cancer risks begin to be significant 8 yr after the onset of pancolitis or 12-15 yr after the onset of left-sided colitis	Colonoscopy with biopsies for dysplasia	Every 1-2 yr These patients are best referred to a center with experience in the surveillance and management of inflammatory bowel disease

HNPCC, Hereditary nonpolyposis colon cancer.

2 years. During each examination, biopsies should routinely be taken at 10- to 12-cm intervals throughout the colon, from grossly normal as well as abnormal-appearing mucosa. Colectomy is indicated for low- or high-grade dysplasia, for patients with difficult-to-control colitis, and for those who cannot comply with routine surveillance.

FAMILIAL ADENOMATOUS POLYPOSIS

Patients from FAP families who have not been tested for an *APC* mutation should begin routine screening at puberty with annual flexible sigmoidoscopy. If polyps are not identified by age 40, then the frequency of examination can be decreased to once every 3 years. However, individuals who express the phenotype require upper endoscopy to examine the periampullary region. Patients with a known genetic mutation or relatives of FAP kindred should undergo colectomy when they develop polyps, because stage-specific survival of colorectal cancer appears to be the same for polyposis patients as for those with sporadic bowel cancers.

LYNCH SYNDROME

Colorectal screening for patients with Lynch syndrome should be done by full colonoscopy, because these individuals are predisposed to develop proximal colonic lesions. The adenoma-to-carcinoma sequence appears to be more rapid in this cohort, so endoscopy should be performed every 1 to 2 years. For individuals with known mutations or family history consistent with the Amsterdam Criteria, screening should begin at age 21.[1] Screening for extracolonic disease should be done as well, including urine cytology, pelvic ultrasound, and periodic endometrial biopsy.

COLORECTAL CANCER STAGING

The prognosis for patients with colorectal cancer is related to the stage of disease at diagnosis and tumor histology, including differentiation, lymphatic invasion, and extent of tumor-free surgical resection margins. In the future, molecular genetic markers may define subsets of patients who are either more or less likely to develop

---

BOX 164-2 American Joint Committee on Cancer—Union Internationale Contre le Cancer Tumor, Node, Metastasis Stage Grouping

PRIMARY TUMOR (T)

TX   Primary tumor cannot be assessed

T0   No evidence of primary tumor

Tis Carcinoma in situ: intraepithelial or invasion of lamina propria*

T1   Tumor invades submucosa

T2   Tumor invades muscularis propria

T3   Tumor invades through the muscularis propria into pericolorectal tissues

T4a Tumor penetrates to the surface of the visceral peritoneum†

T4b Tumor directly invades or is adherent to other organs or structures†,‡

REGIONAL LYMPH NODES (N)

NX   Regional lymph nodes cannot be assessed

N0   No regional lymph node metastasis

N1   Metastasis in 1-3 regional lymph nodes

N1a Metastasis in 1 regional lymph node

N1b Metastasis in 2-3 regional lymph nodes

N1c Tumor deposit(s) in the subserosa, mesentery, or nonperitonealized pericolic or perirectal tissues without regional nodal metastasis

N2   Metastasis in 4 or more regional lymph nodes

N2a Metastasis in 4-6 regional lymph nodes

N2b Metastasis in 7 or more regional lymph nodes

PRIMARY TUMOR (T)

M0   No distant metastasis

M1   Distant metastasis

M1a Metastasis confined to one organ or site (e.g., liver, lung, ovary, nonregional node)

M1b Metastases in more than one organ/site or the peritoneum

---

*Tis included cancer cells confined within the glandular basement membrane (intraepithelial) or mucosal lamina propria (intramucosal) with no extension through the muscularis mucosae into the submucosa.

†Direct invasion in T4 includes invasion of other organs or other segments of the colorectum as a result of direct extension through the serosa, as confirmed on microscopic examination (e.g., invasion of the sigmoid colon by a carcinoma of the cecum) or, for cancer in a retroperitoneal or subperitoneal location, direct invasion of other organs or structures by virtue of extension beyond the muscularis propria (i.e., respectively, a tumor on the posterior wall of the descending colon invading the left kidney or lateral abdominal wall; or a mid or distal rectal cancer with invasion of prostate, seminal vesicles, cervix, or vagina).

‡Tumor that is adherent to other organs or structures, grossly, is classified cT4b. However, if no tumor is present in the adhesion, microscopically, the classification should be pT1-4a depending on the anatomical depth of wall invasion. The V and L classifications should be used to identify the presence or absence of vascular or lymphatic invasion, whereas the PN site-specific factor should be used for perineural invasion.

TABLE 164-4 American Joint Committee on Cancer—Union Internationale Contre le Cancer Tumor, Node, Metastasis Staging of Colon and Rectal Cancer

ANATOMIC STAGE	PROGNOSTIC GROUPS		
Stage	T	N	M
0	Tis	N0	M0
I	T1	N0	M0
	T2	N0	M0
IIA	T3	N0	M0
IIB	T4a	N0	M0
IIC	T4b	N0	M0
IIIA	T1-T2	N1/N1c	M0
	T1	N2a	M0
IIIB	T3-T4a	N1/N1c	M0
	T2-T3	N2a	M0
	T1-T2	N2b	M0
IIIC	T4a	N2a	M0
	T3-T4a	N2b	M0
	T4b	N1-N2	M0
IVA	Any T	Any N	M1a
IVB	Any T	Any N	M1b

From Edge SB, Byrd DR, Compton CC, et al, editors: *AJCC Cancer Staging Manual*, ed 7. New York, 2010, Springer-Verlag.
Note: cTNM is the clinical classification, pTNM is the pathologic classification. The y prefix is used for those cancers that are classified after neoadjuvant pretreatment (e.g., ypTNM). Patients who have a complete pathologic response are ypT0N0cM0 that may be similar to Stage Group 0 or I. The r prefix is to be used for those cancers that have recurred after a disease-free interval (rTNM).

---

tumor recurrence, which would lead to more rational application of adjuvant multimodality treatment.[36,37] However, use of such molecular markers remains investigational at this time.

The tumor, node, and metastasis (TNM) staging system of the American Joint Committee on Cancer (AJCC) and International Union Against Cancer (UICC) is the standard colorectal cancer staging system. The seventh edition of the *AJCC Cancer Staging Manual*, published in 2010, is outlined in Box 164-2 and Table 164-4.

The letters "c" and "p" are used as prescripts to denote clinical and pathologic staging, respectively. The prescript "y" is used to denote posttreatment staging of a tumor (e.g., ypT2N1M0 represents a pathologically staged tumor extending into the muscularis propria, with metastases noted in one to three regional lymph nodes, in a patient who received preoperative treatment).

In colorectal carcinomas, the staging category pTis (carcinoma in situ) denotes either malignant cells that are confined by glandular basement membrane (intraepithelial carcinoma) or invade beyond the basement membrane into the mucosal lamina propria (intramucosal carcinoma). The terms "high-grade dysplasia" and "intraepithelial carcinoma" are often used synonymously. The definition of invasive colorectal cancer, that is, pT1, includes tumor cell invasion through the muscularis mucosae and into the submucosa, where abundant lymphatics are located. This is in contrast to the definition of other gastrointestinal and solid tumors, in which invasion below the lamina propria is considered malignant.

There are several other nuances and subtleties in the TNM staging system. Extramural tumor deposits are classified as N1c. pT4 refers to tumor extension into adjacent organs or structures, penetration of the parietal peritoneum with or without involvement of an adjacent structure, or free perforation into the peritoneal cavity.

As is true for most epithelial cancers, the presence of metastases in regional lymph nodes has a significant impact on survival. Proper staging and treatment of

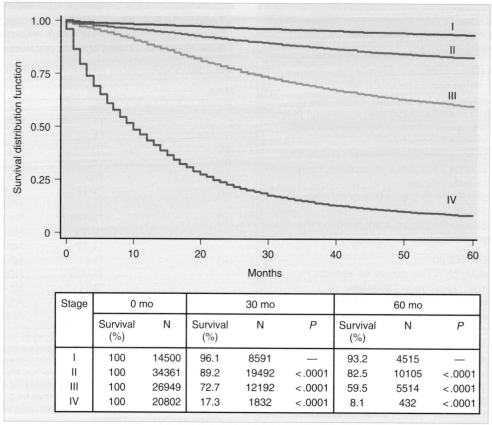

Stage	0 mo		30 mo			60 mo		
	Survival (%)	N	Survival (%)	N	P	Survival (%)	N	P
I	100	14500	96.1	8591	—	93.2	4515	—
II	100	34361	89.2	19492	<.0001	82.5	10105	<.0001
III	100	26949	72.7	12192	<.0001	59.5	5514	<.0001
IV	100	20802	17.3	1832	<.0001	8.1	432	<.0001

FIGURE 164-4 Five-year survival by American Joint Committee on Cancer, fifth edition, system stages I–IV *(upper)*. Outcome of colorectal cancer by stage *(lower)*. (From O'Connell JB, Maggard MA, Ko CY: Colon cancer survival rates with the new AJCC 6th edition staging. *J Natl Cancer Inst* 96:1420, 2004.)

colorectal cancer requires adequate lymphadenectomy. In a study of T3 tumors, Goldstein et al[38] illustrated the relationship between staging accuracy and lymphadenectomy: lymph node metastases were noted in 85% of cases when 15 or more nodes were recovered but in only 22% when fewer than 15 were identified in the specimen. Furthermore, within the cohort of patients who did not demonstrate nodal metastases, survival was greatest in the subgroup with high lymph node recovery. Although there are many factors related to the number of nodes examined, including extent of resection and diligence of the pathologist, these data support the concept that proper oncologic resection is associated with improved outcome. Based on this study and others, it has been recommended that at least 12 lymph nodes be examined in order to accurately stage colorectal cancer patients.[39]

Alternative methods for detecting very small amounts of metastatic disease have been developed, including molecular biology–based techniques and immunohistochemistry. Recent studies have shown that a polymerase chain reaction (PCR)–based assay can distinguish patients with occult nodal disease and higher risk of recurrence from those with histologic and molecularly negative lymph nodes.[40] Occult nodal disease identified on molecular analysis is currently not part of the seventh edition of the AJCC/UICC TNM staging N1. The use of sentinel node biopsy for intestinal malignancy remains investigational. Study results are discordant, and one cooperative group study noted an unacceptably high false-negative rate (negative sentinel lymph node with positive nonsentinel lymph nodes), indicating that this may not be valid in colorectal cancer.[41] The inconsistent results, and the fact that lymphadenectomy remains a component of colorectal resection, has limited the use of sentinel node analysis.

The relationship between pathologic stage of disease and outcome is depicted in Figure 164-4.[42] In addition to bowel wall penetration and lymph node status, other pathologic features that have been shown to predict outcome are listed in Box 164-3. Lymphovascular invasion is associated with nodal and distant disease as well as independent predictors of survival. If data are corrected for nodal involvement and histologic differentiation, prognosis in patients with colorectal cancer—in contrast to patients with many other solid tumors—is not influenced by the size of the primary lesion.

TREATMENT OF PRIMARY COLON AND RECTAL CARCINOMA

The mainstay of therapy for locoregional colon and rectal carcinoma is surgery. In colon cancer, adjuvant chemotherapy is administered to reduce the risk of

BOX 164-3 Selected Pathologic Prognostic Factors in Colorectal Cancer

Adjacent organ involvement (colon)
Radial margin (rectum)
Degree of differentiation
Blood vessel invasion
Lymphatic vessel invasion
Perineural invasion
Immune response
DNA content
Proliferative index
Allelic loss of chromosome 18q (DCC)
KRAS mutation
MMR deficiency

recurrence, which usually appears as distant failure. In rectal cancer, neoadjuvant combined-modality therapy, including chemotherapy and radiation, is administered to improve resectability, aid in sphincter preservation, and reduce local as well as distant recurrence. Adjuvant chemotherapy is administered primarily to reduce the risk of distant recurrence.

In treating colorectal cancer, it is critical to understand that surgical dissection of the primary tumor is limited to those patients for whom cure is realistically possible, or to those with symptomatic lesions resulting in acute obstruction or clinically significant bleeding. For patients who present with synchronous primary and incurable metastatic disease, resection of the primary tumor is not routinely indicated. Advances in systemic chemotherapy (which are outlined later) have greatly increased the likelihood of tumor control through medical management, and chemotherapy can be routinely started with an asymptomatic or minimally symptomatic primary in place. There is no need to "prepare such a patient for chemotherapy" by performing palliative resection of a primary tumor that does not actively require palliation. In fact, resection of a primary lesion in the setting of metastatic disease is significantly associated with morbidity and mortality. A large review of Medicare/SEER data for patients age 65 and older reported that resection of a synchronous primary tumor was associated with a 30-day postoperative mortality of 10%.[43]

SURGERY

The basic tenet of performing colorectal cancer surgery with curative intent is to remove the primary lesion with adequate margins, along with regional lymph nodes. Determining the extent of lymphadenectomy is based on a thorough understanding of anatomy and the lymphatic spread of intestinal cancer, and is one of the most challenging aspects of cancer surgery.

The regional lymphatics of the colon have been well described.[44] Abundant lymphatic capillaries are found in the submucosa, and efferent vessels proceed peripherally through the circular and longitudinal layers of the muscularis propria, communicating with a clearly defined subserosal plexus. Lymphatic flow in the subserosal network is principally circumferential. Longitudinal

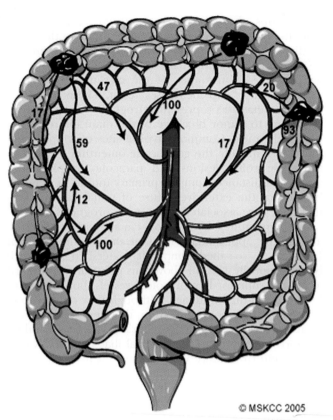

FIGURE 164-5 Lymphatic drainage for colon cancer. (From Memorial Sloan-Kettering Cancer Center, 2005.)

intramural lymphatic spread is generally limited to 2 cm, which explains the general rule of obtaining a 5-cm proximal and distal intestinal margin during surgery. The majority of subserosal lymphatics pass into the mesentery to the paracolic lymph nodes. Under normal circumstances, lymph flow within the colon mesentery proceeds centrally, in an orderly fashion, from smaller to larger collecting lymphatics, and eventually to the root of the mesentery. Lymphatic vessels are closely associated with the vascular pedicles, and the centrally directed flow proceeds along the nearest (or most immediately accessible) route to the apex of the mesentery. Thus, we can conveniently describe the pathways of lymphatic flow by the appropriate vascular pedicle, including the ileocolic, right colic, and midcolic routes of the superior mesenteric system and the left colic, sigmoidal, and superior rectal routes of the inferior mesenteric system (Figure 164-5).

Although there are many variations in the arrangement of lymph nodes along the pathways of flow, three roughly separable groups can be identified. First-echelon lymph nodes are paracolic, associated with the marginal vessel of Drummond. These nodes are the most numerous and, in surgical therapy, the most important. Second-echelon, or intermediate, lymph nodes are located in the mesentery at the level of the division of mainstem blood vessels into peripheral branches. Third-echelon nodes, represented by the central or principal nodes, are closest to the root of the mesentery and are associated with takeoff of the major vascular pedicles. Cancer emboli generally take the most direct route to regional lymph nodes; thus, there is a stepwise progression centrally from the paracolic nodes adjacent to tumor, to the intermediate nodes along the most contiguous mesenteric vascular pedicle, and finally to the main or principal lymph nodes at the apex of the mesentery. However, variations and "skip metastases" exist. These unusually situated metastases represent retrograde lymphatic flow secondary to tumor blockage of the main efferent lymphatic channels. Common atypical sites of lymph node metastases include the gastrocolic omentum, related to transverse colon lesions and paracolic lymph nodes noted at a distance from the primary tumor. In general, because of the extensive nature of nodal disease, skip metastases are associated with a poor prognosis.[44]

In the rectum, at about 7 to 8 cm above the anal verge and at the approximate level of the middle valve of Houston, a so-called lymphatic watershed exists: all lymph from the rectum above this point drains upward along the superior hemorrhoidal vessels, but below this level there is dual drainage. Although flow remains predominately superior in direction, there may be independent or associated drainage laterally along the middle hemorrhoid vessels to the internal iliac chain of lymph nodes, and from there via retroperitoneal vessels to the paraaortic nodes. Very distal lesions can drain along the superficial perineal lymphatics, with flow directed toward the superficial inguinal lymph nodes.

Regardless of the location of the primary tumor, the goal of surgery is to remove it with adequate intestinal margins, en bloc with regional lymph nodes. As noted, longitudinal spread along the colon rarely extends beyond 2 cm, and this has been the rationale for resecting 5 cm of normal intestine proximal and distal to the lesion. In practice, however, the length of intestinal resection is generally determined by devascularization from lymphadenectomy. Lymph nodes at risk for metastases include those along the primary vascular pedicle closest to the tumor as well as adjacent vessels. These secondary routes have been well described and are summarized in Figure 164-5. There is a tendency to extrapolate from these studies and perform radical or extended lymph node resections in hopes of improving patient outcome; however, this is not borne out in practice. For example, "high ligation" of the inferior mesenteric artery at its takeoff from the aorta has not been shown to improve outcome[45]; it is instead associated with increased perioperative morbidity, including autonomic nerve injury and associated sexual and bladder dysfunction. Operative strategies and lymphadenectomy for colorectal cancer are outlined in Figure 164-6.

The widespread application of sphincter-sparing techniques, including low anterior resection with coloanal anastomosis, especially in combination with combined-modality therapy (chemoradiation), allows most patients to avoid abdominoperineal resection and permanent colostomy. The technique of intersphincteric dissection is increasingly used to gain distal margin and avoid a permanent colostomy.[46] In intersphincteric dissection, the internal sphincter (a continuation of the rectal muscularis propria) is resected with the rectum, allowing for an additional 1 cm of distal margin (Figure 164-7). Following this procedure, patients rely on the external sphincter for continence. These technical advances now allow sphincter preservation for the majority of rectal cancer patients, reserving abdominoperineal resection for those patients with poor preoperative function and those with tumors extending into the external sphincter complex.[47] The functional sequelae and quality of life associated with ultralow coloanal anastomosis has become the center of research.[48] Creation of a reservoir such as a colonic J-pouch or coloplasty is advocated whenever technically feasible, as it appears to improve short-term (and possibly long-term) function.[49]

The increasingly common application of these sphincter-saving techniques has renewed interest in defining the necessary length of distal bowel margin. Although 5 cm of distal rectum was originally thought necessary,[50] 2 cm is now widely accepted as sufficient.[51] More recent studies have indicated that even shorter margins may be adequate, especially if there is significant tumor regression in response to combined-modality therapy.[52] Possibly of more importance than the length of distal intestine removed beyond the tumor is the status of the lateral and circumferential resection margins. Clearly these margins have been overlooked in the past, yet they are as critical as the distal margin in terms of tumor recurrence.[53]

Not surprisingly, studies have shown a relationship between quality of surgical technique and outcome. Blunt pelvic dissection can result in local recurrence rates as high as 25%. Conversely, appropriate mesorectal excision (mesorectal excision at least 5 cm below a high rectal lesion, and total mesorectal excision for middle/low rectal cancers) is associated with local failure rates ranging from 5% to 10%.[54,55] Careful attention must be given to all margins, including the circumferential resection margin.[53] As might be expected, surgeon and hospital volume appear to influence the outcome of colorectal cancer surgery.[56]

Special Circumstances

Surgical Treatment of Hereditary Bowel Cancer. Surgical options for patients with hereditary colorectal cancer syndromes include both therapeutic and prophylactic procedures. In patients with FAP, the most common operations include total abdominal colectomy with ileorectal anastomosis, and total proctocolectomy with either ileal pouch–anal anastomosis or end ileostomy. Total abdominal colectomy with ileorectal anastomosis is reserved for individuals with minimal rectal disease that can be controlled endoscopically. The advantages of ileorectal anastomosis include a less complex surgical procedure, relatively normal postoperative bowel function, and preservation of bladder and sexual function. However, the remaining rectum requires frequent surveillance, as the risk of developing rectal cancer ranges from 10% to 50%,[57] with 40% to 75% of patients eventually requiring rectal resection. The advantage of total proctocolectomy with ileal pouch–anal anastomosis includes complete elimination of the at-risk colorectal mucosa. However, this is a more complex procedure with an associated risk of bladder and sexual dysfunction postoperatively, as well as worse (although generally acceptable) bowel function. Total proctocolectomy with end

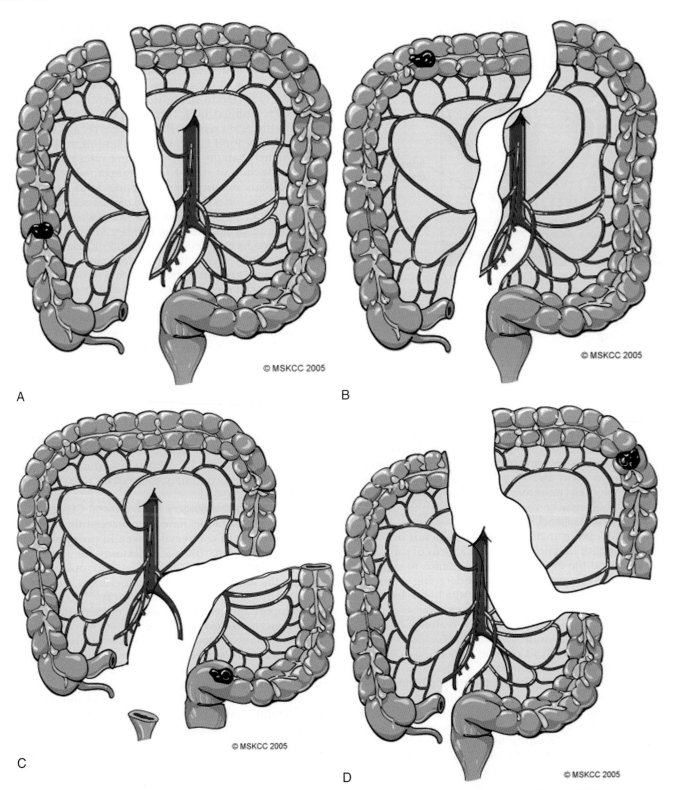

FIGURE 164-6 Operative strategies for colorectal cancer. (From Memorial Sloan-Kettering Cancer Center, 2005.)

ileostomy is usually reserved for patients presenting with advanced rectal cancer, or for those who are unwilling or unable to undergo an ileal pouch–anal anastomosis.

The surgical management of Lynch syndrome patients depends on initial presentation. Lynch syndrome patients who present with cancer or polyps not amenable to endoscopic removal should be considered for total abdominal colectomy with ileorectal anastomosis. Other options include segmental resection followed by frequent endoscopic surveillance, and enrollment in chemoprevention trials. Women, especially those who have completed childbearing, should be considered for total abdominal hysterectomy with bilateral salpingo-oophorectomy. Lynch syndrome patients presenting with rectal cancer

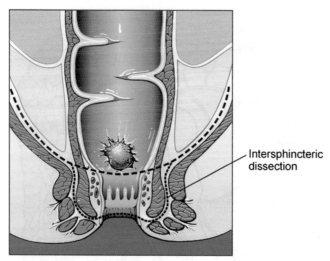

Intersphincteric dissection

FIGURE 164-7 The technique of intersphincteric resection allows for additional distal margin for tumors located at the anorectal ring. (From Rullier E, Laurent C, Bretagnol F, et al: Sphincter-saving resection for all rectal carcinomas: the end of the 2-cm rule. *Ann Surg* 241:465, 2005.)

should be considered for total proctocolectomy with ileal pouch–anal anastomosis. Less preferable options that may nevertheless be appropriate for select patients include segmental rectal resection followed by frequent endoscopic surveillance. At-risk individuals with no colonic manifestations should be monitored closely with frequent endoscopic surveillance; because penetrance is only 80%, as many as 20% will not develop the phenotype. In select circumstances, prophylactic total abdominal colectomy may be reasonable (see Chapter 163).

Surgery for Malignant Polyps. The treatment of superficial carcinomas or malignant polyps depends on tumor location, depth of bowel invasion if a focus of carcinoma is found, and the amenability of the tumor to complete endoscopic removal. Patients undergoing complete removal of pedunculated polyps which on histologic examination reveal superficial carcinoma with clear margins and no high-risk pathologic features, can often be closely observed without formal colectomy. On the other hand, medically fit patients undergoing complete removal of superficial tumors or polyps demonstrating positive margins or high-grade pathologic features such as lymphovascular/perineural invasion, poor differentiation, or single cell infiltrate, are at increased risk for regional nodal metastases, and in these cases formal intestinal resection is warranted.

Local Excision of Rectal Cancer. Local excision (transanal excision and transanal endoscopic microsurgery) of rectal cancers has recently gained popularity. The appeal is considerable, including rapid surgical recovery, minimal morbidity, and preservation of bowel function. However, more recent data suggest that extreme caution, careful patient selection, and a full discussion of potential risks and benefits are warranted before embarking on this approach. Generally this procedure is reserved for patients with superficial rectal adenocarcinoma (T1 or T2) that occupies less than one-third of the bowel circumference, demonstrates no palpable or radiologically documented perirectal nodes, and is located within 10 cm of the anal verge. Although the early results of local excision were encouraging, more recent studies with long-term followup data consistently show high rates of recurrence and poorer survival than would be expected in the setting of early rectal cancer.[58] This is exemplified by a recent report of 125 patients treated with local excision. Rates of local recurrence were 17% and 28% for T1 and T2 rectal lesions, respectively, much higher than the local recurrence rates reported for radical resection of stage I rectal cancer.[59] The explanation for high relapse rates following local excision is multifactorial, but is clearly related to the issue of regional lymph nodes. Local excision does not assess, remove, or treat potential lymph node metastases. Although patients are screened by endorectal ultrasound or magnetic resonance imaging (MRI) with rectal coil before undergoing local excision, a recent study found that nodal metastases from superficial rectal lesions (T1 and T2) are generally small and very difficult to detect preoperatively.[60] Of even more concern are reports noting that local recurrences are not uniformly amenable to salvage surgery.[61] In fact, the two largest series on salvage surgery for recurrent rectal cancer following local excision show that relapse is generally diagnosed when disease is quite advanced, at which time extended multiorgan resection is usually required. Overall survival after salvage surgery is disappointingly low, especially when one considers the early stage of the initial lesion.[61,62] Improved staging modalities are clearly needed to identify optimal candidates for local excision. Until then, patients should be fully informed of the current limitations of local excision (see Chapter 165).

Minimally Invasive Surgery for Colorectal Cancer. Minimally invasive techniques have been successfully employed in the treatment of colorectal cancer. In prospective randomized series, laparoscopic colectomy for cancer has demonstrated oncologic equivalence to open surgery and has the advantages of smaller incisions, less discomfort, and quicker postoperative recovery.[63-65] Overall, the data support the use of minimally invasive surgery for colon cancer. However, it should be stressed that all of these studies involve surgeons who have extensive experience with laparoscopic colectomy. Some of the available data regarding the "learning curve" for laparoscopic colectomy indicates that a surgeon must perform 30 to 50 cases to become proficient enough to avoid and/or effectively handle complications or conversions, and make efficient use of operating time. These data stress the importance of a surgical mentor, as well as knowledgeable use of laparoscopic-assisted procedures, such as hand-assisted surgery, in the learning curve.

There is considerably less available data on laparoscopic rectal resection for cancer. Laparoscopic total mesorectal excision has been described; however, this is a much more demanding procedure technically because of the confines of the bony pelvis and the limitations of current stapling technology, especially when attempting sphincter preservation.[66] As the field continues to advance, however, the full potential of minimally invasive rectal cancer resection should be realized (see Chapter 178).

CHEMOTHERAPY

Adjuvant Therapy of Colon Cancer

Until the late 1980s, trials of adjuvant chemotherapy in colon cancer had been largely unsuccessful. This was likely due to the fact that they were far too small (often as few as 30 to 50 patients per arm) to detect the subtle benefits that chemotherapy can offer. In the first adequately sized study, involving more than 900 patients, those who received 1 year of 5-fluorouracil (5-FU) plus levamisole (an agent thought to have immune-modulatory effects but later shown to be inactive) had a risk reduction of 33% compared with those receiving surgery only.[67] Further studies demonstrated that 6 months of chemotherapy had essentially the same benefit as 12 months, and that 5-FU plus leucovorin (folinic acid) was as active as 5-FU plus levamisole or 5-FU plus levamisole and leucovorin (LV). Thus, 6 months of 5-FU/LV became standard practice for all stage III patients who did not have a medical contraindication to this treatment.[68]

As will be discussed later, during the late 1990s and the early part of this decade a number of drugs were shown to have clinically meaningful activity in metastatic colorectal cancer. This led to studies to evaluate whether incorporation of such agents into the adjuvant setting would be useful in increasing the cure rate. Of all the drugs tried thus far, however, only oxaliplatin has shown benefit. The lack of benefit demonstrated by other agents remains poorly explained, but serves as a cautionary note about the need to complete adjuvant trials before adopting new agents into the adjuvant setting.

Oxaliplatin Regimens. Oxaliplatin is a platinum-based antineoplastic compound with essentially no nephrotoxicity. Neurotoxicity, myelosuppression, nausea, vomiting, and diarrhea are its main toxicities. Oxaliplatin has minimal antitumor activity by itself, but has shown greater activity when combined with 5-FU/leucovorin. In the pivotal MOSAIC (Multi-center International Study of Oxaliplatin/5-Fluorouracil/Leucovorin in the Adjuvant Treatment of Colon Cancer) trial, a total of 2246 patients (of whom 60% were stage III and 40% stage II), were randomized to postoperative 5-FU/LV by 48-hour infusion every other week, plus/minus a 2-hour infusion of oxaliplatin.[69,70] (This regimen of oxaliplatin, 5-FU, and leucovorin given every other week with infusional 5-FU is known by the acronym FOLFOX.) Five-year disease-free survival (DFS) was 73.3% for the FOLFOX group compared with 67.4% in the 5-FU/LV group ($P = 0.003$). Six-year overall survival rates were 72.9% for those receiving FOLFOX versus 68.7% for those receiving 5-FU/LV ($P = 0.023$). No improvement in overall survival was seen with the addition of oxaliplatin in patients with stage II disease. The outcome of this trial established FOLFOX as the (current) routine standard treatment for patients with stage III colon cancer.

Long-term neurotoxicity is a major concern in oxaliplatin therapy. The toxicities seen in the FOLFOX arm included a 12% incidence of grade 3 sensory neuropathy, which remained at grade 3 in 1% of patients at the time of their 1-year followup. Twenty-seven percent of those receiving oxaliplatin in the MOSAIC trial had some residual neurotoxicity 1 year after the end of treatment, and 11% had some residual neurotoxicity after 4 years of followup. (If such toxicity has not resolved after 4 years, it is unlikely to resolve fully and may therefore be permanent.)

The National Surgical Adjuvant Breast and Bowel Project (NSABP) C-07 trial evaluated the addition of oxaliplatin to a weekly schedule of 5-FU/LV by brief intravenous bolus injection (as opposed to infusion), and randomly assigned 2407 patients with stage II or III colon cancer (71% with stage III disease) to half a year of weekly bolus 5-FU/LV, with or without oxaliplatin administered on weeks 1, 3, and 5 of every 8-week cycle (known as the FLOX regimen).[71] The 3-year DFS in the FLOX arm was 77%, versus 72% in the 5-FU/LV arm. This represents a 21% risk reduction. The weekly bolus schedule of 5-FU/LV used here is known to cause a substantial amount of diarrhea, and hospitalizations for diarrhea/dehydration were required for 5% of patients receiving FLOX and 3% receiving 5-FU/LV.

Studies of the oral fluoropyrimidines capecitabine and tegafur-uracil (UFT) have demonstrated that each is an acceptable alternative to parenteral 5-FU/LV in the adjuvant setting. In a study powered to evaluate the noninferiority of capecitabine compared with the Mayo Clinic bolus 5-FU/LV schedule, noninferiority was demonstrated.[72] Similar results (noninferiority of an oral fluoropyrimidine versus Mayo Clinic 5-FU/LV) were shown in the NSABP C-06 trial of the oral agent UFT plus oral leucovorin (although UFT is not commercially available in the United States).[73] However, because the standard regimen in the adjuvant setting is no longer 5-FU/LV alone, use of these oral agents is limited.

More recently, the combination of oral capecitabine plus parenteral oxaliplatin (CapeOx) has been compared with parenteral 5-FU/LV. This trial has only been reported in abstract form at the time of this writing. Preliminary reports show a modest but statistically significant improvement in 3-year DFS for patients in the CapeOx arm.[74] It is important to remember that CapeOx requires a motivated, reliable patient willing to maintain compliance with the complex medication schedule. These patients will require intravenous oxaliplatin, so it is not a matter of oral versus intravenous chemotherapy. Whether parenteral FOLFOX or parenteral plus oral CapeOx is more convenient for the patient is a matter of conjecture, and it is likely that opinions on this will vary.

Negative Trials. As outlined later in the section on metastatic disease, irinotecan, bevacizumab, and cetuximab are all active agents in metastatic colorectal cancer. All of these, however, have failed to show benefit in the adjuvant setting, and none have a role in treating anything but stage IV disease.

Irinotecan. The CALGB studied the addition of irinotecan to bolus 5-FU/LV. This trial demonstrated no clinical benefit, and a higher rate of early death was seen in the irinotecan-containing arm, as were significant increases in grade severity and life-threatening neutropenia.[75] Similarly disappointing results were seen with the FOLFIRI regimen (irinotecan plus a 48-hour infusion of 5-FU/LV). Two studies done in Europe combining irinotecan with 48-hour 5-FU infusion demonstrated no benefit.[76,77] An additional study of 5-FU/LV plus/minus irinotecan in patients with resected liver metastases also showed no benefit with irinotecan.[78]

Bevacizumab. A phase III trial in the metastatic setting using irinotecan, 5-FU, and leucovorin plus/minus bevacizumab showed a 4.7-month median survival benefit to the group receiving bevacizumab. Following this, the NSABP conducted a 2700-patient randomized trial of FOLFOX versus FOLFOX plus bevacizumab. Thus far, this trial has only been reported in abstract form. It is a negative trial, having failed to meet its prespecified primary endpoint of improved 3-year DFS.[79] There was an interesting but not clinically relevant improvement in DFS at 1 year, suggesting that indefinite continuation of bevacizumab might offer some benefit; however the toxicity and expense of such prolonged bevacizumab exposure make the use of such an approach unreasonable. At this time, there is no role for bevacizumab in the adjuvant treatment of colon cancer.

Cetuximab. Trials in metastatic colorectal cancer had shown that cetuximab was an active agent. The National Cancer Institute (NCI) cooperative groups therefore conducted a phase III trial of FOLFOX plus/minus cetuximab in patients with stage III colon cancer. Well after the trial had started, it became clear that tumors with mutations in the *KRAS* gene were insensitive to cetuximab. The trial was therefore amended to enroll only those patients whose tumors had wild-type, or non-mutated *KRAS*. The results of the trial, presented only in abstract form thus far, show no benefit and some increased toxicity with the addition of cetuximab.[80] Thus, cetuximab, and presumably the very similar agent panitumumab, should not be used in the adjuvant setting.

Stage II Colon Cancer

Stage II colon cancer has a reasonably good chance of surgical cure, with 72% to 85% overall survival. This is one of the most controversial areas in terms of treatment. In general, the evidence is not compelling that chemotherapy offers any meaningful improvement in the cure rate for low-risk stage II colon cancer. For patients with "high-risk" stage II—defined by the presence of either a T4 primary lesion, clinical obstruction, perforation, poorly differentiated histology, or inadequate lymph node sampling (<10 nodes)—risk of relapse is actually higher than the risk of relapse for patients with stage IIIA disease. Therefore, high-risk stage II patients who do not have contraindications to chemotherapy are routinely treated with adjuvant chemotherapy. An analysis in the MOSAIC trial demonstrated no benefit to adding oxaliplatin to treatment of stage II patients; however, an exploratory analysis suggested improved outcome with FOLFOX for high-risk stage II patients.[81] Thus, oxaliplatin should not be used for good-risk stage II patients if the decision in made to offer chemotherapy.

Molecular Markers

At the time of this writing, we do not have any fully validated markers to assist us in selecting patients who either do or do not need chemotherapy, or specific chemotherapy agents, in the adjuvant setting. The Eastern Cooperative Oncology Group (ECOG) E5202 trial is evaluating the role of chemotherapy in higher-risk stage II colorectal cancer patients, as defined by absence of high microsatellite instability (MSI) and intact 18q status. Patients with microsatellite stable disease and/or loss of heterozygosity (LOH) at chromosome 18q are assigned to treatment with modified FOLFOX-6 and randomized to receive or not receive bevacizumab, whereas patients with high MSI and no 18q LOH are assigned to the observation-alone arm. Accrual is currently ongoing.

Some studies have suggested that tumors with high MSI, as detected either by direct measurement or by demonstration of MMR deficiency on immunohistochemical staining, do not benefit or may even suffer a detriment from 5-FU/LV. However, an analysis of MSI from archival tissues in four NSABP adjuvant chemotherapy trials demonstrated no prognostic correlation, and no trend toward a correlation between high MSI and overall survival ($P = 0.67$).[82] More recently, Sargent et al reported on 457 stage II or III colon cancer patients with available tumor samples who were randomized to 5-FU-based chemotherapy versus observation in NCI cooperative group trials.[83] Fifteen percent of these patients were found to have MMR-deficient tumors. In individuals with MMR-deficient tumors, no benefit from 5-FU in terms of DFS was seen. In the stage II patients with MMR-deficient tumors, treatment with 5-FU appeared to be associated with decreased overall survival. These data support the use of MMR evaluation in stage II patients and suggest that single-agent fluoropyrimidine should not be used in patients with MMR-deficient tumors. As oxaliplatin was not available and therefore was not used in the patients studied, these data do not comment on the role of MMR in impacting the efficacy of FOLFOX or other oxaliplatin-containing regimens.

A quantitative multigene assay has been explored as a possible predictor of the potential benefit, or lack thereof, of chemotherapy.[84] Although this assay did demonstrate an ability to characterize patients along prognostic lines, it failed to identify who should or should not receive chemotherapy. Therefore, it provides no basis for decision making and is not recommended in the management of stage II colon cancer at this time.

Summary and Clinical Recommendations

The FOLFOX regimen is the current regimen of choice for stage III and high-risk stage II patients. The CapeOx and FLOX regimens appear to be acceptable alternatives. Trials of irinotecan, bevacizumab, and cetuximab have been negative in the adjuvant setting, and these agents should therefore not be used in adjuvant treatment. In those patients to be treated with fluoropyrimidine alone, 5-FU/LV, or the oral fluoropyrimidines capecitabine or UFT plus leucovorin appear to be reasonable options. Adjuvant chemotherapy for stage II colon cancer remains a complex and controversial topic. All stage II patients should have a medical oncology consultation for a frank discussion of the potential benefits and risks (see Chapter 175).

RECTAL CANCER

The management of local and locoregionally advanced rectal cancer differs from the management of colon cancer in that radiation therapy plays a major role.

Patient evaluation should include either endorectal ultrasound or pelvic MRI, as the initial treatment decision is based on the T stage determined by one of these modalities. In general, if the patient has a T1 or T2 rectal primary without unequivocal evidence of nodal metastases, initial resection is warranted. The exception would be a patient with a distal tumor for whom a sphincter-sparing procedure might be facilitated by tumor regression, in which case preoperative chemoradiotherapy would be indicated. If, however, the preoperative workup indicates either a T3 or T4 primary and/or positive lymph nodes, preoperative chemoradiation is warranted. Many older uncontrolled trials allowed for some differences of opinion on this issue. However, the German Rectal Trial, published in 2004, provides level 1 evidence in favor of preoperative chemoradiotherapy in anything other than T1 or T2 lesions, rendering previous arguments to the contrary moot.[85] This trial, though showing no statistically significant difference in overall survival, showed improved local control (which is the goal of radiation therapy) and decreased toxicity when preoperative rather than postoperative chemoradiotherapy was used.

At present, no studies have demonstrated the superiority of any chemotherapy regimen other than single-agent 5-FU when combined with concurrent radiation therapy. Most trials suggest that oral capecitabine is an acceptable alternative to parenteral 5-FU, although the results of the definitive R-04 trial on this matter are pending. It should be noted that oral chemotherapy requires a motivated, reliable, and compliant patient if it is to be accomplished safely and successfully.

A treatment plan including preoperative pelvic radiation therapy plus chemotherapy also includes postoperative chemotherapy, beginning 4 to 6 weeks after surgery and lasting approximately 4 months. It is imperative to note, and to discuss in advance with the patient, that absolutely no finding intraoperatively will obviate the necessity for postoperative chemotherapy. Even if a pathologic complete response is noted at operation, postoperative chemotherapy must be given as initially planned. Pathologic complete response is an indication of the results of radiation plus chemotherapy; it indicates nothing about the effect of chemotherapy on micrometastatic disease. To fully minimize the chance of death from distant metastatic disease, the full, planned course of postoperative chemotherapy must be given. Extrapolating from the data on colon cancer, postoperative oxaliplatin-containing regimens such as FOLFOX are typically used in the setting of rectal cancer postoperatively. The data thus far do not support routine incorporation of oxaliplatin into concurrent chemoradiotherapy regimens (see Chapter 175).[86]

TREATMENT OF SYSTEMIC METASTATIC (STAGE IV) DISEASE

From the late 1950s until the mid-1990s, chemotherapy for colorectal cancer was limited to 5-FU. Between 1996 and 2004, five new agents received regulatory approval (irinotecan, capecitabine, oxaliplatin, cetuximab, and bevacizumab). We have been stuck in the doldrums of drug development for colorectal cancer ever since. With the exception of panitumumab, which differs only trivially from cetuximab and does not open up any novel treatment paradigms, nothing new has become available.

Fluorouracil (5-FU), patented in 1957, remains the single most active and important drug in the treatment of colorectal cancer. It is a sobering reality that all drugs developed since have essentially been failures when compared to preclinical expectations. All of these agents were designed to replace 5-FU. None, however, has demonstrated single-agent superiority. As a result, the fallback strategy of drug development has been employed: drugs that have failed to show any ability to displace 5-FU have been combined with it, and the resulting regimens show evidence of superiority over single-agent 5-FU alone.

The first such agent to be developed was the topoisomerase I (topo I) inhibitor, irinotecan. A randomized trial of irinotecan/5-FU/leucovorin (IFL) versus 5-FU/leucovorin alone demonstrated modest superiority for the IFL regimen.[87] This trial used 5-FU on a weekly bolus injection schedule. A parallel trial conducted in Europe used an every-other-week infusion schedule of 5-FU, with similar results.[88]

At the same time, investigators working with the third-generation platinum compound oxaliplatin showed that the combination of oxaliplatin plus 2-day infusions of 5-FU/LV (FOLFOX) every other week was superior to the 5-FU/LV regimen alone.[89] These trials, however, while demonstrating improvements in response rate and progression-free survival, failed to show a statistically significant survival benefit; because of this, approval of oxaliplatin in the United States was delayed for several years.

Subsequently, a randomized intergroup trial (N9741) of irinotecan plus bolus 5-FU/LV (IFL), versus oxaliplatin plus infusional 5-FU (FOLFOX), showed a higher response rate and longer time to tumor progression for the FOLFOX arm.[90] Survival on the FOLFOX arm was superior; however, the meaning of these survival data is difficult to interpret because second-line irinotecan was widely available to the FOLFOX patients, whereas second-line oxaliplatin was not widely available to the IFL patients (oxaliplatin was not approved for use in the United States at that time). Second-line irinotecan has been shown to confer a survival advantage,[91] and survival has been correlated with the availability of all active drugs.[92]

Overall, the N9741 trial did show the FOLFOX regimen to be preferable to the IFL regimen. Unfortunately, this was largely misinterpreted as evidence of the superiority of oxaliplatin over irinotecan, which is not a correct interpretation. In fact, what the trial most likely shows is the superiority of infusional over bolus 5-FU. Two randomized studies comparing first-line FOLFOX (infusional 5-FU/leucovorin plus oxaliplatin) versus FOLFIRI (infusional 5-FU/LV plus irinotecan) indicate that response rate, time to tumor progression, and overall survival were virtually the same, regardless of which regimen was used first.[93,94] The conclusion of the aggregate of these trials is that FOLFOX or FOLFIRI are equally acceptable in the front-line management of metastatic colorectal cancer.

A large phase III trial compared FOLFOX to the combination of capecitabine plus oxaliplatin (CapeOx), demonstrating that these two regimens were comparable in efficacy and similar in overall degree of toxicity.[95] Thus, FOLFOX, FOLFIRI, or CapeOx are acceptable standard front-line combination regimens. Capecitabine has also been the focus of a large trial comparing sequential use of single agents to combinations. In this trial, patients treated with sequential single agents experienced overall survival similar to that achieved with combination regimens.[96] The FOCUS trial, which compared front-line infusional 5-FU/leucovorin to front-line FOLFOX and FOLFIRI, also showed no survival benefit by using combination therapy as initial treatment.[97] These trials indicate the importance of individualization of care. Clearly, some patients can be spared the toxicity of combination regimens without detriment, whereas others, especially those with rapidly progressing and/or symptomatic disease, are more likely to benefit from the higher response rates achieved with combination therapies.

Bevacizumab is a monoclonal antibody that binds to vascular endothelial growth factor (VEGF). It was initially hoped that bevacizumab would have meaningful single-agent antitumor activity, but this turned out not to be the case. Bevacizumab does appear to add to the efficacy of some chemotherapeutic regimens, however. In a randomized, double-blind, placebo-controlled trial, IFL plus bevacizumab was superior to IFL plus placebo, with a 4.7-month improvement in overall survival, a 4.4-month improvement in progression-free survival, and a 35% to 45% improvement in response rate.[98] The addition of bevacizumab to front-line oxaliplatin-based therapy has been somewhat less successful. In a very large, randomized, placebo-controlled trial of either CapeOx or FOLFOX plus either bevacizumab or placebo,[99] progression-free survival was significantly improved statistically, but the incremental benefit was a modest 1.4 months. Overall survival was also improved by 1.4 months, which did not reach statistical significance. In addition, the response rate with bevacizumab was virtually identical to that of placebo.

Cetuximab and panitumumab are monoclonal antibodies that target the epidermal growth factor receptor (EGFR). Although they have never been (and likely never will be) compared head to head, they appear to be extremely similar and have very similar activity profiles. Panitumumab is associated with a lower incidence of hypersensitivity reactions.

Initial studies of cetuximab demonstrated a 22.5% response rate in irinotecan-refractory colorectal cancer when cetuximab was given in combination with continued irinotecan,[100] and a single-agent response rate of 10.5%.[101] These activity levels were subsequently confirmed in a randomized trial. Panitumumab was also shown to have a 10% response rate as a single agent in a similar patient population.[102] Subsequently, it was demonstrated that both of these agents had potential efficacy only in cancers characterized by a wild-type (nonmutated) *KRAS* gene. *KRAS* mutational analysis has now

become standard practice, and neither cetuximab nor panitumumab should be offered to patients whose tumors have mutated *KRAS*.[103,104] The major side effect of both of these anti-EGFR monoclonal antibodies is an acne-like skin rash. Studies have now consistently shown that, for reasons that remain unclear, skin rash is tightly linked to antitumor activity, and only those patients with moderate to severe skin rashes benefit from these agents. Management of the skin rash is difficult, however. Oral antibiotics appear to improve it somewhat, but topical agents other than moisturizers have not demonstrated convincing usefulness thus far.

Studies using either cetuximab or panitumumab with first-line FOLFOX or FOLFIRI regimens have now been reported.[105-107] Activity, as expected, is confined to those patients with wild-type *KRAS* tumors; in several studies, patients with mutated *KRAS* who receive anti-EGFR agents actually have a worse outcome than the control arm.[106,107] Given that only those patients who react with substantial skin rash benefit from this approach, its practical utility in first-line management is somewhat limited. Patients with *KRAS* wild-type tumors, and those whose metastatic disease is potentially convertible to resectability by a substantial regression in tumor size, are reasonable candidates for consideration of front-line combination chemotherapy plus an anti-EGFR inhibitor, as this strategy has been shown to improve response rates.

Given the demonstrated activity of bevacizumab and the anti-EGFR agents with chemotherapy, there was logical enthusiasm for combining anti-VEGF and anti-EGFR strategies. A small, randomized phase II study demonstrated the feasibility of this strategy[108]; however, two large randomized trials, one with CapeOx-bevacizumab plus/minus cetuximab[109] and the other with FOLFOX-bevacizumab plus/minus panitumumab,[110] each showed that there was not only *no* benefit to adding an anti-EGFR agent to a regimen of chemotherapy plus bevacizumab, but that there was actually a harmful effect: the dual antibody regimens had worse outcomes than the control arms. Therefore, concurrent use of bevacizumab plus anti-EGFR agents is not recommended (see Chapter 175).

CHEMOTHERAPY WITH SURGERY FOR METASTATIC DISEASE

Resection of stage IV disease confined to liver or lung has become accepted standard practice. The role of chemotherapy in such surgical strategies continues to be defined. As noted earlier, a randomized trial of 5-FU/LV plus/minus irinotecan after liver resection showed no benefit for the irinotecan-containing arm.[78] However, this study did not address the merits of chemotherapy versus no chemotherapy. In the first trial to address this issue with reasonable power, patients with clinically resectable liver metastases were randomly assigned to surgery alone versus surgery with 3 months of preoperative FOLFOX and 3 months of postoperative FOLFOX.[111] Of the patients who actually underwent an R0 resection, those who received chemotherapy had a statistically significant improvement in 3-year DFS; however, the actual improvement was 9.2%, a substantially smaller margin than had been hoped for. Nevertheless, in patients whose disease has not progressed through FOLFOX chemotherapy, use of FOLFOX in the perioperative setting appears to be appropriate.

Previously, the assumption had been made that any therapy demonstrating activity in unresected stage IV disease would be a reasonable adjuvant therapy in resected stage IV disease. This concept requires reexamination, however. As noted earlier, irinotecan,[78] bevacizumab,[79] and cetuximab[80] (and, by extrapolation, panitumumab) have all been shown to be ineffective in resected stage III patients: none eradicated micrometastases in these patients. As it is difficult to see how these agents could be expected to eradicate micrometastases in the stage IV setting with any greater efficacy than in stage III, it would seem difficult to justify their use following resection of stage IV disease. In terms of preoperative therapy, it is important to distinguish between (1) the true neoadjuvant setting (in which disease is clearly resectable, and in which case these agents would not appear to have any more role than they would in postoperative use) and (2) disease that is not believed to be resectable but rather *potentially convertible* to resectability in the setting of a sufficient antitumor response. In such cases, use of an anti-EGFR agent with chemotherapy, use of an irinotecan-containing regimen, and use of an irinotecan-containing regimen with bevacizumab would appear to be reasonable considerations. It should be noted that bevacizumab did not improve the response rate or degree of tumor shrinkage in a 1400-patient randomized trial with oxaliplatin-based chemotherapy.[99] Bevacizumab does appear to improve the response rate with irinotecan-based therapy, so if shrinkage of gross metastatic disease for the purpose of converting a patient from unresectable to resectable is the goal of treatment, the use of an irinotecan-plus-bevacizumab-containing combination would seem reasonable. It should also be noted that bevacizumab does impede wound healing, and its half-life is approximately 21 days. Therefore, it is recommended that bevacizumab be discontinued at least 6 weeks prior to any planned major surgery (see Chapter 175).

COLORECTAL CANCER POSTRESECTION FOLLOWUP

Eighty percent of patients who recur after curative resection of colon and rectal carcinomas do so within 3 years. Therefore, any posttreatment plan should include regular followup during at least these 3 years. An additional biologic precept in designing followup should take into account the efficacy of therapy once recurrent disease is identified. It is important to note that the role of surveillance is to identify recurrent disease that can be resected with true curative intent; early identification of asymptomatic, incurable disease is exceedingly unlikely to improve outcome, as there are neither data nor a compelling rationale to believe that outcome would be improved by earlier institution of noncurative treatment, such as systemic chemotherapy. These facts dictate the schedule summarized in Figures 164-8 and 164-9.[112]

In general, if a patient is a candidate for resection of recurrent disease (e.g., hepatic resection), serum CEA testing should be performed every 3 to 6 months for 2 years then every 6 months for a total of 5 years after resection of the primary tumor. Chest, abdomen, and pelvis CT is recommended annually for 3 years for patients at high risk for recurrence. Positron emission tomography–computed tomography (PET-CT) scan is not routinely recommended. Colonoscopy should be performed 1 year after surgery or 3 to 6 months after surgery if not performed preoperatively because of an obstructing lesion, and then 3 years later, and then every 5 years, unless findings or specific risk factors dictate more frequent evaluations.

Another important aspect of followup is instruction of the patient. Specific and nonspecific signs and symptoms that should initiate a patient's return for routine history, physical examination, and appropriate diagnostic studies should be detailed. When these signs and symptoms are not present, and because palliation is generally the only goal in treating most recurrences, there is little benefit in attempting to define recurrence early. Nevertheless, it is suggested that a clinical history and physical examination be performed every 3 to 6 months for the first 3 postoperative years, and at least annually for the next 2 years. Routine oncologic followup and surveillance is typically considered completed after approximately 5 years, and routine diagnostic imaging, CEA monitoring, or other oncologic followup is not typically recommended.

Colonoscopic surveillance, however, is routinely recommended to continue indefinitely. This is because the rationale for colonoscopy in perioperative staging and followup is not to identify recurrent cancer, and the yield in diagnosing isolated suture line recurrence by either endoscopy or guaiac testing of stool is low. The major reason for using colonoscopy is to identify synchronous or metachronous bowel tumors, usually polyps. As patients are exposed more uniformly to followup endoscopy after primary colorectal cancer resection, the incidence of metachronous lesions seems to be increasing.[112-114] Whatever the ultimate incidence of metachronous bowel lesions, however, patients with sentinel colorectal carcinomas are unquestionably at significant risk of developing metachronous polyps. If these polyps are discovered and removed, the risk of subsequent development of colon and rectal cancer decreases. Adequate screening to rule out synchronous lesions at the time of primary surgery or later, and serial followup every 3 to 5 years to ensure a cancer- and polyp-free colon, should be a mandatory part of any postoperative surveillance program for colorectal cancer patients.

TUMOR MARKERS

Carcinoembryonic antigen (CEA) remains the prototypical solid tumor marker. Despite its lack of specificity, if used correctly CEA testing is a valuable addition to the process of clinical decision making in patients diagnosed with colon or rectal carcinoma. However, it is not an appropriate screening test. Whether sampled once or serially, CEA cannot be used in the differential

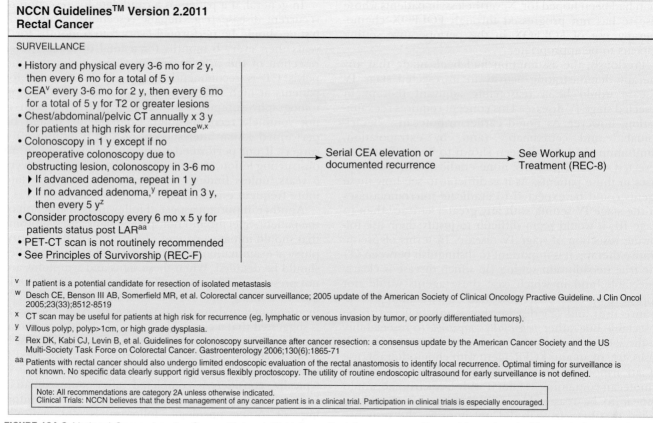

diagnosis of an unknown-but-suspected bowel problem or malignancy. Nevertheless, when CEA concentrations are determined before primary tumor resection, they may be of additional prognostic value; this is particularly true in patients with stage II disease, for whom elevated preoperative CEA is a poor prognostic marker and may influence the decision regarding whether or not to administer adjuvant chemotherapy.

Serial CEA values obtained postoperatively are a potentially effective means of monitoring response to therapy. A postoperative CEA titer serves as a measure of the completeness of tumor resection. It should be remembered, however, that the half-life of CEA is 7 to 14 days; therefore, postoperative baselines are best established several weeks after resection. If a preoperatively elevated CEA value does not fall to normal within 2 to 3 weeks after surgery, it is likely that (1) the resection was incomplete or (2) occult metastases are present. A rising trend in serial CEA values from a normal postoperative baseline (<5 ng/mL) may predate any other clinical or laboratory evidence of recurrent disease by 6 to 9 months.

Serial CEA values tend to roughly parallel tumor regression or progression during treatment for metastatic disease. The majority of patients who respond to treatment show a decline in CEA levels. Rising CEA levels are usually incompatible with tumor regression. However, the actual utility of these measurements is limited, as decisions to continue or discontinue a chemotherapy

regimen should rarely (if ever) be made on the basis of a rising CEA alone.

There are no data to guide an optimal schedule of CEA monitoring after potentially curative colorectal resection. A reasonable strategy is to obtain CEA levels every 3 to 6 months for the first 3 years postoperatively and every 6 months for the fourth and fifth postoperative year. The available data do not suggest that continued CEA monitoring after 5 years is of significant benefit. Colonoscopy is recommended at 1 year following resection, and then 3 years after that, and then every 5 years thereafter. Routine computed tomography (CT) scans and chest radiography have not been shown to improve survival; thus, formal evidence-based recommendations on CT or radiographic imaging studies cannot be made, although annual CT scans for the first 3 to 5 years are a frequent and reasonable practice.

A newly elevated CEA level should first be repeated to confirm the finding or rule out laboratory error. A confirmed new elevation should be further evaluated with a full-body CT scan and, if this is negative, a colonoscopy. In considering workup of an elevated CEA level, it is important to keep in mind that the goals of this screening are to identify potentially curable patients: individuals with surgically resectable metastatic disease. Isolated liver, lung, or ovarian metastases are potentially curable with surgery, as are some local anastomotic recurrences. Identification of asymptomatic but incurable disease, such as peritoneal metastases or retroperitoneal lymph

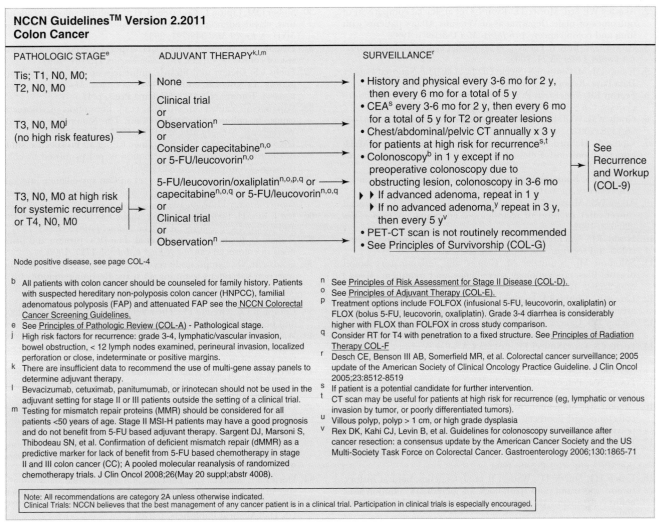

FIGURE 164-9 National Comprehensive Cancer Network Guidelines: Colon cancer surveillance. (Reproduced with permission from Colon cancer version 2.2011, 11/18/10. Copyright National Comprehensive Cancer Network, Inc, 2010. All rights reserved.)

nodes, is of essentially no benefit and does not contribute to the patient's overall well-being. There is no evidence that early initiation of systemic chemotherapy for incurable metastatic disease results in a better outcome. Thus, the role of CEA monitoring and postoperative imaging is to help identify patients with resectable (and therefore curable) disease.

"Second look" surgery in the absence of an identified curable lesion on imaging studies is no longer recommended, because it is extremely unlikely to show curable disease. In later application of radioimmunologic scanning techniques using either external or intraoperative gamma-scanning,[115] the weak link remains lack of any effective systemic therapy even when recurrent disease is found early.

Serial CEA rise will show the steepest slope if liver or lung is the first or only site of recurrence. Specific diagnostic tests to confirm recurrence in the liver or lung are now preferable to so-called blind, CEA-directed second-look procedures.[116] At present, only patients manifesting recurrence of colorectal carcinoma as defined, isolated liver, lung, ovarian, or anastomotic metastases

should undergo surgery. Therefore, it is recommended that postoperative monitoring of CEA be reserved for patients who would be candidates for resection of these potentially curable metastases should they occur. As is the case with other followup testing, the optimal frequency of serial CEA monitoring has not been established.[116]

PET scanning has been recommended by some as a tool for workup of elevated CEA. It should be remembered, however, that identification of asymptomatic, unresectable disease is unlikely to improve long-term outcome, and may actually increase the patient's anxiety. In the setting of negative, high-quality, current CT and/ or MRI scans, most surgeons would be reluctant to operate on the basis of a positive PET scan alone. For this reason, the true contribution of PET to management of an elevated postresection CEA is questionable.

REFERENCES

1. Jemal A, Siegel R, Xu J, et al: Cancer statistics, 2010. *CA Cancer J Clin* 60:277, 2010.

2. Akerley WL 3rd, Moritz TE, Ryan LS, et al: Racial comparison of outcomes of male Department of Veterans Affairs patients with lung and colon cancer. *Arch Intern Med* 153:1681, 1993.

3. Parkin DM, Bray F, Ferlay J, et al: Global cancer statistics, 2002. *CA Cancer J Clin* 55:74, 2005.

4. Jessup JM, McGinnis LS, Steele GD Jr, et al: The National Cancer Data Base. Report on colon cancer. *Cancer* 78:918, 1996.

5. Fearon ER, Vogelstein B: A genetic model for colorectal tumorigenesis. *Cell* 61:759, 1990.

6. Grady WM: WCIMP and colon cancer gets more complicated. *Gut* 56:1498, 2007.

7. Lipton L, Halford SE, Johnson V, et al: Carcinogenesis in MYH-associated polyposis follows a distinct genetic pathway. *Cancer Res* 63:7595, 2003.

8. Sandler RS: Epidemiology and risk factors for colorectal cancer. *Gastroenterol Clin North Am* 25:717, 1996.

9. Atkin WS, Morson BC, Cuzick J: Long-term risk of colorectal cancer after excision of rectosigmoid adenomas. *N Engl J Med* 326:658, 1992.

10. Heald RJ: Synchronous and metachronous carcinoma of the colon and rectum. *Ann R Coll Surg Engl* 72:172, 1990.

11. Solomon MJ, Schnitzler M: Cancer and inflammatory bowel disease: Bias, epidemiology, surveillance, and treatment. *World J Surg* 22:352, 1998.

12. Lavery IC, Chiulli RA, Jagelman DG, et al: Survival with carcinoma arising in mucosal ulcerative colitis. *Ann Surg* 195:508, 1982.

13. Sacher DB: Cancer in Crohn's disease: Dispelling the myths. *Gut* 35:1507, 1994.

14. Fuchs CS, Giovannucci EL, Colditz GA, et al: A prospective study of family history and the risk of colorectal cancer. *N Engl J Med* 331:1669, 1994.

15. Powell SM, Petersen GM, Krush AJ, et al: Molecular diagnosis of familial adenomatous polyposis. *N Engl J Med* 329:1982, 1993.

16. Nugent KP, Spigelman AD, Phillips RK: Life expectancy after colectomy and ileorectal anastomosis for familial adenomatous polyposis. *Dis Colon Rectum* 36:1059, 1993.

17. Brensinger JD, Laken SJ, Luce MC, et al: Variable phenotype of familial adenomatous polyposis in pedigrees with 3′ mutation in the APC gene. *Gut* 43:548, 1998.

18. Lynch HT, Smyrk TC, Watson P, et al: Genetics, natural history, tumor spectrum, and pathology of hereditary nonpolyposis colorectal cancer: An updated review. *Gastroenterology* 104:1535, 1993.

19. Vasen HF, Mecklin JP, Khan PM, et al: Hereditary non-polyposis colorectal cancer. *Lancet* 338:877, 1991.

20. Aarnio M, Sankila R, Pukkala E, et al: Cancer risk in mutation carriers of DNA-mismatch-repair genes. *Int J Cancer* 81:214, 1999.

21. Lindor NM, Rabe K, Petersen GM, et al: Lower cancer incidence in Amsterdam-I criteria families without mismatch repair deficiency: Familial colorectal cancer type X. *JAMA* 293:2028, 2008.

22. Scott RJ, McPhillips M, Meldrum CJ, et al: Hereditary nonpolyposis colorectal cancer in 95 families: Differences and similarities between mutation-positive and mutation-negative kindreds. *Am J Hum Genet* 68:118, 2001.

23. Shashidharan M, Smyrk T, Lin KM, et al: Histologic comparison of hereditary nonpolyposis colorectal cancer associated with MSH2 and MLH1 and colorectal cancer from the general population. *Dis Colon Rectum* 42:722, 1999.

24. Haggitt RC, Reid BJ: Hereditary gastrointestinal polyposis syndromes. *Am J Surg Pathol* 19:871, 1986.

25. Giardiello FM, Welsh SB, Hamilton SR, et al: Increased risk of cancer in the Peutz-Jeghers syndrome. *N Engl J Med* 316:1511, 1987.

26. Jass JR, Williams CB, Bussey HJ, et al: Juvenile polyposis—a precancerous condition. *Histopathology* 13:619, 1988.

27. Laken SJ, Petersen GM, Gruber SB, et al: Familial colorectal cancer in Ashkenazim due to a hypermutable tract in APC. *Nat Genet* 17:79, 1997.

28. Prior TW, Chadwick RB, Papp AC, et al: The I1307K polymorphism of the APC gene in colorectal cancer. *Gastroenterology* 116:58, 1999.

29. Rozen P, Shomrat R, Strul H, et al: Prevalence of the I1307C APC gene variant in Israeli Jews of differing ethnic origin and risk for colorectal cancer. *Gastroenterology* 116:54, 1999.

30. Sieber OM, Lipton L, Crabtree M, et al: Multiple colorectal adenomas, classic adenomatous polyposis, and germ-line mutations in MYH. *N Engl J Med* 348:791, 2003.

31. Hyman NH, Anderson P, Blasyk H: Hyperplastic polyposis and the risk of colorectal cancer. *Dis Colon Rectum* 47:2101, 2004.

32. Fuchs CS: Dietary and lifestyle influences on colorectal carcinogenesis. In Saltz LB, editors: *Colorectal Cancer: Multimodality Management.* Totowa, NJ, 2002, Humana Press, p 47.

33. Winawer SJ, Zauber AJ, Ho MN, et al: Prevention of colorectal cancer by colonoscopic polypectomy. The National Polyp Study Workgroup. *N Engl J Med* 329:1977, 1993.

34. Hixson LJ, Fennerty MB, Sampliner RE, et al: Prospective study of the frequency and size distribution of polyps missed by colonoscopy. *J Natl Cancer Inst* 82:1769, 1990.

35. Zauber AG, Winawer SJ, Bond J, et al: Can surveillance intervals be lengthened following colonoscopic polypectomy? [Abstract] *Gastroenterology* 112:A50, 1997.

36. Jen J, Kim H, Piantadosi S, et al: Allelic loss of chromosome 18q and prognosis in colorectal cancer. *N Engl J Med* 331:213, 1994.

37. Shibata D, Reale MA, Lavin P, et al: The DCC protein and prognosis in colorectal cancer. *N Engl J Med* 335:1727, 1996.

38. Goldstein NS: Lymph node recoveries from 2427 pT3 colorectal resection specimens spanning 45 years: Recommendations for a minimum number of recovered lymph nodes based on predictive probabilities. *Am J Surg Pathol* 26:179, 2002.

39. Compton CC, Greene FL: The staging of colorectal cancer: 2004 and beyond. *CA Cancer J Clin* 54:295, 2004.

40. Waldman SA, Hyslop T, Schulz S, et al: Association of GUCY2C expression in lymph nodes with time to recurrence and disease-free survival in pN0 colorectal cancer. *JAMA* 301:745, 2009.

41. Bertagnolli M, Miedema B, Redston M, et al: Sentinel node staging of resectable colon cancer: Results of a multicenter study. *Ann Surg* 240:624, 2004.

42. O'Connell JB, Maggard MA, Ko CY: Colon cancer survival rates with the new American Joint Committee on Cancer sixth edition staging. *J Natl Cancer Inst* 96:1420, 2004.

43. Temple LK, Hsieh L, Wong WD, et al: Use of surgery among elderly patients with stage IV colorectal cancer. *J Clin Oncol* 22:3475, 2004.

44. Herter FP, Slanetz CA: Patterns and significance of lymphatic spread from cancer of the colon and rectum. In Weiss L, Gilbert HA, Ballon SC, editors: *Lymphatic system metastases.* Boston, 1980, GK Hall Medical Publishers, p 275.

45. Pezim ME, Nicholls RJ: Survival after high or low ligation of the inferior mesenteric artery during curative surgery for rectal cancer. *Ann Surg* 200:729, 1984.

46. Weiser MR, Quah HM, Shia J, et al: Sphincter preservation in low rectal cancer is facilitated by preoperative chemoradiation and intersphincteric dissection. *Ann Surg* 249:236, 2009.

47. Rullier E, Laurent C, Bretagnol F, et al: Sphincter-saving resection for all rectal carcinomas: The end of the 2-cm distal rule. *Ann Surg* 241:465, 2005.

48. Temple LK, Bacik J, Savatta SG, et al: The development of a validated instrument to evaluate bowel function after sphincter-preserving surgery for rectal cancer. *Dis Colon Rectum* 48:1353, 2005.

49. Hallbrook O, Pahlman L, Krog M, et al: Randomized comparison of straight and colonic J pouch anastomosis after low anterior resection. *Ann Surg* 224:58, 1996.

50. Goligher JC, Dukes CE, Bussey HJ: Local recurrences after sphincter saving excisions for carcinoma of the rectum and rectosigmoid. *Br J Surg* 39:199, 1951.

51. Wilson SM, Bears OH: The curative treatment of carcinoma of the sigmoid, rectosigmoid, and rectum. *Ann Surg* 183:556, 1976.

52. Moore HG, Riedel E, Minsky BD, et al: Adequacy of 1-cm distal margin after restorative rectal cancer resection with sharp mesorectal excision and preoperative combined-modality therapy. *Ann Surg Oncol* 10:80, 2003.

53. Quirk P, Durdey P, Dixon MF, et al: Local recurrence of rectal adenocarcinoma due to inadequate surgical resection: Histopathological study of lateral tumour spread and surgical excision. *Lancet* 2:996, 1986.

54. Enker WE, Thaler HT, Cranor ML, et al: Total mesorectal excision in the operative treatment of carcinoma of the rectum. *J Am Coll Surg* 181:335, 1995.

55. Heald RJ, Moran BJ, Ryall RD, et al: Rectal cancer: The Basingstoke experience of total mesorectal excision, 1978-1997. *Arch Surg* 133:894, 1998.

56. Schrag D, Cramer LD, Bach PB, et al: Influence of hospital procedure volume on outcomes following surgery for colon cancer. *JAMA* 284:3028, 2000.

57. Rodriguez-Bigas MA, Petrelli NJ: Management of hereditary colon cancer syndromes. In Saltz LB, editor: *Colorectal Cancer: Multimodality Management*, Totowa, NJ, 2002, Humana Press, p 99.

58. Gimbel MI, Paty P: A current perspective on local excision of rectal cancer. *Clin Colorectal Cancer* 4:26, 2004.

59. Blumberg D, Paty P, Picon AI, et al: Stage I rectal cancer: Identification of high-risk patients. *J Am Coll Surg* 186:574, 1998.

60. Landmann RG, Wong WD, Hoepfl J, et al: Can endorectal ultrasound (ERUS) correctly determine nodal stage in patients considered for local excision? [Abstract] In: Program and Abstracts of the American Society of Colon and Rectal Surgeons 2005 Annual Meeting, April 30-May 5, 2005, Philadelphia, Poster 14, p. 326.

61. Weiser MR, Landmann RG, Wong WD, et al: Surgical salvage of recurrent rectal cancer after transanal excision. *Dis Colon Rectum* 48:1169, 2005.

62. Hermsen PE, Nonner J, De Graaf EJ, et al: Recurrences after transanal excision or transanal endoscopic microsurgery of T1 rectal cancer. *Minerva Chir* 65:213, 2010.

63. Delgado S, Lacy AM, García Valdecasas JC, et al: Could age be an indication for laparoscopic colectomy in colorectal cancer? *Surg Endosc* 14:22, 2000.

64. Jayne DG, Guillou PJ, Thorpe H, et al: Randomized trial of laparoscopic-assisted resection of colorectal carcinoma: 3-year results of the UK MRC CLASICC Trial Group. *J Clin Oncol* 25:3061, 2007.

65. The COlon cancer Laparoscopic or Open Resection Study Group: Laparoscopic surgery versus open surgery for colon cancer: Short-term outcomes of a randomised trial. *Lancet Oncol* 6:477, 2005.

66. Weiser MR, Milsom JW: Laparoscopic total mesorectal excision with autonomic nerve preservation. *Semin Surg Oncol* 19:396, 2000.

67. Laurie JA, Moertel CG, Fleming TR, et al: Surgical adjuvant therapy of large bowel carcinoma: An evaluation of levamisole and the combination of levamisole and fluorouracil. *J Clin Oncol* 7:1447, 1989.

68. Haller DG, Catalano PJ, Macdonald JS, et al: Phase III study of fluorouracil, leucovorin, and levamisole in high-risk stage II and III colon cancer: Final report of Intergroup 0089. *J Clin Oncol* 23:8671, 2005.

69. Andre T, Boni C, Mounedji-Boudiaf L, et al: Oxaliplatin, fluorouracil, and leucovorin as adjuvant treatment for colon cancer. *N Engl J Med* 350:2343, 2004.

70. Andre T, Boni C, Navarro M, et al: Improved overall survival with oxaliplatin, fluorouracil, and leucovorin as adjuvant treatment in Stage II or III colon cancer in the MOSAIC Trial. *J Clin Oncol* 27:3109, 2009.

71. Kuebler JP, Wieand HS, O'Connell MJ, et al: Oxaliplatin combined with weekly bolus fluorouracil and leucovorin as surgical adjuvant chemotherapy for Stage II and III colon cancer: Results from NSABP C-07. *J Clin Oncol* 25:2198, 2007.

72. Twelves C, Wong A, Nowacki MP, et al: Capecitabine as adjuvant treatment for stage III colon cancer. *N Engl J Med* 352:2696, 2005.

73. Lembersky BC, Wieand HS, Petrelli NJ, et al: Oral uracil and tegafur plus leucovorin compared with intravenous fluorouracil and leucovorin in stage II and III carcinoma of the colon: Results from National Surgical Adjuvant Breast and Bowel Project Protocol C-06. *J Clin Oncol* 24:2059, 2006.

74. Haller D, Tabernero J, Maroun J, et al: 5LBA First efficacy findings from a randomized phase III trial of capecitabine + oxaliplatin vs. bolus 5-FU/LV for stage III colon cancer (NO16968/XELOXA study) 7:4, 2009.

75. Saltz LB, Niedzwiecki D, Hollis D, et al: Irinotecan fluorouracil plus leucovorin is not superior to fluorouracil plus leucovorin alone as adjuvant treatment for Stage III colon cancer: Results of CALGB 89803. *J Clin Oncol* 25:3456, 2007.

76. Ychou M, Raoul J-L, Douillard J-Y, et al: A phase III randomised trial of LV5FU2 + irinotecan versus LV5FU2 alone in adjuvant high-risk colon cancer (FNCLCC Accord02/FFCD9802). *Ann Oncol* 20:674, 2009.

77. Van Cutsem E, Labianca R, Bodoky G, et al: Randomized phase III trial comparing biweekly infusional fluorouracil/leucovorin alone or with irinotecan in the adjuvant treatment of Stage III colon cancer: PETACC-3. *J Clin Oncol* 27:3117, 2009.

78. Ychou M, Hohenberger W, Thezenas S, et al: A randomized phase III study comparing adjuvant 5-fluorouracil/folinic acid with FOLFIRI in patients following complete resection of liver metastases from colorectal cancer. *Ann Oncol* 20:1964, 2009.

79. Wolmark N, Yothers G, O'Connell MJ, et al: A phase III trial comparing mFOLFOX6 to mFOLFOX6 plus bevacizumab in stage II or III carcinoma of the colon: Results of NSABP Protocol C-08. *J Clin Oncol* 27:(suppl; Abstract LBA4), 2009.

80. Alberts SR, Sargent DJ, Smyrk CJ, et al: Adjuvant mFOLFOX6 with or without cetuxiumab (Cmab) in KRAS wild-type (WT) patients (pts) with resected stage III colon cancer (CC): Results from NCCTG Intergroup Phase III Trial N0147. *J Clin Oncol* 28:(suppl; Abstract CRA3507), 2010.

81. de Gramont A, Boni C, Navarro M, et al: Oxaliplatin/5FU/LV in adjuvant colon cancer: Updated efficacy results of the MOSAIC trial, including survival, with a median follow-up of six years. *J Clin Oncol* 25:Abstract 4007, 2007.

82. Kim GP, Colangelo LH, Wieand HS, et al: Prognostic and predictive roles of high-degree microsatellite instability in colon cancer: A National Cancer Institute-National Surgical Adjuvant Breast and Bowel Project Collaborative Study. *J Clin Oncol* 25:767, 2007.

83. Sargent DJ, Marsoni S, Monges G, et al: Defective mismatch repair as a predictive marker for lack of efficacy of fluorouracil-based adjuvant therapy in colon cancer. *J Clin Oncol* 28:3219, 2010.

84. Kerr D, Gray R, Quirke P, et al: A quantitative multigene RT-PCR assay for prediction of recurrence in stage II colon cancer: Selection of the genes in four large studies and results of the independent, prospectively designed QUASAR validation study. *J Clin Oncol* 27: abstr 4000, 2009.

85. Sauer R, Becker H, Hohenberger W, et al: Preoperative versus postoperative chemoradiotherapy for rectal cancer. *N Engl J Med* 351:1731, 2004.

86. Gerard J-P, Azria D, Gourgou-Bourgade S, et al: Comparison of two neoadjuvant chemoradiotherapy regimens for locally advanced rectal cancer: Results of the phase III trial ACCORD 12/0405-Prodige 2. *J Clin Oncol* 28:1638, 2010.

87. Saltz LB, Cox JV, Blanke C, et al: Irinotecan plus fluorouracil and leucovorin for metastatic colorectal cancer. Irinotecan Study Group. *N Engl J Med* 343:905, 2000.

88. Douillard JY, Cunningham D, Roth AD, et al: Irinotecan combined with fluorouracil compared with fluorouracil alone as first-line treatment for metastatic colorectal cancer: A multicentre randomised trial. *Lancet* 355:1041, 2000.

89. de Gramont A, Figer A, Seymour M, et al: Leucovorin and fluorouracil with or without oxaliplatin as first-line treatment in advanced colorectal cancer. *J Clin Oncol* 18:2938, 2000.

90. Goldberg RM, Sargent DJ, Morton RF, et al: A randomized controlled trial of fluorouracil plus leucovorin, irinotecan, and oxaliplatin combinations in patients with previously untreated metastatic colorectal cancer. *J Clin Oncol* 22:23, 2004.

91. Cunningham D, Pyrhonen S, James R, et al: Randomised trial of irinotecan plus supportive care versus supportive care alone after fluorouracil failure for patients with metastatic colorectal cancer. *Lancet* 352:1413, 1998.

92. Grothey A, Sargent D, Goldberg RM, et al: Survival of patients with advanced colorectal cancer improves with the availability of fluorouracil-leucovorin, irinotecan, and oxaliplatin in the course of treatment. *J Clin Oncol* 22:1209, 2004.

93. Tournigand C, Andre T, Achille E, et al: FOLFIRI followed by FOLFOX6 or the reverse sequence in advanced colorectal cancer: A randomized GERCOR study. *J Clin Oncol* 22:229, 2004.

94. Colucci G, Gebbia V, Paoletti G, et al: Phase III randomized trial of FOLFIRI vs FOLFOX4 in the treatment of advanced colorectal cancer: A multicenter study of the Grupo Oncologico Italia Meridionale. *J Clin Oncol* 23:4866, 2005.

95. Cassidy J, Clarke S, Diaz-Rubio E, et al: Randomized phase III study of capecitabine plus oxaliplatin compared with fluorouracil/folinic acid plus oxaliplatin as first-line therapy for metastatic colorectal cancer. *J Clin Oncol* 26:2006, 2008.

96. Koopman M, Antonini NF, Douma J, et al: Sequential versus combination chemotherapy with capecitabine, irinotecan, and oxaliplatin in advanced colorectal cancer (CAIRO): A phase III randomised controlled trial. *Lancet* 370:135, 2007.

97. Seymour MT, Maughan TS, Ledermann JA, et al: Different strategies of sequential and combination chemotherapy for patients with poor prognosis advanced colorectal cancer (MRC FOCUS): A randomised controlled trial. *Lancet* 370:143, 2007.

98. Hurwitz H, Fehrenbacher L, Novotny W, et al: Bevacizumab plus irinotecan, fluorouracil, and leucovorin for metastatic colorectal cancer. *N Engl J Med* 350:2335, 2004.

99. Saltz LB, Clarke S, Diaz-Rubio E, et al: Bevacizumab in combination with oxaliplatin-based chemotherapy as first-line therapy in metastatic colorectal cancer: A randomized phase III study. *J Clin Oncol* 26:2013, 2008.

100. Saltz L, Rubin M, Hochster H, et al: Cetuximab (IMC-C225) plus irinotecan (CPT-11) is active in CPT-11-refractory colorectal cancer (CRC) that expresses epidermal growth factor receptor (EGFR). *J Clin Oncol* 20:Abstract 7, 2001.

101. Saltz LB, Meropol NJ, Loehrer PJ, Sr, et al: Phase II trial of cetuximab in patients with refractory colorectal cancer that expresses the epidermal growth factor receptor. *J Clin Oncol* 22:1201, 2004.

102. Hecht JR, Patnaik A, Berlin J, et al: Panitumumab monotherapy in patients with previously treated metastatic colorectal cancer. *Cancer* 110:980, 2007.

103. Amado RG, Wolf M, Peeters M, et al: Wild-type KRAS is required for panitumumab efficacy in patients with metastatic colorectal cancer. *J Clin Oncol* 26:1626, 2008.

104. Karapetis CS, Khambata-Ford S, Jonker DJ, et al: K-ras mutations and benefit from cetuximab in advanced colorectal cancer. *N Engl J Med* 359:1757, 2008.

105. Van Cutsem E, Kohne C-H, Hitre E, et al: Cetuximab and chemotherapy as initial treatment for metastatic colorectal cancer. *N Engl J Med* 360:1408, 2009.

106. Douillard J-Y, Siena S, Cassidy J, et al: Randomized, phase III trial of panitumumab with infusional fluorouracil, leucovorin, and oxaliplatin (FOLFOX4) versus FOLFOX4 alone as first-line treatment in patients with previously untreated metastatic colorectal cancer: The PRIME study. *J Clin Oncol* 28:4697, 2010.

107. Bokemeyer C, Bondarenko I, Makhson A, et al: Fluorouracil, leucovorin, and oxaliplatin with and without cetuximab in the first-line treatment of metastatic colorectal cancer. *J Clin Oncol* 27:663, 2009.

108. Saltz LB, Lenz H-J, Kindler HL, et al: Randomized phase II trial of cetuximab, bevacizumab, and irinotecan compared with cetuximab and bevacizumab alone in irinotecan-refractory colorectal cancer: The BOND-2 study. *J Clin Oncol* 25:4557, 2007.

109. Tol J, Koopman M, Cats A, et al: Chemotherapy, bevacizumab, and cetuximab in metastatic colorectal cancer. *N Engl J Med* 360:563, 2009.

110. Hecht JR, Mitchell E, Chidiac T, et al: A randomized phase IIIB trial of chemotherapy, bevacizumab, and panitumumab compared with chemotherapy and bevacizumab alone for metastatic colorectal cancer. *J Clin Oncol* 27:672, 2009.

111. Nordlinger B, Sorbye H, Glimelius B, et al: Perioperative chemotherapy with FOLFOX4 and surgery versus surgery alone for resectable liver metastases from colorectal cancer (EORTC Intergroup trial 40983): A randomised controlled trial. *Lancet* 371:1007, 2008.

112. Nava HR, Pagana TJ: Postoperative surveillance of colorectal carcinoma. *Cancer* 49:1043, 1982.

113. Nivatvongs S, Fryd DS: How far does the proctosigmoidoscope reach? A prospective study of 1000 patients. *N Engl J Med* 303:380, 1980.

114. Reasbeck PG: Colorectal cancer: The case for endoscopic screening. *Br J Surg* 74:12, 1987.

115. Tuttle SE, Jewell SD, Mojzisik CM, et al: Intraoperative radioimmunolocalization of colorectal carcinoma with a hand-held gamma probe and MAb B72.3: Comparison of in vivo gamma probe counts with in vitro MAb radiolocalization. *Int J Cancer* 42:352, 1988.

116. Staab HJ, Anderer FA, Hornung A, et al: Doubling time of circulating CEA and its relation to survival of patients with recurrent rectal cancer. *Br J Cancer* 46:773, 1982.

Local Excision of Rectal Cancer

Jennifer L. Irani | Ronald Bleday

Despite recent improvements in patient awareness and compliance with screening modalities, rectal cancer continues to be a significant medical and social problem worldwide. It is estimated that in 2010, approximately 40,000 new cases of rectal cancer will be diagnosed, and 51,400 deaths will be attributed to colon and rectal cancer in the United States alone. Abdominoperineal resection (APR) has been the traditional treatment for *distal* rectal adenocarcinomas and continues to be the standard to which all other operations for the treatment of rectal cancer must be compared. This procedure involves the en bloc removal of the tumor, rectum, sphincter complex, and surrounding lymph nodes, leaving the patient with a permanent colostomy. The 5-year survival rates after an APR by stage range from 78% to 100% for stage I, 45% to 73% for stage II, and 22% to 66% for stage III.[1-4] Despite radical resection of both the tumor and surrounding tissue, recurrence rates, including local recurrences, remain roughly 20%, ranging from 8.5% for stage I disease to 28.6% for stage III disease with surgery alone.[5] These variations in recurrence rates can be attributed to such variables as tumor location within the rectum, surgical technique, and the addition of adjuvant therapy.

Although APR is the mainstay of therapy for distal rectal cancer, it is associated with significant morbidity and mortality. A recent review of the literature showed that mortality rates for APR range from 0% to 6.3%,[6,7] with some studies having a 61% incidence of postoperative complications.[3] The majority of these complications are urinary and perineal wound infections with rates as high as 50% and 16%, respectively.[8] APR also leads to a significant change in body image and social habits. In a patient survey performed in 1983 by Williams and Johnston,[9] 66% of patients complained of significant leaks from their stoma appliances, 67% experienced sexual dysfunction, and only 40% of patients who were working preoperatively returned to their jobs following their operation. Some advocate for ultra-low anterior resections in patients with distal rectal cancer in order to avoid a permanent colostomy. These procedures, however, lead to significant functional issues and do not seem to improve the quality of life compared with the APR. These complications and quality-of-life issues, coupled with improvements in patient selection secondary to innovations in preoperative imaging modalities such as endorectal magnetic resonance imaging (eMRI), 3T MRI, and ultrasound, have led to a renewed interest in local treatment of rectal cancers with the hope of achieving similar survival rates with less morbidity and mortality compared with APR.

PREOPERATIVE EVALUATION

Proper patient selection remains the key to successful local excision of rectal cancers. The retrospective literature shows that there is a direct correlation between local recurrence and specific pathologic tumor features, including depth of invasion, lymphatic invasion, histologic grade, and most importantly negative margins at the time of resection. In the past, preoperative evaluation relied solely on a digital rectal examination, which was found to demonstrate depth of invasion with some degree of accuracy.[10,11] More recent studies have refuted this evidence.[12] Today imaging studies can more accurately predict preoperative stage of rectal cancers, and these techniques include endorectal ultrasound (ERUS), eMRI, and 3T MRI.

Preoperative evaluation begins with a thorough history and physical examination, taking care to note sphincter function, as local excision in the setting of poor preoperative sphincter function may be inappropriate. A digital rectal examination should be performed to assess the distance of the tumor from the anal verge, as well as its size and mobility. Tumors amenable to local excision should be less than 4 cm in diameter and occupy less than 40% of the bowel circumference (Box 165-1). The distance of the tumor from the dentate line is crucially important to judge resectability: tumors less than 5 cm from the dentate are amenable to transanal resection, whereas tumors in the middle third of the rectum may require a transcoccygeal approach or transanal endoscopic microsurgery (TEM). Immobile tumors are likely transmural and, thus, not amenable to local excision. The overall health of the patient must be taken into account, as patients who are considered medically unfit for a major resection are often good candidates for local excision.

ENDORECTAL ULTRASOUND, ENDORECTAL MRI, AND 3T MRI

ERUS was introduced as a means of preoperatively staging small rectal cancers during the 1990s. ERUS remains very operator dependent and there is a significant learning curve, but in experienced hands ERUS can determine depth of tumor invasion reliably. In 1993, Solomon reported a sensitivity of 97% and a specificity of 87% in determining the depth of invasion with ERUS.[13] Garcia-Aguilar et al found that ERUS was not as useful for determining the exact stage, with an overall accuracy of only 59%. However, ERUS was very useful for differentiating tumors localized within the rectal wall that are amenable to local excision, from those that extend into

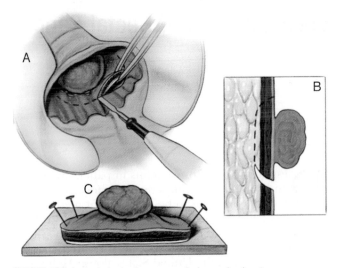

FIGURE 165-1 **A,** A 1- to 2-cm margin is marked out circumferentially on the rectal mucosa. **B,** A full-thickness excision is carried out with dissection into the perirectal fat. **C,** The specimen is oriented for the pathologist in order to accurately identify all margins.

the perirectal fat, and require radical resection and adjuvant chemoradiation.[14] Garcia-Aguilar et al also found that the accuracy of ERUS in detecting lymph node metastases ranged from 60% to 80%.[14]

3T MRI and eMRI are also being used to determine the depth of invasion of the primary rectal tumor. 3T MRI is the preferred preoperative evaluation method at our institution. As with ERUS, there is a significant learning curve in performing and reading MRI.[15] Kim et al found that the overall accuracy of eMRI for staging depth of invasion and nodal metastases was 81% and 63%, respectively.[16] They also found eMRI to have a sensitivity of 78.5% and a specificity of 41.9% making it more sensitive but less specific than ERUS in their study.[16]

Computed tomography (CT) has also been used to evaluate small rectal cancers; however, it is not as accurate as ERUS or MRI in evaluating the depth of invasion. Thus, the use of CT is not recommended for the evaluation of the primary tumor. CT is still valuable in the initial evaluation of the patient with low rectal cancer because of its ability to detect evidence of distant metastases. Posteroanterior and lateral chest radiographs are useful for the same reason.

It is our recommendation that each institution select a modality that it prefers and concentrate the experience into one person's or one team's hands so as to maximize accuracy and consistency of results. Proper decision making and patient selection for the use of local excision or local excision with adjuvant therapy is dependent on reliable and reproducible imaging. We prefer 3T MRI. In our hands, it is less operator dependent than ERUS and provides us significantly more information on the mesorectal tissues than ERUS.

TECHNIQUE

Historically, there are three approaches to local excision of rectal cancer: transanal, transcoccygeal, and transsphincteric. The transsphincteric approach has been associated with fecal incontinence secondary to sphincter dysfunction and thus has fallen out of favor. Recently a newer technique, transanal endoscopic microsurgery (TEM), has provided a minimally invasive option for local excision that also allows the operator to reach lesions that are located more proximally and would have required a transcoccygeal or transsphincteric approach in the past.

TRANSANAL EXCISION

Local excision is accomplished via a transanal approach in the majority of patients with low rectal cancers. In our prospective study of 48 local excisions for rectal cancer, 33 were performed using a transanal approach.[17] Before local excision, we still prefer that all patients receive a complete mechanical bowel preparation the day before surgery with intravenous antibiotics given within 1 hour of surgery. The use of the full bowel prep facilitates in keeping the field free of stool while operating and keeps stool from coming across the area in the first day post-procedure. However, a more limited left-sided bowel preparation can also be used. After induction of anesthesia, the patient is placed in the prone jackknife position, with the buttocks taped apart. A pudendal nerve block should then be administered, which aids in the control of postoperative discomfort and more importantly relaxes the sphincter complex. A Pratt bivalve retractor is then used to dilate the anus and expose the lesion. Once adequate visualization has been obtained, traction sutures are placed 1 to 2 cm distal to the tumor, and the limits of dissection are marked on the mucosa using electrocautery. This line of dissection should be approximately 1 to 2 cm from the border of the tumor circumferentially. If visualization is not initially adequate, serial traction sutures are used to prolapse the lesion into the field of view. Next, the electrocautery is used to make a full-thickness incision along the previously marked mucosa (Figure 165-1). Upon completion of this incision, the perirectal fat should be visible beneath the lesion to confirm a full-thickness excision. In anterior lesions, care must be taken not to injure the back wall of the vagina in women, or the prostate in men. The lesion is then excised leaving visible perirectal fat at the base of the lesion. We prefer to close the defect in the bowel wall transversely using interrupted 3-0 Vicryl sutures.

Complications after transanal excisions include urinary retention, urinary tract infections, delayed hemorrhage, infections of the perirectal and ischiorectal space, and fecal impactions. However, the overall incidence of these complications is quite low.[17]

TRANSCOCCYGEAL EXCISION

The transcoccygeal approach is used preferentially over the transanal approach for larger, more proximal lesions. It was originally popularized by Kraske, who found it beneficial when operating on lesions within the middle or distal third of the rectum. This approach is especially useful for lesions on the posterior wall of the rectum, but it can certainly be used for anterior or lateral lesions as well. In our series, the transcoccygeal approach was used where the distal margin was approximately 4.8 cm from the dentate line as compared to 3.0 cm for the transanal approach.[17]

Again we prefer that all patients have a mechanical bowel preparation the day before surgery with antibiotics given within 1 hour of the procedure. The patient is placed in the prone jackknife position with the buttocks taped apart after the induction of general anesthesia. The tape will be released for closure in order to facilitate the approximation of the subcutaneous tissues and skin. An incision is made in the posterior midline adjacent to the sacrum and coccyx down to the upper border of the posterior aspect of the external sphincter (Figure 165-2). The coccyx, which along with the anal coccygeal ligament, lies immediately deep to the skin and subcutaneous tissue, is removed to improve exposure. The levator ani muscles will now be visible at the base of the wound and should be separated in the midline, exposing a membrane that resides just outside of the perirectal fat. Division of this membrane allows for complete mobilization of the rectum within the extraperitoneal pelvis.

For posterior-based lesions, the distal margin of the tumor can be palpated via a rectal examination, and then the mesorectum and rectum are transected at a point 1 to 1.5 cm distal to the tumor (Figure 165-3). The excision is then completed with a 1-cm margin surrounding the lesion. For posterior lesions, the transcoccygeal approach allows for the removal of perirectal nodes that lie in the surrounding mesorectal tissue. For anterior lesions, a posterior proctotomy is made, and then the

lesion is approached under direct vision, again excising the lesion down to the perirectal fat with a 1-cm margin (Figures 165-4 and 165-5). Following removal, the specimen is reoriented for the pathologist and all the rectal incisions are closed in either a longitudinal or transverse manner to avoid narrowing of the rectum, using an

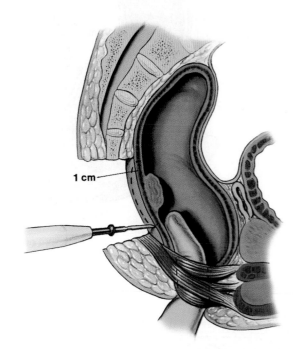

FIGURE 165-3 For posteriorly based lesions, after the rectum has been exposed, the surgeon can palpate the distal margin of the tumor then choose the dissection margin greater than 1 cm away from the margin for the initial proctotomy. The dissection is then completed under direct vision.

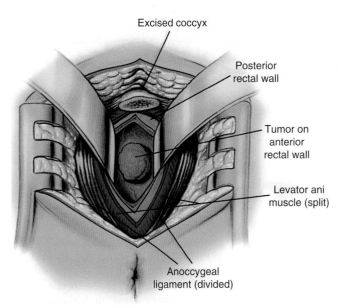

FIGURE 165-4 For anterior lesions, the posterior full rectum is opened and the full-thickness excision is completed through the proctotomy.

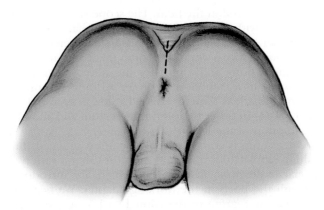

FIGURE 165-2 Incision line for the transcoccygeal approach.

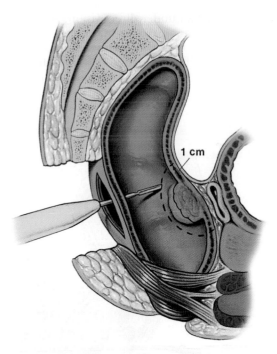

FIGURE 165-5 The coccyx is excised, the levator split (but not divided) in the midline, and the rectum is mobilized. After mobilization, the posterior wall of the rectum can be opened to expose an anterior lesion.

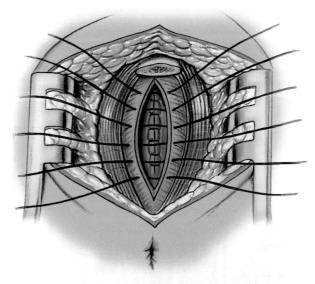

FIGURE 165-6 The anterior and posterior walls of the rectum are closed in one layer in either a longitudinal or transverse fashion so that the lumen is not significantly narrowed.

absorbable suture (Figure 165-6). An air test should be performed, filling the operative field with sterile saline, and insufflating air in the rectum in order to check for air leaks in the suture line. Once these air leaks are controlled, the levator ani is reapproximated in the midline, and the anal coccygeal ligament is reattached to the sacrum.

An uncommon but severe complication of this procedure is the development of a fecal fistula that extends from the rectum to the posterior midline incision. The incidence of this complication ranges from 5% to 20%, and most heal after temporary diversion of the fecal stream via a loop ileostomy or colostomy.[17-19]

Although the Kraske technique is rarely used, it is important to appreciate the technique. It can be best applied for small posterior midrectal cancers. The technique provides a significant amount of mesorectal fat along with the accompanying nodes, allowing for accurate staging of most lesions. The approach can also be used for palliation with more advanced lesions, and the approach in general can be used to access lesions, both benign and malignant, of the midrectum. As TEM (see Transanal Endoscopic Microsurgery, later) becomes widely popular, the Kraske approach may become obsolete.

TRANSSPHINCTERIC EXCISION

The transsphincteric approach developed by York and Mason involves the complete division of the sphincters and the posterior wall of the rectum. The procedure starts similarly to the Kraske transcoccygeal approach except that the levator ani and the external sphincter muscles are divided in the midline. These muscles are carefully tagged so that they can be reapproximated exactly at the end of the procedure. Care must be taken to remain in the midline to avoid the nerve supply to the sphincters that lie in a posterolateral position bilaterally. Once the lesion is removed, the rectum, sphincters, and overlying musculature are closed in a careful stepwise manner. This procedure has an increased risk of incontinence secondary to sphincter dysfunction. Because the exposure provided from this approach is similar to that from the Kraske procedure, which carries less risk of incontinence, there are very few indications for this technique.

TRANSANAL ENDOSCOPIC MICROSURGERY

TEM was first described in 1984.[20] The surgery is performed with the use of a special resectoscope that is 4 cm in diameter and available in lengths of both 12 and 20 cm. The scope is inserted with an obturator in place, which is then removed and replaced with an airtight glass faceplate. The rectum is then manually insufflated, such as in rigid sigmoidoscopy, and the lesion is identified and centered in the field. The scope is then secured in position with the aid of a support arm that is attached to the operating table. The glass faceplate is then removed and replaced with a working adapter that contains several instrument ports and a port for the stereoscope that is connected to a camera and projected onto a monitor. Carbon dioxide is then insufflated at low pressure (10 to 15 cm H_2O) in order to distend the rectum and allow for visualization of the lesion (Figure 165-7).[21]

Once setup is complete, the operation proceeds in a fashion similar to a transanal excision using a variety of special endoscopic instruments, which are introduced through the ports in the working adapter. We begin by marking the margin of resection 1 to 1.5 cm circumferentially around the lesion using electrocautery. The

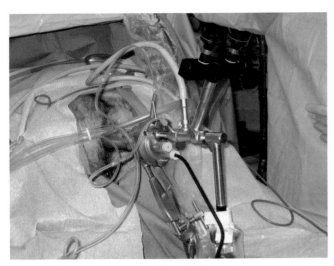

FIGURE 165-7 Positioning of the operating proctoscope and operating instruments for transanal endoscopic microsurgery. The lesion needs to be in the lower quarter of the field. For anterior lesions, the patient is placed in the prone position as shown.

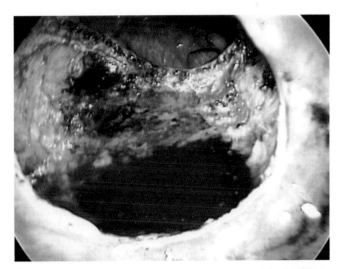

FIGURE 165-9 A full-thickness excision has been performed into the perirectal fat. The defect can be closed primarily or left open.

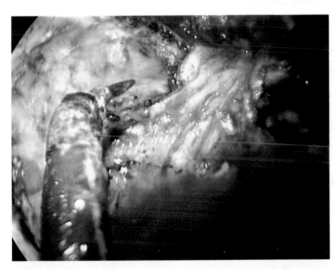

FIGURE 165-8 Transanal endoscopic microsurgery as seen under the camera of the operating proctoscope. A cautery needle-tip dissector is used for the excision. Care needs to be taken to recognize whether the peritoneal cavity has been entered.

lesion is then grasped and the excision proceeds along the previously marked line through the full thickness of the rectal wall and into the perirectal fat. The specimen is removed by temporarily removing the faceplate after complete excision. The defect is then closed using 3-0 polydiaxanone suture in a continuous or interrupted fashion (Figures 165-8 and 165-9).[21]

TEM allows for local excision of proximal rectal lesions that are not accessible via the transanal, transsphincteric, or transcoccygeal approaches. Despite favorable results of this relatively new technique, it is just now gaining in popularity. Barriers to it use are the expense of the equipment, lack of familiarity with the equipment and setup, and complexity of the TEM operating system. However,

with the increased use of screening colonoscopy, smaller rectal lesions are being detected more frequently. The TEM system allows for a minimally invasive approach for early midrectal cancers.

OUTCOMES

When local excision was initially reintroduced, it was reserved for patients who either refused a colostomy or were deemed medically unfit for a radical operation secondary to any of a number of comorbidities. Morson et al published one of the earliest series on local excision of rectal cancer in 1977.[22] In this series, he reported 143 cases of low rectal cancers treated via local excision. At the time of excision, 91 of these lesions were found to have negative margins, and in the patients with negative margins only 2 suffered local recurrence, whereas one had a distant recurrence, yielding a crude 5-year survival of 82%. However, for the 69 patients with positive margins, 13 suffered a local recurrence and there was 1 distant recurrence, yielding a crude 5-year survival of only 60%. Of note, 115 of the 143 carcinomas were noted to be T1 lesions. These results prompted a renewed interest in local excision as they showed that local recurrence and survival rates were similar to those of APR, while the morbidity was greatly reduced.

RETROSPECTIVE STUDIES

Most reports of local excision for rectal cancer are small retrospective reviews from single institutions. The results of these studies are difficult to generalize and to interpret. The length of followup varies from study to study, and many combine patients with tumors of different depth, positive margins, and different forms of local therapy, including snare cautery and fulguration. Multiple retrospective studies, including studies from the University of Minnesota, Mayo Clinic, and Memorial Sloan-Kettering Cancer Center[23-25] have been presented and published with no standard entrance criteria, no standard preoperative imaging criteria, no standards for use of adjuvant therapy, and no standard followup regimen. The studies also span decades, with patients from 20 years ago being evaluated together with patients operated on recently. Therefore, the results and conclusions from such retrospective studies should be looked on with some skepticism. Although recent studies have more rigorous selection and study criteria, it is unlikely that anything short of a prospective, randomized clinical trial will clarify the precise risks and benefits of local excision for early rectal cancer.

A selection of retrospective reviews report a local recurrence rate of 5% to 33% and 5-year survival rates of 57% to 100%.[25-30] For a more detailed description of some of these studies, please review Table 165-1. These studies demonstrate that patients with superficial tumors and negative margins at the time of resection have low recurrence rates and a very good prognosis. Although some of these studies are flawed and not conclusive, they do suggest that local excision may provide adequate oncologic control with considerably lower morbidity and mortality rates than APR for select distal rectal cancers.

The data seem to support the use of local excision for T1 tumors with good histology (no lymphovascular invasion, well differentiated, low grade, and no tumor budding). Outcome is best when resection margins are negative for tumor. Although many studies show differences in local recurrence, higher with local excision compared with radical resection, most do not show an overall survival difference, likely owing to the excellent prognosis of T1 rectal cancer. You et al used the National Cancer Database to compile data from 997 institutions comparing local excision alone versus radical surgery for T1 and T2 tumors. Although local recurrence was higher after local excision, the 5-year overall survival was not influenced by the type of procedure performed for T1 tumors.[31] The data on the use of local excision alone for T2 cancers, even when completely excised and properly staged, demonstrates that local excision alone is inadequate therapy. Not only is local recurrence higher in patients with T2 tumors treated with local excision, but overall survival is lower also. Interestingly, the disease-specific survival did not differ between patients with T2 tumors treated with local excision versus standard

TABLE 165-1 Series of Local Excision Alone—Retrospective Series

Author	No. of Patients	Treatment Arms	Followup	Recurrence Local	Survival
You, 2007[31]	765 (601 T1, 164 T2)	765 LE	Median of 76 mo for T1 and 68 mo for T2	T1: 12.5% T2: 22.1%	T1: 77.4% (overall 5-yr survival) T2: 67.6% (overall 5-yr survival)
Mellgren, 2000[32]	108 (69 T1, 39 T2)	108 TA	Median, 53 mo	T1: 18% T2: 47%	T1: 72% (overall 5-yr survival) T2: 65% (overall 5-yr survival)
Nascimbeni, 2004[33]	70 T1	70 LE	Median, 97 mo	6.6%	72% (overall 5-yr survival)
Endresth, 2005[34]	35 T1	35 TA	Range, 24-97 mo	12%	70% (overall 5-yr survival)
Koscinski, 2003[29]	58 (26 T1 and 32 T2)	47 TA, 6 TC, 5 TEM	Mean of 48 mo for T1 and 59 mo for T2	T1: 5% T2: 28%	T1: 100% (5-yr actuarial survival probability) T2: 84.4% (5-yr actuarial survival probability)
Horn, 1989[35]	38 (17 T1, 14 T2, 7 requiring APR after LE)	3 endoscopic polypectomy, 35 TA, 5 salvage APR	Median, 50 mo	T1: 0% T2: 43%	T1: 100% T2: 82.6%
Gall, 1992[36]	84 (54 T1, 19 T2, 11 T3) via LE 383 APR	16 endoscopic polypectomy, 68 LE, 383 APR	Median, 77.5 mo	T1: 11% (LE), 0% (APR) T2: 22% (LE), 5% (APR)	T1 – 74 ± 15% (LE), 100%-2% (APR) T2 – 68 ± 24% (LE), 76 ± 11% (APR)
Morson, 1977[22]	143 (115 T1, 20 T2, 7 T3)	143 LE Only 91 with negative margins		2/91 (2%) with negative margins 13/69 (19%) with positive margins	Corr. 5-yr of 100% with negative margins Corr. 5-yr of 83%-96% with positive margins
Whiteway, 1985[37]	46 (13 T1, 18 T2, 15 T3)	46 TA and TSp 27 for cure, 6 disseminated disease 13 for high risk		Approximately 8 (17%)	Cancer-specific survival of 87%

APR, Abdominoperineal resection; *LE,* local excision; *TA,* transanal excision; *TC,* transcoccygeal excision; *TSp,* transsphincteric excision; *TEM,* transanal endoscopic microsurgery.

resection.[31] Controversy remains as to what other therapy should be offered. Some surgeons feel that all T2 patients should proceed to a radical resection, whereas others think adjuvant chemoradiation either before or after excision will suffice.

ADJUVANT THERAPY

Local recurrence continues to be a major source of morbidity and mortality following both local excision and radical resection for rectal cancer. The major risk factors for recurrence include the depth of invasion of the primary tumor, positive surgical margins, histologic grade of the tumor, and the presence of tumor in the regional lymph nodes. The addition of adjuvant or neoadjuvant radiation has been shown to decrease these local recurrence rates, and there is increasing evidence that chemoradiation may have a beneficial effect on survival. This has led to recommendations by the National Institutes of Health stating that all patients with stage II or higher rectal cancer should be treated with adjuvant chemoradiation.

One of the major shortcomings of local excision is the inability to pathologically assess the regional lymph nodes. Microscopic disease can be present in the regional lymph nodes in up to 12% of T1 lesions, 22% of T2 lesions, and 58% of T3 and T4 lesions.[38,39] This microscopic disease may lead to local recurrence if left untreated. These findings have caused many observers to advocate for the use of postoperative radiation following

local excision in an attempt to eradicate any nodal disease, especially in more aggressive tumors with some of the risk factors previously mentioned. It also further emphasizes the need for preoperative ERUS or 3T/eMRI in order to identify patients with nodal disease who may be inappropriate for local excision.

Unfortunately, most studies involving local excision combined with pre- or postoperative chemoradiation are small, retrospective, single-institution studies. The patient population, radiation and chemotherapy protocols, and tumor characteristics are highly variable between these studies (Table 165-2), and thus, 5-year survival rates range from 33% to 100%. However, local recurrence rates are decreased when compared to local excision alone; ranging from 0% to 15% for T1 and T2 lesions, and 0% to 20% for T3 lesions.

PROSPECTIVE STUDIES

Unfortunately, there are very few prospective studies of local excision for distal rectal adenocarcinoma with or without chemoradiotherapy (Table 165-3). We treated 48 patients with rectal adenocarcinoma via local excision, using postoperative chemoradiation for all T2 and T3 lesions. Over a mean followup period of 40.5 months, we found an overall survival of 93.8%, with recurrence rates by stage of 9.5% for T1 lesions, 0% for T2 lesions, and 40% for T3 lesions. Of note, local recurrence was seen in 3 of 5 patients with lymphatic invasion and 2 of 2 patients with positive margins at the time of local

TABLE 165-2 Local Excision Plus XRT—Retrospective Series

Author	No. of Patients	Treatment Arms	Followup	Local Recurrence	Survival
Wong, 1993[7]	25	21 TA, 4 endoscopic polypectomy or fulguration All got 50 Gy XRT postoperation	Median, 72 mo (minimum of 36 mo)	6/25 (24%)	Crude 5-yr survival of 96%
Mendenhall, 2008[30]	67 (34 T1, 12 T2, 2 T3, 19 no stage data)	65 TA, 2 TC 48 received 45-60 Gy XRT postoperation	Median, 65 mo (6-273 mo)	T1 = 11% T2-3 = 25%	T1 = 76% T2-3 = 77%
Bailey, 1992[40]	63 (35 T1, 18 T2, 10 T3)	63 LE 34 XRT at 45-50 Gy	Median, 44 mo (12-130 mo)	4/53 (7.5%)	Crude 5-yr survival of 74.3%
Chakravarti, 1999[27]	99 (58 T1, 41 T2)	52 LE alone 47 LE plus 45-64.8 Gy XRT (45 postoperation, 2 preoperation); 33 also had 5-FU	Median, 51 mo (4-162 mo)	LE alone = 11% T1, 67% T2 LE + CRT = 0% T1, 15% T2	Relapse-free 5-yr survival LE alone = 80% T1, 33% T2 LE + CRT = 65% T1, 76% T2
Paty, 2002[25]	125 (74 T1, 51 T2)	125 LE 31 received 45-54 Gy and 15 of them got 5-FU	Median, 80.4 mo	T1 = 17% T2 = 26%	10-yr survival of 74% for T1 and 72% for T2
Willett, 1994[41]	56 (34 T1, 22 T2)	45 TA or TSp, 10 TC, 1 fulguration 30 received 45 Gy postoperation XRT Since 1986, received 5-FU	Median, 48 mo	Since 1985, 0/20 patients after chemoradiation	Actuarial 5-yr recurrent-free survival of 72%

CRT, Chemoradiation therapy; 5-FU, 5-fluorouracil; LE, local excision; TA, transanal excision; TC, transcoccygeal excision; TSp, transsphincteric excision; XRT, radiation therapy.

TABLE 165-3 Local Excision Plus Adjuvant Therapy—Prospective Series

Author	No. of Patients	Treatment Arms	Followup	Local Recurrence	Survival
Ota, 1992[42]	46	LE Postoperative XRT (53 Gy) 5-FU for 7 T3, 1 T2	Median, 36 mo (18-73 mo)	3/46 (6.5%) All T3	Overall 3-yr survival of 93%
Bleday, 1997[17]	48 (21 T1, 21 T2, 6 T3)	Postoperative XRT 54 Gy and 5-FU/500 mg/m² day 1-3, 28-30 for T2, T3 lesions	Mean, 40.5 mo	4/48 (8%)	Overall 3-yr survival of 93.8%
Steele, 1999[43]	110 (59 T1, 51 T2)	Postoperative XRT 54 Gy and 5-FU/500 mg/m² day 1-3, 29-31 for T2 lesions	Mean, 48 mo	T1 = 3/59 (5.1%) T2 = 7/51 (13.7%)	Overall 6-yr survival of 85%
Greenberg, 2008[44a]	110 (59 T1, 51T2)	Postoperative XRT 54 Gy and 5-FU/500 mg/m² day 1-3, 29-31 for T2 lesions	Median, 85 mo	T1 = 8% T2 = 18%	Overall 10-yr survival T1 = 84% T2 = 66%

5-FU, 5-Fluorouracil; *LE*, local excision; *XRT*, radiation therapy.

excision. From our results, we concluded that surgery alone was adequate for T1 lesions, whereas T2 lesions required a combination of surgery and chemoradiation, provided there were negative margins and no lymphatic involvement. If either of these characteristics were present, however, we recommended the addition of chemoradiation for T1 lesions and radical resection for T2 lesions.

Ota et al published their results from a study of 46 patients with a median followup time of 36 months. In their study, all patients received postoperative radiation, whereas T3 patients received chemotherapy in addition to their radiation treatments. Their results were similar to ours, with a 6.5% local recurrence rate and a 3-year survival rate of 93%.[42]

Steele et al published a multicenter, prospective trial of local excision for rectal cancer in 110 patients. All of these patients were thoroughly screened preoperatively to ensure that their tumors were within 10 cm of the dentate line, less than 4 cm in size, and involved less than 40% of the circumference of the bowel wall. Furthermore, all patients had to be N0M0, and statistical analyses were only performed on patients with negative margins at the time of resection. Patients were treated with postoperative chemoradiation only if they had T2 lesions. They published survival rates of 87% and 85% for T1 and T2 lesions, respectively, with an overall survival rate of 85%. They also found an overall disease-free survival rate of 78%, with 84% for T1 lesions and 71% for T2 lesions.[43]

To evaluate the long-term oncologic response of distal rectal cancers to local excision, Greenberg et al[44a] analyzed the 10-year results from the CALGB prospective, multiinstitutional study originally published by Steele et al.[43] With a median followup of 7.1 years, 10-year rates of overall survival were 84% for patients with T1 and 66% for patients with T2 rectal cancer. Disease-free survival was 75% for T1 and 64% for T2 disease. Local recurrence rates for patients with T1 and T2 lesions were 8% and 18%, respectively, and rates of distant metastases were 5% for T1 and 12% for T2 lesions. Among those patients who had recurrences, the median time to recurrence was 3.9 years for patients with T1 lesions and 1.95 years for

patients with T2 lesions. The results of this study show that local excision for patients with T1 disease is associated with comparable rates of local recurrence, overall survival, and disease-free survival as historic controls after radical resection.[44a] The outcomes for T2 patients, however, have significant room for improvement.

Preliminary results of a phase II trial (ACOSOG Z6041) of neoadjuvant chemoration and local excision for T2N0 rectal cancer reveal high pathologic complete response rates and negative resection margins, however, high complication rates. Garcia-Aguilar et al[44b] accrued 90 patients, 79 of whom completed neoadjuvant capecitabine and oxaliplatin during radiation (62 patients completed both chemotherapy and radiotherapy per protocol). Seventy-seven underwent local excision. Thirty-four patients (44%) had a pathologic complete response and 49 (64%) tumors were downstaged (ypT0-1). Of the 5 local excision specimens that contained lymph nodes, one T3 tumor had a positive node. Only one patient had a positive margin. Toxicity necessitated a protocol decrease in capecitabine and radiation dosage. Overall, 33 patients (39%) developed grade ≥3 complications. Long-term oncologic outcomes are forthcoming.

TRANSANAL ENDOSCOPIC MICROSURGERY

Although TEM is still a relatively new technique, it is likely to have at least equal, if not better, outcomes as traditional transanal excision, and perhaps even standard total mesorectal excision, in the properly selected patient.[45-47] There are a few small, single-institution, retrospective and prospective studies describing the use and outcomes of TEM for the excision of rectal cancer (Table 165-4). In general, these studies show survival and recurrence rates ranging from 83% to 100% and 0% to 27% respectively. These rates are equivalent to those seen for transanal excision, but again comparison is difficult because of the differences in patient population, adjuvant therapy, and tumor characteristics. Some studies comparing TEM with transanal excision show fewer specimens with positive resection margins using the TEM technique, which some attribute to better visualization with TEM.[45,47] Even when the initial capital cost of the

TABLE 165-4 Transanal Endoscopic Microsurgery

Author	No. of Patients	Treatment Arms	Followup	Local Recurrence	Survival
Lezoche, 2002[48]	35 (all T2)	All had preoperative 50-Gy XRT then TEM	Median, 38 mo (24-96 mo)	1/35 (2.85%)	Probability of survival at 96 mo = 83%
Farmer, 2002[49]	49 (36 Tis, 10 T1, 3 T2, 1 T3)	All TEM	Median, 33 mo (20-48 mo)	2/49 (5.6%) 1 patient had a salvage APR	1 death from disseminated cancer Survival = 97.9%
Zimuddin, 2000[21]	21 (7 Tis, 9 T1, 5 T2)	All TEM	Mean, 15 mo	0% for T0 and T1 20% for T2	100% for all grades
de Graaf, 2002[50]	76 (32 Tis, 21 T1, 18 T2, 5 T3)	All TEM	Median, 10 mo, mean 13.9 mo (1-52 mo)	Tis = 0%, T1 = 10%, T2 = 33%, and T3 = 0%	1 patient died, yielding overall survival of 98.7%
Lezoche, 2008[46]	70 (T2)	All had preoperative 50-Gy XRT plus 5-FU, then 35 TEM 35 Lap TME	Median, 84 mo	5.7% TEM 2.8% Lap TME	Probability of survival 94% TEM 94% Lap TME
Lee, 2003[51]	74 (52 TI, 22 T2) 100 (17 T1, 83 T2) = Total 174	74 TEM 100 radical surgery	Mean, 31 mo	TEM: 4.1% T1, 19.5% T2 Radical surgery: 0% T1, 9.4% T2 (T1 $P = 0.95$, T2 $P = 0.04$)	5-yr survival TEM: T1 100%, T2 94.7% Radical surgery: T1 93%, T2 96% (T1 $P = 0.07$, T2 $P = 0.48$)

APR, Abdominoperineal resection; *5-FU*, 5-fluorouracil; *Lap TME*, laparoscopic total mesorectal excision; *LE*, local excision; *TEM*, transanal endoscopic microsurgery; *XRT*, radiation therapy.

TEM equipment is taken into account, cost analyses of TEM versus open procedures have shown TEM to be extremely cost-effective.[52,53]

NEOADJUVANT CHEMORADIOTHERAPY

Advanced rectal cancer is currently treated with neoadjuvant chemoradiation followed by radical resection. It is natural to hypothesize that patients could benefit from the known tumoricidal effects of preoperative chemoradiation prior to local excision.[54] Initial studies are small, retrospective, single-institution, and without rigorous entry or study criteria.[55,56] Nevertheless, many authors are showing similar local recurrence and survival rates with the use of preoperative therapy as those seen after conventional surgery in T2 and T3 rectal cancer patients.[46,56] Specifically, excellent results have been shown in patients who achieve a pathologic complete response to preoperative chemoradiation, again highlighting the importance of proper patient selection (Table 165-5).[57-60] Currently a phase II trial (ACOSOG Z6041) is ongoing studying the outcome of small distal T2N0Mx patients treated with neoadjuvant chemoradiation and local excision. Long-term oncologic results will not be known for several years.[54]

ALGORITHM FOR LOCAL EXCISION OF RECTAL CANCER

Patient selection
- Mobile tumor less than 4 cm in diameter, less than 40% of the bowel circumference, within 5 cm of the dentate line (Table 165-6)

- Significant medical comorbidities making radical excision unacceptable even for patients with T3 lesions

Preoperative imaging
- ERUS or eMRI/3T MRI dependent on institutional preference
- T1 or T2 tumors with no signs of locoregional nodal metastases
- CT scan to assess for distant metastases

Chemoradiotherapy
- T1 lesions completely excised but with unfavorable histology
- T2 lesions (adjuvant or neoadjuvant chemoradiotherapy)

Followup
- Office visits with physical exam, carcinoembryonic antigen (CEA), and proctoscopy every 3 months for the first 2 years and then every 6 months until 5 years
- CT scans of the abdomen and pelvis at 12 months, then annually for 3 years or with an increase in CEA or change in symptoms
- Colonoscopy at 1 year following surgery and then every 3 to 5 years
- Radical resection as salvage for any local recurrence

SUMMARY

Rectal cancer remains a significant cause of morbidity and mortality worldwide. Studies have shown that local excision for favorable T1 cancers, and local excision combined with adjuvant chemoradiation in select T2 cancers, can yield similar rates of survival and recurrence when compared with radical resection. This is accomplished with shorter hospital stays, fewer complications,

TABLE 165-5 Local Excision Plus Neoadjuvant Therapy

Author	No. of Patients	Treatment Arms	Followup	Local Recurrence	Survival
Lezoche, 2005[55]	100 (54 T2, 46 T3)	Preoperative 50.4-Gy XRT (25 patients also got 5-FU) followed by TEM	Median, 55 mo	5% (cumulative probability of local recurrence at 90-mo followup was 5%)	Cancer-specific survival at 90-mo followup: 92% for T2, 85% for T3
Lezoche, 2008[46]	35 (T2)	Preoperative 50-Gy XRT plus 5-FU then TEM	Median, 84 mo	5.7%	Overall survival: 72% Probability of survival: 94%
Guerrieri, 2008[56]	196 (51 T1, 84 T2, 61 T3)	All T2 and T3 got preoperative 50.4-Gy XRT, some also got 5-FU, all underwent TEM	Median, 81 mo	0% T1 6% T2 5% T3	Rectal cancer-specific survival: 100% pT1 90% pT2 77% for pT3
Callender, 2010[57]	520 (T3N0M0 or T3N1M0)	All got preoperative 45-, 50.4-, or 52.5-Gy XRT and 5-FU, then 47 LE (6 TC, 41 TA) (12 had prohibitive comorbidity, 15 refused TME, 15 had complete clinical response, 5 unknown) 473 TME (141 APR, 332 LAR)	Median, 63 mo (LE) Median, 59 mo (TME)	10.6% LE 7.6 % TME (*P* = 0.52)	No significant difference in disease-specific survival or overall survival between the LE and TME groups
Nair, 2008[58]	44 (10 T2N0, 22 T3N0, 11 T2/-T3N0, 1 unknown)	All got preoperative 50.4-Gy XRT and 5-FU, then TA (15 medically unfit, 29 refused radical surgery) 5 pPR underwent immediate radical surgery (70% had cCR, 57% pCR)	Median, 64 mo	9% (3 patients after LE only, 1 patient after LE immediately followed by radical resection)	Overall 5-yr survival: 84% T2/T3N0 81% T2/T3N1

APR, Abdominoperineal resection; *5-FU*, 5-fluorouracil; *LAR*, lower anterior resection; *LE*, local excision; *TA*, transanal excision; *TC*, transcoccygeal excision; *TEM*, transanal endoscopic microsurgery; *TME*, total mesorectal excision; *XRT*, radiation therapy.

TABLE 165-6 Treatment Recommendations following Initial Resection

T STAGE	LOW RISK*	HIGH†
T1	No further treatment	Adjuvant chemoradiation
T2	Adjuvant or Neoadjuvant chemoradiation	Radical resection
T3	Radical resection	Radical resection

*Low risk: well or moderately differentiated with no evidence of lymphatic or vascular invasion.
†High risk: poorly differentiated or lymphatic invasion or vascular invasion.

and greater patient satisfaction. Strict selection criteria remain extremely important as local excision should not be offered to patients with transmural or regional nodal involvement. Also, larger tumors, even recurrent disease, may always be treated with salvage APR, but the outcomes of such treatment are not fully known.

REFERENCES

1. Enker WE, Laffer UT, Block GE: Enhanced survival of patients with colon and rectal cancer is based upon wide anatomic resection. *Ann Surg* 190:350, 1979.
2. Localio SA, Eng K, Gouge TH, et al: Abdominosacral resection for carcinoma of the midrectum: Ten years experience. *Ann Surg* 188:475, 1978.
3. Rosen L, Veidenheimer MC, Coller JA, et al: Mortality, morbidity, and patterns of recurrence after abdominoperineal resection for cancer of the rectum. *Dis Colon Rectum* 25:202, 1982.
4. Walz BJ, Lindstrom ER, Butcher HR Jr, et al: Natural history of patients after abdominal-perineal resection. Implications for radiation therapy. *Cancer* 39:2437, 1977.
5. McCall JL, Cox MR, Wattchow DA: Analysis of local recurrence rates after surgery alone for rectal cancer. *Int J Colorectal Dis* 10:126, 1995.
6. Rothenberger DA, Wong WD: Abdominoperineal resection for adenocarcinoma of the low rectum. *World J Surg* 16:478, 1992.
7. Wong CS, Stern H, Cummings BJ: Local excision and post-operative radiation therapy for rectal carcinoma. *Int J Radiat Oncol Biol Phys* 25:669, 1993.
8. Pollard CW, Nivatvongs S, Rojanasakul A, et al: Carcinoma of the rectum. Profiles of intraoperative and early postoperative complications. *Dis Colon Rectum* 37:866, 1994.
9. Williams NS, Johnston D: The quality of life after rectal excision for low rectal cancer. *Br J Surg* 70:460, 1983.
10. Mason AY: President's address. Rectal cancer: The spectrum of selective surgery. *Proc R Soc Med* 69:237, 1976.
11. Nicholls RJ, Mason AY, Morson BC, et al: The clinical staging of rectal cancer. *Br J Surg* 69:404, 1982.
12. Rafaelsen SR, Kronborg O, Fenger C: Digital rectal examination and transrectal ultrasonography in staging of rectal cancer. A prospective, blind study. *Acta Radiol* 35:300, 1994.
13. Solomon MJ, McLeod RS: Endoluminal transrectal ultrasonography: Accuracy, reliability, and validity. *Dis Colon Rectum* 36:200, 1993.

14. Garcia-Aguilar J, Mellgren A, Sirivongs P, et al: Local excision of rectal cancer without adjuvant therapy: A word of caution. *Ann Surg* 231:345, 2000.
15. Drew PJ, Farouk R, Turnbull LW, et al: Preoperative magnetic resonance staging of rectal cancer with an endorectal coil and dynamic gadolinium enhancement. *Br J Surg* 86:250, 1999.
16. Kim NK, Kim MJ, Yun SH, et al: Comparative study of transrectal ultrasonography, pelvic computerized tomography, and magnetic resonance imaging in preoperative staging of rectal cancer. *Dis Colon Rectum* 42:770, 1999.
17. Bleday R, Breen E, Jessup JM, et al: Prospective evaluation of local excision for small rectal cancers. *Dis Colon Rectum* 40:388, 1997.
18. Christiansen J: Excision of mid-rectal lesions by the Kraske sacral approach. *Br J Surg* 67:651, 1980.
19. Killingback M: Local excision of carcinoma of the rectum: Indications. *World J Surg* 16:437, 1992.
20. Beuss GTR, Gunther M: Endoscopic operative procedures for the removal of rectal polyps. *Coloproctology* 6:254, 1984.
21. Azimuddin K, Riether RD, Stasik JJ, et al: Transanal endoscopic microsurgery for excision of rectal lesions: Technique and initial results. *Surg Laparosc Endosc Percutan Tech* 10:372, 2000.
22. Morson BC, Bussey HJ, Samoorian S: Policy of local excision for early cancer of the colorectum. *Gut* 18:1045, 1977.
23. Hahnloser D, Wolff BG, Larson DW, et al: Immediate radical resection after local excision of rectal cancer: An oncologic compromise? *Dis Colon Rectum* 48:429, 2005
24. Mellgren A, Goldberg J, Rothenberger DA: Local excision: Some reality testing. *Surg Oncol Clin N Am* 14:183, 2005.
25. Paty PB, Nash GM, Baron P, et al: Long-term results of local excision for rectal cancer. *Ann Surg* 236:522; discussion 529, 2002.
26. Benson R, Wong CS, Cummings BJ, et al: Local excision and postoperative radiotherapy for distal rectal cancer. *Int J Radiat Oncol Biol Phys* 50:1309, 2001.
27. Chakravarti A, Compton CC, Shellito PC, et al: Long-term follow-up of patients with rectal cancer managed by local excision with and without adjuvant irradiation. *Ann Surg* 230:49, 1999.
28. Gonzalez QH, Heslin MJ, Shore G, et al: Results of long-term follow-up for transanal excision for rectal cancer. *Am Surg* 69:675, 2003.
29. Koscinski T, Malinger S, Drews M: Local excision of rectal carcinoma not-exceeding the muscularis layer. *Colorectal Dis* 5:159, 2003.
30. Mendenhall WM, Morris CG, Rout WR, et al: Local excision and postoperative radiation therapy for rectal adenocarcinoma. *Int J Cancer* 96:89, 2001.
31. You YN, Baxter N, Stewart A, et al: Is the increasing rate of local excision for stage I rectal cancer in the United States justified? *Ann Surg* 245:726, 2007.
32. Mellgren A, Sirivongs P, Rothenberger DA, et al: Is local excision adequate therapy for early rectal cancer? *Dis Colon Rectum* 43:1064; discussion 1071, 2000.
33. Nascimbeni R, Nivatvongs S, Larson DR, et al: Long-term survival after local excision for T1 carcinoma of the rectum. *Dis Colon Rectum* 47:1773, 2004.
34. Endreseth BH, Myrvold HE, Romundstad P, et al: Transanal excision vs. major surgery for T1 rectal cancer. *Dis Colon Rectum* 48:1380, 2005.
35. Horn A, Halvorsen JF, Morild I: Transanal extirpation for early rectal cancer. *Dis Colon Rectum* 32:769, 1989.
36. Gall FP: Update of the German experience with local excision of rectal cancer. *Surg Oncol Clin N Am* 1:99, 1992.
37. Whiteway J, Nicholls RJ, Morson BC: The role of surgical local excision in the treatment of rectal cancer. *Br J Surg* 72:694, 1985.
38. Brodsky JT, Richard GK, Cohen AM, et al: Variables correlated with the risk of lymph node metastasis in early rectal cancer. *Cancer* 69:322, 1992.
39. Rosenthal SA, Yeung RS, Weese JL, et al: Conservative management of extensive low-lying rectal carcinomas with transanal local

40. Bailey HR, Huval WV, Max E, et al: Local excision of carcinoma of the rectum for cure. *Surgery* 111:555, 1992.
41. Willett CG, Compton CC, Shellito PC, et al: Selection factors for local excision or abdominoperineal resection of early stage rectal cancer. *Cancer* 73:2716, 1994.
42. Ota DM: M.D. Anderson Cancer Center Experience with Local Excision and Multimodality Therapy for Rectal Cancer. *Surg Oncol Clin N Am* 1:147, 1992.
43. Steele GD Jr, Herndon JE, Bleday R, et al: Sphincter-sparing treatment for distal rectal adenocarcinoma. *Ann Surg Oncol* 6:433, 1999.
44a. Greenberg J, Shibata D, Herndon JE 2nd, et al: Local excision of distal rectal cancer: An update of cancer and leukemia group B 8984. *Dis Colon Rectum* 51:1185, 2008.
44b. Garcia-Aguilar J, Shi Q, Thomas CR Jr, et al: A phase II trial of neoadjuvant chemoradiation and local excision for T2N0 rectal cancer: Preliminary results of the ACOSOG Z6041 trial. *Ann Surg Oncol* 19:384, 2012.
45. Christoforidis D, Cho HM, Dixon MR, et al: Transanal endoscopic microsurgery versus conventional transanal excision for patients with early rectal cancer. *Ann Surg* 249:776, 2009.
46. Lezoche G, Baldarelli M, Guerrieri M, et al: A prospective randomized study with a 5-year minimum follow-up evaluation of transanal endoscopic microsurgery versus laparoscopic total mesorectal excision after neoadjuvant therapy. *Surg Endosc* 22:352, 2008.
47. Moore JS, Cataldo PA, Osler T, et al: Transanal endoscopic microsurgery is more effective than traditional transanal excision for resection of rectal masses. *Dis Colon Rectum* 51:1026; discussion 1030, 2008.
48. Lezoche E, Guerrieri M, Paganini AM, et al: Long-term results of patients with pT2 rectal cancer treated with radiotherapy and transanal endoscopic microsurgical excision. *World J Surg* 26:1170, 2002.
49. Farmer KC, Wale R, Winnett J, et al: Transanal endoscopic microsurgery: The first 50 cases. *Austr N Z J Surg* 72:854, 2002.
50. de Graaf EJ, Doornebosch PG, Stassen LP, et al: Transanal endoscopic microsurgery for rectal cancer. *Eur J Cancer* 38:904, 2002.
51. Lee W, Lee D, Choi S, et al: Transanal endoscopic microsurgery and radical surgery for T1 and T2 rectal cancer. *Surg Endosc* 17:1283, 2003.
52. Maslekar S, Pillinger SH, Sharma A, et al: Cost analysis of transanal endoscopic microsurgery for rectal tumours. *Col Dis* 9:229, 2007.
53. Middleton PF, Sutherland LM, Maddern GJ: Transanal endoscopic microsurgery: A systematic review. *Dis Colon Rectum* 48:270, 2005.
54. Kim CJ, Yeatman TJ, Coppola D, et al: Local excision of T2 and T3 rectal cancers after downstaging chemoradiation. *Ann Surg* 234:352; discussion 358, 2008.
55. Lezoche E, Guerrieri M, Paganini AM, et al: Long-term results in patients with T2-3 N0 distal rectal cancer undergoing radiotherapy before transanal endoscopic microsurgery. *Br J Surg* 92:1546, 2005.
56. Guerrieri M, Baldarelli M, Organetti L, et al: Transanal endoscopic microsurgery for the treatment of selected patients with distal rectal cancer: 15 years experience. *Surg Endosc* 22:2030, 2008.
57. Callender GG, Das P, Rodriguez-Bigas MA, et al: Local excision after preoperative chemoradiation results in an equivalent outcome to total mesorectal excision in selected patients with T3 rectal cancer. *Ann Surg Oncol* 17:441, 2010.
58. Nair RM, Siegel EM, Chen DT, et al: Long-term results of transanal excision after neoadjuvant chemoradiation for T2 and T3 adenocarcinomas of the rectum. *J Gastrointest Surg* 12:1797; discussion 1805, 2008.
59. Kim E, Hwang JM, Garcia-Aguilar J: Local excision for rectal carcinoma. *Clin Colorectal Cancer* 7:376, 2008.
60. Borschitz T, Wachtlin D, Mohler M, et al: Neoadjuvant chemoradiation and local excision for T2-3 rectal cancer. *Ann Surg Oncol* 15:712, 2008.

Transanal Endoscopic Microsurgery

Neil J. Mortensen | Roel Hompes

Approximately 30 years after the introduction of transanal endoscopic microsurgery (TEM) by Buess et al,[1] it has become the treatment of choice for large benign rectal lesions and a valuable option for well-selected malignant rectal tumors. TEM was initially designed in an effort to improve the results for local excision of rectal adenomas.[2] The Parks transanal excision is safe and straightforward; however, the limited access with restricted views and range (lower rectum) are major drawbacks. The inadequate exposure leads to less precise excisions with higher rates of specimen fragmentation and positive resection margins, accounting for the high rates of local recurrence.[3] The posterior local approaches, Kraske (suprasphincteric/transsacral) or Mason (transsphincteric), offer access for larger and also more proximal rectal lesions, but their use is sporadic because these procedures are technically challenging and are associated with significant postoperative morbidity rates.[4,5] In contrast, lesions throughout the entire rectum are accessible with the TEM instrumentation, and the stable platform allows for accurate dissection with adequate resection margins.[3,6]

For rectal cancer, total mesorectal excision (TME) in combination with autonomic nerve preservation (ANP), as described and popularized by Heald in the 1980s, is considered the criterion standard.[7] A meticulously executed TME by an appropriately trained surgeon, with short- or long-course neoadjuvant radiotherapy if indicated, leads to a marked decrease in local recurrence rates. However, this oncologic excellence comes at a cost, with well-documented significant postoperative morbidity and mortality. Despite the dramatic improvements in surgical technique, the reported incidence of long-term functional sequelae such as postoperative bowel, urinary, and sexual dysfunction still range from 30% to 40%, 0% to 12%, and 20% to 50%, respectively.[8-10] These functional sequelae, with their negative impact on daily living and quality of life will become more of a consideration, especially because the earlier detection and advances in the treatment of rectal cancer have improved survival rates. Data from the UK National Bowel Cancer Screening Programme show that 35% of screen-detected cancers are tumor-node-metastasis (TNM) stage I, as compared to 10% before the introduction of screening.[11] The approach to management of early colorectal cancer is therefore becoming more important from a public health perspective. For these early-stage cancers, there is evidence that radical surgery is overtreatment and that local excision with preservation of the rectum is adequate.[12,13] The challenge that lies within this concept of "trading off" oncologic excellence for less morbidity and

functional preservation is to identify these early rectal cancers and provide patients with an accurate prognosis of their risk of local recurrence.

In this chapter, we will describe the TEM technique, the selection of suitable candidates for its use, and provide outcome data of TEM for benign and malignant rectal tumors.

PATIENT SELECTION

Selection of patients appropriate for TEM is essential to preserve the low morbidity rates and gain maximal oncologic success. The preoperative workup is more or less the same for benign and malignant lesions and will be discussed later.

BENIGN DISEASE

TEM has proven to be safe and even superior to transanal excision of rectal adenoma (RA).[3] Theoretically, it should be technically feasible to resect rectal lesions situated up to 20 cm posteriorly, 15 cm laterally, and 12 cm anteriorly from the anal verge, without entering the peritoneal cavity. The feasibility of TEM for RA throughout the entire rectum was assessed in a prospective analysis by a Dutch group.[6] There were no exclusion criteria for referred RA, and TEM was intended in all RA. Conversion was necessary in 9.6% of patients (34/353) and depended on distance from the anal verge ($P = 0.007$) and was more common in circumferential lesions ($P = 0.001$). However, conversion rates decreased with increasing experience over time. They concluded that nearly all RA can be removed safely with TEM throughout the entire rectum. The key for success is that small, midrectal lesions are probably more suited to start off with than the more bulky, circumferential high or very distal lesions. At the beginning of the surgeon's learning curve, these cases are also best scheduled as the last case so that time is not a concern.

MALIGNANT DISEASE

The same criteria for "TEM-ability" apply for malignant lesions, which ideally are lesions lying in the extraperitoneal rectum and of a size amenable to TEM. The main concern with this approach is that potentially involved lymph nodes are not removed, and therefore TEM for rectal cancer is still controversial and is not regarded by all clinicians as an oncologic procedure with intent to cure.

The main emphasis therefore lies in identifying those early rectal cancers with the lowest probability of lymph node metastases (LNM). Depth of tumor invasion is a

TABLE 166-1 Histopathologic Features of Low- and High-Risk Early Rectal Cancer

	Low-risk ERC	High-risk ERC
ABSOLUTE FACTORS		
Morphology	Polypoid	Ulcerated
	Sessile	Flat raised
Tumor grade	G1-G2	G3-G4/signet ring
Depth of invasion	Haggitt 1-3	Haggitt 4
	pT1sm1	pT1sm2-3
Lymphovascular invasion	No	Yes
Resection margin	R0	Rx or R1
RELATIVE FACTORS		
Tumor budding	–	+
Mucinous histology	–	+
Position in distal 1/3 rectum	–	+
Tumor size	<3-4 cm	>3-4 cm
Cribriform-type structural atypia	–	+

potent predictor of LNM, as in situ carcinomas do not have the potential for metastatic spread because of paucity of lymphatics within the colorectal mucosa.[14] T1 cancers have 0% to 15% probability of LNM, versus 16% to 28% in T2 tumors.[15] T1 tumors with a low risk (5%) of lymph node involvement have diameters less than 3 cm, are well to moderately differentiated, and show no tumor budding or lymphovascular invasion.[12,16] High-risk lesions, on the other hand, have a high risk of LNM (27%) and thus these are less favorable cancers for local excision and should be offered radical surgery as primary treatment. T1 lesions can be further subdivided by level of submucosal invasion, better known as the Kikuchi classification.[17] Lymph node involvement is 1% to 3% for sm1 (low risk) and 8% and 23% for sm2 and sm3 lesions (high risk), respectively.[18] The guidelines of the Association of Coloproctology of Great Britain and Ireland recommend further treatment for any TEM specimen exhibiting any of the aforementioned high-risk features.[8] An overview of these and other less well known (relative) risk factors are shown in Table 166-1.

Other tumors that may be removed by TEM are carcinoids, and patients with malignant tumors, who are not curable or are an anesthetic risk (American Society of Anesthesiologists [ASA] grade 3 or 4), may undergo palliative resections. A further indication is the reexcision of a site where a malignant polyp has been snared and where the margin is not clear or very close.

MISCELLANEOUS

Other indications cited as case reports or small series include rectourethral fistula repair, rectovaginal fistula repair, rectal prolapse repair, and strictureplasties.[19,20] These are, however, mere anecdotal reports and have not achieved widespread popularity.

PREOPERATIVE WORKUP

All patients should get a standard preoperative workup to determine suitability for a local excision. Assessment of the rectal lesion by the operating surgeon at any stage

of the preoperative assessment is vital. A meticulous proctologic examination should be performed in the clinic or office setting, including a digital rectal evaluation, and rigid rectoscopy along with adequate biopsies if feasible. Lesions should be classified according to the location from the dentate line (in centimeters), size, and perceived depth of rectal wall penetration. Preoperative colonoscopy should also be performed, especially in tumors that are too high for assessment by digital rectal examination. With the rectum insufflated, it is easier to determine the circumferential extent and with instillation of some water, which acts as a reference point, the exact quadrants that are involved can be determined. Synchronous lesions are excluded, and at the same time large villous lesions can be debulked to allow better access to the base of the lesions at the time of TEM.

The staging process is not complete without radiologic imaging. Endorectal ultrasound and magnetic resonance imaging (MRI) provide further information on local extension of rectal wall invasion (T-stage) and lymph node involvement (N-stage). Endorectal ultrasound has the highest accuracy at the moment for staging early rectal cancer, whereas MRI staging is superior in imaging the locally advanced tumors and involved mesorectal nodes. The accuracy of MRI for LNM can be improved by the use of lymphotrophic contrast agents, because size alone is a poor predictor.[21,22] Both these techniques should be seen as complementary rather than competitive.

Although perhaps questionable for benign lesions, the pre-TEM MRI is still valuable as a baseline examination should the lesion be malignant on definitive histology, and also provides the surgeon with images regarding the fat cushion anterior to the rectum. Chest and abdominopelvic computed tomography (CT) are mainly useful to exclude distant metastatic disease for malignant lesions of the rectum. The role of positron emission tomography (PET) for local and regional staging of rectal cancer is limited, and should be reserved for evaluation of local recurrence or doubtful mesorectal nodes.

Although preoperative staging is essential, it is not always accurate, and underestimation of extent of tumor or overstaging is not uncommon. Histologic assessment of the specimen is critical, because this is the most important factor for predicting the risk of lymphatic spread and the need for further treatment (see later).

TRANSANAL ENDOSCOPIC MICROSURGERY TECHNIQUE

ANESTHESIA AND POSITIONING

General anesthesia is preferable, as a more stable pneumorectum is obtained. Regional anesthesia can be a practical alternative for patients not fit to have a general anesthesia.

The bulk of the lesion should be always kept at six o'clock in the operation field, so the patient is positioned accordingly: lithotomy for posteriorly located lesions, lateral decubitus for lesions on the sidewall, and extreme jackknife position with the legs apart for anterior lesions. As with all surgery, discussion and preoperative planning

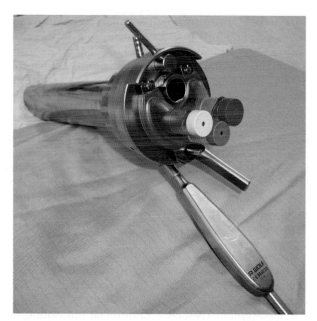

FIGURE 166-1 Rectoscope with facepiece and capped rubber sleeves through which the instruments and optics can be inserted.

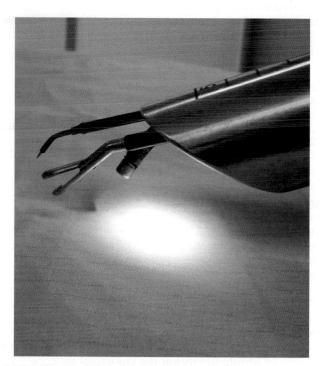

FIGURE 166-2 Tissue graspers angulated to the right and downwards; high-frequency cautery knife angulated to the left and downwards; suction device angulated downwards.

with anesthetic colleagues is essential in order to weigh up the risks and benefits of a given anesthetic technique and position.

EQUIPMENT

The TEM rectoscope is 40 mm in diameter and is either 12 or 20 cm in length. At the surgeon's end, the rectoscope is sealed with a gastight, removable facepiece. This has four ports, one for the magnifying stereoscopic optic and three for instruments (Figure 166-1). The stereoscopic optic provides a true three-dimensional view with perceptible depth of field, resolution, and sixfold magnification. An accessory endoscope can be connected that will display to a separate monitor the surgical field, which is invaluable for teaching. Unlike laparoscopic equipment, the lens is equipped with a separate irrigation channel for cleaning that is activated by a foot pedal. Once the pneumorectum is established, the intrarectal pressure is autoregulated at a pressure of 12 to 15 mm Hg by constant-flow carbon dioxide insufflation. Instruments differ from laparoscopic surgery by incorporating an angulation close to the working end, which increases triangulation otherwise lost by the narrow working channel and helps negotiate the curve of the rectum produced by the shape of the sacrum (Figure 166-2). It also reduces instrument clashing.

PROCEDURE

Once the patient is stable on the table, an anal block (20 mL of 0.5% bupivacaine) aids relaxation of the sphincters and provides additional postoperative analgesia. After a gentle dilating digital rectal examination, the well-lubricated rectoscope is inserted and the lesion is identified. Once the rectoscope is advanced into the desired position, it is locked into position and then fixed to the table using a Martin arm (Figure 166-3). All tubes are connected and the pneumorectum is established.

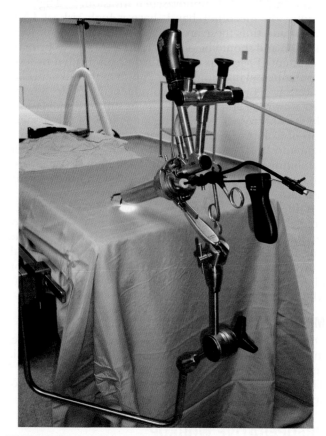

FIGURE 166-3 Rectoscope (20 cm long) fixed to the operating table by means of a Martin arm.

The margin of clearance is marked with diathermy making eschar dots, the size of which will depend to some extent on the nature of the lesion in question. All lesions should be excised with at least a 1-cm margin of normal mucosa, although a 5-mm margin is acceptable for benign lesions. A resection involving the full thickness of the rectal wall is preferred, as partial-thickness excisions are associated with a sixfold increase in the risk of an involved margin.[4] However, a partial-thickness excision may be acceptable if the lesion is known to be benign, or if the procedure is done with the intent of compromise, disease-controlling palliation, or as a prelude to adjuvant therapies. Mixed partial- and full-thickness excisions can be undertaken either to preserve the internal anal sphincter where a lesion encroaches on the upper anal canal or to prevent perforation into the peritoneal cavity for more proximal lesions. Full-thickness excision carries a risk of perforation, and the height of the most proximal point of the lesion to the anal verge, and therefore the likelihood of that area being peritonealized or not, must be considered. In practice, this means lesions up to 20 cm from the dentate line posteriorly, 15 cm laterally, and 10 to 12 cm anteriorly.

The dissection is usually started distal to the lesion in the midline of the surgical field by incising the rectal wall progressively until the perirectal fat is reached. Where the lesion lies just above the dentate line, the initial plane of dissection is submucosally, by incising the rectal wall onto the internal sphincter muscle. These extremely distal lesions can be difficult to excise by TEM, because of frequent loss of pneumorectum and bleeding from hemorrhoidal vessels. Once the surgical plane is identified, the dissection is continued orally and from the patient's left to right, dissecting tissue behind the lesion onto the proximal resection margin. It is necessary to dissect close to the rectal wall to avoid damaging the vaginal wall and urethra or to avoid accidental entry into the peritoneal cavity. Where the posterior rectum has been incised, it may be possible to take a lymph node sample for analysis.[23] The diagnostic value of mesorectal sampling has not been evaluated, and doing this may compromise future completion/salvage resection.

If there is bleeding during dissection, the bleeding vessel is best controlled by compression with the tip of an instrument and then coagulated with the tip of the suction device or grasped with a forceps and coagulated. Serious bleeding most often indicates that dissection has been performed deeply into the perirectal fat or mesorectum and may be reduced by the use of energy devices, such as the Harmonic Scalpel.

Inadvertent perforation of the rectum is a major risk and is associated with sepsis and the theoretical risk of tumor seeding into the peritoneal cavity. Defects should be closed as soon as possible to avoid the "aerosol" of microbes and potentially viable tumor cells. If the defect is large or fecal soiling is suspected, a laparoscopic lavage of the pelvis should be considered. This will allow not only dilution of microbes but a "leak test" can also be performed.

After retrieval of the specimen, the defect produced by resection should be rinsed with a copious amount of disinfectant fluid to prevent abscess formation and the theoretical possibility of tumor implantation. The wound can be closed by a transverse continuous absorbable monofilament 2-0 suture, but the dehiscence rate is high, especially for those lesions closest to the anal verge. To facilitate closure, the endoluminal pressure is reduced to 10 to 12 mm Hg. Instead of tying a knot to secure the suture, a silver clip is pressed onto the thread to lock the suture. Closure of the defect is easier when sewing from right to left, and aborally to orally. Stay sutures may help with alignment, and changing the direction of suturing (orally to aborally) may help to get better access, especially for closure of the left side of the defect. The sutures are short (8 cm), as excess length will impair suturing.

The specimen should be handled with care and is pinned out on a piece of cork with detailed information for the pathologist concerning preoperative staging and/or neoadjuvant treatment and orientation of the specimen. Ideally, the specimen should be sent fresh.

POSTOPERATIVE CARE

POSTOPERATIVE INSTRUCTIONS

Patients are sent back to the ward with a urinary catheter and a rectal Foley catheter (32 French) that will drain residual rinsing fluid and serves to detect postoperative bleeding at an early stage. Both catheters can be removed the following morning.

Patients are immediately started on a clear liquid diet and progress to a regular diet if tolerated. If no complications arise, the patient is discharged on the first postoperative day. A short course of oral antibiotics may be prescribed at the discretion of the operating surgeon.

POSTOPERATIVE COMPLICATIONS

Complication rates after TEM are generally low, ranging from 5% to 10%. In a review by Middleton et al, the overall morbidity rate was reported to be 10.3%.[24] The most common complications are minor and include pain, bleeding, fever, and urinary retention. Other less frequent, more serious complications are intra- or transmural abscess formation, fistulas to perineum or vagina, and rectal strictures. Post-TEM fever and urinary retention usually tend to resolve in the first 24 hours after surgery. In case of ongoing fever and/or other signs of sepsis, intravenous antibiotics and radiologic imaging should be considered.

Wound breakdown can lead to pelvic sepsis, and if conservative management with antibiotics fails, an examination under anesthesia of the rectum should be performed for local drainage and, in a worst case scenario, a diversion colostomy or ileostomy may be necessary. Wound dehiscence can also occur at a later stage, and symptoms usually include anal pain, frequency/urgency, and a foul-smelling rectal discharge. Treatment options at this stage are administration of daily enemas with antibiotics and analgesics and/or a medical colostomy, and if these fail a diversion colostomy or ileostomy. Wound dehiscence is more frequent in patients who had neoadjuvant radiotherapy, and the use of hyperbaric oxygen therapy, in particular, may be beneficial and could prevent stoma formation in these patients.

The anal sphincter is significantly dilated by the 4-cm TEM-scope, so transient fecal incontinence is present in nearly all patients undergoing TEM. The duration of the sphincter weakness is found to correlate with the duration of the procedure, but usually recovers.[25] Functional data have shown that incontinence symptoms tend to be resolved after 6 months and that quality of life and even the functional scores may improve after tumor removal.[26]

SURVEILLANCE AND TREATMENT STRATEGIES

If the lesion is benign, followup is as for other adenomata and includes surveillance endoscopy at 1 and 3 years postoperatively; further interval depends on local findings. Patients will also be seen in clinic with additional rigid sigmoidoscopy at 3, 6, 18, and 24 months.

Decisions after local excision of rectal cancer with curative intent depend predominantly on the histopathologic characteristics of the resection specimen. But the patient's wishes and comorbidities should also be considered. The risk of leaving viable tumor, for instance in unidentified lymph node metastasis, must be balanced against the morbidity and mortality of radical surgery, which may be unnecessary. Many patients will have considerable comorbidity, and avoiding radical surgery will be attractive for patient and surgeon.

In general, low-risk early rectal cancers may be followed up closely, and high-risk early rectal cancers should be offered completion radical surgery. The term *completion surgery* is preferred to the often quoted *salvage surgery*, as salvage has negative connotations implying recovering a situation from a wrecked state. In fact, TEM may be considered an excisional biopsy, and oncologic outcomes of completion surgery following TEM with high-risk histology are comparable to primary radical surgery alone.[12,27] Completion surgery may be offered post-TEM without compromising oncology, but from a technical viewpoint the TEM resection may compromise subsequent surgery. There may be a tendency to avoid restorative resection in favor of abdominoperineal excision where the TEM resection has been in the lower third of the rectum, especially in cases of wound breakdown. There is no particular consensus on timing of surgery, beyond a desire to allow the initial inflammation of the TEM resection to settle, and consideration of the timing of adjuvant therapy.

Although recurrence rates following local excision in carefully selected cases should be low, it is imperative that those that "fail" treatment should be identified at the earliest opportunity. In some patients, there may have been a tradeoff between the oncologic benefits and operative risks of radical surgery. There is little consensus on followup schedules after local excision of an early rectal cancer. Recurrences usually occur within the first 2 years after resection, so investigation should be rigorous in this time period. The Oxford protocol is consensus-led and consists of followup in clinic and flexible endoscopy at 3-month intervals for the first year, and thereafter every 6 months for up to 5 years. Pelvic MRI is performed at 3, 9, and 24 months postoperatively, and a CT of the chest, abdomen, and pelvis is performed annually for 3 years. At present, PET-CT is not routinely recommended but is used to resolve uncertainty if local recurrence is suspected on MRI or CT. Although not part of our protocol, carcinoembryonic antigen levels can be determined every 3 to 6 months for 2 years, then every 6 months for a total of 5 years in patients who are potential candidates for resection of isolated metastasis. Endorectal ultrasound is used by many units but it can lack the clear baseline reference images of MRI and be hard to reproduce.

In patients with significant comorbidities that preclude major abdominal surgery, completion surgery may not be an option for "high-risk" early rectal cancer or pT2 disease. For these patients, adjuvant radiotherapy may be a reasonable compromise, provided that they are sufficiently counseled because the benefit of adjuvant radiotherapy and/or chemotherapy following TEM is not well known. Regarding adjuvant radiotherapy after TEM, Duek et al hint at some benefit.[28] Twelve patients with T2 rectal adenocarcinoma who had undergone radiotherapy after TEM remained disease free after a median followup of 3 years, whereas a 50% recurrence rate was seen in 4 patients who refused adjuvant treatment.

RESULTS

PATIENTS WITH BENIGN DISEASE

Although both TEM and transanal excision are safe procedures, a systematic review by Middleton et al found a lower morbidity rate after TEM versus transanal excision (10.3% versus 17%, respectively).[24] A recent large prospective analysis of two matched groups (TEM vs. transanal excision) came to the same findings, with significant lower morbidity after TEM (5.3% vs. 10%).[3]

Middleton et al also showed a low recurrence rate of 5% after local excision of rectal adenoma by TEM.[24] Some of the studies reviewed in his manuscript and other more recent series will be further discussed here. In our department, TEM has been used for local excision of rectal lesions since 1993, and over a period of 12 years 148 patients with rectal adenomas were treated.[29] In the majority of cases (84%), a complete excision could be achieved (R0). Histologically proven local recurrence rate after resection of rectal adenomas was 7.6%, with a median time to recurrence of 23 months (range, 6.5 to 123). Radical surgery to deal with this local recurrence was necessary in only two patients, thus avoiding radical surgery in 77 of 79 patients (97%) in whom the tumor was too high for a conventional transanal excision. Guerrieri et al reported on the pooled analysis of 588 adenomas resected by TEM after a median followup of 44 months. The recurrence rate was 4.3% and in most cases recurrences could be managed by re-TEM (87%).[30] De Graaf et al compared two matched groups of RA after Parks' per anal resection (PAR) (n = 43) and TEM (n = 216), and reported a significantly lower recurrence rate after TEM (23.3% vs. 3.7%).[3] They reported incomplete excision as the main factor responsible for the difference in local recurrence between these two techniques. Clear margins were observed in 50% after PAR and 88% after TEM, whereas tumor fragmentation (leading to significantly more unclear margins) occurred in 23.8% and 1.4%, respectively. Whitehouse analyzed risk factors for recurrence in 146 resections of RA by TEM.[31] After a median followup of 23 months, the local recurrence rate was 4.8%, and only microscopic involvement of the resection margin was found to be significantly associated with local recurrence. However, not all incomplete excisions seem to recur, and this could be due to the definition of an R1 margin (within 1 mm of margin) and the fulguration effect of diathermy on the resection margin.[32] This implies that in selected cases, early and regular surveillance could be implemented, whereas others might need reexcision.

PATIENTS WITH MALIGNANT DISEASE

Early Rectal Cancer

Early rectal cancer is defined as invasive adenocarcinoma spreading into, but not beyond, the submucosa (T1 in TNM classification) and this in the absence of lymph node disease. TEM seems to be the procedure of choice for local excision of early rectal cancers, and if patients are selected appropriately, recurrence rates and survival can be similar to those after radical surgery. However, reported recurrence rates in the literature range from 0% to 20.8% and indicate the importance of appropriate patient selection.[12,13,29,33-38] The only prospective randomized analysis by Winde et al revealed no significant difference in local recurrence (4% vs. 0%) or 5-year survival (96%) between TEM and radical surgery, respectively, for uT1N0 rectal cancer.[35] However, TEM proved to be the safest technique, with lower early and late morbidity. Borschitz et al reported on the long-term outcome in 84 patients with pT1 rectal cancer.[36] The group of patients with low-risk pathologic characteristics (and R0 resection) had a local recurrence rate of 6% and 10-year disease-free survival of 89%. The local recurrence rate in the high-risk group was considerably higher (39%); however, this was reduced to 6% after early completion surgery and resulted in a 10-year disease-free survival of 93%. In the study by Heintz et al, 103 consecutive patients with T1 rectal cancer were treated by TEM ($n = 58$) or radical surgery ($n = 45$), and outcome stratified again according to low- or high-risk lesions.[37] No difference was observed in local recurrence and 5-year disease-free survival in the groups with low-risk T1 carcinoma. In the group of high-risk T1 cancers, the recurrence rate was higher in the TEM group (33% vs. 18%), although actuarial 5-year survival was similar. In both the low-risk and high-risk groups, all the recurrences were observed in patients with involved resection margins. The resection margin was obviously only involved after TEM and was higher in the group of high-risk cancers (42% vs. 22%). Interestingly, none of the patients in the group with low-risk T1 carcinoma undergoing radical surgery developed lymph node metastases, whereas 36% of patients in the high-risk group had involved lymph nodes. Both these features underscore the necessity for radical surgery in the treatment of high-risk early rectal cancers. In an effort to determine the impact of margin status, De Graaf et al prospectively analyzed the outcome after TEM ($n = 80$) and radical surgery ($n = 75$) for T1 rectal cancer with standardized histopathologic assessment of the specimens.[38] Of the 80 patients, only 3 had an initially positive

excision margin, and had a re-TEM with no evidence of residual tumor tissue. After radical surgery, no local recurrence was observed and although all patients after TEM had a negative excision margin, local recurrence was still 24%. In 80% of patients with a local recurrence, salvage surgery was performed. Overall and cancer-free survival was similar in both groups: 75% versus 77% and 90% versus 87% after TEM versus radical surgery, respectively. Bach et al reported on the outcome of 487 patients who underwent a TEM procedure for rectal cancer.[12] The majority of patients had a pT1 tumor ($n = 253$) and were subclassified using the submucosal staging system (sm1 to sm3). Sm1 tumors were least likely to recur, with a local recurrence rate of 3% to 4% for smaller lesions. The calculated hazard ratio for local recurrence was 2.74 for pT1sm2-3 tumors versus sm1.

Invasive Rectal Cancer

The role of TEM in the management of T2-3 rectal cancer remains controversial and is not routinely used. High local recurrence rates are reported when TEM alone is used in the treatment for more advanced rectal cancers.[12,39-41] This is of course no surprise, because of the high risk of lymph node involvement in T2-3 rectal cancer.

For T2 lesions, this was shown in a study by Borschitz et al, who reported unacceptably high local recurrence rates for low- and high-risk T2 rectal adenocarcinoma of 29% and 50%, respectively.[40] All patients who were fit enough to undergo completion surgery were offered this option, and local recurrence rate in this group was significantly reduced to 7%. In a retrospective analysis of T1 and T2 rectal cancer treated with TEM ($n = 74$) or radical surgery ($n = 100$), Lee et al observed no difference in recurrence rates and 5-year survival rates in the T1 group.[41] In patients with T2 cancers, the TEM group (19.5%) showed a significantly higher recurrence rate than the radical surgery group (9.4%); however, this did not translate into a significant difference in 5-year survival rates. It has been suggested that in the case of local excision for a T2 rectal cancer, and assuming that further surgery is not an option, the patient could be offered adjuvant radiotherapy.[42] The same option was explored by Duek et al, who reported no recurrence in patients who had undergone radiotherapy after TEM for a T2 cancer ($n = 12$), whereas 50% recurrence was seen in patients who refused radiotherapy ($n = 4$) after a median followup of 3 years.[28]

There is also mounting evidence of the benefit of neoadjuvant chemoradiotherapy in combination with local excision for some more advanced rectal cancers (T2-3).[13,33,43] Lezoche et al recently reported on the outcome of 84 patients with T2 rectal cancer after high-dose radiotherapy and subsequent TEM.[13] Before initiation of the radiotherapy, a safety margin of normal mucosa around the tumor was marked with a tattoo. The TEM procedure involved a full-thickness excision of the rectal wall within the marked area and included a large amount of perirectal tissue. After a median followup period of 97 months, 4 patients experienced a local recurrence (4.7%) and 2 patients a distant metastases. In 2 patients, the local recurrence was extraluminal and both died of metastatic disease (only 1 patient had salvage surgery). The remaining 2 patients with mucosal recurrence underwent salvage surgery and were alive and disease free at the end of the followup period. The patients who experienced a recurrence were low or non-responders to neoadjuvant treatment. Disease-free survival rate at the end of the followup period was 93%.

Guerrieri et al studied 196 patients with T1-3N0 rectal cancer (51 T1, 84 T2, and 61 T3) undergoing TEM.[33] All patients staged preoperatively as T2-3 underwent preoperative high-dose radiotherapy. The definitive histologic examination revealed a complete pathologic response in 34 patients, 25 within the T2 group and 9 patients in the T3 group. At a median followup of 81 months, the local failure rate was 4.1% (5 pT2 and 3 pT3) and the rectal cancer-specific survival was 90% for pT2 and 77% for pT3. For pT1 cancers, none of the patients developed a local recurrence.

CONCLUSION

From the data available in the literature and from our own experience, we can conclude that TEM is a safe and effective treatment of rectal adenoma, with favorable results in comparison to conventional transanal excision. It is paramount that negative resection margins are achieved, because this seems to be the major factor responsible for local failure. If lesions are incompletely resected, the patient should be offered early re-TEM or should be followed very closely and at short intervals.

Local excision for early rectal cancer is at the moment still a challenging field, full of conflicting evidence and priorities. On one hand, the quality of radical surgery has improved in the past few decades, but bowel cancer screening programs and heightened public awareness will increase the proportion of cancers presenting at an early stage. Insight into tumor behavior through molecular analyses will improve and may reach a point where individual tumor profiles allow more tailored treatment. This will fuel demand for less radical and morbid surgery.

Currently TEM can be considered as a first-line therapy for T1 rectal cancer without any adverse pathologic findings (low-risk pT1). High-risk early rectal cancers mandate further treatment in the form of completion surgery and/or adjuvant (chemo)radiotherapy to prevent high local failure rates. TEM may also be appropriate for T2-3 lesions that have undergone neoadjuvant chemoradiotherapy with a good clinical response. Patients with a poor response should ideally undergo radical surgery rather than TEM, unless they refuse radical surgery or are medically unfit for major surgery (compromise/palliation). However, the use of TEM in advanced rectal cancer should be limited to a select group of patients and should be within the boundaries of a trial. We must await the results of randomized controlled trials to make any further recommendations.

REFERENCES

1. Buess G, Hutterer F, Theiss J, et al: A system for transanal endoscopic rectum operation. *Chirurgica* 55:677, 1984.
2. Buess G, Theiss R, Gunther M, et al: Endoscopic operative procedure for the removal of rectal polyps. *Coloproctology* 84:254, 1984.
3. De Graaf EJ, Burger JW, van Ijsseldijk AL, et al: Transanal endoscopic microsurgery is superior to transanal excision of rectal adenomas. *Colorectal Dis* 13:762, 2011.
4. Onaitis M, Ludwig K, Perez-Tamayo A, et al: The Kraske procedure: a critical analysis of a surgical approach for mid-rectal lesions. *J Surg Oncol* 94:194, 2006.
5. Qiu HZ, Lin GL, Xiao Y, et al: The use of posterior trans-sphincteric approach in surgery of the rectum: A Chinese 16-year experience. *World J Surg* 32:1776, 2008.
6. De Graaf EJ, Doornebosch PG, Tetteroo GWM, et al: Transanal endoscopic microsurgery is feasible for adenomas throughout the entire rectum: A prospective study. *Dis Colon Rectum* 52:1107, 2009.
7. Heald RJ, Husband EM, Ryall RD: The mesorectum in rectal cancer surgery—the clue to pelvic recurrence? *Br J Surg* 69:613, 1982.
8. Association of Coloproctology of Great Britain and Ireland: Guidelines for the Management of Colorectal Cancer (3rd edn). 2007. http://www.library.nhs.uk/theatres/Viewresource.aspx?resID=31479
9. Nesbakken A, Nygaard K, Bull-Njaa T, et al: Bladder and sexual dysfunction after mesorectal excision for rectal cancer. *Br J Surg* 87:206, 2000.
10. Kim NK, Aahn TW, Park JK, et al: Assessment of sexual and voiding function after total mesorectal excision with pelvic autonomic nerve preservation in males with rectal cancer. *Dis Colon Rectum* 45:1178, 2002.
11. Ellul P, Fogden E, Simpson CL, et al: Downstaging of colorectal cancer by the National Bowel Cancer Screening Programme in England: First round data from the first centre. *Colorectal Dis* 12:420, 2010.
12. Bach SP, Hill J, Monson JR, et al: A predictive model for local recurrence after transanal endoscopic microsurgery for rectal cancer. *Br J Surg* 96:280, 2009.
13. Lezoche G, Guerrieri M, Baldarelli M, et al: Transanal endoscopic microsurgery for 135 patients with small nonadvanced low rectal cancer (iT1-iT2, iN0): Short- and long-term results. *Surg Endosc* 25:1222, 2011.
14. Day DW, Jass JR, Price AB, et al: Epithelial tumours of the large intestine. In *Morson and Dawson's Gastrointestinal pathology*, ed 4, Oxford, 2003, Blackwell Science, p 551.
15. Sengupta S, Tjandra JJ: Local excision of rectal cancer: What is the evidence? *Dis Colon Rectum* 44:1345, 2001.
16. Ganai S, Kanumuri P, Rao RS, et al: Local recurrence after transanal endoscopic microsurgery for rectal polyps and early cancers. *Ann Surg Oncol* 13:547, 2006.
17. Kikuchi R, Takano M, Takagi K, et al: Management of early invasive colorectal cancer. Risk of recurrence and clinical guidelines. *Dis Colon Rectum* 38:1286, 1995.
18. Nascimbeni R, Burgart LJ, Nivatvongs S, et al: Risk of lymph node metastasis in T1 carcinoma of the colon and rectum. *Dis Colon Rectum* 45:200, 2002.
19. Bochove-Overgaauw DM, Beerlage HP, Bosscha K, et al: Transanal endoscopic microsurgery for correction of rectourethral fistulae. *J Endourol* 20:1087, 2006.
20. Baatrup G, Svensen R, Ellensen VS: Benign rectal strictures managed with transanal resection—a novel application for transanal endoscopic microsurgery. *Colorectal Dis* 12:144, 2010.
21. Beets GL, Beets-Tan RG: Pretherapy imaging of rectal cancers: ERUS or MRI? *Surg Oncol Clin N Am* 19:733, 2010.
22. Thrall JH: Nanotechnology and medicine. *Radiology* 230:315, 2004.
23. Mentges B, Buess G, Schafer D, et al: Local therapy of rectal tumours. *Dis Colon Rectum* 39:886, 1996.
24. Middleton PF, Sutherland LM, Maddern GJ: Transanal endoscopic microsurgery: A systematic review. *Dis Colon Rectum* 48:270, 2005.
25. Kennedy ML, Lubowski DZ, King DW: Transanal endoscopic microsurgery excision: Is anorectal function compromised? *Dis Colon Rectum* 45:601, 2002.
26. Doornebosch PG, Gosselink MP, Neijenhuis PA, et al: Impact on transanal endoscopic microsurgery on quality of life and functional outcome. *Int J Colorectal Dis* 23:709, 2008.
27. Hahnloser D, Wolff BG, Larson DW, et al: Immediate radical resection after local excision of rectal cancer: An oncologic compromise? *Dis Colon Rectum* 48:429, 2005.
28. Duek SD, Issa N, Hershko DD, et al: Outcome of transanal endoscopic microsurgery and adjuvant radiotherapy in patients with T2 rectal cancer. *Dis Colon Rectum* 51:379, 2008.

29. Bretagnol F, Merrie A, George B, et al: Local excision of rectal tumours by transanal endoscopic microsurgery. *Br J Surg* 94:627, 2007.
30. Guerrieri M, Baldarelli M, Morino M, et al: Transanal endoscopic microsurgery in rectal adenomas: Experience of six Italian centres. *Dig Liver Dis* 38:202, 2006.
31. Whitehouse PA, Tilney HS, Armitage JN, et al: Transanal endoscopic microsurgery: Risk factors for local recurrence of benign rectal adenomas. *Colorectal Dis* 8:795, 2006.
32. Ganai S, Kanumuri P, Rao RS, et al: Local recurrence after transanal endoscopic microsurgery for rectal polyps and early cancers. *Ann Surg Oncol* 13:547, 2006.
33. Guerrieri M, Baldarelli M, Organetti L, et al: Transanal endoscopic microsurgery for the treatment of selected patients with distal rectal cancer: 15 years experience. *Surg Endosc* 22:2030, 2008.
34. Christoforidis D, Cho HM, Dixon MR, et al: Transanal endoscopic microsurgery versus conventional transanal excision for patients with early rectal cancer. *Ann Surg* 249:776, 2009.
35. Winde G, Nottberg H, Keller R, et al: Surgical cure for early rectal carcinomas (T1). Transanal endoscopic microsurgery vs. anterior resection. *Dis Colon Rectum* 39:969, 1996.
36. Borschitz T, Heintz A, Junginger T: The influence of histopathologic criteria on the long-term prognosis of locally excised pT1 rectal carcinomas: Results of local excision (transanal endoscopic microsurgery) and immediate reoperation. *Dis Colon Rectum* 49:1492, 2006.
37. Heintz A, Morschel M, Junginger T: Comparison of results after transanal endoscopic microsurgery and radical resection for T1 carcinoma of the rectum. *Surg Endosc* 12:1145, 1998.
38. De Graaf EJ, Doornebosch PG, Tollenaar RA, et al: Transanal endoscopic microsurgery versus total mesorectal excision of T1 rectal adenocarcinomas with curative intention. *Eur J Surg Oncol* 35:1280, 2009.
39. Zacharakis E, Freilich S, Rekhraj S, et al: Transanal endoscopic microsurgery for rectal tumors: the St. Mary's experience. *Am J Surg* 194:694, 2007.
40. Borschitz T, Heintz A, Junginger T: Transanal endoscopic microsurgery of pT2 rectal cancer: Results and possible indications. *Dis Colon Rectum* 50:292, 2007.
41. Lee W, Lee D, Choi S, et al: Transanal endoscopic microsurgery and radical surgery for T1 and T2 rectal cancer. *Surg Endosc* 17:1283, 2003.
42. Chakravarti A, Compton CC, Shellito PC, et al: Long-term follow-up of patients with rectal cancer managed by local excision with and without adjuvant irradiation. *Ann Surg* 230:49, 1999.
43. Borschitz T, Wachtlin D, Mohler M, et al: Neoadjuvant chemoradiation and local excision for T2-3 rectal cancer. *Ann Surg Oncol* 15:712, 2008.

Operations for Colorectal Cancer: Low Anterior Resection

Vassiliki Liana Tsikitis | Alfred M. Cohen

Because 70% to 80% of patients with rectal cancer have disease beyond the rectal wall through either direct extension or lymphatic spread, most patients require radical resection.[1] Optimal oncologic and functional results require a precise surgical approach, selectively integrated with adjuvant radiotherapy and chemotherapy.

Rectal cancer surgery is a local-regional therapy, but the oncologic efficacy of such surgery is based principally on its rate of local control.[2] The pelvis is a common site of recurrence, which is a major cause of complications and death.[3] Pain secondary to nerve invasion, perineal breakdown, and obstruction, along with bleeding and fistulization, often creates an unmanageable problem. Salvage therapy is limited in most cases and provides incomplete and temporary palliation.[4] The attitude that pelvic recurrence is best prevented should prevail and help guide the choice of operation and conduct of the pelvic dissection.

The major risk factors for relapse, both local and distant, are the number of involved regional lymph nodes, the extent of transmural penetration, and tumor grade.[5,6] Two observations strongly implicate inadequate surgical resection as a major cause of pelvic recurrence. First, involvement of the lateral or circumferential margin of resection strongly correlates with subsequent local recurrence.[7] Conventional resection yields a positive lateral margin in 25% of cases, with local recurrence developing in approximately 80% of these patients. Second, a clear lateral margin on serial section correlates with local control. Studies from the United Kingdom and Germany have demonstrated that the frequency of local recurrence varies among individual surgeons, from less than 10% to more than 50%.[8,9] The surgeon's operative technique and ability to achieve a negative circumferential margin are strong determinants of local control.[10]

A common practice in pelvic surgery is "blunt" dissection, which is associated with a high risk for mesorectal or rectal perforation.[11] Heald et al[9,10] advocated total mesorectal excision (TME) in conjunction with low anterior resection (LAR) as the optimal surgical treatment of low rectal cancer. This technique involves removal of the entire rectal mesentery, including that distal to the tumor, as an intact unit. TME requires precise dissection in an areolar plane outside the visceral fascia that envelops the rectum and its mesentery. In contrast to conventional blunt dissection techniques, the envelope that encompasses the pelvic tissue is removed intact, without the risk for mesorectal or rectal perforation that is frequently associated with blunt dissection along the rectosacral fascia. This approach maximizes the likelihood of obtaining a negative lateral or peripheral margin. In addition, TME facilitates nerve preservation, enables complete hemostasis, and emphasizes gentle handling to avoid tearing or disrupting the smooth outer surface of the mesorectum. In a large series of patients treated by rectal resection with TME, MacFarlane et al[12] reported only a 5% local failure rate without the use of radiotherapy. Although such technical strategies are not fully proved, there is increasing evidence to support the conclusion that TME does improve local control. TME has been shown to achieve a negative circumferential margin in 93% of resected specimens.[13] In addition, other surgeons using similar TME techniques have reported local failure rates of less than 10% for transmural or node-positive rectal cancer.[14-16] These data are quite compelling, but all of these reports represent a select group of patients; patients who underwent abdominoperineal resection were excluded, and some patients who received adjuvant radiation therapy were included. Most important, the patients reported are those who have undergone a "potentially curative" operation. Hence, patients with close tangential or lateral margins may be excluded from such reports. Although no randomized trial of TME has been performed, TME has been evaluated prospectively in Sweden, where it has been introduced through a formal preceptorship-based training program. A 5-year prospective audit revealed a local recurrence rate of 7% after the addition of TME as opposed to a historical control rate of 23%.[16] These data are summarized in Table 167-1.

Inherent in reports on TME is the use of sharp mesorectal excision. This technique involves cautery and scissors dissection in the well-defined plane outside the mesorectal visceral fascial lining, which is the "only plane" definable during precise pelvic surgery. We perceive this to be the most important aspect of optimization of pelvic surgery. TME as a component of sharp mesorectal excision may be appropriate for mid- and low rectal cancer but not for all rectal cancer. Sharp mesorectal excision is appropriate for all patients.

In the United States, attempts to reduce local recurrence and to improve survival rates have emphasized postoperative adjuvant chemotherapy and radiation therapy. Randomized trials have shown convincingly that for transmural or node-positive rectal cancer treated with conventional surgery, the addition of adjuvant therapy improves outcome. The combination of postoperative chemotherapy and radiation therapy further improves local control and increases overall survival rates.[17,18] In 1990, a National Institutes of Health consensus conference report on rectal cancer recommended combined

TABLE 167-1 Results of Total Mesorectal Excision for Rectal Cancer

Series	n	Radiation Therapy	Local Failure (%)	Survival (%)
Cawthorne et al,[13] 1990	122	n = 7	7	NS
MacFarlane et al,[12] 1993	135	None	5	78
Enker and Cranor,[15] 1995	204	<33%	6	77
Arbman et al,[16] 1996	128	n = 3	7	68
Zaheer et al,[14] 1998	514	None	7	78

NS, Not stated.

postoperative chemotherapy and radiation therapy as the standard of care for patients with stage II (*transmural node-negative*) and III (*node-positive*) rectal cancer.[19]

The National Surgical Adjuvant Breast and Bowel Project (NSABP) RO-1 trial compared surgical resection alone with adjuvant chemotherapy or radiation therapy. The data demonstrated a survival benefit with single-modality adjuvant chemotherapy. Current adjuvant therapy trials are testing how to best combine chemotherapy and radiation therapy with regard to drug selection, dose, sequence, and timing to optimize results. The benefits of continuous venous 5-fluorouracil infusion along with leucovorin, levamisole, or both versus the bolus delivery of 5-fluorouracil are under study in separate cooperative group trials in the United States.

Several studies have suggested that postoperative radiation therapy has a considerable long-term detrimental impact on bowel function. With computed tomography (CT) or ultrasonography, the presence of extensive hepatic metastases can be excluded preoperatively. In addition, endorectal ultrasound provides objective information with regard to transmural spread. The use of a preoperative chemoradiation strategy is becoming increasingly common. Whether preoperative adjuvant therapy offers better local control, as previously indicated in a trial of preoperative versus postoperative radiotherapy from Sweden,[20,21] was tested by the German cooperative group. They confirmed the efficacy of the preoperative (neoadjuvant) sequence.[22]

Left unanswered is whether adjuvant local-regional radiotherapy is necessary in the setting of optimal resective surgery. A two-arm randomized study of TME with or without *short-course, high-fraction* (25 Gy in five fractions) preoperative radiotherapy for resectable rectal cancer was performed in the Netherlands.[23] Participation in this trial was limited to surgeons trained in TME who had performed five operations with a member of the monitoring committee. Preoperative radiation reduced local failure by one-half, despite TME. The greatest benefit was in the node-positive patients.

With increasing emphasis on cost-effectiveness and quality-of-life issues, the incremental, but costly, benefit of adjuvant radiation therapy in patients undergoing optimal resection will have to be clearly redefined. Data

are persuasive that the use of postoperative chemoradiation after conventional resection has a profound negative impact on late bowel function.[24] There are few data regarding the impact of preoperative irradiation on late bowel function, particularly at the most common U.S. doses and fractions.

GOALS AND TERMINOLOGY

The goals of operative treatment of patients with rectal cancer are to cure cancer locally (within the pelvis) and to minimize risk with regard to sphincter loss and bowel, bladder, and sexual dysfunction. Many of the aspects of surgical resection that are described later will affect the success of all of these goals. The issues related to conduct of rectal cancer resection and the risk for local recurrence apply primarily to patients with mid and low rectal cancer, that is, cancers at or below the peritoneal reflection. The upper third of the rectum, commonly from 11 to 15 cm from the anal verge, is at considerably reduced risk for local recurrence. Patients with cancer of the upper part of the rectum or rectosigmoid are generally treated initially by surgical resection, and adjuvant therapy follows the colon cancer postoperative paradigm. Sphincter-preserving resections of the rectum are referred to as *anterior resection, low anterior resection* (LAR), or *low anterior resection with coloanal reconstruction*. In general, anterior resection refers to resection of the sigmoid or rectosigmoid and may involve mobilization of the presacral plane and the anterior plane. LAR is used to refer to anterior resection combined with complete clearance of the pelvic side walls. In this chapter, the technique refers only to patients undergoing LAR with a sutured or, more commonly, a stapled reconstruction in the low pelvis. Reconstruction involving a coloanal anastomosis is discussed in Chapter 169. A stapled reconstruction at the pelvic floor should not be referred to as a *coloanal anastomosis*.

PATIENT SELECTION

All patients with rectal cancer should receive preoperative chest radiography and CT scan of the abdomen and pelvis to rule out metastatic disease. In the selection of patients suitable for a sphincter-preserving approach, tumor size, differentiation, and location are all taken into account. Low-lying anaplastic or poorly differentiated cancers generally require abdominoperineal resection and chemoradiation therapy. Bulky transmural tumors just above the anorectal ring also frequently require complete proctectomy. The location of the tumor is determined by digital rectal examination and visualization with a rigid sigmoidoscope, usually with the patient in the left lateral decubitus position. The distance from the anal verge or the dentate line is determined. The most important distance is that related to the upper portion of the anal canal, generally referred to as the *anorectal ring*. In a slender patient, particularly a woman, a cancer that is easily palpable but several centimeters above the anorectal ring may be amenable to LAR with a stapled reconstruction. In other patients, as discussed later, this technique is not feasible. An additional tumor feature that determines the likelihood for sphincter preservation is its circumferential location. A tumor 2 to 3 cm above the anorectal ring posteriorly, after total mesorectal mobilization, will frequently be 5 to 6 cm above the anorectal ring when traction is applied. However, an anteriorly located tumor has very little cephalad mobility after mesorectal mobilization.

In addition to these tumor factors involved in allowing a sphincter-preserving approach, there are a number of aspects related to the individual patient. Body habitus and gender are pivotal. A slender woman is the ideal patient. Sphincter preservation in a heavy man with a large prostate and an anterior-based tumor is always problematic, even with cancer in the midrectum. For many such patients, bowel continuity is best restored by coloanal reconstruction. Sphincter preservation is generally precluded in men with a history of prostate cancer treated by either external-beam radiation therapy, brachytherapy seed implantation, or radical prostatectomy.

Patients with extensive diverticulosis or previous left colectomy may not be amenable to LAR and restoration of bowel continuity because of inadequate length of good-quality proximal bowel. There are also rare patients with an incomplete marginal artery of the colon. However, most often an inadequate marginal artery represents an iatrogenic intraoperative complication from excess tension on the bowel. Finally, patients should not undergo very low reconstruction in the presence of poor resting and squeezing anal canal pressure.

PREOPERATIVE RADIATION THERAPY

Patients with locally advanced transmural rectal cancer that is tethered or fixed should be evaluated for preoperative radiation therapy. This is usually combined with 5-fluorouracil–based concurrent chemotherapy, both as a radiosensitizer and as an adjuvant for disseminated disease. In addition, there is a subset of patients with relatively early, but very low, cancer in whom preoperative radiation therapy is used to facilitate sphincter preservation. The appropriate adequate distal margin to achieve an excellent clinical response remains unclear in a patient with an early cancer who receives preoperative radiation therapy; 5 mm may be acceptable. However, it is completely unacceptable to divide through cancer in an unrealistic attempt at sphincter preservation. Frozen-section control of the distal and lateral specimen margins is important before proceeding with restoration of bowel continuity. An incisional biopsy at the start of the operation does not provide adequate data for determination of the ability to achieve tumor clearance.

MANAGEMENT OF OBSTRUCTING CANCER

There are many patients with radiologic or even endoscopic suggestion of obstruction by an upper rectal or rectosigmoid cancer that clinically causes little interference with bowel function. Such patients may undergo elective resection. In the presence of a locally advanced rectal cancer with symptomatic obstruction, patients should undergo a preliminary diversion, receive chemoradiation therapy, and then undergo rectal resection. All

such patients should be extensively evaluated preoperatively with chest radiography and computed tomography or ultrasonography, or both, of the liver. A diverting stoma can be created laparoscopically or with a limited laparotomy. A low sigmoid loop colostomy is advantageous in that it will be outside the radiation field and can permit a two-stage operation with resection of the colostomy as part of LAR after the completion of radiation therapy. A left-sided transverse colostomy is to be avoided because of the potential for interference with colon mobilization for reconstruction. If a right-sided transverse colostomy is performed, care must be taken to not damage the middle colic vessels, which are necessary for the reconstruction. Distal loop ileostomy is also acceptable. Finally, laser ablation with endoscopically placed endoluminal stents that traverse the tumor can facilitate emptying of the bowel and subsequent bowel cleansing in preparation for later excision.

EXTENT-OF-RESECTION ISSUES

DISTAL MURAL MARGINS

For many decades, a 5-cm distal mucosal/mural margin was recommended, but a considerable body of data now does not support this rule.[25] Distal spread may occur by direct submucosal extension or, less likely, via intramural lymphatics. Serial histologic sections of the bowel wall distal to resected specimens reveal that a large majority of patients have no distal spread. Only 2.5% of patients will have spread of more than 2 cm, and such spread almost always occurs in patients with anaplastic or poorly differentiated node-positive cancer. There appears to be no correlation between the risk for local recurrence and a distal margin in excess of 2 cm. Much of these data refer to pathologic and not surgical distances. Aggressive stretch on the specimen can double the pathologic length. During the past decade the general rule of a 2-cm distal margin has been challenged.[26,27] A 1-cm tumor-free distal margin following preoperative combined-modality therapy and total mesorectal excision ensures removal of all local disease in the majority of rectal cancer cases.[27]

DISTAL MESORECTAL MARGIN

The information provided earlier concerning TME focused on intact removal of the lymph node packet and is based on data showing distal spread of positive lymph nodes beyond the gross tumor.[28] As with distal mural spread, such extension is relatively uncommon but occurs more frequently with high-grade tumors associated with multiple positive lymph nodes. In patients with upper rectal cancer, TME is not appropriate because the risk for lymph node metastasis in the low mesorectum is extremely low and TME may result in a relatively ischemic rectal stump. For such patients, a 5-cm clearance of mesorectum below the gross tumor is adequate. The mesorectum must be divided at a right angle to the point below the tumor selected for bowel division. Most patients with midrectal cancer will have the entire lymph node packet removed through complete mesorectal excision, which facilitates lateral margin clearance and sphincter reconstruction by clearing the distal muscular tube.

PROXIMAL VASCULAR LIGATION

The oncologic benefits of inferior mesenteric artery ligation with clearance of the high lymph node and periaortic lymph nodes are minimal or nil.[29,30] In the series reported by Grinnell,[29] there were no 5-year survivors in patients with positive nodes along the inferior mesenteric artery. However, "high ligation" is frequently necessary for adequate colon mobilization in patients undergoing restorative procedures, as discussed later.

LATERAL MESORECTAL MARGINS

The issue of sharp mesorectal excision was discussed previously. The lateral margins, which involve the posterior and anterior planes of the coronal dissection, as well as the lateral planes of the sagittal dissection, are under the control of the operating surgeon. Tumors that are tethered to a side wall require much more extensive lateral dissection, as discussed in sections that follow.

LATERAL PELVIC LYMPH NODES

A few surgical groups remove the internal iliac or lateral pelvic lymph nodes, particularly in patients with locally advanced cancer, because of data supporting the occurrence of lateral lymph node spread in a small subset of patients. However, the impact of such extended lateral dissection on local control and survival is unclear. Lateral dissection is frequently associated with increased sexual and bladder dysfunction. It is unlikely that such lateral lymph nodes truly represent "regional" lymph nodes, and in general they should not be included as part of the standard technique of LAR.

SYNCHRONOUS ORGAN RESECTION

Bilateral salpingo-oophorectomy to remove occult ovarian metastases and to prevent primary ovarian cancer remains controversial. Approximately 3% to 5% of patients with colorectal cancer will have synchronous ovarian metastases and will benefit by resection. The benefit associated with the removal of grossly normal ovaries is small at best.

Management of patients with a large fibroid uterus remains problematic. Routine total abdominal hysterectomy under such circumstances should be avoided because of the increased risk for a rectovaginal fistula. Data suggest that a considerable number of subclinical anastomotic leaks occur after LAR, and in the presence of a synchronous vaginal closure, some of these leaks will become clinically apparent with the development of a rectovaginal fistula, which is a serious problem, particularly in an irradiated patient. An alternative to total abdominal hysterectomy in such women is supracervical hysterectomy.

In women with anteriorly based rectal cancer that is tethered to the posterior aspect of the vagina, a concurrent posterior vaginectomy is appropriate. The surgeon should not feel compelled to routinely perform total abdominal hysterectomy with the posterior vaginectomy. High rectal cancer with transmural involvement in the cul-de-sac may require posterior pelvic exenteration, which involves clearing both ureters, extensively mobilizing the bladder, and taking all lateral and posterior tissues with the uterus, cervix, and upper part of the vagina. This procedure is equivalent to "radical hysterectomy" with rectal resection and is the only way to completely surgically excise the cul-de-sac. Rectal reconstruction is certainly feasible in many such patients, and abdominoperineal resection may not add anything to the oncologic cure.

In irradiated patients or those undergoing sphincter reconstruction, any vaginal defect must be closed. Such closure is most easily performed with either an omental flap or, more commonly, a rectus abdominis flap. Except in very young women, the rectus flap may exclude skin. The anterior fascia is left intact, and the muscle and peritoneum are taken over the full length of the muscle. This flap is very durable and is based on the inferior epigastric vessels. The flap is rotated 180 degrees, and the peritoneum is sewn to the vaginal defect through a perineal approach. In younger women, a formal myocutaneous flap is used.

CONCOMITANT HEPATOBILIARY SURGERY

In patients with symptomatic gallstones, cholecystectomy at completion of the rectal reconstruction is appropriate. If the splenic flexure has been mobilized, the cholecystectomy can be performed without extending the incision and with very little incremental complication. Resection of hepatic metastasis during the same operation has been shown to be equally safe. Best results are demonstrated from experienced centers where synchronous resections of colon and rectal cancers with liver metastases have similar morbidity as staged procedures.[31,32] However, most of those studies involve a higher number of colon cancer than rectal cancer cases with liver metastases. Hepatic resection is appropriate in selected patients and in general only if it will not add major morbidity.

RELEVANT PELVIC ANATOMY

The essence of performing an optimal operation for mid- or low rectal cancer is to dissect sharply with scissors, cautery, or both in defined anatomic planes. The *mesorectum* is not a true mesentery, but it is the common terminology used to describe the node-bearing fatty tissue that surrounds the extraperitoneal rectum. It is covered by a visceral fascia. Between this visceral fascia and the lateral pelvic wall is an areolar plane, the identification of which is essential for sharp mesorectal excision. Posteriorly, the visceral and lateral or parietal fasciae fuse into the "rectosacral fascia." This fascia tethers the posterior aspect of the rectum into the sacral hollow, and division of this structure is required for LAR. Anteriorly, the perirectal fat abuts the Denonvilliers fascia. The Denonvilliers fascia envelops the seminal vesicles and fuses with the prostate fascia. In women, the perirectal fat abuts the rectovaginal septum.

In the upper part of the pelvis posterior to the superior hemorrhoidal vessel is nerve-bearing tissue located within the Waldeyer fascia. The sympathetic nerve trunks reside within this plane. The main parasympathetic nerve trunk necessary for erection and orgasm is S3. This nerve exits in the midpelvis just distal to the piriformis muscle in the horizontal portion of the sacrum and lies just medial to the parietal pelvic fascia. The parasympathetic and sympathetic nerves fuse into a plexus along the pelvic side wall and then extend anterolaterally into the seminal vesicles, prostate, and the vaginal or penile structures.

GENERAL ISSUES RELATED TO LOW ANTERIOR RESECTION

BOWEL PREPARATION

In the absence of high-grade obstruction, full mechanical and oral antibiotic preparation was thought necessary to reduce the risk for postoperative wound infection. A recent Cochrane review[33] challenges the utility of mechanical bowel preparation for elective colorectal resections; however, the data retrieved from "the rectal group" only contained 275 participants. The authors of the Cochrane review conclude that collaborative, properly designed multicenter randomized controlled trials are needed to address the safety and clinical effectiveness of mechanical bowel preparation. Such preparation may still be done on an outpatient basis, except in the elderly or in patients with obstruction. Bowel cleansing is performed by restricting patients to a clear liquid diet for 36 hours and by the use of cathartics. Oral antibiotics may be administered the afternoon and evening before surgery. Intravenous antibiotics are administered once, approximately 30 minutes before making the skin incision.

OPEN SURGERY

The general standard of care for rectal resection involves laparotomy and general exploration, mobilization, and resection, followed by reconstruction. The role of laparoscopically assisted surgery will be discussed later in the chapter.

INITIAL EXPLORATION

As a routine, careful evaluation of the liver, gallbladder, stomach, colon, and peritoneal surfaces is performed. In women, careful assessment of the ovaries and uterus is appropriate. The exact locoregional extent of disease is now determined. The high iliac nodes, inferior mesenteric artery nodes, and periaortic nodes are clinically evaluated.

PELVIC DISSECTION

The conduct and sequence of the operation are described later. However, adequate positioning of the patient, appropriate instruments, and the use of self-retaining retractors and a fiberoptic headlight are important elements in performing optimal pelvic surgery.

OPERATIVE TACTICS

PATIENT POSITION

The patient is placed in the modified lithotomy position (Figure 167-1), with the thigh in approximately 15%

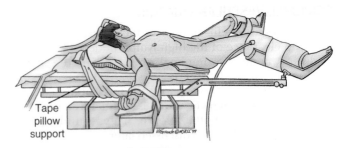

FIGURE 167-1 Appropriate patient position for low anterior resection. To prevent patient slippage when in the Trendelenburg position, a pillow is placed under the nape of the neck. Shoulder supports are not required. Care must be taken to avoid arm hyperextension.

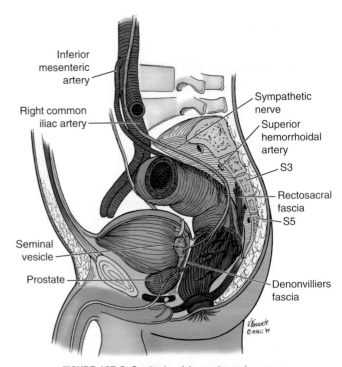

FIGURE 167-2 Sagittal pelvic anatomy in a man.

flexion. Care should be taken to avoid the development of peroneal palsy as a result of the stirrups or leg compression boots. In general, a special support under the sacrum is not necessary unless coloanal reconstruction or abdominoperineal resection is being contemplated. The rectum is suctioned, and a urinary catheter is placed and draped either over or under the leg. In women, complete vaginal irrigation and preparation are necessary.

Traditionally, pelvic surgery has been performed with the patient in a steep Trendelenburg position. With the use of appropriate self-retaining retractors, however, such positioning is no longer necessary and is frequently counterproductive. The Trendelenburg position may be helpful for the initial pelvic dissection, but for the distal dissection, the reverse Trendelenburg position is preferable.

SAGITTAL ANATOMY

In the pelvis, the sympathetic nerves lie posterior to the mesorectal visceral fascia (Figure 167-2). However, at the

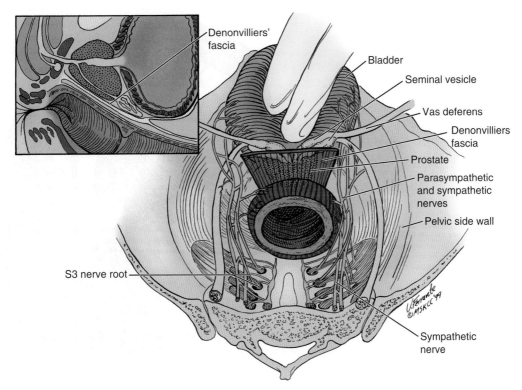

FIGURE 167-3 Transverse midpelvic anatomy in a man.

level of the aortic bifurcation and above, the nerves are perilously close to the inferior mesenteric artery. They must be sharply separated and pushed posteriorly to avoid nerve damage.

The rectosacral fascia represents a well-defined fusion of the parietal and visceral fasciae in the midpelvis. During LAR, this fascia, which frequently extends between S3 and S5, must be sharply separated with scissors and cautery to allow full clearance of the pelvic floor to the level of the anorectal ring posteriorly.

In men, the Denonvilliers fascia is a crucial anterior anatomic structure. It envelops the seminal vesicles, extends along the prostate, and fuses with the lowermost portion of the prostatic capsule. It can be quite dense and protects the prostate from direct invasion by anteriorly based cancer. The anterior dissection in men should be performed anterior to the Denonvilliers fascia. As with the rectosacral fascia posteriorly, separation of the prostatic capsule and the Denonvilliers fascia requires sharp dissection.

TRANSVERSE MIDPELVIC ANATOMY

The Denonvilliers fascia is shown lifted from the rectum and overlying the seminal vesicles in Figure 167-3. The S3 nerve roots, which are usually just distal to the piriformis muscle, may lie along the parietal pelvic fascia or be separate and more medial. Merging of the sympathetic and parasympathetic nerves is demonstrated.

VASCULAR SUPPLY TO THE RECTUM AND LEFT COLON

The left colic branch arises 3 to 4 cm from the origin of the inferior mesenteric artery, then gives off sigmoid branches, and finally continues as the superior hemorrhoidal artery, as illustrated in Figure 167-4. Not shown in this figure are the middle hemorrhoidal arteries, which are small branches that arise from the internal iliac (hypogastric) artery at the level of the S3 nerves. There are important additional collateral vessels via the inferior hemorrhoidal artery that pass from the levatores cephalad along the distal aspect of the rectum. These vessels support the distal portion of the bowel after LAR.

The arch of Riolan is a common variant that represents an ascending branch of the inferior mesenteric artery (see Figure 167-4). Most commonly, it does not join the proximal middle colic but passes to the marginal artery at the splenic flexure. It may replace the left colic artery. When mobilizing the left colon, such an ascending vessel should not be divided unless absolutely necessary for colon length.

SYMPATHETIC NERVES

The sympathetic nerves are necessary for antegrade ejaculation. As mentioned, they lie in a plane posterior to the lymphatic and nodal pedicle. At the sacral promontory, left and right trunks separate and pass along the high pelvic side wall. Patients with high rectal cancer and extensive lateral spread may require resection of the sympathetic nerves along the pelvic side wall to obtain adequate clearance.

SIGMOID MOBILIZATION FROM THE LEFT

After completion of routine exploration, placement of the retractors, and packing of the bowels (or our preference, evisceration of the small bowel over the right hypochondrium), the initial dissection involves sigmoid

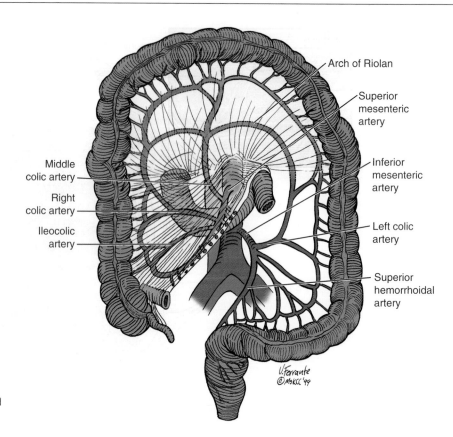

FIGURE 167-4 Arterial supply to the rectum and colon.

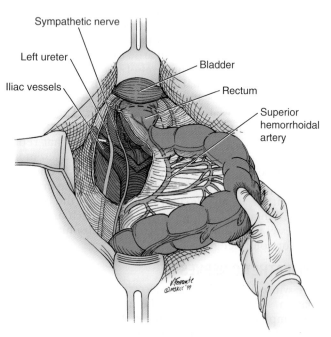

FIGURE 167-5 Mobilization of the sigmoid colon from the left.

mobilization on the left (Figure 167-5). The apex of the sigmoid is frequently tethered near the internal ring. The sigmoid is fully mobilized to its apex, and the lower portion of the left colon is mobilized. With retraction anteriorly and to the right, tissue overlying the left common iliac artery is opened, and the opening is extended down into the pelvis. Care should be taken to

incise only the peritoneum at this point in the procedure. The ureter is now identified. The peritoneal opening is extended further into the pelvis. At this point, the sigmoid is aggressively pulled anteriorly and to the right, and the soft tissue between the superior hemorrhoidal vessels and the Waldeyer fascia is separated. Clearance along the bony sacrum at the level of the promontory will divide the sympathetic nerves. The appropriate plane is more anterior and just posterior to the superior hemorrhoidal vessels, which arch over the anterior aspect of the sacrum when the sigmoid is placed at appropriate tension.

SIGMOID MOBILIZATION FROM THE RIGHT

The sigmoid colon is now lifted anteriorly and to the left, and the retroperitoneum is inspected to identify the right ureter (Figure 167-6). Cautery is used to incise the peritoneum near the right common iliac artery, and the incision is extended down the right pelvic side wall medial to the ureter. At this point, the correct depth of dissection is unclear. If the left-sided mobilization has proceeded to the midline, the operating surgeon can place a hand beneath the superior hemorrhoidal from the left. The sigmoid colon and the superior hemorrhoidal vessels are encompassed by the index and middle fingers and the thumb, and the vascular pedicle is lifted away from the Waldeyer fascia. Cautery dissection is carried out from the right until the tissue over the sacral promontory is exposed. At this point, the sympathetic nerves remain posterior. No further pelvic dissection should be performed until the proximal portion of the colon is divided.

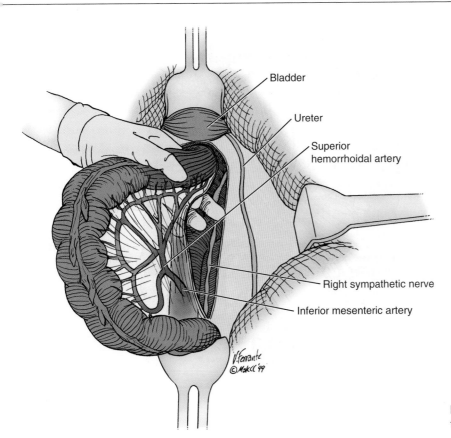

Bladder

Ureter

Superior
hemorrhoidal artery

Right sympathetic nerve

Inferior mesenteric artery

FIGURE 167-6 Mobilization of the sigmoid colon from the right.

LEFT COLON MOBILIZATION WITH STRONG TRACTION ON THE LEFT COLON

The entire left colon is now mobilized. A common mistake is to extend the dissection superiorly along the "white line of Toldt" to the level of the spleen. An initial dissection along this line should proceed more medially, directly over the midpoint of the kidney, and then around the splenic flexure. Essential to facilitate this dissection is identification of the Gerota fascia. It is quite apparent when one has transgressed this fascia because perinephric fat will be poking through the fascia.

The extent of colonic mobilization depends on the quality and redundancy of the left and sigmoid colon and the length and location of the rectum and the rectal tumor. It is always best to err on the side of full mobilization rather than having to reposition all the retractors at the end of the operation to gain additional length. There are three components entailed in mobilization of the left colon and splenic flexure. The initial component involves lifting the left colon from the Gerota fascia and mobilizing the colon via retroperitoneal and splenic flexure mobilization. The second component is actual division of the vessels. Ligation of the inferior mesenteric artery and inferior mesenteric vein will gain considerable additional length. The third component is division of the transverse colon mesentery as it runs underneath the pancreas. This step provides complete mobilization of the colon to the level of the middle colic artery (Figure 167-7). Although this technique affords the operating surgeon a more capacious descending colon for reconstruction, such extensive mobilization may result in

autonomic denervation of the bowel with subsequent spasm and bowel dysfunction.

BOWEL DIVISION AND DISTAL TRACTION

After mobilization of the splenic flexure, the proximal colon and blood supply to the rectosigmoid should be divided before any pelvic dissection commences. With care being taken in regard to the sympathetic nerves, either the superior hemorrhoidal or the inferior mesenteric artery is ligated and divided. The proximal sigmoid or the junction of the descending colon and sigmoid is then divided. If a lengthy pelvic dissection is likely, it is best to divide the bowel with a stapler and worry about the reconstruction at a later time. For routine midrectal cancer that is going to be stapled, a purse-string clamp or a purse-string stapler can be placed proximally, and a clamp or staple line can be placed distally. If a side-to-end or a pouch reconstruction is under consideration, then again, just a linear staple line is placed. The colon is divided. For the pelvic dissection, more important than retractors is anterior traction with a clamp on the bowel and the mesorectum.

INITIAL POSTERIOR DISSECTION

With aggressive traction on the bowel and its mesentery, the sympathetic nerves will be apparent and can be cleared along their length by either spreading with scissors or the use of cautery. The nerves should be separated from the mesorectum laterally. The pelvis is then entered with spreading of scissors between the sympathetic nerves passing through the Waldeyer fascia and through the areolar tissue until the bony pelvis is

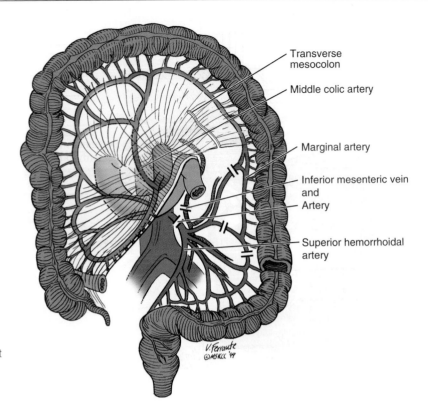

Transverse mesocolon

Middle colic artery

Marginal artery

Inferior mesenteric vein and Artery

Superior hemorrhoidal artery

V. Ferrante ©MSKCC '99

FIGURE 167-7 Vascular division to obtain maximum proximal colon length. The marginal artery is present in almost all patients. Loss of this artery is usually iatrogenic as a result of aggressive traction on the bowel.

identified. The operation then proceeds 4 to 5 cm along the sacrum posteriorly to the level of the rectosacral fascia. No attempt at side wall dissection or anterior dissection is made at this time. By sweeping the ureters and the sympathetic nerves laterally, the fascia overlying the piriformis is identified. This should be the limit of the lateral dissection at this time. With spreading of scissors in this very easily separable areolar plane between the visceral fascia overlying the mesorectum and the bony pelvis posteriorly, dissection proceeds rather briskly at this point in the operation (Figure 167-8). Appropriate retraction on the rectal specimen and the use of a St. Marks or Parks retractor and a fiberoptic headlight facilitates this dissection. Care is always taken to avoid injury to the sacral vessels, which may be in the midline or slightly off midline and have a tendency to be tented up into this areolar tissue.

DIVISION OF THE RECTOSACRAL FASCIA

At the level of S3-5, multiple slips of thin fascia pass from the parietal fascia posteriorly into the visceral mesorectal fascia. These are the rectosacral fascia fibers. At this point, further spreading with scissors will identify the levators. This is best accomplished approximately 1 to 2 cm off midline. The patient should be placed in a neutral or reverse Trendelenburg position. The levators are now cleared on both sides while staying on the surface of the levator fascia. The midline raphe is divided with cautery. Care must be taken to not enter the rectum at this stage. Unless the entire rectum is mobilized to the anus, a very low reconstruction will not be feasible.

At this point, the main parasympathetic nerves should be identified and dissected anteriorly (Figure 167-9). By sweeping up the side walls with heavy closed scissors in a "wiping motion," the main S3 nerve trunks become quite apparent. Traction on the mesorectum anteriorly after exposure of the levators distal to these nerves facilitates such identification. Cautery and scissors are used to clear these nerves for approximately two-thirds of their length anteriorly. Small branches will be seen and can be clipped and divided or gently cauterized. The full side wall dissection is not completed until the anterior dissection has been accomplished.

ANTERIOR DISSECTION IN WOMEN

The most important aspect of the anterior dissection in a woman who has not previously undergone hysterectomy is traction on the fundus of the uterus (Figure 167-10). The assistant standing between the patient's legs lifts the uterus anteriorly and inferiorly. Traction is then placed on the rectal specimen superiorly. A hand is pressed posteriorly on the upper part of the rectum, and this defines the peritoneum in the pouch of Douglas. Cautery is used to help open this plane. The dissection proceeds along the length of the vagina. Meticulous dissection is required at this point to avoid damage to the very thin-walled posterior vagina. In a woman who has previously undergone hysterectomy, two fingers are placed in the apex of the vagina to help define the appropriate plane along the posterior rectovaginal septum. In a woman with a lengthy vagina, a gauze pad on a clamp will be helpful. This dissection should proceed under direct vision with cautery and scissors to at least 90% of the length of the vagina. With large, lengthy scissors, the fatty tissue anterolateral to the rectum is cleared so that the levators are exposed both anteriorly and posteriorly. Only after this portion is completed will the pelvic side walls be dissected. At this point, the rectum will have

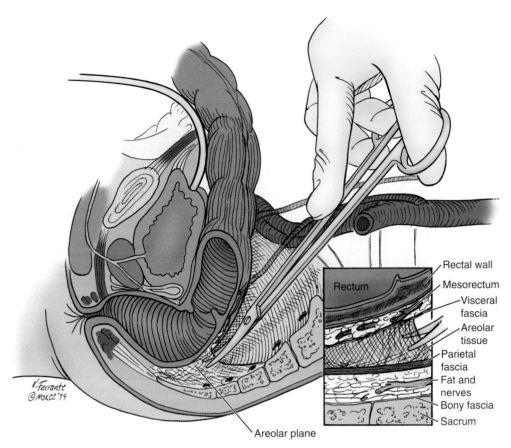

Rectal wall
Rectum
Mesorectum
Visceral fascia
Areolar tissue
Parietal fascia
Fat and nerves
Bony fascia
Sacrum

Areolar plane

FIGURE 167-8 Sharp dissection in the areolar plane outside the mesorectal envelope.

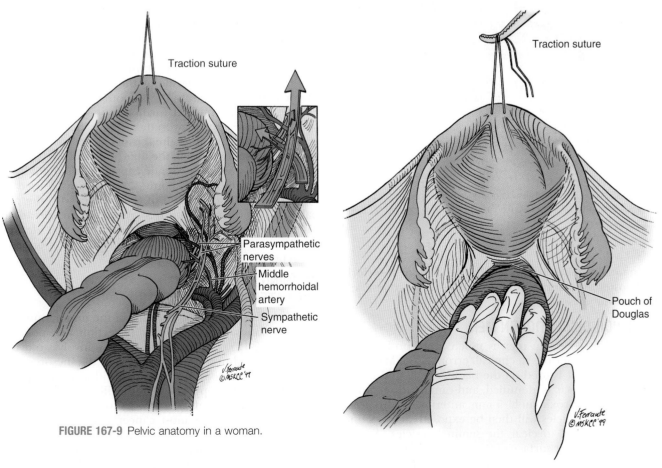

Traction suture

Traction suture

Parasympathetic nerves

Middle hemorrhoidal artery

Sympathetic nerve

Pouch of Douglas

FIGURE 167-9 Pelvic anatomy in a woman.

FIGURE 167-10 Anterior exposure in a woman.

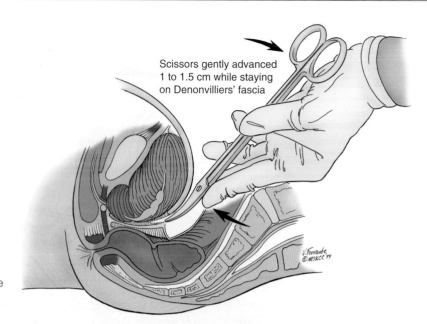

FIGURE 167-11 Anterior dissection in a man, with the Denonvilliers fascia separated from the prostatic capsule.

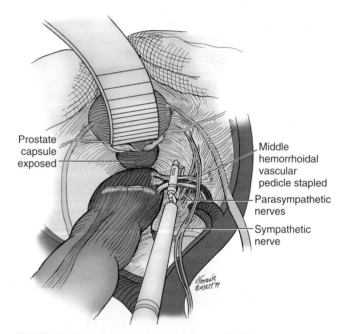

FIGURE 167-12 Division of the "lateral ligaments" (neurovascular pedicle) with a laparoscopic vascular stapler while protecting the autonomic nerves.

been totally mobilized down to the pelvic floor anteriorly and posteriorly, and the levators will be visible completely around the mesorectum.

ANTERIOR DISSECTION IN MEN

Anterior dissection in men is much more problematic and prone to serious technical error. A St. Marks or similar retractor is used on the bladder. The fold in the anterior cul-de-sac is identified, and cautery dissection is performed approximately 5 mm anterior to this fold. The seminal vesicles will then be exposed. Scissors and cautery are used to clear the seminal vesicles. At this point, the anterior surface of the Denonvilliers fascia will be quite clear. The patient should be placed in the

reverse Trendelenburg position to facilitate access to the plane of dissection, and the St. Marks retractor is used to lift the seminal vesicles while the operator assistant's hand pushes posteriorly on the upper part of the rectum. Bleeding from this area is controlled with either a lengthy ball-tipped coagulator or argon beam coagulation. Further separation of the Denonvilliers fascia from the prostatic capsule is best accomplished with scissors dissection (Figure 167-11). Lengthy scissors with the fingers as a fulcrum are used to actually press aggressively against the prostate. Despite leading to certain anxiety on the part of the operating surgeon, it is actually the safest maneuver. The tips of the scissors are gently advanced 1 to 1.5 cm while staying anterior (dorsal) to the Denonvilliers fascia along the prostate capsule. A finger is used to identify the smooth prostatic capsule. Scissors are then pushed further at this point, and by spreading, the entire prostate will be cleared. While staying 1 cm off midline, the scissors are pushed further past the prostate to break the attachment of the Denonvilliers fascia with the prostatic capsule. This should not be done bluntly. At this point, a finger can be used to confirm that the distal end of the urethra with the palpable catheter has been cleared. As in women, spreading with the scissors in the anterolateral plane will identify the levators anteriorly and join it with the posterior dissection.

DEFINING AND DIVIDING THE LATERAL ATTACHMENTS

Based on the extent and laterality of the tumor, multiple sagittal planes for the lateral dissection are possible (Figure 167-12). The most conservative involves moving medially to within the visceral fascia of the mesorectum. This is appropriate in a young man with a small superficial tumor on the opposite side. It will be the safest way to protect the sympathetic and parasympathetic nerves but is inadequate for most cancer patients. The most common dissection is along the parietal fascia, which is directly on the medial portion of the S3 nerve. For bulky tumors adherent to the side wall in which sympathetic and parasympathetic nerve trunks are intentionally sacrificed, the plane of dissection is along the vascular adventitia of the internal iliac vessels. On rare occasion, most commonly for recurrent cancer, the plane lateral to the vessels is used.

The main S3 nerve trunks are generally quite easy to identify in the first 2 to 3 cm as they exit the sacrum and, hence, easy to protect. The problematic area is the point where these autonomic trunks merge with the sympathetic nerves and then sweep anterolaterally toward the seminal vesicles. Hence, the strategy used is posterior dissection followed by anterior dissection, which leaves just the side wall under direct vision to allow clearance of these nerves. The options at this point are gentle cautery clearance, clips, and (our preference) placement of multiple vascular staples with a laparoscopic instrument, which provides bidirectional hemostasis between six rows of fine vascular staples (see Figure 167-12).

LEVEL OF DISTAL TRANSECTION

At this point, the rectum will be fully mobilized from the posterior, anterior, and lateral attachments. A decision where to divide the rectum and mesentery is made at this time. These are two separate issues that were discussed previously. Whichever is chosen for the individual patient, the rectum cannot be divided until it is clear of all fatty tissue. If TME has been performed, the distal 4 to 5 cm of rectum is already entirely clear and is just a muscular tube. Management of the distal portion of the rectum will then depend on whether one is going to hand-sew, staple, or perform a coloanal reconstruction. If staple reconstruction is going to be performed, a decision regarding a purse-string or "double-staple" technique[34] will have to be made. If an upper rectal cancer is being resected, some mesentery will be left. The distal part of the rectum must be clear in all patients before division.

In dealing with an early cancer, a cancer within an adenoma, or an irradiated patient who has had a complete or nearly complete response, sigmoidoscopic assessment of the actual location of the tumor should be performed at this time to clearly identify the appropriate level of transection.

TECHNIQUE OF DISTAL BOWEL MANAGEMENT

If at all possible, before rectal division the distal part of the rectum may be irrigated free of cancer cells. There are considerable general oncologic principles to support this approach, but no randomized clinical data. Irrigation is probably less important when the patient has received full-dose preoperative radiation therapy. Before rectal division, it is important to place either a right-angle clamp or a staple line on the rectum. One should irrigate distally at that point and then place another staple line or purse-string clamp suture below this initial clamp. It serves no purpose to place a staple line or a right-angle clamp, irrigate the rectum, and then divide *above* this clamp because tumor cells will almost certainly be entrapped at the clamp or staple line. Whether saline, water, or a cytotoxic agent is used for irrigation is probably a personal preference. We use nothing more than saline to dilute out any tumor cells by irrigating with 50 mL six to eight times. Division of the distal portion of the bowel is then performed, as discussed in the next

section. For surgeons who do not perform this operation on a daily basis, placement of a linear staple line across the bowel and then proceeding with the double-staple technique is probably the most reliable method. A high-quality linear stapling device that allows the pin to be placed before firing the stapler must be used (Figure 167-13). The pin allows the stapler to be pushed aggressively down into the pelvis without the rectum slipping out the open end of the stapler. For a very low staple line, the assistant may use a fist in the perineum to push from below.

COLORECTAL RECONSTRUCTION

The rectum may be reconstructed with sutures or staples and with an end-to-end, side-to-end, or a colon J-pouch side-to-end technique. If suturing is performed, a Baker anastomosis using a side-to-end technique is most reliable (Figure 167-14). Below a right-angle clamp, the posterior aspect of the rectum is opened and a single layer of interrupted sutures is then placed, facilitated by a fiberoptic headlight. The bowel is then divided anteriorly, and a single layer of anterior sutures is placed. This was a traditional approach for reconstruction for many years before the advent of surgical staples, and it is highly effective with adequate visualization. The side-to-end technique obviates the size discrepancy issue. Surgical stapling with intraluminal circular staples has become the standard for most LAR procedures. If at all possible, transanal placement of the stapler is most appropriate. The preferred approach is the double-staple technique, which is described extensively in the next section.

In the absence of diverticular disease and a capacious left colon, an end-to-end technique is quite satisfactory. The largest intraluminal stapler that will comfortably fit is appropriate. It is important to determine ahead of time what the anus will accept. Although the colon may be capacious, the patient may have had an anal stricture that prohibits placement of a large stapler per anus. For patients with diverticulosis, a side-to-end technique is preferable. An increasing body of data support the use of a 6- to 8-cm colon J pouch in patients undergoing a very low reconstruction or a coloanal reconstruction. Construction of such a J pouch is described in the chapter on coloanal reconstruction. If low rectal reconstruction with a stapled pouch is performed, the anvil is sewn into the apex of the J, identical to a standard side-to-end approach.

DOUBLE-STAPLE TECHNIQUE

The double-staple technique for most surgeons solves the fecal contamination problem and the size discrepancy issues associated with an end-to-end double–purse-string approach. Once the staple line has been placed across the rectum, confirmation of hemostasis is obtained, and a moist pack is left in the pelvis. The anvil is removed from the appropriately sized stapler and placed into the distal end of the colon (see Figure 167-13). Whether using a purse-string stapling device or a hand-sewn purse-string technique, it is important that the colon be cleared over the edge of the anvil to avoid stapling through any vascular appendices epiploicae. Hemostasis in the pelvis is now confirmed, and the stapler is placed transanally and up the rectum. The pin is opened and positioned so

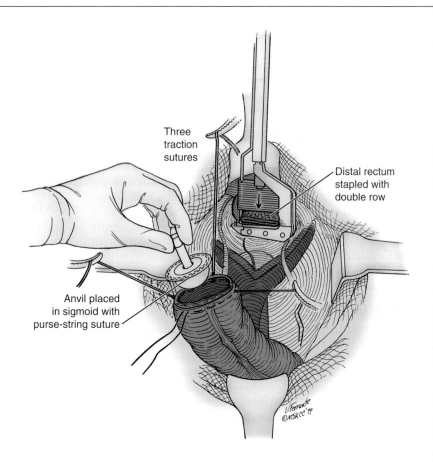

FIGURE 167-13 The "double-staple" technique.

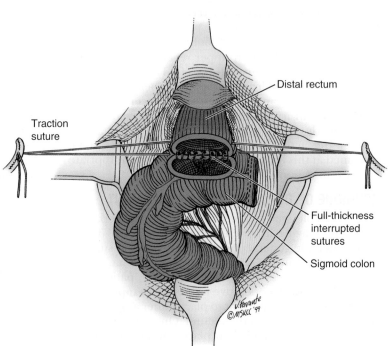

FIGURE 167-14 Sutured side-to-end anastomosis. This approach obviates problems with size discrepancy between the colon and midrectum.

that it peeks out just anterior or posterior to the staple line (Figure 167-15). Every effort should be made to avoid coming directly through the staple line because it will tear as the staples catch on the plastic bar. A long electrosurgical tip in cutting mode is used to allow the stapler pin to be advanced. The pointed pin is removed,

with care taken to not puncture a sacral vein. A long Kelly clamp is used to hold the anvil pin and insert it into the stapler cartridge. Before closure of the stapler, the proximal part of the bowel is checked for the correct 360-degree rotation, and the prostate/vagina and proximal colonic appendices epiploicae are confirmed to be

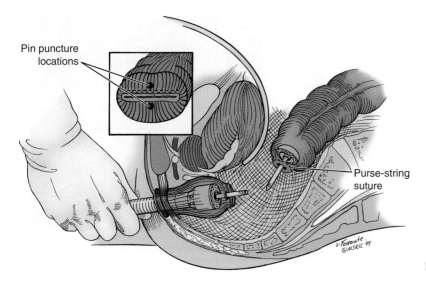

Pin puncture
locations

Purse-string
suture

FIGURE 167-15 The "double-staple" technique.

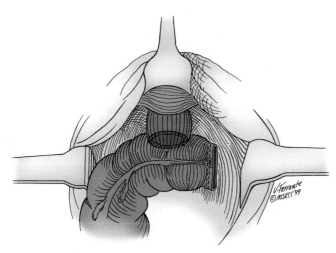

FIGURE 167-16 Stapled side-to-end anastomosis. The anvil is placed out the side of the proximal part of the bowel, after which the end is stapled closed. The circular staple line and the linear closure line should be approximately 2 cm apart to avoid ischemia of intervening tissue.

away from the staple line. The stapler is tightened completely, fired, and then gently removed. Figure 167-16 demonstrates the double-staple technique for a side-to-end reconstruction.

The presence of two intact "doughnuts" is confirmed. It is important to not start "spinning" the anvil because if there is an incomplete doughnut, one cannot identify the 360-degree location of the defect. The absence of a complete doughnut does not mandate a diversion; it is possible to have stapled correctly with an incomplete doughnut. The reverse is also true. The anastomosis should be palpated from below and then air injected transanally with saline instilled into the pelvis to look for an air leak. Frequently, bubbles are trapped in the pelvis, so before injecting air into the rectum, the saline in the pelvis should be jostled to try to break up any air pockets. The operating surgeon pinches the colon proximal to the anastomosis to avoid filling the colon with air during this process, while making sure that sufficient distention

is present. If a minor air leak is noted, the test should be repeated, and if confirmed, the patient can undergo sigmoidoscopy. If there is only a minimal defect in nonirradiated patients with good bowel preparation, it is usually adequate to just temporarily divert with an ileostomy or a colostomy. Of course, if at all possible, a few sutures should be placed, but this may not be feasible. The use of excess traction on these stapled anastomoses to try to identify a defect is frequently very disruptive and may destroy the entire anastomosis. One must judge how aggressively to pursue trying to actually suture the leak. A large leak requires the placement of sutures or complete revision of the anastomosis.

A policy of routine diversion with either colostomy or loop ileostomy is not recommended. Even with the increasing use of TME, routine diversion for a low anastomosis is uncommon. At the Memorial Sloan-Kettering Cancer Center, a leak rate of 4% and an overall mortality rate of 0.6% with the selective use of diversion has been reported.[35] The leak rate is identical in irradiated and nonirradiated patients. A recent metaanalysis demonstrated that patients who have received neoadjuvant radiation benefit from routine diverting loop ileostomy construction.[36]

We prefer to place a closed-suction drain in the pelvis in all patients. Randomized data do not demonstrate a reduction in pelvic abscess rates, but the numbers of LAR patients in these studies are too few to reach a definitive conclusion.

LAPAROSCOPIC LOW ANTERIOR RESECTION

Laparoscopic colonic resections have been proven by controlled randomized trials to benefit patients.[37,38] Patients in the laparoscopic-assisted group benefit from earlier recovery of bowel function, decreased intraoperative blood loss, less postoperative pain, and reduced length of hospital stay. Disease-free and overall survival, as well as time to recurrence, are similar in the laparoscopic-assisted and open colectomy groups,[37-39] supporting the equivalence of laparoscopy to the standard open colectomy for all stages of colon cancer. Despite the increasing acceptance of laparoscopic colonic resections, laparoscopic resection of rectal cancer still requires careful review. In rectal resections, surgical integrity of total mesorectal excision is one of the most important predictors of local recurrence; therefore, concerns of being able to perform a technically demanding procedure laparoscopically were raised. Advocates of laparoscopic surgery report that improved optics during a laparoscopic approach gives the opportunity to the operating surgeon to clearly visualize fascial planes within the pelvis. Single-institution studies have shown that laparoscopic resection of rectal cancers is as safe as the open approach. Results suggest that patients do benefit from laparoscopic rectal resections with less operative blood loss, decreased use of pain medications, speedier postoperative recovery, and overall similar morbidity and mortality.[40-44] The CLASSICC trial[39,45] offers the most validated evidence on laparoscopic rectal resections; nevertheless, that study questioned the efficacy of laparoscopic rectal resections with higher rates of positive circumferential radial margins in the laparoscopic group compared with the open surgery group and high conversion rates of 29%. However, recent studies do report much lower conversion rates ranging from 3% to 10%.[40-42] Currently two large randomized controlled trials are being conducted in Europe and the United States evaluating the equivalence of laparoscopic rectal resections to open rectal resections: COLOR II and the ACOSOG-Z6051, correspondingly.

Because laparoscopic rectal resections are technically demanding, advocates of robotic surgery suggest that this new technology may offer a less demanding alternative to laparoscopic resection with better optics. Since the report of da Vinci system–assisted colectomy, robotic-assisted colorectal surgery has been shown to be safe and feasible.[46] However, as with laparoscopic surgery, further prospective controlled trials are needed to establish robotic-assisted rectal surgery comparable to open rectal surgery.

TECHNICAL ASPECTS OF LAPAROSCOPIC APPROACH

The same oncologic principles of the open surgical resection are followed during the laparoscopic-assisted approach. The patient is placed in lithotomy position with both patients' arms tucked to the side with thumbs up and palms facing the patients' hips, and the shoulders are padded. After sufficient pneumoperitoneum is established, the abdomen is carefully explored. The left colon is mobilized through a medial to lateral approach where the left ureter is safely identified and protected at all times. The inferior mesenteric pedicle is divided and the sigmoid colon is fully mobilized to facilitate rectal retraction. We proceed with posterior dissection of the rectum with sharp dissection, and the sympathetic plexus is visualized and protected (Figure 167-17). The anterior and lateral dissection of the rectum is continued with traction and countertraction and sharp dissection following the same principles as described in the open approach. A Pfannenstiel incision is used to exteriorize the specimen and then the anastomosis takes place. For further discussion of laparoscopic surgery in rectal cancer patients, see Chapter 178.

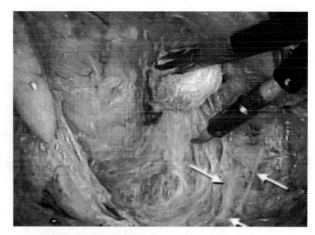

FIGURE 167-17 Right superior hypogastric plexus.

POSTOPERATIVE MANAGEMENT

Routine nasogastric suction is not required. However, persistent nausea and vomiting requiring nasogastric tube placement will develop in approximately 10% of patients 2 to 3 days after surgery. In the absence of major intestinal distress, a clear liquid diet may be started in the early postoperative days, with advancement to a low-fat, low-fiber diet over the next 2 days. If a pelvic drain is placed, it may be removed after 3 to 4 days. If daily drainage exceeds several hundred milliliters, a sample should be sent for determination of creatinine in the fluid to rule out a bladder or ureteral leak before drain removal. The urinary catheter is removed on the second or third postoperative day. Most patients are ready for discharge on the sixth or seventh day. Recently enhanced postoperative recovery programs[47] in experienced centers have introduced a multidisciplinary approach to a "fast-track" clinical pathway after colonic resections that result in fewer complications, a reduction in hospital stay and therefore a reduction in cost, and a quicker return to work and daily activities. However, further corroboration of these data is needed from multicenter national studies.

When a diverting stoma is present, the patient should be educated regarding management, and home nursing care every few days for the first few weeks should be arranged. If postoperative adjuvant therapy is not required, a water-soluble contrast enema is performed before the stoma is closed at 6 to 8 weeks. If adjuvant therapy is used, closure is generally deferred.

Bowel function is frequently problematic after LAR. Cluster bowel movements are probably related to the denervation associated with mobilization of the colon and division of the inferior mesenteric artery. Frequency and urgency may be due to anastomotic stricture, neorectal spasm, or the effect of radiation. Gentle fiber supplementation after meals and antispasmodic medication before meals may be required for many months. After all chemotherapy is complete, patients should begin a low-fat, high-fiber diet. Lactose intolerance is frequently worse after surgery and chemotherapy. Perineal burning is related to fecal contamination. The use of soothing "baby wipes" after each bowel movement is crucial to avoid skin irritation. Early staple line strictures are aggressively dilated with digital examination 3 to 4 weeks after surgery and repeated monthly as needed. Late, persistent strictures may require intraluminal cautery strictureplasty; if more than 10 cm from the anus, balloon dilation is effective. A high-fiber diet is essential after stricture dilation to maintain the patency of the anastomotic lumen.

REFERENCES

1. Parker SL, Tong T, Bolden S, et al: Cancer statistics, 1996. *CA Cancer J Clin* 46:5, 1996.
2. Scholefield JH, Northover JM: Surgical management of rectal cancer. *Br J Surg* 82:745, 1995.
3. Gunderson LL, Sosin H: Areas of failure found at reoperation (second or symptomatic look) following "curative surgery" for adenocarcinoma of the rectum. Clinicopathologic correlation and implications for adjuvant therapy. *Cancer* 34:1278, 1974.
4. Tschmelitsch J, Kronberger P, Glaser K, et al: Survival after surgical treatment of recurrent carcinoma of the rectum. *J Am Coll Surg* 179:54, 1994.
5. Fielding LP, Phillips RK, Fry JS, et al: Prediction of outcome after curative resection for large bowel cancer. *Lancet* 2:904, 1986.
6. Chapuis PH, Dent OF, Fisher R, et al: A multivariate analysis of clinical and pathological variables in prognosis after resection of large bowel cancer. *Br J Surg* 72:698, 1985.
7. Adam IJ, Mohamdee MO, Martin IG, et al: Role of circumferential margin involvement in the local recurrence of rectal cancer. *Lancet* 344:707, 1994.
8. Phillips RK, Hittinger R, Blesovsky L, et al: Local recurrence following "curative" surgery for large bowel cancer: I. The overall picture. *Br J Surg* 71:12, 1984.
9. Heald RJ: Rectal cancer: the surgical options. *Eur J Cancer* 31A:1189, 1995.
10. Heald RJ, Husband EM, Ryall RD: The mesorectum in rectal cancer surgery—the clue to pelvic recurrence? *Br J Surg* 69:613, 1982.
11. Beart RGRN: Anterior resection of the rectum. *Mastery of Surgery* 2010:15717.
12. MacFarlane JK, Ryall RD, Heald RJ: Mesorectal excision for rectal cancer. *Lancet* 341:457, 1993.
13. Cawthorne SJ, Parums DV, Gibbs NM, et al: Extent of mesorectal spread and involvement of lateral resection margin as prognostic factors after surgery for rectal cancer. *Lancet* 335:1055, 1990.
14. Zaheer S, Pemberton JH, Farouk R, et al: Surgical treatment of adenocarcinoma of the rectum. *Ann Surg* 227:800, 1998.
15. Enker WE, Thaler HT, Cranor ML, et al: Total mesorectal excision in the operative treatment of carcinoma of the rectum. *J Am Coll Surg* 181:335, 1995.
16. Arbman G, Nilsson E, Hallbook O, et al: Local recurrence following total mesorectal excision for rectal cancer. *Br J Surg* 83:375, 1996.
17. Krook JE, Moertel CG, Gunderson LL, et al: Effective surgical adjuvant therapy for high-risk rectal carcinoma. *N Engl J Med* 324:709, 1991.
18. O'Connell MJ, Martenson JA, Wieand HS, et al: Improving adjuvant therapy for rectal cancer by combining protracted-infusion fluorouracil with radiation therapy after curative surgery. *N Engl J Med* 331:502, 1994.
19. NIH consensus conference. Adjuvant therapy for patients with colon and rectal cancer. *JAMA* 264:1444, 1990.
20. Pahlman L, Glimelius B, Graffman S: Pre- versus postoperative radiotherapy in rectal carcinoma: An interim report from a randomized multicentre trial. *Br J Surg* 72:961, Dec 1985.
21. Frykholm GJ, Glimelius B, Pahlman L: Preoperative or postoperative irradiation in adenocarcinoma of the rectum: Final treatment results of a randomized trial and an evaluation of late secondary effects. *Dis Colon Rectum* 36:564, 1993.
22. Sauer R, Becker H, Hohenberger W, et al: Preoperative versus postoperative chemoradiotherapy for rectal cancer. *N Engl J Med* 351:1731, 2004.
23. Kapiteijn E, Marijnen CA, Nagtegaal ID, et al: Preoperative radiotherapy combined with total mesorectal excision for resectable rectal cancer. *N Engl J Med* 345:638, 2001.
24. Kollmorgen CF, Meagher AP, Wolff BG, et al: The long-term effect of adjuvant postoperative chemoradiotherapy for rectal carcinoma on bowel function. *Ann Surg* 220:676, 1994.
25. Williams NS: The rationale for preservation of the anal sphincter in patients with low rectal cancer. *Br J Surg* 71:575, 1984.
26. Rullier E, Laurent C, Bretagnol F, et al: Sphincter-saving resection for all rectal carcinomas: The end of the 2-cm distal rule. *Ann Surg* 241:465, 2005.
27. Guillem JG, Chessin DB, Shia J, et al: A prospective pathologic analysis using whole-mount sections of rectal cancer following preoperative combined modality therapy: Implications for sphincter preservation. *Ann Surg* 245:88, 2007.
28. Reynolds JV, Joyce WP, Dolan J, et al: Pathological evidence in support of total mesorectal excision in the management of rectal cancer. *Br J Surg* 83:1112, 1996.
29. Grinnell RS: Results of ligation of inferior mesenteric artery at the aorta in resections of carcinoma of the descending and sigmoid colon and rectum. *Surg Gynecol Obstet* 120:1031, 1965.
30. Pezim ME, Nicholls RJ: Survival after high or low ligation of the inferior mesenteric artery during curative surgery for rectal cancer. *Ann Surg* 200:729, 1984.
31. Chua HK, Sondenaa K, Tsiotos GG, et al: Concurrent vs. staged colectomy and hepatectomy for primary colorectal cancer with synchronous hepatic metastases. *Dis Colon Rectum* 47:1310, 2004.
32. Martin R, Paty P, Fong Y, et al: Simultaneous liver and colorectal resections are safe for synchronous colorectal liver metastasis. *J Am Coll Surg* 197:233; discussion 241, 2003.
33. Guenaga KK, Matos D, Wille-Jorgensen P: Mechanical bowel preparation for elective colorectal surgery. *Cochrane Database Syst Rev* 1:CD001544, 2009.
34. Griffen FD, Knight CD Sr, et al: The double stapling technique for low anterior resection. Results, modifications, and observations. *Ann Surg* 211:745; discussion 751, 1990.
35. Enker WE, Merchant N, Cohen AM, et al: Safety and efficacy of low anterior resection for rectal cancer: 681 consecutive cases from a specialty service. *Ann Surg* 230:544; discussion 552, 1999.
36. Birgisson H, Pahlman L, Gunnarsson U, et al: Late gastrointestinal disorders after rectal cancer surgery with and without preoperative radiation therapy. *Br J Surg* 95:206, 2008.
37. A comparison of laparoscopically assisted and open colectomy for colon cancer. *N Engl J Med* 350:2050, 2004.
38. Veldkamp R, Kuhry E, Hop WC, et al: Laparoscopic surgery versus open surgery for colon cancer: Short-term outcomes of a randomised trial. *Lancet Oncol* 6:477, 2005.
39. Guillou PJ, Quirke P, Thorpe H, et al: Short-term endpoints of conventional versus laparoscopic-assisted surgery in patients with colorectal cancer (MRC CLASICC trial): Multicentre, randomised controlled trial. *Lancet* 365:1718, 2005.
40. Kim SH, Park IJ, Joh YG, et al: Laparoscopic resection for rectal cancer: A prospective analysis of thirty-month follow-up outcomes in 312 patients. *Surg Endosc* 20:1197, 2006.
41. Ng SS, Leung KL, Lee JF, et al: Laparoscopic-assisted versus open abdominoperineal resection for low rectal cancer: A prospective randomized trial. *Ann Surg Oncol* 15:2418, 2008.
42. Pugliese R, Di Lernia S, Sansonna F, et al: Laparoscopic resection for rectal adenocarcinoma. *Eur J Surg Oncol* 35:497, 2009.
43. Scheidbach H, Schneider C, Konradt J, et al: Laparoscopic abdominoperineal resection and anterior resection with curative intent for carcinoma of the rectum. *Surg Endosc* 16:7, 2002.
44. Staudacher C, Di Palo S, Tamburini A, et al: Total mesorectal excision (TME) with laparoscopic approach: 226 consecutive cases. *Surg Oncol* 16:S113, 2007.
45. Jayne DG, Guillou PJ, Thorpe H, et al: Randomized trial of laparoscopic-assisted resection of colorectal carcinoma: 3-year results of the UK MRC CLASICC Trial Group. *J Clin Oncol* 25:3061, 2007.
46. Park YA, Kim JM, Kim SA, et al: Totally robotic surgery for rectal cancer: From splenic flexure to pelvic floor in one setup. *Surg Endosc* 24:715, 2010.
47. Kehlet H: Fast-track colorectal surgery. *Lancet* 371:791, 2008.

Abdominoperineal Resection of the Rectum for Cancer

Dimitrios Avgerinos | Joseph E. Martz | Warren E. Enker

Abdominoperineal resection (APR) of the rectum, first popularized by Miles, has undergone progressive anatomic changes to evolve into the present operation.[1-3] From the original Miles resection, which probably was the equivalent of the present resection for inflammatory bowel disease, to the bilateral en bloc radical pelvic lymphadenectomy that is currently practiced in Japan, various surgical investigators have designed operations intended to circumvent all of the local and regional (i.e., pelvic) spread that may be associated with primary rectal cancer. The operation that we describe is an APR performed according to the dissection principles of total mesorectal excision (TME) with autonomic nerve preservation (ANP).[4] APR is a cancer operation that is focused on the curative resection of distal rectal cancers with regional disease, on maintaining local control and with the goal of achieving negative circumferential margins of resection, particularly at the level of the levator ani.[5] The vast majority of surgeons perform APR as an open procedure. Nevertheless, recent advances in minimally invasive surgery have allowed surgeons to apply greater use of laparoscopy to colon and rectal surgery.

INDICATIONS FOR THE OPERATION

APR is the procedure of choice for invasive carcinomas of the distal rectum where there is inadequate room for a negative distal margin and where sphincter preservation may be compromised by direct sphincter invasion. APR is also indicated for persistent or recurrent epidermoid carcinomas of the anal canal (after initial chemotherapy and radiation), for some rare lesions of the anorectum (e.g., melanoma), for sarcomas that arise from the levator ani and involve the anal canal, for locally advanced (i.e., bulky rectal tumors), for some chordomas, and for most resectable patients with recurrent rectal carcinoma. Where indicated, as in some anal and low rectal cancers, some surgeons may add either an en bloc or a separate pelvic lymphadenectomy for gross pelvic side-wall nodal disease. In some cases, patients with a primary rectal cancer, presenting with poor function, that is, incontinence, are better served by an APR, from a functional standpoint, even if a sphincter-preserving operation might be performed (see later).

PREPARATION OF THE PATIENT

STAGING

It is important to stage the patient as accurately as possible. Preoperative staging should include a physical examination, rigid proctosigmoidoscopy in the left lateral recumbent position, documenting the location of the tumor as measured in centimeters proximal to the anal verge, as well as other features such as the configuration of the tumor (sessile, ulcerated, exophytic, circumferential), its location along the rectal circumference, the presence or absence of extramural palpable disease (i.e., mesorectal nodes), attachment to the vagina or prostate or direct sphincter invasion and whether there was prior pelvic surgery or radiation therapy. Preoperative colonoscopy is indicated to rule out synchronous cancers.

Additional elements of staging (e.g., complete blood cell count, liver function tests, and carcinoembryonic antigen values) and chest radiography are indicated. A computed tomographic (CT) scan of the chest and abdomen assists in documenting the presence of distant metastases.

Recent findings suggest that high-definition or high-resolution magnetic resonance imaging (MRI) is now the standard of care for defining locoregional disease prior to neoadjuvant radiation and chemotherapy and in the evaluation of treatment prior to surgery. Such studies, when read by gastrointestinal imaging experts, are particularly adept at defining the relationship of direct extension or of nodal disease to the endopelvic fascia or the potential involvement of the circumferential resection margin.[6]

PREOPERATIVE CONSULTATION WITH THE PATIENT AND FAMILY

The surgeon should confer with the patient and family to explain such issues as the rationale in support of the operation, the role of APR versus sphincter preservation, the use of adjuvant therapy, the risks of surgery, and the potential benefits. The patient should have a thorough understanding of the long-term consequences of APR (i.e., the nature of a colostomy) and of the possibilities of changes or losses in both sexual and urinary function, particularly in older patients. A particularly important concern is the issue of bowel function after a very distal low anterior resection (LAR) or a coloanal anastomosis versus an APR with a permanent colostomy. Many studies have now shown that patients who achieve only poor function after a sphincter-preserving operation have a far worse lifestyle than patients who are taking care of a permanent end sigmoid colostomy. Often, such patients suffer from varying degrees of daytime or nighttime incontinence, incomplete evacuations, cluster movements, periodicity and, in some cases, sleepless nights. Long pleasure trips are compromised by stops at public bathrooms, often with unpleasant and embarrassing consequences. In contrast, an end left-sided stoma may need emptying and skin care, but may be far more manageable with less interference with normal life, on many levels. Where a choice for sphincter-preservation versus APR exists in a very distal rectal cancer, and the patient is seeking advice regarding sphincter preservation, this difficult issue, which will be decided by the surgeon's intraoperative judgment during the operation, must be openly shared with the patient and family prior to surgery. This subject may benefit from repeated discussions prior to surgery.

Providing patients with appropriate reading materials and supportive consultations with enterostomal nurses or connecting such patients with other patients who have undergone an APR has proved most helpful to their cognitive as well as emotional preparation.

Other patient and family concerns, such as the average length of stay, home care after discharge, dietary preparation, avoidance of aspirin (unless medically indicated), and other issues, are reviewed, and a written brochure containing perioperative information is provided to the patient. In the age group of patients with rectal cancer, a complete preoperative medical evaluation is often necessary because of coexisting medical conditions such as heart disease, hypertension, and diabetes, among others. In 25% to 40% of patients, obesity may play a significant role in their operation, their recovery, and as a major factor in their long-term outcomes. Autologous or family blood and sperm donations are considered rare elective choices, as appropriate.

Prior to operation, patients are taught coughing, deep breathing, incentive spirometry, splinting of wounds, methods of analgesia, leg exercises, and upright positioning in bed in an ongoing effort to minimize complications that can include atelectasis, pneumonia, and deep vein thrombophlebitis.

PREOPERATIVE BOWEL PREPARATION

Mechanical bowel preparation is accomplished in the elective, unobstructed patient. A low-fiber diet is maintained for several preoperative days, and a 24-hour mechanical preparation includes the use of citrate of magnesia and bisacodyl tablets or one-half gallon of polyethylene glycol solution with bisacodyl tablets on the day before surgery. Partially obstructed patients may benefit from longer and gentler preparation, including greater reliance on enemas. The occasional older, infirm, or obstructed patient may require hospitalization. Prophylactic antibiotics are administered intravenously within 1 hour prior to the incision and are repeated after 3 hours of surgery. Postoperative doses are not indicated. Some surgeons successfully use anti–mu opioid inhibitors to reduce the likelihood of narcotic-associated ileus.

POSITION OF THE PATIENT

The operation is performed with the patient in the lithotomy-Trendelenburg position with the legs supported on Allen hydraulic stirrups, with sacral and lumbar support provided by a gel pad.[7] The popliteal fossae and the tibial tuberosities are supported and padded to avoid peroneal or tibial nerve palsies and compartment syndromes. Sequential compression boots are helpful in preventing deep vein thrombophlebitis. The perineum is draped into the sterile field, but it is kept separate from the abdominal field by a supplementary drape that may be removed intraoperatively. The anus is closed with a watertight suture to minimize contamination. The bladder is catheterized within the sterile field. If the patient has a locally advanced primary tumor (i.e., marginally resectable or adjacent organ invasion) or a recurrent tumor in the pelvis and/or has undergone extensive preoperative radiation and/or prior pelvic surgery, indwelling ureteral catheters are considered helpful during the dissection. They are not used except for the specific indications cited. In cases of recurrent or locally advanced disease requiring lengthy dissections, consideration may be given to leaving the patient in a supine position, shifting to stirrups only when necessary to avoid compartment syndromes.

In recent times, some authors have repositioned patients for the perineal phase of the APR, in order to facilitate the perineal dissection. The aim is to achieve negative circumferential or lateral margins at the level of the levator ani. Surgeons have reported using the prone position[8] or the on-table, knee-chest position[9] with bolsters for support. We have used the Andrews spine surgery operating table setup in the knee-chest position, first transferring the patient from the supine position on the operating table to a stretcher, and rotating the patient back onto the Andrews table to achieve a formal or a right-angle knee-chest position, with good results.

ABDOMINOPERINEAL RESECTION FOR ADENOCARCINOMA OF THE RECTUM

An APR is thought of by most surgeons as the operation performed when there simply is no sphincter-preserving option available because of the distal location of the primary tumor. Evidence suggests that in most instances, APR may be the appropriate operation for distal rectal cancer and is not just an amputation of the rectum as a last resort. During the 1990s, sufficient evidence accrued to suggest that low rectal cancer (0 to 5 cm from the anal verge) represents a biologically more aggressive disease than cancer of the midrectum.[4] It has been repeatedly demonstrated in the surgical literature that the 5-year survival rate of patients requiring an APR is significantly less than the survival rate of patients who can be treated with sphincter preservation.[4,7] These results do not reflect a purely technical issue, such as skill of sphincter preservation or of avoiding positive margins, as poorer survival has been observed even in the hands of surgeons who are normally successful at avoiding APR.

Clinicopathologic findings support these observations. Lymph node–clearing studies demonstrate that compared to patients with midrectal cancers, patients with low rectal cancer have a higher incidence of positive mesorectal lymph nodes, a higher incidence of lateral pelvic node involvement, a higher overall incidence of pelvic recurrence in Duke B and C cases, and a lower 5-year survival rate.[10] A higher incidence of pulmonary metastases and a proportionately lower incidence of liver metastases are observed than are seen in cases of midrectal cancer, indicating a higher likelihood of low rectal cancer spreading systemically via the internal iliac vessels, as opposed to the liver via the inferior mesenteric circulation.[4] Adverse pathologic findings (e.g., poor degree of differentiation, extramural venous spread, venous invasion, lymphatic vascular invasion, perineural invasion, and nonnodal implants) are also more common in the mesorectum of patients with low rectal cancers.[7,10-12] Thus, in patients with low rectal cancers, APR may prove to be the best means of clearing the pelvis of all regional cancer specifically, and not just an amputation of last resort or an operation based solely on the inability to perform a low anterior resection (LAR). Other pathologic observations of the contents of the mesorectum support complete removal of the mesorectum, for at least 5 cm beyond the distal edge of the primary tumor in conjunction with any rectal excision, regardless of the height of the lesion.[10] Careful attention to the issues that govern the complete resection of all pelvic disease is warranted by these observations.

Where sphincter preservation can be accomplished, Hida et al have demonstrated that 20% of patients with T3 lesions harbor lymph node metastases as far as 4 cm distal to the lowest palpable edge of the tumor.[10] Under such circumstances, at least 4 cm of the mesorectum, distal to the lowest palpable edge of the primary tumor, are removed with the specimen, determining the distal margin of resection.

PRINCIPLES OF TOTAL MESORECTAL EXCISION WITH AUTONOMIC NERVE PRESERVATION

The principles of TME have been extensively reviewed elsewhere.[4,7,13-15] The overwhelming majority of regional disease contributing to the spread of rectal cancer is contained within the mesorectum,[5,7,10,11] which is defined by the boundaries of the visceral layer of the pelvic fascia.[11] The goal of surgery for rectal cancer, whether sphincter preserving or not, is the resection of the rectum and the mesorectum as a single unit, contained within the visceral layer of the pelvic fascia, with intact circumferential margins uninvolved by cancer. Although there has been professional interest in the extent of resection for years, including issues such as high ligation and the question of pelvic lymphadenectomy, the most important current focus of surgical standards in rectal cancer is the need to adopt a uniform, standardized extent of pelvic dissection. These standards are necessary to accomplish a resection of all regional disease encompassed within the mesorectum and surrounded by negative or uninvolved circumferential margins, that is, an R0 resection. The operation must result in a reproducible pathological specimen with an R0 resection, pathologically negative circumferential margins of 2 mm or more, and a macroscopically smooth and shiny visceral fascia enveloping the mesorectum indicating no evidence of mesorectal violation.[5]

The more experience that is gained worldwide, the clearer is the evidence that the results of TME as a standardized operation for rectal cancer contrast sharply with those of nonstandardized operations. In a multisurgeon series[15] from the University of Leiden that involved consecutive, unselected patients with Duke B or C rectal cancers, TME was associated with a 69% 5-year survival rate versus 42% for nonstandardized resections, and the 5-year incidence of pelvic failure after TME was 8% versus 40% after nonstandardized operations. Other studies have produced similar results.[7,16,17]

To accomplish this goal, the surgeon must become familiar with a precise sharp dissection along the plane that separates the visceral from the parietal layers of the pelvic fasciae, producing the specimen of rectum and mesorectum with an intact and uninvolved visceral layer of the fascia, a dissection that preserves the autonomic nervous structures of the pelvis. Some have referred to this plane using descriptive adjectives, such as the "holy plane" (Heald) or the "extrafascial plane" (Hill), but in view of the fact that it is the only pelvic areolar plane that separates visceral from parietal structures, we prefer to describe this plane as the concentric areolar tissue plane that is found outside of the contours of the visceral layer and medial to the parietal layers of the pelvic fascial planes that cover the autonomic nerves plexuses (Figure 168-1). In a cross-sectional schematic view of the pelvis, this plane is the equivalent of one of the rings in a target, with the rectum and mesorectum located centrally.

There are several key technical points associated with the successful accomplishment of this dissection, as listed here and discussed in the following sections:

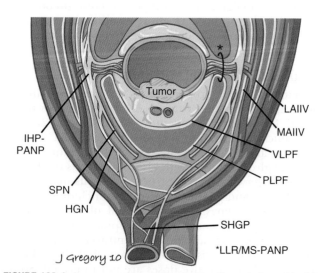

FIGURE 168-1 A cross section of the rectum through the midpelvis outlining the various layers of the pelvic fasciae. *HGN,* Hypogastric nerves; *IHP-PANP,* inferior hypogastric plexus or lateral segment of the lateral ligament of the rectum; *LLR* or *MS PANP,* so-called lateral ligament of the rectum, or the medial segment of the pelvic autonomic nerve plexus (PANP)*; *MAIIV* and *LAIIV,* medial and lateral adventitiae of the internal iliac vessels, respectively; *SHGP,* superior hypogastric plexus; *SPN,* sacral parasympathetic nerves; *VLPF* and *PLPF,* visceral and parietal layers of the pelvic fascia, respectively. (Redrawn from Enker WE, Kafka NJ, Martz J: Planes of sharp dissection for primary, locally advanced, or recurrent rectal cancer. *Semin Surg Oncol* 18:19, 2000.)

1. Initial entry into the retrorectal space
2. Identification of the superior hypogastric nerves and the inferior hypogastric plexus (IHP), referred to by some as the pelvic autonomic nerve plexuses (PANPs)
3. Separation of the posterior visceral compartment from the anterior visceral compartment (e.g., the rectovaginal septum in the female and Denonvilliers fascia in the male)[18]
4. Isolation of the medial segment of the lateral ligament and preservation of the pelvic splanchnic nerves, also known as sacral parasympathetic nerves
5. Mobilization of the distal rectum in relation to the levator ani (i.e., complete mobilization of the rectum)
6. In the case of APR, the perineal dissection including resection of the levator is carried out as close as possible to the bony margins of the pelvic side walls. Wide resection of the levator ani muscles to ensure no violation of the cancer has been practiced for years, as previously published.[19] Although some have recently referred to this operation as a "cylindrical" APR,[20] the operation described in this chapter has been practiced by us for the past 3 to 4 decades.

INITIAL ENTRY INTO THE RETRORECTAL SPACE

The inferior mesenteric artery (IMA), the sigmoid mesentery, and the sigmoid colon have been divided, and the "rectal" specimen is held upward and forward under traction. Just posterior to the superior rectal veins and artery, the plane between the hypogastric nerves and the outer edge of the mesorectum is entered, separating retroperitoneal from mesenteric structures at the level of the sacral promontory. From the promontory, distally, the pelvic dissection is in progress and is performed entirely using sharp technique, along with traction and countertraction at all levels of the dissection, until the anal hiatus of the levator ani is reached. The sine qua non of all rectal cancer surgery is this complete mobilization of the rectum. The mesorectum and the hypogastric nerves are sharply separated from each other, by dissection within the areolar plane that separates the visceral from the parietal pelvic fasciae circumferentially (Figure 168-2). Dissection with a medium-length pair of Metzenbaum scissors is most expedient, although in the teaching setting, dissection with a right-angle clamp and cauterization of all small branches of the hypogastric nerves leading from the main trunk to the mesorectum is commonly practiced. To avoid injury to the hypogastric nerves, the surgeon must appreciate that these nerves routinely enter the outermost layer of the visceral fascia at the level of the rectosigmoid, only to diverge laterally again toward the pelvic side wall as the main trunks of the autonomic nerves and the IHP.[21] In either an open or a laparoscopic APR, care must be taken to avoid contact with the autonomic nerves when using energy-producing dissecting instruments. Such energy may be globally dispersed to these nerves and may render them fibrotic and functionless. The dissection continues, distally, with a deep St. Mark's retractor holding the rear of the mesorectum forward, while the assistant simultaneously maintains upward traction on the specimen.

At this point, the retrorectal space is open dorsal to or behind the mesorectum and between the lateral

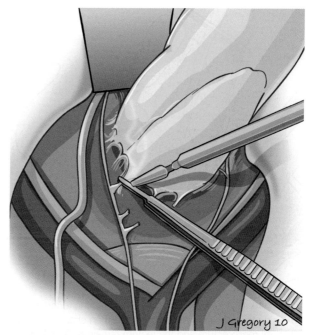

FIGURE 168-2 Dissection between the left hypogastric nerve (covered by the parietal fascia) and the visceral layer of the pelvic fascia. Separation of these structures allows one to enter the plane between the visceral and the parietal layers of the pelvic fascia, proceeding caudad. (Redrawn from Enker WE: Total mesorectal excision with sphincter and autonomic nerve preservation in the treatment of rectal cancer. *Curr Tech Gen Surg* 5:1, 1996.)

ligaments. At or slightly above the level of S3, in the midline, one encounters the rectosacral fascia. This structure is divided sharply (Figure 168-3). This important act constitutes one of the major differences between TME and conventional surgery, as the surgeon performing a conventional resection is dissecting down the retrorectal plane bluntly and encounters the rectosacral ligament as a significant obstruction to further progress. To avoid disrupting the presacral venous plexuses, a surgeon moves the bluntly dissecting hand forward, often rupturing instead, into the mesorectum just where positive nodes or other pathologic findings are most likely to be found, that is, to or proximal to the level of the primary tumor in the rectum.[7] A portion of the violated mesorectum remains, attached to the sacrum, and constitutes the nidus for persistent (i.e., "recurrent") cancer that presents as a local recurrence, clinically within 2 years.[22] By contrast, in TME, all dissection is performed sharply, and the sharp division of the rectosacral fascia ensures that the mesorectal specimen remains intact as well as surrounded by the visceral layer of the pelvic fascia as one passes this point in the dissection. After the rectosacral fascia is sharply divided, the pelvis opens widely to view distally or caudad, and further elements of dissection become possible under direct vision. Dissection is facilitated by a deep St. Mark's retractor. In cases where a sphincter-preserving operation was advisable, this same hindrance to further blunt dissection at the level of the rectosacral fascia is what frequently prompts a decision to perform an APR, whereas further sharp dissection down the presacral plane would have

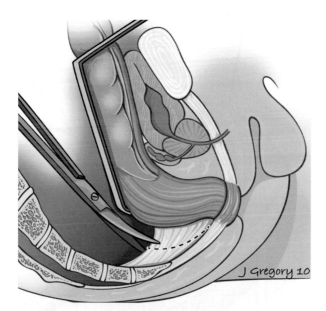

FIGURE 168-3 The rectosacral fascia or ligament is found midway down along the curvature of the sacrum. When sharply divided, the integral mesorectum and the rectum remain an intact unit of primary tumor and potential mesorectal lymph node spread, as the node-bearing fat is not violated. Once the ligament is sharply divided, the distal pelvis is much easier to dissect sharply. In this illustration, at or just proximal to the level of the coccyx, the blending visceral and parietal fasciae are being divided with care to avoid injury to the mesorectum viscerally and care is taken in dividing the nerves to the levator ani muscles parietally. (Redrawn from Enker WE: Total mesorectal excision with sphincter and autonomic nerve preservation in the treatment of rectal cancer. *Curr Tech Gen Surg* 5:1, 1996.)

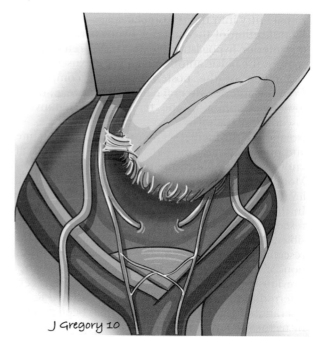

FIGURE 168-4 Circumferential sharp dissection frees the visceral from the parietal layers of the pelvic fascia. Included within the most medial layer of the parietal fascia are the pelvic autonomic nerves and the plexuses. The medial segment of the plexus is a neurovascular bundle to the rectum, the so-called lateral ligament. This may be divided sharply along the outer edge of the mesorectum, preserving the autonomic nerves and sexual and urinary functions. (Redrawn from Enker WE: Total mesorectal excision with sphincter and autonomic nerve preservation in the treatment of rectal cancer. *Curr Tech Gen Surg* 5:1, 1996.)

mobilized the rectum sufficiently to perform the sphincter-preserving operation. The TME dissection is much easier and more open to view in the slender patient with a gynecoid pelvis and a posterior tumor, as opposed to an obese patient, particularly in a narrow android pelvis with an anterior tumor.

INDICATION OF THE HYPOGASTRIC NERVES, THE INFERIOR HYPOGASTRIC PLEXUSES, AND THE SACRAL PARASYMPATHETIC NERVES: THE PELVIC AUTONOMIC NERVES AND PLEXUSES

As the nerves are dissected away from the mesorectum, the complete course of the hypogastric nerves becomes evident, leading to the IHP-PANP, the lateral portion of the so-called lateral ligament (Figure 168-4).[23] As the posterior dissection reaches the level of S3, one may observe the anterior nerve roots of the parasympathetic nerves as they exit from the sacral foramina, bilaterally. Particularly in the gynecoid pelvis, an antegrade dissection of these nerves anterolaterally and medial to the IHP-PANPs may be possible and expedient. More commonly, particularly in the narrow android pelvis, one must first shift to the anterior dissection between the rectum and seminal vesicles, to surround the rectum/mesorectum with dissected spaces and leave the dissection of the sacral nerves and the medial segments of the lateral ligaments to a later point.

SEPARATION OF ANTERIOR AND POSTERIOR COMPARTMENTS

Forward or anterior traction is now applied to the genitourinary tract. Often, the hand-held St. Mark's retractor proves to be superior to the self-retaining retractor at this point in the dissection, providing both upward and forward retraction. In women, upward traction on the uterus or gently held Allis clamps on the vagina may also help define the rectovaginal septum.

Countertraction is maintained by the nondominant hand as downward (i.e., posterior) pressure on the anterior rectum and anterior traction is applied to the vagina, seminal vesicles, and other structures caudad. Either in the open case or in a hand-assisted laparoscopic case (HALS), for optimum benefit, the fingertips provide countertraction within millimeters of the site to be sharply dissected. If the peritoneum of the cul-de-sac has not been fully incised, it is completely incised now. The plane between the rectum and the genitourinary tract is developed sharply. In the case of the female pelvis, sharp dissection leaves a nonviolated full-thickness wall of the vagina with intact blood supply. Unless the vagina needs to be sacrificed as an involved adjacent organ, the vascularity of the posterior vaginal wall must not be disturbed by an ill-conceived sense of radicality, namely, dissection within the wall of the vagina to obtain a "wide" anterior margin. Especially following neoadjuvant radiation, such an intramural dissection can lead to a late rectovaginal

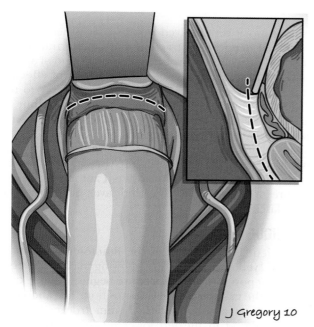

FIGURE 168-5 The anterior dissection in the pelvis of a male is facilitated by a St. Mark's retractor. The dissection begins between the seminal vesicles and the Denonvilliers fascia (*inset*) and returns to the rectoprostatic interface distal to the junction of Denonvilliers fascia and the prostatic capsule. Denonvilliers fascia remains attached to the rectum as the specialized portion of the visceral layer of the pelvic fascia covering the anterior margin of the mesorectum. (Redrawn from Enker WE: Total mesorectal excision with sphincter and autonomic nerve preservation in the treatment of rectal cancer. *Curr Tech Gen Surg* 5:1, 1996.)

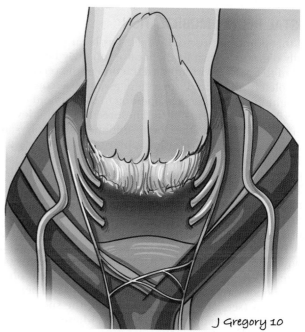

FIGURE 168-6 The neurovascular bundle to the rectum (the medial segment of the lateral ligament) has been divided, the visceral layer of the fascia is intact overlying the back wall of the mesorectum, and the pelvic autonomic plexuses remain intact. (Redrawn from Enker WE: Total mesorectal excision with sphincter and autonomic nerve preservation in the treatment of rectal cancer. *Curr Tech Gen Surg* 5:1, 1996.)

fistula because of combined surgical and radiation-induced necrosis. The dissection continues down to the pelvic floor or the anal hiatus in the levator ani.

In the male patient, the technique of dissection continues in the same manner. The anterior plane is begun by incising the cul-de-sac, and after both seminal vesicles are outlined, the plane of dissection shifts anteriorly to encompass Denonvilliers fascia, separating the rectum and the mesorectum from the genitourinary structures until the junction of Denonvilliers fascia and the prostatic capsule. Further dissection continues distally between the mesorectal fat and the prostate capsule, staying as wide as possible anteriorly (Figure 168-5). This may prove very difficult in the face of obesity, an android pelvis, or an anteriorly situated tumor.

LATERAL LIGAMENTS

After the anterior and posterior dissections have been completed, the remaining dissections are lateral and anterolateral. The anatomy has been well demonstrated by Sato and Sato.[23] The retraction is changed to provide the surgeon with optimal views of the lateral pelvic side wall. Excellent lighting is needed, as are extra-long instruments, including suction cannulas (e.g., Cooley), DeBakey forceps, and dissecting instruments. The rectum is retracted medially by the first assistant. On either side of the table, the surgeon (who is ipsilateral) dissects, while the assistant retracts toward himself or herself, providing visibility of the edge of the mesorectum and the

dissection plane. All dissection is performed sharply, along the areolar plane previously described, under direct vision, with careful hemostasis. The dissection is performed between the lateral edge of the mesorectum and the medial edge of the IHP-PANP, preserving the intact plexus. The goal is to *identify* both the medial segment of the lateral ligament as well as the entire plexus or lateral segment, *dividing only* the medial segment containing the neurovascular branches of the PANP and the middle rectal artery, which are the only structures that are headed directly to the rectum. This dissection preserves the lateral portion of the IHP-PANP that is integrating the fibers of the pelvic autonomic nervous system into functional bundles. These bundles head anteriorly to supply the genitourinary system for both sexual and urinary functions (Figure 168-6).[23] The sacral parasympathetic nerve or nerves (S3 and S4 or the "nervi erigentes") may be observed leading directly from the sacral foramen of S3 to the IHP or the PANP along the pelvic side wall and should be preserved unless there is a need to take the nerves to achieve a tumor-free margin. Once the dissection has separated the edge of the mesorectum from the IHP-PANP, the levator ani become visible, approximately 3 to 4 cm distally. The same dissection is completed on the opposite side of the pelvis. Optimally with two experienced surgeons this may be achieved by switching who dissects and who retracts, before finalizing the pelvic or abdominal side of the procedure with complete mobilization to the pelvic floor.

DISTAL RECTAL MOBILIZATION

At this point, the rectum, which has been circumferentially dissected down to the levator ani, may be elevated out of the pelvis. With upward traction of the rectum, the completely mobilized specimen assumes a completely straight line from the anal opening to the sigmoid colon. The final attachments of the mesorectum to the levator ani, particularly in the lower midline posteriorly, are divided sharply. An occasional bleeder may be grasped with forceps and cauterized, where the visceral and parietal layers of the pelvic fascia seem to fuse in the midline. This fusion plane is the only known remnant of Waldeyer's fascia, as used in current nomenclature.[21,24] In the patient with a midrectal cancer, which is treatable by low anterior resection, the rectum is divided at this point in the operation. In the patient with a low rectal cancer, the abdominopelvic portion of the operation is now complete and the surgeon proceeds with the perineal phase of the operation. Some technical aspects of the perineal dissection (see later), such as handling the specimen as a guide to dissection, do not apply where a two-team approach is used.

THE LAPAROSCOPIC ABDOMINOPERINEAL RESECTION

Advances in minimally invasive surgery have allowed the application of the laparoscopic approach to distal rectal cancers that require an APR. The extraperitoneal location of the rectum and the fact that the majority of the dissection for a distal cancer may be performed via the perineum, the absence of an anastomosis, and the ability to perform the pelvic dissection along normal tissue planes are potential advantages of the laparoscopic approach. Another advantage is the fact that with the use of laparoscopic port sites, a midline or transverse lower abdominal incision is not needed. The only other abdominal incision needed is the left lower quadrant site that will serve for positioning of the end sigmoid colostomy. Patients with recurrent rectal cancer, bulky lesions, or adjacent organ involvement should not be offered a laparoscopic approach to APR.

The short-term as well as the cancer-related safety of the laparoscopic technique has been studied extensively over the past few years in patients whose operations are following the same principles and guidelines, whether open or closed. Overall survival, isolated pelvic recurrence rates, and disease-free survival rates have been similar for the open and laparoscopic techniques. No differences in the distance from mesorectal tumor to the lateral or circumferential margin(s) or the number of harvested lymph nodes have been reported. Advantages include a shorter length of stay and decreased time to ambulation, and earlier return to work or to normal activities of daily living for patients undergoing laparoscopic colorectal surgery.[25,26] Nevertheless, complication rates associated with the laparoscopic technique per se have involved increased perineal wound infection rates and/or inferior long-term sexual function outcomes.[27,28] These inferior sexual function outcomes are likely the

result of two as yet unsolved laparoscopic issues: the lack of optimal deep pelvic traction and countertraction at the site of dissection, a problem of leverage and of appropriate instrumentation, and, in the absence of effective retraction, the transmission of damaging energy to the pelvic autonomic nerves, from the energy output of current dissecting/coagulation or welding instruments. In the absence of vigorous medial rectal retraction, the damage that is secondary to energy sources occurs while dissecting in the plane between the visceral fascia, covering the mesorectum and the adjacent autonomic nerves that are only covered by the thin layer of the parietal pelvic fascia.

TECHNIQUE

The patient is positioned in the lithotomy position in Allen, or "yellow fin," stirrups, allowing maximum versatility in leg position. The procedure begins with the knee height in the maximal downward position. The abdomen is entered via a subumbilical 10-mm trocar. A 5-mm trocar is placed in the left lower quadrant two fingerbreadths superior and medial to the anterior iliac spine. Placement is intended to avoid injury to the inferior epigastric vessels. In the obese patient with a widened distance between the iliac crests, the surgeon benefits from placing the trocar in a slightly more medial position. An additional 5-mm trocar is placed four fingerbreadths superior. In the right lower quadrant, a 12-mm trocar is placed two fingerbreadths superior and medial to the anterior iliac spine, with an additional 5-mm trocar placed superior to this (Figure 168-7).

The procedure begins with a thorough inspection of the abdomen for evidence of metastatic disease with a

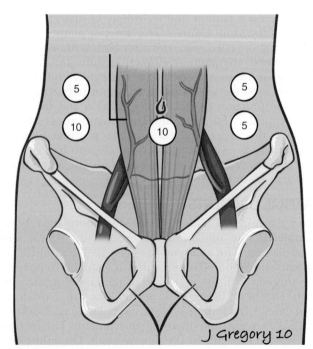

FIGURE 168-7 Trocar placement for the laparoscopic abdominoperineal resection. The inferior trocar is placed two fingerbreadths superior and medial to the anterior iliac spine.

30-degree-angled 10-mm scope. The intraperitoneal surfaces, liver, and the pelvic side wall, where visible, are inspected. The steps of the procedure can be outlined as follows, mimicking the open procedure in many respects:

1. Vascular division of the inferior mesenteric vessels
2. Division of the sigmoid colon
3. TME of the rectum
4. Creation of the colostomy
5. Completion of the proctectomy via the perineum

Many surgeons, while preferring to divide the distal sigmoid, laparoscopically, continue to perform the majority of the pelvic as well as the perineal dissection via an open perineal approach. The cephalocaudal pelvic dissection or the perineal pelvic dissection leaves a lot of room for excellent surgery by whatever route is most comfortable in the hands of the operating surgeon.

The initial dissection begins with the ventral and lateral traction of the sigmoid colon with a bowel grasper and the identification of the inferior mesenteric artery (IMA). The overlying peritoneum should be scored with the mesentery separated off the retroperitoneum from the level of the sacral promontory. The left ureter and gonadal vessels are identified. Their identification can be facilitated by lighted ureteral stents in a surgeon's early laparoscopic experience with the medial-to-lateral dissection approach. The division of the vascular pedicle with the LigaSure device or Endo-GIA vascular staplers is performed about 2 cm distal to the origin of the IMA (Figure 168-8). The inferior mesenteric vein is similarly identified in the medial-to-lateral mobilization of the sigmoid mesentery and divided at the corresponding level.

After dividing the vascular pedicle, the remaining mesentery is mobilized and a window is created posterior to the colon wall. The bowel is divided with the endoscopic linear stapler, and the remaining mesentery is then divided.

Although performed laparoscopically, the rest of the procedure is conducted in the same way as the open technique. Additional retraction may be obtained via the placement of an extracorporeal Prolene suture into the pelvis or by the use of a fan retractor. This Prolene suture is placed with a Keith needle via a suprapubic puncture site. This may be useful in securing a large uterus, providing enhanced anterior retraction of the rectum. In larger tumors and in the difficult android pelvis, the pelvic dissection is often facilitated by a Pfannenstiel incision. This allows for the preservation of much of the advantages of the laparoscopic procedure while ensuring an adequate mesorectal dissection.

After completion of the abdominal portion of the procedure, the colostomy may be created via a separate circular incision in the left rectus sheath. Prior to entering the peritoneum, the distal colon should be grasped using a bowel grasper via a right-sided port and delivered into the stoma site incision. The colon should not be matured until the completion of the procedure. If the pneumoperitoneum is to be reestablished, it may require the placement of Vaselinized packing at the stoma site to prevent excessive air leakage. The perineal operator can then complete the proctectomy and delivery of the specimen (see earlier).

THE PERINEAL DISSECTION

The perineal dissection is based on several goals: the complete resection of the rectum and the mesorectum, the anatomic resection of the surrounding fat of the ischiorectal space, and the most lateral, that is, the widest possible circumferential resection of the levator muscles possible in each patient. Learning or performing a proper perineal dissection can be a daunting chore, especially in the muscular android pelvis.

POSITIONS OF THE PATIENT FOR THE PERINEAL PHASE OF THE OPERATION HAVE BEEN REVIEWED (See Earlier)[9]

The perineal phase begins with an outline of the cutaneous incision. The landmarks for complete resection are the perineal body anteriorly, the palpable tip of the coccyx posteriorly, and the medial palpable edges of the ischial tuberosities laterally (Figure 168-9).[19] The entire dissection may be performed using the cautery device, and few if any sutures are used for hemostasis, except in relation to the puborectalis muscles or to the prostate capsule. The incision is made in the skin and deepened to the subcutaneous fat circumferentially. In the lithotomy position, the two posterior quadrants (3 to 6 o'clock and 6 to 9 o'clock) are incised first, so minor blood loss from the upper half of the incision does not obscure the field. The skin edges of the specimen are grasped in the midline with Lahey clamps, which may be tied together with a sponge or an umbilical tape and used for retraction.

Self-retaining retractors or skin-retracting sutures are used where possible. Various rotating blades are used together with a T-shaped prototype of a self-retaining retractor in conjunction with the Thompson retractor

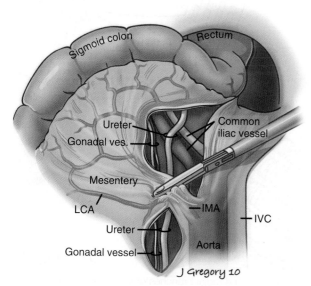

FIGURE 168-8 The division of the vascular pedicle is performed about 2 cm distal to the origin of the inferior mesenteric artery. The vascular pedicle may be divided with the LigaSure device or Endo-GIA vascular staplers. *IMA,* Inferior mesenteric artery; *IVC,* inferior vena cava; *LCA,* left colic artery.

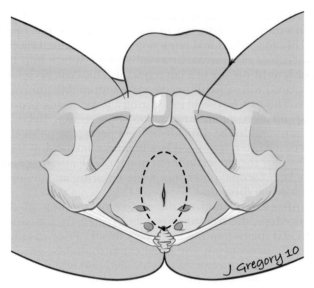

FIGURE 168-9 The topographic landmarks for the perineal dissection. The skin should be incised where one can palpate the medial edges of the ischial tuberosities laterally, the coccyx dorsally, and at the level of the perineal body ventrally. (Adapted from Enker WE: Cancer of the rectum: Operative management and adjuvant therapy. In Fazio VW, editor: *Current therapy in colon and rectal surgery*. Ontario, 1990, BC Decker, p 120.)

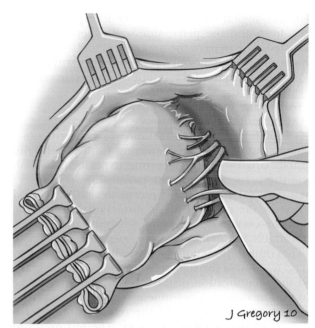

FIGURE 168-10 The radial branches of the pudendal nerves are located running toward the rectum and across the ischiorectal space. They may be appreciated as violin strings by palpation between thumb and index finger. (Adapted from Enker WE: Cancer of the rectum: Operative management and adjuvant therapy. In Fazio VW, editor: *Current therapy in colon and rectal surgery*. Ontario, 1990, BC Decker, p 120.)

system. Alternatively, temporary, widely placed sutures may retract the skin and subcutaneous tissues radially.

The dissection is deepened until the puborectalis muscles are noted. The transverse perineus muscle is superficial. The ischiorectal fat may be divided with the cautery or entered with a clamp just below the puborectalis muscles until the levator ani are reached. A finger follows this path and then curls dorsally, toward the coccyx. Anterior to the finger, strong bands, or "violin strings," may be felt traversing the ischiorectal space bilaterally (Figure 168-10).[19] These fibers represent the radial branches of the pudendal nerves, whose fibers are going to the anal sphincter. Each nerve is accompanied by its blood supply, and when cut, bleeding from these vessels can suffuse through the fat and obscure the field. A clamp is passed under each of these vessels, identifying it and separating it from the surrounding fat. The vessel and nerve are grasped using forceps or another clamp and cauterized and divided medial to the prominent eschar (Figure 168-11). When all of the branches have been divided circumferentially, the levators may be exposed and the dissection proceeds to the next step.

In the posterior midline, the anococcygeal raphe is divided, and the anococcygeal ligament is dissected to the coccyx. The levator attachment to the coccyx is divided sharply, and the pelvis is entered, signaled by a small collection of blood or fluid. The levators are swept over the index finger and divided as close to the pelvic side wall as possible (Figure 168-12). Although the levators may be preserved for pelvic floor closure in surgery for inflammatory bowel disease, in cancer surgery they are divided widely and if this step has been properly performed, the remaining levators should not be available for pelvic floor closure. The levator ani are a presumed pathway for lymphatic spread for rectal carcinomas

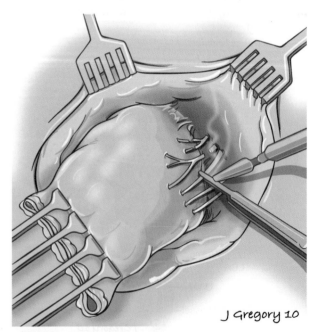

FIGURE 168-11 The radial branches of the pudendal nerves are isolated and cauterized, avoiding ligation of the ischiorectal fat. (Adapted from Enker WE: Cancer of the rectum: Operative management and adjuvant therapy. In Fazio VW, editor: *Current therapy in colon and rectal surgery*. Ontario, 1990, BC Decker, p 120.)

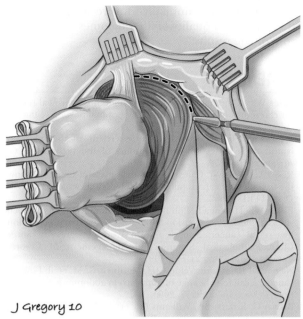

J Gregory 10

FIGURE 168-12 The levator ani muscles are divided with a finger initially passed inside the pelvis in the midline dorsally. The levators are divided from the 2 o'clock to the 10 o'clock position as close to the pelvic side walls as the pelvis will allow. Wide dissection of the levator ani results in no "coning" defect at the level of the levator ani muscles, what is currently being referred to as the "cylindrical" abdominoperineal resection (APR), leading to the lowest possible risk of inadequate or positive circumferential margins. In an APR for cancer, the surgeon should not be able to close the levator defect by approximating the remaining levator muscles. In our hands, this is not a new operation but one that we have practiced for the past three or more decades. (Adapted from Enker WE: Cancer of the rectum: Operative management and adjuvant therapy. In Fazio VW, editor: *Current therapy in colon and rectal surgery*. Ontario, 1990, BC Decker, p 120.)

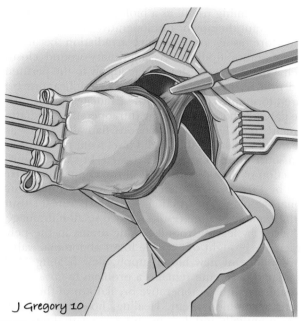

J Gregory 10

FIGURE 168-13 The puborectalis muscles are divided, and the specimen can be removed. (Adapted from Enker WE: Cancer of the rectum: Operative management and adjuvant therapy. In Fazio VW, editor: *Current therapy in colon and rectal surgery*. Ontario, 1990, BC Decker, p 120.)

to the iliac lymph node chain. Once the levators have been divided from the 2 o'clock to the 10 o'clock position, the retrorectal space is open. The specimen may now be passed from the abdominal to the perineal dissector via the posterior opening. The dissection continues anteriorly, guided by the easier handling that the delivered specimen allows. If possible, the rectum and the prostate are separated in the midline using a blunt instrument such as a Kelly clamp. The final attachments of the rectum to the perineum are the puborectalis muscles, which are the medial fascicles of the pelvic diaphragm (Figure 168-13). Although they are coronally oriented in the intact pelvis, they are obliquely situated in the perineum, when the specimen is passed to the perineum. The puborectalis muscles may be divided with the cautery, or with clamps, and if needed, heavy absorbable sutures may be used to each of four puborectalis heads.

COLOSTOMY

The end sigmoid colostomy is constructed using a transrectus defect in the left lower abdominal wall. The skin opening of the colostomy has been optimally chosen and marked by the enterostomal therapist or surgeon before

the operation with the patient sitting upright to avoid skin folds. A superior method for avoiding parastomal hernia is the extraperitoneal colostomy, ascribed to Goligher, in which the sigmoid colon is tunneled out to the abdominal defect extraperitoneally. The skin and subcutaneous tissues are excised as usual, and the anterior rectus sheath is either excised or cut in the cruciate fashion. The rectus muscle is split, and the posterolateral corner of the rectus fascia is identified. The edge of the rectus sheath is opened gently and carefully by spreading with a clamp, and a plane is created between the transversalis fascia and the peritoneum. If a defect is created in the peritoneum, it may be repaired. The colon is "tunneled" out through this channel, and the peritoneum is sutured to the psoas fascia. The colostomy is brought out so that it rests on the abdominal wall with no tension. The mucocutaneous junction is matured at the end of the case, after skin closure. If an extraperitoneal colostomy is not possible, the lateral defect is closed securely to avoid an interval peristomal hernia.

CLOSURE OF THE PELVIC FLOOR AND BIOLOGIC SPACERS

After hemostasis and irrigation, the perineal floor is closed in two layers—one of Scarpa fascia and the other of dermis or dermis and skin—using absorbable sutures. Particularly in the irradiated pelvis and perineum, an attempt is made to fill the pelvis with an omental pedicle, importing neovasculature or fresh blood supply to promote healing in the irradiated field. The cecum may be used frequently to fill the pelvis excluding the small bowel. Increasingly, a rectus muscle or myocutaneous flap is becoming useful as a biologic spacer either after neoadjuvant therapy or intraoperative radiation therapy or before using postoperative irradiation because of intraoperative findings. As a primary wound closure, such a flap brings fresh vascular supply to the perineum and primary healing with far fewer complications compared to simple closure.[29] In the irradiated patient or in the patient who is undergoing intraoperative irradiation, a rectus muscle or myocutaneous flap also serves as a means of excluding the small bowel from the pelvis and as a source of neovasculature as well. In cases requiring resection of the posterior wall of the vagina, reconstruction by a rectus myocutaneous flap also provides a functional vaginal reconstruction as well as perineal closure, with dramatic healing results. Closed suction drainage is achieved by leaving round Silastic drains in the pelvis, which are brought out via the lower abdominal wall. In the absence of new blood supply, slow healing of the irradiated perineum remains a problem in 25% to 50% of patients, with postoperative breakdown of the wound being a common event. Healing, however, does take place eventually and does not interfere with the resumption of systemic chemotherapy. Unlike the persistent perineal wound healing problems associated with Crohn disease, these wounds do heal, but they may represent a continuing problem of an uncomfortable, open wound requiring dressing changes for several months.

ADJACENT ORGAN INVOLVEMENT

About 10% of rectal cancers exhibit some form of adjacent organ invasion, involvement, or adherence, which is sufficient to raise concerns about the circumferential margins. Resection along the standard planes could cut across tumor, violating all principles of curative therapy. This event has a catastrophic outcome, significantly raising the local recurrence rates and dramatically reducing the chances of survival to about one-fourth of the survival rate that would be predicted by stage alone.

Proper management of adjacent organ involvement requires en bloc resection of the adjacent organ and reconstruction, wherever involvement is suspected. Although the entire subject is beyond the scope of this chapter, examples of this approach include the en bloc posterior vaginectomy and reconstruction of the posterior vaginal wall and perineum and the varying degrees of pelvic exenteration. Reconstruction is successfully accomplished by the use of a rectus myocutaneous flap.

SUMMARY

APR of the rectum performed in accordance with the principles of TME and autonomic nerve preservation is the operation of choice for low-lying primary rectal cancers that do not meet the criteria for local or for sphincter-preserving therapy, for pelvic recurrences of rectal cancers, and for a variety of other malignant anorectal diseases. The concept of wide perineal resection remains crucial and is enjoying a current revival in rectal cancer circles. Modern concepts have reduced both the morbidity and the mortality rates of the procedure since its introduction in the early part of the 20th century.

Recent advances in minimally invasive surgery may have further improved quality-of-life outcomes without affecting oncologic results.

REFERENCES

1. Miles WE: A method of performing abdomino-perineal resection for carcinoma of the rectum and the terminal portion of the pelvic colon. *Lancet* 2:379, 1908.
2. Stearns MW Jr, Deddish MR: Five-year results of abdomino-pelvic lymph node dissection for carcinoma of the rectum. *Dis Colon Rectum* 2:169, 1959.
3. Rosi PA, Cahill WJ, Carey J: A ten-year study of hemicolectomy in the treatment of carcinoma of the left half of the colon. *Surg Gynecol Obstet* 114:15, 1962.
4. Enker WE, Havenga K, Polyak T, et al: Abdominoperineal resection via total mesorectal excision and autonomic nerve preservation in low rectal cancer: Symposium on World Progress in Surgery-Clinico-pathological Staging and Management of Colorectal Cancer. *World J Surg* 21:715, 1997.
5. Nagtegaal ID, van de Velde CJH, Marijnen CAM, et al: Low rectal cancer: A call for a change of approach in abdominoperineal resection. *J Clin Oncol* 23:9257, 2005.
6. Brown G, Kirkham A, Williams GT, et al: High resolution MRI of the anatomy important in total mesorectal excision of the rectum. *AJR Am J Roentgenol* 182:431, 2004.
7. Enker WE, Thaler HT, Cranor ML, et al: Total mesorectal excision in the operative treatment of carcinoma of the rectum. *J Am Coll Surg* 181:335, 1995.
8. Holm T, Ljung A, Haggmark T, et al: Extended abdominoperineal resection with gluteus muscle flap reconstruction of the pelvic floor for rectal cancer. *Br J Surg* 94:232, 2006.
9. van Dijk TH, Wiggers T, Havenga K: Abdominoperineal resection for rectal cancer: Reducing the risk of local recurrence. *Semin Colon Rectal Surg* 21:81, 2010.
10. Hida JI, Yasutomi M, Maruyama T, et al: Lymph node metastases detected in the mesorectum distal to carcinoma of the rectum by the clearing method: Justification of total mesorectal excision. *J Am Coll Surg* 184:584, 1997.
11. Reynolds JV, Joyce WP, Dolan J, et al: Pathological evidence in support of total mesorectal excision in the management of rectal cancer. *Br J Surg* 83:1112, 1996.
12. Hida JI, Yasutomi M, Tokoro T, et al: Examination of nodal metastases by a clearing method supports pelvic plexus preservation in rectal cancer surgery. *Dis Colon Rectum* 42:510, 1999.
13. Enker WE: Potency cure and local control in the operative treatment of rectal cancer. *Arch Surg* 127:1396, 1992.
14. Enker WE, Havenga K, Martz J: Operative complications in pelvic surgery. In Winchester DP, Jones RS, Murphy GP, editors: *Cancer surgery for the general surgeon.* Philadelphia, Lippincott, 1999, Williams & Wilkins, p 71.
15. Havenga K, Enker WE, Heald RJ, et al: Improved survival and local control after total mesorectal excision or D3 lymphadenectomy in the treatment of primary rectal cancer: An international analysis of 1141 patients. *Eur J Surg Oncol* 25:368, 1999.
16. Enker WE: Safety and efficacy of low anterior resection for rectal cancer: Six hundred eighty-one consecutive cases from a specialty service. *Ann Surg* 230:544, 1999.
17. MacFarlane JK, Ryall RDH, Heald RJ: Mesorectal excision for rectal cancer. *Lancet* 341:457, 1993.
18. Enker WE: Total mesorectal excision with sphincter and autonomic nerve preservation in the treatment of rectal cancer. *Curr Tech Gen Surg* 5:1, 1996.
19. Enker WE: Cancer of the rectum: Operative management and adjuvant therapy. In Fazio VW, editor: *Current therapy in colon and rectal surgery.* Toronto, 1990, BC Decker, Inc., p 120.
20. West N, Finan PJ, Anderin C, et al: Evidence of the oncological superiority of cylindrical abdominoperineal excision for low rectal cancer. *J Clin Oncol* 26:3517, 2008.
21. Havenga K, DeRuiter MC, Enker WE, et al: Anatomical basis of autonomic nerve-preserving total mesorectal excision for rectal cancer. *Br J Surg* 83:384, 1996.
22. Quirke P, Durdey P, Dixon MF, et al: Local recurrence of rectal adenocarcinoma due to inadequate surgical resection:

Histopathological study of lateral tumor spread and surgical excision. *Lancet* 1:996, 1986.

23. Sato K, Sato T: The vascular and neuronal composition of the lateral ligament of the rectum and the rectosacral fascia. *Surg. Radiol Anat* 13:17, 1991.

24. Church JM, Raudkivi PJ, Hill GL: The surgical anatomy of the rectum: A review with particular relevance to the hazards of rectal mobilization. *Int J Colorect Dis* 2:158, 1987.

25. Fleshman JW, Wexner SD, Anvari M, et al: Laparoscopic versus open abdominoperineal resection for cancer. *Dis Colon Rectum* 42:7, 1999.

26. Kockerking F, Scheidbach H, Schneider C, et al: Laparoscopic abdominoperineal resection: Early postoperative results of a prospective study involving 116 patients. *Dis Colon Rectum* 43:11, 2000.

27. Jayne DG, Brown JM, Thorpe H, et al: Bladder and sexual function following resection for rectal cancer in a randomized clinical trial of laparoscopic versus open technique. *Br J Surg* 92:1124, 2005.

28. Quah HM, Jayne DG, Eu KW, et al: Bladder and sexual dysfunction following laparoscopically assisted and conventional open mesorectal excision for cancer. *Br J Surg* 89:1551, 2002.

29. Small T, Friedman DJ, Sultan M: Reconstructive surgery of the pelvis after surgery fro rectal cancer. *Semin Surg Oncol* 18:259, 2000.

Coloanal Anastomosis and Intersphincteric Resection

Jérémie H. Lefèvre | Yann Parc

The goal of coloanal anastomosis (CAA) is to preserve the anal sphincter and restore bowel continuity after total removal of the rectum. This operation was originally described for rectal cancer,[1] but it has since been widely used not only for malignant and benign tumors of the rectum but also for complex rectovaginal fistulas, hemangiomas, and radiation proctitis.

Because tumor deposits or metastatic lymph nodes can be found in the mesorectum for 2 to 5 cm (very rare) below the lower edge of the tumor,[2] the necessity of performing total mesorectal excision is widely accepted for the treatment of cancers of the *lower* rectum. In contrast, distal intramural spread of rectal cancer rarely exceeds 1 cm. In patients in whom the spread exceeds 1 cm, advanced disease commonly occurs, with multiple positive lymph nodes and distant metastases.[3] Importantly, anterior resection with a margin of 1 cm distal to the tumor is associated with 5-year survival and local recurrence rates similar to those for abdominoperineal resection (APR).[4] Therefore, for the surgical treatment of cancer of the lower portion of the rectum, a distal margin of 1 cm is sufficient, provided all of the mesorectum has been removed. For some cancers of the distal third of the rectum, a 1-cm margin can be obtained below the lower edge of the tumor, but the level of bowel transection renders intrapelvic anastomosis technically difficult or impossible. In these situations, bowel continuity can be restored with CAA. In other situations, the rectum is transected a few centimeters above the level of the levator ani muscles, and a double-stapled low colorectal anastomosis is technically feasible. However, some surgeons advocate both total mesorectal and total rectal excision with CAA for the treatment of all low rectal cancers. To respect the 1-cm margin oncologically and preserve the sphincter, when the extension of the tumor is limited to the muscular layer in cases of very low rectal cancer, a partial resection of the upper part of the internal sphincter can be performed.[5,6]

After total rectal resection and straight CAA, the concomitant loss of rectal reservoir function results in increased frequency, urgency, and fecal incontinence.[7] As our group[8] and Lazorthes et al[9] suggested, and as was demonstrated in several comparative studies,[10-15] the frequency of these troublesome symptoms can be decreased by adding a colonic pouch anastomosed directly to the anal canal.

In this chapter, we describe the technical aspects of hand-sewn, stapled colonic pouch–anal anastomosis, coloplasty, side-to-end anastomosis, and intersphincteric resection and provide data about the oncologic and functional results of these procedures.

OPERATIVE TECHNIQUE

PREPARATION FOR COLOANAL ANASTOMOSIS

Preoperative Preparation

A mechanical bowel preparation is performed the day before surgery, and systemic antibiotics are administered within 1 hour before the incision. Appropriate deep venous thrombosis prophylaxis is recommended.

The patient is positioned to allow a combined abdominal and perineal approach. The legs are placed in Lloyd-Davis stirrups, and the hips are flexed 30 degrees. A Foley catheter is placed in the bladder.

For laparoscopic surgery, the right thigh is extended by 10 to 20 degrees to facilitate the use of the lower right operative trocar. The patient is attached to the table with straps to be able to move the table without risking sliding of the patient on the table.

Incision for Laparotomy

The abdomen is opened through a midline incision that extends to the pubic symphysis.

Incision and Trocar Placement for Laparoscopy

A 1-cm vertical incision is performed 2 to 3 cm above the umbilicus. A 10-mm optical trocar is inserted and insufflation begun. Two 5-mm trocars are then inserted on the right midclavicular vertical line, one around MacBurney point and one 10 cm above. When required, a 5-mm trocar can be placed on the left midclavicular vertical line 5 cm under the ribs. A 12-mm trocar is inserted above the pubis in the midline, where a 5-cm incision will be performed to extract the rectum (Figure 169-1).

Abdominal Exploration

The abdominal cavity is explored to assess for ascitic fluid, invasion of mesenteric or paraaortic lymph nodes, peritoneal carcinomatosis, resectability of the tumor, and liver metastasis.

Division of the Inferior Mesenteric Vessels and Colon Mobilization

The inferior mesenteric artery (IMA) is ligated and divided about 2 cm from the aorta to preserve the autonomic nerves, which split around its origin. If the decision to perform APR can be made only intraoperatively, the rectal dissection is performed first and mobilization of the left colon is performed later. If, however, CAA is planned, the inferior mesenteric vein is transected at its termination, below the body of the pancreas near the ligament of Treitz, because this provides the greatest amount of mobility of the splenic flexure. It is helpful for the surgeon to be positioned between the patient's legs to take down the splenic flexure. Complete mobilization of the left colon is performed to ensure adequate length of viable bowel and to avoid any traction on the anastomosis. The descending colon, the splenic flexure, and the left portion of the transverse colon are mobilized, and the superior left colic artery is divided to provide further length (Figure 169-2). The left ureter is identified by locating the intersigmoidal fossa at the root of the sigmoid mesentery; it is dissected laterally away from the origin of the IMA.

When the procedure is performed by laparoscopy, the dissection is started by the ligation of the inferior mesenteric vein just under the pancreas (Figure 169-3).

The left colon mesentery is mobilized from the middle where the vein was divided from attachments to the splenic flexure. The transverse colon mesentery is divided to create access to the lesser sac. Thus, the insertion of the transverse colon mesentery is freed from the pancreas from the midline to the splenic flexure to mobilize completely the left transverse colon. To finalize this mobilization, the omentum is divided from the transverse colon from the midline to the left. Then, the origin of the IMA is found by dividing the upper part of the mesorectum from the promontory (Figure 169-4).

The left ureter is found and left behind to mobilize the sigmoid mesentery under the origin of the IMA. The IMA is then divided and the lateral attachments of the colon are then divided.

Total Mesorectal Excision

The sigmoid colon is lifted anteriorly to allow visualization of the IMA as it becomes the superior hemorrhoidal artery. The tissue just posterior to the vessel contains the hypogastric nerves. Sharp dissection allows preservation of these nerves and entrance into the perfect presacral plane for total mesorectal excision. Sharp dissection is extended downward around the curve of the sacrum in the midline, past the coccyx, and forward in front of the anococcygeal raphe. The lateral attachments are mobilized by extending the plane of dissection forward from

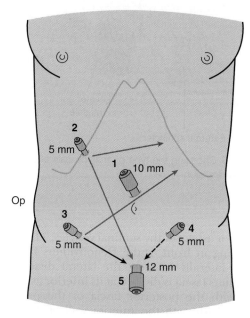

FIGURE 169-1 Trocar placement for laparoscopic approach.

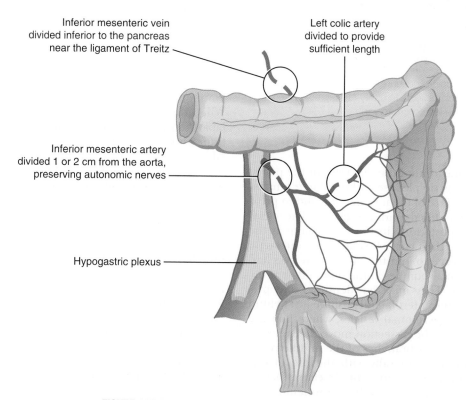

FIGURE 169-2 Division of the inferior mesenteric vessels.

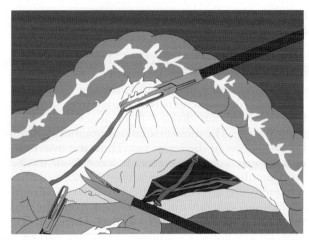

FIGURE 169-3 Laparoscopic procedure: dissection of the inferior mesenteric vein.

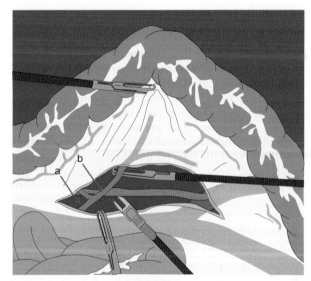

FIGURE 169-4 Laparoscopic procedure: dissection of the inferior mesenteric artery. Inferior mesenteric artery (a). Sigmoid artery after the division with the left colic artery (b).

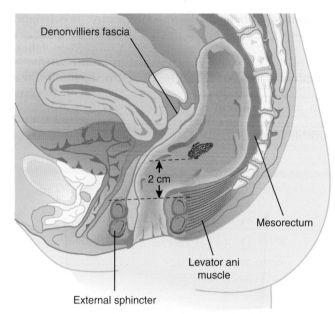

FIGURE 169-5 Choosing the type of anastomosis after rectal mesorectum excision.

the posterior midline around the side walls of the pelvis. The inferior hypogastric plexuses, which curve tangentially around the surface of the mesorectum and in proximity to it, are identified and preserved. The nervi erigentes lie more posteriorly in the same plane as the presacral nerves and then curve forward from the sacral foramina and converge to join the presacral nerves and form the neurovascular bundles at the outer edge of the Denonvilliers fascia. They must be identified and preserved, especially in the anterolateral position just behind the lateral edges of the seminal vesicles, where they are in danger of injury. As the dissection moves deeper into the pelvis, one or two tiny branches of the middle rectal vessels may be divided, generally with the use of diathermy coagulation. In men, anterior dissection begins with a transverse incision through the peritoneum anterior to the peritoneal reflection to descend straight to the superior aspect of the seminal vesicles. The dissection moves along in front of the Denonvilliers fascia and is extended laterally to meet the lateral dissection. The Denonvilliers fascia is divided at its inferior aspect, where it fuses with the posterior fascia of the prostate and contact is made with the anterior wall of the last centimeter of the rectum before it enters the levator ani muscle. In women, anterior dissection begins with a transverse incision at the bottom of the peritoneal reflection and moves along the posterior aspect of the cervix and the vagina down to the level of the levator ani.

When the operation is performed by laparoscopy, the dissection of the mesorectum can then be conducted either by laparoscopy or via a limited midline incision or Pfannenstiel incision based on the difficulty of the case. When the dissection is performed by laparoscopy, as by laparotomy this dissection starts by the posterior dissection. Thus, lateral dissections are conducted with a specific attention for the urogenital innervations, some reports showing worse sexual function after laparoscopic dissection.[16] To finish the dissection, the anterior part is performed last.

Choosing the Type of Anastomosis

At this stage, the whole mesorectum has been fully mobilized (Figure 169-5).

If the tumor extends through the bowel wall into the levator ani, abdominoperineal resection must be performed. On the other hand, if a right-angled rectal clamp can be applied below the lower border of the tumor, a sphincter-saving operation can probably be considered. If division of the rectum 2 cm below the edge of the tumor leaves 1 cm or more of rectum above the levator ani, a stapled anastomosis (colorectal or coloanal) is feasible. A hand-sewn CAA will need to be used if the distance between the level of resection and the upper border of the anal sphincter does not allow the use of a stapling device. This is the case for very low rectal tumors when the remaining anal canal is too short after rectal resection to admit the circular stapler, or when a TA stapler cannot be safely applied 2 cm below the tumor.

An alternative method of sphincter preservation for very distal lesions is to approach the tumor from the perineum first. This technique allows complete mobilization of distal perirectal tissues without the "cone-down effect" that can occur when working in the distal pelvis via the abdomen (see the nonmucosectomy technique later).

If a "sufficient" margin cannot be obtained between the distal edge of the tumor and the upper part of the sphincter, but that a sufficient margin can be achieved between the distal edge of the tumor and the dentate line, an intersphincteric resection can be attempted. In such cases, it is impossible to apply a right-angled clamp below the lower border of the tumor, but with a rectal examination it can be perceived that a resection of part of the internal sphincter will allow a distal margin of 1 cm. The dissection can then be started in the abdomen by dividing the upper part of the internal sphincter from the levator ani. However, the main part of the dissection is performed during the perineal dissection.

HAND-SEWN COLONIC POUCH–ANAL ANASTOMOSIS

Mucosectomy of the Rectal Stump

If it is technically feasible, after full mobilization of the rectum and mesorectum, the muscular wall of the rectum is transected circumferentially at the level of the anorectal ring (Figure 169-6). The mucosa will be visible but should not be incised. If impossible, this will be performed via a perineal approach.

Transanal exposure is obtained with two Gelpi retractors applied perpendicular to each other on the external sphincter or with a Lone Star retractor. A solution of saline with epinephrine (1:1,000,000) is injected into the submucosa to balloon it up and float the mucosa away from the underlying muscle. A circumferential mucosectomy is then carried out from the dentate line up to the stapled-over end of the rectum (Figure 169-7). The specimen is then removed. Hemostasis of the muscular stump and the lower portion of the pelvis is easily achieved when the specimen has been removed and after irrigation with warm saline.

Nonmucosectomy Technique

The patient is put in the prone jackknife position and a Lone Star retractor is placed. The tumor or residual ulceration (after chemoradiotherapy) is palpated and a margin 2 cm distal to this point is marked with the cautery circumferentially. The most distal position that can be used is the dentate line. A full-thickness incision is made with the cautery through the internal sphincter into the intersphincteric plane and advanced circumferentially. The edges of the rectum (specimen side) are grasped with wide-mouthed Allis clamps. The dissection is continued proximally with blunt and sharp dissection in the intersphincteric plane to the distal part of the rectum with the help of small Deaver retractors (Figure 169-8). Once maximal length is achieved, the specimen side of the rectum is oversewn to prevent spillage of the tumor and stool. A sponge is inserted in the anal canal

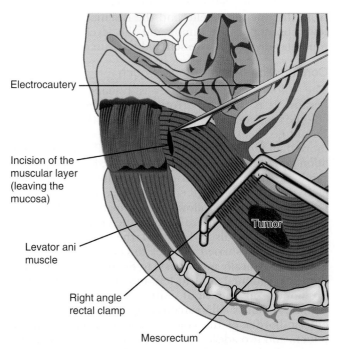

FIGURE 169-6 Hand-sewn coloanal anastomosis showing incision of the muscular layer of the rectum at the level of the levator ani muscle.

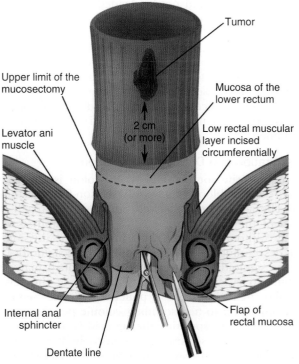

FIGURE 169-7 Mucosectomy of the rectal stump.

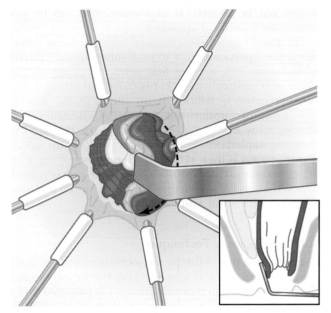

FIGURE 169-8 Preparation of the "intersphincteric space" is facilitated by assistance from the "abdominal surgeon." (From Schiessel R, Novi G, Holzer B, et al: Technique and long-term results of intersphincteric resection for low rectal cancer. *Dis Colon Rectum* 48:1858, 2005.)

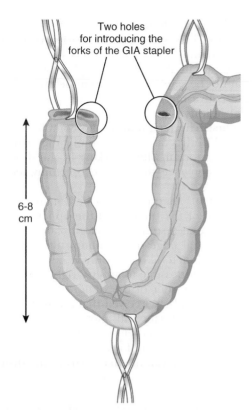

FIGURE 169-9 Preparation of the colonic J reservoir for a hand-sewn coloanal anastomosis.

and the patient is placed in the lithotomy position for the abdominal procedure.

Intersphincteric Dissection

As already described, transanal exposure is obtained with two Gelpi retractors applied perpendicular to each other on the external sphincter or with a Lone Star retractor. No saline solution should be used as the mucoa and muscular should not be divided. A circumferential division of the mucosa and internal sphincter is then carried out from the dentate line or the point considered to be at 1 cm below the lower border of the tumor. The anterior part of the dissection may represent a challenge, especially for the urethra in male patients. To facilitate such dissection, a rigid guide can be placed in the urethra. Once the abdominal dissection plan is found, the specimen can be mobilized through the abdomen.

Preparation and Division of the Colon

A suitable site for division of the colon is chosen to ensure a good blood supply and a tension-free anastomosis. The apex of the planned pouch should reach the level of the lower border of the pubic symphysis very easily without traction. The usual site for division is the descending colon just proximal to the sigmoid. Use of the sigmoid colon to construct the pouch may contribute to evacuatory problems because of the severe motility dysfunction of a pouched sigmoid segment in comparison to a descending colonic pouch.[17] Moreover, in Western societies, the sigmoid is often affected by diverticular disease or surrounded by fatty epiploic appendices, which may complicate pouch construction. In addition, the sigmoid colon may have been in the radiation field and therefore not be optimal for anastomosis; always try to use *nonirradiated* descending colon instead. The colon is divided after the application of a TA 55 stapling device, and the stapled end is oversewn with continuous 4-0 suture. The specimen is removed from the operative field, and the distance between the lower border of the tumor and the level of the distal muscular division is assessed and measured.

Construction of the Colonic Pouch

The colonic pouch for CAA is J shaped, principally because it is easy to perform. The optimal size for a colonic reservoir is not known. However, these reservoirs should be small, with each limb of the pouch being no more than 9 cm in length; otherwise, difficulty in evacuation and sometimes constipation occur. In a prospective randomized study, similar clinical results were obtained at 1 year with a small (5 cm) or a large (10 cm) pouch, but with long-term followup, constipation and evacuation problems were more likely in the group with a large reservoir.[18] The distal 15 cm of the colon is brought together in a J-shaped manner to construct the pouch. Each limb typically measures 6 to 8 cm. The descending limb is positioned on the left and the efferent limb is positioned on the right, with the mesentery placed behind. A pair of Allis forceps is applied on the antimesenteric border of the colon at the apex of the future pouch, and two additional Allis forceps are placed at the base of the pouch: one on the stapled end of the colon and the other on the descending limb of the pouch (Figure 169-9).

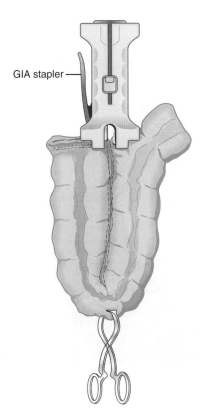

FIGURE 169-10 Creation of a colonic J pouch without apical colotomy.

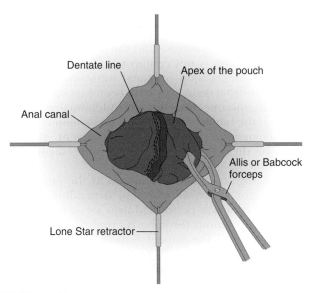

FIGURE 169-11 The apex of the pouch is drawn through the anus.

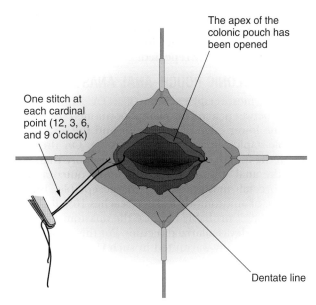

FIGURE 169-12 Hand-sewn coloanal anastomosis.

Two adjacent holes are made by stab puncture on the antimesenteric border of each limb of the pouch at an equal distance from the top, close to the Allis forceps. The two forks of a GIA stapler (50 or 90) are introduced into the lumen of the colon, each through one hole, toward the apex of the pouch (Figure 169-10).

Before firing, it is necessary to check that the mesocolon of the pouch is away from the stapler. The bowel is then everted to expose the remaining bridge, which is divided by application of a GIA 50 stapler. The pouch is inverted, the Allis forceps are removed, and the hole is closed with continuous 4-0 polyglycolic acid suture. In this manner, the pouch is totally closed with no risk for septic contamination of the pelvis during its descent to the anal canal. Moreover, the size of the hole that will be made at the apex of the pouch for the anastomosis will be chosen to exactly fit the diameter of the anal canal.

Coloanal Anastomosis

The apex of the pouch is brought to the anus with a Babcock forceps introduced through the anal stump (Figure 169-11). During this maneuver, care should be taken to not twist the colon around its mesentery. To facilitate descent of the pouch, the genitourinary organs should be lifted with a hand or retractor, and the pouch should be gently pushed from above.

The pouch is then anchored to the anal sphincter with four stitches of absorbable suture, each at one cardinal point just above the mucosal section. The apex of the pouch is then opened, and the mucosa of the anal canal is anastomosed to the full thickness of the colon with the use of interrupted 4-0 polyglycolic acid suture (Figure 169-12).

Four stitches are initially placed at 3, 6, 9, and 12 o'clock, and then an additional one or two stitches are added to each of the quadrants thus formed. The perianal retractors are removed, and a small drain is inserted through the anastomosis into the reservoir and will be left in place for 24 to 48 hours to reveal any bleeding in the pouch, obviate the risk for pouch distention by blood clots, and facilitate treatment of such hemorrhage by saline irrigation.

Drainage, Loop Stoma, and Postoperative Care

Two multiperforated closed-suction drains are usually placed in the pelvis posterior and anterior to the pouch. We strongly advocate routine construction of a diverting stoma simply because anastomotic leakage after total mesorectal excision and an ultralow anastomosis causes dramatic complications.[14,19,20] We usually prefer a loop ileostomy over a colostomy because there is no risk of traction on the anastomosis and the blood supply to the descending colon is not compromised. However, some surgeons prefer a loop proximal transverse colostomy because the distal ileum may have been exposed to radiation during preoperative therapy. Additionally, prior to closure, if the mobilized colon and mesocolon compress the duodenojejunal junction, the ligament of Treitz should be divided to avoid postoperative small bowel obstruction.

The nasogastric tube is removed at the end of the procedure or the next morning, depending on how much dissection was performed near the stomach. Appropriate deep venous thrombosis prophylaxis should be maintained until the patient is fully ambulatory. The urinary catheter is generally removed on the third postoperative day. The pelvic suction drains are removed 24 to 48 hours after surgery.

The stoma is closed in 6 to 8 weeks and after a water-soluble contrast study performed through the efferent limb of the stoma has shown satisfactory healing of the pouch and the anastomosis. If a leak is observed, the stoma should be left in place for an additional few weeks and the contrast study repeated.

STAPLED COLONIC POUCH–ANAL ANASTOMOSIS

After total mesorectal excision, if a TA stapler can be applied between a rectal clamp positioned 1 or 2 cm below the lower edge of the tumor and the levator ani, a double-stapled anastomosis is possible. On the other hand, if the length of the rectal stump is more than 3 cm above the anal sphincter, the functional outcome after low colorectal anastomosis will be acceptable, but the incidence of anastomotic leakage reaches 10% to 15% in most series,[19,21] probably because the anastomosis is performed on a devascularized rectum. For this reason, fecal diversion is usually warranted in such cases.

Division of the Rectum

A right-angled rectal clamp is applied below the lower edge of the tumor (Figure 169-13). The lower portion of the rectum is washed with a povidone-iodine solution. Though not proven, this may be helpful in decreasing the risk for anastomotic recurrence as a result of viable tumor cells being trapped within the stapled line. The rectal clamp is used to horizontally align the rectum and facilitate positioning of a terminal anastomosis stapling device (TA 30 or 55, Roticulator 55 or 30) or linear stapler (Tx or Contour) on the lower part of the rectum at the level of the levator ani. On closing the instrument before firing, care must be taken to include only the rectum (and nothing else) within the stapler. After firing, the rectum is divided, the specimen is removed from the pelvis, and the distal margin on the specimen is assessed.

Construction of the Pouch

The colon is divided at the junction of the descending and sigmoid colon after the application of a TA 55 stapling device, and the stapled end is oversewn with continuous 4-0 suture. Six to 9 cm proximal to the colonic end, a 1-cm opening is created on the antimesenteric

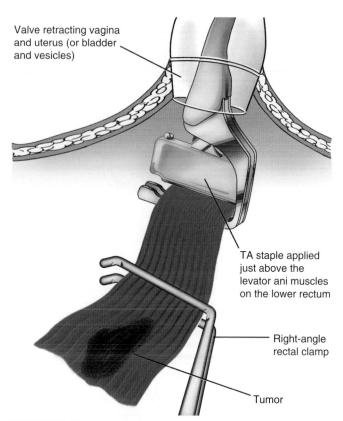

Valve retracting vagina and uterus (or bladder and vesicles)

TA staple applied just above the levator ani muscles on the lower rectum

Right-angle rectal clamp

Tumor

FIGURE 169-13 Double-stapled coloanal anastomosis. A TA stapler is applied at least 2 cm below the lower edge of the tumor, at the level of the levator ani muscle.

border of the colon. The forks of a GIA 50 or 90 stapler are inserted into each limb, and a stapled side-to-side anastomosis is performed between the two limbs to create the pouch (Figure 169-14).

A simple over-and-over continuous purse-string suture of 0 or 2-0 nylon or polypropylene (Prolene) is placed around the hole where the GIA stapler was inserted. The anvil of a circular stapler (EEA 28/31 or ILS 29/33) is disconnected from the stapler and introduced into the hole, and the purse-string suture is tightened.

Coloanal Anastomosis

The body of the circular stapler is introduced into the anus, aided by lubricant and the assistant's fingers. The spindle is slowly advanced and should perforate the rectal wall just posterior to the linear TA stapled line. The two halves of the stapler (anvil and body) are approximated (Figure 169-15) and the instrument is closed, with great care taken to not catch adjacent structures such as the posterior wall of the vagina or the seminal vesicles. The gun is fired when the gap is within the recommendations. The stapler is carefully removed and the rings are checked. They should be identified from both the rectal and the colonic sides. The distal (anorectal) ring should be sent for pathologic examination. If both anastomotic rings are intact, it is not necessary to test the anastomosis because the fecal stream will be diverted regardless. If either ring is incomplete, proctoscopy should be performed to determine whether sutures are required to close a significant defect.

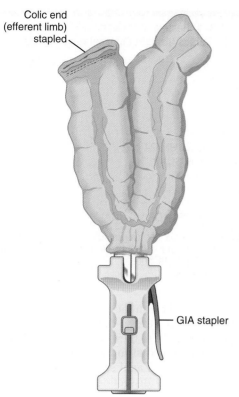

FIGURE 169-14 Double-stapled coloanal anastomosis: preparation of the colonic J pouch.

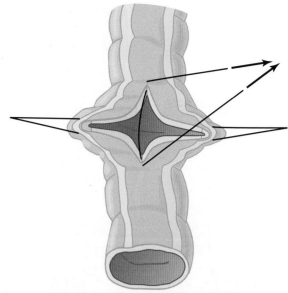

FIGURE 169-16 Stay sutures are placed midway between the colotomy on each side so that the longitudinal opening can be closed in transverse fashion. The next suture is a seromuscular stitch placed in the middle to line up the closure. This middle suture is not tied until the remainder of the row is placed. Next, starting at each end and working toward the middle, seromuscular sutures of 2-0 polyglycolic acid are placed to close the colotomy. (From Fazio VW, Mantyh CR, Hull TL: Colonic "coloplasty": Novel technique to enhance low colorectal or coloanal anastomosis. *Dis Colon Rectum* 43:1448, 2000.)

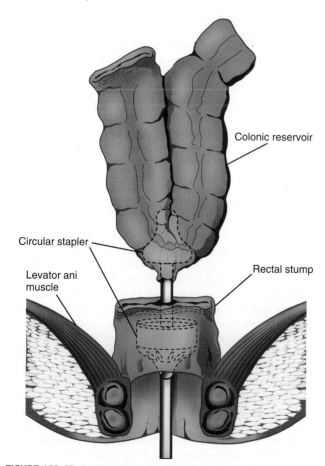

FIGURE 169-15 Double-stapled coloanal anastomosis with a colonic J pouch.

Drainage, stoma, and postoperative care are similar to those for a hand-sewn anastomosis. A randomized study has compared 20 patients with stapled J-pouch anastomoses to 17 patients with hand-sewn J-pouch anastomoses and demonstrated that the stapled coloanal anastomosis was significantly faster than hand-sewn anastomosis and has similar functional results.[22]

Transverse Coloplasty

There are several circumstances in which a colonic pouch cannot be constructed, including a narrow pelvis, severe diverticulosis, inadequate colonic length, and sometimes metastatic disease or other technical problems.[23] An alternative method was devised by Fazio et al[24] in which a reservoir is created just proximal to the anastomosis by adapting the Heineke-Mikulicz strictureplasty technique used for the small bowel (Figure 169-16). The colotomy can be closed with either sutures or a stapler. Functional results have been similar to those of the colonic J pouch.[25,26] Technically, the reservoir is easier to construct and is less bulky than the colonic J pouch.

Side-to-End Anastomosis

An alternative to the J pouch is the side-to-end coloanal anastomosis.[27,28] This technique is easier than the J pouch and can be performed with a circular stapling device or manually. After TME, the anvil of the circular stapler is placed 3 to 4 cm from the end of the divided bowel. A circular stapler is then introduced through the anus and fired to create the anastomosis.

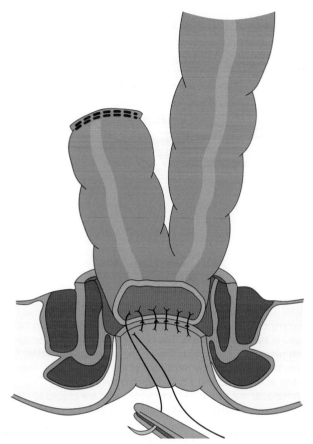

FIGURE 169-17 Side-to-end hand-sewn coloanal anastomosis.

In case of mucosectomy and transanal approach, the colon is pulled through the anus and a stitch is placed 4 cm from the end of the colon with a long remaining thread. The colon is then pushed into the abdominal cavity and by pulling on the string, the colon is positioned correctly to perform a side-to end anastomosis manually as previously described (Figure 169-17).

Laparoscopy

Laparoscopic surgery for rectal cancer is now gaining acceptance among many U.S. surgeons. It has been embraced by European surgeons for the past decade. A randomized study, the CLASICC trial, has reported results after 3 years of followup showing no differences in terms of oncologic results, whereas in the first report more tears of the mesorectum were observed after laparoscopic dissection.[29,30] Moreover, although a number of studies have reported that laparoscopic proctectomy is safe and even provides good functional and oncologic results,[31-35] the American Society of Colon and Rectal Surgeons in its recently revised practice parameters[36] has not endorsed the use of laparoscopy for rectal cancer at this time.

FUNCTIONAL RESULTS

Complete rectal excision followed by reconstruction with an ultralow colorectal anastomosis or a straight CAA results in a greatly reduced reservoir capacity and an alteration in the continence mechanism. The association

BOX 169-1 Results of Metaanalysis of Colonic Reservoirs Versus Straight Coloanal Anastomosis

No. of studies	35
No. of patients	2240
SCA	1066
JP	1050
CP	124
Complications	No difference
No. less frequent BM/24 hr (JP + CP versus SCA)	
6 mo	1.88
1 yr	1.35
2 yr	0.74
Fecal urgency (JP + CP vs. SCA)	Less prevalent

From Heriot AG, Tekkis PP, Constantinides V, et al: Meta-analysis of colonic reservoirs versus straight coloanal anastomosis after anterior resection. *Br J Surg* 93:19, 2006.
BM, Bowel movement; *CP,* coloplasty; *JP,* J pouch; *SCA,* straight coloanal.

of increased bowel frequency, urgency of defecation, and minor fecal leakage (the so-called anterior resection syndrome) is seen in 5% to 60% of patients.[7,37-39] The mechanism underlying this dysfunction is complex but involves a decrease in internal anal sphincter tone secondary to the trauma of pelvic dissection and anal dilation and a loss of the rectal reservoir. A colonic pouch may increase reservoir capacity and act as a pressure relief in which the high intraluminal pressure generated within the relatively noncompliant colon is dissipated before it reaches the anal canal.

The functional outcome after a colon pouch–anal anastomosis has been shown to be superior to that of a straight CAA or an ultralow CAA. Earliest reports[8,9] were confirmed in initial randomized trials.[11,13,14,40] A metaanalysis has compared the functional results of 2240 patients from the collected series (Box 169-1).[41] A reduction in bowel frequency and a decreased incidence of urgency are observed in all studies. The functional results of colon pouch–anal anastomosis are comparable to those obtained with a low colorectal anastomosis.[42,43] The functional superiority of the colonic J pouch is greatest within the first year after surgery[44] but is still sustained over the long term.[42,45]

The major drawback of the pouch is fecal retention secondary to poor evacuation. In our series,[9,46] this was observed in 20% of patients; these patients required enemas or suppositories to defecate. The combination of smaller J pouches (5 rather than 10 cm long) constructed from the descending rather than the sigmoid colon may help overcome these problems.[18]

A recent randomized multicenter trial has compared the functional issues of the three types of anastomosis (straight CAA, J pouch, and coloplasty).[47] After anterior resection, patients were grouped to either a J pouch–eligible group or a J pouch–ineligible group. In the J pouch–eligible group, patients were randomized to receive either a J pouch of 5 cm or a coloplasty (CP-1) and those not eligible for a J pouch were randomized to receive either a coloplasty (CP-2) or a straight CAA. Two hundred ninety-seven patients were included and evaluated in the study (115 J pouch, 109 CP-1, 35 straight

CAA, and 38 CP-2). An improvement in the number of total daily bowel movements was observed from 4 months to 24 months after surgery in all of the four groups. The J pouch group had a significantly lower number of total daily movements compared with CP-1 (2 [2-3] vs. 3 [2-4], $P = 0.007$). The CP-2 group had a similar result as the straight CAA group ($P = 0.94$). Patients with a J pouch also wore fewer pads than patients with a CP-1 (54% vs. 70%, $P = 0.02$). Finally, the J pouch reduced significantly the number of clustering episodes when compared with a coloplasty ($P < 0.03$). The comparison of a coloplasty (CP-2) with a straight CAA did not reveal any differences between procedures. The authors concluded that for a patient who was eligible to receive a J pouch, this procedure should be preferred to coloplasty. For patients who cannot have a pouch, coloplasty seemed not to improve the bowel function over that with a straight CAA.[47] A subanalysis of these four groups to determine the influence of preoperative radiotherapy (PRT) was also performed.[48] Two hundred eleven patients with PRT were compared to 153 nonirradiated patients. Radiotherapy had no influence on surgical morbidity, on the rate of anastomotic leakage, or on the global morbidity rate. Global bowel function was evaluated in 297 patients. The analysis of the impact of both the PRT and the reconstruction technique (J pouch vs. coloplasty) showed that patients with a J pouch had better results in the number of bowel movements at 4, 12, and 24 months (2.5 ± 1.3 vs. 4.2 ± 4.9 at 24 months, $P = 0.011$), in the frequency of urgency at 24 months ($P < 0.001$), in the use of pads at 24 months ($P = 0.006$), and in the use of antidiarrheal drugs at 24 months ($P = 0.006$). These results confirm the beneficial effect of the J pouch, especially for patients with a rectal cancer treated with neoadjuvant radiotherapy.

Concerning the side-to-end anastomosis (STE CAA), a prospective randomized trial has compared 50 patients with a J pouch to 50 patients with an STE CAA.[28] The functional results were similar (incontinence score, number of bowel movements, drug use, pad, etc.). At 12 months, there was, however, a tendency toward worse results in the group with a side-to-end anastomosis (lower rate of patients able to defer defecation more than 30 minutes (47% vs. 68%, $P = 0.052$), more patients with anal burning (16% vs. 5%, $P = 0.09$), and more patients feeling that bowel function adversely affects daily life (30% vs. 16%, $P = 0.13$).

Finally, intersphincteric resections (IRS) have been studied by our group with a retrospective study of 83 patients.[49] The mean number of bowel movements per day was 2.3 ± 1.3, 29% had nocturnal defecation, and 46% wore protective pads. Using the Wexner score, 41% of patients were fully continent (score = 0) and 24% were incontinent with a mean score of 15. In multivariate analysis, the only influencing factor on continence was the use of preoperative radiotherapy.

CONCLUSION

Low anterior resection with total mesorectal excision and CAA eradicates low rectal cancers while preserving sphincter function and providing oncologic results similar to those of APR and low anterior colorectal anastomosis. The functional results of straight CAA are far from perfect, particularly in terms of bowel frequency and urgency. The addition of a colonic reservoir or coloplasty markedly decreases the frequency of defecation without increasing morbidity and should therefore be the option of choice. The long-term results of colon pouch–anal anastomosis are good, but spontaneous evacuation continues to be a problem that may alter quality of life.

REFERENCES

1. Parks AG: Transanal technique in low rectal anastomosis. *Proc R Soc Med* 65:975, 1972.
2. Quirke P, Durdey P, Dixon MF, et al: Local recurrence of rectal adenocarcinoma due to inadequate surgical resection. Histopathological study of lateral tumour spread and surgical excision. *Lancet* 2:996, 1986.
3. Shirouzu K, Isomoto H, Kakegawa T: Distal spread of rectal cancer and optimal distal margin of resection for sphincter-preserving surgery. *Cancer* 76:388, 1995.
4. Williams NS: The rationale for preservation of the anal sphincter in patients with low rectal cancer. *Br J Surg* 71:575, 1984.
5. Schiessel R, Novi G, Holzer B, et al: Technique and long-term results of intersphincteric resection for low rectal cancer. *Dis Colon Rectum* 48:1858; discussion 1865, 2005.
6. Schiessel R, Rosen HR: Preservation and restoration of sphincter function in patients with rectal cancer. *Can J Gastroenterol* 14:423, 2000.
7. Paty PB, Enker WE, Cohen AM, et al: Long-term functional results of coloanal anastomosis for rectal cancer. *Am J Surg* 167:90; discussion 94, 1994.
8. Parc R, Tiret E, Frileux P, et al: Resection and colo-anal anastomosis with colonic reservoir for rectal carcinoma. *Br J Surg* 73:139, 1986.
9. Lazorthes F, Fages P, Chiotasso P, et al: Resection of the rectum with construction of a colonic reservoir and colo-anal anastomosis for carcinoma of the rectum. *Br J Surg* 73:136, 1986.
10. Nicholls RJ, Lubowski DZ, Donaldson DR: Comparison of colonic reservoir and straight colo-anal reconstruction after rectal excision. *Br J Surg* 75:318, 1988.
11. Seow-Choen F, Goh HS: Prospective randomized trial comparing J colonic pouch-anal anastomosis and straight coloanal reconstruction. *Br J Surg* 82:608, 1995.
12. Ortiz H, De Miguel M, Armendariz P, et al: Coloanal anastomosis: Are functional results better with a pouch? *Dis Colon Rectum* 38:375, 1995.
13. Kusunoki M, Shoji Y, Yanagi H, et al: Function after anoabdominal rectal resection and colonic J pouch–anal anastomosis. *Br J Surg* 78:1434, 1991.
14. Hallbook O, Pahlman L, Krog M, et al: Randomized comparison of straight and colonic J pouch anastomosis after low anterior resection. *Ann Surg* 224:58, 1996.
15. Ho YH, Tan M, Seow-Choen F: Prospective randomized controlled study of clinical function and anorectal physiology after low anterior resection: Comparison of straight and colonic J pouch anastomoses. *Br J Surg* 83:978, 1996.
16. Morino M, Allaix ME, Giraudo G, et al: Laparoscopic versus open surgery for extraperitoneal rectal cancer: A prospective comparative study. *Surg Endosc* 19:1460, 2005.
17. Seow-Choen F: Colonic pouches in the treatment of low rectal cancer. *Br J Surg* 83:881, 1996.
18. Lazorthes F, Gamagami R, Chiotasso P, et al: Prospective, randomized study comparing clinical results between small and large colonic J-pouch following coloanal anastomosis. *Dis Colon Rectum* 40:1409, 1997.
19. Karanjia ND, Corder AP, Bearn P, et al: Leakage from stapled low anastomosis after total mesorectal excision for carcinoma of the rectum. *Br J Surg* 81:1224, 1994.
20. Matthiessen P, Hallbook O, Rutegard J, et al: Defunctioning stoma reduces symptomatic anastomotic leakage after low anterior

resection of the rectum for cancer: A randomized multicenter trial. *Ann Surg* 246:207, 2007.

21. Dehni N, Schlegel RD, Cunningham C, et al: Influence of a defunctioning stoma on leakage rates after low colorectal anastomosis and colonic J pouch-anal anastomosis. *Br J Surg* 85:1114, 1998.

22. Laurent A, Parc Y, McNamara D, et al: Colonic J-pouch-anal anastomosis for rectal cancer: A prospective, randomized study comparing handsewn vs. stapled anastomosis. *Dis Colon Rectum* 48:729, 2005.

23. Harris GJ, Lavery IJ, Fazio VW: Reasons for failure to construct the colonic J-pouch. What can be done to improve the size of the neorectal reservoir should it occur? *Dis Colon Rectum* 45:1304, 2002.

24. Fazio VW, Mantyh CR, Hull TL: Colonic "coloplasty": Novel technique to enhance low colorectal or coloanal anastomosis. *Dis Colon Rectum* 43:1448, 2000.

25. Mantyh CR, Hull TL, Fazio VW: Coloplasty in low colorectal anastomosis: Manometric and functional comparison with straight and colonic J-pouch anastomosis. *Dis Colon Rectum* 44:37, 2001.

26. Ulrich A, Z'Graggen K, Schmitz-Winnenthal H, et al: The transverse coloplasty pouch. *Langenbecks Arch Surg* 390:355, 2005.

27. Machado M, Nygren J, Goldman S, et al: Functional and physiologic assessment of the colonic reservoir or side-to-end anastomosis after low anterior resection for rectal cancer: A two-year follow-up. *Dis Colon Rectum* 48:29, 2005.

28. Machado M, Nygren J, Goldman S, et al: Similar outcome after colonic pouch and side-to-end anastomosis in low anterior resection for rectal cancer: A prospective randomized trial. *Ann Surg* 238:214, 2003.

29. Guillou PJ, Quirke P, Thorpe H, et al: Short-term endpoints of conventional versus laparoscopic-assisted surgery in patients with colorectal cancer (MRC CLASICC trial): Multicentre, randomised controlled trial. *Lancet* 365:1718, 2005.

30. Jayne DG, Guillou PJ, Thorpe H, et al: Randomized trial of laparoscopic-assisted resection of colorectal carcinoma: 3-year results of the UK MRC CLASICC Trial Group. *J Clin Oncol* 25:3061, 2007.

31. Dulucq JL, Wintringer P, Stabilini C, et al: Laparoscopic rectal resection with anal sphincter preservation for rectal cancer: Long-term outcome. *Surg Endosc* 19:1468, 2005.

32. Barlehner E, Benhidjeb T, Anders S, et al: Laparoscopic resection for rectal cancer: Outcomes in 194 patients and review of the literature. *Surg Endosc* 19:757, 2005.

33. Tsang WW, Chung CC, Li MK: Prospective evaluation of laparoscopic total mesorectal excision with colonic J-pouch reconstruction for mid and low rectal cancers. *Br J Surg* 90:867, 2003.

34. Rullier E, Sa Cunha A, Couderc P, et al: Laparoscopic intersphincteric resection with coloplasty and coloanal anastomosis for mid and low rectal cancer. *Br J Surg* 90:445, 2003.

35. Lujan J, Valero G, Hernandez Q, et al: Randomized clinical trial comparing laparoscopic and open surgery in patients with rectal cancer. *Br J Surg* 96:982, 2009.

36. Tjandra JJ, Kilkenny JW, Buie WD, et al: Practice parameters for the management of rectal cancer (revised). *Dis Colon Rectum* 48:411, 2005.

37. Karanjia ND, Schache DJ, Heald RJ: Function of the distal rectum after low anterior resection for carcinoma. *Br J Surg* 79:114, 1992.

38. Miller AS, Lewis WG, Williamson ME, et al: Factors that influence functional outcome after coloanal anastomosis for carcinoma of the rectum. *Br J Surg* 82:1327, 1995.

39. Lewis WG, Holdsworth PJ, Stephenson BM, et al: Role of the rectum in the physiological and clinical results of coloanal and colorectal anastomosis after anterior resection for rectal carcinoma. *Br J Surg* 79:1082, 1992.

40. Sailer M, Fuchs KH, Fein M, et al: Randomized clinical trial comparing quality of life after straight and pouch coloanal reconstruction. *Br J Surg* 89:1108, 2002.

41. Heriot AG, Tekkis PP, Constantinides V, et al: Meta-analysis of colonic reservoirs versus straight coloanal anastomosis after anterior resection. *Br J Surg* 93:19, 2006.

42. Dehni N, Tiret E, Singland JD, et al: Long-term functional outcome after low anterior resection: Comparison of low colorectal anastomosis and colonic J-pouch-anal anastomosis. *Dis Colon Rectum* 41:817; discussion 822, 1998.

43. Benoist S, Panis Y, Boleslawski E, et al: Functional outcome after coloanal versus low colorectal anastomosis for rectal carcinoma. *J Am Coll Surg* 185:114, 1997.

44. Joo JS, Latulippe JF, Alabaz O, et al: Long-term functional evaluation of straight coloanal anastomosis and colonic J-pouch: Is the functional superiority of colonic J-pouch sustained? *Dis Colon Rectum* 41:740, 1998.

45. Lazorthes F, Chiotasso P, Gamagami RA, et al: Late clinical outcome in a randomized prospective comparison of colonic J pouch and straight coloanal anastomosis. *Br J Surg* 84:1449, 1997.

46. Berger A, Tiret E, Parc R, et al: Excision of the rectum with colonic J pouch-anal anastomosis for adenocarcinoma of the low and mid rectum. *World J Surg* 16:470, 1992.

47. Fazio VW, Zutshi M, Remzi FH, et al: A randomized multicenter trial to compare long-term functional outcome, quality of life, and complications of surgical procedures for low rectal cancers. *Ann Surg* 246:481; discussion 488, 2007.

48. Parc Y, Zutshi M, Zalinski S, et al: Preoperative radiotherapy is associated with worse functional results after coloanal anastomosis for rectal cancer. *Dis Colon Rectum* 52:2004, 2009.

49. Chamlou R, Parc Y, Simon T, et al: Long-term results of intersphincteric resection for low rectal cancer. *Ann Surg* 246:916; discussion 921, 2007.

Recurrent and Metastatic Colorectal Cancer

Kellie L. Mathis | Heidi Nelson

Proper surgery and the administration of adjuvant and neoadjuvant therapies of colon and rectal cancers aim to minimize the risk of development of locally recurrent or metastatic disease. Despite best efforts, relapse of disease still occurs in significant numbers of patients (30% to 50%). Historically, the presence of either locally recurrent or metastatic disease signified an incurable condition. Increasingly, it is recognized that focal relapses can be managed surgically with curative intent. Early detection of disease relapse with appropriate postoperative surveillance programs can identify treatable recurrences, thereby increasing rates of secondary cures. Focal recurrences involving the liver, lung, and locoregional recurrences have the greatest potential for cure if localized and of limited extent at the time of presentation. The discussion of the management of liver metastases from colorectal cancer is outlined in Chapter 171. Therefore, the focus of this chapter is on the detection and management of locoregional and pulmonary recurrences after the treatment of primary colorectal cancer.

TUMOR RELAPSE

INCIDENCE OF RECURRENT DISEASE

According to data from the Surveillance Epidemiology and End Results (SEER) project from 1999 to 2006, 5-year overall survival across all colorectal cancer stages is 65%. It varies from 90% in patients with localized (stage I to II) disease to 69.5% for those with disease that has spread to the lymph nodes (stage III).[1] In a population-based study of 2657 patients by Manfredi et al, the incidence of any recurrence after curative resection for colon cancer was 9.9% at 1 year, 26.2% at 3 years, and 31.5% at 5 years. Five-year recurrence rates ranged from 9.3% for stage I tumors to 56.1% for stage III disease. Locoregional recurrence occurred in 12.8% of patients at 5 years, and distant metastases occurred in 26% of patients at 5 years. Distant sites of disease included the liver in 45%, lung in 10%, brain in 2%, bone in 2%, and other sites in 4%. Multiple organs were involved in 19% of patients with distant metastases.[2] In a similar population-based study during the same time period, the author group reported the incidence of local recurrence after curative resection for rectal cancer (682 patients) as 9.1% at 1 year and 22.7% at 5 years. The 5-year local recurrence rate was 10% for stage I cancer and 41% for stage III.[3] The likelihood of relapse was historically believed to be highest within the first 2 years after resection, but recent reports suggest that the median time to recurrence is increasing, especially for rectal cancers,[4,5] and surveillance beyond 5 years may be necessary.

FACTORS THAT INFLUENCE RECURRENCE

A large number of risk factors have been associated with relapse of colorectal cancer, including tumor-related and technical factors (Box 170-1).

Tumor Stage

The extent of disease, or tumor stage, is to date the single most important factor that predicts relapse and survival. The American Joint Committee on Cancer (AJCC) Colorectal Cancer Staging system is shown in Box 170-2, and survival by TN categorization is shown in Table 170-1. The risk of local recurrence is increased when the tumor has invaded beyond the confines of the bowel wall (T3 to T4) or involves nodes (N+) and is highest in patients with both.[6]

Other Tumor-Related Factors

Certain histologic features have been correlated with aggressive behavior, including poor tumor differentiation, mucin production, and venous or lymphatic invasion. Involvement of circumferential margins of resection is also prognostic for both rectal and colon carcinoma.[7] Other poor-risk indicators include bowel obstruction, perforation, and tumor adherence to other local organs.[6,8]

Molecular Features

Many molecular markers have also been found to predict aggressive tumor behavior; these include aneuploidy, the presence of mutant p53, and loss of heterozygosity at chromosome 18q. High microsatellite instability phenotype, which is present in approximately 20% of colorectal carcinomas, has been associated with improved prognosis. Conversely, the presence of low microsatellite instability has been associated with a worse prognosis.[9-12]

Technical Factors

Although tumor-related factors remain the main determinants of prognosis for colon carcinoma, technical factors also influence rates of both local recurrence and overall survival for patients with rectal carcinoma. Local recurrence rates after rectal cancer resections range from 4% to 40%,[3,13] which is at least partially dependent on the individual operating surgeon.[6,13] Some authors have shown increased local recurrence rates in tumors in the distal rectum, possibly related to increased technical difficulty. At a minimum, it is evident that wide anatomic resection of the tumor—in all dimensions, including mesorectal, radial (circumferential), distal bowel, and en bloc resection of adherent organs—is critical.

In 2000, a consensus panel was convened to discuss surgical guidelines for colon and rectal cancer in order to bring together the best evidence to balance oncologic results with functional outcomes. The summary of their recommendations is shown in Table 170-2. All margins should be negative. For rectal cancers, a minimum distal margin of 2 cm is ideal and a margin of more than 1 cm is acceptable where the tumor is not locally advanced and abdominoperineal resection (APR) is the only alternative. Circumferential margins should be as wide as possible, ideally greater than 2 mm. Bowel margins of at least 5 cm proximally and distally are considered standard for colon cancers, and lymphadenectomy to the origin of the primary feeding vessel is considered appropriate.[14]

Of all the surgical techniques reviewed and considered significant, none has received more attention than the concept of mesorectal clearance.[15] In Scandinavian countries, the implementation of appropriate mesenteric clearance, referred to as *total mesorectal excision* (TME), has reduced local recurrence rates and improved survival.[16] In all cases, sharp dissection should be performed in the areolar tissue behind the mesentery, just in front of the sacrum and particularly at the level of Waldeyer fascia. The fascia propria should be removed intact with proper rectal dissection. Therefore, a total mesorectal excision is advised for all cancers of the distal rectum for which APR or low anterior resection and coloanal anastomosis are planned. In the management of more proximal rectal cancers, it seems reasonable to use a margin of approximately 4 cm of distal mesorectum as a benchmark,[14] because tumor deposits in the mesorectum are rarely reported 4 cm beyond the tumor. Despite optimization of surgical techniques, adjuvant radiation treatment remains an independent factor reducing the incidence of local relapse.[17]

DETECTION OF RELAPSES

Key to the detection of relapses is the implementation of surveillance guidelines. Detection of recurrent disease is the first step; confirmatory tests are then used to delineate the extent of disease and the suitability for resection and adjuvant therapies.

BOX 170-1 Factors Associated With a High Risk of Relapse for Colorectal Cancer

TUMOR FACTORS
Disease stage
High-grade tumor (poorly differentiated)
Tumor location
Obstruction/perforation
Venous invasion
Perineural invasion
Mucin production
Diminished stromal immune reaction
Aneuploidy
Mutant *p53* gene expression
Low microsatellite instability

TECHNICAL FACTORS
Inadequate resection margins (radial, distal, mesorectal)
Implantation of exfoliated cells
Tumor location (tumors in pelvis and splenic flexure are anatomically and technically more difficult)

BOX 170-2 Pathologic TNM Staging Nomenclature

PRIMARY TUMOR (T)

Tx	Primary tumor cannot be assessed
T0	No evidence of primary tumor
Tis	Carcinoma in situ: intraepithelial or invasion of lamina propria
T1	Tumor invades submucosa
T2	Tumor invades muscularis propria
T3	Tumor invades through the muscularis propria into the subserosa or into nonperitonealized pericolic or perirectal tissues
T4a	Tumor penetrates the surface of the visceral peritoneum
T4b	Tumor directly invades or is histologically adherent to other organs or structures

REGIONAL LYMPH NODES (N)

Nx	Regional lymph nodes cannot be assessed
N0	No regional lymph node metastasis
N1a	Metastasis in 1 regional lymph nodes
N1b	Metastasis in 2 to 3 regional lymph nodes
N1c	Extranodal cancer cell deposits
N2a	Metastasis in 4 to 6 regional lymph nodes
N2b	Metastasis in 7 or more regional lymph nodes

DISTANT METASTASIS (M)

Mx	Distant metastases cannot be assessed
M0	No distant metastasis
M1a	Distant metastasis to 1 site
M1b	Distant metastasis to more than 1 site

AJCC STAGE GROUPINGS

Stage 0	Tis, N0, M0
Stage I	T1, N0, M0
	T2, N0, M0
Stage IIA	T3, N0, M0
Stage IIB	T4a, N0, M0
Stage IIIA	T1, N1, M0
	T2, N1, M0
	T1, N2a, M0
Stage IIIB	T3, N1, M0
	T4a, N1, M0
	T2, N2a, M0
	T3, N2a, M0
	T1, N2b, M0
	T2, N2b, M0
Stage IIIC	T4a, N2a, M0
	T3, N2b, M0
	T4a, N2b, M0
	T4b, N1, M0
	T4b, N2, M0
Stage IVA	Any T, Any N, M1a
Stage IVB	Any T, Any N, M1b

Used with the permission of the American Joint Committee on Cancer, Chicago, Illinois. The original source for this material is the *Cancer Staging Manual, Seventh Edition.*

TABLE 170-1 Observed 5-Year Survival by TN Category, Using SEER Reports

Stage	OBSERVED 5-YEAR SURVIVAL (%)	
	Rectum	Colon
T1N0	82	80
T2N0	78	76
T3N0	66	68
T4aN0	56	62
T4bN0	46	48
T1-2N1	70	72
T1N2a	72	64
T2N2a	58	64
T3N1a	56	58
T4aN1a	54	52
T3N1b	50	52
T1N2b	54	52
T4aN2a	46	44
T4aN1b	46	44
T23N2a	44	44
T2bN2b	42	52
T3N2b	32	30
T4N2b	24	16
T4bN1	24	26
T4bN2a	16	16
T4bN2b	12	14

Data from Gunderson LL, Jessup JM, Sargent DJ, et al: Revised TN categorization for colon cancer based on national survival outcomes data. *J Clin Oncol* 28:264, 2010.

SURVEILLANCE GUIDELINES

A 2007 Cochrane review of eight randomized trials that investigated the impact of intensive surveillance strategies confirmed a significant survival advantage at 5 years in patients participating in more intensive surveillance after curative resection of colorectal cancer. Moreover, the group with more intensive followup had more frequent operations with curative intent as well.[18] Additional metaanalyses of these trials have confirmed reduction in death rates and in some cases cost-effectiveness of intensive surveillance strategies.[18,19] Unfortunately, each of the surveillance strategies within the eight trials was unique, and it is not clear which specific component(s) of the proposed surveillance programs is most responsible for improving survival. Several cancer and specialty societies, including the American Society of Colon and Rectal Surgeons (ASCRS), the American Society of Clinical Oncology (ASCO), and the National Cancer Comprehensive Network (NCCN) have published guidelines for surveillance strategies (Table 170-3).[19-21] Each strategy is unique, but there are several generalities among the ASCO and NCCN guidelines, including frequent examinations with CEA measurement, annual chest and abdominal CT scans for 3 years, and colonoscopy. The ASCRS guidelines do not recommend routine chest and abdominal imaging, but given the recent Cochrane review, they will likely be updated to include these studies in the future.

History and Physical Examination

Symptoms of recurrence might include abdominal, pelvic, perineal, or sciatic pain; change in bowel habits; obstruction; anorexia; weight loss; malaise; and rectal

TABLE 170-2 Summary of Surgical Guidelines for Treatment of Colon and Rectal Cancer

Location of Cancer	Surgical Guideline and Grade of Recommendation
Colon	Lymphadenectomy should extend to the level of the origin of the primary feeding vessel; suspected positive lymph nodes outside the standard resection should be removed when feasible (grade C).
	Bowel margins ≥5 cm proximally and distally should be used (grade D).
	Laparoscopic colectomy for cancer should be confined to clinical trials (grade D). We suggest newer guidelines would accept laparoscopic colectomy as an alternative option with grade A evidence.
Rectum	The ideal bowel margin is ≥2 cm distally and ≥5 cm proximally, measured fresh with the use of full thickness; the minimally acceptable distal margin for sphincter preservation is 1 cm (grade B).
	Lymphovascular resection of the rectum should include a wide anatomic resection of the mesorectum, including the mesorectal fascia propria and ≥4 cm of clearance distal to the tumor and proximal ligation of the primary feeding vessel (grade C).
	Extended lateral lymphatic dissection cannot be supported on current evidence (grade C).
	Length of bowel cannot be supported as an important surgical variable (grade D).
Colon and rectum	En bloc resection should be performed for tumors adherent to local structures (grade B).
	Inadvertent bowel perforation increases the risk of recurrence and should be avoided (grade B).
	Thorough abdominal exploration for metastatic and locally advanced primary and lymph node disease should be performed (grade D).
	The no-touch technique is debated with little evidence to support it (grade C).
	Bowel washout may have theoretical benefits in rectal cancer, but such benefits have not been proven (grade C).
	Ovaries grossly involved with tumor should be removed; prophylactic oophorectomy cannot be supported (grade D).

From Nelson H, Petrelli N, Carlin A, et al: Guidelines 2000 for colon and rectal cancer surgery. *J Natl Cancer Inst* 93:591, 2001.

TABLE 170-3 Surveillance Recommendations

Parameter	ASCRS (2004)[19]	ASCO (2005)[20]	NCCN (2008)[21]
History and physical examination	Minimum of 3 times per yr for 2 yr	Every 3-6 mo for 3 yr; then every 6 mo to 5 yr	Every 3-6 mo for 2 yr; then every 6 mo to 5 yr
CEA	Minimum of 3 times per yr for 2 yr	Every 3 mo for 3 yr*	Every 3-6 mo for 2 yr; then every 6 mo to 5 yr[†]
Chest screening	Insufficient evidence to recommend for or against	CT chest every year for 3 yr[‡]	Chest CT every year for 3 yr[§]
Colonoscopy	At 3-yr intervals	At 3 yr and if results are normal, then every 5 yr	At 1 yr, 3 yr, and 5 yr if negative, then every 5 yr
CT of abdomen/pelvis	Not recommended	Every year for 3 yr[§]	Every year for 3 yr[¶]

Modified from Tsitikis VL, Malireddy K, Green EA, et al: Postoperative surveillance recommendations for early stage colon cancer based on results from the clinical outcomes of surgical therapy trial. *J Clin Oncol* 27:3672, 2009.
ASCO, American Society of Clinical Oncology; *ASCRS,* American Society of Colon and Rectal Surgeons; *CEA,* carcinoembryonic antigen; *CT,* computed tomography; *NCCN,* National Comprehensive Cancer Network.
*If the patient is a candidate for surgery or systemic therapy.
[†]If the patient is a potential candidate for further intervention.
[‡]For patients who are at higher risk of recurrence and who could be candidates for curative intent surgery.
[§]CT scan may be useful for patients at high risk for recurrence (e.g., lymphatic or venous invasion by tumor or poorly differentiated tumors).
[¶]Colonoscopy in 1 year except if no preoperative colonoscopy due to obstructing lesion, colonoscopy in 3-6 months; if abnormal, repeat in 1 year; if no advanced adenoma (villous polyp, polyp >1 cm, or high-grade dysplasia), repeat in 3 years, then every 5 years.

bleeding or discharge. Physical examination may reveal the presence of advanced disease (e.g., mass on abdominal, rectal, vaginal, or perineal examination or the presence of an enlarged supraclavicular node). Unfortunately, when signs and symptoms arise, the relapse is often at a late stage and beyond the hope of cure. Furthermore, these symptoms often present in the interval between routine followup appointments. The history and physical examination does, however, provide valuable information on the general health status of the patient, which is vital in determining the suitability for aggressive resection. And these visits can also be important in counseling patients regarding increased cancer risk in family members and the need for screening for additional cancers.

Laboratory and Imaging Studies

Of all of the available tests, the chest radiograph would seem to be the most rational because of its low cost and potential to detect asymptomatic but resectable lesions. However, the impact of surveillance chest radiographs on survival has been limited when tested in prospective studies.[19] CT of the chest is recommended annually for the first 3 years following primary tumor resection by ASCO and NCCN.

Routine blood cell counts and chemistries are not helpful. Liver function tests are rarely abnormal, and when they are, this often indicates the presence of extensive, unresectable disease.

It is reasonable to obtain a computed tomographic (CT) scan of the abdomen and pelvis 6 to 12 months after surgery to serve as a baseline study and then repeat the CT scan at 6- to 12-month intervals for 2 to 3 years. The ASCRS guidelines for surveillance after colorectal cancer resection advise against routine abdominal CT, but the Cochrane review suggested a survival benefit in patients who underwent liver imaging compared with those who did not.[18]

Endoscopy

The aim of endoscopy is the detection of anastomotic recurrences and metachronous lesions, the latter being more common. Full colonoscopy is required to detect metachronous lesions, but the frequency of surveillance colonoscopies remains the subject of debate. It is influenced by variables such as age of cancer onset, genetic predisposition, and other risk factors. For average-risk patients, a colonoscopy at 1 and 5 years seems the most common practice. ASCRS guidelines suggest colonoscopy at 3-year intervals.[19] For patients with genetic susceptibilities, the interval should be 1 to 2 years depending on the certainty and magnitude of the risk. Also, patients who did not receive a preoperative colonoscopy (because of emergency presentation, obstruction, etc.) should undergo colonoscopy as early as feasible after resection.

For patients with high-risk tumors, especially of the rectum, it is reasonable to perform more frequent examinations of the anastomosis using flexible sigmoidoscopy. This technology may allow the identification of the rare anastomotic recurrence or the more frequently occurring extrarectal recurrence. Extraluminal recurrences from residual lymphatic tissue represent the apparent origins of most locoregional pelvic recurrences. The role of endoscopic ultrasound (EUS) to detect extraluminal recurrences in the followup of patients with a colorectal anastomosis is currently being studied.

Carcinoembryonic Antigen Test

When the carcinoembryonic antigen (CEA) test was introduced, it received a great deal of attention because of its simplicity. Frequent monitoring of CEA levels was advocated and found to be effective in detecting the presence of local and liver recurrence before the disease became clinically apparent. In a recent metaanalysis of 20 studies, the overall sensitivity and specificity of CEA for detecting colorectal cancer recurrence was 64% and

90%, respectively.[22] Despite this, CEA monitoring as a part of surveillance is currently recommended by most societies as it is the only known tumor marker.

Positron Emission Tomography

Positron emission tomography (PET), an imaging modality based on the detection of 2-(^{18}F)-fluoro-2-deoxyglucose, is not recommended for routine use in colorectal cancer surveillance. However, several authors have reported its use for the detection of recurrent colorectal carcinoma. Contemporary series report a sensitivity to detect local recurrences at the primary colorectal resection site of approximately 90% and the superiority of PET over other imaging modalities in the detection of local and extrapelvic recurrences.[23] In addition, one group suggests that PET can be 87% accurate in detecting locally recurrent rectal carcinoma even in a previously irradiated field.[24] PET has also been combined with CT, providing both anatomic and metabolic information. In one report, with the addition of CT to PET, the specificity increased from 29% to 64% for pelvic recurrences and from 68% to 87% for extrapelvic recurrences compared to PET alone.[25] Although PET scans have been advocated for use in asymptomatic patients to detect recurrence, the role of PET as a surveillance tool following curative treatment of colorectal carcinoma is not currently recommended.

PET may play a greater role as a confirmatory study in verifying the presence of a recurrence in the setting of a rising CEA or equivocal imaging studies. However, as discussed later, a positive finding on PET scan is not equivalent to histology and is not sufficient evidence to proceed to surgical exploration.

CONCLUSION

The aim of any postoperative followup strategy should be early detection of resectable disease. These efforts should be focused on identifying (1) tumors of favorable prognosis (i.e., slow growing); (2) sites of disease amenable to resection for cure (i.e., locoregional, hepatic, and pulmonary); and (3) patients who are a good risk, vigorous, and motivated who would be suitable for extensive resection.

LOCOREGIONAL RECURRENCE

The algorithm in Figure 170-1 summarizes our clinical approach to disease recurrence. Locoregional recurrences account for 5% to 19% of colon cancer and 7% to 33% of rectal cancer relapses.[2,3,26,27] Of these, only approximately 30% are resectable with curative intent.[28] This section focuses on locally recurrent *rectal* cancer, because most of the strategies for diagnosis and therapy can be similarly applied to locally recurrent colon cancers.

Patients with untreated locally recurrent rectal cancer live a median of 5 months.[28] Radiation therapy alone is rarely curative and in some studies prolongs survival to a median of 7 to 15 months.[28,29] In contrast, complete resection of locally recurrent disease can be accomplished in some patients with mean survival times of 33 to 59 months and a long-term 5-year survival rate of up to 30%.[28,30]

The patient presenting with only locally recurrent rectal cancer and no demonstrable extrapelvic disease presents a challenge because of the difficulty achieving adequate exposure and surgical access in the pelvis. Furthermore, these recurrences typically involve multiple organs and structures, which require extensive resection in an attempt to achieve histologically negative margins. Whether extensive surgery is possible or even reasonable requires judgment on the part of the surgeon. A number of factors should be carefully considered, including the overall health status of the patient, the status of extrapelvic disease, and the extent of local pelvic disease.

PREOPERATIVE EVALUATION AND PATIENT SELECTION

General Health

In the approach to repeat resection, it is imperative that the patient and physician understand the extent and magnitude of the endeavor. The ideal patient should be in good health; such extended resection in combination with preoperative chemoradiotherapy is not appropriate for patients who are in poor health, with American Society of Anesthesiologists classification IV or V, as well as most patients with classification III.

Exclusion of Extrapelvic Disease

Once it is determined that the patient is suitable for surgery, the next step is to confirm that the locoregional recurrence is isolated. In addition to physical examination and standard surveillance tests outlined earlier, a CT scan of the abdomen and pelvis will help to assess the presence of extrapelvic disease. Evaluation of the liver can be further supplemented by hepatic ultrasound, magnetic resonance imaging (MRI), or PET scan when the CT scan detects a suspicious but nondiagnostic finding. In cases of a borderline chest radiograph, a chest CT scan should be obtained. The identification of small indeterminate nodules is common and problematic; PET can also be useful in these patients. These tests for metastatic disease are performed before preoperative radiation and chemotherapy and repeated again just before surgery. This provides additional reassurance that patients with aggressive disease that may have metastasized in the interim will be identified, thus avoiding noncurative surgery.

Evaluation of the Presence and Extent of Local Disease

It may be particularly challenging to prove resectability of a lesion because it is often difficult to differentiate between recurrent tumor and postoperative changes. Evaluation begins with a physical examination of the rectum and vagina. Next, endoscopy and CT with or without MRI are performed. There are generally three ways of differentiating postoperative changes from recurrent tumor. The first is to document a change in the lesion, such as increase in size, over time; the second is invasion of adjacent organs; and finally, the third is histologic evidence obtained from biopsies. Histologic evidence may be obtained from a luminal or mucosal aspect

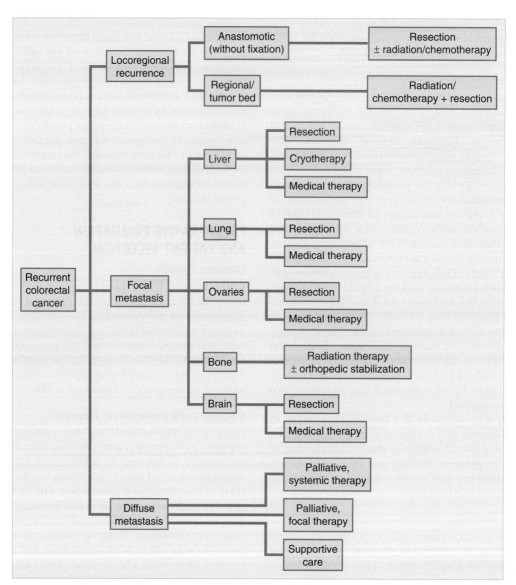

FIGURE 170-1 Flow chart of therapeutic options for recurrent colorectal cancer. (Modified from Frizelle F, Nelson H: Recurrent colon cancer. In Wexner SD, Vernava AM, editors: *Clinical decision making in colorectal surgery*. New York, 1995, Igaku-Shoin, p 390.)

of the recurrence, although this presentation is least common. Extraluminal lesions that are palpable through the perineum or rectum or vagina may be biopsied transrectally or transvaginally. All other tumors are generally amenable to biopsy with CT guidance. Occasionally, pelvic disease is suspected because of a rising CEA level with no obvious recurrence by imaging. In such situations, histologic proof should be sought prior to considering surgery. Exploratory pelvic surgery should be discouraged in the absence of imaging findings because the CEA elevation could be due to extrapelvic disease or elevated for a reason unrelated to recurrent rectal cancer. Furthermore, the only way to exclude a pelvic recurrence is to explore the entire pelvis down to the level of the pelvic floor. This is often an extraordinary task and even when possible, it is often difficult to distinguish scar from tumor even using frozen-section histology. Some tumors produce nodular or discrete recurrences, whereas others can have ill-defined limits and be infiltrative or sheet-like

in nature; the determination of borders and resectability can, accordingly, be difficult. Histologic evidence of recurrence and radiographic imaging suitable for defining the extent and boundaries of a pelvic recurrence are essential.

Resectability

Locoregional recurrences can extend anteriorly, posteriorly, laterally, or in a combination of directions. In addition, any of the organs in and around the pelvis may be involved, including intestinal, urologic, gynecologic, bony, and vascular structures. When assessing locoregional recurrences, two factors are important: fixation and anatomic location. The combination of these two factors determines resectability (Figure 170-2). Suzuki et al originally categorized the extent of local recurrence based on the degree of fixation with F0 indicating no fixation and F1 to F3 indicating one to three sites of fixation, respectively.[31] We have modified this scheme for F0

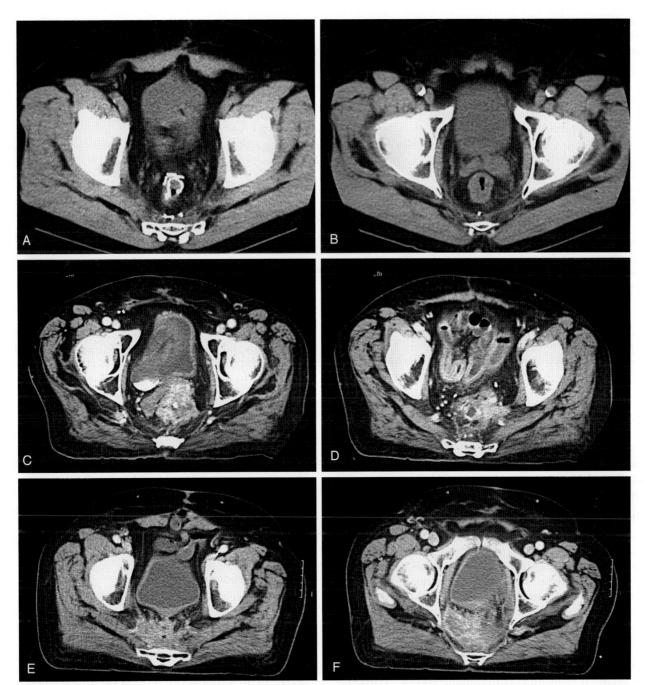

FIGURE 170-2 Classification of local recurrence according to fixation. **A** and **B** are examples of no fixation (F0). **A,** The stapled low anterior anastomosis is easily visualized on CT scan. **B,** Distal to the anastomosis is a perianastomotic recurrence; there is no evidence of fixation to local organs or structures. Complete resection with negative margins would be anticipated. **C** and **D** are examples of fixed resectable (FR). **C,** Single-site fixation to anterior structures such as the bladder, as illustrated, or gynecologic structures can typically be resected with negative margins. **D,** Lateral pelvic side wall fixation can be resected, but margins will often be close or microscopically positive. **E** and **F** are examples of fixed, not resectable (FNR). **E** and **F,** Two images from the same patient illustrate posterior fixation (**E**) and anterior fixation (**F**) in addition to lateral side wall involvement, rendering this recurrence unresectable.

to indicate when the tumor is not fixed, FR to indicate when the tumor is fixed but resectable, and FNR to indicate when the tumor is fixed and not resectable. FR is further subdivided by noting the anatomic extent of the fixation (anterior, posterior, and lateral) because this allows the determination of the extent of resection that will be required. Anteriorly fixed lesions may require a hysterectomy and/or a partial or complete cystectomy,

and in lesions with posterior fixation, a sacrectomy may be necessary.

Despite this classification, it is not always possible to predict resectability before surgery. Some indicators predict that curative surgery with negative resection margins is not likely possible (Box 170-3). For example, unless there is infiltration of the trigone of the bladder at the insertion of the ureters to the bladder, bilateral

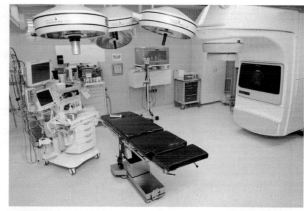

FIGURE 170-3 The intraoperative electron radiation therapy suite, showing the equipment, operating room table, and linear accelerator.

ureteric obstruction usually indicates a bulky tumor that has invaded the lateral pelvic side walls. This indicates that disease is present at the level of the pelvic inlet, suggesting circumferential disease, and generally the large circumferential tumor that extends to the pelvic side wall should be considered unresectable. For relapses that involve the sacrum, lesions that are central and distal to S2 can be removed with a distal sacrectomy. Nerve root involvement of S1 or S2 or evidence of invasion of the sacrum at the level of S1 and S2 typically indicates unresectable disease. Sacrectomy proximal to S2 results in sacroiliac joint instability, and although it is technically feasible to internally fix this, it is not warranted for cases of locally recurrent rectal cancer. Lesions above S2 and unilateral are occasionally treated with resection of the anterior sacral table. Any tumor with a component of bone involvement both above and below S2 is not resectable.

TRIMODALITY THERAPY

The cornerstone of treatment for locally recurrent rectal cancer with a curative intent is surgery. However, surgery alone results in a high local and systemic failure rate. This has been the rationale for a multimodality approach to the treatment using preoperative radiation therapy plus concomitant chemotherapy and maximal resection for local control and chemotherapy to address the possibility of systemic failure.

Preoperative Radiation Therapy and Chemotherapy

Although it provides symptomatic relief, radiation therapy alone does not result in any significant chance of cure; furthermore, as stated earlier, surgery alone in cases of locally advanced rectal cancer gives rise to high relapse rates. When combined, radiation therapy and surgery reduce local recurrence rates and increase resectability.[17] Similarly, when used in the scenario of locally recurrent cancer, radiation therapy has been shown to improve results. In addition, the demonstration that combined fluorouracil-based chemoradiotherapy further improves results for primary rectal cancer prompted us to use a similar regimen in patients undergoing treatment for recurrent disease. As an added modality to avoid or reduce dose-related toxicity while improving local control, we combine external beam radiation therapy (EBRT) plus chemotherapy with intraoperative electron radiation therapy (IOERT). IOERT offers the advantages of tumor-directed therapy with limited normal tissue exposure and single-fraction, high biologic equivalence with improved local control in high-risk sites.

A full course of external beam radiation (5040 cGy) with protracted venous infusion 5-fluorouracil (5-FU) chemotherapy ($225 \text{ mg/m}^2/24 \text{ hr}$) is administered preoperatively to patients who have not had previous pelvic radiation therapy. Patients who have received previous adjuvant radiotherapy in the treatment of their primary tumor are treated with 1000 to 3000 cGy of preoperative radiation plus 5-FU–based chemotherapy when possible. The safety and feasibility of re-radiation to the pelvis has been established.[32] Maximum synergy between full-dose preoperative external beam and intraoperative radiation occurs if the two are completed within a 4- to 8-week interval. For patients receiving a full course of treatment with doses of approximately 5040 cGy, a 3- to 5-week rest period before surgery and IOERT is standard. Restaging is performed before the procedure is undertaken.

Operative Procedures

It is imperative that the first step in planning for surgery of this magnitude includes an extensive discussion and explanation of the planned procedure with the patient and relatives. Sphincter-saving surgery is most often not indicated in cases of local recurrence. Therefore, within the discussion must be the acceptance of a permanent colostomy. In addition, an ileal conduit or a sacrectomy (or both) in situations of anterior or posterior fixation may be required.

Patients undergo a mechanical and antibiotic bowel preparation the night before surgery. At our institution, all patients with locally recurrent rectal cancers are scheduled for surgery in a dedicated IOERT suite. This suite within the operating room complex houses the standard operating room equipment, a linear accelerator, and special anesthetic equipment that allows movement of the anesthetized patient from operating to radiating stations (Figure 170-3). In addition, remote controls allow monitoring of the patient outside the suite in a lead-shielded room while radiation is delivered.

The patient is placed in the combined position. Special care is taken to ensure that the calves are not resting on the stirrups because prolonged operating times can result in compartment syndrome or venous thrombosis. Nearly all patients receive ureteral stents; the 0-degree cystoscope is used to instrument the bladder, and the 70-degree scope is used to inspect the bladder for mucosal or extrinsic abnormalities. On occasion, direct bladder invasion is detected cystoscopically; this information can help guide the extent of surgery. No. 5 French ureteral stents are inserted using the 30-degree cystoscope, and these are secured to a Foley catheter.

A lower midline incision is used to provide optimal pelvic exposure, as well as to facilitate the possible use of rectus abdominis myocutaneous flap. Care is exercised to preserve the inferior epigastric vessels when it is anticipated that a transpelvic rectus abdominis flap may be used. Exploration includes an examination of the liver, peritoneum, omentum, ovaries, retroperitoneum, and wound to confirm the absence of extrapelvic disease because this would contraindicate radical resection. Very rarely, exceptions may be made in very young patients who have limited pelvic and liver disease where the pelvic recurrence and liver metastases are each synchronously resected for curative potential (R0).

We use a self-retaining ring retractor. The small bowel is packed superiorly for pelvic exposure. Because these operations are lengthy, care must be taken to avoid pressure from a retractor on the retroperitoneal/pelvic tissues; femoral nerve injuries have been described, implicating prolonged retractor pressure as a causative factor. Because pelvic fibrosis is the rule, the dissection starts at the bifurcation of the aorta so a safe fascial plane is found to guide the posterior dissection down to the pelvic floor (Figure 170-4, A). The iliac arteries and veins are coursed from the aorta and cava to the branching of the internal and external branches. Below the common and external branches of the iliac arteries, the vessels can be ligated without concern for ischemia. Knowledge of the location of these vessels prevents most of the risk for exsanguination and the need for vascular bypass; at the same time, it facilitates identification of the safest posterior and lateral planes. In the same way, the ureters are identified from the pelvic brim and followed by anterior dissection to the level of their insertion into the bladder. It is usually necessary to trace the ureters right to their insertion into the bladder so the lateral dissection can be performed safely. Ureter dissection is more extensive when a cystectomy or sacrectomy is contemplated; it is essential for the construction of an ileal conduit and for the prevention of injury during the posterior dissection, respectively.

Nonfixed Lesions. The recurrence of F0 lesions after local excisions or low anterior resection may require nothing more than a simple completion APR. The main difference between this and the standard APR is the added difficulty in dissection due to fibrosis and postoperative changes in anatomy. Distinction between fibrosis and tumor infiltration is difficult at best. In such circumstances, particularly when it occurs outside the realm of planned resection (sacral promontory and lateral pelvic side walls), frozen-section histology should be performed. If tumor cells are seen within the samples of diffuse or extensive "fibrosis," complete resection with negative margins is not feasible.

Fixed-Resectable, Anterior Lesions. Anterior lesions demonstrate the greatest diversity between men and women. In women, anterior fixation may require little more than en bloc resection of the rectum, uterus, and posterior wall of the vagina. In contrast, anterior fixation in a narrow male pelvis is more likely to require cystectomy or cystoprostatectomy. Caution should be exercised for lesions that are directly invading the trigone or prostate because these are often circumferential and "after the fact" are found not to be completely resectable. It is perhaps the tissue planes at and below the seminal vesicles that allow for ease of circumferential tumor spread. Pelvic MRI or PET-CT fusion studies show promise for better delineation of tumor extent in these cases.

For anterior lesions, partial cystectomy may be sufficient in some cases to accomplish negative margins. However, it may be preferable to perform total cystectomy and ileal conduit for heavily irradiated bladders where tissues are unlikely to allow for proper healing and acceptable postoperative functional results.

Fixed-Resectable, Posterior Lesions. The ideal procedure for tumors with posterior fixation and bone involvement is a distal sacrectomy. If sacral resection is considered it should be distal to S2-S3. Having said that, true sacral invasion is uncommon and sacral resection is rarely indicated. A resection more proximal than S2 may require stabilization of the sacroiliac joints with internal fixation and other reconstructive methods and is not indicated. Furthermore, by limiting the resection to the S2-3 level, the preservation of one S3 root is generally possible. This is usually sufficient to preserve bladder function. Best results in terms of margins and risk of recurrence can be expected for central lesions, that is, those without a pelvic side wall component.

Distal sacrectomy consists of four stages: (1) the anterior resection procedures, (2) the posterior resection procedures, (3) IOERT, and (4) pelvic reconstruction. Anterior procedures are performed with the patient in the lithotomy position. The abdominal cavity is explored before pelvic dissection. As described earlier, to minimize the risk of inadvertent injury due to anatomic displacement, dissection of the ureters and iliac vessels begins at the level of the aortic bifurcation (see Figure 170-4, A and B) and progresses deep into the pelvis. The posterior plane is generally the safest place to begin but is limited to the level of the tumor. Anterior and lateral resection planes are dissected with adherent organs, and structures are removed en bloc with the posterior-based tumor. A frozen-section biopsy at the level of posterior fixation ensures that a negative sacral margin is achievable. In addition, the top of the sacral resection margin is scored, a maneuver that facilitates identification of the level of posterior sacral transection.

With resectability established, the remainder of the anterior and lateral dissections is completed, leaving the tumor attached only to the sacrum posteriorly. The internal iliac artery and veins are ligated bilaterally if sacral transection proximal to S3-4 is anticipated (see Figure 170-4, C); this reduces blood loss during sacrectomy. Either an omental or a rectus abdominis flap (Figure 170-5) is mobilized and transposed into the pelvis for subsequent retrieval and reconstruction during

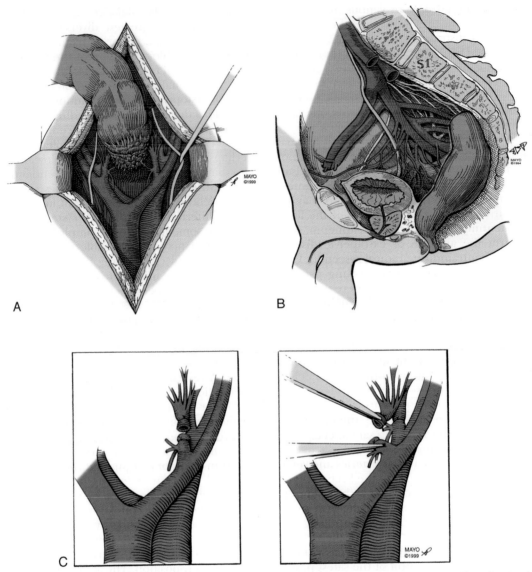

A

B

C

FIGURE 170-4 A, Broad view of pelvic dissection. The iliac vessels are dissected from the level of the aortic bifurcation to at least the origin of the internal iliac branches. The ureters are located and followed from the pelvic brim to their insertion into the bladder. Once the vessels and ureters are located, it is safe to proceed with the posterior dissection, commencing at the sacral promontory. **B,** Anterior approach (operative anatomy of pelvic structures). The anterior procedure provides assurance that no extrapelvic disease is present and provides several preparatory steps for the sacral resection, including anterior and lateral dissection, proximal sacral margin delineation, parasacral vascular ligation, gastrointestinal and/or urinary stoma formation, and omental or rectus abdominis flap creation. **C,** Bilateral internal iliac artery and vein ligation is performed if sacral transection proximal to S3-4 is expected. The artery typically must be ligated and divided to provide exposure to the internal iliac vein. The vein can be ligated without transection. (Copyright Mayo Foundation, 1999.)

the posterior procedure. The gastrointestinal or urinary stomas are fashioned before closure of the abdomen. This completes the anterior procedures.

The patient is repositioned prone, and a posterior midline incision is made over the lower lumbars and sacrum to the coccyx. If sacrectomy is performed simultaneous with APR en bloc, then the elliptical anal excision is incorporated with the proximal sacrum incision. The gluteus is dissected to expose the entire sacrum. This exposure facilitates the division of the sacrotuberous and sacrospinous ligaments (Figure 170-6, *A*). With care taken to protect the sciatic and pudendal nerves, the piriformis muscle is divided (Figure 170-6, *B*). Division of this muscle allows the endopelvic fascia to be entered.

Once the pelvic floor is opened, palpation from behind allows identification of the level of sacral transection as previously determined by frozen sections that confirmed the absence of tumor. The orthopedic surgeon next performs the laminectomy, dural sac ligation, and bony transection. The pelvic surgeon assists in completing the lateral pelvic side wall dissection, taking care to protect the ureters, bladder, and urethra. Intraoperative irradiation, as described later, is performed next, followed by wound closure with or without flap reconstruction.

Intraoperative Delivery of Electron Beam Radiation Therapy. Once the specimen is resected, it is reviewed by the pathologist, surgeon, and radiation oncologist to

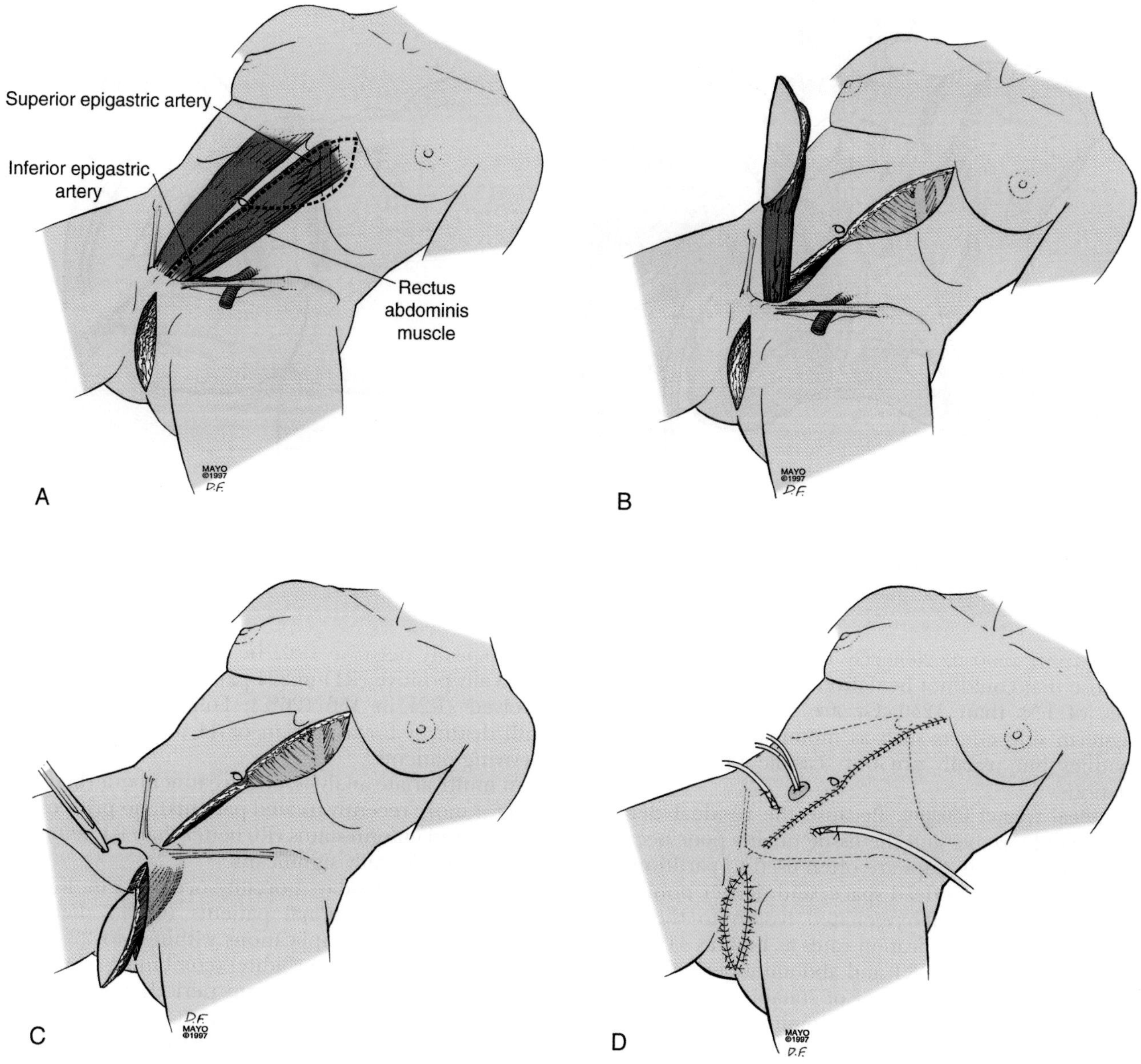

FIGURE 170-5 Rectus abdominis myocutaneous flap pelvic closure. This series of drawings illustrates the perineal positioning of a rectus flap. The same technique is used for sacrectomy wounds—only that the flap is left in the pelvis at the end of the anterior (abdominal) procedures and pulled through the posterior defect and sutured after the sacrectomy and intraoperative electron radiation therapy are completed. **A,** Once perineal resection is complete, the skin paddle is designed to match the size of the defect. The harvest site for the skin paddle is determined based on the direct perforators from the underlying rectus abdominis muscle. **B,** The myocutaneous flap and associated skin paddle are raised and include the anterior fascia of the rectus sheath. The blood supply is provided by the inferior epigastric artery. **C,** The flap is delivered through the pelvis to the perineal defect. Care is taken to avoid stretching or torsion on the inferior epigastric blood supply. **D,** The skin paddle is secured with interrupted sutures, and the abdominal fascia and skin are reapproximated. (Copyright Mayo Foundation, 1997.)

determine margins and the need for IOERT. As indicated, additional biopsies may be required to define sites of marginal resection. When IOERT is required, a Lucite applicator is positioned in the pelvis to target the tissues at risk (Figure 170-7). The applicator is selected for size (typically 5 to 8 cm in diameter) and shape (typically circular and 30 degrees beveled). The patient is then positioned under the linear accelerator. Between 1000 and 2000 cGy is delivered depending on the extent of margin involvement and the dose of preoperative EBRT.

If full-dose preoperative EBRT of 5040 cGy was achieved, a dose of 1000 to 1250 cGy is recommended for less than or equal to microscopic residual disease (R0 or R1); 1500 to 1750 cGy for gross residual disease less than 2 cm in size (R2); and 2000 cGy is reserved for unresected or gross residual disease of more than 2 cm in size (R2). These single-dose radiation treatments are biologically equivalent to 1.5 to 2.5 times the same quantity of EBRT fractions.[13] If the preoperative EBRT dose was limited to 2000 to 3000 cGy because of prior EBRT, the IOERT dose

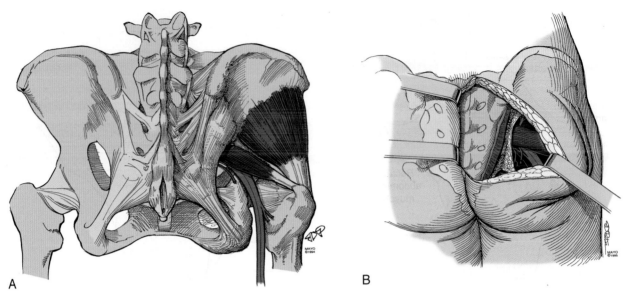

FIGURE 170-6 Operative techniques, posterior approach showing anatomic relationships **(A)** and operative anatomy **(B).** To remove the sacral tumor posteriorly, the gluteus must be dissected from the sacrum, and the sciatic nerve identified. The sacrotuberous and sacrospinous ligaments, piriformis muscle, and endopelvic fascia are divided, and then the dural sac is ligated and sacrum transected. (Copyright Mayo Foundation, 1994.)

ranges from 1500 to 2000 cGy to account for some of the dose that could not be delivered with EBRT. IOERT doses of less than 1250 cGy are less likely to cause long-term side effects such as motor and sensory neuropathies but usually are not feasible in retreatment situations.

Perineal Wound Closure. Because the residual defects are generally sizable and the tissue quality poor because of prior irradiation, flaps are often used to partition the pelvis, obliterate the dead space, and deliver nonirradiated vascularized well-oxygenated tissues to the area. Perineal wound complication rates as high as 41% have been reported after EBRT and abdominoperineal resection.[33] If the omentum is not of suitable size or consistency, the vertical rectus abdominis myocutaneous (VRAM) flap is preferred, especially for sacrectomy wounds (see Figure 170-5).[34] In addition, the rectus is versatile and can be used to reconstruct a narrowed or shortened vagina after extensive resection. A vaginal tube can be constructed from a spiral configuration of the rectus attached to a short cuff at the introitus or from a folded flap reconstructing the anterior or posterior defects. Sexual function can be acceptable after flap-vaginal reconstruction.[35] Patients undergoing VRAM reconstruction have fewer wound complications (abscess, wound dehiscence) than those undergoing primary closure or thigh flaps. Abdominal wall complications are rare after VRAM harvest.[36]

Results of Trimodality Treatment for Locally Recurrent Disease

In the largest experience with long-term followup reported to date, 607 patients with locally recurrent rectal cancers were treated at our institution between 1981 and 2008 with the multimodality approach we have described. All patients underwent maximal resection with the administration of IOERT. The margins were histologically negative (R0) in 227 cases (37%), microscopically positive (R1) in 224 patients (37%) and grossly involved (R2) in 156 (26%). Followup was complete until death or for a median of 44 months for the 194 surviving patients.

At multivariate analysis, only treatment era (better survival for more recently treated patients), no prior chemotherapy, and margin status (R0 better than R1 better than R2) were statistically significant.[37]

Morbidity. Thirty-day mortality occurred in 1 patient (0.2%) and 5 additional patients (0.8%) died from treatment-related complications within 3 to 22 months of surgery. Overall morbidity (combining short- and long-term throughout followup period) was 50%. The most frequent causes of morbidity were wound-related complications in 20% of patients, gastrointestinal obstruction or fistula in 14%, ureteral obstruction in 10%, and peripheral neuropathy in 7%.[37]

Additional reports of patients undergoing similar multimodality therapy for recurrent rectal cancers describe similar rates of short-term morbidity (17% to 40%) and mortality (0% to 2%).[31,38]

Cancer Outcomes. In this study by Haddock et al, the median survival was 36 months, and the 5- and 10-year survival estimates were 30% and 16%, respectively. Patients undergoing potentially curative resection (R0) had longer 5-year overall survival compared with patients with residual disease (R1 and R2). Central relapse (within the IOERT field) occurred in only 14% of patients at 5 years. Local relapse within the external beam radiation field was observed in 28% of patients at 5 years, and distant relapse had occurred in 53% by 5 years. All forms of relapse were more common in patients with subtotal resection (R1 and R2) than in patients with R0 resection.[37] Although the highly selected use of IOERT precludes definitive conclusions regarding its specific contribution to cancer outcomes, the encouraging

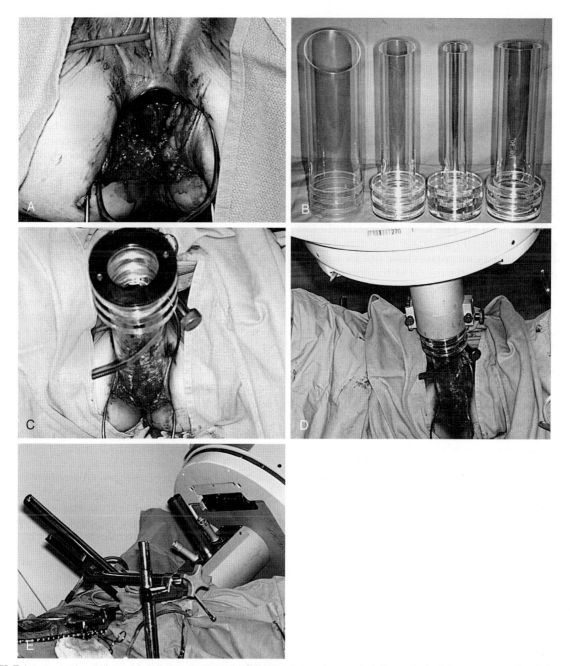

FIGURE 170-7 Intraoperative delivery of radiation therapy. **A,** Once the tumor is resected, the pathologist, surgeon, and radiation oncologist examine the closest margins and determine the site and extent of tumor bed risk. Sites of recurrence deep in the pelvis are often best approached with a perineal port for radiation therapy. **B,** A Lucite applicator is selected to fit the surgical field at risk for failure of local control. Several sizes and shapes are available with varying degrees of bevel to accommodate the field of radiation. **C to E,** The applicator is placed into the field, stabilized to the operating table, and connected to the linear accelerator.

cancer outcomes in this series of patients support its continued use.

Locally Recurrent Colon Carcinoma. It is estimated that approximately 10% to 20% of patients with resected colon cancer present with an isolated locoregional recurrence amenable to surgical resection. The role of multimodality treatment for this specific indication is not considered as standard of care. However, in one study of 73 patients with locally recurrent colon carcinoma treated with a combination of chemotherapy, EBRT, and surgical excision followed by IOERT there was a 5-year survival of 24.7%. More specifically, the 5-year survival rate in the

subset of 38 patients with R0 resection was 37.4%.[39] Although this specific treatment strategy and in particular the use of IOERT cannot be easily applied on a widespread basis, these data demonstrate once more the validity of an aggressive approach to treat locally recurrent colorectal carcinoma in select patients.

Summary

Patients who otherwise enjoy good health and who present with isolated locally recurrent tumors may be candidates for trimodality therapy with EBRT, chemotherapy (concomitant with EBRT and maintenance following resection), repeat resection, and IOERT. The possibility of cure and the extent of resection, including anterior and posterior exenteration, are determined by the anatomic location and degree of tumor fixation. When achievable with negative margins or microscopic residual disease, the use of resection and trimodality therapy that includes IOERT is associated with acceptable 5-year survival rates and acceptable morbidity.

PULMONARY METASTASIS

The liver is the most common site of colorectal metastasis, and the management of hepatic lesions is discussed separately in Chapter 171. The lung is the second most common site of colorectal metastasis. Less than 10% of patients with pulmonary metastases have disease isolated to the lungs, and only 2% of patients with colorectal lung metastases are candidates for metastasectomy. The basic management is described here. In general, favorable outcomes can be anticipated when lesions are isolated or in only one lung lobe and can be completely resected in an otherwise healthy individual.

PATIENT SELECTION

No formal guidelines exist with regard to pulmonary surveillance after resection of colorectal carcinoma. Most lung metastases are initially seen on plain chest radiographs. Once detected, a CT scan of the thorax is necessary to evaluate the resectability of the lesion and to detect other smaller lesions. At the same time, a metastatic workup should be done to exclude extrathoracic lesions in the manner as outlined earlier. General guidelines for pulmonary resection for metastatic disease include the following: disease should be limited, preferably three or fewer lesions; all disease must be amenable to complete resection; and patients must be in good health with good pulmonary function and pulmonary reserve.

RESULTS OF PULMONARY RESECTION

Pulmonary resection for metastasis can be performed with low mortality and high success rates, with contemporary 5-year survival rates in the range of 27% to 41%.[40-42] Analogous to hepatic metastases, there is an inverse relationship between the number of metastases and survival outcomes.[41,43] Other prognostic factors include maximal size of the largest lesion,[42] mediastinal or thoracic lymph node involvement,[41] and in some series prethoracotomy CEA level.[41] In the Mayo Clinic series of 139 patients, 71% had solitary lesions. The authors reported an operative mortality rate of 1.4%, a 5-year survival rate of 31%, and a 20-year survival rate of 16%.[40] Interestingly, the disease-free interval is not consistently a predictor of survival.[41-43] In the report by Onaitis et al, there was no difference in oncologic outcomes between those treated with thoracoscopic procedures versus standard thoracotomy.[43] The role of adjuvant therapy after resection of pulmonary metastasis is not established, because there is no evidence that systemic therapies reduce the high risk of subsequent relapse in these patients. Repeat resection of recurrent pulmonary

metastasis has been described, with survival being very similar to that for the first resection.[44]

SUMMARY

Although pulmonary metastases are less common than hepatic secondary tumors, it is worthwhile identifying isolated pulmonary lesions amenable to resection. In addition, not only do first resections have a reasonable 5-year survival outcome, but repeat resections for recurrent metastatic lesions are also associated with a reasonable chance for cure. The most important criterion for good outcome is patient selection. Isolated resectable lesions in patients with good health and good pulmonary reserve are key to this outcome.

ISOLATED METASTASES—OTHER SITES

The bone and brain are much less often involved with focal metastatic lesions. These lesions typically manifest in the setting of diffuse disease and are rarely curable. Bone metastases are usually treated with internal fixation as required for stabilization and irradiation for palliation of pain and to control disease. In cases of solitary brain metastases in a nonvital region, resection and postoperative irradiation are reasonable. When surgical resection is not indicated, steroids plus irradiation serve to palliate the process.[45]

Peritoneal carcinomatosis is present in approximately 10% of patients presenting with colorectal cancer and median survival is 7 months.[46] It was previously considered to be an incurable disease and treated with palliative therapies only. In recent years, cytoreductive surgery followed by hyperthermic intraperitoneal chemotherapy (HIPEC) has been used with some success. A phase III randomized trial comparing maximal cytoreductive surgery and HIPEC to systemic chemotherapy with palliative surgery for colorectal cancer with peritoneal carcinomatosis showed improved survival in the HIPEC group (median survival, 22.3 vs. 12.6 months).[47] The United States Military Cancer Institute in conjunction with the American College of Surgeons Oncology Group is conducting a phase III protocol comparing overall survival in patients with peritoneal carcinomatosis from colorectal cancer undergoing either cytoreductive surgery with HIPEC versus systemic chemotherapy.

DIFFUSE METASTASES

In the presence of diffuse disease, no curative options are available. However, the importance and complexity of palliative therapies should not be overlooked or underestimated. Management should be refocused toward the short-term goals of improving quality of life and prolonging life where appropriate. Toward the end of life, the physician should facilitate the family and individual in coping with chronic illness and the concept of death and at the same time in alleviating disabling symptoms.

CHEMOTHERAPY AGENTS

5-Fluorouracil (5-FU) has been the mainstay of palliative chemotherapy for unresectable colorectal cancer for many years. However, in the past 2 decades, newer agents have demonstrated activity against metastatic colorectal carcinoma in a number of phase III trials, namely irinotecan and oxaliplatin. The addition of irinotecan to the standard regimen of 5-FU and leucovorin, referred to as the FOLFIRI regimen, has resulted in a statistically significant survival benefit compared with the standard treatment alone.[48] Similarly, the addition of oxaliplatin to 5-FU and leucovorin (FOLFOX regimen) improved survival over 5-FU and leucovorin alone.[49] This area of investigation is rapidly evolving as monoclonal antibodies are being tested in combination with more traditional chemotherapeutic agents.

TARGETED THERAPIES

Drugs that selectively target specific molecular pathways involved in tumorigenesis or tumor progression are referred to as targeted therapies. Monoclonal antibodies are one example. These have been used in combination with traditional chemotherapy agents to improve control of metastatic disease. Bevacizumab is a humanized monoclonal antibody directed against the vascular endothelial growth factor (VEGF) ligand. The addition of bevacizumab to both irinotecan and oxaliplatin regimens has shown survival benefits. In a recent trial on 813 patients with previously untreated metastatic colorectal carcinoma, the median overall survival in the subgroup treated with FOLFIRI plus bevacizumab was 20.3 months compared with 15.6 months in the group treated with the FOLFIRI regimen alone.[50] In another report in patients with advanced colorectal cancer, the addition of bevacizumab to the FOLFOX regimen increased the median overall survival from 10.8 to 12.9 months.[51] Prominent side effects of bevacizumab are hypertension, gastrointestinal perforations, wound complications, and thromboembolic events. Other anti-VEGF agents in clinical development include vatalanib (PTK787/ZK), a selective tyrosinase inhibitor, and Angiozyme, which catalyzes the mRNA encoding the VEGF receptors.

Cetuximab is an FDA-approved chimeric humanmouse antibody directed against the endothelial growth factor receptor (EGFR). A group of 1217 patients with metastatic colorectal carcinoma were randomized to receive a combination of FOLFIRI and cetuximab versus FOLFIRI alone. Response rate and progression-free survival were significantly greater in the combination arm although no survival benefits were noted.[52] Interestingly, patients with a KRAS mutation do not respond to cetuximab, whereas those with wild type KRAS do.[52] Other EGFR inhibitors currently under investigation include panitumumab (ABX-EGF), gefitinib (ZD 1839), and erlotinib (OSI 774).

Recent innovations in the medical treatment of metastatic colorectal carcinoma have already significantly improved the survival of this patient population. As several new agents and combinations of agents are being developed and tested, further improvements and establishment of newer standards of care are anticipated.

OTHER PALLIATIVE TREATMENTS

Later in the course of the disease, palliation is focused entirely on relieving symptoms, either surgically or medically. Surgery has historically been the mainstay of treatment to relieve bowel obstruction, but in recent years self-expanding metal stents have been increasingly used as an alternative to emergent surgery. An analysis of 54 studies with a total of 1198 patients showed technical and clinical success rates of 94% and 91% for intraluminal stents, respectively. Major complications included perforation (4%), stent migration (12%), and reobstruction (7%), with a stent-related mortality of 0.6%.[53] Although stents have been most often used to allow colonic decompression and bowel preparation followed by surgery, their use to palliate symptoms and avoid colostomy in patients with unresectable primary or recurrent colorectal cancer has also been proven effective.[54] The use of stents to promptly resolve colorectal obstruction and allow a more rapid initiation of chemotherapy is also attractive although data on this approach are still limited. Medical therapies, including narcotic agents, antidepressants, local nerve blocks, and epidural analgesic pumps, can be used to relieve pain and improve coping abilities. Finally, patients and family often need reassurance and assistance with end-of-life issues; they must never feel abandoned.

CONCLUSION

Colorectal cancer relapse, although often complex in presentation, can best be considered and categorized as resectable for possible cure or not. Where the former is possible, long-term survival can be achieved, specifically for isolated lesions in the liver, lungs, and locoregional sites. For relapses in local and regional sites, results appear to be improved with the use of multimodality therapy, including EBRT plus concomitant 5-FU–based chemotherapy, in addition to maximal resection and IOERT. These results may be further enhanced by the introduction of new systemic adjuvant therapies with different mechanisms of actions that are aimed at reducing the risk of systemic failure. In the meantime, a focus of efforts on surveillance and early detection of high-risk but resectable sites may improve outcomes for locally recurrent and/or metastatic disease. When presented with cases of diffuse disease, clinical efforts should not be abandoned but rather refocused on improving quality of life.

REFERENCES

1. Surveillance Epidemiology and End Results. SEER Stat Fact Sheets: Colon and Rectum. Available at: http://seer.cancer.gov/statfacts/html/colorect.html. Accessed September 17, 2010.
2. Manfredi S, Bouvier AM, Lepage C, et al: Incidence and patterns of recurrence after resection for cure of colonic cancer in a well defined population. *Br J Surg* 93:1115, 2006.
3. Manfredi S, Benhamiche AM, Meny B, et al: Population-based study of factors influencing occurrence and prognosis of local recurrence after surgery for rectal cancer. *Br J Surg* 88:1221, 2001.
4. Platell CFE: Changing patterns of recurrence after treatment for colorectal cancer. *Int J Colorectal Dis* 22:1223, 2007.
5. Sadahiro S, Suzuki T, Ishikawa K, et al: Recurrence patterns after curative resection of colorectal cancer in patients followed for a minimum of ten years. *Hepatogastroenterology* 50:1362, 2003.
6. Porter GA, Soskolne CL, Yakimets WW, et al: Surgeon-related factors and outcome in rectal cancer. *Ann Surg* 227:157, 1998.

7. Dresen RC, Gosens MJ, Martijn H, et al: Radical resection after IORT-containing multimodality treatment is the most important determinant for outcome in patients treated for locally recurrent rectal cancer. *Ann Surg Oncol* 15:1937, 2008.

8. Stocchi L, Nelson H, Sargent DJ, et al: Impact of surgical and pathologic variables in rectal cancer: A United States community and cooperative group report. *J Clin Oncol* 19:3895, 2001.

9. Dresen RC, Peters EEM, Rutten HJT, et al: Local recurrence in rectal cancer can be predicted by histopathological factors. *Eur J Surg Oncol* 35:1071, 2009.

10. Kohonen-Corish MRJ, Daniel JJ, Chan C, et al: Low microsatellite instability is associated with poor prognosis in stage C colon cancer. *J Clin Oncol* 23:2318, 2005.

11. Soreide K, Janssen EAM, Soiland H, et al: Microsatellite instability in colorectal cancer. *Br J Surg* 93:395, 2006.

12. Cunningham D, Atkin W, Lenz H-J, et al: Colorectal cancer. *Lancet* 375:1030, 2010.

13. Stocchi L, Wolff BG: Operative techniques for radical surgery for rectal carcinoma: Can surgeons improve outcomes? *Surg Oncol Clin N Am* 9:785; discussion 799, 2000.

14. Nelson H, Petrelli N, Carlin A, et al: Guidelines 2000 for colon and rectal cancer surgery. *J Natl Cancer Inst* 93:583, 2001.

15. Heald RJ, Moran BJ, Ryall RD, et al: Rectal cancer: The Basingstoke experience of total mesorectal excision, 1978-1997. *Arch Surg* 133:894, 1998.

16. Wibe A, Moller B, Norstein J, et al: A national strategic change in treatment policy for rectal cancer—implementation of total mesorectal excision as routine treatment in Norway. A national audit. *Dis Colon Rectum* 45:857, 2002.

17. Kapiteijn E, Marijnen CA, Nagtegaal ID, et al: Preoperative radiotherapy combined with total mesorectal excision for resectable rectal cancer. *N Engl J Med* 345:638, 2001.

18. Jeffery M, Hickey BE, Hider PN: Follow-up strategies for patients treated for non-metastatic colorectal cancer. *Cochrane Database Syst Rev* 1:CD002200, 2007.

19. Anthony T, Simmang C, Hyman N, et al: Practice parameters for the surveillance and follow-up of patients with colon and rectal cancer. *Dis Colon Rectum* 47:807, 2004.

20. Desch CE, Benson AB 3rd, Somerfield MR, et al: Colorectal cancer surveillance: 2005 update of an American Society of Clinical Oncology practice guideline. *J Clin Oncol* 23:8512, 2005.

21. NCCN colon cancer clinical practice guidelines in oncology. *J Natl Compr Cancer Network* 1:1, 2008.

22. Tan E, Gouvas N, Nicholls RJ, et al: Diagnostic precision of carcinoembryonic antigen in the detection of recurrence of colorectal cancer. *Surg Oncol* 18:15, 2009.

23. Watson AJM, Lolohea S, Robertson GM, et al: The role of positron emission tomography in the management of recurrent colorectal cancer: A review. *Dis Colon Rectum* 50:102, 2007.

24. Moore HG, Akhurst T, Larson SM, et al: A case-controlled study of 18-fluorodeoxyglucose positron emission tomography in the detection of pelvic recurrence in previously irradiated rectal cancer patients. *J Am Coll Surg* 197:22, 2003.

25. Kau T, Reinprecht P, Eicher W, et al: FDG PET/CT in the detection of recurrent rectal cancer. *Int Surg* 94:315, 2009.

26. Galandiuk S, Wieand HS, Moertel CG, et al: Patterns of recurrence after curative resection of carcinoma of the colon and rectum. *Surg Gynecol Obstet* 174:27, 1992.

27. McDermott FT, Hughes ES, Pihl E, et al: Local recurrence after potentially curative resection for rectal cancer in a series of 1008 patients. *Br J Surg* 72:34, 1985.

28. Bakx R, Visser O, Josso J, et al: Management of recurrent rectal cancer: A population based study in greater Amsterdam. *World J Gastroenterol* 14:6018, 2008.

29. Allum WH, Mack P, Priestman TJ, et al: Radiotherapy for pain relief in locally recurrent colorectal cancer. *Ann R Coll Surg Engl* 69:220, 1987.

30. Hahnloser D, Nelson H, Gunderson LL, et al: Curative potential of multimodality therapy for locally recurrent rectal cancer. *Ann Surg* 237:502, 2003.

31. Suzuki K, Dozois RR, Devine RM, et al: Curative reoperations for locally recurrent rectal cancer. *Dis Colon Rectum* 39:730, 1996.

32. Das P, Delclos ME, Skibber JM, et al: Hyperfractionated accelerated radiotherapy for rectal cancer in patients with prior pelvic irradiation. *Int J Radiat Oncol Biol Phys* 77:60, 2010.

33. Bullard KM, Trudel JL, Baxter NN, et al: Primary perineal wound closure after preoperative radiotherapy and abdominoperineal resection has a high incidence of wound failure. *Dis Colon Rectum* 48:438, 2005.

34. Radice E, Nelson H, Mercill S, et al: Primary myocutaneous flap closure following resection of locally advanced pelvic malignancies. *Br J Surg* 86:349, 1999.

35. D'Souza DN, Pera M, Nelson H, et al: Vaginal reconstruction following resection of primary locally advanced and recurrent colorectal malignancies. *Arch Surg* 138:1340, 2003.

36. Butler CE, Gundeslioglu AO, Rodriguez-Bigas MA: Outcomes of immediate vertical rectus abdominis myocutaneous flap reconstruction for irradiated abdominoperineal resection defects. *J Am Coll Surg* 206:694, 2008.

37. Haddock M, Miller R, Nelson H, et al: Combined modality therapy including intraoperative electron irradiation for locally recurrent colorectal cancer. *Int J Radiat Oncol Biol Physics* 79:143, 2011.*

38. Heriot AG, Byrne CM, Lee P, et al: Extended radical resection: The choice for locally recurrent rectal cancer. *Dis Colon Rectum* 51:284, 2008.

39. Taylor WE, Donohue JH, Gunderson LL, et al: The Mayo Clinic experience with multimodality treatment of locally advanced or recurrent colon cancer. *Ann Surg Oncol* 9:177, 2002.

40. McAfee MK, Allen MS, Trastek VF, et al: Colorectal lung metastases: Results of surgical excision. *Ann Thorac Surg* 53:780; discussion 785, 1992.

41. Pfannschmidt J, Muley T, Hoffmann H, et al: Prognostic factors and survival after complete resection of pulmonary metastases from colorectal carcinoma: Experiences in 167 patients. *J Thorac Cardiovasc Surg* 126:732, 2003.

42. Vogelsang H, Haas S, Hierholzer C, et al: Factors influencing survival after resection of pulmonary metastases from colorectal cancer. *Br J Surg* 91:1066, 2004.

43. Onaitis MW, Petersen RP, Haney JC, et al: Prognostic factors for recurrence after pulmonary resection of colorectal cancer metastases. *Ann Thorac Surg* 87:1684, 2009.

44. McCormack PM, Burt ME, Bains MS, et al: Lung resection for colorectal metastases. 10-year results. *Arch Surg* 127:1403, 1992.

45. Mahmoud N, Bullard Dunn K: Metastasectomy for stage IV colorectal cancer. *Dis Colon Rectum* 53:1080, 2010.

46. Jayne DG, Fook S, Loi C, et al: Peritoneal carcinomatosis from colorectal cancer. *Br J Surg* 89:1545, 2002.

47. Verwaal VJ, van Tinteren H, van Ruth S, et al: Predicting the survival of patients with peritoneal carcinomatosis of colorectal origin treated by aggressive cytoreduction and hyperthermic intraperitoneal chemotherapy. *Br J Surg* 91:739, 2004.

48. Saltz LB, Cox JV, Blanke C, et al: Irinotecan plus fluorouracil and leucovorin for metastatic colorectal cancer. Irinotecan Study Group. *N Engl J Med* 343:905, 2000.

49. de Gramont A, Figer A, Seymour M, et al: Leucovorin and fluorouracil with or without oxaliplatin as first-line treatment in advanced colorectal cancer. *J Clin Oncol* 18:2938, 2000.

50. Hurwitz H, Fehrenbacher L, Novotny W, et al: Bevacizumab plus irinotecan, fluorouracil, and leucovorin for metastatic colorectal cancer. *N Engl J Med* 350:2335, 2004.

51. Saltz LB, Lenz H-J, Kindler HL, et al: Randomized phase II trial of cetuximab, bevacizumab, and irinotecan compared with cetuximab and bevacizumab alone in irinotecan-refractory colorectal cancer: The BOND-2 study. *J Clin Oncol* 25:4557, 2007.

52. Van Cutsem E, Kohne C-H, Hitre E, et al: Cetuximab and chemotherapy as initial treatment for metastatic colorectal cancer. *N Engl J Med* 360:1408, 2009.

53. Sebastian S, Johnston S, Geoghegan T, et al: Pooled analysis of the efficacy and safety of self-expanding metal stenting in malignant colorectal obstruction. *Am J Gastroenterol* 99:2051, 2004.

54. Hunerbein M, Krause M, Moesta KT, et al: Palliation of malignant rectal obstruction with self-expanding metal stents. *Surgery* 137:42, 2005.

---

*Reference 37: This study represents the largest series to date for patients with recurrent rectal cancer treated with multimodality therapy, n = 607.

Resection and Ablation of Metastatic Colorectal Cancer to the Liver

Sarah Y. Boostrom | David M. Nagorney | Florencia G. Que

In this chapter, we address the management of hepatic metastases from colorectal cancer. Our primary aim is to provide a practical algorithm of treatment options for various clinical situations encountered by surgeons. Within this overview, the advantages and disadvantages of therapeutic alternatives are presented in some detail, to facilitate management of these often complex clinical situations and, more importantly, to benefit the patient's care.

Metastatic colorectal carcinoma in the liver is a significant clinical problem. Nearly 70% of the approximate 150,000 persons who develop colorectal carcinoma yearly in the United States will harbor hepatic metastases *eventually*. Approximately 25% of these patients have metastases that are recognized at the initial clinical presentation of the primary tumor, and in another 45% of the patients, metastases are diagnosed subsequently. Nearly 50% of the patients with hepatic metastases harbor disease in the liver only, and these patients are the focus for hepatic resection. Currently, hepatic resection of colorectal metastases (CRM) is the treatment of choice for patients with resected or resectable primary and regional disease if all gross liver disease can be excised. However, ablation of hepatic metastases evolves as either an alternative or adjunct to re-resection if primary and regional disease as well as all gross liver disease can be excised.

PATIENT SELECTION

Many controversies exist about the treatment of liver metastases from colorectal carcinoma. These include effectiveness and response to adjuvant and neoadjuvant chemotherapy, the timing of resection for synchronous metastases, disappearing tumors, and the operative indications for multiple metastases and extrahepatic metastases.[1] As these factors affect the prognosis of these patients, they also affect patient selection, timing of surgical intervention, and ultimately their outcomes. To start with, the selection of patients with CRM for hepatic resection includes the patient's fitness for surgery, the stage of the primary tumor, the extent of the hepatic metastases, the intent of the resection, and response to neoadjuvant chemotherapy.

The morbidity associated with hepatic resection directly relates to patient selection. Although a number of factors are considered in the surgical decision making, a recent study of 747 hepatectomies revealed that the incidence of postoperative complications was statistically increased and influenced by the American Society of Anesthesiologists (ASA) score, the presence of hepatic steatosis, the extent of resection, and an associated extrahepatic procedure. Interestingly, age was found not to be an independent predictor of increased morbidity.[2] Thus, the clinical performance status of the patient and the comorbidities of the major organ systems should permit resection with an expected mortality risk of less than 5%.

Patients considered for resection should be evaluated with computed tomography (CT) or magnetic resonance imaging (MRI) and in some cases, also a positron emission tomography (PET) scan. Temporally, CRM present in three clinical situations: synchronously with the primary cancer, metachronously after resection of the primary cancer, and metachronously after previous hepatic or pulmonary resection of CRM. Technical advances in both liver and colonic surgery have enabled simultaneous resection of the primary colorectal cancer and liver metastases to be performed safely in patients with synchronous tumors. Undertaking concurrent resection of the primary colorectal cancer and hepatic metastases requires thorough preoperative hepatic imaging, thus allowing for evaluation of the intrahepatic extent of disease and also to exclude extrahepatic disease. Furthermore, preoperative imaging allows for determining the number and distribution of liver lesions as well as defining the biliary and vascular structures. Lastly, Karoui et al found that in 33 patients with bilobar synchronous colorectal liver metastases who were candidates for two-stage hepatectomy, combined resection of the primary tumor and first-stage hepatectomy may reduce the number of procedures and allow optimization of chemotherapy administration, thus possibly improving outcome.[3] A recent publication by de Haas et al suggests that combining colorectal resection with limited hepatectomy is safe in patients with synchronous tumors and is associated with less cumulative morbidity than a delayed procedure. However, the combined strategy may have a negative impact on disease-free survival.[4] In patients with synchronous CRM who would benefit from neoadjuvant treatment of the primary lesion, a "reverse" approach of resecting the metastasis and then treating with chemotherapy radiation first and the colorectal surgery last appears feasibly safe and minimizes "vanishing" liver metastasis.[5]

The stage of the primary cancer clearly affects the decision to resect the hepatic metastases. Although boundaries are expanding, candidates for hepatic resection must have had complete excision of the primary cancer without gross residual extrahepatic metastatic disease. If the primary cancer is not controllable, resection of metastatic colorectal cancer is not indicated. Standard resection of the primary cancer with gross tumor-free margins of resection and appropriate regional lymphadenectomy is the goal of the colonic or rectal resection. Confirmation of an adequate locoregional resection allows a surgeon who is considering reoperation to focus on an evaluation of the metastases and not the primary cancer. If objective documentation of an adequate resection of the primary cancer is lacking, further evaluation of the site of the origin of the primary cancer is performed. Although an inadequate resection of the primary cancer does not exclude reoperation for metastatic disease, the patient must be informed of potentially decreased survival caused by residual primary disease. Indeed, the surgeon who is undertaking hepatic resection must stress that re-excision of the residual primary cancer may be required or that resection of metastases may be aborted because unresectable residual primary cancer may be found at exploration, even if the hepatic metastases themselves are resectable. Surgeons to whom patients are referred for resection of hepatic metastases must be cognizant of the possibility that an inadequate resection of the primary cancer has been performed and act accordingly.

Assessment of the adequacy of the primary operation depends in part on the origin of the primary colorectal tumor. In brief, the risk of locoregional recurrence of primary colorectal carcinoma correlates with the tumor, node, metastases (TNM) stage. Risk of locoregional recurrence is greatest for advanced T and N stage. Careful imaging evaluation of the primary and regional tumor site is indicated in patients who have had locally advanced-stage cancers.

Additional primary tumor factors that may be relevant to patient selection for the resection of hepatic metastases are the intraoperative features of the primary tumor and the operative technique used to resect the tumor. For example, patients with large colorectal tumors with invasion into or adherence to adjacent structures, or colorectal tumors that are "peeled off" from adjacent pelvic structures or major vascular structures with tumor extending to the microscopic margins may benefit from postoperative adjuvant irradiation and chemotherapy in an attempt to gain optimal local control. In general, such adjuvant treatment precedes surgery for hepatic metastases and subsequent restaging before hepatic resection, inclusive of positron emission scintigraphy or PET scanning, is performed. Other factors that warrant consideration in patient selection for reoperation are factors that predispose the patient to progression of peritoneal disease, such as division of adhesions between the primary tumor and adjacent structures, fracture of the tumor during resection, and incisional or wedge biopsy of hepatic metastases. Gross spillage of tumor during resection of the primary cancer usually dictates a longer period of observation before reoperation for hepatic metastases to allow detection of intraperitoneal disease progression. Finally, hepatic resection for metastases should rarely be undertaken if any extrahepatic metastases exist, exclusive of regional lymph node or limited pulmonary metastases. Focal extrahepatic disease that is concurrently resectable is currently considered only a relative contraindication to resection. Concurrent contraindications to resection of hepatic metastases include distant metastases, including peritoneal carcinomatosis, osseous or brain metastases, extraabdominal lymph node metastases, and multiple unresectable pulmonary metastases. Extensive liver metastases, including multiple bilobar metastases or involvement of both the afferent and efferent vasculature, are also contraindications to resection.

The extent of hepatic metastatic disease affects patient selection for liver resection. In brief, adequate hepatic reserve in patients without chronic liver disease can be assumed if only two anatomically adjacent segments are preserved after resection. If cirrhosis is present, the extent of resection is reduced, and ablation may assume a larger therapeutic role. Extensive hepatic steatosis without cirrhosis also limits the extent of hepatic resection. Portal vein embolization (PVE) of the lobe of anticipated resection (to induce hypertrophy of the planned remnant) is indicated when initial remnant volume is marginal.

FACTORS DETERMINING RESECTABILITY

Resection or ablation of metastases should never put the liver at risk for irreversible dysfunction. The aim of liver resection is to remove all disease to a negative margin, while preserving sufficient liver volume and function with adequate inflow and outflow. The extent of resection depends on the size of the metastases, the intrahepatic site, and the relationship of the tumor to major afferent and efferent vasculature and bile ducts.

Resectability of CRM to the liver has evolved over the past decade, primarily because of improvements in chemotherapy and surgical technique. Historically, subgroups of patient populations with large tumor numbers, large tumor size, lymph node involvement, or extrahepatic pulmonary disease were considered unresectable. However, newer chemotherapy protocols are allowing for a decrease in disease burden, thus allowing for restaging and an attempt at curative resection. The downside to neoadjuvant chemotherapy, however, is that, as Vauthey et al have shown, there is a 20% incidence of steatohepatitis in association with irinotecan-based chemotherapy and a 19% incidence of sinusoidal injury after treatment with oxaliplatin.[6] Ribero et al also found that the addition of bevacizumab reduced the incidence and severity of oxaliplatin-related sinusoidal injury while improving clinical response to the chemotherapy.[7] Other series have reported a higher rate of sinusoidal injury and an increase in perioperative blood transfusions and surgical complications in patients who received preoperative chemotherapy than those who did not.[8]

RISK-SCORING SYSTEMS

To aid in determining who will benefit most from surgical intervention, several risk scoring systems have been developed. The aims of these scoring systems are to optimize patient selection for hepatic resection and to stratify patients for the need of adjuvant therapies. Independent risk factors such as carcinoembryonic antigen (CEA) level, tumor size, and tumor number have been reported to predict outcome after resection of colorectal liver metastases. Different authors have used different variables and cutoff values to discriminate between patient groups with different prognoses. For example, scoring systems proposed by Schindl et al (*n* = 131) uses Dukes stage of colorectal cancer, number of liver metastases, CEA levels, albumin, and alkaline phosphatase levels[9]; Ueno et al ($n = 85$) includes aggressiveness of primary tumor, early liver metastases, and number of liver metastases[10]; and Lise et al ($n = 135$) includes percentage of liver invasion, metastases to lymph nodes at the primary tumor site, number of liver metastases, preoperative glutamic pyruvic transaminase levels, and type of liver resection.[11] However, because such scoring systems have been developed on small study populations, their clinical utility has not been established. Three other scoring systems were developed on large patient populations. In a multicenter study, Nordlinger et al, through a national collective registry of 1513 patients, developed a prognostic scoring system based on seven identified risk factors: age more than 60 years, primary cancer extending into serosa, positive regional lymph nodes, liver metastases confirmed within 24 months of the primary cancer, CEA levels, size of metastasis more than 5 cm, and less than 1-cm resection margin of the metastases.[12] Three risk groups were defined: low risk (zero to two risk factors), intermediate risk (three to four risk factors), and high risk (five to seven risk factors).[12] In a similar method, Fong et al, through a single-institution study of 1001 patients, devised a system based on node-positive primary cancer, hepatic metastases confirmed within 12 months of the primary cancer, more than one metastasis, size of metastasis more than 5 cm, and CEA level greater than 200 ng/mL.[13] Six risk groups were stratified by the sum of the individual prognostic variables.[13] Iwatsuki et al, also through a single-institution study of 230 patients, proposed a risk score based on more than three hepatic metastases, size of metastasis more than 8 cm, hepatic metastases confirmed within up to 30 months of the primary cancer, and bilobar hepatic metastases.[14] Five risk grades were stratified based on the sum of the individual prognostic variables: grade 1 being no risk factor present to grade 5, including patients with four risk factors.[14] These staging systems were based on multivariate survival analysis and reflected the prognosis. Nagorney et al[15] proposed a Mayo risk-scoring system with 662 patients and found that survival was stratified best by the Fong scoring system[13] and least by that of Iwatsuki[14] and Nordlinger.[12] The proposed Mayo model performed only marginally better than the Fong,[13] Iwatsuki,[14] and Nordlinger[12] systems in discriminating high/low risk of death from disease. All three models were only marginally better than chance alone in predicting disease-specific survival and recurrence.[15]

More recently, additional work has shown that in a number of malignancies, including colorectal carcinoma, the host's inflammatory response to tumor (IRT) plays a significant role in determining prognosis. In particular, an elevated (>10 mg/L) preoperative C-reactive protein (CRP) or a neutrophil to lymphocyte ratio (>5:1) has been associated with poorer cancer-specific survival. Malik et al, through a single-institution study of 700 patients, developed a prognostic scoring system based on two factors: more than eight metastases and the absence or presence of IRT.[16] Patients received a score of 0 if they had fewer than eight metastases and the absence of an IRT, a score of 1 if they had eight or more metastases or

IRT, and a score of 2 if they had eight or more metastases and an IRT. With this simplified scoring system, they were able to stratify patients into a relatively good prognosis of 49% if the score was 0, 34% if the score was 1, and 0% if the score was 2. In addition, they noted that the magnitude of the CRP elevation predicted worsening prognosis.[16]

MARGINS

Although a 1-cm margin has historically been considered appropriate to reduce the risk of intrahepatic recurrence at the margins of resection, because of more effective chemotherapy, recent data suggest that microscopically free resection margins continue to allow for improved survival when compared to positive margins. Pawlik et al reviewed 557 patients who underwent hepatic resection for CRM and determined that a positive margin was associated with an increased risk of recurrence. However, patients with negative margins experienced similar recurrence rates regardless of negative margin measurement. Thus, they concluded that a predicted margin of less than 1 cm should not exclude patients from being a candidate for surgical resection.[17] Margins, whether 1 cm or microscopic, however, should never risk damage to major hepatic vasculature. In addition, resection margins can be extended with the use of radiofrequency ablation (RFA) or cryoablation.

NUMBER OF METASTASES

The number of metastases is also no longer a contraindication provided adequate liver volume remains following resection. Weber et al concluded that resection in patients with four or more CRM can achieve long-term survival and that the number of hepatic metastases alone should not be used as a sole contraindication to resection.[18] Similarly, although long-term prognosis in patients with metastases to lymph nodes is unfavorable, hepatic resection combined with lymphadenectomy may be beneficial in occasional patients whose disease has been downstaged or completely eliminated clinically by chemotherapy and can be resected completely. Extrahepatic disease is usually associated with poorer survival. However, recent data report 5-year survivals of up to 50% in patients undergoing resection of isolated pulmonary metastases.[19] The Mayo data, when reported many years ago before advancements in chemotherapy, described 5- and 10-year survival of 30% and 16%, respectively, in patients undergoing both hepatic and pulmonary resection for CRM, thus concluding that resection of extrahepatic metastases in highly selected patients is safe and can improve overall survival.[20] Furthermore, recent reports suggest that patients with synchronous presentation of metastatic disease to the liver and lungs have similar survival after resection to those patients presenting with metachronous disease.[21] Timing of resection in patients presenting with synchronous disease, however, should allow for liver resection before lung resection to permit complete pulmonary function prior to lung resection. In addition, hepatic resection before lung resection allows for surgical inspection of the abdomen, ruling out advanced disease. Peritoneal metastases are considered by most advanced centers to be a contraindication to surgical resection. Although there are limited data reporting a small survival advantage of combined resection and intraperitoneal chemotherapy, this is not standard of care and is not routinely practiced.

DISAPPEARING TUMORS

Despite the evidence favoring hepatectomy when feasible, many medical oncologists prefer to continue systemic chemotherapy to maximal benefit, resulting in a population of patients with small residual nodules without uptake on fluoro-2-deoxy-D-glucose positron emission tomography (FDG-PET).[22] The debate rages over whether to resect lesions based on pretreatment localization or to observe closely and only resect areas of defined recurrence.

Benoist et al[23] examined whether a complete radiographic response indicated a cure of hepatic colorectal cancer liver metastases. In their series, they identified 38 of 586 patients with colorectal liver metastases who had "disappearance" of at least one metastases following chemotherapy. These 38 patients had 183 metastases of which 66 "disappeared" after chemotherapy. At the time of surgery, 20 of 66 (30%) tumors that had "disappeared" on preoperative imaging had macroscopic disease. An additional 12 of 15 "disappearing" tumors that were resected had microscopic disease identified on pathology. Twenty-three of 31 tumors that were labeled as "disappearing" and left in situ recurred during followup. Overall, a true pathologic response was achieved in only 17% of patients. Based on these results, the authors suggest that when feasible the site of the lesion that "disappeared" should be resected.

Auer et al[24] reported their experience treating 435 patients with colorectal liver metastases. Thirty-nine patients (9%) had a total of 118 disappearing lesions following chemotherapy. Sixty-eight disappearing liver metastases were resected, and 50 were followed clinically. Seventy-five (66%) disappearing liver metastases were true complete responses; 44 pathologic complete responses were found after resection, and 31 durable clinical responses were determined at the 1-year followup or later. In their series, a clinical response was independently associated with hepatic arterial infusion chemotherapy, inability to detect the disappearing metastases on MRI, and normalization of CEA.

Thus, 4% to 13% of patients with liver metastases from colorectal cancer will have a complete response following neoadjuvant chemotherapy. Of this subgroup, true complete response rates are reported between 17% and 65%. When patients with a true pathologic clinical response undergo resection, 5-year survival rates are reported as high as 75% by two independent groups.[8]

GENERAL PRINCIPLES AND PREPARATION FOR RESECTION

Resection or ablation of metastases should never put the liver at risk for irreversible dysfunction. The extent of resection will depend on the size of the metastases, intrahepatic site, and on the relationship of the tumor to major afferent and efferent vasculature and bile ducts. In patients with deeply seated metastases, formal anatomic resections are indicated. Moreover, metastatic disease manifesting indistinct margins mandates formal resection. A 1- to 2-cm margin is considered appropriate to reduce the risk of intrahepatic recurrence at the margins of resection. However, margins of resection should never risk damage to major hepatic vasculature. The afferent and efferent vasculature of the liver remnant must be protected scrupulously.

The liver parenchyma can be transected by a variety of methods: compression (finger fracture or digitoclasis, clamp fracture, or Kellyclasis staples), contact (Cavitron Ultrasonic Aspirator [Cavitron Corporation, Long Island, NY]), or thermal (electrocautery, laser, RFA). Each approach has advantages and disadvantages. Most methods disrupt parenchyma to expose vessels and bile ducts for ligation. A new method (TissueLink [TissueLink Medical, Inc, Dover, NH] and Harmonic Scalpel [Ethicon Endo-Surgery, Inc, Cincinnati, Ohio]) fuses small vessels and ducts. Although the extent of parenchymal necrosis adjacent to the transection plane varies among techniques, such devitalized parenchyma is not clinically significant. Vessels or ducts of diameter larger than 2 mm generally require ligation with suture or clips. Major hepatic or portal veins are best occluded securely with the use of vascular staples or alternatively a running monofilament permanent suture.

ANATOMY

Safe hepatic resection depends on a clear understanding of the hepatic anatomy. Although hepatic regenerative capacity and metabolic reserve permit many types of resections, resection based on preservation of residual anatomic integrity best reduces the operative risk and optimizes function. Couinaud's[25] description of hepatic anatomy highlights the anatomic features of the liver relevant to resection and in adults provides anatomic terminology that is clinically useful. Figure 171-1 details the ligamentous, segmental, and vascular anatomy of the liver that are important factors to consider for liver resection. Although the regenerative capacities and metabolic reserve of the liver are great, hepatic resection based on anatomic considerations reduces operative risk and optimizes postoperative liver function. In general, anatomic resections are preferable oncologically to ensure cancer-free margins and to lower the risk of potential sites for intrahepatic spread. The major anatomic features of the liver relevant to resection have been detailed elsewhere.[25]

The hilar plate is the extension of a vasobiliary sheath that is particularly relevant to hepatic resection (Figure 171-2). The vasobiliary sheath represents a fusion of the endoabdominal fascia around the bile ducts, portal vein, and hepatic artery at the porta hepatis. These fibrous sheaths invest the components of the pedicles from the portal vein bifurcation to the sinusoids. By contrast, the hepatic veins lack endoabdominal fascial investment and, consequently, are more fragile than their portal counterparts. The density of the vasculobiliary sheaths decreases as the pedicles extend intrahepatically. At the hepatic hilus, these sheaths fuse to form plates

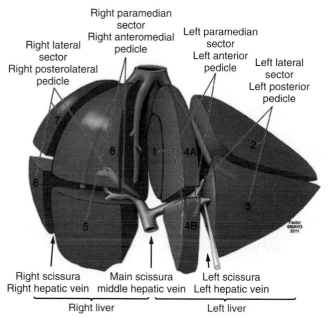

FIGURE 171-1 Hepatic anatomy: eight segments in the liver (segment 4 is divided into 4A and 4B). The major inflow and outflow is labeled as well as the sectoral anatomy. (Reproduced with permission of the Mayo Foundation.)

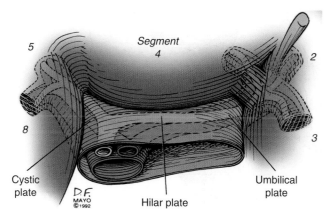

FIGURE 171-2 The fascial plates of the liver hilus, which represent a fusion of endoabdominal fascia around the portal structures. The fascial plate at the liver base is formed by three plates—cystic, hilar, and umbilical—which fuse with ill-defined boundaries. (The numbers refer to the hepatic segments.) (Reproduced with permission of the Mayo Foundation.)

that surround the portal pedicles, both anteriorly and posteriorly. Three primary hepatic plates are recognized: the cystic, the hilar, and the umbilical plates (see Figure 171-2). Recognition of the vasculobiliary sheaths and the hepatic plates facilitates precise access to the hilar structures. Division of these plates is needed to expose and mobilize the portal pedicle during resection.

PREOPERATIVE CARE

The preoperative preparation for patients undergoing hepatic resection is similar to that undertaken for any major pancreaticobiliary procedure. Coagulation profiles are corrected and prophylactic antibiotics

directed at upper gastrointestinal tract flora are administered. Importantly, if jaundice or cholangitis and bile duct obstruction are present, biliary decompression by endoscopic or percutaneous intubation is preferred to improve hepatic function and control infection. Biliary drainage is established for the anticipated hepatic remnant. In general, major hepatic resection is not undertaken unless the total serum bilirubin is nearly normal and clinical infection is controlled.

A major complement to the safety of hepatic resection is anesthetic management. The maintenance of low central venous pressure (5 to 7 mm Hg) reduces parenchymal blood loss via small hepatic veins. Large-bore intravenous access for rapid transfusion is also essential.

The major pitfalls or danger points with hepatic resection include hemorrhage from hepatic or portal veins or hepatic arteries; air embolism from hepatic venous injury; injury to the biliary ductal system with postoperative obstruction or fistula formation; portal or hepatic vein compromise with subsequent ischemia or postsinusoidal portal hypertension, respectively; prolonged vascular inflow occlusion leading to refractory hepatic ischemia or hepatic injury; and injury to the diaphragm, inferior vena cava, or intestine.

SURGICAL TECHNIQUE

INCISION AND EXPOSURE

For open resections, whether performing the resection laparoscopically or open, obtaining adequate exposure is critical to safe resection. Laparoscopic liver resections are covered elsewhere and will not be discussed.

A bilateral subcostal incision or a right subcostal incision with a vertical extension to the xiphoid process affords wide exposure for any hepatic resection (Figure 171-3). A long midline incision provides a satisfactory alternative, particularly for limited resections of segments II through VI or if the patient has a narrow or acute costal angle. Tumors that involve segments VII or VIII or extended lobar resections are approached more safely through a bilateral subcostal incision, which permits better exposure and control of the hepatic vein/inferior vena cava junction. Rarely, a right thoracic extension (thoracoabdominal incision) may be necessary for safe exposure of large bulky tumors that involve segments VII and VIII or those that require inferior caval reconstruction. All perihepatic adhesions are divided. Any adherent diaphragm is excised with the metastasis. The liver is mobilized by complete division of its ligamentous attachments (i.e., coronary, falciform, and triangular ligaments) (Figure 171-4). The thin gastrohepatic omentum is incised adjacent to the hepatoduodenal ligament. The foramen of Winslow is opened in anticipation of subsequent inflow vascular occlusion. An upper hand or chain retractor should be used to elevate the rib cage anteriorly and cephalad. Additional retractors may be used to retract the remaining viscera caudally.

PARENCHYMAL TRANSECTION

The hepatic parenchyma is transected by the method of personal preference. Each method disrupts the

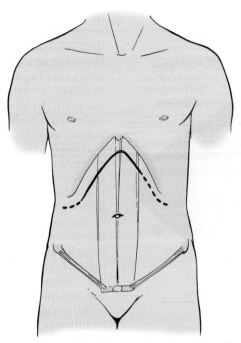

FIGURE 171-3 The standard subcostal incision extending to the anterior axillary lines bilaterally. (Reproduced with permission of the Mayo Foundation.)

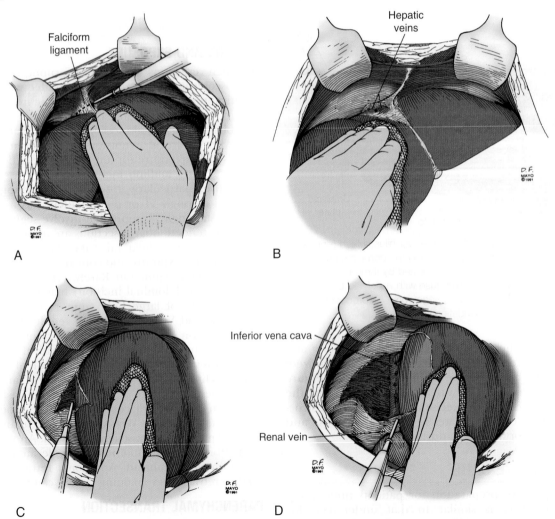

FIGURE 171-4 **A,** Mobilization of the liver is initiated by dividing the falciform ligament. **B,** Division of the falciform ligament is extended to the hepatic veins posteriorly. **C,** The liver is rotated medially to divide the right coronary and triangular ligaments, exposing the bare area of the liver. **D,** Complete division of the right coronary and triangular ligaments exposes the right lateral aspect of the inferior vena cava. Multiple short hepatic veins are visible after complete exposure. (Reproduced with permission of the Mayo Foundation.)

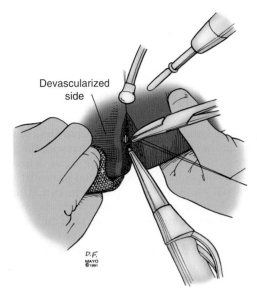

FIGURE 171-5 Parenchymal transection of the liver. The hepatic parenchyma is transected in the standard fashion with compression of the parenchyma manually along both sides of the planned transection plane. The parenchyma may be divided with an ultrasonic aspirator (as shown here) or by other methods. Vessels and bile ducts along the devascularized side or specimen side of the liver are clipped. The vessel and bile duct along the opposite side (the patient's side) of the liver are suture ligated for permanent and secure closure and to avoid artifact on postresection liver imaging. (Reproduced with permission of the Mayo Foundation.)

parenchyma to expose vessels or ducts for ligation or cauterization. Hemorrhage is reduced by digital compression of the liver on each side of the transection plane. Both the surgeon and the assistant compress the parenchyma on opposing sides of the transection plane (Figure 171-5). Typically, the assistant surgeon maintains hemostasis by electrocautery or clips. An additional assistant maintains field exposure by suctioning bile or blood from the transection interface. Bile ducts or vessels with diameter larger than 2 mm are clamped with metal clips or ligated with suture. Suture ligation of remnant vessels or ducts reduces artifacts during postoperative imaging. After local hemostasis and bile stasis are obtained, the abdomen is closed. Closed low-pressure suction drainage is optional.

TYPES OF SURGICAL TREATMENT OF HEPATIC METASTASES

Multiple terms have been used to describe various hepatic resections. The current recommendations for formal terminology have been proposed and are referenced for review.[26a]

WEDGE RESECTIONS

Wedge resections (i.e., nonanatomic resections) are performed without reference to segmental or sectoral anatomy. Wedge resections typically are subsegmental and frequently cross intersegmental planes and are well tolerated by the liver because they are used for small peripheral, nonhilar tumors. Wedge resections are usually performed with a minimum of blood loss, even without inflow vascular occlusion.

ANATOMIC UNISEGMENTAL AND POLYSEGMENTAL RESECTIONS

Anatomic resections of a single liver segment or multiple contiguous liver segments require identification and ligation of the segmental vascular biliary pedicles for accurate anatomic demarcation of the segment or segments. Portal and segmental pedicles are best approached by dissection from the hilus to the appropriate pedicle or by direct rapid parenchymal transection along an estimated intersegmental plane with ultrasound guidance. Dissection from the hilum is most applicable for anterior liver segments. Dissection along an intersegmental plane is more appropriate for ligation of the posterior hepatic segments II, VII, and VIII. Both approaches are facilitated by temporary inflow vascular occlusion to reduce hemorrhage and by the use of the ultrasonic aspirator to rapidly expose the pedicles through the intervening parenchyma. Alternatively, methylene blue may be injected into the segmental or portal pedicle using ultrasound guidance, which provides visual identification of the anatomic segmental or sectoral anatomy. Total vascular isolation of the liver may be required rarely for large tumors. If so, the infrahepatic suprarenal and suprahepatic inferior vena cava are excluded to permit occlusion by vascular clamps or tapes.

LOBAR RESECTIONS

Lobar resections are polysegmental resections based on the primary right and left portal pedicles. The risk of blood loss is reduced significantly by ligation of the appropriate lobar hepatic arterial and portal venous branches before parenchymal transection. In addition, ligation of the corresponding hepatic vein before parenchymal transection further reduces blood loss. Major lobar resections can be extended either anatomically or nonanatomically. Anatomic extensions are performed by resecting the involved liver segments adjacent to the principal plane and nonanatomic extensions by subsegmentectomy.

The liver is mobilized fully for all lobar resections. Cholecystectomy is performed either en bloc with the resected lobe (if adherent to the tumor) or before parenchymal transection to facilitate exposure of the hilar structures. The lobar hepatic artery is ligated initially. The right hepatic artery generally traverses the triangle of Calot. Pericholedochal lymph nodes are excised to further expose the bile duct, portal vein, and hepatic artery and for staging. For a right lobectomy, the right lateral aspect of the hepatoduodenal ligament is incised longitudinally just posterior to the bile duct (Figure 171-6). The right hepatic artery, regardless of the origin, is always found lateral to the common hepatic duct or inferior to the right main hepatic duct, where it enters the liver parenchyma.

The left hepatic artery is approached through the lesser sac through the left lateral aspect of the hepatoduodenal ligament after division of the gastrohepatic omentum. The main left hepatic artery is generally found

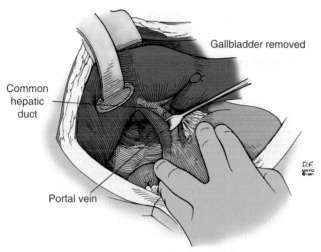

FIGURE 171-6 Exposure of the hepatic hilus for vascular control before major hepatic resection. Cholecystectomy facilitates exposure of the major vessels of the liver at its hilus. The peritoneum along the right lateral aspect of the hepatoduodenal ligament is incised, and the bile duct is retracted medially and superiorly using a vein retractor. The major portal vessels can then be identified. (Reproduced with permission of the Mayo Foundation.)

just inferior to the base of the round ligament as it enters the left lobe between segments III and IV anterior to segment I (Figure 171-7). When present, an accessory left hepatic artery arising from the left gastric artery courses through the gastrohepatic omentum and is often divided during division of the gastrohepatic omentum for resections of the left lobe. Lymphatic vessels around the hepatic arteries are ligated before division to reduce postoperative lymphatic drainage. Regardless of the type of lobectomy performed, the artery that supplies the lobe of the resection is occluded temporarily, whereas the artery to the opposite lobe is palpated to ensure patency of the arterial supply to the hepatic remnant. After blood flow to the hepatic remnant is appropriately confirmed, the lobar artery is doubly ligated with heavy silk and divided.

A similar approach is used for right hepatic artery ligation, although the right hepatic artery is exposed to the right aspect of the hepatoduodenal ligament (Figure 171-8). The bile duct is retracted anteriorly with a vein retractor to expose the portal venous bifurcation. Again, the right portal vein is exposed to the right of the hepatoduodenal ligament, and the left portal vein is exposed to the left of the hepatoduodenal ligament. The main

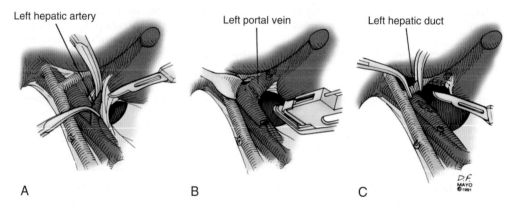

FIGURE 171-7 Vascular and biliary control before left hepatectomy is best obtained through the gastrohepatic omentum along the left lateral aspect of the hepatoduodenal ligament. Initially, the left hepatic artery is ligated at its origin. **A,** The left main artery enters the liver just below the falciform ligament. **B,** The left main portal vein, which courses toward the left shoulder, is transected with a vascular stapler. **C,** Finally, the left main bile duct is transected and ligated. (Reproduced with permission of the Mayo Foundation.)

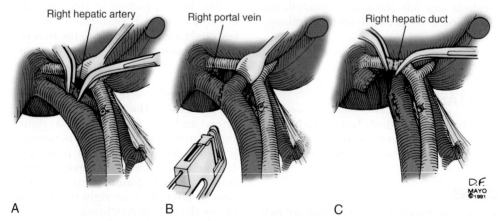

FIGURE 171-8 Exposure of the right hepatic artery and right main portal vein branch is best obtained through the right lateral aspect of the hepatoduodenal ligament. The bile duct is retracted medially and superiorly with a vein retractor. **A,** The right main hepatic artery is identified and divided between clamps. **B,** The right main portal vein branch is exposed and transected with a vascular stapler. **C,** After clear identification, the right main bile duct is divided. (Reproduced with permission of the Mayo Foundation.)

left portal vein branch always bifurcates from the right main branch at an approximately 90-degree angle and courses anterolaterally.

Occasionally, two major branches of the right portal vein—anterior and posterior—may arise separately without a common trunk, resulting in a portal vein trifurcation. The appropriate lobar portal vein branch is freed from the surrounding lymphoareolar tissue and is ligated with a vascular stapler or a running vascular suture after division between clamps (see Figures 171-7 and 171-8). A simple suture ligature is not used on the portal vein because ligature dislodgemeny can result in immediate life-threatening hemorrhage. After division of the lobar blood supply, a clear line of vascular demarcation along the principal hepatic plane between the lobes confirms appropriate and complete lobar vascular ligation (Figure 171-9). Parenchymal transection can be initiated at this time or after ligation of the hepatic vein (depending on the size of the tumor and the tumor–hepatic vein relationship). After the blood supply to the liver has been controlled, the hepatic veins may be approached safely.

During a right lobectomy, multiple short hepatic veins between the inferior vena cava and the paracaval segments are ligated to prevent avulsion during anterior retraction of the liver. Ligation starts caudally and proceeds cephalad. Occasionally, a large right inferior hepatic vein enters the inferior vena cava from the posterior aspect of segment VI. Either staples or a running suture closure for secure ligation of this vein is preferred to simple ligature. To expose the main right hepatic vein, the hepatocaval ligament bridging segments I and VII is divided (Figure 171-10). A moderate-sized vein frequently traverses this ligament, and its presence should be anticipated before division. The main right hepatic vein, which has an extrahepatic component of 1 to 2 cm, is dissected from the inferior vena cava and the overlying liver. Unless large metastases preclude access, the right hepatic vein can almost always be transected with a vascular stapler before parenchymal transection. After division, the parenchymal side is ligated with a running vascular suture before parenchymal transection.

During left lobectomy, ligation of the main left hepatic vein, which usually joins the middle hepatic vein before entering the vena cava, can be deferred until parenchymal transection is complete because extrahepatic exposure is technically more difficult. Although the middle hepatic vein can be ligated during either right or left lobectomy, preservation reduces postoperative hepatic congestion and the volume of postoperative serous drainage. Alternatively, compression of the left hepatic vein at the confluence of the middle and left hepatic veins by a vascular clamp can be used to reduce hemorrhage from the hepatic venous branches along the interface of the liver during transection.

The parenchymal transection is guided by the zone of vascular demarcation and intraoperative ultrasonography. Parenchyma is transected by the surgeon's method of choice (Figure 171-11). Major bile ducts are ligated with permanent suture. Injection of the cystic duct stump or main bile duct can be performed with saline or a dilute methylene blue solution to exclude occult bile leaks along the transection interface. Bile leaks are closed

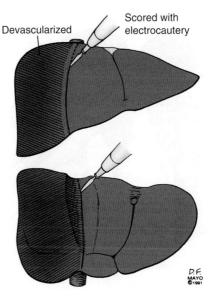

FIGURE 171-9 After completion of hilar ligation of the major lobar hepatic vessels, the interface between the vascularized and devascularized portions of the liver is evident. The planned transection plane is marked with cautery immediately adjacent to the devascularized portion of the liver. (Reproduced with permission of the Mayo Foundation.)

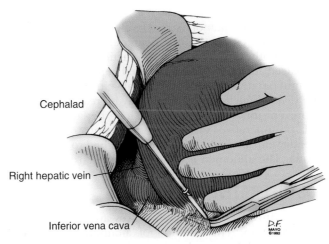

FIGURE 171-10 Transection of the right main hepatic vein. Access to the right main hepatic vein extrahepatically can best be achieved only after full mobilization of the right lobe. Frequently, a thick band of tissue extends from the caudate lobe to segment VII, just inferior to the right hepatic vein. Complete division of the retrocaval ligament is required for adequate extrahepatic exposure of the main right hepatic vein in its junction with the inferior vena cava. (Reproduced with permission of the Mayo Foundation.)

with sutures or clips. After parenchymal transection, topical hemostatic agents are used as needed. In general, persistent, diffuse interface hemorrhage or oozing results from elevated central venous pressure due to excessive intraoperative crystalloid, colloid, and blood product transfusion or, rarely, due to various causes of right heart failure. Compression of the transection interface and reduction in the central venous pressure by vasodilators or by decreasing the rate of fluid infusion and diuresis

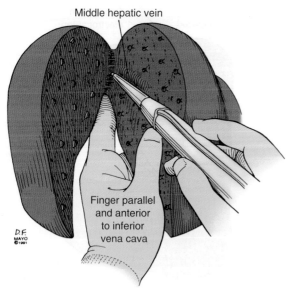

Middle hepatic vein

Finger parallel
and anterior
to inferior
vena cava

FIGURE 171-11 Parenchymal transection is continued throughout the liver with vascular biliary structures ligated as necessary. The surgeon's orientation for appropriate parenchymal transection can be maintained by using the index finger as a guide. (Reproduced with permission of the Mayo Foundation.)

will reduce such hemorrhage. Development of a coagulopathy requires blood component therapy, liver packing, and normothermia. If preferred, a suction drain or drains are placed adjacent to the transected hepatic surface and brought out dependently and laterally through the flank. The divided falciform ligament may be reapproximated to prevent torsion of a small left lobe hepatic remnant and postoperative vascular compression of the left hepatic vein. The omentum is not attached to the parenchyma. The abdomen is closed in a standard fashion.

POSTOPERATIVE CARE

Postoperative care generally involves appropriate fluid administration. The addition of albumin to standard crystalloid solutions reduces postoperative weight gain and maintains adequate urine output. Most hepatic resections are associated with a mild acidosis and coagulation abnormalities in the immediate postoperative period. Neither acid-based abnormalities nor coagulation deficits are corrected postoperatively unless they are clinically significant. Urinary output is monitored until hemodynamic stability has been maintained for 24 hours. Postoperative epidural analgesia markedly improves pulmonary function and pain control.

COMPLICATIONS OF HEPATIC RESECTION AND THEIR MANAGEMENT

INTRAOPERATIVE COMPLICATIONS

Hemorrhage is the most common intraoperative complication. It results from major vessel trauma along the transection interface or from coagulopathy. Inflow occlusion or total hepatic vascular isolation has dramatically reduced abrupt life-threatening hemorrhage from trauma to the major hepatic vasculature. A simple Pringle maneuver with an appropriate-sized vascular clamp or loop snare easily controls hemorrhage from either the portal vein or the hepatic arteries. Traumatic injury to the extrahepatic bile duct from a vasculature clamp is rare. The noncirrhotic liver tolerates warm ischemia periods for more than 1 hour without permanent long-term consequence. Ischemia/reperfusion injury may be reduced by intermittent occlusion. Although ischemic hepatic injury is reflected by elevations of serum aspartate transaminase and bilirubin and prolongation of the prothrombin time, these changes reverse to normal within 7 to 10 days.

Diffuse hemorrhage from the transection interface usually results from elevation of the central venous pressure greater than 12 to 15 mm Hg. Continuous intraoperative monitoring of the central venous pressure and volume replacement to maintain central venous pressures between 5 and 8 mm Hg reduces this operative risk of hemorrhage but allows the maintenance of adequate systemic hemodynamics. Vasodilators may also be required. Persistent interface hemorrhage is treated best by coagulation with electrocautery, the argon beam coagulator, tissue link, or by compression with laparotomy pads and topical hemostatic agents. Should interface bleeding persist after the use of these techniques, intraoperative evaluation for coagulopathy must be undertaken. An intraoperative thromboelastogram should be obtained and abnormal coagulation profiles should be corrected with blood products as indicated.

The last significant intraoperative complication is air embolus from hepatic vein damage. Although a potentially life-threatening source of cardiac arrhythmias and ventilation/perfusion defects, early recognition is possible through careful anesthetic monitoring. The techniques for anesthetic monitoring for venous air embolism include precordial Doppler sonography, right heart catheterization, capnography from mass spectroscopy, transcutaneous oxygen probes, and transesophageal echocardiography. Doppler sonography and transesophageal echocardiography are the most sensitive, whereas abnormalities of capnographic mass spectrometry provide the most practical recognition of venous air embolism. With an increasing volume of air embolism, initial gas exchange abnormalities are supplanted by deteriorating systemic hemodynamics. Venous air embolism should be suspected initially by decreases in arterial oxygen tension, transcutaneous oxygen pressure, and fractional end-tidal concentrations of carbon dioxide and an increase in fractional end-tidal concentration of nitrogen. If undetected, the arterial carbon dioxide tension and transcutaneous carbon dioxide pressures will increase rapidly. Advanced signs include a precordial machinery murmur, visible air in the hepatic vein or inferior vena cava, and a decrease in cardiac output and blood pressure. Treatment consists of placing the patient in a Trendelenburg position, suture closure of the hepatic vein, and aspiration of the intracardiac air through a central venous pressure catheter with positive-pressure ventilation.

POSTOPERATIVE COMPLICATIONS

Postoperative hemorrhage usually arises from displaced vascular clips or ligatures. Recognition should be obvious by depressed hemodynamics or bloody abdominal drainage. Any concurrent coagulopathy should be at least partially corrected before reoperation for control of hemorrhage.

Serosanguineous drainage through intraabdominal drains is expected postoperatively. The volume of drainage may vary widely. Large-volume drainage may require isotonic fluid replacement to maintain fluid and electrolyte balance in the postoperative period. In general, abdominal drains can be removed safely regardless of the volume unless the drainage is bilious. Usually, even high-output drainage volumes are resorbed rapidly through the peritoneum without the formation of focal fluid collections or ascites. In patients with cirrhosis, drains should be avoided after hepatic resection because of protracted ascitic fluid drainage. Moreover, secondary infection of the ascites, which is associated with prolonged drainage, will be avoided.

Bilious drainage through the intraabdominal drains or after puncture of loculated perihepatic fluid collections is indicative of a biliary injury. Most injuries are best managed conservatively by continuous closed-suction drainage until they resolve. Minor fistulas (<100 mL/day) usually resolve with continuous suction drainage. Major fistulas (>200 mL/day) warrant cholangiographic evaluation and biliary stenting to speed resolution. Major fistulas may require Roux-en-Y hepaticojejunostomy for definitive repair. Reoperation for repair of biliary fistula is indicated rarely unless there has been complete disruption of the major bile duct from the remnant liver and a complete absence of bilioenteric bile flow.

A perihepatic intraabdominal abscess may occur after any hepatic resection. Careful hemostasis and bile stasis after resection will reduce perihepatic fluid accumulation and the risk of infection. Percutaneous drainage of abscesses is the treatment of choice.

Finally, hepatic insufficiency or failure can occur after hepatic resection. Hepatic failure usually occurs in patients with chronic hepatic diseases and cirrhosis or after extended polysegmental resection. The most common cause of hepatic insufficiency after hepatic resection is inadequate residual functional reserve. The treatment of this cause of hepatic failure is simply supportive. Preoperative PVE is indicated in patients in whom small hepatic remnants are anticipated. Orthotopic liver transplantation provides the only curative solution for refractory postoperative hepatic failure caused by inadequate reserve. However, even in selected patients, the risk associated with orthotopic liver transplantation for the salvage of hepatic failure induced by resection is exceedingly high and contraindicated in the presence of metastatic cancer, albeit resected.

Correctable causes of hepatic insufficiency should be sought postoperatively. Correctable causes of hepatic failure postoperatively include major bile duct obstruction and efferent or afferent vascular compromise as a result of vascular thrombosis or vessel narrowing. Bile duct obstruction should be suspected by steadily increasing total and direct serum bilirubin levels.

Endoscopic retrograde or magnetic resonance cholangiography best defines the location and extent of the injury, but only the former technique permits therapeutic intervention. Percutaneous transhepatic cholangiography is less useful postoperatively because of delayed proximal bile duct dilation and altered hepatic position after resection. Potentially correctable major hepatic vasculature injuries include portal and hepatic vein thromboses. Color flow Doppler ultrasonography is the best screening technique if suspected. Definitive imaging by angiography, magnetic resonance imaging, or computed tomographic angiography further defines the extent and vascular damage caused by thrombus. Once thromboses are recognized, reoperation for thrombectomy and repair of the venous damage that precipitated the thrombus are indicated. Systemic thrombolytic agents are contraindicated because of recent operative intervention. Anticoagulants (heparin and warfarin [Coumadin]) are useful to prevent recurrent thrombosis. Additional aspects important to mention in the surgical resection of hepatic colorectal metastases are sinusoidal obstruction syndrome (SOS) and chemotherapy associated steatohepatitis (CASH). Specifically, oxaliplatin has been shown to be associated with sinusoidal dilation while irinotecan is associated with steatohepatitis, the latter of which is associated with increased operative risk and mortality. Thus the extent of resection as well as other patient factors and chemotherapy administered, should be taken into account prior to liver resection.[26b]

NONRESECTIONAL SURGERY FOR HEPATIC METASTASES

HEPATIC ARTERY INFUSION

Hepatic artery infusional chemotherapy has been used for unresectable hepatic metastases for colorectal carcinoma and as adjuvant therapy after hepatic resection. Although combination systemic chemotherapy has produced objective responses in only a minority of patients and has had significantly improved patient survival rates compared with no therapy or single-agent chemotherapy, systemic chemotherapy remains primarily palliative. Alternatively, regional chemotherapy for unresectable metastases has proven to be more effective. The theoretical rationale for regional or hepatic artery infusional chemotherapy is based on the nearly exclusive arterial blood supply of the metastases from the hepatic artery and first-pass drug clearance kinetics, which support high local hepatic concentrations of the drug with reduced systemic toxicity. Multiple studies have compared the use of regional hepatic arterial infusion of 5-fluorodeoxyuridine (5-FUDR) with systemic 5-fluorouracil (5-FU). Metaanalyses of these trials have shown that (1) objective tumor response rates are significantly greater for regional 5-FUDR than for systemic 5-FU treatment[27] and (2) there is minimal or no improvement in overall survival. The use of regional infusional chemotherapy improved median survival times by only 3.2 months compared with systemic chemotherapy. The data from individual trials may bias outcomes because many patients randomized to regional therapy did not complete therapy because of technical problems with the infusion pump or toxicity. Subset analyses of the patients who actually received regional therapy suggests improved survival compared with those treated systemically. Further trials of regional infusion of 5-FUDR are being carried out in an attempt to reduce associated toxicity and to address the role of concurrent systemic chemotherapy as an adjunct after the resection of metastases.

Complications of intrahepatic arterial chemotherapy can be divided into two broad groups: (1) pump-related (technical) complications and (2) chemotherapy-related complications.[6] Pump-related complications of intrahepatic arterial chemotherapy include pump malfunctions, pump site infections, and chemotherapy-related complications, including hematologic and gastrointestinal toxicities. Gastrointestinal toxicity includes nausea, vomiting, and diarrhea, which occur infrequently with hepatic artery infusion of 5-FUDR. When diarrhea does occur, misperfusion of chemotherapy to the gastrointestinal tract through an improperly placed catheter or hepatic arterial collateral vessels should be suspected. The most common problems of hepatic artery infusion therapy are gastroduodenal ulceration and hepatotoxicity. Ulcer disease usually results from misperfusion of the stomach and duodenum via small collateral branches of the hepatic artery or the right gastric artery and are preventable by careful division of these collateral vessels during pump placement. Hepatobiliary toxicity is the most problematic toxicity. The bile ducts are particularly sensitive to regional chemoperfusion because like the hepatic metastases, bile ducts derive their blood supply almost exclusively from the hepatic artery. Clinically, biliary toxicities manifest as an elevation in the aspartate aminotransferase, alkaline phosphatase, and bilirubin levels, as well as cholangiographic biliary sclerosis mimicking sclerosing cholangitis. Hepatotoxicity is manifested by hepatitis. Dose reduction of 5-FUDR and concurrent corticosteroid perfusion through the pump may reduce hepatobiliary toxicity.

CRYOABLATION

Frequently, either the extent or location of hepatic metastases precludes safe resection. Cryoablation offers a technically sound and biologically rational approach for the treatment of such liver metastases.[28] The reputed advantages of cryoablation versus resection of hepatic metastases are the avoidance of the inherent risks of resection over the technical ease and safety of the cryoablation with its potentially similar efficacy. Cryosurgery is an ablative procedure based primarily on the chemicophysiologic sequelae of rapid freeze-thaw cycles on cellular membranes. To achieve a total cell kill, tissue temperatures of $-50°$ C or below are required. Repetitive freeze-thaw cycles increase the probability of complete tissue destruction. Thawing should be completed before the onset of the next freeze cycle for maximum cytotoxic potential. Various cryounits are commercially available and differ primarily by type of cryogen and probes and rapidity of freeze-thaw cycles. In brief, the technique for cryoablation is simple. The liver is mobilized, and

the metastases are located. Depending on the size of the metastases, an appropriate-sized cryoprobe is placed through the metastases, and cryoablation is initiated under ultrasonographic guidance. The cryoprobe is removed, and the cryotract is packed with a hemostatic agent.

Intraoperative ultrasonography is essential for effective cryoablation. Ultrasonography provides (1) accurate positioning of cryoprobes within the metastases to avoid injury to major bile ducts and vessels, (2) accurate monitoring of the freeze-thaw process with a clear demonstration of the freeze-front, and (3) detection of occult hepatic metastases. For large tumors, multiple concurrent probes speed treatment.

Potential intraoperative complications of hepatic cryosurgery include accidental freezing of adjacent tissues, cracking of the liver parenchyma, bleeding due to the introduction of trotter probes, hypothermia and related cardiac arrhythmias, nitrogen embolism, bile duct or major vascular injury, and renal failure from myoglobinuria. Insulation of the diaphragm, bowel, and skin from the liver with laparotomy packs prevents accidental cryoinjury to adjacent structures. Bleeding from the probe tract is rarely a problem and can be easily controlled by packing the cryotract with hemostatic material. Large vessels tolerate cryotherapy extremely well without rupture or occlusion because of the continued dissipation of thermal energy by the flow of blood. In contrast, large bile ducts are extremely vulnerable to cryoinjury, and caution should be exercised in treating tumors located near the hilum. After cryosurgery, a transient elevation of liver enzymes and a mild leukocytosis may occur, but they should normalize within 1 week. Carcinoembryonic antigen levels will remain elevated for approximately 6 weeks. Patients are commonly febrile for 3 to 4 days after cryoablation but respond promptly to treatment with indomethacin. Pleural effusions, subphrenic abscesses, or bile collections occur rarely.

Survival rates after cryoablation for unresectable metastases approach 60% at 2 years with median survival times of 25 to 32 months.[28,29] To date, the outcome of cryoablation alone for hepatic metastases from colorectal carcinoma has been promising. Survival rates have ranged from 15% to 35% at 5 years. Whether survival after cryoablation will be equivalent to resection is yet undetermined. No randomized, controlled trials have been performed to compare these treatments. Adjuvant chemotherapy (regional or systemic) has been used frequently with cryoablation in an effort to improve outcome. Adjuvant cryoablation has been used concurrently with resection for the treatment of small, deep-seated hepatic metastases during major hepatectomy, and consequently, has extended the role of resection in some patients who were otherwise unresectable.

HYPERTHERMIA

In contrast to cryoablation, focal hyperthermia also has tumor ablative potential. The technology for focal delivery of hyperthermic temperatures capable of tumor destruction has been developed using microwave, radiofrequency, and laser techniques. The general technique of hyperthermic ablation is similar to cryoablation. An applicator or probe is inserted into the tumor guided by ultrasound imaging. Ablation cycles are usually not repeated. Monitoring of the destruction zone by ultrasound is less accurate than cryoablation for some of these modalities because echogenicity changes minimally with heat. Interstitial laser ablation has involved the use of the neodymium-doped yttrium-aluminum-garnet (Nd:YAG) laser, primarily because of its light emission wavelength. Biologic response depends on wavelength, intensity, exposure time, and absorption characteristics of the tissue. The current major advantages of hyperthermic ablation include ease of application, both percutaneous and open applicability, accuracy, retreatment potential, and decreased hospitalization time. Disadvantages include delivery unit expense, variable reaction time monitoring, and size of maximum destruction zones.

The use of radiofrequency ablation (RFA), as either a primary or adjunct modality, has proven the most versatile of ablative techniques[30] and is currently the most widely used by surgeons and interventional radiologists. The advantages of RFA include (1) tumor necrosis for metastases adjacent to vasculature that, if resected, would jeopardize postresection function; (2) tumor necrosis for deep, small (≤3 cm) metastases that, if resected, would require removal of significant tissue volume and jeopardize function; (3) tumor necrosis of metastases (3 to 5 cm) in patients with underlying chronic liver diseases or cirrhosis; and (4) enlargement of postresection margins. The disadvantages of RFA include: (1) high recurrence rate for large tumors (>5 cm); (2) necrosis of adjacent structures—major bile ducts, stomach, duodenum, colon, and diaphragm; (3) delayed tumor recurrence on late (>3 years) followup[31]; and (4) metastases must be clearly visible by imaging.

Radiofrequency ablation can be performed percutaneously or at laparoscopy or laparotomy. RFA generally is associated with minimal morbidity and rarely with mortality. Currently, RFA is used primarily as an adjunct to resection or as primary therapy when resection is precluded regardless of cause. Although initial outcomes with RFA (<3 years) were similar to those of resection in patients with similar primary and metastatic cancer characteristics, late outcomes (5 years) are unknown and evidence-based data are unavailable.

PROGNOSTIC DETERMINANTS

Hepatic resection of metastatic colorectal cancer to the liver has become the treatment of choice for selected patients. Overall 5-year survival rates consistently range between 25% and 40% (Table 171-1).[12,17,31-34] Operative mortality rates are usually 4% or less. Perioperative morbidity rates range from 15% to 20%. Indications for resection of hepatic metastases include any hepatic metastases that can be resected with cancer-free margins provided that a functional hepatic remnant can be maintained. Concurrent resections are now indicated provided surgical expertise for both colorectal and hepatic surgery is available, all other resectability criteria are fulfilled, and the patient's intraoperative condition permits extending the operation for hepatic resection. The only outcome difference overall is the negative impact of

"synchronous" metastases. Such resections are favored when encountered to allow prompt initiation of the potent chemotherapy now available.

Focal extrahepatic peritoneal disease that is concurrently resectable was previously thought to be a contraindication to resection but is now considered only a relative contraindication. Concurrent contraindications to resection of hepatic metastases include distant metastases (including peritoneal carcinomatosis, osseous or brain metastases, extraabdominal lymph node metastases, and multiple, unresectable pulmonary metastases); extensive liver metastases (multiple, bilobar metastases, metastatic involvement of both the afferent and efferent vasculature, and medically unresponsive metastases); and prohibitive comorbidity inclusive of hepatic insufficiency.

Many surgeons have postulated that overall survival rates for patients with hepatic metastases for colorectal cancer could be increased by refining patient selection for resection or by neoadjuvant chemotherapy leading to resection of initially unresectable metastases. If clinical factors with consistent prognostic value were identifiable, resection should be encouraged for patients with a high probability of survival. Moreover, if effective adjuvant chemotherapy after hepatic resection becomes established, the treatment of hepatic metastases could be further stratified by survival risk based on these prognostic factors and response to adjuvant therapy. Potential prognostic factors have been culled from various patient, primary tumor, and metastatic disease characteristics from literature reports. In addition, the relationship of survival to medical and surgical intervention has been examined. Associations between potential prognostic factors and survival have been based on the analysis of overall or disease-free survival data.[13] Factors that have a statistical correlation to survival are shown in Table 171-1. Because Table 171-1 is simply a tabulation of prognostic factors abstracted from individual reports, the strength of survival correlation varied among factors. There was no single factor other than incomplete resection that absolutely and reliably precluded survival. Hepatic resection of metastatic colorectal cancer should be the primary treatment approach unless all gross disease is not resectable. Current risk-scoring systems permit stratification of expected outcomes and identify patients with low probability of survival. However, these systems do not identify patients whose survival is certain and preclude consideration for adjuvant therapy.

RECURRENCE AND REPEAT HEPATIC RESECTION

Recurrence (or reappearance) of tumor after potentially curative liver resection usually involves the liver, lungs, and peritoneal cavity. In the French multicenter study, 1013 of 1569 patients (65%) with accessible followup data developed recurrent disease. The liver was involved in 63% of patients with recurrences, which included nearly 47% of patients with recurrent disease limited to the liver. Metastatic disease after hepatectomy occurred in 70% of the 607 patients from the U.S. Registry of

TABLE 171-1 Clinicopathologic Factors Adversely Associated With Survival in Patients Who Underwent Hepatic Resection for Metastatic Colorectal Cancer

Patient Clinical Findings	Primary Colorectal Cancer	Pathologic Findings in Metastatic Colorectal Cancer	Interventional Findings
Age ≥70 yr	TNM stage 3	Percent replacement (extent) ≥50%	Margins of resection
Male gender	Histologic grade: high	Bilobar distributions	≤1 cm
Symptoms: jaundice, pain	to undifferentiated	Number ≥4	Nonanatomic hepatic
Performance status <50%	Primary site: Rectum	Satellite configuration	resection
	Colorectal venous	Size ≥1 cm	Perioperative blood
	invasion	Perihepatic lymphatic metastases	transfusions
	Tumor DNA aneuploidy	Extrahepatic metastases	
		Serum carcinoembryonic antigen level ≥30 ng/mL	
		Tumor DNA aneuploidy	
		Intrahepatic vascular invasion	
		Intrahepatic biliary invasion	
		Synchronous recognition ≤1 yr from primary	

Hepatic Metastases.[30] Three hundred sixteen patients had recurrence in a single organ: 149 (47%) in the liver, 73 (23%) in the lung, 30 (10%) local, and 61 (19%) in other sites. These patterns of recurrence after hepatic resection for metastatic colorectal cancer have been confirmed repeatedly. Given the frequency of isolated hepatic progression, repeat hepatic resection has been often performed.[35,36] Interestingly, reports have consistently shown that survival after repeat resection is equal to that after the initial hepatic resection, and predictors of survival are similar to those for the first hepatic operation: 5-year survival rates of 25% to 30% can be expected after repeat hepatic resection. These findings warrant assessment for resection in all patients with recurrent hepatic metastases after hepatic resection.

SALVAGE HEPATECTOMY

The main cause of unresectability is achieving a balance between resection of the entire tumor burden while leaving sufficient residual functional liver parenchyma (at least 30% of initial liver parenchyma) for survival. The definition of unresectability depends on many factors, not the least of which is the surgical expertise and support care at the medical facility. Theoretical prognostic factors and technical factors of unresectability of hepatic metastases are essentially determined by factors that affect the amount of postresection functional hepatic mass; the most important of these are tumor location, number of metastases, and bilobar disease.

PROGNOSTIC FACTORS INFLUENCING RESECTABILITY

Some subgroups of patients with negative prognostic factors such as lymph node involvement, large number of tumors (≥4), large size of metastases (>10 cm), or extrahepatic disease have been historically considered unresectable. However, recent studies suggest that all of these criteria treated with newer chemotherapy protocols, which are improving long-term survival, are also

Table 171-2 Survival Estimates

Modality	Author	Publication Year	5-Year Survival *3-Year (%)
Surgical resection	Adson[32]	1984	25
	Fong[33]	1997	38
	Scheele[34]	1995	38
	Choti[37]	2002	58
	Hur[38]	2009	50
RFA	Aloia[39]	2006	27
	Jakobs[40]	2006	68*
	Abitabile[41]	2007	57*
	Hur[38]	2009	25
Resection + RFA	Abdalla[31]	2004	36
Resection + Adjuvant therapy (FOLFOX/FOLFIRI)	Liu[42]	2010	54
Unresectable converted to resectable and resected	Bismuth[43]	1996	40
	Tanaka[44]	2003	38
	Adam[45,46]	2004	33
Recurrent followed by resection	de Jong[47]	2009	32
	van der Pool[48]	2009	35

RFA, Radiofrequency ablation.

able to downstage patients to allow for an attempt at curative resection. (Table 171-2). Patients who successfully underwent downstaging with neoadjuvant chemotherapy and then resection have similar survival rates to those patients who were resectable at their initial presentation. Historically, 1- to 2-cm margins were considered the criterion standard for resection of hepatic metastases. A recent study has examined the relationship of measured margins of hepatic resection for CRM to survival and local recurrence[49] and suggested that a smaller margin (2 mm) may be as effective. Histopathology of resected specimens showed that micrometastases in the surrounding liver were present in 2% of patients and were found within 4 mm of the margin. The incidence of definitive recurrence at the surgical margin was 13.3%, 2.8%, and 0% if the margin was <2 mm, 2 to 4 mm, and 5 mm or wider, respectively. Resective margins can be extended with the use of RFA or cryoablation provided the ablation zone does not affect major ducts or vessels. In general, at least a 1-cm margin is preferred.

Lastly, extrahepatic disease is usually associated with poorer survival. Nevertheless, long-term survival is reported in a significant number of patients when complete resection of extrahepatic disease is achieved, particularly with pulmonary metastases. With control of the primary disease prior to pulmonary resection, 5- and 10-year survivals of 30% and 16%, respectively, can be expected.[19,20] Similarly, although long-term prognosis in patients with metastases to lymph nodes is unfavorable, hepatic resection combined with lymphadenectomy may be beneficial in occasional patients whose disease has been downstaged or completely eliminated clinically by chemotherapy and can be resected completely.[32]

STRATEGIES FOR IMPROVING RESECTABILITY

Strategies for improving resectability are based on clinical response to neoadjuvant chemotherapy to downstage disease stage and increase postresection hepatic reserve in combination with cytodestructive modalities such as RFA. Novel chemotherapeutic regimens combining 5-FU, folinic acid, and oxaliplatin or irinotecan with or without Avastin have been proven to increase both patient survival and quality of life. In fact, response to chemotherapy before hepatic resection may become a major selection factor for resection. A recent study[45] demonstrated that patients with tumor progression on chemotherapy had a poorer outcome, even after potentially curative hepatectomy. Tumor stabilization or a decrease in tumor burden during chemotherapy was associated with long-term survival. Five-year survival was 37%, 30%, and 8% for patients with objective tumor response, tumor stabilization, and tumor progression, respectively. (Control of metastatic disease before surgery may be crucial for a chance of prolonged remission in patients at high risk for progression after resection.)

If the anticipated functional hepatic volume after hepatic resection is considered marginal, strategies utilizing hepatic regeneration can transform some patients from unresectable to resectable. Portal vein embolization and staged resection are two such treatment modalities. Portal vein embolization of the planned hepatic resection allows hypertrophy of the remnant liver and has been demonstrated to allow more patients with previously unresectable liver tumors to undergo successful resection.[50] Portal vein embolization is indicated when the functional liver remnant is estimated at less than 30% of initial functional hepatic volume in which hepatic failure is a leading cause of postoperative death. Portal vein embolization of the resection volume induces contralateral compensatory hypertrophy of the hepatic remnant, thus decreasing the risk of postoperative liver failure. Once hypertrophy of the remnant liver volume has plateaued, usually 4 to 6 weeks postprocedure, hepatic resection can be performed. Pre-resectional selective PVE may increase the rate of resection in such

patients by 20%.[51] Their 5-year survival is 40%, similar to the survival rate of patients who did not require selective PVE. Importantly, tumor volume may also increase to a similar extent as the remnant, which emphasizes that PVE must be used selectively.[52] Lastly, cryotherapy and RFA can be used efficiently during operation for resection to recruit patients to treatment who would not be resected otherwise. Initial treatment outcomes and complication rates were similar for either ablative technique, but local recurrence was higher for cryoablation.[53] Currently, ablation is limited by large size of metastases, proximity to major vessels and bile ducts, and loss of tumor definition by chemotherapy. Thus, RFA can be used in conjunction with resection for multiple metastases to allow selection of patients with otherwise unresectable lesions.

Two-stage hepatectomy consists of sequentially resecting hepatic metastases that would otherwise be unresectable because of insufficient hepatic reserve. This option is usually reserved for patients with multiple bilobar metastases responsive to chemotherapy. The initial hepatic resection for metastases is performed on the planned remnant liver, which allows it to hypertrophy in the absence of metastasis. The second hepatic resection for metastases is performed after restaging to exclude interim progression and is intended to be curative. After the initial liver resection, surgery is deferred 6 weeks to allow the early regeneration of the remnant liver, though Vauthey et al showed growth of liver.[6] Postoperative chemotherapy, consisting of the same proven chemotherapy that the patient responded to previously, is continued for further response. The second hepatectomy should only be performed if there is no interim tumor progression and significant hepatoxicity from chemotherapy has not occurred. Clinical data suggest that disease-free survival can be achieved in some patients.[54]

The usefulness of aggressive multimodality therapy including neoadjuvant combination chemotherapy to downstage hepatic metastases and techniques to increase postresection hepatic reserve (selective PVE, second resection, and ablation) to allow salvage of patients otherwise considered unresectable is best shown by the studies from the Paul Brousse Hospital.[46] The outcome of 1104 of 1439 patients (77%) with CRM who were initially unresectable were treated with combination chemotherapy consisting of 5-fluorouracil, leucovorin combined with oxaliplatin, irinotecan, or both. Responses of the nonresectable patients were assessed after every four courses for resection. Of the 1104 patients treated, 138 patients (12.5%) were considered "good responders" and underwent hepatic resection after an average of 10 cycles. Liver resection was combined with PVE, ablative treatment, or second-stage hepatectomy in 42 patients (30%), and resection of extrahepatic disease was performed in 41 patients (30%). Operative mortality was less than 1% and after a mean followup of 48.7 months, 111 of the 138 (80%) patients developed tumor recurrence. Some patients developed recurrence in the liver only (29%), extrahepatic (9%), or both hepatic and extrahepatic (43%). Hepatic-only recurrences (52 patients) were treated by repeat hepatectomy, whereas 42 patients with extrahepatic resection were resected. Survival in these two groups was 33% and 23% at 5 and 10 years, respectively. Disease-free survival was 22% and 17% at 5 and 10 years, respectively. Patients whose hepatic metastases were initially resectable had 5- and 10-year survival of 48% and 30%, respectively.

In conclusion, improvements in combination chemotherapy leading to downstaging of metastatic disease and modalities to induce selective hypertrophy of the remnant liver in patients who would otherwise not be candidates for hepatic resection can now permit hepatic resection with curative intent in selective responsive patients.

REFERENCES

1. Minagawa M, Yamamoto J, Kosuge T, et al: Simplified staging system for predicting the prognosis of patients with resectable liver metastasis: Development and validation. *Arch Surg* 142:269; discussion 277, 2007.
2. Belghiti J, Hiramatsu K, Benoist S, et al: Seven hundred forty-seven hepatectomies in the 1990s: An update to evaluate the actual risk of liver resection. *J Am College Surg* 191:38, 2000.
3. Karoui M, Vigano L, Goyer P, et al: Combined first-stage hepatectomy and colorectal resection in a two-stage hepatectomy strategy for bilobar synchronous liver metastases. *Br J Surg* 97:1354, 2010.
4. de Haas RJ, Adam R, Wicherts DA, et al: Comparison of simultaneous or delayed liver surgery for limited synchronous colorectal metastases. *Br J Surg* 97:1279, 2010.
5. Mentha G, Roth AD, Terraz S, et al: "Liver first" approach in the treatment of colorectal cancer with synchronous liver metastases. *Dig Surg* 25:430, 2008.
6. Vauthey JN, Marsh RDW, Cendan JC, et al: Arterial therapy of hepatic colorectal metastases. *Br J Surg* 83:447, 1996.
7. Ribero D, Wang H, Donadon M, et al: Bevacizumab improves pathologic response and protects against hepatic injury in patients treated with oxaliplatin-based chemotherapy for colorectal liver metastases. *Cancer* 110:2761, 2007.
8. Thomay A, Charpentier K: Optimizing resection for "responding" hepatic metastases after neoadjuvant chemotherapy. *Journal of Surgical Oncology* Published online 23 Aug N/A:N/A, 2010.
9. Schindl M, Wigmore SJ, Currie EJ, et al: Prognostic scoring in colorectal cancer liver metastases: Development and validation. *Arch Surg* 140:183, 2005.
10. Ueno H, Mochizuki H, Hatsuse K, et al: Indicators for treatment strategies of colorectal liver metastases. *Ann Surg* 231:59, 2000.
11. Lise M, Bacchetti S, Da Pian P, et al: Patterns of recurrence after resection of colorectal liver metastases: Prediction by models of outcome analysis. *World J Surg* 25:638, 2001.
12. Nordlinger B, Jaeck D, Guiget M: Multicentric retrospective study by the French Surgical Association. In Nordlinger B, Jaeck D, editors: *Treatment of hepatic metastases of colorectal cancer.* New York, 1992, Springer-Verlag, p 129.
13. Fong Y, Fortner J, Sun RL, et al: Clinical score for predicting recurrence after hepatic resection for metastatic colorectal cancer: Analysis of 1001 consecutive cases. *Ann Surg* 230:309; discussion 318, 1999.
14. Iwatsuki S, Dvorchik I, Madariaga JR, et al: Hepatic resection for metastatic colorectal adenocarcinoma: A proposal of a prognostic scoring system. *J Am College Surg* 189:291, 1999.
15. Zakaria S, Donohue JH, Nagorney DM, et al: Hepatic resection for colorectal metastases: Value for risk scoring systems? *Ann Surg* 246:183, 2007.
16. Malik HZ, Prasad KR, Halazun KJ, et al: Preoperative prognostic score for predicting survival after hepatic resection for colorectal liver metastases. *Ann Surg* 246:806, 2007.
17. Pawlik TM, Scoggins CR, Zorzi D, et al: Effect of surgical margin status on survival and site of recurrence after hepatic resection for colorectal metastases. *Ann Surg* 241:715, 2005.
18. Weber SM, Jarnagin WR, DeMatteo RP, et al: Survival after resection of multiple hepatic colorectal metastases. *Ann Surg Oncol* 7:643, 2000.
19. Miller G, Biernacki P, Kemeny NE, et al: Outcomes after resection of synchronous or metachronous hepatic and pulmonary colorectal metastases. *J American College Surg* 205:231, 2007.
20. Headrick JR, Miller DL, Nagorney DM, et al: Surgical treatment of hepatic and pulmonary metastases from colon cancer. *Ann Thorac Surg* 71:975; discussion 979, 2001.
21. Shah SA, Haddad R, Al-Sukhni W, et al: Surgical resection of hepatic and pulmonary metastases from colorectal carcinoma. *J Am College Surg* 202:468, 2006.
22. Adams RB, Haller DG, Roh MS: Improving resectability of hepatic colorectal metastases: Expert consensus statement by Abdalla, et al. *Ann Surg Oncol* 13:1281, 2006.
23. Benoist S, Brouquet A, Penna C, et al: Complete response of colorectal liver metastases after chemotherapy: Does it mean cure? *J Clin Oncol* 24:3939, 2006.
24. Auer RC, White RR, Kemeny NE, et al: Predictors of a true complete response among disappearing liver metastases from colorectal cancer after chemotherapy. *Cancer* 116:1502, 2010.
25. Couinaud C: *Surgical anatomy of the liver revisited.* Paris, 1989, Denk.
26a. Terminology Committee of the International Hepato-Pancreato-Biliary Association: IHPBA Brisband 2000 Terminology of Liver and Anatomy Resections. *HPB* 2:333, 2000.
26b. Vauthey JN, Pawlik TM, Ribero D, et al: Chemotherapy regimen predicts steatohepatitis and an increase in 90-day mortality after surgery for hepatic colorectal metastases. *J Clin Oncol* 1:24, 2006.
27. Meta-Analysis Group in Cancer: Reappraisal of hepatic Arterial infusion in the treatment of nonresectable liver metastases from colorectal cancer. *J Nat Cancer Inst* 8:252, 1996.
28. Ravikumar TS: The role of cryotherapy in the management of patients with liver tumors. *Adv Surg* 30:281, 1996.
29. Korpan NN: Hepatic cryosurgery for liver metastases. Long-term follow-up. *Ann Surg* 225:193, 1997.
30. Hughes KS, Simon R, Songhorabodi S, et al: Resection of the liver for colorectal carcinoma metastases: A multi-institutional study of patterns of recurrence. *Surgery* 100:278, 1986.
31. Abdalla EK, Vauthey J-N, Ellis LM, et al: Recurrence and outcomes following hepatic resection, radiofrequency ablation, and combined resection/ablation for colorectal liver metastases. *Ann Surg* 239:818; discussion 825, 2004.
32. Adson MA, van Heerden JA, Adson MH, et al: Resection of hepatic metastases from colorectal cancer. *Arch Surg* 119:647, 1984.
33. Fong Y, Cohen AM, Fortner JG, et al: Liver resection for colorectal metastases. *J Clin Oncol* 15:938, 1997.
34. Scheele J, Stang R, Altendorf-Hofmann A, et al: Resection of colorectal liver metastases. *World Journal of Surgery* 19:59, 1995.
35. Fernandez-Trigo V, Shamsa F, Sugarbaker PH: Repeat liver resections from colorectal metastasis. Repeat Hepatic Metastases Registry. *Surgery* 117:296, 1995.
36. Nordlinger B, Vaillant JC: Repeat resections for recurrent colorectal liver metastases. *Cancer Treat Res* 69:57, 1994.
37. Choti MA, Sitzmann JV, Tiburi MF, et al: Trends in long-term survival following liver resection for hepatic colorectal metastases. *Ann Surg* 235:759, 2002.
38. Hur H, Ko YT, Min BS, et al: Comparative study of resection and radiofrequency ablation in the treatment of solitary colorectal liver metastases. *Am J Surg* 197:728, 2009.
39. Aloia TA, Vauthey J-N, Loyer EM, et al: Solitary colorectal liver metastasis: Resection determines outcome. *Arch Surg* 141:460; discussion 466, 2006.
40. Jakobs TF, Hoffmann RT, Trumm C, et al: Radiofrequency ablation of colorectal liver metastases: Mid-term results in 68 patients. *Anticancer Res* 26:671, 2006.
41. Abitabile P, Hartl U, Lange J, et al: Radiofrequency ablation permits an effective treatment for colorectal liver metastasis. *European J Surg Oncol* 33:67, 2007.
42. Liu J-H, Hsieh Y-Y, Chen W-S, et al: Adjuvant oxaliplatin- or irinotecan-containing chemotherapy improves overall survival following resection of metachronous colorectal liver metastases. *Int J Colorectal Dis* 25:1243, 2010.
43. Bismuth H, Adam R, Levi F, et al: Resection of nonresectable liver metastases from colorectal cancer after neoadjuvant chemotherapy. *Ann Surg* 224:509; discussion 520, 1996.
44. Tanaka K, Adam R, Shimada H, et al: Role of neoadjuvant chemotherapy in the treatment of multiple colorectal metastases to the liver. *Br J Surg* 90:963, 2003.

45. Adam R, Pascal G, Castaing D, et al: Tumor progression while on chemotherapy: A contraindication to liver resection for multiple colorectal metastases? *Ann Surg* 240:1052; discussion 1061, 2004.

46. Adam R, Delvart V, Pascal G, et al: Rescue surgery for unresectable colorectal liver metastases downstaged by chemotherapy: A model to predict long-term survival. *Ann Surg* 240:644; discussion 657, 2004.

47. de Jong MC, Mayo SC, Pulitano C, et al: Repeat curative intent liver surgery is safe and effective for recurrent colorectal liver metastasis: Results from an international multi-institutional analysis. *J Gastrointest Surg* 13:2141, 2009.

48. van der Pool AEM, Lalmahomed ZS, de Wilt JHW, et al: Local treatment for recurrent colorectal hepatic metastases after partial hepatectomy. *J Gastrointest Surg* 13:890, 2009.

49. Kokudo N, Miki Y, Sugai S, et al: Genetic and histological assessment of surgical margins in resected liver metastases from colorectal carcinoma: Minimum surgical margins for successful resection. *Arch Surg* 137:833, 2002.

50. Nordlinger B, Sorbye H, Glimelius B, et al: Perioperative chemotherapy with FOLFOX4 and surgery versus surgery alone for resectable liver metastases from colorectal cancer (EORTC Intergroup trial 40983): A randomised controlled trial. *Lancet* 371:1007, 2008.

51. Azoulay D, Castaing D, Smail A, et al: Resection of nonresectable liver metastases from colorectal cancer after percutaneous portal vein embolization. *Ann Surg* 231:480, 2000.

52. Kokudo N, Tada K, Seki M, et al: Proliferative activity of intrahepatic colorectal metastases after preoperative hemihepatic portal vein embolization. *Hepatology* 34:267, 2001.

53. Adam R, Hagopian EJ, Linhares M, et al: A comparison of percutaneous cryosurgery and percutaneous radiofrequency for unresectable hepatic malignancies. *Arch Surg* 137:1332; discussion 1340, 2002.

54. Adam R, Laurent A, Azoulay D, et al: Two-stage hepatectomy: A planned strategy to treat irresectable liver tumors. *Ann Surg* 232:777, 2000.

Neoplasms of the Anus

Elizabeth C. Wick | Jonathan E. Efron

The goal of this chapter is to review the anatomy of the anal and perianal area and to discuss the neoplasms of this region. Anal and perianal malignancies are rare and account for about 2% of all lower gastrointestinal tract cancers. They include squamous cell carcinoma (SCC) of the anal canal and margin, the precursor lesions of SCC, anal dysplasia, as well as the rare perianal tumors, which include melanoma, basal cell carcinoma, verrucous carcinoma, and Paget disease.

ANATOMY

The anal area is divided into the anal canal and anal margin. The "surgical" anal canal and the "anatomic" anal canal have distinct definitions. The surgical anal canal begins at the anorectal ring or levator ani muscles and extends to the anal verge (Figure 172-1). The anal verge is the most inferior aspect of the anal sphincter muscle and represents the transition between anoderm and normal skin. The anal canal measures 2 to 6 cm and is usually longer in men than in women. The internal anal sphincter (continuation of the outer longitudinal muscle of the rectal wall) and the external anal sphincter (continuation of the puborectalis muscle) encircle the anal canal and control fecal continence. The anatomic anal canal is defined as the short segment covered by squamous mucosa that extends from the dentate line to the anal verge.

The dentate line marks the transition between the columnar epithelium of the intestine and the squamous epithelium of the anal canal. The mucosa of the most superior aspect of the surgical anal canal (between the anorectal ring and the dentate line) can have rectal, transitional urothelial-like and/or squamous characteristics. In this area, squamous metaplasia is a normal histologic variant. This region is sometimes termed the anal transition zone (ATZ) and is particularly susceptible to infection with human papillomavirus (HPV). It is now recognized that the length of the ATZ is highly variable and, in fact, it can actually extend a few centimeters into the lower rectum.

The anal margin begins at the anal verge and extends in a 5-cm radius around the anus. It can be completely visualized when gentle traction is placed on the buttocks.[1] Anoscopy is not necessary to visualize the complete anal margin. Histologically, it is characterized by stratified squamous epithelium. Frequently the pathologist can identify skin appendages such as apocrine glands on biopsy to help differentiate specimens from the canal and margin.

The perianal region has two channels for lymphatic drainage. In the anal canal, lesions above the dentate line drain through the superior rectal lymphatics into the inferior mesenteric lymph nodes as well as through the middle and inferior rectal lymphatics to the internal iliac nodes. Lesions around the dentate line and the perianal skin drain into the inferior rectal lymphatics to the inguinal nodes.

The histology of the anal region is diverse and therefore a variety of different cancers may arise. The vast majority of anal malignancies are squamous cell in origin, with the anal canal lesions usually being nonkeratinizing and the anal-margin lesions being keratinizing. Melanoma can arise in the anal canal or the anal margin, and basal cell carcinoma can occur at the anal margin as well. Verrucous carcinoma and Paget disease are only seen in the anal-margin area.

SQUAMOUS CELL CANCER OF THE ANUS

EPIDEMIOLOGY

Anal cancer is a rare malignancy of the gastrointestinal tract. It is projected that 5260 new cases will be diagnosed and 720 people will die from anal cancer in 2010.[2] Over the past 30 years, there has been a steady rise in the incidence of anal cancer. Risk factors are infection with HPV, cigarette smoking, infection with human immunodeficiency virus (HIV), anal receptive intercourse, history of vulvar or cervical cancer, sexual promiscuity, and immunosuppression after organ transplantation.[3] Historically, women were at increased risk but, in a recent analysis of the National Cancer Institute Surveillance Epidemiology and End Results (SEER) database, the incidence of anal cancer was seen to be similar in men and women. This may be a reflection of the gender imbalance in HIV infection, one of the leading risk factors for anal cancer.[4] The incidence of anal cancer in HIV-positive patients has risen since the adoption of highly active antiretroviral therapy (HAART). This is likely a reflection of the fact that HAART prolongs survival in patients with HIV but does not affect the rate of anal cancer in this population. In the SEER database, the median age at diagnosis was 60 years and the overall 5-year survival was 66%.[5] Patients with localized disease have a good prognosis (5-year survival approaching 80%), but in patients with lymphatic or distant spread at the time of diagnosis, survival is significantly worse, being 60% and 31%, respectively, at 5 years.[2]

Histologically, anal cancer is an SCC. As mentioned earlier, the area of the anal transition zone can harbor different variants of squamous epithelium, including cloacogenic, transitional, and basaloid epithelium. Today, cloacogenic, transitional, basaloid, and mucoepidermoid carcinomas of the anal canal are grouped under SCCs

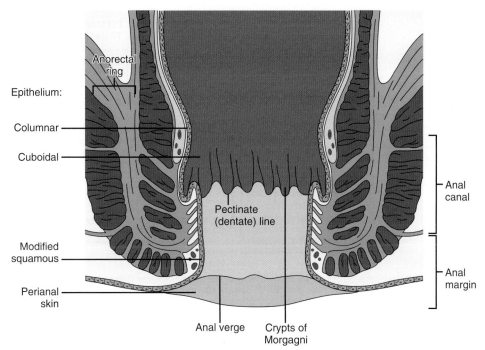

Epithelium:

Columnar

Cuboidal

Modified squamous

Perianal skin

Anorectal ring

Pectinate (dentate) line

Anal canal

Anal margin

Anal verge   Crypts of Morgagni

FIGURE 172-1 Perianal anatomy.

because their treatment and prognosis are similar to that for SCC.[6]

DIAGNOSIS

Most patients present with rectal bleeding and pain. Because these symptoms are nonspecific, patients are frequently misdiagnosed as having a benign anorectal condition such as hemorrhoids.

Initial evaluation should consist of a thorough history including risk factors for anal cancer and a complete physical examination with detailed evaluation of the inguinal lymph nodes, digital rectal examination, and anoscopy with biopsy (if not previously done). Important features to note during the rectal examination are the size of the lesion, its relationship to the anal sphincters, and any evidence of invasion of surrounding structures such as the vagina in women. Sometimes the area will be too painful to examine and/or biopsy in the office, in which case, an examination under anesthesia should be done (Figures 172-2 and 172-3).

Additional symptoms such as incontinence, change in bowel habits, pelvic pain, and rectovaginal or rectovesical fistulas are ominous. These symptoms suggest advanced malignancy with infiltration into the sphincters or penetration into the rectal wall.[7] A Mayo Clinic series of 188 patients demonstrated tumor invasion past the mucosa in 88% of such patients.[8]

STAGING

Staging of anal cancer is based on the size of the primary, involvement of regional lymphatics, and the presence or absence of distant metastatic disease (Table 172-1). As described earlier, the size of the primary is based on physical examination findings. Initial examination of the lymph nodes is done by physical examination but further evaluation by CT scan of the abdomen and pelvis is

mandatory because all of the draining lymph nodes are not palpable. Lymph nodes larger than 1 cm are considered to be positive for purposes of staging and treatment. Chest computed tomography (CT) is done to evaluate for distant sites of disease because the lymphovascular drainage of the anus is systemic and the most common site of distant disease is the lung. Positron emission tomography–CT (PET-CT) is now being used to stage and monitor patients with anal cancer. PET-CT may be more sensitive than CT for identifying lymph nodes containing metastatic disease, particularly those that are not enlarged, thus increasing the accuracy of clinical staging. PET-CT diagnosed involved lymph nodes in 17% and 24% of people who were deemed not to have lymph node involvement by physical examination and CT, respectively.[9] Small studies have recently reported that high fluorodeoxyglucose (FDG) uptake in tumors may be a biomarker that predicts more aggressive tumor biology including shorter disease-free interval and higher rate of persistent or recurrent disease after chemoradiation therapy.[10] Endoanal ultrasound has been used to assess tumor depth and sphincter involvement, but the ultrasound results have not affected treatment plans and, thus, presently, ultrasound staging is not routinely recommended.

TREATMENT

Historically, anal cancer was treated with abdominal perineal resection (APR). This was associated with significant morbidity (mainly urinary/sexual dysfunction and wound complications) and poor locoregional control of the disease. Because local recurrences can be difficult to treat, some surgeons even advocated very wide excision with flap closure at the time of the initial resection. Reported 5-year survival rates with radical surgery alone ranged from 30% to 71%, with the local recurrence rate

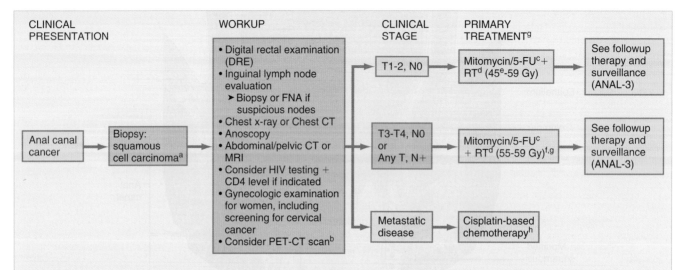

CLINICAL PRESENTATION	WORKUP	CLINICAL STAGE	PRIMARY TREATMENT[g]	

Anal canal cancer → Biopsy: squamous cell carcinoma[a] →

WORKUP:
- Digital rectal examination (DRE)
- Inguinal lymph node evaluation
  ➤ Biopsy or FNA if suspicious nodes
- Chest x-ray or Chest CT
- Anoscopy
- Abdominal/pelvic CT or MRI
- Consider HIV testing + CD4 level if indicated
- Gynecologic examination for women, including screening for cervical cancer
- Consider PET-CT scan[b]

CLINICAL STAGE / PRIMARY TREATMENT:
- T1-2, N0 → Mitomycin/5-FU[c]+ RT[d] (45[e]-59 Gy) → See followup therapy and surveillance (ANAL-3)
- T3-T4, N0 or Any T, N+ → Mitomycin/5-FU[c] + RT[d] (55-59 Gy)[f,g] → See followup therapy and surveillance (ANAL-3)
- Metastatic disease → Cisplatin-based chemotherapy[h]

[a]For melanoma histology, see the NCCN Melanoma Guidelines, for adenocarcinoma, see the NCCN Rectal Cancer Guidelines.
[b]PET-CT scan does not replace a diagnostic CT. The routine use of a PET-CT scan for staging or treatment planning has not been validated.
[c]See Principles of Chemotherapy ANAL-A.
 Ajani JA, Winter KA, Gunderson LL, et al: Fluorouracil, mitomycin, and radiotherapy vs fluorouracil, cisplatin, and radiotherapy for carcinoma of the anal canal: A randomized controlled trial. *JAMA* 299:914, 2008. In a randomized trial, the strategy of using neoadjuvant therapy with 5-FU + cisplatin followed by concurrent therapy with 5-FU + cisplatin + RT was not superior to 5-FU + mitomycin + RT.
[d]See Principles of Radiation Therapy ANAL-B.
[e]Reevaluate at 45 Gy, if persistent result, consider increasing to 55-59 Gy.
[f]Include bilateral inguinal/low pelvic nodal regions based upon estimated risk of inguinal involvement.
[g]Patients with anal cancer as the first manifestation of HIV, may be treated with the same regimen as non-HIV patient. Patients with active HIV/AIDS-related complications or a history of complications (e.g., malignancies, opportunistic infections) may not tolerate full-dose therapy or may not tolerate mitomycin and require dosage adjustment or treatment without mitomycin.
[h]Cisplatin/5-fluorouracil recommended for metastatic disease. If this regimen fails, no other regimens have shown to be effective.
 See Principles of Chemotherapy ANAL-A.

Note: All recommendations are category 2A unless otherwise indicated.
Clinical Trials: NCCN believes that the best management of any cancer patient is in a clinical trial. Participation in clinical trials is especially encouraged.

FIGURE 172-2 National Comprehensive Cancer Network guidelines for the treatment of anal cancer (Anal-1). (From National Comprehensive Cancer Network Clinical Practice Guidelines in Oncology: Anal Carcinoma, version 1.2011. National Comprehensive Cancer Network, Inc.)

varying from 18% to 45%.[11] In a Mayo Clinic series of 188 patients treated for anal cancer between 1950 and 1976, APR was performed in 118 of these patients. Their 5-year survival rate was 71%.[8]

In 1974, Nigro et al described the use of relatively low-dose radiotherapy (30 Gy over a 3-week period) in combination with low-dose 5-FU and mitomycin C (MMC) (5-FU infused for 4 days during the first week of radiation therapy and MMC given as a bolus dose on day 1) in an attempt to render three unresectable tumors amenable to resection. All three patients obtained complete remission, and in the two who accepted APR 6 weeks later, no residual tumor was found.[12] Followup studies found similar results with combined-modality therapy (CMT) for anal cancer.[13-15] The technique was refined over the next 10 years, and routine radical surgery gave way to excision of the primary site after completion of CMT.[16] In uncontrolled studies, management of anal cancer with radiation therapy alone or CMT was comparable to surgery with respect to local control and survival. Five multiinstitutional randomized trials have laid the foundation for the current CMT of anal cancer (Table 172-2). The UK Coordinating Committee on Cancer Research (UKCCCR) reported the results of 585 patients with anal cancer randomly assigned to receive 45 Gy of radiation therapy or 45 Gy of radiation with continuous-infusion 5-FU in weeks 1 and 5 and MMC in week 1. Patients were

evaluated at 6 weeks for response. Those with a good response received a radiation boost and those with a poor response proceeded to salvage surgery. Patients receiving CMT had a 46% reduction in the risk of local failure as compared to the patients receiving radiation alone, although early morbidity was higher in the CMT patients as compared to radiation-alone patients. Despite improvement in local control, CMT did not improve overall survival.[17] The European Organisation for Research and Treatment of Cancer (EORTC) randomized 110 patients to a similar regimen of 5-FU, MMC, and radiation and again found that CMT improved local control and led to a longer colostomy-free interval but did have survival advantage as compared to radiation therapy alone.[18] The Radiation Therapy Oncology Group (RTOG) and Eastern Cooperative Oncology Group (ECOG) tested the role of MMC in CMT on disease-free and overall survival in anal cancer. Three hundred ten patients were randomized to 45 to 54.4 Gy radiation therapy and infusional 5-FU in week 1 with or without MMC in weeks 1 and 5. The addition of MMC was associated with improved disease-free survival (73% vs. 51%) and lower colostomy rates, at the expense of significantly higher toxicity.[19]

Based on the success of cisplatin-based therapy in head and neck squamous cell cancers and the significant toxicity associated with MMC, the U.S.

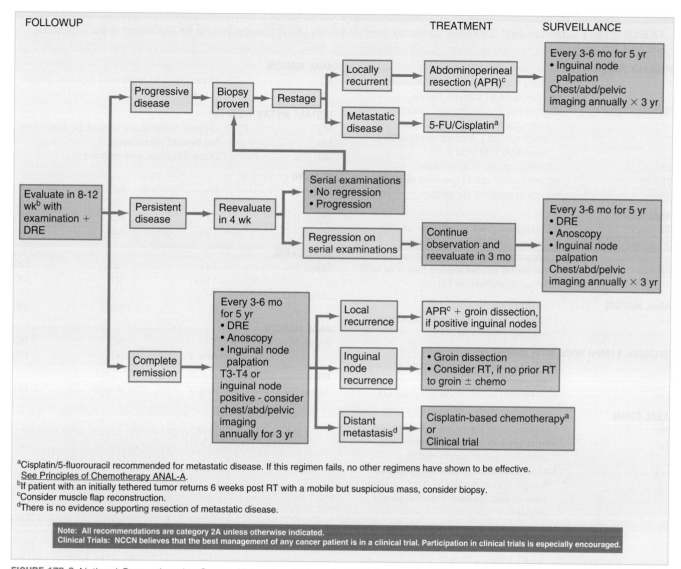

FOLLOWUP · TREATMENT · SURVEILLANCE

aCisplatin/5-fluorouracil recommended for metastatic disease. If this regimen fails, no other regimens have shown to be effective. See Principles of Chemotherapy ANAL-A.
bIf patient with an initially tethered tumor returns 6 weeks post RT with a mobile but suspicious mass, consider biopsy.
cConsider muscle flap reconstruction.
dThere is no evidence supporting resection of metastatic disease.

Note: All recommendations are category 2A unless otherwise indicated.
Clinical Trials: NCCN believes that the best management of any cancer patient is in a clinical trial. Participation in clinical trials is especially encouraged.

FIGURE 172-3 National Comprehensive Cancer Network guidelines for the followup of anal cancer (Anal-3). (From National Comprehensive Cancer Network Clinical Practice Guidelines in Oncology: Anal Carcinoma, version 1.2011. National Comprehensive Cancer Network, Inc.)

Gastrointestinal Intergroup trial RTOG 98-11 compared radiation therapy (45 to 59 Gy) with 5-FU and MMC to radiation therapy with 5-FU and cisplatin. Unlike prior studies, the chemotherapy in the 5-FU/cisplatin arm was structured as induction chemotherapy. No difference was seen in the overall or disease-free survival and, in fact, the patients in the 5-FU/cisplatin arm required more colostomy procedures.[5] Because of the structure of this trial, it is unclear if the increased need for colostomies in the 5-FU/cisplatin arm was related to the use of cisplatin or the "neoadjuvant" approach. Trials are underway to further study the role of cisplatin in treating anal cancer and to define the role of "neoadjuvant" and "adjuvant" chemotherapy in combination with radiation therapy for anal cancer. The U.K. ACT II trial studied 900 patients with anal cancer treated with either 5-FU/MMC or 5-FU/cisplatin and radiation. Based on early results with a median of 3 years' followup, there is no difference in complete response.

Intensity-Modulated Radiation Therapy

The radiation therapy component of the CMT is the source of much morbidity. Traditionally, the delivery of radiation treatments is based on CT-guided or three-dimensional images of the pelvis (conformal radiation therapy). Intensity-modulated radiation therapy (IMRT) was introduced in the late 1990s as a means to deliver very focused radiation therapy, so as to limit the dose to healthy organs (small bowel, vagina, bladder, and femoral heads) and to administer precise, escalating doses of radiation to areas of concern. Early results using IMRT for the treatment of anal cancer showed comparable local control and disease-free survival as conformal radiation with lower intestinal and cutaneous complications.[20] The Radiation Therapy Oncology Group (RTOG) recently completed a prospective phase 2 study of 5-FU, MMC, and IMRT for anal cancer to determine the treatment-related toxicity and disease-related outcomes, and the results will soon be published. Currently, many

TABLE 172-1 American Joint Committee on Cancer Seventh Edition (2010) Staging System for Carcinoma of the Anal Canal and Anal Margin

PRIMARY TUMOR (T)

Tx	Primary tumor cannot be assessed
T0	No evidence of primary tumor
Tis	Carcinoma in situ (Bowen disease, high-grade squamous intraepithelial lesions (HSIL), anal intraepithelial neoplasia II-III (AIN II-III)
T1	>2 cm in greatest dimension
T2	>2 cm but <5 cm in greatest dimension
T3	>5 cm in greatest dimension

ANAL CANAL

T4	Invading adjacent structures: vagina, urethra, or bladder (involvement of the sphincter muscle alone, rectal wall, or perirectal subcutaneous tissue or skin is not classified as T4)

ANAL MARGIN

T4	Invading deep extradermal structure: skeletal muscle or bone

REGIONAL LYMPH NODE INVOLVEMENT (N)

Nx	Regional lymph nodes cannot be assessed
N0	No regional lymph node involvement

ANAL CANAL

N1	Metastases to perirectal lymph nodes
N2	Metastases to unilateral internal iliac and/or inguinal lymph nodes
N3	Metastases to perirectal and inguinal lymph nodes and/or bilateral internal iliac and/or bilateral inguinal lymph nodes

ANAL MARGIN

N1	Metastases to ipsilateral inguinal lymph nodes

DISTANT METASTASES (M)

Mx	Distant metastases cannot be assessed
M0	No distant metastases
M1	Distant metastases present

STAGING

Stage 0	Tis	N0	M0
Stage I	TI	N0	M0
Stage II	T2	N0	M0
	T3	N0	M0

ANAL CANAL

Stage IIIA	T4	N0	M0
	T1-3	N1	M0
Stage IIIB	T4	N1	M0
	Any T	N2,3	M0

ANAL MARGIN

Stage III	T4	N0	M0
	Any T	N1	M0

BOTH

Stage IV	Any T	Any N	M1

centers have transitioned to using IMRT when possible for anal cancer.

FOLLOWUP AND SURVEILLANCE

The best timing for biopsy of apparent residual disease after completing CMT has not been well defined. Tumors will continue to regress after the completion of CMT. The current recommendation is to evaluate patients 8 to 12 weeks after completing CMT with digital rectal examination. During this examination, it should be determined if the patient has (1) complete regression, (2) persistent disease, or (3) progressive disease (Figure 172-4). Post-treatment biopsies should not be routinely performed unless there is suspicion of recurrence or disease continues to progress. Once the disease regresses, patients are usually followed at 3- to 6-month intervals with digital examination, anoscopy, and physical examination of the inguinal nodes for 5 years. For patients with a history of T3 or T4 disease or lymph node involvement, annual CT scans of the chest, abdomen, and pelvis should be considered. If there is persistent disease at 8 to 12 weeks, then the patient should be reevaluated every 4 weeks to document regression. If there is no regression after 12 to 16 weeks or progressive disease, salvage therapy with either further CMT or APR is required. Prior to considering salvage therapy, it is critical to rule out metastatic disease. Half of the CMT therapy failures can be classified as persistent and half as recurrent disease. Although PET-CT is sometimes used for surveillance, its precise role has not been defined. Presently, surveillance with PET-CT is not part of the National Comprehensive Cancer Network (NCCN) guidelines for management of anal cancer.

SALVAGE SURGERY

Residual tumor is treated by either radical surgery (see Figure 172-4) or further CMT. Both the UKCCCR and the RTOG/ECOG trials described earlier studied the role of additional CMT therapy for patients with persistent disease.[19] In the UKCCR trial, 24 patients who were found to have residual disease after initial CMT were given a radiation boost with 9.0 Gy to the tumor bed and repeat infusion of 5-FU and cisplatin. Half of the patients treated for persistent disease showed a complete response and were disease-free after the additional CMT.

Initial studies of the role of salvage APR for patients who fail CMT have been disappointing, with long-term survival of less than 24% to 53%. Ghouti et al examined their success in 36 patients who underwent salvage APR

TABLE 172-2 Trials on Combined-Modality Therapy for Anal Canal Squamous Cell Carcinoma

Author	Year	N	Complete Response Rate (%)	Five-Year Survival Rate (%)
Cummings et al	1984	30	98	70
Greenall et al	1985	18	72	78
Sischy	1985	29	89.6	81
Meeker et al	1986	19	88	87.5
Nigro	1987	104	91	81
Tviet et al	1989	24	87.5	58
Sischy et al	1989	79	90	73
Cummings et al	1991	57 RT only	56	61
		66 RT + 5-FU	60	62 (disease-free)
		69 CMT	86	55
Lopez et al	1991	33	88	79
Tanum et al	1991	106	84	72
Rich et al	1993	58	89	94
Allal et al	1993	68	67.5	65.5
Smith et al	1994	42	73.8	90
Martenson et al	1995	52	74	58
Doci et al	1996	35	94	94
Martenson et al	1996	19	68	NR
Arnott et al	1996	279 RT only	30	58 (3-yr)
		238 CMT	39	65 (3-yr)
Flam et al	1996	145 RT + 5-FU	86	51 (disease-free)
		146 CMT	92.2	73 (disease-free)
Bartelink et al	1997	52 RT only	54	40
		51 CMT	80	60
Ceresoli et al	1998	35	100	71

Adapted from Sato H, Koh K, Bartolo DCC: Management of anal canal cancer. *Dis Colon Rectum* 48:1301, 2005.
CMT, Combined radiation therapy and chemotherapy with 5-fluorouracil (5-FU) and mitomycin C (MMC); *RT*, radiation therapy.

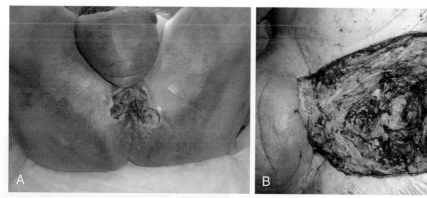

FIGURE 172-4 Recurrent squamous cell carcinoma of the anal canal. Preexcision **(A)** and postexcision **(B)**.

after either failure of CMT or local recurrence of anal cancer.[21] The 5-year survival rate in the immediate failure group was 60.7%, with a 71.5% rate in the recurrence group. The 5-year disease-free survival rates were 31.1% and 48.2%, respectively. Of note, some form of recurrence developed in 64% of the patients at 30 months. The perineal wound complication rate in this study was 70%, which corresponds with other studies that have shown an increase in the wound complication rate with the use of neoadjuvant chemoradiation therapy.[22] Consequently, some authors are advocating routine primary closure of APR defects with rectus flap reconstruction. Chessin et al performed a case-control series comparing

perineal wound closure performed primarily or with rectus abdominis flaps. The wound complication rate was significantly higher in the primary closure group (44.1% vs. 15.8%).[23] The gracilis muscles can also be used as reconstruction flaps for large perineal wounds.

No randomized trials have compared salvage CMT with local resection or APR. Salvage CMT provides the same benefits as primary CMT, namely, sphincter preservation. The results of subsequent APR after salvage CMT have not been examined, but serious consideration should be given to primary wound closure with a muscle flap in view of the significant risk for perineal wound breakdown.

ANAL DYSPLASIA

Anal dysplasia is becoming a more common condition that can occur both in the anal canal and at the anal margin. The terms Bowen disease, anal intraepithelial neoplasia (AIN) I, II, and III, and squamous carcinoma cell in situ have all been used to describe anal dysplasia. The recent edition of the American Joint Committee on Cancer manual has recommended simplifying the classification scheme to either low-grade squamous intraepithelial lesions (LSIL) or high-grade squamous intraepithelial lesions (HSIL).[1] Differentiation between LSIL and HSIL is based on specific histologic features: nuclear-to-cytoplasmic ratio and relationship of atypical cells with respect to the basement membrane. The definition of LSIL includes AIN I and HSIL includes Bowen disease, AIN II, and AIN III. In the past, Bowen disease or squamous cell carcinoma in situ was usually diagnosed as an incidental finding by pathologists after another anorectal procedure, commonly excisional hemorrhoidectomy. The recommended treatment for Bowen disease was detailed mapping of the anal canal followed by wide local excision and skin grafting.[24] This procedure was associated with very high morbidity as well as high recurrence rates (23% in one report). Recent detailed pathologic studies of patients with Bowen disease demonstrated that these lesions were indistinguishable from HSIL and all had histologic evidence of HPV infection.[25]

Anal squamous intraepithelial lesion (SIL) is associated with the human papillomavirus (HPV) infection and anal condyloma. HPV is the cause of almost all cervical cancers and the majority of anal cancers. In a population-based study using the SEER database, 77.9% of anal cancers and 65.5% of anal dysplasia were considered HPV-associated.[26] HPV types can be further classified based on their potential for malignant transformation. In general, low-risk types (6, 11, 16, and 39) are associated with anal warts and high-risk types (16, 18, 58, and 45) are associated with LSIL, HSIL, and anal cancer.[25] HPV is the most common sexually transmitted disease and infection is associated with sexual promiscuity and the presence of other venereal diseases. Anoreceptive intercourse is not necessary for transmission. In heterosexual patients, anal and perianal infection occurs because the virus pools in the vagina or at the base of the penis and from there it can spread to the perianal region. Patients with a compromised cellular immune system are at higher risk of developing chronic infection. This includes patients with human immunodeficiency virus (HIV), solid organ transplant recipients, and those with autoimmune diseases.[27,28]

The incidence of SIL in HIV-positive males who engage in anal receptive intercourse has been documented to be as high as 52% in some series.[29] Indeed, the overall incidence of SIL in males engaging in anal receptive intercourse is thought to be 35 per 100,000, and this figure doubles in the same population that is also HIV positive.[29,30] A study by Palefsky et al found that in patients who are HIV positive, engage in anoreceptive intercourse, and are taking highly active antiviral therapy, 81% had some form of anal dysplasia and 52% had HSIL.[30] The clinical features of SIL are not well defined,

and most patients are asymptomatic with the diagnosis made during the diagnosis and/or treatment of anal condyloma. The rate of detection of SIL in patients who undergo resection of anal condyloma ranges from 28% to 35%. This figure can rise as high as 60% in HIV-positive individuals.[31-33] Novel screening techniques, such as anal cytology and high-resolution anoscopy, have been investigated over the past 20 years in high-risk populations.[34] Such screening has been prompted by the high incidence of SIL in HIV-positive patients and the fact that SIL is essentially asymptomatic and undetectable to the naked eye. Anal cytologic examination uses techniques similar to cervical Pap smears and requires brushing of the anal canal and verge. Palefsky et al demonstrated a 69% sensitivity of detecting dysplasia in HIV-positive patients versus a 47% sensitivity in HIV-negative patients. Increasing the number of visits and screening procedures enhanced the sensitivity of the test.[35] A diagnosis of SIL should be followed up with a detailed evaluation of the perianal and anal region.

High-resolution anoscopy requires an operating microscope, acetic acid, and Lugol's iodine. First, the anal margin and anal canal are coated with 3% acetic acid and then examined using the microscope. Areas infected with HPV will be white and have characteristic vascular markings. Lugol's iodine is then applied; areas of HSIL do not absorb the Lugol's iodine and will remain pale. Areas of LSIL and normal tissue will turn brown/black from the Lugol's iodine (Figure 172-5). The areas of suspected HSIL should be biopsied to confirm the diagnosis and then ablated with either electrocautery or infrared coagulation. The goal is to achieve a superficial burn in the areas of HSIL while preserving uninvolved regions. Using this technique, HSIL can be eradicated from immunocompetent patients. Recurrence is common in HIV-positive patients; thus, close followup is important. After treatment, patients should be followed with anal Pap smears at 3-month intervals.[25,36-38]

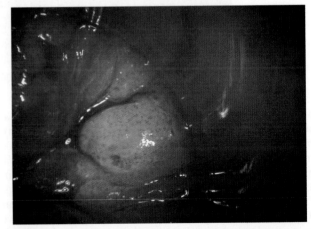

FIGURE 172-5 High-resolution anoscopy of high-grade squamous intraepithelial lesions. Areas of dysplasia appear white with characteristic vascular markings after the application of 3% acetic acid. (Courtesy J. Michael Berry, University of California, San Francisco.)

An alternative treatment for HSIL is immunomodulation. Reports on the use of immunotherapy, which involves the application of 5% imiquimod (Aldara) cream, topical 5% 5-fluorouracil (5-FU), or a combination of the two to the anal area are limited to small case series. Imiquimod is an immunomodulator that enhances interferon's activity. Several case reports have documented complete resolution of HSIL when treated with imiquimod cream or both imiquimod and 5-FU.[39,40] Kreuter et al reported on 10 HIV-positive patients who were also infected with HPV serotype 16, had various grades of AIN, and were treated with 5% imiquimod cream. The cream was applied three times a week for 4 months; side effects included erythema and burning at the initiation of therapy. Most patients had complete resolution or downgrading of the AIN.[41]

PERIANAL LESIONS

Perianal neoplasms are rare, accounting for 3% to 4% of all anorectal neoplasms. The most common lesions are SCC of the anal margin, melanoma, Paget disease, basal cell carcinoma, and verrucous carcinoma. These lesions are frequently initially misdiagnosed as benign perianal conditions, resulting in delays in definitive treatment.

ANAL-MARGIN SQUAMOUS CELL CARCINOMA

SCC of the anal margin is more akin to SCC in other cutaneous locations as opposed to SCC of the anal canal. Differentiating the two is partially dependent on the physician's understanding of the perianal anatomy. On the biopsy, the pathologist can also usually differentiate the two based on the presence of skin appendages and keratinization in anal-margin SCC. Anal-margin SCC are firm, erythematous lesions that may have central ulcers and/or heaped-up edges. Usually patients are asymptomatic but sometimes they complain of pruritus, pain, and drainage. Staging is done with a combination of physical examination with focus on the size of lesion in question and chest, abdomen, and pelvis CT to evaluate involvement of the femoral and inguinal lymph nodes (Figure 172-6). Anal-margin cancers most commonly spread to the inguinal lymph nodes. Risk of nodal involvement is correlated to the size of the primary lesion.[16,42] One series reported that 24% of lesions between 2 and 5 cm had involved lymph nodes, whereas 67% of lesions larger than 5 cm had involved lymph nodes. The treatment of anal-margin cancer is distinct from anal canal cancer. Small lesions (T1, N0) are treated similar to other cutaneous SCC with wide local excision (1-cm margin). For lesions that are close to the anal sphincter, wide local excision can compromise the sphincters and fecal continence. In these cases, radiation therapy is an alternative to APR. Patients with larger lesions and/or sphincter or lymph node involvement are best treated by CMT.[16] Patients with lesions larger than 2 cm should also receive radiation to the inguinal region, whereas the pelvic nodes should be included in the case of tumors larger than 5 cm.

BASAL CELL CARCINOMA

Although basal cell carcinoma (BCC) is the most common skin malignancy, perianal lesions are rare, accounting for less than 0.1% to 0.2% of perianal tumors. Risk factors for non–sun-exposed BCC have not been clearly defined but it is postulated that immunosuppression and ionizing radiation may be important in the pathogenesis of these lesions. Most BCCs are located at the anal margin and have heaped-up edges and central ulceration. They are usually superficial and rarely metastasize to regional lymph nodes. The treatment is local excision with a 0.5- to 1-cm margin.

It is important to obtain histologic confirmation to distinguish these lesions from a basaloid carcinoma which is a subtype of squamous cell carcinoma.

ANAL MELANOMA

Anal melanoma is a rare tumor and usually presents with advanced disease. There were 256 new cases of anorectal melanoma documented in the National Cancer Database between 1985 and 1994.[43] Anal melanoma is more commonly seen in women, and the median age at diagnosis is 60 years. Most patients seek medical attention for perianal discomfort or bleeding per rectum. Frequently the lesions are misdiagnosed as hemorrhoids and treated conservatively before the diagnosis is made. Interestingly, up to 25% of lesions can be amelanotic, making the diagnosis especially challenging.

The treatment of anorectal melanoma has been controversial. Historically, APR was advocated but it is increasingly recognized that radical resection does not impact the course of the disease. Local excision is usually sufficient for control of the locoregional disease. The Mayo Clinic reviewed their experience with 50 patients with anal melanoma and found 5-year and disease-free survival rates of 22% and 16%, respectively.[44] In this series, patients continued to die of their disease up to 11 years after initial diagnosis. No survival benefit was found between those who underwent APR (19% disease free at 66 months to 20 years) and those who were treated by local excision (18% disease free with a followup of 66 months to 44 years). Other groups have reviewed their experience with anal melanoma and similarly found no survival advantage with radical resection. The one study to the contrary is from the Memorial Sloan-Kettering group. They reviewed their experience (85 patients were treated between 1929 and 1993) and found that although overall survival was poor (17% at 5 years), of the patients with resectable disease, those treated with APR had improved long-term survival compared with those treated with local excision.[45] A recent analysis of the SEER database (1982 to 2002) identified 109 patients who underwent surgery for anal melanoma and found similar median survivals with local excision and APR (28 vs. 17 months, $P = 0.3$). Patients with localized disease as compared to regional disease tended to have improved 5-year survival (43.1% vs. 12.5%, $P = NS$).[46] A systematic review of 14 series of anal melanoma patients identified no survival advantage in patients treated with APR.[47] Sentinel lymph node mapping has been integrated into the

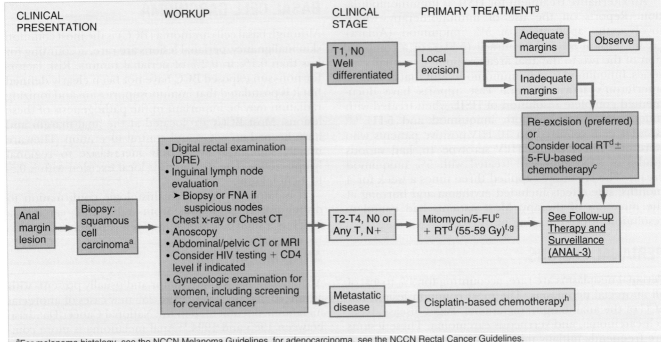

CLINICAL PRESENTATION — WORKUP — CLINICAL STAGE — PRIMARY TREATMENT[g]

- Anal margin lesion → Biopsy: squamous cell carcinoma[a]

- Digital rectal examination (DRE)
- Inguinal lymph node evaluation
  - ➤ Biopsy or FNA if suspicious nodes
- Chest x-ray or Chest CT
- Anoscopy
- Abdominal/pelvic CT or MRI
- Consider HIV testing + CD4 level if indicated
- Gynecologic examination for women, including screening for cervical cancer

T1, N0 Well differentiated → Local excision → Adequate margins → Observe; Inadequate margins → Re-excision (preferred) or Consider local RT[d] ± 5-FU-based chemotherapy[c]

T2-T4, N0 or Any T, N+ → Mitomycin/5-FU[c] + RT[d] (55-59 Gy)[f,g] → See Follow-up Therapy and Surveillance (ANAL-3)

Metastatic disease → Cisplatin-based chemotherapy[h]

[a]For melanoma histology, see the NCCN Melanoma Guidelines, for adenocarcinoma, see the NCCN Rectal Cancer Guidelines.
[c]See Principles of Chemotherapy ANAL-A.
 Ajani JA, Winter KA, Gunderson LL, et al: Fluorouracil, mitomycin, and radiotherapy vs fluorouracil, cisplatin, and radiotherapy for carcinoma of the anal canal: A randomized controlled trial. *JAMA* 299:914, 2008. The strategy of using neoadjuvant therapy with 5-FU + cisplatin followed by concurrent therapy with 5-FU + cisplatin + RT was not superior to 5-FU + mitomycin + RT.
[d]See Principles of Radiation Therapy ANAL-B.
[f]Include bilateral inguinal/low pelvic nodal regions based upon estimated risk of inguinal involvement.
[g]Patients with anal cancer as the first manifestation of HIV, may be treated with the same regimen as non-HIV patient. Patients with active HIV/AIDS-related complications or a history of complications (eg, malignancies, opportunistic infections) may not tolerate full-dose therapy or may not tolerate mitomycin and require dosage adjustment or treatment without mitomycin.
[h]Cisplatin/5-fluorouracil recommended for metastatic disease. If this regimen fails, no other regimens have shown to be effective.
 See Principles of Chemotherapy ANAL-A.

Note: All recommendations are category 2A unless otherwise indicated.
Clinical Trials: NCCN believes that the best management of any cancer patient is in a clinical trial. Participation in clinical trials is especially encouraged.

FIGURE 172-6 National Comprehensive Cancer Network guidelines for the treatment of anal-margin cancer (Anal-2). (From National Comprehensive Cancer Network Clinical Practice Guidelines in Oncology: Anal Carcinoma, version 1.2011. National Comprehensive Cancer Network, Inc.)

management of cutaneous melanoma but is not proven helpful in staging anal melanoma. The efficacy of adjuvant chemotherapy and/or radiation after local excision is unproven but there is an encouraging report of 23 patients who received radiation after local excision. Although overall survival was not improved, local and nodal recurrence was lower.[48] In conclusion, anal melanoma is usually a systemic disease at the time of presentation and it is rare that it can be cured by surgery. Therefore, quality of life is an important consideration and, in most cases, local excision should be done if feasible and the presence of any metastatic disease should be ruled out prior to any surgical intervention.

BUSCHKE-LÖWENSTEIN TUMORS

Verrucous carcinoma of the anal region is also known as giant condyloma acuminata or Buschke-Löwenstein tumors. These large lesions were first described by Buschke and Löwenstein in 1925. They can affect any area of the anogenital region and are locally aggressive,

leading to significant morbidity. The lesions are HPV related, with HPV-6 and HPV-11 being the most common variants identified. Although traditionally verrucous carcinoma are considered benign, large lesions can harbor small foci of invasive cancer. Coinfection with HIV may increase the risk of malignant transformation. Excision is the standard for treatment. Usually this can be accomplished with simple or staged excisions, but APR is sometimes necessary because of proximity of the lesion to the anal sphincters. A few case reports have noted that chemotherapy and radiation can cause regression of these lesions, but further study is necessary.[49,50]

PAGET DISEASE

Perianal Paget disease is a rare intraepithelial adenocarcinoma. Patients with perianal Paget present with pruritus and, occasionally, bleeding, a palpable lump, soiling, or a change in bowel habits. Examination usually reveals an erythematous or whitish gray, scaling, rash-like lesion with well-demarcated edges. The appearance can be similar to eczema. The disease generally occurs in patients older than 60 years and is found equally in men and women. Management begins with biopsy of the perianal skin lesion to establish the diagnosis. Therapy is determined on the basis of the local extent of the lesion and whether an associated adenocarcinoma is present. Workup for associated colorectal malignancy should include colonoscopy, although an article by Sarmiento et al[51] in which 13 patients with anal Paget disease were described revealed that even though 4 had associated malignancies, none of them were visceral. The true extent of the lesion may not be obvious macroscopically. Beck and Fazio advocated mapping of the perianal area with punch biopsies 1 cm from the lesion prior to planned excision.[24] Alternatively, margins can be evaluated by intraoperative frozen section. Perianal Paget disease is associated with visceral malignancies (adnexal and gastrointestinal). If the Paget lesion is isolated, wide local excision with skin graft or advancement flap reconstruction is performed. The extent of the disease may be difficult to identify grossly. Paget disease has a high rate of local recurrence, so close surveillance is necessary after treatment.

CONCLUSION

The management of anal malignancies has changed dramatically over the past 40 years. These changes are based on both the development of improved nonoperative therapies and a better understanding of some of the associated disorders that may predispose to the development of anal carcinoma. A comprehensive understanding of the anatomy and the pathogenesis of the disorder are required to appropriately manage these conditions.

REFERENCES

1. Wolff BG, Fleshman JW, Beck DE, et al, editors: *The ASCRS Textbook of Colon and Rectal Surgery*, New York, 2007, Springer Science and Business Media LLC.
2. http://www.cancer.gov/cancertopics/types/anal.
3. Chang GJ, Berry JM, Jay N, et al: Surgical treatment of high-grade anal squamous intraepithelial lesions: A prospective study. *Dis Colon Rectum* 45:453, 2002.
4. Grulich AE, Li Y, McDonald A, et al: Rates of non-AIDS-defining cancers in people with HIV infection before and after AIDS diagnosis. *AIDS* 16:1155, 2002.
5. Ajani JA, Winter KA, Gunderson LL, et al: Fluorouracil, mitomycin, and radiotherapy vs fluorouracil, cisplatin, and radiotherapy for carcinoma of the anal canal: A randomized controlled trial. *JAMA* 299:1914, 2008.
6. Longacre TA, Kong CS, Welton ML: Diagnostic problems in anal pathology. *Adv Anat Pathol* 15:263, 2008.
7. Cummings BJ: Anal cancer. *Int J Radiat Oncol Biol Phys* 19:1309, 1990.
8. Boman BM, Moertel CG, O'Connell MJ, et al: Carcinoma of the anal canal. A clinical and pathologic study of 188 cases. *Cancer* 54:114, 1984.
9. Czito BG, Willett CG: Current management of anal canal cancer. *Curr Oncol Rep* 11:186, 2009.
10. Kidd EA, Dehdashti F, Siegel BA, et al: Anal cancer maximum F-18 fluorodeoxyglucose uptake on positron emission tomography is correlated with prognosis. *Radiother Oncol* 95:288, 2010.
11. Sato H, Koh PK, Bartolo DC: Management of anal canal cancer. *Dis Colon Rectum* 48:1301, 2005.
12. Nigro ND, Vaitkevicius VK, Considine B Jr: Combined therapy for cancer of the anal canal: A preliminary report. *Dis Colon Rectum* 17:354, 1974.
13. Cummings B, Keane T, Thomas G, et al: Results and toxicity of the treatment of anal canal carcinoma by radiation therapy or radiation therapy and chemotherapy. *Cancer* 54:2062, 1984.
14. Greenall MJ, Quan SH, Urmacher C, et al: Treatment of epidermoid carcinoma of the anal canal. *Surg Gynecol Obstet* 161:509, 1985.
15. Meeker WR Jr, Sickle-Santanello BJ, Philpott G, et al: Combined chemotherapy, radiation, and surgery for epithelial cancer of the anal canal. *Cancer* 57:525, 1986.
16. Papillon J, Chassard JL: Respective roles of radiotherapy and surgery in the management of epidermoid carcinoma of the anal margin. Series of 57 patients. *Dis Colon Rectum* 35:422, 1992.
17. Epidermoid anal cancer: Results from the UKCCCR randomised trial of radiotherapy alone versus radiotherapy, 5-fluorouracil, and mitomycin. UKCCCR Anal Cancer Trial Working Party. UK Co-ordinating Committee on Cancer Research. *Lancet* 348:1049, 1996.
18. Bartelink H, Roelofsen F, Eschwege F, et al: Concomitant radiotherapy and chemotherapy is superior to radiotherapy alone in the treatment of locally advanced anal cancer: Results of a phase III randomized trial of the European Organization for Research and Treatment of Cancer Radiotherapy and Gastrointestinal Cooperative Groups. *J Clin Oncol* 15:2040, 1997.
19. Flam M, John M, Pajak TF, et al: Role of mitomycin in combination with fluorouracil and radiotherapy, and of salvage chemoradiation in the definitive nonsurgical treatment of epidermoid carcinoma of the anal canal: Results of a phase III randomized intergroup study. *J Clin Oncol* 14:2527, 1996.
20. Salama JK, Mell LK, Schomas DA, et al: Concurrent chemotherapy and intensity-modulated radiation therapy for anal canal cancer patients: A multicenter experience. *J Clin Oncol* 25:4581, 2007.
21. Ghouti L, Houvenaeghel G, Moutardier V, et al: Salvage abdominoperineal resection after failure of conservative treatment in anal epidermoid cancer. *Dis Colon Rectum* 48:16, 2005.
22. Bullard KM, Trudel JL, Baxter NN, et al: Primary perineal wound closure after preoperative radiotherapy and abdominoperineal resection has a high incidence of wound failure. *Dis Colon Rectum* 48:438, 2005.
23. Chessin DB, Hartley J, Cohen AM, et al: Rectus flap reconstruction decreases perineal wound complications after pelvic chemoradiation and surgery: A cohort study. *Ann Surg Oncol* 12:104, 2005.
24. Beck DE, Fazio VW, Jagelman DG, et al: Perianal Bowen's disease. *Dis Colon Rectum* 31:419, 1988.
25. Chang GJ, Welton ML: Human papillomavirus, condylomata acuminata, and anal neoplasia. *Clin Colon Rectal Surg* 17:221, 2004.
26. Watson M, Saraiya M, Ahmed F, et al: Using population-based cancer registry data to assess the burden of human papillomavirus-associated cancers in the United States: Overview of methods. *Cancer* 113:2841, 2008.
27. Kong CS, Welton ML, Longacre TA: Role of human papillomavirus in squamous cell metaplasia-dysplasia-carcinoma of the rectum. *Am J Surg Pathol* 31:919, 2007.
28. Ogunbiyi OA, Scholefield JH, Raftery AT, et al: Prevalence of anal human papillomavirus infection and intraepithelial neoplasia in renal allograft recipients. *Br J Surg* 81:365, 1994.
29. Palefsky JM, Holly EA, Hogeboom CJ, et al: Virologic, immunologic, and clinical parameters in the incidence and progression of anal squamous intraepithelial lesions in HIV-positive and HIV-negative homosexual men. *J Acquir Immune Defic Syndr Hum Retrovirol* 17:314, 1998.
30. Palefsky JM, Holly EA, Efirdc JT, et al: Anal intraepithelial neoplasia in the highly active antiretroviral therapy era among HIV-positive men who have sex with men. *AIDS* 19:1407, 2005.
31. Chin-Hong PV, Palefsky JM: Natural history and clinical management of anal human papillomavirus disease in men and women infected with human immunodeficiency virus. *Clin Infect Dis* 35:1127, 2002.
32. Metcalf AM, Dean T: Risk of dysplasia in anal condyloma. *Surgery* 118:724, 1995.
33. Carter PS, de Ruiter A, Whatrup C, et al: Human immunodeficiency virus infection and genital warts as risk factors for anal intraepithelial neoplasia in homosexual men. *Br J Surg* 82:473, 1995.
34. Berry JM, Palefsky JM, Jay N, et al: Performance characteristics of anal cytology and human papillomavirus testing in patients with high-resolution anoscopy-guided biopsy of high-grade anal intraepithelial neoplasia. *Dis Colon Rectum* 52:239, 2009.

35. Palefsky JM, Holly EA, Hogeboom CJ, et al: Anal cytology as a screening tool for anal squamous intraepithelial lesions. *J Acquir Immune Defic Syndr Hum Retrovirol* 14:415, 1997.

36. Stier EA, Goldstone SE, Berry JM, et al: Infrared coagulator treatment of high-grade anal dysplasia in HIV-infected individuals: An AIDS malignancy consortium pilot study. *J Acquir Immune Defic Syndr* 47:56, 2008.

37. Pineda CE, Berry JM, Jay N, et al: High-resolution anoscopy targeted surgical destruction of anal high-grade squamous intraepithelial lesions: A ten-year experience. *Dis Colon Rectum* 51:829; discussion 835, 2008.

38. Jay N, Berry JM, Hogeboom CJ, et al: Colposcopic appearance of anal squamous intraepithelial lesions: Relationship to histopathology. *Dis Colon Rectum* 40:919, 1997.

39. Diaz-Arrastia C, Arany I, Robazetti SC, et al: Clinical and molecular responses in high-grade intraepithelial neoplasia treated with topical imiquimod 5%. *Clin Cancer Res* 7:3031, 2001.

40. Gutzmer R, Kaspari M, Vogelbruch M, et al: Successful treatment of anogenital Bowen's disease with the immunomodulator imiquimod, and monitoring of therapy by DNA image cytometry. *Br J Dermatol* 147:160, 2002.

41. Kreuter A, Hochdorfer B, Stucker M, et al: Treatment of anal intraepithelial neoplasia in patients with acquired HIV with imiquimod 5% cream. *J Am Acad Dermatol* 50:980, 2004.

42. Papillon J, Mayer M, Montbarbon JF, et al: A new approach to the management of epidermoid carcinoma of the anal canal. *Cancer* 51:1830, 1983.

43. Chang AE, Karnell LH, Menck HR: The National Cancer Data Base report on cutaneous and noncutaneous melanoma: A summary of 84,836 cases from the past decade. The American College of Surgeons Commission on Cancer and the American Cancer Society. *Cancer* 83:1664, 1998.

44. Thibault C, Sagar P, Nivatvongs S, et al: Anorectal melanoma—an incurable disease? *Dis Colon Rectum* 40:661, 1997.

45. Yeh JJ, Shia J, Hwu WJ, et al: The role of abdominoperineal resection as surgical therapy for anorectal melanoma. *Ann Surg* 244:1012, 2006.

46. Kiran RP, Rottoli M, Pokala N, et al: Long-term outcomes after local excision and radical surgery for anal melanoma: Data from a population database. *Dis Colon Rectum* 53:402, 2010.

47. Homsi J, Garrett C: Melanoma of the anal canal: A case series. *Dis Colon Rectum* 50:1004, 2007.

48. Ballo MT, Gershenwald JE, Zagars GK, et al: Sphincter-sparing local excision and adjuvant radiation for anal-rectal melanoma. *J Clin Oncol* 20:4555, 2002.

49. Haque W, Kelly E, Dhingra S, et al: Successful treatment of recurrent Buschke-Lowenstein tumor by radiation therapy and chemotherapy. *Int J Colorectal Dis* 25:539, 2010.

50. Armstrong N, Foley G, Wilson J, et al: Successful treatment of a large Buschke-Lowenstein tumour with chemo-radiotherapy. *Int J STD AIDS* 20:732, 2009.

51. Sarmiento JM, Wolff BG, Burgart LJ, et al: Paget's disease of the perianal region: An aggressive disease? *Dis Colon Rectum* 40:1187, 1997.

Retrorectal Tumors

Eric J. Dozois

The retrorectal space is the location for a wide spectrum of rare tumors. Pathology in this region ranges from simple benign cysts that may be approached by a single surgeon familiar with pelvic anatomy, to complex malignant lesions involving multiple pelvic structures requiring a multidisciplinary surgical team for effective management. Improvements in imaging modalities, coupled with neoadjuvant chemoradiation, and the realization that multidisciplinary teams are required for optimal treatment, have led to better outcomes in this challenging group of patients.

ANATOMIC CONSIDERATIONS

Given the bony confines of the pelvis and its complex anatomy, tumors arising in the retrorectal space are in proximity to multiple structures. Evaluation and management requires an understanding of the anatomic relationships of the pelvic soft tissues and neurologic and osseous structures. The retrorectal space is a potential space that can accommodate large masses, leading to displacement of pelvic organs (Figure 173-1). The mesorectum forms the anterior border of this space, and the anterior aspect of the sacrum forms the posterior border. Superiorly, the space extends to the peritoneal reflection and inferiorly to the rectosacral fascia.[1] The lateral boundaries are demarcated by the lateral ligaments, the ureters, and the iliac vessels. The retrorectal space itself contains loose connective tissue, the middle sacral artery, superior hemorrhoidal vessels, and branches of sympathetic and parasympathetic nerves. Vascular and neural structures originate or traverse in proximity to this area and may give rise to, or be involved by, retrorectal tumors (Figure 173-2).

Knowledge of sacral root function is of particular importance in order to counsel patients adequately regarding potential functional sequelae. If all sacral roots on only one side are sacrificed, normal anorectal function is preserved and sphincter-sparing operations may be considered if oncologically appropriate. Likewise, if only the upper three sacral roots (S1 to S3) remain intact on either side of the sacrum, the patient will still exhibit spontaneous defecation and control of anorectal contents. If both S3 roots are removed or damaged, anal incontinence and difficult defecation will result, and a permanent colostomy is indicated.[2] The need for sacrectomy requires the surgical team be familiar with the anatomy of the sacrotuberous and sacrospinous ligaments (Figure 173-3), sciatic nerve, piriformis muscle (Figure 173-4), and the thecal sac and sacral nerve roots (Figure 173-5). Our practice has been to incorporate the skills of both an oncologic orthopedic surgeon and a spine surgeon to assist in this regard. When the majority

of the sacrum is removed, pelvic stability will be maintained if more than half of the S1 vertebral body is preserved. As stress fractures to this remnant may occur if preoperative radiation has been utilized, preservation of spinopelvic stability may require fusion.

INCIDENCE AND CLASSIFICATION

Retrorectal tumors are rare (incidence <1%) and few surgeons will encounter them unless they practice at specialized referral centers.[3,4] Any tissue type within, or adjacent to the retrorectal space, may give rise to benign or malignant lesions. The most comprehensive classification of retrorectal masses considers each potential cell line.[5] The author has modified and updated the classification schemes previously described to subcategorize tumors into malignant and benign status, as this has significant clinical implications (Box 173-1). In general, two-thirds are congenital in origin, of which a further two-thirds are developmental cysts, and the next most common masses are neurogenic tumors.[6] Developmental cysts may originate from any of the three germ layers and include epidermoid and dermoid cysts, enterogenous cysts, tailgut cysts, and teratomas. Teratomas are the most common presacral tumor in children. Cystic lesions are seen most commonly in women and most solid lesions are either chordomas or sarcomas.[6] Malignancy is more common in men, even though most retrorectal tumors occur in women.

CLINICAL PRESENTATION AND DIAGNOSIS

HISTORY AND PHYSICAL EXAMINATION

Symptoms are frequently absent or nonspecific and retrorectal tumors may be discovered incidentally on routine pelvic or rectal examination. Pain, if present, is typically vague and of long duration, in the perineum, low back, or both. Classically, this pain is aggravated by sitting and ameliorated by standing or walking. Pain is an ominous sign, being present more commonly when the lesion is malignant than benign (88% vs. 39%).[6] The vague nature of the pain may even have eluded diagnosis to the point that the patient has been previously referred to a psychiatrist. Constipation, urinary and fecal incontinence, and sexual dysfunction are usually symptoms of advanced tumors with sacral nerve involvement.

Occasionally, patients will complain of persistent perianal discharge and their symptoms may have previously been attributed to perianal fistula or pilonidal disease. Several circumstances should alert the examiner to the possibility of a retrorectal cystic lesion as a cause of this presentation: repeated operations for "anal fistula,"

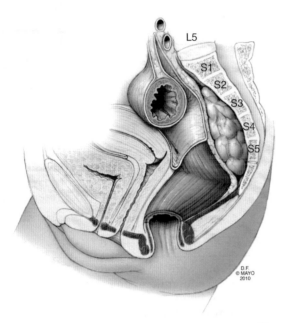

FIGURE 173-1 Retrorectal mass displacing pelvic organs. (By permission of Mayo Foundation for Medical Education and Research. All rights reserved.)

inability to uncover a primary source of infection at the dentate line, recurrent infection of the retrorectal space without obvious cause, presence of a postanal dimple, and fullness and fixation of the precoccygeal area.[1]

A careful physical examination should focus on the perineum and rectum. Evidence of a postanal dimple should be sought, but is rare. In most patients, a digital rectal examination will reveal the presence of an extra-rectal mass, displacing the rectum anteriorly. The overlying rectal mucosa is usually smooth and mobile; absence of this feature overlying the mass is suggestive of prior infection of a cystic lesion that has discharged through the rectum, or of advanced malignancy. The rectal examination is also important in evaluating for fixation and determining the level of the tumor in relation to the coccyx and other structures such as the prostate. Neurologic evaluation focused on the sacral nerves and musculoskeletal reflexes may indicate the presence of sacral nerve involvement.

INVESTIGATIONS

Retrorectal masses should undergo detailed evaluation with computed tomography (CT) and/or magnetic resonance imaging (MRI). Plain radiographs of the sacrum will identify bone expansion and destruction, calcification, and soft tissue–occupying masses, but are not pathognomonic of a specific tumor type. These features

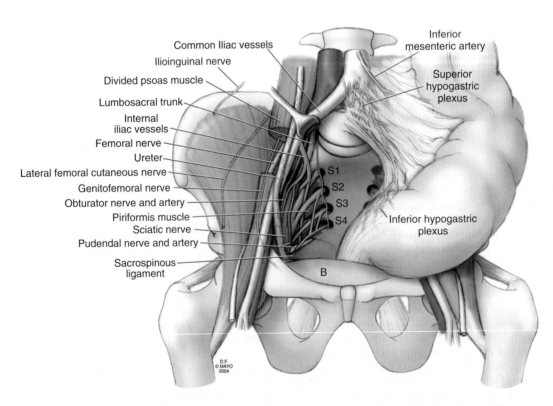

FIGURE 173-2 Vascular and neural anatomy of retrorectal space. (By permission of Mayo Foundation for Medical Education and Research. All rights reserved.)

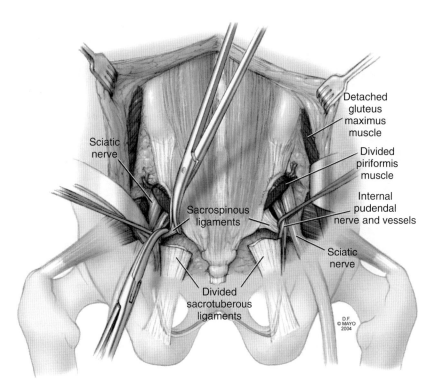

FIGURE 173-3 Anatomy of posterior sacrum: sacrotuberous and sacrospinous ligaments. (From Dozois EJ, Jacofsky DJ, Dozois RR: Presacral tumors. In *The ASCRS textbook of colon and rectal surgery*. New York, 2007, Springer, p 511.)

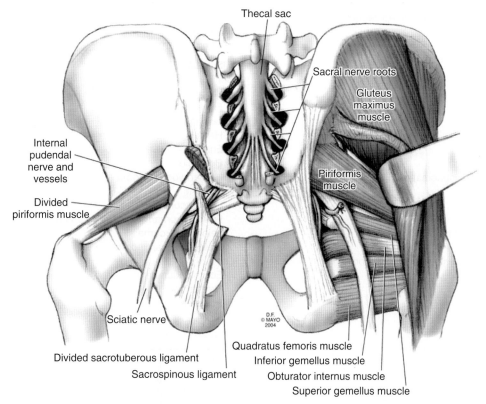

FIGURE 173-4 Anatomy of posterior sacrum: piriformis muscle and sciatic and pudendal nerves. (From Dozois EJ, Jacofsky DJ, Dozois RR: Presacral tumors. In *The ASCRS textbook of colon and rectal surgery*. New York, 2007, Springer, p 502.)

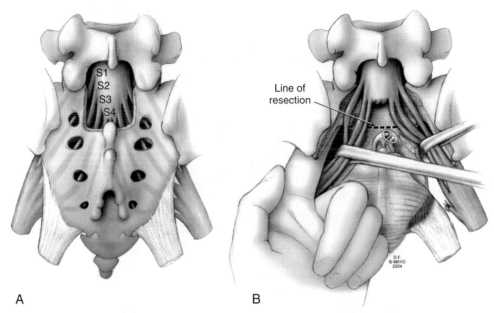

A   B

FIGURE 173-5 Anatomy of posterior sacrum: thecal sac **(A)** and nerve roots **(B).** (From Dozois EJ, Jacofsky DJ, Dozois RR: Presacral tumors. In *The ASCRS textbook of colon and rectal surgery.* New York, 2007, Springer, p 511.)

BOX 173-1 Classification of Retrorectal Tumors

CONGENITAL
Benign
   Developmental cysts (teratoma, epidermoid, dermoid,
      mucus-secreting)
   Duplication of rectum
   Anterior sacral meningocele
   Adrenal rest tumor
Malignant
   Chordoma
   Teratocarcinoma

NEUROGENIC
Benign
   Neurofibroma
   Neurilemoma (Schwannoma)
   Ganglioneuroma
Malignant
   Neuroblastoma
   Ganglioneuroblastoma
   Ependymoma
   Malignant peripheral nerve sheath tumors

OSSEOUS
Benign
   Giant cell tumor
   Osteoblastoma
   Aneurysmal bone cyst

Malignant
   Osteogenic sarcoma
   Ewing sarcoma
   Myeloma
   Chondrosarcoma

MISCELLANEOUS
Benign
   Lipoma
   Fibroma
   Leiomyoma
   Hemangioma
   Endothelioma
   Desmoid
   Hemangiopericytoma
Malignant
   Liposarcoma
   Fibrosarcoma/malignant fibrous histiocytoma
   Leiomyosarcoma
   Metastatic carcinoma
Other
   Ectopic kidney
   Hematoma
   Abscess

are commonly seen with chordoma, as bone destruction is present in a third of patients. Bone destruction, however, may also be seen with benign tumors such as giant cell tumors, neurilemoma, aneurysmal bone cysts, and osteochondroma.[6] A "scimitar" sign on sacral views is a classic feature seen in association with anterior sacral meningocele, a diagnosis that should be confirmed with myelography or MRI with gadolinium.

CT imaging distinguishes whether tumors are cystic, solid, and mixed (solid and cystic components). Moreover, CT imaging determines if other pelvic structures such as the bladder, uterus, ureters, or rectum are involved. Cortical bone destruction is also demonstrated by CT, whereas MRI is superior in evaluation of marrow involvement. MRI, by improving soft tissue resolution, is quite helpful in planning the extent of resection of adjacent structures. Spinal imaging is best performed by MRI, which may demonstrate meningocele, nerve root, and foraminal involvement by tumor and thecal sac compression. MR angiogram or venogram may add additional information regarding vascular involvement and indicate the need for a vascular surgeon to be a member of the multidisciplinary surgical team. Endoanal ultrasound may be helpful in determining the relationship of a retrorectal mass to the wall of the rectum. These lesions are often completely separate from the rectum, but infection, transrectal biopsy, or malignancy may result in involvement of the rectal wall.

ROLE OF PREOPERATIVE BIOPSY

Whether or not to biopsy a presacral mass has previously been a hotly debated topic, fueled by the lack of information available on these rare tumors. Some authors have stated that preoperative biopsy is contraindicated in the case of any presacral tumor considered resectable,[6-8] whereas others have stated that all solid or mixed solid/cystic tumors should be biopsied prior to surgical intervention.[9-12] Advances in preoperative imaging techniques and neoadjuvant therapy have clarified the issue and the need for biopsy is predicated on whether the result will change preoperative or operative management.

Simple cystic lesions usually need not be biopsied as results will not alter management. The situation may be very different, however, for solid and heterogeneously cystic lesions. Patients with tumors that respond to neoadjuvant chemoradiation (Ewing sarcoma, osteogenic sarcoma, and neurofibrosarcoma) will benefit from biopsy and appropriate preoperative adjuvant therapy. Tumors that attain very large proportions, such as desmoid tumors, may be more readily excised if some degree of tumor regression is obtained with radiation. In the author's opinion, the most important role of biopsy, apart from determining the need for neoadjuvant therapy, is for surgical planning. For oncologic resection that may include pelvic organ resection, sacrectomy, and amputation, multidisciplinary team planning and discussion with the patient depend heavily on the preoperative diagnosis obtained by biopsy.

When a biopsy is to be performed it must be performed correctly. Transrectal or transvaginal biopsy should be avoided for several reasons. If malignancy is present, excision of the rectum and/or vagina may not be necessary, but becomes mandated if the biopsy tract traverses these organs. In the presence of a cystic lesion, transrectal biopsy introduces the risk of infection, rendering subsequent attempts at excision more difficult because of distortion of embryologic tissue planes, which in turn increase the risk of recurrence and collateral injury. Inadvertent biopsy of a meningocele may result in the disastrous complications of meningitis and death. If tissue diagnosis of a retrorectal mass is required, a needle biopsy should be performed by an experienced radiologist and within the field of the proposed area of resection so that the needle tract may be excised en bloc with the specimen at the time of operation. Either the transperineal or parasacral approach may be considered depending on the anticipated field of resection (Figure 173-6). It is imperative to discuss the case with a radiologist familiar with evaluation of pelvic tumors and with an appreciation of the intended operative approach.

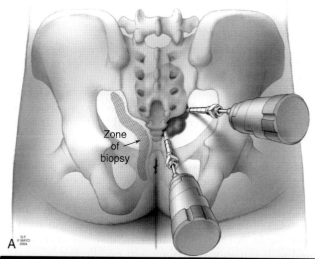

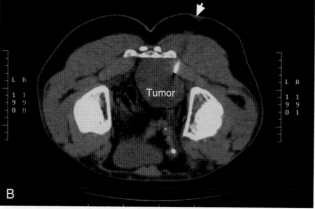

FIGURE 173-6 Preoperative biopsy technique showing ideal zone of needle path **(A),** and CT scan demonstrating appropriate direction of biopsy tract **(B).** (From Dozois EJ, Jacofsky DJ, Dozois RR: Presacral tumors. In *The ASCRS textbook of colon and rectal surgery.* New York, 2007, Springer, p 511.)

TABLE 173-1 Features of Retrorectal Cysts

Cyst Type	Tissue Type	Distinguishing Features	Mechanism of Formation	Female:Male Ratio
Dermoid cyst	Keratinizing stratified squamous epithelium	+/– sweat glands, hair follicles, sebaceous cysts	Failure of separation of cutaneous ectoderm from neural ectoderm	F > M
Epidermoid cyst	Keratinizing stratified squamous epithelium	No skin appendages	Failure of separation of cutaneous ectoderm from neural ectoderm	F > M
Enterogenous cyst (duplication cyst)	Squamous or columnar epithelium	Well-defined muscular wall with myenteric plexus; +/– villi or crypts	Sequestration of the developing hindgut	F > M
Tailgut cyst	Squamous or glandular columnar or transitional or mixture	Smooth muscle may be present, but not well defined; no myenteric plexus	Remnants of embryonic primitive gut	3 : 1
Teratoma	Contains tissue from each of the germ layers	May contain hair, bone, teeth		F > M

TUMOR-SPECIFIC FEATURES

DEVELOPMENTAL CYSTS (Table 173-1)

Epidermoid and Dermoid Cysts

These cysts result from abnormal closure of the ectodermal tube of the fetus.[13] Epidermoid and dermoid cysts both exhibit keratinizing stratified squamous epithelium, whereas epidermoid cysts bear no skin appendages. Dermoid cysts may exhibit characteristic sweat glands, hair follicles, or sebaceous cysts and have an intraspinal component.[14]

Dermoid and epidermoid cysts are more common in women and may be associated with a postanal dimple or sinus. An infection rate of up to 30% has been noted, in which case the cysts present as retrorectal or perirectal abscesses. Communication between an abscess and a postanal dimple may result in a false diagnosis of perianal fistula. A recurrently infected cyst has been associated with squamous carcinoma in middle age.[3]

Enterogenous Cysts

Enterogenous cysts (duplication cysts of the rectum) are thought to result from sequestration of the developing hindgut. They may be lined by squamous epithelium (like dermoid and epidermoid cysts) or columnar epithelium (like tailgut cysts). They differ from these other entities by having a well-defined muscular wall with a myenteric plexus. Villi or crypts are also commonly found in intestinal duplications but not tailgut cysts (TGC), and malignancy has been reported.[15,16]

Tailgut Cysts

Multiple terms have been used to describe TGC, including cystic hamartoma and postanal gut cyst. These retrorectal cysts are thought to originate from remnants of the embryonic primitive gut that extends into the transient true tail that develops in the human embryo between 35 and 56 days of gestation before regressing.[15] Despite their

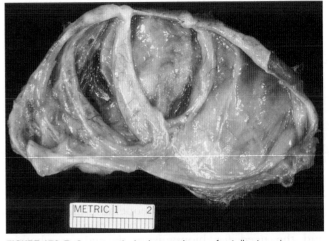

FIGURE 173-7 Gross pathologic specimen of a tailgut cyst revealing multicystic, multiloculated appearance.

rare nature, the pathologic features of TGC have been well described. The masses are multicystic and multilocular (Figure 173-7). They are lined by squamous, glandular columnar, or transitional epithelium, all three of which may be present in the same specimen.[17] Presence of the latter two epithelial types excludes the diagnosis of dermoid and epidermoid cysts, which contain squamous epithelium only. Although smooth muscle may be identified in the specimen, a well-defined muscular wall with myenteric plexus should be absent in order to exclude the possibility of a duplication cyst. The majority of TGC have been reported in adults, with few reports of these lesions being detected in neonates.[18] Presence of calcification on imaging is common in teratomas and generally eliminates the diagnosis of TGC but may occur in the presence of malignant degeneration.[15] CT imaging reveals a well-defined, homogeneous mass, with preservation of adjacent fat planes and often keratinous debris within the cysts (Figure 173-8).[19]

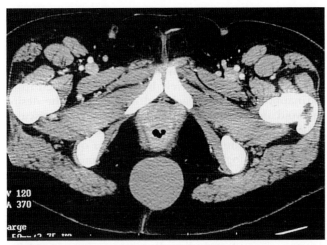

FIGURE 173-8 Typical computed tomographic appearance of a tailgut cyst.

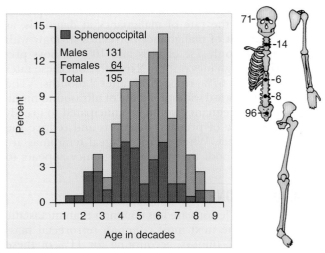

FIGURE 173-9 Distribution of chordomas, showing predilection for sacrococcygeal and sphenooccipital sites. (From Dahlin DC: *Bone tumors: General aspects and data on 6,221 cases*, ed 3. Springfield, Ill, 1978, Charles C. Thomas.)

Malignant degeneration of tailgut cysts was 13% in a recent series from the Mayo Clinic, and should always be considered.[11] The majority of reported malignancies have been adenocarcinomas.[15,17,20-23] Presacral carcinoid tumors have also been described in association with TGC,[24,25] leading to the speculation that these carcinoids arise from neuroendocrine cells in presacral hindgut rests.[26]

NEUROGENIC TUMORS

Neurogenic tumors include all of the following; schwannomas, ganglioneuromas, ganglioneuroblastomas, neurofibromas, neuroblastomas, ependymomas, and malignant peripheral nerve sheath tumors (neurofibrosarcoma, malignant schwannomas, neurogenic sarcomas). In a recently published Mayo Clinic series of neurogenic tumors of the pelvis, schwannomas were the most common benign tumor, and malignant peripheral nerve sheath tumors, the most common malignant lesions.[12] Benign schwannoma are typically solitary, well-circumscribed, encapsulated tumors.[27] Malignant transformation of schwannomas is rare.[28] Differentiating between benign and malignant neurogenic tumors preoperatively can be challenging without a tissue biopsy as imaging alone is not adequate for this differentiation, and in these patients, a preoperative biopsy is paramount to guide operative approach (nerve sparing vs. nerve resection).

SACROCOCCYGEAL CHORDOMAS

Sacrococcygeal chordomas are the most frequently encountered malignant tumor of the retrorectal space. They are believed to originate from the primitive notochordal tissues either from the nuclei pulposi or from abnormal rests. This explains their location anywhere along the spinal column with a predilection for the sphenooccipital and the retrorectal regions (Figure 173-9).[29]

Chordomas are seen mostly in men and rarely before the age of 30 years. Patients may be asymptomatic or present with a long-standing history of vague pain mostly in the perineal area characteristically aggravated by sitting and ameliorated by standing or walking.[30-32] Advanced, large tumors may cause constipation, fecal and urinary incontinence, and sexual dysfunction. Anterior and lateral views of the sacrum demonstrate bone destruction and a soft tissue–occupying mass. Other tumors less likely to cause bony destruction include giant cell tumors, schwannomas, aneurysmal bone cysts, and osteochondromas.[30] Transrectal biopsies must be avoided, as curability will be compromised because of introduction of infection and the necessity for proctectomy.[31] If the diagnosis remains unclear after imaging, a transperineal or parasacral biopsy within the field of impending surgical resection is indicated.

TERATOMA AND TERATOCARCINOMA

Presacral teratoma is the most common teratoma seen in infancy and is seen more commonly in females.[33,34] Presacral teratomas typically contain tissue from each germ layer, although the degree of differentiation may vary. The more well differentiated the elements are, with recognizable hair, bone or teeth for example, the more likely the tumor is to be benign. As with other retrorectal masses, benign lesions are usually cystic, whereas malignant degeneration appears to result in solid components.

Teratomas may be confined to the pelvis, or may extend superiorly into the presacral space or downward with an externally visible component. Altman classified these tumors in infants into four types depending on the relative representation of external and intrapelvic components.[33] Type IV tumors are entirely presacral with no external component. These differences in presentation explain why more than 50% of infants were diagnosed on the day of birth in a series from 1974; 18% were not diagnosed within the first 6 months of life. This impacted significantly on the rate of malignancy at diagnosis, as the development of malignancy correlates strongly with age in infants; only 7% of girls and 10% of boys presented with malignancy prior to 2 months, but these rates rose to 48% and 67%, respectively after 2 months.[33] The current trend toward widespread use of ultrasound monitoring during pregnancy would be anticipated to greatly increase the rate of prenatal diagnosis and reduce the risk of malignancy. When sacrococcygeal teratomas are found in adulthood, the risk of malignancy appears to be low.[34]

OSSEOUS LESIONS

Primary osseous lesions are less common than metastatic ones, but are the next most common retrorectal mass after neurogenic tumors, accounting for 11% of these lesions. There is a male predominance of 2:1, and half of these masses are malignant: Ewing sarcoma, myeloma, and osteogenic sarcoma.[6] Malignant lesions are represented by such tumors as giant cell tumor, aneurysmal bone cyst, and osteochondroma.[6] Bone destruction is a frequent accompanying feature of such tumors, even those that are benign, and frequently present with pain.

MISCELLANEOUS LESIONS

Miscellaneous lesions in this region include metastatic lesions, inflammatory changes/abscess related to Crohn disease or diverticulitis, hemangiopericytomas, hematomas, and pelvic ectopic kidneys. Carcinoid tumors are unusual but have been reported, but most represent direct extension or metastatic spread from rectal carcinoids.[35] Rarely, presacral tumors will present as part of a congenital syndrome such as the Currarino syndrome, which is a combination of presacral mass, anorectal malformations, and sacral anomalies.[36] In the Currarino syndrome, the most frequent component of the presacral mass is meningocele, but teratomas have been identified in 20% to 40% of reported cases.[37,38]

SURGICAL INTERVENTION AND APPROACH

RATIONALE

Retrorectal tumors, once diagnosed, should be treated surgically and this rationale is based on several observations.[1,6] The lesion may be malignant, or progress to malignancy from a benign state. Anterior sacral meningocele may become infected and result in meningitis if left untreated. Cystic lesions are also at risk of becoming infected, which renders subsequent excision more difficult and increases the risk of recurrence. Retrorectal masses in young women may continue to grow and result in dystocia.

There are several circumstances that may result in less than optimal management of these tumors. Given the vague symptoms that often accompany these tumors, patients may present with advanced disease, with a large mass affecting multiple pelvic structures. Many surgeons are reluctant to approach such rare and complex lesions with which they have little experience, and others may not be familiar with the techniques that allow for a complete resection. Some may be aware of older data describing poor outcomes after resection of chordomas, and thus adopt a defeatist attitude, and not be familiar with the improved outcomes that may be attained with an aggressive surgical approach. The outcome may be compromised preoperatively by biopsies obtained from an inappropriate approach. Intraoperatively, the desire to avoid injury to the rectal wall, or to neurovascular structures, results in a misguided attempt to limit the extent of resection, which compromises oncologic outcomes.[12] Oncologic and functional outcomes can be optimized, however, if an experienced, multidisciplinary team approaches these tumors, especially complex malignant lesions.[39]

THE MULTIDISCIPLINARY TEAM

An experienced multidisciplinary team is essential for optimal outcomes in patients with malignant retrorectal tumors. Preoperatively, members will include an experienced radiologist, medical oncologist, radiation oncologist, and anesthesiologist. The surgical team must be appropriate for the intended resection. Smaller benign lesions are comfortably dealt with solely by a colorectal surgeon specifically trained to manage these lesions. Suspected osseous and neurogenic lesions, especially those extending to the upper half of the sacrum, should be approached by a multidisciplinary team comprising a colorectal surgeon, orthopedic oncologic surgeon, and a spine surgeon or neurosurgeon. Additional expertise may be required of colleagues in vascular surgery, urology, and plastic surgery. Postoperatively, the team may also require the skills of a rehabilitation therapist. Referral of patients to experienced centers is essential to decrease morbidity and maximize oncologic outcomes.

TECHNICAL APPROACH

There are three possible approaches to the resection of a retrorectal tumor: anterior-only (transabdominal), posterior-only (perineal or parasacral), or combined anterior-posterior approach. Accurate preoperative imaging is vital in defining the relationship of the tumor to the sacrum and the margins of resection. Small low-lying lesions below S3 may be removed with a posterior-only approach through a parasacral/paracoccygeal incision. Tumors extending above S3 should be approached either from the abdomen alone or with a combined anterior and posterior approach, depending on the need for concomitant sacral resection (Figure 173-10).

The approach used determines patient positioning and prepping. Another factor to be considered is the need for reconstruction and soft-tissue coverage, where the plastic surgeon plays a vital role. Although a transabdominal rectus abdominis myocutaneous (TRAM) flap is often the flap of choice, occasionally a gracilis flap may be used and the patient's skin prep should be planned accordingly.

Tumors Located Below S3—The Posterior Approach

The patient is placed in the prone jackknife position and the buttocks are taped apart. An incision is made over the lower sacrum and coccyx down to the anoderm,

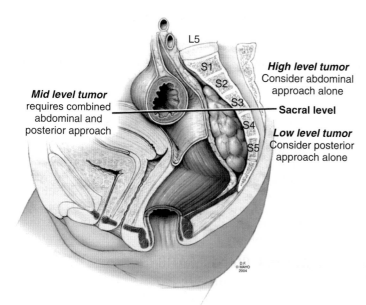

FIGURE 173-10 Determination of anterior, posterior, or combined anterior-posterior approach based on level of tumor in relation to sacral bodies (From Dozois EJ, Jacofsky DJ, Dozois RR: Presacral tumors. In *The ASCRS textbook of colon and rectal surgery*. New York, 2007, Springer, p 509.)

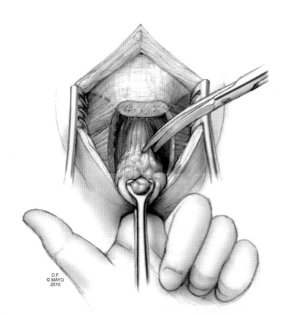

FIGURE 173-11 Use of finger to assist tumor extraction off rectum via perineal approach. (From Dozois EJ, Jacofsky DJ, Dozois RR: Presacral tumors. In *The ASCRS textbook of colon and rectal surgery*. New York, 2007, Springer, p 509.)

being cautious to avoid damage to the sphincter complex. Coccygectomy can facilitate exposure and resection of large tumors. The lesion can then be dissected in a plane between the retrorectal fat and the tumor. A pseudocapsule is often encountered that facilitates safe dissection from the surrounding tissues, including the rectal wall. In the case of very small lesions, especially if cystic, the surgeon may double-glove the nondominant hand and, with the index finger in the anal canal and lower rectum, push the lesion outward, away from the depths of the wound (Figure 173-11). This technique facilitates dissection of the lesion away from the wall of the rectum

without entry into the rectal lumen. Prior infection of a cystic lesion may obliterate the plane between the cyst wall and the rectum. A portion of the rectal wall may be excised with the specimen and the defect closed in two layers. If necessary, the lower sacrum and coccyx can also be excised en bloc with the tumor, if indicated.

Combined Anterior-Posterior Approach

If the upper extension of the tumor is above the S3 level, an anterior-posterior approach is preferred. The patient is usually positioned in the supine position. If resection of the rectum is to be combined with reestablishment of bowel continuity, a carefully padded, combined synchronous (modified dorsal lithotomy) position is used. Other positions, such as the "sloppy lateral" position have also been described to facilitate a two-team approach to the combined anterior and posterior resection.

The abdominal cavity is entered through a lower midline incision and the peritoneal cavity is carefully explored to rule out disseminated disease. After mobilization of the lower sigmoid, the presacral space is entered just below the promontory and the posterior mesorectum dissected off the sacral fascia down to the level of the upper extension of the tumor. The lateral stalks are also separated from the tumor. If the tumor can be separated safely from the posterior rectum, the lesion is dissected free in a plane anterior to the mass between its capsule and the mesorectum. Posterior to the tumor, if a plane exists between the lesion and the sacrum, this too is carefully developed. Isolated tumors, without invasion of adjacent organs, may be dissected free circumferentially in this manner and removed. If the tumor is bulky, it may compress and displace the rectum, making attempts at dissection between the tumor and the rectum risky. In this event, we favor excision of the rectum en bloc with the tumor. If the lesion is benign, or if it is considered to have a low risk of recurrence despite being malignant, reestablishment of bowel continuity may be considered, with a protective diverting loop ileostomy if indicated by low level of anastomosis and preoperative irradiation. If the tumor extends high on the sacrum, with evidence of invasion so that both S3 roots and even S2 nerve roots will need to be sacrificed, excision of the rectum en bloc with the mass may facilitate resection, avoids tumor cell spillage, and is appropriate in the patient who will be rendered incontinent. In this situation, the upper rectum is transected above the level of the tumor, using a cutting stapler and distally its anterior and lateral attachments are completely freed to the level of the pelvic floor. An end sigmoid colostomy is established.

Resection of large complex tumors may result in substantial loss of blood. This may occur from friable, irradiated pelvic vessels, or from the sacrectomy itself. Thus, when a major sacrectomy is contemplated, ligation of the middle sacral artery and the internal iliac vessels and its branches helps reduce blood loss. Preservation of the anterior division of the internal iliac artery, which gives off the inferior gluteal artery, reduces the risk of perineal and gluteal necrosis. The assistance of a vascular surgeon is invaluable for this step, especially in the presence of an irradiated field. It is helpful to mobilize the ureters, together with supporting tissues, and suspend them laterally away from the planned margin of the sacrectomy, employing a fine absorbable suture through the paraureteral tissues.

With extended sacral excision, especially when radiation is an integral part of the treatment, a well-vascularized musculocutaneous flap derived from the rectus abdominis can be used to close the perineum. The flap can be mobilized at this point in the procedure and placed in the deep pelvis to be accessed later via the perineal wound and used for closure. To protect both the flap and other vital structures during the perineal portion of the procedure, a barrier of thick plastic sheeting or laparotomy pads is placed immediately in front of the sacrum, to be removed after resection of the sacrum.

After closure of the abdominal incision and creation of the stoma, the patient is moved into the prone position. A midline incision is made over the sacrum and coccyx down to the anus, the anococcygeal ligament is transected and the levators retracted bilaterally. If the rectum is to be preserved, its posterior aspect is separated from the tumor. The orthopedic surgeon can then proceed with dissection of the gluteus maximus muscles on both sides, transection of the sacrospinous and sacrotuberous ligaments, and division of the piriformis muscles to expose the sciatic nerves. An osteotomy is then carried out at the S3 level or even higher after exposing and preserving if at all possible at least one S3 nerve root. The neural sac may need to be ligated. In this fashion, the tumor can be removed en bloc with the attached sacrum, coccyx, and involved sacral nerve roots, with or without the rectum.

Laparoscopic Approaches for Presacral Tumor Resection. Recently, there have been reports using minimally invasive laparoscopic techniques as an approach for presacral tumor resection.[40-42] If the anterior portion of a combined anterior-posterior approach can be done

laparoscopically (rectum divided, colostomy made, tumor partially mobilized, and vasculature ligated), it should decrease the morbidity of the overall operation significantly. Lengyel et al described a laparoscopic approach to treat advanced rectal cancer with similar surgical steps to the malignant presacral tumor laparoscopic resection.[42] It was performed in two phases: a laparoscopic abdominal phase with the patient in the modified Lloyd-Davies position, followed by a transsacral phase with the patient in the prone jackknife position. The key features of the abdominal (laparoscopic) component were lateral-to-medial mobilization of the rectum, ligation of the inferior mesenteric vessels, careful identification and preservation of the pelvic nerves and sacral nerve roots, and division of the colon with construction of the colostomy and completion of the proctectomy.

FOLLOWUP CONSIDERATIONS

To assess for recurrence in cases of benign tumors, an annual visit that includes a digital rectal examination should be scheduled. If digital rectal examination reveals a mass, a CT scan is done. Further, we recommend a baseline CT at 1 year following surgery and then repeated at every 5 years, even if the physical examination is normal.

In the case of malignant tumors, the patients are followed more closely, with particular attention to local recurrence and pulmonary metastasis. An annual pelvic MRI and chest CT scan are performed for the first 5 years. If the patient has the rectum in place, annual digital rectal examination with possible anoscopy is performed by the colorectal surgeon. Patients are offered repeat resection for locally advanced tumors and for pulmonary metastasis if all disease can be removed operatively.

RESULTS

Malignant Tumors

Results of surgical treatment depends on the natural behavior of the tumor and the adequacy of resection. In malignant cases, if wide margins are not achieved, or if the tumor is violated, the local recurrence rate is high and the outcome is poor. In general, most malignant tumors reported in the literature have had a poor prognosis, but many such tumors had been incompletely resected or excised piecemeal.[6,12] Kaiser et al found that local recurrence rate increased from 28% to 64% if the tumor was violated in patients with chordomas.[43]

Fuchs et al have reported one of the largest series of sacral chordoma.[44] Fifty-two patients underwent surgical treatment for sacrococcygeal chordoma in a 21-year period. At an average of 7.8 years of followup, 23 patients were alive with no evidence of disease. Twenty-three patients (44%) had local recurrence. The rate of recurrence-free survival was 59% at 5 years and 46% at 10 years. The overall survival rates were 74%, 52%, and 47% at 5, 10, and 15 years, respectively. The most important predictor of survival was a wide margin.

On the other hand, surgical management of nonchordoma malignant retrorectal tumors has only been reported in small series or single case reports, and therefore limited data exist on the long-term oncologic outcomes.[6,45] In a recent analysis of retrorectal sarcomas at our institution (unpublished data), 37 patients underwent resection, 84% had an R0 margin, and 16% an R1.[39] Overall, 76% of the patients required en bloc resection of adjacent pelvic organs and bony structures. The most frequent sarcomas found were malignant peripheral nerve sheath tumors and chondrosarcomas. Intraoperative radiation therapy was administered to 22% of patients. Overall survival at 2, 5, and 10 years was 75%, 55% and 47%, respectively. Disease-free survival at 5 years was 51%.

Cody et al reported their experience with malignant presacral tumors.[45] Excision of these tumors was described as "en bloc" or "in fragments," and 48% developed local recurrence. Survival at 5, 10, 15, and 20 years was 69%, 50%, 37%, and 20%, respectively. Lev-Chelouche et al reported on 21 patients with malignant presacral tumors.[7] No patients underwent preoperative biopsy. Nearly all patients had a palpable lesion on rectal examination. Fifteen of 21 malignant lesions were completely excised. Most recurrences were seen in patients with incomplete resection and 50% of these died of disease. Wang et al reported their series of 22 patients with malignant presacral tumors.[46] Tumor size ranged from 1.5 to 40 cm. No patients underwent preoperative biopsy. Five patients had complete resection and 17 had incomplete resection. The overall 5-year survival rate for malignant tumors was 41%. Postoperative chemotherapy and radiotherapy was used in selected patients. Bohm et al reported their series of 24 patients with congenital presacral tumors.[47] In their series, 4 patients had chordomas and 20 had developmental cysts. Three of four chordoma patients had recurrence at 25, 32, and 55 months. Patients with recurrence presented with pain and neurologic disturbance. Complete local reexcision was done in the 3 patients with recurrence.

Few data exist regarding the outcomes in patients undergoing surgery for presacral tumors of neurogenic origin. The largest surgical series reported to date of pelvic neurogenic tumors included several in the presacral space.[12] In that series, 89 patients were identified, of whom 44 were male. Median age was 38 years. Malignant lesions were found in 43 patients (48%). Schwannomas were the most common benign tumor (61%) and malignant peripheral nerve sheath tumors the most common malignant lesion (81%). Malignant tumors had histopathologic evidence of infiltration of surrounding structures in 49% of cases. Intralesional resection was the most common surgical technique for both benign and malignant tumors. Five-year local recurrence rates for benign and malignant lesions were 35.9% and 35.0%, respectively. Survival in those with malignant lesions at 1, 5, and 10 years was 79.5%, 47.9%, and 29.6%, respectively. Five-year disease-free survival for malignant tumors was 25.9%.

Congenital Cystic Lesions

In general, cystic lesions can be completely excised via a posterior approach. Large cystic lesions such as teratomas extending high into the pelvis can be excised via a combined abdominal-perineal approach. There continues to be some debate as to whether or not a coccygectomy needs to be done for all resections of congenital cystic lesions.[48] Several authors advocate coccygectomy, stating that this approach improves surgical exposure and decreases the risk of recurrence as the coccyx may harbor a nidus of totipotential cellular remnants that may later evolve into a recurrent cyst.[16,34] The concern of increased recurrence though is not supported by any published data. In fact, some authors state that if the cyst is not adherent to the coccyx, and can be removed entirely without coccygectomy, the coccyx should be left in place.[47] Probably, the cyst itself, and not the coccyx per se, harbors the aberrant remnants of the postanal gut leading to the formation of the cyst, and if the cyst is not adherent to the coccyx, there would be no advantage to a coccygectomy. It is clear from our recent series that our approach followed this perspective, and most surgeons elected to preserve the coccyx unless en bloc resection was required for malignancy or if the cyst was densely adherent to the coccyx.[11]

In a past Mayo Clinic series, 49 congenital cystic lesions were described including 15 epidermoid cysts, 16 mucus-secreting cysts, 15 teratomas, 3 teratocarcinomas, and 2 meningoceles.[6] Average cyst size ranged from 4 to 7 cm. Almost all cystic lesions were treated with a posterior approach. Of 66 patients with benign tumors, 10 had recurrence (4 had giant cell tumors, 6 had congenital benign cysts), most of which were treated successfully with reexcision. Recently, we updated our experience in the surgical management of tailgut cysts.[11] Thirty-one patients were identified and complete cyst excision was achieved in all patients, using a posterior (20/31), anterior (9/31), or combined (2/31) approach. Coccygectomy or distal sacrectomy was performed in 26% of the patients. Malignant transformation was present in 4 patients (13%), adenocarcinoma in 3, and carcinoid in 1. A fistula to the rectum was found in 4 patients (13%). One benign recurrence was detected during followup.

Lev-Chelouche et al reported on 21 benign presacral lesions.[7] Complete excision of benign lesions was possible in all cases with no recurrences during the 10-year followup. Singer et al reported on 7 patients with presacral cysts (6 females, 1 male).[47] All patients had previously been misdiagnosed and treated for pilonidal cysts, perirectal abscesses, fistula in ano, psychogenic disorder, proctalgia fugax, and posttraumatic or postpartum pain before the correct diagnosis was made. Patients underwent an average of 4.1 prior operative procedures. All patients were successfully treated with resection through a parasacrococcygeal approach after the correct diagnosis was made with CT fistulogram.

ALGORITHM

At our institution, we have established a decision-making algorithm to guide the management of retrorectal tumors (Figure 173-12).

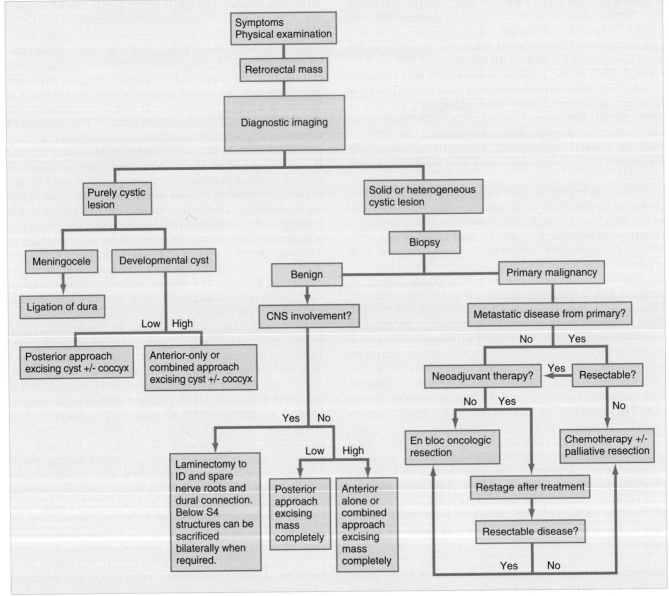

FIGURE 173-12 Algorithm to guide the management of retrorectal tumors. (From Dozois EJ, Jacofsky DJ, Dozois RR: Presacral tumors. In *The ASCRS textbook of colon and rectal surgery.* New York, 2007, Springer, p 512.)

REFERENCES

1. Dozois RR: Retrorectal tumors: Spectrum of disease, diagnosis and surgical management. *Perspect Colon Rectal Surg* 3:241, 1990.
2. Gunterberg B, Kewenter J, Petersen I, et al: Anorectal function after major resections of the sacrum with bilateral or unilateral sacrifice of sacral nerves. *Br J Surg* 63:546, 1976.
3. Spencer RJ, Jackman RJ: Surgical management of precoccygeal cysts. *Surg Gynecol Obstet* 115:449, 1962.
4. Whittaker LD, Pemberton JD: Tumors ventral to the sacrum. *Ann Surg* 107:96, 1938.
5. Uhlig BE, Johnson RL: Presacral tumors and cysts in adults. *Dis Colon Rectum* 18:581, 1975.
6. Jao SW, Beart RW Jr, Spencer RJ, et al: Retrorectal tumors: Mayo Clinic experience, 1960-1979. *Dis Colon Rectum* 28:644, 1985.
7. Lev-Chelouche D, Gutman M, Goldman G, et al: Presacral tumors: A practical classification and treatment of a unique and heterogeneous group of diseases. *Surgery* 133:473, 2003.
8. Milsom JW, Fazio VW, et al: Our approach to the management of congenital presacral tumors in adults. *Int J Colorectal Dis* 8:134, 1993.
9. Eilber FR: Expert commentary on Dozois RR. Retrorectal tumors: Spectrum of disease, diagnosis and surgical management. *Perspect Colon Rectal Surg* 3:241, 1990.
10. Hughes DE, Lamb J, Salter DM, et al: Fine-needle aspiration cytology in a case of chordoma. *Cytpoathology* 3:129, 1992.
11. Mathis KL, Dozois EJ, Grewal MS, et al: Malignant risk and surgical outcomes in presacral tailgut cysts. *Br J Surg* 97:575, 2010.
12. Dozois EJ, Wall JC, Spinner RJ, et al: Neurogenic tumors of the pelvis: Clinicopathologic features and surgical outcomes using a multidisciplinary team. *Ann Surg Oncol* 16:1010, 2009.
13. Cardell BS, Laurance B: Congenital dermal sinus associated with meningitis. Report of a fatal case. *Br Med J* 2:1558, 1951.
14. Bale PM: Sacrococcygeal developmental abnormalities and tumors in children. *Perspect Pediatr Pathol* 1:9, 1984.
15. Hjermstad BM, Helwig EB: Tailgut cysts. Report of 53 cases. *Am J Clin Pathol* 89:139, 1988.

16. Springall RG, Griffiths JD: Malignant change in a retrorectal duplication. *J R Soc Med* 83:185, 1990.

17. Lim K-E, Hsu W-C, Wang C-R: Tailgut cyst with malignancy: MR imaging findings. *AJR Am J Roentgenol* 170:1488, 1998.

18. Antao B, Lee AC, Gannon C, et al: Tailgut cyst in a neonate with anal stenosis. *Eur J Pediatric Surg* 14:212, 2004.

19. Johnson AR, Ros PR, Hjermstad BM: Tailgut cyst: Diagnosis with CT and sonography. *AJR Am J Roentgenol* 147:1309, 1986.

20. Marco V, Fernandez-Layos M, Autonell J, et al: Retrorectal cyst-hamartomas. Report of two cases with adenocarcinoma developing in one. *Am J Surg Pathol* 6:707, 1982.

21. Maruyama A, Murabayashi K, Hayashi M, et al: Adenocarcinoma arising in a tailgut cyst: Report of a case. *Surg Today* 28:1319, 1998.

22. Graadt van Roggen JF, Welvaart K, de Roos A, et al: Adenocarcinoma arising within a tailgut cyst: Clinicopathological description and follow up of an unusual case. *J Clin Pathol* 52:310, 1999.

23. Schwarz RE, Lyda M, Lew M, et al: A carcinoembryonic antigen-secreting adenocarcinoma arising within a retrorectal tailgut cyst: Clinicopathological considerations. *Am J Gastroenterol* 95:1344, 2000.

24. Schnee CL, Hurst RW, Curtis MT, et al: Carcinoid tumor of the sacrum: Case report. *Neurosurgery* 35:1163, 1994.

25. Song DE, Park JK, Hur B, et al: Carcinoid tumor arising in a tailgut cyst of the anorectal junction with distant metastasis: A case report and review of the literature. *Arch Pathol Lab Med* 128:578, 2004.

26. Horenstein MG, Erlandson RA, Gonzalez-Cueto DM, et al: Presacral carcinoid tumors. Report of three cases and review of the literature. *Am J Surg Pathol* 22:251, 1998.

27. Daneshmand S, Youssefzadeh D, Chamie K, et al: Benign retroperitoneal schwannoma: A case series and review of the literature. *Urology* 62:993, 2003.

28. Woodruff JM, Selig AM, Crowley K, et al: Schwannoma (neurilemoma) with malignant transformation. A rare, distinctive peripheral nerve tumor. *Am J Surg Pathol* 18:882, 1994.

29. Dahlin DC: *Bone tumors: General aspects and data on 6,221 cases*, ed 3. Springfield, IL, 1978, Charles C. Thomas, p 329.

30. Chandawankar RY: Sacrococcygeal chordoma: Review of 50 consecutive patients. *World J Surg* 20:717, 1996.

31. Samson IR, Springfield DS, Suit HD, et al: Operative treatment of sacrococcygeal chordoma: A review of twenty-one cases. *J Bone Joint Surg Am* 75:1476, 1993.

32. Rich TA, Schiller A, Suit HD, et al: Clinical and Pathologic review of 48 cases of chordoma. *Cancer* 56:182, 1985.

33. Altman RP, Randolph JG, Lilly JR: Sacrococcygeal teratoma: American Academy of Pediatrics Surgical Section Survey-1973. *J Pediatr Surg* 9:389, 1974.

34. Miles RM, Stewart GS: Sacrococcygeal teratomas in adults. *Ann Surg* 179:676, 1974.

35. Luong TV, Salvagni S, Bordi C: Presacral carcinoid tumour. Review of the literature and report of a clinically malignant case. *Dig Liver Dis* 37:278, 2005.

36. Pendlimari R, Leonard D, Dozois EJ: Rare malignant neuroendocrine transformation of a presacral teratoma in patient with Currarino syndrome. *Int J Colorectal Dis* 11:1383, 2010.

37. Currarino G, Coln D, Votteler T: Triad of anorectal, sacral, and presacral anomalies. *AJR Am J Roentgenol* 137:395, 1981.

38. Kochling J, Pistor G, Marzhauser Brands S, et al: The Currarino syndrome—hereditary transmitted syndrome of anorectal, sacral and presacral anomalies. Case report and review of the literature. *Eur J Pediatr Surg* 6:114, 1996.

39. Dozois EJ, Jacofsky DJ, Billings BJ, et al: Surgical approach and oncologic outcome following multidisciplinary management of rectal sarcomas. *Ann Surg Onc* 18:983, 2011.

40. Gunkova P, Martinek L, Dostalik J, et al: Laparoscopic approach to retrorectal cyst. *World J Gastroenterol* 14:6581, 2008.

41. Konstantinidis K, Theodoropoulos GE, Sambalis G, et al: Laparoscopic resection of presacral schwannomas. *Surg Laparosc Endosc Percutan Tech* 15:302, 2005.

42. Lengyel J, Sagar PM, Morrison C, et al: Multimedia article. Laparoscopic abdominosacral composite resection. *Dis Colon Rectum* 52:1662, 2009.

43. Kaiser TE, Pritchard DJ, Unni KK: Clinicopathologic study of sacrococcygeal chordoma. *Cancer* 53:2574, 1984.

44. Fuchs B, Dickey ID, Yaszemski MJ, et al: Operative management of sacral chordoma. *J Bone Joint Surg Am* 87:2211, 2005.

45. Cody HS III, Marcove RC, Quan SH: Malignant retrorectal tumors: 28 years' experience at Memorial Sloan-Kettering Cancer Center. *Dis Colon Rectum* 24:501, 1981.

46. Wang JY, Hsu CH, Changchien CR, et al: Presacral tumor: A review of forty-five cases. *Am Surg* 61:310, 1995.

47. Singer MA, Cintron JR, Martz JE, et al: Retrorectal cyst: A rare tumor frequently misdiagnosed. *J Am Coll Surg* 196:880, 2003.

48. Izant RJ Jr, Filston HC: Sacrococcygeal teratomas. Analysis of forty-three cases. *Am J Surg* 130:617, 1975.

Rare Colorectal Malignancies

Paul J. McMurrick | Peter W.G. Carne | Michael Johnston |

William D. Wallace

The vast majority of malignancies of the large bowel are derived from surface epithelial cells, predominately adenocarcinoma. However, up to 2% to 5% of colorectal cancers (CRC) are pathologically distinct and include tumors of neuroendocrine, lymphoid, and mesenchymal origin.[1-3]

This chapter addresses malignancies of the large bowel derived from non–surface epithelial cells. Extrarectal malignancies of the pelvis and anal canal are discussed in other chapters.

These lesions frequently represent a diagnostic and management challenge, as they are rarely seen by individual medical practitioners and are often associated with a poor prognosis. Because of the uncommon nature of these lesions, most of the literature supporting management strategies is based on small case series with few large population-based studies.

CLASSIFICATION

Generally, rare colorectal malignant lesions are classified by the tissue of origin (Table 174-1).

NEUROENDOCRINE/CARCINOID TUMORS

The inclusive term *neuroendocrine tumor* (NET) has been adopted by the World Health Organization (WHO) to encompass the broad spectrum of neuroendocrine neoplasms, including carcinoids.

Neuroendocrine tumors may occur throughout the gastrointestinal (GI) tract, but most commonly they affect the appendix (38%), small intestine (29%), and colorectum (21%).[4] Recent data from the United States, the United Kingdom, and Scandinavia have demonstrated a steady rise in incidence of gastrointestinal NETs over the past three decades and a change in anatomic distribution with a relative increase in rectal lesions.[4-6] These findings may, in part, be explained by improvements in diagnosis and adoption of standardized histologic diagnostic criteria. Despite the reported increased incidence, colorectal NETs remain rare, with colonic lesions accounting for approximately 0.3% and rectal lesions for 1% of all CRCs.

Neuroendocrine tumors have positive reactions to immunohistochemical markers of neuroendocrine cells including neuron-specific enolase, chromogranin, and synaptophysin. Serum chromogranin A can be used as a tumor marker for surveillance of patients following treatment. Surgery represents the primary curative modality for these tumors.

CLASSIFICATION OF NEUROENDOCRINE TUMORS

Gastrointestinal NETs are classified using the WHO criteria[7,8] according to their degree of differentiation and histologic features such as proliferation rate or tumor grade. The distinction of well-differentiated from poorly differentiated NETs is a key component of this classification, as the clinical behavior and management strategy are distinct between the two categories. Well-differentiated NETs often are slow growing, while poorly differentiated NETs are usually highly aggressive. To prevent confusion between classification systems, the term *carcinoid tumor*, being synonymous with well-differentiated NET, is still included in the WHO system, while *malignant carcinoid* is synonymous with poorly differentiated neuroendocrine carcinoma. The most recent WHO classification lists the following subgroups of neuroendocrine tumor: NET grade 1 (carcinoid), NET grade 2, NET grade 3 (large cell or small cell type).

COLORECTAL NEUROENDOCRINE TUMORS

Well-differentiated NETs may be secretory or "functioning" for a variety of hormones and biogenic amines, such as serotonin, histamine and kallikrein, which are responsible for the carcinoid syndrome. This syndrome describes an array of symptoms including nausea, vomiting, diarrhea, flushing, and bronchoconstriction and can be associated with cardiac abnormalities. Carcinoid syndrome occurs primarily in the setting of liver metastases because of failure of hepatic metabolism of neuroendocrine substances. Rarely, when venous blood from the tumor enters the systemic circulation directly, the carcinoid syndrome may occur in the absence of liver metastases. Patients with colorectal NETs are, however, much less likely to produce vasoactive substances than those with NETs in other locations.

Patients with colorectal NETs are at significant risk of synchronous and metachronous cancers. Synchronous tumors appear to be predominately in the GI tract, occurring at a rate of approximately 8% to 40%, whereas metachronous tumors usually occur outside the GI tract and have a reported incidence of up to 22.6%.[9] Overall, the risk of a second cancer is 31%. In 2010, the American Joint Cancer Committee produced a TNM classification for the first time (Table 174-2). This will be of assistance in future studies of NETs of the GI tract and help in the assessment of newer treatments as they become available.

IMAGING

Endoscopic appearance is usually that of a submucosal mass (Figure 174-1). Endoscopic ultrasonography (EUS)

TABLE 174-1 Classification of Rare Tumors of the Large Intestine

PRIMARY TUMORS

Epithelial	Neuroendocrine
	Squamous cell carcinoma
Lymphoid	Lymphoma
	Plasmacytoma
Mesenchymal	Gastrointestinal stromal
	Liposarcoma
	Leiomyosarcoma
	Rhabdomyosarcoma
	Malignant fibrous histiocytoma
	Angiosarcoma
	Fibrosarcoma
	Schwannoma
Other	Melanoma
	Kaposi sarcoma
SECONDARY TUMORS	Breast
	Lung
	Kidney
	Melanoma
	Bladder

Adapted from Corman ML: *Colon and rectal surgery*, ed 4. Philadelphia, 1998, Lippincott Williams & Wilkins.

TABLE 174-2 TNM Classifications of Gastrointestinal Tract NETs

TX	Tumor unable to be assessed
T0	No evidence of tumor
T1	Tumor invades lamina propria or submucosa, ≤2 cm in size
T1a	Tumor <1 cm in size
T1b	Tumor 1-2 cm in size
T2	Tumor invades muscularis propria, or >2 cm in size with invasion of lamina propria or submucosa
T3	Tumor invades through muscularis propria into subserosa or into nonperitonealized pericolic or perirectal tissue
T4	Tumor invades peritoneum or other organs
NX	Regional lymph nodes unable to be assessed
N0	No regional lymph node metastases
N1	Regional lymph node metastases
M0	No distant metastases
M1	Distant metastases
Stage 1	T1N0M0
Stage 2a	T2N0M0
Stage 2b	T3N0M0
Stage 3a	T4N0M0
Stage 3b	Any TN1M0
Stage 4	Any T, Any N, M1

From Edge SE, Byrd DR, Carducci MA, et al: *AJCC cancer staging manual*, ed 7. New York, 2010, Springer.

is useful to accurately assess tumor size, depth of invasion, and lymph node involvement in rectal lesions. As there is a very small risk of metastatic spread with rectal NETs smaller than 2 cm, CT imaging rarely adds to clinical information for small, EUS-evaluated tumors. It is,

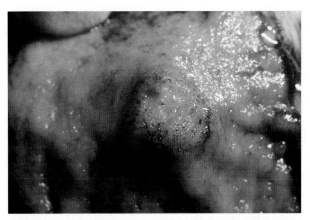

FIGURE 174-1 Carcinoid tumor presenting as a submucosal mass.

however, recommended to exclude metastases, especially for larger or more invasive lesions. Magnetic resonance imaging (MRI) may also be of benefit in this setting.

Somatostatin receptor scintigraphy (octreotide scan) is useful to assess whether known metastatic tumors express somatostatin receptors; however, there is little evidence that routine scintigraphy improves the sensitivity of standard imaging staging techniques.

Tumor Markers

Serum chromogranin A is a useful tumor marker for monitoring patients with metastatic disease or for surveillance following treatment of early-stage lesions. It should be noted that spuriously high levels can be seen in patients taking proton pump inhibitors, chronic gastritis, renal insufficiency, and other inflammatory diseases.[10] As colorectal NETs infrequently secrete serotonin or other bioactive hormones, the routine measurement of serum serotonin or urinary 5-hydroxyindolacetic acid (5-HIAA) is not recommended.[11]

COLONIC NEUROENDOCRINE TUMORS (CARCINOIDS)

Colonic NETs frequently present at an advanced stage, with nodal or distant metastases. They are more commonly found in the proximal colon and are often large at the time of diagnosis. Presentation is often in the seventh decade of life and may be with an abdominal mass, large bowel obstruction, rectal bleeding, or other nonspecific symptoms. Carcinoid syndrome is only rarely seen.

Segmental resection forms the mainstay of management of this rare tumor, similar to the management of colonic adenocarcinoma. Five-year survival rates range from 76% in the setting of localized disease to 44% and 30% in patients with regional or metastatic disease, respectively.[5] Synchronous NETs are rare; however, second primary malignancies occur at a rate of 25% to 40%.

RECTAL NEUROENDOCRINE TUMORS (CARCINOIDS)

Rectal NETs are more common than colonic NETs. Presenting symptoms include rectal bleeding, constipation, pain, and tenesmus; however, they are often an incidental finding, diagnosed on endoscopic assessment performed for other indications. Peak incidence is in the fifth to seventh decades of life. Most rectal NETs arise in the midrectum, 5 to 10 cm from the anal verge, and are submucosal in location.[11,12]

In contrast to colonic lesions, most rectal NETs (80%) are small (<1 cm) localized lesions with low risk of metastases, and overall 5-year survival is up to 88%.[5] In the absence of metastatic disease, a 92% 5-year survival rate is reported; this is reduced to 44% with nodal metastases and 7% with distant metastases. Rectal NETs larger than 2 cm metastasize in around 60% to 80% of cases.[11]

Surgery remains the only curative therapeutic modality. Treatment will depend on tumor size and depth of invasion. T1 tumors can be treated successfully with curative intent by local excision. Small (≥2 cm) T2 tumors invading the muscularis propria can also be treated with local excision when lymph node metastases have been excluded. Transanal endoscopic microsurgery is a very useful technique for local excision of rectal carcinoids. Tumors larger than 2 cm, those invading the muscularis propria, or those with lymph node involvement should undergo an oncologic resection (anterior resection or abdominoperineal resection). Adjuvant chemotherapy and radiotherapy are not curative and should not be administered outside of a clinical trial.

FOLLOWUP

Patients with invasive NETs can have recurrence many years after successful treatment. The utility of long-term surveillance is, however, unknown. For low-risk neoplasms (stage 1), the likelihood of recurrence is so low that radiologic imaging is probably not warranted. For more advanced lesions, radiologic surveillance may be useful. Recurrences may occur many years after the diagnosis and long-term followup may be required. Serum chromogranin A levels may also be a useful tool in the followup of these patients.

TREATMENT OF METASTATIC DISEASE

Data on the treatment of metastatic colorectal NET are lacking, and current treatments are based on data from the treatment of metastatic NET from other primary sites in the GIT. Treatment options include somatostatin analogues, interferon-α, hepatic arterial embolization, and cytoreductive surgery. As the course of patients with regional or distant metastatic disease may be indolent, attempts should be made to resect all of the tumor if possible.

Somatostatin analogues (e.g., octreotide) have been primarily indicated for treatment of carcinoid syndrome in the setting of metastatic disease; however, there is some evidence to suggest an additional inhibitory effect on tumor growth in midgut NETs.[13] Tumors or metastases are considered to be most responsive to octreotide when lesions are shown to be somatostatin receptor positive on scintigraphy.

Interferon-α has some antisecretory and antiproliferative effects and has also been used in the setting of advanced metastatic disease in midgut NETs.[14] Other investigational therapies include radiolabeled somatostatin analogues and angiogenesis inhibitors. Given the lack of evidence for the treatment of metastatic colorectal NETs, participation in clinical trials is recommended.

NEUROENDOCRINE CARCINOMAS

This group of malignant neuroendocrine tumors is rare and highly aggressive. A single large tertiary referral center reported 38 cases over a 23-year period.[15] Presentation is with advanced disease in 65% to 85% of cases. Prognosis is therefore often poor, with a series from Memorial Sloan-Kettering reporting a median survival of 10.4 months.[15] Treatment of this uncommon malignancy is not clearly established. Surgery is the primary curative modality; however, radiotherapy and chemotherapy may also play a role.

SQUAMOUS CELL CARCINOMA

Squamous cell carcinoma (SCC) of the colon and rectum is extremely rare, comprising approximately 0.1 to 1 per 1000 colorectal cancers.[3,16] To make the diagnosis, it is necessary to exclude (1) cranially extending anal canal squamous cell carcinoma, (2) squamous cell carcinoma in a fistulous tract, and (3) metastatic squamous cell carcinoma. Because of its rarity and poor understanding, considerable controversy exists with regard to its pathogenesis. Several theories of pathogenesis have been proposed, including focal squamous differentiation within adenocarcinoma, malignant change in persistent ectopic embryonal ectodermal cells, or squamous metaplasia resulting from abnormal stimulation such as ulcerative colitis, schistosomiasis, or human papillomavirus (HPV). These tumors are found most commonly in the right colon or rectum.[17] Presenting symptoms are similar to those of colorectal adenocarcinoma.

Resection would appear to be the predominant curative treatment modality and the operation will depend on the level at which the tumor has arisen and the presence of coexisting disease. Adjuvant radiation and chemotherapy have also been used in various combinations. Because of the rarity of these tumors, data relating to adjuvant treatment modalities are lacking; however, complete pathologic responses after neoadjuvant chemoradiation have been noted in at least one series of rectal SCCs.[16] The long-term prognosis of this tumor is similarly difficult to comment on because of the limited number of cases described in the literature. It does appear to be poor when compared to adenocarcinoma; however, long-term survivors have been reported and 5-year survival in one series has been reported at 49%.[2]

PRIMARY LYMPHOMA OF THE COLON AND RECTUM

Extranodal lymphoma, although rare, is most frequently found in the gastrointestinal tract, predominantly in the small bowel or stomach. The large intestine is the site of 10% to 20% of GI lymphoma, with the cecum and rectum the most common locations.[18] Primary colonic lymphoma is reported to account for 0.1% to 0.5% of all colorectal cancers.

The most common subtype of colonic lymphoma is diffuse large B-cell lymphoma, although T-cell lymphoma is more common in Far Eastern countries. Unlike gastric mucosa-associated lymphoid tissue (MALT) lymphoma, there is no association with *Helicobacter pylori* in colonic MALT-type lesions.

Presentation is usually in the sixth decade of life, most commonly in males, and symptoms can be nonspecific. There is a higher incidence in immunosuppressed patients and an association between human immunodeficiency virus positivity and anorectal lymphoma. Weight loss and abdominal pain are the most frequent complaints with or without a change in bowel habit or rectal bleeding. Tumors can be bulky, and a palpable mass may be apparent on physical examination. Computed tomography (CT) will demonstrate the extent of disease and exclude distant nodal disease. Differentiating primary colorectal lymphoma from adenocarcinoma may prove difficult on imaging alone, and endoscopic biopsy should be performed.

Treatment involves a multidisciplinary approach using surgery, radiation therapy, and chemotherapy to a variable extent. There is a paucity of quality evidence to guide optimum therapy and certainly a lack of randomized trials comparing different modalities. Surgical resection is usually advocated for localized disease to prevent complications such as perforation, obstruction, or hemorrhage. Multiagent chemotherapy is used in most cases and forms the basis of treatment for most moderate- to high-grade lymphomas. Radiotherapy has been used with some success in the adjuvant setting for rectal lymphoma, and some authors have reported complete clinical response after combination chemoradiotherapy.[19]

Prognosis of colorectal lymphoma is generally worse than gastric or small bowel lymphoma and will depend on stage at presentation and histologic grade. Overall 5-year survival rates range from 27% to 55%.[20]

MESENCHYMAL TUMORS OF THE RECTUM

Tumors of the mesenchyme of the rectum are rare, with the most common being a gastrointestinal stromal tumor (GIST). Originally, leiomyomas and leiomyosarcoma were reported as more common, but recent advances in immunohistochemistry techniques have allowed for better classification. Rarer tumors include malignant fibrous histiocytoma, liposarcoma, malignant schwannoma, hemangiopericytoma, and rhabdomyosarcoma. The interstitial mesenchymal stem cells may differentiate into smooth muscle cells and, when mutated, give rise to a GIST, leiomyoma, or sarcoma. Most mesenchymal tumors present incidentally or with a mass effect. They rarely cause bleeding but may be found incidentally with hemorrhoids or similar perianal conditions.

All rectal tumors should be biopsied because treatment modalities differ. The biopsy site and direction of the incision should always be planned with future resection in mind.

Mesenchymal tumors are well imaged in the pelvis with MRI. Endorectal ultrasonography may be useful for demonstrating invasion if the tumor is appropriately located. Malignant tumors are generally positron emission tomographic (PET) avid and are well staged using this modality in combination with CT scanning.

GASTROINTESTINAL STROMAL TUMORS

GISTs were originally mistakenly classified as leiomyomas, leiomyosarcomas, or smooth muscle tumors arising from the mesenchyme of the gut and divided with some difficulty histologically into benign and malignant tumors. It is now thought they arise from the interstitial cells of Cajal (ICC) or their precursors—the interstitial mesenchymal cells. Generating slow electrical waves, the interstitial cells of Cajal are intercalated between the intramural neurons and the effector smooth muscular cells to form a gastroenteric pacemaker system, which regulates peristalsis.

The interstitial cells of Cajal express CD117, which is a product of the *c-kit* protooncogene (Figure 174-2). This gene encodes a tyrosine kinase receptor that is involved in regulation of cell proliferation. Mutation of this protooncogene leads to a state of continuous activation of the tyrosine kinase receptor complex resulting in unchecked proliferation and a malignant GIST.

Immunohistochemistry is the mainstay of diagnosis at present, with positive expression of CD117 being a major diagnostic criterion. The cell surface hemopoietic progenitor antigen CD34 is also expressed by GISTs and has been used as a diagnostic marker; however, it may be less sensitive than CD117. The differential diagnosis includes schwannoma and leiomyoma, which stain more for the smooth muscle marker SMA and with desmin. Differentiating a GIST from a subclass called gastrointestinal autonomic nerve (GAN) tumors can be achieved by staining for neuron-specific enolase and skeinoid.

Epidemiology

GISTs are approximately 10 times more common than true leiomyomas and sarcomas but still, in the largest population study to date, occur in only 0.68 per 100,000 people per annum.[21,22] The average age at presentation is approximately 60 years with a slight male preponderance. Eighty percent are diagnosed in individuals older than 50 years of age. The majority of GISTs occur in the

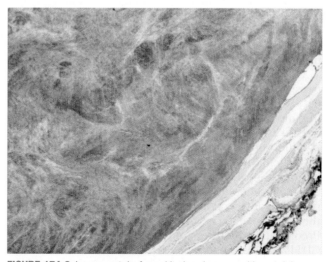

FIGURE 174-2 Immunostain for *c-kit* showing a positive staining consistent with gastrointestinal stromal tumor. Note the pushing but not invasive margin, suggesting that this tumor is benign.

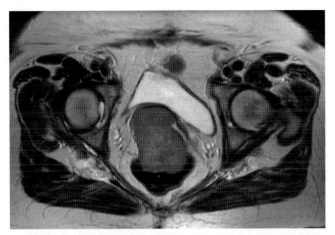

FIGURE 174-3 Moderate-sized rectal gastrointestinal stromal tumor on T2-weighted MRI showing homogeneous texture and pushing margin.

stomach (51%) and small intestine (36%), with the colon making up 7% of tumors and the rectum 5%.[21] A small percentage occur in the omentum, mesentery, and retroperitoneum.

Approximately 10% to 30% of GISTs are malignant, with differentiation from benign tumors being made by the diagnosis of metastases or demonstration of invasion on clinical presentation, imaging, or pathology.

Presentation, Diagnosis, and Investigation

GISTs of the colon and rectum are rare and often present incidentally during investigations for other conditions. Those with symptoms may describe rectal bleeding from focal ulceration, rectal or pelvic pain, tenesmus, or obstruction or a rectal mass. Endoscopy may reveal a submucosal mass.

The most common imaging modalities used to diagnose colorectal GISTs are CT, MRI, or EUS (Figure 174-3). Contrast-enhanced CT is useful to evaluate morphology, local invasion, and distant metastases, with most lesions appearing as extraluminal or intramural well-defined lesions. Similarly, GISTs can be well characterized on T2-weighted MRI images as homogeneous isointensity masses without necrosis or hemorrhage and by enhancement with gadolinium. MRI also allows for planning of surgery, with good definition of tumor margins seen.

Of malignant GISTs, 20% present with distant metastases, 20% with regional metastases, and the remaining 60% with localized disease. Most GISTs are PET avid, and this modality may be useful in assessing for metastatic disease as well as response to medical therapy.

Differentiation from leiomyomas and sarcomas may be difficult, and primary excision is recommended for intraperitoneal GISTs, with resection of the involved colon. If abdominoperineal excision is likely to be required for resection of a tumor around the anorectum, then biopsy can be performed through skin to be excised. Preoperative biopsies and histologic confirmation of CD117 expression may be useful, as sarcomas of the anorectum may be treated with preoperative radiation therapy, the use of which has been associated with worse prognosis in GISTs.

Management

Medical Therapy. In recent years, specific therapy aimed at inhibiting the tyrosine kinase receptor on GISTs has been developed. Imatinib mesylate is a specific tyrosine kinase receptor inhibitor, which selectively blocks the constitutive activity of *c-kit* in GIST cells, halting excessive proliferation. It was initially approved for treatment of unresectable or metastatic disease although now it forms a major component of multidisciplinary treatment as adjuvant therapy. Treatment arrests growth and may result in subsequent regression but it is not directly tumoricidal; 80% of malignant tumors respond, but subsequent resistance to therapy is not uncommon. There is some evidence to suggest that GISTs with specific mutations of *c-kit* (those involving exon 11) are associated with an enhanced response to tyrosine kinase receptor inhibitors.[23] Resistance to imatinib treatment may develop as further mutations in the tumor genome arise.[24] Increasing dosage or switching to another tyrosine kinase inhibitor such as sunitinib can lead to continued response.[25] Complications of therapy include cerebral edema, retinal changes, pleural and pericardial effusions, and bone marrow suppression.

Radiation therapy and conventional chemotherapeutic agents are not effective in the treatment of GISTs.

Surgery. Surgery remains the mainstay of treatment for localized disease. The main principle is to achieve clear margins, and this can usually be performed by wedge or segmental resection. Recurrence is related to positive margins, so clearance should be obtained in length of colon or rectum as well as radially, with consideration given to the associated morbidity. Care must be taken not to enter or rupture the tumor itself because contamination almost certainly results in implantation and dissemination of malignant tumors. GISTs do not metastasize via lymphatics, and therefore lymphadenectomy is unnecessary. Differentiation between malignant and benign GISTs intraoperatively can be difficult unless invasion has been noted. If malignancy is suspected, a 2-cm margin of normal tissue is regarded as adequate by most authors. Small rectal GISTs (<2 cm) with no evidence of invasion on MRI or EUS may be treated by full-thickness excision by transanal endoscopic microsurgery, provided satisfactory margins can be obtained. Transanal excision is considered inadequate for rectal GISTs growing outside the rectum and for larger rectal tumors, in order to achieve a 2-cm margin. Exenterative surgery may be required to achieve a R0 resection. There is little evidence beyond anecdotal experience that this 2-cm margin improves survival, but it allows for good clearance without encountering tumor during surgery. Local recurrence of rectal GIST has been shown to be reduced by radical resection compared to local excision in at least one study.[26]

Neoadjuvant treatment with imatinib to achieve tumor shrinkage has shown encouraging results and gained popularity recently. Preoperative treatment may allow less extensive surgery to achieve R0 resection in large rectal lesions with better postoperative functional outcome.[27] Response to neoadjuvant therapy can be measured by a decrease in size and density on CT or MRI imaging; however, PET/CT may be more accurate because of its ability to assess metabolic activity. Maintenance medical therapy may be used even in localized disease or if radical surgery is deemed excessively morbid or risky from the patient's perspective. Surveillance with CT/PET is recommended, with an increase in metabolic activity often being evident before any change in size of a lesion. This may help decisions regarding dosage or a change in therapy to sunitinib. It is advised, however, if surgery is contemplated, that organs invaded on pretreatment imaging should be included in the resection regardless of posttreatment imaging outcome. Similarly, localized recurrent disease may be pretreated before attempting further radical surgery.

Prognosis

Without evidence of invasion or high-grade activity, those GISTs designated as benign have a good prognosis, with little recurrence reported with local excision.

Malignant GISTs have an overall 5-year survival of 45% in population-based studies. Good prognosis can be predicted by (1) the grade of tumor (<5 mitoses per high-power field), (2) the presence of skeinoid fibers, and (3) size smaller than 5 cm. Even with early surgical treatment, there is a high risk of hepatic and local recurrence, and recurrence rates of up to 50% have been reported.[28] There is emerging evidence for the use of adjuvant

therapy, and mutational status can help predict response to imatinib in extensive or metastatic disease.[29]

LEIOMYOMA AND LEIOMYOSARCOMA

Leiomyoma and leiomyosarcoma are rare tumors that comprise less than 0.1% of all rectal malignancies. They are the second most common mesenchymal GI tumor after GISTs. They are true smooth muscle tumors and show smooth muscle differentiation on light microscopy. Colorectal smooth muscle tumors tend to be polypoidal, whereas upper GI tract lesions tend to be more intramural in location.[30] In contrast to GISTs, *c-kit* mutations are largely absent and they are immunohistochemically negative for CD117 or CD34 markers but will have positive staining for smooth muscle markers, such as actin and desmin.

Rectal lesions can be evaluated by MRI, endorectal ultrasonography, and CT/PET (Figure 174-4). Malignancy may be suspected by size of tumor, irregularity, and mixed echogenicity with cystic spaces and echogenic foci. Grading is based on the number of mitoses present in 50 high-power fields. A large size of tumor and the presence of necrosis indicate a poorer prognosis.

Benign tumors can be excised locally. Low-grade malignant tumors may be excised with a margin of 1 cm of normal tissue. Good survival has also been obtained

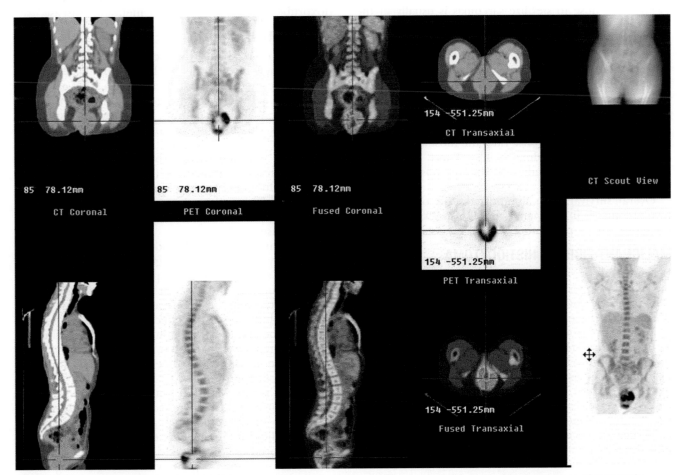

FIGURE 174-4 CT/PET scan showing rectal leiomyosarcoma with central inactive core (likely necrosis) and no evidence of metastatic disease.

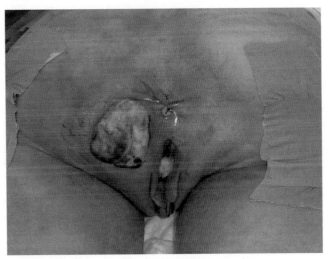

FIGURE 174-5 Necrotic leiomyosarcoma of the rectum after neoadjuvant radiation, invading the skin and vagina.

for small malignant tumors (<5 cm) with local resection and postoperative brachytherapy. High-grade leiomyosarcomas are best resected with a 4-cm margin, although a smaller margin may be adequate after neoadjuvant radiotherapy, as unlike GISTs they are moderately radiosensitive. This is preferable in the pelvis because a 4-cm margin will often require pelvic exenteration (Figure 174-5). The dose to sterilize sarcomas is usually in the order of 60 Gy, a toxic dose to both the rectum and small bowel; however, most irradiated tissue will be removed at the time of the resection. As with the treatment of rectal cancer, there is a significant leak rate after high-dose radiation for restorative surgery and wound problems are common with abdominoperineal resection, so preemptive flap closures should be considered.

Chemotherapy has been used for metastatic disease with a 15% to 20% response rate, the most active agents being ifosfamide and doxorubicin. There is little evidence to suggest that adjuvant therapy postoperatively confers any benefit.

Overall survival for small reported series of rectal leiomyosarcomas is in the vicinity of 50% to 70% at 3 years for those tumors presenting without metastases.

MALIGNANT FIBROUS HISTIOCYTOMA

Because of the rarity of this tumor, little is known regarding its pathogenesis. The cell of origin is thought to be the fibroblast and tumors previously characterized as fibrosarcoma have been included in this group. Controversy still surrounds the classification of these tumors, with the World Health Organization now designating malignant fibrous histiocytoma (MFH) a subclass of pleomorphic sarcomas.

Occurrence in the rectum is rare with few reported cases,[31] and tumors arising in the bony pelvis adjacent to the rectum are more common. Surgical resection as for colorectal adenocarcinoma is considered to be the most effective treatment, although the optimal treatment protocol has not been universally clarified. Malignant fibrous histiocytomas are moderately sensitive to radiation therapy and should be managed in a multidisciplinary

setting. Neoadjuvant radiation may enable a less radical operation to be performed to achieve R0 resection, which in the pelvis is important for limitation of morbidity. Total dose is usually in the order of 60 Gy, with 45 Gy given before surgery and the remainder as a boost after surgery.

Chemotherapy is of little benefit, although imatinib, used in the treatment of malignant GISTs, has been shown to be effective in animal models. Prognosis generally reflects histologic grade. Patients treated without metastases with low-grade tumors have 5-year survival rates in excess of 60%, whereas high-grade tumors have a 20% to 25% survival.

LIPOSARCOMA

Liposarcomas of the colorectum are exceedingly rare, and there are few reports of their occurrence. Their clinical and pathologic behavior can be predicted only by comparison with the behavior of liposarcoma in other parts of the body. Malignancy is suspected by size and fixation and should prompt biopsy. They have been excised with small (<1 cm) margins without reports of recurrence. Metastatic disease is rare, but multicentricity is not uncommon so other lesions should be sought using clinical examination and CT scan, particularly to look at the retroperitoneum where large tumors can be present asymptomatically. Limited success has been achieved with chemotherapy using anthracycline (e.g., doxorubicin) and ifosfamide for metastatic disease.

RHABDOMYOSARCOMA

Rhabdomyosarcomas of the rectum and perianal region are extremely rare tumors in children but even rarer in adults. The median age of presentation is 4 years, with usual clinical features involving a mass or suspected perianal abscess. They are more common in individuals affected by Li-Fraumeni syndrome and neurofibromatosis type I.

Tumors are well imaged by MRI and staged with CT and clinical examination. PET scanning has a high sensitivity for metastases, and in combination with CT a reduced false-positive rate. Lymph node metastases occur in approximately 10% of patients without metastatic disease.

Rhabdomyosarcomas should be managed in a multidisciplinary setting because surgery is not always required. All tumors should undergo biopsy, and diagnosis is made with immunohistochemistry or electron microscopy.

These tumors are moderately radiation sensitive, requiring high doses for effective tumor kill, but this dose can be reduced with combination chemotherapy. Multiple agents have been shown to be effective, with the most common regimen used being vincristine, actinomycin D, and cyclophosphamide.

Surgery is often morbid, with wide excision margins required to prevent recurrence. More recently, reports of the use of radiofrequency ablation in combination with neoadjuvant therapy have emerged, but this has not been explored well in the pelvis.

Overall prognosis is poor, with lesions arising in the pelvis and particularly from mucosal sites having survival figures of less than 50%.

SCHWANNOMA OF COLON AND RECTUM

Schwannomas are rare tumors derived from the cells of neural sheath. Gastrointestinal schwannomas are most commonly encountered in the stomach, and few cases of colorectal tumors have been reported in the medical literature.[32] They present as polyps or intramural masses and can present with rectal bleeding if mucosal ulceration is present. Differentiation from other mesenchymal tumors such as GIST can be difficult, particularly on radiologic imaging.

They can be categorized according to their histologic appearance into spindle cell, epithelioid, and plexiform subtypes with some clinicopathologic differences.[33] The majority of tumors show indolent behavior; however, a clinical spectrum to frank malignancy exists. Local recurrence is not uncommon. Treatment is usually by segmental anatomic resection and there is insufficient data to guide the use of adjuvant therapy.

OTHER MISCELLANEOUS TUMORS

PRIMARY AND SECONDARY MELANOMA OF THE LARGE INTESTINE

Anorectal melanoma is an uncommon condition associated with a very poor prognosis. The anorectum is the third most common site for primary melanoma after the skin and retina and it accounts for 0.2% to 3% of melanoma.[34] It has been hypothesized that many reported cases of primary melanoma in fact represent metastatic spread in patients in whom the primary lesion has never been identified or has spontaneously regressed, although a small number of cases seem to demonstrate indication of primary growth in the large bowel. Unlike cutaneous melanoma where exposure to ultraviolet radiation is a recognized risk factor, there are limited data regarding contributing factors for anorectal melanoma.

Anorectal melanoma can affect patients of any age, and presenting symptoms are typical for many anorectal conditions, including bleeding, pruritus, tenesmus, or discomfort. Lesions may appear as a mass in the anal canal or rectum and may be mistaken for a polyp or hemorrhoid. In contrast to cutaneous melanoma, lesions are often not pigmented. Up to 38% of patients are found to have metastases at the time of presentation.[35] Radiologic evaluation is by CT, MRI, and endorectal ultrasonography.

Histopathologic staining is typical of melanoma (Figure 174-6), with tumor cells arranged in nests and positive staining for melanosome protein HMB-453. Treatment of primary anorectal melanoma is usually by standard radical anatomic resection, after exclusion of metastatic disease (Figure 174-7); however, local resection is considered a valuable alternative. Most studies published to date have not shown a significant difference in outcome between radical surgery and local excision.[36] There is no evidence to support inguinal lymphadenectomy, as it does not appear to affect survival and is associated with increased morbidity.

Prognosis of patients with anorectal melanoma remains dismal despite potentially curative radical

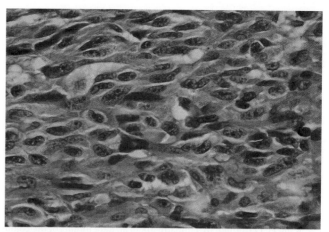

FIGURE 174-6 Hematoxylin–eosin stain of primary rectal melanoma.

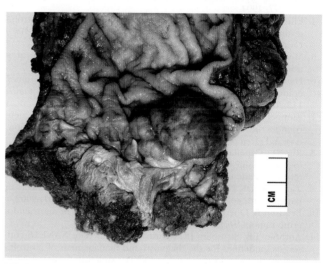

FIGURE 174-7 Abdominoperineal resection specimen of primary melanoma of the lower one-third of the rectum. Macroscopically, the lesion appeared indistinguishable from adenocarcinoma of the rectum. Preoperative ultrasonography demonstrated T3 penetration.

surgery. Outcome is related to stage at presentation, with overall 5-year survival of 6% to 28%.[36] The exact role for adjuvant therapy is uncertain, as there are limited data available. Chemotherapeutic agents used for cutaneous melanoma are usually employed in anorectal disease. A detailed review of literature relating to melanoma metastatic to the colon from the Mayo Clinic[37] indicated that fewer than 100 cases of isolated metastases have been reported in the literature. The average interval between primary presentation and the development of a clinically significant colonic secondary lesion was more than 7 years. One- and 5-year survival rates were 37% and 21%, respectively, for resected patients. Nodal status and presentation with either bowel obstruction or perforation were associated with a reduction in survival time.

BUSCHKE-LÖWENSTEIN TUMORS

Buschke-Löwenstein tumors have been reported fewer than 50 times. First described in 1925, the term refers to a locally invasive, rapidly growing variant of condylomata acuminata, with deep penetration of local tissues. They are associated with HPV-6 and HPV-11.[38] The histology is similar to that of simple condylomata acuminata with an orderly arrangement of the epithelial layers. The basement is maintained intact, and cell polarity is preserved. The major difference between condylomata acuminata and the Buschke-Löwenstein tumor lies in the tendency of the latter to downward growth, simulating malignant invasion. Cure is obtained by early and radical excision; radiation therapy may assist in local control.

REFERENCES

1. Cuffy M, Abir F, Longo WE: Management of less common tumors of the colon, rectum, and anus. *Clin Colorectal Cancer* 5:327, 2006.
2. Kang H, O'Connell JB, Leonardi MJ, et al: Rare tumors of the colon and rectum: A national review. *Int J Colorectal Dis* 22:183, 2007.
3. DiSario JA, Burt RW, Kendrick ML, et al: Colorectal cancers of rare histologic types compared with adenocarcinomas. *Dis Colon Rectum* 37:1277, 1994.
4. Ellis L, Shale MJ, Coleman MP: Carcinoid tumors of the gastrointestinal tract: Trends in incidence in England since 1971. *Am J Gastroenterol* 105:2563, 2010.
5. Modlin IM, Lye KD, Kidd M: A 5-decade analysis of 13,715 carcinoid tumors. *Cancer* 97:934, 2003.
6. Hauso O, Gustafsson BI, Kidd M, et al: Neuroendocrine tumor epidemiology: Contrasting Norway and North America. *Cancer* 113:2655, 2008.
7. Kloppel G, Perren A, Heitz PU: The gastroenteropancreatic neuroendocrine cell system and its tumors: The WHO classification. *Ann N Y Acad Sci* 1014:13, 2004.
8. Rindi G, Capella C, Solcia E: Introduction to a revised clinicopathological classification of neuroendocrine tumors of the gastroenteropancreatic tract. *Q J Nucl Med* 44:13, 2000.
9. Tichansky DS, Cagir B, Borrazzo E, et al: Risk of second cancers in patients with colorectal carcinoids. *Dis Colon Rectum* 45:91, 2002.
10. Eriksson B, Oberg K, Stridsberg M: Tumor markers in neuroendocrine tumors. *Digestion* 62:33, 2000.
11. Anthony LB, Strosberg JR, Klimstra DS, et al: The NANETS consensus guidelines for the diagnosis and management of gastrointestinal neuroendocrine tumors (NETs): Well-differentiated NETs of the distal colon and rectum. *Pancreas* 39:767, 2010.
12. Wang AY, Ahmad NA: Rectal carcinoids. *Curr Opin Gastroenterol* 22:529, 2006.
13. Ducreux M, Ruszniewski P, Chayvialle JA, et al: The antitumoral effect of the long-acting somatostatin analog lanreotide in neuroendocrine tumors. *Am J Gastroenterol* 95:3276, 2000.
14. Kolby L, Persson G, Franzen S, et al: Randomized clinical trial of the effect of interferon alpha on survival in patients with disseminated midgut carcinoid tumours. *Br J Surg* 90:687, 2003.
15. Bernick PE, Klimstra DS, Shia J, et al: Neuroendocrine carcinomas of the colon and rectum. *Dis Colon Rectum* 47:163, 2004.
16. Nahas CS, Shia J, Joseph R, et al: Squamous-cell carcinoma of the rectum: A rare but curable tumor. *Dis Colon Rectum* 50:1393, 2007.
17. Frizelle FA, Hobday KS, Batts KP, et al: Adenosquamous and squamous carcinoma of the colon and upper rectum: A clinical and histopathologic study. *Dis Colon Rectum* 44:341, 2001.
18. Crump M, Gospodarowicz M, Shepherd FA: Lymphoma of the gastrointestinal tract. *Semin Oncol* 26:324, 1999.
19. Bilsel Y, Balik E, Yamaner S, et al: Clinical and therapeutic considerations of rectal lymphoma: A case report and literature review. *World J Gastroenterol* 11:460, 2005.
20. Wong MT, Eu KW: Primary colorectal lymphomas. *Colorectal Dis* 8:586, 2006.
21. Tran T, Davila JA, El-Serag HB: The epidemiology of malignant gastrointestinal stromal tumors: An analysis of 1,458 cases from 1992 to 2000. *Am J Gastroenterol* 100:162, 2005.
22. Nilsson B, Bumming P, Meis-Kindblom JM, et al: Gastrointestinal stromal tumors: The incidence, prevalence, clinical course, and prognostication in the preimatinib mesylate era—a population-based study in western Sweden. *Cancer* 103:821, 2005.
23. Heinrich MC, Corless CL, Demetri GD, et al: Kinase mutations and imatinib response in patients with metastatic gastrointestinal stromal tumor. *J Clin Oncol* 21:4342, 2003.
24. Gounder MM, Maki RG: Molecular basis for primary and secondary tyrosine kinase inhibitor resistance in gastrointestinal stromal tumor. *Cancer Chemother Pharmacol* 67:S25, 2011.
25. Demetri GD, van Oosterom AT, Garrett CR, et al: Efficacy and safety of sunitinib in patients with advanced gastrointestinal stromal tumour after failure of imatinib: A randomised controlled trial. *Lancet* 368:1329, 2006.
26. Changchien CR, Wu MC, Tasi WS, et al: Evaluation of prognosis for malignant rectal gastrointestinal stromal tumor by clinical parameters and immunohistochemical staining. *Dis Colon Rectum* 47:1922, 2004.
27. Wasserberg N, Nunoo-Mensah JW, Beart RW Jr, et al: Is there a role for neoadjuvant treatment with Gleevec for large rectal gastrointestinal stromal tumors? *Int J Colorectal Dis* 22:981, 2007.
28. Reddy RM, Fleshman JW: Colorectal gastrointestinal stromal tumors: A brief review. *Clin Colon Rectal Surg* 19:69, 2006.
29. Gomes AL, Bardales RH, Milanezi F, et al: Molecular analysis of c-Kit and PDGFRA in GISTs diagnosed by EUS. *Am J Clin Pathol* 127:89, 2007.
30. Agaimy A, Wunsch PH: True smooth muscle neoplasms of the gastrointestinal tract: Morphological spectrum and classification in a series of 85 cases from a single institute. *Langenbecks Arch Surg* 392:75, 2007.
31. Bosmans B, de Graaf EJ, Torenbeek R, et al: Malignant fibrous histiocytoma of the sigmoid: A case report and review of the literature. *Int J Colorectal Dis* 22:549, 2007.
32. Braumann C, Guenther N, Menenakos C, et al: Schwannoma of the colon mimicking carcinoma: A case report and literature review. *Int J Colorectal Dis* 22:1547, 2007.
33. Miettinen M, Shekitka KM, Sobin LH: Schwannomas in the colon and rectum: A clinicopathologic and immunohistochemical study of 20 cases. *Am J Surg Pathol* 25:846, 2001.
34. Chang AE, Karnell LH, Menck HR: The National Cancer Data Base report on cutaneous and noncutaneous melanoma: A summary of 84,836 cases from the past decade. The American College of Surgeons Commission on Cancer and the American Cancer Society. *Cancer* 83:1664, 1998.
35. Podnos YD, Tsai NC, Smith D, et al: Factors affecting survival in patients with anal melanoma. *Am Surg* 72:917, 2006.
36. Heeney A, Mulsow J, Hyland JM: Treatment and outcomes of anorectal melanoma. *Surgeon* 9:27, 2011.
37. Tessier DJME, Young-Fadock T, Wolff BG: Melanoma metastatic to the colon: Case series and review of the literature with outcome analysis. *Dis Colon Rectum* 46:441, 2003.
38. Grussendorf-Conen EI: Anogenital premalignant and malignant tumours (including Buschke-Lowenstein tumours). *Clin Dermatol* 15:377, 1997.

Adjuvant and Neoadjuvant Therapy for Colorectal Cancer

Steven R. Alberts | Jason A. Call | Christopher L. Hallemeier |

Robert C. Miller

An estimated 103,000 cases of colon cancer and 40,000 cases of rectal cancer are diagnosed annually in the United States. More than 50,000 patients will die annually from colorectal cancer.[1] Adjuvant and neoadjuvant chemotherapy as well as radiation therapy have the potential to improve survival and locoregional control in patients who undergo potentially curative resection. For colon cancer, where local recurrence risks are typically minimal, adjuvant therapy is delivered with multiagent systemic therapy with the intent of reducing the risks of nodal or systemic recurrence. For rectal cancer, where patients are at increased risk of both local and distant failures, adjuvant and neoadjuvant regimens that are combinations of both radiation therapy and chemotherapy may reduce the risk of recurrence.

ADJUVANT THERAPY FOR COLON CANCER

A long history of clinical trials assessing the potential benefit of adjuvant therapy for resected adenoma of the colon exists.[2] Initial trials established the significant benefit of adjuvant therapy following surgery over surgery alone. Subsequent trials have focused on refining that benefit through the manner in which chemotherapy is provided and by exploring the potential benefit of new drugs.

RECURRENCE RATE

The recurrence rate of colon and rectal cancer has been well established through prior trials that had included surgery-only arms. Using databases from completed randomized trials, the risk of recurrence can be determined by the level of tumor invasion and number of lymph nodes involved by metastatic disease through pooled analyses.[3] For stage 2 colon cancer, the risk of recurrence, with appropriate lymph node assessment, is in the range of 20% at 5 years with surgery alone, whereas the risk for stage 3 colon cancer is much higher.[4]

In determining the benefit of adjuvant therapy, randomized clinical trials historically used overall survival (OS) as the primary endpoint. More recently, disease-free survival (DFS) has become an accepted surrogate for overall survival and has served as the primary endpoint in more recent trials. A metaanalysis of 18 randomized trials involving 20,898 patients found that the 3-year DFS is closely correlated with 5-year OS.[5]

STAGE 3 COLON CANCER

The added benefit of adjuvant chemotherapy for resected stage 3 colon cancer over surgery alone has been established in multiple prior randomized trials.[2] These trials most commonly used 5-fluorouracil (5-FU) in combination with either leucovorin (LV) or levamisole. Many of these trials also included patients with stage 2 colon cancer, making the interpretation of some trials more difficult in regard to the subgroup of patients with stage 3 colon cancer. Based on the evidence of significant benefit from adjuvant therapy, the more recent generation of trials has assessed the role of newer chemotherapy drugs, such as oxaliplatin and irinotecan, as well as targeted agents. The drugs oxaliplatin and irinotecan both provide additional benefit in the setting of metastatic colorectal cancer when added to 5-FU and LV.

The use of oxaliplatin in adjuvant therapy was first assessed in the phase III randomized trial MOSAIC.[6] In this trial, patients with resected stage 2 or 3 colon cancer were randomized to either 5-FU and LV alone or in combination with oxaliplatin (Table 175-1). The 5-FU was given as a bolus on days 1 and 2 followed by a 22-hour infusion on each of these 2 days every 2 weeks (LV5FU2). Oxaliplatin was given as a 2-hour infusion on day 1 (FOLFOX4). The trial design required that a total of 12 cycles of therapy be administered as tolerated to conform to the standard practice of giving 6 months of 5-FU and LV. The primary endpoint for this trial was DFS. The trial accrued 2246 patients from 146 centers in 20 countries. For patients receiving FOLFOX4, the probability of DFS at 3 years was 78.2%, whereas patients receiving LV5FU2 had a 3-year DFS of 72.9%. This represented a significant improvement in DFS with a hazard ratio of 0.77 (95% confidence interval [CI], 0.65 to 0.91; P = 0.002). In a subgroup analysis, a significant benefit was seen for patients with stage 3 colon cancer, but not those with stage 2 (see Table 175-1). The DFS benefit of FOLFOX4 over LV5FU2 translated into a significant improvement in overall survival at 6 years when analyzed for all patients entered into the trial and for patients with stage 3 colon cancer.[7]

A separate phase III trial was conducted by the National Surgical Adjuvant Breast and Bowel Project (NSABP). NSABP clinical trial C-07 differed from MOSAIC in that it used a bolus regimen of 5-FU and LV, either alone (FULV) or in combination with oxaliplatin (FLOX).[8] The results of this trial were comparable to those reported for MOSAIC. With 2407 eligible patients, the 3-year DFS rate for FLOX was 76.1% compared with 71.8% for FULV (see Table 175-1). The hazard ratio was 0.80 (95% CI, 0.69 to 0.93; P = 0.0034). The specific DFS rate for stage 3 patients in this trial has not been reported.

TABLE 175-1 Recent Randomized Phase III Clinical Trials of Adjuvant Therapy for Resected Colon Cancer

Clinical Trial	Regimens	Stage	Disease-Free Survival			Overall Survival		
OXALIPLATIN-BASED REGIMENS								
MOSAIC[6,7]	LV5FU2 vs. FOLFOX4		LV5FU2	FOLFOX	P value	LV5FU2	FOLFOX	P value
	(N = 2246)	Overall	72.9%	78.2%	0.02	76%	78.5%	0.046
		Stage 3 (60%)	65.2%	72.2%	—	68.7%	72.9%	0.023
		Stage 2 (40%)	84.3%	87.0%	—	86.8%	86.9%	0.986
NSABP C-07[8]	FULV vs. FLOX		FULV	FLOX	0.0034	FULV	FLOX	—
	(N = 2407)	Overall	71.8%	76.1%		NS	NS	
		Stage 3	—	—		—	—	
		Stage 2	—	—		—	—	
IRINOTECAN-BASED REGIMENS								
CALGB 89803[12]	FULV vs. IFL		FULV	IFL	P value	FULV	IFL	P value
	(N = 1264)	Stage 3	69%	66%	0.85	71%	68%	0.74
PETACC-3[10]	LV5FU2 vs. FOLFIRI	Stage 3	LV5FU2	FOLFIRI		LV5FU2	FOLFIRI	
	(N = 2094)		60.7%	62.9%	0.1059	71.3%	73.6%	0.0942
Accord02[11]	LV5FU2 vs. FOLFIRI	Stage 3	LV5FU2	FOLFIRI		LV5FU2	FOLFIRI	
	(N = 400)		60%	51%	0.22	67%	61%	0.26
TARGETED THERAPY								
NSABP C-08[13]	FOLFOX ± Bevacizumab		FOLFOX	FOLFOX + Bev	P value	FOLFOX	FOLFOX + Bev	P value
	(Bev) (N = 2672)	Overall	75.5%	77.4%	0.15	—	—	—
		Stage 3 (75.1%)	—	—		—	—	
		Stage 2 (24.9%)	—	—		—	—	
NCCTG N0147[14]	FOLFOX ± Cetuximab (Cmab) (N = 1863)	Stage 3	FOLFOX	FOLFOX + Cmab		FOLFOX	FOLFOX + Cmab	
			74.6%	71.5%	0.08	87.3%	85.6%	0.15

Based on the primary endpoint for MOSAIC and NSABP C-07, the combination of oxaliplatin, 5-FU, and LV, in either the FOLFOX4 or FLOX regimen, should be considered as the standard options for patients with resected stage 3 colon cancer. The two combinations differ primarily in the manner in which they are given and in selected side effects. FLOX has the potential advantage of not requiring an infusion pump and of a lower cumulative dose of oxaliplatin. The lower dose of oxaliplatin resulted in a lower rate of oxaliplatin-induced peripheral neuropathy compared to that observed with the use of FOLFOX4. However, FLOX is more likely to cause a severe enteropathy.[9] It is also important to note that the FOLFOX4 regimen has been modified in subsequent adjuvant trials. The currently used combination (mFOLFOX6) does not use a bolus of 5-FU on day 2 and uses a 46-hour infusion of 5-FU after the bolus dose on day 1.

Although oxaliplatin has improved the likelihood of DFS and OS, the drug irinotecan has not provided similar benefits despite its benefit to patients with metastatic colorectal cancer. In a randomized phase III trial (PETACC-3) of 2094 patients with resected stage 3 colon cancer, patients were randomized to either LV5FU2 alone or in combination with irinotecan (FOLFIRI).[10] Based on both 3- and 5-year DFS rates, no meaningful difference was seen with the addition of irinotecan to LV5FU2. In the analysis of the primary endpoint of DFS, the hazard ratio was 0.90 (95% CI, 0.79 to 1.02; $p = 0.106$). This trial did not stratify patients based on

T stage, resulting in a greater number of patients with T4 tumors being enrolled in the FOLFIRI arm. In an exploratory analysis following completion of the trial, an adjustment for the imbalance in T stage suggested a possible benefit to the use of FOLFIRI.

Although the results of the PETACC-3 trial suggested a possible benefit to the use of irinotecan for resected stage 3 colon cancer, two other trials failed to show any benefit. In the Accord02 trial, patients deemed to be at high risk (N2 disease or N1 disease with obstruction or perforation) were randomized to either LV5FU2 or FOLFIRI.[11] The 3-year DFS was 60% for patients receiving LV5FU2 compared with 51% for those receiving FOLFIRI. This trial also did not stratify patients according to T stage as well as N stage. By accounting for this imbalance, the hazard ratio changed from 1.12 to 0.98, showing no evidence of any benefit.

In the third trial, led by the Cancer and Leukemia Group B (CALGB), the bolus regimen FULV was compared to the bolus 5-FU and LV with the addition of irinotecan (IFL).[12] CALGB 89803 enrolled 1264 patients with resected stage 3 colon cancer. The 3-year DFS rate for patients receiving FULV was 69% compared with 66% for patients receiving IFL. The 5-year OS rate was 71% and 68%, respectively, for FULV and IFL. Based on this trial and the results of PETACC-3 and Accord02, there appears to be no role for irinotecan in adjuvant therapy for resected stage 3 colon cancer.

Two additional phase III adjuvant trials have been reported that explored the potential benefit of targeted therapy in combination with chemotherapy. In NSABP C-08 patients were either randomized to chemotherapy alone, using the mFOLFOX6 regimen, or to mFOLFOX6 with bevacizumab.[13] In this trial, mFOLFOX6 and bevacizumab were given for 12 cycles followed by an additional 6 months of bevacizumab. Patients receiving bevacizumab had a similar outcome in regard to those receiving mFOLFOX6 alone (see Table 175-1) with a hazard ratio of 0.89 and P value of 0.15.

In a separate trial (N0147) led by the North Central Cancer Treatment Group (NCCTG), patients with resected stage 3 colon cancer were randomized to either mFOLFOX6 for 12 cycles or mFOLFOX6 combined with the epidermal growth factor receptor (EGFR) inhibitor cetuximab for 12 cycles.[14] In this trial, randomization to one of the two treatment arms was restricted to patients with wild-type KRAS given evidence that patients with mutated KRAS-expressing tumors do not benefit from EGFR-directed antibodies, including cetuximab. In this trial, the addition of cetuximab did not show any added benefit to chemotherapy alone (hazard ratio [HR] = 1.21; $p = 0.08$).

Stage 2 Colon Cancer

The role of adjuvant chemotherapy in stage 2 colon cancer remains uncertain. Various risk factors have been identified that correlate to an increased risk of recurrence. These risk factors include T4 tumors, undifferentiated tumors, lymphovascular invasion, obstruction, perforation, and inadequate lymph node assessment. More recently, molecular markers or panels of markers have been used to identify patients at increased risk of recurrence. However, the ability of these markers or panels to predict benefit from adjuvant therapy has not been validated in a prospective trial.

Evidence of potential benefit of adjuvant therapy has been primarily established through subgroup analyses of trials enrolling patients with both stage 2 and 3 colon cancer. In MOSAIC (see Table 175-1), 40% of the patients enrolled had stage 2 colon cancer. For patients with study-defined high-risk stage 2 colon cancer (T4, occlusion/perforation, poorly differentiated tumor, venous invasion, and <10 examined lymph nodes), a nonsignificant trend toward improved 5-year DFS was observed.[7] A similar analysis was not performed in NSABP C-07. In the randomized phase III trial Quick and Simple and Reliable (QUASAR), 3239 patients with resected colon or rectal cancer were randomized to either 5-FU and LV or observation following surgery.[15] In the subgroup of patients ($n = 2146$) with stage 2 colon cancer, a reduction in the risk of recurrence was seen with a hazard ratio of 0.82 (95% CI, 0.63 to 1.08).

Given the lack of any prospectively performed and completed phase III trials for stage 2 colon cancer, the use of pooled analyses has also been used to determine if adjuvant therapy may be of benefit. In a pooled analysis of NSABP clinical trials C-01 through C-05, an assessment of the potential benefit of 5-FU and LV following surgery versus surgery alone was made.[16] A total of 1255 patients with stage 2 colon cancer were enrolled in one of these five trials. The pooled analysis showed a significant trend of benefit for both OS (HR = 0.58, 95% CI, 0.48 to 0.71;

$p < 0.0001$) and DFS (HR = 0.68, 95% CI, 0.57 to 0.81; $p < 0.0001$).

With the available information, there remains uncertainty about the potential benefit of adjuvant therapy for resected stage 2 colon cancer. As this is a heterogeneous group of patients, the use of markers of high risk will likely be needed to determine those patients most likely to derive benefit from adjuvant therapy.

RADIOTHERAPY FOR RESECTED COLON CANCER

In contrast to rectal cancer, radiotherapy is infrequently used for adjuvant therapy for colon cancer. Although the anatomic confines of the pelvis potentially limit the adequacy of lateral and distal margins during resection of rectal carcinomas, this is far less likely to be the case for colon carcinomas. A large, randomized clinical trial in locally advanced (T3N1 or T3N2) colon cancers of the ascending or descending colon or those adherent to adjacent normal organs demonstrated no difference in survival between groups that received either fluorouracil and levamisole alone versus those that received radiotherapy in addition to fluorouracil and levamisole.[17]

ADJUVANT THERAPY FOR RECTAL CANCER

RATIONALE

Although surgery alone for stage I rectal cancer can result in rates of local relapse of less than 5%, patients with locoregionally advanced disease (T3-4 or with positive regional nodes) have less favorable outcomes with surgery as monotherapy. Because of their location in the pelvis, advanced tumors of the rectum, located between fusion of the taenia and the puborectalis ring, are less surgically accessible compared with tumors in the colon. Although the peritoneal lining covers the front and sides of the upper rectum and the anterior portion of the middle rectum, it is reflected away to leave the lower rectum without any peritoneal lining to prevent local tumor spread.[18] As a result, surgery alone for patients with either positive lymph nodes or T3-4 primary disease is associated with local relapse rates of 12% to 50% at 5 years.[19]

Endorectal ultrasound is currently a standard as a staging modality in the preoperative evaluation of patients with rectal cancer. This modality can aid in selecting patients suitable for neoadjuvant therapy. Fine-needle aspiration may also be used for sampling of visualized nodes under ultrasound guidance. Magnetic resonance imaging (MRI) is likewise useful in the preoperative evaluation of patients with rectal cancer and will likely become the staging modality of choice. The MERCURY study group prospectively staged 408 patients with MRI preoperatively to assess the ability of preoperative MRI to predict clear resection margins.[20] Margins were defined as being "potentially affected" if they showed tumor within 1 mm of the mesorectal margin. Such a definition had a 92% specificity for predicting a negative margin, a sensitivity of 59%, and an 88% accuracy. When comparing results for the group undergoing primary surgery with or without short-course radiotherapy, assessment with MRI had a better accuracy (92%) compared with digital rectal examination (70%).

Fluropyrimidines, such as 5-FU or capecitabine, have been used as a radiosensitizing agent in rectal cancer as discussed later. Several clinical trials have addressed the dosing and administration of this agent for the use in chemoradiation of rectal cancer. Some interest in recent years has focused on the orally administered agent capecitabine. It has been used widely as a radiosensitizing agent for rectal cancer, although not with robust data from clinical trials to support its replacement of standard 5-FU. This drug is converted to 5-FU by enzymatic activation in vivo. Capecitabine may have a therapeutic advantage of having a higher conversion to 5-FU within colorectal tumor cells as these cells have a greater concentration of thymidine phosphorylase.[21] There are some preliminary data that this agent may be safe and effective for use in preoperative chemoradiation.[22] The NSAPB R04 trial is currently testing capecitabine (825 mg/m^2 orally twice daily 5 days during each week of radiation randomized) as an alternative to standard PVI 5-FU (with both agents being tested with and without oxaliplatin).

ADJUVANT THERAPY

Adjuvant radiotherapy has been applied to patients at high risk (T3-4 or with positive regional nodes) of relapse after surgery. A postoperative approach has the advantage of being able to select patients who may benefit from additional treatment based on pathologic findings. Such a strategy has been shown to be beneficial when combined with postoperative chemotherapy.[23-26] One trial, performed by the NCCTG tested the addition of chemotherapy to postoperative radiotherapy for deeply invasive or node-positive rectal cancers.[23] Radiotherapy was delivered to a dose of 4500 to 5040 cGy. Patients receiving chemotherapy began with semustine 130 mg/m^2 (single dose) orally along with 5-FU (300 mg/m^2/day on days 1 to 5 and 400 mg/m^2/day for 5 days starting day 36). Radiation was started 4 weeks after the initial two cycles of chemotherapy, and 5-FU was given by rapid infusion 500/mg/m^2 for 3 days during weeks 1 and 5 of radiation. This was again followed by more chemotherapy after radiation consisting of semustine 100 mg/m^2 (single dose) orally with 5-FU 300 mg/m^2/day for 5 days and then 5-FU was repeated at a dose of 400 mg/m^2/day for 5 days 1 month later. The combined approach reduced the local recurrence by 46% ($P = 0.036$), the distant recurrence by 37% ($P = 0.011$), and the overall death rate by 36% ($P = 0.025$).

After establishing adjuvant chemoradiation as beneficial in the setting of locoregionally advanced rectal cancer, a multiinstitutional effort led by the NCCTG was undertaken to improve on the outcomes of bolus 5-FU.[27] Six hundred patients with rectal tumors either involving the perirectal fat or adjacent organs or who had regional lymph nodes found to be positive after a potentially curative resection were randomized to one of four arms. All arms had systemic chemotherapy administered both before and after adjuvant chemoradiation. Arm 1 had systemic therapy with 5-FU and semustine and radiation with concurrent bolus 5-FU. Arm 2 had the same systemic chemotherapy but the 5-FU during radiation was done as protracted venous infusion (PVI). Arm 3 had treatment with 5-FU without semustine before and after

chemoradiation and the 5-FU during radiation was a bolus injection. The last group (arm 4) had 5-FU without semustine and radiation that was given with concomitant PVI 5-FU. Those assigned to 5-FU systemic therapy without semustine received a higher dose of rapid infusion 5-FU (500 mg/m^2 day on days 1 to 5 and 36 to 40 with two more 5-day infusions at a dose of 450 mg/m^2/day after radiation) than in the arms that did also receive semustine. Radiation was to a total dose of 5040 to 5400 cGy. The bolus 5-FU given during radiation was at a dose of 500 mg/m^2/day on 3 consecutive days on both weeks 1 and 5 of radiation. In contrast, patients assigned to PVI were planned to receive 5-FU 225 mg/m^2/day by infusion into a central venous line throughout radiation. Although the results showed no benefit for the combination of 5-FU and semustine, there did exist a difference in the two methods of chemoradiation. PVI improved the relapse-free survival ($P = 0.01$) and overall survival ($P = 0.005$) compared to bolus injection 5-FU. There was also a difference in the pattern of severe toxicity, with diarrhea being more common in the PVI group; however, leukopenia was more common in the bolus 5-FU group.

An intergroup trial published by Smalley et al (GI INT 0144) looked at replacing the two 5-day courses of bolus 5-FU before and after postoperative chemoradiation with either PVI 5-FU 300 mg/m^2/day for 42 days (still using the PVI during radiation) or a regimen of two cycles of bolus 5-FU, leucovorin, and levamisole before and after radiation (with bolus 5-FU and leucovorin during radiation).[28] Neither arm provided additional benefit in terms of relapse-free or OS when compared to bolus 5-FU before and after chemoradiation with PVI 5-FU. Grade 3 to 4 hematologic toxicity was very low (4%) in the arm treated with only PVI chemotherapy. The intergroup trial published by Tepper et al was also unable to show any benefit to adding leucovorin, levamisole, or both to a bolus 5-FU strategy.[29]

NEOADJUVANT THERAPY

Radiation therapy delivered in a neoadjuvant fashion has several theoretical advantages over postoperative therapy. By delivering radiation before definitive surgery, there is the potential to decrease tumor seeding at the time of surgery, and some tumors that may require sacrifice of the sphincter may experience a response adequate to allow a sphincter-preserving approach. In addition, postoperative radiation may be less effective in the relatively hypoxic postoperative pelvis, which may render malignant cells more resistant to radiation. Moreover, toxicity may be increased because the small bowel often falls into the pelvis, which is the area targeted for radiation. Given these reasons, there have been many trials investigating the role of neoadjuvant chemoradiation.

The EORTC performed a large randomized trial of various combinations of chemotherapy and with neoadjuvant radiotherapy.[30] Eligible patients had resectable T3 or T4 rectal cancer and were randomized to one of 4 arms. The first arm received neoadjuvant radiotherapy alone to 45 Gy to the posterior pelvis over 5 weeks. Arm 2 received the same radiation plus preoperative chemotherapy delivered as 5-day courses of fluorouracil (350 mg/m^2/day) with leucovorin (20 mg/m^2/day) during the first and fifth weeks of radiation. The third arm received both preoperative radiotherapy and postoperative chemotherapy (four courses of the same chemotherapy as arm 2 given every 3 weeks), and the fourth arm received preoperative chemoradiotherapy in addition to postoperative chemotherapy. The 5-year overall survival for the entire group was 65.2% and did not differ significantly between the groups that received preoperative or postoperative chemotherapy. All chemotherapy arms were effective in decreasing the local recurrence (8.7%, 9.6%, and 7.6% in arms 2, 3, and 4, respectively) compared with radiation alone (17.1%).

There have been two randomized trials performed, one in Germany and one by the NSABP, that compared preoperative and postoperative chemoradiation.[31,32] Sauer et al reported the results of the trial from the German Rectal Cancer Study Group where 803 patients with clinically staged T3 or T4 tumors or positive nodal disease were randomized to both preoperative chemoradiation with 5040 cGy in 28 fractions along with PVI 5-FU (1000 mg/m² /day over 120 hours during weeks 1 and 5 of radiation) and postoperative chemotherapy (four 5-day cycles of 5-FU) or postoperative chemoradiation that differed only by the addition of another 540-cGy boost.[31] Total mesorectal excision (TME) was performed either within 6 weeks after preoperative treatment or was followed by adjuvant treatment 1 month postoperatively in the postoperative arm. Eighteen percent (staged with endorectal ultrasound and computed tomography preoperatively) of patients in the postoperative arm were found to have stage I disease at the time of surgery and did not receive chemoradiation. The primary outcome of OS did not differ significantly at 5 years between the preoperative (76%) and postoperative (74%) groups. However, these authors noted several advantages for the preoperative arm. Local recurrence improved to 6% compared to 13% at 5 years (P = 0.006). In a comparison of patients who did receive radiotherapy, preoperative delivery improved the rate of any acute grade 3 or 4 toxicity from 40% to 27% (P = 0.001) and any late toxicity from 24% to 14% (P = 0.01). This difference was not apparent, however, when including all patients regardless of whether they actually received radiation. Among patients who were deemed to require an abdominoperineal resection (116 in the preoperative group and 78 in the postoperative group), 39% in the preoperative group were able to undergo a sphincter-preserving approach, whereas this was only 19% in the postoperative group (P = 0.004). Thus, the authors proposed the preoperative approach as the preferred method as it was associated with a better toxicity profile, improved local control, and improved sphincter preservation for low-lying tumors.

The second trial of preoperative radiation compared with postoperative radiation was reported by Roh et al.[32] This trial also enrolled patients with clinically staged T3 or T4 or node-positive disease and randomized eligible patients to either preoperative or postoperative chemoradiation regimens. Radiotherapy consisted of 4500 cGy in 25 fractions to the pelvis with a 540-cGy boost. In the preoperative group, patients were treated with one cycle of 5-FU 500 mg/m² and leucovorin 500 mg/m² given once per week for 6 weeks followed by radiation with

cycles 2 and 3 of chemotherapy (consisting of 5-FU 325 mg/m² and leucovorin 20 mg/m² for 5 days during weeks 1 and 5 of radiation). In the postoperative arm, the same three cycles of chemotherapy were given before and during radiation but were not started until after definitive surgery (type defined by the treating physician). Both arms received an additional four cycles of chemotherapy (each given with 5-FU 500 mg/m² and leucovorin 500 mg/m² given once per week for 6 weeks) either after the surgery in the preoperative arm or after adjuvant chemoradiation in the postoperative arm. The protocol only accrued 267 of the planned 900 patients and was closed early. However, these authors were able to note an improvement in DFS with preoperative chemoradiation (64.7% vs. 53.4% at 5 years, P = 0.011) and a trend toward better overall survival for the patients treated preoperatively (74.5% vs. 65.6% at 5 years, P = 0.065).

SHORT-COURSE PREOPERATIVE RADIOTHERAPY

Although a long course of radiation combined with chemotherapy has been commonly used in North America, a second method of preoperative treatment for advanced rectal cancer has been to deliver radiotherapy without chemotherapy in an abbreviated (hypofractionated) fashion. Such a regimen delivering 25 Gy in five daily fractions can be performed with a short interval (1 week) to surgery. Investigators from Sweden performed a randomized trial in which 908 patients with resectable, nonmetastatic rectal cancer were assigned to either receive treatment with radiation (25 Gy in five fractions) before surgery or to undergo surgery with no additional therapy.[33] Long-term results (median followup of 13 years) demonstrated that preoperative hypofractionated radiation alone improved overall survival from 30% to 38% (P = 0.008), cancer-specific survival from 62% versus 72% (P = 0.03), and local failure from 26% to 9% (P < 0.001).

Short-course preoperative radiation has also been shown to be effective in the setting of TME. Kapiteijn and others from the Dutch Colorectal Cancer Group randomly assigned 1805 eligible patients with resectable rectal cancer to receive 25 Gy in five fractions followed by TME or TME alone.[34] Although the overall survival was 82% in both arms at 2 years, radiation improved the local failure rate at 2 years for patients in which all macroscopic tumor was removed from 8.2% to 2.4% (P = 0.01).

Also, the MRC and NCI-Canada performed a randomized trial of short-course preoperative radiotherapy to postoperative chemoradiotherapy in which 92% of patients underwent TME.[35] Six hundred seventy-four patients were randomized to receive 25 Gy in five fractions preoperatively and 676 patients received postoperative treatment. Postoperative treatment consisted of 45 Gy in 25 fractions given concurrently with 5-FU (either as a continuous infusion or a weekly regimen with leucovorin) and was only given in the event the patient had involvement of the circumferential margins of resection

(≤1 mm). Preoperative radiation reduced the rate of local recurrence from 10.6% to 4.4% at 3 years. DFS at 3 years also improved from 77.5% to 71.5%, although overall survival was similar between the two groups. This adds to the data on the efficacy of short-course preoperative radiation alone. However, because the trial did not call for treatment of many patients who met the classic criteria for adjuvant therapy (T3-4 or node positive), it is difficult to draw conclusions on the superiority of preoperative short-course radiation compared with postoperative chemoradiation.

One study looked at outcomes of short-term preoperative radiation alone versus standard-dose preoperative radiation plus chemotherapy. The Polish Colorectal Study Group tested neoadjuvant chemoradiation to short-course preoperative radiation (25 Gy in five fractions) in patients with resectable clinically staged T3 and T4 tumors.[36] The chemoradiation involved 5040 cGy of radiation at 180 cGy per fraction combined with chemotherapy (leucovorin 20 mg/m^2/day and 5-FU 325 mg/m^2/day given as rapid infusion on 5 consecutive days during weeks 1 and 5 of radiotherapy). Adjuvant chemotherapy was optional. Acute toxicity was higher in patients treated with chemoradiation at a rate of 18.2% compared with 3.2%. Local recurrence was similar at 9% in the short-course preoperative arm and 14.2% in the chemoradiation arm ($P = 0.170$). There was no significant difference in overall survival, DFS, or late toxicity.

LOCAL EXCISION AND RADIATION THERAPY

Low-lying rectal cancers have conventionally been managed with an abdominoperineal resection (APR). In an effort to spare patients the potential morbidity of such an approach (colostomy, alterations in urinary and sexual function), various sphincter-preserving approaches with surgery or radiation have been attempted.

Endocavitary radiation has been used either alone or in combination with brachytherapy or external beam radiotherapy; this technique is not widely used currently.[37] Investigators have also studied local excision with adjuvant therapy most commonly done postoperatively. Some multiinstitutional experience has been obtained testing the role of local excision with or without postoperative therapy. The RTOG performed a phase II trial of conservative surgery followed by postoperative treatment.[38] This trial focused on patients who would have otherwise required an APR, with the proximal extent 10 cm or less from the anal verge and tumor size less than 4 cm. Surgery (gross total resection) was to be performed by either a transanal, transsacral or transcoccygeal approach with en bloc removal of the tumor and full-thickness excision of the rectal wall. Postoperative treatment was dictated by the pathologic results of the tumor as is shown in Table 175-2 along with corresponding local-regional failure rates for each group. Chemotherapy consisted of 5-FU 1000 mg/m^2/day for 96 hours given for two cycles. Local-regional failure was 4% for all T1 tumors, 16% for T2 tumors, and 23% for all T3 tumors.

Greenberg et al reported on long-term outcomes of CALGB 8984, a trial designed to assess outcomes after local excision for distal rectal tumors.[39] Patients with

TABLE 175-2 Postoperative Treatment After Limited Surgery for Distal Rectal Cancers on RTOG 89-02

Group Characteristics	N	Treatment	Local-Regional Recurrences*
≤3 cm, grade 1-2, T1, margins clear ≥ 3 mm, normal CEA, no ALI or VSI	14	Observation	1 (7%)
Margins ≥ 3 mm, did not meet criteria above	18	Radiation 50-56 Gy + 5-FU	2 (11%)
Margins < 3 mm, did not meet criteria above	33	Radiation 59.4-65 Gy + 5-FU	5 (15%)

CEA, Carcinoembryonic antigen; *LI*, lymphatic invasion; *N*, number of patients; *VSI*, vascular space invasion.
*Including isolated local-regional recurrence with or without distant recurrence.

cancers T1-2, N0 within 10 cm of the dentate line, less than 4 cm in dimension and occupying less than or equal to 40% of the bowel circumference were eligible in the setting of an R0 resection. The trial included 110 eligible patients. Surgery was performed by either a transanal, transsphincteric, or transrectal approach. Patients with T1 tumors were observed without any further treatment, whereas T2 tumors received 5400 cGy in 30 fractions along with 5-FU 500 mg/m^2 on days 1 to 3 and 29 to 31 of radiation. Ten-year overall survival was 84% for T1 lesions and 66% for T2 lesions ($P = 0.04$). There was also a trend observed for DFS being worse with those treated for T2 lesions (10-year rate of 75% vs. 64%, $P = 0.07$). Corresponding local recurrence rates at 10 years was 8% and 18% for T1 and T2, respectively. On the basis of these results, the authors recommended radical excision with TME as being standard for patients with T2 lesions.

Although the aforementioned data indicate that select patients with early localized tumors (small, T1, grade 1 to 2, occupying a small portion of the rectal circumference, negative margins by >3 mm, N0, and no angiolymphatic or perineural invasion) may appropriately be treated with local excision alone, other patients should undergo resection. Results with adjuvant therapy may not overcome the limitations of local excision for patients with risk factors. ACOSOG has completed a trial of preoperative chemoradiotherapy followed by local excision for T2 tumors (ACOSOG Z6041), but the results have not yet been reported.

SUMMARY

Recommended indications and regimens for neoadjuvant/adjuvant radiation or chemoradiation in rectal cancer are displayed in Boxes 175-1 and 175-2. Generally, if patients have T3 or T4 tumors or positive regional lymph nodes before surgery, then neoadjuvant chemoradiation or short-course radiation alone can be used. Some tumors may be rendered amenable to a sphincter-sparing approach by means of full-course chemoradiation as suggested by the data from the German Rectal Cancer Study Group trial.[31] Patients who undergo surgery

> **BOX 175-1** Current Indications for Neoadjuvant/Adjuvant Radiation or Chemoradiation for Rectal Cancer
>
> - Stage T3 or T4
> - Node-positive tumors
> - Conversion of a distal rectal tumor to one amenable to a sphincter-sparing operation

> **BOX 175-2** Current Treatment Regimens for Neoadjuvant/Adjuvant Radiation or Chemoradiation for Rectal Cancer
>
> - Preoperative chemoradiation: 5040 cGy in 28 fractions of external beam radiotherapy with concurrent 5-FU (bolus or continuous venous infusion) or capecitabine oral chemotherapy, followed by resection in approximately 1 month, and consideration of postoperative adjuvant chemotherapy
> - Preoperative radiation alone: 5 Gy × 5 fractions
> - Postoperative chemoradiation: two cycles systemic therapy (5-FU or oxaliplatin based chemotherapy followed by 5040-5400 cGy in 28-30 fractions of external beam radiotherapy with concurrent 5-FU (bolus or continuous venous infusion) or capecitabine oral chemotherapy, followed by consideration of two further cycles of systemic therapy

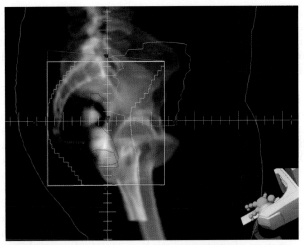

FIGURE 175-2 Lateral beam's eye view of radiotherapy treatment portal used in neoadjuvant radiochemotherapy for locally advanced rectal cancer.

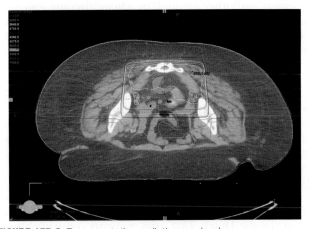

FIGURE 175-3 Representative radiotherapy isodose curve distribution used in neoadjuvant radiochemotherapy for locally advanced rectal cancer.

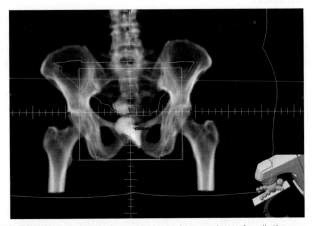

FIGURE 175-1 Posterior-anterior beam's eye view of radiotherapy treatment portal used in neoadjuvant radiochemotherapy for locally advanced rectal cancer.

without preoperative therapy and are found to have high-risk features such as T3 or T4 or positive nodes should be offered adjuvant chemoradiation. Typical radiotherapy portals used in the neoadjuvant or adjuvant treatment of rectal cancer are shown in Figures 175-1 and 175-2. Figure 175-3 demonstrates a typical radiotherapy dose distribution within the pelvis during such therapy.

TOXICITY OF ADJUVANT PELVIC RADIOTHERAPY FOR RECTAL CANCER

The addition of adjuvant therapy to the surgical treatment of rectal cancer has resulted in significant improvements in local-regional tumor control, freedom from distant metastases, and overall survival; however, these improvements in outcome come at the cost of increased risk of acute and late toxicity.

ACUTE GASTROINTESTINAL TOXICITY

In patients receiving adjuvant therapy for rectal cancer, enteritis and proctitis, manifested primarily by increased stool frequency, is the major form of acute toxicity. In an NCCTG trial involving adjuvant radiotherapy for rectal cancer, 53% of the patients treated with concurrent pelvic radiotherapy and 5-FU experienced acute diarrhea.[23,40] Severe or life-threatening diarrhea occurred in 22% of patients. Additionally, patients report a broad range of bowel changes during adjuvant therapy, including increases in nocturnal bowel movements, fecal incontinence, clustering (multiple bowel movements in 30 minutes), urgency, cramping, and blood in stools.[41] Upper gastrointestinal toxicity, namely stomatitis and nausea, are common as well.[42]

Acute gastrointestinal injury due to adjuvant therapy is a result of intestinal mucosal injury via direct cytotoxic effects on epithelial stem cells, apoptosis of microvascular endothelial cells, and induction of inflammatory cytokines. Damage to the intestinal villi leads to loss of ability to absorb nutrients and water, resulting in diarrhea and other bowel function changes.

Mild acute gastrointestinal toxicity can be managed with diet modification and the use of antidiarrheal agents such as loperamide. Diarrhea refractory to these measures may require chemotherapy dose reductions/discontinuation and/or radiotherapy treatment breaks. Octreotide has modest efficacy in the treatment of radiotherapy- and/or chemotherapy-induced diarrhea. Aggressive supportive care with parenteral volume repletion and correction of electrolyte abnormalities is crucial as acute gastrointestinal toxicity can occasionally be fatal. Currently, there are no agents of proven efficacy in the prevention of acute enteritis because of adjuvant therapy other than reducing the volume of bowel mucosa treated.

ACUTE NONGASTROINTESTINAL TOXICITY

Adjuvant radiotherapy and/or chemotherapy can also cause clinically significant toxicity in other organ systems. Fatigue is a common complaint in patients undergoing adjuvant combined-modality therapy. Cytopenias are common because of bone marrow suppression from systemic therapy and irradiation of hematologic progenitor cells in the pelvic bones. Oxaliplatin can cause peripheral neuropathy in a dose-dependent manner. Urinary frequency and urgency can occur as a result of irradiation of the urinary bladder. Dermatologic toxicities can include erythema and desquamation in the radiotherapy treatment field as well as fluoropyrimidine-induced desquamation on the hands and feet.

In some randomized studies, the administration of preoperative radiotherapy increased perioperative morbidity. In the Dutch TME trial, patients receiving short-course preoperative radiotherapy (25 Gy/5 fractions) had a higher median blood loss during surgery and a higher incidence of perineal complications, compared with those who did not receive preoperative radiotherapy.[34] Operative mortality was not significantly different between the two groups. However, in the German Rectal Cancer Study Group trial, in which patients with locally advanced rectal cancer were randomized to immediate surgery followed by postoperative adjuvant therapy versus preoperative concurrent conventionally fractionated radiotherapy and chemotherapy, the rates of in-hospital mortality, anastomotic leakage, delayed sacral wound healing, postoperative bleeding, and ileus were similar in the two groups.[31]

LATE GASTROINTESTINAL TOXICITY

In patients with rectal cancer treated with resection and adjuvant therapy, chronic alteration in bowel function is common. Kollmorgen et al conducted a matched cohort study examining bowel function in patients with locally advanced rectal cancer without evidence of disease recurrence 2 to 5 years after low anterior resection and either no adjuvant therapy or adjuvant concurrent conventionally fractionated radiotherapy and chemotherapy.[43] Patients who received adjuvant therapy reported more bowel movements per day (median, 7 vs. 2; $P < 0.001$)

and higher rates of clustering of bowel movements (42% vs. 3%, $P < 0.001$), nighttime bowel movements (46% vs. 14%, $P < 0.001$), incontinence (56% vs. 7%, $P < 0.001$), and inability to defer defecation more than 15 minutes (78% vs. 19%), compared with those who did not receive adjuvant therapy. In a long-term followup (median, 5.1 years) of the Dutch TME trial, patients receiving short-course preoperative radiotherapy (25 Gy/5 fractions) reported increased rates of fecal incontinence (62% vs. 38%, $P < 0.001$), anal blood loss (11% vs. 3%, $P = 0.004$), and impact of bowel function on activities of daily living, compared with those who did not receive preoperative radiotherapy.[44]

LATE NONGASTROINTESTINAL TOXICITY

Adjuvant radiotherapy may increase the risk of late complications to other pelvic structures. In the MRC/NCIC randomized study for patients with operable rectal cancer, men receiving short-course preoperative radiotherapy (25 Gy/5 fractions) reported significantly higher rates of sexual dysfunction at 2 years after randomization than those receiving selective postoperative radiotherapy.[45,46] There was no difference in urinary complaints between these two cohorts. Elderly women receiving adjuvant radiotherapy for rectal cancer were observed to have slightly increased risk of pelvic bone or femoral neck fractures.[47]

SUMMARY

In patients with locally advanced rectal cancer, the addition of adjuvant chemotherapy and/or radiotherapy increases the incidence and severity of acute and late toxicities over that observed with surgery alone. Refinements in patient selection for therapies, development of novel systemic agents, advances in radiotherapy treatment delivery, and improvements in supportive care may all contribute to reducing these toxicities.

ADJUVANT CHEMOTHERAPY FOR RECTAL CANCER

In addition to a fluoropyrimidine given with radiation, most patients will also receive postoperative adjuvant chemotherapy. As noted earlier, patients receiving postoperative radiation have typically received two cycles of chemotherapy prior to combined chemotherapy and radiation based on the approach used in the clinical trial INT 0114.[29] Two additional cycles of chemotherapy are then given after the completion of the radiation. Patients receiving preoperative radiation have typically received 4 to 6 months of adjuvant chemotherapy. All randomized phase III trials for rectal cancer to date have used 5-FU alone or in combination with either leucovorin or levamisole. No completed trials have assessed the added benefit of oxaliplatin in combinations such as FOLFOX or FLOX. Support for the use of regimens such as FOLFOX in rectal cancer has been extrapolated from adjuvant colon cancer trials. Given the benefit of oxaliplatin-containing regimens in colon cancer over 5-FU and leucovorin alone, most practice guidelines now support the use of adjuvant FOLFOX for resected rectal cancer.

Although the optimal number of cycles of FOLFOX has yet to be defined, patients are typically given 8 to 12 cycles of adjuvant FOLFOX.

REFERENCES

1. Jemal A, Siegel R, Xu J, Ward E: Cancer statistics. *CA Cancer J Clin* 60:277, 2010.
2. Chau I, Cunningham D: Adjuvant therapy in colon cancer: Current status and future directions. *Cancer Treat Rev* 28:223, 2002.
3. Gill S, Loprinzi CL, Sargent DJ, et al: Pooled analysis of fluorouracil-based adjuvant therapy for stage II and III colon cancer: Who benefits and by how much? *J Clin Oncol* 22:1797, 2004.
4. Chang GJ, Rodriguez-Bigas MA, Skibber JM, et al: Lymph node evaluation and survival after curative resection of colon cancer: Systematic review. *J Natl Cancer Inst* 99:433, 2007.
5. Sargent DJ, Patiyil S, Yothers G, et al: End points for colon cancer adjuvant trials: Observations and recommendations based on individual patient data from 20,898 patients enrolled onto 18 randomized trials from the ACCENT Group. *J Clin Oncol* 25:4569, 2007.
6. Andre T, Boni C, Mounedji-Boudiaf L, et al, Multicenter International Study of Oxaliplatin/5-Fluorouracil/Leucovorin in the Adjuvant Treatment of Colon Cancer: I. Oxaliplatin, fluorouracil, and leucovorin as adjuvant treatment for colon cancer. *N Engl J Med* 350:2343, 2004.
7. Andre T, Boni C, Navarro M, et al: Improved overall survival with oxaliplatin, fluorouracil, and leucovorin as adjuvant treatment in stage II or III colon cancer in the MOSAIC trial. *J Clin Oncol* 27:3109, 2009.
8. Kuebler JP, Wieand HS, O'Connell MJ, et al: Oxaliplatin combined with weekly bolus fluorouracil and leucovorin as surgical adjuvant chemotherapy for stage II and III colon cancer: Results from NSABP C-07. *J Clin Oncol* 25:2198, 2007.
9. Kuebler JP, Colangelo L, O'Connell MJ, et al: Severe enteropathy among patients with stage II/III colon cancer treated on a randomized trial of bolus 5-fluorouracil/leucovorin plus or minus oxaliplatin: A prospective analysis. *Cancer* 110:1945, 2007.
10. Van Cutsem E, Labianca R, Bodoky G, et al: Randomized phase III trial comparing biweekly infusional fluorouracil/leucovorin alone or with irinotecan in the adjuvant treatment of stage III colon cancer: PETACC-3. *J Clin Oncol* 27:3117, 2009.
11. Ychou M, Raoul JL, Douillard JY, et al: A phase III randomised trial of LV5FU2 + irinotecan versus LV5FU2 alone in adjuvant high-risk colon cancer (FNCLCC Accord02/FFCD9802). *Ann Oncol* 20:674, 2009.
12. Saltz LB, Niedzwiecki D, Hollis D, et al: Irinotecan fluorouracil plus leucovorin is not superior to fluorouracil plus leucovorin alone as adjuvant treatment for stage III colon cancer: Results of CALGB 89803. *J Clin Oncol* 25:3456, 2007.
13. Allegra CJ, Yothers G, O'Connell MJ, et al: Phase III trial assessing bevacizumab in stages II and III carcinoma of the colon: Results of NSABP protocol C-08. *J Clin Oncol* 29:11, 2011.
14. Alberts SR, Sargent DJ, Nair S, et al: Effect of oxaliplatin, fluorouracil, and leucovorin with or without cetuximab on survival among patients with resected stage III colon cancer. *JAMA* 307:1383, 2012.
15. Quasar Collaborative Group, Gray R, Barnwell J, et al: Adjuvant chemotherapy versus observation in patients with colorectal cancer: A randomised study. *Lancet* 370:2020, 2007.
16. Wilkinson NW, Yothers G, Lopa S, et al: Long-term survival results of surgery alone versus surgery plus 5-fluorouracil and leucovorin for stage II and stage III colon cancer: Pooled analysis of NSABP C-01 through C-05. A baseline from which to compare modern adjuvant trials. *Ann Surg Oncol* 17:959, 2010.
17. Martenson JA, Willett CG, Sargent DJ, et al: Phase III study of adjuvant chemotherapy and radiation therapy compared with chemotherapy alone in the surgical adjuvant treatment of colon cancer: Results of Intergroup Protocol 0130. *J Clin Oncol* 22:3277, 2004.
18. Edge SB, Byrd DR, Compton CC, et al, editors: *American Joint Committee on Cancer, and American Cancer Society. AJCC cancer staging manual*, ed 7, New York, 2010, Springer-Verlag.
19. Gunderson LL, Sargent DJ, Tepper JE, et al: Impact of T and N stage and treatment on survival and relapse in adjuvant rectal cancer: A pooled analysis. *J Clin Oncol* 22:1785, 2004.
20. Brown G, Daniels IR, Heald RJ, et al: Diagnostic accuracy of preoperative magnetic resonance imaging in predicting curative resection of rectal cancer: Prospective observational study. *Br Med J* 333:779, 2006.
21. Schuller J, Cassidy J, Dumont E, et al: Preferential activation of capecitabine in tumor following oral administration to colorectal cancer patients. *Cancer Chemother Pharmacol* 45:291, 2000.
22. Kim J-S, Kim J-S, Cho M-J, et al: Preoperative chemoradiation using oral capecitabine in locally advanced rectal cancer. *Int J Radiat Oncol Biol Phys* 54:403, 2002.
23. Krook JE, Moertel CG, Gunderson LL, et al: Effective surgical adjuvant therapy for high-risk rectal carcinoma. *N Engl J Med* 324:709, 1991.
24. Wolmark N, Wieand HS, Hyams DM, et al: Randomized trial of postoperative adjuvant chemotherapy with or without radiotherapy for carcinoma of the rectum: National Surgical Adjuvant Breast and Bowel Project Protocol R-02. *J Natl Cancer Inst* 92:388, 2000.
25. Gastrointestinal Tumor Study Group: Prolongation of the disease-free interval in surgically treated rectal carcinoma. *N Engl J Med* 312:1465, 1985.
26. Tveit KM, Guldvog I, Hagen S, et al: Randomized controlled trial of postoperative radiotherapy and short-term time-scheduled 5-fluorouracil against surgery alone in the treatment of Dukes B and C rectal cancer. *Br J Surg* 84:1130, 1997.
27. O'Connell MJ, Martenson JA, Wieand HS, et al: Improving adjuvant therapy for rectal cancer by combining protracted-infusion fluorouracil with radiation therapy after curative surgery. *N Engl J Med* 331:502, 1994.
28. Smalley SR, Benedetti JK, Williamson SK, et al: Phase III trial of fluorouracil-based chemotherapy regimens plus radiotherapy in postoperative adjuvant rectal cancer: GI INT 0144. *J Clin Oncol* 24:3542, 2006.
29. Tepper JE, O'Connell M, Niedzwiecki D, et al: Adjuvant therapy in rectal cancer: Analysis of stage, sex, and local control—Final report of intergroup 0114. *J Clin Oncol* 20:1744, 2002.
30. Bosset JF, Collette L, Calais G, et al: Chemotherapy with preoperative radiotherapy in rectal cancer. *N Engl J Med* 355:1114, 2006.
31. Sauer R, Becker H, Hohenberger W, et al: Preoperative versus postoperative chemoradiotherapy for rectal cancer. *N Engl J Med* 351:1731, 2004.
32. Roh MS, Colangelo LH, O'Connell MJ, et al: Preoperative multimodality therapy improves disease-free survival in patients with carcinoma of the rectum: NSABP R-03. *J Clin Oncol* 27:5124, 2009.
33. Folkesson J, Birgisson H, Pahlman L, et al: Swedish rectal cancer trial: Long lasting benefits from radiotherapy on survival and local recurrence rate. *J Clin Oncol* 23:5644, 2005.
34. Kapiteijn E, Marijnen CAM, Nagtegaal ID, et al: Preoperative radiotherapy combined with total mesorectal excision for resectable rectal cancer. *N Engl J Med* 345:638, 2001.
35. Sebag-Montepore D, Stephens RJ, Steele R, et al: Preoperative radiotherapy versus selective postoperative chemoradiotherapy in patients with rectal cancer (MRC CR07 and NCIC-CTG C016): A multicentre, randomised trial. *Lancet* 373:811, 2009.
36. Bujko K, Nowacki MP, Nasierowska-Guttmejer A, et al: Long-term results of a randomized trial comparing preoperative short-course radiotherapy with preoperative conventionally fractionated chemoradiation for rectal cancer. *Br J Surg* 93:1215, 2006.
37. Gerard JP, Chapet O, Ortholan C, et al: French experience with contact x-ray endocavitary radiation for early rectal cancer. *Clin Oncol* 19:661, 2007.
38. Russell AH, Harris J, Rosenberg PJ, et al: Anal sphincter conservation for patients with adenocarcinoma of the distal rectum: Long-term results of Radiation Therapy Oncology Group protocol 89-02. *Int J Radiat Oncol Biol Phys* 46:313, 2000.
39. Greenberg JA, Shibata D, Herndon JE, et al: Local excision of distal rectal cancer: An update of Cancer and Leukemia Group B 8984. *Dis Colon Rectum* 51:1185, 2008.
40. Miller RC, Sargent DJ, Martenson JA, et al: Acute diarrhea during adjuvant therapy for rectal cancer: A detailed analysis from a randomized intergroup trial. *Int J Radiat Oncol Biol Phys* 54:409, 2002.
41. Haddock MG, Sloan JA, Bollinger JW, et al: Patient assessment of bowel function during and after pelvic radiotherapy: Results of a prospective phase III North Central Cancer Treatment Group clinical trial. *J Clin Oncol* 25:1255, 2007.

42. Krook JE, Moertel CG, Gunderson LL, et al: Effective surgical adjuvant therapy for high-risk rectal carcinoma. *N Engl J Med* 324:709, 1991.

43. Kollmorgen CF, Meagher AP, Wolff BG, et al: The long-term effect of adjuvant postoperative chemoradiotherapy for rectal carcinoma on bowel function. *Ann Surg* 220:676, 1994.

44. Peeters KC, van de Velde CJ, Leer JW, et al: Late side effects of short-course preoperative radiotherapy combined with total meso-rectal excision for rectal cancer: Increased bowel dysfunction in irradiated patients—a Dutch colorectal cancer group study. *J Clin Oncol* 23:6199, 2005.

45. Stephens RJ, Thompson LC, Quirke P, et al: Impact of short-course preoperative radiotherapy for rectal cancer on patients' quality of life: Data from the Medical Research Council CR07/National Cancer Institute of Canada Clinical Trials Group C016 randomized clinical trial. *J Clin Oncol* 28:4233, 2010.

46. Sebag-Montefiore D, Stephens RJ, Steele R, et al: Preoperative radiotherapy versus selective postoperative chemoradiotherapy in patients with rectal cancer (MRC CR07 and NCIC-CTG C016): A multicentre, randomised trial. *Lancet* 373:811, 2009.

47. Baxter NN, Habermann EB, Tepper JE, et al: Risk of pelvic fractures in older women following pelvic irradiation. *JAMA* 294:2587, 2005.

Radiation Injuries to the Rectum

George Singer | Theodore J. Saclarides

The benefits of radiotherapy are well established for primary as well as recurrent genitourinary and anorectal malignancies; however, radiation injury to healthy tissues within the lower abdomen and pelvis can be severe. Two hundred thousand cases of prostatic, bladder, testicular, cervical, endometrial, and rectal cancer are diagnosed annually each year, and half of these are candidates for radiotherapy. Many of these patients will experience altered gastrointestinal function because of damage to the small and large bowel. The rectum, in particular, because of its fixed nature within the pelvis and its proximity to the targeted area, is the most frequently injured organ. Patients with mild to moderate radiation proctitis can experience tenesmus, urgency, bleeding, diarrhea, and incontinence. Severe rectal complications of pelvic radiation include hemorrhagic proctitis, rectovaginal fistulas, and anorectal strictures.[1] This chapter will review medical and surgical treatments of radiation injury of the rectum (Box 176-1).

INCIDENCE OF COMPLICATIONS

The German physicist Wilhelm Roentgen discovered x-rays in 1895. A mere 2 years after this discovery, David Walsh described the first case of radiation enteritis in a person working in an x-ray lab who complained of abdominal pain and diarrhea and whose symptoms improved with the use of a lead barrier.[2] The first clinical report of severe intestinal injury following radiotherapy for cancer was described in 1917,[3] and 13 years later a paper was published describing proctitis in a group of patients receiving pelvic radiotherapy.[4] It is now known that radiation damages the lipid layer of cell membranes, proteins, and cellular DNA, with the worst damage occurring in cells with a high mitotic rate, such as intestinal mucosa. Multiple factors can predispose a patient to radiation proctitis, including diabetes mellitus, hypertension, collagen vascular disease, and concomitant or previous chemotherapy. Most patients will improve with temporary cessation of radiotherapy, fluid resuscitation, diet modification, and antidiarrheal medications. Most symptoms resolve within months after completion of therapy. A small number of patients will need more aggressive therapy.[1]

Radiation doses for prostate cancer are higher than for other malignancies and are the most frequent cause of radiation proctitis. Advances in external beam radiation such as three-dimensional conformal radiotherapy (3D CRT) and intensity-modulated radiotherapy (IMRT) have made it possible to give higher doses without increasing late complications to the rectum. Radiation doses can also be limited with brachytherapy, where carefully implanted needles deliver radiation directly into the prostate. Despite these advances, 80% of patients treated with radiotherapy for prostate cancer will experience rectal bleeding within 3 years and 8% of patients will need treatment for chronic complications.[5] One percent of patients will develop severe complications such as hemorrhage, obstruction, fistula, and perforation. Risk factors include widening of the radiation field to include pelvic lymph nodes, diabetes mellitus, prior pelvic surgery, and split-course rather than continuous-course radiation.[6]

Although smaller radiation doses are used for other pelvic malignancies, complications are still seen. One-third of patients will experience proctitis after cervical radiation.[7] One study found that 7% of patients undergoing curative radiotherapy for endometrial cancer developed severe complications at 3 years' followup. Chemotherapy and radiotherapy have become mainstay treatments for anal cancer and provide both high cure rates and the ability to preserve the anus and sphincter. However, one study found that 15% of patients who had received radiotherapy for anal cancer developed severe complications after 10 years of followup. Risk factors for injury included involvement of both the anal canal and anal margins, higher radiation doses, and local excision performed before radiation.[8]

ACUTE RADIATION PROCTITIS

Acute radiation proctitis occurs during or within the first 6 weeks following radiotherapy. Symptoms include discomfort, diarrhea, tenesmus, mucoid discharge, and rectal bleeding. When endoscopy is performed, the mucosa can appear dusky, inflamed, and edematous, with a poorly visible vascular pattern. The tissue is not markedly friable and ulcers are infrequently seen.[9] Histopathology demonstrates hyperemia, edema, and inflammatory cell infiltration of the mucosa, which can progress to crypt abscesses, sloughed epithelial cells, and ulceration.[10]

CHRONIC RADIATION PROCTITIS

The first signs of chronic radiation proctitis occur 9 to 15 months following radiotherapy, but may develop after more than 2 years and rarely up to 30 years later.[11] Bleeding is the most common symptom. Workup should be patient directed. A complete blood count (CBC) should be obtained to evaluate for anemia and inflammation/infection as well as an abdominal radiograph to look for small bowel obstruction. Evaluation must include endoscopy to rule out tumor recurrence. Computed tomography (CT) scan should be considered to rule out metastatic

---

BOX 176-1 **Management of Radiation-Induced Rectal Bleeding**

1. Initial workup
   a. Patient directed, beginning with a history and physical
   b. Laboratory studies including a complete blood count
   c. CT imaging as clinically warranted to exclude metastatic disease
   d. Endoscopy with biopsies as clinically warranted to exclude recurrent malignancy
2. Nonoperative management
   a. Mild cases may be observed with supportive therapy, e.g., hydration
   b. Drug therapy
   c. Hyperbaric oxygen
   d. Aqueous formaldehyde
   e. Argon plasma coagulation
3. Operative management
   a. Reserved for the most refractory cases of rectal bleeding
   b. Individualized therapy with the benefits of surgery weighed against the potential morbidity of major abdominal/pelvic surgery
   c. Age, comorbid illnesses, presence of recurrent malignancy, and function of sphincter taken into consideration
   d. Acute radiation changes allowed to subside as possible

---

disease. On endoscopic evaluation, the mucosa appears pale and friable, with multiple, continuous telangiectasias. Ulcers of the anterior wall can be seen in 10% of patients although many of these are asymptomatic. Biopsy should be done judiciously because of the risk of fistulization and directed at the posterior and lateral walls if possible to avoid areas of increased radiation. Histopathology demonstrates variable regeneration of the rectal tissue with a thickened, fibrotic submucosa, large abnormal fibroblasts, endarteritis, and tissue ischemia.[12]

NONOPERATIVE MANAGEMENT

The surgeon should be well-versed in the nonoperative management of radiation proctitis, particularly hemorrhagic proctitis, because this is the most common symptom requiring evaluation and treatment. Although treatment of mild cases is generally supportive, sometimes consisting only of hydration, many of the more severe cases may be referred to a surgeon. No specific treatment may be needed for mild rectal bleeding, in which case symptoms may resolve spontaneously. One study found that 35% of patients with mild bleeding stopped bleeding within 6 months.[13] For radiation-induced strictures, stool softeners can be helpful for mild obstructive symptoms. Balloon or Savary-Gilliard dilators may be used for those who do not respond to stool softeners provided that the segments of strictured bowel are short. The risk of perforation is increased when dilating long or angulated strictures.[14] Surgery may be needed for high-grade obstruction.

For hemorrhagic proctitis, diversion of the fecal stream by loop ileostomy or colostomy without proctectomy has had mixed results and complete cessation of rectal bleeding is infrequently observed.[15] Studies have looked at prophylactic medications given during radiation, but success has not been uniformly seen. Oral sucralfate, a drug thought to have a favorable effect on epithelial-associated microvascular injury, was not found to produce a statistical difference in symptom resolution and was associated with increased rates of rectal bleeding. Another study of 26 patients with moderate and severe proctitis who were given oral sucralfate twice daily until bleeding stopped or treatment was considered a failure found that the frequency of rectal bleeding decreased by 77% at 4 weeks and 92% at 16 weeks.[16] Other studies have shown a beneficial effect of oral sucralfate when given to treat diarrhea, increasing the consistency and decreasing the frequency of bowel movements.[17]

One of the most promising treatments is amifostine, which acts as a radioprotectant. Intracellular oxidation of amifostine yields an active metabolite that scavenges free radicals, thus stabilizing cellular DNA. One study that randomized 100 patients with advanced inoperable rectal cancer to external beam radiation with or without amifostine showed a statistically significant decrease in the number of patients who developed moderate and severe complications if they had taken amifostine. The study also found no evidence of tumor protection.[18] Other studies have looked at the efficacy of sulfasalazine[19] and aminosalicylates,[20] well established in treating idiopathic ulcerative colitis, finding mixed results for radiation proctitis. Finally, a small study of prophylactic use of misoprostol suppositories found beneficial effects in 9 of 16 patients.[21]

Many studies have assessed treatment of rectal bleeding that occurs during or after completion of radiotherapy. Some have shown benefit with topical butyrate,[22] oral metronidazole,[23] oral vitamin A,[24] and a combination of oral vitamins C and E.[25] Other studies have shown no benefit with pentosan phosphate,[26] short-chain fatty acid enemas,[27] and pentoxyphylline.[28] Larger, randomized, placebo-controlled studies are needed to elucidate possible benefits of these medications.

In those patients where initial conservative therapy fails to control rectal bleeding, more aggressive therapy is available. Four modalities have been extensively studied, including hyperbaric oxygen, topical formalin, laser ablative therapy, and argon plasma coagulation (APC).

Hyperbaric oxygen has proven efficacy in treating refractory foot ulcers for patients with diabetes mellitus[29] and other conditions. It is theorized that hyperbaric oxygen overcomes chronic tissue hypoxia in radiation-damaged tissues and with repeated sessions induces growth of regenerative tissue, capillaries, and epithelium. It is generally well tolerated but is limited by being expensive and not widely available. Multiple studies have shown its efficacy in radiation proctitis. One study of 120 patients with refractory radiation proctitis randomized to hyperbaric oxygen therapy or a sham procedure showed a clinical response of 89% versus 63%, respectively.[30] Unfortunately, successful therapy may take multiple sessions. One study found that 5 of 5 patients stopped bleeding but required 18 to 60 treatments.[31]

Aqueous formaldehyde, or formalin, is perhaps the most established therapy for chronic hemorrhagic proctitis. Formalin treats rectal bleeding by inducing coagulative tissue necrosis on contact. Initially used for the treatment of hemorrhagic cystitis, multiple studies via various applications have shown it to be an easy, inexpensive, well-tolerated, and effective treatment for hemorrhagic proctitis. Formalin is, however, extremely irritating to the anoderm and contact with it should be avoided. It may be prudent to remove residual formalin from the rectum with a normal saline flush following the procedure. Formalin is also not without its own serious complications which, although rare, include fistula and bowel necrosis requiring bowel resection and sometimes colostomy.[32] One study instilled 20 mL of 5% formaldehyde into the rectum during flexible sigmoidoscopy without sedation and found that 13 of 23 patients (65%) needed only one session to stop bleeding and 4 of 20 patients stopped with a second session (overall, 74%) after an average followup of 23 months.[33] Another study treated 100 patients with a 10% buffered solution of formalin via a cotton-tip applicator during outpatient office proctoscopy, with an overall 93% success rate after an average 3.5 sessions at 2- to 4-week intervals.[34] Finally, a smaller study found cessation of hemorrhagic proctitis in 12 of 16 patients following instillation of 30 to 50 mL of formalin followed by a 60-mL normal saline flush. One patient required three treatments before cessation and 3 patients continued to have intermittent bleeding, although none required additional transfusions.[35]

Laser ablative therapy, though effective, has been shown to require multiple treatments[36] and has been replaced by APC as a treatment of therapy-resistant radiation proctitis. APC is an efficacious treatment modality; one study found that 39 of 40 patients with refractory hemorrhagic proctitis were successfully treated with APC after one to two treatments; although after 3 to 30 months' followup, most patients still experienced mild bleeding but did not require transfusion. The one patient who failed therapy responded to formalin treatment and none of the patients required surgery.[37] Another study of 12 patients who had previously failed formalin therapy found that 6 achieved complete cessation of bleeding, whereas 4 had symptomatic improvement; 2 continued to have bleeding from the sigmoid colon.[38] Although neither of these two studies documented any serious complications of treatment, a third study found that 2 of 15 patients developed rectal strictures, which responded to dilation in both cases.[39]

In summary, hyperbaric oxygen has been used successfully but in a limited capacity. Availability and cost may limit its utility. Formalin instillation and APC also show promise; patients who fail one of these modalities may be treated with the other with a reasonable degree of success.

OPERATIVE TREATMENT

Operative treatment of the radiated rectum is reserved for the most refractory cases and for complications such as high-grade obstruction, perforation, fistula, and persistent bleeding. The benefits of surgery must be weighed against complications of major pelvic surgery. For low-risk patients, the best treatment for rectal strictures and fistulas is proctectomy with reanastomosis. However, operative treatment must be individualized; age, presence of comorbid illnesses, presence of locally recurrent or widely metastatic disease, and function of the sphincter must be taken into consideration. Preoperative management, again, should include endoscopy and possible biopsy to rule out recurrent malignancy. When possible, any acute radiation changes should be given time to subside before repair.

Anal manometry can assess the native rectum's ability to function as a storage reservoir by measuring intrarectal pressure and assessing sensation after instillation of sequential volumes of air in a balloon placed into the rectal vault. Patients with normal function should be able to feel 15 to 30 mL of air, have the urge to defecate at 90 mL, and be able to tolerate up to 200 mL without excessive discomfort. A noncompliant, irradiated rectum cannot accommodate increasing volumes without inappropriate elevation of intrarectal pressure. Patients may experience significant discomfort shortly after the threshold is reached for defecation. These findings may argue for a resectional procedure rather than local repair of a rectovaginal fistula or anorectal stricture.

Once surgery is chosen, the surgeon must select the best operative approach. For most cases of hemorrhagic proctitis, a transabdominal resection (proctectomy) is needed. For a rectovaginal fistula or rectal stricture, location determines the best operative approach. A local perineal approach may be preferred for disease of the distal rectum and anal canal. High rectovaginal fistulas and strictures with loss of rectal compliance are best fixed via a transabdominal approach. Lastly, restoration of intestinal continuity may or may not be possible and is determined by preexisting sphincter dysfunction, health of the distal bowel margin, and the skill of the surgeon. Generally, options include proctectomy with end colostomy; proctectomy with coloanal straight anastomosis, colonic J-pouch, or coloplasty; ileocecal reservoir; or sigmoid colon overlay patch. Patients who are not candidates for an extensive resection may benefit from a proximal diverting ostomy as the sole form of treatment. Fecal diversion alone has its limitations (e.g., if one is treating hemorrhagic proctitis, bleeding may continue). When treating a rectovaginal fistula, the patient will continue to have mucoid (albeit not feculent) discharge through the anus. Proximal diversion of the fecal stream should always be performed if impaired healing of a distal anastomosis is a concern; postoperative contrast studies of the distal colon should be obtained before reversal. Preoperative management includes a thorough bowel cleansing, intravenous antibiotics, marking of the potential stoma sites if used, and deep vein thrombosis prophylaxis, Foley catheter, and sometimes ureteral stents to assist in identification of ureters during pelvic dissection.

PROXIMAL SIGMOID ONLAY PATCH

The proximal sigmoid onlay patch or Bricker-Johnson procedure is rarely used to treat rectovaginal fistulas and rectal strictures, having been replaced with the colonic reservoir made during proctectomy. It is included for historical completeness. The procedure consists of division of the rectosigmoid junction, debridement of the fistula or stricture, and suturing of the open end of the sigmoid colon to the debrided edges of the rectal injury. In this method, a loop is created to which the proximal colon is anastomosed. The procedure requires temporary fecal diversion. Benefits of this procedure are avoidance of a proctectomy and its associated blood loss and construction of a loop of sigmoid colon than can perform as a reservoir. However, the diseased rectum is left in place and brings with it risk of anastomotic leak, bleeding, and stenosis. Studies have shown no advantage of the proximal sigmoid onlay patch to proctectomy and coloanal anastomosis with or without construction of a colonic J-pouch.[40]

PROCTECTOMY

Proctectomy begins with the mobilization of the sigmoid and descending colon. The splenic flexure may need to be mobilized to obtain sufficient length of bowel. The rectum is dissected down to the pelvic floor and the rectovaginal septum is entered to separate the rectum from the vagina. The left colic artery and inferior mesenteric vein are ligated at the inferior border of the pancreas to allow for mobilization of the colon. The proximal point of colon transection is at an area of the left colon where the bowel is soft and supple and is free of muscular hypertrophy and radiation changes. One must confirm blood supply to the proximal colon by checking capillary refill at the cut edge; if blood supply is questionable, the distal transverse colon should be used as the proximal limb. The distal point of transection should be at the pelvic floor, leaving only 1 to 2 cm of rectum. The proximal limb is then anastomosed to the short rectal cuff using either staplers or a hand-sewn technique. If the new anastomosis is close to the vaginal fistula, the vagina can be repaired in layers and omentum should be interposed between the two viscera.

ILEOCECAL-ANAL ANASTOMOSIS

In a variation of the ileoanal anastomosis, an ileocecal segment is isolated on its lymphovascular pedicle, rotated, and anastomosed to the anorectal stump, thus creating a reservoir that functions as a neorectum (Figures 176-1 and 176-2). One study found that two patients treated in this manner showed good-quality defecation with good tolerances to volume and compliance on anal manometry.[41] A larger study of 30 patients treated with preservation of the anal sphincter found normal continence in 19 of 23 patients although there was a high rate of postoperative hemorrhage, small bowel obstruction, pelvic and perianal sepsis, and anastomotic stricture.[42]

COLONIC J-POUCH ANAL ANASTOMOSIS

The colonic J-pouch anal anastomosis consists of proctectomy in the usual manner with construction of a colonic J-pouch, which is then anastomosed to the anorectal stump. After mobilization of the left colon and splenic flexure in the usual manner, a stapling device is used to create a colonic reservoir from a 5- to 6-cm segment of the distal colon, thereby increasing the storage capacity of the neorectum. Larger pouches are

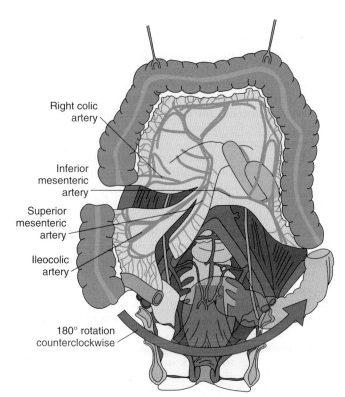

FIGURE 176-1 The ileocecal segment that will function as a neorectum.

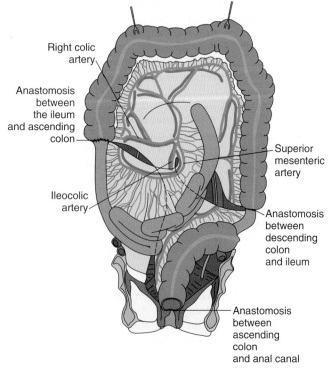

FIGURE 176-2 Ileocecal-anal anastomosis.

associated with difficult evacuation. The pouch is then stapled or hand-sewn to the anorectal stump (Figures 176-3 and 176-4) and is protected with a temporary loop ileostomy. One study of 40 patients randomized to either colonic J-pouch or straight coloanal anastomosis found

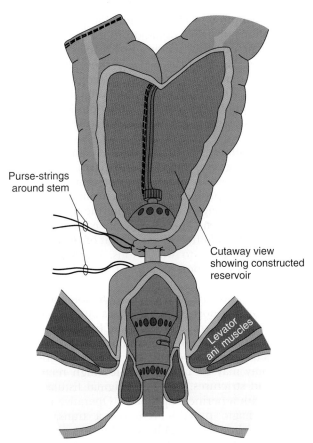

FIGURE 176-3 Having completed the colonic J-pouch, an EEA end-to-end anastomosis (EEA) stapler is inserted through the anus thus creating the colonic J-pouch to anal canal anastomosis.

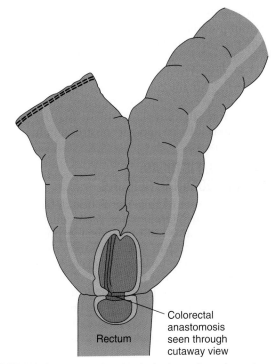

FIGURE 176-4 The completed colonic J-pouch anal anastomosis.

significant improvements in the frequency of defecation at 3, 12, and 24 months; less clustering of stools at 3 and 12 months; and less frequent incontinence in the first year. No significant difference in the complication rate was found.[43]

COLOPLASTY

Coloplasty was first described in 2000 as an alternative to colonic J-pouch for increasing the storage capacity of the neorectum.[44] Coloplasty begins with an 8- to 10-cm longitudinal colotomy between the taenia 4 to 6 cm from the distal cut end of the colon, which is then closed in a transverse fashion using a single layer of interrupted absorbable sutures (Figure 176-5). The distal cut end of the colon is then stapled or hand-sewn to the anal cuff and protected with a loop ileostomy. There have been multiple studies comparing coloplasty to colonic J-pouch and straight coloanal anastomosis. One study of 20 patients with coloplasty, 16 with colonic J-pouch, and 17 with straight coloanal anastomosis found similar complication rates but a significant difference in function between the groups. The coloplasty group had 2.6 bowel movements per day compared with 3.1 in the colonic J-pouch and 4.5 in the straight coloanal anastomosis groups. Furthermore, the coloplasty and colonic J-pouch groups tolerated greater volumes and had increased compliance on anal manometry compared to the straight coloanal anastomosis group.[45] Another study of 40

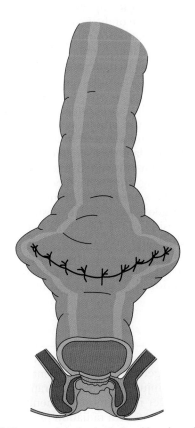

FIGURE 176-5 The completed coloplasty with coloanal anastomosis.

consecutive patients randomized to coloplasty or colonic J-pouch found similar rates of complications, resting and squeezing pressures, and neorectum volumes on manometry; however, the coloplasty group had increased sensitivity and decreased frequency, with 2.0 bowel movements compared to 2.75 in the colonic J-pouch group.[46] Because of the size of the created neorectum and the mesentery that accompanies the bowel, coloplasty may be an especially good alternative to J-pouch construction in patients with a narrow pelvis.

RECTOVAGINAL FISTULAS: NONTRANSABDOMINAL REPAIRS

The location of a rectovaginal fistula best determines the operative technique. Options for repair include transanal, transvaginal, and transperitoneal approaches; the basic principles of repair are the same regardless of which is chosen. These include (1) excluding recurrent cancer as the cause of the fistula; (2) allowing time for acute changes to subside before repair; (3) excising the fistula and interposing healthy tissue between the repaired vagina and the rectum; and (4) considering diversion of the fecal stream for large or recurrent fistulas.

Transanal fistulectomy begins with the patient in the prone jackknife position. A trapezoidal flap of mucosa, submucosa, and circularis muscle whose base is twice as wide as its top (to ensure adequate blood supply) is mobilized to a point several centimeters above the fistula. The rectal opening of the fistula is part of the flap but it is excised. After the flap is elevated, the rectovaginal septum is closed and the flap advanced and sutured into place. The vaginal side of the fistula is left open to permit drainage.[47] In a variation of this procedure, a transanal sleeve advancement flap (similar to the one previously described but with a circumferential sleeve of rectum) is advanced to cover the fistula site after excision of the fistula tract.[48]

Transvaginal and transperineal fistulectomies begin with the patient in the lithotomy position. The vaginal mucosa is incised and elevated in all directions around the fistula. The fistula is then excised, debrided, and the rectovaginal septum is inverted into the rectum with a series of purse-string sutures. Finally, the vaginal mucosa is closed over the septum. The transperineal approach affords the surgeon improved exposure of the fistula tract. After excision of the fistula tract via episioproctotomy, the vaginal and rectal walls are closed in layers without tension, and healthy tissue (e.g., Martius flap) can be interposed between the two closures. One should note that a previously irradiated perineum may not heal well.

SUMMARY

The rectum is both fixed within the pelvis and is in proximity to areas targeted for radiation, making it the most frequent organ injured by radiotherapy. Radiotherapy for prostate cancer is the most frequent cause of radiation proctitis. Patients with radiation proctitis can experience mild to moderate tenesmus, urgency, bleeding, diarrhea, and incontinence. Bleeding is the most common symptom of chronic radiation proctitis. Severe complications of pelvic radiation to the rectum include hemorrhagic proctitis, rectovaginal fistulas, and anorectal strictures. Most injuries occur in the acute phase and respond to temporary cessation of radiotherapy, fluid resuscitation, diet modification, and antidiarrheal medications. Evaluation of chronic radiation proctitis must include endoscopic evaluation to rule out tumor recurrence.

Oral sucralfate is currently the best studied medication for treating rectal bleeding and diarrhea. Amifostine holds promise as a treatment because of its radioprotective effects. Few problems become chronic, and most of these can be managed with formalin therapy and argon plasma coagulation. Formalin is an easy, inexpensive, well-tolerated, and effective treatment of rectal bleeding usually requiring one to two sessions. Argon plasma coagulation is also a good treatment modality for these patients.

The operative treatment of radiation proctitis is reserved for the most refractory cases and for complications such as high-grade obstruction, fistula, and uncontrolled hemorrhage. Anal manometry can assess the native rectum's ability to function as a storage reservoir. Proctectomy may be undertaken for high rectovaginal fistulas and strictures. Low rectovaginal fistulas can be repaired with a perineal approach. Operative treatment of hemorrhagic proctitis requires a transabdominal resection of the rectum. Elderly and infirm patients may best benefit from a well-constructed end colostomy alone. Proctectomy can be accompanied by end colostomy or various techniques to restore continuity such as straight anastomosis, colonic J-pouch, coloplasty, or ileocecal reservoir. Coloplasty may have improved function compared to colonic J-pouch anastomosis without increasing complication rate; however, both are preferable to a straight coloanal anastomosis without a reservoir. If continuity is restored, temporary fecal diversion is recommended to protect the anastomosis.

REFERENCES

1. Mahmoud NN, Fry RD: Radiation injury to the small and large bowel. In Cameron JL: *Current surgical therapy 9.* Philadelphia, 2008, Mosby, p 205.
2. Walsh D: Deep tissue traumatism from Roentgen ray exposure. *Br Med J* 2:272, 1897.
3. Franz K, Orth J: Falleiner: Roentgen shading. *Klin Wochenschr* 45:662, 1917.
4. Buie LA, Malmgren GE: Factitial proctitis. *Trans Am Proctol Soc* 29:80, 1930.
5. Moore EM, Magrino TJ, Johnstone PA: Rectal bleeding after radiation therapy for prostate cancer: Endoscopic evaluation. *Radiology* 217:215, 2000.
6. Schultheiss TE, Lee WR, Hung MA, et al: Late GI and GU complications in the treatment of prostate cancer. *Int J Radiat Oncol Biol Phys* 37:3, 1997.
7. Huang EY, Lin H, Hsu HC, et al: High external parametrial dose can increase the probability of radiation proctitis in patients with uterine cervix cancer. *Gynecol Oncol* 79:406, 2000.
8. Allal AS, Mermillod B, Roth AD, et al: Impact of clinical and therapeutic factors on major late complications after radiotherapy with or without concomitant chemotherapy for anal carcinoma. *Int J Radiat Oncol Biol Phys* 39:1099, 1997.
9. Gelfand MD, Tepper M, Katz LA, et al: Acute irradiation proctitis in man. *Gastroenterology* 54:401, 1968.

10. Trier JS, Browning TH: Morphologic response of human small intestinal to x-ray exposure. *J Clin Invest* 45:194, 1996.

11. Anderson RE: Radiation injury. In Kissane JM, editor: *Anderson's pathology*. St Louis, 1985, CV Mosby, p 239.

12. White DC: *An atlas of radiation histopathology*. Technical Information Center, Office of Public Affairs, US Energy Research, and Development Administration TID-26676:141, 1975.

13. Gilinsky NH, Burns DG, Barbezat GO, et al: The natural history of radiation-induced proctosigmoiditis: An analysis of 88 patients. *Q J Med* 52:40, 1983.

14. Triadafilopoulos G, Sarkisian M: Dilatation of radiation-induced sigmoid stricture using sequential Savary-Gilliard dilators. A combined radiologic-endoscopic approach. *Dis Colon Rectum* 33:1065, 1990.

15. Zimmerman DD, Gosselink MP, Briel JW, et al: The outcome of transanal advancement flap repair of rectovaginal fistulas is not improved by an additional labial fat flap transposition. *Tech Coloproctol* 6:37, 2002.

16. Kochhar R, Sriram PV, Sharma SC: Natural history of late radiation proctosigmoiditis treated with topical sucralfate. *Dig Dis Sci* 44:973, 1999.

17. Hendrickson R, Franzen L, Littbrand B: Effects of sucralfate on acute and late bowel discomfort following radiotherapy of pelvic cancer. *J Clin Oncol* 10:969, 1992.

18. Liu T, Liu Y, He S, et al: Use of radiation with or without WR-2721 in advanced rectal cancer. *Cancer* 69:2820, 1992.

19. Goldstein F, Khoury J, Thornton JJ: Treatment of chronic radiation enteritis and colitis with salicylazosulfapyridine and systemic corticosteroids. A pilot study. *Am J Gastroenterol* 65:201, 1976.

20. Baum CA, Biddle WL, Miner PB Jr: Failure of 5-aminosalicylic acid enemas to improve chronic radiation proctitis. *Dig Dis Sci* 34:758, 1989.

21. Khan AM, Birk JW, Anderson JC, et al: A prospective randomized placebo-controlled double blinded pilot study of misoprostol rectal suppositories in the prevention of acute and chronic radiation proctitis symptoms in prostate cancer patients. *Am J Gastroenterol* 95:1961, 2000.

22. Vernia P, Fracasso PL, Casale V, et al: Topical butyrate for acute radiation proctitis: Randomized, crossover trial. *Lancet* 356:1232, 2000.

23. Cavcic J, Turcic J, Martinac P, et al: Metronidazole in the treatment of chronic radiation proctitis: Clinical trial. *Croat Med J* 41:314, 2000.

24. Karamanolis G, Triantafyllou K, Tsiamoulos Z, et al: Argon plasma coagulation has a long-lasting therapeutic effect in patients with chronic radiation proctitis. *Endoscopy* 41:529, 2009.

25. Kennedy M, Bruninga K, Mutlu EA, et al: Successful and sustained treatment of chronic radiation proctitis with antioxidant vitamins E and C. *Am J Gastroenterol* 96:1080, 2001.

26. Pilepich MV, Paulus R, St Clair W, et al: Phase III study of pentosanpolysulfate (PPS) in treatment of gastrointestinal tract sequelae of radiotherapy. *Am J Clin Oncol* 29:132, 2006.

27. al-Sabbagh R, Sinicrope FA, Sellin JH, et al: Evaluation of short-chain fatty acid enemas: Treatment of radiation proctitis. *Am J Gastroenterol* 91:1814, 1996.

28. Venkitaraman R, Price A, Coffey J, et al: Pentoxifylline to treat radiation proctitis: A small and inconclusive randomised trial. *Clin Oncol (R Coll Radiol)* 20:288, 2008.

29. Löndahl M, Katzman P, Nilsson A, et al: Hyperbaric oxygen therapy facilitates healing of chronic foot ulcers in patients with diabetes. *Diabetes Care* 33:998, 2010.

30. Clarke RE, Tenorio LM, Hussey JR, et al: Hyperbaric oxygen treatment of chronic refractory radiation proctitis: A randomized and controlled double-blind crossover trial with long-term follow-up. *Int J Radiat Oncol Biol Phys* 72:134, 2008.

31. Mayer R, Klemen H, Quehenberger F, et al: Hyperbaric oxygen—an effective tool to treat radiation morbidity in prostate cancer. *Radiother Oncol* 61:151, 2001.

32. Luna-Perez P, Rodriguez-Ramirez SE: Formalin instillation for refractory radiation-induced hemorrhagic proctitis. *J Surg Oncol* 80:41, 2002.

33. Cullen SN, Frenz M, Mee A: Treatment of haemorrhagic radiation-induced proctopathy using small volume topical formalin instillation. *Aliment Pharmacol Ther* 23:1575, 2006.

34. Haas EM, Bailey HR, Farragher I: Application of 10 percent formalin for the treatment of radiation-induced hemorrhagic proctitis. *Dis Colon Rectum* 50:213, 2007.

35. Saclarides T, King DG, Franklin JL, et al: Formalin instillation for refractory radiation induced hemorrhagic proctitis: Report of 16 patients. *Dis Colon Rectum* 39:196, 1996.

36. Taylor JG, Disario JA, Bjorkman DJ: KTP laser therapy for bleeding from chronic radiation proctopathy. *Gastrointest Endosc* 52:353, 2000.

37. Venkatesh KS, Ramanujam P: Endoscopic therapy for radiation proctitis-induced hemorrhage in patients with prostatic carcinoma using argon plasma coagulator application. *Surg Endosc* 16:707, 2002.

38. Tijandra JJ, Sengupta S: Argon plasma coagulation is an effective treatment for refractory hemorrhagic radiation proctitis. *Dis Colon Rectum* 44:1759, 2001.

39. Tam W, Moore J, Schoeman M: Treatment of radiation proctitis with argon plasma coagulation. *Endoscopy* 32:667, 2000.

40. Bricker EM, Johnston WD, Patwardhan RV: Repair of postirradiation damage to colorectum: A progress report. *Ann Surg* 193:555, 1981.

41. von Flue MO, Degen LP, Belinger C, et al: The ileocecal reservoir for rectal replacement in complicated radiation proctitis. *Am J Surg* 172:335, 1996.

42. Faucheron JL, Rosso R, Tiret E, et al: Soave's procedure: The final sphincter-saving solution for iatrogenic rectal lesions. *Br J Surg* 85:962, 1998.

43. Lazorthes F, Chiotasso P, Gamagami RA, et al: Late clinical outcome in a randomized prospective comparison of colonic J pouch and straight coloanal anastomosis. *Br J Surg* 84:1449, 1997.

44. Fazio VW, Mantyh CR, Hull TL: Colonic "coloplasty": Novel technique to enhance low colorectal or coloanal anastomosis. *Dis Colon Rectum* 43:1448, 2000.

45. Mantyh CR, Hull TL, Fazio VW: Coloplasty in low colorectal anastomosis: Manometric and functional comparison with straight and colonic J-pouch anastomosis. *Dis Colon Rectum* 44:37, 2001.

46. Furst A, Suttner S, Agha A, et al: Colonic J-pouch vs. coloplasty following resection of distal rectal cancer: Early results of a prospective, randomized, pilot study. *Dis Colon Rectum* 46:1161, 2003.

47. Hudson CN: Rectovaginal fistula: Vaginal repair. In Fielding LP, Goldberg SM, editors: *Rob and Smith's operative surgery: Surgery of the colon, rectum, and anus*, ed 5. Boston, 1993, Butterworths, p 852.

48. Marchesa P, Hull TL, Fazio VW: Advancement sleeve flaps for treatment of severe perianal Crohn's disease. *Br J Surg* 85:1695, 1998.

PART FIVE

Techniques and Pearls

Antibiotics, Approaches, Strategy, and Anastomoses

Jan Rakinic | Steven Tsoraides

Whatever you do may seem insignificant, but it is most important that you do it.

Gandhi

The successful outcome of surgical intervention depends on preparation. The surgeon's preparation for handling surgical emergencies—memorization of emergency protocols, experience in similar situations—must be accomplished long before the patient in extremis presents. Preparation for elective surgical intervention affords the advantage of proper preoperative evaluation of patient and disease extent, as well as the opportunity to modify some risk factors, with the goal of improving the patient's outcome. Appropriate assessment of the patient's history and performance status, deliberate consideration of the procedure planned, and a thorough understanding of the technical aspects and associated risks of the procedure planned are vital for success. Operative risks and benefits must be presented to the patient. The possibility of infection, hemorrhage, anastomotic dehiscence, disease recurrence, degree of alteration in bodily function or appearance, injury to or involvement of adjacent structures, and possible nerve damage resulting in weakness, paralysis, or genitourinary dysfunction should all be discussed. The therapeutic relationship is most sound when patient and surgeon are in concordance regarding anticipated outcomes.

PREPARING THE PATIENT FOR SURGERY: MANAGING RISKS

CARDIOPULMONARY AND OTHER MEDICAL RISKS

The incidence of comorbidities increases as the American population ages, elevating the risks associated with surgical intervention. A major portion of morbidity encountered after colorectal procedures is due to underlying comorbid conditions unrelated to the disease process being addressed surgically. Although beyond the scope of this chapter, it is understood that indicated medical evaluation(s) are required before elective major

surgery. Most Americans over the age of 50 will undergo a symptom-directed cardiac evaluation. Pulmonary evaluation is also performed as indicated by history and/or symptoms. Other disease processes, such as glucose intolerance of varying degree, obesity, renal or hepatic impairment, venous thromboembolic disease, sedentary lifestyle, and the physical deconditioning often associated with these entities all impact the cumulative risk of major surgical intervention. Discussion of these risks, as well as the expected postoperative management, is an important part of preparing the patient for the planned surgical procedure and recovery period. Preprocedure counseling is an important component of Early Recovery After Surgery programs (discussed later in this chapter), which have been designed to shorten hospital stays, improve patient care, reduce complications, and lower costs. Counseling prepares patients for a process that may be appreciably different than the process they may have experienced previously or been told about by friends or family members. Reframing patients' expectations in a proactive way allows patients to know that they can exert positive effects on their own recovery.

INFECTIOUS RISKS

Prehospital Bathing

Surgical site infection (SSI) is a serious complication that can lead to a prolonged hospital stay and higher costs. Prehospital bathing or showering with skin antiseptics has been proposed as a safe, cost-efficient way to decrease postoperative SSIs. However, a metaanalysis of seven trials, encompassing more than 10,000 patients, failed to show clear evidence that bathing with chlorhexidine in the prehospital setting provided any benefit over other wash products.[1]

Bowel Preparation: Mechanical Bowel Washout

Studies in the 1970s showed that fecal washout significantly decreased infectious complications after elective bowel resection. Nonabsorbable polyethylene glycol (CoLyte, GoLYTELY) is used widely, as are combinations of laxatives and purgatives. Clinically significant electrolyte disturbances occur infrequently with these regimens. The most common side effect is mild dehydration caused by inadequate oral fluid replacement. Use of carbohydrate-electrolyte rehydration solutions can diminish this transient intravascular volume contraction.[2] Oral sodium phosphate, used commonly for bowel preparation, is now known to carry a risk of further renal impairment in patients with existing renal insufficiency, and is currently recommended for use only in patients younger than 60 with no evidence of renal impairment.[3] Mannitol, historically used for colonic lavage, is metabolized by colonic flora with the production of hydrogen gas, and explosions have been reported during both open and endoscopic procedures. Mannitol is now used rarely for bowel washout.

Resection of the right colon without mechanical washout has long been acknowledged safe, whereas left colon resection without mechanical washout has been debated for some time. A number of reports have suggested that mechanical bowel preparation may be associated with higher rates of anastomotic leak and infectious complications.[4] Others have found generally equivalent outcomes for prep and no prep. In 2009 the Cochrane Collaboration published an update on mechanical bowel preparation in patients undergoing elective colorectal surgery.[5] Five new trials were added to this second update of the review, bringing the total number of included trials to 14 (4821 participants). No statistically significant difference was found when comparing patients who had undergone mechanical bowel preparation with those who had not with respect to anastomotic leak, mortality rates, peritonitis, need for reoperation, wound infection, or other nonabdominal complications, prompting the authors to conclude that there is no evidence that mechanical bowel preparation improves the outcome for patients. However, several studies have shown interesting results in certain subgroups of colectomy patients. A multicenter randomized trial from the Netherlands that included 1354 patients undergoing elective colorectal resection found no difference in rates of anastomotic leak, wound infection, fascial dehiscence, urinary tract infection, or pneumonia between prepped and unprepped groups. However, of those patients with anastomotic leak, significantly fewer abscesses occurred when mechanical bowel prep had been performed compared to no prep.[6] Additionally, a randomized controlled trial from Australia that included a high percentage of ultralow anastomoses reported that bowel washout was associated with fewer anastomotic leaks requiring reoperation than preparation with a single phosphate enema.[7] It may be that specific risks vary among subgroups of colorectal surgery patients.

There remain situations in which bowel washout may be desirable. During laparoscopic colon resection, manipulation and identification of pathology may be easier if the colon is empty of feces. Bowel washout may also be indicated if intraoperative colonoscopy is considered.

Oral Antibiotics

A Cochrane review encompassing 182 trials of preoperative antibiotic use between 1980 and 2007 found that combined oral and intravenous antibiotic prophylaxis significantly lowered surgical wound infection rate.[8] However, the authors noted that the studies were quite heterogeneous, making comparison a challenge. Many patients find the oral antibiotic regimen difficult to tolerate. Three hundred consecutive patients were randomized to receive either three doses of oral neomycin/erythromycin, one dose, or none before elective colorectal resection; all received mechanical washout and parenteral antibiotics. Compared with patients who received no oral antibiotics, patients who received three doses experienced significantly more nausea and vomiting ($P < 0.0005$), and patients who received any oral antibiotics had significantly more abdominal pain ($P < 0.077$). No differences were seen in wound infection, dehiscence, urinary tract infections, pneumonia, postoperative ileus, or intraabdominal abscess.[9] A retrospective case-controlled study at a tertiary care Veterans Administration hospital revealed that patients given preoperative oral antibiotics prior to elective colon resection had nearly three times the rate of postoperative *Clostridium difficile* colitis as patients who did not receive oral antibiotics (7.4% vs. 2.6%; $P = 0.03$).[10] Wound infection rates did not differ between the two groups. Among American surgeons who use bowel washout, most omit preoperative oral antibiotics, believing they offer no additional benefit above that conferred by parenteral antibiotics.

Parenteral Antibiotics

The immediate preoperative administration of parenteral antibiotics decreases the incidence of wound infections following elective colon surgery. This remains true in the absence of additional oral antibiotics. However, these benefits disappear if parenteral antibiotics are given *after* surgery has begun, implying that therapeutic tissue levels must be achieved before making the incision. Infectious complications increase when the anastomosis is in the extraperitoneal rectum or when operative time exceeds 3 hours; antibiotics should be readministered during lengthy procedures. Some surgeons administer three doses of parenteral antibiotics, adding two postoperative doses to the standard preoperative dose. A few reports have suggested that this may be associated with a lower incidence of wound infection; a Cochrane review did not demonstrate a benefit to administration of three doses of antibiotics.[8]

Clostridium difficile colitis, a well-recognized complication of antibiotic use, was first identified in conjunction with clindamycin use, but now is most commonly associated with cephalosporins. *C. difficile* colitis has been reported following administration of virtually every antibiotic currently in use. The incidence after elective gastrointestinal surgery has been estimated at 1.2%, with patients undergoing resections of the colon, small bowel, and stomach at highest risk.[11] Diagnosis can be elusive, with as many as 15% to 20% of patients testing negative when toxin enzyme immunoassay is used. Newer polymerase chain reaction methods for diagnosis have a sensitivity of 100% and specificity of 96%. Treatment consists of appropriate supportive care, the discontinuation (if possible) of all other antibiotics, and the administration of oral metronidazole, as the parenteral route is less effective. Oral vancomycin, with its increased risk and expense, is indicated for patients who do not respond to metronidazole or who are extremely ill. Up to 25% of patients require retreatment because of recurrence. Vancomycin may be delivered by enema when the oral route is unavailable or ineffective; stool "transplants" using healthy family members as donors have been reported as a method to reintroduce normal colonic flora.[12] Patients who are very ill or do not respond to medical treatment often require urgent abdominal colectomy; the mortality rate is quite high.[13]

Operative Skin Preparation

Hair removal from the surgical site should be as minimal as possible, using electric clippers rather than a razor to minimize skin abrasion, which increases the risk of wound infection. The surgical site may then be prepared using one of several techniques. Povidone-iodine preparation has been employed for years. Alcohol-based preparations such as Chloraprep (2% chlorhexidine and 70% isopropyl alcohol) or Duraprep (iodine povacrylex in isopropyl alcohol) have recently become more widely used. Chlorhexidine-alcohol was found to be superior to povidone-iodine in one study[14]; another found a higher incidence of SSIs using chlorhexidine-alcohol as compared to iodine povacrylex and povidone-iodine.[15] Both alcohol-based preparations must be allowed to dry for full effectiveness; considering this, an interesting study showed that saline removed chlorhexidine from skin, whereas iodine povacrylex remained intact.[16] However, no clear advantage for any of these agents has yet been definitely demonstrated.

Topical Antibiotics and Antiseptics

Intraincisional, intraluminal, and intraperitoneal antibiotics and antiseptics have been recommended periodically as a method to prevent wound infection. Any benefit of such topical antibiotic application is difficult to determine as parenteral antibiotics are always administered in these studies. There is no evidence supporting routine intraperitoneal antibiotic irrigation in elective colon surgery. Although povidone-iodine has been instilled into the colonic lumen as a topical "instant" bowel preparation, this technique is not widely practiced in the United States.

VENOUS THROMBOEMBOLIC RISK

Up to 10% of patients undergoing colorectal surgery suffer venous thromboembolic events (VTEs). Patients with cancer or inflammatory bowel disease are at particular risk, as are those with a previous history of VTE. Additional parameters associated with increased risks of embolic events are many, including prolonged operative time, multiple preoperative blood transfusions, preoperative hospitalization, and obesity (Table 177-1).[17] The incidence of postoperative VTE is decreased by 50% or more when appropriate prophylactic measures are instituted preoperatively; the initiation of prophylaxis *postoperatively* is far less effective. The eighth edition of the American College of Chest Physicians' Evidence-Based Clinical Practice Guidelines for prevention of venous thromboembolism recommends that patients

TABLE 177-1 VTE Risk Factors and Estimated Relative Risk

VTE Risk Factor	Estimated Relative Risk
Major surgery or major trauma	5-200
History of VTE	50
Age >50 yr	5
Age >70 yr	10
Cancer	5
Hospitalization for major medical illness	5
Antiphospholipid antibodies	2-10
Pregnancy	7
Estrogen therapy	2-5
Estrogen receptor modulators	3-5
Obesity	1-3
Antithrombin deficiency	25
Protein C or S deficiency	10
Factor V Leiden mutation	5-50

Adapted from Bates SM, Ginsberg JS: Treatment of deep vein thrombosis. *N Engl J Med* 351:268, 2004.

undergoing major general surgery have thromboprophylaxis with a low-molecular-weight heparin, low-dose heparin, or fondaparinux.[18] Each of these recommendations is supported by Grade 1A evidence. Low-molecular-weight heparin has the advantage of once-daily administration and a lower risk of heparin-induced thrombocytopenia. In studies of patients undergoing colorectal surgical procedures, both low-molecular-weight heparin and low-dose unfractionated heparin have been shown to reduce the incidence of VTE.[19]

Persuasive evidence suggests that the hypercoagulable state induced by surgery persists for at least 14 days, and perhaps 1 month, after surgery. Investigation of a national managed-care database found that patients undergoing orthopedic or abdominal surgery remained at risk for VTE after discharge, with the median time to VTE being 51 days.[20] Rasmussen et al performed a metaanalysis of trials evaluating prolonged thromboprophylaxis in patients after major abdominal or pelvic surgery, concluding that 1 month of thromboprophylaxis with low-molecular-weight heparin significantly reduced the risk of VTE compared to treatment only while in the hospital, without increasing the bleeding complications.[21] Although not current standard practice, long-term postoperative prophylaxis should be considered for patients at elevated risk for postoperative VTE.

ENHANCED RECOVERY AFTER SURGERY

Enhanced recovery after surgery (ERAS, or Fast Track) programs have been used for years in colorectal surgery. Individual programs differ in details, but share the goals of shortened hospital stay, improved patient care, reduced complications, and lowered costs. Discharge goals are identical to those used for patients managed conventionally. The most common elements in the pre-, intra-, and postoperative phases are shown in Table 177-2, along with the advantages gained by each element. A number of studies have shown that ERAS programs reduce hospital stay with no increase in morbidity, mortality, or

TABLE 177-2 Most Common Elements of Early Recovery After Surgery Programs

Phase	Measure	Advantage Gained
Preoperative	Counseling	Avoids anxiety; prepares patients for program and recovery
	No bowel prep	Avoids fluid, electrolyte alterations; possibly fewer surgical site injuries
	Avoid opioid/sedative premedications	Avoids delay in postoperative mobilization and oral fluid tolerance
	carbohydrate-rich fluids	Reduces postoperative insulin resistance, accelerates recovery and discharge
Intraoperative	Avoid fluid overload	Decreases aggravation of ileus and impaired wound healing
	Normothermia	Fewer wound infections, cardiac complications, transfusion needs
	Hyperoxia	
Postoperative	Selective use of nasogastric tubes	Less postoperative fever, atelectasis, pneumonia
	Early ambulation	Less insulin resistance and muscle loss, better oxygenation, lowers venous thromboembolic event risk
	Early feeding	Sooner return of GI function
	Early catheter removal	Facilitates earlier ambulation

Adapted from K Lassen, M Soop, J Nygren, et al: Consensus review of optimal perioperative care in colorectal surgery. Enhanced recovery after surgery group recommendations. *Arch Surg* 144:961, 2009.

readmission rates.[22] Although the laparoscopic approach shares some of these advantages when compared to standard open surgery, no additional benefit is identified when the laparoscopic approach is included with an ERAS program.[23]

Recovery after colectomy is often delayed by postoperative ileus. Many factors contribute to this, and several of the elements of ERAS programs decrease the duration of ileus experienced. Alvimopan, a peripherally acting *mu*-opioid receptor antagonist, blocks peripheral opioid receptors but does not cross the blood-brain barrier, allowing postoperative opioids to remain effective against pain while diminishing the effect on the *mu* receptors in the gut. Treatment must be started preoperatively. Alvimopan has been shown to decrease the duration of postoperative ileus without compromising opioid analgesia and is associated with a shorter length of stay.[24] No increase in morbidity has been reported with this regimen.

SAFETY ISSUES

OPERATING ROOM MEASURES PRIOR TO INCISION

A number of elements reducing patient risk warrant attention in the operating theater before the operative procedure begins. The surgical site is often marked by the surgeon in the preoperative phase to prevent wrong-site surgery, although this is less of a concern in abdominal procedures. Sequential compression devices or pneumatic stockings must be placed *and turned on* before the induction of anesthesia to gain the benefit of venous thrombosis reduction. The surgeon must ensure that antibiotics have been infused, and that standard or low-molecular-weight heparin has been administered, if appropriate. The choice of airway management is made based on the procedure, positioning, patient factors, and the anesthesiologist's clinical judgment.

The patient is properly positioned. Care must be taken to protect the arms from excessive abduction. If the

prone jackknife position is used, special attention must be given to the airway, face, and eyes. Lithotomy or modified lithotomy positioning in Allen stirrups requires attention to the fibular head to prevent compression injury to the common peroneal nerve. When arms are tucked, the elbows must be properly padded to prevent ulnar nerve damage, and the hands must be protected from mobile hardware during position adjustments. Care must be exercised in securing the patient to the table when anticipating position changes to assist in gravity retraction of intraabdominal contents. A suctioned bean-bag placed under the patient may help with secure positioning in these instances.

CHOICE OF SURGICAL APPROACH

LAPAROSCOPIC COLON RESECTION

Laparoscopic colon resection, with intracorporeal or extracorporeal anastomosis, is discussed at length in Chapter 178. The extent of resection must be appropriate for the disease process and is identical whether performed laparoscopically or open. This approach is best suited for patients who have not had extensive abdominal surgery and do not have significant pulmonary embarrassment. However, surgeons skilled in this approach, in partnership with anesthesia colleagues who understand and accept the challenge, have safely extended the employment of this approach. Limitations of this approach include unrecognized injuries to adjacent organs because of limited visibility and longer operative times. Surgeons who acquire this skill in practice have encountered a steep learning curve; trainees learning laparoscopic skills in residency do not experience this challenge in the same way.

ROBOTIC AND ROBOTIC-ASSISTED RESECTION

Robotic and robotic-assisted resection is in its infancy in colorectal surgery. The robotic approach seems particularly useful when the operative field is small, structures are closely juxtaposed, and precision is vital, such as dissection in a narrow pelvis and identification of a nervous plexus.[25] Most reports include relatively few cases that have been carefully selected; these reports agree that the technique is safe and feasible, although operative time is longer, and the additional expense is of concern.

NATURAL ORIFICE TRANSLUMINAL ENDOSCOPIC SURGERY

The goal of natural orifice transluminal endoscopic surgery (NOTES) is to perform surgical procedures in the peritoneum and other body spaces by gaining entry through a natural body orifice and traversing the wall of the gastrointestinal tract, omitting the need for any incision in the abdominal wall. There remain major fundamental goals that must be addressed before NOTES will be ready for wider clinical use, including prevention of infection, instrument development, creation of a multitasking platform, reliable techniques for closure of the iatrogenic incision into the lumen of intraperitoneal organs, and the ability to recognize and manage intraperitoneal complications such as hemorrhage and other adverse events.[26] Most clinical case reports to date have used a hybrid technique that accesses the peritoneal cavity through the vagina, which presents less of a closure issue.

TRANSANAL RESECTION TECHNIQUES

Classic *transanal excision* of rectal lesions, although simple in concept, can prove quite challenging in practice. This approach carries less operative morbidity than transabdominal surgery, but has several technical limitations. The anus is unavoidably stretched to some degree, which can produce alterations in continence, sometimes persistent. Exposure and visibility are limited, making it difficult to access lesions that are more than 4 to 6 cm from the dentate line. (These approaches are discussed at length in Chapter 165.)

Transanal Endoscopic Microsurgery

Transanal endoscopic microsurgery (TEM) extends the boundaries of the classic transanal approach by using a 40-mm-diameter operating rectoscope with sixfold magnification and ports for the manipulation of laparoscopic-type instruments. This technique has been used to resect rectal lesions as high as 24 cm from the anal verge, with acceptable morbidity and mortality. The main drawbacks of TEM are the cost and complexity of the equipment. There also are postoperative alterations in anorectal physiology that appear to persist. However, adequate continence is satisfactorily preserved in most patients.[27]

Evaluation of the role for transanal and TEM excision of rectal cancer continues. Local recurrence rates for histologically proven T1 cancers with an absence of poor prognostic indicators (such as lymphovascular invasion, poor differentiation on histopathology, aneuploidy, or evidence of lymph node involvement on physical examination or imaging) have been reported as widely variable,[28,29] and results of salvage resection after local recurrence have been disappointing.[29] The adjunct roles of radiation and chemotherapy remain controversial.

Transanal Single Port Microsurgery

There have been several recent case reports of successful transanal excision of rectal lesions using a laparoscopic port inserted into the anus.[30] Although early experience shows this approach to be safe in selected patients, and utilizes instrumentation already available at most hospitals, larger multicenter studies should be undertaken for evaluation of the application and safety of this technique.

LAPAROTOMY

Laparotomy is the approach that all others must be compared to when evaluating results. Other approaches must be shown to be as effective and safe. Resection for cancer must adhere to the same principles of oncologic surgery despite the approach employed. Laparotomy remains the approach of choice in most colorectal emergencies that require operative intervention, as well as many cases of recurrent colorectal cancer.

INCISIONS

A vertical midline incision through the linea alba is the incision of choice for colorectal surgery as it is rapidly made, may be easily extended to provide unlimited access to the abdominal cavity, and is swiftly and safely closed. The main disadvantage of the midline approach is a 5% to 10% incidence of incisional hernia. A 2005 Cochrane review reported that transverse incisions have a lower incidence of incisional hernia, cause less pain, and are associated with fewer pulmonary complications[31]; other studies have found no difference in pain or complications. Oblique incisions in the lower quadrants provide reasonably good exposure of the appendix and proximal right colon on the right and of the sigmoid and rectosigmoid colon on the left. Low anterior resection can be performed through a Pfannenstiel incision when the patient's body habitus permits. However, this incision affords limited access to the remainder of the peritoneal cavity. Paramedian incisions were popular in the past, probably because the incidence of ventral herniation seemed lower than that after a midline incision. However, the hernia incidence increases as distance from the midline decreases. Drawbacks of the paramedian approach include more time to enter the peritoneal cavity, more blood loss while the incision is being made, and longer time for the layered closure. Authors tend to agree that the optimal incision remains the surgeon's choice, with consideration of the disease, planned procedure, and patient's body habitus.

Closure of abdominal incisions should follow the surgical principles of gentle tissue handling and proper hemostasis. Results from studies using human cadaveric fascia in suture pullout tests suggest that sutures used to close the abdominal wound should optimally be spaced 10 to 15 mm apart.[32] A recent metaanalysis of elective midline laparotomy closure revealed significantly lower hernia rates when a continuous, slowly absorbable suture material was used[33] when compared to interrupted sutures and rapidly absorbable or braided suture materials.[34] A number of reports have evaluated prophylactic reinforcement of incisions felt to be at high risk for hernia formation with various forms of mesh,[35] including stoma sites[36]; herniation rates appear to be lower, but other wound complications occur that must be managed.[35] Longer followup of patients with prophylactic mesh placement at the time of incision closure or stoma creation may elucidate the risks and benefits of this approach.

RESECTION—EXTENT, INTENT, AND PALLIATIVE THERAPY

When the colon is resected for inflammatory bowel disease, diverticulitis, or other benign conditions, less bowel and mesentery are resected than when operating for cancer. In resecting the colon or rectum for carcinoma, the main vascular supply of the cancer-bearing segment is divided at or close to its origin, which by definition devascularizes a larger portion of the bowel, above and below the site of the tumor. The mesentery supporting the pathway of lymphatic drainage is excised en bloc with the bowel. Straightforward resections are well described in several texts and will not be reproduced here.

COLON OBSTRUCTION

PATHOPHYSIOLOGY OF OBSTRUCTION AND GOALS OF TREATMENT

Acute obstruction of the colon requires prompt relief. Distention of the colon is associated with increased intraluminal pressure, which decreases colonic wall blood flow and shunts blood preferentially to the muscularis propria and away from the mucosa, compromising mucosal integrity. Potential sequelae include colonic perforation and sepsis. The small bowel may be dilated if the ileocecal valve is incompetent. Large-volume third-space fluid losses occur, resulting in hypovolemia and electrolyte imbalances. Progressive abdominal distention provokes respiratory embarrassment. The goal of intervention in patients is relief of the obstruction and treatment of the underlying cause, if clinically indicated, at the same procedure. Management depends on both the cause and the location of the obstruction. Peritonitis requires urgent exploration regardless of the cause. A sigmoid or cecal colonic volvulus may be reduced by sigmoidoscopy or colonoscopy, permitting an elective approach for definitive therapy. Inflammatory lesions, such as diverticulitis and Crohn disease, may improve with intensive medical therapy, bowel rest, and nutritional support, allowing resection on an elective basis, particularly when the obstruction is partial. Aside from simple diversion, nearly all cases of acute colonic obstruction managed operatively are approached via laparotomy as colonic distention and potential fecal spillage are difficult to manage laparoscopically.

RESECTABLE, POTENTIALLY CURABLE OBSTRUCTING COLORECTAL CANCERS

Right colonic obstruction often presents clinically as a small bowel obstruction, and the colon distal to the obstruction may be empty. Management consists of right colectomy, with primary ileocolonic anastomosis or formation of end ileostomy as clinically indicated. Morbidity rates are quite acceptable. The remainder of the colon must be evaluated for synchronous lesions at an appropriate time. Intraoperative palpation of the colon is known to miss lesions, even with full mobilization of both flexures.

The historical approach for left-sided obstruction included three stages. The initial step was fecal diversion for relief of obstruction. A colostomy is generally performed; closed-loop obstruction results when an ileostomy is constructed in the patient with a competent ileocecal valve. Interval resection of the lesion followed when clinically indicated. Lastly, the stoma was closed. This approach carried excessive morbidity and mortality rates and is rarely indicated today. Current management is usually resection of the obstructing lesion with end stoma (a *Hartmann procedure*), or resection with immediate anastomosis, with or without a proximal loop stoma. The Hartmann procedure is chosen when patients are very ill or when other circumstances such as anemia, hypotension, hypoalbuminemia, and steroid medications make anastomosis inadvisable. Evaluation of the proximal colon should take place within a reasonable period. One must recall that closure of a Hartmann procedure requires a formal laparotomy. It is reported that up to 50% of patients after Hartmann never come to stoma closure because of comorbidities.

Total abdominal colectomy with either ileostomy or ileorectal anastomosis may also be performed in left-sided obstruction. Advantages include removal of the disease process, no requirement for a bowel preparation or investigation for synchronous lesions, easy irrigation of the rectum before anastomosis if one is performed, and avoidance of a stoma if ileoproctostomy is performed. The rectum must be free of disease and suitable for anastomosis, which can be easily assessed in the operating room with either rigid or flexible sigmoidoscopy. Operative morbidity and mortality are acceptable, even in elderly patients; however, the postoperative bowel alterations are tolerated poorly by some patients. Intraoperative colonic lavage proponents argue that the technique allows urgent resections to be more limited, promoting better postoperative colonic function. Drawbacks of intraoperative colonic lavage include patient hypothermia, requirement for operating room personnel experienced in the technique, and prolongation of the operation. Because most operations for obstruction are urgent, patients may be expected to be less than fit, making it difficult to justify the additional time and potential morbidity of intraoperative colonic lavage.

Pelvic malignancies often have contiguous involvement of adjacent structures, necessitating en bloc removal of disease, even if resection may be palliative. The simplest case is rectal cancer that involves one or more loops of small bowel. For patients with more complex involvement, such as bladder, vagina, pelvic side wall, sacrum, prostate, or pelvic vasculature, preoperative planning for a team approach may include specialists in urology, gynecologic oncology, orthopedic or neurosurgery, plastic surgery, vascular surgery, radiation oncology, and wound/ostomy nursing specialists.

MANAGEMENT STRATEGIES IN UNRESECTABLE CANCERS

Up to 20% to 30% of those with colorectal cancer present with unresectable disease. The patient's nutritional state is compromised, and many have additional serious comorbidities as well. Fecal diversion has often been used in this setting but carries the risks associated with anesthesia, surgery, and stoma care, while doing little to alleviate cancer-related bleeding or pain. The obstructing lesion may be bypassed, sparing the patient a stoma, but other operative risks remain, bowel habits are frequently altered, and again, complications other than obstruction are not addressed. Surgical resection of the primary lesion has long been felt to produce results superior to bypass alone in patients with unresectable disease who are fit enough to tolerate surgery. However, as more experience is gained with nonoperative management, this approach has been reevaluated.

Neodymium:yttrium-aluminum-garnet or diode laser energy can be used endoluminally to recanalize obstructing lesions in patients considered poor surgical candidates. Large series have shown this approach to be effective, less costly, and less morbid than standard palliative surgical treatment. Laser energy also successfully manages bleeding from unresectable cancers.[37,38]

Endoscopic stenting of obstructing colon lesions is safe and leads to earlier hospital discharge and lower costs than surgical palliation.[39,40] If necessary, this may be preceded with laser recanalization or bleeding treatment. Several types of stent have been used; the most common is the self-expanding bare metal mesh stent. Most reports describe stenting in the left colon and rectum, but stents can also be safely placed in the proximal colon. Morbidity rates are acceptably low in most series, consisting chiefly of stent dislodgement or migration, bowel perforation, and reobstruction from tumor ingrowth during the patient's remaining life span.[41] Though infrequent, these complications are quite serious, almost always requiring surgical intervention, and associated with a high morbidity rate.

MEDICAL TREATMENT OF LOCALLY ADVANCED STAGE IV DISEASE

Several recently published studies present persuasive evidence that intensive medical treatment with chemotherapy, and radiation when indicated, results in avoidance of surgical or endoscopic intervention in the majority of patients with stage IV colorectal cancer.[42,43] Ballian et al also showed that findings at colonoscopy could not predict if near-obstructing lesions would progress to complete obstruction during treatment.[42] This approach has the potential to avoid significant procedure-related morbidity in most stage IV patients, and perhaps also provide a better quality of life during disease management.

ANASTOMOSES

Intestinal anastomoses are fashioned in a variety of ways, with the specific technique used largely a function of

surgeon preference. Hand-sewn anastomoses have become less common with the proliferation of intestinal stapling devices. Nevertheless, knowledge of the techniques for creating a hand-sewn anastomosis remains a key part of surgical education, as every surgeon will have a stapler misfire sometime in his or her career. Sutureless anastomotic techniques have not gained wide acceptance in the United States despite initial favorable reports.

SUTURED ANASTOMOSES

Many types of absorbable and nonabsorbable suture material have been used in intestinal anastomoses. Good surgical technique, including gentle handling of the bowel, adequate hemostasis, meticulous approximation of well-vascularized bowel, and a tension-free anastomosis are more important than the choice of suture material. Two-layer anastomoses are common, with some technical variations. The inner layer is usually an absorbable 3-0 or 4-0 running full-thickness stitch, and the outer layer is an inverting, usually 3-0, seromuscular stitch, which may be running or interrupted, absorbable or nonabsorbable. The outer posterior row is placed first (Figure 177-1). The inner row is then placed, posterior

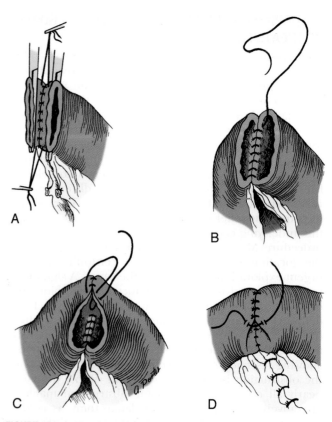

FIGURE 177-1 Two-layer, hand-sewn, end-to-end anastomosis. **A,** Placement of posterior outer layer of Lembert stitches. **B,** Inner posterior layer, shown as continuous, but may also be interrupted. **C,** Inner anterior layer, shown here as Connell stitch. **D,** Outer anterior layer of Lembert seromuscular stitches. (From Zinner MJ, Schwartz SI, Ellis H, editors: *Maingot's abdominal operations*, ed 10. Stamford, Conn, 1997, Appleton & Lange.)

wall first, followed by the anterior wall. The anterior outer row is the last completed.

One-layer anastomoses are preferred by some surgeons. A full-thickness technique, interrupted (Figure 177-2, *A*) or running (Figure 177-2, *B*), with absorbable or nonabsorbable suture is common for hand-sewn colorectal anastomoses. An interrupted inverting seromuscular technique can also be used for small bowel, colon, or colorectal anastomoses, with silk, polyglycolic acid (Vicryl), or polyglycolitic acid (Dexon), size 3-0 or 4-0 (Figure 177-3). Both single-layer methods produce secure anastomoses with rates of stricture and leak comparable to those of the two-layer technique. Hand-sewn coloanal or ileal pouch–anal anastomoses are usually

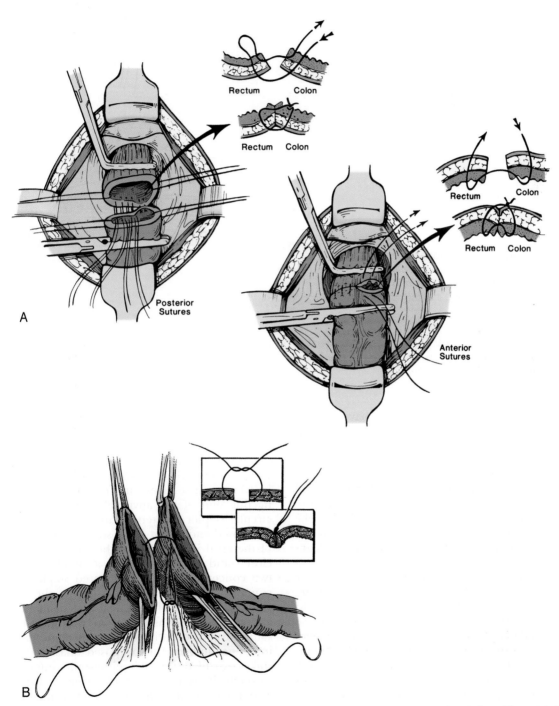

FIGURE 177-2 One-layer, full-thickness, end-to-end, hand-sewn low anterior anastomosis. **A,** Interrupted technique. The posterior row is placed first, with knots tied on the mucosal side. The anterior row is then placed. Knots may be tied on the mucosal or serosal side. **B,** Continuous technique. The suture is begun on the posterior wall, with the knot tied on the serosal side. The suture is continued in a running fashion. (**B** from Max E, Sweeney WB, Bailey HR, et al: Results of 1,000 single-layer continuous polypropylene intestinal anastomoses. *Am J Surg* 162:461, 1991.)

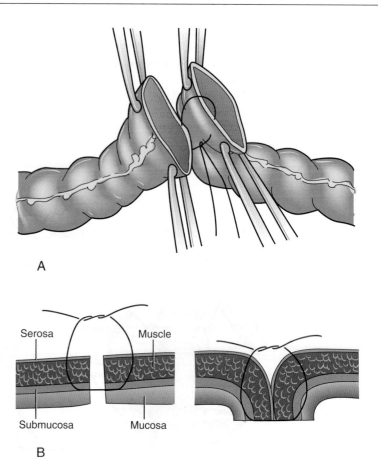

FIGURE 177-3 One-layer seromuscular anastomosis.
A, Operative appearance. The posterior row is placed first.
B, Detail of stitch placement. Care is taken to invert the
mucosa, which is not incorporated into the suture.

fashioned with one layer of interrupted absorbable sutures, with each suture incorporating the full thickness of both components of the anastomosis.

STAPLED ANASTOMOSES

Modern surgical gastrointestinal staplers have evolved from the first 1950s-era Russian prototypes. Staplers can be used to construct anastomoses in any portion of the gastrointestinal tract, and many techniques have been described. Stapled and sutured anastomoses have been extensively compared. A Cochrane review of colorectal anastomoses found no superiority of one type of anastomosis over another.[44] A later Cochrane review of ileocolic anastomosis found that stapled functional end-to-end ileocolic anastomoses were associated with fewer leaks than hand-sewn ileocolic anastomoses.[45]

The **linear stapling-cutting devices** place two linear double rows of staggered staples and divide the tissue between the two double rows. These staplers are used to divide the bowel with closure of both sides. This device can also be used to fashion a side-to-side (functional end-to-end) anastomosis (Figure 177-4), with the resultant enterotomy closed by application of a **linear stapler** (see Figure 177-7), which places two linear staggered rows of staples. Excess tissue is removed with a scissor, as this stapling device does not contain a knife. The linear stapling-cutting devices for laparotomy are available in several lengths between 50 and 100 mm and in two staple heights. The linear staplers are available in several lengths from 30 to 90 mm, and in two staple heights. Variations

include a linear stapler with a reticulating head, and a stapling-cutting device with a handle fashioned after the classic linear stapler.

Circular staplers are used to construct end-to-end or end-to-side anastomoses. The stapler (Figure 177-5) consists of a tubular body and a detachable anvil. The body of the stapler is most often passed per anus to the end of the rectal stump, which has been closed with a purse-string stitch (Figure 177-6) or a linear stapler (Figure 177-7). The anvil is secured within the proximal bowel by tying a purse-string suture securely around the connecting end of the anvil. The spike contained in the circular stapler is extended under direct vision through the closed end of the rectal stump. The connecting end of the anvil is placed onto the spike, and the stapler is closed and fired, producing a circular anastomosis of two concentric rows of staggered staples. The stapler contains a circular knife that excises the excess tissue. Colorectal, coloanal, and ileal pouch–anal anastomoses are commonly constructed in this way. The circular stapler can also be introduced through an enterotomy into one limb of the proposed anastomosis, with the spike extruded through either the intestinal wall or through the stapled or purse-stringed closed end. The anvil is secured into the other limb of the intended anastomosis. The anvil is placed onto the stapler spike as usual, and the stapler is closed and fired, and then extracted. The enterotomy used to introduce the circular stapler must be closed separately—often with the linear stapler.

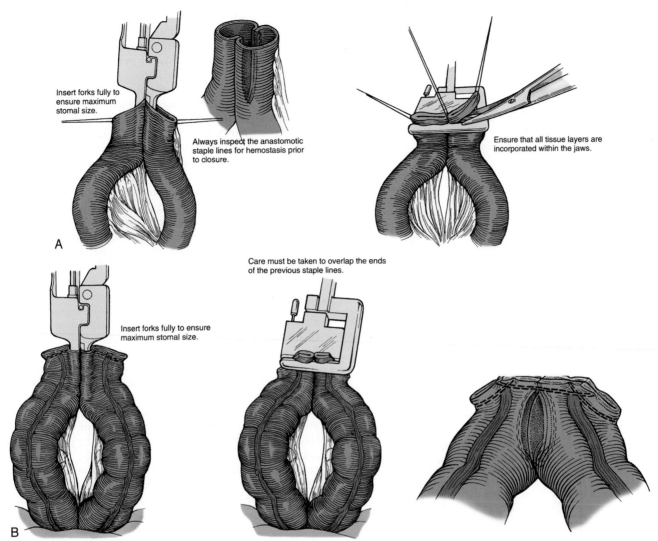

FIGURE 177-4 A, Side-to-side (functional end-to-end) small bowel anastomosis performed with the linear-cutting stapler. The enterotomy is closed with a linear stapler. **B,** Side-to-side (functional end-to-end) colonic anastomosis done with the linear-cutting stapler. The enterotomy is closed with a linear-type stapler. (From Zinner MJ, Schwartz SI, Ellis H, editors: *Maingot's abdominal operations*, ed 10. Stamford, Conn, 1997, Appleton & Lange.)

SUTURELESS ANASTOMOSES

The earliest reported compression device for bowel anastomosis was the Murphy button of the 1920s. Biofragmentable compression devices have been used in intestinal anastomosis for more than 15 years, and though results are good,[46] the devices have not become widely used in the United States. Other methods of compression anastomosis are being developed, including magnetic devices[47] and nickel-titanium alloy shape-memory devices.[48] Various glues have been studied in animal model intestinal anastomosis; however, safety is not yet acceptable for clinical use. Studies of intestinal anastomoses performed in rats using *n*-butyl-2-cyanoacrylate, synthetic glue, showed that glued anastomoses had lower bursting pressures, higher stricture rates, and significantly more inflammatory response than sutured anastomoses.[49] Laser-welded anastomoses have shown some early promise in experimental studies, and further investigation is ongoing.

ANASTOMOSIS OR STOMA?

A satisfactory anastomosis is likely to result if all of the following questions can be answered in the affirmative regardless of the anastomotic technique used. Is the patient stable? Is the resection complete? Is hemostasis satisfactory? Has all debris been removed from the proposed anastomotic site? Are both ends of the intestine healthy and well vascularized? Will the proposed anastomosis be tension free? Leak rates of 2% to 5% after intraperitoneal colonic anastomoses and 5% to 10% after colorectal anastomoses are expected. However, if the patient becomes unstable intraoperatively, rapidly performed diversion is indicated, and continuity may be reestablished at a subsequent appropriate time. In the event of peritonitis with fecal or purulent soilage of the peritoneal cavity, resection of the diseased segment with fecal diversion remains the standard of care. If the proximal bowel is not able to hold sutures or staples, diversion is necessary. Risk factors for poor

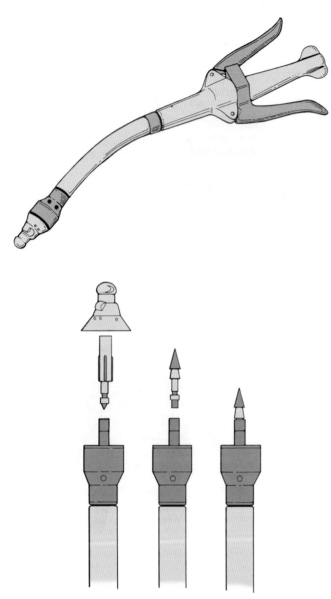

FIGURE 177-5 Circular-type staplers. Note detachable anvil and snap-on trocar.

outcome—intraperitoneal contamination, peritonitis, emergency operation, and septic patient—should overrule the desire to spare the patient from the difficulty of living with a stoma, even temporarily.

Anastomosis may present a challenge when the proximal and distal bowel diameters differ significantly. A side-to-side anastomosis (functional end-to-end) is often performed in this setting (see Figure 177-4). An end-to-side anastomosis can also be constructed using the end of the dilated segment to the side of the normal segment of bowel. An end-to-end anastomosis may be fashioned by transecting the normal bowel at an angle, with the longer end at the mesenteric side to preserve blood supply, and anastomosing this to the transected larger segment.

In the absence of an anastomotic leak, the mortality rate after colorectal resection is 2%; with a leak, mortality is as high as 10%. Function and oncologic outcome are also worse after pelvic anastomotic leak.[50] When the risk for anastomotic leak is elevated, and the patient would be unlikely to survive such a complication, consideration of the patient's general status should guide the surgical choice. If the patient's clinical performance is unlikely to improve sufficiently to allow closure of a diverting stoma to be considered in the future, the patient will be best served by a well-planned end stoma. However, if the patient's clinical situation can logically be expected to improve, anastomosis with proximal diversion is a valid option. Creation of a proximal diverting stoma has been shown to decrease complications associated with a pelvic anastomotic leak, although there is no mortality advantage.[51] The loop stoma is usually closed 10 to 12 weeks after the initial procedure. Still, some patients never improve sufficiently for stoma closure to be undertaken. This highlights the importance of meticulous planning for and performance of every stoma, because some stomas intended to be temporary will become lifelong.

IMPROVING SURGICAL CARE

Following pilot studies in the Veterans Administration healthcare system and 14 academic institutions, the American College of Surgeons' National Surgical Quality Improvement Program (NSQIP) invited participation by private sector hospitals across the country in 2004. The goal of the program is measurement and improvement of the quality of surgical care in the United States. Evaluation of data collected between 2005 and 2007 showed that 66% of hospitals improved with respect to risk-adjusted mortality and 82% improved in risk-adjusted complication rates. Although hospitals that had initially performed worse had more likelihood of improvement, better-performing hospitals also showed improvement.[52]

Information gleaned from the database has in some instances highlighted additional areas of patient care that can benefit from redirection of improvement efforts. Evaluation of outcomes for elderly (>75 years) patients undergoing upper gastrointestinal tract, hepatobiliary, pancreatic, or colorectal operations over a 2-year period showed that after adjusting for differences in preoperative comorbidities, perioperative morbidity was 1.2 to 2 times higher, and mortality was 2.9 to 6.7 times higher than that observed in younger patients. The elderly were significantly more likely to have cardiac, pulmonary, and urologic complications, whereas SSIs, postoperative bleeding events, DVTs, and rates of return to the operating room did not differ.[53] This information can help hospitals focus improvement efforts for elderly patients in specific high-risk areas. Similarly, an outcomes comparison of nonemergency versus emergency operations in 142 hospitals over 3 years revealed that hospitals with favorable outcomes after nonemergency colorectal resections do not necessarily have similar outcomes for emergency operations.[54] This suggests that hospitals examine their emergency surgery procedures to identify areas of concern, and focus quality improvement efforts appropriately.

As the reality of "pay for performance" looms nearer, the ability for surgeons to evaluate outcomes and identify areas that would benefit from focused efforts at improvement is a tool as powerful and revolutionary as any

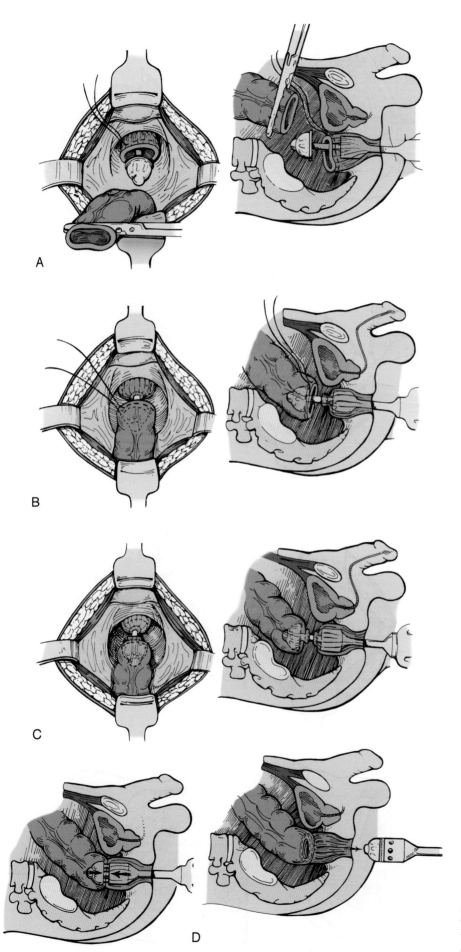

FIGURE 177-6 Stapled low anterior resection with proximal and distal purse-string sutures. **A,** The stapler is passed gently transanally until the anvil protrudes from the sectioned edge of the rectum. The distal purse string is secured around the inferior edge of the anvil shaft. **B,** The proximal colon is placed onto the anvil. **C,** The proximal purse string is tied around the upper end of the anvil shaft. **D,** The stapler is closed to the desired degree and fired, completing the anastomosis. The stapler is then gently withdrawn.

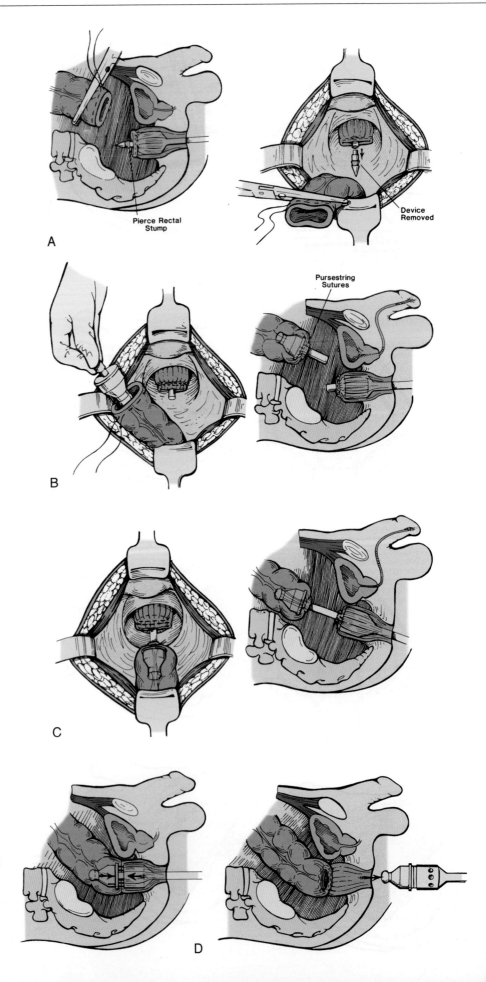

FIGURE 177-7 Stapled low anterior anastomosis performed with double-stapled technique. **A,** The stapler is passed transanally to the end of the rectal stump. The instrument is slowly opened; the trocar pierces the end of the stump, which has been closed by an application of the linear stapler. **B,** The anvil is placed into the proximal bowel and tied into place with a purse-string suture. **C,** The anvil is snapped onto the shaft of the stapler. **D,** The stapler is closed to the desired degree and fired, completing the anastomosis. The stapler is then gently withdrawn.

technologic advance to date. Participation in surgeon-led efforts to improve the performance of our profession and keep our patients safe is a clear demonstration of the commitment of surgeons to deliver care of the highest quality.

ANNOTATED REFERENCES

Contant CME, Hop WCJ, van 't Sant HP, et al: Mechanical bowel preparation for elective colorectal surgery: A multicentre randomized trial. *Lancet* 370:2112, 2007.

Slim K, Vicaut E, Panis Y, et al: Meta-analysis of randomized clinical trials of colorectal surgery with or without mechanical bowel preparation. *Br J Surg* 91:1125, 2004.

These papers, a randomized multicenter trial (Contant et al) and a literature review (Slim et al) of bowel washout vs. no washout before elective colorectal resection, include 2885 patients. The results do not show any advantage to bowel washout prior to elective colorectal surgery. Disadvantages to washout include patient inconvenience, fluid and electrolyte alterations, and cost. Several studies have noted that complications of anastomotic leak are lower after bowel washout, but the numbers in these groups are small. While risks may differ in very low anastomoses, the data is not yet clear. Omission of bowel washout is also a component of enhanced recovery after resection programs, which have been shown to safely accelerate recovery after elective bowel surgery and reduce costs.

Doornebosch PG, Ferenschild FT, deWilt JH, et al: Treatment of recurrence after transanal endoscopic microsurgery (Tem) for T1 rectal cancer. *Dis Colon Rectum* 53:1234, 2010.

Tsai BM, Finne CO, Nordenstam JF, et al: Transanal endoscopic microsurgery resection for rectal tumors: Outcomes and recommendations. *Dis Colon Rectum* 53:16, 2010.

The debate over transanal excision of early rectal cancer continues. Technologic advances have allowed surgeons to push the limits of resection, but the lower morbidity of a transanal or TEM resection must be weighed against higher local recurrence rate and salvage rates that are disappointingly low. Considering the poor outcome of even highly selected T1 rectal cancers, these papers have provided important data that questions the role of transanal/TEM excision of rectal cancer.

Spyropoulos AC, Hussein M, Lin J, Battleman D: Rates of symptomatic venous thromboembolism in US surgical patients: A retrospective administrative database study. *J Thromb Thrombolysis* 28:458, 2009.

The current practice of working toward outcome improvement via systems-based approaches has led to intense scrutiny of many areas where improvement is possible, and expected. Decrease of venous thromboembolic events (VTE) has been identified as one such outcome. The data discussed in this paper suggest that current VTE-prophylaxis guidelines may be insufficient, as there remains a risk for VTE beyond the acute hospital phase that is not currently routinely addressed. The authors provide persuasive evidence that VTE prophylaxis should be continued for 30 days after hospital discharge in patients at elevated risk.

Basse L, Jakobsen DH, Bardram L, et al: Functional recovery after open versus laparoscopic colonic resection: A randomized, blinded study. *Ann Surg* 241:416, 2005.

Lassen K, Soop M, Nygren J, et al: Consensus review of optimal perioperative ccare in colorectal surgery. *Arch Surg* 144:961, 2009.

Enhanced recovery after surgery (ERAS) programs have been proven to shorten hospital stays, improve patient care, reduce complications, and lower costs. While measures contained in most ERAS programs are often employed in postoperative care, it appears that the program as a whole provides the greatest benefit. No additional benefit has been proven when the laparoscopic approach is included with an ERAS program; however, most laparoscopic surgeons already employ many of the measures in ERAS programs.

Ballian N, Mahvi DM, Kennedy GD: Colonoscopic findings and tumor site do not predict bowel obstruction during medical treatment of stage IV colorectal cancer. *Oncologist* 14:580, 2009.

Poultsides GA, Servais EL, Saltz LB, et al: Outcome of primary tumor in patients with synchronous state IV colorectal cncer receiving combination chemotherapy without surgery as initial treatment. *J Clin Oncol* 27:3379, 2009.

Surgeons have long preferred resection of the primary in Stage IV disease in reasonably fit patients due to concerns about potential bleeding and obstructive complications. As newer chemotherapy agents began to prolong survival in Stage IV patients, these concerns initially appeared magnified. These reports demonstrate the validity of nonoperative management for this group of patients, with decreased treatment-related morbidity and perhaps also an improved quality of life.

REFERENCES

1. Webster J, Osborne S: Preoperative bathing or showering with skin antiseptics to prevent surgical site infection. *Cochrane Database Syst Rev* 2:CD004985, 2007.
2. Noblett SE, Watson DS, Huong H, et al: Pre-operative oral carbohydrate loading in colorectal surgery: A randomized controlled trial. *Colorectal Dis* 8:563, 2006.
3. Russmann S, Lamerato L, Motsko SP, et al: Risk of further decline in renal function after the use of oral sodium phosphate or polyethylene glycol in patients with a preexisting glomerular filtration rate below 60 ml/min. *Am J Gastroenterol* 103:2707, 2008.
4. Slim K, Vicaut E, Panis Y, et al: Meta-analysis of randomized clinical trials of colorectal surgery with or without mechanical bowel preparation. *Br J Surg* 91:1125, 2004.
5. Guenaga KKFG, Matos D, Wille-Jorgensen P: Mechanical bowel preparation for elective colorectal surgery. *Cochrane Database Syst Rev* 1:CD001544, 2009.
6. Contant CME, Hop WCJ, van't Sant HP, et al: Mechanical bowel preparation for elective colorectal surgery: A multicentre randomized trial. *Lancet* 370:2112, 2007.
7. Platell C, Barwood N, Makin G: Randomized clinical trial of bowel preparation with a single phosphate enema or polyethylene glycol before elective colorectal surgery. *Br J Surg* 93:427, 2006.
8. Nelson RL, Glenny AM, Song F: Antimicrobial prophylaxis for colorectal surgery. *Cochrane Database Syst Rev* 1:CD001181, 2009.
9. Espin-Basany E, Sanchez-Garcia JL, Lopez-Cano M, et al: Prospective, randomized study on antibiotic prophylaxis in colorectal surgery. Is it really necessary to use oral antibiotics? *Int J Colorectal Dis* 20:542, 2005.
10. Wren SM, Ahmed N, Jamal A, et al: Preoperative oral antibiotics in colorectal surgery increase the rate of *Clostridium difficile* colitis. *Arch Surg* 140:752, 2005.
11. Zerey M, Paton BL, Lincourt AE, et al: The burden of *Clostridium difficile* in surgical patients in the United States. *Surg Infect (Larchmt)* 8:557, 2007.
12. Bakken JS: Fecal bacteriotherapy for recurrent *Clostridium difficile* infection. *Anaerobe* 15:285, 2009.
13. Sailhamer EA, Carson K, Chang Y, et al: Fulminant *Clostridium difficile* colitis: Patterns of care and predictors of mortality. *Arch Surg* 144:433, 2009.

14. Darouiche R, Wall MJ Jr, Itani KMF, et al: Chlorhexidine-alcohol versus povidone-iodine for surgical-site antisepsis. *N Engl J Med* 362:18, 2010.

15. Swenson BR, Hedrick TL, Metzger R, et al: Effects of preoperative skin preparation on postoperative wound infection rates: A prospective study of 3 skin preparation protocols. *Infect Control Hosp Epidemiol* 30:964, 2009.

16. Stahl JB, Morse D, Parks PJ: Resistance of antimicrobial skin preparations to saline rinse using a seeded bacteria model. *Am J Infect Control* 35:367, 2007.

17. Bates SM, Ginsberg JS: Clinical practice. Treatment of deep-vein thrombosis. *N Engl J Med* 351:268, 2004.

18. Geerts WH, Bergqvist D, Pineo GF, et al: Prevention of venous thromboembolism: American College of Chest Physicians evidence-based clinical practice guidelines (8th edition). *Chest* 133:381S, 2008.

19. Bergqvist D: Venous thromboembolism: A review of risk and prevention in colorectal surgery patients. *Dis Colon Rectum* 49:1620, 2006.

20. Spyropoulos AC, Hussein M, Lin J, et al: Rates of symptomatic venous thromboembolism in US surgical patients: A retrospective administrative database study. *J Thromb Thrombolysis* 28:458, 2009.

21. Rasmussen MS, Jorgensen LN, Wille-Jorgensen P: Prolonged thromboprophylaxis with low molecular weight heparin for abdominal or pelvic surgery. *Cochrane Database Syst Rev* 1:CD004318, 2009.

22. Lassen K, Soop M, Nygren J, et al: Consensus review of optimal perioperative care in colorectal surgery. *Arch Surg* 144:961, 2009.

23. Basse L, Jakobsen DH, Bardram L, et al: Functional recovery after open versus laparoscopic colonic resection: A randomized, blinded study. *Ann Surg* 241:416, 2005.

24. Ludwig K, Enker WE, Delaney CP, et al: Gastrointestinal tract recovery in patients undergoing bowel resection: Results of a randomized trial of alvimopan and placebo with a standardized accelerated postoperative care pathway. *Arch Surg* 143:1098, 2008.

25. D'Annibale A, Morpurgo E, Fiscon V, et al: Robotic and laparoscopic surgery for treatment of colorectal diseases. *Dis Colon Rectum* 47:2162, 2004.

26. Karimyan V, Sodergren M, Clark J, et al: Navigation systems and platforms in natural orifice transluminal endoscopic surgery (NOTES). *Int J Surg* 7:297, 2009.

27. Jin Z, Yin L, Xue L, et al: Anorectal functional results after transanal endoscopic microsurgery in benign and early malignant tumors. *World J Surg* 34:1128, 2010.

28. Doornebosch PG, Ferenschild FT, deWilt JH, et al: Treatment of recurrence after transanal endoscopic microsurgery (TEM) for T1 rectal cancer. *Dis Colon Rectum* 53:1234, 2010.

29. Tsai BM, Finne CO, Nordenstam JF, et al: Transanal endoscopic microsurgery resection for rectal tumors: Outcomes and recommendations. *Dis Colon Rectum* 53:16, 2010.

30. Lorenz C, Nimmesgern T, Back M, et al: Transanal single port microsurgery (TSPM) as modified technique of transanal endoscopic microsurgery (TEM). *Surg Innov* 17:160, 2010.

31. Brown SR, Goodfellow PB: Transverse versus midline incisions for abdominal surgery. *Cochrane Database Syst Rev* 4:CD005199, 2005.

32. DesCoteaux JG, Temple WJ, Huchcroft SA, et al: Linea alba closure: Determination of ideal distance between sutures. *J Invest Surg* 6:201, 1993.

33. Diener MK, Voss S, Jensen K, et al: Elective midline laparotomy closure: The INLINE systematic review and meta-analysis. *Ann Surg* 251:843, 2010.

34. Ruchinski J, Margolis M, Panagopoulos G, et al: Closure of the abdominal midline fascia: Meta-analysis delineates the optimal technique. *Am Surg* 67:421, 2001.

35. El-Khadrawy OH, Moussa G, Mansour O, et al: Prophylactic prosthetic reinforcement of midline abdominal incisions in high-risk patients. *Hernia* 13:267, 2009.

36. Wijeyekoon SP, Gurusamy K, El-Gendy K, et al: Prevention of parastomal herniation with biologic/composite prosthetic mesh: A systematic review and meta-analysis of randomized controlled trials. *J Am Coll Surg* 211:637, 2010.

37. Jakobs R, Miola J, Eickhoff A, et al: Endoscopic laser palliation for rectal cancer—therapeutic outcome and complications in eighty-three consecutive patients. *Z Gastroenterol* 40:551, 2002.

38. Courtney ED, Raja A, Leicester RJ: Eight years experience of high-powered endoscopic diode laser therapy for palliation of colorectal carcinoma. *Dis Colon Rectum* 48:845, 2005.

39. Carne PW, Frye JN, Robertson GM, et al: Stents or open operation for palliation of colorectal cancer: A retrospective, cohort study of perioperative outcome and long-term survival. *Dis Colon Rectum* 47:1455, 2004.

40. Tilney HS, Lovegrove RE, Purkayastha S, et al: Comparison of colonic stenting and open surgery for malignant large bowel obstruction. *Surg Endosc* 21:225, 2007.

41. Fernandez-Esparrach G, Bordas JM, Giraldez MD, et al: Severe complications limit long-term clinical success of self-expanding metal stents in patients with obstructive colorectal cancer. *Am J Gastroenterol* 105:1087, 2010.

42. Ballian N, Mahvi DM, Kennedy GD: Colonoscopic findings and tumor site do not predict bowel obstruction during medical treatment of stage IV colorectal cancer. *Oncologist* 14:580, 2009.

43. Poultsides GA, Servais EL, Saltz LB, et al: Outcome of primary tumor in patients with synchronous stage IV colorectal cancer receiving combination chemotherapy without surgery as initial treatment. *J Clin Oncol* 27:3379, 2009.

44. Lustosa SA, Matos D, Atallah AN, et al: Stapled versus handsewn methods for colorectal anastomosis surgery. *Cochrane Database Syst Rev* 3:CD003144, 2001.

45. Choy PY, Bissett IP, Docherty JG, et al: Stapled versus handsewn methods for ileocolic anastomosis. *Cochrane Database Syst Rev* 9:CD004320, 2011.

46. Forde KA, Goodell KH, DellaBadia M: A 10-year single-institutional study of the biofragmentable anastomosis ring. *Am J Surg* 191:483, 2006.

47. Jamshidi R, Stephenson JT, Clay JG, et al: Magnamosis: Magnetic compression anastomosis with comparison to suture and staple techniques. *J Pediatr Surg* 44:222, 2009.

48. Tulchinsky H, Kashtan H, Rabau M, et al: Evaluation of the NiTi shape memory BioDynamix ColonRing in colorectal anastomosis: First in human multi-center study. *Int J Colorectal Dis* 25:1453, 2010.

49. Bae K-B, Kim S-H, Jung S-J, et al: Cyanoacrylate for colonic anastomosis; is it safe? *Int J Colorectal Dis* 25:601, 2010.

50. Law WL, Choi HK, Lee YM, et al: Anastomotic leakage is associated with poor long-term outcome in patients after curative colorectal resection for malignancy. *J Gastrointest Surg* 11:8, 2007.

51. Montedori A, Cirocchi R, Farinella E, et al: Covering ileo- or colostomy in anterior resection for rectal carcinoma. *Cochrane Database Syst Rev* 5:CD006878, 2010.

52. Hall BL, Hamilton BH, Richards K, et al: Does surgical quality improve in the American College of Surgeons National Surgical Quality Improvement Program: An evaluation of all participating hospitals. *Ann Surg* 250:363, 2009.

53. Bentrem DJ, Cohen ME, Hynes DM, et al: Identification of specific quality improvement opportunities for the elderly undergoing gastrointestinal surgery. *Arch Surg* 144:1013, 2009.

54. Ingraham AM, Cohen ME, Bilimoria KY, et al: Comparison of hospital performance in nonemergency versus emergency colorectal operations at 142 hospitals. *J Am Coll Surg* 210:155, 2010.

Laparoscopic Colorectal Surgery

David A. Etzioni | Tonia M. Young-Fadok

Laparoscopic techniques in colorectal surgery are the natural result of the successful application of laparoscopy in biliary surgery. Following its introduction in the late 1980s,[1,2] laparoscopic cholecystectomy rapidly became the standard of care; success with this procedure has led naturally to the application of minimally invasive techniques to other intraabdominal organs.

Although it is difficult to state with certainty when the first laparoscopic colorectal resection was performed, a study by Jacobs et al is likely the first significant series of such procedures.[1] This initial report was appropriately cautious, but was prescient in stating that laparoscopic colonic surgery "has the potential to be as popular as laparoscopic cholecystectomy." In the 2 decades since this initial experience was published, laparoscopic colorectal surgery has become an accepted standard of care for patients requiring a wide array of colon and rectal operations.

The development of laparoscopic colorectal surgical techniques has involved the accumulation of experience with a broad range of approaches. Initially the laparoscopic approach was used for procedures such as simple mobilization and colotomy to remove benign lesions. Over time, laparoscopic techniques were applied to the full spectrum of colorectal operations, with encouraging results.

Outcomes with laparoscopic colorectal surgery have not been universally positive. Early in the advent of laparoscopic colon surgery, reports of tumor implantation at the site of minimal access incisions prompted a period of reflection in this rapidly growing area.[2] An influential report published in 1996 by Johnstone et al identified 35 cases of port site recurrences among patients undergoing laparoscopic or thoracoscopic surgery for malignancy.[3] Based on this report (as well as others) and a growing concern over the safety of colorectal surgery, there emerged the need for well-conducted randomized controlled trials to compare outcomes achieved with laparoscopic versus open approaches.

The field of laparoscopic colon surgery reached maturity with the publication of the Clinical Outcomes of Surgical Therapy (COST) trial in 2004.[4] In this study, 872 patients undergoing right, left, or sigmoid colectomy were randomized to laparoscopic versus open surgery. With a median followup of 4.4 years, there were no differences between the two groups in terms of recurrence rates. Concerns over surgical site implantations were quenched, with less than 1% of patients in either arm experiencing this complication.

Since the publication of results from the COST trial, multiple randomized controlled trials have documented the success of laparoscopic techniques in a variety of contexts. Laparoscopic colectomy is increasingly a focus

of training within accredited colorectal training programs. Athough the technique is certainly becoming more widely applied, it is very difficult to ascertain the proportion of colectomies that are performed laparoscopically, and there are two main reasons for this. First, there are no population-based databases that accurately designate a colectomy according to whether it was performed using laparoscopic versus open techniques. Second, there are issues related to what actually constitutes a laparoscopic procedure. If a procedure is performed that uses laparoscopy to allow for a smaller incision, is this procedure laparoscopic or laparoscopy-assisted? Many leaders in laparoscopic colorectal surgery are proponents of a hand-assisted approach, which is minimally invasive but generally invokes a larger incision than a "straight" laparoscopic approach.

As surgeons have become more comfortable performing laparoscopic colectomies, the extension of the technique to rectal surgery is natural, if not inevitable. Rectal operations, however, incur a set of pragmatic difficulties that make laparoscopic approaches more challenging. Relative to the abdomen, the pelvis is more confined, thereby restricting the extent to which the rectum can be mobilized. Given the initial concerns raised over the risks of implantation with laparoscopic colectomies for cancer, the surgical community has moved forward at a measured pace in examining the outcomes of laparoscopic versus open approaches for rectal cancer.

In this chapter, we review current knowledge regarding the application of laparoscopic surgical techniques in performing colorectal operations. Throughout, we will specifically highlight the results from a growing number of randomized trials in order to supply evidence, rather than opinion, regarding the benefits and challenges of laparoscopic versus open approaches. Despite the obvious distinctions between an operation that is performed laparoscopically as opposed to open, it should be acknowledged that relative to traditional (open) surgery, laparoscopy is a different technique, not a different procedure. The indications and scope of operation should be similar. To the extent that laparoscopy allows for an identical operation to be performed while incurring a lower rate of complications and/or improved patient outcomes, the approach becomes preferable.

OUTCOMES WITH MINIMAL ACCESS VS. OPEN COLORECTAL SURGERY

The benefits of laparoscopy in colorectal surgery were not always assured. Early reports of laparoscopy-assisted colectomy did not show clear advantages, and this was an initial cause of concern.[5,6] Even the early reports from the COST study demonstrated marginal benefits of laparoscopic over open surgery.[7] Considering the increased complexity, expense, and operative time that are generally associated with a laparoscopic procedure, is the procedure justified?

The potential benefits of laparoscopic colectomy include shorter duration of postoperative ileus, reduced pain, decreased need for analgesics, earlier introduction of diet, shorter length of hospital stay, and improved cosmetic appearance. These benefits are countered by longer operative times, the expense of laparoscopic equipment, and a long learning curve. It would seem intuitive that these benefits and detriments could be easily measured in the context of a well-conducted randomized trial. In this section, we review the evidence regarding outcomes experienced by patients who undergo surgery using minimal access versus open techniques for colorectal surgery. As mentioned previously, there is significant difficulty in categorizing (dichotomously) a surgical procedure as having been performed laparoscopically (vs. not). We will therefore include data regarding several different types of comparative studies.

THE LAPAROSCOPIC LEARNING CURVE

In order to interpret the literature regarding the benefits of laparoscopic (vs. open) colorectal surgery, the concept of a learning curve needs to be discussed. It is unreasonable to expect that surgeons' initial efforts with laparoscopic surgical techniques would yield the same experience as that of a trained and/or seasoned laparoscopic surgeon. Several studies have examined the laparoscopic "learning curve," documenting significant improvements in performance, especially with regard to the time required to complete the operation.[8,9]

Each of the large laparoscopic trials had clear criteria that each participating surgeon had to meet regarding their expertise with the approach. In the COST trial, each surgeon had to have performed at least 20 laparoscopic colon resections, and also submit a video that demonstrated appropriate technique.[7] In the ongoing American College of Surgeons Oncology Group (ACOSOG) Z6051 trial, participating surgeons need experience with 20 laparoscopic colon and rectal operations (each) and also must submit a video.[10]

An important question also arises regarding the occurrence of complications throughout the learning curve. Several studies have investigated the relationship between the likelihood of complications at different points in the learning curve. Ozturk et al analyzed a body of 200 hand-assisted operations and found that during the course of this series, operative times shortened considerably but there were no changes in rates of complications.[11] Kiran et al found that although operative times were longer early in the learning curve, that this did not translate into increased costs (other than operative time) or higher rates of complications.[12] The learning curve appears to be of greatest concern in terms of the duration of the operation (and associated costs) but not in terms of complications or other facets of cost or quality of care.

The character of the learning curve may also be different between hand-assisted laparoscopy and "straight" laparoscopic approaches. In a randomized comparison of hand-assisted versus open colectomy, the former resulted in decreased postoperative ileus, shorter length of stay, and smaller incisions with no difference in operative time or complications.[13] Randomized trials comparing hand-assisted with straight laparoscopic techniques found similar functional results with fewer conversions in the former group.[14-16] By allowing surgeons without extensive laparoscopic experience to perform laparoscopic colectomy, it has been suggested that a hand-assisted approach may be more readily learned than a straight laparoscopic approach.

OPERATIVE TIME

Although there exists some variation in the definition of "operative time," the term is most commonly defined as the time between starting an incision and the completion of skin closure. In general, most studies report longer operative times for laparoscopic colorectal procedure relative to a procedure done with an open incision. In prospective randomized trials, this difference has ranged from 20 to 60 minutes longer in the laparoscopic arm.[4,17,18] With experience, operative times do decrease and may become comparable, particularly in the more simple segmental colectomies, such as right and sigmoid resections. There is also evidence that the learning curve has a long tail—operative times are noted to improve gradually even after initial proficiency is achieved.[19]

RETURN OF GASTROINTESTINAL FUNCTION

Return of gastrointestinal function is often the rate-limiting step governing the time at which patients can be safely discharged after a colorectal resection. Several of the major randomized trials examining laparoscopic versus open colorectal resection have documented a clear benefit of laparoscopic surgery over open surgery in terms of resumption of bowel function (Table 178-1).

The underlying factors behind these findings are multifactorial, including less intraoperative bowel manipulation, reduced exposure of the peritoneal cavity to air, less requirement for narcotics, and other unidentified factors. It is worth noting that in canine and porcine models, the return of gastrointestinal motility is demonstrably quicker after laparoscopic intervention.[24-26] The shorter duration of postoperative ileus seems to translate into earlier introduction of liquids and solid food after laparoscopic colectomy.

DURATION OF HOSPITALIZATION

The overall length of stay after a colorectal resection is a composite endpoint that encompasses a broad array of factors. For most patients, the most important of these factors is return of bowel function, but other factors such as complications (especially reoperation), social factors, and the reacquisition of the ability to perform activities of daily living are also important. Intuitively, a minimally invasive surgical approach has the capacity to positively affect each of these factors and thereby engender a shorter length of stay. In Table 178-2, we review the differences in lengths of stay between patients undergoing a minimally invasive versus open approach as seen in the major randomized controlled trials.

TABLE 178-1 Return of Postoperative Gastrointestinal Function: Results of Randomized Controlled Trials

Study	Sample Size	ILEUS (hr)		ILEUS (%)		TIME TO FIRST BOWEL MOVEMENT		TIME TO RESUMPTION OF ANY DIET		TIME TO RESUMPTION OF NORMAL DIET	
		Lap	Open	Lap	Open	Lap	Open	Lap	Open	Lap	Open
COLOR, 2005[20]	1082					3.6 d	4.6 d				
CLASICC, 2005[*, 17]	498					5 d	6 d			5 d	6 d
Braga et al, 2007[21]	226							2.1 d	3.0 d		
Liang et al, 2007[22]	268	48 h	96 h								
COREAN, 2010[23]	340			10.0%	12.9%					85.0 h	93.0 h

Lap, Laparoscopic.
*Figures represent actual treatment (not intention to treat).

TABLE 178-2 Length of Stay After Colorectal Resection: Results of Randomized Controlled Trials

	Operation	Sample Size	MEAN LENGTH OF STAY	
			Laparoscopic	Open
Lacy et al, 2002[18]	Colon cancer (other than transverse)	219	5.2 d	7.9 d
COST, 2004[4]	Right, left, sigmoid colectomy	853	5 d*	6 d*
COLOR, 2005[20]	Right, left, sigmoid colectomy	1082	8.2 d	9.3 d
CLASICC, 2005[17]	Colon cancer (other than transverse)	794	11 d*,†	9 d*,†
Braga et al, 2007[21]	Right colectomy	226	5.4 d	6.4 d
Liang et al, 2007[22]	Left colectomy	269	9.0 d	14.0 d
Braga et al, 2010[27]	Left colectomy	268	7.0 d	8.7 d

*Value represents a median value.
†Value represents findings from intention-to-treat analysis.

It would be simplistic to believe that these shorter lengths of stay are absolutely the result of the surgical approach used. Patients undergoing laparoscopic surgery may have different expectations regarding their health and discharge criteria. However, the more rapid return of gastrointestinal function seen with minimally invasive surgery (see Table 178-1) supports the real benefit of laparoscopic surgery in reducing length of stay.

Clearly, however, bowel function is not the only determinant of duration of hospitalization. The wide variation in mean length of stay shown in Table 178-2 attests to this fact. An increasing amount of attention has been paid recently to fast-track patient care protocols; these protocols have the capacity to work synergistically with a minimally invasive approach to reduce lengths of stay.[28-31] Their benefit is best considered an adjunct to either open or laparoscopic surgery.

POSTOPERATIVE PAIN

Patient experience of postoperative pain is an important endpoint that is notoriously difficult to standardize and measure. Pain levels vary throughout the day, especially in relationship to physical activity, and are also specifically affected by the dose and recency of administered opioids. Therefore, most assessments of postoperative pain focus on the use of opioid medications—both the quantity administered and the duration over which they are used.

In Table 178-3, randomized trials where postoperative pain was specifically analyzed are shown. In the majority of these studies, laparoscopic procedures are associated with decreased pain and/or a decreased amount/duration of opioid use.

POSTOPERATIVE PULMONARY FUNCTION

Postoperative compromise of pulmonary function is a well-recognized phenomenon, and the degree of compromise is related closely to the severity of postoperative pain. Appropriate pain control permits deep breathing and use of incentive spirometry devices. None of the large randomized trials reported a distinct analysis of pulmonary function, but evidence from several smaller trials hints at some benefit to postoperative pulmonary function with a laparoscopic approach. These trials are shown in Table 178-4.

QUALITY OF LIFE

Quality of life is a challenging endpoint to assess. Any discussion of the impact of a surgical intervention on quality of life necessarily begins with a review of the mechanisms by which it is measured. Several different instruments are commonly used to assess quality of life. Of these, the Short Form 36 (SF-36) questionnaire is the most widely used, composed of 36 questions aimed at quantifying an individual's overall well-being. Each of these 36 questions is answered based on a discrete scale,

TABLE 178-3 Assessments of Postoperative Pain: Results of Randomized Controlled Trials

	Operation	Sample Size	Findings
Schwenk et al, 1998[32]	Right colectomy, left colectomy, anterior resection, APR	60	Lowered opioid use in laparoscopic group
Milsom et al, 2001[33]	Resection for ileocolic Crohn disease	60	No difference in opioid use
COST, 2004[4]	Colectomies (other than transverse)	863	Decreased duration of opioid use in laparoscopic group
Liang et al, 2007[22]	Left colectomy	269	Lower pain scale scores in laparoscopic group
COREAN, 2010[23]	Low rectal resection	340	Lower pain scale scores in laparoscopic group

TABLE 178-4 Assessments of Postoperative Pulmonary Function: Results of Randomized Controlled Trials

	Operation	Comparison Groups	Sample Size (Total)	Findings
Milsom et al, 1998[34]	Right or sigmoid colectomy	Laparoscopic vs. open	109	Faster return to baseline FEV_1 and FVC in laparoscopic group
Schwenk et al, 1999[35]	Right colectomy, anterior resection, APR	Laparoscopic vs. open	60	Higher FVC and FEV_1 on postoperative day 1 in laparoscopic group
Milsom et al, 2001[33]	Ileocolic resection for Crohn disease	Laparoscopic vs. open	60	Faster recovery of FVC and FEV_1 in laparoscopic group

and the results are converted to a "score" in eight domains including general quality of life, physical function, role function, social function, bodily pain, mental health, and vitality. Other instruments, including the Quality of Life Questionnaire for Cancer (QLQ-C30) and the Quality of Life Questionnaire for Colorectal Cancer (QLQ-CR38) have questions that are more specifically targeted at cancer-related symptoms and related functional impairments.

Quality of life outcomes were analyzed in reports from the COlon carcinoma Laparoscopic or Open Resection (COLOR) trial (285 patients).[36] This study used the QLQ-C30 instrument, and found significantly higher scores in the domains of social function and role function at 2 to 4 weeks postoperation. An Italian study examining 268 patients undergoing laparoscopic versus open left colectomy also reported quality-of-life outcomes using the SF-36.[27] That study found significant improvements in domains of general health, physical functioning, and social functioning 6 months after surgery.

The SF-36 and QLQ-C30 scales are considered quite broad, in that they encompass a broad range of physical, mental, and social/emotional factors that impact quality of life. Because these instruments are broad, they are potentially insensitive to issues related to postoperative pain and recovery. The COST study (872 patients) used a different set of mechanisms that were specifically targeted at symptoms and functional status[7]: first, a scale called the Symptoms Distress Scale; second, a brief five-item quality-of-life index; and third, a straightforward estimation of health on a scale from 0 to 100 (0 = *death* and 100 = *perfect health*). The results of the quality-of-life assessments in the COST study were surprising—using each of these three techniques, there were no significant differences between the laparoscopic and the open arms.

Why does minimally invasive surgery engender such a marginal impact on patient quality of life? The answer is likely related to the nature of how quality of life is conceptualized and measured. Inherently, a patient's self-report of his or her quality of life encompasses a broad range of factors—the measurement is *multidimensional*. Other factors (that have little or nothing to do with the size of a patient's incision) are probably more important to our patients' *overall* quality of life than the surgical approach used or the short-term outcomes experienced. Also, the measurements of quality of life are *dimensionless*—there is no way to utilize a score on an SF-36 scale in a decision-making algorithm that encompasses tradeoff. How important is it to improve a patient's physical functioning score by 10%? These types of questions cannot be answered. It is our belief that the positive impact of minimally invasive surgery is underestimated by the quality-of-life outcomes reported to date. The other documented benefits of the approach are more truly representative of its advantages.

ONCOLOGIC OUTCOMES

Whatever benefits are achieved through a minimally invasive approach should not come at the expense of the oncologic intent of the operation. As mentioned earlier, reports of a higher risk of wound implantation in laparoscopic colon resections for cancer resulted in an impetus to closely study the technique and its outcomes. Wound recurrences are only one oncologic outcome—what is known about the long-term outcomes of a minimally invasive versus an open approach to colorectal cancer?

In Table 178-5 are listed the results of the major randomized trials examining oncologic outcomes with laparoscopic versus open resection for colorectal cancer. Several of these studies have reported long-term

TABLE 178-5 Oncologic Outcomes: Results of Randomized Controlled Trials

	Operation(s)	Sample Size	Duration of Followup	Outcome(s) Analyzed
COST, 2004[4]	Colon cancer (other than transverse)	872	Median 4.4 yr	No difference in recurrence rates
CLASICC, 2005[17]	Colorectal cancer (other than transverse)	794	Short-term	No differences in rates of positive circumferential radial margin
Liang et al, 2007[22]	Left colon cancer	269	Median 40 mo	No difference in recurrence rates
Lacy et al, 2008[37]	Colon cancer (other than transverse)	219	Median 95 mo	Higher overall survival, cancer-related survival, and disease-free survival in laparoscopic group
COLOR, 2009[38]	Right or left colon cancer	1248	Median 52 mo	No difference in overall survival or disease-free survival
CLASICC, 2010[39]	Colorectal cancer (other than transverse)	794	Median 56 mo	No difference in overall survival, disease-free survival, local recurrence, or distant recurrence
COREAN, 2010[23]	Low rectal cancer	340	Minimum 3 mo	No differences in rates of positive circumferential resection margin or macroscopic quality of mesenteric resection

TABLE 178-6 Costs of Treatment: Results of Randomized Controlled Trials

	Operation	Sample Size	Findings
Targarona et al, 2002[15]	Resection for lesions in left or right colon	54	Equivalent costs
Liang et al, 2002[40]	Sigmoid resection	42	Higher costs in laparoscopic group
Salkeld et al, 2004[41]	Rectopexy	39	Lower costs in laparoscopic group
Leung et al, 2004[42]	Rectosigmoid resection	337	Higher costs in laparoscopic group
CLASICC Trial, 2006[43]	Right colectomy, left colectomy, anterior resection, APR	682	Equivalent costs
Braga et al, 2007[21]	Right colectomy	226	Higher costs in laparoscopic group
Braga et al, 2010[27]	Left colectomy	268	Equivalent costs

outcomes only in the past 1 to 2 years. None of these studies found inferior results in the laparoscopic group; one study[37] found improved survival in the laparoscopic group. The two studies that examined margin status and quality of total mesorectal excision in rectal cancer resections both found that the laparoscopic and open approaches yielded similar specimens.[20,23] These findings strongly imply that laparoscopic approaches are noninferior in terms of their oncologic outcomes.

COSTS OF TREATMENT

In general, laparoscopic colorectal procedures are associated with higher operating room and equipment costs compared with open procedures. To a variable extent, these higher costs are offset by reductions in lengths of stay. Several of the major randomized laparoscopic trials reported cost data as an outcome, and these are tabulated in Table 178-6.

These findings may underestimate the actual impact of a successful minimally invasive surgery program on a financial bottom line. None of the trials listed in Table 178-6 incorporates a societal perspective, which is arguably the most important. After a minimally invasive

operation (relative to an open procedure), patients experience less pain and their return to work or activities of daily living is quicker. It is a reasonable speculation that the requirement for assistance from families or other caretakers is less. These indirect costs are generally not included in calculations of the relative expense inherent in a laparoscopic versus open approach.

Ideally, a laparoscopic operation would yield better outcomes *and* be cost-saving. To date, this does not appear to clearly be the case. Laparoscopic colorectal resections generate a higher expense than an open procedure. Absent additional advances in procedures that either shorten operative time or minimize equipment costs, the procedures are best considered more expensive than a traditional open operation.

COMPLICATIONS

Data suggest that rates of complications are similar with laparoscopic colorectal operations relative to open operations.[4,17,20-23,27] Despite the size and quality of these trials, it is difficult to say whether there is a difference in the types of complications that occur. Intuitively, the smaller incision size inherent in laparoscopic procedures would result in lower rates of wound infection/wound discharge—this has only been borne out in one trial.[23] Other complications, including anastomotic leakage, abscess, bleeding, and reoperation occur with comparable frequency.

FUTURE OF LAPAROSCOPIC COLORECTAL SURGERY

In many ways, it appears that the vast majority of what can be delivered by minimally invasive colorectal surgery has already arrived. Colectomies are routinely performed using incisions that are just large enough to permit extraction of the specimen and extracorporeal anastomosis. Some surgeons employ a completely intracorporeal approach, but it is our opinion that this approach is unnecessarily time-consuming and technically demanding because removal of a specimen for pathologic examination mandates an incision of modest size.

In what ways can we expect laparoscopic colorectal surgery to evolve in the future? In this section, we will review several directions in which the field may advance in the near future.

DISSEMINATION

As mentioned in the introduction, there is no accurate way to estimate the proportion of colorectal operations in the United States that are currently performed laparoscopically. It is a certainty, however, that the proportion of colorectal operations performed laparoscopically is increasing.

The reasons underlying this trend deserve some mention. Laparoscopic colorectal operations are increasingly an integral part of formal training in colorectal surgery. In a similar vein, it is worth noting how difficult it is to acquire familiarity with the technique outside the context of a formal training program. Although the majority of colorectal operations are performed by general surgeons[44] (not certified in colorectal surgery), each general surgeon performs a relatively small number of colorectal resections each year. According to data from the American Board of Surgery, over half of general surgeons perform fewer than 12 colectomies per year.[45] This low volume may make it difficult for many surgeons to ascend the learning curve within a reasonable time period. Assuming that half of presenting cases are even amenable to a laparoscopic approach, and reducing the learning curve to 40 rather than 50 cases, it would still require 8 years to ascend the learning curve, making an additional assumption that the learning curve retains the same characteristics despite the paucity of cases. This situation prompts the call for means of shortening the learning curve (e.g., simplified step-by-step approaches or hand-assisted approaches) or careful credentialing procedures for surgeons who perform these operations.

LAPAROSCOPIC PROCTECTOMY

Relative to colectomies, operations for rectal cancer introduce an additional level of complexity. The confines of the bony pelvis, particularly in men and obese patients, result in specific challenges for even the most experienced laparoscopic surgeon. Neoadjuvant treatment with chemoradiation further contributes to these difficulties because of the distorted tissue planes that result from radiation.

Early results from the CLASICC trial raised concern over the rate of positive radial margins.[17] Among patients undergoing low anterior resection, positive circumferential radial margins were noted in 12% (12/129 patients) who underwent a laparoscopic operation, compared with 6% (4/64 patients) who had an open operation. Although these findings did not reach statistical significance, concerns over the quality of the technique were part of the impetus behind a randomized trial of laparoscopic techniques for rectal cancer in the United States.

The American College of Surgeons Oncology Group (ACOSOG) Z6051 study is intended to address these concerns. This study is a multicenter, randomized controlled trial of patients with T1-T3N1 or T3N0M0 rectal cancers within the lowest 12 cm of the rectum.[10] Its primary endpoint is an estimation of the quality of the operation, estimated through the status of circumferential margins and the completeness of the mesorectal excision. The ACOSOG Z6051 study is not yet completed, but since its inception results from the open versus laparoscopic surgery for mid- or low rectal cancer after neoadjuvant chemoradiotherapy (COREAN trial) have been reported.[23] This study (340 patients) found no differences in the rates of positive radial margins or completeness of mesorectal excision between laparoscopic and open treatment arms. These findings are encouraging in their implication that the laparoscopic technique does not compromise the oncologic aspects of the operation.

ROBOTIC SURGERY

The use of a robot in colorectal surgical procedures was first described in 2003.[46] Robotic technology has much to offer surgeons who perform laparoscopic colorectal operations. The optics are superb, and often include a binocular camera that enables a three-dimensional view. More importantly, the instrumentation allows greater articulation and stability than do conventional laparoscopic instruments.

Robotic surgery has been a focus of significant attention, especially in the areas of urologic and rectal surgery. Many (if not most) major academic surgical centers have a robotic surgical device and a cadre of surgical faculty with a dedicated interest in its use and results. The technique is not widely used in colonic surgery, because of the need to operate in multiple quadrants of the abdomen (in robotic surgery, this leads to a time-consuming maneuver of dedocking and redocking the device), and because stapling devices obviate the need for intraoperative suturing. To date, there have been no significant randomized trials reporting a direct comparison between robotic and nonrobotic laparoscopic approaches to rectal cancer treatment, but several series have documented excellent results with the use of this new technology.

Given the apparent benefits of robotic surgery, there are only two reasons *not* to use a robotic device for rectal surgery. First is the question of cost—the expense of these devices is nontrivial. Although the cost per procedure is difficult to standardize, the outright purchase price of the robot is approximately $2 million, and the cost of annual service fees are more than $150,000 per year. Second, using the device involves an additional learning curve. Some have found that the learning curve is easier as the instrumentation more closely approximates what the human hand can accomplish. Nevertheless, the transition from open to robotic surgery or from laparoscopic to robotic surgery requires an additional investment of time and resources from the interested surgeon. Additionally, despite the purported benefit of making the dissection easier, no study to date has shown a reduction in operative time.

Is the promise of robotic surgery worth the cost? Several authors have wondered this question out loud.[46-51] The degree to which robotic surgery will become part of the standard of care for rectal surgery is unknown at this time. Given the increasing scrutiny of comparative effectiveness and cost containment, proponents of robotic surgery will be asked to justify this capable but expensive technology.

SINGLE-INCISION LAPAROSCOPIC COLORECTAL SURGERY

As experienced laparoscopists continue their efforts to minimize the number and size of their incisions, there exists a natural boundary to what can be achieved: one incision, only large enough for specimen extraction. Single-incision laparoscopic colectomy (SILC) represents this concept—the use of a single hiatus in the abdominal wall through which insufflation, visualization, dissection, and specimen extraction/anastomosis all occur.

The procedure is technically demanding, primarily the result of clustering instruments within a single working port. Several innovations in the devices used have facilitated the approach, making it increasingly practical. SILC surgery is still in its infancy, although a growing number of case reports have documented its feasibility for a range of operations, including colectomy,[52-55] proctectomy,[54-56] and ileoanal procedures.[52,55,57]

How does SILC compare with other laparoscopic approaches in terms of patient outcomes? No randomized trials have been performed to date comparing SILC to traditional laparoscopic techniques. Given the relatively small benefit seen from laparoscopic surgery (compared with open surgery or hand-assisted surgery), it is unlikely that even a large trial will demonstrate a clear benefit. The role of SILC surgery in the spectrum of laparoscopic techniques is for now promising, but uncertain.

TECHNICAL ASPECTS OF LAPAROSCOPIC COLORECTAL SURGERY

COLORECTAL CANCER RESECTIONS

Careful preoperative planning and attention to detail are critical in any cancer operation. Expertise with laparoscopic colorectal techniques is so important that the American Society of Colon and Rectal Surgeons (ASCRS)

and the Society of American Endoscopic and Gastrointestinal Surgeons (SAGES) have jointly endorsed credentialing recommendations and SAGES has published "Guidelines for Laparoscopic Resection of Curable Colon and Rectal Cancer."[58] We highly recommend all surgeons who are acquiring familiarity with minimally invasive techniques for treating colorectal cancer to review these guidelines. A series of steps for performing laparoscopic right colectomy and laparoscopic low anterior resection are shown in Boxes 178-1 and 178-2. The elements of a sigmoid resection are incorporated within an anterior resection, with some minor modification.

PLANNING

Preoperative evaluation includes staging, assessment of comorbidities, and decision regarding the operative approach, whether laparoscopic or open. Cross-sectional imaging with computed tomography (CT) or magnetic resonance imaging (MRI) is essential in order to know the extent of locoregional invasion, as well as the presence of any metastatic disease (known or suspected). The necessity of chest CT is controversial, but recommended by professional guidelines and should therefore be performed routinely.[59] For patients with rectal cancer, staging

---

BOX 178-1 Steps for a Right Colon Resection

1. Instruments: three 5-mm trocars and one 12-mm trocar, 30-degree or flexible scope, endoscopic graspers, electrocautery scissors, vessel sealing device
2. Position: supine or lithotomy, safely secured to bed for steep airplaning/Trendelenburg, sequential compression devices (Figure 178-1)
3. Port placement: four trocars (supraumbilical, suprapubic, right and left lower quadrant), (diamond shape)
4. Trendelenburg, right side up: retract small bowel out of pelvis
5. Elevate cecum anteriorly and cephalad, and incise peritoneum around base of cecum and terminal ileal mesentery from pelvic brim to aortic bifurcation (Figure 178-2); identify and protect right ureter
6. Retract cecum medially and incise the right lateral peritoneal reflection to the hepatic flexure (Figure 178-3)
7. Retract hepatic flexure caudad and divide the hepatocolic attachments (Figure 178-4)
8. To divide the ileocolic pedicle intracorporeally, traction is placed upward on the mesentery near the ileocecal junction to place the pedicle under tension. The mesenteric windows cephalad and caudad are opened, the vascular pedicle is isolated, and the vessels are ligated and transected; the right branch of the middle colic artery also can be transected
9. The supraumbilical port site incision is extended around the umbilicus to 4 to 6 cm (Figure 178-5); a ring drape or other form of wound protection is used for cancer cases; the terminal ileum and right colon are exteriorized, and resection and anastomosis are performed (Figure 178-6)
10. The fascia of any 12-mm port and the periumbilical incision are closed

BOX 178-2 Steps for a Low Anterior Resection

1. Equipment: two 12-mm trocars and two 5-mm trocars, 30-degree or flexible scope, endoscopic graspers, electrocautery scissors, and vessel sealing device
2. Position: low lithotomy, secured to bed for steep airplaning/Trendelenburg, sequential compression devices
3. Port placement: four trocars (diamond shape) (Figure 178-7)
4. Trendelenburg, left side up: remove small bowel from pelvis. Retract sigmoid medially, divide left lateral peritoneal reflection in the avascular plane, and identify and protect the left ureter; mobilize sigmoid and descending colon in the retroperitoneal plane to the aortic bifurcation medially and to the splenic flexure proximally
5. Reverse Trendelenburg, left side up: mobilize the splenic flexure; for cancer, the omentum should be removed with the appropriate part of transverse colon, and the splenocolic attachments can be divided and the splenic flexure and omentum swept off the retroperitoneum; for a low anterior resection, if only mobilization of the flexure is required, the omentum may be retained and dissected off the distal transverse colon
6. The presacral plane is entered by pulling up on the sigmoid and extending the left-sided dissection at the pelvic brim distally and scoring the left pararectal peritoneum; dissection continues medially and distally; the right pararectal peritoneum is scored and the dissection in the presacral plane is joined with that from the left (Figures 178-8 and 178-9)
7. In cancer, intraoperative endoscopy may be required to mark the distal margin; the mesorectum is cleared at the chosen level with the vessel sealing device; the rectum is transected with a laparoscopic linear articulated stapler (Figure 178-10)
8. Dissection continues proximally in the presacral space over the sacral promontory, and the base of the inferior mesenteric artery is isolated and divided; the inferior mesenteric vein is encountered cephalad and may be divided if required for a tension-free anastomosis
9. The specimen is exteriorized via a 4- to 6-cm periumbilical incision (Figure 178-11); the remaining proximal sigmoid mesentery and proximal division of the bowel is divided; a purse-string suture is placed on the proximal margin, securing the head of an EEA stapler
11. The bowel is returned to the abdominal cavity, the incision is closed, and pneumoperitoneum is reestablished; the head of the stapler is docked onto the handle inserted via the anus (Figure 178-12)
12. All port sites >5 mm are closed with fascial sutures

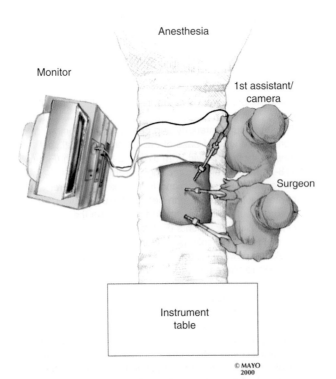

FIGURE 178-1 Patient and staff positioning and trocar placement for right hemicolectomy. (From Young-Fadok TM, Nelson H: Laparoscopic colectomy. In Baker RJ, Fischer JE, editors: *Mastery of surgery*, ed 4. Philadelphia, 2001, Lippincott Williams & Wilkins, p 1581. Copyright Mayo Foundation.)

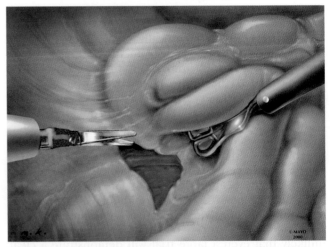

FIGURE 178-2 Retraction of cecum and terminal ileum cephalad while opening peritoneum in "groove" at base of small bowel mesentery. (From Young-Fadok TM, Nelson H: Laparoscopic colectomy. In Baker RJ, Fischer JE, editors: *Mastery of surgery*, ed 4. Philadelphia, 2001, Lippincott Williams & Wilkins, p 1581. Copyright Mayo Foundation.)

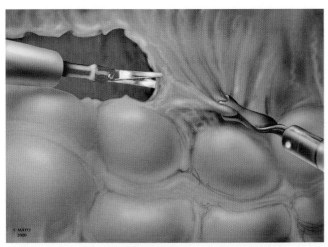

FIGURE 178-3 Retraction of ascending colon medially and opening of right lateral peritoneal reflection. (From Young-Fadok TM, Nelson H: Laparoscopic colectomy. In Baker RJ, Fischer JE, editors: *Mastery of surgery*, ed 4. Philadelphia, 2001, Lippincott Williams & Wilkins, p 1581. Copyright Mayo Foundation.)

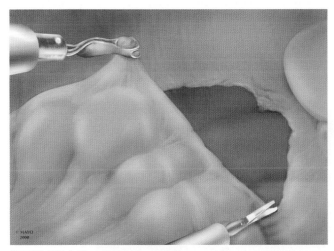

FIGURE 178-4 Elevation of hepatic flexure obliquely toward feet and anterior abdominal wall to expose correct retroperitoneal plane and the duodenum. (From Young-Fadok TM, Nelson H: Laparoscopic colectomy. In Baker RJ, Fischer JE, editors: *Mastery of surgery*, ed 4. Philadelphia, 2001, Lippincott Williams & Wilkins, p 1581. Copyright Mayo Foundation.)

may also include an endorectal ultrasound, with the possibility of preoperative chemoradiation for stage II or III tumors.

The informed consent discussion preceding a laparoscopic colorectal operation should encompass the same discussion as would an open operation; additionally, the possibility of conversion needs to be plainly stated; patients should not be promised a laparoscopic approach. The exact site of the cancer must be confirmed, and synchronous tumors must be excluded—both of these goals are accomplished well by an experienced endoscopist. Colonoscopic tattooing is helpful if performed correctly. India ink or alternative dye must be injected into the submucosa in three or four quadrants around the lesion to avoid the site of tattooing being obscured by

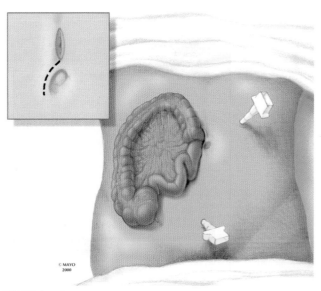

FIGURE 178-5 Enlargement of supraumbilical port site incision around umbilicus to allow exteriorization of whole right colon from terminal ileum to midtransverse colon. (From Young-Fadok TM, Nelson H: Laparoscopic colectomy. In Baker RJ, Fischer JE, editors: *Mastery of surgery*, ed 4. Philadelphia, 2001, Lippincott Williams & Wilkins, p 1581. Copyright Mayo Foundation.)

the mesentery or attachments to the retroperitoneum. Intraoperative endoscopy is best avoided because of associated bowel distention, although colonoscopy using carbon dioxide may minimize (not eliminate) this issue.[60]

PATIENT POSITIONING

Patient positioning is critical in laparoscopic colorectal surgery. With appropriate steps to stabilize the patient on the operating room gurney, steep positioning allows gravity to function effectively as a retractor. For all laparoscopic colorectal operations other than a right colectomy, the patient is placed in low lithotomy position. This position allows for a surgeon or assistant to stand between the legs. Extremities should be carefully padded at all pressure points. Specific attention is given to securing the patient to the bed in order to avoid slipping during surgery—this can be done according to surgeon preference, using either "eggshell" foam, beanbag, or other technique. Once the patient is secured, a stable patient position should be confirmed by tilting the table in all directions, prior to draping, to ensure that the patient will not move with changes in bed position.

OPERATIVE TECHNIQUE

An appropriate oncologic resection for colon cancer includes proximal and distal resection margins, proximal ligation of the primary vascular pedicle(s) along with intervening mesentery, and en bloc resection of locally advanced adherent colorectal tumors. The use of a minimally invasive approach does not imply a deviation from accepted oncologic principles. En bloc resection of a T4 tumor invasive into an adjacent organ may be attempted by an experienced surgeon, but in less experienced hands should prompt an open approach if discovered on preoperative imaging and indicates conversion if found

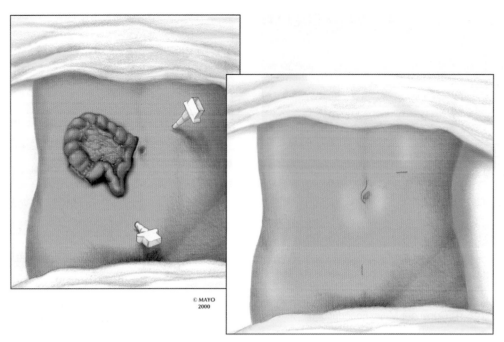

FIGURE 178-6 Extracorporeal creation of side-to-side stapled anastomosis and return to the abdominal cavity with closure of incisions. (From Young-Fadok TM, Nelson H: Laparoscopic colectomy. In Baker RJ, Fischer JE, editors: *Mastery of surgery*, ed 4. Philadelphia, 2001, Lippincott Williams & Wilkins, p 1581. Copyright Mayo Foundation.)

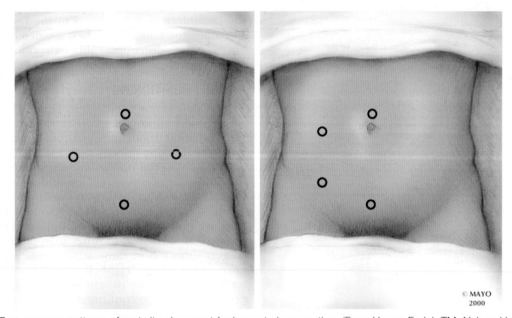

FIGURE 178-7 Two common patterns of port site placement for low anterior resection. (From Young-Fadok TM, Nelson H: Laparoscopic colectomy. In Baker RJ, Fischer JE, editors: *Mastery of surgery*, ed 4. Philadelphia, 2001, Lippincott Williams & Wilkins, p 1581. Copyright Mayo Foundation.)

intraoperatively. Published guidelines exist for open rectal cancer surgery, including a distal margin of 1 to 2 cm and mesorectal excision with radial clearance.[61]

LAPAROSCOPIC APPROACHES FOR DIVERTICULAR DISEASE

Minimally invasive surgical techniques are well employed in performing the spectrum of surgical procedures required for diverticular disease. Sigmoid colectomy, left colectomy, and diverting ileostomy/colostomy are all eminently feasible in most cases. Although colectomy is occasionally required for diverticular bleeding, this indication is rare, and we will focus our discussion on considerations specific to colectomy for diverticulitis.

ELECTIVE COLECTOMY

Elective colectomy for patients with serial episodes of self-limited, medically treated diverticulitis is performed

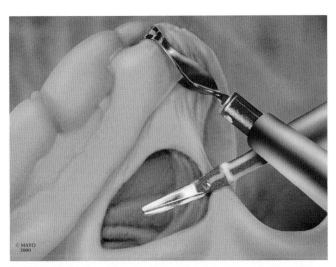

FIGURE 178-8 Entry into superior portion of presacral space from the right side of the rectum, joining prior dissection from left side. (From Young-Fadok TM, Nelson H: Laparoscopic colectomy. In Baker RJ, Fischer JE, editors: *Mastery of surgery*, ed 4. Philadelphia, 2001, Lippincott Williams & Wilkins, p 1581. Copyright Mayo Foundation.)

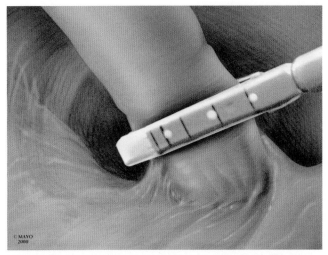

FIGURE 178-10 Transection of rectum with laparoscopic linear stapler. (From Young-Fadok TM, Nelson H: Laparoscopic colectomy. In Baker RJ, Fischer JE, editors: *Mastery of surgery*, ed 4. Philadelphia, 2001, Lippincott Williams & Wilkins, p 1581. Copyright Mayo Foundation.)

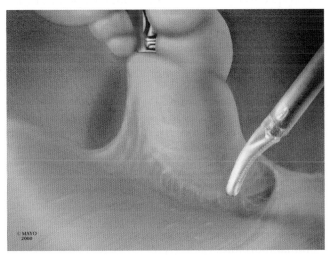

FIGURE 178-9 Dissection in presacral space with retraction of rectum anterosuperiorly. (From Young-Fadok TM, Nelson H: Laparoscopic colectomy. In Baker RJ, Fischer JE, editors: *Mastery of surgery*, ed 4. Philadelphia, 2001, Lippincott Williams & Wilkins, p 1581. Copyright Mayo Foundation.)

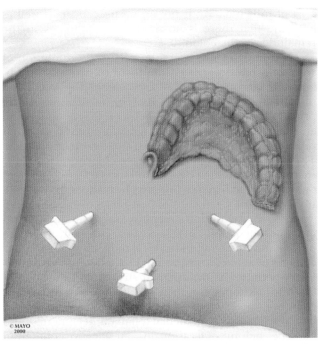

FIGURE 178-11 Exteriorization of the mobilized/transected sigmoid colon and proximal rectum. (From Young-Fadok TM, Nelson H: Laparoscopic colectomy. In Baker RJ, Fischer JE, editors: *Mastery of surgery*, ed 4. Philadelphia, 2001, Lippincott Williams & Wilkins, p 1581. Copyright Mayo Foundation.)

more than 20,000 times per year in the United States.[62] The specific threshold—the number of episodes a patient has had—after which a surgeon should recommend this procedure has evolved over time, but is still quite vague. Recommendations from the ASCRS published in 2006 state simply (and ambiguously) that after two episodes, the decision to perform a colectomy should be made on a "case by case basis."[63] Other research using decision models advocate a more conservative approach, waiting until four or more episodes.[64] The correct threshold is not easily determined, given how little is actually known about the natural history of the disease. Importantly, however, the use of laparoscopic surgery should not

change a surgeon's propensity to offer colectomy to a patient with serial episodes of diverticulitis.

When an elective laparoscopic sigmoid colectomy is planned for a patient with recurrent diverticulitis, several steps should be undertaken. First, the patient's entire history of radiographic investigations should be reviewed. It is imperative that the surgeon plan resection of all components that have been shown to be inflamed during prior episodes. Second, a complete colonic evaluation is

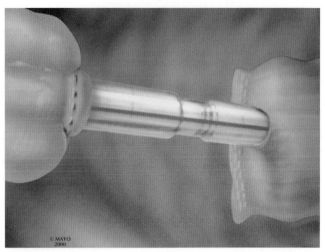

FIGURE 178-12 Docking of anvil of stapler onto handle. (From Young-Fadok TM, Nelson H: Laparoscopic colectomy. In Baker RJ, Fischer JE, editors: *Mastery of surgery*, ed 4. Philadelphia, 2001, Lippincott Williams & Wilkins, p 1581. Copyright Mayo Foundation.)

necessary. This serves the dual purpose of ensuring the area of inflammation is not an occult cancer, as well as ensuring that there is no significant pathology in the remainder of the colon.

The timing of the operation relative to resolution of symptoms has never been the focus of dedicated study, but it is customary to wait 6 weeks in the hope that inflammation will resolve, thereby facilitating a safe primary anastomosis. Fistulas between the sigmoid colon and skin, bladder, uterus, or vagina are rare but do not represent a contraindication to a laparoscopic approach. The most common of these fistulas—colovesical fistulas—require only minimal dissection to separate the sigmoid colon from the bladder, followed by bladder decompression with a Foley catheter for 5 to 7 days to allow healing.

Preoperative or intraoperative ureteral stent placement may be helpful in select cases, especially when the preoperative imaging indicates significant phlegmonous changes or anatomic distortion. Lighted stents are unnecessary because the firm tubular structure of the stent in the retroperitoneum usually can be detected at laparoscopy, but some surgeons prefer them. A combination of lateral-to-medial and medial-to-lateral techniques also may be helpful. Occasionally, an elective operation uncovers a severity of disease that is greater than suspected. In these cases, a low threshold for conversion is prudent. Hartmann operation or primary anastomosis with proximal diverting loop ileostomy is reasonable in situations where the proximal and/or distal bowel segments are actively inflamed.

ACUTE DIVERTICULITIS

Patients with acute diverticulitis who fail to respond readily to appropriate conservative treatment (bowel rest, intravenous antibiotics) and those who demonstrate signs of sepsis should undergo an urgent operation. Findings of free perforation and fecal peritonitis or extensive purulent peritonitis are absolute contraindications to laparoscopy. Complete exploration and clearance of contaminated material are not possible using laparoscopy and should prompt conversion to an open operation. In the absence of these findings, a laparoscopic approach is clearly feasible

LAPAROSCOPIC LAVAGE FOR ACUTE DIVERTICULITIS

One of the more recent areas of interest—and concomitant controversy—involves the use of laparoscopic lavage for patients requiring surgery for acute diverticulitis. The technique is somewhat variable in early reports, but generally includes a laparoscopic exploration, lavage, wide drainage, and (sometimes) an effort to repair any area of perforation.[65-67] In these series, Hinchey stage IV (feculent) peritonitis was a contraindication to the approach and dictated a conversion to a traditional resection.

Following these early reports, Myers at al reported the results of a prospective multiinstitutional study of 100 patients.[68] Eight patients with feculent (Hinchey stage IV) perforated diverticulitis causing generalized peritonitis underwent laparotomy and Hartmann resection. Laparoscopic lavage was performed in the other 92 patients, with morbidity and mortality rates of 4% and 3%, respectively. Two patients developed a pelvic abscess postoperatively, requiring intervention. Only 2 patients presented with recurrent diverticulitis at a median followup of 36 months. The authors concluded that laparoscopic management of perforated diverticulitis with generalized (purulent) peritonitis is feasible, with a low recurrence risk in the short term.

In another recent study, Franklin et al reported 40 patients undergoing laparoscopic lavage and placement of drains in complicated diverticulitis and diverticulitis without fecal peritonitis.[69] The average operative time was 62 minutes and there were no conversions. Just more than 50% underwent elective interval sigmoid colectomy, and none of the remaining patients required surgical intervention after 96 months' followup. The authors note that this approach avoids a colostomy, allows elective interval sigmoidectomy, and was associated with minimal morbidity.

Alamili et al performed a review of the literature that included eight studies—none randomized—reporting 213 patients with acute complicated diverticulitis managed by laparoscopic lavage.[70] Mean age was 59 years and most patients had Hinchey stage III disease. Conversion to laparotomy occurred on 6 patients (3%), and the complication rate was 10%. Mean hospital stay was 9 days. After mean followup of 38 months, 38% underwent elective sigmoid resection. Potential benefits were acknowledged but larger studies were recommended.

The appropriate place of laparoscopic lavage in the treatment of acute diverticulitis is still uncertain. To date, there have been no randomized or multiinstitutional studies that directly compare the technique to traditional laparoscopic or open approaches. It is hoped that this will change with the completion of the Dutch "LADIES" trial, a five-armed trial that will examine the role of the Hartmann operation for diverticulitis with fecal peritonitis and lavage versus Hartmann operation versus resection with primary anastomosis for all other cases (Figure 178-13).[71]

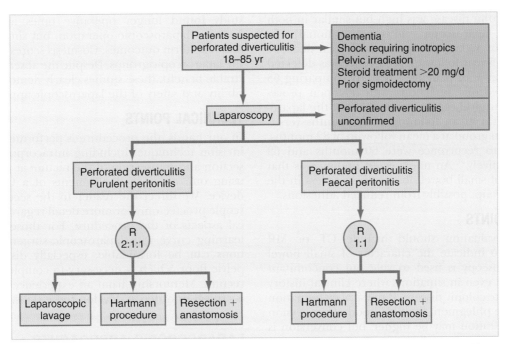

FIGURE 178-13 Study profile for the Dutch LADIES trial. (From Swank HA, Vermeulen J, Lange JF, et al: The LADIES trial: Laparoscopic peritoneal lavage or resection for purulent peritonitis and Hartmann procedure or resection with primary anastomosis for purulent or faecal peritonitis in perforated diverticulitis (NTR2037). *BMC Surg* 10:29, 2010.)

TECHNICAL POINTS (FOR ACUTE OR ELECTIVE SIGMOID COLECTOMY)

A laparoscopic sigmoid resection should involve an extent of resection that follows established guidelines. The proximal division of the sigmoid should occur in soft, pliable tissue; distal resection should occur in the peritonealized portion of the rectum, distal to the point where the taeniae have coalesced. Diverticulitis is known to recur after sigmoid resection—the only factor that is widely accepted as preventive of such recurrence is anastomosis within the rectum.[72,73] This requires an intracorporeal anastomotic technique, either using an end-to-end stapling device or a hand-sewn approach through an open abdominal incision. An extracorporeal anastomosis cannot fulfill these requirements.

LAPAROSCOPIC APPROACHES FOR CROHN DISEASE

A complete discussion of the indications for surgical treatment in patients with Crohn disease is found in Chapters 159 and 161. These indications are briefly summarized as situations in which disease activity is symptomatic and refractory to maximal medical management. Laparoscopic approaches to patients who require surgical treatment for Crohn disease are challenged by the manifestations of a chronic inflammatory disease process. This may include adhesions from prior surgery or inflammation, fistulous attachments between abdominal elements, shortened mesentery, and fragile viscera.

In a prospective randomized trial, 60 patients were assigned to conventional or laparoscopic resection, although study design was unconventional because randomization occurred after an initial diagnostic laparoscopy to assess feasibility of a laparoscopic resection.[33] The laparoscopic arm showed benefits in terms of restoration of pulmonary function, morbidity, and length of stay. Oral intake was not started for 3 days to evaluate nutritional parameters and likely obviated any potential differences in length of stay between laparoscopic and open groups (5 vs. 6 days; not significant). In another study, a case-matched series of laparoscopic versus open ileocolostomy for Crohn disease showed that mean length of stay was 4.1 days for laparoscopy patients compared with 6.7 days for open procedure patients; the operative times were the same, and laparoscopy resulted in reduced costs.[74]

Other retrospective studies consistently report quicker return of bowel function, earlier tolerance of oral diet, and reduced postoperative pain, which combine to produce a shorter length of stay compared with traditional open procedures.[33,74-78] In these studies, the conversion rates range from 10% to 20%, with the proportion of complex cases (abscess, fistula, or reoperative surgery) ranging from 40% to 50%.

One concern regarding laparoscopic surgery has been the potential to miss more proximal areas of small bowel disease. This concern was raised by the observation that many laparoscopic surgeons were examining the proximal small bowel by performing an "instrument-over-instrument" inspection, passing the small bowel between two instruments while inspecting it. Tactile feedback regarding subtle lesions was missing. Several longer-term studies have shown no excess incidence of recurrent disease in laparoscopic cases. In one series with mean long-term followup of 39 months, 32 patients undergoing laparoscopic ileocolic resection were compared with 29 patients undergoing open resection.[79] The incidence of recurrent Crohn disease was high but similar in both groups (48% laparoscopic, 44% conventional). In another series of 39 laparoscopic and 53 open ileocolic resections with 5-year followup, recurrence was detected in 27% versus 29% of patients.[80] A study comparing 63 laparoscopic ileocolic resections with 50 open procedures showed surgical recurrence in 9.5% of the laparoscopic group at a mean followup of 63 months versus 24% in the open group at a mean followup of 82 months. Median times to recurrence were 60 months and 62 months, respectively.[81] An unexpected finding was that the incidence of small bowel obstruction was less in the laparoscopic group, possibly from reduced adhesions.

TECHNICAL POINTS

Preoperative evaluation should include CT or MR enterography to indicate the character of small bowel disease. Colonoscopy is used to rule out concomitant colonic disease, even in situations where clinical history does not indicate colonic disease. If physical examination finds a palpable phlegmon, the likelihood of conversion to an open operation may be higher, but conversion is not inevitable.

Patients can be positioned in either supine or lithotomy position. At the beginning of the procedure, it is helpful to ensure that the small intestine is completely mobilized out of the pelvis, as pelvic fixation makes an extracorporeal anastomosis impossible.[82] Mobilization of the entire right colon (including hepatic flexure), even if only the cecum is affected, permits easier exteriorization and facilitates a wide side-to-side stapled anastomosis if that is the surgeon's preference. The use of a small periumbilical incision as the extraction site allows for easy extraction of the mobilized bowel because it overlies the ileocolic pedicle. In addition, use of this incision allows the entire small bowel to be exteriorized and examined for areas of synchronous disease.

Operations for isolated ileocolic Crohn disease are appropriate for surgeons early in their laparoscopic learning curve. An uncomplicated ileocolic resection requires only intracorporeal mobilization, with or without vascular pedicle division, and the resection and anastomosis are performed extracorporeally. Occasionally, the mesentery associated with the resection is inflamed and fragile—this should immediately prompt any surgeon to obtain adequate exposure in order to facilitate control of the mesenteric blood vessels.

LAPAROSCOPIC APPROACHES FOR ILEOANAL POUCH PROCEDURES

Laparoscopic surgery has an evolving role in the management of ulcerative colitis and familial adenomatous polyposis (FAP). Total abdominal colectomy, proctocolectomy, proctectomy, and ileoanal pouch–anal anastomosis (IPAA) are all feasible in the hands of an experienced laparoscopic surgeon.

A recent review by the Cochrane Collaborative analyzed the collected experience of 11 trials (including one randomized trial[83]) consisting of 607 patients undergoing an IPAA for either FAP or ulcerative colitis.[84] This study found longer operative times among patients having a laparoscopic operation, but similar short-term and long-term outcomes. Cosmesis scores were higher in the laparoscopic groups. Despite the absence of a demonstrable benefit, these studies clearly demonstrate the feasibility and safety of the laparoscopic approach.

TECHNICAL POINTS

In our hands, the procedure is performed using a four-incision technique, including intracorporeal pelvic dissection and transection of the rectum at the pelvic floor using one or more deployments of a GIA-30 stapling device. We direct the reader to the section on laparoscopic proctectomy for more detail regarding the technical aspects of the procedure. For those early in their learning curve with laparoscopic surgery, these operations can be formidable, especially dissection to the pelvic floor, which is necessary to completely excise the rectum. Mentorship from an experienced laparoscopist is critical in order to develop these skills.

LAPAROSCOPIC APPROACHES FOR RECTAL PROLAPSE

Several different transabdominal operations are widely used for rectal prolapse, including rectopexy, rectosigmoid resection, mesh fixation, and combinations thereof. Each of these components is technically feasible using a laparoscopic approach.[85] Mobilization of the rectum for rectal prolapse is an ideal procedure by which to learn the laparoscopic technique of rectal mobilization. These patients are usually relatively thin, with a mesorectum that is already hypermobile. The experience used in performing these operations can be extended to other procedures, such as laparoscopic proctocolectomy or total mesorectal excision for rectal cancer.

The advantages of laparoscopic procedures for rectal prolapse appear similar in character to those seen with other operations. There has only been one small randomized trial that directly compared outcomes with laparoscopic versus open approach for rectal prolapse. Solomon et al randomized 40 patients, and found that operative time was longer in the laparoscopic group (153 minutes vs. 102 minutes; $P < 0.01$).[86] The average hospital stay was shorter (3.9 days vs. 6.6 days; $P < 0.01$), and a mean cost savings of £357 per patient was subsequently shown in the laparoscopic group.[41] Other nonrandomized studies have yielded similar findings. Case series have shown that with the laparoscopic approach operative times are longer,[87] length of stay is shorter,[87,88] and the conversion rate is acceptable (less than 10%).[87-89]

A complete assessment of the outcomes of the laparoscopic approach needs to encompass long-term followup. Unfortunately, the technique is new enough that long-term followup is relatively sparse. In a large series of 117 patients with a mean followup of 62 months, the rate of recurrent full-thickness prolapse was only 2.5%, although there was an 18% rate of mucosal prolapse.[90] Other studies have documented recurrence rates that are noninferior to open operations using mesh fixation.[85,89]

TECHNICAL ISSUES

The laparoscopic approach to rectal prolapse is generally composed of three main elements: rectal mobilization, rectosigmoid resection, and rectopexy. Rectal mobilization and resection are performed according to the steps previously described for anterior resection. The anastomosis can be constructed according to surgeon preference, usually using an end-to-end anastomotic stapling device. An alternative to this is to mobilize the left colon and retrieve the redundant colon through a transverse muscle-splitting incision in the left abdomen. Resection and hand-sewn anastomosis can then be accomplished, encompassing an amount of colon that allows for a straightened rectosigmoid entering the low pelvis. The rectopexy is then performed below the level of the anastomosis.

If rectopexy is performed, there are several techniques by which to accomplish fixation. Intracorporeal suturing may be used to affix the lateral rectal peritoneum to the sacrum; alternatively, this step has been simplified further by the availability of laparoscopic tacking devices, which are effective at securing the pararectal tissues to the sacral promontory.

SUMMARY

Evidence has accumulated that the laparoscopic approach provides outcomes that are equivalent or superior to an open operation for a broad spectrum of colorectal procedures. As the field continues to evolve, surgeons are gaining increasing experience with more complex procedures, including total abdominal colectomies and low pelvic dissection. These advances expand the spectrum of indications that are appropriate for laparoscopic approach and the numbers of patients who potentially benefit from the technique.

Looking toward the future, there are several directions in which the field may progress. Robotic surgery, SILC, and other techniques have the capacity to offer added benefits to patients, but their true potential is as yet unproven. Surgeons engaged in pushing the envelope should continue to rigorously analyze their outcomes to allow the field to move forward with due attention to the principles of evidence-based medicine.

REFERENCES

1. Jacobs M, Verdeja JC, Goldstein HS: Minimally invasive colon resection (laparoscopic colectomy). *Surg Laparosc Endosc* 1:144, 1991.
2. Berends FJ, Kazemier G, Bonjer HJ, et al: Subcutaneous metastases after laparoscopic colectomy. *Lancet* 344:58, 1994.
3. Johnstone PA, Rohde DC, Swartz SE, et al: Port site recurrences after laparoscopic and thoracoscopic procedures in malignancy. *J Clin Oncol* 14:1950, 1996.
4. A comparison of laparoscopically assisted and open colectomy for colon cancer. *N Engl J Med* 350:2050, 2004.
5. Bokey EL, Moore JW, Keating JP, et al: Laparoscopic resection of the colon and rectum for cancer. *Br J Surg* 84:822, 1997.
6. Wexner SD, Cohen SM, Johansen OB, et al: Laparoscopic colorectal surgery: A prospective assessment and current perspective. *Br J Surg* 80:1602, 1993.
7. Weeks JC, Nelson H, Gelber S, et al: Short-term quality-of-life outcomes following laparoscopic-assisted colectomy vs open colectomy for colon cancer: A randomized trial. *JAMA* 287:321, 2002.
8. Bennett CL, Stryker SJ, Ferreira MR, et al: The learning curve for laparoscopic colorectal surgery. Preliminary results from a prospective analysis of 1194 laparoscopic-assisted colectomies. *Arch Surg* 132:41; discussion 45, 1997.
9. Simons AJ, Anthone GJ, Ortega AE, et al: Laparoscopic-assisted colectomy learning curve. *Dis Colon Rectum* 38:600, 1995.
10. Soop M, Nelson H: Laparoscopic-assisted proctectomy for rectal cancer: On trial. *Ann Surg Oncol* 15:2357, 2008.
11. Ozturk E, da Luz Moreira A, Vogel JD: Hand-assisted laparoscopic colectomy: The learning curve is for operative speed, not for quality. *Colorectal Dis* 12:e304, 2010.
12. Kiran RP, Kirat HT, Ozturk E, et al: Does the learning curve during laparoscopic colectomy adversely affect costs? *Surg Endosc* 24:2718, 2010.
13. Kang JC, Chung MH, Chao PC, et al: Hand-assisted laparoscopic colectomy vs open colectomy: A prospective randomized study. *Surg Endosc* 18:577, 2004.
14. Litwin DE, Darzi A, Jakimowicz J, et al: Hand-assisted laparoscopic surgery (HALS) with the HandPort system: Initial experience with 68 patients. *Ann Surg* 231:715, 2000.
15. Targarona EM, Gracia E, Garriga J, et al: Prospective randomized trial comparing conventional laparoscopic colectomy with hand-assisted laparoscopic colectomy: Applicability, immediate clinical outcome, inflammatory response, and cost. *Surg Endosc* 16:234, 2002.
16. Hand-assisted laparoscopic surgery vs standard laparoscopic surgery for colorectal disease: A prospective randomized trial. HALS Study Group. *Surg Endosc* 14:896, 2000.
17. Guillou PJ, Quirke P, Thorpe H, et al: Short-term endpoints of conventional versus laparoscopic-assisted surgery in patients with colorectal cancer (MRC CLASICC trial): Multicentre, randomised controlled trial. *Lancet* 365:1718, 2005.
18. Lacy AM, Garcia-Valdecasas JC, Delgado S, et al: Laparoscopy-assisted colectomy versus open colectomy for treatment of non-metastatic colon cancer: A randomised trial. *Lancet* 359:2224, 2002.
19. Waters JA, Chihara R, Moreno J, et al: Laparoscopic colectomy: Does the learning curve extend beyond colorectal surgery fellowship? *JSLS* 14:325, 2010.
20. Veldkamp R, Kuhry E, Hop WC, et al: Laparoscopic surgery versus open surgery for colon cancer: Short-term outcomes of a randomised trial. *Lancet Oncol* 6:477, 2005.
21. Braga M, Frasson M, Vignali A, et al: Open right colectomy is still effective compared to laparoscopy: Results of a randomized trial. *Ann Surg* 246:1010; discussion 1014, 2007.
22. Liang JT, Huang KC, Lai HS, et al: Oncologic results of laparoscopic versus conventional open surgery for stage II or III left-sided colon cancers: A randomized controlled trial. *Ann Surg Oncol* 14:109, 2007.
23. Kang SB, Park JW, Jeong SY, et al: Open versus laparoscopic surgery for mid or low rectal cancer after neoadjuvant chemoradiotherapy (COREAN trial): Short-term outcomes of an open-label randomised controlled trial. *Lancet Oncol* 11:637, 2010.
24. Bessler M, Whelan RL, Halverson A, et al: Controlled trial of laparoscopic-assisted vs open colon resection in a porcine model. *Surg Endosc* 10:732, 1996.
25. Bohm B, Milsom JW, Fazio VW: Postoperative intestinal motility following conventional and laparoscopic intestinal surgery. *Arch Surg* 130:415, 1995.
26. Hotokezaka M, Combs MJ, Schirmer BD: Recovery of gastrointestinal motility following open versus laparoscopic colon resection in dogs. *Dig Dis Sci* 41:705, 1996.
27. Braga M, Frasson M, Zuliani W, et al: Randomized clinical trial of laparoscopic versus open left colonic resection. *Br J Surg* 97:1180, 2010.
28. Lloyd GM, Kirby R, Hemingway DM, et al: The RAPID protocol enhances patient recovery after both laparoscopic and open colorectal resections. *Surg Endosc* 24:1434, 2010.
29. Bosio RM, Smith BM, Aybar PS, et al: Implementation of laparoscopic colectomy with fast-track care in an academic medical center: Benefits of a fully ascended learning curve and specialty expertise. *Am J Surg* 193:413; discussion 415, 2007.
30. Raue W, Haase O, Junghans T, et al: "Fast-track" multimodal rehabilitation program improves outcome after laparoscopic sigmoidectomy: A controlled prospective evaluation. *Surg Endosc* 18:1463, 2004.

31. Senagore AJ, Duepree HJ, Delaney CP, et al: Results of a standardized technique and postoperative care plan for laparoscopic sigmoid colectomy: A 30-month experience. *Dis Colon Rectum* 46:503, 2003.

32. Schwenk W, Bohm B, Muller JM: Postoperative pain and fatigue after laparoscopic or conventional colorectal resections. A prospective randomized trial. *Surg Endosc* 12:1131, 1998.

33. Milsom JW, Hammerhofer KA, Bohm B, et al: Prospective, randomized trial comparing laparoscopic vs. conventional surgery for refractory ileocolic Crohn's disease. *Dis Colon Rectum* 44:1; discussion 8, 2001.

34. Milsom JW, Bohm B, Hammerhofer KA, et al: A prospective, randomized trial comparing laparoscopic versus conventional techniques in colorectal cancer surgery: A preliminary report. *J Am Coll Surg* 187:46; discussion 54, 1998.

35. Schwenk W, Bohm B, Witt C, et al: Pulmonary function following laparoscopic or conventional colorectal resection: A randomized controlled evaluation. *Arch Surg* 134:6; discussion 13, 1999.

36. Janson M, Lindholm E, Anderberg B, et al: Randomized trial of health-related quality of life after open and laparoscopic surgery for colon cancer. *Surg Endosc* 21:747, 2007.

37. Lacy AM, Delgado S, Castells A, et al: The long-term results of a randomized clinical trial of laparoscopy-assisted versus open surgery for colon cancer. *Ann Surg* 248:1, 2008.

38. Buunen M, Veldkamp R, Hop WC, et al: Survival after laparoscopic surgery versus open surgery for colon cancer: Long-term outcome of a randomised clinical trial. *Lancet Oncol* 10:44, 2009.

39. Jayne DG, Thorpe HC, Copeland J, et al: Five-year follow-up of the Medical Research Council CLASICC trial of laparoscopically assisted versus open surgery for colorectal cancer. *Br J Surg* 97:1638, 2010.

40. Liang JT, Shieh MJ, Chen CN, et al: Prospective evaluation of laparoscopy-assisted colectomy versus laparotomy with resection for management of complex polyps of the sigmoid colon. *World J Surg* 26:377, 2002.

41. Salkeld G, Bagia M, Solomon M: Economic impact of laparoscopic versus open abdominal rectopexy. *Br J Surg* 91:1188, 2004.

42. Leung KL, Kwok SP, Lam SC, et al: Laparoscopic resection of rectosigmoid carcinoma: Prospective randomised trial. *Lancet* 363:1187, 2004.

43. Franks PJ, Bosanquet N, Thorpe H, et al: Short-term costs of conventional vs laparoscopic assisted surgery in patients with colorectal cancer (MRC CLASICC trial). *Br J Cancer* 95:6, 2006.

44. Etzioni DA, Cannom RR, Madoff RD, et al: Colorectal procedures: What proportion is performed by American board of colon and rectal surgery-certified surgeons? *Dis Colon Rectum* 53:713, 2010.

45. Hyman N: How much colorectal surgery do general surgeons do? *J Am Coll Surg* 194:37, 2002.

46. Delaney CP, Lynch AC, Senagore AJ, et al: Comparison of robotically performed and traditional laparoscopic colorectal surgery. *Dis Colon Rectum* 46:1633, 2003.

47. Awad MM, Fleshman JW: Robot-assisted surgery and health care costs. *N Engl J Med* 363:2174; author reply 2176, 2010.

48. Barbash GI, Glied SA: New technology and health care costs—the case of robot-assisted surgery. *N Engl J Med* 363:701, 2010.

49. Delaney CP, Senagore AJ, Ponsky L: Robot-assisted surgery and health care costs. *N Engl J Med* 363:2175; author reply 2176, 2010.

50. Ibrahim AM, Makary MA: Robot-assisted surgery and health care costs. *N Engl J Med* 363:2175; author reply 2176, 2010.

51. Shukla PJ, Scherr DS, Milsom JW: Robot-assisted surgery and health care costs. *N Engl J Med* 363:2174; author reply 2176, 2010.

52. Chambers WM, Bicsak M, Lamparelli M, et al: Single-incision laparoscopic surgery (SILS) in complex colorectal surgery: A technique offering potential and not just cosmesis. *Colorectal Dis* 13:393, 2010.

53. Merchant AM, Lin E: Single-incision laparoscopic right hemicolectomy for a colon mass. *Dis Colon Rectum* 52:1021, 2009.

54. Law WL, Fan JK, Poon JT: Single-incision laparoscopic colectomy: Early experience. *Dis Colon Rectum* 53:284, 2010.

55. Gash KJ, Goede AC, Chambers W, et al: Laparoendoscopic single-site surgery is feasible in complex colorectal resections and could enable day case colectomy. *Surg Endosc* 25:835, 2010.

56. Bege T, Lelong B, Esterni B, et al: The learning curve for the laparoscopic approach to conservative mesorectal excision for rectal cancer: Lessons drawn from a single institution's experience. *Ann Surg* 251:249, 2010.

57. Geisler DP, Condon ET, Remzi FH: Single incision laparoscopic total proctocolectomy with ileopouch anal anastomosis. *Colorectal Dis* 12:941, 2010.

58. Society of American Gastrointestinal and Endoscopic Surgeons: Guidelines for laparoscopic resection of curable colon and rectal cancer. http://www.sages.org/publication/id/32/, Accessed May 1, 2011.

59. Engstrom PF, Arnoletti JP, Benson AB 3rd, et al: NCCN Clinical Practice Guidelines in Oncology: Colon cancer. *J Natl Compr Canc Netw* 7:778, 2009.

60. Nakajima K, Lee SW, Sonoda T, et al: Intraoperative carbon dioxide colonoscopy: A safe insufflation alternative for locating colonic lesions during laparoscopic surgery. *Surg Endosc* 19:321, 2005.

61. Tjandra JJ, Kilkenny JW, Buie WD, et al: Practice parameters for the management of rectal cancer (revised). *Dis Colon Rectum* 48:411, 2005.

62. Etzioni DA, Mack TM, Beart RW Jr, et al: Diverticulitis in the United States: 1998-2005: Changing patterns of disease and treatment. *Ann Surg* 249:210, 2009.

63. Rafferty J, Shellito P, Hyman NH, et al: Practice parameters for sigmoid diverticulitis. *Dis Colon Rectum* 49:939, 2006.

64. Salem L, Veenstra DL, Sullivan SD, et al: The timing of elective colectomy in diverticulitis: A decision analysis. *J Am Coll Surg* 199:904, 2004.

65. O'Sullivan GC, Murphy D, O'Brien MG, et al: Laparoscopic management of generalized peritonitis due to perforated colonic diverticula. *Am J Surg* 171:432, 1996.

66. Faranda C, Barrat C, Catheline JM, et al: Two-stage laparoscopic management of generalized peritonitis due to perforated sigmoid diverticula: Eighteen cases. *Surg Laparosc Endosc Percutan Tech* 10:135; discussion 139, 2000.

67. Taylor CJ, Layani L, Ghusn MA, et al: Perforated diverticulitis managed by laparoscopic lavage. *Austr N Z J Surg* 76:962, 2006.

68. Myers E, Hurley M, O'Sullivan GC, et al: Laparoscopic peritoneal lavage for generalized peritonitis due to perforated diverticulitis. *Br J Surg* 95:97, 2008.

69. Franklin ME Jr, Portillo G, Trevino JM, et al: Long-term experience with the laparoscopic approach to perforated diverticulitis plus generalized peritonitis. *World J Surg* 32:1507, 2008.

70. Alamili M, Gogenur I, Rosenberg J: Acute complicated diverticulitis managed by laparoscopic lavage. *Dis Colon Rectum* 52:1345, 2009.

71. Swank HA, Vermeulen J, Lange JF, et al: The LADIES trial: Laparoscopic peritoneal lavage or resection for purulent peritonitis and Hartmann's procedure or resection with primary anastomosis for purulent or faecal peritonitis in perforated diverticulitis (NTR2037). *BMC Surg* 10:29, 2010.

72. Thaler K, Baig MK, Berho M, et al: Determinants of recurrence after sigmoid resection for uncomplicated diverticulitis. *Dis Colon Rectum* 46:385, 2003.

73. Benn PL, Wolff BG, Ilstrup DM: Level of anastomosis and recurrent colonic diverticulitis. *Am J Surg* 151:269, 1986.

74. Young-Fadok TM, HallLong K, McConnell EJ, et al: Advantages of laparoscopic resection for ileocolic Crohn's disease. Improved outcomes and reduced costs. *Surg Endosc* 15:450, 2001.

75. Alabaz O, Iroatulam AJ, Nessim A, et al: Comparison of laparoscopically assisted and conventional ileocolic resection for Crohn's disease. *Eur J Surg* 166:213, 2000.

76. Bemelman WA, Slors JF, Dunker MS, et al: Laparoscopic-assisted vs. open ileocolic resection for Crohn's disease. A comparative study. *Surg Endosc* 14:721, 2000.

77. Evans J, Poritz L, MacRae H: Influence of experience on laparoscopic ileocolic resection for Crohn's disease. *Dis Colon Rectum* 45:1595, 2002.

78. Duepree HJ, Senagore AJ, Delaney CP, et al: Advantages of laparoscopic resection for ileocecal Crohn's disease. *Dis Colon Rectum* 45:605, 2002.

79. Tabet J, Hong D, Kim CW, et al: Laparoscopic versus open bowel resection for Crohn's disease. *Can J Gastroenterol* 15:237, 2001.

80. Bergamaschi R, Pessaux P, Arnaud JP: Comparison of conventional and laparoscopic ileocolic resection for Crohn's disease. *Dis Colon Rectum* 46:1129, 2003.

81. Lowney JK, Dietz DW, Birnbaum EH, et al: Is there any difference in recurrence rates in laparoscopic ileocolic resection for Crohn's disease compared with conventional surgery? A long-term, follow-up study. *Dis Colon Rectum* 49:58, 2006.

82. Young-Fadok TM, Nelson H: Laparoscopic right colectomy: Five-step procedure. *Dis Colon Rectum* 43:267; discussion 271, 2000.

83. Maartense S, Dunker MS, Slors JF, et al: Hand-assisted laparoscopic versus open restorative proctocolectomy with ileal pouch anal anastomosis: A randomized trial. *Ann Surg* 240:984; discussion 991, 2004.

84. Ahmed Ali U, Keus F, Heikens JT, et al: Open versus laparoscopic (assisted) ileo pouch anal anastomosis for ulcerative colitis and familial adenomatous polyposis. *Cochrane Database Syst Rev* 1:CD006267, 2009.

85. D'Hoore A, Cadoni R, Penninckx F: Long-term outcome of laparoscopic ventral rectopexy for total rectal prolapse. *Br J Surg* 91:1500, 2004.

86. Solomon MJ, Young CJ, Eyers AA, et al: Randomized clinical trial of laparoscopic versus open abdominal rectopexy for rectal prolapse. *Br J Surg* 89:35, 2002.

87. Kairaluoma MV, Viljakka MT, Kellokumpu IH: Open vs. laparoscopic surgery for rectal prolapse: A case-controlled study assessing short-term outcome. *Dis Colon Rectum* 46:353, 2003.

88. Boccasanta P, Venturi M, Reitano MC, et al: Laparotomic vs. laparoscopic rectopexy in complete rectal prolapse. *Dig Surg* 16:415, 1999.

89. Lechaux D, Trebuchet G, Siproudhis L, et al: Laparoscopic rectopexy for full-thickness rectal prolapse: A single-institution retrospective study evaluating surgical outcome. *Surg Endosc* 19:514, 2005.

90. Ashari LH, Lumley JW, Stevenson AR, et al: Laparoscopically-assisted resection rectopexy for rectal prolapse: Ten years' experience. *Dis Colon Rectum* 48:982, 2005.

More than one million individuals in the United States and Canada live with some type of intestinal stoma. These stomas are typically constructed as one of the last components of a long and challenging surgical procedure. Although created in only a few short minutes, permanent stomas must function for the remainder of the ostomate's lifetime.

The creation of a stoma is a technical exercise. Like most undertakings, if done correctly, the stoma will usually function well with minimal complications for the remainder of the ostomate's life. Conversely, if created poorly, stoma complications are common and can lead to years of misery. Intestinal stomas are in fact enterocutaneous anastomoses and all the principles that apply to creation of any anastomosis (i.e., using healthy intestine, avoiding ischemia and undue tension) are important in stoma creation.

INDICATIONS

Stomas are created either as a temporary means of fecal diversion when an anastomosis is unsafe or unwise, or as permanent orifices for the passage of excrement (stool or urine) when surgical resection prohibits the body's normal orifices from accomplishing these tasks. In this chapter, we will discuss the creation of ileostomies and colostomies.

Permanent colostomies are nearly always created from the sigmoid or descending colon, usually in association with distal bowel resection. Colostomies proximal to the splenic flexure typically function poorly, are often placed in locations difficult for ostomates to manage, and are at high risk for complications. If a permanent colostomy is contemplated using the transverse or ascending colon, the surgeon should strongly consider resecting the remaining large bowel and creating an end ileostomy. Common indications for a colostomy are listed in Box 179-1.

With the development and general acceptance of the ileal pouch–anal anastomosis (IPAA), permanent ileostomies are far less common than they were 25 years ago. Nonetheless, permanent ileostomies are often created for inflammatory bowel disease, familial adenomatous polyposis, multiple synchronous colorectal cancers, and a variety of other miscellaneous disorders. Poor anal function, comorbid diseases, or quality of life considerations may make an ileostomy preferable to more complex reconstructive options in selected patients.

Temporary diverting stomas are usually created in association with distal bowel resections when anastomosis is unsafe or to protect a distal anastomosis when operative conditions or comorbidities make proximal diversion of the fecal stream prudent.

Traditionally, three types of diverting stomas predominate: end sigmoid colostomy, transverse loop colostomy, and loop ileostomy.

PREOPERATIVE CONSIDERATIONS

Patients undergoing either elective or emergency surgery in which the creation of an abdominal stoma is a possibility should be adequately prepared preoperatively. Emergent surgery dictates a more rapid preparation than elective surgery, but stoma considerations must not be neglected.

Many patients are unsure as to what a colostomy or ileostomy is. A few minutes of preoperative education by the surgeon combined with printed material is very helpful. In addition, if available, all patients should meet with an enterostomal therapist (ET). The ET can provide specific information regarding stoma appliances, dietary and clothing alterations, and pouch management. Most importantly, the ET will help select the appropriate abdominal wall site for the future stoma. Appropriate stoma placement decreases postoperative complications and may improve the ostomate's well-being for years following surgery. Bass et al showed that preoperative counseling and marking by an ET prior to surgery improves postoperative quality of life.[1]

In addition to meeting with an ET, patients scheduled for stomal surgery often benefit from the opportunity to meet with other ostomates. Prior patients now well adjusted to life with a stoma provide an excellent, "non-medical" source of information and are often glad to share their experience with new ostomates. In addition, local chapters of the United Ostomy Association and the Crohn and Colitis Foundation may be of benefit in this area.

Patients should be marked prior to surgery. An abdominal surgeon should be able to locate and mark stoma sites. In most circumstances, marking is simple, straightforward, and only requires a few minutes. Three abdominal wall landmarks outline the "ostomy triangle" (Figure 179-1): The anterior superior iliac spine, the pubic tubercle, and the umbilicus. The stoma should lie within this triangle overlying the rectus muscle, generally at the site of an infraumbilical bulge in the abdominal wall. A site should be located on a flat segment of the abdominal wall 5 cm away from bony prominences, the umbilicus, prior surgical scars, or skin folds. Once the site has been selected and marked, the patient should sit up to ensure any new skin folds do not interfere with the stoma site. The patient's beltline should be identified and avoided if possible as this decreases postoperative clothing restrictions.

Special circumstances may require additional consideration. In obese individuals, a large pannus may

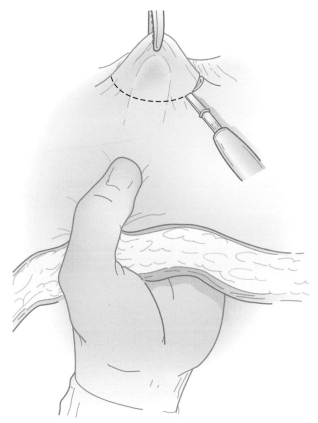

FIGURE 179-2 A disc of skin is excised at the stoma site.

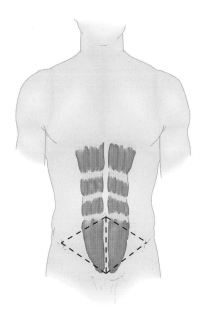

FIGURE 179-1 The ostomy triangle is defined by the anterior superior iliac spine, the umbilicus, and the pubic tubercle on the right and left sides of the abdominal wall for ileostomy and colostomy placement, respectively.

preclude stoma placement below the umbilicus. The pannus is often thicker in this area and may also hide the stoma from the patient's vision, making management difficult. Patients confined to a wheelchair should be marked while in their chair in order to avoid unanticipated postoperative difficulties. As mentioned, despite these restrictions, the stoma should pass through the rectus abdominal muscle in order to decrease the complications of parastomal hernia and stomal prolapse. In complex or potentially problematic cases, a stoma site can be marked and the stoma appliance left in place for 24 hours in order to determine the accuracy of preoperative placement.

OPERATIVE TECHNIQUES

END ILEOSTOMY

End ileostomies are routinely performed in association with either partial or total colorectal resections. Exposure is generally through a midline incision and the stoma is created after performing the indicated bowel resection. The premarked stoma site (usually in the right lower quadrant) is excised (Figure 179-2). A skin disc the size of a quarter is removed sparing all subcutaneous fat, as this fat is helpful to support the stoma in the postoperative period. The fat is then separated with scissors or cautery to expose the anterior rectus sheath. The sheath is incised vertically with a curved Mayo scissors for 3 to 4 cm (Figure 179-3). The incision can then be extended in a cruciate fashion laterally for 1 cm if desired. Medial extension should be avoided as this brings the stoma incision in proximity with the midline incision and may make the midline closure more difficult. The rectus abdominis muscle is split in the direction of its fibers to expose the posterior sheath. With the nondominant hand protecting the underlying viscera, the posterior sheath is bluntly opened with the Mayo scissors and the defect is enlarged to admit two fingers (Figure 179-4).

After the abdominal wall defect has been created, the ileum is prepared. Any residual retroperitoneal attachments are divided to facilitate passage of the bowel through the abdominal wall without tension. The mesentery may be cleared from the terminal 5 to 6 cm of the ileum. Care is taken to leave a 1-cm strip of mesentery with the ileum, as this generally carries a vessel paralleling the ileal wall and will prevent stomal ischemia (Figure 179-5). The ileum is then oriented with the cut mesenteric edge cephalad and passed through the previously created defect in the abdominal wall. The ileum should protrude 5 to 6 cm beyond skin level and appear pink and well perfused. The lateral ileal gutter may be closed if desired to prevent small bowel obstruction secondary to small bowel rotating around the ileostomy. This is done by suturing the free edge of the ileal mesentery

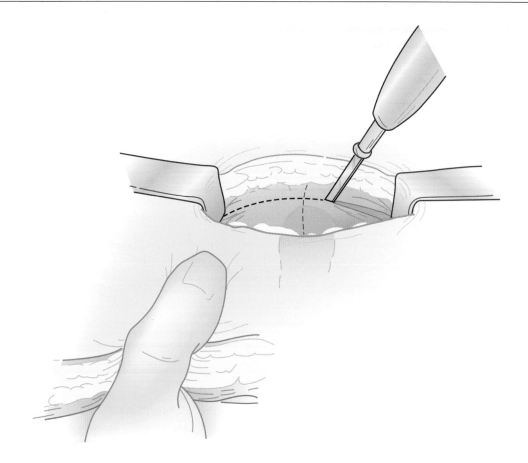

FIGURE 179-3 The anterior rectus sheath is opened vertically. It may be extended laterally in a cruciate "T" fashion if desired. Medial extension should be avoided.

(taking care to avoid blood vessels feeding the stoma) to the abdominal wall lateral to the midline incision up to the falciform ligament. There is no need to suture the ileum to the posterior fascia of the abdominal wall as this has not been shown to decrease the risk of prolapse or hernia. The abdominal incision is then closed in routine fashion including the skin.

The incision is protected to prevent contamination with intestinal contents and the staple line removed from the ileum. Ileostomies must be everted and matured to prevent serositis and skin irritation because of the caustic nature of the ileal effluent. This is accomplished by "tripartite" sutures containing dermis, the seromuscular layer of the bowel at the fascial level, and full-thickness bites of the cut edge of the ileum (Figure 179-6). Three or four of these everting sutures are placed first without tying. After all the everting sutures have been placed, they are tied while general traction is placed within the lumen of the ileum by an Allis clamp to facilitate eversion. After the stoma has been everted, the enterocutaneous anastomosis is completed with sutures between the cut edge of the ileum and dermis. The bowel should appear pink and protrude 2 to 3 cm beyond the abdominal skin.

END COLOSTOMY

As previously discussed, left-sided end colostomies are usually created in association with distal colorectal resection. The lateral attachments of the colon are transected along the white line of Toldt until sufficient colon is mobilized to create a colostomy that protrudes from the abdominal wall and can be matured without tension. Once the colon has been sufficiently mobilized, the stoma site is prepared and the abdominal wall defect created similar to that described for end ileostomy. The only differences are that the premarked stoma site is usually in the lower left quadrant and the cutaneous and fascial openings may need to be slightly larger to facilitate unrestricted passage of the colon through the abdominal wall.

After the trephine site has been successfully created, the colon is oriented without twisting and passed through the abdominal wall. Again, the colon should protrude beyond the abdominal skin and appear well perfused. There is no need to close the lateral gutter or to suture the colon to the posterior abdominal fascia as neither of these maneuvers have been shown to prevent parastomal hernia or prolapse. Alternatively, a "retroperitoneal colostomy" can be created by tunneling the colon under the posterolateral peritoneum and exiting through the previously created stoma site. This has been associated with decreased rates of parastomal herniation and prolapse, but the increased technical demands with its creation have limited its utility.

Once the abdominal incision has been closed and protected, the colostomy can be matured. Colostomies may be sutured without eversion as distal colonic contents are not irritating to the surrounding skin.

Meagher et al have devised a technique helpful in creating an end sigmoid colostomy in patients with a thick abdominal wall. The stoma site is created in standard fashion. A small wound protector (used in laparoscopic specimen extraction) is then inserted into the stoma trephine and opened maximally. The bowel is then passed through the wound protector. The inner ring of the wound protector is transected and removed. The remaining wound protector is brought out externally. The authors suggest this technique decreases spillage and minimizes bowel trauma during stoma exteriorization, particularly in the obese patient.[2]

DIVERTING STOMAS

As previously mentioned, diverting stomas are created to divert the fecal stream away from the "downstream" intestine. Diverting stomas consist of three types: loop ileostomy, loop colostomy, and end loop stomas. In the past, the most common loop stoma created was the transverse loop colostomy, popularized for the treatment of complicated diverticular disease and for protection of distal anastomoses. The transverse loop colostomy is often a poorly tolerated stoma with high complication rates and, therefore, has largely been replaced by the loop ileostomy. Additionally, anywhere a loop ileostomy or a loop colostomy is planned, an end loop ileostomy or end loop colostomy can be performed at the surgeon's discretion.

LOOP ILEOSTOMY

The loop ileostomy is generally created in association with distal bowel resection. After the resection and/or anastomosis have been completed, a segment of terminal ileum is selected. The most distal segment of the terminal ileum that will reach the abdominal wall without tension is selected. This generally corresponds to a segment 20 to 30 cm proximal to the ileocecal valve or from an ileoanal reservoir. The ileum is encircled with a Penrose drain or umbilical tape after its mobility has been ensured.

An abdominal wall defect is created as previously described for an end ileostomy. The defect may need to be slightly larger to accommodate both loops of bowel, which, by necessity, pass through the abdominal wall in a loop stoma. Before passing the ileum through the abdominal wall, proper orientation is ensured and the

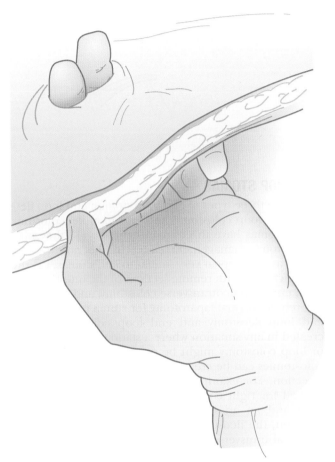

FIGURE 179-4 The stoma site admits two fingers.

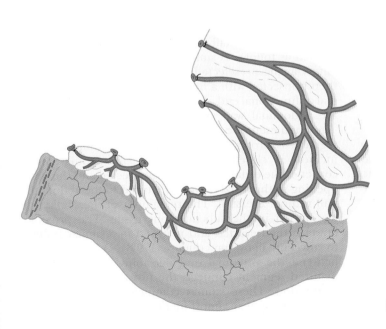

FIGURE 179-5 The ileum is prepared for ileostomy creation.

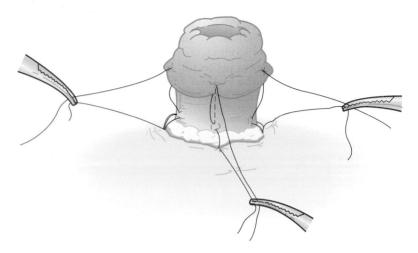

FIGURE 179-6 "Tripartite bites" between the dermis, the seromuscular layer of the bowel wall at the fascial level, and full thickness of the cut edge evert the stoma.

distal end is marked with a suture in order to prevent maturation of the incorrect segment after the abdominal incision has been closed. The ileal loop is passed through the abdominal wall without twisting and should protrude 4 to 5 cm beyond the abdominal skin. The midline incision is closed appropriately and protected with a cutaneous drape. The distal aspect of the ileum just above the abdominal wall is transected along approximately 80% of its circumference (from mesentery to mesentery). The distal end is then matured with simple sutures between the full-thickness terminal bowel and dermis. These sutures are placed close to one another in order to "reserve" the majority of the stoma site for the functional, proximal stoma.

Once the distal end has been sewn to the abdominal skin, the proximal end is everted. Three "tripartite" bites are taken between the dermis, the seromuscular layer of the ileum 5 cm proximal to the transected end, and a full-thickness bite of the open end of the ileum. Once the three sutures have been placed, they are tied with gentle traction applied to an Allis clamp within the lumen to facilitate eversion. Maturation is completed with two additional sutures between the dermis and the full thickness of the terminal ileum (Figure 179-7). The loop stoma should protrude adequately, with its functional end occupying approximately 80% of the trephine circumference. Unless undue tension is present, a support rod is generally not necessary.

LOOP COLOSTOMY

A loop sigmoid colostomy may be created in order to prevent the fecal stream from reaching the rectum and anus in cases of incontinence, severe anorectal infection, or for proximal protection after complex anal reconstruction. This stoma is essentially created in identical fashion to that of a loop ileostomy with the exception that the stoma is commonly placed in the left lower quadrant. Eversion is not strictly necessary because of the noncaustic nature of the effluent from the left colon. However, in many circumstances, an end loop stoma as described in the following section is easier to create and functions better than the standard loop colostomy.[3]

END LOOP STOMAS

There are three types of end loop stomas: end loop ileostomy, end loop colostomy, and end loop ileocolostomy. These stomas have three main benefits: (1) they often make stoma management easier in the postoperative period as they appear very similar to end stomas, (2) they can be created with remote sections of the intestine, such as an end loop ileotransverse colostomy, and (3) they do not require formal laparotomy for stoma takedown. The end loop ileostomy and end loop colostomy can be created in any situation where a standard loop ileostomy or loop colostomy might be performed. End loop ileocolostomies can be created in association with intestinal resection. For example, a right colectomy may be performed for right colon trauma or for right colon ischemia and an anastomosis is deemed unwise. In this situation, the ileostomy and the transected edge of the proximal transverse colon can be brought through one single stoma site, avoiding the need for a second stoma and laparotomy at the time of stoma takedown.

End Loop Ileostomy

Following intestinal resection and creation of an appropriate abdominal wall defect, the end loop ileostomy is created as follows: A small defect is created in the mesentery at the preselected ileal stomal site. The bowel is then transected with a linear stapling device. The proximal or functional end of the ileostomy is brought through the abdominal wall as for a standard end ileostomy. The antimesenteric corner of the distal, nonfunctional segment is brought through the same stoma site. The incision is closed appropriately. The antimesenteric corner of the distal staple line is transected and the small opening in the distal bowel is matured to the abdominal wall without eversion. The remainder of the staple line lies buried in the subcutaneous tissue. The proximal bowel is then everted and matured in a similar fashion to any end ileostomy (Figure 179-8). A single suture between the proximal end ileostomy and the distally matured segment connects the two and completes the maturation. These stomas completely divert the fecal stream and appear almost identical to end ileostomies.

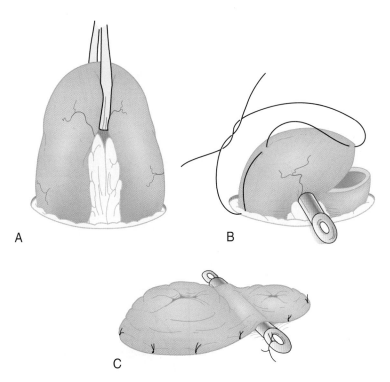

A

B

C

FIGURE 179-7 Creation of a loop ileostomy with support rod.

End Loop Colostomy

The end loop colostomy is created with a preselected segment of the sigmoid colon. It is mobilized appropriately and passed through the previously created abdominal wall defect similar to that of an end loop ileostomy. The abdominal incision is closed appropriately. The end colostomy is matured in a similar fashion to that of the end loop ileostomy. As previously mentioned for loop colostomies, the proximal end may be everted but a flush colostomy may also be created.

End Loop Ileocolostomy

This stoma can be performed in association with resection of the right colon when an anastomosis is unsafe. Following resection, the terminal ileum is prepared as for any routine end ileostomy. Often a stoma site will have to be created in the right upper quadrant in order to facilitate passage of the ileostomy and the distal transverse colon through the same abdominal aperture. Once the stoma site has been created, the terminal ileum is brought through the abdominal wall similar to an end ileostomy. The stapled-off end of the proximal transverse colon is brought through the abdominal wall defect. The mesenteric defect can be closed as with any standard colon resection.

Following this, the abdominal incision is closed in routine fashion. The antimesenteric corner of the transverse colon staple line is then transected and matured without eversion to the abdominal wall stoma site. Cutaneous sutures should be placed in proximity in order to save the majority of the stoma site for the ileostomy. Once this has been completed, the staple line is resected from the terminal ileum and the ileum matured as for a standard end ileostomy (Figure 179-9). The final suture

between transverse colon and the ileum is placed to complete the maturation.

This stoma has the previously mentioned advantages of avoiding a second stoma site for a mucous fistula. In addition, because the terminal ileum and transverse colon are in close approximation through the same stoma site, stoma takedown can be later performed directly through a parastomal incision without the need for a formal laparotomy. This may significantly decrease subsequent morbidity and recovery time after the subsequent stoma takedown.

Laparoscopic Ileostomy

If an ileostomy is needed in conjunction with a laparoscopic bowel resection (protection of a low anastomosis) or an ileostomy alone is needed (diversion proximal to complex anovaginal fistula repair or anal canal reconstruction), it can be easily created laparoscopically. Principles that apply to open ileostomy creation also apply when the operation is performed laparoscopically. The site should be selected according to the patient's body habitus and functional needs.

If a colectomy in conjunction with the ileostomy is essential, then ileostomy siting should be considered at the time of trochar placement. A trochar can certainly be placed through the future stoma trephine, but sites adjacent to the trephine within the footprint of the stoma appliance should be avoided. Trochars in place for the colectomy or proctectomy can be used to perform the intracorporeal components of the ileostomy creation.

If the ileostomy is created without any additional abdominal surgery, then only two ports are commonly necessary: one at the umbilicus for the camera and a second through the stoma site to manipulate the

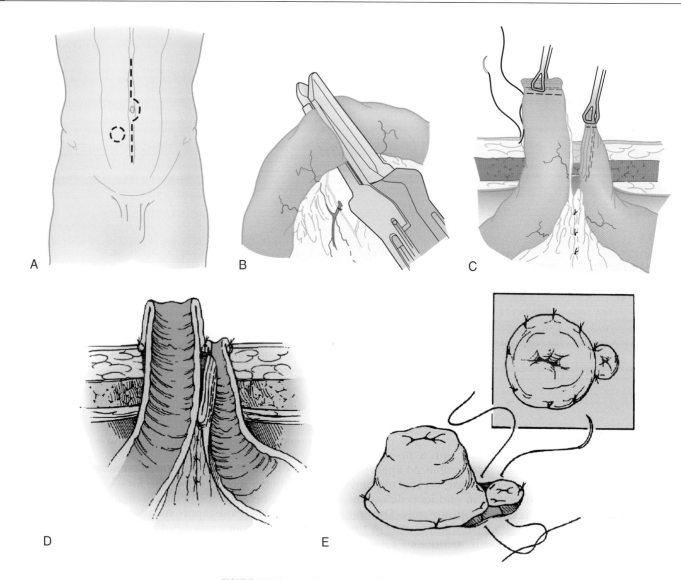

FIGURE 179-8 Creation of an end loop ileostomy.

terminal ileum. Under either circumstance, the operative principles are similar.

The terminal ileum is located just proximal to the ileocecal valve. The bowel is followed retrograde until a segment that easily reaches the abdominal wall at the stoma site is identified. Pneumoperitoneum should be deflated when assessing ileal length, as the abdomen will not be distended when the ileostomy is created or in use. Ileal mobilization is rarely required. Extreme care should be taken to ensure proper orientation of the bowel. The proper loop of bowel is grasped with a grasper through the stoma trephine and proximal and distal bowels carefully identified. If an additional port is available, the tip of a marking pen is grasped with a laparoscopic grasper and the distal end marked just beyond the grasper. (This is not possible if the two-port technique is used.)

Pneumoperitoneum is released and the stoma trephine is created in standard fashion around the grasper. The loop is then eviscerated carefully without twisting. Once this is done, pneumoperitoneum is reestablished and proper orientation is confirmed. (This is *essential* as

creating an ileostomy from the distal limb is highly problematic for the patient [because it can lead to an unanticipated mechanical small bowel obstruction] and very embarrassing for the surgeon.) Once proper orientation is confirmed, the stoma can be matured in standard fashion. A loop, end-loop, or end ileostomy can be created as indicated based on the clinical setting. After completion of stoma maturation, pneumoperitoneum is reestablished, proper orientation confirmed, and the abdominal cavity is checked for bleeding.

Laparoscopic Colostomy

Similar to ileostomy, all types of colostomies can be performed laparoscopically. Sigmoid colostomy is most common. Techniques are very similar to the creation of laparoscopic ileostomies. If trocars have been placed for rectosigmoid resection, no additional ports will be needed. If a colostomy is performed without other abdominal surgery, then three or four ports may be necessary. A camera port is placed through the umbilicus. Two ports are placed in the right midabdomen and the

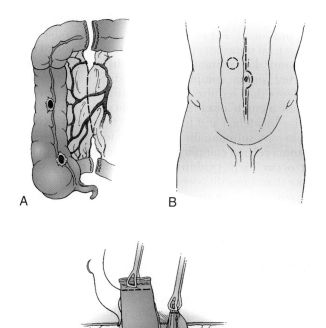

FIGURE 179-9 Creation of an end loop ileocolostomy.

right lower quadrant, respectively. A fourth port may be placed through the previously marked stoma site, if colonic mobilization is required. If the colostomy is created in conjunction with an abdominoperineal resection or sigmoid resection, mobilization is often already completed at this point. Occasionally, additional descending colon mobilization is necessary to create a stoma without tension.

If no colonic resection has been performed, then the sigmoid and descending colon will require mobilization. The sigmoid colon is retracted medially through the right midabdomen port, and the lateral peritoneal reflection is retracted laterally through the "stoma" port. The lateral attachments are then taken down with scissors or cautery through the right lower quadrant port. Once mobilization is complete, pneumoperitoneum is released and the colon checked for length. Again, the distal end is marked with a marker tip attached to a grasper (if distal resection has not been performed) after orientation has been carefully confirmed.

Pneumoperitoneum is then decompressed and the stoma trephine created in standard fashion. The colon is brought through the abdominal wall defect without twisting and the stoma matured with standard technique. As with ileostomy, end, end loop, or loop colostomy can all be created laparoscopically. After stoma completion, pneumoperitoneum is reestablished, orientation confirmed, and the abdominal wall cavity checked for bleeding.

ANTIADHESION BARRIERS AND STOMAS

Some authors have advocated the use of carboxymethyl cellulose and sodium hyaluronate when creating temporary loop stomas in order to facilitate ostomy reversal.[4,5] Very little is known about this, and it has not been subject to the rigors of a clinical trial. Authors suggest that wrapping the ileum at the time of stoma creation will minimize adhesions between the stoma and the abdominal wall, making stoma takedown easier. One study by Kawamura et al suggests shorter operative times in the antiadhesion group,[4] whereas a similar study by Tang et al does not.[5]

The technique is described as follows. The loop selected is eviscerated and a large sheet of Seprafilm is cut in half. The proximal and distal limbs of the bowel and their adjacent mesentery are wrapped in a "sushi roll" style. After the barrier has adhered, the loop is brought through the abdominal wall at the preselected site and the stoma matured in standard fashion. The utility of this technique remains unproven, but minimizing adhesions between the ileum and the abdominal wall should, in concept, make dissection at the time of ileostomy takedown easier.

ENTEROSTOMAL THERAPY

A dedicated ET's contribution to the long-term quality of life of an ostomate is simply immeasurable. Such therapists provide preoperative counseling, early postoperative education and guidance, and act as a long-term resource for individuals with stomas. They supply information on appliance choices, local support groups such as the United Ostomy Association and the Crohn's and Colitis Foundation, suggest dietary or clothing modifications that may alleviate stoma-related problems, and aid in the management of skin problems, parastomal hernias, prolapse, and other complications. In most situations, an ET or surgical nurse will provide detailed postoperative education for a new ostomate. However, if this support is unavailable, it is the surgeon's responsibility to ensure the patient is educated in appliance management.

The appliance must be emptied frequently enough to avoid overfilling and dislodgement of the pouch. This is determined by the location of the stoma and the patient's natural bowel pattern. Ileostomies are usually emptied four to six times per day, with colostomies emptied once or twice per day or even once every other day. The entire appliance only needs to be changed every 4 to 7 days. The exact details vary from individual to individual, but a common technique for changing a typical one-piece system is explained in Box 179-2.

Pouches should generally be changed when the stoma is least active, which is often after a period of fasting. The time will vary from individual to individual, but changing the appliance when the stoma is less active avoids the need to control fresh output during the procedure.

The noise and odor of gas emitted from a stoma are a major concern to most ostomates. Anything that causes gas before creation of the stoma is likely to create gas following its construction. Gas comes from two sources: swallowed air and bacterial breakdown of ingested foodstuffs, particularly carbohydrates. The amount of

---

BOX 179-2 Stoma Care

1. Gather all supplies.
2. Gently remove soiled pouch by pushing down on skin while lifting up on pouch. Discard soiled pouch in odor-proof plastic bag. *Save tail closure.*
3. Clean stoma and peristomal skin with water; pat dry. *If indicated*, shave or clip peristomal hair.
4. Use stoma-measuring guide or established pattern to determine size of stoma. *Presized pouch:* Check to be sure pouch opening is correct size. Order new supplies if indicated. *Cut-to-fit-pouch:* Trace correctly sized pattern onto back of barrier or pouch surface and cut stomal opening to match pattern. Once stomal shrinkage is complete, this step may be omitted and preparation of the clean pouch may be completed before the soiled pouch is removed.
5. Apply skin barrier paste around the stoma. (*Tip:* wet finger to facilitate paste application.) An alternative approach is to apply skin barrier paste to the aperture in the prepared pouch or barrier. Allow paste to dry. *Optional:* Apply skin sealant to skin that will be covered by tape. Allow to dry.
6. Remove paper backing from pouch or barrier to expose adhesive surface; center pouch opening over stoma and press into place. Attach closure. *Optional:* Apply tape strips to "picture frame" the pouch-skin junction.

From Lavery IC, Erwin-Toth P: Stoma therapy. In Cataldo P, MacKeigan J, editors: *Intestinal stomas.* New York, 2004, Marcel Dekker, p 65.

---

swallowed air can be minimized by avoiding the use of straws, excessive talking while eating, chewing gum, and smoking. Each individual can best identify which foods lead to gas production, but beans, broccoli, onions, brussel sprouts, beer, and dairy products in lactose-deficient individuals are common culprits. Avoiding these foods is a personal choice, but will decrease the quantity and odor of stomal flatus. Yogurt, parsley, and orange juice have been associated with decreased odor. Odor-proof pouches, charcoal filters, and pouch deodorants (such as commercial deodorants, mouthwash, and perineal deodorants) may also help. Orally ingested deodorants are also available and include bismuth subgallate and chlorophyllin complex. However, the most important key to preventing odor is good peristomal hygiene and creating a leak-proof seal at the time of appliance change.

A period of adjustment occurs in all ostomates, but attention to detail at the time of appliance change combined with minor dietary and clothing modifications, should make a stoma completely unnoticeable to all except the ostomate's closest acquaintances. In addition, abdominal stomas should not preclude participation in almost any physical activity.

COMPLICATIONS

Despite modest advances in surgical technique and enterostomal therapy, complications after stoma creation remain extremely common. The rate of stoma-specific complications in the literature varies quite widely, ranging from 10% to 70% depending on the methodology of the study, the length of followup, and the definition of a complication.[6-10] For example, virtually all ostomates will have at least transient episodes of minor peristomal irritation, and skin irritation is often the most commonly reported stoma complication. Studies only reporting problems that require revisional surgery will obviously indicate a much lower rate of complications. As such, the relative incidence and frequency of the specific complications vary substantially from series to series.

Stoma-related complications may be classified as those that occur early (within 1 month of surgery) or late (more than 1 month postoperatively). The most common early complications are peristomal skin irritation, leakage, high output, and ischemia. The most commonly reported late complications include parastomal hernia, prolapse, obstruction, and stenosis.

INCIDENCE

There is no universally accepted criteria for what constitutes a "complication." As such, adverse events associated with stoma creation may be quite mild, such as transient skin irritation or leakage, or require major revisional surgery as may be the case for parastomal hernia or necrosis. In a 20-year retrospective review of 1,616 patients in the Cook County Hospital database, Park et al reported a 34% incidence of complications, 28% being early and 6% classified as late.[6] The most common early complications were skin irritation (12%), pain associated with poor stoma location (7%), and partial necrosis (5%). The most common late complications were also skin irritation (6%), prolapse (2%), and stenosis (2%). Of note, complications varied greatly by service, with ostomies created by general surgeons associated with a 47% complication rate, whereas the complication rate for colorectal surgeons was 32%. Duchesne et al retrospectively reviewed 164 ostomates cared for at Charity Hospital in New Orleans.[7] The overall complication rate was 25%; 38% of the complications were early and 62% were late. As is typically the case, ileostomies were associated with a higher complication rate than colostomies. The most common complications were necrosis (22%), prolapse (22%), skin irritation (17%), and stenosis (17%). Risk factors for complications included inflammatory bowel disease, ischemic colitis, and increased body mass index. As others have observed,[8] obesity markedly increased the risk of skin irritation. Of particular note was the sixfold decrease in stoma complications when an ET was involved in the patient's care.

Saghir et al retrospectively reviewed 121 stoma patients and reported a 67% complication rate, 41% of which were considered minor and 26% were considered major.[9] Nine of the patients (7%) required revisional surgery. Complications were associated with older age, increased medical comorbidities, and an ostomy created by other than a colorectal surgeon.

Life table analyses have been performed both for patients undergoing ileostomies[11] and colostomies.[12] The cumulative probability of a complication after creation of an end ileostomy in 150 patients was 68% at 20 years. There was a 34% cumulative risk of skin problems, which tended to diminish over time. Twenty-three percent of patients developed a bowel obstruction. Of note in this series, patients undergoing an ileostomy for ulcerative colitis had a higher risk of complications than those undergoing an ileostomy for Crohn disease. Most other studies find the opposite to be true. The actuarial risk of a colostomy complication was 58.1% at 13 years.[12] The cumulative probability of revisional surgery was 17% at 11 years. The most common complications were hernia (37%), obstruction (14%), prolapse (12%), and stenosis (7%).

Both patient-specific and technical factors contribute to stoma complications. Preoperative consultation with an ET, or at least preoperative stoma marking, reduces the incidence of stoma-related complications.[1]

SKIN IRRITATION/LEAKAGE

Skin irritation is very common among patients with a stoma. In a review of 610 patients, it was by far the most common early local complication.[8] The problem is far more commonly seen in patients with an ileostomy owing to the liquid, caustic effluent[13]; this highlights the need for proper technique when an ileostomy is created. Nugent et al described the results of a study utilizing quality-of-life questionnaires in 391 ostomates.[14] Fifty-one percent reported problems with a "rash" and 36% had experienced leakage, both of which were much more commonly seen with ileostomies than colostomies. Thirty percent of patients with a colostomy and 55% with an ileostomy had experienced a reaction to the adhesive. However, only 8% of ostomates reported a substantial degree of difficulty associated with skin irritation.

Although a minor degree of skin irritation on occasion is probably inevitable, most significant cases of skin irritation are potentially preventable. Preoperative marking by an ET can help ensure proper siting and a secure fit. Appropriate location and careful appliance fitting minimize the noxious, irritating effect that can be associated with leakage or unprotected peristomal skin (Figure 179-10). Patients also need to be monitored for allergic reactions to the components of the appliance.

Particular attention must be paid to older patients who may have limitations in eyesight or dexterity. Patients with a high-output stoma are at particular risk for skin

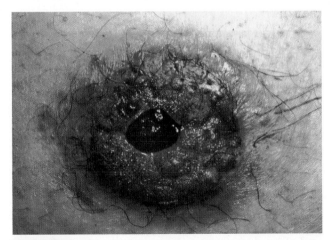

FIGURE 179-10 Skin irritation around the stoma site from a poorly fitting appliance.

irritation and ulceration if they do not have an appropriately fitted appliance. Obesity has been frequently reported to be associated with an increased risk of skin irritation, likely owing to technical problems with stoma construction.[15] Consideration should be given to placing the stoma in the upper abdomen where there is typically much less subcutaneous fat and the patient can see it much more readily.

The patient should be instructed to avoid creams or ointments that may interfere with the adherence of their appliance. In the postoperative period, a stoma will tend to become less edematous and the abdomen becomes less distended. As such, it is quite common to need to "downsize" the appliance at the first postoperative visit to minimize exposed skin. Changing a stoma too frequently may lead to excessive wear and tear on the parastomal skin; on the other hand, too long an interval between changing the appliance may be associated with erosion of the protective barrier.

Even with the help of an excellent ET, specific skin infections may occur. Fungal overgrowth is evident when there is a bright red rash around the stoma with associated satellite lesions. This is typically easily treated by dusting the parastomal skin with an appropriate antifungal powder or an oral agent in refractory cases. If the dermatitis conforms precisely to the outline of the stoma appliance, then an allergic reaction to the wafer or other component of the appliance is likely the culprit. Peristomal skin irritation may also be associated with reactivation of inflammatory bowel disease.

Fortunately, most cases of skin irritation and leakage are readily managed by conservative means. However, a redundant pannus, surgical scars, or creases with poor stoma siting may result in the need for revisional surgery. Revising the site of the stoma or combined abdominal wall recontouring and stoma revision may be necessary.[16]

HIGH-OUTPUT STOMAS

For obvious reasons, a high-output state is typically described in association with an ileostomy rather than a colostomy. Marked diarrhea and dehydration occur in 5% to 20% of ileostomy patients, with the greatest risk occurring in the early postoperative period. An ileostomy usually functions by the third or fourth postoperative day.[17] The output typically peaks on the fourth postoperative day, with an output of up to 3.2 L reported. Because the ostomy effluent is rich in sodium, hyponatremia can be a problem. The particular window of vulnerability for dehydration appears to be between the third and eighth postoperative day. In time, the small bowel typically adapts with mucosal hyperplasia and there is a steady decrease in ostomy output. However, patients with an ileostomy, particularly those who have had concomitant small bowel resection, are at risk to become dehydrated. Most often, this is easily managed by oral rehydration with one of the commonly available sports drinks. However, patients who have lost considerable absorptive surface owing to previous bowel resection and/or those with recurrent/residual Crohn disease are at particular risk. In addition to the loss of absorptive surface area, ileal resection also removes the fat or complex carbohydrate stimulation of the so-called ileal brake, which slows gastric emptying and small bowel transit.[18] Fluid and electrolyte maintenance in these patients may require a period of parenteral hydration and nutrition.

Clostridium difficile enteritis is an increasingly reported cause of ileostomy diarrhea, especially in patients who have had a total colectomy for inflammatory bowel disease.[19] The typical presentation is ileostomy diarrhea followed by ileus. This condition has been associated with a high mortality, although early recognition and treatment appears to be associated with better outcomes.[20]

Ileostomy diarrhea may be treated in its milder forms with oral fiber supplements or cholestyramine, which can thicken secretions. Histamine receptor antagonists or proton pump inhibitors are often useful in reducing gastric fluid secretion, especially in the first 6 months after surgery when hypergastrinemia is most severe.[21] Often, antimotility agents (e.g., loperamide or diphenoxylate) or opiates (e.g., codeine or tincture of opium) may be required to slow intestinal transit. In refractory cases, somatostatin analogue has been used with some success. Somatostatin reduces salt and water excretion and slows gastrointestinal tract motility. However, its clinical usage has met with variable results.[22] Special mention is made of patients with a high ostomy required to treat complications of an anastomotic leak. Good results have been reported with exteriorizing the leak and reinfusing the ostomy effluent into the downstream limb until gastrointestinal continuity can be restored. This has led to weaning parenteral nutrition in a substantial number of patients.[23]

A related problem in patients with an ileostomy is the development of urinary stones. The obligatory loss of fecal water, sodium, and bicarbonate reduces urinary pH and volume.[24] Whereas approximately 4% of the general population develop urinary stones, the incidence in patients with an ileostomy is approximately twice that. Whereas uric acid stones comprise less than 10% of the calculi in the general population, they comprise 60% of stones in ileostomy patients. There is also an increase in the incidence of calcium oxalate stones.[25]

BOWEL OBSTRUCTION

Life table analyses suggest that bowel obstruction is a rather common complication of ostomy creation. Twenty-three percent of patients with an ileostomy ultimately develop bowel obstruction.[11] Adhesions are probably the most common cause, but small bowel volvulus or internal hernia may be the culprit. Although it is frequently mentioned that suture of the mesentery to the lateral abdominal wall may prevent volvulus or obstruction, retrospective analyses have not shown any benefit to this maneuver.[11,12] Treatment is not dissimilar to other patients presenting with a mechanical small bowel obstruction.

However, special note must be made of food bolus obstruction. Many patients with an ileostomy may develop signs and symptoms of bowel obstruction owing to the accumulation of poorly digested foodstuffs (e.g., popcorn, peanuts, and fresh fruits and vegetables). A careful history may reveal dietary indiscretions. Further, the possibility of a food bolus obstruction should be considered in any patient with an ileostomy who has

radiologic evidence of a distal obstruction. A red rubber catheter may be inserted gently into the ostomy and saline irrigation initiated. If suspicious concretions begin to pass into the stoma, the irrigations may be carefully repeated until the obstruction is relieved.

ISCHEMIA

Edema and venous congestion are very common after stoma creation owing to mechanical trauma and compression of the small mesenteric venules as they traverse the abdominal wall. This is typically self-limiting and requires no treatment.[26] However, ischemia may be related to tension on the mesentery or excessive mesenteric division, particularly in obese patients or those undergoing emergency surgery.[27] A common error is dividing the sigmoidal vessels to obtain the length to allow a colostomy to reach the skin. In these cases, the inferior mesenteric vessels should instead be divided proximally and/or the splenic flexure mobilized, preserving the sigmoid arcades.

If ischemia becomes apparent, a glass test tube or flexible endoscope may be inserted into the stoma. If the stoma is viable at fascial level, then the patient may be carefully observed. However, if there is question about the viability of the stoma at the fascial level, immediate laparotomy and stoma revision is required. Early ischemia is seen in 1% to 10% of colostomies and 1% to 5% of ileostomies.[28]

PARASTOMAL HERNIA

Parastomal hernia is probably the most common stoma complication requiring operative intervention (Figure 179-11). A parastomal hernia develops in 2% to 28% of patients with an end ileostomy and 4% to 48% with an end colostomy.[29] The occurrence of these hernias increases with time[30]; as such, the reported incidence depends greatly on the length of followup. Most patients with a parastomal hernia can be managed expectantly or with a belted appliance; however, patients with unrelenting pain, obstruction, or difficulty maintaining an appliance generally require surgical repair.

Patient-specific factors such as obesity, advanced age, and chronic obstructive pulmonary disease appear to increase the risk of parastomal herniation.[10] From the

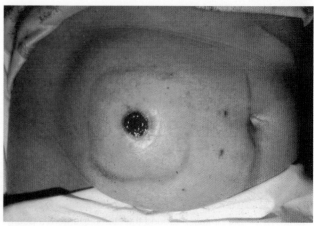

FIGURE 179-11 Large parastomal hernia.

technical standpoint, making the smallest possible opening in the abdominal wall without making the stoma ischemic seems prudent. However, many of the other "preventive" measures such as lateral space closure, fascial fixation, or stoma placement through the rectus muscle, appear to have no effect on the incidence of these hernias. The use of prosthetic mesh prophylactically, especially in the sublay position, may reduce the risk of parastomal herniation.[31,32]

Unfortunately, the results of surgical correction have historically been poor, highlighting the importance of careful patient selection and prudent attempts at conservative management in patients without clear indications for surgery. In one of the largest reported series, 63% of patients developed a recurrent hernia and 63% had at least one complication.[33] The most commonly described techniques are direct repair, stoma relocation, and mesh repair. The recurrence rate with mesh repairs (0% to 33%) clearly appears to be lower than that of direct repair (46% to 100%), or stoma relocation (76%).[29,34,35]

A wide variety of mesh repairs have been described, but it remains uncertain what type of mesh should be used and what the optimal position is for placement. The intraperitoneal or underlay mesh repair, championed by Sugarbaker, has probably been associated with the most encouraging results.[36] Intraabdominal pressure tends to keep the mesh in place. One benefit of the intraperitoneal technique is that a concomitant incisional hernia may be repaired at the same time. Various laparoscopic techniques have been successfully utilized for intraperitoneal mesh placement.[37-39] Concerns have been expressed about the long-term risk of mesh erosion, prompting interest in the use of biologic mesh materials.[40,41]

Mesh may also be placed using an extraperitoneal fascial onlay technique.[42,43] A curvilinear lateral incision is made outside the outline of the stoma wafer. The hernia sac is entered and omentum and bowel are reduced. An onlay mesh is secured to the fascial defect. The advantage of this technique is that it avoids a major intraperitoneal procedure, making it attractive in patients who are poor candidates for laparoscopy/laparotomy. However, the recurrence rate with this procedure is undoubtedly much higher than with underlay placement of the mesh.

STENOSIS

Stoma stenosis may result from ischemia, excessive tension, retraction, or recurrent inflammatory bowel disease. The reported incidence is typically less than 10%.[12]

Mild asymptomatic stenosis does not require any treatment. Skin-level stenosis is readily treated with local procedures such as a Z- or W-plasty,[44] whereas those associated with Crohn disease usually require formal bowel resection. Timing of surgery is an important consideration in patients with a retracted and/or stenotic stoma. Fourteen percent of colostomies and 12% of ileostomies develop retraction within 3 weeks of surgery[45]; many of these will develop a stenosis, ultimately requiring revision. With good enterostomal therapy (e.g., use of a convex pouch) and temporizing measures such as gentle

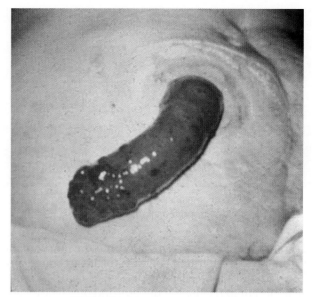

FIGURE 179-12 Prolapsed ileostomy.

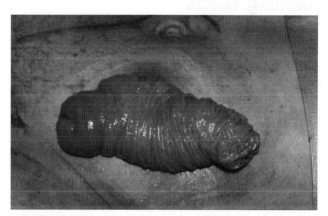

FIGURE 179-13 Large prolapse of a transverse loop colostomy.

digital dilation, the acute inflammatory response is permitted to subside. This facilitates the ability to perform a local revision at a later date when the bowel and mesentery are less friable and rigid.

PROLAPSE

The risk of stoma prolapse has been reported to be 11.8% at 13 years (Figure 179-12).[12] Transverse loop colostomies are especially notorious for prolapse (Figure 179-13); the efferent limb is virtually always the offending cause. Although somewhat controversial, this is a primary reason why loop ileostomy is commonly preferred to loop colostomy for temporary fecal diversion.[46,47] Although often advocated, mesenteric fixation or lateral space closure do not appear to reduce the incidence of stoma prolapse.

Although the prolapse is often unsettling to the patient or healthcare providers, asymptomatic prolapse requires no treatment, especially if the stoma is temporary. When the prolapse causes ischemia, obstruction, or pouching problems, surgical intervention is warranted and usually straightforward. The stoma is freed up from the abdominal wall and the bowel delivered until taut.

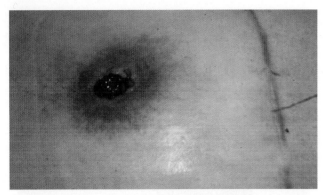

FIGURE 179-14 The characteristic "blue hue" of peristomal varices is visible only after removing the stoma appliance.

The redundant bowel is amputated and the mucocutaneous border reestablished. In cases of incarcerated prolapse without advanced ischemia, sugar can be applied as a desiccant to facilitate reduction and obviate the need for urgent surgery.[48]

PERISTOMAL VARICES

Stomal varices may cause life-threatening hemorrhage. The varices occur at the level of the mucocutaneous border of the ostomy secondary to the anastomoses between the high-pressure portal venous system and the low-pressure subcutaneous veins of the abdominal wall.[49] The diagnosis is suspected in ostomates with serious liver disease and confirmed by the typical purplish hue or "caput medusae" of the peristomal skin. Common scenarios include extensive liver metastases after abdominoperineal resection for rectal cancer or sclerosing cholangitis in a patient who has undergone total proctocolectomy with ileostomy for ulcerative colitis. A high index of suspicion is critical and the stoma wafer must be removed to allow for skin inspection (Figure 179-14).[50]

Patients with very short life expectancies (e.g., extensive liver metastases) may be treated by mucocutaneous disconnection; the stoma is freed up to the level of fascia, thereby dividing the portosystemic connections. Recent reports suggest that percutaneous coil embolization may be another option in this subgroup.[51] Because these anastomoses typically re-form within 1 year, more definitive solutions are required in most patients. More durable options include surgical shunts, transjugular intrahepatic portosystemic shunts (TIPS), or liver transplantation, based on life expectancy and the status of the associated liver disease.

SUGGESTED READINGS

Carne PW, Robertson GM, Frizelle FA: Parastomal hernia. *Br J Surg* 90:784, 2003.

Cottam J, Richards K, Halsted A, et al: Results of a nationwide prospective audit of stoma complications within three weeks of surgery. *Colorectal Dis* 9:834, 2007.

Israelsson LA: Parastomal hernias. *Surg Clin N Am* 88:113, 2008.

Lavery IC, Erwin-Toth P: Stoma therapy. In Cataldo P, MacKeigan J, editors: *Intestinal stomas.* New York, 2004, Marcel Dekker, p 65.

REFERENCES

1. Bass EM, Pino AD, Tan A, et al: Does preoperative stoma marking and education by the enterostomal therapist affect outcome? *Dis Colon Rectum* 40:440, 1997.
2. Meagher AP, Owen G, Gett R: Multimedia article. An improved technique for end stoma creation in obese patients. *Dis Colon Rectum* 52:531, 2009.
3. Unti JA, Abcarian H, Pearl RK, et al: Rodless end-loop stomas—A seven year experience. *Dis Colon Rectum* 34:999, 1991.
4. Kawamura YJ, Kakizawa N, Tan KY, et al: Sushi-roll wrap of Seprafilm for ileostomy limbs facilitates ileostomy closure. *Tech Coloproctol* 13:211, 2009.
5. Tang CL, Seow-Choen F, Fook-Cong S, et al: Bioresorbable adhesion barrier facilitates early closure of the defunctioning ileostomy after rectal excision: A prospective, randomized trial. *Dis Colon Rectum* 46:1200, 2003.
6. Park JJ, Del Pino A, Orsay CP, et al: Stoma complications: The Cook County Hospital experience. *Dis Colon Rectum* 42:1575, 1999.
7. Duchesne JC, Wang YZ, Weintraub SL, et al: Stoma complications: A multivariate analysis. *Ann Surg* 68:961, 2002.
8. Pearl RK, Prasad LM, Orsay CP, et al: Early local complications from intestinal stomas. *Arch Surg* 120:1145, 1985.
9. Saghir JH, McKenzie FD, Leckie DM: Factors that predict complications after construction of a stoma: A retrospective study. *Eur J Surg* 167:531, 2001.
10. Arumugam PJ, Bevan L, MacDonald L, et al: A prospective audit of stomas—analysis of risk factors and complications and their management. *Colorectal Dis* 5:49, 2003.
11. Leong AP, Londono-Schimmer EE, Phillips RK: Life table analysis of stomal complications following ileostomy. *Br J Surg* 81:727, 1994.
12. Londono-Schimmer EE, Leong AP, Phillips RK: Life table analysis of stomal complications following colostomy. *Dis Colon Rectum* 37:916, 1994.
13. Makela JT, Turku PH, Laitinen ST: Analysis of late stomal complications following ostomy surgery. *Ann Chir Gynaecol* 86:305, 1997.
14. Nugent KP, Daniels P, Stewart B, et al: Quality of life in stoma patients. *Dis Colon Rectum* 42:156974, 1999.
15. Leenen LPH, Kuypers JH: Some factors influencing the outcome of stoma surgery. *Dis Colon Rectum* 32:500, 1989.
16. Evans JP, Brown MH, Wilkes GH, et al: Revising the troublesome stoma: Combined abdominal wall recontouring and revision of stomas. *Dis Colon Rectum* 46:122, 2003.
17. Tang CL, Yunos A, Leong AP, et al: Ileostomy output in the early postoperative period. *Br J Surg* 82:607, 1995.
18. Nehra V, Camilleri M, Burton D, et al: An open trial of octreotide long-acting release in the management of short bowel syndrome. *Am J Gastroenterol* 96:1494, 2001.
19. Wood M, Hyman N, Hebert J, et al: Catastrophic *Clostridium difficile* enteritis in a pelvic pouch patient. *J Gastroint Surg* 1:350, 2008.
20. Lundeen SJ, Otterson MF, Binion DG, et al: *Clostridium difficile* enteritis: An early postoperative complication in inflammatory bowel disease patients after colectomy. *J Gastrointest Surg* 11:138, 2007.
21. Buchman AL, Scolapio J, Fryer J: AGA technical review on short bowel syndrome and intestinal transplantation. *Gastroenterology* 124:111, 2003.
22. Szilagyi A, Shrier I: Systematic review: The use of somatostatin or octreotide in refractory diarrhea. *Aliment Pharmacol Ther* 15:1889, 2003.
23. Calicis B, Parc Y, Caplin S, et al: Treatment of postoperative peritonitis of small bowel origin with continuous enteral nutrition and succus entericus reinfusion. *Arch Surg* 137:296, 2002.
24. Christie PM, Knight GS, Hill GL: Comparison of relative risks of urinary stone formation after surgery for ulcerative colitis: Conventional ileostomy *vs.* J-pouch. A comparative study. *Dis Colon Rectum* 39:50, 1996.
25. Christie PM, Knight GS, Hill GL: Metabolism of body water and electrolytes after surgery for ulcerative colitis conventional ileostomy *versus* J-pouch. *Br J Surg* 77:149, 1990.
26. Cottam J, Richards K, Hasted A, et al: Results of a nationwide prospective audit of stoma complications within 3 weeks of surgery. *Colorectal Dis* 9:834, 2007.
27. Robertson I, Eung E, Hughes D, et al: Prospective analysis of stoma related complications. *Colorectal Dis* 7:279, 2005.

28. Shellito PC: Complications of abdominal stoma surgery. *Dis Colon Rectum* 41:1562, 1998.

29. Carne PW, Robertson GM, Frizelle FA: Parastomal hernia. *Br J Surg* 90:784, 2003.

30. Mylonakis E, Scarpa M, Barolla M, et al: Life table analysis of hernia following end colostomy construction. *Colorectal Dis* 3:334, 2001.

31. Janes A, Cengiz Y, Israelsson LA: Randomized clinical trial of the use of a prosthetic mesh to prevent parastomal hernia. *Br J Surg* 91:280, 2004.

32. Gögenur I, Mortensen J, Harvald T, et al: Prevention of parastomal hernia by placement of a polypropylene mesh at the primary operation. *Dis Colon Rectum* 46:1131, 2006.

33. Rubin MS, Schoetz DJ Jr, Matthews JB: Parastomal hernia. Is stoma relocation superior to fascial repair? *Arch Surg* 129:413, 1994.

34. Cheung MT, Chia NH, Chiu WY: Surgical treatment of parastomal hernia complicating sigmoid colostomies. *Dis Colon Rectum* 44:266, 2001.

35. Steele SR, Lee P, Martin MJ, et al: Is parastomal hernia repair with polypropylene mesh safe? *Am J Surg* 185:436, 2003.

36. Sugarbaker PH: Peritoneal approach to prosthetic mesh repair of paraostomy hernias. *Ann Surg* 201:344, 1985.

37. Stelzner S, Hellmich G, Ludwig K: Repair of paracolostomy hernias with a prosthetic mesh in the intraperitoneal onlay position: Modified Sugarbaker technique. *Dis Colon Rectum* 47:185, 2004.

38. Hansson BME, Bleichrodt RP, de Hingh IH: Laparoscopic parastomal hernia repair using a keyhole technique results in a high recurrence rate. *Surg Endosc* 23:1456, 2009.

39. Mancini GJ, McClusky DA 3rd, Khaitan L, et al: Laparoscopic parastomal hernia repair using a nonslit mesh technique. *Surg Endosc* 21:1487, 2007.

40. Steele SR, Lee P, Martin MJ, et al: Is parastomal hernia repair with polypropylene mesh safe? *Am J Surg* 185:436, 2003.

41. Ellis CN: Short-term outcomes with the use of bioprosthetics for the management of parastomal hernias. *Dis Colon Rectum* 46:1118, 2008.

42. Hansson BME, van Nieowenhoven EJ, Bleichrodt RP: Promising new technique in the repair of parastomal hernia. *Surg Endosc* 17:1789, 2003.

43. Amin SN, Armitage NC, Abercrombie JF, et al: Lateral repair of parastomal hernia. *Ann R Coll Surg Engl* 83:206, 2001.

44. Beraldo S, Titley G, Allan A: Use of W-plasty in stenotic stoma: A new solution for an old problem. *Colorectal Dis* 8:715, 2006.

45. Cottam J, Richards K, Hasted A, et al: Results of a nationwide prospective audit of stoma complications within 3 weeks of surgery. *Colorectal Dis* 9:834, 2007.

46. Edwards DP, Leppington-Clarke A, Sexton R, et al: Stoma-related complications are more frequent after transverse colostomy than loop ileostomy: A prospective randomized clinical trial. *Br J Surg* 88:360, 2001.

47. Rondelli F, Reboldi P, Rulli A, et al: Loop ileostomy versus loop colostomy for fecal diversion after colorectal or coloanal anastomosis: A meta-analysis. *Int J Colorectal Dis* 24:479, 2009.

48. Shapiro R, Chin EH, Steinhagen RM: Reduction of an incarcerated, prolapsed ileostomy with the assistance of sugar as a desiccant. *Tech Coloproctol* 14:269, 2010.

49. Fucini CF, Wolff BG, Dozois RR: Bleeding from peristomal varices: Perspectives on prevention and treatment. *Dis Colon Rectum* 34:1073, 1991.

50. Spier BJ, Fayyad AA, Lucey MR, et al: Bleeding stomal varices: Case series and systematic review of the literature. *Clin Gastroenterol Hepatol* 6:346, 2008.

51. Naidu SG, Castle EP, Kriegshauser JS, et al: Direct percutaneous embolization of bleeding stomal varices. *Cardiovasc Intervent Radiol* 33:201, 2010.

CHAPTER 180

Surgery in the Immunocompromised Patient

Carlos E. Pineda | George J. Chang | Mark L. Welton

The immunocompromised state is characterized by defects in the system of defense against infections and malignancy and is classified as primary (as in immunodeficiency syndromes) or secondary (as in acquired states). Impaired immune function may thus result from genetic disorders, malnutrition, injury, disease, cancer therapy, inflammatory diseases, or pharmacologic manipulation. Advances in transplantation, oncology, and the treatment of acquired immunodeficiency syndrome (AIDS) have increased the life expectancy of these patients, and thus the population of patients with impaired immunologic function has enlarged. Immunocompromised patients who have problems that require surgical attention are more likely to experience a delay in diagnosis and an increased mortality rate compared with patients without immune defects. Because an increasing number of surgical patients are immunocompromised, it is important to recognize and to understand the immunocompromised state to properly manage these patients.

MECHANISMS OF IMMUNODEFICIENCY

Host defense mechanisms are broadly characterized as innate and adaptive. Innate immunity represents the first line of defense and includes a set of barriers (mechanical, chemical, and biologic) as well as cells and preexisting molecules that act immediately on contact with an infectious agent. Adaptive immunity, also known as acquired immunity, is based on activity of T and B cells and allows for immune responses that are more focused and intense than those of the innate immune system.[1] Primary and acquired defects in these defenses may occur.

Table 180-1 lists the most common primary immunodeficiencies and their sequelae. Patients with primary immune defects are more likely to have infectious complications that require medical, rather than surgical, treatment compared with patients with acquired deficiencies. With combined cellular and humoral defects, severe, life-threatening infections with opportunistic organisms such as cytomegalovirus (CMV), *Pneumocystis jiroveci*, or *Candida* may occur. Secondary immunodeficiency is caused by immunosuppressive medication administered to patients after transplantation, with inflammatory bowel disease (IBD), cancer, cancer therapies, injury, or malnutrition. Common causes of acquired immunodeficiency in surgical patients are summarized in Box 180-1.

PHARMACOLOGIC THERAPY

One of the most common causes of immunosuppression in surgical patients occurs when immunosuppressive drug therapy is administered to patients for transplantation, anticancer therapy, or IBD. Other diseases that are treated with pharmacologic immunosuppression include autoimmune disorders such as rheumatoid arthritis and scleroderma. Pharmacologic immunosuppression may occur due to corticosteroid therapy, lymphocyte inhibition, cytotoxic and antimetabolite chemotherapy, or cytokine regulation. Immunosuppressive drugs commonly used for solid organ transplantation and IBD, along with their mechanisms of action, are listed in Table 180-2. The net effect is down-regulation of the cellular immune response with a resultant increased susceptibility to bacterial infection, impairment of wound healing, and increased risk for some malignancies (e.g., skin cancers, cervical and anal cancers, and non-Hodgkin lymphomas). Furthermore, these immunosuppressive agents cause hepatotoxicity, nephrotoxicity, and bone marrow suppression, which pose additional problems for the management of these patients.

CANCER AND CANCER THERAPY

Defects in both T- and B-cell–mediated immunity are associated with advanced cancer. This occurs primarily as a result of the malignancy and secondarily as a result of the oncologic therapy. Tumorigenesis may be associated with impaired cytokine production and lymphokine-activated killer cell development. The secondary causes of immunosuppression include the effects of chemotherapy and radiation therapy on the bone marrow and intestinal mucosa. These therapies cause bone marrow suppression with neutropenia or pancytopenia and can result in profoundly impaired immune function. Lymphocytes are the most radiosensitive immune cells. Thus, irradiation is associated with lymphocyte dysfunction and resultant defects in humoral and cell-mediated immunity.

Chemotherapy and radiation also have deleterious effects on barrier defenses. Both radiation and chemotherapy can cause mucosal sloughing or ulceration in the gastrointestinal tract, leading to weakened barrier defenses and an increased risk for bacterial transmigration. Finally, these immunosuppressed patients with cancer often have indwelling catheters through which chemotherapy is delivered and that allow bacterial access through the skin.

MALNUTRITION AND INJURY

Prolonged starvation is associated with both humoral and cellular immune defects with reduced immunoglobulin production and T-cell proliferation in response to immunogens. Macrophage and neutrophil defects may also occur. Wound healing is impaired. Trauma and injury cause similar immune defects, especially in cellular immunity.

Burns are among the injuries that cause the most dramatic immunosuppression. They cause defects in humoral and cellular immunity similar to traumatic injury, in addition to loss of epithelial barriers. In severe burns, immunoglobulin levels reach their nadir on the second to third day, and depletion of IgG, an important opsonizing antibody, correlates with septic complications.[2] As a result, approximately 50% of the mortality of patients in burn units are from infection.

ACQUIRED IMMUNODEFICIENCY SYNDROME

The pathogenesis of AIDS immunosuppression begins with the binding of the human immunodeficiency virus (HIV) virions to the CD4 lymphocytes (also known as helper T cells) via an interaction between the gp120 viral envelope protein and the CD4 cell surface molecule. The viral core components, consisting of a single-stranded RNA particle and the reverse transcriptase, become internalized in the target CD4 cell. Within the cell, the single-stranded viral RNA becomes transcribed into double-stranded DNA, which incorporates into the host genome and is subsequently expressed to yield infectious viral progeny that are released with cell lysis. In progressive HIV infection, the amount of virus increases and the number of CD4 cells decreases. CD4 lymphocytes are

TABLE 180-1 Common Causes of Primary Immunodeficiency

Defect	Sequelae
IgA or IgM deficiency syndromes	Bacterial infections
Hypogammaglobulinemia	Staphylococcal and encapsulated bacterial infections; increased risk for lymphoma, leukemia, and gastric carcinoma
Complement defects	Bacterial infections and increased risk for death from sepsis
T-cell defects	Fungal and viral infections
Natural killer cell defects	Viral infections
Combined cellular/humoral deficiency	Fungal, viral, opportunistic infections; graft-versus-host disease
Leukocyte adhesion molecule defects	Bacterial infections, abnormal antibody responses to infection
Phagocytic dysfunction	Bacterial and fungal infections

BOX 180-1 Common Causes of Acquired Immunodeficiency in Surgical Patients

Diabetes mellitus
Age
Cancer
Chemotherapy
Inflammatory bowel disease
Liver disease
Malnutrition
Radiation
Renal failure
Thermal injury
Transplantation
Splenectomy

TABLE 180-2 Commonly Encountered Immunosuppressive Drugs in Transplantation and Inflammatory Bowel Disease

Agent	Route	Mechanism of Action
Corticosteroids	PO/IV/PR	Inhibit cytokine production and secretion, particularly IL-2 by T cells; may also have other effects
Cyclosporine	PO/IV	Binds to cyclophilin, thus inhibiting calcineurin-mediated gene activation; results in decreased IL-2 production and T-cell proliferation
Tacrolimus	PO/IV	Binds to FK-binding protein, causing inhibition of calcineurin
Sirolimus	PO	Binds to nuclear FK-binding protein, inhibits T-cell cycle progression
Azathioprine	PO/IV	Antimetabolite
Mycophenolate mofetil	PO/IV	Inhibits purine synthesis
OKT3	IV	Murine monoclonal antihuman antibody to CD3+ T cells; targets T-cell proliferation
ALG/ATG	IV	Polyclonal antilymphocyte or antithymocyte globulin; targets T-cell proliferation
Basiliximab, daclizumab	IV	Monoclonal antibodies to CD25 (high-affinity IL-2 receptors expressed on activated T lymphocytes); targets T-cell activation and proliferation
Infliximab	IV	Chimeric monoclonal antibody to TNF-α
Experimental		
Anti–IL-12	SC	Inhibits Th1 response
Adalimumab	IV	Humanized monoclonal antibody to TNF-α
Fontolizumab	IV	Anti–interferon-γ monoclonal antibody
Natalizumab	IV	Anti–α4-integrin monoclonal antibody, inhibits leukocyte migration
Visilizumab	IV	Anti-CD3 monoclonal antibody

IL, Interleukin; IV, intravenous; PO, oral; PR, per rectum; SC, subcutaneous; TNF, tumor necrosis factor.

important in the host cellular immune system. The depletion of these cells results in the impairment of cytotoxic lymphocyte and natural killer cell responses.

Infection with HIV results in a broad spectrum of immunocompromise from mild to severe. Because of the progressive nature of their disease, patients with AIDS (CD4 count <200, or history of opportunistic infections), in contrast with other immunocompromised patients, become more immunosuppressed with time. In patients with AIDS, the absolute CD4 lymphocyte count has been considered to be the best marker for the degree of immunodeficiency. However, significant progress has been made in the quantitative diagnosis of HIV. The HIV viral RNA load can be quantified, and it may be a more sensitive indicator of HIV progression and predictor of death than is the CD4 count.

THERAPEUTIC APPROACH TO IMMUNOCOMPROMISED PATIENTS

STEROIDS

Since 1949, when Hench et al first described the beneficial effects of cortisone in patients with rheumatoid arthritis, hundreds of indications for the use of steroid therapy have been described. These include the treatment of inflammatory conditions such as ulcerative colitis and Crohn disease, the treatment and prevention of graft rejection in organ transplantation, the treatment of chronic obstructive pulmonary disease, and the treatment of collagen vascular diseases. Administration of steroids has effects on immune defenses and the hypothalamic-pituitary-adrenal (HPA) axis that are now well established. Steroid therapy is a common reason for immunocompromise in surgical patients. It is thus important to identify patients who receive or have received steroid therapy and to understand how this may affect their perioperative management.

IMMUNOSUPPRESSION

Corticosteroids have many antiinflammatory effects that make them potent immunosuppressants. These antiinflammatory effects are also the mechanisms through which the complications of steroid therapy occur. Much of their activity is initiated at the molecular level via binding to cytoplasmic glucocorticoid receptors.[3] The steroid-receptor complex migrates to the nucleus, where it acts by affecting gene transcription. The net effects are inhibition of cytokine gene transcription and secretion, particularly interleukin (IL)-1, IL-6, and tumor necrosis factor by macrophages and IL-2 by T cells. Furthermore, macrophage activation and mobilization are inhibited, as is endothelial adhesion molecule expression.

Steroids increase exposure to pathogens by diminishing the barrier function of the gut mucosa through decreased mucosal turnover and regeneration. They also cause atrophy of the gut lymphoid elements and thinning of the bowel wall.[4]

IMPAIRED WOUND HEALING

The inhibitory effects of corticosteroids on wound healing were first described in 1950, but the cellular events were not known until the 1960s. Steroids have two major effects on wound repair: (1) inhibition of initial inflammation and (2) inhibition of matrix metalloproteinases and collagen synthesis. These effects are seen clinically as increased rates of postoperative complications in patients who receive corticosteroids. Dehiscence or incisional hernia after intraperitoneal surgery in steroid-treated patients has been reported to be as high as 13% versus 2% for nonsteroid-treated patients.[5] Among patients with Crohn disease, the postoperative complication rate has been reported to be significantly higher among patients treated with long-term steroid therapy.[6] An animal model of chronic steroid use demonstrated a significant decrease in the bursting strength of colonic anastomoses with steroid therapy.[7] Finally, in a multivariate analysis of women with Crohn who underwent rectovaginal fistula repair, smoking and use of steroids were found to be independent predictors of repair failure ($P = 0.04$).[8]

Despite these studies, controversy persists over the effects of steroid administration on clinical outcomes after bowel surgery and the need for protective fecal diversion. A review of 692 patients at the Cleveland Clinic found no difference in septic complications in patients receiving corticosteroids compared with those not receiving steroids if a protective loop ileostomy was created at the time of ileal pouch–anal anastomosis. However, the authors did note a significant increase in septic complications in the steroid group compared with the nonsteroid group when the fecal stream was not diverted.[9] In contrast, Schrock et al[10] reported no difference in the clinically detectable rate of leakage after colonic anastomoses in patients who had received steroids. A more recent review at the same authors' institution confirmed the observation that there was no increase in the morbidity rate associated with primary anastomosis in a selected group of patients receiving less than 40 mg of prednisone per day.[11] However, high-dose steroids do appear to have significant adverse effects on bowel anastomoses. In a review of 606 patients who underwent left-sided colonic resection, infectious complications were higher in steroid-treated patients, but anastomotic leak rates were similar.[12] Our preferred technique is to reserve primary anastomosis for patients who have a technically uncomplicated operation and are on limited doses of steroids. Diversion is performed in those with technical complications and in those who have had significant steroid exposure. In a recent survey of North American colorectal surgeons, an ileoanal pouch anastomosis with fecal diversion is performed in 73%, 90%, and 82% of patients who are not on steroids, are on 10 mg of prednisone a day, and on 40 mg of prednisone a day, respectively.[13]

ALTERED HORMONAL RESPONSE TO STRESS

Increased secretion of cortisol from the zona fasciculata of the adrenal cortex in response to adrenocorticotropic hormone (ACTH) released from the anterior pituitary gland is an essential component of the surgical stress response. The nonstressed human adrenal gland secretes approximately 10 mg of cortisol per day.[14] After major surgery, the stressed adrenal gland secretes 75 to 150 mg of cortisol during the first 24 hours. It has since been demonstrated that hormonal responses to graded surgical stress reflect the degree of surgical stress and that the effects are transient; ACTH levels return to normal within 24 hours, whereas cortisol reaches normal levels 48 to 72 hours after surgery.[14]

The most accurate way to evaluate the capacity of the adrenal cortex to respond to stress is the rapid ACTH stimulation test. After a baseline cortisol level is obtained, 25 units (250 µg) of synthetic ACTH (Cosyntropin, Cortrosyn) is administered intravenously, and serial plasma cortisol determinations are made at 30 and 60 minutes. A normal response is an increase in the plasma cortisol level of at least 7 µg/dL above baseline or an absolute ACTH-induced rise in plasma cortisol to more than 20 µg/dL.

STRESS-DOSE STEROIDS

In 1952, Fraser et al first reported a case of postoperative hypotension and death caused by perioperative withdrawal from glucocorticoid therapy. This was followed by a similar report by Lewis in 1953, which also gave recommendations for perioperative glucocorticoid treatment for patients on chronic steroid therapy. Those recommendations, a roughly fourfold increase in glucocorticoid dosage, became the standard of therapy until recently. Adrenal insufficiency in a patient on chronic steroids usually manifests as hypotension, abdominal pain, nausea, vomiting, fever, and dehydration and can progress to hypovolemic shock. Concomitant electrolyte abnormalities, caused by mineralocorticoid insufficiency, are unusual. Adrenal insufficiency is an uncommon complication after surgery in patients on chronic steroid therapy.[15]

Despite the low incidence of secondary adrenal insufficiency, some authors have advocated the use of screening tests for adrenocorticoid insufficiency, such as the synthetic ACTH stimulation test, to determine the need for perioperative so-called stress-dose steroids in surgical patients. This would apply to any patient who has received corticosteroid therapy within the year before surgery, because recovery of the HPA axis may take up to 1 year after steroid withdrawal.[16] Recommendations for patients with HPA axis dysfunction are summarized in Table 180-3.

Over the past 20 years, understanding of adrenal cortical responses to surgery and anesthesia has improved, and an increasing body of evidence challenges the standard recommendations for perioperative corticosteroid coverage in patients on chronic steroid therapy. In a study of adrenalectomized monkeys treated with replacement corticosteroids for 4 months and then subjected to cholecystectomy, no difference in outcome was observed between animals receiving only physiologic doses of steroids and those receiving supraphysiologic stress-dose steroids.[17] However, an increased mortality rate was associated with subphysiologic steroid replacement. Another study of 40 renal transplant patients admitted to the hospital with significant physiologic stress such as sepsis or surgery observed no increase in mortality, hospital stay, or eosinophilia associated with simple replacement steroid therapy without stress-dose therapy. In this group, the synthetic ACTH stimulation test overestimated the incidence and degree of clinically significant adrenal dysfunction compared with other biochemical determinants, such as serum ACTH, urinary free cortisol, or serum cortisol.[18] Similar findings were reported in a double-blinded study of stress-dose steroids in patients with abnormal Cosyntropin stimulation tests with hemodynamic parameters as endpoints.[19] Together, these studies suggest that supraphysiologic steroid supplementation in surgical patients is unnecessary and that physiologic cortisol replacement may be sufficient even for patients undergoing major procedures.

Despite these data, a survey of practice patterns among fellows of the American Society of Colon and Rectal Surgeons demonstrated that the majority (84% of 307 survey responders) of surgeons still administer perioperative stress-doses of steroids. This is partly due to the difficulty in applying the limited data to the spectrum of patients that include those on low-dose steroids such as for transplantation and those on very high antiinflammatory doses of steroids such as for IBD. It is our practice to administer a perioperative steroid bolus for patients on long-term chronic steroid therapy, followed by a rapid taper. Patients on low doses of short duration or those undergoing minor operations (i.e., takedown of loop ileostomy) receive their usual replacement dose. Although a complete discussion of this subject is beyond the scope of this chapter, Box 180-2 lists some of the common physiologic and metabolic effects of acute adrenal insufficiency.

IMMUNOSUPPRESSION FOR TRANSPLANTATION

Generalized T-cell immunosuppression remains the mainstay of posttransplantation immunosuppression. Agents are directed at various steps in T-cell activation,

TABLE 180-3 Recommendations for Perioperative Steroid Replacement Therapy

Degree of Surgical Stress	Steroid Dose
Minor	25 mg hydrocortisone or equivalent, then resume normal dose
Moderate	50-75 mg/day hydrocortisone or equivalent for 1 to 2 days, then resume usual dose as clinical course dictates
Major	100-150 mg/day hydrocortisone or equivalent for 2 to 3 days, then resume usual dose as clinical course dictates

BOX 180-2 Common Manifestations of Acute Adrenal Insufficiency

Pyrexia (fever)
Tachycardia
Hypotension
Hyponatremia
Hyperkalemia
Elevated urinary sodium
Decreased urinary potassium

including gene transcription, DNA synthesis, cell cycling, and T-cell receptor function. Most current immunosuppressive regimens involve triple therapy with corticosteroids, cyclosporine or tacrolimus, and azathioprine or mycophenolate mofetil. The detrimental effects of corticosteroids on wound healing are well known. No demonstrable effect on wound healing, however, has been shown with cyclosporine, azathioprine, tacrolimus, or mycophenolate mofetil.[20] However, sirolimus and everolimus (mammalian target of rapamycin [mTOR]) do cause significant impairment in wound healing.[21] Everolimus has been found to cause a significant decrease in the breaking strength of intestinal anastomoses and fascia in rats that persists up to 4 weeks.[22]

Transplantation immunosuppression is directed at the cellular immune response and results in a significant impairment in the host's ability to fight bacterial and viral infections. Fifty to 75% of transplant recipients have one or more episodes of bacterial infection, and 30% to 60% have one or more serious viral infections after transplantation.[23] Most common infectious complications, such as bronchitis after lung transplantation and urinary tract infection after renal transplantation, can be treated medically. However, transplant patients may be more likely to develop serious perioperative infectious complications that require reoperation. Appropriate perioperative antibiotic prophylaxis should be administered, and steroid prophylaxis should be given as previously outlined.

During the perioperative period, maintenance immunosuppression should be continued. If the patient does not have a functioning gastrointestinal tract, intravenous preparations may be administered, but the transplant pharmacist should be consulted to determine equivalent dosing based on bioavailability. Daily monitoring of serum trough levels of agents such as cyclosporine and tacrolimus is necessary to prevent inadequate immunosuppression or drug toxicity.

IMMUNOSUPPRESSION FOR INFLAMMATORY BOWEL DISEASE

IBD is a common reason for pharmacologic immunocompromise in patients seen by general and colorectal surgeons. Often these patients have medically refractory disease or fulminant colitis associated with high-dose steroids, other immunosuppressive agents, and malnutrition at the time of evaluation by the surgeon. A complete discussion of the evaluation and management of patients with IBD occurs in Chapter 159. As with immunosuppression for transplantation, perioperative steroid replacement needs should be considered when operating on patients with IBD. Surgical interventions in patients with IBD are broadly categorized based on the indication as emergent or elective. In the emergent setting, the goal of treatment is life saving and may be in the setting of fulminant colitis with chronic ulcerative colitis or acute bowel obstruction or perforation with Crohn disease. Priorities in the management of these patients are the same as for those without immunocompromise for IBD—patients should be thoroughly evaluated for a medical cause of their acute abdominal symptoms (e.g., acute CMV or *Clostridium difficile* colitis in a patient with chronic

ulcerative colitis) while undergoing resuscitation. Surgical therapy should not be unnecessarily delayed and should be directed at treating the acute problem. In the elective setting treatment can be definitive. Of concern is the potential risk for increased perioperative morbidity in these patients. However, even in toxic and fulminant colitis in immunosuppressed patients, complications after subtotal colectomy are related to the severity of the inflammatory bowel disease and not the immunosuppressed state.[24] Furthermore, even restorative proctocolectomy with ileal pouch–anal reconstruction has been shown to be safely performed in patients on immunosuppressive therapy for IBD.[25]

CANCER IMMUNOSUPPRESSION

Malignancy may cause or be a result of immunosuppression. Advanced malignancies are associated with defects in T- and B-cell function. Drug toxicities, tumor burden, and cytokine release cause malnutrition, which further suppresses the patient. There are additional direct immunosuppressive effects of cancer therapies. Whole-body radiation may result in profound immunosuppression from bone marrow depression and resultant pancytopenia. It also has local effects on barrier defenses such as the skin or intestinal mucosa. The majority of chemotherapeutic agents also cause some degree of myelosuppression that may respond poorly to granulocyte-colony-stimulating factor (G-CSF). The resultant pancytopenia renders the cancer patient markedly susceptible to opportunistic infections, particularly during chemotherapy administration, when bone marrow suppression is the greatest.

Severe neutropenia is defined as an absolute neutrophil count less than $500/mm^3$ and is associated with severe immunosuppression. The magnitude of the neutropenia is directly related to the patient's risk for infection and mortality. An important consideration in the evaluation of patients with chemotherapy-induced myelosuppression is the timing of the nadir of the leukocyte count. Most myelotoxic chemotherapeutic agents result in the nadir of neutropenia at approximately 10 to 14 days following drug administration. Approaching this nadir, the patient is at the highest risk for perioperative complications; however, when the counts have begun to recover, the patient's risk may improve. Further consideration can be given to the velocity of the rise in counts. In selected circumstances, it may be possible to provide supportive care through this severely neutropenic state and delay surgical intervention until the neutrophil count has recovered to be greater than $500/mm^3$.

Neutrophil count recovery may be accelerated by the use of G-CSF (filgrastim, pegfilgrastim), which has been shown to decrease the duration and severity of neutropenia, the incidence of infections and febrile neutropenia, the duration of neutropenia-related hospitalization, and antibiotic use.[26] The role of colony-stimulating factors in the management of surgical disease in the setting of neutropenia is unclear; however, improved outcome has been demonstrated for patients with pneumonia, cellulitis, abscess, or sinusitis.[27] Preoperative administration of filgrastim in high-risk patients (American Society of Anesthesiologists [ASA] grades III and IV) did reveal a decrease in the rate of infectious and non-infectious complications, and a decrease in length of stay compared with placebo in a prospective randomized trial.[28]

SURGICAL RISK ASSESSMENT IN PATIENTS WITH ACQUIRED IMMUNODEFICIENCY

As the understanding of HIV infection and its treatment has improved, the complication rates in patients with HIV who undergo surgery have decreased. More recently, the introduction of highly active antiretroviral therapy (HAART) has revolutionized the management of HIV-infected individuals. HAART regimens use combinations of three or more antiretroviral agents and result in maintenance of immunologic function and reduced morbidity and mortality in HIV-infected patients.[29] However, the exact surgical risks associated with HIV infection are unknown because HIV infection exists as a spectrum or continuum. For example, during the early stages of HIV infection, the helper T-cell (CD4) level may be near normal, and the patient therefore has a relatively intact immune system. Later, as the disease progresses and the CD4 cell count falls below 300 cells/mm^3, patients may experience self-limited illnesses such as mild to moderate skin and respiratory tract infections. Patients with AIDS as defined by the Centers for Disease Control and Prevention (CD4 cell counts <200 cells/mm^3) may experience opportunistic and uncommon infections that present in unusual manners. Higher rates of operative morbidity and mortality occur in these patients, as well as in patients with postoperative viral loads greater than 75,000 RNA copies/mL.[30-32]

Harris and Schecter observed that the presence of AIDS-related abdominal pathology conferred a three- to fourfold increased operative morbidity risk and increased the associated average mortality rate from 15% to 44%.[33] The best predictor of increased operative risk in these patients is the patient's cardiopulmonary, renal, endocrine, and nutritional reserve status and not the absolute CD4 T-cell count. Other poor prognostic factors included an active opportunistic infection, serum albumin level of less than 2.5 g/dL, and the presence of concurrent organ failure. Although the literature regarding surgical complications in HIV-infected patients is largely retrospective, descriptive, and based on small numbers of patients, there is general agreement that HIV infection by itself is not the determinant risk factor; rather, the overall clinical status of the patient determines the surgical risk.

SPECIFIC SURGICAL PROBLEMS IN IMMUNOCOMPROMISED PATIENTS

Acute abdominal pain in the immunocompromised patient presents a particular challenge to the surgeon. In addition to the myriad conditions affecting immunocompetent patients in general, these patients are also susceptible to conditions such as opportunistic or drug-related gastroenteritis, pancreatitis, kidney stones, gastrointestinal lymphoma, Kaposi sarcoma, and neutropenic enterocolitis. The workup is frequently made more difficult by

the lack of specific inflammatory responses, delayed or absent signs of peritoneal inflammation, and the possibility of concurrent pathology.[30]

The initial evaluation and care of the immunocompromised patient (airway, breathing, and circulation) are no different than those of the immunocompetent patient in this regard. Once the patient has been adequately resuscitated, a careful history should be taken, and a careful physical examination should be performed. The severity of symptoms and signs in immunocompromised patients who present with catastrophic complications may be much lower than expected in an immunocompetent patient. A full laboratory workup, including a complete blood cell count, urinalysis, plain radiographs of the chest and abdomen, electrocardiogram, blood cultures, and CMV serology, should be obtained. A chemistry panel that includes liver function tests and amylase should be obtained as indicated. Computed tomography (CT) should be liberally used as a part of the diagnostic workup because the physical examination and laboratory data are often unreliable. Despite these measures, uncertainty about the diagnosis is common. The decision for surgical treatment depends on the underlying diagnosis. In general, the indications for acute surgical interventions in the immunocompromised patient are no different than for those patients with an intact immune system, with few exceptions (e.g., neutropenic typhlitis). Therefore, the surgeon must have a high degree of clinical suspicion for significant pathology despite seemingly minimal physical findings.

ACUTE APPENDICITIS

Acute appendicitis is a common abdominal surgical problem in both immunocompromised and immunocompetent patients. The evaluation of an immunocompromised patient in whom acute appendicitis is suspected proceeds as it would for an immunocompetent patient. A high index of suspicion may help to avoid delays in diagnosis. The safety of emergency surgery for acute appendicitis in severely immunocompromised patients has been described with a mortality rate less than 10%.[34,35] However, the pediatric surgical literature has reported success with nonoperative management of acute appendicitis in neutropenic patients that are otherwise stable.[36] A similar approach with close observation and intravenous antibiotics may be possible in highly selected adult patients with severe neutropenia, early signs of acute appendicitis without any evidence of systemic sepsis, and in whom recovery of the neutropenia is anticipated during the following 24 to 48 hours, though several anecdotal reports show a good outcome with appendectomy.[37] Few differences are observed in clinical findings and perioperative morbidity and mortality rates between non-HIV and HIV patients without AIDS.[30]

ENTERIC OR COLONIC COMPLICATIONS

Colonic complications that lead to perforation in the immunocompromised patient are catastrophic and often fatal.[38] Common causes of bowel perforation include diverticulitis, infectious colitides (particularly CMV colitis), malignancy, foreign body, and trauma. Less common causes include neutropenic enteritis and in patients who have undergone kidney transplant for polycystic kidney disease who have diverticular disease.[38] However, the management of the immunocompromised patient with pneumoperitoneum requires a tailored approach that considers the underlying disease biology, clinical presentation, and prognosis.[39]

DIVERTICULAR DISEASE

Patients who are immunocompromised are at a high risk for complications associated with diverticulitis and can have a more fulminant course and more frequently require surgical intervention.[40,41] Heart, lung, and heart-lung transplant patients have been found to have a substantially increased risk of developing severe diverticulitis requiring surgical intervention compared to nontransplant patients. However, surgery has been proven safe with a low mortality rate.[42] Kidney transplant recipients have been considered to be at a particular risk because of an association between polycystic kidney disease and diverticulosis. Because of this association, pretransplantation screening for diverticulosis in patients has been advocated by some, though there is no evidence to support a pretransplantation colectomy in asymptomatic patients.[43] The mortality of freely perforated diverticulitis in kidney transplant patients has decreased significantly in recent decades from greater than 60% to approximately 10%. This decrease in mortality has been attributed to more widespread use of steroid-sparing agents.[44] Immunosuppression can make the abdominal examination less reliable, confounding the assessment and resulting in reports of increased morbidity and mortality rates with conservative management. Moreover, the disease could be advanced at presentation. We favor a conservative approach that recognizes the limitations of the physical examination and uses early imaging (e.g., CT scan) rather than prophylactic colectomy or urgent laparotomy. As with immunocompetent patients, the immunocompromised patient with a pericolic abscess is better treated with CT-guided drainage, resection, and primary anastomosis than with urgent exploration, colectomy, and stoma formation.

INFECTIOUS COLITIDES

Immunocompromised patients are susceptible to the same range of infectious diseases of the gastrointestinal tract as immunocompetent patients. However, management of infectious diseases in this population is often complicated by delayed or late presentation. In addition, opportunistic pathogens, such as *C. difficile*, *Cryptosporidium*, and CMV can supervene.[45] Infections of the large bowel usually cause diarrhea, which may be bloody or contain mucus, and can produce fever or abdominal pain. In transplant recipients, mycophenolate mofetil can cause severe diarrhea and abdominal pain, mimicking infectious enterocolitis. The workup of a patient with suspected infectious colitis should include a complete history, especially recent travel, unusual ingestions suspect for food poisoning, similar illnesses among family members, recent hospitalizations, and treatment with antibiotics. It should also include testing for fecal leukocytes, *C. difficile* toxin, CMV culture, and stool cultures for bacteria, ova, and parasites. Selective endoscopic evaluation may be useful to obtain tissue or cultures and to establish the extent of colonic involvement. Radiographic imaging may be necessary to assess the degree of colonic involvement and to examine for evidence of necrosis or perforation. Regardless of the cause of the enteritis, early diagnosis and institution of medical therapy or surgical intervention are critical to prevent progression to necrosis or perforation.

CMV is the most common infectious complication of solid organ transplantation or HIV infection. It is also a common pathogen in patients with IBD. Symptoms include fever, weight loss, diarrhea, and hematochezia or melena. Endoscopic examination reveals patches of characteristic ulcers that mimic mucosal ulcerative colitis. CMV infection affects the arterioles of the gastrointestinal tract, resulting in bowel wall ischemia and perforation.[30] Medical therapy for CMV enteritis includes high-dose ganciclovir (5 mg/kg every 12 hours, usually for 14 days). Control of the diarrhea with loperamide or octreotide can be initiated after therapy with ganciclovir has been instituted.[46]

C. difficile infection occurs in relationship with antibiotic use and results from a proliferation of the toxin-producing strains of *C. difficile*, a gram-positive anaerobic organism. The toxins produce mucosal damage and inflammation. Patients typically present with watery diarrhea, fever, and leukocytosis. Abdominal pain and tenderness are also common. Some patients develop toxic megacolon. Symptoms can occur both during antibiotic administration or weeks to months after the cessation of treatment. The diagnosis is made by rapid immunoassays that test for antigens or toxins in the stool or with polymerase chain reaction (PCR) testing. These tests are inexpensive and easy to perform but should be discouraged in asymptomatic patients. If confirmation is needed, tissue culture assay can be performed with biopsy samples from a sigmoidoscopic or colonoscopic examination, although testing should not delay therapy when clinically indicated.[47] When the toxin binds to the bowel wall, it affects the mucosa, creating the inflammation and plaque-like membranes seen endoscopically. This has led to the name *pseudomembranous colitis*. However, these may not be present in immunocompromised patients.[48] Fecal leukocytes, although not specific for *C. difficile* colitis, are present about 50% of the time.

The mainstay of therapy involves cessation of the offending antibiotics, supportive care, and the administration of oral vancomycin or metronidazole, which are highly effective against *C. difficile*. Metronidazole (250 mg four times a day) administered for 10 to 14 days is the first line of therapy because it is less expensive and resistant organisms are uncommon. Vancomycin (125 mg four times a day) or even bacitracin (25,000 U four times a day) can be administered if treatment with metronidazole fails. Oral vancomycin is not systemically absorbed and reaches high levels in the colon. For patients who are unable to tolerate an oral dose because of abdominal surgery or ileus, intravenous metronidazole is effective, with bactericidal levels of the drug in the stool. Cholestyramine to bind the bacterial toxin or vancomycin enemas have both been reported in the treatment of refractory *C. difficile* colitis. Vancomycin dosage is 500 mg in 100 mL of saline every 6 hours as a retention enema. Rifaximin has recently been proposed for patients who have experienced a second or third recurrence. Studies of the use of probiotics have been inconclusive and are currently not routinely recommended.[47] Lastly, fulminant colitis develops in up to 13% of solid organ transplant patients, thus requiring surgical intervention at a higher rate when compared to immunocompetent patients.[49]

Cryptosporidiosis is a common cause of diarrhea in immunosuppressed patients and healthcare workers. Transmission is via the fecal-oral route and can be acquired through zoonosis. Sporozoites attach firmly to the mucosa, causing an inflammatory cell infiltrate in the lamina propria. Patients present with fever, abdominal pain, and watery diarrhea. Colonic biopsy, acid-fast staining, or auramine-phenol staining of the stool reveals oocysts. The disease is self-limiting, lasting about 2 weeks. The treatment is supportive with rehydration. No medication is known to be effective for immunocompromised patients. Though quite rare, there have been patients with advanced HIV with cryptosporidiosis who developed pneumatosis cystoides intestinalis which led to intestinal perforation.[50]

STEROID-INDUCED GASTROINTESTINAL PERFORATION

First reported in 1950, acute gastrointestinal perforation is a well-documented complication of chronic steroid therapy. In these patients, the lesions are often in unusual locations or result in perforation in an otherwise normal colon.[51] Mortality rates have been reported to be as high as 85% to 100%. Delay in treatment is an important reason for the high mortality rates and is associated with steroid doses of more than 20 mg of prednisone per day.[52,53] The inhibition of the inflammatory response results in a decreased tendency to wall off perforating lesions. These factors lead to a greater frequency of free perforation as well as a reduced peritoneal protective response to soilage in patients who receive chronic corticosteroid therapy. Furthermore, steroids may impair mucosal regeneration and cause atrophy of the lymphoid elements with thinning of the bowel wall.[4]

NEUTROPENIC ENTERITIS

Neutropenic enteritis (typhlitis or neutropenic enterocolitis) is a potentially life-threatening complication in patients receiving cytotoxic chemotherapy and in patients with aplastic anemia or cyclic neutropenia. It is a disease typically of the cecum, ascending colon, and terminal ileum and associated with varying degrees of mucosal and submucosal necrosis, hemorrhage, and ulceration. Originally described by Wagner and associates as a complication of childhood leukemia, neutropenic enteritis occurs most commonly in patients receiving high-dose chemotherapy for either hematologic or solid-organ malignancies. An increased association with chemotherapeutic agents used in the treatment of leukemias and lymphomas (i.e., cytosine arabinoside, vincristine, doxorubicin, methotrexate, cyclophosphamide, etoposide, daunomycin, and prednisone) has been observed, but high doses of virtually any myelotoxic regimen can cause neutropenic enteritis. It can also occur after high-dose chemotherapy and autologous stem cell transplantation for solid tumors. The clinical presentation usually consists of the triad of fever, abdominal pain, and diarrhea in a neutropenic patient. Other symptoms include nausea, vomiting, hematochezia, and abdominal distention. Symptoms generally occur approximately 7 to 9 days after the onset of neutropenia (10 to 14 days after initiation of chemotherapy). A rapid course suggests a more virulent form of the disease. The differential diagnosis includes other causes of acute abdominal pain, such as appendicitis, diverticulitis, ischemic colitis, pseudomembranous colitis, inflammatory bowel disease, and chemotherapy-induced gastroenteritis.[54]

Laboratory studies are generally not useful in making the diagnosis, although positive blood cultures with a variety of gram-positive and gram-negative species have been reported. Plain radiographs may show a paucity of gas in the right lower quadrant with dilated small bowel loops, thumbprinting, pneumatosis intestinalis, or free air. However, plain radiographs may be completely normal in mild cases. Ultrasound and CT are significantly more sensitive than plain radiographs in establishing the diagnosis. Findings include bowel wall thickening, a fluid-filled, dilated cecum, ascites, a periintestinal inflammatory mass, pericolic fluid or inflammatory changes in the pericolic soft tissues, pneumatosis, or free air. CT is particularly useful in the followup evaluation of the patient whose clinical condition has not improved despite the resolution of neutropenia; occult retroperitoneal perforation or advanced bowel necrosis may be identified. Barium enema and colonoscopy may precipitate perforation and should not be used.[54]

The optimal treatment of neutropenic enteritis is aggressive medical therapy consisting of bowel rest, nasogastric suction, hydration, broad-spectrum intravenous antibiotics, and close observation. In general, the clinical course does not improve until after the neutrophil count begins to recover. Recombinant granulocyte colony-stimulating factor has thus been used to quicken recovery. Close observation with CT scanning is important if the patient's clinical course is not improving. Surgery is recommended for patients who meet the following criteria: (1) free intraperitoneal perforation, (2) persistent intestinal bleeding despite resolution of neutropenia and coagulopathy, and (3) clinical deterioration despite maximal medical care, suggesting uncontrolled sepsis. Resection with stoma is recommended in these cases, given the high anastomotic leak rate in patients with leukopenia. Furthermore, all necrotic tissue should be removed. Lastly, chemotherapy should not be reinstituted until patients have recovered completely from the enteritis.[54]

ANORECTAL COMPLICATIONS

Anorectal problems are challenging clinical dilemmas in immunocompromised patients, particularly in those who are neutropenic or have AIDS. Symptoms usually include pain, ulceration, discharge, incontinence, bleeding, mass, or tenesmus. Both benign and malignant pathologic processes cause these symptoms. Common

TABLE 180-4 Common Anorectal Infections in the Immunocompromised Patient

Causative Organism or Condition	Manifestations
Neisseria gonorrhoeae	Nonulcerating proctitis with a mucopurulent discharge
Syphilis	Primary chancre may be single or multiple, painful or painless; may be confused with fissures; immunocompromised patients may have a prolonged interval between acute infection and seroconversion
Chlamydia proctitis and lymphogranuloma venereum (LGV)	Severe proctitis with ulceration may result from LGV; serologic responses may be impaired in immunocompromise, so tests should be performed on rectal swabs or mucosal biopsy samples
Herpes simplex virus	Perianal clusters of vesicles coalesce and ulcerate; may develop into a persistent ulcerative lesion
Human papillomavirus (HPV)	Multiple types, associated with "benign" genital warts (HPV-6, -11, -42) or with the development of high-grade dysplasia and anal cancer (HPV-16, -18, -33); may result in condylomatous, papular, or keratotic lesions; intraanal disease is common, so proctoscopy is essential

communicable anorectal pathogens are similar to those occurring in immunocompetent patients (Table 180-4). Other noncommunicable causes of anal disease include abscess, fistula, perirectal infections, hemorrhoids, fissures, ulcers, and tumors. These lesions are significant problems in the neutropenic patient but may occur in patients with less severe immunocompromise and in patients who are immunocompetent. The workup for anorectal lesions should include a thorough history, inspection, digital rectal examination, anoscopy, and proctoscopy with biopsy samples because immunocompromised patients are at an increased risk for developing both rectal and anal cancers.

Suppurative anal disease in immunocompromised patients requires incision and drainage. In cases of deep perirectal infections, after a thorough examination under anesthesia that includes anoscopy and rigid proctosigmoidoscopy, a CT scan may help to delineate the extension of the abscess and identify the presence of any undrained pus if there is clinical suspicion. Perianal sepsis in immunocompromised patients may have little or no purulent drainage because the patient's immune system is unable to mount a significant inflammatory response.

Anorectal surgery can be safely performed in HIV-positive patients with a low rate of complications (5%). However, in patients with CD4-lymphocyte counts of less than 200, delayed wound healing may occur.[31] The management of anorectal suppurative disease in severely immunocompromised patients should liberally utilize

long-term drainage strategies including draining setons and meticulous perianal care to avoid skin maceration.

MALIGNANCIES IN THE IMMUNOCOMPROMISED PATIENT

An increased incidence of squamous cell carcinoma of the skin, non-Hodgkin lymphoma, Kaposi sarcoma, cervical carcinoma in situ, and carcinoma of the anogenital region occurs in immunosuppressed patients.[55] Moreover, patients with immunocompromise are subject to the same risk for common malignancies that affect the general population. Additionally, there has been an increase in the incidence of lymphomas in the postcyclosporine era compared with the precyclosporine era. Other medications associated with lymphomas include the use of OKT3 and tacrolimus. Two factors—immunosuppression and oncogenic viruses—appear to be important in the pathogenesis of many malignancies in immunosuppressed patients (e.g., Epstein-Barr virus for lymphomas and human papillomavirus [HPV] for anal and cervical squamous cell carcinomas). Because these malignancies occur at an average of 5 years after the initiation of immunosuppression for transplantation, the surgeon may be asked to evaluate a patient with abdominal complications of lymphoma or with anogenital or hepatobiliary lesions. The appropriate transplant physician should be consulted, and reduction in or cessation of immunosuppression should be considered.[55]

Adverse immunologic effects also occur with cancer chemotherapy, malnutrition, and acquired immunodeficiency. In addition, some of the genetic factors that predispose a patient to a primary malignancy may play a role in the development of a secondary malignancy. Radiation therapy is another important contributor to secondary carcinogenesis. Leukemias and lymphomas are common secondary malignancies, followed by carcinomas of the thyroid, breast, lung, and stomach and sarcomas of soft tissue and bone. Childhood cancer survivors have a sixfold increased risk of developing a secondary malignancy.[56]

In transplant recipients, carcinomas of the skin and lips are the most common, particularly after kidney transplant. Compared with the frequencies of these squamous cell carcinomas in the general population, the incidence is 65 to 250 times higher. The lesions are more likely to be multiple in location and aggressive. Patients with multiple tumors, tumors on the head, extracutaneous tumors, advanced age, poor differentiation, tumor thickness greater than 5 mm, and invasion of underlying tissues have poor prognosis.[55] Kaposi sarcoma is the most common malignant tumor in patients with AIDS. Gastrointestinal tract lesions are usually asymptomatic but can cause abdominal pain, weight loss, nausea, bleeding, obstruction, perforation, intussusception, ulceration, or protein-losing enteropathy. The lesions look similar to Crohn disease on endoscopy but are located in the submucosa. Gastrointestinal involvement of Kaposi sarcoma portends a poor prognosis and therapy is aimed at palliation, stopping disease progression, and improving symptoms.[57]

Anal neoplasms are more common in immunocompromised patients. In a Danish population study, there was a markedly increased incidence of anal cancer in patients with HIV, history of solid organ transplant, and hematologic malignancies. A moderate increased incidence was noted in patients with the following autoimmune diseases: Crohn disease, psoriasis, polyarteritis nodosa, and Wegener granulomatosis.[58]

Prediction of the biology and planning for the treatment of tumors of the perianal region is dependent on precise localization of the tumor with respect to anal landmarks such as the dentate line, the anal verge, and the anal sphincters. These landmarks define two classes of perianal neoplasms: tumors of the anal margin and tumors of the anal canal. The Histologic Typing of Intestinal Tumors (adopted by the World Health Organization) defines the anal canal as extending from the upper to the lower border of the internal anal sphincter (from the pelvic floor to the anal verge). The anal margin extends from the anal verge (the junction of the highly specialized epithelium of the anoderm with the hair-bearing perianal skin) to 5 to 6 cm from this point. Squamous cell tumors of the anal margin are well-differentiated, keratinizing tumors that behave similarly to squamous cell tumors of the skin elsewhere. Tumors of the anal canal are aggressive high-grade tumors with significant risk for metastasis.

HPV has been implicated as a causative agent in the development of anal cancer. As in the cervix, HPV types 16 and 18 appear to be causally related to the development of high-grade dysplasia and anal cancer, whereas types 6 and 11 cause common genital warts and low-grade dysplasia.[59]

These parallels to cervical disease have led investigators to explore the use of anal Papanicolaou smears and high-resolution anoscopy (magnified examination of the anus with a colposcope or operating microscope) as a method of detecting and destroying high-grade lesions in high-risk patients before the development of cancer.[59] If high-grade disease is found, referral for surgical excision or ablation is recommended. The anal canal is painted with acetic acid and examined circumferentially with an operating microscope or colposcope. Vascular changes characteristic of severe dysplasia are noted, and the distribution of disease in the anus is mapped. For indeterminate lesions, the anal canal can be painted with Lugol solution and mapped again. Lugol solution is a concentrated (10%) iodine solution that stains glycogen stores in nondysplastic tissues a dark brown/black. Low-grade dysplasia stains partially, and high-grade disease does not take up the solution, leaving it mahogany in color. The dysplastic disease is destroyed with electrocautery, while attempting to spare as much normal tissue as possible to prevent anal stenosis. This therapy can also be performed in the office for low-volume disease and treated with infrared coagulator ablation.[59]

SUMMARY

Advances in the medical care of the immunocompromised patient have increased life expectancies and therefore increased the likelihood that these patients will require intervention by a general surgeon. The management of the acutely ill immunocompromised patient should first include the standard survey of the airway, breathing, and circulation before an exhaustive effort is undertaken to establish a diagnosis. Immunocompromised patients are susceptible to the same diseases that occur in immunocompetent patients but are also susceptible to opportunistic diseases. The surgeon must maintain a high index of suspicion and realize that the physical examination and laboratory studies may be unreliable or misleading. However, it should be emphasized that the immunocompromised state in and of itself is rarely a contraindication to a necessary surgical procedure; rather, the overall clinical presentation should be considered on an individual basis, and the therapy should be tailored to each patient.

REFERENCES

1. Melvold RW, Sticca RP: Basic and tumor immunology: A review. *Surg Oncol Clin N Am* 16:711, 2007.
2. Moran K, Munster AM: Alterations of the host defense mechanism in burned patients. *Surg Clin North Am* 67:47, 1987.
3. Rhen T, Cidlowski JA: Antiinflammatory action of glucocorticoids—new mechanisms for old drugs. *N Engl J Med* 353:1711, 2005.
4. Penn I, Brettschneider L, Simpson K, et al: Major colonic problems in human homotransplant recipients. *Arch Surg* 100:61, 1970.
5. Reding R, Michel LA, Donckier J, et al: Surgery in patients on long-term steroid therapy: A tentative model for risk assessment. *Br J Surg* 77:1175, 1990.
6. Post S, Betzler M, von Ditfurth B, et al: Risks of intestinal anastomoses in Crohn's disease. *Ann Surg* 213:37, 1991.
7. Furst MB, Stromberg BV, Blatchford GJ, et al: Colonic anastomoses: Bursting strength after corticosteroid treatment. *Dis Colon Rectum* 37:12, 1994.
8. El-Gazzaz G, Hull T, Mignanelli E, et al: Analysis of function and predictors of failure in women undergoing repair of Crohn's related rectovaginal fistula. *J Gastrointest Surg* 14:824, 2010.
9. Ziv Y, Church JM, Fazio VW, et al: Effect of systemic steroids on ileal pouch-anal anastomosis in patients with ulcerative colitis. *Dis Colon Rectum* 39:504, 1996.
10. Schrock TR, Deveney CW, Dunphy JE: Factors contributing to leakage of colonic anastomoses. *Ann Surg* 177:513, 1973.
11. Parangi SBS, Lehman E: Restorative proctocolectomy without diverting ileostomy is safe. *Gastroenterology* 112:A1464, 1997.
12. Tresallet C, Royer B, Godiris-Petit G, et al: Effect of systemic corticosteroids on elective left-sided colorectal resection with colorectal anastomosis. *Am J Surg* 195:447, 2008.
13. de Montbrun SL, Johnson PM: Proximal diversion at the time of ileal pouch-anal anastomosis for ulcerative colitis: Current practices of North American colorectal surgeons. *Dis Colon Rectum* 52:1178, 2009.
14. Jung C, Inder WJ: Management of adrenal insufficiency during the stress of medical illness and surgery. *Med J Aust* 188:409, 2008.
15. Salem M, Tainsh RE Jr, Bromberg J, et al: Perioperative glucocorticoid coverage. A reassessment 42 years after emergence of a problem. *Ann Surg* 219:416, 1994.
16. Livanou T, Ferriman D, James VH: Recovery of hypothalamo-pituitary-adrenal function after corticosteroid therapy. *Lancet* 2:856, 1967.
17. Udelsman R, Ramp J, Gallucci WT, et al: Adaptation during surgical stress. A reevaluation of the role of glucocorticoids. *J Clin Invest* 77:1377, 1986.
18. Bromberg JS, Alfrey EJ, Barker CF, et al: Adrenal suppression and steroid supplementation in renal transplant recipients. *Transplantation* 51:385, 1991.
19. Glowniak JV, Loriaux DL: A double-blind study of perioperative steroid requirements in secondary adrenal insufficiency. *Surgery* 121:123, 1997.
20. Goldberg M, Lima O, Morgan E, et al: A comparison between cyclosporin A and methylprednisolone plus azathioprine on bronchial healing following canine lung autotransplantation. *J Thorac Cardiovasc Surg* 85:821, 1983.

21. Roine E, Bjork IT, Oyen O: Targeting risk factors for impaired wound healing and wound complications after kidney transplantation. *Transplant Proc* 42:2542, 2010.

22. Willems MC, van der Vliet JA, de Man BM, et al: Persistent effects of everolimus on strength of experimental wounds in intestine and fascia. *Wound Repair Regen* 18:98, 2010.

23. Johnston TD, Katz SM: Special considerations in the transplant patient requiring other surgery. *Surg Clin North Am* 74:1211, 1994.

24. Stewart D, Chao A, Kodner I, et al: Subtotal colectomy for toxic and fulminant colitis in the era of immunosuppressive therapy. *Colorectal Dis* 11:184, 2009.

25. Zmora O, Khaikin M, Pishori T, et al: Should ileoanal pouch surgery be staged for patients with mucosal ulcerative colitis on immunosuppressives? *Int J Colorectal Dis* 22:289, 2007.

26. Dale DC: Colony-stimulating factors for the management of neutropenia in cancer patients. *Drugs* 62:1, 2002.

27. Ozer H, Armitage JO, Bennett CL, et al: 2000 update of recommendations for the use of hematopoietic colony-stimulating factors: Evidence-based, clinical practice guidelines. American Society of Clinical Oncology Growth Factors Expert Panel. *J Clin Oncol* 18:3558, 2000.

28. Bauhofer A, Plaul U, Torossian A, et al: Perioperative prophylaxis with granulocyte colony-stimulating factor (G-CSF) in high-risk colorectal cancer patients for an improved recovery: A randomized, controlled trial. *Surgery* 141:501, 2007.

29. Kress KD: HIV update: Emerging clinical evidence and a review of recommendations for the use of highly active antiretroviral therapy. *Am J Health Syst Pharm* 61:S3, 2004.

30. Saltzman DJ, Williams RA, Gelfand DV, et al: The surgeon and AIDS: Twenty years later. *Arch Surg* 140:961, 2005.

31. Dua RS, Wajed SA, Winslet MC: Impact of HIV and AIDS on surgical practice. *Ann R Coll Surg Engl* 89:354, 2007.

32. Deneve JL, Shantha JG, Page AJ, et al: CD4 count is predictive of outcome in HIV-positive patients undergoing abdominal operations. *Am J Surg* 200:694; discussion 699, 2010.

33. Harris HW, Schecter WP: Surgical risk assessment and management in patients with HIV disease. *Gastroenterol Clin North Am* 26:377, 1997.

34. Chirletti P, Barillari P, Sammartino P, et al: The surgical choice in neutropenic patients with hematological disorders and acute abdominal complications. *Leuk Lymphoma* 9:237, 1993.

35. Skibber JM, Matter GJ, Pizzo PA, et al: Right lower quadrant pain in young patients with leukemia. A surgical perspective. *Ann Surg* 206:711, 1987.

36. Wiegering VA, Kellenberger CJ, Bodmer N, et al: Conservative management of acute appendicitis in children with hematologic malignancies during chemotherapy-induced neutropenia. *J Pediatr Hematol Oncol* 30:464, 2008.

37. Forghieri F, Luppi M, Narni F, et al: Acute appendicitis in adult neutropenic patients with hematologic malignancies. *Bone Marrow Transplant* 42:701, 2008.

38. Catena F, Ansaloni L, Gazzotti F, et al: Gastrointestinal perforations following kidney transplantation. *Transplant Proc* 40:1895, 2008.

39. Badgwell B, Feig BW, Ross MI, et al: Pneumoperitoneum in the cancer patient. *Ann Surg Oncol* 14:3141, 2007.

40. Goldberg HJ, Hertz MI, Ricciardi R, et al: Colon and rectal complications after heart and lung transplantation. *J Am Coll Surg* 202:55, 2006.

41. Klarenbeek BR, Samuels M, van der Wal MA, et al: Indications for elective sigmoid resection in diverticular disease. *Ann Surg* 251:670, 2010.

42. Qasabian RA, Meagher AP, Lee R, et al: Severe diverticulitis after heart, lung, and heart-lung transplantation. *J Heart Lung Transplant* 23:845, 2004.

43. Hwang SS, Cannom RR, Abbas MA, et al: Diverticulitis in transplant patients and patients on chronic corticosteroid therapy: A systematic review. *Dis Colon Rectum* 53:1699, 2010.

44. Dalla Valle R, Capocasale E, Mazzoni MP, et al: Acute diverticulitis with colon perforation in renal transplantation. *Transplant Proc* 37:2507, 2005.

45. Huppmann AR, Orenstein JM: Opportunistic disorders of the gastrointestinal tract in the age of highly active antiretroviral therapy. *Hum Pathol* 41:1777, 2010.

46. Bartels MC, Mergenhagen KA: Octreotide for symptomatic treatment of diarrhea due to cytomegalovirus colitis. *Ann Pharmacother* 45:e4, 2011.

47. Cohen SH, Gerding DN, Johnson S, et al: Clinical practice guidelines for *Clostridium difficile* infection in adults: 2010 update by the Society for Healthcare Epidemiology of America (SHEA) and the Infectious Diseases Society of America (IDSA). *Infect Control Hosp Epidemiol* 31:431, 2010.

48. Nomura K, Fujimoto Y, Yamashita M, et al: Absence of pseudomembranes in *Clostridium difficile*-associated diarrhea in patients using immunosuppression agents. *Scand J Gastroenterol* 44:74, 2009.

49. Riddle DJ, Dubberke ER: *Clostridium difficile* infection in solid organ transplant recipients. *Curr Opin Organ Transplant* 13:592, 2008.

50. Davies AP, Chalmers RM: Cryptosporidiosis. *BMJ* 339:b4168, 2009.

51. Warshaw AL, Welch JP, Ottinger LW: Acute perforation of the colon associated with chronic corticosteroid therapy. *Am J Surg* 131:442, 1976.

52. ReMine SG, McIlrath DC: Bowel perforation in steroid-treated patients. *Ann Surg* 192:581, 1980.

53. Nakashima H, Karimine N, Asoh T, et al: Risk factors of abdominal surgery in patients with collagen diseases. *Am Surg* 72:843, 2006.

54. Davila ML: Neutropenic enterocolitis. *Curr Opin Gastroenterol* 22:44, 2006.

55. Zafar SY, Howell DN, Gockerman JP: Malignancy after solid organ transplantation: An overview. *Oncologist* 13:769, 2008.

56. Bhatia S, Constine LS: Late morbidity after successful treatment of children with cancer. *Cancer J* 15:174, 2009.

57. Arora M, Goldberg EM: Kaposi sarcoma involving the gastrointestinal tract. *Gastroenterol Hepatol (N Y)* 6:459, 2010.

58. Sunesen KG, Norgaard M, Thorlacius-Ussing O, et al: Immunosuppressive disorders and risk of anal squamous cell carcinoma: A nationwide cohort study in Denmark, 1978-2005. *Int J Cancer* 127:675, 2010.

59. Pineda CE, Welton ML: Management of anal squamous intraepithelial lesions. *Clin Colon Rectal Surg* 22:94, 2009.

Anorectal Anomalies

Scott A. Engum | Jay L. Grosfeld

Anorectal malformations (ARMs) are relatively common congenital anomalies. The first report of surgical correction by performance of an anoplasty was by Amussat in 1835. Stephens performed the first objective studies with ARM and proposed an initial approach to separate the rectum and urinary system in 1953.[1] Several surgical techniques have been proposed since this time, with the main objective being to protect and use the puborectalis sling. In 1982, deVries and Peña described a new operative approach—posterior sagittal anorectoplasty (PSARP).[2,3] With this approach, it became possible to correlate the external appearance of the perineum with the operative findings and subsequent clinical outcome. A detailed history on ARM is beyond the scope of this chapter and can be found in a review by Grosfeld in 2006.[4]

The cause of ARM is unknown. The vast majority of experience in the management of these problems has been obtained at specialized children's hospitals that deal with disorders of the newborn. The reported incidence of anorectal anomalies ranges from 1:3500 to 1:5000 live births. Some families have a genetic predisposition, with ARMs noted in succeeding generations. The estimated risk for a couple having a second child with an ARM is approximately 1%.[5] The majority of anorectal atresias are not detected prenatally. The counseling and management of pregnancy with a lower abdominal cystic mass in the fetus must take into consideration differential diagnoses including ARM. Malformations occur more commonly in boys than girls (1.4:1 to 1.6:1)[6,7]; however, this may vary according to the level of the defect, because the majority of females have low (rectovestibular fistula)[8] rather than high lesions.

EMBRYOLOGY

The gastrointestinal tract develops from the embryonic gut, which is composed of an epithelium of endodermal origin surrounded by cells of the mesoderm. Cell signaling between these two tissue layers appears to play a critical role in coordinating patterning and organogenesis of the gut and its derivatives. Studies have shown that sonic hedgehog signals are essential for organogenesis of the mammalian gastrointestinal tract and suggest that mutating members of this signaling pathway may be involved in the occurrence of human gastrointestinal malformations.[9-12]

Although numerous efforts have been made to understand the abnormal processes that produce ARMs, neither the normal nor the abnormal development of the hindgut and cloaca is fully understood. Most theories to explain the disturbance in embryogenesis resulting in ARMs are mainly speculative. There is general agreement that the cloaca is seen in the 12- to 15-day embryo. The *cloacal membrane* is defined as that area between the primitive streak and the body stalk where endoderm and ectoderm fuse without intervening mesoderm. The allantois is an extension of gut endoderm that becomes part of the bladder and extends up to the amnion. The allantois marks the ventrocephalic limits of the cloaca. Cloacal folds (or genital folds) are mesoblastic proliferations that surround the cloacal membrane.

The mesonephric ducts join the superior lateral wall of the cloaca just inside the cloacal membrane at 28 days of gestation. The cloaca is at that point a large chamber into which the hindgut enters superiorly and the tailgut exists inferiorly. Just in front of the hindgut, the allantois projects ventrally and superiorly. The ventral body wall develops and displaces the upper end of the cloaca. Anal tubercles (mesoblastic structures) form on both sides of the cloaca at its junction with the tailgut and impinge on the lumen at this junction. The anal tubercles fuse centrally, displacing the cloacal orifice of the involuting tailgut dorsally away from the cloacal membrane.[13]

The urorectal septum descends to demarcate the cloaca into a ventral urogenital sinus and a dorsal hindgut. Investigations utilizing the Carnegie Embryological Collection and three-dimensional modeling have suggested that the urogenital sinus and anorectum form early and are separated by the urorectal septum as a passive structure. There does not seem to be septation or differentiation of the cloaca itself.[14,15] Others have illustrated that a delay of tailgut regression, an abnormal and massive apoptotic cell death involving the posterior cloacal wall, and underdevelopment of the dorsal aspect of the cloaca and its membrane may also contribute to a culmination of aberrations that result in a spectrum of ARMs.[16] By the middle of the seventh week of gestation, the anus and rectum are completely divided from the urogenital tract. The anal membrane then involutes and becomes perforate. The mesodermal perineal body extends to the level of the anal folds (hillocks). The cloaca completely divides, and no external cloaca exists. The anal tubercles unite behind the cloaca and form a U-shaped fold dorsally and laterally between the tail and the anus. The dorsal cloacal wall evaginates just above the level where the anal tubercle impinges on the lumen at the future site of the crypts and columns of Morgagni. The anorectal musculature becomes defined and arises from the third sacral to the first coccygeal myotonic hypomeres, starting at the eighth week of gestation.[17] The anal portion of the rectum is initially long and is of endodermal origin (hindgut origin). In the ninth week of gestation, the external sphincter, levator ani (particularly the puborectalis muscle), and even the ganglia and plexuses of the rectum are well defined.

In the 55-mm fetus, the anal portion of the rectum is reduced in length and gradually becomes shorter and broader. According to studies of human embryos in the Carnegie collection by deVries and Friedland,[13] no proctodeum is observed. This finding contradicts the time-honored role of the anal pit (or proctodeum of ectodermal origin) in the development of the anal canal as demonstrated in other mammalian species (e.g., chick embryo). Furthermore, it brings into question the theory that ARMs are the result of a failure of the anal pit (proctodeum) to become continuous with the hindgut cavity. Additional studies in human embryos are required to further elucidate the exact cause of the myriad of anorectal anomalies.

CLASSIFICATION

ARMs are classified according to their anatomic level of presentation and gender. Ladd and Gross proposed the original types I through IV malformation classification system in 1934. Several modifications of this system were subsequently proposed, in large part based on embryologic observations. Smith,[18] in addition to Stephens and Smith,[19] developed an important classification at an international workshop on ARMs in 1970 (Table 181-1). This system was based on whether the lesions were located low (translevator), at an intermediate level, high (supralevator), or whether it was a miscellaneous type. This culminated in 11 different lesions noted in males and 16 in females. Although this classification was used extensively (particularly in Australia and New Zealand), it was considered too complex and detailed by many pediatric surgeons.

In 1984, Stephens and Smith[20] and others developed the Wingspread classification to address only commonly observed anorectal anomalies (Table 181-2). This classification used similar terms and was based on anatomic levels but excluded other important anomalies such as rectocloacal defects and anterior ectopic anus. There were 7 different lesions in males and 10 in females, with the cloacal malformations listed separately under the new classification system.

In 1995, Peña[21] proposed a more recent classification system in which the lesions are grouped according to gender and whether a colostomy is indicated in the management (Table 181-3). This system further classifies the anomalies according to the differences in treatment and prognosis.

The Krickenbeck conference[22] (26 international authorities on congenital malformations of the organs of the pelvis and perineum) in 2005 determined that the international Wingspread classification is still useful in the choice of the surgical approach. However, to develop a system for comparable followup studies, a modification of the classification of Peña according to the type of the fistula and including rare/regional variants was proposed (Table 181-4). The major clinical groups were classified as perineal (cutaneous) fistulas, rectourethral fistulas (prostatic and bulbar), rectovesical fistulas, vestibular fistulas, cloacal malformations, patients with no fistula, and anal stenosis. Rare/regional variants were subclassified as pouch colon, rectal atresia/stenosis, rectovaginal fistulas,

TABLE 181-1 International Classification of Anorectal Anomalies (1970)

Level	Male	Female
HIGH DEFORMITIES (SUPRALEVATOR)		

Anorectal agenesis	Without fistula
	With fistula
	  Rectovesical
	  Rectourethral
		Without fistula
		With fistula
		  Rectovesical
		  Rectovaginal (high)
		  Rectocloacal

Rectal atresia, male and female		
INTERMEDIATE DEFORMITIES (SUPRALEVATOR AND TRANSLEVATOR)		

Anal agenesis	Without fistula
	With fistula
	  Rectobulbar
		Without fistula
		With fistula
		  Rectovaginal (low)
		  Rectovestibular

Anorectal stenosis		
LOW DEFORMITIES (INFRALEVATOR)		

At normal anal site	Covered anus:
	  complete
	Anal stenosis
		Covered anus:
		  complete
		Anal stenosis

At perineal site	Anterior perineal anus Anocutaneous fistula (Covered anus: incomplete)	Anterior perineal anus Anocutaneous fistula (Covered anus: incomplete)
At vulvar site		Vulvar anus Anovulvar fistula Anovestibular fistula

Data from Stephens FD, Smith ED: *Anorectal malformations in children.* Chicago, 1971, Year Book.

H-type fistulas, and others. This new international classification enables the different operative procedures to be more comparable to each other than with the Wingspread classification.

Regardless of the classification system used, lesions are characterized as to whether they occur as high-lying, intermediate, or low-lying anomalies with or without an associated fistula from the hindgut. High-lying lesions indicate that the end of the rectal atresia is located in a supralevator location above the pubococcygeal line. Intermediate lesions indicate that the end is in a translevator position between the pubococcygeal line and the lower sacrum. Low-lying (infralevator) lesions indicate that the end of the rectal atresia has passed beyond the level of the levator (through the puborectalis) to a position below the lowest portion of the ischium (Figure 181-1).

Using the Wingspread classification system, Holschneider et al[7] found that 47% of anorectal defects were

TABLE 181-2 Wingspread Classification of Anorectal Anomalies (1984)

Level	Male	Female
High	Anorectal agenesis	Anorectal agenesis
	With rectoprostatitis	With rectovaginal fistula
	Without fistula	Without fistula
	Rectal atresia	Rectal atresia
Intermediate	Rectobulbar urethral fistula	Rectovestibular fistula
		Rectovaginal fistula
	Anal agenesis without a fistula	Anal agenesis without a fistula
Low	Anocutaneous fistula	Anovestibular fistula
	Anal stenosis*	Anocutaneous fistula
		Anal stenosis*
		Cloacal malformations
	Rare malformations	Rare malformations

Developed by Stephens FD, et al: Symposium on Anorectal Abnormalities, Wingspread Report, 1984, Racine, Wisc.
*Previously called *covered anus*.

TABLE 181-3 Peña Classification of Anorectal Malformations

Category	Criteria
MALES	
No colostomy	Perineal fistula
Colostomy	Rectourethral fistula
	Bulbar
	Prostatic
	Rectovesical fistula (bladder neck)
	Imperforate anus without fistula
	Rectal atresia
FEMALES	
No colostomy	Perineal fistula
Colostomy	Vestibular fistula
	Persistent cloaca (<3 cm or >3 cm common channel)
	Imperforate anus without fistula
	Rectal atresia

From Peña A: Anorectal malformations. *Semin Pediatr Surg* 4:35, 1995.

TABLE 181-4 Standards for Diagnosis: International Classification (Krickenbeck)

Major Clinical Groups	Rare/Regional Variants
Perineal (cutaneous) fistula	Pouch colon
Rectourethral fistula	Rectal atresia/stenosis
Prostatic	Rectovaginal fistula
Bulbar	H fistula
Rectovesical fistula	
Vestibular fistula	
Cloaca	
No fistula	
Anal stenosis	

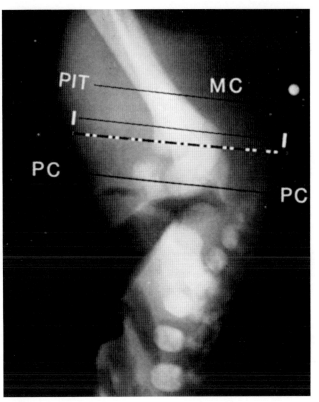

FIGURE 181-1 Lateral invertogram in a patient with anorectal agenesis and a rectourethral fistula. Air shadow is above the pubococcygeal line (PC). Air is noted anteriorly in bladder. I is the line of the ischial ossification site (the level of translevator lesion), whereas MC is the mucocutaneous line, the level of low (infralevator) lesions. PIT indicates the anal dimple. (From deVries PA: The surgery of anorectal anomalies: Its evolution with evaluations of procedures. *Curr Probl Surg* 21:1, 1984.)

low, 14% were intermediate, 36% were high, and 1% of patients had cloacal anomalies. More than 80% of patients have a fistulous connection to the genitourinary tract or perineum (Figure 181-2). Eighty percent of boys with high rectal atresia have a fistula to the urethra at the level of the verumontanum, and 6% have fistula to the bladder.[23] In instances of imperforate anus with a recto-urethral fistula, the fistula opens in the lower posterior urethra (bulbar portion) or in the upper posterior urethra (prostatic portion). Those with a bulbar fistula typically have well-functioning sphincters and an intact sacrum, whereas those with a prostatic fistula experience a higher incidence of sacral anomalies and poorly functioning sphincter mechanisms. In boys with a low-lying lesion, 70% have an anocutaneous fistula that presents anterior to the external sphincter along the midline raphe of the perineal body as it extends up to the scrotum (Figure 181-3).

In girls, the easiest way to clinically assess the anatomy is by direct visualization during physical examination of the perineum in the lithotomy position. Girls present with variants of the normal three perineal orifices: (1) urethra, vagina, and a third opening that represents an imperforate anus with associated perineal or rectofourchette/vestibular fistula (Figure 181-4); (2) two

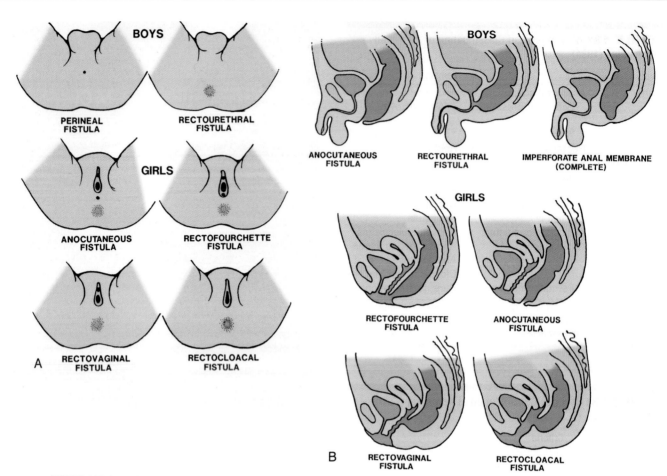

FIGURE 181-2 A, Perineal appearance of anorectal anomalies in boys and girls. **B,** The lateral view of the same defects.

openings (the urethra and vagina) with an imperforate anus and a rectovaginal fistula; and (3) one perineal opening, an imperforate anus with a cloaca, and associated vesicocloacal and rectocloacal fistulas (Figure 181-5). Of the girls with high anomalies, 80% have an associated fistula (usually to the lower third of the vagina), whereas more than 93% with low rectal atresia have a fistula. In females, a rectovestibular fistula is quite common and is located where the rectum opens in the vestibule of the genitalia. These patients typically have a normal sacrum and well-developed sphincteric mechanism. A *persistent cloaca* is defined as a defect in which the rectum, vagina, and urethra enter into one common channel that opens into the perineum as a single orifice. Peña[21] described two cloacal groups: those that have a common channel shorter than 3 cm and the other with a common channel longer than 3 cm. When the channel is shorter than 3 cm, it can usually be repaired via a posterior sagittal approach, whereas a defect with a longer channel presents a more complex anomaly that typically requires a laparotomy and posterior sagittal approach.

Imperforate anus without a fistula in either sex is unusual and accounts for approximately 5% of the entire group. In this instance, the atretic rectum is typically located within 2 cm of the skin of the perineum. These infants usually have a good sacrum and muscle complex. Instances of low imperforate anus in infants with Down syndrome (trisomy 21) are less likely to have an associated fistula. Rectal atresia and stenosis represent a unique defect in which the infant has an intact anal canal with normal sphincter and sacral development along with normal external anatomy; however, when a tube is passed into the rectum, an obstruction is identified that is related to an atresia noted between the anal canal and the rectum.

Congenital pouch colon (CPC), congenital short colon, or pouch colon syndrome[24,25] is an unusual malformation associated with anorectal malformation usually of the high variety in which all or part of the colon is replaced by a pouch-like dilation, which communicates distally with the urogenital tract via a fistula. The association of CPC and rectal atresia is very rare. This condition has been given recognition in the Krickenbeck classification and included under rare anomalies. Spriggs[26] first described the pouch colon anomaly in 1912 and its first detailed description came from Trusler[27] in 1959. This condition is much more common in northern India and neighboring areas than it is in the rest of the world, comprising up to 13.3% of all anorectal malformations and up to 26% of high anomalies.[28,29] There are various hypotheses proposed concerning the etiology of this condition; however, only the theory of intrauterine obliteration of the inferior mesenteric artery[30] substantiates the association of CPC and rectal atresia. A recent evaluation by Gangopadhyay et al[31] looking at the in vitro physiologic functions of the CPC shows that there is a poor

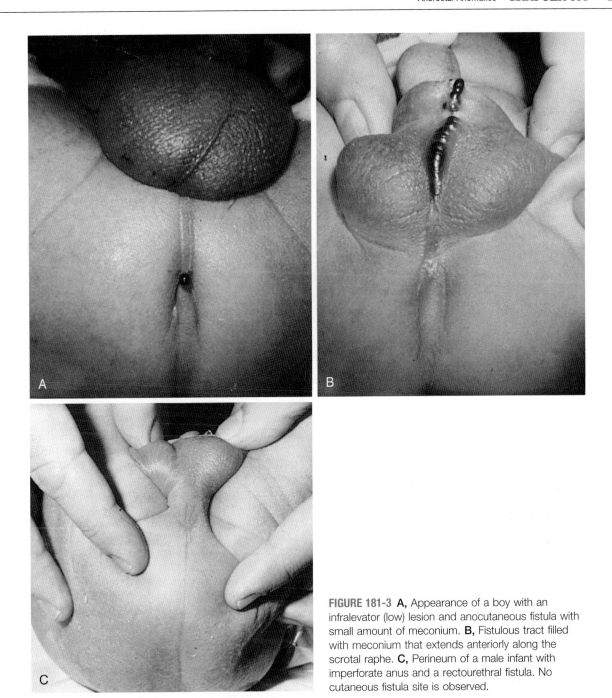

FIGURE 181-3 **A,** Appearance of a boy with an infralevator (low) lesion and anocutaneous fistula with small amount of meconium. **B,** Fistulous tract filled with meconium that extends anteriorly along the scrotal raphe. **C,** Perineum of a male infant with imperforate anus and a rectourethral fistula. No cutaneous fistula site is observed.

neuromuscular development in the CPC. It is theirs and others' conclusion that CPCs have faulty neuromuscular development and cannot function properly as a reservoir for feces and lead to stasis and infection.[32]

ASSOCIATED ANOMALIES

GENITOURINARY TYPES

The association between imperforate anus and abnormalities of the genitourinary system is well recognized. The incidence of genitourinary lesions increases as the level of rectal descent decreases; that is, high imperforate anus is associated with the greatest number of abnormalities. Urologic malformations are present in 40% to 52% of males with high anomalies and in 48% of females with high anomalies.[6,33] For the low and intermediate groups, the incidence of urinary malformations was 21% and 14%, respectively[6]; however, females with cloacal malformations may have genitourinary anomalies in 81% of cases.[34]

The most common anomaly noted is an absent kidney, followed by vesicoureteric reflux. An accurate and thorough investigation must be completed using an abdominal ultrasound and voiding cystourethrogram (VCUG) to minimize long-term morbidity.

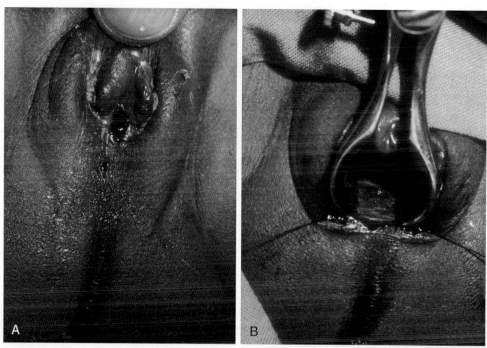

FIGURE 181-4 Perineal examinations in two different girls show the presence of imperforate anus with a rectofourchette fistula **(A),** and a rectovaginal fistula **(B).**

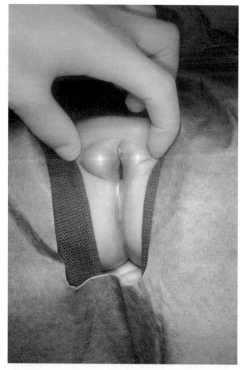

FIGURE 181-5 Female perineum showing a cloaca.

SACRAL AND SPINAL TYPES

The coexistence of spinal and sacral abnormalities in patients with imperforate anus has been well established. Segmentation anomalies, sacral agenesis, or both may occur. In addition, the underlying spinal cord may contain occult dysraphic lesions. The overall incidence of lumbosacral anomalies (noted on plain radiograph)

in patients with imperforate anus ranges from 30% to 44% but is more common in high lesions (48% to 54%) than in low lesions (15% to 27%).[35-37] Spinal cord abnormalities, including a low-lying conus medullaris, a thickened fatty filum terminale, and a cord lipoma, have been observed in 18% to 50% of patients.[35,37-39] Typically, the incidence of spinal lesions is somewhat higher in cases of high rectal atresia and high-lying imperforate anus (44% vs. 27%).[40] There is a correlation between the degree of sacral development and the final functional prognosis. After surgical correction of the ARM, some patients suffer late-onset urinary and/or fecal incontinence and/or orthopedic symptoms and can be related to a tethered cord, which is present in 10% to 52% of cases.[41-44] Tethered cord symptoms include dysfunction of the anal sphincters with fecal incontinence, neurovesical dysfunction, gait disturbance, and spastic abnormalities of the lower extremities.[45,46] The onset of symptoms is variable but usually occurs in childhood and may be slowly progressive. Some have demonstrated that a tethered cord is more common in patients with a high lesion (50%)[47]; however, there is growing literature to support that the incidence occurs equally among high and low lesions.[48-50] Because of these data, most recommend imaging studies of the spine for all patients. One can order an MRI; however, consideration should be given to ultrasound as it is noninvasive and less expensive. Ultrasound is an ideal screening tool for infants younger than 3 months. Ultrasound is recommended for screening, followed by MRI, to confirm abnormal findings.

OTHER ANOMALIES

In addition to the well-known urologic and spinal anomalies, cardiac lesions coexist in 8% of patients with ARMs, esophageal atresia and/or tracheoesophageal fistula occurs in 6%, and abdominal wall defects are noted in 2%.[51,52] The tendency for some of these lesions to occur concurrently is represented by the acronym VACTERL (i.e., *v*ertebral, *a*nal, *c*ardiac, *t*racheoesophageal, *r*enal, and *l*imb anomalies).[53] An imperforate anus may also be associated with duodenal atresia and, rarely, coexist with aganglionic megacolon; presacral lesions (i.e., Currarino syndrome, teratomas, anterior meningocele)[54-56]; chromosomal syndromes,[57,58] including trisomy 13 to 15, trisomy 16 to 18, Down syndrome (trisomy 21)[59,60]; intestinal atresias[61,62]; congenital short colon (pouch colon syndrome)[28]; colon atresia[63]; and cat-eye syndrome (otic atresia and colobomas).

In 1981, Guido Currarino described a form of caudal regression syndrome with hemisacrum (type IV sacral malformation), anorectal malformation, and presacral mass (anterior meningocele), teratoma, and/or rectal duplication. The Currarino syndrome was observed to segregate in an autosomal dominant manner that often displayed phenotypic variability. As defined in the original reports, patients affected by true Currarino syndrome always exhibit the typical hemisacrum, with intact first sacral vertebra, which makes this specific sacral anomaly distinct to this syndrome. Genetic studies suggested that a locus involved in normal sacral and anorectal development mapped to the terminal end (q36) of human chromosome 7. Mutations within the HLXB9 homeobox gene have been identified as the cause.[64,65]

PELVIC MUSCULAR ANATOMY AND THE PHYSIOLOGY OF CONTINENCE

We briefly review the normal anatomy of the rectum and pelvic musculature and mechanisms of continence as they are related to congenital disorders to further understand the reconstruction of complex anorectal anomalies. The normal rectum is divided at its angulation by the contraction of the puborectalis muscle into an ampulla above and an anal canal below. The posterior rectal wall is acutely indented by the anterior pull of the puborectalis muscle and overhangs the remainder of the levator diaphragm. The anal canal is surrounded by sphincter muscles and is tethered to a concentrically arranged internal (involuntary) sphincter and an external (voluntary) sphincter. The skin-lined anal canal has intrinsic sensory receptors with conventional nerve endings that detect pain, touch, temperature, tension, and friction. There are no sensory receptors per se in the ampulla, but it is sensitive to distention (stretch). The puborectalis muscle is the key sensor mechanism at the entry of the anal canal from the ampulla.[20] This governs both unconscious and conscious opening and closing of the anal canal and provides warning of impending defecation.

Continence is maintained normally through a combination of resting tone in all the sphincters and both reflex and voluntary contraction of the puborectalis muscle and deep external anal sphincter. The resting tone in the internal sphincter occludes the lumen of the perineal part of the anal canal but relaxes just ahead of the peristaltic contraction in the adjoining ampulla and pelvic portion of the anal canal. As an increase in the intraluminal pressure in the rectum rises to the level of the resting pressure of the anal canal, the spinal reflex operates to maintain closure through contraction of the puborectalis sling and maintains continence during the relaxation phase.[52] Higher propulsion pressure waves in the rectum force the entrance of stool into the anal canal. This activates stretch receptors of the puborectalis and initiates an afferent impulse to the spinal and cortical centers and an awareness of rectal distention. The voluntary sphincters and regulation of anorectal continence are then under conscious control.

The relaxation of the internal sphincter in response to rectal distention in normal patients is referred to as the *rectoanal reflex* and is lacking in patients with Hirschsprung disease. The internal sphincter is under control of the parasympathetic nervous system through the spinal arc at S2, S3, and S4, which contains nerve centers that coordinate rectal peristaltic activity and involuntary (unconscious) sphincter control. The pudendal nerve supplies the sympathetic stimulus that causes constant contraction of the internal sphincter and produces the so-called continent slit shape of the anus. This cortical arc is called into play when increased intraluminal pressure exceeds the resting pressure. The afferent pathway is via the pudendal nerve to the spinal center and cerebral endings in the cortex that activate the efferent pathway that controls the voluntary muscle sphincters.

The entire length of the anal canal is surrounded by voluntary muscles. The funnel-shaped musculature compresses the upper anal canal on three sides by the anterior pull of the puborectalis sling, whereas the barrel-shaped external sphincter squeezes the lower skin-lined aspect of the anal canal. The levator ani muscle complex is composed of four muscles (pubococcygeus, iliococcygeus, puborectalis, and coccygeus). These structures form the complete muscle floor of the pelvis, provide a portal of exit from the anal canal, and prevent herniation of the pelvic contents alongside the canal by blending with the smooth muscle coats of the rectum.

The external sphincter is a barrel-shaped muscle that lies outside the internal sphincter in continuity with the puborectalis sling and surrounds the anal canal from the pectinate line to the anal orifice. Although Stephens and Smith[19] stressed the importance of the puborectalis muscle in regard to the development of continence in patients with imperforate anus, they also considered the internal and external sphincter muscles to be of minimal value. They theorized that the puborectalis provided the main sphincter mechanism available for continence in these cases. deVries and Peña,[2] however, demonstrated that the external sphincter played an important role in the development of fecal continence. In their careful dissections during the performance of posterior sagittal anoplasty for imperforate anus, they failed to detect an isolated puborectalis muscle but referred to a striated muscle complex that represents a fusion of the puborectalis portion of the levator ani and the external sphincter muscle (particularly the deep portion). They further stated that dorsal to the muscle complex are the superficial and subcutaneous external sphincter muscles that extend up to the coccyx as a separate layer of longitudinal muscle fibers. The point at which the external sphincter muscle fuses with the levator muscle marks the beginning of the striated muscle complex.

Many patients with imperforate anus have problems with continence. There is great variability in the presence of striated muscle from patient to patient. Some patients have weak musculature, whereas some have nearly normal muscle. The presence or lack of underlying sacral and neurologic abnormalities also plays a role in the success or failure in any specific case. In addition, a major problem in many cases (particularly in infants with high imperforate anus) is the lack of internal sphincter muscle. The internal sphincter can be identified in some instances of low imperforate anus with an anterior ectopic opening or perineal fistula. When the location of the rectal atresia associated with imperforate anus is higher, however, the important so-called message center for the rectoanal reflex is lacking, leading to the frequent complaint among some of these patients that they are unaware of the presence of feces in the anus, which results in soiling. Sections taken through the site of a rectourethral fistula indicate that the remnant of the internal sphincter muscle may be within the fistula itself. Because most surgical procedures for imperforate anus leave this area in place to reduce the chance of injury to the urethra, the internal sphincter in these cases is often not of use to the patient. In addition, Holschneider et al[66] have noted abnormal innervation patterns in 96% of specimens (fistula/rectal pouch). Of interest was that all fistula tracts were found to be aganglionic, including the adjacent part of the rectum involving the internal sphincter equivalent. It was concluded that partial denervation of the rectum may not be the only cause of stooling abnormalities after definitive repair. Guan et al have shown in experimental animal models that the sensory neurons innervating the levator ani muscle were deficient in ARM[67] and with their previous work on motor neurons suggest that sensory and motor nerve innervation deficiency of the pelvic muscles in ARM patients contributes to the poor anorectal functions. In patients with high imperforate anus, the goal is to perform a procedure as carefully as possible to preserve whatever sphincter and levator muscles are available and to place the rectum within the muscle complex to allow the best opportunity for the development of socially acceptable continence.

INITIAL MANAGEMENT OF THE NEWBORN

MALE INFANT

In male infants with low lesions, increases in rectal intraluminal pressure may not occur for up to 24 hours after birth. Because this is a low-lying cause of neonatal intestinal obstruction, the physician can safely wait 18 to 24 hours to observe for a bulging anal membrane and possible darkening by meconium. One may also note the presentation of an anocutaneous fistula or find meconium present in the median raphe of the scrotum. Remaining patient during the evaluation may minimize

subjecting the neonate to an unnecessary preliminary colostomy. Decompression of the stomach with an orogastric tube limits distal bowel distention and may reduce the ability to make an appropriate clinical decision. Similarly, if the level of descent of bowel gas relative to the anterior inferior edge of the ischium and pubococcygeal line is to be relied on as a guide to determine the level of rectal atresia, one must wait until the rectum is sufficiently distended with air. Because of the contraction of the levator muscle complex that surrounds the rectum, radiographs obtained in normal newborns may suggest a bowel gas appearance consistent with a high supralevator rectal atresia before intraluminal pressure increases sufficiently to force open the distal rectal lumen. All boys with a perineal fistula, bucket handle abnormality, or median raphe fistula are treated with a cutback or anterior perineal anorectoplasty.

If meconium is noted in the urine (Figure 181-6) but is not visible at the perineum, the patient has a flat-appearing bottom with little or no buttock crease, and anal skin features are absent, one can presume there is an associated sacral defect (dysgenesis or agenesis), and the presence of a high anorectal lesion with a rectourinary fistula is almost certain. Because sacral nerve branches S1, S2, and S3 are necessary for anal continence, patients with sacral agenesis unfortunately have little chance to achieve typical fecal continence. A colostomy is typically the initial surgical management in cases with high or intermediate imperforate anus, to divert stool and minimize the risk of reflux of infected urine from the distal pouch into the vas deferens and causing epididymitis.

FEMALE INFANT

In the female patient, an anocutaneous or anovestibular fistula to the posterior fourchette of the vagina is almost always visible in low types of lesions on physical

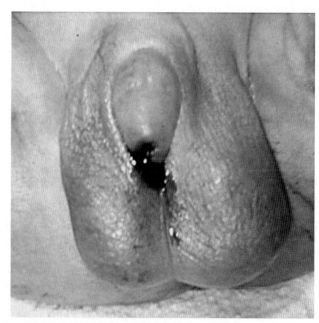

FIGURE 181-6 Meconium is seen coming from the penile urethral orifice. This is consistent with a rectourethral fistula.

examination. If the opening of the bowel cannot be seen, or there is meconium observed coming from the vagina, it is likely there is a high rectovaginal fistula, which usually requires a temporary diverting colostomy and formal reconstruction later. The presence of a single perineal orifice indicates the presence of a cloaca. In the event of a cloaca, a screening abdominal ultrasound is performed. It is important to understand the status of the urologic system prior to colostomy in these patients because it may be necessary to divert the urinary tract. Recommended management of females with an ARM begins with the delineation of the reproductive anatomy as completely as possible. In a recent series of patients treated for imperforate anus with a rectovestibular fistula, 5% had an associated vaginal septum and 9% had an absent vagina.[68] Most pediatric surgeons are aware of the strong association of gynecologic anomalies with a cloacal anomaly, which is cited as 53% to 67% of female patients with uterovaginal anomalies.[69-71] In less complex ARMs such as rectovestibular or rectoperineal fistula, a vaginal septum is the most common anomaly and can be treated during the initial rectal repair. Vaginoscopy should be performed on all girls during the definitive repair of any ARM. If more complex malformations are present, both cystoscopy and vaginoscopy can be performed. Assessment of the internal reproductive anatomy should be performed whenever an intraabdominal procedure is performed. Some prove the patency of the Müllerian system with placement of pediatric feeding tubes in the distal aspect of each fallopian tube and gentle antegrade instillation of saline bilaterally. This assessment can provide reassurance regarding the future outflow of menstrual products. Ultrasound surveillance of the reproductive structures should begin 6 to 9 months after the onset of breast development and continue every 6 to 9 months through menarche.[72]

ALL INFANTS

Unfortunately, a physical examination does not always provide the definitive answer as to which children require a colostomy. Imaging studies have been used to assist in making this decision, including the invertogram[73]; however, as an alternative to holding the infant upside down, a prone cross-table lateral view can be obtained.[74] With this technique, a radiopaque perineal skin marker is taped in place to aid in determining the distance between the end of the rectum and the anal skin site. Other imaging modalities include ultrasonography, magnetic resonance (MR) imaging, VCUG, and lumbosacral radiography. These modalities have been used to determine the level of the distal rectal pouch, to identify the presence of a fistula, and to diagnose any associated congenital anomalies. In the neonate, ultrasound examination of the lumbosacral spine is useful in identifying spinal cord lesions. The puborectalis muscle is a landmark used to distinguish the level of the defect. MR imaging can demonstrate the presence of muscle preoperatively; however, MR may have some limitations in demonstrating the relationship of the distal rectal pouch to the puborectalis muscle and may require sedation and/or a general anesthetic to accomplish in the newborn phase.[75,76] Infracoccygeal ultrasound, on the other hand,

can directly demonstrate the puborectalis muscle in neonates[77] without sedation. It is difficult to accurately depict the puborectalis sling using conventional transperineal ultrasound because this study relies on indirect measurements to reach a conclusion. Reported cutoff values to differentiate low from intermediate and high imperforate anus range from 10 to 25 mm,[78-80] with a recent study stating 15 mm.[81]

In older infants, MR imaging studies are of great value in detecting spine abnormalities. Lumbosacral radiographs are obtained to evaluate the sacral anatomy. Obtaining a renal ultrasound is also useful in detecting associated urinary tract anomalies. A retrograde cystourethrogram is an accurate method of delineating an associated rectourethral fistula in boys. Diagnostic endoscopic evaluation in girls with a cloacal defect is essential before any definitive repair. It demonstrates instances of vaginal septation, vaginal atresia, and duplex uterus and separates high from low cloacal anomalies.

OPERATIVE TECHNIQUE

As a general rule, infants born with low anomalies are treated definitively in the neonatal period. Infants with a complete atretic anal membrane are managed by incising the skin covering (usually seen bulging with meconium behind it) to relieve the obstruction. Anal dilations (using Hegar dilators) for 3 to 6 months result in adequate anal orifice without stenosis. The passage of more-formed stools in later infancy maintains the opening.

ANOCUTANEOUS FISTULA

CUTBACK ANOPLASTY

Infants with an anocutaneous fistula undergo a cutback perineal anoplasty (Figure 181-7). A Y-V technique that creates a U-shaped superficial external sphincter and widened skin orifice is used. The puborectalis and deep external sphincter muscles are carefully identified through electrostimulation and are preserved. A portion of the posterior fistula wall is incised and sutured to the skin edges with interrupted 4-0 absorbable suture. The new anoplasty site should be sized to a No. 10 Hegar dilator. Postoperatively, bowel contents are gently dabbed from the perianal skin with moist cotton balls. Vigorous wiping techniques should be avoided in the first week. Gentle tepid water irrigation can be used after 48 to 72 hours to clean the perineal skin. Daily dilation with a No. 10 Hegar dilator is initiated approximately 10 to 14 days after the procedure and continued for a 6-month period. The dilator size is gradually increased to a No. 13 or 14 dilator.

Although Smith[20] suggested a cutback anoplasty for girls with an anovestibular fistula to the extravaginal fourchette, we believe these patients require either a transplant anoplasty or a minimal PSARP to preserve the perineal body and adequately separate the vaginal and anal orifices as described by Potts et al.[82] Fecal content is passed through the rectofourchette fistula aided by daily dilation, and definitive operative repair can be delayed until the perineal and vaginal tissues become more sturdy. Accurate diagnosis of the level of the rectal atresia

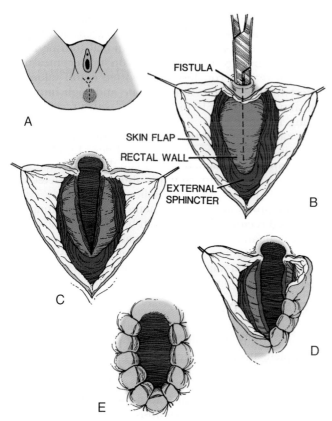

A

FISTULA

SKIN FLAP

RECTAL WALL

EXTERNAL
SPHINCTER

B

C

D

E

FIGURE 181-7 Y-V cutback anoplasty for anal atresia with anocutaneous fistula. After Y incision **(A)**, skin flaps are carefully raised, and the sphincter is identified and preserved **(B)**. The rectal pouch is incised **(C)**, and the edges of the rectum are sutured (full-thickness) to the skin edges **(D and E)**.

is important, because an intermediate-level rectovestibular fistula in a girl is similar to a rectourethral fistula at the level of the verumontanum in a boy and would require a preliminary colostomy. Proponents of anterior sagittal anorectoplasty argue that anal transplantation is performed without the clear identification of muscular anatomy that this procedure provides.[83] However, there are no randomized prospective studies that directly compare the two techniques, and it has been our practice to individualize therapy based on the location of the fistula.

TRANSPLANT ANOPLASTY

Transplant anoplasty is initiated by placing a series of 4-0 silk traction sutures at the 12-, 3-, 6-, and 9-o'clock positions of the fistula opening (Figure 181-8). Using fine curved tenotomy scissors, or electrocautery, the fistula is carefully dissected free close to its wall (in all four quadrants). The anterior dissection in the common wall between the fistula and posterior vaginal wall is usually quite tedious. A fine-tip electrocoagulator, wide-angled magnifying loupes, and small aspirator are useful adjuncts. Once above the level of the fistula site, the anterior and lateral dissection is more easily accomplished. Posteriorly, careful perineal dissection is also required to prevent injury to the striated muscle complex. The superior extent of the posterior dissection is continued superiorly within the puborectalis–deep external

sphincter muscular sling. The site of the new anal orifice is identified by electrical muscle mapping to demonstrate maximum contraction at the pucker site. A skin incision is made at this point, and to join the posterior dissection of the fistula tract within the muscular sling, careful dissection through the center of the subcutaneous and superficial external sphincter muscle is performed. The opening is progressively dilated with Nos. 7, 8, and 9 Hegar dilators. The fistula is then transplanted to the new anal orifice site using the previously placed traction sutures. The fistula site is usually narrow enough to enter this area without tapering. The posterior smooth muscle rectal wall 2.0 cm above the orifice is sutured to the muscle complex with interrupted absorbable sutures to prevent prolapse. Suturing the anal orifice (full thickness) to the edges of the anal skin with interrupted 4-0 absorbable suture completes the anoplasty. The previous fistula site at the fourchette is closed, and an indwelling Foley catheter is left in place for approximately 72 hours to prevent urine from bathing the new suture lines. Alternately, Peña and others approach this lesion by performing a posterior sagittal anoplasty and proximal diverting colostomy in each instance.

ANTERIOR PERINEAL ANORECTOPLASTY

The PSARP has been the mainstay treatment for ARM; however, the anterior perineal anorectoplasty may offer similar outcomes in selected cases. Rectovestibular fistula is the most common form of anorectal anomaly in female patients and the lithotomy position is chosen. The rectal fistula is dissected free and released from the posterior vaginal wall, and the anterior portion of the sphincter muscle is divided through a median perineal skin incision. The rectal fistula is then pulled posteriorly to the center of the sphincter muscle and sutured into place with absorbable interrupted sutures.[83,84] This technique has also been employed for higher lesions but requires considerably more expertise.[85]

HIGH IMPERFORATE ANUS

ARM is one of the major indications for a colostomy in a newborn infant.[86,87] In most patients, colostomy is performed as a temporary procedure before definitive surgical correction of the malformation is completed. A colostomy is recommended in the neonatal period for both boys and girls with anorectal anomalies, excluding those with perineal fistula; however, the use of neonatal pull-through procedures is challenging this long-standing approach. The colostomy often permits a better radiologic definition of the malformation (i.e., distal colostogram), continued growth of the child while waiting for the definitive procedure, and protection of the operative anoplasty site when a corrective procedure has been performed.

CONSTRUCTION OF A COLOSTOMY

Infants with intermediate or high anorectal agenesis or rectal atresia, with or without a fistula to the genitourinary tract, and all patients with cloacal anomalies require an initial colostomy. Most surgeons prefer a sigmoid colostomy for these anomalies, as recommended by

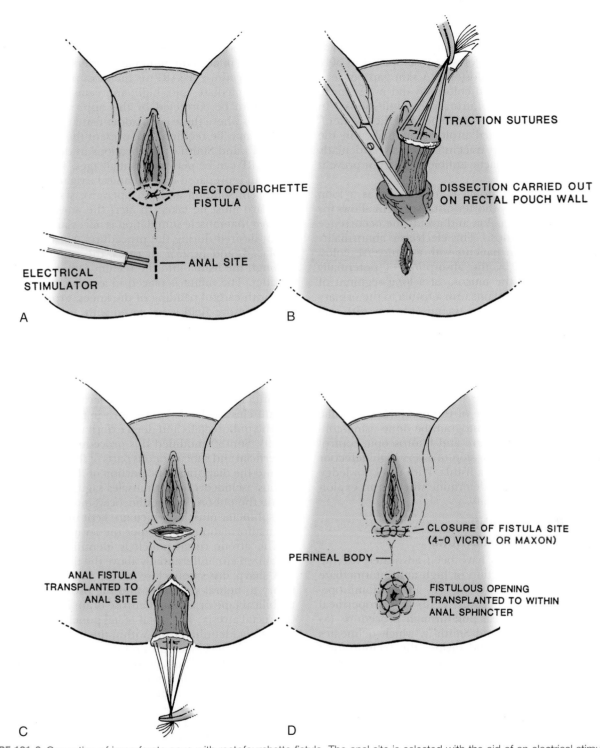

FIGURE 181-8 Correction of imperforate anus with rectofourchette fistula. The anal site is selected with the aid of an electrical stimulator **(A)**. Traction sutures are placed. The fistula is carefully dissected free with tenotomy scissors **(B)**. The traction sutures are used to guide the opening to a transplanted anal location within the sphincter complex. Interrupted 4-0 absorbable sutures are used **(C)**. The fistulous site is closed with interrupted 4-0 suture. Note the preservation of the perineal body **(D)**.

Wilkins and Peña,[88] at the junction of the descending and the sigmoid colon, but some surgeons recommend a right transverse colostomy for infants with a cloacal anomaly. A sigmoid stoma is smaller and more manageable with a decreased tendency to prolapse and more formed stool; it eliminates distal loop fecal impaction; it allows sufficient length of colon distal to the stoma so that subsequent pull-through procedure can be carried out without tension; and it may reduce the risk of urinary tract infections. Most surgeons recommend a divided colostomy to ensure complete fecal diversion and thus potential contamination of the urinary tract and vagina because of spillover of fecal material into the efferent limb and the rectal fistula. Patwardhan et al have recently shown that the incidence of urinary tract infections was 28% in patients with loop colostomy compared to 30% in patients with divided colostomy. A skin gap between the two ends of the divided colostomy did not seem to prevent the development of urinary tract infections.[89] In agreement with the findings of Wiener and Kiesewetter,[90] the incidence of associated urologic anomalies in the patients who had a urinary tract infection was particularly high (71%) and prophylactic antibiotics did not prevent the infections.[89]

Even if the sigmoid stoma is maintained as a loop colostomy, the relatively shorter distal segment allows for irrigation of the distal colon and avoids the occurrence of hyperchloremic acidosis. This electrolyte abnormality is occasionally seen in patients with a transverse colostomy and is caused by the absorption of potentially infected urine from the mucosa of a long segment of unused distal colon.[23] Infants with a fistula to the urinary tract may benefit from urinary tract prophylaxis with oral trimethoprim-sulfamethoxazole. The colostomy is left in place until the time of definitive repair.

Prior to the definitive anorectal procedure, a distal colostogram can be carried out. Peña suggests this is the single most valuable method to accurately study an ARM. This study will demonstrate the location of the blind rectum and identify the site of the rectourinary fistula. Peña recommends the colostogram be done using considerable hydrostatic pressure and fluoroscopic control to minimize the false impression of a very high defect or pure rectal atresia without a fistula. With this knowledge in hand, the surgeon can determine whether an exploratory laparotomy is necessary.

CORRECTION OF HIGH AND INTERMEDIATE MALFORMATIONS

A number of techniques have been advocated for the modern operative correction of high and intermediate anorectal anomalies, including (1) the abdominoperineal pull-through procedure[91]; (2) a sacroperineal or sacroabdominoperineal pull-through procedure (as advocated by Stephens and Smith[19]), which delineates the puborectalis muscle and divides the rectourethral fistula from within the rectal atresia; and (3) in the 1960s, modifications of the Stephens procedure were reported by Kiesewetter[92] and by Rehbein,[93,94] using a submucosal resection that leaves a muscular sleeve from the original rectal atresia in place through which an abdominoperineal pull-through procedure is performed. In 1975, Mollard et al[95,96] advocated the use of an anterior transperineal approach to identify the puborectalis sling and the fistula and then used Kiesewetter's technique to complete the procedure. In 1982, deVries and Peña[2] described the PSARP, a procedure that divides each of the striated muscles in the posterior midline sagittal plane, divides the fistula from within the atretic rectal lumen, and tapers the distal bowel to fit snugly within the muscle complex, which is then reconstituted around the rectum and anoplasty site. More recent innovations by Yokoyama et al[97] and modifications by Smith[20] combine the excellent exposure afforded by the Peña and deVries[3] sagittal

anorectoplasty (which avoids laparotomy and gains excellent exposure to divide the fistula) but keeps the combined puborectalis, pubococcygeus, and deep external sphincter intact and minimally tapers the bowel. The Peña procedure (PSARP) is the most popular operation for intermediate and high anorectal lesions, and all ARMs can be corrected by this approach; however, in instances where there is a bladder fistula, additional laparotomy may be required. We present the Peña operation (PSARP) and Smith's modifications in detail.

PSARP can be performed at all ages. The distal bowel segment is prepared by mechanical irrigation with 0.25% neomycin solution and perioperative systemic antibiotics. Care must be taken to alert the anesthesiologist to the fact that muscle stimulation is necessary and paralysis is not desired during the procedure. A urinary catheter is placed, and in 25% of cases, the catheter may pass through the fistula into the rectum rather than into the bladder. The infant is placed in a prone jackknife position with careful padding of the knees, groin, and chest. The operative field is prepared with an iodophor solution, and appropriate sterile drapes and linens are applied. The proposed anal site is determined by electrical muscle stimulation and marked.

A midline sagittal incision is placed on the lower sacrum just above the coccyx and is carried inferiorly to the anticipated anal site; all of the levator ani and sphincter muscles are divided posteriorly in the midline, including the puborectalis and deep external sphincter (Figure 181-9). Smith[20] modified this procedure by dividing the superficial and subcutaneous parts of the external sphincter and the diaphragmatic portion of the levator (iliococcygeus, ischiococcygeus) muscles sagittally but does not divide the puborectalis, pubococcygeus, and deep external sphincter muscles, which are kept intact. The higher the malformation, the deeper the levator muscle.

The atretic rectal pouch is identified and carefully mobilized circumferentially above the fistula site by blunt and sharp dissection close to the bowel wall to avoid injury to neural structures and the prostatic plexus. An umbilical tape or a small Penrose drain is passed around the rectal atresia. The distal rectal pouch is entered, and the fistula identified from within the lumen. A submucosal plane is developed around the fistula to avoid injury to the seminal vesicles and prostate. The fistula is closed with interrupted 4-0 absorbable sutures. If able, closing additional tissue over the urethral fistula site may minimize the risk of postoperative complications. The atretic rectal pouch is then carefully mobilized, keeping the dissection in the plane of the bowel wall and using a fine-tip electrocoagulator to cauterize multiple vessels (from the middle hemorrhoidal artery) just beyond the rectal wall. In most cases, rectal mobilization is more than adequate through the sacroperineal approach, and a laparotomy is unnecessary.

Once the rectum is fully mobilized, a decision is made concerning the need to taper the rectum. If tapered, the distal bowel is narrowed to comfortably fit within the reconstituted muscle complex without causing injury to the essential muscles. Tapering is accomplished by excising a V-shaped wedge of the posterior wall of the rectal atretic segment and using a two-layered inverting closure

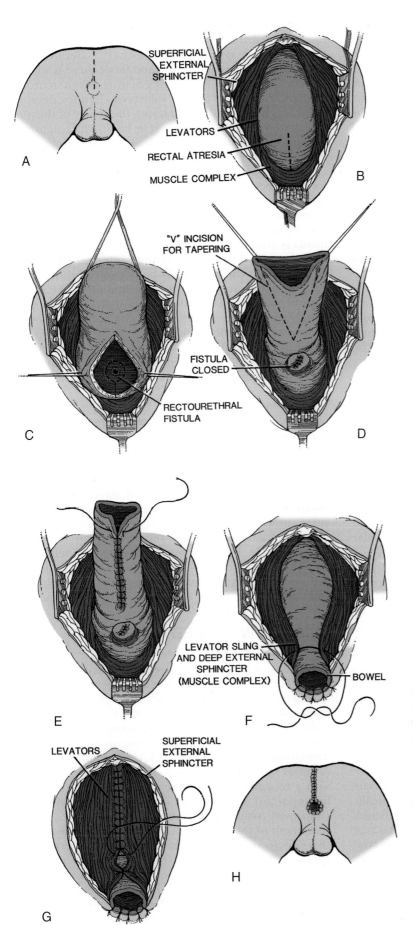

FIGURE 181-9 Posterior sagittal anorectoplasty. In the prone position, an incision is made in the midline from the lower sacrum to the selected anal site **(A).** The levator and sphincter muscles are divided posteriorly in the midline. The rectal pouch is identified **(B).** The pouch is opened, and the rectourethral fistula is identified within the rectal lumen **(C).** Submucosal resection frees the bowel from the fistula, which is closed with interrupted sutures **(D).** The bowel is tapered to a No. 12 Hegar size **(E).** The muscle complex is reconstituted starting at the deepest portion of the puborectalis muscle and the deep external sphincter **(F).** Levators and superficial external sphincters are then reapproximated with interrupted sutures **(G).** The tapered anoplasty is sutured to the skin with interrupted 4-0 absorbable suture **(H).**

with interrupted 4-0 absorbable sutures in the inner and outer layer. It is important to avoid excessive tapering, which may result in a severe stricture. We usually perform the tapering over a No. 12 Hegar dilator.

The tapered rectum is then placed within the divided muscular complex, which is reconstituted around the rectum with fine interrupted absorbable sutures. The deepest suture begins where the distal portion of the levator ani joins the external sphincter layers, bringing the rectum close to the urethra or vagina. Electrical muscle stimulation is used to identify the structures. The wall of the rectum is tacked to the muscle complex in a few places in an attempt to reincorporate the longitudinal smooth muscle of the rectum with the striated muscle complex, causing a tethering effect. The proximal margins of the levators are closed with interrupted suture. The course of the tapered anoplasty then passes more posteriorly to the site of the new anal opening. The anoplasty is completed by securing the end of the tapered bowel (full thickness) to the skin exit with interrupted 4-0 sutures, incorporating the subcutaneous sphincter in the bites. Performing the procedure with slight tension on the anoplasty avoids postoperative prolapse.

In Smith's modification of the Peña procedure, a Penrose drain is passed through the sling below the fistula site, and the tapered bowel is then passed through the sling anterior to the drain with the aid of traction sutures. The distal bowel is placed within the divided levator muscles and superficial and subcutaneous external sphincter muscles, which are accurately reconstituted around the bowel with interrupted 4-0 absorbable sutures. The anoplasty Smith advocated is a skin-lined tract originally credited to H. H. Nixon of London[98,99] that avoids anocutaneous stenosis. Skin closure of the main wound in both techniques is accomplished with subcuticular absorbable sutures and Steri-Strips.

The colostomy is left in place for approximately 2 to 3 months to allow complete healing and adequate dilation of the new anoplasty site. Daily dilations are started at 10 to 14 days after the procedure using Nos. 8, 9, and 10 Hegar dilators initially and then advancing to larger dilators with time (up to a maximum of No. 13 or 14 Hegar size). The parents must be carefully instructed regarding the importance of the dilations, which must be performed on a daily basis at home to avoid stenosis. Frequent followup visits to the surgeon's office after the procedure is necessary to monitor progress, because dilations may be necessary for 6 to 12 months postoperatively.

NEONATAL PULL-THROUGH PROCEDURES

The traditional surgical correction of a high or intermediate imperforate anus in the male infant has typically been a three-stage process. Despite performing a technically perfect operation, there are subsets of children that require significant lifelong bowel management for constipation or incontinence.[8,100] It is unlikely that much can be done to improve the outcome for children with poor prognostic factors (abnormal sacrum, poor perineal musculature, colonic dysmotility, and deficient pelvic innervation).[101] The theoretical basis for early restoration

of gastrointestinal continuity stems from the belief that the neuronal framework for normal bladder and bowel function exists at the time of birth.[102,103] Because neonates are incontinent of urine and feces, there is a learning period in which long-lasting activity-driven neuronal changes take place during neuronal circuitry development.[104] Theoretically, by delaying the repair of the anorectal anomaly, critical time may be lost in which neuronal networks and synapses would have formed resulting in normal or near-normal anorectal function.[105]

Unfortunately, many studies at this time have limited followup because it takes a few years to develop continence. The following advantages of a definitive neonatal procedure are highlighted: (1) there is only a single operation, (2) urinary tract colonization through the fistula is avoided, (3) the potential morbidity of a colostomy is avoided (prolapse, stenosis, retraction, bleeding, etc.), and (4) the fistula can be documented by cystoscopy, thus avoiding other imaging studies.[101] The advantage of avoiding a colostomy especially in developing countries may be an attractive alternative because a colostomy is socially unacceptable, colostomy bags are expensive and difficult to locate, many of the parents are illiterate and cannot manage the colostomy, and these environments usually have no stomal therapists available.[106]

Peña cautioned that some of the most devastating complications that he has seen after a posterior sagittal exploration occurred in patients who underwent posterior sagittal exploration without a precise diagnosis obtained by a distal colostogram. The worst morbidity was observed in instances of high defects (rectal–bladder neck fistulas) while looking for an atretic rectum that could only be found at laparotomy. Peña suggested that surgeons who want to attempt to repair these anomalies in a single-stage approach should develop their own learning curve. Perhaps the first cases that are performed should be relatively low-lying lesions noted on a simple cross-table radiograph taken in the prone position rather than attempting repair of a possible higher lesion that carries higher risks.[101]

MINIMALLY INVASIVE REPAIR OF HIGH IMPERFORATE ANUS

Minimal access surgery has revolutionized the field of surgery in the past decade. The laparoscopically assisted anorectal pull-through (LAARP) for high ARM uses fundamental concepts learned from decades of experience with high ARM repair and additionally incorporates modern technologic advancements in surgical instrumentation and technique.[107] LAARP combines extraordinary anatomic exposure of an infant's deep pelvis with a reconstruction technique that minimizes trauma to important surrounding structures. The advantages (improved visualization, relatively atraumatic proper placement of the pull-through bowel without division of the muscle complex, preservation of the internal anal sphincter fibers within the fistula) essentially allow the surgeon to treat a high lesion similar to a low lesion, are associated with decreased postoperative pain, and potentially reduce the incidence of perineal wound complications.[108]

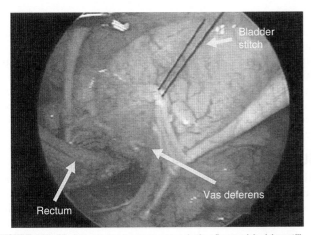

FIGURE 181-10 Although decompressed, the floppy bladder still needs to be retracted anteriorly. In this figure, a percutaneously placed U-stitch is placed through the bladder and is used for retraction, thereby allowing exposure of the deep pelvic structures. (From Sydorak RM, Albanese CT: Laparoscopic repair of high imperforate anus. *Semin Pediatr Surg* 11:217, 2002.)

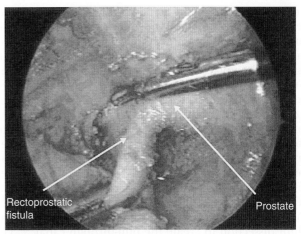

FIGURE 181-11 The completed dissection of the rectoprostatic fistula before division is shown. The upper instrument is pushing up on the prostate and bladder, and the lower instrument is grasping the rectum. (From Sydorak RM, Albanese CT: Laparoscopic repair of high imperforate anus. *Semin Pediatr Surg* 11:217, 2002.)

The infant is positioned horizontally and supine on the operating room table to allow the surgeon and assistant to stand at the patient's head, and, if present, a second surgeon can work at the feet. A total-body sterile preparation is employed from the nipple line to the toes. Preoperative cystoscopy may be helpful in identifying the level of the fistula if not known previously. An indwelling Foley catheter is placed. Local anesthetic may be infiltrated into the subcutaneous tissue around the laparoscopic port sites either preemptively or at the completion of the case. Using an umbilical trocar for camera visualization has not been optimal.[108] Thus the ideal position for the camera port is just to the right of the midline below the liver edge. A 5-mm cannula is introduced 3.0 cm to the right and above the umbilicus. A 30-degree scope is used because this provides excellent visualization of the deep pelvic structures and allows several views of the same structure. Surgeons have utilized either a three- or four-port method using either 3- or 5-mm trocars.

Dissection begins at the level of the peritoneal reflection, and the blood supply to the sigmoid and rectum is preserved. Too high a dissection and sacrifice of these vascular structures may result in ischemia of the distal bowel. In addition, the dissection remains adjacent to the wall of the colon to minimize potential damage to the vas deferens, ureter, urethra, prostate, and pelvic nerves. The bladder despite being decompressed requires retraction (Figure 181-10). Some have used a trocar site for retraction, whereas others have used a transcutaneous bladder stitch that is inserted through the abdominal wall.[108] Once the dissection has reached the level of the bladder neck (Figure 181-11), a bipolar scissors is used to minimize lateral damage to the pelvic nerves. The distal colon is dissected circumferentially, leaving only the fistulous tract connection. The Harmonic Scalpel or endoscopic clips have been used to divide the fistula tract.[107,108] Some surgeons have been concerned that complications related to these methods may result in urethral stricture or recurrent fistula and advocate

division and direct suturing of the fistula tract.[108] Some have utilized a fine flexible endoscope inserted into the rectum through an opening made in the anterior rectal wall during laparoscopically assisted pull-through to facilitate complete excision of the rectal bulbar fistula in the male.[109] Others, after opening the rectal urethral fistula, have inserted a fine catheter with 10-mm calibration and advanced until its tip was seen to emerge at or near the verumontanum by another surgeon performing cystoscopy. The inside measurement from rectal urethral fistula opening to urethral orifice (X) and the outside length (Y) from the rectal urethral fistula opening to end of dissection completion were calculated (X-Y).[110] If (X-Y) was more than 5 mm, the rectal end was further dissected toward the urethra. Followup in this group's patient cohort did not show any evidence of diverticulum formation when studied by ultrasound, urethrography, or MRI. There is more recent discussion about leaving the rectourethral fistula alone and allowing it to close over the urethral/bladder catheter. There is no current long-term followup of this technique to provide further comment.

Once the rectum and the fistula are free, the pelvic musculature can be identified. The classic anatomic arrangement of the puborectalis, resembling a sling-shot, can often be appreciated (Figure 181-12). An assistant can now use a perineal muscle stimulator to identify the location of the central portion of the anorectal muscular complex, and this is marked. Some surgeons have used a laparoscopic muscle stimulator as well to identify the exact position for the pull-through within the abdomen.[111,112] Others have used MRI-guided laparoscopy-assisted anorectoplasty in which they position an MRI-compatible needle at the central site of the parasagittal muscle contraction and confirm with MRI location before the initiation of the procedure. Unfortunately, their procedural time averaged 450 minutes and there was an average of six limited MRIs per patient to advance the needle for localization.[113] In essence, one identifies a direct line between the centers of the internal sphincter (external stimulator) and the levator ani (internal stimulator), thus creating an anatomically correct position of the anorectum through the external anal sphincter. The assistant then places a Veress needle/trocar system transcutaneously through the two slings, and the sheath of the Veress needle is dilated sequentially from a 5- to 12-mm size depending on the size of the bowel and age of the infant. An endo-Babcock is then introduced into the abdomen and the rectum secured and the bowel is then brought out through the pelvic musculature and out onto the perineum (Figure 181-13). Some have utilized intraoperative ultrasound to determine the positioning of the pull-through canal in the pelvic floor muscles.[114] In addition, one can use a mosquito forceps to perform blunt dissection to create the pull-through canal.[115] The anoplasty is then completed with interrupted absorbable

sutures (Figure 181-14). Several rectum-to–presacral fascia sutures can be placed to increase the length of the skin-lined anal canal and to minimize the risk of prolapse. Prolapse has been shown to occur in 9% to 46%[116,117] of patients compared to the 3% rate described in the PSARP procedure.[118] Rectum and pelvis dissection should be as limited as possible in order to minimize section of anatomic attachments between posterior rectum and sacrum.

SURGERY FOR CLOACAL MALFORMATION

The initial treatment of a neonate with a cloacal malformation is to provide drainage of the urinary tract and the colon (colostomy). Intermittent catheterization usually can empty the distended vagina and bladder. Infants with a cloacal anomaly do not require an extensive pelvic laparotomy to assess the anatomy. This assessment can be done endoscopically and radiologically. Ultrasound may detect associated genital anomalies such as hydrocolpos, uterine didelphys, and vaginal anomalies, all making repair more complex. MR imaging of the spinal canal should be performed because a third of these patients have a tethered spinal cord.[119-121] Cloacal reconstruction can be a long and difficult procedure and goes beyond the scope of this chapter, but it is usually deferred until the patient is approximately 1 year old. The surgeon will typically perform endoscopy to specifically determine the length of the common channel. There are two well-characterized groups of cloacas and represent distinctly different challenges. The first consists of a common channel shorter than 3 cm. This is the case in the majority of patients and repair can usually be done via a posterior sagittal approach along with urogenital advancement. The pelvis is approached through a long midsagittal incision and down into the single perineal opening. The rectum or vagina is opened. The goal of this procedure is to separate the rectum from the vagina and, subsequently, the vagina from the urinary tract. The rectum and vagina have a common wall, and the separation of these structures requires a meticulous and time-consuming effort, but this dissection is usually easier than separation of the vagina from the urinary tract. The urogenital sinus (common channel) must be reconstructed to become the new urethra by tubularizing the

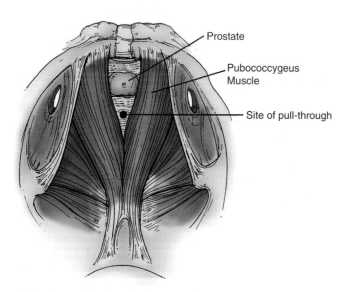

FIGURE 181-12 Laparoscopic visualization of the pelvis after dissection of the rectum out of the pelvis in a typical boy with high imperforate anus and rectourethral fistula. (From Georgeson KE, Inge TH, Albanese CT: Laparoscopically assisted anorectal pull-through for high imperforate anus: A new technique. *J Pediatr Surg* 35:927, 2000.)

Prostate

Pubococcygeus Muscle

Site of pull-through

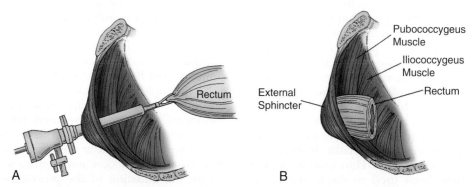

Rectum

Pubococcygeus Muscle

Iliococcygeus Muscle

External Sphincter

Rectum

A

B

FIGURE 181-13 A, Sagittal view of the trocar through the external sphincter and levator ani and pull-through of the rectum. **B,** Position of the rectum after pull-through to the perineal wound. (From Georgeson KE, Inge TH, Albanese CT: Laparoscopically assisted anorectal pull-through for high imperforate anus: A new technique. *J Pediatr Surg* 35:927, 2000.)

tissue (Figure 181-15). The second group has a common channel longer than 3 cm and usually needs a laparotomy and either a vaginal switch maneuver or vaginal replacement with either rectum, colon, or small bowel. The vaginal orifice is sutured to the perineal skin immediately behind the urethra. The perineal body is then reconstructed to the anterior component of the external sphincter. The rectum is then reconstructed as previously described for the PSARP procedure.[122]

POSTOPERATIVE COMPLICATIONS

Although deVries and Peña[2] reported only minor postoperative complications, some authors have described a number of serious complications after the PSARP

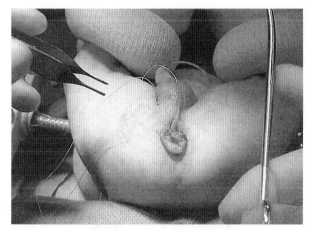

FIGURE 181-14 The pull-through is completed, and the anorectoplasty is being performed. (From Sydorak RM, Albanese CT: Laparoscopic repair of high imperforate anus. *Semin Pediatr Surg* 11:217, 2002.)

procedure. Others[123] have reported major complications in 26% of cases, including sacral wound dehiscence and/or infection, ureteric injury, neurogenic bladder, femoral nerve palsy, leak from the tapered rectoplasty, recurrent urethral fistula, multiple rectocutaneous fistulas, and a supralevator fistula. Most of these complications, however, were related to technical errors and are probably avoidable. Genitourinary complications, including neurogenic bladder, urethral stricture, and urethral diverticulum, have also been observed and may be related to technical errors at the time of the PSARP procedure.

Previous clinical practice has included evaluation for the presence of a tethered cord in those children who have imperforate anus with a high lesion. In a retrospective study, Golonka et al noted that 34.9% of their patients had evidence of a tethered cord. Twenty-six percent of patients had a high lesion compared to 50% having a low lesion. Forty-five percent of the patients with low lesions and a tethered cord had no other lumbosacral anomalies. Thus, early evaluation for tethered cord is advocated for all children with ARM.[124]

REOPERATIVE SURGERY

Reoperation may be considered for a number of reasons, including to achieve improved functional results following a primary procedure, improve pain and discomfort, recurrent fistula, wound dehiscence, persistent anorectal stricture, fecal incontinence, or missing the sling at the first procedure (as detected by MRI). The number of patients who require a reoperation for fecal incontinence has decreased over the years and coincides with the use of the posterior sagittal approach.[125] The most rewarding group of patients to treat are those with previous catastrophic complications, because they enjoy the greatest benefit.

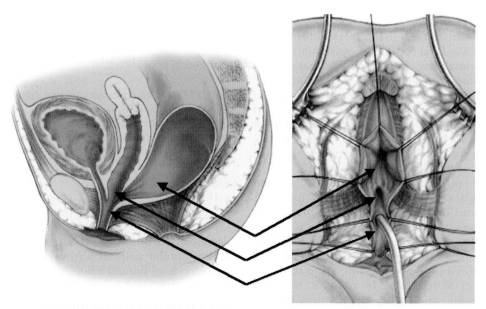

FIGURE 181-15 Female cloaca. *Arrows* indicate common channel, vagina, and distal rectum. The rectum and vagina will be separated, followed by tubularization and reconstruction of urethra, vagina, and rectum. (From Peña A, Levitt MA: Anorectal malformations. In Grosfeld JL, O'Neill JA, Coran AG, Fonkalsrud EW, editors: *Pediatric surgery*, ed 6. Philadelphia, 2006, Mosby.)

Based on Peña's anatomic findings,[125] he speculated that retraction, dehiscence, and acquired rectal atresia were most likely caused by technical errors. In addition, rectal strictures are most likely caused by ischemia of the distal part of the rectum. Some surgeons follow a protocol to dilate the rectum in the operating room rather than have the patient's family perform this at home on a daily basis. This may actually provoke a rectal laceration with further healing with a scar and possible intractable ring of fibrosis. If necessary, revision anoplasty (Y-V, Nixon, diamond flap, and three-flap techniques) can be used.[126,127]

Persistent rectourethral fistulas occur because the repair probably did not address the fistula initially, most likely using a perineal approach rather than a PSARP. Recurrent rectourethral/rectovaginal fistula may result if the fistula is closed but the rectum is not mobilized adequately, resulting in tension on the anterior wall of the rectum.

Posterior urethral diverticulum is typically present when the patient has a transabdominal procedure and the surgeon was unable to reach the fistula. The patient may pass mucus though the urethra or have orchiepididymitis, urinary tract infection, or urinary pseudoincontinence.[125]

Misdiagnosis of a cloaca as a rectovaginal fistula and then repairing only the rectal component of the defect create significant long-term difficulties for subsequent reconstruction. A true congenital rectovaginal fistula is an extremely unusual defect.[21] An acquired vaginal atresia may occur as a result of devascularization of the vagina during separation from the urethra during a cloacal repair. With the use of total urogenital mobilization, the risk of this complication has been reduced.

FUNCTIONAL RESULTS

Because of variability in anatomy and sacral deformity, the wide spectrum of anorectal disorders managed by different surgical techniques, and dissimilar criteria for success, the results are difficult to interpret and compare. As a general rule, the fecal continence rate after the correction of low anomalies is quite good. The anal canal is in its normal anatomic position, and a simple cutback or transplant anoplasty for a low fistula usually results in a good outcome. Unfortunately, the higher the rectal atresia/fistula, typically the worse the functional outcome. In some reports, girls have better fecal continence results than boys. This is possibly due to the increased incidence of low- and intermediate-level anomalies in girls.

The sacral ratio proposed as a method to evaluate the sacrum in patients with imperforate anus is useful in estimating the functional prognosis (Figure 181-16). In general, ratios lower than 0.500 significantly decrease the chance of achieving good bowel function. The measurement of the sacrum is easy to accomplish and eliminates the difficulty frequently experienced in trying to count the number of sacral vertebrae. In addition, by using sacral measurements, one can detect abnormal sacra, which are quite short despite the fact that they may have the normal number of vertebrae.[21] A recent evaluation to test the repeatability and validity of the sacral ratio

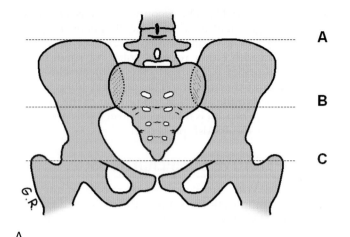

A

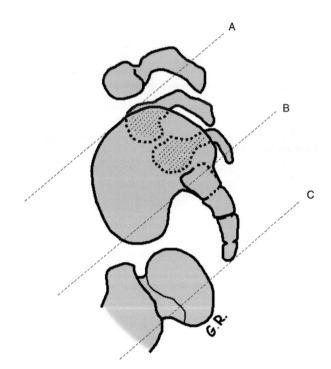

Normal ratio: BC/AB = 0.77

B

FIGURE 181-16 Anteroposterior **(A)** and lateral **(B)** illustrations showing sacral ratio measurement (*dashed lines A, B,* and *C* are shown). (From Peña A, Levitt MA: Anorectal malformations. In Grosfeld JL, O'Neill JA, Coran AG, Fonkalsrud EW, editors: *Pediatric surgery*, ed 6. Philadelphia, 2006, Mosby.)

measurement as a method for detecting sacral abnormalities showed that the sacral ratio has good interobserver and intraobserver repeatability. The mean value for a normal anteroposterior ratio concurred with that described previously by Peña, but the variability of values among similar patients was wide, suggesting this single measure is of limited value in discriminating a normal from an abnormal sacrum.[128]

ASSESSMENT OF CONTINENCE

A number of methods to assess continence have been developed and include subjective (e.g., good, fair, poor),

TABLE 181-5 International Classification (Krickenbeck) for Postoperative Results

1. Voluntary bowel movements	Yes/no
Feeling of urge	Yes/no
Capacity to verbalize	Yes/no
Hold the bowel movement	Yes/no
2. Soiling	Yes/no
Grade 1	Occasionally (once or twice per week)
Grade 2	Every day, no social problem
Grade 3	Constant, social problem
3. Constipation	Yes/no
Grade 1	Manageable by changes in diet
Grade 2	Requires laxative
Grade 3	Resistant to laxatives and diet

numerical (e.g., the Kelly score[129] based on fecal leakage, sensation, and contrast enema findings or the Cleveland Clinic Florida Incontinence Scoring System based on frequency of incontinence for solids, liquids, gas, pad use, and any alterations in lifestyle),[130] and a variety of physiologic evaluations, including balloon anorectal manometry, electrical sphincter muscle mapping, and anorectal angulation. The Krickenbeck conference[22] participants (2005) concluded that a simpler classification for followup studies was needed, and this group developed an international classification (Krickenbeck) for postoperative results (Table 181-5). This score is based on clear definitions of continence parameters; however, it has not yet been validated. Despite numerous technical advances in the surgical repair of ARM, a significant number of children have long-term problems with fecal continence and there is no universally accepted standard scoring system for the evaluation of this problem. Little is known about the psychosocial consequences of this chronic disability, although there is extensive anecdotal evidence that fecal incontinence is the cause of distress to both the child and the family. A long-term evaluation of children with anorectal anomalies by Ludman and Spitz[131] demonstrated that (1) children/adolescents with incontinence are not less well adjusted than those with good bowel control; (2) in children with continence, those with frequent soiling accidents were more likely to be recognized as emotionally disturbed; (3) young girls with incontinence showed significantly more behavioral and internalized problems; (4) parental factors were strongly associated with outcome; (5) incontinent adolescents were not more emotionally disturbed than those with good bowel control; and (6) parental perception of how others would react to a child with fecal incontinence influenced the child's coping behaviors.

OUTCOME IN PATIENTS WITH HIGH IMPERFORATE ANUS

Outcome studies in children with anorectal malformations have been traditionally based on subjective analysis of stool function. Patients historically have been ranked by either the surgeon or parent into three groups: excellent, good, and fair.[132,133] Long-term results for patients with high imperforate anus indicate that an excellent to good result is obtained in approximately 50% of patients,[23,92] whereas the remaining half will have a fair or poor (incontinent) outcome. Scales have been developed to objectively evaluate stool function in children; however, they are primarily used to assess patients with encopresis where children are anatomically normal and have a psychological etiology for their ailment.[134] Mollard et al[95] reported the best results, with 80% of patients being continent. However, this study included only 15 patients. The results of studies suggest that the short-term functional results after the Peña procedure and its modifications have been encouraging, in that good results have been achieved in 70% of patients.[23,135,136] Ultimately, achieving good quality of life is dependent not only on successful surgical interventions but also on other strategies such as psychological counseling, drug therapy, dietary restrictions, and a bowel training program. Brandt et al[137] have shown the usefulness of a 23-question Baylor Continence Scale to differentiate between children who have had a repair for anorectal malformation, children with enuresis, and normal children. In the clinical setting, the 23-question form was difficult to use and a 6-question abbreviated version was just as effective in differentiating the anorectal malformation patients from control patients. Clinical studies show that biofeedback is effective in improving the outcome in those with constipation and fecal soiling. The pathologies of congenital anorectal malformations are complex and mixed and previous biofeedback methods may be unsuitable. Zhengwei et al[138] feel that individualized biofeedback is more suitable for improvement of the clinical outcome and the quality of life in both short- and long-term followup. This technique, however, must be used in concert with other methods and requires patient motivation and compliance. The advent of cutaneous electromyography electrodes and computer-assessed games allows better compliance and acceptance in children. A child must undergo a careful preassessment to ensure the patient and therapist of proper expectations.[139]

CONSTIPATION

Constipation is one of the most frequent sequelae seen in children with imperforate anus. More important, the frequency of constipation does not coincide with the frequency of fecal incontinence. Children with low lesions have a better prognosis in regard to continence but often have a higher incidence of significant constipation than those with high defects. Peña[21] noted that 61.4% of patients with vestibular fistula had constipation, whereas 41.4% of patients with a prostatic fistula and 18.1% with an associated bladder neck fistula had this problem. Some suggest that dissection of the rectal pouch may provoke some degree of denervation of the rectum, decreasing motility, and may contribute to the occurrence of severe constipation (low, 35.7% occurrence; high, 72% occurrence)[140]; however, Peña supported the concept that the degree of rectal ectasia that the patient has initially in the atretic rectal segment predicts the most severe constipation, as may be the case in instances of rectovestibular fistulas. Most of the patients who experience soiling are exhibiting signs of overflow pseudoincontinence (encopresis), provoked by severe constipation. If this is ignored, a megasigmoid may develop, which is associated with a vicious cycle of further constipation and colon enlargement. Aggressive treatment of constipation is warranted, and, if necessary, sigmoid resection may be necessary to eliminate the chronic impaction and cure the overflow pseudoincontinence. Rectal mucosal prolapse is a common condition that is frequently confused with prolapsing hemorrhoids and is mainly the result of constipation and chronic straining. The treatment is based on the severity of symptoms and findings on examination and can range from conservative measures to surgical excision of the prolapsed mucosa. Some have begun utilizing the procedure for prolapsed hemorrhoids first described by Longo in 1998[141] because of less postoperative pain, fewer analgesics, early discharge, less time off work in the adult patient, and less pain at first bowel movement.[142]

TREATMENT OF POSTOPERATIVE FECAL INCONTINENCE

Patients with ARM frequently experience fecal incontinence despite the vigorous efforts of pediatric surgeons to perform a precise anatomic repair. At least 25% of all patients treated with a PSARP procedure still suffer from fecal incontinence.[21] Treatment with enemas, laxatives, and medications are often prescribed by clinicians in an indiscriminate manner and without a demonstrated benefit. Peña et al[143] have shown that this indiscriminate use of therapy not only failed to keep the patient clean but also may actually worsen the patient's condition. Peña has advocated an organized plan for bowel management therapy.

Others have shown that somatic and behavioral factors contribute to the persistence of chronic defecation problems. Treatment of these problems in patients with anal atresia should also include behavioral modification techniques.[144,145] Patients who remain incontinent beyond the age of 5 or 6 years should be evaluated for additional procedures. Careful study of the pelvic musculature and sacral anatomy, the urinary tract, and electrical sphincter mapping should be done before reoperation. These patients typically have an abnormal sacrum, flat perineum, and poor sphincters. There usually is evidence that they were born with a high ARM or cloaca with a common channel longer than 3.0 cm. Their sacral ratio is almost always less than 0.4. Reoperative procedures are most useful for instances of missed muscle complex or a misplaced anal orifice in patients with a good sacrum; however, with the poor prognostic factors noted, reoperation will not improve their situation. The Peña PSARP and the Mollard anterior perineal procedure have been used successfully (in 33% of patients) as secondary operations with good pelvic musculature.[18] It is wise to protect a secondary anoplasty procedure with a proximal diverting colostomy to ensure healing without fecal contamination.[3] Another reason not to reoperate on patients with fecal incontinence is the problem of short colon and, therefore, an incapacity to form solid stool, because these patients often do not gain bowel control regardless of how well their sphincters function. It had previously been believed that children with anorectal disorders would gradually improve their bowel habits with time. However, new data indicate that as the patients grow older, they likely implement their own bowel management programs and do not actually acquire improved bowel function.[21]

In instances of incontinence that occur despite a proper pull-through procedure, a gracilis muscle sling operation may prove useful in achieving voluntary muscle tone and improved control. This latter procedure is useful in 60% to 70% of cases; nevertheless, it is difficult to know exactly when to recommend this type of surgery. Newer options include the artificial bowel sphincter and electrostimulated gracilis neosphincter. At the present time, these surgical options are under investigation in children, and long-term morbidity and outcomes are not yet available.[146-148]

Enemas are often required to ensure complete fecal evacuation after the sling and sphincter procedures. In some instances in which incontinence is inevitable (e.g., sacral agenesis, failure of previous surgical procedures, and reoperation), an end colostomy may be the most appropriate long-term procedure to achieve a socially acceptable status. The Malone antegrade colonic enema (MACE) procedure, in which the appendix,[149] cecal flap, cecostomy tube (Chait),[150-152] or a sigmoid irrigation tube[153] is used as a continent stoma to deliver antegrade enemas, has become a popular alternative to evacuate the colon and to promote cleanliness.[154] When used in patients, the antegrade colonic enema procedure has been one of the most effective means the pediatric surgeon has to achieve socially acceptable continence status. However, this also carries with it some morbidity— especially stomal stenosis, which may occur in 25% to 30% of cases but can be decreased with frequent dilations/ catheterizations and the inlay of skin at the cutaneous stomal anastomosis. The MACE procedure is successful in achieving cleanliness in more than 70% of cases.

GENITOURINARY TRACT

Most patients with an ARM and concomitant sacral agenesis have vesicourethral as well as anorectal dysfunction and have both urinary and fecal incontinence.[8,155] However, in contrast to vesicourethral dysfunction, anorectal dysfunction does not cause functional deterioration of other organs. Significant long-term sequelae can arise from neurogenic lower urinary tract dysfunction, including recurrent urinary tract infection, vesicoureteral reflux (VUR), impaired renal function, and urinary incontinence. Moreover, other problems that can arise from impaired genitourinary innervation include ejaculatory and erectile dysfunction. Operative dissection during surgical treatment of ARM gets perilously close to the ejaculatory system, especially when a rectourethral fistula is present. Therefore, in addition to reconstructing the anorectal anomaly, other major goals in the management of these patients are preservation of renal function, prevention of urinary tract infections, maintenance of sexual function, and treatment of urinary incontinence.[156] Some children do not receive appropriate early urologic treatment; therefore, screening all newborns with ARMs for associated lower urinary tract anomalies and dysfunction along with appropriate urologic management is necessary to prevent urinary tract deterioration.

Spinal dysraphism and neurovesical dysfunction (NVD) frequently are associated in children with ARMs. A significant proportion of these patients also have associated urologic abnormalities, which include VUR, hydronephrosis, or renal agensis.[157] Renal insufficiency and renal failure remain the most significant causes of morbidity and mortality in patients with ARMs.[158] As such, prevention of renal damage remains a high priority. This has led to a recognition of sacral or spinal cord data to predict the risk of urologic problems in patients who demonstrate vertebral anomalies.[159] NVD involves an impaired innervation to the lower urinary tract, which affects both the filling and emptying functions. During the filling phase, detrusor pressure may be increased and the detrusor may be overactive, together with sphincter disturbance and detrusor-sphincter dyssynergy. This may result in incomplete bladder emptying that in turn may be associated with urinary tract infections and subsequent renal damage.[160,161] NVD was seen in 24% of 90 patients with ARM in one series[155] and 18% in another.[162] Among these cases were some patients with a normal sacrum, leading the authors to conclude that a normal radiograph does not exclude the risk of NVD.

An increasing number of young women are facing the prospects of pregnancy and labor having undergone corrective surgery for an anorectal malformation. A basic understanding of the surgical procedure performed, the impact of pregnancy, the suitability of vaginal delivery, and anticipated bladder and bowel dysfunction should all be considered in early pregnancy. The presence of residual problems such as incontinence, soiling, and constipation may aid in making a delivery method decision.

FAMILY DYNAMICS

Having a child with a serious disability can place strain on the whole family. Opinions vary as to the extent a chronic illness or malformation leads to difficulties with psychosocial adjustment and Meijer et al[163] state that the social consequences of chronic illness are not diagnosis specific, but the children with a chronic illness are generally at increased risk for psychosocial problems. Others[164,165] have shown that social functioning of children with juvenile chronic arthritis is remarkably similar to their healthy peers.

Few studies describe the effect of anal malformation on the lives of affected children and their parents. Adolescents with high and low imperforate anus have shown a high frequency of mental (58%) and psychosocial problems (73%), and the strongest predictor of psychosocial outcome was related to the presence of family difficulties[166] and emotional manifestations differ by gender.[167] It has been shown that a high degree of communication is important in reducing stress in children exposed to medical treatment,[168] and children have reported less pain and anxiety if they had been well informed prior to a procedure.[169-171] Interestingly, Ojmyr-Joelsson et al[169] showed that more children with juvenile chronic arthritis (JCA) were reported to have distressing memories than were children with imperforate anus. Children with JCA were older when they experienced

their medical treatment and studies have shown that children need to be around 2 years of age before they can recall experiences of medical procedures and before they can have the narrative skill to report such experiences later.[172] These data may indicate that anal dilations at an early age may create few distressful memories and may support early surgical reconstruction of the anal canal.[173]

Analyzing three families with qualitative methods resembling content analysis referred to as "editing analysis,"[174] Nisell et al[175] showed that the parents' experiences of suffering were overwhelming. Negative emotions displayed sorrow, pain, and disappointment. The parents related that the children had periods of depression and lived in fear of leakage and lack of bowel control and the families' daily lives were constrained as a result of this fear. Relations between parent and child were strained because of stressful treatments. After a MACE operation, there was noted to be a decisive positive change in both patients' and parents' lives.

OUTCOME OF CLOACAL SURGERY

Cloaca, which occurs in approximately 1 of 50,000 births, is the most complex of ARMs, with confluence of the rectum, vagina, and bladder in a urogenital sinus. Functional results for the bowel, the genital tract, and the urinary tract have been uniformly poor. In the current era, a reasonable lifestyle can be accomplished for most of these children with comprehensive surgical planning.[122]

The results of cloacal reconstruction are satisfactory for most patients. Sixty-two percent void spontaneously, 88% are socially clean with bowel control, and 89% have described normal coitus, with six women reported having children.[176] The best results have been achieved in centers where the surgeon has a special interest in this very complex reconstructive surgery and large operative volume.

SUMMARY

In spite of the technical advances in the surgical repair of ARM, the management of patients with variants of imperforate anus is difficult and carries a significant degree of physician responsibility, often requiring long-term followup into adulthood. A concise understanding of the anatomy and the surgical techniques is essential. These are procedures that should not be attempted by the occasional surgeon who rarely deals with neonatal anomalies. Unfortunately, there remain a significant number of patients who undergo attempted anorectal repairs with catastrophic complications. Many of these complications are preventable. One must have a thorough understanding of these malformations and the first operation performed well by an experienced pediatric surgeon most often allows the child the best chance for successful bowel control.

REFERENCES

1. Stephens FD: Imperforate rectum: A new surgical technique. *Med J Aust* 1:202, 1953.

2. deVries PA, Peña A: Posterior sagittal anorectoplasty. *J Pediatr Surg* 17:638, 1982.

3. Peña A, deVries PA: Posterior sagittal anorectoplasty: Important technical considerations and new applications. *J Pediatr Surg* 17:796, 1982.

4. Grosfeld JL: Anorectal malformations (ARM)—A historical overview. In Holschneider AM, Hutson JM, editors: *Anorectal malformations in children*. Berlin, 2006, Springer-Verlag, p 3.

5. Murken JD, Albert A: Genetic counseling in cases of anal and rectal atresia. *Prog Pediatr Surg* 9:115, 1976.

6. Santulli TV, Schullinger JN, Kiesewetter WB, et al: Imperforate anus: A survey from the members of the Surgical Section of the American Academy of Pediatrics. *J Pediatr Surg* 6:484, 1971.

7. Holschneider AM, Pfrommer W, Gerresheim B: Results in the treatment of anorectal malformations with special regard to the histology of the rectal pouch. *Eur J Pediatr Surg* 4:303, 1994.

8. Peña A: Posterior sagittal anorectoplasty: Results in the management of 322 cases of anorectal malformations. *Pediatr Surg Int* 3:94, 1988.

9. Kimmel SG, Mo R, Hui CC, et al: New mouse models of congenital anorectal malformations. *J Pediatr Surg* 35:227, 2000.

10. Jo Mauch T, Albertine KH: Urorectal septum malformation sequence: Insights into pathogenesis. *Anat Rec* 268:405, 2002.

11. Mo R, Kim JH, Zhang J, et al: Anorectal malformations caused by defects in sonic hedgehog signaling. *Am J Pathol* 159:765, 2001.

12. Kim J, Kim P, Hui CC: The VACTERL association: Lessons from the Sonic hedgehog pathway. *Clin Genet* 59:306, 2001.

13. deVries PA, Friedland GW: The staged sequential development of the anus and rectum in human embryos and fetuses. *J Pediatr Surg* 9:755, 1974.

14. Rogers DS, Paidas CN, Morreale RF, et al: Septation of the anorectal and genitourinary tracts in the human embryo: Crucial role of the catenoidal shape of the urorectal sulcus. *Teratology* 66:144, 2002.

15. Paidas CN, Morreale RF, Holoski KM, et al: Septation and differentiation of the embryonic human cloaca. *J Pediatr Surg* 34:877, 1999.

16. Qi BQ, Beasley SW, Frizelle FA: Clarification of the processes that lead to anorectal malformations in the ETU-induced rat model of imperforate anus. *J Pediatr Surg* 37:1305, 2002.

17. Crelin ES: Development of the musculoskeletal system. *CIBA Clin Symp* 33:1, 1981.

18. Smith ED: The identification and management of ano-rectal anomalies. In Smith ED, editor: *Progress in pediatric surgery*, vol 9. Munich, 1976, Urban-Schwarzenberg, p 7.

19. Stephens FD, Smith ED: *Anorectal malformations in children*. Chicago, 1971, Year Book.

20. Smith ED: The bath water needs changing, but don't throw out the baby: An overview of anorectal anomalies. *J Pediatr Surg* 22:335, 1988.

21. Peña A: Anorectal malformations. *Semin Pediatr Surg* 4:35, 1995.

22. Holschneider A, Hutson J, Pena A, et al: Preliminary report on the International Conference for the Development of Standards for the Treatment of Anorectal Malformations. *J Pediatr Surg* 40:1521, 2005.

23. Templeton JM, O'Neill JA Jr: Anorectal malformations. In Ravitch MM, Welch K, Randolph JG, et al, editors: *Pediatric Surgery*, Chicago, 1985, Year Book, p 1022.

24. Singh S, Pathak IC: Short colon malformation with imperforate anus. *Surgery* 71:781, 1972.

25. Wakhlu AK, Tandon RK, Kalra R: Short colon associated with anorectal malformations. *Indian J Surg* 44:621, 1982.

26. Spriggs NJ: Congenital occlusion of the gastrointestinal tract. *Guy Hosp Rep* 776:143, 1912.

27. Trusler GA, Mestel AL, Stephens CA: Colon malformation with imperforate anus. *Surgery* 45:328, 1959.

28. Budhiraja S, Pandit SK, Rattan KM: A report of 27 cases of congenital short colons with imperforate anus: So-called pouch colon syndrome. *Trop Doct* 27:217, 1997.

29. Wardhan H, Gangopadhyay AN, Singhal GD, et al: Imperforate anus with congenital short colon (pouch colon syndrome). *Pediatr Surg Int* 5:124, 1990.

30. Dickenson SJ: Agenesis of the descending colon with imperforate anus. Correlation with modern concepts of the origin of intestinal atresia. *Am J Surg* 113:270, 1987.

31. Gangopadhyay AN, Pandey A, Rastogi N, et al: A study of the functional aberration of the pouch in anorectal malformation associated with congenital pouch colon. *Colorectal Dis* 12:226, 2010.

32. Gangopadhyay AN, Patne SC, Pandey A, et al: Congenital pouch colon associated and anorectal malformation—histopathologic evaluation. *J Pediatr Surg* 44:600, 2009.

33. Parrott TS: Urologic implications of anorectal malformations. *Urol Clin North Am* 12:13, 1985.

34. Zivkovic SM, Krstie ZD, Vukanic DV: Vestibular fistula: The operative dilemma—cutback, fistula transplantation or posterior sagittal anorectoplasty? *Pediatr Surg Int* 6:111, 1991.

35. Long FL, Hunter JV, Mahboubi S, et al: Tethered cord and associated vertebral anomalies in children and infants with imperforate anus: Evaluation with MR imaging and plain radiography. *Radiology* 200:377, 1996.

36. Carson JA, Barnes PD, Tunell WP, et al: Imperforate anus: The neurologic implications of sacral abnormalities. *J Pediatr Surg* 19:838, 1984.

37. Tsakayannis DE, Schamberger RC: Association of imperforate anus with occult spinal dysraphism. *J Pediatr Surg* 30:1010, 1995.

38. Levitt MA, Patel M, Rodriguez G, et al: The tethered spinal cord in patients with anorectal malformations. *J Pediatr Surg* 32:462, 1997.

39. Rivosecchi M, Lucchett MC, Zaccara A, et al: Spinal dysraphism detected by magnetic resonance imaging in patients with anorectal anomalies: Incidence and clinical significance. *J Pediatr Surg* 30:488, 1995.

40. Davidoff AM, Thompson CV, Grimm JK, et al: Occult spinal dysraphism in patients with anal agenesis. *J Pediatr Surg* 26:1001, 1991.

41. Long FR, Hunter JV, Mahboubi S, et al: Tethered cord and associated vertebral anomalies in children and infants with imperforate anus: Evaluation with MR imaging and plain radiography. *Radiology* 200:377, 1996.

42. Jia H, Zhang K, Zhang S, et al: Quantitative analysis of sacral parasympathetic nucleus innervating the rectum in rats with anorectal malformation. *J Pediatr Surg* 42:1544, 2007.

43. Morimota K, Takemota O, Wakayama A: Tethered cord association with anorectal malformation. *Pediatr Neurosurg* 38:79, 2003.

44. Tuuha SE, Aziz D, Drake J, et al: Is surgery necessary for asymptomatic tethered cord in anorectal malformation patients? *J Pediatr Surg* 39:773, 2004.

45. Barkovich AJ: Congenital anomalies of the spine. In Barkovich AJ, editor: *Pediatric neuroimaging*, ed 4. Philadelphia, 2000, Lippincott Williams & Wilkins, p 704.

46. Tsakayannis DE, Shamberger RC: Association of imperforate anus with occult spinal dysraphism. *J Pediatr Surg* 30:1010, 1995.

47. Heij HA, Nievelstein RA, de Zwart I, et al: Abnormal anatomy of the lumbosacral region imaged by magnetic resonance in children with anorectal malformations. *Arch Dis Child* 74:441, 1996.

48. Golonka NR, Haga LJ, Keating RP, et al: Routine MRI evaluation of low imperforate anus reveals unexpected high incidence of tethered spinal cord. *J Pediatr Surg* 37:966, 2002.

49. Mosiello G, Capitanucci ML, et al: How to investigate neurovesical dysfunction in children with anorectal malformations. *J Urol* 170:1610, 2003.

50. Miyasaka M, Nosaka S, Kitano Y, et al: Utility of spinal MRI in children with anorectal malformation. *Pediatr Radiol* 39:810, 2009.

51. Parrott TS, Woodard JR: Importance of cystourethrography in neonates with imperforate anus. *Urology* 13:607, 1979.

52. Hasse W: Associated malformations with anal and rectal atresia. *Prog Pediatr Surg* 9:99, 1976.

53. Khoury MJ, Cordero JR, Greenberg F, et al: A population study of the VACTERL association. *Pediatrics* 71:815, 1983.

54. Kochling J, Pistor G, Marzhauser BS, et al: The Currarino syndrome—hereditary transmitted syndrome of anorectal, sacral and presacral anomalies: Case report and review of the literature. *Eur J Pediatr Surg* 6:114, 1996.

55. Lee SC, Chun YS, Jung SE, et al: Currarino triad: Anorectal malformation, sacral bony abnormality and presacral mass—a review of 11 cases. *J Pediatr Surg* 32:58, 1997.

56. Gegg CA, Vollmer DG, Tullous MW, et al: An unusual case of the complete Currarino triad: Case report, discussion of the literature, and the embryogenic implications. *Neurosurgery* 44:658, 1999.

57. Lam FW, Chan WK, Lam ST, et al: Proximal 10q trisomy: A new case with anal atresia. *J Med Genet* 37:E24, 2000.

58. Wang J, Spitz L, Hayward R, et al: Sacral dysgenesis associated with terminal deletion of chromosome 7q: A report of two families. *Eur J Pediatr* 158:902, 1999.

59. Torres R, Levitt MA, Tovilla JM, et al: Anorectal malformations and Down's syndrome. *J Pediatr Surg* 33:194, 1998.

60. Clarke SA, Van der Avoirt A: Imperforate anus, Hirschsprung's disease, and trisomy 21: A rare combination. *J Pediatr Surg* 34:1874, 1999.

61. Asabe K, Handa N: Anorectal malformation with ileal atresia. *Pediatr Surg Int* 12:302, 1997.

62. Ein SH: Imperforate anus (anal agenesis) with rectal and sigmoid atresia in a newborn. *Pediatr Surg Int* 12:449, 1997.

63. Goodwin S, Schlatter M, Connors R: Imperforate anus and colon atresia in a newborn. *J Pediatr Surg* 41:583, 2006.

64. Belloni E, Martucciello G, Verderio D, et al: Involvement of the HLXB9 homeobox gene in Currarino syndrome. *Am J Hum Genet* 66:312, 2000.

65. Verlinsky Y, Rechitsky S, Schoolcraft W, et al: Preimplantation diagnosis for homeobox gene HLXB9 mutation causing Currarino syndrome. *Am J Med Genet* 134A:103, 2005.

66. Holschneider AM, Ure BM, Pfrommer W, et al: Innervation patterns of the rectal pouch and fistula in anorectal malformations: A preliminary report. *J Pediatr Surg* 31:357, 1996.

67. Guan K, Hui L, Yang F, et al: Defective development of sensory neurons innervating the levator ani muscle in fetal rats with anorectal malformation. *Birth Defects Res A Clin Mol Teratol* 85:583, 2009.

68. Levitt MA, Bischoff A, Breech L, et al: Rectovestibular fistula—rarely recognized associated gynecologic anomalies. *J Pediatr Surg* 44:1261, 2009.

69. Hendren WH: Repair of cloacal anomalies: Current techniques. *J Pediatr Surg* 21:1159, 1986.

70. Pena A, Levitt MA, Hong A, et al: Surgical management of cloacal malformations: A review of 339 patients. *J Pediatr Surg* 39:470, 2004.

71. Raffensperger JG, Ramenofsky ML: The management of a cloaca. *J Pediatr Surg* 8:647, 1973.

72. Breech L: Gynecologic concerns in patients with anorectal malformations. *Semin Pediatr Surg* 19:139, 2010.

73. Wangensteen OH, Rice CO: Imperforate anus: A method of determining the surgical approach. *Ann Surg* 92:77, 1930.

74. Narasimharao KL, Prasad GR, Katariya S, et al: Prone cross-table view: An alternative to the invertogram in imperforate anus. *AJR Am J Roentgenol* 140:227, 1983.

75. Han TI, Kim IO, Kim WS: Imperforate anus: US determination of the type with infracoccygeal approach. *Radiology* 228:226, 2003.

76. Kim IO, Han TI, Kim WS, et al: Transperineal ultrasonography in imperforate anus: Identification of the internal fistula. *J Ultrasound Med* 19:211, 2000.

77. Han TI, Kim IO, Kim WS, et al: US identification of the anal sphincter complex and levator ani muscle in neonates: Infracoccygeal approach. *Radiology* 217:392, 2000.

78. Schuster SR, Teele RL: An analysis of ultrasound scanning as a guide in determination of "high" or "low" imperforate anus. *J Pediatr Surg* 14:798, 1979.

79. Oppenheimer DA, Carroll BA, Shochat SJ: Sonography of imperforate anus. *Radiology* 148:127, 1983.

80. Donaldson JS, Black CT, Reynolds M, et al: Ultrasound of the distal pouch in infants with imperforate anus. *J Pediatr Surg* 24:465, 1989.

81. Haber HP, Seitz G, Warmann SW, et al: Transperineal sonography for determination of the type of imperforate anus. *AJR Am J Roentgenol* 189:1525, 2007.

82. Potts WJ, Riker WL, DeBoer A: Imperforate anus with rectovesical, urethral, vaginal and perineal fistula. *Ann Surg* 140:381, 1954.

83. Doria do Amaral F: Treatment of anorectal anomalies by anterior perineal anorectoplasty. *J Pediatr Surg* 34:1315, 1999.

84. Okada A, Kamata S, Imura K, et al: Anterior sagittal anorectoplasty for rectovestibular and anovestibular fistula. *J Pediatr Surg* 27:85, 1992.

85. Chainani M: The anterior sagittal approach for high imperforate anus: A simplification of the Mollard approach. *J Pediatr Surg* 33:670, 1998.

86. Mollitt DL, Malangoni MA, Ballantine TVN, et al: Colostomy complications in children: An analysis of 146 cases. *Arch Surg* 115:455, 1980.

87. Bishop HC: Colostomy in the newborn. *Am J Surg* 101:642, 1961.

88. Wilkins S, Peña A: The role of colostomy in the management of anorectal malformations. *Pediatr Surg Int* 3:105, 1988.

89. Patwardhan N, Kiely EM, Drake DP, et al: Colostomy for anorectal anomalies: High incidence of complications. *J Pediatr Surg* 36:795, 2001.

90. Wiener ES, Kiesewetter WB: Urologic abnormalities associated with imperforate anus. *J Pediatr Surg* 8:151, 1973.

91. Swenson O, Donnellan WL: Preservation of the puborectalis sling in imperforate anus repair. *Surg Clin North Am* 47:173, 1967.

92. Kiesewetter WB: Imperforate anus: II. The rationale and techniques of the sacro-abdominoperineal operation. *J Pediatr Surg* 2:106, 1967.

93. Rehbein F: Zur operation der hohen Rectumatresis mit Recto-urethral-fistel: Abdomino-sacro-perinealer Durchzur. *Z Kinderchir* 2:503, 1965.

94. Rehbein F: Imperforate anus: Experiences with the abdomino-perineal and abdomino-sacro-perineal pull-through procedures. *J Pediatr Surg* 2:99, 1967.

95. Mollard P, Marechal JM, Jaubert de Beaujen M: Surgical treatment of high imperforate anus with definition of the puborectalis sling by an anterior perineal approach. *J Pediatr Surg* 13:499, 1978.

96. Mollard P, Marechal JM, Jaubert de Beaujen M: Le reperage de la sangle du releveur au cours du traitement des imperforations ano-rectale hautes. *Ann Chir* 16:461, 1975.

97. Yokoyama J, Hyashi A, Ikawa H, et al: Abdominoextended sacroperineal approach in high-type anorectal malformations and a new operative method. *Z Kinderchir* 40:151, 1985.

98. Davies MR, Cywes S: The use of a lateral skin flap perineoplasty in congenital anorectal malformations. *J Pediatr Surg* 19:577, 1984.

99. Nixon HH: A modification of the proctoplasty for rectal agenesis. *Pamietnik I-Go Zjazdu* 10:5, 1967.

100. Hedlund H, Peña A, Rodriguez G, et al: Long-term anorectal function in imperforate anus treated by a posterior sagittal anorectoplasty: Manometric investigation. *J Pediatr Surg* 27:906, 1992.

101. Albanese CT, Jennings RW, Lopoo JB, et al: One-stage correction of high imperforate anus in the male neonate. *J Pediatr Surg* 34:834, 1999.

102. Mueller RS: Development of urinary control in children. *JAMA* 172:1256, 1960.

103. Freeman NV, Burge DM, Soar JS, et al: Anal-evoked potentials. *Z Kinderchir* 31:22, 1980.

104. Nicoll RA, Malenka RC: Contrasting properties of two forms of long-term potentiation in the hippocampus. *Nature* 377:115, 1995.

105. Wiesel TN, Hubel DH: Comparison of the effects of unilateral and bilateral eye-closure on cortical unit response in kittens. *J Neurophysiol* 28:1029, 1981.

106. Adeniran JO: One-stage correction of imperforate anus and rectovestibular fistula in girls: Preliminary results. *J Pediatr Surg* 37:16, 2002.

107. Georgeson KE, Inge TH, Albanese CT: Laparoscopically assisted anorectal pull-through for high imperforate anus—a new technique. *J Pediatr Surg* 35:927, 2000.

108. Sydorak RM, Albanese CT: Laparoscopic repair of high imperforate anus. *Semin Pediatr Surg* 11:217, 2002.

109. Yamataka A, Kato Y, Lee KD, et al: Endoscopy-assisted laparoscopic excision of rectourethral fistula in a male with imperforate anus. *J Laparoendosc Adv Surg Tech* 19:S241, 2009.

110. Koga H, Kato Y, Shimotakahara A, et al: Intraoperative measurement of rectourethral fistula: Prevention of incomplete excision in male patients with high-/intermediate-type imperforate anus. *J Pediatr Surg* 45:397, 2010.

111. Iwanaka T, Arai M, Kawashima H, et al: Findings of pelvic musculature and efficacy of laparoscopic muscle stimulator in laparoscopy-assisted anorectal pull-through for high imperforate anus. *Surg Endosc* 17:278, 2003.

112. Yamataka A, Segawa O, Yoshida R, et al: Laparoscopic muscle electrostimulation during laparoscopy-assisted anorectal pull-through for high imperforate anus. *J Pediatr Surg* 36:1659, 2001.

113. Raschbaum GR, Bleacher JC, Grattan-Smith D, et al: Magnetic resonance imaging-guided laparoscopic-assisted anorectoplasty for imperforate anus. *J Pediatr Surg* 45:220, 2010.

114. Yamataka A, Yoshida R, Kobayashi H, et al: Intraoperative endosonography enhances laparoscopy-assisted colon pull-through for high imperforate anus. *J Pediatr Surg* 37:1657, 2002.

115. Watayo H, Kaneyama K, Ichijo C, et al: Is intraoperative anal endoscopy necessary during laparoscopy-assisted anorectoplasty for high/intermediate type imperforate anus? *J Laparoendosc Adv Surg Tech* 18:123, 2008.

116. Podevin G, Petit T, Mure PY, et al: Minimally invasive surgery for anorectal malformation in boys: A multicenter study. *J Laparoendosc Adv Surg Tech* 19:S233, 2009.

117. Kudou S, Iwanaka T, Kawashima H, et al: Midterm follow-up study of high-type imperforate anus after laparoscopically assisted anorectoplasty. *J Pediatr Surg* 40:1923, 2005.

118. Belizon A, Levitt M, Shoshany G, et al: Rectal prolapse following posterior sagittal anorectoplasty for anorectal malformations. *J Pediatr Surg* 40:192, 2005.

119. Sato Y, Pringle KC, Bergman RA, et al: Congenital anorectal anomalies: MR imaging. *Radiology* 168:157, 1988.

120. Karrer EM, Flannery AM, Nelson MD, et al: Anorectal malformations: Evaluation of associated spinal dysraphic syndromes. *J Pediatr Surg* 23:45, 1988.

121. Warf BC, Scott RM, Barnes PD, et al: Tethered spinal cord in patients with anorectal and urogenital malformations. *Pediatr Neurosurg* 19:25, 1993.

122. Hendren WH: Cloaca, the most severe degree of imperforate anus: Experience with 195 cases. *Ann Surg* 228:331, 1998.

123. Nakayama DK, Templeton JM, Ziegler MM, et al: Complications of posterior sagittal anoplasty. *J Pediatr Surg* 21:488, 1988.

124. Golonka NR, Haga LJ, Keating RP, et al: Routine MRI evaluation of low imperforate anus reveals unexpected high incidence of tethered spinal cord. *J Pediatr Surg* 37:966, 2002.

125. Peña A, Hong AR, Midulla P, et al: Reoperative surgery for anorectal anomalies. *Semin Pediatr Surg* 12:118, 2003.

126. Anderson KD, Newman KD, Bond SJ, et al: Diamond flap anoplasty in infants and children with an intractable anal stricture. *J Pediatr Surg* 29:1253, 1994.

127. Becmeur F, Jofmann-Zango I, Jouin H, et al: Three-flap anoplasty for imperforate anus: Results for primary procedure or for redoes. *Eur J Pediatr Surg* 11:311, 2001.

128. Warne SA, Godley ML, Owens CM, et al: The validity of sacral ratios to identify sacral abnormalities. *BJU Int* 91:540, 2003.

129. Kelly JH: The clinical and radiological assessment of anal continence in childhood. *Aust N Z J Surg* 42:62, 1972.

130. Jorge JM, Wexner SD: Etiology and management of fecal incontinence. *Dis Colon Rectum* 36:77, 1993.

131. Ludman L, Spitz L: Coping strategies of children with feacal incontinence. *J Pediatr Surg* 31:563, 1996.

132. Pena A, Hong A: Advances in the management of anorectal malformations. *Am J Surg* 180:370, 2000.

133. Rintala RJ, Lindahl HG, Rasanen M: Do children with repaired low anorectal malformations have normal bowel function? *J Pediatr Surg* 32:823, 1997.

134. Voskuijl WP, Heijmans J, Heijmans HS, et al: Use of Rome II criteria in childhood defecation disorders: Applicability in clinical and research practice. *J Pediatr Surg* 145:213, 2004.

135. deVries PA, Cox KL: Surgery of anorectal anomalies. *Surg Clin North Am* 65:1139, 1985.

136. Rintala RJ, Lindahl H: Is normal bowel function possible after repair of intermediate and high anorectal malformations? *J Pediatr Surg* 30:491, 1995.

137. Brandt ML, Daigneau C, Graviss EA, et al: Validation of the Baylor continence scale in children with anorectal malformations. *J Pediatr Surg* 42:1015, 2007.

138. Zhengwei Y, Weilin W, Yuzuo B, et al: Long-term outcomes of individualized biofeedback training based on the underlying dysfunction for patients with imperforate anus. *J Pediatr Surg* 40:555, 2005.

139. Berquist WE: Biofeedback therapy for anorectal disorders in children. *Semin Pediatr Surg* 4:48, 1995.

140. Chen CC, Lin CL, Lu WT, et al: Anorectal function and endopelvic dissection in patients with repaired imperforate anus. *Pediatr Surg Int* 13:133, 1998.

141. Longo A: Treatment of hemorrhoids disease by reduction of mucosa and hemorrhoidal prolapse with a circular suturing device: A new procedure. In *Proceedings of the 6th World Congress of Endoscopic Surgery*. Rome, 1998, Monduzzi Editori, p 77.

142. Amortegui JD, Solla JA: Procedure for prolapsed hemorrhoids for treatment of rectal mucosa prolapse following anorectoplasty for imperforate anus. *Am Surg* 74:443, 2008.

143. Peña A, Guardino JM, Tovilla MA, et al: Bowel management for fecal incontinence in patients with anorectal malformations. *J Pediatr Surg* 33:133, 1998.

144. van Kuyk EM, Brugman-Boezeman AT, Wissink-Essink M, et al: Biopsychosocial treatment of defecation problems in children with anal atresia: A retrospective study. *Pediatr Surg Int* 16:317, 2000.

145. Diseth TH, Emblem R: Somatic function, mental health, and psychosocial adjustment of adolescents with anorectal anomalies. *J Pediatr Surg* 31:638, 1996.

146. da Silva GM, Jorge JM, Belin B, et al: New surgical options for fecal incontinence in patients with imperforate anus. *Dis Colon Rectum* 47:204, 2004.

147. Altomare DF, Rinaldi M, Pannarale OC, et al: Electrostimulated gracilis neosphincter for faecal incontinence and total anorectal reconstruction: Still an experimental procedure? *Int J Colorectal Dis* 12:308, 1997.

148. Baeten CG, Konsten J, Heineman E, et al: Dynamic graciloplasty for anal atresia. *J Pediatr Surg* 29:922, 1994.

149. Ellsworth PI, Webb HW, Crump JM, et al: The Malone antegrade colonic enema enhances the quality of life in children undergoing urological incontinence procedures. *J Urol* 155:1416, 1996.

150. Lee SL, Rowell S, Greenholz SK: Therapeutic cecostomy tubes in infants with imperforate anus and caudal agenesis. *J Pediatr Surg* 37:345, 2002.

151. Rivera MT, Kugathasan S, Berger W, et al: Percutaneous colonoscopic cecostomy for management of chronic constipation in children. *GI Endo* 53:225, 2001.

152. Chait PG, Shandling B, Richards HM, et al: Fecal incontinence in children: Treatment with percutaneous cecostomy tube placement—a prospective study. *Radiology* 203:621, 1997.

153. Gauderer MW, Decou JM, Boyle JT: Sigmoid irrigation tube for the management of chronic evacuation disorders. *J Pediatr Surg* 37:348, 2002.

154. Squire R, Kiely E, Carr B, et al: The clinical application of the Malone antegrade colonic enema. *J Pediatr Surg* 28:1012, 1993.

155. Boemers TML, Beek FJA, van Gool JD, et al: Urologic problems in anorectal malformations: I. Urodynamic findings and significance of sacral anomalies. *J Pediatr Surg* 31:407, 1996.

156. Holt B, Pryor JP, Hendry WF: Male infertility after surgery for imperforate anus. *J Pediatr Surg* 30:1677, 1995.

157. Diamond DA, Gosalbez R: Neonatal urologic emergencies. In Walsh PC, Retik AB, Vauhan ED, Jr, et al, editors: *Campbell's Urology*. Philadelphia, 1998, WB Saunders, p 1649.

158. Shaul DB, Harrison EA: Classification of anorectal malformations: Initial approach, diagnostic tests, and colostomy. *Semin Pediatr Surg* 6:187, 1997.

159. Boemers TM, de Jong TP, van Gool JD, et al: Urologic problems in anorectal malformations: II. Functional urologic sequelae. *J Pediatr Surg* 31:634, 1996.

160. Diokno AC, Sonda LP, Hollander JB, et al: Fate of patients started on clean intermittent self-catheterization in the treatment of infants and young children with myelomeningocele and neurogenic bladder dysfunction. *J Urol* 129:1120, 1983.

161. Geraniotis E, Koff SA, Enrile B: The prophylactic use of clean intermittent catheterization in the treatment of infants and young children with myelomeningocele and neurogenic bladder dysfunction. *J Urol* 139:85, 1988.

162. Sheldon C, Cormier M, Crone K, et al: Occult neurovesical dysfunction in children with imperforate anus and its variants. *J Pediatr Surg* 26:49, 1991.

163. Meijer SA, Sinnema G, Bijstra JO, et al: Social functioning in children with chronic illness. *J Child Psychol Psychiatry* 41:309, 2000.

164. Huygen ACJ, Kuis W, Sinnema G: Psychological, behavioral, and social adjustment in children and adolescents with juvenile chronic arthritis. *Ann Rheum Dis* 59:276, 2000.

165. Noll RB, Kozlowski K, Gerhardt C, et al: Social, emotional, and behavioral functioning of children with juvenile rheumatoid arthritis. *Arthritis Rheum* 43:1387, 2000.

166. Siseth T, Emblem R, Vandevik I: Adolescents with anorectal malformations and their families: Examples of hidden psychosocial trauma. *Family Syst Med* 13:215, 1995.

167. Ludman L, Spitz L: Psychosocial adjustment of children treated for anorectal anomalies. *J Pediatr Surg* 30:495, 1995.
168. Schreier H, Ladakakos C, Morabito D, et al: Posttraumatic stress symptoms in children after mild to moderate pediatric trauma: A longitudinal examination of symptom prevalence, correlates, and parent-child symptom reporting. *J Trauma* 58:353, 2005.
169. Ojmyr-Joelsson M, Christensson K, Frenckner B, et al: Children with high and intermediate imperforate anus: Remembering and talking about medical treatment carried out early in life. *Pediatr Surg Int* 24:1009, 2008.
170. Cohen LL, Blount RL, Cohen RJ, et al: Children's expectations and memories of acute distress: Short- and long-term efficacy of pain management interventions. *J Pediatr Psychol* 26:367, 2001.
171. Zelikovsky N, Rodrigue JR, Gidycz CA, et al: Cognitive behavioral and behavioral interventions help young children cope during a voiding cystourethrogram. *J Pediatr Psychol* 25:535, 2000.
172. Peterson C, Rideout R: Memory for medical emergencies experienced by 1- and 2-year-olds. *Dev Psychol* 34:1059, 1998.
173. Levitt MA, Pena A: Outcomes from the correction of anorectal malformations. *Curr Opin Pediatr* 17:394, 2005.
174. Polit DF, Hungler BP: *Essentials of nursing research, methods, appraisals and utilization,* ed 4. Philadelphia, 1997 Lippincott.
175. Nisell M, Ojmyr-Joelsson M, Frenckner B, et al: How a family is affected when a child is born with anorectal malformation. Interviews with three patients and their parents. *J Pediatr Nurs* 18:423, 2003.
176. Hendren WH: Management of cloacal malformations. *Semin Pediatr Surg* 6:217, 1997.

Reoperative Pelvic Surgery

Jonathan Worsey | Victor W. Fazio

Reoperation in the pelvis may be one of the most challenging and daunting situations that confronts the abdominal surgeon. This chapter discusses the applied anatomy and pathophysiology of the pelvis as it pertains to reoperative surgery. A practical approach to preoperative workup and planning is presented, though the main focus examines clinical and technical aspects of these operations. The discussion is in the context of gastrointestinal (GI) surgery, although these principles can be equally applied to urologic or gynecologic surgery.

APPLIED ANATOMY

The term *pelvis* is derived from the Latin term meaning basin and indeed in the anatomic position, the pelvis resembles a forward-tilted basin composed of bone covered with muscle and lined with fascia. This forward angulation of the pelvis limits visualization of the anterior pelvic surface, especially deep in the pelvis, and the unyielding bony margins of the pelvis limit exposure that can be obtained with retraction.

The fascial planes in the pelvis warrant discussion because their correct identification and an appreciation of their relationships is crucial, especially in the reoperative situation where they may have been already disturbed. The pelvic organs are covered with visceral pelvic fascia, which is an extension of the parietal fascia lining the pelvis. The presacral fascia is a condensation of the parietal endopelvic fascia, and breach of this layer may lead to, at best, troublesome bleeding and, at worst, catastrophic bleeding. This is in part due to the avalvular presacral veins that communicate directly with the basivertebral veins. The pelvic sympathetic nerves run downward and laterally across the pelvic brim over this fascia to join the pelvic plexus on the lateral side wall and then supply the anal and urinary sphincters. Initial posterior rectal dissection, if performed sharply and in the right plane, allows relatively easy and safe separation of the fascia propria of the rectum from presacral fascia avoiding these structures. If this plane has previously been entered and especially if the rectum has been resected and replaced with a segment of colon or a small bowel pouch, the plane is much less well defined or even obliterated. This may lead to inadvertent dissection through the presacral fascia, resulting in hemorrhage or damage to the sympathetic trunks. Likewise, anterior to the rectum, a layer of fascia separates the rectum and base of bladder (also the seminal vesicles and prostate in the male), the rectovesical fascia or fascia of Denonvilliers. The significance of this is that the pelvic splanchnic nerves pass anterior to this fascia, which can usually be identified as a shiny white layer and unless there is an anterior rectal cancer, dissection on the rectal side of the plane will protect these important nerves. After anterior mobilization of the distal rectum, this plane may also be difficult to define placing these structures at risk of damage. Important urologic and vascular structures course within the pelvis and are at risk of damage during pelvic reoperation. The distal half of the ureter lies within the pelvis, crossing the pelvic brim at the iliac artery bifurcation and then coursing downward along the lateral pelvic side wall before turning upward and medially to enter the base of the bladder at the pelvic floor. The iliac arteries, veins, and their many tributaries also run throughout the pelvis, providing a rich blood supply for the pelvic organs but also the potential for significant hemorrhage.

PATHOPHYSIOLOGY

A number of changes occur in the pelvis following surgery and these also contribute to the difficulty of subsequent operation. Under normal circumstances, the mobile small bowel and, to a lesser extent, the sigmoid colon fill the rectouterine and rectovesical pouches. After pelvic surgery, adhesions commonly develop fixing the bowel here. In cases where the rectum is removed, the increased space and raw surfaces of the pelvic floor and presacral space often allow multiple loops of small bowel to become firmly entrapped and difficult to mobilize. Development of adhesions around anastomoses or particularly a rectal stump may be very dense and difficult. Another problem seen after mobilization and division of the rectum is its immediate tendency to fall down into the pelvis. Even after division of the more proximal rectum, if the presacral and lateral attachments have been taken down, the stump may disappear into the depths of the pelvis, where it may fold on itself, become fixed, and subsequently be difficult to mobilize. Additionally, a midrectal stump, initially an intraperitoneal structure, may become covered by peritoneum as the distal pelvis reperitonealizes after surgery and may prove exceptionally difficult to find and define.

When the sigmoid colon and rectum are mobilized, it is usual to identify the ureters, particularly the left ureter, at the pelvic brim and upper pelvis where they are at risk of damage. This may involve varying degrees of dissection depending on the ease of identification. Subsequently, the ureters may then assume a much more variable course at the pelvic brim and it is not unusual for a significantly more medial position, sometimes with even fusion to the mesorectum or particularly a rectal stump occurring. Likewise, after previous resection or mobilization of the colon from either gutter, the abdominal portions of the ureters can be encountered surprisingly quickly during lateral abdominal dissection. They may be closely related to the small bowel or its mesentery as they fuse to the retroperitoneum and/or remnants of the mesocolon.

GENERAL MEASURES

DECIDE ON TIMING OF REOPERATION

As with reoperation in the abdomen, if possible, 3 or preferably even 6 months should be allowed before reoperative pelvic surgery is attempted. In cases of benign disease, an even longer interval may be useful when practical, though in the case of persistent or early recurring malignant disease this is unlikely to be possible. Waiting may reduce the difficulty and potential complications attributable to adhesions. Should early reoperative pelvic surgery be required, as in the case of an anastomotic leak or obstruction, there is a window of about 10 to 14 days before the adhesions reach their worst when reexploration may perhaps be undertaken safely. After this, there is a significant risk of iatrogenic injury, and alternative approaches such as percutaneous abscess drainage, proximal fecal diversion, or parenteral nutrition should be contemplated to buy time. Factors that may make adhesions worse include sepsis and irradiation and in the presence of these, if the patient can wait, at least 6 months or perhaps even a year should be allowed (Box 182-1).

PREPARE THE PATIENT

Pelvic reoperation may necessitate prolonged surgery and anesthesia, and careful preoperative patient preparation may help reduce general postoperative complications. The nutritional status of the patient should be addressed, with protein and calorie deficiencies corrected, preferably via the enteral route but parenterally

---

BOX 182-1 Factors Contributing to Difficulty of Reoperative Pelvic Surgery

ANATOMIC FACTORS
Orientation and angulation of pelvis
Unyielding bony margins that cannot be retracted
Narrow male pelvis (android)
Course and relationships of vascular, neural, and urologic structures
Vascular anatomy of sacrum

PATHOPHYSIOLOGIC FACTORS
Tendency of small bowel to fill and become fixed in pelvis postoperatively
Potential for markedly ectopic position of ureters in postoperative pelvis
Tendency of bowel anastomosis or rectal stump to fuse to surrounding structures
Obliteration of critical fascial planes that protect important neurovascular structures
Retraction and folding on itself of a divided and mobilized rectum
Physiologic reperitonealization in the distal pelvis

---

if needed. In older patients, particular attention to cardiopulmonary status is important because bleeding may cause intraoperative blood pressure fluctuations and prolonged anesthetic times, and large incisions may predispose the patient to pulmonary problems. Reoperative pelvic surgery also carries a very high risk of pelvic and lower extremity thromboembolic problems. Appropriate and aggressive prophylaxis must be used especially in the elderly, those with malignancy, and those with other risk factors. Compression stockings are important, though the additional use of pharmacologic anticoagulation is usually mandatory despite concerns regarding perioperative or postoperative bleeding. The preoperative placement of a caval filter should be considered in those at highest risk or where heparin cannot be given. Mechanical bowel preparation and appropriate preoperative antibiotics should be administered even if entering the bowel lumen is not planned, as this may nevertheless occur.

PREOPERATIVE IMAGING STUDIES

The purpose of imaging studies is really twofold: first, in the case of malignant disease, to exclude locally unresectable disease or distant metastatic disease that would preclude a curative resection; second, to provide a preoperative plan of attack, by detailing the pelvic anatomy and identifying normal and abnormal structures and their relationships.

Determining resectability of malignant pelvic disease can be unreliable on clinicopathologic grounds[1] and is improved by using either computed tomographic (CT) scanning and/or magnetic resonance (MR) scanning. In a series of 119 patients from Memorial Sloan-Kettering undergoing reoperation for pelvic recurrence of colon and rectal cancer, only the presence of pelvic side wall involvement and ureteric obstruction was associated with a statistically significantly smaller chance of a complete resection.[2] Conversely, anastomotic and anterior pelvic recurrence proved particularly amenable to curative resections. Positron emission tomographic–computed tomographic (PET-CT) scanning is also routinely performed in the case of malignant pelvic recurrence. It is a sensitive and specific technique for colon and rectal cancer,[3] especially when the size of recurrence is greater than 1 cm. Liver or lung metastases that are not amenable to resection may discourage a now palliative pelvic operation. PET-CT scanning is also useful in distinguishing postoperative changes from locally recurrent malignant disease in the pelvis that can be very difficult with conventional imaging. Others advocate a more selective use of PET-CT scanning, arguing that when baseline and serial CT/MRIs read by experienced GI radiologist are positive or negative for recurrent disease the yield of PET-CT in providing additional information is low. However, when these studies are equivocal, a definitive diagnosis could now be made in half of this group.[3] CT scanning and MR imaging may also provide a road map of pelvic anatomy when the initial operation was performed elsewhere or there has been a significant interval change because of an abscess or anastomotic leak. Standard contrast studies may better define a rectal stump, an anastomotic stricture, or an enterocutaneous fistula.

ANTICIPATE BLEEDING

Blood should be crossmatched, and if clinically indicated, coagulation parameters should be checked. The use of a cell saver in certain circumstances where fecal contamination is not anticipated may be appropriate. The availability at short notice of other clotting agents, such as platelets, fresh-frozen plasma, and cryoprecipitate, is also advisable in case massive transfusion is required. Recently, the use of recombinant factor VIIa has been described in cases of life-threatening hemorrhage complicated by massive blood product replacement or underlying coagulopathy; this may be particularly useful if a sacral resection is anticipated or planned.

ANTICIPATE A LONG, DIFFICULT CASE AND THE NEED FOR OTHER SPECIALISTS

Although the following recommendations sound obvious, having the right operation at the right time of day by the right surgical team may be difficult to arrange but well worth the investment:

1. Schedule the case first and do not plan other difficult cases to follow.
2. Use the most senior help available as anesthesia and assistants, a colleague or partner rather than a new house officer.
3. Forewarn urologic, gynecologic, vascular, and other specialists of the possible need for intraoperative assistance.
4. Give the anesthetist advance notice of the potential for a long and bloody operation, and allow time for the placement of appropriate large bore lines and monitoring devices. Epidural or other neuraxial anesthesia may be helpful in early postoperative pain management and assist in promoting early ambulation and effective pulmonary toilet. Perioperative anticoagulation must be taken into account with these techniques, because of the risk of epidural bleeding.

SPECIFIC MEASURES

PATIENT POSITIONING

Given the potential for a long operation, careful positioning and padding are essential to avoid injury due to pressure or poor position. We place the patient on a beanbag that can be molded to fit the patient and then fixed in position when the air is evacuated. This is especially useful because it stops the patient from slipping down the table when steep Trendelenburg position is applied and it tends to more evenly distribute weight bearing. Do not let the anesthetist talk you into leaving an arm out from the side for better vascular access; allow the time needed before final positioning to place the appropriate lines. Tuck both arms securely at the patient's side even if the patient is obese; otherwise, room to obtain adequate visualization of and access to the pelvis is jeopardized. The legs are placed in carefully positioned and padded Lloyd-Davies or Allen stirrups; the right hip is not overflexed because this will interfere with a self-retaining retractor placed in the most distal aspect of the wound. The patient is prepared from the nipples to the perineum and draped so that access to the perineum can be obtained without contaminating the abdominal field.

OPTIMIZING VISIBILITY AND EXPOSURE

Long midline incisions are routinely used, with the distal end carried on to the pubis and the proximal incision being made as far as needed; it may be necessary to gain initial and safe entry to the abdomen above the umbilicus away from prior dense adhesions or fistulas. Enterocutaneous fistulas are left in place until the bowel around them is fully mobilized to avoid injury to noninvolved bowel. A self-retaining retractor is used, and a C-arm is attached to this to retract the viscera into the upper abdomen. A bladder blade also attaches to the self-retaining retractor, and if properly placed, it should sit snugly against the pubic bone. A large chromic suture is often placed in the dome of the uterus and then tied around the bladder blade to pull the uterus up out of the pelvis. Once the small bowel has been brought up out of the pelvis, placing the patient in Trendelenburg position will help keep the pelvic field clear.

A headlight can be useful, especially with the newer lightweight models using more powerful light sources. In addition, lighted retractors (Figures 182-1 and 182-2) and occasionally the free light cord are most helpful

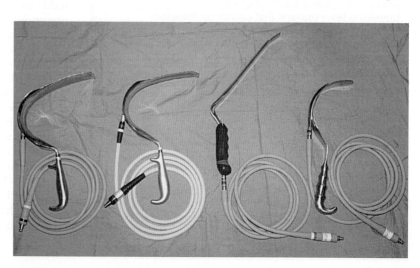

FIGURE 182-1 Commonly used lighted retractors in pelvic surgery. *Left to right:* standard-width deep pelvic retractor, narrow-width deep pelvic retractor, straight-blade retractor (Bright-Track), and lighted Deaver retractor.

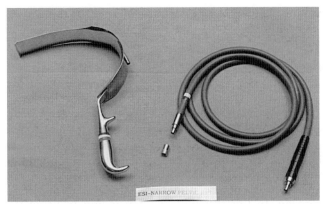

FIGURE 182-2 Close view of narrow pelvic retractor. Unlike the lighted Goligher straight-blade retractor, this allows for vigorous elevation of the prostate and bladder base away from the rectum or the low rectum and mesorectum from the sacrum. (This is Dr. Worsey's [the senior author of this chapter] preferred retractor.)

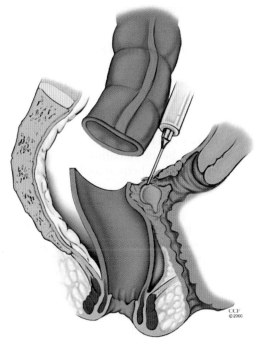

FIGURE 182-3 Schematic showing injection of saline into the scar between rectum-rectal stump and posterior vagina, which may be fused inseparably. A 1- to 2-mm-thick septum can be made into a 7- to 10-mm septum, allowing some cushion against inadvertent rectal or vaginal injury. (Copyright 2000, Cleveland Clinic Foundation.)

deep in the pelvis. The first instrument to be used is often the lighted Deaver retractor. This has a relatively shallow curve and is a short instrument that is ideal for the early part of the posterior rectal dissection, when a broad instrument is of value. It is also of value for the early anterior rectal and bladder exposure and dissection and may be used to good effect with a high splenic flexure mobilization. As the rectal dissection progresses, longer instruments are used, especially in the case of the narrower male pelvis; two additional types of retractors are then used. The Bright-Track instrument is 15 inches long and 1.5 inches wide and is used with the fiberoptic light source. It is ideal for anterolateral retraction of the seminal vesicles and prostate or vagina, deep in the pelvis when bleeding occurs, and the most inferior part of the posterior rectal dissection. The final retractor that is used is a longer and much more curved retractor, with wide- and narrow-blade types. This is especially useful in lifting the rectum forward with some degree of force to accentuate the correct plane of dissection behind the rectum. In addition, it can be used to retract the bladder and prostate or vagina forward to assist with dissection or subsequent hemostasis. Because the light source can get very hot, care must be taken to avoid burning the drapes or, even worse, the patient or surgeon.

CONDUCTING THE OPERATION

Adhesions are taken down carefully, with the preferred technique being to mobilize matted loops of bowel into the wound and then to separate the individual loops. This is not usually possible when a loop or loops of small bowel descend into the pelvis and are fused to the vagina, levators, or anterior sacrum. In this instance, it is best to try to identify the afferent and efferent loops descending into the pelvis and, with a sponge in the nondominant hand, to gently retract the apex of the loop caudad. Sharp dissection is performed close to the bowel wall, and the loop is separated from the dense fibrous adhesions. Enterotomies or myotomies may be unavoidable and should be repaired or resected as appropriate. Once the loops of bowel are delivered into the wound, their separation is not usually too difficult.

On occasion, dissection may be exceedingly difficult owing to grade IV adhesions that fuse the bowel together or to the abdominal wall or owing to the presence of an enterocutaneous fistula. In the case of a fistula to the abdominal wall, the bowel should be mobilized around this, leaving the fistulous connection for last and then detaching it sharply. Dissection of the most dense adhesions may be facilitated by infiltrating the fused area with saline using a small-gauge needle (*hydrodissection*). This preferentially expands the correct plane for dissection and reduces the likelihood of bowel injury and contamination of the field. Sometimes even this cannot overcome the fusion between bowel and the abdominal wall, and here, if a relatively small area is involved, it may be circumvented by leaving the abdominal fascia attached to the bowel. The dissection is carried outside the fascia, returning to the abdominal cavity beyond the area of fusion. Hydrodissection also may be of value in finding a plane between the vagina and the previously mobilized rectum (Figure 182-3). In very difficult and seemingly impossible cases, decide early if the potential for harm is becoming greater than the potential for good and whether temporizing measures such as drain placement or proximal diversion are better options. Further waiting or referral to those with more experience is the sensible approach. Similarly, think carefully before "crossing the Rubicon" when successful completion of the operation is in doubt. Division of the blood supply or damage of bowel that cannot be mobilized or getting into bleeding in an area where adequate exposure is unlikely are examples of this.*

IDENTIFICATION OF PELVIC STRUCTURES

During reoperation, identifying specific anatomic structures may indeed be difficult. If a scarred obliterated pelvis becomes reperitonealized, it may appear at first glance that the entire rectum, bladder, and uterus have been removed because of the deceptive smooth concavity of the pelvis. This may be especially so after the effects of external beam radiation therapy. However, there are specific ways to help identify important pelvic structures.

Ureters

Identification of the ureters may be facilitated by preoperative ureteric stent placement, which we perform frequently for reoperative pelvic surgery. Unfortunately, in the most difficult cases, where the ureter may be kinked or angulated because of adhesions or inflammation, stent placement sometimes cannot be safely undertaken. Furthermore, dense adhesions may make palpation of even stented ureters difficult.

Early identification, with or without stenting, is the key to avoiding ureteric injury. In the densely scarred pelvis, the ureters are found proximally and traced to the pelvis. They may be marked by loosely placed encircling ligatures, and then are constantly referred back to during the conduct of the dissection. Critics of stenting cite increased cost and time and that stents have not been proved to reduce the rates of ureteric injury. However, one of the great disasters of pelvic surgery is the missed ureteric injury, and this is rarely the case with stented ureters, where injury is much more obvious and readily identified. If a stent is not or cannot be placed, the intravenous administration of indigo carmine (5 mL) will turn the urine blue and can help to detect an occult injury leaking urine.

Bladder

There usually is not much difficulty in identifying the bladder, but a couple of points are worthy of mention. If the previous abdominal incision was taken down to the pubis for maximal exposure and the bladder likewise mobilized to allow its anterior retraction, the bladder may be densely adhered beneath the midline fascia in the lower part of the wound. Care is necessary in reentering the abdomen to avoid inadvertent injury to the bladder at this point. After irradiation, there may be a tight restrictive crescent moon–shaped band in the deep pelvis corresponding to a fibrous bladder base, which will adversely affect exposure of the lower rectum. This is improved by placing superficial cautery incisions

in the bladder base, with the entrance of the ureters taken into account, and then stretching this narrow entrance.

Rectal Stump

Depending on the previous operation, this may be conveniently sitting in the lower aspect of the abdominal wound (really the distal sigmoid) or alternatively, out of sight in the depths of the pelvis below a reperitonealized pelvic floor, or anywhere in between. If divided at or just below the sacral promontory, which is commonly done, the stump may be adherent to the presacral fascia, the great vessels, or the ureters, with all being at risk of damage. In this situation, it often is best to begin the rectal dissection lateral to the midrectum in "virgin tissue" and to develop the plane of the mesorectum. Once the peritoneum has been incised, this is facilitated by retracting the rectum medially using the lighted Deaver retractor and then using electrocautery to follow the mesorectum posteriorly to the presacral space, which can more readily be found with this approach. The proximal part of the rectal stump is then mobilized by sharp dissection or electrocautery exactly in the midline over a 1- to 2-cm area to allow development of the plane between the posterior mesorectum and the presacral fascia. The dissection is then kept on the posterior wall of the mesorectum, and attached ureters, sympathetic trunks, or vessels are dissected free. Using the appropriate narrow retractors, the plane is developed to meet the presacral dissection beginning laterally, and this is carried caudad as far as needed. The remainder of the lateral attachments and lateral stalks can then be divided if necessary.

Should there be only a short, nearly invisible rectal stump, its initial identification and subsequent mobilization can be facilitated by placing a large bougie or proctoscope in the rectum. This should be done with some care because it is not uncommon for a stricture to develop in a defunctionalized rectum. With a very low rectal stump, bimanual palpation is a useful technique not only to identify the rectum but also to accurately assess the level of the dissection in relation to the sphincters. Here, an additional sleeve and glove are donned to allow the placement of a finger through the anus into the distal rectum, which is then palpated from above with the other hand (Figures 182-4 and 182-5).

Before any anastomosis is attempted to a defunctionalized rectum, the presence of an occult stricture must be excluded. This can be done either preoperatively or intraoperatively.

Vagina

In reoperative operations, the vagina should always be prepped with povidone-iodine in case it is inadvertently entered. Similar to the rectal dissection, the use of an obturator or a bougie may be extremely helpful in the identification and prevention of injury. The use of hydrodissection in the case of an obliterated rectovaginal plane has been discussed. Occasionally, bimanual palpation with one finger in the rectum and one in the vagina facilitates the separation of the most distal aspects of the rectum and vagina.

---

*In classical times the Rubicon river marked the boundary between the Roman province of Cisalpine Gaul to the north and Italy proper to the south and Roman law forbade any general to cross the river southward with his army to potentially threaten the republic. A Roman general was thus obliged to disband his army before crossing the Rubicon, otherwise both he and his men were guilty of high treason and sacrilege, and automatically condemned to death. This law was famously broken by Julius Caesar in 49 BC who subsequently overthrew the republic and became emperor. (*Wikipedia*).

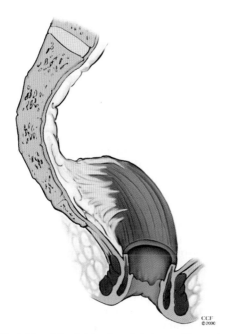

FIGURE 182-4 The difficult (short) rectal stump. Stump length of less than 10 to 12 cm usually means a difficult dissection. Fusion of the stump apex to the low sacrum requires several alternative or composite procedures for safe mobilization. Stump apex leak caused by radiation with chronic sepsis makes for extra difficulty. (Copyright 2000, Cleveland Clinic Foundation.)

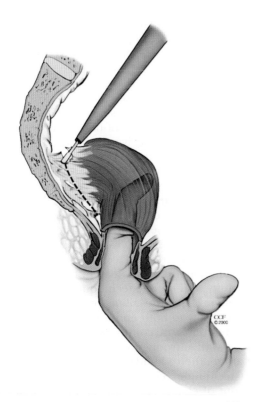

FIGURE 182-5 Electrocautery is kept exactly in the midline and over a short distance of 2 to 3 cm. Bimanual examination with a double-gloved index finger in the rectum may help guide the surgeon in rectal mobilization. (Copyright 2000, Cleveland Clinic Foundation.)

CONTROL OF BLEEDING

The anticipation of significant bleeding and appropriate preoperative crossmatching of blood are essential. Those at risk of clotting disorders should be identified, and appropriate clotting factors should be administered or made available for intraoperative use. The benefits of perioperative heparin must be weighed against the potential for bleeding as mentioned earlier.

The common sites at which pelvic bleeding is encountered are as follows:

1. Presacral and lateral sacral veins: Premature, inadvertent breaching of the presacral or Waldeyer fascia occurs above the S3-S4 level. This is usually caused by blunt dissection in the presacral space, although it may also occur when the fascia is deliberately incised to gain access to presacral masses or occasionally to excise recurrent rectal cancer. Another situation in which this happens is with synchronous abdominal and perineal dissections. If the perineal operator gets ahead of the abdominal operator and breaks through the anococcygeal ligament too posteriorly, the dissection may proceed beneath the rectosacral fascia, shearing the basivertebral branches of the lateral sacral veins.
2. Internal iliac vein: The internal iliac vein is injured if tearing or shearing of branches from the main trunk occurs. Also, in the irradiated pelvis, vascular structures may be covered by such dense indurated and adherent scar tissue that exploratory incisions may lacerate the internal or external iliac veins.
3. Rectovaginal, retroprostatic, and paravesical veins: Bleeding may occur anterolaterally.
4. Pelvis: Arterial bleeding may occur from any of the arterial structures in the pelvis.
5. Sacrum or presacral artery: Bleeding may occur from the cut end of the sacrum or presacral artery if hemisacrectomy is performed.

When significant bleeding occurs, there are a number of general and specific measures that should be initiated depending on the site of bleeding. In general, good lighting, more than one suction, and good exposure are the keys to identifying the source of the bleeding. If the bowel lumen has not been entered, then the cell saver can be used to scavenge shed blood. In extreme cases, the rapid infusion system may be used, although such precipitous bleeding that cannot at least be slowed by direct pressure or packing is unusual.

When bleeding is encountered, the following steps should be taken. If the point of bleeding cannot be identified quickly, use an index finger to apply pressure. Should this fail to stop the bleeding, place packs, inform the anesthetists of the problem, and allow them to catch up with blood loss and send for blood. Optimize light, suction, and exposure and then gently tease out the packs until the bleeding site is seen. If the bleeding site is seen, use a sponge or small cotton pledget on an instrument to control the bleeding because this will allow more room to perform measures to stop the bleeding than if a finger is used. If bleeding occurs from the presacral area, such a maneuver will sufficiently control the bleeding to facilitate more definitive maneuvers. These are the following:

- Apply a suture using a ¾-circle needle (e.g., 2-0 Vicryl on a UR6 needle) if the bleeding is localized and there is sufficient intact fascia on either side to provide tamponade.
- If there is insufficient intact fascia, use a sterile thumbtack with or without some Surgicel secured beneath it. The thumbtack is best driven home using the flat part of a heavy pair of scissors.
- A roll of Surgicel or a 1-cm cube of rectus muscle may be sewn over the bleeding point again using a stout ¾-circle needle.
- If this does not work, then pack the pelvis after applying Surgicel to the bleeding area.

At this point, proceed with the remainder of the operation, returning to check hemostasis in 30 to 60 minutes. If this is satisfactory, suction drains will be left in the pelvis and an omental pedicle brought down to fill the dead space. If there is continued bleeding, additional packs are placed, and the abdomen is closed with the intent of returning to the operating room within 48 hours to remove the packs. Recurrent bleeding after such packing is rare.

If the bleeding cannot be readily controlled, the key to packing is to pack early, before there has been massive blood loss and the vicious downward spiral of coagulopathy and hypothermia has begun. Packs should be firmly placed at the site of bleeding and not roughly stuffed into the pelvis so as to cause shearing of small veins and compound the problem. If a pelvic anastomosis is to be created and the packs need to be left for 24 to 48 hours, the anastomosis should be left until the packs are removed, because a tightly packed pelvis may compromise the blood supply of the proximal bowel and put tension on the newly created anastomosis. Stapling or oversewing of the cut end of bowel and leaving it in the pelvis provide the safest alternative. For less severe bleeding, we have used packing in the presence of an anastomosis without untoward complications such as dehiscence.

Ligation of the internal iliac vein in the case of bleeding from its more distal branches is rarely helpful because of the rich collateral network. Direct injuries to the vein can be managed with ligation above and below the injury. However, in the frozen, irradiated pelvis, mobilization, isolation, and ligation of the vein may be impossible, and either repair with a fine vascular suture or oversewing may be required. To obtain visualization of the injury, pressure may need to be applied above and below the venous injury using a peanut or small swab on an instrument.

Arterial injuries may be treated by ligation or oversewing if bleeding is from small distal branches. Likewise, a single internal iliac artery can usually be ligated without untoward effects. In the case of injury to the external iliac artery, repair must be undertaken. Direct repair with fine vascular sutures can be undertaken with proximal and distal control. Short segments of more significant damage can be excised and the mobilized ends can be reanastomosed safely, but the need for more extensive reconstruction with prosthetic graft creates problems. Because there is likely to be contamination from either intestinal lumen or a focus of infection, anatomic placement of a vascular graft is inadvisable and an extraanatomic graft may be required (usually a femorofemoral crossover graft).

Drainage

We routinely drain the reoperative pelvis. If there has been minimal bleeding and this has been readily controlled, a single Jackson-Pratt or Atraum suction drain will suffice. If, however, there has been significant blood loss, fecal contamination, or both, then sump drains are used and brought out through a separate stab incision rather than the wound. These can be irrigated with normal saline and are usually removed on postoperative day 3.

The omentum is routinely mobilized and brought down the left gutter to fill any dead space in the pelvis or to wrap around or isolate an anastomosis. It is not usually necessary to mobilize the omentum inside the epiploic arcade unless it is short or has been partially removed at a prior operation. One or two sutures are used to hold the omentum in the pelvis or to incorporate it into the perineal wound closure in the case of abdominoperineal resection; otherwise, cephalad migration may occur. Perineal drains are rarely used.

SPECIFIC CLINICAL PROBLEMS

BENIGN

Reversal of Hartmann Procedure

Anastomosis to a closed out-of-circuit rectum, as in the second stage of a Hartmann procedure, is perhaps the commonest pelvic reoperation and may pose a couple of common problems (Figure 182-6, A). First, there may be a midrectal stricture, which makes passage of the stapler impossible. Usually, the serial passage of dilators per rectum remedies this, but occasionally, further rectal resection to healthy rectum is needed. Second, it is tempting to pass the cartridge of the stapler without the anvil per rectum and to drive the trocar through the presumed end of the rectum. However, if the oversewn end of the rectum has much scarring around it, the distal donut may be excessively large and cause tearing of the anastomosis on withdrawal. Similarly, if the trocar is brought through the rectum close to but not at the end, ischemia may develop between the anastomosis and the oversewn end of the rectum, with a risk of subsequent perforation. The variation of technical problems in the fashioning of an anastomosis deep in the pelvis calls for some ingenuity, and no one technique will always be the best. In general, the prevailing principle of ensuring good blood supply to both ends of bowel applies. Thus, if the distal rectum is too contracted to allow for a stapled anastomosis with introduction of the cartridge component per anum, then a hand-sewn anastomosis is perhaps the safest technique. This is appropriate if the rectum has been out of circuit for many months or years. One variation is the side-to-end anastomosis, in which the stapler head is passed through the open end of the distal colon, punching the trocar through the antimesenteric colon wall 5 to 7 cm from the open colonic end. The anvil is inserted into the opened distal rectum, which

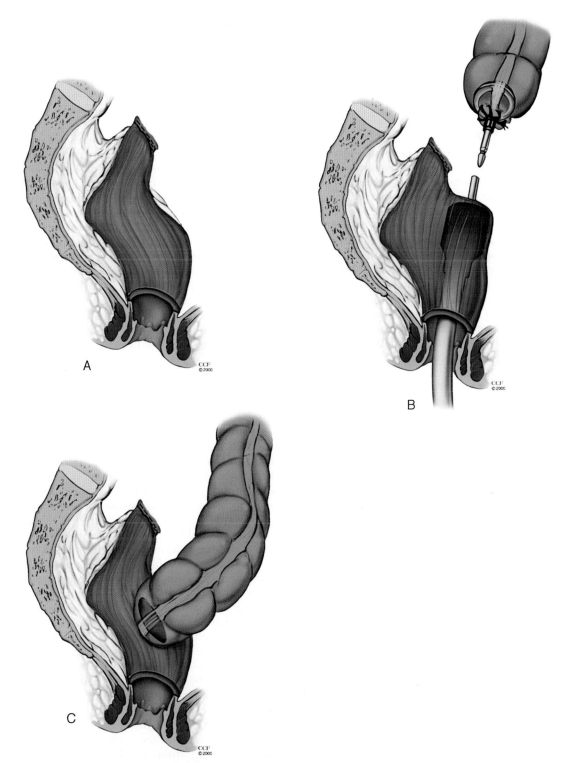

A

B

C

FIGURE 182-6 Reversal of Hartmann operation. A problem with double-stapled operations is that the apex of the stump is scarred and narrowed and tends to "concertina" on the cartridge component **(A)**. This leads to incomplete tissue rings and dehiscence of the anastomosis. The solution is removal of the narrowed apex with anastomosis **(B)** or end colon–to–side of rectum anastomosis **(C)**. (Copyright 2000, Cleveland Clinic Foundation.)

previously had a purse-string suture placed, and the stapled anastomosis is completed (Figure 182-6, *B* and *C*). On withdrawal of the circular stapler, the opened colon end is closed with a linear stapler, the tissue rings are checked, and anastomotic integrity is confirmed by transanal insufflation of dilute povidone-iodine. Care must be taken not to include the back wall of the colon in the circular stapler and staple-shut the colon. Passage of a large clamp proximally through the anastomosis ensures this is not the case.

In case of apparent inadequate colon length due to previous resection and previous splenic flexure mobilization, a few crucial inches of length can be obtained by mobilizing the colon to the hepatic flexure and passing the colon through a mesenteric window between the ileocolic and superior mesenteric vessels. Thus, a retro-ileocolic low rectal anastomosis is made.

Redo Pelvic Pouch Procedure

The redo pelvic pouch procedure perhaps epitomizes the difficulties encountered in benign reoperative pelvic surgery. Not only has there been extensive pelvic dissection with removal of the entire rectum but also a neorectum has been placed into the pelvis whose blood supply is dependent on a single posterior blood vessel—the superior mesenteric artery. The successful performance of this procedure emphasizes the principles discussed earlier. Careful positioning is required to allow initial perineal access to disconnect the pouch-anal anastomosis; then the abdominal phase of the operation and finally reanastomosis to the anal canal below the dentate line are undertaken. Ureteric stents are routinely placed to reduce the chance of inadvertent injury. The pelvic dissection requires sharp mobilization of the pouch, which is usually fused to the presacral fascia, obliterating the anatomic dissection plane. Particular care is required with the posterior dissection to avoid injury to the superior mesenteric artery, which is the major blood supply. Adhesion of the pouch deep within the pelvis requires the careful use of retractors and lighting to allow safe mobilization under direct vision. Bleeding is sometimes a problem, necessitating the maneuvers described earlier. Drainage with either sump or passive drains is combined with mobilization and placement of the omentum deep within the pelvis. Surprisingly, obtaining a tension-free anastomosis is rarely a problem.

The results of a series of redo pelvic pouches at our institution highlight some of the problems that can be encountered with such surgery yet at the same time illustrate the success that can be achieved with experience and a well-organized approach to the reoperative pelvis.

Experience with Redo Pelvic Pouch Operations. From 1983 to 2007, 241 abdominal reconstructions of pelvic pouches were performed with the most common indications being fistula, leak, stricture and pouch dysfunction.[4] Ureteric stent placement was routine and pouches were usually mobilized to the pelvic floor. Although the posterior pelvic mobilization was often difficult, with inadvertent pouch enterotomy being common, this was easily repaired. The early concerns involved attaining sufficient extra length (pouch reach) of the ileum to allow for a tension-free neo-ileal pouch–anal anastomosis; however, this proved to be an unfounded concern.

Seventy-one cases had a new pouch constructed and in 171 cases the original pouch was salvaged. Failure was observed in 29 of these cases with either pouch excision or proximal fecal diversion. Long-term pouch salvage was 85%, and compared to a matched nonrevised pouch group, only daytime leakage, nighttime leakage, and pad usage were significantly higher. All other parameters and quality of life were similar between the groups.

MALIGNANT

Although the general operative principles discussed earlier apply to surgery for recurrent malignancy, more emphasis must be placed on weighing the benefits of surgery against the potential for complications or death. Preoperative imaging and staging are essential to avoid an unnecessary and unhelpful operation. As discussed earlier, PET scanning has become useful in this respect,[3] and the pattern of recurrence in the pelvis may also be predictive of the chance of a complete resection.[2] Palliative resections of recurrent rectal, gynecologic, or urologic carcinomas in the pelvis have been rarely indicated, because control of symptoms is low, with high morbidity and poor long-term survival. However, with the advent of newer biologic chemotherapeutic agents directed against angiogenesis or growth factors, survival with metastatic colon and rectal cancer may be prolonged from historical expectations, and the role of palliative surgery may need to be reevaluated. Preoperative chemotherapy and radiation (if not received earlier) should be considered as it would be for primary rectal cancers, the indications being bulky or advanced disease. As with primary rectal cancer, waiting 4 to 6 weeks before subsequent surgery is recommended.

Reoperation for recurrent rectal cancer is almost always a difficult undertaking. Landmarks may be absent owing to pelvic fibrosis and scarring. Ureteric stents may be impalpable. Distinction between postoperative scarring and radiation effect from recurrent cancer may be difficult. Certain landmarks include the promontory of the sacrum, aorta, aortic bifurcation, and iliac vessels. If some mobility can be imparted to the matted scar around a previous colorectal anastomosis, one is encouraged to go forward. Trial dissection of the presacral space may come to a halt when real or apparent fusion of a midsacral-level colorectal anastomosis—the site of recurrence to the sacrum—is encountered. In such cases, if a sense of partial fusion is obtained, the surgeon may choose to dissect posterior to the Waldeyer fascia. This is a bold step, because shearing of the basivertebral veins from the sacrum may occur, especially if an osteotome is used. However, the surgeon may be rewarded by finding a plane in which a fibrous layer of thickened membrane—or periosteum—is anterior to the sacrum. Bleeding may be dealt with by one of the methods described earlier. It is important to identify situations where such efforts are beyond the capacity to perform a curative operation; these include preoperative sciatic pain, lower limb lymphedema, bilateral ureteric obstruction, retroperitoneal paraaortic lymph node involvement by cancer, and especially fixation of the pelvic mass to the side walls of the pelvis. Although an anastomosis may occasionally be possible, usually distal transection and stapling of the lower rectum or abdominoperineal resection is required.

Radical resection, including exenteration and/or sacral resection, is sometimes indicated in experienced hands at centers with appropriate anesthesia and intensive care support. A standardized algorithmic approach includes accurate preoperative imaging and there are several classification systems of local recurrence depending on site and organ involvement that can help predict the likelihood of a complete, potentially curative resection.[1] As more experience is gained, the extent of resection performed and the ability to achieve a complete resection has increased. Prior absolute contraindications to resection, such as iliac vessel and ureteric involvement have been challenged, with acceptable morbidity and long-term survival.[5,6] A large series of patients from several tertiary Australasian centers[6] demonstrated that with careful preoperative staging and aggressive surgical technique including en bloc resection of involved structures, more than 60% of patients could receive a complete resection with negative margins and a further 25% with only microscopically positive margins. Resection included adjacent organs or structures in more than half the cases; major complications occurred in 27% and there was less than 1% operative mortality. A 5-year cancer-free survival rate of 41.5% was achieved. With these increasingly aggressive resections in often-irradiated fields, myocutaneous flap reconstruction has been advocated as a means to decrease major perineal wound complications because it has been shown to be effective with primary cancer resections.[7]

Intraoperative radiation therapy (IORT) is advocated by some to further improve local control of completely resected recurrent cancer or to treat microscopic or macroscopically positive margins. A dedicated operating room necessary for this will only be feasible at tertiary care centers. In the earlier referenced series of patients from Memorial Sloan-Kettering,[1] 101 of 119 received IORT in a dedicated operating room from a shielded ^{192}Ir source. Doses of 1500 cGy were given with a negative margin, and 1750 cGy was given with a positive margin.

Our experience with reoperation for selected recurrent rectal cancer justifies this approach and relies on accurate preoperative staging and a familiarity with the reoperative pelvis and reconstructive techniques.

OPERATIVE MEASURES TO MAKE SUBSEQUENT PLANNED OR UNPLANNED PELVIC SURGERY EASIER AND SAFER

Although it is rare to perform a planned second operation in the pelvis, the instances where difficulty can be minimized are Hartmann procedures when a subsequent colorectal anastomosis or pelvic pouch is planned. Leaving the rectal stump long by essentially dividing the distal sigmoid and not entering the pelvis prevents a potentially difficult pelvic dissection. If the distal sigmoid

is diseased and there are concerns as to so-called stump blowout, it can be left long enough to suture it above the fascia in the lowermost portion of the wound. Any breakdown here would be in the subcutaneous tissues rather than the peritoneal cavity and easily managed by opening the skin.

Much of the difficulty in reoperative pelvic surgery is the mobilization of small bowel out of the pelvis. Almost any operation in the pelvis allows small bowel to become adherent to the site of surgery, and this is particularly pronounced when a large space is created such as in the case of an abdominoperineal resection. Inflammation due to infection, bleeding, or irradiation is also likely to make the small bowel more firmly adherent. Routine use of an omental pedicle to fill the potential space may reduce this. Further, the liberal use of drains with or without irrigation may lessen the inflammation that promotes adhesions. Seprafilm placed beneath the abdominal wall and even in the pelvis may also help reduce adhesions.

CONCLUSION

Reoperative pelvic surgery may be one of the most challenging procedures that a surgeon can face. However, careful preoperative planning and patient preparation combined with a well-practiced, methodical intraoperative approach may yield rewarding results with acceptable complications.

REFERENCES

1. Mirnezami AH, Sagar PM, Kavanagh D, et al: Clinical algorithms for the surgical management of locally recurrent rectal cancer. *Dis Colon Rectum* 53:1248, 2010.
2. Moore H, Shoup M, Riedel E, et al: Colorectal cancer recurrences: Determinants of resectability. *Dis Colon Rectum* 47:1599, 2004.
3. Staib L, Schirrmeister H, Reske SN, et al: Is ^{18}F-fluorodeoxyglucose positron emission tomography in recurrent colorectal cancer a contribution to surgical decision making? *Am J Surg* 180:1, 2000.
4. Remzi FH, Fazio VW, Kirat HT, et al: Repeat pouch surgery by the abdominal approach safely salvages failed ileal pelvic pouch. *Dis Colon Rectum* 52:198, 2009.
5. Austin KK, Solomon S, Michael J: Pelvic exenteration with en bloc iliac vessel resection for lateral pelvic wall involvement. *Dis Colon Rectum* 52:1223, 2009.
6. Heriot AG, Byrne CM, Lee P, et al: Extended radical resection: The choice for locally recurrent rectal cancer. *Dis Colon Rectum* 51:284, 2008.
7. Butler Charles E, Gundeslioglu A, Ozlem Rodriguez-Bigas Miguel A: Outcomes of immediate vertical rectus abdominis myocutaneous flap reconstruction for irradiated abdomino-perineal fields. *J Am Coll Surg* 206:694, 2008.

Evidence-Based Decision Making in Colon and Rectal Surgery

Najjia N. Mahmoud | Emily Carter Paulson

Evidence-based surgical practice is rapidly becoming synonymous with "quality" care. The areas of evidence in colorectal surgery are immense and diverse. To focus on several topics of recent interest, this chapter focuses on enhanced recovery pathways (ERPs) and some of their components. A discussion of the evidence and controversies around ERPs, or "fast track," protocols is helpful to understand how individual components of care contribute to the overall well-being and recovery of the patient. We chose to focus on ERPs as a group and then parse out some salient components such as need for bowel preparation, antibiotic prophylaxis, and factors relating to postoperative ileus (POI), for further discussion of the evidence.

ENHANCED RECOVERY PATHWAYS

During the past decade, there has been a great deal of interest in postoperative recovery pathways designed to streamline and codify postoperative care following a variety of procedures. Although these protocols differ from hospital to hospital, the literature describes 17 elements that should be included in the ideal ERP (Table 183-1). The main elements include preoperative counseling, avoidance of bowel preparation, no preoperative fasting, opioid-sparing analgesia and midthoracic epidurals, antibiotic prophylaxis, short incisions, no nasogastric tubes, normothermia, operative and postoperative fluid restrictions, no abdominal drains, oral diet at will, and early mobilization. There have been several randomized clinical trials and two recent systematic reviews evaluating these pathways.

A review by Wind et al, published in 2006, included six studies, three randomized controlled trials (RCTs) and three controlled clinical trials, published between 1998 and 2005.[1] These were single-institution studies and the number of ERP elements included ranged from 4 to 12, although all studies included early mobilization and diet. In five of six studies, hospital stay was significantly shorter in the ERP patients and in pooled analysis, the ERP patients had a hospital stay almost 2 days shorter than patients in a traditional pathway (TP). There was no difference seen in the rate of readmissions. One study reported significantly lower morbidity in the ERP group, especially cardiovascular and pulmonary complications. In pooled analysis, this trend was also observed. There was no difference seen in rates of anastomotic leakage or mortality. POI, measured by time to first bowel movement (BM) and tolerance of a solid diet, was reduced in the ERP group. There were mixed results regarding the outcomes of pain and fatigue, with some studies

reporting no difference between ERP and TP groups, whereas others reported increased pain and fatigue in the TP group compared to the ERP group. These authors concluded that ERP programs result in improved recovery after surgery, with a reduction in morbidity rates and hospital stay.

A more recent review published in 2009, by Gouvas et al, evaluated 11 studies—4 RCTs and 7 controlled clinical trials—comparing ERP to TP.[2] In this meta-analysis, primary hospital stay and total hospital stay (including readmission) were significantly lower in the ERP group (weighted mean differences, −2.35 days; $P < 0.00001$ and −2.46 days, $P < 0.00001$, respectively). There were no overall differences in readmission rates or mortality noted across the studies. One study showed a significant reduction in morbidity rates in the ERP patients. The other studies all had a trend in favor of lower morbidity with ERP, but in no other study was that trend significant. Overall, there was no significant difference noted in terms of nasogastric tube reinsertion or pain and fatigue measures, but most studies favored the ERP groups with respect to both of these parameters. These authors conclude that ERPs contribute to a quicker recovery of patients after colorectal surgery and result in lower morbidity and shorter hospital stays.

Overall, there has been a great deal of effort put into designing ERPs based on the best evidence available. In general, there are elements supported by extremely strong evidence, such as no bowel preparation, early initiation of diet and mobilization, and antibiotic prophylaxis (see discussion later), whereas other elements are less well supported. For example, it was once thought that laparoscopic surgery would be key in any ERP. Since 2005, several studies have come to inconsistent conclusions on this topic. There has been no clear difference between patients treated with open versus laparoscopic colon resections when a postoperative ERP is followed. In 2009, the Enhanced Recovery After Surgery (ERAS) Group published a consensus review of optimal perioperative case in colorectal surgery, mentioned earlier.[3] They reviewed the evidence for and made recommendations about 20 ERP elements. Again, the evidence is not robust for all elements, but this is a good summary of the components involved in ERPs for colorectal surgery.

MECHANICAL BOWEL PREPARATION

Mechanical bowel preparation before elective colorectal resection is common practice among general and colorectal surgeons. Removal of stool from the colon before manipulation, resection, and anastomosis is thought to

TABLE 183-1 Components of a Standard Enhanced Recovery Pathway for Colorectal Surgery

ERP Components	Level of Evidence*
Preoperative counseling	Grade B
Preoperative feeding—minimization of fasting	Grade A
Synbiotics	Not discussed in Consensus Review
No bowel preparation	Grade A
No premedication	Grade A
Fluid restriction	Grade A
Perioperative high O_2 concentrations	Not discussed in Consensus Review
Active prevention of hypothermia	Grade A
Epidural analgesia	Grade A
Minimally invasive/transverse incisions	Grade B
No routine use of nasogastric tubes	Grade A
No use of drains above peritoneal reflection	Grade A
Enforced postoperative mobilization	Grade B
Enforced early postoperative feeding	Grade A
Balanced analgesia—multimodal, low/no opioids	Grade A
Standard laxatives and antiemetics	Grade B
Early removal of urinary catheter	Not discussed in Consensus Review

*Level of evidence derived from Lassen K, Soop M, Nygren J, et al: Consensus review of optimal perioperative care in colorectal surgery: Enhanced recovery after surgery group recommendations. *Arch Surg* 144:961, 2009.
Grade A, Based on at least two good-quality randomized controlled trials (RCTs) or one metaanalysis of RCTs with homogeneity; *Grade B,* consensus recommendations based on the best available evidence.

reduce the risk of postoperative complications, including surgical-site and intraabdominal infections as well as anastomotic leak.

Although the practice is widespread, there is no compelling evidence indicating that bowel preparation results in superior outcomes. The majority of RCTs have shown that not only is there no difference in outcome between patients undergoing bowel preparation versus no preparation, but also there may be an increased risk of anastomotic leak following mechanical bowel cleansing.

There are numerous RCTs as well as several meta-analyses examining the efficacy of mechanical bowel preparation. Later, we review several of the largest randomized trials and detail the results of the most thorough metaanalyses in an effort to fully present the existing evidence addressing the efficacy of mechanical bowel preparation.

One of the earliest randomized studies was performed by Burke et al in 1994.[4] In this study, 169 patients undergoing elective left colonic or rectal resection were randomized before surgery to bowel preparation or no bowel preparation. Indications for surgery included carcinoma, diverticular disease, and inflammatory bowel disease, and the operations performed were left colonic resection or reversal of the Hartmann procedure, and anterior resection. Surgical technique was standardized and no patient had a defunctioning colostomy. The

overall morbidity rate, 18%, was similar in the two groups. There were 7 anastomotic leaks: 3 in 39 patients who had undergone bowel preparation and 4 in 36 who had not ($P > 0.9$). Two deaths occurred, both of patients who had received bowel preparation, one secondary to anastomotic leak. These authors concluded that bowel preparation does not influence outcome after elective colorectal surgery.

In the same year, another randomized trial of 149 patients by Santos et al concluded that mechanical bowel preparation is unnecessary and may be harmful in terms of preventing wound infection and anastomotic dehiscence in patients undergoing elective colorectal surgery.[5] Despite this early evidence from RCTs raising doubts regarding the necessity of mechanical bowel preparation, the practice continued to be widespread. A survey study published in 2003 revealed that although 90% of the colorectal surgeons surveyed questioned the importance of mechanical preparation, more than 99% routinely used it.[6]

Since that time, continued controversy over the use of bowel preparation has spawned several more RCTs. In 2007, Pena-Soria et al examined the relationship between bowel preparation and surgical-site infection and anastomotic leak in 97 patients.[7] They found no difference in surgical-site infection between the two groups. They did report, however, that patients receiving bowel preparation had almost twice the frequency of anastomotic dehiscence compared to the nonprepped group (8.3% vs. 4.1%; $P = 0.05$). They concluded that outcomes may be the same or even worse when mechanical bowel preparation is routinely used for colorectal surgery with primary intraperitoneal anastomosis.

The largest randomized trial examining this question was published in 2007 by Contant et al.[8] These authors performed a multicenter randomized trial that included more than 1400 patients at 13 hospitals. Patients were consented to receive either no bowel preparation, which included a regular diet the day before surgery, versus a bowel preparation of either polyethylene glycol or sodium phosphate and a clear liquid diet the day before surgery. In this study, the rate of anastomotic leak, 4.8% in patients who received bowel prep and 5.4% in patients who did not, did not differ significantly between groups ($P = 0.69$). Patients who had mechanical bowel preparation did have fewer abscesses after anastomotic leak than those who did not (0.3% vs. 2.5%; $P = 0.001$). Other complications such as fascial dehiscence, superficial infection, and mortality did not differ between groups. These authors concluded that mechanical bowel preparation before elective colorectal surgery can safely be abandoned.

In an effort to synthesize the results from the almost 20 years of trials examining this issue, several large meta-analyses have combined the data from a number of randomized trials. In 2004, Slim et al analyzed the results of seven randomized trials, including 1454 patients, comparing bowel preparation with no preparation in colorectal surgery.[9] They reported significantly higher rates of anastomotic leak after bowel preparation (5.6% vs. 3.2%; $P = 0.032$). All other end points (wound infection, other septic complications, and nonseptic complications) also favored the no-preparation regimen. Interestingly, a subgroup analysis showed that anastomotic leak was significantly greater after bowel preparation with polyethylene glycol (PEG) compared with no preparation but not after other types of preparation. These authors concluded that there is good evidence to suggest that mechanical bowel preparation using PEG should be omitted before elective colorectal surgery, whereas other bowel preparations should be evaluated by further large randomized trials.

These conclusions were supported by a metaanalysis published in 2010 by Zhu et al that specifically analyzed five RCTs that compared mechanical bowel preparation with PEG to no preparation.[10] They found no significant differences in rates of surgical-site infection, organ space infection, mortality, or anastomotic leak, although there was a tendency toward higher rates of anastomotic leak (odds ratio [OR], 1.78; 95% confidence interval [CI], 0.95 to 3.33; $P = 0.07$), in the PEG group. When the main complications of leak and surgical-site infection were examined together, there were significantly higher rates in the PEG group (OR, 1.76; 95% CI, 1.09 to 2.85; $P = 0.02$). Again, these authors concluded that the use of mechanical bowel preparation with PEG does not lower postoperative complications in elective colorectal surgery and may increase anastomotic leak.

Finally, the largest, and most thorough, metaanalysis was published by Guenaga et al in 2009.[11] These authors analyzed 13 RCTs, including 4777 patients, comparing bowel preparation to no bowel preparation. They found that rates of anastomotic leakage, though slightly higher in the bowel preparation groups, were not significantly different following either low anterior rectal resections or colonic resections. Rates of secondary complications such as wound infection, extraabdominal complications, and others were not different between the two groups. They concluded that there was no statistically significant evidence that patients benefit from mechanical bowel preparation.

Overall, there is sound evidence that omitting mechanical bowel preparation before colectomy is safe. Some argue, however, that bowel prep is still necessary before left-sided colon resections and rectal resections requiring low pelvic anastomoses or when a defunctionalizing diverting ostomy is created. Although there are not as many studies examining this question specifically, there is also evidence that bowel preparation is not required before these resections. In 2005, Bucher et al performed an RCT comparing bowel prep with PEG ($n = 78$) versus no bowel prep ($n = 75$) in patients undergoing only left-sided colectomy or low anterior rectal resection. They concluded that omission of bowel preparation before elective left-sided colorectal surgery was associated with a reduction in the rate of postoperative infectious and extraabdominal complications, and a shorter hospital stay. The previously discussed metaanalysis by Guenaga supports this conclusion as well. That analysis included 275 patients undergoing low anterior resection. Fourteen of 139 (10%) patients who received a bowel prep and 9 of 136 (6.6%) who did not suffered anastomotic leak (OR, 1.73; CI, 0.73 to 4.10).

There are two circumstances, however, where bowel preparation may still be prudent. Small unmarked tumors or suspicion that intraoperative colonoscopy might be required justifies bowel preparation to aid in visualization.

ANTIBIOTIC PROPHYLAXIS

It has long been recognized that antibiotic prophylaxis for patients undergoing surgery on the large intestine reduces the risk of postoperative wound infection. In 1981, Baum et al published the results of a metaanalysis evaluating a series of studies comparing the rate of wound infection in patients receiving antibiotic prophylaxis to patients receiving no prophylaxis.[12] They concluded that the risk of wound infection was so diminished in the prophylaxis group that in the future, studies investigating prophylactic antibiotic use could not ethically include a no-treatment group. Since that time, the use of preoperative antibiotics has become routine, but the choice of antibiotic, the timing of antibiotic dosing, and the use of postoperative therapy continues to defy easy standardization.

There have been hundreds of studies looking at the type of antibiotic used, the timing of antibiotic dosing, and the need for intraoperative redosing and postoperative dosing. These are too numerous to describe in detail in this text. A recent, extensive metaanalysis, published in 2009, sought to distill the results of the RCTs into several coherent conclusions in colorectal surgery.[13] Available evidence was used to confirm the need for prophylaxis, determine what spectrum of bacteria needs to be addressed, and determine the optimal timing and route of antibiotic administration. We will review their findings and the pertinent evidence on which they based their conclusions later.

Most surgeons, based on known reviews of practice patterns, recognize that prophylactic antibiotic dosing is beneficial in patients undergoing large bowel surgery. This practice is clearly supported by a large body of evidence, including 10 placebo-controlled trials in the 1980s. The combined analysis of these trials indicates that prophylactic antibiotics reduce the wound infection rate from 39% to 10%, with all 10 trials individually finding a significant or nearly significant benefit in favor of prophylaxis. There is no debate that antibiotic prophylaxis is standard of care for elective clean-contaminated colorectal surgery procedures.

The type and timing of the antibiotic prophylaxis is more controversial and more diverse across practices. In particular, many prescribe 24 hours of postoperative prophylactic antibiotics or favor redosing of intravenous (IV) antibiotics during lengthy cases. A recent metaanalysis evaluated 25 randomized trials that compared a single preoperative dose of antibiotics to longer duration of dosing. There was no evidence that longer duration of antibiotic dosing reduced the risk of wound infection more than a single preoperative dose. Additionally, the authors looked at 3 studies that specifically examined the recommendation that antibiotics with short half-lives be redosed during long cases.[14-16] Again, no further reduction in wound infection was noted with the additional dosing.

The spectrum of antibiotics used for prophylaxis is another area where practice patterns vary widely. There are, however, many studies that indicate that antibiotics that include coverage for both aerobic and anaerobic bacteria provide the greatest benefit in the reduction of postoperative wound infection. Based on the meta-analysis of existing randomized trials, the addition of anaerobic coverage to a regimen including aerobic coverage reduced wound infections by 45% ($P = 0.008$). Similarly, adding aerobic coverage to a regimen of anaerobic coverage reduced wound infection by almost 60% ($P = 0.002$).

Finally, there have been many studies investigating whether the addition of prophylactic oral antibiotics is effective in reducing wound infections. Three studies compared oral prophylaxis alone to oral and IV prophylaxis alone. When analyzed together, the addition of IV prophylaxis significantly reduced the rate of wound infection by greater than 65%. There have also been studies, however, evaluating the addition of oral prophylaxis to IV prophylaxis. Interestingly, the addition of oral prophylaxis does provide added benefit to the IV prophylaxis, with a significant risk reduction in wound infection of 45%. It is important to note that in each of these studies, all patients received a bowel preparation. It is unclear what role oral antibiotics should continue to play in light of the evidence against the routine use of bowel preparation, discussed earlier. There have been no studies evaluating the efficacy of oral antibiotics in the unprepped colon. If surgeons moved toward a practice of performing colorectal surgery without mechanical bowel preparation, this will be an area that needs further study.

Based on an evaluation of 106 randomized studies that included almost 16,000 patients, Nelson et al made several conclusions regarding the use of prophylactic antibiotics for colorectal surgery.[13] These recommendations supported the conclusion reached by Baum et al in 1981 that there is overwhelming evidence to support the use of antibiotic prophylaxis in patients undergoing colorectal surgery.[12] They also concluded that the antibiotics used should cover both anaerobic and aerobic bacteria. Additionally, the evidence indicates that preoperative dosing of IV antibiotics, preferably approximately 1 hour prior to incision, is imperative. There is no evidence supporting redosing of antibiotics during long cases, or the routine administration of postoperative antibiotics following uncomplicated, elective colorectal surgery. Finally, based on the evidence reviewed in this analysis, it appears that the combination of oral and IV antibiotics provides the optimal prophylactic regimen in patients receiving a bowel preparation. If practice patterns change, based on existing evidence, and bowel preparation is not common practice in the future, the use of oral antibiotic prophylaxis will have to be reexamined.

These conclusions were supported in the Consensus Review of Optimal Peri-operative Care in Colorectal Surgery, a consensus statement published by a large group of European colorectal surgeons, based on a critical appraisal of the available literature.[3] These authors concluded that there was level A evidence (defined as evidence based on two high-quality RCTs or one metaanalysis of RCTs with homogeneity) that patients undergoing colorectal surgery should receive single-dose antibiotic prophylaxis against both aerobes and anaerobes approximately 1 hour before surgical incision.

POSTOPERATIVE ILEUS

POI is a common occurrence following colorectal resection. It not only affects patient comfort but also increases length of stay and cost following surgery. The ability to reduce the incidence of POI has been a topic of great interest in the colorectal literature for years. Factors including resumption of oral intake, mu-opioid agonists, epidural analgesia, and even gum chewing have been explored in randomized trials. The evidence regarding these factors as they relate to POI and recovery following colorectal surgery is discussed later.

POSTOPERATIVE ORAL INTAKE

Resumption of oral intake following colorectal surgery is often the prime factor limiting patient's discharge from the hospital. Traditionally, oral intake has been withheld until patients demonstrate return of bowel function, either by passing flatus or having a BM. Following this conservative pathway, the average patient tolerates a regular diet on day 5 following colorectal resection. Although there is little evidence to support this approach, many still use it to guide postoperative diet management. In reality, there are numerous studies that support the idea that early oral nutrition following colorectal surgery has no deleterious effect on patient outcome and, in fact, can be beneficial in terms of patient satisfaction and length of hospital stay.

More than 15 years ago, Binderow et al performed a small RCT in patients undergoing laparotomy and colon resection, comparing traditional diet advancement with allowance of regular diet on postoperative day 1.[17] These investigators found that a slightly higher percentage of the early diet patients required replacement of a nasogastric tube, but that bowel function as evidenced by return of flatus or BM still occurred at the same time in both groups. Also, in patients who tolerated early oral intake, there was a trend toward shorter hospitalizations. This seminal, small study concluded that early oral intake is possible after laparotomy and colorectal resection.

Several years later, Hartsell et al performed another randomized study, again comparing early institution of oral intake to traditional diet management.[18] In this trial, early oral intake consisted of liquids on postoperative day 1, followed by regular diet as soon as the patient could tolerate a liter of fluid during the day, regardless of flatus or BM. No significant differences were seen in rates of nausea and vomiting or nasogastric tube replacement. There was also no difference noted in length of hospital stay.

In 2007, a randomized trial by Han-Geurts et al compared early institution of oral intake as tolerated by the patient (a "free diet" group) with traditional advancement of diet based on return of bowel function.[19] They observed that more patients in the free diet group required reinsertion of a nasogastric tube (20% vs. 10%, $P = 0.213$) but that this was not statistically significant.

There was no difference observed in the complication rate, and the return of gastrointestinal (GI) function was similar in both groups. A normal diet was tolerated after a median of 2 days in the free diet group compared with 5 days in the conventional group ($P < 0.001$). These authors again showed that early resumption of oral intake does not lead to a significantly increased rate of nasogastric tube reinsertion or complications. The lack of traditional markers of GI functional recovery, namely flatus and BMs, did not affect the tolerance of oral diet. They concluded that there is no reason to withhold oral intake in the early postoperative period following open colorectal surgery.

In 2009, a metaanalysis was published evaluating RCTs published through 2006, which compared traditional diet advancement with early oral intake following colorectal surgery.[20] These authors included 13 RCTs, with a total of 1173 patients. Overall, there were few differences noted between the two treatment groups in terms of complications. There was a trend toward fewer anastomotic dehiscences and shorter hospital stays, by about 1 day, in the early oral intake groups, although these did not reach significance. There was a slightly higher incidence of vomiting noted across the trials in the patients treated with early initiation of oral intake, but again, return of bowel function, recorded as flatus or BM, was unaffected. The conclusion of this metaanalysis, the largest to date, was that there is no advantage to the traditional conservative management of oral intake following colorectal surgery. Finally, in the 2009 Consensus Review, the authors concluded that there was grade A evidence (defined above) supporting the practice of allowing patients to commence an oral diet at will immediately following colorectal surgery.[3]

MU-OPIOID RECEPTOR ANTAGONISTS

Peripherally acting mu-opioid receptor antagonists are a class of agents that specifically block the action of opiates on intestinal mu receptors, thereby mitigating the effects of opioid-induced constipation. To date, there are only two Food and Drug Aministration (FDA)–approved pharmaceuticals in this class: alvimopan and methylnaltrexone bromide.

Alvimopan was approved in May 2008 as an orally administered drug for the treatment of POI. Alvimopan is a novel, selective, peripherally active mu-opioid receptor antagonist. It is administered orally and works by blocking the mu-opioid receptor, minimizing the paralytic effect opiates have on the intestines, while, because it does not cross the blood-brain barrier, having little effect on analgesia. The promise of pharmaceutical reduction of POI has spurred great interest in this and other mu-opioid antagonists in the past decade. During that time, five RCTs have been published investigating the safety of alvimopan and its effect on bowel recovery following abdominal surgery. One pooled analysis of three of these trials was also published.

In 2004, an RCT of 451 patients undergoing bowel resection was performed by Wolff et al.[21] Patients were randomized to receive 6 mg of alvimopan, 12 mg of alvimopan or placebo 2 hours preoperatively and twice a day postoperatively. The time to GI recovery, defined as

tolerance of regular food and passage of a BM, was accelerated with 6 or 12 mg of alvimopan, with a mean difference of 15 hours ($p < 0.005$) and 22 hours ($P < 0.001$), respectively, compared with placebo. In the 12-mg group, time to hospital discharge was also improved by an average of 22 hours compared to placebo ($P = 0.003$). Complications and adverse reactions were not different among the groups. These authors concluded that alvimopan was well tolerated and accelerated GI recovery and time to hospital discharge compared with placebo in patients undergoing bowel resection.

Two subsequent RCTs by Delaney et al and Viscusi et al, respectively, confirmed the findings from this initial trial.[22,23] A pooled analysis of these three trials was performed in 2007 by Delaney.[24] This pooled analysis included more than 1100 patients randomized to 6 mg or 12 mg of alvimopan or placebo in patients who underwent laparotomy and bowel resection. In pooled analysis, alvimopan reduced the time to GI recovery by 12 to 18 hours in both the 6- and 12-mg alvimopan groups compared to placebo. Additionally, the time to placement of a discharge order was reduced compared to placebo by 16 hours ($P < 0.001$) in the 6-mg group and 18 hours ($P < 0.001$) in the 12-mg group. There was no significant difference in opioid use between the groups. Also, the rate of adverse effects was lower in the alvimopan group, with lower rates of nausea and POI.

A more recent trial, published in 2008 by Ludwig et al, compared 12 mg alvimopan to placebo administered before surgery and twice per day afterward in 629 patients undergoing laparotomy and bowel resection.[25] All patients were managed postoperatively with a standard accelerated postoperative pathway that included early ambulation and early institution of oral feeding. In this study, the mean time to recovery of GI function, defined as tolerance of solid food and passage of first BM was accelerated by 20 hours in the alvimopan group ($P < 0.001$), whereas hospital discharge was 17 hours earlier compared to placebo ($P < 0.001$). Additionally, significantly fewer patients who received alvimopan remained in the hospital for 7 postoperative days or longer (18% vs. 30.8%; $P < 0.001$). Alvimopan patients were almost 60% less likely to develop a POI and more than 40% less likely to require nasogastric tube insertion. The overall hospital readmission rates within 10 days of discharge and the anastomotic leak rates were low and comparable between placebo- and alvimopan-treated groups. Finally, the opioid consumption did not differ significantly between the two groups, with the alvimopan group tending to use less morphine than the placebo group (185 morphine sulfate equivalents [MSEs] vs. 219 MSEs; $P = 0.06$). These authors concluded that alvimopan is safe, reduces POI and related morbidity, and accelerates GI tract recovery without compromising pain control.

The most recent RCT of alvimopan was published in 2008 by Buchler et al.[26] Briefly, they evaluated the safety and efficacy of alvimopan (6 and 12 mg every 12 hours) compared to placebo in patients undergoing laparotomy and either small or large bowel resection. Overall, unlike the prior studies, they did not show a significant reduction in time to tolerate solid food and first BM or flatus, although the trend was in favor of alvimopan. Patients in this trial, however, received either opioid patient-controlled analgesia (PCA) or opioids without PCA delivery. In the other trials, all patients received opioid analgesia via a PCA. In this study, the opioid usage differed significantly between the PCA and non-PCA patient groups. For example, in the placebo patients, the PCA group received an average of 92.1 MSEs, whereas the non-PCA group received only 45.3 MSEs. Differences were similar in the alvimopan treatment groups. In the PCA group, return of bowel function and time to first BM were significantly accelerated in the alvimopan treatment groups compared to placebo, whereas in patients treated with intermittent morphine and no PCA, no reductions in mean time to GI recovery were observed. This trial offered a unique perspective on alvimopan usage, suggesting that alvimopan, though safe in all patients, is most useful in patients receiving opioid analgesia in higher total quantities via a PCA.

Despite evidence in favor of the efficacy and safety of alvimopan, several barriers to use remain. It is not clear if alvimopan is as effective in patients receiving nonopioid-based epidural anesthesia. The initial trials of alvimopan for POI specifically excluded the use of epidural analgesia. There is a considerable amount of evidence to support the routine use of nonopioid epidural analgesia for patients undergoing bowel resection. It is also relatively costly to use and cannot be used in the outpatient setting. Analyses show that use results in cost savings as a result of reduction of hospital stay and that a reduction of POI-related complications also occurs. Methylnaltrexone bromide was approved by the FDA in May 2008 in the subcutaneously administered form for the palliation of medically refractory opioid-induced constipation in patients with end-stage disease. It is designed to mitigate the effect of opioids on peripheral receptors without interfering with central nervous system pain relief.

Methylnaltrexone has been formulated in subcutaneous, IV and per os (PO) forms. The IV form has been used in clinical trials assessing its effect on POI as a primary endpoint in open colon resection without epidural anesthesia. The other two forms have been used primarily in the treatment of opioid-induced constipation in opioid–dependent patients. In a phase II randomized, double-blind study of 0.3 mg/kg of methylnaltrexone versus placebo given within 90 minutes of surgery for up to 7 days (but no more than 24 hours after GI recovery), it was found that there was a significant decrease in time to first BM and time to tolerance of food. There was no reduction in hospital length of stay.[27]

In a followup phase III study, with more than 500 patients, 12 or 24 mg of IV methylnaltrexone was administered every 6 hours. Preliminary results failed to demonstrate any improvement in length of stay or GI recovery.[28] Finally, an article published early in 2011 reported the results of two identically designed, multicenter, double-blind, parallel-group, placebo-controlled studies that randomly assigned patients undergoing segmental colectomy (study 1, $N = 515$; study 2, $N = 533$) receiving 12 or 24 mg of methylnaltrexone intravenously or placebo every 6 hours starting within 90 minutes of surgery completion, continuing for up to 10 days or up

to 24 hours after GI recovery. In these studies, there were no differences observed between the groups with respect to time to discharge eligibility, time to hospital discharge, and clinically meaningful events of nausea and vomiting following segmental colectomy.[29] Overall, there were very few adverse events noted in these trials.

POSTOPERATIVE ANALGESIA

There has been debate over the years as to the optimal postoperative analgesia regimen for patients undergoing colon resection, both following laparotomy and laparoscopy. It has long been recognized that intravenous opioids, though effective for pain relief, can prolong POI, delaying return of bowel function and possibly tolerance of a regular diet. As such, there has been interest in using epidural analgesia in the postoperative period. There have been numerous randomized trials comparing epidural and IV analgesia following open colon resection. A few of the largest of these trials, as well as a recent metaanalysis evaluating 16 of these RCTs, are discussed briefly later. Additionally, there have been a few recent studies and reviews examining the same issue following laparoscopic colon resection. These are also discussed briefly at the end of this section.

One of the early randomized trials evaluating the efficacy and safety of epidural analgesia versus intravenous analgesia following colorectal resection was published in 2001 by Carli et al.[30] In this study, patients received either morphine patient-controlled analgesia (PCA) or a bupivacaine and fentanyl infusion via an epidural catheter for 4 days postoperatively. Analgesia was discontinued on postoperative day 4, and acetaminophen and codeine were then used orally as needed. Diet (in this study, liquid and protein drinks were started on all patients on postoperative day 1) and mobilization were the same between the two groups. The cumulative pain score (measured by the visual analog scale [VAS]) was significantly improved in the epidural patients with rest, coughing, and movement on the first 3 postoperative days. Pain scores were the same between groups by day 4. There was no difference in the incidence of postoperative nausea and vomiting between the two groups, but the time from surgery to first flatus and BM was significantly shorter in the epidural group. Twelve of 21 epidural patients passed flatus and 7 of 21 had a BM during the first 2 postoperative days, compared to 4 of 21 ($P = 0.001$) and 1 of 21 ($P = 0.005$), respectively, in the PCA group. Length of stay and rate of complications were the same between the two groups.

A more recent trial, published by Zutshi et al in 2005, evaluated epidural versus intravenous analgesia in patients undergoing laparotomy and bowel resection, all of whom were enrolled in an enhanced recovery program including early ambulation and oral intake.[31] Postoperatively, patients in the epidural group received a continuous infusion of bupivacaine and fentanyl, supplemented by a patient-controlled bolus. The epidural was removed on postoperative day 2 and oral pain medications were offered. Patients in the intravenous group received a PCA that delivered intravenous analgesia on demand and were switched to oxycodone starting 48 hours after surgery. There was no difference in length of stay between the two groups. Although patients in the epidural group passed stool earlier than the PCA group (2 days vs. 4 days), there was no difference in time to tolerance of a regular diet. The epidural patients did have a lower pain score during the first 2 days (mean score, 2.46 vs. 3.33; $P = 0.01$). Additionally, there was no significant difference between groups for quality of life, satisfaction with hospital stay, or return to normal activities at discharge or at postoperative days 10 and 30. These authors concluded that for patients undergoing bowel resection who are enrolled in an enhanced recovery pathway following surgery, epidural anesthesia offers no benefit.

In 2007, Marret et al published a metaanalysis evaluating 16 randomized trials comparing epidural analgesia versus intravenous opioid analgesia after colorectal surgery.[32] More than 800 patients were included in the study, 406 in the epidural group and 400 in the IV group. Length of stay was not significantly different in the two groups across the 13 trials that measured this outcome. Interestingly, in the later studies that employed an enhanced recovery pathway for all patients, length of stay was generally significantly shorter than in studies using a more traditional recovery pathway. As in the previously discussed study, the use of epidural analgesia in patients treated with an enhanced pathway did not shorten length of stay compared to the IV analgesia group. Pain relief, as measured by the VAS in 11 studies, was improved in the epidural groups at 24 and 48 hours. Additionally, in 15 studies, POI was shortened in the epidural groups, by an average of 36 hours. The rate of major postoperative complications was the same between groups, but there was a higher rate of complications such as hypotension and urinary retention in the epidural groups. Overall, this metaanalysis concluded that epidural analgesia does decrease VAS pain score and the duration of ileus, which results in improved patient comfort and facilitates more prompt resumption of oral intake. Despite these benefits, the use of epidural analgesia does not shorten length of hospital stay. Based on this metaanalysis, the authors conclude that hospital stay is most affected by "fast-track postoperative care," regardless of analgesia method used.

Until recently, there were very few studies examining the efficacy of epidural versus intravenous analgesia in patients undergoing laparoscopic colectomy. An article published in 2010 by Levy et al reviewed the eight studies that examined analgesia regimens specifically following laparoscopic colorectal resections.[33] Based on the three randomized trials included, there was no difference in length of stay between the epidural and IV analgesia groups. Although there was heterogeneity in the studies, the average time to tolerance of a regular diet was approximately 1 day shorter in the epidural group (2.8 vs. 3.9 days). The one randomized trial that included time to passage of flatus found the epidural group to have a significantly shorter time to passing flatus (2 vs. 3 days). Similarly, the two RCTs that looked at time to first BM found that this was shorter in the patients receiving epidural analgesia. Both RCTs that evaluated pain as an outcome reported that the visual analog pain scores (1 to 10) were significantly lower in the epidural groups (2.5 vs. 5.4). Overall, there was no difference in the rates of complications and readmissions between the two groups.

These authors concluded that there is still a paucity of data assessing the most appropriate analgesia regimen following laparoscopic colon resection. Again, it appears that epidural analgesia improves pain scores and shortens time to return of bowel function and tolerance of a diet but does not result in shorter lengths of stay or fewer complications.

There may be some disadvantages regarding the routine use of epidural analgesia. Epidural analgesia creates a sympathetic blockade that can lead to hypotension necessitating fluid boluses postoperatively, which could result in edema at the anastomosis.[34] Hypotension may lead to reduced colonic blood flow, impairing anastomotic healing.[35] Also, because epidural analgesia requires an indwelling catheter, it necessitates specialized nursing care and can limit postoperative mobility. An alternative to epidural analgesia is intrathecal analgesia, which is distinguished from epidural analgesia by catheter location within the neuraxis. With the intrathecal approach, the catheter lies within the subarachnoid space, where small quantities of medication have direct access to spinal drug receptor sites. During epidural administration, larger doses of medication must diffuse across the dura to reach these receptors. Some potential advantages of intrathecal analgesia include ease of catheter placement, particularly in the presence of spinal pathology, fewer catheter problems (catheter migration, tip occlusion, etc.), and lower dose requirements, which may reduce side effects and lower drug costs. Additionally, intrathecal analgesia requires a single injection before induction of anesthesia and the analgesia effect can last for up to 24 hours. Compared to epidural analgesia, nursing care is less intensive and specialized, mobility is achieved more rapidly, and the impact on fluid dynamics is minimal. Despite these theoretical advantages, there is a paucity of data regarding intrathecal analgesia and outcomes following colorectal surgery.

In 2010, Virlos et al examined short-term outcomes with intrathecal versus epidural analgesia in laparoscopic colorectal surgery.[36] An observational study of 175 consecutive patients who underwent elective laparoscopic colorectal surgery was performed. Seventy-six patients received epidural analgesia and 99 patients received a single injection of intrathecal analgesia. In this study, patients receiving intrathecal analgesia had a reduced median postoperative pain score (0 vs. 3.5; $P < 0.001$), an earlier return to mobility (1 vs. 4 days; $P < 0.001$), and a shorter hospital stay (4 vs 5 days; $P < 0.001$) than patients receiving epidural analgesia. Other outcomes, including return of bowel function, nausea and vomiting, complications, and readmission, were not different between the two groups. These authors concluded that intrathecal analgesia may have advantages over epidural analgesia in patients undergoing laparoscopic colorectal surgery.

There are no trials reported examining intrathecal analgesia specifically following open colorectal resection. There have also been no randomized trials examining the efficacy of intrathecal versus epidural analgesia following either laparoscopic or open resection. There are clear theoretical advantages of intrathecal analgesia, but the evidence supporting its use is limited. Further randomized trials would be helpful to examine the future role that intrathecal analgesia should play in recovery programs following colorectal resections.

MECHANICAL TREATMENT

Mechanical treatment includes the use of chewing gum in the immediate postoperative period, which hypothetically stimulates the gastrocolic reflex and hormonally induces peristalsis. A systematic review evaluated four published studies on this technique that all used sugarless gum three times a day beginning on postoperative day 1, continuing until the first flatus or BM.[37] Among a total of 158 patients, 78 received chewing gum added to standard care, and 80 received only standard care. The number of patients in each study was small and the results were somewhat mixed. Nevertheless, these studies demonstrated a significant difference between the groups with regard to recovery of bowel function. With combined standard postoperative care and gum chewing, the patients passed flatus 24.3% earlier (weighted mean difference, −20.8 hours; $P = 0.0006$) and had a BM 32.7% earlier (weighted mean difference, −33.3 hours; $P = 0.0002$). They were discharged 17.6% earlier than those having ordinary postoperative treatment (weighted mean difference, −2.4 days; $P < 0.00001$). In the aggregate, there was a 20-hour reduction in the time to bowel recovery. There were no differences between groups with regard to complications, readmissions, or reoperation rates. Chewing gum may provide a safe, relatively harmless method of stimulating bowel motility and reducing the duration of POI.

CONCLUSIONS

As future studies are performed, the appropriate use and necessary elements of postoperative ERPs will be better understood. For now, although it is not clear which recovery pathway is ideal, it is clear that ERPs will play a key role in caring for colorectal surgery patients, particularly as health systems examine ways to reduce hospital length of stay without compromising safety. Old dogmas and traditions, such as prolonged postoperative nothing-by-mouth status and the routine use of bowel preparation, are already being challenged by solid evidence from a multitude of randomized trials. It is hoped that this review, which touches only on a few crucial topics, together with the references included will help guide the reader to evidence-based appropriate and safe management of patients undergoing colorectal resection.

REFERENCES

1. Lassen K, Soop M, Nygren J, et al: Consensus review of optimal perioperative care in colorectal surgery: Enhanced recovery after surgery (ERAS) group recommendations. *Arch Surg* 144:961, 2009.
2. Wind J, Polle SW, Fung Kon Jin PH, et al: Systematic review of enhanced recovery programmes in colonic surgery. *Br J Surg* 93:800, 2006.
3. Gouvas N, Tan E, Windsor A, et al: Fast-track vs. standard care in colorectal surgery: A meta-analysis update. *Int J Colorectal Dis* 24:1119, 2009.
4. Burke P, Mealy K, Gillen P, et al: Requirement for bowel preparation in colorectal surgery. *Br J Surg* 81:907, 1994.
5. Santos JC Jr, Batista J, Sirimarco MT, et al: Prospective randomized trial of mechanical bowel preparation in patients undergoing elective colorectal surgery. *Br J Surg* 81:1673, 1994.
6. Zmora O, Wexner SD, Hajjar L, et al: Trends in preparation for colorectal surgery: Survey of the members of the American Society of Colon and Rectal Surgeons. *Am Surg* 69:150, 2003.
7. Pena-Soria MJ, Mayol JM, Anula-Fernandez R, et al: Mechanical bowel preparation for elective colorectal surgery with primary intraperitoneal anastomosis by a single surgeon: Interim analysis of a prospective single-blinded randomized trial. *J Gastrointest Surg* 11:562, 2007.
8. Contant CM, Hop WC, van't Sant HP, et al: Mechanical bowel preparation for elective colorectal surgery: A multicentre randomised trial. *Lancet* 370:2112, 2007.
9. Slim K, Vicaut E, Panis Y, et al: Meta-analysis of randomized clinical trials of colorectal surgery with or without mechanical bowel preparation. *Br J Surg* 91:1125, 2004.
10. Zhu QD, Zhang QY, Zeng QQ, et al: Efficacy of mechanical bowel preparation with polyethylene glycol in prevention of postoperative complications in elective colorectal surgery: A meta-analysis. *Int J Colorectal Dis* 25:267, 2010.
11. Guenaga KK, Matos D, Wille-Jorgensen P: Mechanical bowel preparation for elective colorectal surgery. *Cochrane Database Syst Rev* 1:CD001544, 2009.
12. Baum ML, Anish DS, Chalmers TC, et al: A survey of clinical trials of antibiotic prophylaxis in colon surgery: Evidence against further use of no-treatment controls. *N Engl J Med* 305:795, 1981.
13. Nelson RL, Glenny AM, Song F: Antimicrobial prophylaxis for colorectal surgery. *Cochrane Database Syst Rev* 1:CD001181, 2009.
14. Carr ND, Hobbiss J, Cade D, et al: Metronidazole in the prevention of wound sepsis after elective colorectal surgery. *J R Coll Surg Edinb* 29:139, 1984.
15. Cuthbertson AM, McLeish AR, Penfold JC, et al: A comparison between single and double dose intravenous Timentin for the prophylaxis of wound infection in elective colorectal surgery. *Dis Colon Rectum* 34:151, 1991.
16. Grundmann R, Burkardt F, Scholl H, et al: One versus three doses of metronidazole/mezlocillin for antibiotic prophylaxis in colon surgery. *Chemioterapia* 6:604, 1987.
17. Binderow SR, Cohen SM, Wexner SD, et al: Must early postoperative oral intake be limited to laparoscopy? *Dis Colon Rectum* 37:584, 1994.
18. Hartsell PA, Frazee RC, Harrison JB, et al: Early postoperative feeding after elective colorectal surgery. *Arch Surg* 132:518; discussion 520, 1997.
19. Han-Geurts IJ, Hop WC, Kok NF, et al: Randomized clinical trial of the impact of early enteral feeding on postoperative ileus and recovery. *Br J Surg* 94:555, 2007.
20. Lewis SJ, Andersen HK, Thomas S: Early enteral nutrition within 24 h of intestinal surgery versus later commencement of feeding: A systematic review and meta-analysis. *J Gastrointest Surg* 13:569, 2009.
21. Wolff BG, Michelassi F, Gerkin TM, et al: Alvimopan, a novel, peripherally acting mu opioid antagonist: Results of a multicenter, randomized, double-blind, placebo-controlled, phase III trial of major abdominal surgery and postoperative ileus. *Ann Surg* 240:728; discussion 734, 2004.
22. Delaney CP, Weese JL, Hyman NH, et al: Phase III trial of alvimopan, a novel, peripherally acting, mu opioid antagonist, for postoperative ileus after major abdominal surgery. *Dis Colon Rectum* 48:1114; discussion 1125; author reply 1127, 2005.
23. Viscusi ER, Goldstein S, Witkowski T, et al: Alvimopan, a peripherally acting mu-opioid receptor antagonist, compared with placebo in postoperative ileus after major abdominal surgery: Results of a randomized, double-blind, controlled study. *Surg Endosc* 20:64, 2006.
24. Delaney CP, Wolff BG, Viscusi ER, et al: Alvimopan, for postoperative ileus following bowel resection: A pooled analysis of phase III studies. *Ann Surg* 245:355, 2007.
25. Ludwig K, Enker WE, Delaney CP, et al: Gastrointestinal tract recovery in patients undergoing bowel resection: Results of a randomized trial of alvimopan and placebo with a standardized accelerated postoperative care pathway. *Arch Surg* 143:1098, 2008.
26. Buchler MW, Seiler CM, Monson JR, et al: Clinical trial: Alvimopan for the management of post-operative ileus after abdominal surgery: Results of an international randomized, double-blind, multicentre, placebo-controlled clinical study. *Aliment Pharmacol Ther* 28:312, 2008.

27. Viscusi E, Rathmell J, Fichera A, et al: A double-blind, randomized, placebo controlled trial of methylnaltrexone (MNTX) for postoperative bowel dysfunction in segmental colectomy patients (Abstract A893). Presented at the American Society of Anesthesiologists Annual Meeting. Atlanta, GA. 2005.

28. Progenics Pharmaceuticals, Inc:—Wyeth and Progenics provide update on phase 3 clinical trial of intravenous methylnaltrexone for postoperative ileus http://www.progenics.com/releasedetail.cfm?releaseid=298721. Accessed April 27, 2011.

29. Yu CS, Chun HK, Stambler N, et al: Safety and efficacy of methylnaltrexone in shortening the duration of postoperative ileus following segmental colectomy: Results of two randomized, placebo-controlled phase 3 trials. *Dis Colon Rectum* 54:570, 2011.

30. Carli F, Trudel JL, Belliveau P: The effect of intraoperative thoracic epidural anesthesia and postoperative analgesia on bowel function after colorectal surgery: A prospective, randomized trial. *Dis Colon Rectum* 44:1083, 2001.

31. Zutshi M, Delaney CP, Senagore AJ, et al: Randomized controlled trial comparing the controlled rehabilitation with early ambulation and diet pathway versus the controlled rehabilitation with early ambulation and diet with preemptive epidural anesthesia/analgesia after laparotomy and intestinal resection. *Am J Surg* 189:268, 2005.

32. Marret E, Remy C, Bonnet F, Postoperative Pain Forum Group: Meta-analysis of epidural analgesia versus parenteral opioid analgesia after colorectal surgery. *Br J Surg* 94:665, 2007.

33. Levy BF, Tilney HS, Dowson HM, et al: A systematic review of postoperative analgesia following laparoscopic colorectal surgery. *Colorectal Dis* 12:5, 2010.

34. Liu SS, Carpenter RL, Mackey DC, et al: Effects of perioperative analgesia technique on rate of recovery after colon surgery. *Anesthesiology* 83:757, 1995.

35. Gould TH, Grace K, Thorne G, et al: Effect of thoracic epidural anaesthesia on colonic blood flow. *Br J Anaesth* 89:446, 2002.

36. Virlos I, Clements D, Benyon J, et al: Short-term outcomes with intrathecal *versus* epidural analgesia in laparoscopic colorectal surgery. *Br J Surg* 97:1401, 2010.

37. Chan MK, Law WL: Use of chewing gum in reducing postoperative ileus after elective colorectal resection: A systematic review. *Dis Colon Rectum* 50:2149, 2007.

Index

Page numbers followed by "f" indicate figures, "t" indicate tables, and "b" indicate boxes.

A

A delta fiber, 1733
A islet cell, 1262
Aachen inguinal hernia classification,
  567-568, 568t
AAST liver injury scale, 1482, 1482t
AAST organ injury scale for upper enteric
  injuries, 680, 680t
AAST pancreatic injury scale, 1236-1237,
  1237t, 1626
ABC transporters, 1297
Abdominal aortic surgery, colonic ischemia
  complicating, 1873-1876, 1875f-1876f
Abdominal approaches
  choice in colorectal surgery, 2219-2220
    laparoscopic colon resection and, 2219
    laparotomy and, 2220
    natural orifice transluminal
      endoscopic surgery and, 2220
    robotic and robotic-assisted resection
      and, 2219-2220
    transanal resection techniques and,
      2220
  in rectal prolapse, 1826-1827
    laparoscopic, 1827
    rectopexy in, 1826, 1826f
    resection in, 1826-1827
    resection-rectopexy in, 1827, 1827f
Abdominal compartment syndrome,
  1486-1487
Abdominal distention
  in colonic volvulus, 1850-1851
  in duplication cyst, 1052-1053
  in meconium ileus, 1053-1054, 1054f
  patient history of, 1741
  in small bowel obstruction, 866
Abdominal esophagus perforation, 482-483
Abdominal examination
  in acute appendicitis, 2023
  in colorectal trauma, 1841-1843
  in small bowel obstruction, 867
  in splenic trauma, 1636
Abdominal exploration
  in aortoenteric fistula, 1095
  coloanal anastomosis and, 2122
  in Crohn disease, 893, 894f
Abdominal incision, 2220-2221
  in Crohn disease, 893, 893f-894f
Abdominal length of sphincter, 195, 196t
Abdominal mass
  in acinar cell carcinoma of pancreas,
    1269-1270
  in acute appendicitis, 2020, 2027
  in aortoenteric fistula, 1094-1095
  in choledochal cyst, 1397
  in colonic intussusception, 1850
  in duplication cyst, 1052-1053
  in gallbladder cancer, 1365, 1369
  in hepatocellular carcinoma, 1568
  in intussusception, 1060
  in solid pseudopapillary tumor of
    pancreas, 1268

Abdominal mass *(Continued)*
  in superior mesenteric artery aneurysm,
    1102
  in transmesenteric hernia, 956
Abdominal pain
  in acinar cell carcinoma of pancreas,
    1269-1270
  in acute appendicitis, 2019
  in acute mesenteric ischemia, 1073
  after bile duct surgery, 1417
  in amebic liver abscess, 1473-1474
  in aortoenteric fistula, 1094-1095
  in autoimmune pancreatitis, 1270-1271
  in biliary dyskinesia, 1333
  in choledochal cyst, 1397
  in chronic pancreatitis, 1135-1136, 1137t
  in colonic intussusception, 1850
  in colonic ischemia, 1868
  in colonic volvulus, 1850-1851
  in colorectal carcinoid tumor, 1023
  in Crohn disease, 883, 1968
  differential diagnosis of, 2022
  in diverticular disease, 1880-1881
  in dumping syndrome, 757-758
  in duplication cyst, 1052-1053
  in foreign body ingestion, 803
  in gastric cancer, 774
  in gastrointestinal lymphoma, 1035
  in gastroparesis, 781
  in hepatocellular carcinoma, 1568
  immunocompromised patient and, 2267
  in intussusception, 1055-1056
  in pancreatic pseudocyst, 1146
  in paraduodenal hernia, 955
  patient history of, 1741
  in pediatric gastric tumor, 817
  in pediatric peptic ulcer disease, 818
  postprandial, 1085
  in primary pancreatic lymphoma,
    1272-1273
  in pyogenic liver abscess, 1466, 1466t
  in radiation enteritis, 990-991
  in sciatic hernia, 619
  in small bowel obstruction, 870f
  in small bowel volvulus, 874
  in solid pseudopapillary tumor of
    pancreas, 1268
  in sphincter of Oddi dysfunction, 1334
  splenic mass and, 1649-1650
  in superior mesenteric artery aneurysm,
    1102
  in ulcerative colitis, 1963
  in Zollinger-Ellison syndrome, 750
Abdominal radiography
  in aortoenteric fistula, 1095-1096
  in jejunoileal atresia, 1050, 1051f
  in meconium ileus, 1053-1054, 1054f
  in obturator hernia, 617f
  in pediatric gastric outlet obstruction,
    810-811, 811f
  in pyogenic liver abscess, 1467
  in sigmoid volvulus, 1851, 1852f

Abdominal radiography *(Continued)*
  in small bowel obstruction, 867-868
  in small bowel volvulus, 874-875
Abdominal trauma
  colorectal injuries in, 1841-1849
    abdominal assessment in, 1841-1843
    anorectal injury and, 1846
    causes of, 1842t
    damage control in surgery for, 1844
    definitive repair and management of,
      1844-1845, 1845f, 1846t
    diagnostic problems in, 1843-1844
    foreign bodies in, 1847
    gradation of injuries in, 1842t
    gunshot wounds in, 1842t
    iatrogenic, 1846-1847
    military injury considerations in,
      1845-1846
    postoperative complications in,
      1847-1848, 1848t
  hepatobiliary injuries in, 1479-1490
    avulsion of liver in, 1488
    bilehemia in, 1488, 1488f
    classification of, 1482, 1482t
    extrahepatic bile duct injuries in,
      1488-1489
    gallbladder injury in, 1488
    hemobilia in, 1487-1488
    historical perspective of, 1479-1480
    initial evaluation in, 1480-1482, 1481f
    major venous bleeding in, 1485
    management algorithm for, 1489f
    mortality from, 1488
    nonoperative management of,
      1486-1487, 1487f
    perihepatic packing and damage
      control strategies in, 1485-1486
    principles of operative treatment in,
      1482-1487, 1483f-1484f
    requirements of adjunctive invasive
      treatment in, 1486-1487
    subscapular hematomas in, 1487
  mesenteric arterial injury in, 961-965
    anatomy and exposure in, 962-964,
      963f-964f
    intraoperative management and repair
      in, 963-964
    lacerations and contusions in, 961-962,
      962f
    outcomes in, 964
  pancreatic injury in, 1234-1240
    diagnosis of, 1234-1235, 1235f
    intraoperative evaluation of,
      1235-1236, 1236f
    operative intervention for, 1236-1239,
      1237f-1238f, 1237t
    postoperative considerations in, 1239,
      1239f
  splenic injury in, 1636-1639
    diagnosis of, 1636-1637, 1637t
    laparoscopic splenectomy in, 1618
    in Nissen fundoplication, 234

Erythema nodosum, 884
Erythrocyte culling, 1612
Erythromycin
  for delayed gastric emptying after
      pancreatic resection, 1283
  for gastroparesis, 973
  hepatocanalicular cholestasis and, 1556
  motilin and, 834
  for postvagotomy gastroparesis, 761
  for pouchitis, 1997
Escherichia coli
  in acute cholangitis, 1347
  in overwhelming postsplenectomy
      infection, 1620, 1652
  in pyogenic liver abscess, 1468-1469
  in splenic abscess, 1656, 1669
ESD; *See* Endoscopic submucosal dissection
Esomeprazole, 218
Esophageal adenocarcinoma, 410
  achalasia and, 352-353
  age, sex, and race distribution of,
      375-377, 377f
  barium studies in, 77, 78f-80f, 82f, 84f
  Barrett esophagus and
    dysplastic, 306-307, 307t
    transformation of squamous mucosa
        into columnar epithelium in, 285
  carcinoembryonic antigen in, 419
  chemotherapy for, 453-454
  detection of, 410-411, 411f
  early endoscopic management of,
      411-414
    efficacy of, 414
    endoscopic mucosal resection in,
        412-413, 413f
    endoscopic submucosal dissection in,
        413-414, 413f
    initial staging in, 411-412, 412f, 412t
    safety of, 414
  endoscopic esophageal ultrasonography
      in, 118-125, 118b
    depth of tumor and, 120-124,
        120f-122f
    determination of metastases and, 124,
        125f
    lymph node involvement and, 122-124,
        123f-124f
    posttherapy stage and, 124-125
    recurrence stage and, 125
  endoscopic evaluation of, 108-109,
      109f-110f
  epidemiology of, 416-417
  etiology of, 417-418
  gastroesophageal reflux disease and, 180
    antireflux surgery and, 182-185, 184f
    medical therapy prevention or
        promotion of cancer and,
        181-182, 183f
    risk indicators for, 181
  genetics of, 382-394, 386t, 387f
    cell cycle control and, 388-389
    columnar metaplasia and Barrett
        esophagus and, 385
    etiology and risk factors and, 382-384,
        383t
    genetic alterations as biomarkers for
        prognosis and, 389-390, 390t-391t
    growth factor signaling and, 386-387
    signal transduction and, 387-388
    sporadic esophageal cancer and,
        384-385, 384f
    targeted therapy and, 390-391
    transcriptional regulation and, 388

Esophageal adenocarcinoma *(Continued)*
  incidence of, 375, 376f
  risk factors for, 377-378, 377t, 417t
  staging of
    AJCC, 118b, 397, 400t
    TNM, 120, 424, 424t
Esophageal ampulla, 69
Esophageal atresia
  annular pancreas and, 1241
  anorectal malformation with, 2278-2279
  embryology of, 33, 36f, 41-42, 43f
Esophageal atresia with tracheoesophageal
    fistula, 509-514
  anatomic classification and risk
      stratification in, 511, 511f
  general overview of, 509-510, 510f
  historical background of, 509
  long-gap esophageal atresia in, 513
  management considerations in, 510-511
  open repair of, 511-512, 511f-512f
  outcome and long-term complications in,
      513-514
  postoperative care in, 513
  thoracoscopic repair of, 512-513, 513f
Esophageal balloon distention and acid
    perfusion, 60, 60f
Esophageal benign tumors, 462-477
  classification of, 464, 464b
  diagnosis of, 463
  endoscopy in, 463
  fibrovascular polyp in, 472, 472t
  granular cell tumor in, 470-471, 470f
  hemangioma in, 471
  historical background of, 462
  incidence of, 462-463
  intramural, 471-472
  medical therapy for, 463
  mesenchymal, 464-470, 464t
    gastrointestinal stromal tumor in,
        469
    leiomyoma in, 465-469, 465f-468f,
        466t-467t
    schwannoma in, 469-470
  observation in, 463
  squamous papilloma in, 472-473, 473f
  surgical treatment of, 463
  symptoms of, 463
Esophageal bypass in caustic esophageal
    injury, 490
Esophageal cancer, 375-381
  age, sex, and race distribution of,
      375-377, 377f
  assessment of symptoms in, 63-64, 63f
  barium studies in, 77-85
    for esophageal duplication cyst, 85
    for evaluation of therapy, 81-83
    for metastatic disease to esophagus, 83,
        84f
    radiologic appearance in, 77, 78f-81f
    for staging, 77-81
  Barrett esophagus and, 379, 417-418
    dysplastic, 306-307, 307t
    transformation of squamous mucosa
        into columnar epithelium in, 285
  changing epidemiology in, 379
  clinical manifestations of, 379-380
  diagnosis of, 419
  endoscopic esophageal ultrasonography
      in, 118-125, 118b
    depth of tumor and, 120-124,
        120f-122f
    determination of metastases and, 124,
        125f

Esophageal cancer *(Continued)*
  lymph node involvement and, 122-124,
      123f-124f
  posttherapy stage and, 124-125
  recurrence stage and, 125
  endoscopic evaluation of, 108-109,
      109f-110f
  endoscopic management of, 410-415
    clinical burden in, 410
    diagnosis and, 410, 411f
    efficacy of, 414
    initial staging and, 411-412, 412f, 412t
    mucosal resection and submucosal
        dissection in, 412-414, 413f
    safety of, 414
  epidemiology of, 416-417
  etiology of, 417-418, 417t
  genetics of, 382-394
    cell cycle control and, 388-389
    columnar metaplasia and Barrett
        esophagus and, 385
    etiology and risk factors and, 382-384,
        383t
    genetic alterations as biomarkers for
        prognosis and, 389-390, 390t-391t
    growth factor signaling and, 386-387
    signal transduction and, 387-388
    sporadic esophageal cancer and,
        384-385, 384f
    squamous cell carcinoma and
        adenocarcinoma and, 383t,
        385-389, 386t, 387f
    targeted therapy and, 390-391
    transcriptional regulation and, 388
  incidence of, 375, 376f
  mortality and prognosis in, 375
  multimodality treatment of, 451-461
    chemoradiation therapy in, 455-459,
        456t-457t
    chemotherapy in, 452-455, 453t, 455t
    radiation therapy in, 451-452,
        452t-453t
    rationale for, 451
  palliative treatment of, 438-450
    alcohol sclerotherapy in, 438-439
    argon beam coagulation in, 443
    bougienage in, 439
    brachytherapy in, 444-445
    chemoradiation in, 445-446
    chemotherapy in, 446
    clinical nurse specialist and, 448-449
    combined radiation therapy in, 445
    endoscopic photodynamic therapy in,
        443-444
    esophageal prostheses in, 439-443,
        441f-442f
    external beam radiotherapy in, 444
    management of terminal patient and,
        448
    Nd:YAG laser electrocoagulation in,
        443
    new agents in, 446-447
    patient assessment in, 438, 439b, 440t
    patient with prominent local symptoms
        and, 447, 447f
    surgical therapy in, 448
  pathology of, 418-419, 418f-419f
  patient evaluation in, 420-422, 420f-421f
  presentation of, 419, 419t
  risk factors for, 377-378, 377t
    Barrett esophagus in, 379
    caustic esophageal injury in, 490
    diet and nutrition in, 378

Methotrexate
  for Crohn disease, 890
  hepatotoxicity of, 1554
  for inflammatory bowel disease, 1972
  for pediatric Crohn disease, 819
Methyldopa hepatotoxicity, 1555
Methylnaloxone, 2313
Methylprednisolone
  after biliary atresia surgery, 1394t
  for idiopathic thrombocytopenic
    purpura, 1661
Metoclopramide
  for delayed gastric emptying after
    pancreatic resection, 1283
  for gastroesophageal reflux disease,
    216-217
  for gastroparesis, 782, 973
  for postvagotomy gastroparesis, 761
Metrizamide; *See* Amipaque
Metronidazole
  for amebic liver abscess, 1475
  for *Clostridium difficile* infection,
    2268-2269
  for Crohn disease, 890
  for diverticular disease, 1888
  for *Helicobacter pylori* infection,
    1042t
  for pouchitis, 1997
Michelassi strictureplasty, 895, 898f
Microflora, colonic, 1729
Microfold cell, 842
Microgastria, 810
Micro-RNAs, esophageal cancer and, 390,
  390t-391t
Microsatellite instability, 2042, 2051
Microsurgical anastomosis, 926
Microvilli, 841-842
Microwave ablation in liver cancer,
  1514-1516, 1516f, 1574
Midazolam
  for endoscopic esophageal
    ultrasonography, 113
  for endoscopic retrograde
    cholangiopancreatography,
    1339-1340
Middle colic artery, 846f, 1070f, 1689f-
  1691f, 1690
  variations in, 1693, 1693f
Middle colic vein, 847f
Middle hemorrhoidal artery, 1690f
Middle hepatic vein, 1427f, 1431
  right extended hepatectomy and,
    1501-1502, 1503f
Middle sacral artery, 1714, 1714f
Middle thoracic esophagus, 395, 396f
Midesophageal diverticulum, 372-373
Midgut volvulus, 807, 808f, 1048
Midline abdominal incision
  closure of, 600
  in hepatic resection, 1492
Midline follicle excision and lateral
  drainage in pilonidal disease, 1836,
  1836f
Midodrine, 1449
Migrating motor complex, 645, 786-787,
  849, 849f
MII; *See* Multichannel intraluminal
  impedance
Milan criteria, 1575, 1576f
Miliary hemangiomatosis, 1864
Military-related colorectal trauma,
  1845-1846
Milk, pruritus ani and, 1934, 1934t

Milligan-Morgan hemorrhoidectomy,
  1899-1900
Milwaukee Classification System of
  sphincter of Oddi dysfunction,
  1334-1335, 1334t-1335t
Minicholecystectomy, 1321
Mini-laparoscopically guided percutaneous
  gastrostomy, 673
Minimal access retroperitoneal pancreatic
  necrosectomy, 1170
Minimally invasive necrosectomy, 1128,
  1129f
Minimally invasive surgery
  in acute and chronic pancreatitis
    complications, 1168-1178
  for infected pancreatic necrosis,
    1168-1170, 1169f
  for pancreatic duct disruption,
    1172-1173
  for pancreatic duct stones, 1174-1176,
    1175f
  for pancreatic duct stricture,
    1168-1170
  for pancreatic pseudocyst, 1170-1172,
    1172f
  in colorectal cancer, 2064
  in gastric resection, 731, 732f
  in gastrointestinal stromal tumor,
    1031-1032, 1031f-1032f
  in high imperforate anus, 2286-2288,
    2287f-2289f
  in pancreatic cancer, 1199-1200
    laparoscopic distal pancreatectomy
      with spleen preservation in,
      1199-1200
    laparoscopic
      pancreaticoduodenectomy in,
      1200
  in pancreatic duct disruption,
    1172-1173
  in pancreatic duct stones, 1174-1176,
    1175f
  in pancreatic duct stricture, 1168-1170
  in pancreatic pseudocyst, 1170-1172,
    1172f
  in short esophagus, 207-208
  splenic, 1618-1625, 1619b
    anatomic considerations in, 1620-1621
    anterior approach in, 1621
    contraindications for, 1619
    hand-assisted laparoscopic splenectomy
      in, 1623-1624
    in hematologic disorders, 1618-1619
    immunization against overwhelming
      postsplenectomy infection in,
      1620
    lateral approach in, 1621-1622
    natural orifice transluminal
      endoscopic surgery in, 1624
    patient selection for, 1619
    postoperative care in, 1624-1625
    preoperative imaging in, 1619
    prophylactic considerations in, 1620
    robot-assisted laparoscopic
      splenectomy in, 1624
    single-port laparoscopic splenectomy
      in, 1624
    surgical complications in, 1625
    in trauma, 1618
Minimally invasive surgery staging of
  esophageal cancer, 422
Miniprobe in endoscopic esophageal
  ultrasonography, 113-114, 114f

Minnesota Multiphasic Personality
  Inventory Assessment, 1788
Minocycline hepatotoxicity, 1555
Minor papilla, 842, 843f
Mirizzi syndrome, 1370
Mitochondrial cytopathy, drug-induced,
  1554
Mitomycin C for anal canal squamous cell
  carcinoma, 2168
Mixed cholangiohepatocellular carcinoma,
  1580-1581, 1581f
Mixed hernia, 494, 495f
Mixed serrated colorectal adenoma,
  2031-2032
Mixed type intraductal papillary mucinous
  neoplasm, 1221
MMR gene mutations, 2042
Model for End-stage Liver Disease, 1525,
  1525t-1526t, 1599, 1599b
Moderate sedation in colonoscopy, 1947
Modified Gilbert inguinal hernia
  classification, 567-568, 568t
Modified Johnson classification of gastric
  ulcers, 709t
Modified Puestow procedure, 1245-1246
Molecular adsorbents recirculating system,
  1540
Molecular biomarkers
  in colorectal cancer, 2066
  in dysplastic Barrett esophagus, 307
Moloney darn, 574-575
Monosaccharides, 859
Morgagni hernia, 506
Morphine-prostigmine provocation test,
  1335
Moskel-Walske-Neumayer strictureplasty,
  895, 896f
Mother and baby choledochoscopy, 1343
Motilin, 646, 782
  in control of small bowel motility, 851,
    851f, 851t
  physiologic functions of, 834, 835t-836t
Motility
  anal canal, 1721
  colonic, 1730-1733
    colonic transit assessment and,
      1730-1731, 1730f
    in healthy person, 1732-1733, 1732f
    heterogeneity in, 1728-1729
    recording techniques for, 1731, 1731f
  duodenal, 836-837, 837t
  gallbladder, 1300-1301
  gastric, 645-646, 781-786
  intestinal, 786-789, 849-852, 849f
    autonomic nervous system control of,
      849-850
    colonic distention and, 852
    enteric nervous system control of, 850,
      850f
    hormonal control of, 850-852, 851f,
      851t
    obesity and, 852
    systemic disease effect on, 852
  rectal, 1720-1721
Motility agents
  for gastroesophageal reflux disease,
    216-217
  for gastroparesis, 782
Motilium; *See* Domperidone
MRC; *See* Magnetic resonance
  cholangiography
MRCP; *See* Magnetic resonance
  cholangiopancreatography

Respiratory complications
  in epiphrenic diverticulum, 367-368
  in esophagectomy, 430, 430t, 537-538,
    544-545
Respiratory inversion point, 195f-196f
Rest syndrome, 769
Retained excluded antrum syndrome, 750
Retinopathy
  after islet allotransplantation, 1260
  after pancreas transplantation, 1257
Retractors in pelvic surgery, 2300-2301,
  2300f-2301f
Retroduodenal artery, 1067
Retrograde bypass in chronic mesenteric
  ischemia, 1087-1088, 1087f-1088f
Retroperitoneal abdomen, 676
Retroperitoneal access to pancreatic
  necrosis, 1159, 1160f
Retroperitoneal hernia, 954
Retropharyngeal hematoma, 327-328
Retroplaced gallbladder, 1296
Retrorectal intussusception, 1804
Retrorectal space, 2177, 2178f
  abdominoperineal resection and,
    2113-2114, 2113f-2114f
Retrorectal tumors, 2177-2189
  anatomic considerations in, 2177,
    2178f-2180f
  endoanal ultrasound of, 1768, 1768f
  enterogenous cysts in, 2182
  epidermoid and dermoid cysts in, 2182
  history and physical examination in,
    2177-2178
  imaging studies in, 2178-2181
  incidence and classification of, 2177,
    2180b
  management algorithm for, 2187, 2188f
  miscellaneous lesions in, 2184
  neurogenic tumors in, 2183
  osseous lesions in, 2184
  preoperative biopsy in, 2181, 2181f
  sacrococcygeal chordomas in, 2183,
    2183f
  surgical treatment of, 2184-2187, 2185f
    combined anterior-posterior approach
      in, 2185-2186
    follow-up considerations in, 2186
    laparoscopic approaches in, 2186
    multidisciplinary team in, 2184
    posterior approach in, 2184-2185,
      2185f
    rationale for, 2184
    results in, 2186-2187
  tailgut cysts in, 2182-2183, 2182f-2183f
  teratoma and teratocarcinoma in,
    2183-2184
Retrosacral fascia, abdominoperineal
  resection and, 2113-2114, 2114f
Retrosternal hernia, 506
Revascularization in acute mesenteric
  ischemia, 1078
Revised Bethesda guidelines for
  microsatellite instability, 2042
Revisional antireflux surgery, 976-977,
  977b
Revisional bariatric surgery, 798-799,
  977-982
  in failed laparoscopic adjustable gastric
    banding, 978-980
  in failed malabsorptive procedure, 982
  in failed Roux-en-Y gastric bypass,
    980-982
  in failed sleeve gastrectomy, 970f, 980

Revisional bariatric surgery (Continued)
  in failed vertical banded gastroplasty,
    977-978
  patient selection in, 977
Revisional pouch surgery in ileal pouch-
  anal anastomosis, 1999-2002, 2000t,
  2001f-2002f
Rex's ramus arcuatus, 1434
RFA; See Radiofrequency ablation
Rfx6 transcription factor, 1121
Rhabdomyoma, esophageal, 471
Rhabdomyosarcoma
  colorectal, 2196
  hepatic, 1582
Riding ulcer, 497
Rifampin
  for antibiotic-soaked prosthetic graft,
    1097-1098
  for pruritus in primary sclerosing
    cholangitis, 1411, 1411t
Rifaximin
  for Clostridium difficile infection,
    2268-2269
  for hepatic encephalopathy, 1449
Right colic artery, 846f, 1689f-1691f, 1690,
  2100f
  variations in, 1692-1693, 1693f
Right colic vein, 847f
Right gastric artery, 1067
  duodenum and, 825f, 826, 827f
  gallbladder and, 1316-1317, 1317f
  stomach and, 638-639, 641f
Right gastric vein, 639, 641f, 847f
Right gastroepiploic artery, 638-639, 641f,
  1067
  esophagogastrostomy and, 522
Right gastroepiploic vein, 639, 641f
Right gastro-omental artery, 846f
Right hemicolectomy, 1861
Right hemiliver, 1432-1433
Right hepatectomy with hilar dissection,
  1499-1500, 1500f-1501f
Right hepatic artery, 1290-1291, 1429
  caterpillar hump anomaly of, 1296,
    1296f
  cholecystectomy-related injury of, 1323
  gallbladder and, 1316-1317, 1317f
  lobar resection and, 2156-2157, 2156f
Right hepatic duct, 1429
  anatomy and embryology of, 1286-1287,
    1287f
  blood supply to, 1290, 1291f
Right hepatic vein, 1427f, 1431
  hepatectomy and, 1498, 1498f
  right lobectomy and, 2157, 2157f
Right lateral sector of liver, 1433
Right lobectomy, 2157, 2157f
Right mesocolic hernia, 1697, 1700f
Right paramedian sector of liver, 1433
Right portal fissure, 1426f, 1432
Right Pringle maneuver, 1432
Right suprarenal vein, 1431
Right thoracoabdominal approach in
  hepatic resection, 1492
Rigid proctosigmoidoscopy, 1746, 1746f
Rigiflex balloon, 359
Rigiflex dilator, 142
Ripstein procedure, 1826, 1826f
Risk assessment in acquired
  immunodeficiency syndrome, 2267
Rituximab
  for autoimmune pancreatitis, 1271-1272
  for intestinal lymphoma, 1042-1043

Robot-assisted laparoscopic splenectomy,
  1624
Robotic rectopexy, 1831
Robotic surgery, 2236-2237
Rockey-Davis in incision in appendectomy,
  2023
Rokitansky-Aschoff sinuses, 1289
Rome II Diagnostic Criteria
  in biliary dyskinesia, 1333, 1334b
  in sphincter of Oddi dysfunction, 1334
Rome III Diagnostic Criteria for functional
  constipation, 1800, 1801b
Rotational flap in anal canal stricture,
  1930-1931, 1932f
Rouvi[ac]ere's sulcus, 1426f, 1430
Roux limb syndrome, 973
Roux stasis syndrome, 707, 718, 765, 786
Roux-en-Y choledochojejunostomy, 695
Roux-en-Y cystojejunostomy, 1171-1172
Roux-en-Y duodenojejunostomy, 943-944
Roux-en-Y esophagojejunoplasty, 532-533,
  533f
  postoperative anastomotic leak in, 930
  in reflux stricture, 212-213, 213f
Roux-en-Y fistula tract-jejunostomy, 1164
Roux-en-Y gastric bypass, 792-796, 794f
Roux-en-Y gastrojejunostomy, 741-742,
  743f-744f
  after distal gastrectomy, 777
  in bile reflux gastritis after Billroth II,
    762, 763f
  blood glucose homeostasis after, 1114
  common bile duct stones after, 1330,
    1330f
  in dumping syndrome, 759, 759f
  in duodenal fistula, 944
  endoscopic antireflux repairs after,
    274-276
  failed, 980-982
  in failed laparoscopic adjustable gastric
    banding, 978
  in failed vertical banded gastroplasty,
    977-978
  intussusception after, 784f, 788
  in reflux stricture, 212-213, 213f
  as remedial operation for end-stage
    benign esophageal disease, 263-264,
    263f
  Roux stasis syndrome after, 786
Roux-en-Y hepaticojejunostomy
  in choledochal cyst, 1400
  in gallbladder cancer, 1366-1367
  in hilar cholangiocarcinoma, 1376-1378
  in iatrogenic bile duct injury repair,
    1386, 1421, 1422f
  in iatrogenic hepatic artery injury,
    1545
Roux-en-Y limb
  in biliary atresia, 1392
  in choledochal cyst, 1394
  in duodenal stump fistula, 944
  in esophagojejunoplasty, 532-533, 533f
  in pancreas transplantation, 1254-1255
  in pancreatic ascites, 1163, 1164f
  in pancreaticojejunostomy, 1197
  in reconstruction in caustic esophageal
    injury, 491
Roux-en-Y pancreaticojejunostomy, 1163,
  1164f
Roux-en-Y reconstruction
  in duodenal ulcer disease, 707, 707f
  in iatrogenic bile duct injury, 1421,
    1422f